KT-171-386

GREEN'S OPERATIVE HAND SURGERY

FIFTH EDITION

VOLUME ONE

David P. Green, MD
Clinical Professor
Department of Orthopaedics
The University of Texas Health Science
 Center at San Antonio
Founding President
The Hand Center of San Antonio
San Antonio, Texas

Robert N. Hotchkiss, MD
Associate Attending Orthopedic
 Surgeon
Hospital for Special Surgery
Director
Alberto Vilar Center for Research of the
 Hand and Upper Extremity
New York, New York

William C. Pederson, MD
Clinical Associate Professor of Surgery
 and Orthopaedic Surgery
The University of Texas Health Science
 Center at San Antonio
Director of Fellowship Training
The Hand Center of San Antonio
San Antonio, Texas

Scott W. Wolfe, MD
Professor of Orthopedic Surgery
Weill Medical College of Cornell
 University
Chief, Hand and Upper Extremity
 Surgery
Attending Orthopedic Surgeon
Hospital for Special Surgery
New York, New York

Illustrator:
Elizabeth Roselius, MS, FAMI

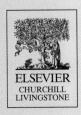

ELSEVIER
CHURCHILL
LIVINGSTONE

ELSEVIER
CHURCHILL
LIVINGSTONE

The Curtis Center
170 S Independence Mall W 300E
Philadelphia, Pennsylvania 19106

GREEN'S OPERATIVE HAND SURGERY   ISBN 0-443-06626-4
Copyright © 2005, 1999, 1993, 1988, 1982 by Elsevier Inc.

VOL 1: P/N 996002403
VOL 2: P/N 996002462

All rights reserved. No part of this publication may be reproduced or transmitted in any form or by any means, electronic or mechanical, including photocopying, recording, or any information storage and retrieval system, without permission in writing from the publisher. Permission may be sought directly from Elsevier's Health Sciences Rights Department in Philadelphia, PA, USA: phone: (+1) 215 238 7869, fax: (+1) 215 238 2239, e-mail: healthpermissions@elsevier.com. You may also complete your request on-line via the Elsevier homepage (http://www.elsevier.com), by selecting 'Customer Support' and then 'Obtaining Permissions'.

NOTICE

Orthopaedic surgery is an ever-changing field. Standard safety precautions must be followed, but as new research and clinical experience broaden our knowledge, changes in treatment and drug therapy may become necessary or appropriate. Readers are advised to check the most current product information provided by the manufacturer of each drug to be administered to verify the recommended dose, the method and duration of administration, and contraindications. It is the responsibility of the licensed prescriber, relying on experience and knowledge of the patient, to determine dosages and the best treatment for each individual patient. Neither the publisher nor the author assumes any liability for any injury and/or damage to persons or property arising from this publication.

International Standard Book Number 0-443-06626-4

Acquisitions Editor: Daniel Pepper
Developmental Editor: Arlene Chappelle
Publishing Services Manager: Tina Rebane
Design Manager: Gene Harris

Printed in the United States of America.

Last digit is the print number: 9   8   7   6   5   4   3   2   1

£275   (5107)

Hand/surgery
Hand Injuries
Hand Deformities

New edition (7th)
2016
Not purchased
2018.

LIBRARY TAUNTON AND SOMERSET HOSPITAL

WE
680
REF

WITHDRAWN

BOOK POCKET
ON NEXT PAGE

SWNHS

C20321060

GREEN'S
OPERATIVE
HAND
SURGERY

FIFTH EDITION

VOLUME ONE

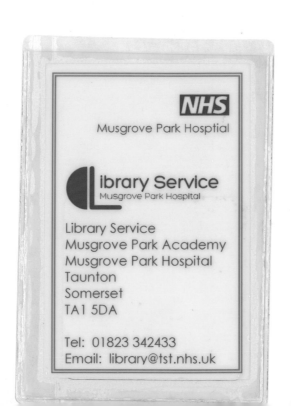

NHS

Musgrove Park Hosptial

Library Service
Musgrove Park Hospital

Library Service
Musgrove Park Academy
Musgrove Park Hospital
Taunton
Somerset
TA1 5DA

Tel: 01823 342433
Email: library@tst.nhs.uk

CONTRIBUTORS

Brian D. Adams, MD
Professor, Orthopaedic Surgery and Biomedical
Engineering, University of Iowa, Iowa City, Iowa
Distal Radioulnar Joint Instability

David W. Altchek, MD
Associate Professor of Clinical Surgery, Weill Medical
College of Cornell University; Associate Attending
Orthopedic Surgeon, Hospital for Special Surgery, New
York, New York
Arthroscopy and the Thrower's Elbow

Peter C. Amadio, MD
Professor of Orthopedics, Mayo Clinic College of
Medicine; Consultant, Department of Orthopedic
Surgery and Surgery of the Hand, Mayo Clinic,
Rochester, Minnesota
Stiff Finger Joints; Fractures of the Carpal Bones

Dimitri J. Anastakis, MD, MEd, FRCS, FACS
Associate Professor, Divisions of Plastic and
Orthopaedic Surgery, Department of Surgery, University
of Toronto; Associate Director, Surgical Services,
University Health Network, Toronto Western Hospital,
Toronto, Ontario, Canada
Free Functioning Muscle Transfers

Douglas M. Anderson, MD
Department of Veterans Affairs, Audie L. Murphy
Memorial Veterans Hospital Division, San Antonio,
Texas
Anesthesia

**George A. Anderson, MBBS, MS Orth, D Orth,
MNAMS Orth, MCh Orth (Liverpool), FAMS-
PNS (Vienna), FACS Orth**
Professor of Orthopaedic Surgery, Head of Dr. Paul
Brand Department of Hand Surgery and Leprosy
Reconstructive Surgery, and Course Director, Hand
Therapy and Leprosy Physiotherapy, Christian Medical
College Hospital, Vellore, Tamil Nadu, India
Ulnar Nerve Palsy

Edward A. Athanasian, MD
Associate Professor of Clinical Orthopedic Surgery,
Weill Medical College of Cornell University; Associate
Attending Orthopedic Surgeon, Hospital for Special
Surgery, and Assistant Attending Surgeon, Memorial
Sloan-Kettering Cancer Center, New York, New York
Bone and Soft Tissue Tumors

Mark E. Baratz, MD
Vice Chairman, Research and Educational Program, and
Director, Division of Hand and Upper Extremities,
Department of Orthopaedic Surgery, Allegheny General
Hospital; Allegheny Orthopaedic Associates, Pittsburgh,
Pennsylvania
Extensor Tendon Injuries

David P. Barei, MD, FRCS(C)
Assistant Professor of Orthopaedics and Sports
Medicine, University of Washington School of
Medicine, Harborview Medical Center, Seattle,
Washington
Fractures of the Distal Humerus

O. Alton Barron, MD
Assistant Clinical Professor of Orthopaedic Surgery,
Columbia College of Physicians and Surgeons; Senior
Attending Hand Surgeon, C. V. Starr Hand Surgery
Center, St. Luke's–Roosevelt Hospital Center, New
York, New York
Dislocations and Ligament Injuries in the Digits

Michael S. Bednar, MD
Associate Professor, Department of Orthopaedic
Surgery and Rehabilitation, Loyola University Health
System, Maywood, Illinois
Congenital Deformities of the Wrist and Forearm

Rolfe Birch, MChir, FRCS
Professor in Neurological Orthopaedic Surgery,
University College London; Visiting Professor,
Department of Academic Neurology, Imperial College,
London; Honorary Consultant Surgeon, Hospital for
Sick Children, London, National Hospital for
Neurology and Neurosurgery, London, Raigmore
Hospital, Inverness, and Birmingham Children's
Hospital; Honorary Surgeon to the Royal Navy,
Peripheral Nerve Injury Unit, Royal National
Orthopaedic Hospital, Middlesex, United Kingdom
Nerve Repair

Allen T. Bishop, MD
Professor of Orthopedic Surgery, Mayo Clinic College
of Medicine; Consultant, Department of Orthopedic
Surgery, and Chair, Division of Hand Surgery, Mayo
Clinic, Rochester, Minnesota
Vascularized Bone Grafting

Martin I. Boyer, MD, MSc, FRCS(C)
Associate Professor, Department of Orthopaedic
Surgery, Chief, Orthopaedic Hand Surgery Service, and
Coordinator, Third and Fourth Year Orthopaedic
Surgery Rotations, Washington University School of
Medicine at Barnes-Jewish Hospital, St. Louis, Missouri
Flexor Tendon Injury (Acute Injuries)

Richard E. Brown, MD, FACS
Clinical Professor, Division of Plastic Surgery, Southern
Illinois University; The Center for Plastic Surgery,
Springfield Clinic, Springfield, Illinois
The Perionychium

Earl Z. Browne, Jr., MD
Section Head, Microsurgery, Department of Plastic
Surgery, The Cleveland Clinic, Cleveland, Ohio
Skin Grafts and Skin Flaps (Skin Grafting)

Michelle Gerwin Carlson, MD
Assistant Professor of Surgery (Orthopedics), Weill
Medical College of Cornell University; Assistant
Attending Orthopedic Surgeon, Hospital for Special
Surgery, New York, New York
Cerebral Palsy

Louis W. Catalano III, MD
Clinical Instructor, Department of Orthopaedic Surgery,
Columbia College of Physicians and Surgeons;
Attending Hand Surgeon, C. V. Starr Hand Surgery
Center, St. Luke's–Roosevelt Hospital Center,
New York, New York
Dislocations and Ligament Injuries in the Digits

Kevin C. Chung, MD, MS, FACS
Associate Professor of Surgery, Section of Plastic
Surgery, Department of Surgery, The University of
Michigan Hand Center, Ann Arbor, Michigan
Skin Tumors

Mark S. Cohen, MD
Professor, Director, Hand and Elbow Section, and
Director, Orthopaedic Education, Department of
Orthopaedic Surgery, Rush University Medical Center,
Chicago, Illinois
Total Elbow Arthroplasty

Struan H. Coleman, MD, PhD
Instructor in Orthopedics, Weill Medical College of
Cornell University; Sports Medicine and Shoulder
Service, Hospital for Special Surgery, New York,
New York
Arthroscopy and the Thrower's Elbow

Randall W. Culp, MD
Associate Professor of Orthopedic, Hand and
Microsurgery, Thomas Jefferson University,
Philadelphia; The Philadelphia Hand Center, P.C.,
King of Prussia, Pennsylvania
Wrist Arthroscopy: Operative Procedures

Timothy R. C. Davis, FRCS, ChM
Special Professor in Trauma and Orthopaedic Surgery,
Nottingham University; Consultant Hand Surgeon,
Queens Medical Centre, Nottingham, United Kingdom
Median Nerve Palsy

Kazuteru Doi, MD, PhD
Clinical Professor, Department of Orthopedic Surgery,
Yamaguchi University School of Medicine, Ube,
Yamaguchi; President, Ogori Daiichi General Hospital,
and Director, Department of Orthopedic Surgery, Ogori
Daiichi General Hospital, Ogori, Yamaguchi, Japan
Traumatic Brachial Plexus Injury

Marybeth Ezaki, MD
Associate Professor of Orthopaedic Surgery, University
of Texas Southwestern Medical Center; Director, Hand
and Upper Extremity Service, Texas Scottish Rite
Hospital for Children, Dallas, Texas
Congenital Contracture

Paul Feldon, MD
Associate Clinical Professor of Orthopaedic Surgery,
Tufts University School of Medicine; Hand Surgical
Associates, Boston, Massachusetts
*Rheumatoid Arthritis and Other Connective Tissue
Diseases*

Diego L. Fernandez, MD
Professor of Orthopaedic Surgery, University of Bern;
Department of Orthopaedic Surgery, Lindenhof
Hospital, Bern, Switzerland
Distal Radius Fractures

Guy Foucher, MD
Professor, Trauma Department, University of Las
Palmas, Gran Canaria, Spain
Vascularized Joint Transfers

Marc Garcia-Elias, MD, PhD
Consultant, Hand Surgery, Institut Kaplan, Barcelona,
Spain
Carpal Instability

William B. Geissler, MD
Professor, Division of Hand and Upper Extremity
Surgery; Chief, Arthroscopic Surgery and Sports
Medicine; Director, Hand and Upper Extremity
Fellowship; Team Consultant, Ole Miss, Department of
Orthopaedic Surgery and Rehabilitation, University of
Mississippi Medical Center, Jackson, Mississippi
Carpal Instability

Günter Germann, MD, PhD
Chairman, Department of Hand, Plastic, and
Reconstructive Surgery, BG-Trauma
Center–Ludwigshafen; Plastic and Hand Surgery,
The University of Heidelberg, Ludwigshafen, Germany
The Burned Hand

Steven Z. Glickel, MD
Associate Clinical Professor of Orthopaedic Surgery, Columbia College of Physicians and Surgeons; Director, C. V. Starr Hand Surgery Center, St. Luke's–Roosevelt Hospital Center, New York, New York
Dislocations and Ligament Injuries in the Digits

Richard D. Goldner, MD
Associate Professor, Department of Orthopaedic Surgery, Duke University Medical Center, Durham, North Carolina
Replantation

David P. Green, MD
Clinical Professor, Department of Orthopaedics, University of Texas Health Science Center at San Antonio; Founding President, The Hand Center of San Antonio, San Antonio, Texas
General Principles; Radial Nerve Palsy

John R. Griffin, MD
Division of Plastic Surgery, Surgery of the Hand, Children's Hospital of Oakland, Oakland, California
Congenital Contracture

Ayan Gulgonen, MD
Istanbul, Turkey
Compartment Syndrome

Douglas P. Hanel, MD
Professor of Orthopaedics and Adjunct Professor of Plastic Surgery, University of Washington; Department of Orthopaedics and Sports Medicine, Harborview Medical Center, Seattle, Washington
Fractures of the Distal Humerus; The Mangled Upper Extremity

Hill Hastings II, MD
Clinical Professor of Orthopaedic Surgery, Indiana University Medical Center; Hand and Upper Extremity Surgeon, The Indiana Hand Center, Indianapolis, Indiana
Wrist Arthrodesis (Partial and Complete)

Vincent R. Hentz, MD
Professor of Surgery, Robert A. Chase Center for Hand and Upper Limb Surgery, Stanford University School of Medicine, Palo Alto, California
Traumatic Brachial Plexus Injury

Robert N. Hotchkiss, MD
Associate Attending Orthopedic Surgeon, Hospital for Special Surgery; Director, Alberto Vilar Center for Research of the Hand and Upper Extremity, New York, New York
Complex Traumatic Elbow Dislocation; Treatment of the Stiff Elbow

Thomas B. Hughes, MD
Drexel University College of Medicine, Department of Orthopaedic Surgery, Allegheny General Hospital, Pittsburgh, Pennsylvania
Extensor Tendon Injuries

Michelle A. James, MD
Assistant Chief of Orthopaedic Surgery, Shriners Hospital for Children, Northern California, Sacramento, California
Congenital Deformities of the Wrist and Forearm

Peter J. L. Jebson, MD
Associate Professor and Chief, Division of Elbow, Hand and Microsurgery, Department of Orthopaedic Surgery, University of Michigan Health System, Ann Arbor, Michigan
Amputations

Karen Johnston Jones, MD
Associate Clinical Professor, Department of Orthopaedic Surgery, The University of Texas Health Science Center at San Antonio; Hand Surgeon, The Hand Center of San Antonio, San Antonio, Texas
Thoracic Outlet Compression Syndrome

Neil F. Jones, MD, FRCS
Professor, Department of Orthopedic Surgery, Division of Plastic and Reconstructive Surgery, University of California, Los Angeles, School of Medicine; Chief of Hand Surgery, UCLA Medical Center, Los Angeles, California
Free Skin and Composite Flaps

Jesse B. Jupiter, MD
The Hansjorg Wyss/AO Professor of Orthopaedic Surgery, Harvard Medical School; Chief, Hand and Upper Extremity Service, Department of Orthopaedic Surgery, Massachusetts General Hospital, Boston, Massachusetts
Fractures of the Proximal Ulna

Morton L. Kasdan, MD, FACS
Clinical Professor of Plastic Surgery, University of Louisville, Louisville, Kentucky
Factitious Disorders

Leonid I. Katolik, MD
Assistant Professor, Department of Orthopaedics and Sports Medicine, University of Washington School of Medicine; Section of Hand, Upper Extremity, and Microvascular Surgery, Harborview Medical Center, Seattle, Washington
Total Elbow Arthroplasty

Robert A. Kaufmann, MD
Assistant Professor, Hand and Upper Extremity Surgery, University of Pittsburgh School of Medicine, Pittsburgh, Pennsylvania
Flexor Tendon Injury (Flexor Tendon Reconstruction); Wrist Arthroscopy: Operative Procedures

Simon P. Kay, FRCS
Professor of Hand Surgery, University of Leeds; Consultant, Plastic and Hand Surgery, Department of Plastic Surgery, St. James's University Hospital, Leeds, United Kingdom
Congenital Deformities of the Hand and Fingers; Congenital Contracture

Mary Ann E. Keenan, MD
Professor of Orthopaedic Surgery, University of
Pennsylvania School of Medicine; Chief, Neuro-
Orthopaedics Service, Hospital of the University of
Pennsylvania, Philadelphia, Pennsylvania
Upper Extremity Dysfunction After Stroke or Brain Injury

Graham J. W. King, MD, MSc, FRCS(C)
Professor, Division of Orthopaedic Surgery, University
of Western Ontario; Hand and Upper Limb Centre, St.
Joseph's Health Centre, London, Ontario, Canada
Fractures of the Head of the Radius

John King, MD
Lakelands Orthopaedic Clinic, Greenwood, South Carolina
Thumb Basal Joint Arthritis

L. Andrew Koman, MD
Vice Chair and Professor, Department of Orthopaedic
Surgery, and Professor, Department of Pediatrics, Wake
Forest University School of Medicine, Wake Forest
University Baptist Medical Center, Winston-Salem,
North Carolina
Complex Regional Pain Syndrome; Vascular Disorders

Scott H. Kozin, MD
Assistant Professor, Department of Orthopaedic
Surgery, Temple University School of Medicine;
Director of Hand Surgery, Shriners Hospital for
Children, Philadelphia, Pennsylvania
*Editor of the Congenital Section; Embryology; Deformities
of the Hand and Fingers; Deformities of the Thumb;
Congenital Contracture*

W. P. Andrew Lee, MD
Professor of Surgery and Chief, Division of Plastic
Surgery, University of Pittsburgh School of Medicine
Pittsburgh, Pennsylvania
Thumb Reconstruction

Michel Leit, MD, MS
Fellow, Department of Orthopaedics, University of
Rochester Medical Center, Rochester, New York
Thumb Basal Joint Arthritis

Graham D. Lister, MB, ChB
Formerly Professor, Department of Surgery, University
of Utah School of Medicine; Formerly Chief, Division
of Plastic and Reconstructive Surgery, University of
Utah Medical Center, Salt Lake City, Utah
*Skin Grafts and Skin Flaps (Skin Flaps); Free Skin and
Composite Flaps*

Dean S. Louis, MD
Active Professor Emeritus, Department of Orthopaedic
Surgery, University of Michigan Health System,
Ann Arbor, Michigan
Amputations; Factitious Disorders

Susan E. Mackinnon, MD, FRCS(C), FACS
Shoenberg Professor of Surgery, and Chief, Division of
Plastic and Reconstructive Surgery, Washington
University School of Medicine, St. Louis, Missouri
Compression Neuropathies

**Govind Narain Malaviya, MB, MS, MSc, FICS,
DHRM**
Deputy Director and Head, Plastic and Reconstructive
Surgery Unit, Central JALMA Institute for Leprosy,
Taj Ganj, Agra, India
Chronic Infections

Ralph T. Manktelow, MD, FRCS(C)
Professor, Division of Plastic Surgery, Department of
Surgery, University of Toronto, Toronto General
Hospital, Toronto, Ontario, Canada
Free Functioning Muscle Transfers

David McCombe, MB, BS, FRACS
Department of Surgery, University of Melbourne;
Department of Orthopaedic Surgery, St. Vincent's
Hospital, Melbourne, Australia
Congenital Deformities of the Hand and Fingers

**Duncan Angus McGrouther, MBChB, FRCS, MSc,
MD**
Professor, Plastic and Reconstructive Surgery Research,
The University of Manchester, Manchester, United
Kingdom
Dupuytren's Contracture

Lewis H. Millender, MD*
Formerly Clinic Professor, Department of Orthopedic
Surgery, Tufts University School of Medicine;
Formerly Assistant Chief, Hand Surgery Service,
New England Baptist Hospital, Boston,
Massachusetts
*Rheumatoid Arthritis and Other Connective Tissue
Diseases*

Steven L. Moran, MD
Assistant Professor of Plastic Surgery, Mayo Clinic
College of Medicine, Rochester, Minnesota
Fractures of the Carpal Bones

Edward A. Nalebuff, MD
Clinical Professor of Orthopaedics, Tufts University
School of Medicine; Chief, Hand Surgery Service,
New England Baptist Hospital, Boston,
Massachusetts
*Rheumatoid Arthritis and Other Connective Tissue
Diseases*

Christine B. Novak, PT, MS
Research Associate Professor, Division of Plastic and
Reconstructive Surgery, Washington University School
of Medicine, St. Louis, Missouri
Compression Neuropathies

Shawn W. O'Driscoll, MD, PhD, FRCS(C)
Professor of Orthopedics, Mayo Clinic College of
Medicine; Consultant, Department of Orthopedics,
Mayo Clinic, Rochester, Minnesota
Recurrent Instability of the Elbow

---

*Deceased

A. Lee Osterman, MD
Professor of Orthopedic and Hand Surgery, Jefferson Medical College of Thomas Jefferson University, Philadelphia; Director, The Philadelphia Hand Center, P.C., King of Prussia, Pennsylvania
Wrist Arthroscopy: Operative Procedures

Mukund R. Patel, MD, FACS
Clinical Associate Professor of Orthopedic Surgery, Downstate Medical Center, State University of New York, Brooklyn; Chief of Hand Surgery, Victory Memorial Hospital, Brooklyn; Senior Attending Hand Surgeon, Maimonides Medical Center, Brooklyn; Staten Island University Hospital, St. Vincent's Catholic Medical Center, Staten Island, New York
Chronic Infections

William C. Pederson, MD
Clinical Associate Professor of Surgery and Orthopaedic Surgery, The University of Texas Health Science Center at San Antonio; Director of Fellowship Training, The Hand Center of San Antonio, San Antonio, Texas
Principles of Microvascular Surgery; Skin Grafts and Skin Flaps (Skin Grafting; Skin Flaps; Coverage of the Elbow); The Management of Snake (Pit Viper) Bites

Katrin Philipp, MD
Resident, Department of Hand, Plastic, and Reconstructive Surgery, Burn Center, BG-Trauma Center, Plastic and Hand Surgery, University of Heidelberg, Ludwigshafen, Germany
The Burned Hand

Gary G. Poehling, MD
Professor and Chair, Department of Orthopaedic Surgery, Wake Forest University School of Medicine, Winston-Salem, North Carolina
Wrist Arthroscopy: Anatomy and Diagnosis; Complex Regional Pain Syndrome

Somayaji Ramamurthy, MD
Professor, Department of Anesthesiology, University of Texas Health Science Center at San Antonio, San Antonio, Texas
Anesthesia

David Ring, MD
Instructor, Orthopaedic Surgery, Harvard Medical School; Hand and Upper Extremity Service, Department of Orthopaedic Surgery, Massachusetts General Hospital, Boston, Massachusetts
Fractures of the Proximal Ulna

Spencer A. Rowland, MD, MS
Clinical Professor, Department of Orthopaedics, The University of Texas Health Science Center at San Antonio, San Antonio, Texas
The Management of Snake (Pit Viper) Bites

David S. Ruch, MD
Professor, Department of Orthopaedic Surgery, Wake Forest University School of Medicine, Winston-Salem, North Carolina
Wrist Arthroscopy: Anatomy and Diagnosis; Vascular Disorders

A. Neil Salyapongse, MD
Plastic and Hand Surgery Associates, Belleville, Illinois
Thumb Reconstruction

Christopher C. Schmidt, MD
Drexel University College of Medicine, and Director, Microsurgical Reconstruction of the Upper Limb, Department of Orthopaedic Surgery, Allegheny General Hospital, Pittsburgh, Pennsylvania
Extensor Tendon Injuries

William H. Seitz, Jr., MD
Director, Hand and Upper Extremity Center, Cleveland Orthopaedic and Spine Hospital at Lutheran, Cleveland, Ohio
Distraction Lengthening in the Hand and Upper Extremity

Frances E. Sharpe, MD
Orthopedic Surgeon, Kaiser Permanente, Fontana Medical Center, Fontana, California
Acute Infections in the Hand; Skin Grafts and Skin Flaps (Coverage of the Elbow)

Alexander Y. Shin, MD
Consultant and Associate Professor of Orthopedic Surgery, Mayo Clinic College of Medicine; Division of Hand Surgery, Department of Orthopedic Surgery, Mayo Clinic, Rochester, Minnesota
Stiff Finger Joints

Beth Paterson Smith, PhD
Associate Professor, and Director, Orthopaedic Research Laboratory, Department of Orthopaedic Surgery, Wake Forest University School of Medicine, Winston-Salem, North Carolina
Complex Regional Pain Syndrome; Vascular Disorders

Thomas L. Smith, PhD
Associate Professor, Department of Orthopaedic Surgery, Wake Forest University School of Medicine, Winston-Salem, North Carolina
Complex Regional Pain Syndrome; Vascular Disorders

Nicole Z. Sommer, MD
Assistant Professor, The Plastic Surgery Institute, Southern Illinois University School of Medicine, Springfield, Illinois
The Perionychium

Dean G. Sotereanos, MD
Professor, Orthopaedic Surgery, Drexel University School of Medicine; Vice Chairman, Department of Orthopaedic Surgery, Allegheny General Hospital, Pittsburgh, Pennsylvania
Complex Traumatic Elbow Dislocation

Peter J. Stern, MD
Norman S. and Elizabeth C. A. Hill Professor and Chairman, Department of Orthopaedic Surgery, University of Cincinnati College of Medicine, Cincinnati, Ohio
Fractures of the Metacarpals and Phalanges

Milan V. Stevanovic, MD, PhD

Professor of Orthopaedics and Surgery, Hand and Microsurgery, and Director, Joseph H. Boyes Microsurgery Laboratory, Keck School of Medicine, Department of Orthopaedic Surgery, University of Southern California, Los Angeles, California

Acute Infections in the Hand; Skin Grafts and Skin Flaps (Coverage of the Elbow)

Alan M. Sugar, MD

Professor of Medicine, Boston University School of Medicine, Boston; Medical Director, HIV/AIDS and Hepatitis Viruses Infection Programs and Infectious Disease Clinical Services, Cape Cod Hospital; Chief, Infection Control Program, Cape Cod Healthcare, Hyannis, Massachusetts

Chronic Infections

John S. Taras, MD

Associate Professor of Orthopedic Surgery, Thomas Jefferson University School of Medicine; Associate Professor of Orthopedic Surgery, and Chief, Hand Surgery, Drexel University School of Medicine; The Philadelphia Hand Center, P.C., Philadelphia, Pennsylvania

Flexor Tendon Injury (Flexor Tendon Reconstruction)

Andrew L. Terrono, MD

Associate Clinical Professor of Orthopaedic Surgery, Tufts University School of Medicine; New England Baptist Hospital; Hand Surgical Associates, Boston, Massachusetts

Rheumatoid Arthritis and Other Connective Tissue Diseases

Matthew M. Tomaino, MD, MBA

Professor of Orthopaedics, and Chief, Division of Hand, Shoulder and Elbow Surgery, University of Rochester Medical Center, Rochester, New York

Thumb Basal Joint Arthritis

James R. Urbaniak, MD

Virginia Flowers Baker Professor and Vice Chairman, Department of Surgery, Duke University Medical Center, Durham, North Carolina

Replantation

Ann E. Van Heest, MD

Associate Professor, Department of Orthopedic Surgery, University of Minnesota; Shriners Hospital–Twin Cities Unit; Pediatric Hand and Upper Extremity Service, Gillette Children's Hospital, Minneapolis, Minnesota

Tetraplegia

Nicholas B. Vedder, MD, FACS

Professor of Surgery and Orthopaedics, and Chief, Division of Plastic Surgery, University of Washington, Seattle, Washington

The Mangled Upper Extremity

Peter M. Waters, MD

Associate Professor of Orthopaedic Surgery, Harvard Medical School; Director, Brachial Plexus and Hand/Upper Extremity Programs, Department of Orthopaedic Surgery, Children's Hospital, Boston, Massachusetts

Pediatric Brachial Plexus Palsy

Fu-Chan Wei, MD, FACS

Professor, Department of Plastic Surgery, Chang-Gung Memorial Hospital; Dean, Medical College, Chang-Gung University, Taipei, Taiwan, Republic of China

Toe-to-Hand Transplantation

Scott W. Wolfe, MD

Professor of Orthopedic Surgery, Weill Medical College of Cornell University; Chief, Hand and Upper Extremity Surgery, and Attending Orthopedic Surgeon, Hospital for Special Surgery, New York, New York

Distal Radius Fractures; Tenosynovitis

PREFACE

The positive acceptance and widespread use of *Operative Hand Surgery* in its previous editions has been most gratifying, but there is always room for improvement and we have tried to make the fifth edition even better. The most noticeable changes for the reader include the following:

1 **Organization.** The entire format and location of chapters have been radically altered. New chapters have been created, deleting relatively obsolete material, introducing new concepts and techniques, and in some instances merging parts of several old chapters into new composites.

2 **Authors.** The major strength of this book has always been the quality of the contributors. Many of the authors who wrote chapters for the first three or four editions are at or near retirement age, but the hand surgery world is blessed with a tremendous pool of exceptional new talent. We have very carefully selected some of these best and brightest to revise old chapters or write new ones, in most instances liberally retaining the core elements of old chapters.

3 **References.** From its conception in 1982, one of the objectives of *Operative Hand Surgery* has been to provide the reader with a comprehensive reference list of virtually everything about a topic that has been written in the English language. Continued adherence to this principle has resulted in an inordinate number of pages being devoted to exhaustive lists of references, which in turn squeezes the amount of space available for text and illustrations. Computer technology has provided a satisfactory compromise: the fifth edition will continue to have comprehensive reference lists for each chapter, but they will reside on a companion CD-ROM. At the end of each chapter, however, the reader will find a list of annotated references compiled by each author, with his or her comments on those articles deemed to be the most important to that subject.

4 **Internet Access.** Another advantage of computer technology makes it possible to have the entire text and all illustrations accessible via the Internet. Not only does this give the reader freer access to the content of the book, but this **e-dition** creates a mechanism to provide more frequent updates than is possible with only the printed version.

5 **Operative Techniques.** Although the emphasis of this book has always been on *operative* treatment, an effort has been made in the fifth edition to incorporate even more specific details of surgical technique. At the same time, attention has not been lessened on the important indications for and alternative methods of specific treatments, and even more has been added regarding expected outcomes.

Perhaps less obvious to the reader, but critical to the ongoing improvement of this book, is the expanded editorial staff. The first two editions of *Operative Hand Surgery* had a single editor; for this fifth edition there have been four, bringing broader expertise and enhanced quality of ideas to the table.

DAVID P. GREEN, MD
ROBERT N. HOTCHKISS, MD
WILLIAM C. PEDERSON, MD
SCOTT W. WOLFE, MD

ACKNOWLEDGMENTS

Over the two-decade life span of *Operative Hand Surgery,* massive changes have taken place in the medical publishing world. Globalization, business mergers, personnel changes, and different priorities have radically altered what goes on behind the scenes in bringing a book to publication. Although some contacts at Elsevier have come and gone, we have been fortunate to have had the steady hand of Developmental Editor Arlene Chappelle guiding, cajoling, and sometimes goading us to complete our assigned tasks in this fifth edition. She has kept us focused on what needed to be done, and we are grateful to her for her clear direction and guidance. Dan Pepper, Acquisitions Editor, inherited this project in mid stream and has been of tremendous help. Tina Rebane, Publishing Services Manager, has done a superb job arranging and overseeing the actual production of this book.

One aspect of medical publishing has not changed—the commitment of very busy surgeons to devote enormous chunks of their time and energy to writing chapters for *Operative Hand Surgery.* We the editors—on behalf of readers of this book and students of hand surgery throughout the world—again express our appreciation to these men and women for their unselfish efforts.

One of our contributors deserves special mention. Scott Kozin took on the unenviable task of section editor for the chapters on congenital abnormalities. From the inception of this book in 1982, that group of chapters has posed the most daunting editorial challenge, probably because the subject virtually defies a clear and precise organizational format. When Dr. Kozin agreed to take on this assignment, he probably did not appreciate its complexity, but despite the predictable difficulty, he stayed the course and saw the job to its completion.

Elizabeth Roselius is one of the major reasons that this book has been successful. She is a world-class medical illustrator whose talents have enhanced numerous books and whose efforts have been widely acknowledged; the first edition of *Operative Hand Surgery* received the Illustrated Medical Book Award, Clinical Text, from the Association of Medical Illustrators. She has added a substantial number of new illustrations for this fifth edition.

Above all, I wish to thank my good friends Bob Hotchkiss, Chris Pederson, and Scott Wolfe. I am grateful to them not only for bringing to the book new insights, but also for assuming an increasingly heavier share of the editorial load.

DAVID P. GREEN, MD

CONTENTS

PART VII
Bone and Soft Tissue Reconstruction

PART VIII
Other Disorders of the Upper Extremity

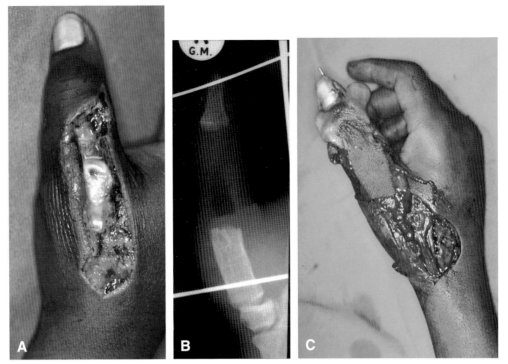

FIGURE 3-15. A 27-year-old man sustained a bite injury to his thumb during an assault. He developed a severe infection of the thumb MP joint, with subsequent spread to the metacarpal head and proximal phalanx. The volar soft tissue, flexor tendon, and neurovascular structures were intact. **A,** Open draining wound with exposed metacarpal head and necrotic proximal phalanx. **B,** Radiograph taken after resection of all necrotic bone. **C,** A free vascularized second toe transfer was used to reconstruct the bone defect, extensor pollicis longus tendon, and soft tissue defect.

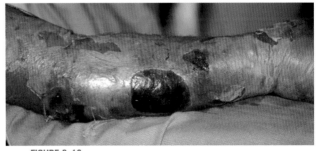

FIGURE 3-18. Characteristic appearance of necrotizing fasciitis.

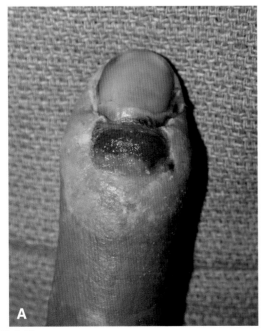

FIGURE 3-16. Osteomyelitis of the middle finger as a complication of pyarthrosis of the DIP joint. **A,** Granulation tissue overlying the DIP joint.

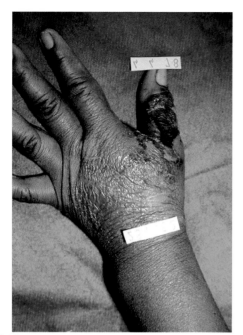

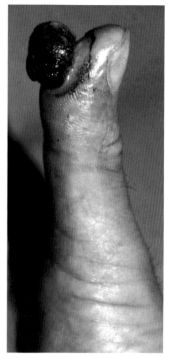

FIGURE 3-19. Cutaneous anthrax. (Courtesy of Dr. Eduardo Gotuzzo, Tropical Medicine Institute, Universidad Peruana Cayetano Heredia, Lima, Peru.)

FIGURE 3-20. Pyogenic granuloma of the thumb.

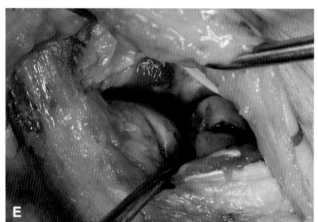

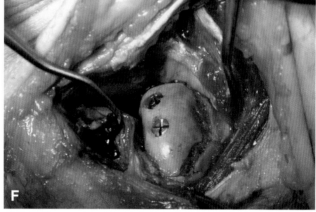

FIGURE 21-9 Capitellar cartilage shear fracture. **E,** Intraoperative photograph of cartilage shear fracture. **F,** Intraoperative photograph demonstrating reduction of the fracture with two 2.0-mm screws and cancellous bone grafting of the radial neck from the lateral epicondyle.

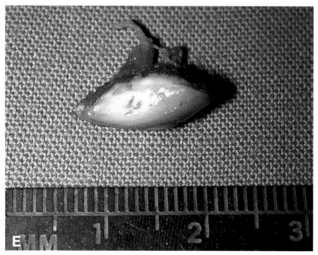

FIGURE 21-16 Excision of fragment of radial head in a 32-year-old man who fell while rollerblading. He had limited prosupination. Studies revealed he had an undisplaced coronoid fracture, a posterior capitellum impression fracture, and a fragment of the radial head anterior to the radial neck. **E,** Attempts to retrieve the fragment arthroscopically failed due to its location distal to the radial head, and an arthrotomy was needed to excise the small fragment.

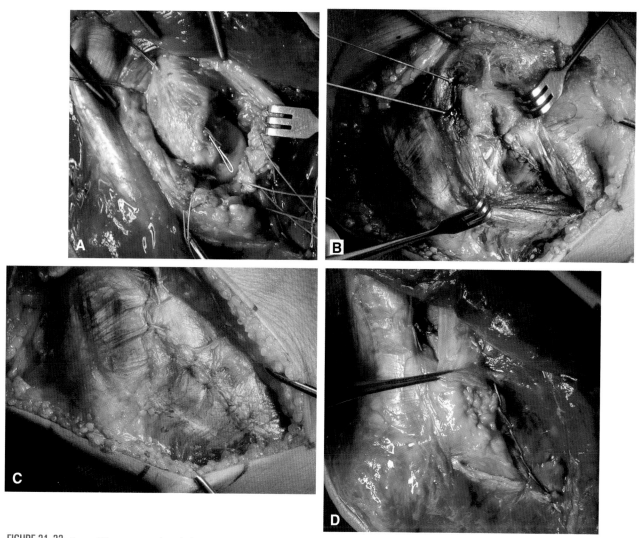

FIGURE 21-22. Lateral ligament repair technique. Method of suture repair of torn or detached lateral collateral ligament complex using sutures through bone tunnels in the lateral epicondyle. **A,** A single hole is drilled at the axis of motion (the center of the arc of curvature of the capitellum) and connected to a hole placed anterior and posterior to the lateral supracondylar ridge. **B,** A locking suture technique is employed to gain a secure hold of the lateral collateral ligament. The interval between the radial and lateral ulnar collateral ligaments and the annular ligament is closed as this suture is brought back to the lateral epicondyle. The ligament sutures are pulled into the holes drilled in the distal humerus while maintaining the forearm in pronation and avoiding varus forces while tying the sutures. **C,** A side-to-side repair of the Kocher interval is used to augment stability. **D,** Alternatively, the fascia of the Kocher interval can be closed as for the ligaments and the repair can be secured to the lateral epicondyle through the aforementioned drill holes.

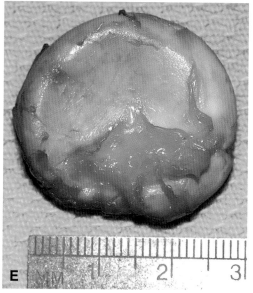

FIGURE 21-26 Osteoarthritis of radial head of a 46-year-old construction worker who had Kirschner wire fixation for a comminuted fracture 4 years previously. **E,** Excision of the radial head and metallic arthroplasty improved his pain and allowed him to return to a supervisory position.

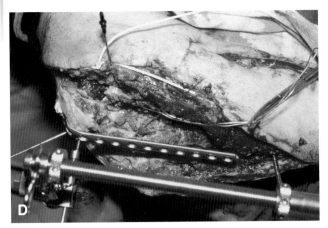

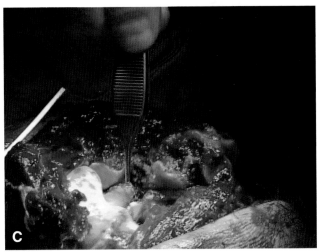

FIGURE 22-8. Anterior (trans-olecranon) fracture-dislocation of the elbow. **D,** The olecranon fragment is held to the trochlea with a stout smooth Kirschner wire. Distraction between this wire and a second distal wire helps realign the intervening fragments. (Copyright © Massachusetts General Hospital Department of Orthopaedic Surgery.)

FIGURE 22-9. Posterior olecranon fracture-dislocation (posterior Monteggia fracture type A). **C,** In this patient the coronoid was fractured into three major fragments: anteromedial, central, and lesser sigmoid notch. (Copyright © Massachusetts General Hospital Department of Orthopaedic Surgery.)

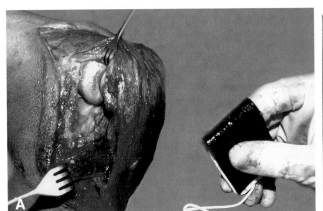

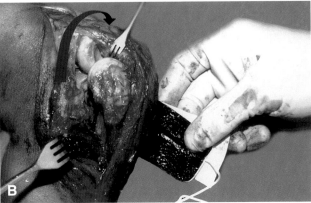

FIGURE 24-10. Tension band wiring. **A,** Tension band wiring is suitable for simple fractures without fracture of the radial head or coronoid or dislocation/subluxation of the ulnohumeral joint. **B,** A technique using anteriorly oriented Kirschner wires, impaction of the proximal ends into the olecranon beneath the triceps insertion, and two small-gauge tension wires can limit hardware-related problems. **C,** Active motion is initiated the morning after surgery. (Copyright © Massachusetts General Hospital Department of Orthopaedic Surgery.)

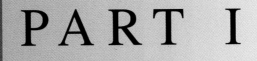

PART I

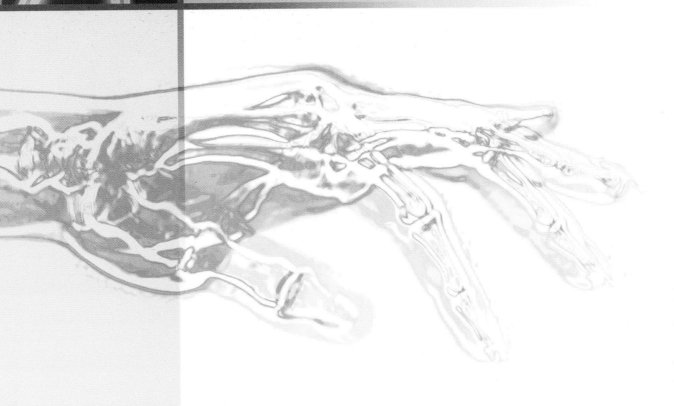

Basic Principles

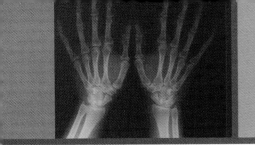

CHAPTER 1

General Principles

David P. Green

Throughout this book the emphasis is on specific details of operative techniques in hand surgery. The purpose of this introductory chapter is to briefly discuss some of the elements that are common to all operations on the hand. The scope of hand surgery is broad and requires a wide range of diverse operative skills. The hand surgeon must be equally facile at suturing together a tiny vessel 1 mm in diameter and fashioning a corticocancellous bone graft into a specific configuration. In all hand surgery procedures, however, one theme is dominant: careful attention to detail and precise, gentle technique are essential for success. In a remarkably prescient article in 1921, Sterling Bunnell[9] emphasized the importance of atraumatic technique in hand surgery. Modern advances in magnification have allowed us to clearly see how damaging to delicate tissues even the most careful and precise attempts at dissection can be. At the same time, refinements in instruments have provided us with improved methods for striving to more nearly achieve the impossible dream of truly atraumatic surgery.

PREOPERATIVE PLANNING

Doing the Correct (and Necessary) Operation

The concept raised in this subheading may sound facetious, but it is not. Knowing what to do when is perhaps the most difficult aspect of becoming a surgeon. Learning specific techniques (e.g., how and where to cut) can often be done in a relatively short time, but developing keen clinical acumen and surgical judgment requires careful attention to the admonitions of respected mentors and years of one's own practice.

In an individual patient, making an accurate diagnosis is the paramount essential first step. Even then, knowing when to intervene surgically is not always an easy decision. The ability to do an operation is not necessarily an indication to do that procedure.

Making a Diagnosis

History and Physical Examination

Trite as it may sound, obtaining a thorough history and performing a meticulous physical examination are the hallmarks of a good diagnostician. Perhaps the best source for learning specific techniques of diagnosis in disorders of the hand is Lister's *The Hand: Diagnosis and Indications*.[30,36]

In my practice, each new patient chart has in it a form for the history and physical examination (Fig. 1-1) that provides a series of reminders for the fellows (and myself) of the pertinent points that must be asked about and examined for. Not all of the blanks need be filled out for every patient, but this repetitive checklist is, I believe, useful in developing good habits. The essential points of the history and physical examination as they pertain to specific conditions are stressed throughout the remainder of this book.

Record Keeping

Probably no surgeons enjoy the paperwork involved in medicine, yet few will deny the importance of clear, comprehensive, and accurate records. From the moment a patient is first seen—in the emergency department, the hospital, or the office—it is absolutely essential that the pertinent facts of the history and clinical examination be recorded accurately.

We have all had the experience of reviewing our own or another physician's records to publish a retrospective clinical study or prepare medicolegal testimony, only to discover that key dates, facts, and figures are missing from carelessly written or dictated notes. Although subjective impressions are important to record, the key to meaningful information in a patient's chart is to have as much objective data as possible. Absolutely essential are specific degrees of joint range of motion and contracture. There are many different ways to record range of motion in the fingers, but I am partial to a method called total active motion (TAM) and total passive motion (TPM) devised in 1977 by the Clinical Assessment Committee (Richard Eaton, chairman) of the American Society for Surgery of the Hand (ASSH). The method is illustrated in the ASSH's small handbook on hand examination and diagnosis,[2] and an example is as follows:

Joint	Active	Passive
Metacarpophalangeal (MP)	10-75	0-90
Proximal interphalangeal (PIP)	30-75	10-95
Distal interphalangeal (DIP)	0-55	0-60
	205	245
	−40	−10
	TAM = 165	TPM = 235

The lack of full extension in each joint is added, and this sum is subtracted from the total amount of flexion. In this example, the patient has a 30-degree extensor lag of the PIP

NAME_____REFERRED BY_____

AGE/HAND DOM/OCCUPATION_____

SIDE INVOLVED___RT ___LEFT ___BOTH

ONSET OF SX_____IF SPECIFIC INJURY, DOI_____

DESCRIPTION OF INJURY

INITIAL SX

SX NOW

WORK STATUS SINCE INJURY: CURRENTLY WORKING ___NO (SINCE_____)
         ___YES (___REGULAR JOB___LIGHT DUTY)

MEDICAL PROBLEMS:
         DIABETIC ___NO ___YES (INSULIN x ____YR/ORAL MEDS x ____ YR)
         OTHER:

TREATMENT TO DATE #X OR HOW LONG: TREATMENT BY: EFFECT:
         ___NONE
         ___SPLINTING
         ___CAST
         ___NSAIDs
         ___THERAPY (TYPE)

         ___INJECTIONS
         ___OTHER:

         ___IMPRESSION:

A

FIGURE 1–1. (**A**) History worksheet.   *Continued*

joint, 10 degrees of which is fixed contracture, whereas motion in the DIP joint is nearly normal. This method has the advantage of being easily reproducible and comparable on subsequent visits when the bottom line number can be compared with a previous figure, but it also allows a quick check of exactly where the major problems remain.

Objective measurements are particularly important, including the circumference of digits to quantitate enlargement, volumetric displacement to monitor swelling of the entire hand, and any other definitive observation that can be used later for comparison. Another measurement that I find particularly informative is the distance between skin creases in a patient with a contracture, especially Dupuytren's (Fig. 1-2).

At the conclusion of the initial examination it is important to try to make a definitive diagnosis because this tends to focus the work-up and treatment plan more clearly. This does not mean that the surgeon needs to fabricate a diagnosis if one is not readily apparent. If a diagnosis cannot be made with reasonable assurance, it is better to defer labeling the patient's condition. The *International Classification of Diseases—Clinical Modification* (ICD-9-CM) has a very specific code for such situations: 729.5 ("Pain in Limb").

The timing of record keeping is important as well. An office note recorded at the time the patient is seen and an operative report dictated immediately after a procedure are likely to contain far more accurate and significant information

PROVOCATIVE TESTS				
CTS		RIGHT		LEFT
	DIRECT COMP.			
	TINEL'S			
	PHALEN'S			
CUBITAL				
	DIRECT COMP.			
	HYPERFLEXION			
NON-ANATOMIC				
	FOREARM			
	ELBOW			
TOS				
	WRIGHT'S			
	ROOS'			

PIP CIRCUM		
	RT	LEFT
II		
III		
IV		
V		

FINGERS		INDEX (II)		LONG (III)		RING (IV)		SMALL (V)	
		Active	Passive	Active	Passive	Active	Passive	Active	Passive
Right									
	MP								
	PIP								
	DIP								
	Subtotal								
	-								
	TAM/TPM								
Left									
	MP								
	PIP								
	DIP								
	Subtotal								
	-								
	TAM/TPM								

2 PT DISCRIM.		DIGIT	RADIAL	ULNAR
RT	THUMB			
	II			
	III			
	IV			
	V			
LT	THUMB			
	II			
	III			
	IV			
	V			

THUMB CMC	Right	Left
Prominence		
Tenderness		
Radial Abd		
Pinch #		
Grip #		
Ext/Abd		
Finklestein		
CMC Grind		

∅ = SUBJECTIVE DIMINUTION

SBRN __NL __ Decreased

DSBUN __NL __ Decreased

B

FIGURE 1–1.—cont'd (**B**) Physical examination worksheet. These worksheets are used in my office to provide a checklist for residents and fellows in developing a reliable and consistent routine of patient evaluation.   *Figure continues on next page.*

than a record dictated days or weeks later. Dictation of the operative note should be considered an integral part of the surgical procedure and is preferably done immediately after the operation, but certainly no later than the day of surgery.

Nonoperative Diagnostic Tools
Doppler Examination

The arterial supply to the hand can be determined easily and accurately by the use of a hand-held Doppler device, which can usually pinpoint an area of vascular occlusion and/or assess arterial flow to the digits. The Doppler probe is used to listen to the radial and ulnar arteries and the arch, as well as the pulps, of each digit. A well-perfused digit should have a strong signal in the pulp. With the probe over the palmar arch, the radial and ulnar artery are sequentially occluded with direct digital pressure. Loss of the signal in the arch signifies occlusion of the nonoccluded vessel. The actual point of occlusion can then often be found by following the course of the vessel with the Doppler pencil probe. By listening to the digital pulps and occluding either the radial or ulnar vessels,

THUMB

Rt		Active	Passive	UCL	RCL
	MP				
	IP				
	Palmar Abd				
	Nail Rotation				
Left					
	MP				
	IP				
	Palmar Abd				
	Nail Rotation				

WRIST

ROM	RIGHT	LEFT	TESTS	RIGHT	LEFT
Extension					
Flexion			PT. MAX. TENDER		
RD			Watson's		
UD			Resisted Pronation		
Pronation			L-T Shear/shuck		
Supination			ECU subluxation		
			DRUJ Instability		

ELBOW

	RIGHT	LEFT
MAX. TENDERNESS		
LAT.EPICONDYLE		
MOBILE WAD		
RADIAL HEAD		
ROM		
FLEX/EXT		
PRO/SUP		
GRIP		
ELBOW FLEXED		
ELBOW EXTENDED		

CERVICAL SPINE

Tenderness		
Flexion		
Extension		
Rotation-R		
Rotation-L		
Reflexes	Right	Left
Biceps		
Triceps		
Strength		
Biceps		
Triceps		

SHOULDER

	Right	Left
Elevation		
Abduction		
Int. Rotation		
Tenderness		
Crepitus		

INTRINSIC TIGHTNESS

	MP EXT.	MP FLEX
II		
III		
IV		
V		

FIGURE 1–1.—cont'd

the dominant artery to that finger can be determined, as well as the presence of an incomplete arch.

Radiographs

Every hand surgeon should have a routine set of standard radiographic views for specific conditions. For example, any patient with a problem involving a single digit must have at least anteroposterior and true lateral views *of the individual digit.* Failure to insist on a true lateral view of the finger itself is a common cause for misdiagnosis. An oblique view often offers additional information, but it should never be accepted in lieu of a true lateral view.

For patients with wrist pain, I have two sets of standard views. If the problem appears to be on the radial side, a so-called scaphoid series is done, which includes (1) a posteroan-terior view in ulnar deviation (to see the scaphoid in profile); (2) an anteroposterior view with fist compression (most likely to show an increased scapholunate gap); (3) a true lateral view (on which the carpal angles can be measured); and (4) an oblique view (to show chip fractures on the dorsum of the carpus and better visualize the distal pole of scaphoid). For patients with pain primarily on the dorsal or ulnar aspects of the wrist, I routinely take three views: (1) a neutral posteroan-terior (necessary to measure ulnar variance); (2) a neutral lateral (to assess carpal alignment); and (3) an oblique (to show the dorsoulnar side of the carpus in profile). (See Chapter 15 for the technique of obtaining true posteroanterior and lateral views.)

Special views are done based on the clinical examination, and many views have been described to show specific struc-

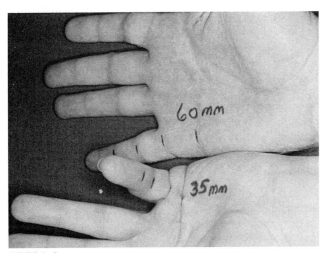

FIGURE 1–2. Measuring the distances between the distal palmar, MP, PIP, and DIP creases in a patient with Dupuytren's contracture (and comparing these with the opposite hand, if normal) provides the surgeon with a very clear image of how much skin deficit has to be "made up" when the finger is straightened. In this example, the distance between the distal palmar crease and the DIP crease is 35 mm in the involved digit and 60 mm in the normal hand.

tures. A few examples are (1) a pisotriquetral view[19] (which is simply a lateral view with 10 to 15 degrees of supination to show this joint in profile); (2) a carpal tunnel view (to show the carpal "pillars," including the hook of hamate and trapezial ridge); (3) Watson's carpometacarpal (CMC) views (to assess carpal boss)[14]; (4) an index CMC view (Fig. 1-3), the best view of the scaphotrapeziotrapezoid joints and trapezoid, which is one of the most difficult areas of the hand to visualize radiographically; and (5) a Brewerton view[6] (to show early erosive or post-traumatic changes beneath the MP collateral ligaments).

Injections

Injections of local anesthetic with or without a corticosteroid serve a dual purpose: (1) to relieve the patient's pain and (2) to provide diagnostic information. Temporary relief of pain after injection is one of the most accurate methods of establishing a diagnosis, and I use local corticosteroid injections frequently in my office. My technique differs slightly from others in that I do not mix the local anesthetic and corticosteroid solutions, for two reasons: (1) injection of the anesthetic alone ensures correct placement of the needle (e.g., in the tendon sheath, carpal tunnel, appropriate joint space) and (2) injection of the corticosteroid superficially can result in hypopigmentation of the skin and/or subcutaneous atrophy, especially in injections for de Quervain's and tennis elbow. Therefore, I first inject only local anesthetic, refill the syringe with corticosteroid (leaving the needle undisturbed; Fig. 1-4), and then inject the corticosteroid directly into the tendon sheath or other intended destination. Although this does not totally eliminate the possibility of untoward local corticosteroid reactions, I believe that it minimizes the likelihood of such. It is important to use lidocaine *without* epinephrine for local and regional anesthesia about the hand.

Bone Scan

Radionuclide imaging with strontium-95 is one of the most useful tools we have to identify occult sites of bone or joint pathology. Bone scans are of no help in nerve or tendon problems, but any joint pathology that evokes inflammation will produce an abnormal bone scan with localized increased uptake. The bone scan is my next step in the work-up in any patient with undiagnosed pain if I suspect that the cause is from the bone or joint. The scan will not tell you *what* is wrong, but it often will reveal *where* the problem is. On many occasions, a "hot" bone scan has prompted me to order a special radiograph that has clearly identified the source of pain.

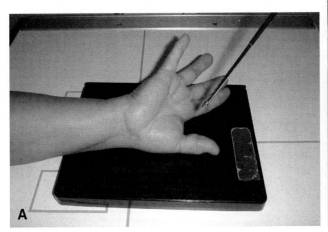

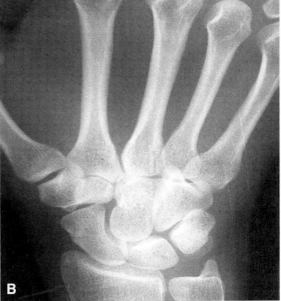

FIGURE 1–3. The index CMC view. **A,** Positioning of the hand is similar to that for a Robert view of the thumb, but with the x-ray beam directed 30 degrees from the central axis (pointer). **B,** Radiograph taken in this position clearly shows the trapezoid and second CMC joint.

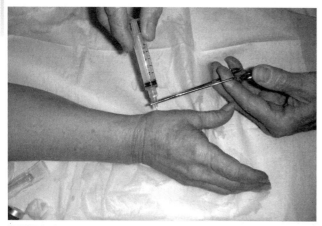

FIGURE 1–4. When injecting a corticosteroid in the hand, it is my practice to localize the joint with local anesthetic, remove the syringe without disturbing the needle, and then inject the corticosteroid solution separately (see text). I carry a hemostat in my coat pocket to facilitate this simple technique.

Computed Tomography

Computed tomography (CT) is the best radiographic way to see precise bony detail. I use CT primarily for (1) identification of occult causes of bone or joint pain, when the routine radiographs are normal or perhaps suggestive of a subtle intra-articular fracture; (2) evaluation of bone structure, such as the Sanders type CT scan[35] for scaphoid nonunion

(Fig. 1-5); and (3) preoperative planning. The latest generation of CT scanners can produce incredibly accurate and realistic three-dimensional images.

Tri-Spiral Tomography ("Polytomes")

Most radiology departments no longer even have the equipment to do polytomes, but these were an important precursor to CT and still provide excellent quality bone detail in those facilities where they are available. Their main advantage was that they could be done with 1- to 2-mm cuts rather than 5 mm, which was the limit in routine tomograms.

Magnetic Resonance Imaging

Magnetic resonance imaging (MRI) can be a very valuable diagnostic tool, but in its present form its use is sometimes abused by inexperienced physicians ordering an MRI even before an adequate physical examination has been done. The value of MRI is very dependent on the quality of the scanner and the expertise of the radiologist, and many scans done today are of limited clinical value because of technical limitations. In my opinion, the main indications of this modality at the present time are when the physician suspects (1) a soft tissue tumor; (2) avascularity (e.g., Kienbock's or Preiser's); or (3) a soft tissue problem such as tendinitis of the extensor carpi ulnaris or an occult ganglion. Without question, however, advances in technology will allow MRI to play an increasingly important role in the diagnosis of hand and wrist problems, especially those involving the soft tissues.

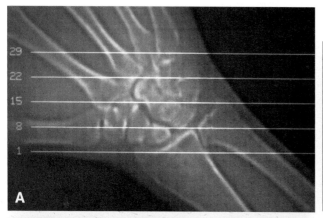

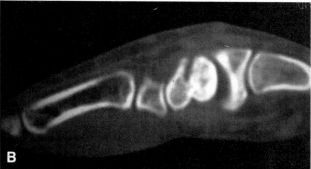

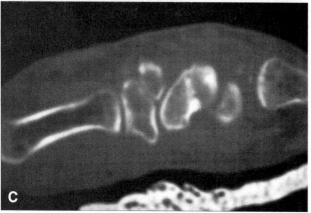

FIGURE 1–5. Sanders[35] has described a simple method for showing a scaphoid "humpback" deformity on CT. **A,** The CT scan is lined up along the axis of the scaphoid itself, not the longitudinal axis of the hand. A typical collapse deformity is shown preoperatively (**B**) and after a volar wedge graft (**C**).

Priorities for Reconstruction

Over the past decade, improved methods of internal fixation and the development of microvascular techniques have enabled surgeons to combine multiple types of tissue repair and reconstruction into a single operation in the very early stages after injury.[17,18] Although the trend has thus been to do as much as possible in the acute trauma setting or shortly thereafter, there are still many patients in whom staged hand reconstruction will be required for a variety of reasons. In such patients, the surgeon must develop a logical plan to achieve the goal of maximum restoration of function. Although each patient presents a unique problem and the plan of management must be developed to suit that particular individual, in general the priorities of reconstruction are as follows: (1) bone and joint stabilization, (2) soft tissue coverage, (3) nerve, and (4) tendon. The details of each of these steps in reconstruction and the principles involved in selecting the appropriate types of surgical procedures are covered in subsequent chapters of this book, but it is perhaps worthwhile here to attempt to put into perspective how those various procedures must be organized into a logical plan of reconstruction.

In most cases, the first priority is to achieve provisional bone and joint stability. With adequate bony stabilization, the soft tissue bed is also stabilized and the risk of secondary infection lessened. Soft tissue coverage is critical early in the reconstructive period, not only to ensure a wound free of infection but also to provide an appropriate cover beneath which subsequent surgical procedures can be done. The type of coverage selected is, of course, dependent on which tissues have been lost and what needs to be replaced in future operations. Newer techniques have enabled hand surgeons to be able to supply bone, tendons, and other tissues concomitantly with the skin coverage.

Definitive stabilization of the bony skeleton must be accomplished before nerve, joint, or tendon operations can be successfully carried out. Because internal fixation of fractures or bone grafting for bony defects usually requires postoperative immobilization, these procedures should not be performed simultaneously with operations that require early movement of adjacent joints unless sufficiently rigid stabilization can be achieved to allow that early motion.

Early repair or grafting of nerves is essential for many reasons: (1) undue delay is likely to compromise ultimate sensory recovery; (2) return of function through reinnervation of specific muscles will determine the future needs for specific tendon reconstruction; (3) restoration of sensibility in the hand is imperative for reasonable function; and (4) return of sensation probably requires the longest period of time to reach its optimum end result.

Before tendon transfers or grafting can be considered, the joints to be moved by those muscle-tendon units must be made as supple as possible. In many instances, this can be accomplished by appropriate exercise therapy and dynamic splinting, but stiff joints that are refractory to these modalities or joints that have been irreparably damaged must be dealt with by soft tissue procedures, arthroplasty, or even arthrodesis.

The final stage in reconstruction is generally aimed at restoration of active motion of joints by appropriate tendon transfers, grafts, or tenolysis.

Tissue Equilibrium

The timing of staged reconstructive procedures (i.e., the interval between operations) cannot be stated in absolute terms. Although in my experience 3 months is a reasonable benchmark to guide the overall planning, this will vary in individual patients and between separate stages in the same patient. More important than a specific time period is the requirement that the soft tissues be as supple as possible and that maximal range of passive motion be reached by appropriate exercise and orthotic modalities. Steindler's "tissue equilibrium" (quoted by Boyes[5]) is an important concept. It implies that soft tissue induration is gone, there is no reaction in the wounds, the joints are supple, and the scars are as soft as they are likely to become. Achieving maximal tissue equilibrium is the most critical factor in the timing of staged reconstruction.

Treatment Objectives

Surgeons must keep their objectives clearly in mind, and these objectives must be realistic. We must take the time necessary to try to help the patient understand these objectives as clearly as possible. Advances in technology and refinements in operative technique have opened up new vistas in hand surgery. Although the range of hand surgery procedures is broad, we must all base our decisions for surgical reconstruction on the axiom, "Do what is needed, not what is possible."

Surgical Judgment

Planning the multiple stages of reconstruction in a severely damaged hand is one of the most difficult and challenging aspects of hand surgery and requires both experience and sound judgment. It is desirable from both the patient's and the surgeon's points of view to have an overall plan in mind, but it is also imperative to allow flexibility in that plan according to the results of the various stages of reconstruction. Knowing when to quit is perhaps the most difficult judgment decision of all. Often the patient and/or the surgeon earnestly desire to restore a hand to normal when that is not possible. Surgeons must keep in mind that "the enemy of good is better," and we must recognize when the chances of worsening a hand that is less than perfect outweigh the likelihood of improving the situation with continued operative intervention.

Surgical Technique

Specific aspects of surgical technique are learned from one's teachers and may vary widely. Certain fundamental principles, however, underlie all techniques. Perhaps the most important of these is what I call "the No. 1 rule of surgery"—start in an area of normal anatomy! In both trauma and reconstructive surgery, the temptation is great for the neophyte surgeon to begin the operation at the site of maximal pathology, which is precisely where the anatomy will be most distorted. Experienced surgeons will virtually always find appropriate virgin tissue planes in normal anatomy and follow these to the site of injury and/or scarring. Strict adherence to this rule will save the surgeon countless hours of difficult and dangerous dissection.

The Operative Game Plan

In designing a specific operation or combination of operations for a given patient, careful preoperative planning is imperative. It is important to combine compatible operations at one sitting to minimize the total number of procedures required to achieve the final objective, particularly in a patient who must undergo multiple stages of reconstruction. At the same time, we must be careful to avoid doing so many procedures at one time that tourniquet and operative time are prolonged and the objectives so broad as to create problems in the postoperative recovery period. It is particularly important that operations requiring diametrically opposed postoperative programs not be done at the same time (e.g., osteotomy of a phalanx and capsulotomy of an adjacent joint), unless sufficiently rigid stabilization of the osteotomy can be achieved to allow early unrestricted range of motion.

The sequential steps of any operation must be carefully thought out in advance by the surgeon to minimize tourniquet time and anticipate any potential problems. It is particularly important to have in mind alternative plans of action in the event that one encounters unexpected findings at the time of surgery. For example, when performing a tenolysis, the surgeon must anticipate the possible need for a type of pulley reconstruction that will not preclude early mobilization. If a tendon or bone graft is to be used, alternative sources must be considered in the event that the predetermined graft is for some reason unsuitable or unavailable. If there is the remotest possibility of needing a graft from another site in the body, that must be taken into consideration when the patient signs the operative permit and in prepping and draping the patient in the operating room.

I have found it particularly worthwhile to sit down the evening before each operation and, in the quiet of my office or study, mentally rehearse the procedures to be performed and methodically think out each step in an attempt to anticipate potential pitfalls and problems. Ask yourself all the "what ifs" you can think of as you rehearse the operation in your mind. Careful attention to detail in the mental preparation of each operation will do much to ensure a successful outcome.

Psychological Impact of Hand Injuries

Surgeons must be aware of the major psychological and emotional impact resulting from hand injury and deformity, and these important aspects of care should not be neglected.[13,20,22-24] Grunert and colleagues[23] reported that an astonishing 94% of patients who sustained severe hand trauma experienced some type of adverse emotional response, including nightmares, flashbacks, affective lability, preoccupation with phantom limb sensations, concentration/attention problems, cosmetic concerns, denial of amputation, and even fear of death. If we ignore these critical—and apparently nearly universal—aspects of hand trauma, we compromise our patient care and limit the results of treatment, no matter how good our technical skills may be.

Although our primary goal is to restore maximum function in the injured hand, we must also do everything we can to assist the patient in learning to live with those residual problems that we cannot make better. In this regard, the hand therapists who work with us can often provide valuable support and guidance for our patients.[21]

PREPPING AND DRAPING

There are almost as many ways to prep and drape a patient for hand surgery as there are hand surgeons. In my opinion, more important than the methods and agents used is that each surgeon select a specific routine and educate his or her own hospital personnel in that technique. Adopting a uniform and standardized method is probably the best way to ensure that each patient receives the same careful attention to detail in skin prepping and draping.

Many studies have compared the efficacy of various agents for skin disinfection, but certainly no consensus exists among surgeons regarding the best method. All the standard antiseptic solutions have been shown to effectively reduce the bacterial flora of the skin; the relative properties, advantages, and disadvantages of the most commonly used disinfectants are listed in Table 1-1.

Skin Preparation

Many years ago, Price[70,71] coined the terms *transient* and *resident* to describe the bacterial flora of the hands. Several

---

Table 1-1
ANTISEPTIC SOLUTIONS

Alcohol	Good immediate skin disinfectant but dries quickly and has less long-term effect[61]
	Ninety-five percent alcohol better than 75% because of dilution by moist skin[56]
Hexachlorophene (pHisoHex)	Forms a film that retains bacteriostatic properties[61]; easily washed off[53]
	Requires multiple applications to be effective[72]
	May be toxic in infants[54]
	Effective against gram-positive, less effective against gram-negative organisms[41,79]
Iodine	Side effects
Alcoholic (tincture)	High incidence of skin irritation (can be lessened by adding iodide)[53,57]
Aqueous (Lugol's solution)	True allergic reactions
Iodophors (Betadine)	Advantages over iodine[57,59,73]
Iodine and polyvinyl pyrrolidine or povidone	Slower release of iodine
	Fewer skin reactions
	Effective against gram-negative and gram-positive organisms
Chlorhexidine (Hibiclens)	Some studies[48,54,66-69,79] have shown it to be superior to Betadine and pHisoHex.
70% alcoholic solution	Repeated washings may have a cumulative effect.[47]

subsequent studies[47,60,65,76] have confirmed Price's observation that most of the bacteria are easily washed off (transient flora) whereas some appear to be almost impossible to eliminate (resident flora). Hann[50] concluded that most of the resident flora are situated around and beneath the fingernails, thus implying that cleaning and trimming of the nails are important parts of the prep routine. Rayan and Flournoy[74] confirmed these findings.

The gamut of skin prep ranges from an elaborate ritual of applying several sequential layers of various soaps and disinfectants to simply painting the hand with an antiseptic solution immediately before surgery.[55,81] Over the past 30 years there have been waves of enthusiasm for various antiseptic agents. Hexachlorophene was at one time thought to be the answer, but that agent was supplanted by the iodophors,[40,46,53,72] and now there appears to be increasingly strong support for chlorhexidine.[48,54,68,69,79] Some studies extol the effectiveness and ease of application of antiseptic sprays in preference to mechanical scrubbing,[39,75] harking back to Lister's carbolic acid spray. Plastic drapes impregnated with iodophor have also been recommended,[44,45] but these are not well suited to hand surgery because of the difficulty in conforming the drape to a hand. Kaul and Jewett[54] commented on the subjective nature of the literature regarding skin disinfection and concluded from their exhaustive review of the literature that "neither the ideal agent nor protocol for surgical scrubbing and skin preparation has yet been devised." In fact, the incidence of infection in the hand is strikingly low (particularly for elective surgical procedures), and it is likely that the type and protocol of the skin preparation is less important than other factors of surgical technique.

For many years I insisted on a complicated ritual of pre-surgical preparation of the patient's hand by the nursing staff the night before or the morning of surgery. This practice has disappeared partly because, in today's world, hand surgery patients are virtually never admitted to the hospital the night before an elective operation but also because it is not necessary. My preferred routine is now a simple 5- to 10-minute povidone-iodine (Betadine) or Hibiclens scrub on the operating room table after the tourniquet has been applied (but not yet inflated).

Patients should be cautioned about scratches and abrasions for a week or so before any elective operation. It is very disconcerting to have to cancel an operation because the patient appears with an infected blister or superficial laceration sustained while working on a car or in the garden a few days earlier. In a working man, especially a mechanic, whose hands are usually covered with grease and multiple superficial skin nicks, it is particularly important to emphasize the need to protect the hand as much as possible before the operation and perhaps have these patients scrub their hands with soap and water nightly for several days before surgery.

Hair Removal

Is hair removal necessary before hand surgery? Although some surgeons routinely shave the arm as part of their skin prep, there is good evidence in the literature now to show that shaving is not only unnecessary but also possibly deleterious.[42,58,78,80] If shaving is desired by the surgeon, it should be done immediately before the operation.[77,78] Even the most careful shaving results in cuts, nicks, and abrasions, and the

longer the time between shaving and surgery, the higher the infection rate.[52] Although at one time I routinely shaved the entire arm in all patients preoperatively, I now limit shaving to small areas where incisions are planned. This is done in the operating room immediately before washing the hand and is simply to avoid the nuisance of having hair in the area where the skin must be incised and subsequently sutured. The mere presence of intact hair on the skin does not appear to be a significant causative factor in wound infections.

Depilatories have been shown to be an effective and probably safer method of preoperative hair removal than shaving.[52,58,77] Despite this, depilatory creams are not widely used, probably because they (1) tend to be messy and take longer, (2) may cause occasional sensitivity reactions,[49] and (3) are reported to incite an inflammatory reaction if they come in contact with an open wound.[38]

Draping

No claim is made here that one method of draping is superior to another, but my own technique is illustrated in Figure 1-6. It is important to cover the hand table with a plastic sheet or other type of waterproof drape to prevent bacterial contamination if the drapes become wet during the procedure. I prefer to prepare and drape the entire arm from fingertips to the distal edge of the tourniquet (protecting the tourniquet with a towel or plastic drape during the preparation to avoid soaking the padding beneath the cuff). The reason for this is to allow maximum exsanguination of the extremity before inflation of the tourniquet.

THE TOURNIQUET

Today the tourniquet is considered an indispensable tool in hand surgery, but its development evolved over several centuries (Table 1-2). Bunnell's emphasis on the need for atraumatic technique in reconstructive surgery firmly established the role of the tourniquet in hand surgery. His rhetorical question "Could a jeweler repair a watch immersed in ink?"[95] has been a favorite quote of hand surgeons for many years.

Inherent Dangers

Although the tourniquet has become universally accepted as an essential instrument in hand surgery, it is not without inherent danger.[93,94] Because the tourniquet is potentially harmful, it is imperative that the surgeon be aware of the dangers and cognizant of the methods to prevent or minimize untoward effects. Most complications are directly related either to the duration of ischemia or to the direct pressure generated by the cuff. It is thought that nerves are more susceptible to mechanical (pressure) injury[167] and muscle more vulnerable to ischemia.[217]

Other Untoward Effects of Ischemia

Reference is occasionally made to a rather ill-defined "post-tourniquet syndrome" characterized by edema, stiffness, pallor, weakness without paralysis, and subjective numbness without objective anesthesia.[137] Several authors have noted that postoperative swelling is increased after operations done under a tourniquet.[186,222,244]

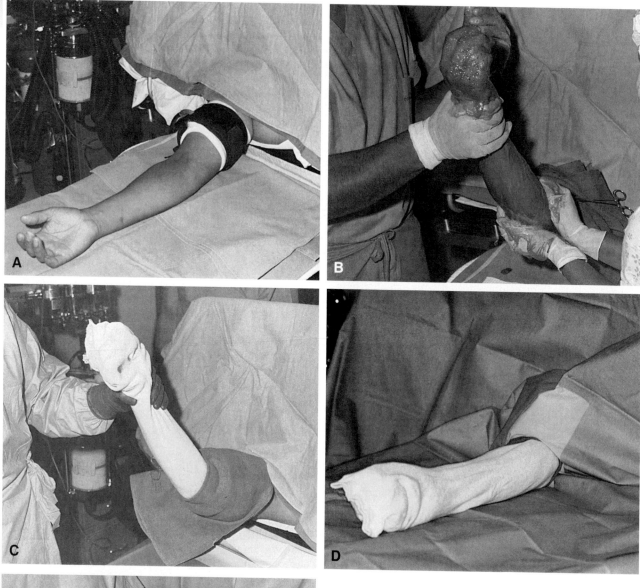

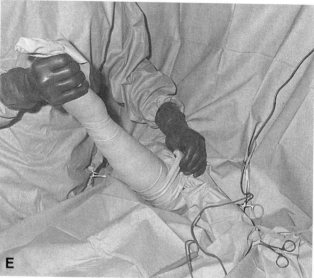

FIGURE 1–6. Prepping and draping the hand. **A,** The tourniquet is wrapped on the arm over several layers of cast padding as high in the axilla as possible. **B,** Prepping the entire extremity from fingertips to the tourniquet allows maximum exsanguination of the limb. Note the towel around the distal edge of the tourniquet to prevent the prep solution from seeping beneath the cuff (a plastic drape with an adhesive edge is now preferred). **C,** A stockinette is applied from fingertips to the tourniquet, and a sterile towel is wrapped around the upper end of the stockinette, where it is clamped with a towel clip. **D,** A fenestrated drape with a cuff of plastic is applied over the limb. Not seen is the important waterproof sheet beneath this layer. **E,** The entire arm is wrapped with a Martin or Ace bandage from fingertips to tourniquet. This is done only after all equipment (e.g., Bovie cord, suction tubing) is in place and all preliminary skin marking and planning is completed.

Table 1-2
HISTORY AND EVOLUTION OF THE TOURNIQUET

600 BC	Sushrutha[194] applied pressure to a main artery with a pebble
1552	Ambroise Paré[151,163] used a ligature to control hemorrhage during a leg amputation.
1674	Morell[227] introduced the field garrote (a cord tightened by twisting a wooden rod).
1718	Jean Louis Petit[151] devised a tourniquet (from the French *tourner* "to turn"), a screw device that applied pressure directly over an artery.
1864	Joseph Lister was probably the first to use a tourniquet for operations other than amputations.
1873	Johann Friedrich August von Esmarch[87,114] used a woven India rubber bandage to exsanguinate a limb before applying a tourniquet (but gave credit to Grandesso-Sylvestri, who had used it in 1871[151]).
1877	An American, Henry Austin Martin, devised the flat rubber bandage familiar to surgeons today[172] but used it to treat stasis ulcers and swelling and never as a tourniquet.
1904	Harvey Cushing introduced the pneumatic tourniquet,[102] primarily for use in craniotomies.

Table 1-3
VENOUS pH IN RESPONSE TO TOURNIQUET ISCHEMIA

Duration (min)	Mean pH	Readjustment Interval* (min)
Preinflation	7.40	
30	7.31	3-5
60	7.19	5-10
90	7.04	10-15
120	6.90	15-20

*Time required to return to preinflation level.

From Wilgis EFS: Observations on the effects of tourniquet ischemia. J Bone Joint Surg Am 53:1343-1346, 1971.

Contrary to what might be expected, venous thrombosis does not appear to be a problem after tourniquet use.[205]

Compartment syndrome has been reported,[172,198] a situation that can cause diagnostic problems, especially if it is combined with post-tourniquet paralysis. Intracompartmental pressure monitoring has been suggested as a way to clarify the diagnosis.[198]

Tourniquet Time

Despite numerous publications based on experimental studies and empirical clinical data, the absolute limits of tourniquet time have never been firmly established or universally accepted. The "safe" duration of tourniquet ischemia suggested in the literature ranges from 45 minutes to 4 hours, with 2 hours being the most widely accepted figure.[95,116,120,125,143,185,192,249,251] There is some rational basis for the 2-hour limit stemming from Wilgis' studies,[248] which showed a progressive acidosis in venous blood distal to the tourniquet in direct proportion to the duration of ischemia (Table 1-3).

Methods to Prolong Safe Tourniquet Time
Reperfusion Breaks ("Breather Periods")
During prolonged operations, most surgeons will wisely deflate and reinflate the tourniquet at periodic intervals. Precisely how often and for how long the tourniquet should be deflated is not known, however. Attempts have been made to demonstrate the duration of ischemia that will produce pathologic changes in skeletal muscle.[194,203,204,206,217,226,238] Wilgis noted that there is an interval of readjustment during which pH values gradually return to normal after release of the tourniquet (see Table 1-3). He used these figures to provide guidelines regarding the "breather period" when extended tourniquet time is required.[248] However, these are merely guidelines, and the truth is that the dilemma has not yet been definitively solved regarding how many (or how often) reperfusion breaks should be taken when very prolonged tourniquet time is required.[103]

Alternating Tourniquets
The late Richard J. Smith and his associates[112,193] introduced an innovative method of prolonging tourniquet time. By using double tourniquet cuffs and alternating these at 1-hour intervals, they reported no permanent adverse sequelae with tourniquet times of up to 4 hours. Their concept was that although this method does not decrease ischemia time, it does prevent continued compression on a localized segment of nerves and vessels.

Hypothermia
Several articles[123,152,218,230,231] have lent support to the suggestion made in 1960 by Paletta and coworkers[199] that hypothermia may reduce the harmful effect of ischemia on tissues. Although most surgeons do not go to the extremes suggested in some of these articles, keeping tissues cool is probably advisable. Periodic irrigation with saline or Ringer's lactate undoubtedly tends to minimize the undesirable drying and warming effects of the operating room lights and prolonged exposure of an open wound.[93]

Conservation of Movement
Obviously, the tourniquet should be regarded by the surgeon as potentially harmful, and every effort should be made to use tourniquet time as efficiently and sparingly as possible.[93,191,248] All preoperative planning, incision marking, and discussion should precede inflation of the tourniquet, and a conscious attempt should be made to work with deliberate speed. Rapid surgery in itself is not necessarily a virtue, but conservation of movement, as advocated by Bunnell,[95] will serve to minimize the potentially harmful effects of tourniquet ischemia.

Tourniquet Pressure
Although relatively uncommon at the present time, post-tourniquet paralysis has been the most frequently recognized complication of tourniquet use. Although the relative roles of ischemia and pressure have been debated,[108,135,192,253] it would appear that direct pressure beneath the cuff is the major causative factor,[118,126,160,169,184,188,196,202,215] but other factors have been implicated.[164]

Measurement of Pressure

Tourniquet paralysis was a more frequent occurrence when the Esmarch (Martin) bandage itself was routinely used as a tourniquet, and it is well documented that these rubber bandages can easily generate pressures far in excess of what is considered safe.[134,184] The incidence of this complication has been significantly reduced but is not entirely eliminated with use of the pneumatic tourniquet. Most of the reported cases appear to have been the result of faulty pressure gauges, although in some cases no recognizable cause was identified.[165,213] The gauges currently used in some commercially available pneumatic tourniquets are subject to significant inaccuracies,[82,127,149,151,253] and routine and regular calibration of each tourniquet before use has been advised.[94,96,97,110,125,127,140,207,243]

Another way to guard against the problem is to install a safety valve in the line between the cuff and the tank to prevent excessive pressure.[140,148,235,246]

Those types of tourniquets using nitrogen or oxygen must be checked periodically to ensure that there is adequate pressure in the tank, and the gas canister in a Kidde-type tourniquet must be replaced whenever the fluid level is low. These checks should be made before commencing an operation to prevent the annoying and troublesome complication of having the cuff deflate during an operation when the tank is depleted. When using the nitrogen tank-type apparatus, the tourniquet must be calibrated on a regular basis, at least daily and preferably before each case. This is easily done with a commercially available test gauge or a standard blood pressure manometer. The modern electric tourniquets with microprocessors require less frequent calibration, and some have a self-test that is activated automatically each time the power switch is turned on.

Cuff Size and Design

The design of the pneumatic cuff has been implicated as a potential source of problems,[90,132,169,196] although the surgeon has little control over this. The appropriate-size cuff should be used for each patient, and in the past the guideline was to use a cuff with a width approximately equal to the diameter of the upper arm. More recent studies have suggested that wider cuffs should be used.[105,139,142,189,190,195] Although wider cuffs may cause increased local pain,[139] it has been shown that lower pressures can be used with a 5-inch cuff than with a 3½-inch cuff.[195] The problem of finding the right cuff size for infants and children was solved by Upton and Mutimer[241] by using disposable blood pressure cuffs, which are commercially available in multiple widths.

A thin layer of soft cast padding is advised to distribute pressure more evenly beneath the cuff and prevent pinching of the skin[99] but is not likely to appreciably alter the direct pressure on the underlying nerves. No more than two to three layers of cast padding are necessary.

Optimum Pressure

The goal of the surgeon should be to use the lowest tourniquet pressure compatible with providing a bloodless field,[131] but controversy exists regarding the "standard" tourniquet pressure. Values ranging from 250 to 300 mm Hg in adults and 150 to 250 mm Hg in children have been suggested in the literature, but slightly higher pressures may be necessary to produce a bloodless field in a patient with an obese arm[242] or hypertension. Several authors have recommended that tourniquet pressure should be set relative to the patient's preoperative systolic pressure, and figures ranging from 20 to 100 mm Hg above systolic pressure have been suggested.[116,158-160,221] Other ways have also been recommended to determine the optimum pressure.[168,192,195,215]

Author's Preferred Method of Tourniquet Use

I prefer and routinely use the microprocessor-controlled (also called computerized) type of tourniquet (Fig. 1-7) originally designed by McEwen[182] and now available commercially. This system has several inherent audio and visual alarms, and a digital gauge provides a constant reading of elapsed (and cumulative) tourniquet time as well as pressure.

Several layers of soft cast padding are wrapped around the upper arm, with care taken to avoid creases or ridges. A 12- or 18-inch cuff will fit nicely on the majority of arms, and it is applied as snugly as possible and as high in the axilla as will fit comfortably. The cuff is connected to the gauge while taking care to avoid kinking and making certain that the connections between tubing and cuff are securely locked.

During the skin preparation, a towel or plastic drape[141,174] should be wrapped around the distal edge of the cuff to prevent seepage of preparation solutions onto the cast padding, because this can result in chemical burns on the skin[92,106,109,125,180] (Fig. 1-8). I prefer to prepare and drape the entire arm as close to the cuff as possible to allow maximal exsanguination.

Some elbow operations can be done with the standard nonsterile tourniquet cuff, but for procedures extending just above the elbow in the region of the distal end of the humerus, I prefer to use a sterile cuff, which allows the entire arm up to and including the axilla to be prepared and draped. A gas-sterilized cuff is then wrapped directly on the arm without cast padding. When this is done, a short length of sterile tubing must be available to connect the cuff to the tourniquet line.

After the completion of draping, the entire arm is wrapped tightly from fingertips to the upper extent of the sterile field with a 4-inch rubber Martin or Ace bandage. In elderly patients and those with rheumatoid arthritis with delicate skin, care must be taken to avoid damage to the skin with the shearing force of the elastic wrap.[158] In limbs with a ganglion, I avoid wrapping the bandage directly over the cyst to prevent rupture. Traditional teaching has been that an elastic wrap should not be used in patients with infections, but for more than 20 years I have routinely exsanguinated infected limbs and have never recognized an untoward reaction from this practice.

Exsanguination should definitely not be done with an elastic wrap in patients with tumors, but there are other ways to at least partially exsanguinate the limb before inflation of the tourniquet. Colville and Small[102] have shown that brachial artery compression just above the elbow for 1 minute with the arm elevated provides an operative field that is almost as bloodless as that achieved with the elastic wrap.

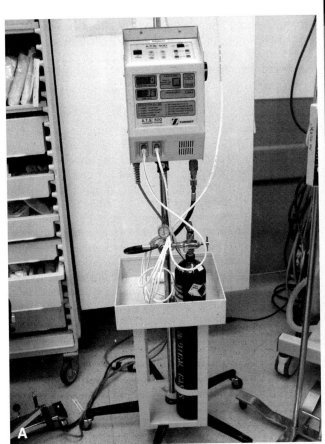
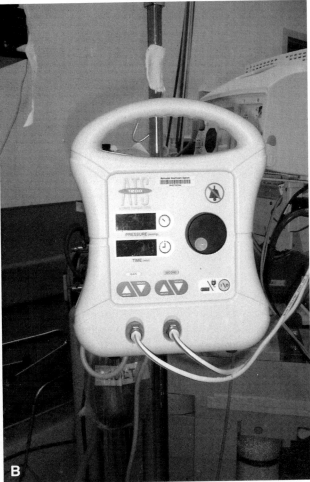

FIGURE 1–7. The tourniquet developed by McEwen and colleagues has digital gauges that provide a constant reading of elapsed (and cumulative) tourniquet time as well as pressure. Older versions of this microprocessor tourniquet were run off a nitrogen tank (**A**), but newer models (**B**) are purely electric. (Courtesy of Zimmer Orthopaedic Surgical Products, Inc.)

"Tourniquet time is precious,"[248] and all skin marking, planning, and discussion should be carried out before inflation of the cuff. I routinely use 250 mm Hg in all adult patients (200 mm Hg in children), but 300 to 350 mm Hg is usually necessary to occlude arterial flow in a particularly muscular or obese arm or in a patient with hypertension. Generally, 50 to 75 mm Hg higher than systolic pressure will suffice. I use 2 hours as my maximum tourniquet time, but if additional tourniquet time is required, I allow an appropriate readjustment interval before reinflation, based on Wilgis' previously cited studies (see Table 1-3). A conscious effort should be made to keep the tissues cool and moist with periodic irrigation of saline or lactated Ringer's throughout, especially in long operations.

A controversial topic in hand surgery is when to deflate the tourniquet. Himel and associates[144] reported less hematoma formation if the tourniquet was deflated and hemostasis achieved than in those cases in which the tourniquet was released after wound closure, but they noted that this decision should be tempered by clinical considerations. Mars and Brock-Utne[176,177] also noted that deflating the tourniquet and gaining hemostasis before closure reduced intracompartmental pressures. At one time I deflated the tourniquet before wound closure in all cases, but now I tend to release it after the dressing has been applied, with certain specific exceptions. If the dissection has been in the region of a major artery, I release the tourniquet before wound closure to be certain that there is not an arterial "pumper," which can result in a significant wound hematoma or even a late false aneurysm.[233] Having had to take two patients with carpal tunnel syndrome back to the operating room on the day of surgery for acute compartment syndromes caused by small, unrecognized arterial bleeders, I now deflate the tourniquet before skin closure in all operations for carpal tunnel syndrome. In addition, I routinely release the tourniquet before closure in all Dupuytren's fasciectomies and in other procedures in which the vascularity of a digit is put at risk during the dissection.

I also make a concerted effort to carefully identify and coagulate small vessels before they are cut during the course of the operation. Use of magnification (2.5× to 4.5× loupes) and bipolar electrocautery greatly facilitates this and minimizes postoperative bleeding and hematoma formation.

If the tourniquet is deflated before closure during a case in which the dissection was carried out in very dense scar tissue, application of epinephrine-soaked sponges can be of benefit in controlling small-vessel ooze. A 1:200,000 solution is easily prepared by adding 1 mL of 1:1000 epinephrine to 200 mL of saline or lactated Ringer's. Keeping in

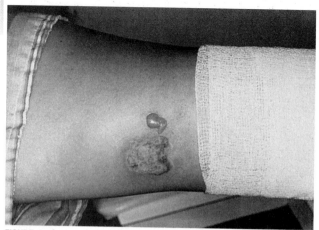

FIGURE 1–8. Leakage of iodophor scrub solution beneath the tourniquet cuff during skin prep can result in partial or even full-thickness skin necrosis, as in this patient.

mind that clotting time is increased as pH drops below 7.2, more than 5 minutes of gentle compression with the epinephrine-soaked sponges may be necessary to ensure adequate cessation of bleeding (see Table 1-2).

Although some surgeons[99] recommend routine removal of the cuff and underlying soft padding immediately after deflation of the tourniquet to prevent ooze secondary to venous constriction, I have rarely found this to be necessary. However, at the completion of the operation, the skin beneath the cuff should be examined for blisters or burns. These are rarely a problem if appropriate padding was applied and care was taken to keep the padding dry during the skin preparation.

Suction drains such as a Hemovac should be used in cases with potential for considerable continuous ooze, but they are not necessary in all cases.

Forearm Tourniquets

Although the tourniquet cuff has traditionally been applied to the upper arm, several reports suggest that forearm tourniquets are safe and reliable. Most authors[101,150,208] have applied a regular pneumatic cuff over padding 5 cm distal to the medial epicondyle, but others[229,250] have used a 12-inch pediatric tourniquet over cast padding just proximal to the wrist. Guirguis and Bell[86,138] wrapped a size 8½ surgical glove around the wrist, although the safety of this was questioned by Hodgson.[147]

Several separate studies[150,175,179] have concluded that the forearm tourniquet is tolerated better than a cuff on the upper arm, but others[119,254] have shown no difference in discomfort between the two sites.

The width of the cuff does not appear to be critical. Margles and colleagues[175] used a standard 12- or 18-inch arm tourniquet (11-cm-wide cuff), but Chan and coworkers[98] preferred a much narrower (5 cm) cuff. A pressure of 75 to 100 mm Hg greater than systolic pressure is recommended for forearm tourniquets.[150,175]

For the hand surgeon who does not routinely use the forearm tourniquet, there may still be specific situations in which this is the best choice, such as in a renal dialysis patient with an arteriovenous shunt in the upper arm or proximal portion

of the forearm. Semer and associates[219] reported no problems in 12 of 14 such patients in whom the routine upper arm cuff was used, but in their other 2 patients the shunt clotted and had to be repaired at the time of surgery. A forearm tourniquet would probably avoid this potential complication. Another reported indication is the patient who has a Norplant subdermal contraceptive device implanted in the medial aspect of the upper arm.[252]

Use of the Tourniquet With Local Anesthesia

Many operations on the hand can be performed quite appropriately under local or regional nerve block anesthesia.[114,155] This does not preclude the use of a pneumatic tourniquet, especially for short procedures. Most patients can tolerate a cuff pressure of 250 mm Hg around the upper arm for about 20 minutes,[197] and this tolerance can be extended with the use of a forearm cuff to approximately 30 minutes. The administration of appropriate preoperative or intraoperative sedation or systemic analgesia will extend the limits significantly.[87,88,104] Dushoff[115] has obtained pain-free ischemia for as long as 60 to 75 minutes by wrapping the entire upper extremity from fingertips to axilla with a sterile rubber bandage after skin preparation and then applying the tourniquet on top of the exsanguinating wrap. Probably the best technique for prolonging tourniquet tolerance is the "ring block," or subcutaneous infiltration of the upper arm with a local anesthetic to block the cutaneous nerves (see Chapter 2). Application of a local anesthetic cream (EMLA) to the skin circumferentially beneath the tourniquet has been shown to be ineffective.[239]

Finger Tourniquets

Occasionally the surgeon may wish to perform a relatively minor procedure on a single finger with some type of tourniquet at the base of the finger. A variety of methods have been described for doing this. Probably the most common technique is to wrap a rubber catheter[146] or a Penrose drain[245] around the base of the finger and clamp it in place with a hemostat, although several studies[128,145,171,220] have shown that excessive pressure can easily be generated with this method. Smellie[223,224] devised a rubber ring tourniquet for the finger (originally latex, later silicone rubber) that is applied with a special instrument called an Elastrator. A similar rubber ring, commercially available as Tourni-cot, comes with a package label warning that "neurovascular damage may result if Tourni-cot is left on the digit longer than one hour."

Exsanguination of the digit before application of the finger tourniquet can also be done in several ways. An assistant (often not available in the setting where finger tourniquets are frequently used) can squeeze the finger while the tourniquet is applied. Wavak and Zook[245] suggested wrapping the digit in a distal-to-proximal direction with a moist 4 × 4-inch gauze sponge opened to its fullest length and folded in half longitudinally. Blumberg[89] and Whitson[247] have used a Penrose drain in similar fashion to a Martin bandage on the finger.

My preferred method for simultaneous exsanguination of the finger and application of a digital tourniquet is that described by Salem.[214] A finger is cut from a sterile rubber glove, stretched over the digit to be operated on, and rolled proximally to form a ring at the base of the finger after cutting off the tip of the glove (Fig. 1-9). Karev's[154] modification of this technique is to apply an entire sterile rubber glove to the patient's hand, snip off the glove tip of the finger to be operated on, and then roll back the glove finger to its base. He noted that the technique is contraindicated in the presence of infection or malignant tumors. This technique has also been endorsed by others,[85,111,122,220] but Whitson[247] noted some disadvantages to the method, not the least of which is that it may be difficult to get the glove on the hand of a sedated patient. Palmer[200] commented that it has the major advantage of being difficult to forget to remove it.

Primarily because of the excessive pressures that can be generated beneath these types of elastic finger tourniquets,[128,134,145,171,220] attempts have been made to devise digital tourniquets with lower and more controllable pressures.[181,237]

Rubber finger tourniquets are probably safe to use for very short operative procedures, but two distinct hazards must be considered by the surgeon: (1) excessive pressure can easily be produced, and (2) do not forget to take it off! Failure to do so will obviously have disastrous results.[100,224,225] One safeguard I employ when using a finger tourniquet in the emergency department or office is to tell both the patient (and the nurse, if one is in attendance) to be sure to remind me to remove the tourniquet before the dressing is applied—but of course I always want to remember this step myself. Others place a small clamp on the finger tourniquet that will require removal during application of the dressing.

Surgical Instruments

The choice of surgical instruments is an individual matter, and surgeons will select those instruments with which they are most comfortable, usually those used during residency and fellowship. In Tables 1-4 through 1-7, I have listed my own basic instrument sets as a frame of reference for new surgeons wishing to have a place to start. I keep my instruments for bone work, tendon transfers, and microsurgical procedures in separate sets to minimize handling; the basic set is used for all cases, and the other supplemental instruments added only when they are needed. Theoretically at least, this protects the instruments from the inevitable abuse that they receive each time they are used, even with careful handling. This system also simplifies the scrub technician's job and reduces the clutter of instruments required for each operation.

A variety of hand tables are commercially available, and each has its own relative advantages and disadvantages. Some hand surgeons prefer to use only an extension from the operating table (e.g., two standard arm boards placed side by side). This eliminates the occasionally annoying table legs and allows the hand table to be raised and lowered more easily, but it frequently does not provide sufficient stability or width for adequate arm support. The "springboard" effect can of course be eliminated with the more standard hand table with legs, which is also wider and provides appropriate arm support, essential features when operating under the microscope.

For the surgeon who works without a cadre of resident assistants, hand-holding devices are essential. The lead hand,

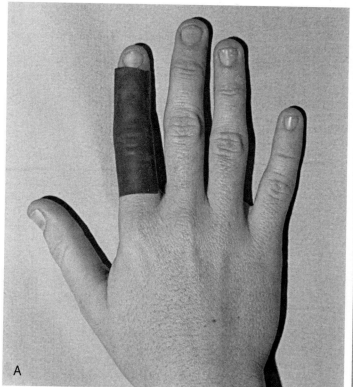
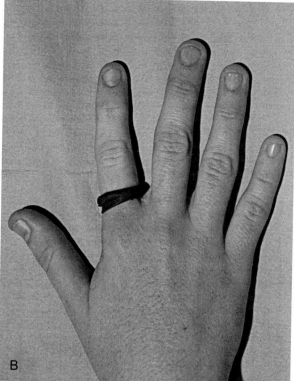

FIGURE 1–9. Salem's[214] method of applying a tourniquet to a single digit is to cut the tip from a sterile glove finger (**A**) and roll it back to the base of the finger (**B**).

Table 1-4
BASIC HAND SURGERY INSTRUMENTS

Scissors

2 pr	Small dissecting scissors (curved strabismus or delicate Metzenbaum)
1 pr	Straight strabismus scissors (suture scissors)
1 pr	Small Metzenbaum scissors
1 pr	Large, curved Mayo scissors
1 pr	Large Formon scissors with serrated edges (e.g., for cutting heavy ligaments)
1 pr	Bandage scissors

Retractors

1 pr	Each of the six types of Meyerding retractors
4	Single skin hooks
2	Small double skin hooks
2	Large double skin hooks
1 pr	Army-Navy retractors
2	Small spring-loaded self-retaining skin retractors (Weck)
2	Small Gelpi self-retaining retractors
1	Small Weitlaner self-retaining retractor

Needle holders

2	Small needle holders
2	Medium needle holders
2	Large needle holders (useful for bending small Kirschner wires

Scalpels

2	Bard-Parker No. 3 knife handles
1	Beaver handle

Forceps

1 pr	Adson delicate-tissue forceps
1 pr	Adson forceps with platforms for tying suture
1 pr	Brown-Adson forceps
1 pr	Small smooth forceps
1 pr	Large smooth forceps
1 pr	6-inch bipolar forceps
1 pr	DeBakey forceps

Clamps

8	Curved mosquito hemostats
2	Fine-tipped mosquito hemostats (Jacobson)
4	Allis clamps
2	Small Kocher clamps
1	Large Kocher clamp
2	Small right-angle clamps

Towel Clips

6	Small towel clips
4	Large towel clips

Elevators

1	Freer periosteal elevator
1	Kleinert-Kutz periosteal elevator
1	Carroll periosteal elevator

Suction Tips

1	Frazier No. 3
1	Frazier No. 5
1	Frazier No. 10

Miscellaneous

1	Metal ruler
1	Carroll finger goniometer
2	Sponge sticks

Table 1-5
BONE INSTRUMENTS

Drill and Accessories

1	Power-operated hand drill (e.g., 3M Minidriver)
4	Sizes of 4- or 6-inch double-pointed Kirschner wires
	0.028 inch
	0.035 inch
	0.045 inch
	0.0625 inch
1	Kirschner wire cutter
2 pr	Needle-nosed pliers (or large needle holders) for bending Kirschner wires
Assorted	Small drill bits
1	Micro-aire saw with assorted blades, burs

Osteotomes

1	Set of mini-osteotomes (2, 4, 6, 8, 10, 12 mm, straight)

Mallet

1	Small mallet

Retractors

1 pr	6-mm mini-Hohmann retractors
1 pr	8-mm mini-Hohmann retractors

Bone Clamps

1	Aesculap fracture reduction clamp
1	Blalock-Kleinert bone reduction forceps
1 ea	Ikuta bone-holding clamps (2 sizes)

Curets

1	Set of small bone curets, sizes 000 through 2

Rongeurs

1	Zaufel-Jansen rongeur
1	Carroll small double-action bone rongeur
1	Liston bone-cutting forceps, straight, 5½ inches ("duckbill")

Gouges

1	Set of small gouges 2, 3, 4, 6, and 8 mm

Miscellaneous

1	Bone awl
1	Small bone hook
1	Large bone hook
1 ea	Bone impactors, three sizes (Sears Craftsman punches)

Table 1-6
TENDON INSTRUMENTS

1	Brand plantaris tendon stripper
1	Brand palmaris tendon stripper
1	Small Kleinert malleable tendon retriever
1	Carroll tendon-pulling forceps
1	Tendon-braiding forceps
1	Large Kelly clamp
1 ea	Hunter prostheses (3, 4, and 5 mm) for sizers
1 set	Meals tenolysis knives

Table 1-7
NERVE REPAIR INSTRUMENTS

2 pr	Dumont forceps, No. 2
2 pr	Dumont forceps, No. 3
1 pr	Microsurgical scissors, curved (dissection)
1 pr	Microsurgical scissors, straight (suture)
1 pr	Barraquer needle holder, curved, delicate
1 pr	Fine-tipped bipolar coagulation forceps
1	Rack for microsurgical instruments

which was apparently invented by Geoffrey Fisk under the influence of Guy Pulvertaft,[15,16] is perhaps the most widely used hand holder and has seen a variety of modifications. The lead hand is ideally suited for working on the palmar surface (Fig. 1-10), but it is less helpful on the dorsum. A rubber band or surgical glove, as suggested by Kilgore,[28] is a simple method of accomplishing the same goal (Fig. 1-11). Strickland's hand surgical table (Fig. 1-12A) is a more elaborate device that incorporates the added features of skin retractors and a built-in drainage system.

Many types of self-retaining retractors are commercially available for exposing the depth of a surgical incision, ranging from a light spring-loaded wire to retract only skin to the heavier Weitlaner and Gelpi retractors for deeper exposure (Fig. 1-13).

Nothing is more frustrating in the operating room than to have instruments that do not work properly. All cutting instruments (e.g., scissors, osteotomes, gouges, curets, tendon strippers) must be sharpened at periodic intervals. The surgeon must set an example for the operating room personnel by using instruments correctly to avoid damage to them and by insisting on proper care and regular maintenance. Common errors are grasping a large needle with a fine needle driver and using delicate scissors to cut heavy structures.

MAGNIFICATION

Magnification has become an essential part of hand surgery, and all hand surgeons should be comfortable in its use. Many years ago Bunnell and Koch, the two major pioneers of hand surgery in the United States, both stressed the importance of atraumatic technique in hand surgery.[9-11,33] No surgery is truly atraumatic, but refinements in magnification have given us an opportunity to more nearly reach that goal. One has only to operate under the microscope to appreciate how destructive even our most precise and careful attempts at surgery are to delicate tissues. At the same time, magnification gives us a decided advantage in attempting to minimize operative trauma.

All hand surgeons should be comfortable with loupes ranging from 2.5× to 4.5× magnification. These are an expensive but necessary part of the surgeon's armamentarium.

The ideal microscope for hand surgery is a double-headed binocular unit with the heads positioned at 180 degrees (i.e., with the surgeon and assistant facing each other across the hand table). The microscope should be easily maneuverable and readily allow change in magnification (6× to 15× is a useful range, although higher magnification is occasionally needed).

The proper place to learn basic microsurgical techniques is in the laboratory, where these difficult skills can be practiced in a quiet, unhurried atmosphere. The operating room, where tourniquet time is precious and multiple attempts at repair are deleterious to results, is not an appropriate environment for one's first attempts at learning the fundamentals of microsurgical techniques.

A more thorough discussion of magnification and microsurgical techniques is found in Chapter 44.

INTRAOPERATIVE RADIOGRAPHY

Bone and joint imaging is frequently needed during hand surgery procedures. Most of this is now done with an image intensifier or one of several widely available portable fluoroscopy machines. Improvements in image quality on the screen and the ability to produce prints of digital images have reduced the need to take regular radiographs on a sterile field. This is still occasionally necessary, and the customary technique is to wrap the cassette in a sterile bag such as a pillow case, Mayo stand cover, or disposable plastic cassette package. The obvious disadvantage of this standard, but somewhat cumbersome, practice is possible contamination of the operative field, and Lynch and Hefferon[31] have shown that loaded x-ray cassettes can be gas-sterilized without damage to the cassette or reduction in quality of the radiographs. Carter[12] suggested the use of presterilized paper-packaged film, similar to dental film but larger in size, which has the added advantage of facilitating exposure of a true lateral view of the finger. The disadvantage of this technique, however, is that the paper-packaged films require significantly greater

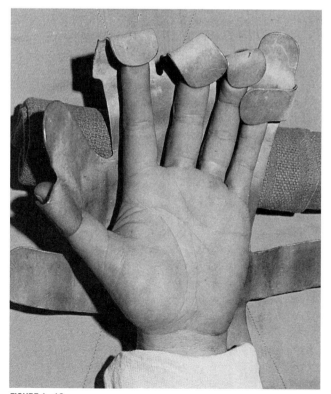

FIGURE 1–10. The lead hand is a most useful device for exposing the volar aspect of the hand.

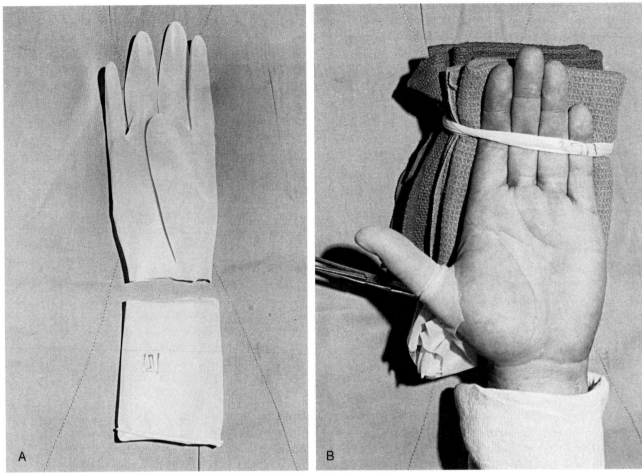

FIGURE 1–11. Kilgore[28] suggested a simple method of holding the hand by using a sterile rubber glove. The proximal part of the glove is cut off (**A**) and used to hold the fingers extended over a stack of towels (**B**). The thumb of the glove is then placed over the patient's thumb and held in place with a Kocher clamp (**B**).

exposure times than does film in a standard cassette, which contains a fluorescent screen.

Radiation Exposure to the Surgeon

Regardless of the type of radiographic imaging used, the precise positioning required in many hand surgery procedures necessitates that the surgeon hold the patient's hand during exposure. Whenever possible, the hand should be pre-positioned and held with some device that allows the surgeon to back away from the field because the primary beam carries a dose rate of more than 100 times that of scattered radiation.[3] Coning down the x-ray beam to visualize only what is necessary will reduce the radiation dose by some 50%.[3] Even with these precautions, however, the hand surgeon is exposed to a certain amount of undesirable radiation. Although hand exposure times are short, the accumulation of many intraoperative radiographs over a lifetime is theoretically harmful.[4] More frequent use of internal fixation in all realms of orthopedics has enhanced this risk. Holding limbs for radiographs has become so commonplace that precautions have lessened and a more cavalier attitude toward repeated irradiation is developing. I fear that the current generation of young hand and orthopedic surgeons is likely to see late radiation problems in the twilights of their careers,

as was seen in earlier generations of physicians and dentists before the hazards of radiation were fully appreciated.

Wearing a lead apron is advisable, but this precaution does not protect the surgeon's hands. For the surgeon who wants to ensure maximum hand protection, gas-sterilized lead gloves can be slipped over rubber surgical gloves when it is necessary to hold the patient's hand for intraoperative radiographs. These are very cumbersome and awkward to use, but the protection provided may be worth the extra trouble. Commercially available "radiation-resistant" surgical gloves are much more convenient, but they offer only minimal shielding (Fig. 1-14).

A significant contribution to the welfare of hand surgeons was made by Eaton and his colleagues on the Roosevelt Hospital Hand Service. The hand holder that they designed for intraoperative radiography (Fig. 1-15) is a most effective device. Even a true lateral radiograph of an individual finger can easily be taken without surgeons having to expose their own hands to potentially harmful radiation.

POSTOPERATIVE CARE

In no other field of surgery does the postoperative management of the patient play so critical a role as it does in

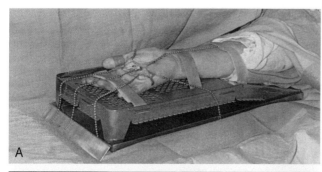

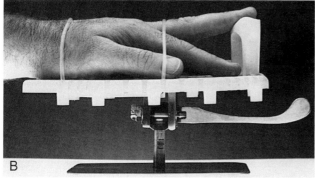

FIGURE 1–12. More elaborate hand-holding devices include (**A**) that designed by Strickland, which incorporates self-retaining retractors and a drainage collection system, and (**B**) the Rotalok surgical hand table, which allows more versatile positioning of the hand.

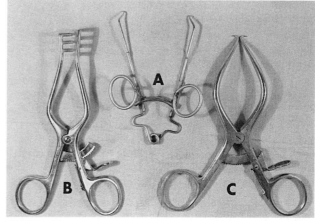

FIGURE 1–13. Many types of self-retaining retractors are available. The three that I find most useful are the light spring-loaded wire for retracting skin available from Weck (**A**) and the Weitlaner (**B**) and Gelpi (**C**) for deeper retraction.

hand surgery. At the risk of sounding a bit trite, it is axiomatic that the postoperative care of the hand is at least as important as the operation itself. From the moment the tourniquet is released, it is the surgeon's goal to return the hand to maximal function in the shortest possible time. To accomplish this, every effort must be taken to minimize postoperative swelling, relieve pain, limit immobilization of the hand to the minimal period commensurate with the goals of the operation,[7] and provide the patient with a very specific exercise program.[8]

Careful attention to detail during application of the postoperative dressing is essential in hand surgery. Although the exact technique of the dressing is almost an art form in itself, there are a number of features of postoperative hand dressings about which most hand surgeons would agree. Even though the term *compression dressing* is frequently used, some surgeons object to this term because they believe

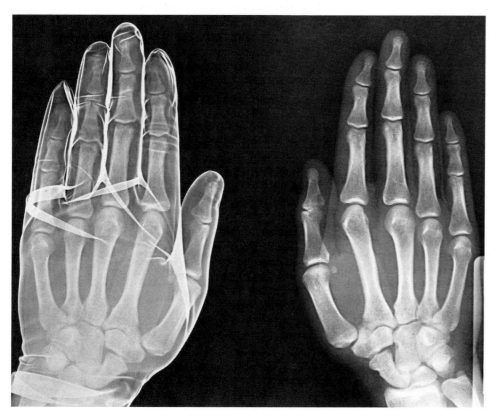

FIGURE 1–14. The "lead-impregnated" gloves that are supposed to protect the hands from radiation during intraoperative use of x-rays in reality provide minimal shielding. Compare the bony detail in the left hand (wearing such a glove) with the unshielded right hand.

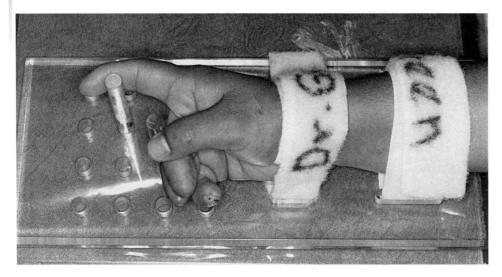

FIGURE 1–15. The x-ray positioning device designed by the Roosevelt Hospital Hand Surgery Service is a significant contribution to the welfare of hand surgeons. This device permits precise positioning of the hand for intraoperative radiography (including a true lateral view of an individual finger, as shown here) without the surgeon having to hold the patient's hand.

that it connotes a tight elastic bandage wrapped about the hand. A better term is perhaps *conforming dressing,* which implies a uniform degree of pressure on the entire hand. It must be snug enough to help control capillary oozing but not too tight to restrict venous return. The finger webs must be separated sufficiently to prevent maceration but not stuffed with so much gauze padding that excessive pressure is applied to the digital nerves. Usually some type of plaster splint is incorporated into the dressing. Neatness is important because the patient may judge the quality of the operation by the external appearance of the dressing. Plaster and blood stains on the digits and proximal portion of the arm should be wiped clean before the patient leaves the operating room.

The position of the various joints will, of course, be dictated by the operative procedure, and the preferred positions for postoperative immobilization are discussed for each of the various procedures described throughout this book. Unless the operation demands some other specific configuration of the hand, the generally preferred positions for immobilization of the hand are (1) the wrist in moderate (30 to 45 degrees) extension; (2) the MP joints in 50 to 75 degrees of flexion, rarely if ever in full extension; and (3) the PIP joints in nearly full extension.[26,27]

It is generally agreed that postoperative elevation of the hand is desirable to minimize edema, although even this time-honored concept has been questioned.[32] Elevation does not mean that the hand should be dangled from a hook like a side of beef in a meat locker. Rather, the elbow should be supported comfortably on the bed or a pillow and the hand merely suspended to prevent its falling into a horizontal position. Likewise, when the patient is out of bed, the hand should never be allowed to assume a dependent position. My instructions to the nursing personnel, the patient, and the patient's family are very simple: *keep the hand higher than the elbow.* If the patient uses a sling, it should be of a type that allows the hand to be elevated comfortably above the elbow (Fig. 1-16) rather than having the hand in a dependent position with the forearm aligned horizontally across the chest. Tegtmeier[37] has shown that the higher the hand, the lower the venous pressure, and that acute flexion of the elbow does not increase venous pressure. It is not necessary to maintain the entire upper extremity in a static, predetermined position, and, in

fact, specific exercises should be given to prevent stiffness and discomfort in the elbow and shoulder.

Elevation of the hand at home in bed can be accomplished in a variety of ways. Carter designed a commercially available support that is bulky but effective (Fig. 1-17). Provost[34] suggested an ingeniously simple method that requires no special equipment or added expense. His technique is so effective that an illustration (Fig. 1-18) is given to each of my patients on discharge from the hospital or outpatient surgery suite.

Most hand surgery operations are painful, and control of postoperative pain is the first step in patient rehabilitation. Relatively potent narcotics are usually required in the immediate postoperative period, and failure to respond to the usual dosages may be related to excessively tight bandages. I have found that patients frequently do not relate their pain specifically to a tight bandage, and yet splitting the circumferential wrap may give significant relief of pain. Some surgeons inject long-acting local anesthetic agents (bupivacaine

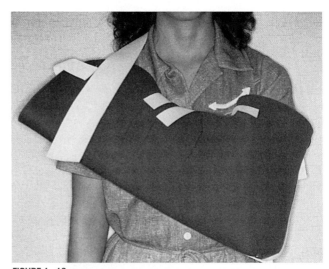

FIGURE 1–16. Proper use of a sling during the postoperative period permits the hand to be held higher than the elbow rather than the forearm lying horizontally across the body.

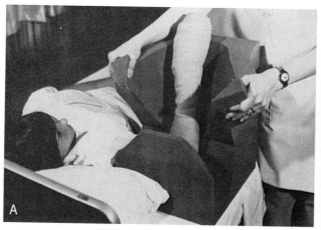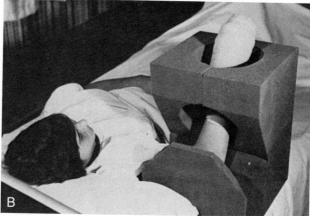

FIGURE 1–17. **A** and **B,** Carter designed a commercially available hand support that is bulky but effective.

[Marcaine]) into the wound at the time of closure as an adjunct to pain control.

Are ice packs necessary or even desirable? These are used routinely by many surgeons, and even though I used them for many years, I no longer do so. Some patients seem to like ice packs, but I doubt seriously that the amount of cold that penetrates a large, bulky dressing has any significant effect in reducing postoperative swelling. Moreover, the atten-tion required to maintain the ice packs in proper position and the frequent changes necessary to keep them cold occa-sionally cause concern that exceeds their potential benefit.

Do proteolytic enzymes have any therapeutic role in the prevention or reduction of edema? Although some studies have suggested a beneficial effect,[1,29] it is my impression that such agents are infrequently used by the majority of hand surgeons. They may, however, be a useful adjunct in patients

ELEVATION OF THE HAND

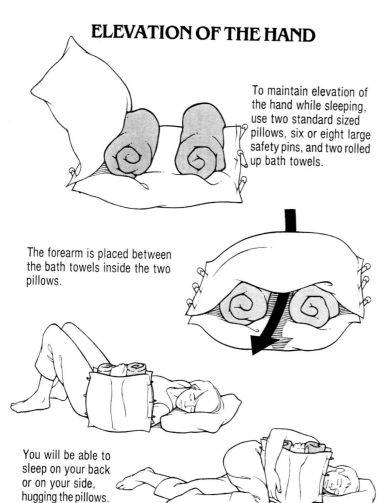

To maintain elevation of the hand while sleeping, use two standard sized pillows, six or eight large safety pins, and two rolled up bath towels.

The forearm is placed between the bath towels inside the two pillows.

FIGURE 1–18. All postoperative and emergency department patients in my practice receive this sheet of instructions for elevation of the hand at home, an ingeniously simple technique suggested by Provost.[34]

You will be able to sleep on your back or on your side, hugging the pillows.

with massive crush injuries, in whom severe swelling is inevitable. Perioperative corticosteroids given either intravenously or as a Medrol (methylprednisolone) DosePak may also be beneficial in such patients if there is no specific contraindication to their use, such as diabetes or infection.

Rehabilitation of the patient after hand surgery is frequently a complex problem requiring the combined efforts of surgeon and therapist. Hand surgeons and hand therapists should have a symbiotic relationship,[21] which means that the efforts of each are made better by the other. Close communication is essential to ensure that they agree on general principles of management and that specific items of information are shared regarding individual patients.

In addition to the specific recommendations made by each author or authors relative to the various operations described in this book, the reader is referred to the many excellent books now available on hand rehabilitation.

ANNOTATED REFERENCES

2. American Society for Surgery of the Hand: The Hand—Examination and Diagnosis, 2nd ed. New York, Churchill Livingstone, 1983.

About 20 years ago, this little handbook was put together by a committee of the ASSH, and since then it has been translated into several languages. For the hand surgeon who teaches medical students or paramedical personnel, this pocket-sized manual is the perfect place to have them start.

18. Godina M: Early microsurgical reconstruction of complex trauma of the extremities. Plast Reconstr Surg 78:285-292, 1986.

Marco Godina of the former Yugoslavia was among the first to advocate multiple-tissue reconstruction in the acute trauma setting. Although he died at a relatively young age, he was a true pioneer and gifted surgeon who set the stage for further developments in microsurgical trauma reconstruction.

21. Green DP: Symbiosis: The hand therapist–hand surgeon relationship. J Hand Ther 8:2-4, 1995.

The relationship between surgeon and therapist should be one in which both are made better by the other, and through which the patient receives the best possible care. Specific ways to achieve this harmony are presented in this address given to the American Society of Hand Therapists.

22. Grunert BK, Devine CA, Matloub HS, et al: Flashbacks after traumatic hand injuries: Prognostic indicators. J Hand Surg [Am] 13:125-127, 1988.

Few surgeons give sufficient thought to the major psychological impact of hand injuries on many patients. This study suggests that virtually all patients with serious trauma to the hand cope with significant emotional problems.

30. Lister G: The Hand: Diagnosis and Indications. New York, Churchill Livingstone, 1993.

This superb book, now in its fourth edition in conjunction with Dr. Paul Smith, is a well-illustrated storehouse of clinical pearls and is probably the best source for reviewing a broad spectrum of physical examination of the hand.

157. Klenerman L: The tourniquet in surgery. J Bone Joint Surg Br 44:937-943, 1962.

Over a period of 20 years, Klenerman published more articles on the tourniquet than any other single individual. This particular one is probably the best historical review of the use of the tourniquet in the literature.

248. Wilgis EFS: Observations on the effects of tourniquet ischemia. J Bone Joint Surg Am 53:1343-1346, 1971.

These studies done by Wilgis more than 30 years ago form the basis for how often and how long the tourniquet should probably be deflated during prolonged cases.

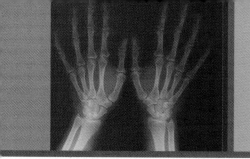

CHAPTER 2

Anesthesia

Somayaji Ramamurthy and Douglas Anderson

nesthesia for hand surgery can be provided by various techniques. General anesthetic techniques do not differ very much from those for other parts of the body, but regional anesthetic techniques have special application in anesthetizing the upper extremity. These techniques, the pharmacology of local anesthetics, and special conditions and problems associated with hand surgery are discussed in this chapter.

REGIONAL ANESTHESIA

General anesthesia is safe and has its own advantages, but we believe regional nerve block is the anesthetic technique of choice for surgery on the upper extremity.

Regional anesthesia causes less disturbance of general body physiology than any other type of anesthesia. It has little effect on body metabolism, respiration, and circulation and on function of the liver, kidney, and other organs.[6] This is of great importance when anesthetizing patients who poorly tolerate the stress imposed by general anesthesia. Patients with severe cardiovascular, respiratory, or renal disease are able to tolerate regional anesthesia for the upper extremity without any untoward effects.[29]

Regional anesthesia is the only method of anesthesia that will prevent all afferent impulses from the site of surgery from reaching the central nervous system. This may be of importance in preventing further vasoconstriction induced by noxious impulses. Regional anesthesia relieves pain and also induces vasodilation in the extremity, thus preventing tissue hypoxia.[29]

Advantages of regional anesthesia include the following[2,31,67]:

- Emergency procedures in patients with a full stomach present the serious hazard of aspiration of gastric contents, which can result in aspiration pneumonia with high morbidity and mortality. A patient can be safely anesthetized by a regional block and remain awake with intact protective reflexes.
- Upper extremity blocks, especially the axillary technique, can be safely used in outpatient surgery.[29]
- Postoperative nausea, vomiting, atelectasis, drowsiness, restlessness, and other complications of general anesthesia are avoided.

- Postoperative nursing care is decreased, and the majority of our hand surgery patients are sent directly to their room or to the outpatient observation room without going through the recovery room.
- At times, such as during emergencies, peripheral blocks permit one physician to administer more than one anesthetic and the patients can be monitored by a less-skilled professional.
- Regional block anesthesia permits patients to remain awake if they do not wish to lose consciousness.
- For patients with fractures of the cervical vertebrae and other serious airway problems, regional anesthetic techniques offer a significant advantage in avoiding movement of the neck and endotracheal intubation.
- Postoperative analgesia is provided, especially when longer-acting anesthetics are used.
- Prolonged analgesia and sympathetic blockade can be provided with continuous block techniques.
- In patients with a history of malignant hyperpyrexia, regional blocks using either ester-type or amide local anesthetics are likely to prevent the development of this condition.

Despite these advantages, regional blocks may not be widely used for several reasons. From the surgeon's point of view, the time required to perform nerve blocks and the delay until anesthesia is complete are too long, and the incidence of unsatisfactory anesthesia is high, often requiring the administration of supplemental general anesthesia. From the anesthesiologist's point of view, particularly if anesthesiology training has provided little opportunity to develop expertise in regional anesthetic techniques, fear of failure may be an important deterrent. This is especially so if the block is to be carried out in the presence of an eager, inquisitive resident or an impatient, pacing surgeon. Fear of litigation because of the possibility of neurologic complication further decreases the use of regional blocks. From the patient's point of view, multiple needle sticks and paresthesias are objectionable and the prospect of being "wide awake" during surgery may be frightening.[243]

If regional anesthesia is to be satisfactory to the patient, it is critical for the surgeon and the anesthesiologist to agree in advance that this is the best form of anesthesia for the patient, so that there is no apparent disagreement when each of them discusses the choices of anesthesia with the patient.

REGIONAL VS. GENERAL ANESTHESIA

In spite of the advantages of regional anesthesia, several factors may exist that prevent its use.

- Time constraints
- Lack of familiarity to the anesthesiologist
- Fear of failure
- Concern about complications
- Patient desire to be completely unaware during the procedure
- Each of these problems can be overcome with appropriate planning.

The patient's apprehension about being awake during administration of the block and surgery and the fear of pain from these procedures may be alleviated by (1) appropriate counseling about the advantages of regional block anesthesia by the surgeon before the patient's admission; (2) supportive reinforcement by the anesthesiologist during the preanesthetic visit, when details of the particular techniques can be explained, including the drugs that will be used to allay apprehension, minimize discomfort, and produce light sleep; and (3) judicious choice of adjunctive preoperative and intraoperative medications to provide tranquility, amnesia, and sleep. If all these practices are carried out, a patient will usually prefer regional anesthesia.[6,29,243]

Principles of Application

Once it is established that regional anesthesia is the technique of choice, the particular type of block and the local anesthetic agent to be used are determined by evaluating the patient's physical status and consulting with the surgeon about the surgical procedure.

A preanesthetic visit is extremely important for success of the block procedure because it permits the physician to establish rapport with the patient and explain the anesthetic procedure. Patients are more likely to cooperate when they are well informed; hence, the details of the procedure are explained to the patient and consent is obtained. Consent for regional anesthesia for surgery is obtained before the patient has received premedication. When the patient is a minor, consent is obtained after discussion with the parents.

Preanesthetic sedation is important to allay apprehension before and during the block. Various combinations of barbiturates, opioids, tranquilizers, and anticholinergics are preferred by individual physicians. Opioids are used if the patient has a painful surgical problem; they also decrease the discomfort produced during the block. In young, healthy adults, some clinicians prefer opioids such as morphine, 0.1 mg/kg, or meperidine (Demerol), 1 mg/kg, along with a minor tranquilizer such as hydroxyzine (Vistaril), 1 mg/kg, or midazolam (Versed), 0.03 to 0.07 mg/kg, given intramuscularly 1 hour before the anticipated time of the procedure to provide amnesia, sedation, and a cooperative and comfortable patient. Benzodiazepines may also be of benefit in preventing central nervous system toxicity from local anesthetic agents.[58,60,61] We prefer not to use anticholiner-

gics, especially scopolamine, in the elderly to avoid dry mouth, excitement, and restlessness. When required, anticholinergics such as atropine or glycopyrrolate (Robinul) can be administered intravenously. The combination of midazolam, 1 mg intravenously, and methadone, 5 mg intravenously, given just before the block provides an excellent combination of medications for adequate sedation and analgesia in most patients.

When the patient arrives in the operating room or block room, an intravenous infusion is started with an indwelling cannula. The rate of infusion is adjusted to an amount that just keeps the line open, because large volumes of intravenous fluid are likely to distend the bladder and make the patient uncomfortable.

After monitoring the patient's blood pressure and heart rate to establish baseline values and assess the cardiovascular effect of the preoperative drugs, further sedation is achieved as necessary by the use of incremental doses of midazolam, 1 mg, and/or fentanyl (Sublimaze), 0.025 mg. A very effective alternative to fentanyl is methadone, 5 mg intravenously.[205,237] An intravenous drip of propofol (Diprivan), 10 mg/mL (10 to 50 µg/kg/min), may also be used. Administration of these drugs is likely to provide postoperative amnesia in addition to making the patient comfortable. A new drug, dexmedetomidine (Precedex), is available for easily titrated sedation and analgesia bolus, 1 mg/kg over 10 min and 0.2 to 0.7 µg/kg/hr, without respiratory depression. It is an α_2 agonist, like clonidine, but has a much shorter duration of action and is administered by continuous intravenous infusion. It is used for sedation and analgesia in the intensive care unit setting as well as for perioperative use.[12,17]

Nerve blocks should never be carried out unless equipment for immediate resuscitation and treatment is available for the management of any complication that may arise during the procedure. This includes a means of ventilation, an airway, bag and mask, endotracheal tube, laryngoscope, suction apparatus, and drugs such as midazolam, ephedrine, epinephrine, and atropine. Because some regional techniques are associated with a small risk of inadvertent spinal or epidural anesthesia, with an associated possibility of hypotension, it is helpful to have medication available that is effective for treating severe hypotension, such as phenylephrine (Neo-Synephrine), vasopressin, or norepinephrine.

All regional blocks are performed with appropriate aseptic precautions. The skin is sterilized by using an organic iodine spray, and sterile gloves are used while performing blocks.

IMPORTANT PRINCIPLES

- Appropriate use of sedation can provide sufficient intraoperative comfort for patients who "don't want to be aware of anything going on."
- All patients require appropriate monitoring during the block and the surgical procedure.
- Emergency equipment including any equipment needed for endotracheal intubation must be immediately available.

Intraoperative Management

Excellent anesthesia of the upper extremity in itself does not guarantee ideal surgical conditions or patient comfort. Patients who are uncomfortable might move the rest of their body and interfere with the operative procedure. It is difficult for any patient to be on a perfectly flat table for any length of time without experiencing some discomfort of the back. To avoid this problem, the operating table is slightly flexed at the back and knees. This is possible when arm boards are used by the hand surgeon. If a hand table is used, flexion of the operating table will interfere with the stability of the hand table. In this case, placing a small pillow under the knees will prevent back discomfort. A pillow placed under the head increases the patient's comfort. Regardless of the local anesthetic agent, it still takes some time for the maximum effect of anesthesia to develop. During this time, if the level of anesthesia is checked frequently or the arm is washed without warning, the patient is still likely to have sensation and may lose confidence in the block analgesia and become very apprehensive. After completion of the block, a minimum of 20 minutes is necessary for peak analgesia to develop. Good analgesia should be established before washing of the wound, painful manipulation, or the start of surgery. Even when good analgesia exists, some proprioception is likely to be intact and the patient may experience vague pressure sensations. For these reasons, it is necessary to continue to allay the patient's apprehension. Adequate sedation can be achieved by using midazolam, fentanyl, and a drip of 1.0% propofol along with a 50:50 or 60:40 nitrous oxide/oxygen mixture. Opioid analgesics are especially useful in patients with rheumatoid arthritis, who are likely to have pain and discomfort in other parts of the body; however, oversedation may result in respiratory depression and an obstructed airway.

Local Anesthetic Pharmacology

Because many local anesthetic agents are available, it is possible to use the appropriate agent for the requirements of the individual case, including the anticipated duration of surgery, the type of motor block needed, and patient allergy to anesthetic agents. Knowledge of the pharmacology of the local anesthetic agents is essential for proper use of these agents.

Action

Local anesthetics produce a temporary block of conduction by interfering with the sodium channels,[53,58] thus preventing the development of an action potential.

Classification

Local anesthetic agents can be classified into two groups according to their structure: esters and amides. There are differences between the two that are clinically very important.

Metabolism

Esters are very rapidly hydrolyzed by plasma pseudocholinesterase; of these, chloroprocaine is the most rapidly hydrolyzed local anesthetic agent. Because absorbed chloroprocaine is very quickly metabolized by plasma pseudo-

---

LOCAL ANESTHETIC AGENTS

ESTERS

- Chloroprocaine (Nesacaine)
- Cocaine
- Procaine (Novocain)
- Tetracaine (Pontocaine)

AMIDES

- Lidocaine (Xylocaine)
- Mepivacaine (Carbocaine, Polocaine)
- Bupivacaine (Marcaine, Sensorcaine)
- Prilocaine (Citanest)
- Etidocaine (Duranest)
- Levobupivacaine (Chirocaine)
- Ropivacaine (Naropin)

---

cholinesterase, the blood level of the drug does not rise significantly and therefore does not cross the placental barrier. For this reason, chloroprocaine is one of the local anesthetic drugs of choice in pregnant women. Amides are broken down intracellularly in the liver cells. This is a longer process, and hence amides are more likely to accumulate and produce a systemic reaction with repeat doses.[53,58]

Allergic Responses

Allergic responses[8,53,58] to local anesthetics are rare. After the physician obtains a thorough history, vasovagal reactions and reactions to epinephrine can be identified. If the patient gives a history of true allergy with urticaria, wheezing, and so on, it is very likely that the patient has an allergic response to an ester compound. Intradermal tests using small quantities are useful. If there is no reaction, the agent can be used safely. A positive reaction can be false positive.

An allergic response to amide compounds is extremely rare, and these compounds can be safely used if the patient is allergic to an ester compound. The use of amides from multiple-dose vials may result in an allergic reaction because of the presence of the preservative methylparaben, which is structurally similar to esters and can produce allergic reactions in patients who are allergic to ester local anesthetics.

Preservatives are added to multiple-dose vials to retard bacterial growth. Multiple-dose vials are more economical, especially when small volumes of drug are used. However, most physicians prefer to use single-dose ampules or vials to avoid the preservatives and the possibility of bacterial contamination. The unused portion should be discarded. Single-dose vials are preferable because the glass particle contamination associated with the use of ampules can be avoided.

Pharmacokinetics

Local anesthetic agents injected into tissue are taken up by the circulation, thus terminating their action. The drugs are distributed in body tissues, the esters being broken down by plasma pseudocholinesterase and the amides metabolized in the liver cells. In the plasma, local anesthetics are bound to plasma protein to a varying degree. Eighty-five to 90% of bupivacaine, levobupivacaine, etidocaine, and ropivacaine are bound to protein in the blood, as opposed to 65% of lidocaine.[53,58] High protein binding explains the drugs' long duration of action in the tissues and also the fact that less free drug is available to cross the placental barrier to the fetus. Hence, bupivacaine is widely used in obstetric anesthesia and is one of the preferred local anesthetic drugs for pregnant patients. Metabolic products of the local anesthetics are excreted by the kidney.

Etidocaine is highly fat soluble and produces an excellent motor block, which may last longer than the sensory block. This sometimes results in a painful, paralyzed arm in the postoperative period.

Alkalinization

Alkalinization of local anesthetics to improve anesthesia onset time has been attempted with brachial plexus blocks but has produced conflicting results. The principle is that raising the pH increases the percentage of local anesthetic present in the nonionized free-base form. It is this form that crosses the nerve cell membrane to reach the site of action of local anesthetics. In a placebo-controlled study evaluating the alkalinization of mepivacaine for an axillary block, Quinlan and colleagues noted that alkalinization had no significant effect on the development of analgesia. However, it did shorten the onset of anesthesia in several nerve distributions and shortened the time to onset of paralysis.[175] For mepivacaine and lidocaine, 1 mL of 8.4% sodium bicarbonate is added for every 10 mL of local anesthetic. For bupivacaine, 0.1 mL of sodium bicarbonate is added for every 10 mL of local anesthetic.

Toxicity

Local Contact Toxicity[53,58]
Local anesthetics used in clinical concentrations have minimal irritating effects on the nerves, skin, and fat. Their negligible neurotoxicity is demonstrated by complete

recovery of function after regional blocks, as well as after histologic studies via intraneural injection.[58]

Systemic Toxicity
Because local anesthetics are not metabolized at the site of injection, they can produce systemic effects once they enter the circulation. Systemic effects depend on the blood level of the anesthetic. Toxic blood levels are reached when the local anesthetic is injected intravascularly or when large doses of drugs are used. Table 2-1 lists the recommended maximum doses of various agents in healthy young adults. Toxicity may be seen with lower doses in elderly patients, critically ill patients, and patients with multiorgan system disease. Moore and associates[160,162] have reported using 400 mg of bupivacaine (80 mL of 0.5%) without any systemic toxicity. Blood levels for this seemingly high dose were below the toxic level even when bupivacaine was injected for intercostal blocks.

Toxicity from systemic absorption of local anesthetics is a very rare occurrence. Significant complications from local anesthetics are usually the result of injecting them into unplanned locations (e.g., intravenous, intrathecal). The practice of recommending a single maximum dose of any local anesthetic makes little sense given the fact that blood levels vary significantly not only with the dose but also the location (e.g., intercostal vs. epidural).

Ropivacaine is a new amide local anesthetic that appears to have less cardiac toxicity than bupivacaine.[77,153,165,181,198] Ropivacaine differs from bupivacaine in having a three-carbon side chain instead of a four-carbon side chain. It is about 40% less potent. It is associated with a lower arrhythmogenic potential than bupivacaine and at similar doses shows less evidence of depression of cardiac conductivity and contractility.[109,198] One study[135] showed that bupivacaine at a dose of 6 mg/kg caused similar hemodynamic effects but slightly more effect on QRS interval duration than ropivacaine at 4 mg/kg in piglets. Ropivacaine ,when compared in equipotent doses, may have slightly less effects in terms of arrhythmias, effects on cardiac conduction (PR interval or QRS), and possibly less negative inotropy, but whether these small differences are clinically significant remains uncertain. In a concentration of 0.5% it has been

Table 2-1
CHARACTERISTICS OF COMMONLY USED DRUGS

Generic Name (Trade Name)	Concentration (mg/dL)		Maximum Dose (mg/kd)*	Approximate Duration
	Infiltration	**Nerve Block**		
Procaine (Novocain)	0.75	1.5-3	10-14	45-90 min, short acting
Chloroprocaine (Nesacaine)	0.75	1.5-3	12-15	
Lidocaine (Xylocaine)	0.5	1-2	8-11	1.5-3 hr, medium duration
Mepivacaine (Carbocaine)	0.5	1-2	8-11	
Tetracaine (Pontocaine)	0.05	0.15-0.2	2	
Bupivacaine (Marcaine)	0.25	0.25-0.5	2.5-3.5	3-10 hr, long acting
Etidocaine (Duranest)	0.5	0.5-1	4-5.5	
Ropivacaine (Naropin)	0.25	0.25-0.5	2.5-3.5	

*Higher doses with the use of 1:200,000 epinephrine.

shown to be an effective agent for brachial plexus blockade,[99,102] with an onset and duration of action similar to that of bupivacaine 0.5%. Ropivacaine 0.25% is similar in onset and duration to bupivacaine 0.25%, but the frequent need for supplementation with both of these agents makes them less desirable if a dense sensory and motor block is desired.[104]

Levobupivacaine (Chirocaine) is the L-isomer of bupivacaine. Bupivacaine is delivered commercially as a racemic mixture. There is some evidence that the D-isomer may be slightly more cardiotoxic than the L-isomer, with the racemic mixture being intermediate in cardiac toxicity. One study[14] involving human volunteers receiving intravenous infusions of bupivacaine and levobupivacaine showed a slight decrease in negative inotropic effect (a decrease in ejection fraction of −2.50 for levobupivacaine versus −4.29% for bupivacaine; $P = .024$), which was statistically significant but probably not clinically significant. In a study[86] looking at the effects of local anesthetics on canine cardiotoxicity the researchers concluded that significantly higher concentrations of ropivacaine than levobupivacaine were required to produce comparable myocardial depression. The cardiac effect of levobupivacaine did not differ from that of bupivacaine. Chang and colleagues[42] compared the effects of injecting bupivacaine, levobupivacaine, and ropivacaine directly into the coronary arteries of sheep and found no significant differences in the cardiac effects of these three drugs. This study found that the lethal dose of levobupivacaine in conscious sheep was significantly less than that of bupivacaine. Graf and coworkers[83] found that racemic bupivacaine had more effect on the arteriovenous conduction than levobupivacaine but less than that of the R-isomer. All other direct cardiac effects were the same for both isomers.

There is little doubt that bupivacaine, levobupivacaine, and ropivacaine can all be used successfully clinically. The two newer drugs were introduced to reduce the cardiac toxicity of bupivacaine. They have no demonstrable other clinical benefit. Given the significantly greater cost of ropivacaine and levobupivacaine and the rarity of the occurrence of cardiac toxicity of bupivacaine, we tend to agree with D'Angelo,[55] who in an editorial wrote that the two newer drugs may not be worth their increased cost.

Prevention of Systemic Reaction

The following measures may be used to prevent or minimize systemic reactions to local anesthetic agents.[58]

LOCAL ANESTHETIC TOXICITY

- Allergy to local anesthetics is rare, especially to the amide group.
- Systemic toxicity can be fatal.
- Severe systemic toxicity is quite rare.
- Bupivacaine in high concentrations and high doses is more dangerous if inadvertently injected intravenously than are levobupivacaine or ropivacaine.

Avoidance of Intravascular Injection. Unintentional intravascular injection, the most common cause of convulsions, can be avoided by careful intermittent aspiration before injecting large quantities of local anesthetic agents. This is very important when using 25-gauge or smaller needles, because blood return is very slow. Inability to aspirate blood does not prevent intravascular injection, and intravascular injection is by far the most common mechanism for systemic toxicity. Injection of small boluses of local anesthetic, followed by a brief period of observation before giving additional boluses, is the safest preventive technique.

Use of the lowest possible dose and concentration of local anesthetic is recommended, thus avoiding toxic blood levels (see Table 2-1).

Use of Epinephrine. Epinephrine used in 1:200,000 concentration produces vasoconstriction. Besides prolonging the duration of anesthesia, it delays vascular uptake and lowers the peak blood level, thus reducing the toxicity of the local anesthetic agent. To avoid compromising the blood supply of the digits, epinephrine should not be used in digital blocks.[1,58,117,190] Epinephrine is also avoided in patients with ischemic heart disease. The maximum total dose of epinephrine in healthy adults is kept below 0.25 mg to avoid systemic reaction to the epinephrine itself. This allows the use of 50 mL of the solution along with epinephrine in 1:200,000 concentration. This concentration of the solution is prepared by adding 0.05 mg (or 0.05 mL of 1:1000 concentration) epinephrine to each 10 mL of the local anesthetic. If there is any doubt about the exact amount to be used, it is better to use a commercially available local anesthetic that already contains epinephrine to avoid unintentional excessive doses of epinephrine. Disadvantages of the commercial mixture are the low pH necessary to keep the epinephrine stable and the heat lability of the epinephrine when autoclaved. The low pH causes injection of the solution to be more painful and may also decrease the effectiveness of the local anesthetic agent. Alkalinization alleviates these problems.

Benzodiazepine Premedication. Barbiturates are ineffective in the prevention of local anesthetic toxicity. DeJong and Heavner have shown that diazepam elevates the convulsive threshold for intravenous lidocaine if given as a premedication 1 hour before the experiment.[60,61] Likewise, pretreatment with midazolam has also been shown to be effective in raising the convulsive threshold for lidocaine, bupivacaine, and etidocaine.[59,220]

Fractionate the Dose. Similar to the practice of giving no more than 3 to 5 mL of local anesthetic when we perform epidural anesthesia, it is probably advisable to fractionate the dose in other situations, pausing briefly to look for signs of inadvertent intravascular injection or spinal anesthesia. Metallic taste, numbness around the mouth, ringing in the ears, and twitching of the face indicate intravascular placement of the needle.[53,58] Tachycardia (or hypertension without tachycardia in patients on β blockers) within 30 seconds of injection of 3 mL of a local anesthetic mixture with epinephrine at 1:200,000 is indicative of intravascular placement of the needle.

PREVENTION OF SYSTEMIC TOXICITY

- Avoid intravascular injection.
- Use epinephrine to slow systemic absorption.
- Use benzodiazepine as a premedication.
- Fractionate the dose.

Signs and Symptoms of Systemic Toxicity

Systemic toxicity can be due to unintentional intravascular injection or drug overdose. Reaction to epinephrine is sometimes confused with local anesthetic toxicity. Intravascular injection produces convulsion during the injection itself, whereas epinephrine produces palpitations and restlessness usually 1 to 2 minutes after completion of the injection. Reaction to an overdose develops approximately 20 minutes after the injection, when peak blood levels are reached. Early symptoms of overdose are headache, ringing in the ears, numbness in the tongue and mouth, twitching of facial muscles, and restlessness. As the blood levels increase, generalized convulsions can result. This is followed by respiratory arrest due to the toxic effect of the drug on the respiratory center in the medulla.

Cardiovascular system depression results in bradycardia; impaired conduction, which leads to asystole; and vascular dilatation, which further decreases the blood pressure.[58]

Treatment of Toxic Reactions

If convulsions start, it is important to prevent injury to the patient, establish the airway, and ventilate the patient. Hyperventilation with oxygen often terminates the convulsion by reducing the $Paco_2$,[62] especially with unintentional intravascular injection. No further treatment may be needed because the blood level is rapidly reduced by redistribution of the drug.

A small dose of intravenous benzodiazepine (diazepam, midazolam) or 50 to 100 mg of thiopental (Pentothal) or propofol is likely to terminate the convulsion. High doses of thiopental may produce additional cardiovascular and central nervous system depression. Propofol (50-100 mg IV) quickly terminates most seizures.[46,96,119] Usually, cardiovascular system depression does not present a problem. If hypotension is noted, intravenous infusion of fluids, elevation of the legs, and vasopressors such as ephedrine will

SIGNS AND SYMPTOMS OF TOXICITY

CENTRAL NERVOUS SYSTEM

- Change in mental status: lethargy, confusion
- Seizures

HEMODYNAMIC

- Abrupt change in heart rate, blood pressure, or electrocardiogram

TREATMENT OF SYSTEMIC TOXICITY OF LOCAL ANESTHETICS

SEIZURES

- Usually a seizure that results from too high a plasma concentration of local anesthetic is brief and self-limited.
- A single dose of propofol (40 to 60 mg IV) or midazolam (1 to 2 mg IV) is often all that is necessary along with supporting the patient's airway and administering oxygen.
- Intubation is usually not required.

CARDIOVASCULAR

- Observe the electrocardiogram closely and treat arrhythmias appropriately.

correct the hypotension by vasoconstriction and stimulation of the heart.[53,58] The cardiovascular toxicity associated with bupivacaine, however, may cause more prolonged and difficult resuscitation.[7] Cardiovascular toxicity from inadvertent intravascular injection of bupivacaine is exceedingly rare. More often, seizures occur. Bretylium has been shown to be more effective than lidocaine for the treatment of bupivacaine-induced cardiac arrhythmias,[124] and even cardiopulmonary bypass has been used to treat resistant ventricular fibrillation associated with bupivacaine toxicity.[139] Some studies[66,193] suggest that milrinone may be effective in reversing the cardiovascular depression (reduction in cardiac output) from bupivacaine.

Techniques of Regional Anesthesia

The important regional anesthetic techniques are brachial plexus block at different levels, peripheral nerve blocks at the elbow and wrist, digital blocks, and intravenous regional anesthesia. Brachial plexus anesthesia is the most important technique because of the common use of pneumatic tourniquets, which usually cannot be tolerated for more than 20 to 30 minutes without anesthesia of the whole arm.

Cervical Epidural Anesthesia/Analgesia

Cervical epidural anesthesia is a simple, safe, and effective method for providing anesthesia or analgesia. Lack of familiarity with the technique has prevented many anesthesiologists from taking advantage of this useful method.

Technique. We prefer the paramedian approach for this technique. The method is the same as the paramedian approach for epidural anesthesia at the lumbar or thoracic levels. With the patient sitting, after sterile prep and drape, the C6-C7 or C7-T1 interspaces are usually selected. About 1 cm lateral to the selected interspace the Tuohy needle is inserted, and a paramedian approach using loss of resistance with air or saline is used. A catheter is inserted 3 to 4 cm into the epidural space.

The distance from the skin to the cervical epidural space at the C7-T1 interspace was 4.81 ± 0.81 cm (mean ± SD) using a midline approach. The distance correlates with body weight.

Complications. Pulmonary complications are the major concern for some people. Respiratory effects are measurable but usually minor,[39,211] especially if lower concentrations of local anesthetic are chosen (0.25% to 0.375% bupivacaine). As with an interscalene or supraclavicular block, if the patient is a "pulmonary cripple," the local anesthetic (choice, dose, and concentration) needs to be adjusted accordingly.

Benefits. Excellent analgesia is easily obtained for a wide variety of situations,[16,35,88,134] including surgery involving the shoulder or any part of the upper extremity.

Unilateral (Lateral) Cervical Epidural. It is possible to obtain a unilateral cervical epidural block by a minor adjustment of the usual technique aiming slightly lateral to the midline.[35,134]

Brachial Plexus Block

 ## Anatomy

The brachial plexus is formed by the union of the anterior rami of the lower cervical nerves (C5 to C8) and the first dorsal nerve (Fig. 2-1). Familiarity with the perineural structures that surround and accompany the brachial plexus as it leaves the vertebral column on its course to the upper arm is as important as knowledge of the formation and distribution of the neural plexus itself. Palpable muscular and vascular landmarks allow accurate location of the plexus percutaneously. An appreciation of the fascial relationships is absolutely essential because this is the basis for all the perivascular techniques.[243,244]

After leaving the intervertebral foramina, the anterior primary rami of the nerves destined to become the brachial plexus travel in the gutter formed by the anterior and posterior tubercles of the corresponding transverse processes of

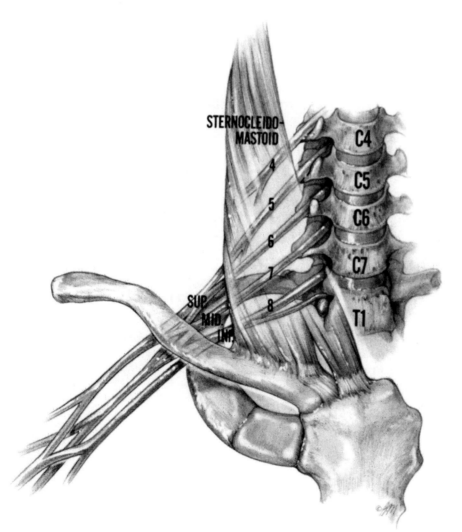

FIGURE 2-1. Brachial plexus showing the relationship of the roots, trunks, divisions, and cords to bony landmarks.

the cervical vertebrae (see Fig. 2-1). After leaving the transverse process, the roots of the plexus descend in front of the middle scalene muscle, which arises from the posterior tubercles of the transverse processes of the lower six cervical vertebrae. The insertion of this muscle on the first rib is separated from that of the anterior scalene muscle by the subclavian groove, on which the artery and the inferior trunk of the brachial plexus will pass. The anterior scalene muscle arises from the anterior tubercles of the transverse processes of the third, fourth, fifth, and sixth cervical vertebrae and inserts on the scalene tubercle of the first rib, thus separating the subclavian artery from the subclavian vein (Fig. 2-2).

The fascia covering both scalene muscles is derived from the prevertebral fascia, which splits to invest these muscles and then fuses again at their lateral margins to form an enclosed interscalene space (Fig. 2-3). Therefore, as the roots leave the transverse processes, they emerge between two walls of the fascia covering the anterior and middle scalene muscles. In their descent toward the first rib to form the trunks of the plexus, the roots may be considered to be "sandwiched" between the anterior and middle scalene muscles, the fascia of which serve as a sheath of the plexus.

As the trunks approach the first rib, they are arranged (as their designations imply—superior, middle, and inferior) one above the other vertically, not one next to the other horizontally as depicted in so many texts (see Fig. 2-2).[243,244]

As the trunks of the plexus cross the first rib, they are joined by the subclavian artery, which lies in a plane anterior to the trunks, so that the inferior trunk lies behind the artery in the subclavian groove, with the middle and superior trunks located above the level of the vessel. At this level the artery and trunks are moving laterally across the ribs and invaginate the scalene fascia to form the "subclavian perivascular space," which is continuous medially and superiorly with the interscalene space and inferiorly and laterally with the axillary perivascular space (Fig. 2-4).[243,244]

The important concept is that there is a continuous, fascia-enclosed, perineural and perivascular space extending from the cervical transverse processes to several centimeters beyond the axilla; this space has been divided into an axillary perivascular space, a subclavian perivascular space, and an interscalene space (see Fig. 2-4). The existence of such a continuous perineural space renders brachial plexus blockade simple. The space described may be entered at any level, and the volume of anesthetic injected at that level will

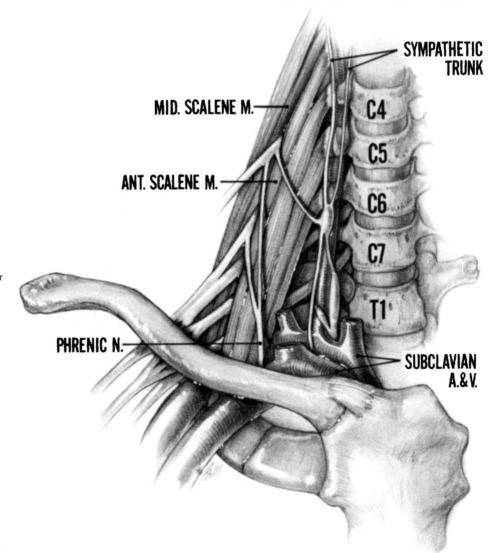

FIGURE 2-2. Muscular and vascular relationships of the brachial plexus.

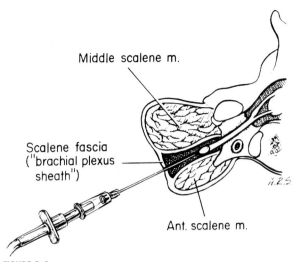

FIGURE 2-3. Brachial plexus sheath bounded by the scalene muscles.

Middle scalene m.

Scalene fascia ("brachial plexus sheath")

Ant. scalene m.

determine the extent of anesthesia. Thus, the technique to be used in any case should be determined on the basis of the surgical site, the required level of anesthesia, and the physical status and habitus of the patient.

The upper medial aspect of the arm is not anesthetized by any brachial plexus block technique, because this area is innervated by the intercostobrachial nerve (T2). This nerve can be blocked by the subcutaneous infiltration of 3 to 5 mL of local anesthetic across the axillary artery for anesthesia before surgery or tourniquet placement.[156,242-244,246]

The brachial plexus can be blocked at the level of the roots, trunks, cords, or peripheral branches. At each level the block has distinct advantages, disadvantages, complications, and distribution of anesthesia.

Kulenkampf[130] and Hirschel[107] were the first to describe a percutaneous method of blocking the brachial plexus. Their technique consisted of injecting local anesthetic around the brachial plexus as it crosses the first rib via a supraclavicular approach. Various modifications have been described since their original report in an attempt to increase the success rate and reduce the rate of complications.[26,28,91,144,156,172]

Conventional Supraclavicular Block

The most widely used type of supraclavicular block was described and popularized by Bonica and coworkers[26] and Moore and associates.[156,159,161] The block is accomplished by finding the first rib with a needle introduced through the skin 0.5 cm above the midpoint of the clavicle and injecting the local anesthetic solution between the rib and the skin. The needle is walked along the first rib from the lateral border of the anterior scalene muscle to the anterior border of the middle scalene muscle. When paresthesias are encountered, 8 to 10 mL of local anesthetic solution is injected to a

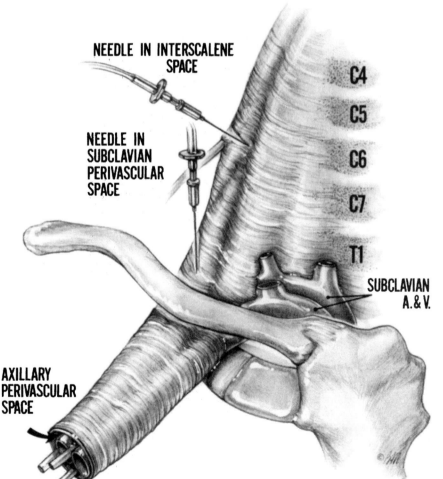

NEEDLE IN INTERSCALENE SPACE

NEEDLE IN SUBCLAVIAN PERIVASCULAR SPACE

C4
C5
C6
C7
T1

SUBCLAVIAN A. & V.

AXILLARY PERIVASCULAR SPACE

FIGURE 2-4. Sheath enclosing the cervical and brachial plexus and the subclavian artery and vein, the "subclavian perivascular space." This is a key concept in the technique of brachial plexus block anesthesia (see text).

total volume of 40 to 50 mL. An attempt is made to elicit paresthesias referred to different parts of the arm, especially the thumb and fingers.[155,158] Satisfactory anesthesia was reported in 91.9% of 1100 cases in which this technique was used.[26] Ultrasonographic guidance with a 7.5-MHz probe has been used to visualize the plexus and avoid pleural or vascular penetration. This technique may increase the safety and efficacy of the supraclavicular block.[121] A more modern variation of this technique includes the use of a nerve stimulator. As with an interscalene approach, a twitch obtained in a deltoid muscle provides adequate anesthesia for shoulder surgery. A twitch involving the pectoralis major muscle also provides adequate block of the brachial plexus. If a twitch is not easily obtained with the classic supraclavicular approach, one can switch to the subclavian perivascular approach (using a very minor modification of the classic supraclavicular technique). If a twitch is not obtained with either of these methods, we can often obtain a good brachial plexus block by simply injecting local anesthetic on top of the first rib at several locations.

Advantages.   This technique produces rapid, reliable anesthesia in expert hands for most of the surgical procedures of the upper extremity and has minimal side effects and complications. Combined with a superficial cervical plexus block, it is excellent for shoulder surgery.

The block is performed with the arm at the side, thus avoiding movement in painful conditions. It produces anesthesia for manipulation and procedures on the upper part of the arm.

Disadvantages.   The first rib is the backstop in this technique for preventing a pneumothorax.[156-158] The midpoint of the clavicle frequently does not correspond to the first rib, and the needle may puncture the cupula of the lung and produce a pneumothorax. The incidence of pneumothorax is 0.5% to 6% with this technique according to older data.[158]

More recent references have cited fairly larger series in both adults and children with no incidents of pneumothorax.[79a,170] We believe that the concern about pneumothorax is considerably overstated. If we are careful to avoid inserting a needle medial to the medial border of the first rib, there should be no pneumothorax. By intentionally starting out aiming the needle more laterally, and using confirmatory landmarks in addition to the middle of the clavicle (palpating the subclavian artery near the middle of the clavicle and tracing the interscalene groove down to the area where we plan to insert the needle), we have not seen any instances of pneumothorax.

Phrenic nerve block occurs in 40% to 60% of patients[155] because of the spread of local anesthetic to the anterior surface of the anterior scalene muscle. This is rarely symptomatic. The patient complains of difficulty in breathing but is still able to expand the chest wall; the feeling is primarily due to decreased afferent impulses from the diaphragm. Radiographic confirmation may be made by obtaining two chest radiographs, one taken after inspiration and one after expiration and noting diaphragmatic movement between the two films.

A double-exposure radiographic technique may also be used to diagnose phrenic nerve block.[103] In this technique the patient is instructed to take a full, deep inspiration and the first image is taken; this is then followed by complete expiration, after which the second image is recorded on the same film, thus allowing easy evaluation of diaphragmatic movement between inspiration and expiration. Usually no treatment is required for phrenic nerve block, although decreases in pulmonary function do occur. Bilateral block in an emphysematous patient may produce difficulty in breathing, cyanosis, and restlessness and may require ventilatory support.[30,156] When the local anesthetic action wears off all the symptoms disappear.

Horner's syndrome is characterized by ptosis, miosis (constriction of the pupil), and anhidrosis, or absence of sweating on the ipsilateral side of the face. It occurs in 70% to 90% of the patients[156] because of the spread of local anesthetic to the cervical sympathetic chain. Symptoms disappear when the block dissipates, and no treatment is required. If necessary, the ocular symptoms can be reversed with one drop of 10% phenylephrine in the eye.[251]

Perivascular Brachial Blocks

In 1964, Winnie and Collins[247] described the perivascular approaches to brachial plexus block. The important concept is that the fascial sheath is continuous from the transverse processes to several centimeters beyond the axilla, that is, from the roots of the plexus to the major nerves of the upper arm. The existence of such a space, which Winnie confirmed radiographically, makes the brachial block very simple.[243,246] The space may be entered at any level, and the volume of anesthetic injected at that level will determine the extent of anesthesia.[132,252] Recommended volumes are listed in Table 2-2. The local anesthetic solution diffuses within the sheath and anesthetizes the various parts of the plexus, as opposed to the physician having to find nerves with multiple needle sticks as described in the classic technique. The single-injection techniques of perivascular blocks minimize the skill and experience required to perform a successful block, markedly reduce the time required to perform the block, and certainly enhance safety by reducing such complications as intravascular injection and postinjection neuropathies, which are known to be a function of the number of injections. Obviously, patients also prefer one stick instead of many.[243,246]

There are three convenient levels at which the plexus may be blocked in this manner: (1) interscalene at the level of the roots, (2) subclavian perivascular at the level of the trunks and the subclavian artery, and (3) axillary perivascular in the axilla or via an infraclavicular approach at the level of the cords.

Interscalene Technique.   The interscalene space is above the cupula of the lung and the subclavian artery, between the fascia covering the anterior and middle scalene muscles (Fig. 2-5). The space is entered to perform the block in the following manner.[242,243,246] The patient is in the dorsal recumbent position, with the head turned slightly to the side opposite that to be blocked. The patient is asked to elevate the head to make the sternocleidomastoid muscle prominent, and the index and middle fingers of the physician are placed behind the posterior border of the clavicular head of the muscle. Then the patient is asked to bring the head down and relax. The fingers of the physician now lie on the anterior

Table 2-2
GUIDE TO DETERMINE VOLUME IN PERIVASCULAR ANESTHESIA

Age (yr)	Male Patients		Female Patients		Formula to Determine Volume (mL)	Concentration (Lidocaine or Mepivacaine)
	Height (inches)	Volume (mL)	Height (inches)	Volume (mL)		
Birth	21	4	20	4		
1	30	6	30	6	Height ÷ 5	0.7-0.8
2	36	7	36	7		
3	40	8	40	8		
4	43	9	43	9		
5	46	12	45	11		
6	49	12.5	48	12	Height ÷ 4	0.8-0.9
7	52	13	51	12.5		
8	54	14	53	13		
9	56	18.5	55	18		
10	58	19	57.5	19		
11	60	20	60	20		
12	62	21	63	21	Height ÷ 3	0.9-1.0
13	65	22	65	22		
14	68	23	66	22		
15	70	23	66	22		
16	71	25	66	22		
After maximum growth	70 or more	Use formula	66 or more	Use formula	Height ÷ 2	1.0-1.5

scalene muscle. The groove between the anterior and the middle scalene muscles is identified by rolling the fingers laterally.[204,242,243,246] A 3.8-cm 22-gauge short-beveled needle is introduced between the fingers on the interscalene groove at the level of the cricoid cartilage (i.e., the level of the sixth cervical transverse process). The direction of the needle is perpendicular to all planes of the side of the neck (i.e., medial, dorsal, and slightly caudad) (see Fig. 2-5). The needle is advanced until a paresthesia is elicited or the transverse process is contacted, in which case the needle is walked on the transverse process in an anteroposterior direction to elicit a paresthesia. When paresthesias are elicited, the desired volume of local anesthetic is injected. A 20-mL volume of local anesthetic produces anesthesia of the brachial plexus as well as the lower cervical plexus, but anesthesia in the ulnar nerve distribution is delayed and occasionally absent. A 40-mL volume produces complete anesthesia of both the cervical and brachial plexuses. It has been shown that when performing this block for shoulder procedures, a paresthesia elicited toward the shoulder does produce an effective block.[187] It is currently more common to use a nerve stimulator than to try to elicit paresthesias.

Advantages. This block is easy to perform, even in obese people, whereas landmarks for the other techniques may not be palpable. The technique is ideal for manipulations and procedures of the upper arm and shoulder, where a high level of anesthesia is obtained with small volumes.

Pneumothorax is commonly thought to be less likely because of the level of insertion of the needle, but it can occur. When infection or malignancy is present in the arm, this technique can be used because it is performed above the level of the lymph nodes.[242,246]

This technique is applicable in children and intoxicated, uncooperative adults because movement is unlikely to injure any important structures at this level.[241,245]

Disadvantages. The main disadvantage of this block is the slow onset or absence of anesthesia in the ulnar nerve distribution. This can be offset by either increasing the volume to 40 mL or, when small volumes of local anesthetics have to be used, by blocking the ulnar nerve separately at the elbow.

Subarachnoid, epidural, and vertebral artery injections are theoretically possible, and several cases have been reported in the literature,[75,131,189,203,206] but the caudad direction of the needle, if carefully observed, should prevent the needle from advancing very far between the transverse processes and thus avoid these complications. Sympathetic block[203] is very rare with this technique. Phrenic nerve block may occur as a result of diffusion of local anesthetic cephalad to involve the more proximal cervical roots (C3, C4, C5) or because of placement of local anesthetic outside the brachial plexus sheath, anterior to the anterior scalene muscle. Urmey and McDonald demonstrated decreases in pulmonary function (decreases in forced vital capacity and

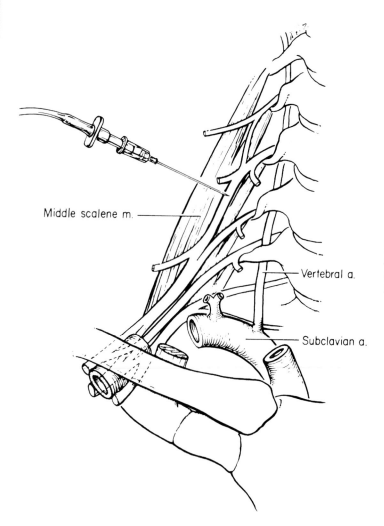

Middle scalene m.

Vertebral a.

Subclavian a.

FIGURE 2-5. Interscalene technique. Note the caudad direction of the needle to avoid complications (see text). (From Winnie AP: Regional anesthesia. Surg Clin North Am 55:861-892, 1975.)

forced expiratory volume in 1 second of 27 ± 4.3% and 26.4 ± 6.8%, respectively) in patients with unilateral hemidiaphragmatic paralysis caused by interscalene block.[225] Interscalene blocks should be avoided in patients in whom the opposite hemidiaphragm is already paralyzed.

Subclavian Perivascular Block.[246] The subclavian perivascular space is entered close to the subclavian artery, between the anterior and middle scalene muscles (Fig. 2-6). The interscalene groove is identified in the same manner as described for the interscalene technique, but the physician's finger slides down the groove and the subclavian artery is palpated. A 3.8-cm 22-gauge short-beveled needle is inserted directly caudad, dorsally tangential to the artery (see Fig. 2-6). If the artery is not palpable, the needle is inserted along the anterior surface of the middle scalene muscle where the nerve trunks are located in the interscalene groove. As the needle is advanced, it is likely to touch one of the three trunks and elicit a paresthesia. If the trunks are missed, the first rib will be encountered. Most of the time a paresthesia is elicited before the needle touches the rib. If possible, a middle trunk (C7) paresthesia should be elicited because this is associated with the highest incidence of success in producing surgical anesthesia of all three trunks.[100] When the paresthesia is encountered, 20 to 40 mL of the local anesthetic solution is injected. Twenty milliliters in the subclavian perivascular space gives the same extent of

anesthesia as 40 mL in the axillary perivascular space and provides anesthesia of the brachial plexus and the lower part of the cervical plexus. Transarterial techniques in which the local anesthetic is deposited after puncturing the subclavian artery and either advancing through or withdrawing from the artery are not effective for subclavian perivascular block.[101] This is in contrast to axillary blocks, where transarterial techniques are effective and frequently used.

Advantages. This block is very easy to perform once the landmarks are located. Small volumes of local anesthetic provide excellent anesthesia, which is established very rapidly. Because this block provides excellent anesthesia so easily, the authors have difficulty in convincing trainees to learn any other approach once they are exposed to the subclavian perivascular approach. Subarachnoid, epidural, and vertebral artery injections are practically impossible.[243,244,246,247]

Disadvantages. Symptomatic nerve block is extremely rare and is seen in fewer than 2% of the patients; it requires patient reassurance but no treatment.

Recurrent laryngeal nerve block, which results in hoarseness of the voice, is seen in 1% of the cases and only on the right side because the recurrent laryngeal nerve loops around the subclavian artery on the right and the arch of the aorta on the left.

Parascalene Technique. Another technique called the parascalene approach has been described.[233] The landmarks are the same as those for the subclavian perivascular approach. The needle is inserted from the anterior scalene muscle posteriorly toward the middle scalene. Although no serious complications have been reported, this technique is not very different from the subclavian perivascular approach.

Plumb Bob Technique. With the "plumb bob" technique, the needle is introduced at the midpoint of the clavicle and directed perpendicular to the skin in a posterior direction.[32] With the patient supine, this direction would be directly toward the floor, following the line of insertion that a plumb bob would generate. If necessary, the needle can be rotated in small steps in a more caudad direction until twitch with a nerve stimulator (or a paresthesia) is elicited. An advantage of this technique is that the incidence of pneumothorax should be low because the advancing needle encounters fibers of the brachial plexus before it encounters the dome of the diaphragm. The success rate of this technique is similar to that of other supraclavicular techniques. One disadvantage of this technique is that the brachial plexus cords are approached in a perpendicular plane and the needle may have to be redirected before encountering one of the cords.

The Intersternocleidomastoid Approach. Pham-Dang and colleagues[173] described a modification of the supraclavicular block that involved aiming the needle between the two heads of the sternocleidomastoid (SCM) muscle and aiming laterally. The needle is inserted at a point "on the inner border of the SCM clavicular head, two fingerbreadths (3 cm) above the sternal notch. The midpoint of the clavicle was marked. After a skin wheal was raised, the stimulating needle was directed caudally, dorsally, and laterally toward the midpoint of the clavicle, passing behind the SCM clavicular head and forming a 40- to 50-degree angle with the plane of the operating table." The success rate was 93%. The authors believed the approach was especially useful for placing a catheter for postoperative pain control.

Posterior Approach to the Brachial Plexus

Several references have been published describing a posterior approach to the brachial plexus. The technique[234] using a nerve stimulator starts with a patient sitting with the head bent forward. At a point 3 cm lateral to the C6-7 interspace, a 110-mm insulated needle is advanced perpendicular to the skin until an appropriate twitch is elicited, usually at a depth of about 6 cm. Rucci and colleagues[191] compared the distribution of the block for this approach with the traditional lateral approach and found significant differences. Dagli and associates[54] reported a high incidence of inadequate anesthesia for forearm or hand surgery with the posterior approach. Variously called a posterior approach to the interscalene block or a cervical paravertebral approach, it is advocated as an excellent method for placing a catheter for a continuous block technique.[23]

Infraclavicular Approaches to the Brachial Plexus

Infraclavicular Blocks. In previously described infraclavicular approaches, physicians attempted to reach the

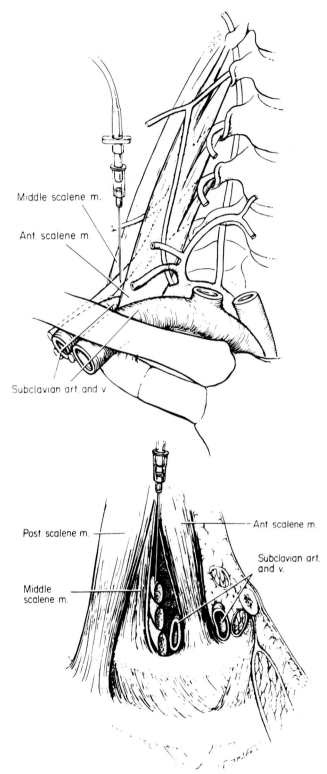

FIGURE 2-6. Subclavian perivascular technique. Note the caudad direction of the needle and its relation to the middle scalene muscle. (From Winnie AP: Regional anesthesia. Surg Clin North Am 55:861-892, 1975.)

Middle scalene m.

Ant. scalene m.

Subclavian art. and v.

Post. scalene m.

Middle scalene m.

Ant. scalene m.

Subclavian art. and v.

Although not impossible, pneumothorax is relatively rare. As long as the needle is directed directly caudad along the scalene muscles, it is likely to touch the rib on which these muscles are inserted. If the needle is directed too far medially or laterally, it may puncture the cupula of the lung and result in pneumothorax.

TYPES OF BRACHIAL PLEXUS BLOCK ABOVE THE CLAVICLE

INTERSCALENE

- Anterior
- Posterior

SUPRACLAVICULAR

- Classic (conventional)
- Plumb bob
- Parascalene
- Intersternocleidomastoid
- Subclavian perivascular

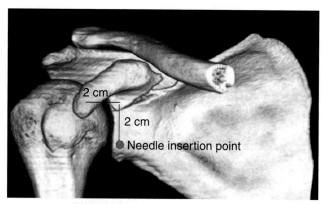

FIGURE 2-7. Landmarks for coracoid block.

plexus above the clavicle with a needle introduced below the clavicle and directed toward Chassaignac's tubercle; this method has all the disadvantages of the supraclavicular techniques. It is important to note that block failure is likely if we accept stimulation of the musculocutaneous nerve as an end point because this nerve is not adjacent to the rest of the brachial plexus in this area.

Raj Approach. Raj and coworkers[178] described an infraclavicular technique in which the needle is directed away from the chest wall, thus avoiding a pneumothorax. The technique consists of introducing an 8-cm, 22-gauge spinal needle 2.5 cm below the midpoint of the clavicle and directing the needle toward the brachial artery.[178,207] A nerve stimulator is used to locate the plexus cords by looking for contraction of the muscles around the elbow or the wrist.[154,176,178] When maximum contractions are obtained, 30 mL of local anesthetic solution is injected.

Paracoracoid Approach Variants. In the *vertical infraclavicular approach* the point of needle insertion is the deltopectoral fossa directed vertically at the bottom of the fossa straight back at an angle of 90 degrees toward the axillary crease. If unable to elicit a twitch, the needle is directed at an angle of 45 degrees toward the coracoid process. The success rate for blocking cutaneous innervation of the hand and forearm was 89% in the study of Jandard and colleagues.[116]

In the *lateral infraclavicular approach* the coracoid is still used as a landmark. The needle is inserted along the sagittal plane until contact is made with the coracoid process. The needle is withdrawn and reinserted directly below the coracoid process until the brachial plexus is stimulated with a nerve stimulator. Forty milliliters of local anesthetic is given. In a study comparing this block with an axillary block, the success rate for this approach was 100% compared with 85% for the axillary block group. Furthermore, the musculocutaneous nerve block was denser in the lateral infraclavicular block group, and also the thoracodorsal, axillary, and medial brachial cutaneous nerves were blocked.[120]

The *coracoid technique* involves inserting the needle 2 cm medial and 2 cm caudad to the coracoid process and

then going straight back. The technique is safe and effective (Fig. 2-7).[238]

Advantages. The benefit of this approach is the ability to easily place a catheter for a continuous block. It provides a good block of all the nerves supplied by the brachial plexus.

Pneumothorax, subarachnoid and epidural injections, phrenic block, cervical sympathetic block, and recurrent laryngeal block are virtually impossible because the needle is directed away from all these structures.

Disadvantages. At the site of the injection the brachial plexus cords are located deeply beneath the pectoralis major and minor muscles; thus a long needle is needed for the block. Whenever long needles are required, technical difficulty increases and accuracy of placement of the solution suffers. However, with experience, these disadvantages can be overcome.[178]

Axillary Block. Blocking the major nerves at the level of the third part of the axillary artery is the most common technique for providing anesthesia for hand surgery. Because the artery and nerves are superficial, the simplicity of the technique and the absence of major complications are responsible for the wide acceptance of this technique.*

 ## Anatomy

The brachial plexus cords form three major nerves at the level of the third part of the axillary artery. With the shoulder abducted, the median nerve lies in front of and slightly above the artery, the ulnar nerve in front and slightly below it, and the radial nerve behind it. The axillary vein lies medial to the artery. The nerves, artery, and vein are enclosed in a fascial sheath, which is part of the same sheath that surrounds the rest of the brachial plexus (Fig. 2-8). The musculocutaneous nerve leaves the sheath of the plexus at

*See references 3, 11, 28, 36, 37, 43, 56, 57, 89, 107, 114, 123, 128, and 161.

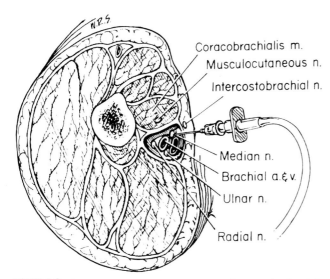

FIGURE 2-8. Cross-sectional view showing the needle properly placed for an axillary perivascular block. Note that the tip of the needle lies superiorly tangential to the artery and vein. (From Winnie AP: Regional anesthesia. Surg Clin North Am 55:861-892, 1975.)

the level of the coracoid process and lies within the substance of the coracobrachialis muscle at the level where the usual axillary block is performed. The axillary nerve also leaves the sheath at the level of the coracoid process. When a small volume of local anesthetic agent is used, these nerves are not anesthetized.

There are many modifications of the original block described by Hirschel in 1911.[107] All of these are performed with the arm abducted to 90 degrees with slight external rotation.

Arterial Puncture Technique. Because nerves surround the axillary artery, many physicians deliberately puncture the artery with a 3.8-cm 22-gauge needle. When arterial blood is aspirated, the needle is withdrawn slowly until blood can no longer be aspirated. The needle is then presumed to be outside the artery but still in the axillary sheath, and 40 to 50 mL of local anesthetic is injected. The escaping blood may interfere with the quality of anesthesia.

The preferred technique is to puncture the artery, aspirate blood, and slowly advance the needle through the artery; the local anesthetic solution is injected when blood can no longer be aspirated.[156] After completion of the injection, the needle is withdrawn and digital pressure is applied to avoid hematoma formation, which may interfere with the anesthesia block by preventing access of the local anesthetic solution to the nerves and causing dilution and hydrolysis of the local anesthetic agent. The same procedure can be followed when the artery is punctured unintentionally. Many clinicians inject half of the anesthetic after passing the needle through the artery and the other half just after withdrawing the needle from the artery.[98] This technique may quicken onset of the block.

Paresthesia Technique. The physician seeks paresthesias by exploring with a needle above and then below the artery. With each paresthesia discovered, 10 to 20 mL of local anesthetic is injected.[156] It is relatively easy to elicit ulnar and median nerve paresthesias but difficult to elicit radial nerve paresthesias because this nerve is located behind the artery. This is a very reliable method of obtaining anesthesia, but it is sometimes difficult to elicit paresthesias. There has been some concern about possible damage to the nerve when paresthesias are elicited,[201,202] especially when epinephrine-containing solutions are used.[200]

Nerve Stimulator Technique. A peripheral nerve stimulator can be used to localize nerves within the axillary sheath. The specific muscle twitch that is elicited identifies the nerve being stimulated. Potential advantages of this technique include the avoidance of arterial puncture with possible hematoma formation, the absence of paresthesia elicitation (and the theoretic risk of subsequent nerve damage), and the usefulness of this technique in an anesthetized or uncooperative patient. The negative terminal of the nerve stimulator should be attached to the stimulating electrode because stimulation requires more current when the needle is positive.[222] The positive terminal of the nerve stimulator is attached to an electrode on the side of the chest opposite the arm that is being anesthetized. Localization of the brachial plexus with the nerve stimulator is equally effective at the interscalene, supraclavicular, and axillary sites.[185]

Infiltration Technique. No attempts are made to identify the sheath or the nerves in this technique. The tissues between the humerus and the skin on either side of the artery are infiltrated with multiple insertions of the needle. This method is useful when landmarks are not palpable and other methods are not applicable.[156]

Thompson and Rorie[215] believe that in the axillary sheath the presence of septa creates multiple compartments and thus inhibits the spread of local anesthetic when it is deposited as a single injection. They recommend using a 1.5-cm 25-gauge needle and depositing 10 mL of local anesthetic above and below the artery. The needle is redirected three times on each side of the artery. If paresthesias are obtained, 3 mL of local anesthetic is injected. The procedure is repeated above or below the artery if the initial block produces inadequate analgesia. Other authors have not observed septa[231] or have found them to be functionally incomplete and not a barrier to the spread of local anesthetic.[171] The high success rate noted with some single-injection techniques also mitigates against the functional significance of these septa.[48]

The small needle and small volume of local anesthetic used may decrease the pain of the injection and reduce the chance of local anesthetic toxicity.

A 1.5-cm needle may not be long enough for many patients. This is likely to produce inadequate analgesia, especially in the radial nerve distribution.

Perivascular Approach. Burnham[36,37] described the currently popular technique of injecting a local anesthetic above and below the artery by identifying the entry into the axillary sheath when the characteristic "click" is felt. In 1961, deJong,[56] on the basis of dissections, calculated that a minimal volume of 42 mL of local anesthetic is necessary to block the musculocutaneous nerve that leaves the sheath at the level of the coracoid process. Winnie and coworkers[243,246,248] confirmed this radiologically and popularized the single-injection technique of axillary block. They have also described various maneuvers to promote central spread of the local anesthetic solution to consistently block the musculocutaneous nerve.[246,248] Winnie's perivascular technique[243,246] consists of entering the sheath superiorly, tangential to the artery with the needle in a cephalad direction, thus avoiding the axillary vein. Digital pressure distal to the needle promotes central spread of the solution. Winnie and coworkers have also shown the superiority of digital pressure[246,248] to the tourniquet technique described by Eriksson.[76] Soon after completion of the injection, the arm is adducted to relieve compression of the sheath by the head of the humerus, thus promoting proximal spread of the solution.[246,248]

The perivascular concept can be used with any method of identifying placement of the tip of the needle in the axillary sheath. Thus arterial puncture, paresthesia, nerve stimulation, or fascial click can be used to confirm placement of the needle in the sheath; in all the maneuvers just described, 30 to 40 mL of local anesthetic is injected to promote central spread of the solution.

Double-Injection Technique. Many clinicians prefer to inject 15 to 20 mL of local anesthetic above and below the artery.[36,37,74] Correct placement of the needle in the sheath is confirmed as described earlier for the perivascular technique. Two injections may hasten the onset of block.

Axillary blocks are easy to perform because of the superficial, palpable landmarks. Pneumothorax, phrenic nerve block, stellate ganglion block, subarachnoid or epidural injection, and other complications of supraclavicular techniques are virtually impossible. These features make it the technique of choice when performing bilateral blocks and in patients with emphysema.

This technique is suitable for children and uncooperative patients, and it is the method of choice for outpatient anesthesia in cases in which pneumothorax and phrenic block could produce serious problems.[29,30]

The double-injection technique cannot be used when passive abduction of the arm is not possible. The volume of local anesthetic necessary is frequently higher than that needed for supraclavicular techniques.

The musculocutaneous nerve may be missed when a small volume of local anesthetic is used. This nerve can be anesthetized by increasing the volume and using the perivascular approach.[243,246] When the volume has to be minimized, the musculocutaneous nerve can be blocked by injecting 5 mL of local anesthetic solution into the substance of the coracobrachialis muscle,[243,246] which is above the axillary artery. The nerve can also be identified with the aid of a nerve stimulator[154] by producing contraction of the biceps muscle.

Very rarely, vascular insufficiency or insufficient venous drainage of the arm can result after arterial or venous puncture in the axilla.[150,183]

The Midhumeral Approach. This approach involves stimulating at the midhumeral level the musculocutaneous, radial, median, and ulnar nerves separately.[72] One study comparing this method with a conventional axillary block found an 84% success rate and more frequent complete

TYPES OF BRACHIAL PLEXUS BLOCKS BELOW THE CLAVICLE

- Axillary block
- Midhumeral
- Infraclavicular:
  - Raj
  - Paracoracoid variants:
    - Vertical infraclavicular block
    - Lateral infraclavicular
    - Coracoid

motor block with this approach compared with a 54% success in the axillary block group.

Catheter Techniques. The insertion of a catheter allows repeated injections of local anesthetic for long surgical procedures. In addition, continuous infusions of analgesic concentrations of local anesthetic may be administered for postoperative pain relief. A blunt-tipped needle and catheter set (Contiplex) may be used, with identification of a "fascial click" to signify entrance into the brachial plexus sheath. The proper position of the catheter may be tested by injecting 2 to 4 mL of cold (refrigerated, 4° to 6°C) normal saline through the catheter. This will elicit a short, but distinct cold paresthesia in the arm and/or hand and thereby indicate correct positioning of the catheter. Alternatively, paresthesia or nerve stimulator techniques may be used to identify correct placement of the advancing needle. A perivenous technique has also been reported in which the neurovascular sheath is identified by fluoroscopy. Five milliliters of contrast agent is injected into an arm vein to opacify the axillary vein.[174] The Contiplex cannula is then advanced at an angle of approximately 30 degrees to the skin in the direction of the vein until an audible "pop" and loss of resistance are felt. Additional contrast medium injected into the cannula confirms accurate positioning of the cannula.

In summary, the axillary block and its variants are probably best used for surgery distal to the elbow. Infraclavicular blocks are good for continuous techniques. Supraclavicular approaches and cervical epidural anesthesia are good for any procedure from the shoulder or any place on the upper extremity.

Blocks Around the Elbow

Blocks around the elbow are rarely performed, even though it is possible to produce anesthesia of the forearm and the hand by blocking the median, ulnar, radial, and lateral and medial antebrachial cutaneous nerves. Reasons for the infrequent use of such blocks are overlap of the distribution of the nerves and the variation in their distribution, which necessitates multiple nerve blocks, except in operative procedures in the little finger, in which an ulnar block alone is sufficient.

An upper arm tourniquet is used in most hand operations, but it is not tolerated well for more than 20 to 30 minutes. Therefore, even if analgesia at the surgical site exists, the patient will experience tourniquet pain. Instead of using multiple blocks at the elbow, the same volume of local anesthetic solution can be used to produce anesthesia of the whole arm by brachial plexus block. However, individual blocks can be extremely useful for supplementing the brachial plexus block when anesthesia is incomplete. Diagnostic nerve blocks at the elbow are useful for evaluating nerve lesions and median-to-ulnar crossover.[74]

Ulnar Nerve Block

An ulnar nerve block is the most useful block for supplementing supraclavicular techniques of brachial plexus block because ulnar nerve anesthesia is frequently missed. The nerve is blocked behind the medial epicondyle, where it is palpable, by using a 1.5-cm, 25-gauge needle and 5 mL of local anesthetic agent. It is very important to avoid impaling the nerve on the bone to prevent damage to the nerve.

Median Nerve Block

The median nerve is posteromedial to the brachial artery just above the elbow joint. The nerve is blocked by introducing a 3.8-cm, 22-gauge short-beveled needle medial to the brachial artery, slightly above the level of a line drawn between the epicondyles. The nerve is identified by paresthesias or by using a nerve stimulator.[154] Five to 10 milliliters of a local anesthetic is injected.

Radial Nerve Block

The radial nerve can be blocked 3 to 4 cm above the lateral epicondyle, where it is close to the distal end of the humerus after piercing the lateral intermuscular septum. A 3.8-cm, 22-gauge needle is introduced at this level, paresthesias are sought (or a nerve stimulator is used to identify the nerve), and 5 to 10 mL of a local anesthetic solution is injected.

Medial and Lateral Antebrachial Cutaneous Nerve Block

The medial[68] and lateral[57] antebrachial cutaneous nerves can be blocked by a subcutaneous ring around the elbow.

Wrist Blocks

Wrist blocks are very useful and are commonly used by hand surgeons to produce anesthesia.[51,65,71,73]

Advantages. Wrist blocks are simple to perform. The nerve supply of the extrinsic muscles of the hand are still preserved, thus enabling the patient to move the fingers, although the intrinsic muscles are paralyzed.

Disadvantages. Use of a tourniquet limits the duration of surgery to 20 to 30 minutes in most patients. Methods of prolonging this period of tourniquet tolerance are discussed

later in this chapter. The ability of the patient to move is likely to be a disadvantage in uncooperative patients.

Median Nerve Block

 ## Anatomy

The median nerve lies between the palmaris longus and the flexor carpi radialis tendons (Fig. 2-9).

Technique. A 1.5-cm, 25-gauge needle is inserted between the palmaris longus and the flexor carpi radialis tendons at the level of the ulnar styloid process or the proximal crease of the wrist. In the absence of the palmaris longus, the needle is inserted on the ulnar side of the flexor carpi radialis tendon. When paresthesias are encountered, 5 mL of local anesthetic is injected. Care must be taken to inject the anesthetic solution around the nerve rather than directly within the substance of the nerve.

An alternative method of blocking the median nerve at the wrist that does not require eliciting paresthesias is that described by Green[85] for injecting the carpal tunnel (Fig. 2-10). A 3.8-cm, 25-gauge needle is inserted into the carpal tunnel from a point just ulnar to the palmaris longus tendon (or in line with the fourth ray if no palmaris is present). With the wrist in slight dorsiflexion, the needle is advanced at approximately a 30-degree angle to the skin and aimed in a slightly radial direction, with the carpal tunnel entered just beneath the transverse carpal ligament (see Fig. 2-10A). If paresthesias are inadvertently elicited, the needle is withdrawn and redirected more deeply to avoid direct injection of the nerve itself.

Five to 7 milliliters of 2% lidocaine is then injected while the surgeon palpates the palm at the distal edge of the carpal tunnel with a finger of the opposite hand. If the needle is in the carpal tunnel, a slight bulge distal to the edge of the ligament (see Fig. 2-10B) will indicate correct placement of the needle within the carpal tunnel. As the lidocaine diffuses throughout the carpal tunnel, the median nerve is blocked.

Finally, Delaunay and coworkers[65] described wrist blocks for carpal tunnel repair. For the median nerve block they suggested 10 mL of local anesthetic (0.5% bupivacaine and 2% lidocaine mixed in equal volumes) deposited 16 mm deep medial to the flexor carpi radialis tendon 6 cm above the wrist crease. For the ulnar nerve, 8 mL of local anesthetic is placed under the flexor carpi ulnaris tendon at a depth of 9 to 10 mm and at 6 cm above the wrist crease.

Ulnar Nerve Block

 ## Anatomy

The ulnar nerve at the level of the wrist has already given off the dorsal cutaneous branch. The ulnar nerve lies immediately radial to the flexor carpi ulnaris tendon (Fig. 2-11). The ulnar artery, which must be avoided, lies radial to the

---

BLOCKS AROUND THE ELBOW

- Ulnar nerve block
- Median nerve block
- Radial nerve block
- Medial and lateral antebrachial cutaneous nerves

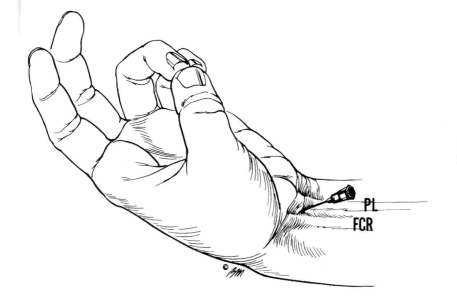

FIGURE 2-9. Wrist block—median nerve. PL, palmaris longus; FCR, flexor carpi radialis.

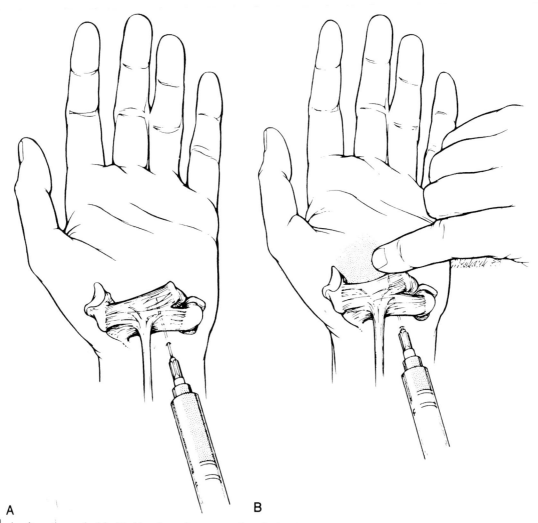

A   B

FIGURE 2-10. An alternative method for blocking the median nerve at the wrist that does not require the elicitation of paresthesias (see text for details of the technique). (From Green DP: Diagnostic and therapeutic value of carpal tunnel injection. J Hand Surg [Am] 9:850-854, 1984.)

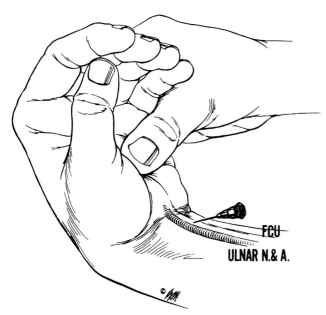

FIGURE 2-11. Wrist block—ulnar nerve. Note that the nerve lies between the artery and the flexor carpi ulnaris (FCU) tendon.

nerve. The anatomy is easy to remember because the nerve and artery maintain the same relationship they have at the elbow, that is, the nerve coming from the medial side and the artery more laterally.

Technique. The nerve is blocked by inserting a 1.5-cm, 25-gauge needle at the level of the proximal crease of the wrist, just radial to the flexor carpi ulnaris tendon, which is made prominent by active flexion of the wrist. When a paresthesia is encountered, 5 mL of local anesthetic is injected, again taking care to avoid injecting anesthetic solution directly into the nerve.

The dorsal cutaneous nerve can be blocked by subcutaneous infiltration of 5 mL of a local anesthetic agent beginning from the site where the ulnar nerve was blocked and extending the infiltration to the midpoint of the dorsum of the wrist.

Superficial Branch of Radial Nerve Block

 Anatomy

This nerve is purely sensory at this level; distal to the radial styloid it divides into multiple terminal branches.

Technique. Subcutaneous infiltration of 5 to 7 mL of a local anesthetic agent starting radial to the radial artery and extending around to the midpoint of the dorsum of the wrist blocks this nerve.

Digital Nerve Block

 Anatomy

Each digit is supplied by four nerve branches, two dorsal and two palmar, that run along the respective sides of the digit. Sensibility on the dorsum of the digits distal to the proximal interphalangeal joints differs in the ulnar and median nerve areas (Fig. 2-12).

Ring Block
A circumferential block around the base of the digit is not recommended because gangrene can result even if no vasopressor drug has been injected with the local anesthetic.[1,196]

WRIST BLOCKS

- Ulnar nerve block
- Median nerve block
- Superficial radial nerve block

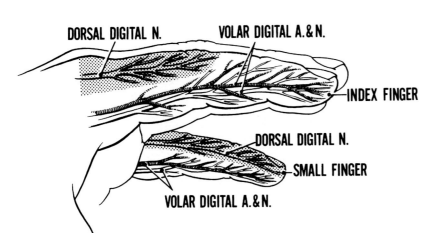

FIGURE 2-12. Relationship and distribution of the digital nerves. Note that in the small finger the dorsal digital nerve extends to the top of the digit; in the median nerve distribution the volar nerve supplies the dorsum of the digit distal to the proximal interphalangeal joint.

Volar Approach

The volar approach is the authors' preferred technique because it is proximal to the common digital arterial communications, whose collateral system obviates the complication of vascular compromise.[1] A skin wheal is made directly over the flexor tendon just proximal to the distal palmar crease (Fig. 2-13), and 2 to 3 mL of a local anesthetic, without epinephrine, is injected on each side of the flexor tendons, where the digital neurovascular bundles are located. This technique is simple and effective; its only disadvantage is that the palmar skin is quite tender and thus injection via this route is rather painful.

Dorsal Approach

An alternative, less painful method of blocking the digital nerves is from the dorsum of the finger (Fig. 2-14). This approach has the added advantage of allowing block of the dorsal nerves without a second needle stick. A 1.5-cm, 25-gauge needle is inserted toward the side of the extensor tendon just proximal to the web. A skin wheal is made and 1 mL of anesthetic solution is injected superficial to the extensor hood to block the dorsal nerve. The needle is then advanced toward the palm until its tip is palpable beneath the volar skin at the base of the finger, just distal to the web. Another 1 mL of anesthetic solution is injected here to block the volar digital nerve.

Before removing the needle, it is redirected across the extensor tendon to the opposite side of the finger, and a small skin wheal is made overlying the other dorsal digital nerve. The needle is then withdrawn and reintroduced into the skin wheal on the opposite side of the finger, and the same technique is repeated.

Care must be taken to use small amounts of anesthetic agent with this method and avoid creating a circumferential ring block, which can result in vascular impairment of the digit.[1,194]

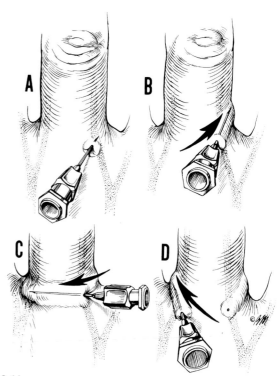

FIGURE 2-14. Digital nerve block—dorsal approach. Care must be taken to be sure that the anesthetic is not injected entirely circumferentially around the finger.

DIGITAL NERVE BLOCKS

- Ring block
- Volar block
- Dorsal block
- Flexor tendon sheath

Flexor Tendon Sheath Technique

Satisfactory anesthesia for a single finger can be obtained by the injection of 2 mL of anesthetic agent into the flexor tendon sheath at the level of the distal palmar crease or metacarpophalangeal flexion crease. Chiu[45] has shown with cadaveric dye injections that complete anesthesia of the digit is easily accomplished with this technique, which has the advantages of a single needle stick and relatively rapid onset.

Local Infiltration

Local infiltration of the skin and subcutaneous tissue is carried out when anesthesia is required in very small areas. It is also useful for supplementing minor inadequacies of a regional block. Extensive local infiltration is not preferred by many hand surgeons because of the distortion of anatomy and the pain caused by multiple needle sticks. However, local edema can be minimized by the addition of 1 mL of hyaluronidase (Wydase) to 20 to 30 mL of local anesthetic agent.

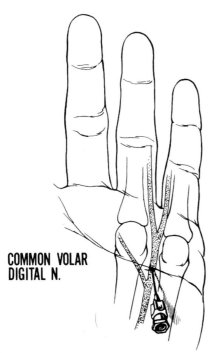

COMMON VOLAR DIGITAL N.

FIGURE 2-13. Digital nerve block—palmar approach.

Intravenous Regional Anesthesia

Intravenous regional block (Bier block[11]) is a very simple technique for producing anesthesia and requires little expertise or prior experience.*

Technique. A dual tourniquet is placed on the upper part of the arm on the side to be blocked. An intravenous infusion is started with a 20- or 22-gauge plastic cannula or a butterfly needle, which is then taped in place. The arm is elevated and exsanguinated with an Esmarch bandage, starting from the fingers all the way to the tourniquet. Thorough exsanguination is the most important part of the technique. Without it the anesthesia is likely to be spotty, the operative field bloody, and the patient likely to have early tourniquet pain. After exsanguination, the proximal tourniquet is inflated and the Esmarch bandage removed. If the patient has a painful extremity, the exsanguination can be accomplished without moving the arm by using an inflatable splint.[249] The local anesthetic solution is then slowly injected through the cannula. Lidocaine, 3 mg/kg given as 0.5% without preservative, provides very satisfactory anesthesia within 4 to 6 minutes and lasts as long as the tourniquet is inflated. The proximal tourniquet is left inflated for 20 minutes or until the patient notices some discomfort; then the distal tourniquet is inflated, and after making sure of its inflation, the proximal tourniquet is deflated. Because the distal tourniquet is applied over the anesthetized area, the patient is not likely to experience any discomfort for about 40 minutes. At the completion of the operative procedure, the tourniquet is deflated for 15 seconds, reinflated for 30 seconds, and deflated again, especially if the duration of anesthesia was 20 minutes or less.[58] If the procedure lasts longer than 40 minutes, the tourniquet can be safely deflated without reinflation.[58] Fifty percent of the local anesthetic is still bound to the tissues for 30 minutes. If additional anesthesia is needed within 30 minutes of tourniquet deflation, only half the original dose is given.[58] For prolonged procedures on the hand, the cannula can be inserted into a cubital vein and left in place and the anesthesia reestablished by repeat injection of the local anesthetic after re-exsanguination.[33]

A second-wrap technique in which a sterile Esmarch bandage is reapplied before making the incision is said to produce a more nearly bloodless operating field and improve anesthesia for the tourniquet by squeezing the local anesthetic solution proximally.[92]

Advantages. Technically, an intravenous regional block is very easy to perform and is suitable for outpatient surgery.[84] Bilateral blocks can be done safely.

Rapid return of motor function enables the surgeon to evaluate the results of the procedure. Some surgeons prefer to use this technique when performing a flexor tenolysis, such as in patients with rheumatoid arthritis. After completion of the operative dissection, the tourniquet is released. After waiting 10 to 15 minutes for ischemic paralysis to wear off, the patient is able to actively move the fingers and thus allow the surgeon to more accurately evaluate the completeness of the tenolysis.[151]

Disadvantages. Even with use of the double cuff, *pain caused by the tourniquet* limits the use of this procedure in operations lasting more than 1 hour. Continuous techniques,[33] thorough exsanguination,[73] and the second-wrap technique may overcome this disadvantage.[92]

There may be *problems with tourniquet release.* When the tourniquet is released,[168] a large bolus of anesthetic enters the systemic circulation; the level peaks within 1 minute and falls rapidly thereafter.[58,194,218,221] This brief elevation of the local anesthetic blood level may produce systemic toxic reactions, including convulsions and cardiac irregularities.[58,235] The longer the tourniquet remains inflated, the lower the anesthetic blood level. About one third of the original dose is washed out within a few minutes after cuff deflation.[58] If the cuff is released for 15 seconds, reinflated, and then released again, it will lower the peak blood level and decrease the possibility of systemic reaction. However, if tourniquet pressure is decreased gradually, when it reaches a pressure below arterial and above venous pressure the resulting venous engorgement is likely to interfere with the operative procedure. When the pressure drops below venous pressure, local anesthetic enters the circulation and produces toxic blood levels.

Loss of anesthesia after cuff deflation may occur. If the surgeon wants to attain hemostasis and then close the wound, there is only 5 to 10 minutes of post-deflation analgesia, which may be inadequate in some procedures. In such cases, supplementation of anesthesia by other methods may be required.[210] If bupivacaine, 0.25% to 0.375%, has been used instead of lidocaine, a more prolonged analgesia (20 minutes to 3 hours) may be obtained after tourniquet release.[160,230,235] However, as a result of reports of several deaths after the use of bupivacaine[94,95] and its known cardiotoxicity, the use of bupivacaine for intravenous regional techniques is no longer recommended.

Muscle relaxation is not complete with this block, and movement may interfere with the procedure. Anesthetic action, along with the analgesia produced by ischemia, usually produces good relaxation. If total muscle paralysis is desired, small quantities of relaxants such as vecuronium (Norcuron), 1 mg, or pancuronium (Pavulon), 1 mg, can be added to the local anesthetic mixture to produce regional relaxation. When a quantity of relaxant as small as this enters the systemic circulation, it is insufficient to produce any problems; an exception is a patient with myasthenia gravis, in whom small doses of relaxants can produce respiratory paralysis.

Problems with equipment may occur. Equipment must be tested and the tourniquet calibrated before use. Once the tourniquet is inflated, the local anesthetic is injected only after absence of the radial pulse is confirmed.

If the proximal and distal cuffs are not properly identified and labeled as such, tourniquet pain is likely to be a problem. Constant vigilance is necessary to make sure that the equipment is in working order and to avoid accidental disconnection and deflation of the cuff.[168]

Exsanguination may *spread infection or tumor cells* proximally, and most hand surgeons consider intravenous regional anesthesia to be contraindicated in the treatment of hand infections or tumors, even though this technique has been used in the presence of infection.[228] Erroneous injection of a foreign substance may result in severe tissue damage.[140]

---

*See references 5, 18, 22, 52, 53, 58, 69, 84, 92, 109, 177, 221, and 228.

GENERAL ANESTHESIA

General anesthesia is usually preferred in children; in adults during bilateral procedures when a bone, tendon, or nerve graft is to be taken from the lower extremity; in prolonged procedures; in uncooperative patients; and in patients who refuse regional techniques. Short procedures in adults and some children can be managed well with mask anesthesia, especially with the presently used inhalation agents, thus avoiding endotracheal intubation.

Prolonged procedures, airway problems, and positions of the patient other than supine usually require endotracheal intubation.

Inhalation Agents

Currently, isoflurane, desflurane, and sevoflurane with or without nitrous oxide are used as inhalational agents.[49,152]

Advantages. These agents are nonexplosive and produce smooth induction and emergence. Anesthetic planes can be changed rapidly and easily.

Disadvantages. There is some concern about possible halothane-associated hepatitis with repeated usage.[49,152] Intraoperative use of epinephrine with halothane or enflurane may produce ventricular arrhythmias, but the use of small doses without encountering problems has been reported.[49,180] Nitrous oxide by itself does not produce sufficient analgesia for operative procedures, but it is used along with other inhalational and intravenous agents.

Intravenous Agents

Thiopental, methohexital, etomidate, and propofol are ultra-short-acting agents that are usually administered for induction of general anesthesia.[49,152] Hypotension caused by vasodilation and respiratory depression are disadvantages to the use of intravenous agents. Opioids are usually added for intraoperative and postoperative analgesia and may be supplemented with muscle relaxants if muscle relaxation is required for the procedure.

Fentanyl (Sublimaze), 0.05 mg/mL, is a commonly used opioid that is inexpensive and fairly effective.

Remifentanil (Ultiva) is a newer, ultra-short-duration (<10 min) narcotic that can be rapidly titrated to effect. It is excellent for procedures that will not last long. It has significant potential for respiratory depression or other adverse effects and should only be used by anesthesiologists. Because of its short duration of action, plans should be implemented for postoperative analgesia before the remifentanil wears off.

Ketamine produces a state of dissociation in which analgesia is present while at the same time the patient maintains adequate ventilation and protective reflexes. It, like methadone, is a *N*-methyl-D-aspartate (NMDA)-receptor antagonist and has been suggested as a good supplement to reduce postoperative pain.[70,87,133]

Advantages. Ketamine can be administered intramuscularly (4 to 5 mg/kg) and is a very useful agent in children as a preliminary anesthetic agent. Three to four minutes after a single intramuscular injection, an intravenous infusion can be started and any anesthetic, including regional technique, can be employed. Ketamine, given immediately before induction and/or during general anesthesia, has been shown in several studies[63,133,149,163] to reduce postoperative pain. Perhaps this is explained by the NMDA-receptor antagonism by ketamine. Other studies[81,110] have failed to demonstrate this effect, perhaps because the doses used were too small.

Disadvantages. Dreams and postanesthetic hallucinations can be very unpleasant, especially in adults. Blood pressure and heart rate increases can be detrimental in patients with cardiovascular system disease. Excessive secretion, irritation of the airway, coughing spasms, and airway obstruction may result in prolonged procedures. If ketamine is combined with other medications such as a benzodiazepine, psychological effects are usually not a problem.[103]

Clonidine has been used to improve hemodynamic stability, reduce the amount of other anesthetic agents needed, and improve postoperative analgesia.[34,105,167] Clonidine can cause bradycardia and a modest reduction of blood pressure that is related to the dose administered.

Dexmedetomidine (Precedex) is an α_2-receptor agonist that appears to be useful for sedation and analgesia.[12,113,115] An intravenous loading dose of 1 µg/kg over 20 minutes is followed by a constant infusion of 0.2 to 0.7 µg/kg/hr. The dose required is significantly reduced if other medications are also administered.

In recent years the use of a laryngeal mask airway and spontaneous respiration during general anesthesia has been increasingly common. This technique is especially suited for brief cases.[118,219] When the laryngeal mask airway is used, the potential complications of endotracheal intubation[4,141] can be avoided. Spontaneous respiration during the case avoids complications of muscle relaxants and may reduce the incidence of intraoperative awareness.[44,97,195]

SPECIAL SITUATIONS

Patient Cooperation

Procedures such as tenolysis, tendon grafts, and capsulotomies may require preservation of the patient's complete ability of active finger movement. In these cases, anesthetic procedures other than general and brachial plexus blockade are preferred.

CURRENT INHALATIONAL ANESTHETICS

- Forane
- Sevoflurane
- Desflurane
- Nitrous oxide

Neuroleptanalgesia with Local Infiltration

Hunter and associates[112] have described the technique of using fentanyl-droperidol (Innovar) with local anesthetic infiltration. After starting an intravenous injection and positioning the patient comfortably, incremental doses of fentanyl-droperidol are injected intravenously to produce neuroleptanalgesia. This is characterized by a patient who has analgesia, is somnolent and oblivious to the surroundings, but is still capable of responding to instructions. In this state, the patient will be able to move his or her fingers on command but has increased pain tolerance. This state is maintained by additional small increments of fentanyl (0.025 mg). The procedure is carried out under local infiltration or digital block. More proximal blocks (e.g., the wrist) are avoided to preserve the tone of the intrinsic muscles, although they can be used when intrinsic muscle paralysis does not interfere with the procedure.[50,51,71,73] The procedure is ordinarily performed with local anesthesia, and the patient is well sedated with fentanyl-droperidol. To allow for active movement of the patient's fingers, it is necessary to deflate the tourniquet and wait 10 to 15 minutes to permit reversal of the ischemic paralysis. The surgeon should inform the anesthesiologist 10 to 15 minutes before deflation of the tourniquet is desired so that a proper level of analgesia may be reached.

Advantages. This technique is a significant advance in hand surgery because it takes some of the guesswork out of procedures such as tendon grafts and tenolysis. A much more accurate assessment of the operation can be done before the wound is closed.

Disadvantages. Prolonged procedures produce discomfort because of the tourniquet, position, and pain from the operative site.

Ischemic paralysis from the tourniquet is likely to interfere with the later part of the procedure, and an appropriate interval (10 to 15 minutes after 1 hour of tourniquet time) must pass.

Oversedation sometimes occurs and patient cooperation is lost. This can be reversed with intravenous naloxone (Narcan), 0.4 mg, if necessary. Hypotension, respiratory depression, and chest wall rigidity can occur with the use of neuroleptanalgesia. More recently, midazolam (0.5- to 1.0-mg increments) has been substituted for droperidol because of the long duration of action associated with large doses of droperidol. Recently, in spite of the long history of the safe use of droperidol in millions of patients, a "black-box" warning[80] from the U.S. Food and Drug Administration has urged caution with the use of droperidol. A small number of cases of polymorphic ventricular tachycardia and death have occurred apparently associated with the use of droperidol.

Intravenous Regional Block

Intravenous regional (Bier block) anesthesia can also be used in a similar manner to allow active motion by the patient, but the amount of additional dissection or suturing that can be done after release of the tourniquet is more limited than with the technique of neuroleptanalgesia

described here. Analgesia can be reinstituted if a continuous technique is used.[33]

Bilateral Procedures

Monitoring
Blood pressure is monitored by placing an appropriate-sized cuff on one of the thighs or around the forehead while using superficial temporal artery compression.[214]

Intravenous Line
An intravenous line can be established in one of the lower extremities. However, we prefer external jugular vein cannulation because of the incidence of thrombophlebitis and because of the long distance the drugs have to travel from the injection site near the anesthesiologist when a lower extremity vein is used.

Regional Block
Bilateral brachial plexus blocks can be performed. An axillary block is performed on at least one side to avoid the possibility of bilateral pneumothorax and phrenic block. A general anesthetic is usually chosen, except when regional anesthesia is specifically indicated.

Tourniquet Tolerance

Patients are not usually able to tolerate the tourniquet well for more than 20 to 30 minutes without a major block or general anesthesia. With a dual-cuff tourniquet, intravenous regional anesthesia can be extended up to 60 minutes.

There are, however, reports claiming long-term tourniquet inflation without patient discomfort.[71,73,126,230] Thorough exsanguination is emphasized. In addition, thorough exsanguination of the area where the tourniquet is to be applied is claimed to improve tourniquet tolerance.[73] The addition of sodium bicarbonate to the local anesthetic may also decrease the incidence of tourniquet-associated pain.[213]

Subcutaneous local anesthetic infiltration in the area of cuff application is reported to increase tourniquet tolerance.[190,230] The technique consists of subcutaneously injecting about 20 mL of a local anesthetic solution, such as 0.5% to 1% lidocaine, with a 22-gauge needle in the area over which the cuff is to be placed. Successful use of a forearm tourniquet with subcutaneous local anesthetic infiltration and a wrist block for procedures below the wrist has been reported.[230]

Rheumatoid Arthritis

Arthritic patients undergo multiple surgical procedures, and such procedures are preferably done with regional anesthesia. Extra care should be taken to keep the patients comfortable on the operating table. Rheumatoid patients are also likely to have airway problems because of ankylosis of the temporomandibular joint and decreased mobility of the cervical spine. Endotracheal intubation may be difficult or impossible, and this is handled better if recognized preoperatively.

Patients with rheumatoid arthritis are also often taking corticosteroids, and parenteral supplementation may be necessary intraoperatively and postoperatively to cover their inability to produce adequate amounts of corticosteroid in response to the stress.[49,152]

Bleeding and Clotting Disorders

Regional anesthesia is contraindicated when a prolonged bleeding or clotting time exists because of the possibility of hematoma formation.[147] If for any reason a brachial plexus block is strongly indicated, axillary block may be preferable[30] because the needle track is accessible and can be compressed to prevent a hematoma. The American Society of Regional Anesthesia and Pain Medicine has issued some guidelines for the safe use of regional anesthesia in patients with impaired coagulation systems.[111]

Low-Molecular-Weight Heparin (LMWH). Preoperative low doses of LMWH require us to wait at least 12 hours before we can perform spinal or epidural anesthesia. Higher (treatment) doses cause a 24-hour delay before such neuraxial procedures. Postoperative LMWH should not be given for at least 24 hours after spinal or epidural anesthesia. Epidural catheters should not be removed for at least 12 hours after the previous dose of LMWH. Subsequent doses of LMWH should be held for at least 2 hours after removal of the catheter.

IMPLICATIONS OF ANTICOAGULANT THERAPY

LOW-MOLECULAR-WEIGHT HEPARIN

Preoperative

- Prophylactic doses require at least a 12-hour delay before neuraxial techniques.
- Therapeutic doses mandate a 24-hour delay.

Postoperative

- Wait at least 24 hours to start LMWH after a neuraxial technique.
- Wait at least 12 hours after the previous dose to remove an epidural catheter.

COUMADIN

- International Normalized Ratio should be less than 1.5 to remove an epidural catheter.

ANTIPLATELET AGENTS

Delay from Time of Last Dose to Neuraxial Anesthetic Technique

- Ticlopidine: 14 days
- Clopidogrel: 7 days
- Abciximab: 24 to 48 hours
- Eptifibatide and tirofiban: 4 to 8 hours

Coumadin. Coumadin should be held for at least 4 to 5 days before surgery if it has been a chronic medication. The International Normalized Ratio should be checked before surgery and should be less than 1.5 to allow safe removal of an epidural catheter.

Antiplatelet Agents. Ticlopidine should be discontinued at least 14 days before spinal anesthesia. Clopidogrel should be held for at least 7 days. Neuraxial techniques should be delayed at least 24 to 48 hours for abciximab and 4 to 8 hours for eptifibatide and tirofiban.

Pregnancy

Elective procedures are usually not done during pregnancy. Emergency surgery requiring anesthesia presents two problems: (1) the likelihood of initiating labor due to stress, especially hypotension and interference with uterine blood flow and (2) possible drug-induced fetal defects, especially in the first trimester.

The anesthetic technique of choice is regional anesthesia with the smallest quantity of drug, preferably with a peripheral block or local infiltration. The local anesthetic drugs of choice are chloroprocaine, which because of rapid hydrolysis has low blood levels, thus keeping the drug unavailable for transfer across the placenta, and bupivacaine, which because most of it is protein bound allows very little drug to be in the free state to cross the placenta.[53,58] Significant cardiotoxicity has been reported after the injection of 0.75% bupivacaine.[7,182]

We prefer to avoid using tranquilizers such as diazepam for sedation because of their unknown fetal effects. Morphine, 1 to 2 mg intravenously, or fentanyl, 0.025 to 0.050 mg, is preferred.

Infection and Malignancy

The presence of infection with involved lymph nodes in the axilla or supraclavicular area is usually considered to be a contraindication to use of the brachial plexus technique. However, Moore[156] uses these blocks if the infection is controlled with antibiotics. Winnie[242,243,246] recommends use of the interscalene technique, which is done above the level of these lymph nodes. Insertion of the needle near malignant lymph nodes should be avoided.

Local anesthetic agents are less effective when injected into an inflamed area because of the increased acidity of the tissues. The increased hydrogen ion concentration decreases the proportion of the local anesthetic base form, which is necessary to penetrate the tissue barriers to reach the nerves.[53,58] Under these circumstances a regional block away from the inflamed areas is preferred.

Pediatric Surgery

General anesthesia is usually used with children. Occasionally, regional anesthesia can be used[13,38,47,142,253] by appropriately sedating the patient. Intramuscular ketamine, 4 to 5 mg/kg, is very useful for this purpose. Regional techniques can also be used in conjunction with a general anesthetic for the purpose of providing postoperative analgesia.

Either the axillary or interscalene technique can be used. A nerve stimulator is very helpful for identifying proper placement of the needle.[154] Volumes and concentrations of local anesthetics are listed in Tables 2-1 and 2-2.

Prolonged Procedures

Peripheral nerve blocks using bupivacaine, ropivacaine, and etidocaine provide analgesia for 8 to 10 hours and are ideal for this purpose. If a short-acting local anesthetic wears off during the operative procedure, the block can be repeated, especially with the supraclavicular techniques. Anesthesia is established immediately because some local anesthetic is already present in the neural tissues. If analgesia is desired for longer periods, continuous techniques with cannulas can be used.* A variety of continuous techniques may be used, including the interscalene, supraclavicular, infraclavicular, subclavian perivascular, or axillary techniques. An infraclavicular block has the advantage of relatively deep catheter insertion with minimal catheter movement. A special cannula-over-needle and catheter set for continuous plexus anesthesia is available (Contiplex, Burron Medical, Inc.). Using sterile technique, the brachial plexus sheath is identified by paresthesias, fascial click, or loss of resistance or with the assistance of a nerve stimulator. The catheter may be passed directly into the fascial sheath, or the space may be distended first with a small volume of local anesthetic solution. To maintain stability of the catheter and promote proximal spread of the local anesthetic, the catheter is introduced through the cannula a distance of several centimeters. A technique has also been described in which a guide wire is passed into the sheath and a catheter is advanced over the guide wire.[10] Once in place, the catheter is secured by suturing it to the skin or using a transparent adhesive dressing. The absence of intravascular placement is verified by careful aspiration before each injection.

Analgesia can be maintained by periodic injections of local anesthetic or by continuous infusion with an infusion pump. Bupivacaine 0.25%, is likely to provide complete analgesia and sympathetic blockade, either postoperatively or in the management of chronic pain syndrome.[11,148] This may also facilitate faster wound healing.[125]

Nerve Injury

There is a reluctance among some physicians to administer regional anesthesia to patients undergoing repair of nerves or with a previous history of nerve damage. They are concerned about the possibility of the anesthetic technique being blamed for worsening the disease or for unsatisfactory results of the repair.

We do not hesitate to use regional anesthetic techniques under these circumstances as long as the neurologic deficit is well documented. If a postoperative neurologic deficit develops, a thorough neurologic examination and electromyogram done soon after surgery and again 3 weeks later are likely to be helpful in establishing whether the neurologic deficit was preexistent (see the later section on Neurologic Complications).

When considering the choice of regional versus general anesthesia, it is of interest to note that brachial plexus injury after anesthesia and surgery is more common after general than regional anesthesia.[129,245] Kroll and colleagues examined the American Society of Anesthesiologist's Closed Claims Study database (1541 claims reviewed) to define the role of nerve damage in the spectrum of anesthesia-related injury that leads to litigation.[129] The majority of the 53 patients who sustained brachial plexus injury received general anesthesia.[128] Anesthetic-related causes of brachial plexus injury in this study included the use of shoulder braces and head-down position (three claims), suspension of the patient's arms on a bar (two claims), other obvious malpositions (four claims), and regional anesthesia technique (two claims).[129]

Equipment

We prefer to perform blocks with an immobile (rigid) needle[241,246] that consists of a short-beveled point with a clear plastic hub (for early recognition of blood) attached to intravenous extension tubing that is connected to a syringe. With this arrangement, aspiration and injection can be performed without moving the needle.

Most nerve blocks are now performed using insulated needles and an appropriate nerve stimulator. Insulated needles (such as Stimuplex-DIG; B. Braun Medical, Bethlehem, PA) permit precise localization of the nerves to be blocked without requiring paresthesias or patient cooperation. A nerve stimulator (such as Braun stimulator pulse frequency, 1 to 2 Hz; pulse width, 100 μsec) is used to obtain an optimum endpoint (adequate motor response of an appropriate muscle group) at an amplitude of less than 0.5 mA. Braun has manufactured a newer nerve stimulator, the Stimuplex HNS11 Peripheral Nerve Stimulator, that permits adjustment of the stimulus pulse duration to 0.1 msec, 0.3 msec, or 1.0 msec.

The larger the amplitude at which a twitch is elicited, the slower the onset of nerve block in general. An acceptable twitch may be obtained even if the tip of the needle is near the nerve, but the tip needs to be in the same fascial plane for success. Although some individuals stress the importance of a particular motor response,[20] others believe that the most important factor is to achieve a motor response from a muscle innervated by the nerve to be blocked at a sufficiently low amplitude of current. For example Vloka and associates[232] reported 100% success when the amplitude is 0.4 mA or less. Several cases have been reported[164,226] in which a paresthesia was elicited without a motor twitch while using a nerve stimulator for regional anesthesia. Paresthesia without muscle contraction can occur.[226] Use of nerve stimulation to perform interscalene block with a B bevel needle can still produce nerve injury.[186] Persistent phrenic nerve paralysis after interscalene brachial plexus block under general anesthesia has resulted in nerve injury.[19]

Broken Needles

Broken needles can produce serious complications by migrating and impaling important structures. Therefore,

---

*See references 10, 25, 64, 78, 127, 148, 166, 179, 184, 188, 192, 197, 199, 217, 223, 224, 229, 240, and 246.

their removal is recommended.[24,157,208] In some instances the very search for the needle can damage tissue.[208] The likelihood of needle breakage can be reduced by (1) examining the needle before use; (2) avoiding very short needles that are inserted all the way under the skin, thus making the broken part inaccessible; and (3) using needles with a security bead.[208] The bead is located on the shaft a short distance away from the hub so that the needle cannot be advanced all the way to the hub, which is the site where the needle most commonly breaks. If it does break, a small segment of the needle stays outside the skin and can be easily removed. In addition, not forcing the needle against the bone, avoiding directional change with a deeply placed needle, and replacing bent needles can help prevent broken needles.

Neurologic Complications after Peripheral Nerve Blocks

Serious prolonged neurologic complications after peripheral nerve blocks using small needles and commonly used concentrations of local anesthetic agents are extremely rare. Occasionally, however, painful paresthesias develop in the postoperative period. These may occur either spontaneously or be elicited by pressure on the site of the nerve block or by abduction of the arm. In most cases they tend to disappear in a period of weeks or months, although occasional reports have noted prolonged paresthesias lasting for more than a year.

Nerve injury after nerve block and surgery may be due to various causes such as mechanical trauma produced by the nerve block needle, position of the arm, or nerve damage secondary to the surgical procedure itself. Chemical toxicity from the injected local anesthetic is very unlikely, but accidental use of high concentrations of epinephrine or contaminants such as metal ions, phenol, alcohol, or sterilizing agents may produce nerve damage. Ischemia of the nerve after prolonged tourniquet use is also a possible cause of nerve injury after nerve block and surgery.

Among these various causes, mechanical trauma produced by the needle or secondary to intraneural injection is a factor that should be considered when performing peripheral nerve blocks. Selander and associates[201] have reported a 2% incidence of postoperative paresthesia in patients in whom paresthesias were elicited during performance of the block. In animal experiments[200] they found that use of a short-beveled needle (45 degree) will significantly reduce the risk of nerve injury when compared with a standard 14-degree bevel. A gentle approach in eliciting paresthesias by using a short-beveled needle with the bevel parallel to the nerve fascicles is likely to minimize damage to the nerve. Intraneural injections can damage a nerve by producing excessive endoneural pressure, but it is very unlikely that this is a significant factor in clinical practice because as soon as the injection of local anesthetic is begun the nerve is pushed away. However, in certain special circumstances, such as if a nerve is impaled against the bone (e.g., the ulnar nerve at the elbow) or when corticosteroid is injected beneath the epineurium, nerve damage can occur.[145]

Winchell and Wolfe[239] reported a 0.36% incidence of postblock neuropathy after brachial plexus block techniques in 854 patients. In the three patients in whom painful paresthesias developed, none had permanent nerve damage. There are other occasional case reports of prolonged block or nerve damage after brachial plexus block techniques.[15,82,136]

In 35 years of performing regional anesthesia, one of us (SR) has encountered five patients who were referred for post-block pain complications. One patient's pain disappeared after a heavy cast was removed from the arm. Another patient had a cervical radiculopathy proximal to the site of the block that was thought to be secondary to rheumatoid arthritis of the cervical spine. In two patients, after neurologic evaluation and electrodiagnostic investigation, the site of the nerve damage was localized at a level below the elbow; these patients had received axillary blocks and there was no evidence of nerve damage above the elbow. In one patient, electrodiagnostic studies confirmed that the problems were preexistent. These latter three patients all had extensive explorations in an attempt to establish an arteriovenous shunt for renal dialysis.

Recently, three cases of severe permanent neurologic injury after axillary block anesthesia from a single hand surgeon's practice were reported.[209] Two of these blocks were performed on the same day by the same anesthesiologist, thus implying some technique-related factor. The third case involved an indwelling axillary catheter. This author also reported the results of a survey of axillary block complications sent to the membership of the American Society for Surgery of the Hand. Of 800 respondents, 65% reported seeing minor, transient complications in their practice and 21% had seen a major neurologic complication. Unfortunately, the data reported here are based solely on physician survey. A very large prospective study is needed to more accurately determine the incidence of neurologic complications after brachial plexus blocks.

Evaluation and Treatment

Because of the low incidence of neurologic complications after peripheral blocks and the likelihood of spontaneous disappearance of the symptoms in most patients, there is not a significant amount of information regarding the management of these patients. Electrodiagnostic evaluations, if done within 3 weeks of the injury, may be helpful in establishing preexisting pathology if there is evidence of denervation of muscles. Electromyography should be repeated 3 weeks after the block and surgery. If a patient had normal preoperative electrodiagnostic studies or a normal electromyogram soon after surgery but an abnormal electromyogram developed 3 weeks after performance of the block, then the block or surgical procedure may be the cause of the nerve damage. We believe that early performance of electrodiagnostic studies along with thorough

---

NEUROLOGIC COMPLICATIONS

- Neurologic complications can occur after regional or general anesthesia.
- The mechanisms of injury are sometimes obscure.
- With appropriate precautions the frequency of nerve injury after nerve blocks is quite low.

neurologic evaluation will be of great benefit in establishing the cause of the problem.

Because most postblock symptoms disappear within a few weeks, no treatment may be necessary other than reassurance. However, if the symptoms persist or are severe to begin with, sympathetic blocks and physical therapy may be of benefit, especially if the patient has signs of reflex sympathetic dystrophy. If the symptoms become chronic, patients should be evaluated in a manner similar to other chronic pain patients, where psychological elements, secondary gain, and other factors are taken into consideration, including a work-up for reflex sympathetic dystrophy.

Compartment Syndromes

Cases of compartment syndrome resulting from regional anesthesia have almost all been from the inadvertent injection of hypertonic saline during intravenous regional anesthesia.[93,143,232] Concern about regional anesthesia masking compartment syndrome is probably unjustified but may lower the threshold for measurement of compartment pressures. The diagnosis of compartment syndrome based on the presence or absence of pain or weakness is fraught with hazard. We need to be alert to the possibility of a compartment syndrome[9,169] and a willingness to measure compartment pressures when any doubt exists. Uslu and colleagues[227] reported that measuring the pressure between a cast and the skin surface reliably tracks compartment pressure for diagnosis for compartment syndrome.

ANNOTATED REFERENCES

23. Boezaart AP, de Beer JF, du Toit C, van Rooyen K: A new technique of continuous interscalene nerve block. Can J Anaesth 46:275-281, 1999.

    This reference discusses a new posterior approach of continuous interscalene block. Compared with the usual approach of Winnie, the success rate was higher and the complication rates were lower. There were no phrenic nerve blocks and no Horner's syndrome. None of the catheters accidentally fell out.

27. Bouaziz H, Narchi P, Mercier FJ: Comparison between conventional axillary block and a new approach at the midhumeral level. Anesth Analg 84:1058-1062, 1997.

    The success rate of the block, as well as the incidence of complete motor blockade, was greater with the midhumeral approach compared with the axillary approach. In this method, four nerves are located with a nerve stimulator and blocked. Times to perform the blocks, mean maximum plasma lidocaine concentration, and time to peak concentration were not different between groups. The success rate of the block, as well as the incidence of complete motor blockade, was greater with the midhumeral approach compared with the axillary approach. However, the onset time to complete anesthesia of the upper extremity was shorter in the axillary approach.

35. Buchheit T, Crews JC: Lateral cervical epidural catheter placement for continuous unilateral upper extremity analgesia and sympathetic block. Reg Anesth Pain Med 25:313-317, 2000.

    This study describes unilateral cervical epidural anesthesia. The authors reported the use of a laterally directed catheter in the cervical epidural space to produce unilateral analgesia for acute and chronic pain. The report mentioned

application of this technique in 30 patients with good results. The authors used contrast dye, patient symptoms, and Horner's syndrome to document predominantly unilateral effects.

65. Delaunay L, Chelly JE: Blocks at the wrist provide effective anesthesia for carpal tunnel release. Can J Anaesth 48:656-660, 2001.

    This article describes the technique for median and ulnar nerve blocks at the wrist and their application for carpal tunnel surgery. After 10 minutes, 9% of patients required supplementation of the median nerve and 32% required supplementation of the ulnar nerve. Seventy-five percent of patients reported mild or no pain from the blocks.

79a. Franco CD, Viera ZE: 1,001 subclavian perivascular brachial plexus blocks: Success with a nerve stimulator. Reg Anesth Pain Med 25:41-46, 2000.

    This is a report of an extensive case series using supraclavicular block without a single pneumothorax or major complication: 97.2% of the blocks were successful, and 1.6% were incomplete and needed supplementation. This success rate is identical to that reported by Riegler and colleagues. This block is safe and effective.

111. ASRA guidelines for regional anesthesia. Available at http://www.asra.com/items_of_interest/consensus_statements/index.iphtml.

    American Society of Regional Anesthesia guidelines for regional anesthesia in the presence of coagulopathy. These guidelines are especially useful for deciding when to perform spinal anesthesia or when to remove an epidural catheter after low molecular heparin and how long to wait after stopping antiplatelet medications.

129. Kroll DA, Caplan RA, Posner K, et al: Nerve injury associated with anesthesia. Anesthesiology 73:202-207, 1990.

    The authors examined the American Society of Anesthesiologists Closed Claims Study database to examine how significant nerve injury was during anesthesia. Fifteen percent of the claims were for anesthesia-related nerve injury, both during general as well as regional anesthesia. Ulnar nerve injury was especially common. The mechanisms of nerve injury are often unclear. This report helps make it clear that although there have been reports of rare nerve injury after regional anesthesia, it is also an uncommon problem that can occur after general anesthesia.

160. Moore DC, Bridenbaugh LD, Bridenbaugh PO, Thompson GE: Bupivacaine hydrochloride: A summary of investigational use in 3274 cases. Anesth Analg 50:856-872, 1971.

    An important report of a large series of cases using rather large doses of bupivacaine for several blocks including intercostals, epidural, and sciatic femoral blocks, which would be expected to produce some of the highest blood levels of bupivacaine. In spite of this, there was minimal toxicity and blood levels were below the toxic range. These authors' extensive experience with bupivacaine indicate that the low doses often advocated are unnecessarily stringent and make blocks more difficult.

161. Moore DC, Bridenbaugh LD, Eather KF: Block of the upper extremity: Supraclavicular approach versus axillary approach. Arch Surg 90:68-72, 1965.

    A good comparison study of supraclavicular versus axillary blocks. The authors make the point that the supraclavicular block is the most versatile (it can be done even when the patient cannot abduct his or her arm), has the most extensive spread of analgesia, and requires less volume. The concern about pneumothorax is vastly overstated and is not a real issue if the person performing the block has been trained properly.

164. Mulroy MF, Mitchell B: Unsolicited paresthesias with nerve stimulator: Case reports of four patients. Anesth Analg 95:762-763, 2002.

There has been a supposition that by using a nerve stimulator we could avoid paresthesias and thereby possibly prevent some cases of nerve injury. This report discusses four cases in which paresthesias were obtained before a motor twitch was ever seen. It is not uncommon to elicit paresthesias unintentionally when using a nerve stimulator. Use of a nerve stimulator does not protect from unintentional contact of a nerve with the needle.

185. Riegler FX: Brachial plexus block with the nerve stimulator: Motor response characteristics at three sites. Reg Anesth 17:295-299, 1992.

This interesting report states that there is no difference between the minimum current at which we see motor twitch at the three sites studied. They also reported highest success rate (97%) with supraclavicular block, intermediate success with interscalene (91%), and 79% with axillary block.

187. Roch JJ, Sharrock NE, Neudachin L: Interscalene brachial plexus block for shoulder surgery: A proximal paresthesia is effective. Anesth Analg 75:386–388, 1992.

Some people have felt that to have success with an interscalene block we need to obtain paresthesia that extends to the hand. This study found that, for shoulder surgery, paresthesia to the deltoid area is sufficient.

225. Urmey WF, McDonald M: Hemidiaphragmatic paresis during interscalene brachial plexus block: Effects on pulmonary function and chest wall mechanics. Anesth Analg 74:352-357, 1992.

This study described phrenic block with unilateral diaphragm paralysis in every patient receiving interscalene block with significant changes in pulmonary function. This leads to the conclusion that this block should probably be avoided in patients with severe chronic lung disease. A unilateral phrenic nerve block is rarely a significant problem even for patients with lung disease.

238. Wilson JL, Brown DL, Wong GY, et al: Infraclavicular brachial plexus block: Parasagittal anatomy important to the coracoid technique. Anesth Analg 87:870-873, 1998.

This is a detailed anatomic study of the paracoracoid approach to the infraclavicular block. The authors suggest a needle insertion site 2 cm medial and 2 cm caudad to the coracoid process. They found that the mean distance from the skin to the anterior wall of the axillary artery was about 4 cm. This is another promising technique that seems especially well suited for continuous brachial plexus block.

239. Winchell SW, Wolfe R: The incidence of neuropathy following upper extremity nerve blocks. Reg Anesth 10:12-15, 1985.

The authors reported a 0.36% incidence of postblock neuropathy after brachial plexus block techniques in 854 patients. In the three patients in whom painful paresthesias developed, none had permanent nerve damage.

246. Winnie AP: Perivascular techniques of brachial plexus block. *In* Plexus Anesthesia. Philadelphia, WB Saunders, 1990, vol 1.

A description of perivascular methods of brachial plexus block. This excellent text provides a complete discussion of all of the perivascular techniques described by Winnie.

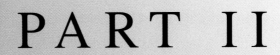

PART II

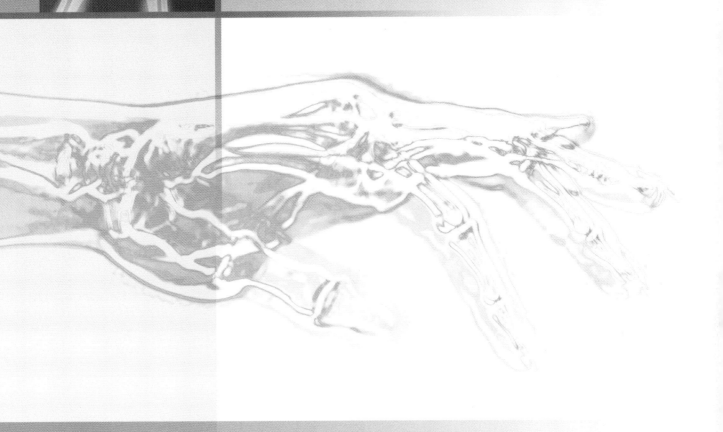

Hand

CHAPTER 3

Acute Infections in the Hand

Milan V. Stevanovic and Frances Sharpe

GENERAL PRINCIPLES

Hippocrates' principles for the treatment of hand infections are fundamentally valid today. *Wounds were kept clean with frequent changes of wine-soaked dressings. Dressings were kept loose "so as not to intercept the pus, but to allow it to flow away freely."*[59,99] Coupled with these early principles is the pioneering work of Dr. Alan Kanavel, a Chicago general surgeon who treated hand infections in the preantibiotic era. Much of our current understanding of the pathogenesis and treatment of hand infections must be credited to his extensive dissections and innovative injection studies. Through these studies, he demonstrated the potential spaces of the hand and the pathogenesis of infection. From this, he developed the surgical principles that remain the cornerstone of modern treatment of hand infections.[93]

Hand infections can result in severe disabilities, including stiffness, contracture, and amputation. These complications have been significantly reduced through the introduction of antibiotic therapy in conjunction with surgical treatment. Although antibiotics have dramatically reduced the morbidity associated with hand infections, their use does not supplant the need for expedient and proper surgical intervention.[24] Several factors influence the outcome of hand infections. These include the location of the infection, infecting organism, timing of treatment, adequacy of surgical drainage, efficacy of antibiotics, and health status and immunocompetence of the host.[64,78,79]

Host factors play a determining role in the severity and duration of infection. There are many medical conditions that reduce the host defenses. Malnutrition, alcoholism, autoimmune diseases, chronic corticosteroid use, and human immunodeficiency virus (HIV) infection are some of the comorbidities to be considered. Yet, the most prevalent disease with associated immunosuppression is diabetes mellitus, which affects 5% to 7% of the adult population of the United States.[56,73]

Although early and superficial infections may respond to nonsurgical management, most acute infections of the hand represent surgical emergencies. The swelling and edema result in increased tissue pressure and can cause ischemia and tissue necrosis by a process resembling compartment syndrome. For example, in septic flexor tenosynovitis, Schnall and associates showed increased pressures in the flexor tendon sheath sufficient to cause ischemia and tendon necrosis.[177] Furthermore, toxins produced by the offending pathogen can cause vascular thrombosis and tissue death. Patients with necrotizing fasciitis and gas gangrene need *immediate* surgical care.

Types of Infections

Cellulitis is an infection of the subcutaneous tissue, which is often diffuse and can be associated with lymphangitis. It is caused by a single organism, usually *Staphylococcus aureus* or β-hemolytic *Streptococcus.* Lymphangitic streaking is more commonly seen with β-hemolytic streptococcal infections. It generally has a more distal nidus and spreads proximally. It is a non–pus-forming infection and as such is treated nonsurgically. If the cellulitis is not responding to intravenous therapy over 24 to 48 hours, this often suggests the formation of pus *(abscess)* and more serious infection. Cellulitis requires hospital admission and close monitoring for response to antibiotic therapy. A specific type of staphylococcal infection is the *staphylococcal scalded skin syndrome,* primarily a disease of young children that results from an exfoliative toxin-producing staphylococcal organism. A high index of suspicion and early differentiation of this process from other skin conditions is important to treatment outcome. When this process occurs in adults, it is associated with a high mortality rate, usually because of serious underlying illness, such as kidney failure or immunosuppression.[40,102] Detection of the exfoliative toxin is required for diagnosis. New immunologic methods allow for more rapid detection.[103] Prompt antibiotic therapy and local wound care are the mainstay of management. *Necrotizing fasciitis* is a serious life-threatening infection that may initially resemble cellulitis. Although purulence is not present, a watery discharge may be seen. The remainder of infections are generally pus forming and are discussed in detail in the remainder of the chapter.

The authors would like to thank **Dr. Robert Neviaser** for the use of portions of his text and drawings from the previous editions of this chapter.

Patient Evaluation

The initial evaluation and management in the emergency department should include a thorough medical history, assessment of risk factors for immunocompromise, and evaluation of tetanus immunization status. Appropriate tetanus prophylaxis should be administered based on immunization history and time of the last booster shot. Hyperimmunoglobulin and tetanus toxoid booster are given if the patient has not had a series of tetanus immunization. Clinical evaluation of the affected extremity should include examination for fluctuance, warmth, edema, redness, tenderness, and lymphangitis or lymphadenopathy. Areas of cellulitis should be marked on the skin so that progression or regression of the infections process can be monitored. If an open draining wound is present, a specimen should be sent for aerobic and anaerobic culture. Blood cultures should be taken in febrile patients. Blood should be drawn for a complete blood cell count and to evaluate the erythrocyte sedimentation rate (ESR), C-reactive protein (CRP), electrolytes, and random blood glucose value. Radiographs are obtained to evaluate for foreign body, gas within the soft tissues, underlying fracture, septic joint, or osteomyelitis.

When a patient presents with an area of fluctuance, this should be provisionally treated with aspiration or decompression until formal surgical débridement is performed. The fluid should be sent for culture. For patients who do not clearly have an abscess, aspiration may be useful to identify a deep pyogenic infection. Swollen painful joints should be aspirated with caution. The site of aspiration should not be over an area of cellulitis. The fluid should be sent for culture. Joint fluid analysis with cell count, glucose, and protein levels can be obtained if adequate specimen is available. If the joint aspirate is not clearly pyogenic, antibiotics are withheld. Nonsteroidal anti-inflammatory drugs (NSAIDs) may be given to both treat the patient and help distinguish between an inflammatory process and sepsis. If the presentation is suggestive of an inflammatory process, antibiotics are withheld while the response to NSAIDs is observed. When infection is suggested, empirical antibiotic therapy should be started in the emergency department after results of cultures are obtained.

Differentiating between an infectious and inflammatory process can be difficult. The suspicion of one process over the other depends on many factors, including the patient's history, presence of underlying diseases, and clinical presentation. When to withhold antibiotic therapy can be a diagnostic challenge, and the use of antibiotics in some circumstances may be done more to treat the physician's anxiety than the patient's disease. Overnight observation in the hospital while antibiotics are withheld allows the disease process to be closely monitored and allows treatment to be changed if the anticipated improvement is not evident with NSAID therapy alone. When the level of suspicion for an infectious process is low, a corticosteroid dose pack may be used. The patient is re-evaluated in 24 to 48 hours. If the process is noninfectious, the process will be nearly resolved. It may take years to develop the clinical experience to recognize these different processes, and even the experienced eye can mistake these two conditions.

Patients with severe infections such as necrotizing fasciitis or gas gangrene or who are immunocompromisd, including diabetics, should be immediately treated with broad-spectrum antibiotic therapy.

Treatment Principles

Most procedures should be performed under tourniquet control. The arm should be elevated for several minutes before inflating the tourniquet. In the setting of an acute infection, exsanguination with an elastic wrapping is contraindicated, owing to the increased likelihood of bacteremia. Surgical drainage should be done through a large incision. The incision should be planned such that it can be extended in any direction, in the event that the extent of the problem is greater than anticipated. Longitudinal incisions across a flexion crease should be avoided when possible. Because most infected wounds are left open, surgical incisions should be planned to minimize the exposure of blood vessels, nerves, and tendons.

Excision of all necrotic tissue is imperative to infection control.[179] In the 1800s, Louis Pasteur noted that it is the environment and not the bacterium that allows the propagation of infection.[23] Specimens for cultures and Gram stain should be obtained. Those specimens sent for pathologic analysis should include the appropriate information to the pathologist, which may more quickly identify fungal and mycobacterial infections. Copious irrigation reduces the bacterial load. Most wounds can be left open, with moist gauze covering the exposed surfaces. Small wounds with a tendency to heal quickly should be kept open with a gauze wick. Neviaser, in previous editions of this chapter, emphasized the use of closed irrigation of infections. This technique has been used with success by many surgeons. It is described in various sections of this chapter, but it is not our preferred method. Multiple débridements may be necessary to control infection. Amputation may be necessary to eradicate infection. Functional results may be improved by amputation of a stiff, contracted, and painful digit. In cases of severe infection such as necrotizing fasciitis or gas gangrene, amputation may be a life-saving procedure.

Postoperatively, loose soft dressings are applied. A short period of immobilization for 24 to 48 with a splint may afford some pain relief to the patient. Early mobilization in the first 24 hours, under the guidance of a hand therapist, reduces some of the morbidity such as edema, stiffness, and contracture associated with severe hand infections.

The most common infecting organisms are *Staphylococcus* and *Streptococcus* species.[8,54,107,110,193] Many infections, especially those caused from bite wounds, those associated with gross contamination, or those seen in diabetics are often mixed species. Empirical antibiotic therapy should be tailored toward the most likely offending pathogen. Broad-spectrum antibiotic therapy should be considered. An infectious disease specialist is a valuable resource in patient management. This individual is familiar with the hospital-specific antibiotic-resistant organisms and can direct antibiotic therapy and follow outpatient intravenous therapy.

Nosocomial Infections

The hand is a very well vascularized region, making it less vulnerable to postoperative infection than other anatomic sites. *S. aureus* is the most common pathogen in clean surgical procedures.[27,182] The use of perioperative intravenous antibiotics within 2 hours preceding surgery has greatly reduced the incidence of postsurgical infections in general orthopedic practice.[36] However, the role of perioperative antibiotics in elective hand surgery is less clear.[86] For surgical procedures that involve the bone or joint, we routinely give intravenous prophylaxis.* Nosocomial infections include not only surgical site infections, but postoperative pneumonia, urinary tract infections, and gastrointestinal infections often related to antibiotic use. The organisms involved are often resistant pathogens, and an infectious disease specialist can help in tailoring the proper management of these infections.

COMMON HAND INFECTIONS

Acute Paronychia

Paronychia is the most common infection in the hand.[21,29,54,90,96,222] It is generally treated by primary care physicians, although refractory cases are often seen by the hand surgeon. Acute paronychia involves the soft tissue fold around the fingernail. It usually results from the bacterial inoculation of the paronychial tissue by a sliver of nail or hangnail, by a manicure instrument, or through nail biting. The disruption of the barrier between the nail fold and the nail plate allows the introduction of bacteria into the tissue bordering the nail (Fig. 3-1). Although most paronychia are mixed infections, the most common infecting organism is *S. aureus*.[20,22]

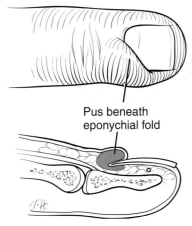

Pus beneath
eponychial fold

FIGURE 3-1. Inflamed paronychium and eponychium shown with pus extending below the eponychial fold.

---

*Editor's note (DPG): I strongly disagree with the practice of giving "prophylactic" antibiotics for all clean bone and joint cases in the wrist and hand. This is not only unnecessary but harmful in the long term, creating super-resistant bacteria. In my practice I do not administer perioperative antibiotics in clean, elective cases unless there is a specific indication to do so. Unfortunately, many orthopedic surgeons give antibiotics indiscriminately purely as a defensive measure, fearing that if the patient does get an infection and no antibiotics were given, a plaintiff's attorney will cite this as inappropriate care.

Clinical Presentation/Preoperative Evaluation

Erythema, swelling, and tenderness immediately adjacent to the nail are the hallmarks of the early clinical presentation. If left untreated, an abscess may form along the nail fold. The abscess may extend below the nail plate, either partially or completely, or it can track volarly into the pulp space.[115,165,181] Because of the continuity of the nail fold with the eponychial tissue overlying the base of the nail, the infection can extend into this region and may continue around to the fold on the opposite side of the fingernail. This rather unusual occurrence is called a "runaround infection." Infection involving the entire eponychium, as well as one lateral fold, is known as an *eponychia*. An eponychia is usually manifested as a collection of pus beneath the proximal portion of the nail in the region of the lunula. It is extremely rare to see both lateral folds and the dorsal tissue infected in the same digit.

Radiographs and laboratory examination are not necessary in uncomplicated cases with early clinical findings. However, patients who have not responded to initial treatment or who present with significant swelling or abscess should be evaluated for underlying systemic diseases such as diabetes. The patient's history and examination will direct the need for wound cultures for atypical organisms, radiographs to evaluate for foreign body or osteomyelitis, and laboratory evaluation.

Pertinent Anatomy

The nail complex consists of the nail bed, nail plate, and perionychium. The nail bed, which lies below the plate, consists of the germinal and sterile matrices. The germinal matrix is responsible for the majority of nail growth. The proximal portion of the nail sits below the nail fold. The border tissue surrounding the nail is the perionychium. The eponychium is the thin layer of tissue extending from the nail wall onto the nail plate. The hyponychium is the mass of keratin just distal to the sterile matrix, below the distal nail plate. This area of the nail complex is highly resistant to infection.[96,222]

Treatment Options

In the very early stages, this infection can be treated by soaks in a warm solution, systemic oral antibiotics, and rest of the affected part.[42] If there is a superficial abscess, treatment can be carried out without anesthesia and should consist of opening the thin layer of tissue over the abscess with a sharp blade directed away from the nail bed and matrix. Drainage of the abscess is performed where the abscess most nearly approaches the surface (Fig. 3-2). The patient is counseled regarding high-risk activities, such as nail biting and manicures.

More extensive infection requires individualized treatment based on the extent of the lesion. Surgical decompression is best carried out under digital block anesthesia at the level of the metacarpal head with plain lidocaine (no epinephrine). If the perionychial fold and the adjacent part of the eponychium are involved, the perionychium and skin adjacent to the nail fold are released. If the perionychial infection involves the pulp, the incision should be deep enough to fully drain the abscess. Infection that travels below the nail plate requires removal of a portion of the nail. If the entire nail matrix is involved, then the entire nail

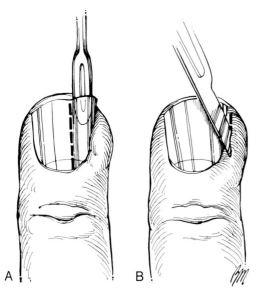

FIGURE 3-2. A, Elevation and removal of one fourth of the nail to decompress the perionychium. **B,** Incision of the perionychial fold with the blade directed away from the nail bed and matrix.

is removed. Purulence below the nail plate can cause pressure on the germinal matrix, resulting in ischemia of the germinal matrix and temporary or permanent arrest of nail growth.[222]

Operative Methods

The perionychial sulcus is elevated from the nail gently by a flat, blunt instrument such as the flat portion of a malleable or metal probe or a Freer elevator. Sharp incision may be used as well. The incision is directed away from the nail bed to avoid injury to the nail bed and subsequent growth abnormality. The incision may be extended proximally along the nail fold, as far proximally as is necessary (Fig. 3-3A and B). It is generally sufficient to carry the incision only to the proximal edge of the nail, but it may extend as far proximally as the distal interphalangeal (DIP) joint. As an alternative, the perionychium may be incised parallel to the sulcus, again extending the incision as far proximally as necessary.

When abscess or fluctuance is found below the eponychium and a single incision does not adequately expose or decompress the involved tissues, a parallel incision along the opposite nail fold is made, allowing the eponychium and nail fold to be elevated and reflected above the nail plate (see Fig. 3-3C to E).

When the abscess extends below the nail plate, a portion of the nail plate should be removed. The amount and location of nail removal depends on the location and extent of involvement below the nail. If the area of fluctuance lies adjacent to the perionychium, a flat blunt probe or Freer elevator is used to separate the affected portion of the nail plate from the nail bed. The nail plate is then cut with a small scissors and removed. In the rare case where the

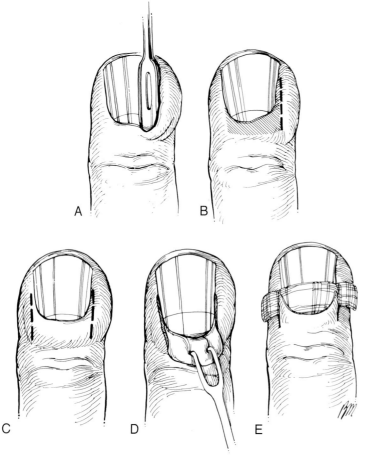

FIGURE 3-3. A, Elevation of the eponychial fold with a flat probe to expose the base of the nail. **B,** Placement of an incision to drain the paronychia and elevate the eponychial fold for excision of the proximal third of the nail. **C** to **E,** Incisions and procedure for elevating the entire eponychial fold with excision of the proximal third of the nail. A gauze pack prevents premature closure of the cavity.

eponychium is infected and pus is present only below the proximal portion of the nail, the eponychium and nail plate are elevated through a single or double incision. The proximal third of the nail plate is carefully removed. Only when the nail is entirely separated from the underlying matrix is it necessary to remove the entire nail plate. After decompression, the area of abscess is irrigated. The wound is left open with a small thin piece of gauze that allows the wound to stay open and drain.

Authors' Preferred Method of Treatment

No one treatment should be used exclusively, because there are cases in which each is applicable. We prefer to treat early infections nonsurgically with oral antibiotics and soaks two to three times per day in a solution of warm water and povidone-iodine (Betadine) at a ratio of 10 parts water to

1 part povidone-iodine. If the patient is allergic to topical povidone-iodine, warm normal saline may be used.

Surgical treatment depends on the location and extent of the perionychial infection. Generally, we release along the perionychial sulcus, extending proximally to the level of the nail base. Double incisions are reserved for more extensive eponychial involvement, or when removal of the proximal portion of the nail is planned. Removal of any portion of the nail is done only when the area of abscess extends below the nail plate. Removal of the entire nail is necessary only when the entire nail plate is separated from the nail matrix by abscess.

Postoperative Management and Expectations

Postoperatively, the patient is given oral antibiotics for 7 to 10 days, depending on the severity of the infection. Dressings are changed two to three times per day, coinciding with soaking of the affected finger in a dilute solution of povidone-iodine for 15 to 20 minutes. We discontinue packing or wicking the wound at 3 to 4 days. Occlusive dressings can lead to skin maceration and should be avoided. Early motion is emphasized to prevent stiffness.

Improvement is noted in most acute cases of paronychia in 3 to 4 weeks with appropriate management; however, some tenderness and hypersensitivity around the surgical scars can be expected for several months. Nail deformity can occur either as a result of the infection or after minimal surgical injury to the nail matrix. Patients with an underlying medical illness may require a longer time for healing and recovery or require additional surgery. This population likewise has a higher risk of recurrent infection.

Complications are rare but do occur. Nail deformity can occur either from the infection itself or from inadvertent injury to the nail matrix from decompression. The risk of injury is minimized by gently separating the nail plate from the underlying matrix and by directing the scalpel blade away from the matrix when incising around the nail bed.[29,90] Persistent infection despite appropriate treatment may be due to inadequate surgical decompression and drainage or inadequate antibiotic coverage. If the infection is not resolving at 1 week, radiographs to evaluate for osteomyelitis, cultures with antibiotic sensitivities, and repeat surgical débridement may be necessary. Robbins found that the most frequent complication of a paronychia was extension to the pulp space through a sinus at the side of the nail. This occurred in approximately 13.5% of patients treated in his series from the 1950s.[165] The occurrence today is rare owing to improved antibiotic therapy and more aggressive surgical treatment. In children with long-standing paronychia, infection can lead to bone involvement and epiphyseal separation.[165]

Misdiagnosis of a paronychia can occur, particularly confusion of perionychial infection with herpetic whitlow. Distinguishing herpetic whitlow from a bacterial infection is important. Incision and drainage of herpetic whitlow is contraindicated and can result in systemic viral infection and/or bacterial suprainfection.[4]

Chronic Paronychia

Clinical Presentation and Preoperative Evaluation

Chronic paronychia characterized by chronically indurated and rounded eponychium is a distinct clinical problem from

---

CRITICAL POINTS: ACUTE PARONYCHIA

INDICATION

- Perionychial or eponychial infection with abscess

PREOPERATIVE EVALUATION

- None required in healthy individual with acute infection
- Laboratory evaluation in diabetics or immunocompromised patients
- Radiographs if long-standing infection or no improvement with conventional therapy

PEARLS

- Careful evaluation for infection residing below the nail plate or in finger pulp

TECHNICAL POINT

- Incise with blade facing away from nail bed to reduce risk of injury to matrix.

PITFALLS

- Misdiagnosis as herpetic whitlow (see page 87)
- Failure to recognize underlying osteomyelitis
- Underlying systemic illness or atypical organism leading to refractory infection

POSTOPERATIVE CARE

- Seven to 10 days of oral antibiotics
- Daily soaks in dilute povidone-iodine solution
- Early finger range of motion

acute paronychia. The chronic inflammation is accompanied by repeated episodes of inflammation and drainage. If left untreated, this results in thickening and grooving of the nail plate. This problem is more common in middle-aged women, with a female-to-male ratio of 4:1.[3,7,194,195] Frequent water immersion, particularly in detergents and alkali solutions, is a predisposing condition. Housewives, bartenders, dishwashers, nurses, swimmers, and children who suck their fingers are often affected. It also more commonly affects patients with diabetes and psoriasis.[7,29,90,196] Cultured organisms include gram-positive cocci, gram-negative rods, *Candida,* and mycobacterial species.[20,126,131,194,196,197]

Pertinent Anatomy and Pathophysiology

Chronic paronychia begins with separation between the nail plate and the dorsal soft tissue covering the nail plate, including the cuticle, eponychium, and nail fold. This leads to colonization usually by staphylococcal organisms. Subsequent infection, by *Candida albicans* and/or colonic organisms, leads to chronic inflammation and recurrent exacerbations with episodic increased erythema and drainage. This chronic inflammation leads to fibrosis and thickening of the eponychium, with resultant decrease in vascularity to the dorsal nail fold. The decreased vascularity reduces the resistance to minor bacterial insults, allowing for recurrent episodes of symptomatic exacerbations.[7,29,96,194,196]

Treatment

Conservative therapies for chronic paronychial infection have included topical corticosteroids, oral and topical antibiotics, and oral and topical antifungal agents. Although reducing exposure to moist environments and chemical irritants may be helpful, these treatments alone have been unsuccessful in a large number of cases.[7,29,95]

Operative Treatment

Eponychial marsupialization is the most common surgical treatment for the chronic paronychium.[3,7,95,96] Under digital block anesthesia and tourniquet control, a crescent-shaped incision is made beginning 1 mm proximal to the distal edge of the eponychial nail fold and extending proximally for 3 to 5 mm. Some authors recommend removal of all thickened tissue. Others have found a 3-mm margin adequate to achieve equal results. The crescent should be symmetrically

shaped and extend to the edge of the nail fold on each side (Fig. 3-4). The crescent of tissue is removed down to but not including the germinal matrix. The wound is left open and allowed to drain. If nail deformity is present, removal of the nail has been reported to improve the cure rate and reduce the risk of recurrence.[7]

Authors' Preferred Methods of Treatment

We have found eponychial marsupialization an effective treatment for this condition. We agree with Bednar and Lane[7] that a 3-mm crescent of tissue is adequate and removal of all thickened tissue is not critical to the outcome. Special care is used to avoid injury to the germinal matrix. The removed tissue is sent for bacterial, fungal, and mycobacterial culture. The remaining tissue is sent for pathologic examination. Nail removal is performed when a nail deformity is present. Wounds are covered with Xeroform gauze. When the nail is removed, Xeroform gauze is placed in the nail bed and nail fold as well.

Patients are counseled regarding exposure to moist environments. Predisposing systemic conditions, such as diabetes and psoriasis, are medically controlled. We evaluate for activities that may lead to mycobacterial exposures, such as home aquariums or terrariums, marine work, or aviary exposure.

Postoperative Management and Expectations

The postoperative dressing is removed at 48 to 72 hours by soaking in 3% hydrogen peroxide solution. The patient is instructed to soak the area three times per day in dilute povidone-iodine solution. This continues until 2 days after all drainage has stopped. Oral antibiotics are given for 2 weeks. If cultures are negative or the organism is not sensitive, the antibiotic therapy is discontinued at 3 to 5 days.

Most chronic paronychial infections resolve with marsupialization. Systemic or topical antibiotics or antifungal agents are often not required. Wound healing by secondary intention occurs over 3 to 4 weeks. Scar sensitivity is more common than in acute paronychia and may persist for

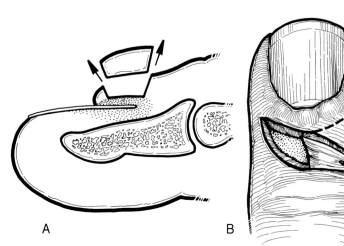

FIGURE 3-4. Eponychial marsupialization for chronic paronychia. **A,** Lateral view showing the area of wedge-shaped excision. Undisturbed matrix is stippled. **B,** Dorsal view of the crescent-shaped area of excision extending to the margins of the nail folds on each side.

A   B

CRITICAL POINTS: CHRONIC PARONYCHIA

INDICATION

- Chronic eponychial infection

PREOPERATIVE EVALUATION

- Thorough work-up and social history for contributing factors
- Laboratory evaluation in diabetics or immunocompromised patients
- Radiographs if never taken

PEARLS

- Nail removal in conjunction with marsupialization if nail deformity is present

TECHNICAL POINT

- Protect the germinal matrix during marsupialization.

PITFALLS

- Misdiagnosis with tumor or cyst
- Unrecognized systemic illness
- Failure to correct environmental factors

POSTOPERATIVE CARE

- Ten to 14 days of oral antibiotics, if cultures are positive and sensitive
- Consider oral antifungal medications
- Daily soaks in dilute povidone-iodine solution
- Early finger range of motion

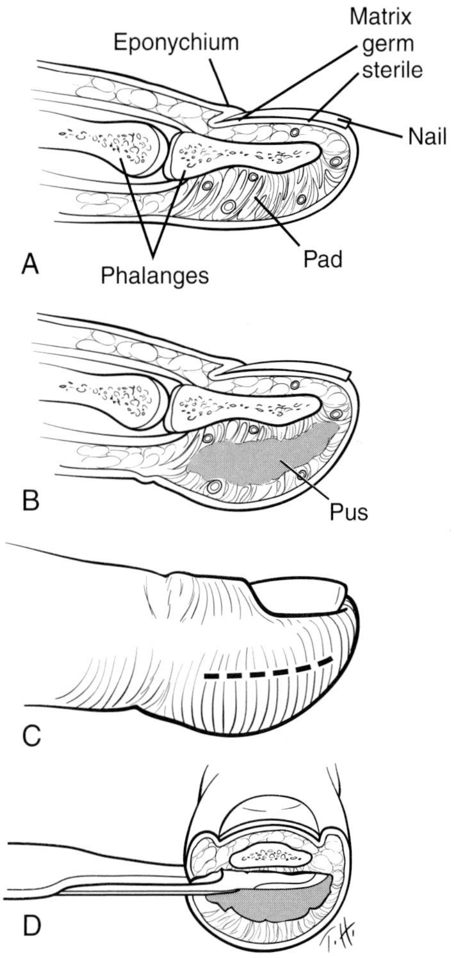

FIGURE 3-5. A, Cross section of the distal fingertip, showing the septated anatomy of the pad. **B,** Collection of pus within the finger pulp space. **C,** Incision for drainage of felon. **D,** The incision should include all of the involved septal compartments.

several months. Nail deformity is also more common than in treatment of acute paronychia. Six to 12 months may be required for nail growth, and residual deformity cannot be assessed until that time. Recurrence rates are higher if the patient does not correct environmental factors or if systemic diseases are not medically controlled. In the event of recurrence, re-marsupialization and nail removal should be done.

Felon

The term *felon* probably has its roots from the Latin *fel,* meaning "bile" or "venom."[125] A felon is a subcutaneous abscess of the distal pulp of a finger or thumb (Fig. 3-5). However, not all abscesses of the distal phalanx are felons. Superficial infections of the most distal part of the pulp skin are known as "apical infections." Apical infections are distinct from the felon in that the palmar pad is not involved.[114] The term *felon* should be reserved for those infections involving multiple septal compartments and causing compartment syndrome of the distal phalangeal pulp. The most commonly cultured organism from felons is *S. aureus.* Infections from gram-negative organisms have also been reported. These are

uncommon and more typically seen in immunocompromised patients or diabetics.[8,16,29,90]

Clinical Presentation and Evaluation

Felons account for 15% to 20% of all hand infections.[114,165] A felon is characterized by severe throbbing pain, tension, and swelling of the entire distal phalangeal pulp. The pulp space is exquisitely tender, but the associated swelling does not extend proximal to the DIP flexion crease, unless the joint or tendon sheath is involved. With the progression of swelling and tension, there is compromised venous return, leading to microvascular injury and development of necrosis and abscess formation. There is often, but not always, a penetrating injury, such as a wood splinter, glass sliver, or minor cut, preceding a felon. "Fingerstick felons" can be seen in diabetics, who repeatedly traumatize the fingertip for blood tests.[155] Once the felon has developed, the patient may attempt a decompression with a knife or needle. The pain and swelling usually develop rapidly. The expanding abscess breaks down the septa and can extend toward the phalanx and produce osteitis or osteomyelitis, or it can extend toward the skin and cause necrosis and a sinus somewhere on the palmar surface of the digital pulp. If such spontaneous, although inadequate, decompression does not occur, it is possible that the digital vessels will be obliterated and a slough of the tactile pulp will result. Other complications of an untreated felon include sequestration of the diaphysis of the distal phalanx, pyogenic arthritis of the DIP joint, and flexor tenosynovitis from proximal extension, although the last is quite rare.[16,165]

Pertinent Anatomy

Kanavel studied the anatomy of the fingertip through multiple sagittal and coronal sections of cadaveric fingers. He described the anatomy of the distal pulp as a "closed sac connective tissue framework, isolated and different from the rest of the finger."[93] Multiple vertical trabeculations divide the pulp of the distal phalanx into a latticework of separate septal compartments. The trabeculae attach the periosteum of the distal phalanx to the epidermis, giving the fingertip structural support and stabilizing the pulp during pinch and grasp. The septal interstices are filled with fat globules and eccrine sweat glands, which open onto the epidermis and provide an access for surface bacteria to enter the pulp space. The digital arteries run parallel to the distal phalanx, giving off a nutrient branch to the epiphysis before entering the pulp space. The diaphysis is supplied principally from volar nutrient vessels from the terminal branches of the digital arteries. The terminal branches of the digital nerve are parallel and palmar to the digital arteries. They arborize extensively within the pulp of the distal phalanx, providing fine tactile discrimination. The highest concentration of sensory receptors in the hand is the volar aspect of the distal phalanx.

Felons may begin with penetrating wounds of the distal pulp or as bacterial contamination of the fat pad through the eccrine sweat glands. Inflammation and cellulitis lead to local vascular congestion, which is aggravated by the closed septal anatomy of the pulp. If left untreated, tissue necrosis and abscess formation follow, resulting in further microvascular impairment.[16] The increased pressure within the pulp as a "closed sac" results in a clinical situation resembling a compartment syndrome. The ischemia of the pulp causes severe ischemic pain in the densely innervated pulp. Blood supply to the periosteum and diaphysis is compromised more than the blood supply to the skin, leading to bone necrosis and sequestration before spontaneous decompression of the felon through the skin. Infection or necrosis of the epiphysis is rarely seen, most likely owing to the preservation of the epiphyseal nutrient artery, which arises from the digital artery proximal to the closed space of the distal pulp and is therefore preserved.[29]

Treatment

Treatment of the felon should be directed toward preserving the function of the distal phalanx. These functions include fine tactile sensibility and a stable durable pad for pinch. In the early cellulitic phase, it may be possible to treat the felon with elevation, antibiotics, and soaks. Several days of immobilization may make the patient more comfortable. Surgical drainage is indicated when there is fluctuance in the pulp. Although it may be difficult to assess fluctuance, it is usually present if the process has been ongoing for more than 48 hours. The basic tenets of all approaches are to avoid injury to the digital nerve and vessels, use an incision that will not leave a disabling scar, keep exploration distal enough

so that the flexor tendon sheath is not violated and an iatrogenic tenosynovitis is not produced, and provide adequate drainage.

Operative Treatment

Several surgical incisions have been described; some of these are of historic interest only and are no longer recommended. Surgery may be performed under digital block anesthesia or under general anesthesia. A tourniquet is helpful for visualization. Regardless of the type of incision, surgical decompression requires thorough removal of necrotic tissue, irrigation, and wound management to allow continued drainage of the abscess cavity. To keep the wound open and draining, one may choose a thick coating of zinc oxide (Kilgore et al.[97]; Canales et al.[29]) or a gauze wick. The first dressing change is done at 24 to 48 hours. Authors' opinions vary as to how long the wound is kept open with a wick drainage. Two to 5 days should be adequate for most cases depending on the severity of infection. Soaking in dilute povidone-iodine solution as described earlier is initiated after the first dressing change and continued until wound closure by secondary intention.

Fish Mouth Incision. The fish mouth, or alligator mouth, incision (Fig. 3-6A) is designed parallel to the volar margin of the distal phalanx. The incision begins distal to the insertion of the flexor digitorum profundus (FDP) tendon. This is approximately in line with the most proximal visible portion of the nail. The incision is continued distally, staying parallel to the volar edge of the underlying phalanx as it curves around the fingertip onto the opposite side and terminating at a point identical to the starting one. The entire volar flap is carefully raised from the phalanx with a knife until the abscess is encountered. A thin instrument, such as tenotomy scissors or a small mosquito clamp, is then inserted into the cavity. The vertical septa are ruptured bluntly to ensure that no pocket of pus has been missed.[19,24]

Although this incision has been recommended for severe infections, it has virtually no place in the treatment of this lesion. Often it leaves an unsightly tender scar. It can also compromise circulation, producing a slough of the tactile pad. Destruction of all of the vertical septa results in a bulbous mobile pad, which makes it difficult for the patient to pick up objects.[29,90,97,114,138,165]

"J" or Hockey Stick Incision. An incision is made just dorsal to the midlateral line on the ulnar side of the finger, starting at a point 1 cm distal to the level of the flexion crease of the DIP joint. The incision is extended distally, following a plane close to the junction of the pad and the nail bed and around the fingertip to the corner of the nail on the opposite side of the digit (see Fig. 3-6B). The pulp tissue and septa are separated from the periosteum of the phalanx, thus allowing all septa to be opened for drainage.[114,165] The best indication for using this incision is an extensive or severe abscess. Even with a severe infection, this incision is seldom necessary. Because it crosses the fingertip it, too, can produce a sensitive, disabling scar at the fingertip.

Through-and-Through Incisions. Through-and-through drainage was described by Brown.[22] This technique starts as a hockey stick incision. In addition, a 1-cm counter-incision is made on the radial side to establish through-and-through drainage (see Fig. 3-6C). This is achieved by rupturing the vertical trabeculae in the pulp and spreading it with a pointed clamp.

This approach is rarely needed because adequate drainage can be achieved by a single incision. Therefore, a second, or counter, incision is usually superfluous. Although, as initially described, the skin incision is carried across the ulnar tip of the finger, adequate drainage and access to the abscess cavity can be achieved with two lateral incisions that end proximal to the fingertip.

Volar Incision. Bolton originally recommended a volar transverse incision (see Fig. 3-6D).[16] After the site of greatest tenderness and tension has been localized by palpation with the tip of a probe, a transverse incision 4 to 5 mm long is made over the site of a central abscess. The knife should be allowed to penetrate only the dermis while a clamp is used to spread the subcutaneous tissue, minimizing the risk to the digital nerves. If a volar sinus is present, an elliptical incision is made at its location to excise the necrotic edges of the tract. Satisfactory drainage can be obtained through this incision. However, this approach never gained popularity because of the risk of injury to the digital nerves and vessels.

Kilgore described an alternative volar approach (see Fig. 3-6E) using a longitudinal palmar incision in the midline of the tactile pad.[29,90,97] The skin is sharply divided in the midline over the site of maximum tension. The incision should not cross the DIP flexion crease. A small scissors or clamp is used to bluntly delineate the abscess cavity. Dissection outside the abscess cavity is not recommended. Particular attention should be paid to avoid penetration of the flexor tendon sheath or joint capsule, which can result in iatrogenic pyarthrosis or septic flexor tenosynovitis.

Proponents of the volar approach maintain that the incision characteristically results in a thin, fine and painless scar. Additionally, the structural integrity of the palmar pad is better maintained and the risk of injury to the digital nerves and vessels is minimized.

Unilateral Longitudinal Incision. Although it is preferred to place the incision on the side opposite the pinching surface, the incision should always be placed on the side of maximal tenderness. When possible, the incision is made on the ulnar side of the second to fourth digits and on the radial side in the thumb and small finger. The incision is started dorsal to and 0.5 cm distal to the DIP joint flexion crease. It is continued distally in line with the volar margin of the distal phalanx, but it does not cross over the fingertip (see Fig. 3-6F). The incision is deepened along a plane just volar to the palmar cortex of the phalanx until the abscess is entered. The opening in the cavity is enlarged until adequate evacuation is achieved.[13,34,138]

Authors' Preferred Methods of Treatment

There are a few situations in which nonsurgical management can be applied. This is in the very early presentation of the acute felon. However, the felon is more typically a very rapidly developing process, and, by the time of presentation, the pulp is tensely swollen and exquisitely tender. This requires surgical decompression whether fluctuance is present or not. We prefer to perform surgery under digital block anesthetic with sedation. A forearm tourniquet is used. The extremity is exsanguinated by elevation. The surgical incision is made longitudinally over the point of maximal tenderness. When the point of maximal tenderness is located in the middle of the pulp, we use the longitudinal volar incision described by Kilgore and colleagues.[97] When the point of tenderness is on the side of the pulp, we use the unilateral longitudinal incision described earlier. All involved septa should be opened and a wound culture is taken. The distal phalanx must be examined with a probe. A rough or softened surface indicates bone involvement, which requires débridement of the softened or necrotic bone. After thorough débridement and irrigation,

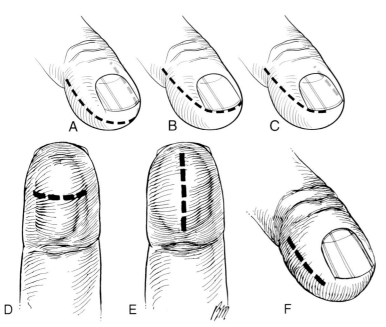

FIGURE 3-6. Incisions for drainage of felons. **A,** Fish mouth incision. This approach is associated with significant complications and should *not* be used. **B,** Hockey stick incision. The incision begins in the midaxial line, aims for the corner of the nail, and passes across the finger in the natural line between skin and nail matrix (see text). **C,** Abbreviated hockey stick incision with counter-incision on the opposite side. An alternative to the full hockey stick incision is to make this incision shorter and make a second incision on the opposite side of the pulp *(faint dotted line).* **D,** Volar drainage is useful if the abscess points volarward, but this incision risks injury to the digital nerves. **E,** Alternative volar approach. There is less risk to the digital nerves, but the incision should not touch or cross the DIP joint flexion crease. **F,** Unilateral longitudinal approach. This incision is the authors' preferred method for treatment of most felons.

CRITICAL POINTS: FELON

INDICATION

- Tense pulp space infection with or without fluctuance

PREOPERATIVE EVALUATION

- Patient history of recent injury and social history
- Laboratory evaluation in diabetics or immunocompromised patients
- Radiographs to evaluate for foreign body or osteomyelitis

PEARLS

- Incision made at point of maximal tenderness

TECHNICAL POINTS

- Avoid incisions crossing the fingertip or DIP flexion crease.
- Protect the digital nerves and vessels.
- Do not violate the flexor tendon sheath.

PITFALLS

- Misdiagnosis as herpetic whitlow (see page 87)
- Unrecognized osteomyelitis
- Incomplete decompression of all involved septa
- Iatrogenic septic flexor tenosynovitis
- Creation of an unstable pulp

POSTOPERATIVE CARE

- Intravenous antibiotic therapy for 5 to 7 days, longer if bone is involved (in hospitalized patients)
- Patients treated in an outpatient setting usually do not require intravenous antibiotics
- Gauze wick for at least 72 hours
- Soaks three times per day in dilute povidone-iodine solution
- Early finger range of motion

the wound is kept open with a thin gauze wick and a sterile dressing is applied. The first dressing change is done between 12 and 24 hours.

Postoperative Management and Expectations

The setting of the drainage procedure (office, emergency department, or operating room) and whether the patient needs to be hospitalized depends on the severity of the infection and the reliability of the patient. In our county hospital patients, we prefer to admit the patients and give intravenous antibiotics until a favorable response to therapy is seen. Oral antibiotics can be used when the infection is controlled. Bone involvement requires longer intravenous therapy. The choice of antibiotic depends on the cultured organism and its antibiotic sensitivity. Because most felons are caused by

S. aureus, initial antibiotic therapy should cover this organism. Factors such as underlying disease, injury mechanism, or contributing occupational or social history may influence antibiotic choice. Dressings are changed two to three times per day. At the time of dressing change, the patient soaks the affected finger in a solution of dilute povidone-iodine for 15 to 20 minutes. Packing or wicking of the wound is discontinued after 3 to 5 days. Occlusive dressings are not used because they often result in skin maceration. Early motion is emphasized to prevent stiffness.

Most felons recover in 3 to 4 weeks with appropriate management. The length of treatment and recovery depends on the severity of the infection and the presence of bone involvement. Tenderness and hypersensitivity around the surgical scars and of the entire pulp can be expected for several months from surgery. In some patients this may be a permanent finding. Pulp deformity, most commonly pulp atrophy, occurs frequently and is permanent. Pulp instability can occur in patients where the infection has involved all of the vertical septa, regardless of the incision used. This will often resolve over time but may take 6 months to a year. In cases of osteomyelitis with large bone loss, nail deformity may occur owing to loss of underlying bone support of the nail matrix, resulting in a short finger with a short nail. In some cases with severe bone involvement amputation should be considered.

Complications of treatment include recurrence of infection, usually as a result of inadequate bone débridement. In these cases, repeat surgical débridement and prolonged organism-specific antibiotic therapy will usually be sufficient. However, amputation may be necessary for refractory infection. Iatrogenic septic flexor tenosynovitis has been reported. Appropriate treatment involves repeat débridement and surgical decompression and irrigation of the flexor tendon sheath, as described later.

Pyogenic Flexor Tenosynovitis

Pyogenic flexor tenosynovitis is a closed-space infection of the flexor tendon sheath of the fingers or thumb. The purulence within the flexor tendon sheath destroys the gliding mechanism, rapidly creating adhesions that lead to marked limitation of tendon function and severe loss of motion. It can also destroy the blood supply, producing tendon necrosis. Early treatment is of paramount importance in limiting the morbidity associated with this diagnosis. Untreated disease and late diagnosis or presentation can lead to devastating disability in hand function. The incidence and serious sequelae of bacterial tenosynovitis are less frequent, owing to early recognition and the availability of appropriate antibiotic therapy. The most common organisms responsible for disease include *S. aureus* and β-hemolytic *Streptococcus. Pasteurella multocida* is frequently cultured in infections caused by animal bites. A wider host of organisms should be considered in immunocompromised patients, who have yielded positive cultures for *Eikenella corrodens, Listeria monocytogenes,* and mixed gram-positive and gram-negative infections.

Clinical Presentation and Preoperative Evaluation

Most patients present with a history of penetrating trauma, typically over the volar aspect of the proximal interphalangeal

(PIP) or DIP joint. A small puncture wound, often from a foreign body or animal, can inoculate the tendon sheath. Hematogenous septic flexor tenosynovitis is rare. When this occurs, disseminated gonococcal infections are the most frequent.[101,171] Levy recommended that hematogenous tenosynovitis should be treated as disseminated gonorrhea until final culture results are available.[110]

Kanavel[93] initially described three cardinal signs of acute flexor tenosynovitis. He later added a semi-flexed posture of the digit as the fourth sign. All four signs need not be present, especially in the early course of the disease. Kanavel's four cardinal signs are:

1. A semi-flexed position of the finger
2. Symmetrical enlargement of the whole digit (fusiform swelling)
3. Excessive tenderness limited to the course of the flexor tendon sheath
4. Excruciating pain on passively extending the finger. The pain should be experienced along the flexor sheath and not localized to a particular joint or abscess.

There are different opinions as to which signs are most clinically useful.[15,93,147,148,159] Kanavel[93] believed that excessive tenderness along the tendon sheath was the most important clinical sign. Polen[159] and Boles and Schmidt[15] agreed that palpation and tenderness along the sheath was a more reliable and reproducible sign. Neviaser[147] believed the most reproducible clinical sign is pain with passive extension. We believe that both of these findings are useful and in combination help distinguish pyogenic flexor tenosynovitis from local abscess or pyarthrosis. Findings in the thumb and small finger may be more subtle, because these fingers have a mechanism of autodecompression through the radial and ulnar bursae.

Laboratory evaluation should include a complete blood cell count. The ESR and CRP may be useful in monitoring the disease process. However, these may be elevated in noninfectious inflammatory processes as well. Radiographs should be taken to evaluate for retained foreign body, underlying pyarthrosis, osteomyelitis, or unrecognized trauma, such as fracture.

There are several conditions that may mimic acute pyogenic flexor tenosynovitis. The differential diagnosis includes herpetic whitlow, felon, pyarthrosis, local abscess, and inflammatory diseases such as rheumatoid arthritis or gout. Herpetic whitlow and felon, as already described, present a different clinical picture, typically with more distal findings. Herpetic whitlow is not associated with the tenseness and swelling that is found in pyogenic flexor tenosynovitis and classically presents with small skin vesicles. Pyarthrosis can more closely resemble an infection of the flexor sheath, because there is commonly pain with passive joint motion and the digit is held in a flexed posture. Unlike flexor synovitis, the location of the traumatic injury is usually on the dorsal surface of the finger, the swelling is more localized around the joint, and pain with palpation is not present along the entire tendon sheath.

In cases in which the clinical presentation is not clear or there is a clinical suspicion of a nonseptic acute tenosynovitis as may be seen in gout, rheumatoid arthritis, or acute stenosing tenosynovitis, aspiration of the tendon sheath should be done. The aspiration is done with a 20- to 22-gauge needle along the flexor sheath from the A1 pulley to the DIP joint in the area of maximal tenderness. If the aspiration is negative, NSAID therapy is initiated. The patient should be closely monitored in the first 24 hours. Depending on patient reliability, this can be done on an inpatient or outpatient basis.

Pertinent Anatomy

Knowledge of the anatomy of the flexor tendon sheaths, bursae, and deep spaces of the forearm is important in understanding the presentation and possible spread of infection in the hand. The flexor tendon sheath, as described by Doyle,[46, 47] is a double-walled structure with a visceral and parietal layer. The visceral layer is closely adherent to the tendon and is the epitenon. The parietal layer lies adjacent to the pulley system. These two layers are hollow tubular structures connected proximally and distally, creating a closed system. In the fingers, the sheaths begin in the palm at the level of the metacarpal neck and end distally just proximal to the DIP joint. In the small finger, there is usually continuity between the flexor sheath and the ulnar bursa, which extends to a point just proximal to the transverse carpal ligament. In the thumb, a similar connection is seen with the radial bursa, which also extends proximal to the transverse carpal ligament.[38,46,93,147,148,173] Proximally, the radial and ulnar bursae have a potential space of communication. This is known as the space of Parona, which lies between the fascia of the pronator quadratus muscle and FDP conjoined tendon sheath. This site of connection between the thumb and small fingers through the radial and ulnar bursae gives rise to the "horseshoe abscess," in which a flexor sheath infection of the thumb or small finger tracks proximally to the wrist and then ascends along the opposite side flexor sheath. Although this is the most commonly described connection, many variations of flexor sheath anatomy exit. This was elegantly described by Scheldrup in 1951.[173] These potential variations and sites of interconnection should be kept in mind to direct appropriate treatment.

The flexor tendons receive their nutrient supply from direct vascular supply and diffusion from the synovial fluid.[31] When bacteria inoculate the flexor sheath, the synovial fluid becomes the nutritional source for the bacteria. The host has limited ability to defend against the bacterial proliferation, owing to the poor vascularity within this closed system. The bacterial proliferation leads to increased volume and pressure within the tendon sheath. Schnall and coworkers demonstrated pressures exceeding 30 mm Hg in more than 50% of flexor sheath infections. This high pressure likely contributes to the pathogenesis of the disease process by obstructing arterial blood supply of the flexor tendons through the vincular system. This can quickly result in tendon necrosis and subsequent rupture. Appropriate and urgent management of flexor tendon sheath infections is imperative in preventing these unwanted complications.

Treatment

There is a narrow range of indications for nonsurgical treatment of pyogenic flexor tenosynovitis. Rarely do patients present with early clinical findings, which may be manageable with antibiotic therapy. Those patients who present within the first 24 hours of the onset of symptoms and have mild pain, mild swelling, and show only partial expression of one or two of Kanavel's signs may be initially treated with intravenous administration of antibiotics. A loose dressing and a dorsal block splint are applied to place the hand at rest. The extremity is elevated. The patient is monitored with close clinical observation in an inpatient hospital setting. If the clinical symptoms are not improving in the first 12 hours, surgical treatment is indicated. Nonsurgical management should seldom be considered in the diabetic or immunocompromised patient.

Before antibiotic therapy is initiated, an aspiration of the tendon sheath is done to obtain material for culture. The aspiration is performed with a 20- to 22-gauge needle. The aspirate can be performed anywhere between the palmodigital crease and the DIP flexion crease. The aspiration should be performed away from any areas of superficial cellulitis. A small amount of saline may be necessary to lavage the sheath to obtain a specimen for culture. If frank pus is encountered on the aspiration, nonsurgical treatment should not be pursued. Patients who present with a local cellulitis along the volar surface of the finger may also have a septic flexor tendon sheath. If nonsurgical treatment is considered, great care must be taken in aspirating the sheath, to prevent inadvertent inoculation of the sheath through the cellulitic subcutaneous tissue.

We should keep in mind that purulent tenosynovitis rapidly destroys the gliding mechanism within the flexor tendon sheath. Delayed or inadequate treatment increases the formation of adhesions within the sheath, permanently limiting tendon excursion and ultimately limiting finger range of motion.

Operative Treatment

Several surgical approaches have been described for the treatment of pyogenic flexor tenosynovitis. Some of these are of historic interest only. Most describe various incisions for proximal and distal exposure of the flexor tendon sheath and various irrigation methods and solutions.

There have been two principal surgical approaches to treatment of flexor tendon sheath infections. The first is through a midlateral incision along the infected finger (Fig. 3-7A). This was described by several authors in the 1940s.[48,53,54,115] Early descriptions of the midlateral incision involved proximal opening of the sheath at the proximal phalanx and distal opening of the sheath at the middle phalanx. Flynn[54] described a wide exposure of the flexor sheath through a midlateral incision. He also recommended that the proximal sheath should be opened through a separate 1.5-cm longitudinal incision at the level of the proximal flexor sheath. Entin[48] emphasized that successful treatment of a flexor sheath infection requires complete exposure of the sheath. In the thumb, index, and small fingers, this can be accomplished through a single extended midlateral incision. For the long and ring fingers, this is done through two incisions: a midlateral incision along the affected digit and a separate incision at the base of the finger just distal to the palmar crease.[48]

Other authors believed that wide exposure of the tendon sheath led to significant postoperative scarring and stiffness of the involved finger. To address this problem, a number of methods were described that were designed to limit exposure of the tendon sheath. Louden and colleagues,[115] in the mid 1940s, described treatment of early flexor tendon sheath infections with a single distal transverse incision just proxi-

mal to the DIP flexion crease. The tendon sheath is opened at this level, and fluid is allowed to egress. Irrigation of the tendon sheath is accomplished by placement of a needle at the proximal extent of the tendon sheath and syringe irrigation (see Fig. 3-7B). Carter and colleagues reported good results with two transverse incisions placed at the proximal and distal ends of the flexor sheath.[33] They modified the technique that had been described in the early 1940s by Marsden[54] by using hydrogen peroxide and oxytetracycline as an irrigating solution (see Fig. 3-7C). Polen used this technique; however, he used the site of abscess or site of local maximum tenderness as the distal egress for the irrigation solution.[159] Besser, in 1976, described a single incision at the proximal edge of the flexor sheath. A catheter is introduced and sutured into position. A small volume of antibiotic-containing irrigant was placed into the sheath every hour. This technique was described more for a postsurgical infection of the tendon sheath than for acute pyogenic flexor tenosynovitis.[11]

With both types of incisions, the sheath is opened proximally and distally and irrigated using a proximally placed catheter. Some authors would add a distally placed egress catheter as well[54] (see Fig. 3-7D). Irrigation solutions included penicillin, which was the principal antibiotic available at the time. As early as the 1940s, some authors would leave an indwelling catheter, which was used to intermittently irrigate the tendon sheath over 48 to 72 hours. Carter and colleagues[33] were the first to describe continuous irrigation of severe tendon sheath infections.

Neviaser popularized a limited midlateral incision, with opening of the tendon sheath distal to the A4 pulley. The proximal tendon sheath is exposed in the distal palm, and a catheter is placed for continuous irrigation[147,148] (see Fig. 3-7D).

Through-and-Through Intermittent Antibiotic Irrigation. An incision is made near and parallel to the DIP flexion crease.[33] The tendon sheath is visualized by retracting both neurovascular bundles to their respective sides. The sheath is opened through a transverse incision to allow fluid to drain. A second transverse incision is made in the region of the distal palm, just proximal to the A1 pulley. The flexor tendon sheath just proximal to the A1 pulley is exposed and opened. A polyethylene catheter with holes cut along its length is inserted well into the sheath. A syringe is attached to the catheter, and antibiotic containing saline is used to copiously irrigate the tendon sheath from proximal to distal. Fluid should egress from the distal incision. The tendon sheath is irrigated until the distal fluid egress is clear. The catheter may be sutured in place so that irrigation can be repeated on the following day. In severe infections a continuous drip is attached to the catheter and run at one drop per second for 24 to 48 hours. Then the catheters are removed and exercises started.

Closed Tendon Sheath Irrigation. As described by Neviaser,[146a,147,148] a zigzag incision is made in the distal area of the palm over the proximal end of the sheath. The sheath is opened at the proximal margin of the A1 pulley. A second incision is made on the ulnar midaxial side of the finger in the middle and distal segments. Access to the distal end of the sheath is obtained through a plane dorsal to the digital artery and nerve. The sheath is resected distal to the A4 pulley. A 16-gauge polyethylene catheter with a single opening at its end is inserted under the A1 pulley in the palm for a distance of 1.5 to 2 cm (see Fig. 3-7D). The catheter is sutured to the skin and the wound closed around it. The sheath is copiously irrigated with saline. A small drain is brought from the tendon through the skin distally and sutured to the skin. The wound is closed around the drain. The system is flushed again to test its patency. The hand is dressed and splinted, with the catheter brought out of the dressing and connected to a 50-mL syringe. The dressing is arranged so that the drain can be seen distally. The system is tested just before the patient leaves the operating suite. Postoperatively, the sheath is flushed manually with 50 mL of sterile saline every 2 hours for 48 hours. At this time the digit is inspected. If signs of infection have abated, the catheter and drain are removed, the wounds dressed lightly to avoid impending motion, and exercises started. If any doubt exists, the irrigation may be continued for an additional 24 hours. Complete motion can be expected in a week.

In the thumb, the proximal part of the sheath is exposed through a thenar crease incision. The distal centimeter of the transverse carpal ligament is incised to allow access to passage of the flexor pollicis longus (FPL) through the wall of the canal into the thenar eminence. The catheter is placed in this opening. Neviaser emphasized that the advantages of this technique include thorough mechanical irrigation of the sheath, accurate placement of the catheter, primary wound healing, and rapid return of function with minimal inconvenience to the patient.[146a,147]

Authors' Preferred Methods of Treatment

Decompression of the septic flexor tendon sheath begins with a midlateral incision. The incisions are designed to avoid scarring on the pinching surface of the fingers. In the index, middle, and ring fingers the incision is placed on the ulnar border, and in the thumb and small finger it is placed on the radial side. The incision is made dorsal to Cleland's ligament (see Fig. 3-7A). The incision extends from the middle of the distal phalanx to just proximal to the web space. The dissection is carried out dorsal to the neurovascular bundle and down to the flexor tendon sheath. This allows decompression of the swollen finger, decreasing compartment pressure. The tendon sheath is opened distal to the A4 pulley. The sheath must be opened enough to allow the easy egress of fluid or pus, typically 4 to 6 mm. Cultures are taken from the tendon sheath effluent. A 1.5- to 2.0-cm transverse volar incision made proximal to the A1 pulley is usually sufficient to expose the proximal flexor sheath. This incision can be easily extended proximally or distally as a Bruner-type incision to allow greater exposure of the tendon sheath if it is necessary. The tendon sheath is opened proximally. If fluid for culture was not obtained distally, cultures should be taken from the proximal sheath. If hypertrophic synovitis is seen, synovial biopsy is recommended. Pathologic examination should include fungal and mycobacterial stains (see Chapter 4).

A 14- or 16-gauge intravenous catheter or a No. 5 pediatric feeding tube is introduced into the tendon sheath and advanced 1.5 to 2.0 cm into the sheath. Syringe irrigation

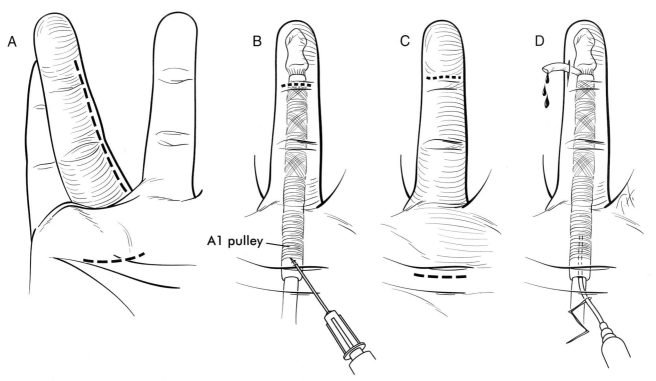

A1 pulley

FIGURE 3-7. Incision for drainage of tendon sheath infections. **A,** Open drainage incisions through the midaxial approach. **B,** Sheath irrigation with distal opening of the sheath and proximal syringe irrigation. **C,** Incisions for intermittent through-and-through irrigation. **D,** Closed tendon sheath irrigation technique.[146a]

with copious amounts of antibiotic containing normal saline is done. The fluid should be seen to egress from the distal opening in the tendon sheath. The tendon sheath should be irrigated until clear fluid is seen distally. We generally prefer to continue irrigating until 400 to 600 mL of irrigant is used.

If we encounter difficulty in irrigating, the catheter is first repositioned. Mobilizing the superficialis and profundus tendons and placing the catheter dorsal to the tendons may allow easy flow of solution. Thickened tenosynovium may impede flow, and a limited proximal synovectomy may be necessary.

CRITICAL POINTS: PYOGENIC FLEXOR TENOSYNOVITIS

INDICATION

- Septic flexor tenosynovitis

PREOPERATIVE EVALUATION

- Clinical examination is the hallmark of diagnosis.
- Laboratory evaluation may include uric acid and rheumatoid factor in addition to complete blood cell count, depending on suspicion of nonpyogenic process.
- Radiographs

PEARLS

- Pain with palpation along flexor tendon sheath and pain with passive extension are most useful in diagnosing early disease.
- Urgent surgical treatment especially in a patient with diabetes or immunocompromise reduces the morbidity associated with this infection.

TECHNICAL POINTS

- Perform early decompression with complete midlateral incision of the finger.
- Incise dorsal to Cleland's ligament.
- Irrigate the sheath until the effluent is clear.
- Use wick to keep the proximal and distal incisions open.

PITFALLS

- Delayed surgical treatment
- Inadequate decompression
- Injury of the digital neurovascular structures

POSTOPERATIVE CARE

- Intravenous antibiotics
- Pain management to allow early range of motion
- First dressing change between 8 and 12 hours
- Soaks in dilute povidone-iodine solution three times per day
- Repeat débridement and irrigation in 48 hours if Kanavel's signs not resolving

Any wounds on the volar surface of the finger should be débrided. Even small puncture wounds, particularly those caused by cat bites, should be débrided and irrigated. In cases in which there is a large volar wound and opening in the tendon sheath at a site of abscess, the irrigant may primarily be flowing out of the abscess site. In this situation, following the débridement of the volar wound, the irrigation catheter can be placed into the tendon sheath at the site of abscess and the distal tendon sheath can be further irrigated.

Postoperative Management and Expectations

Postoperatively, the wounds are left open. A wet gauze wick is placed into the wounds to allow continued drainage. A bulky dressing is applied. The hand is elevated, and the patient is continued on intravenous antibiotics. The first dressing change should be done at 12 to 24 hours. At this time the patient begins soaking in a dilute solution of povidone-iodine, as described earlier. Early motion is initiated. Therapist supervision may be necessary. It is important to keep this wound open to allow drainage. If left alone, the palmar wound will close almost immediately. Therefore, moist gauze wicks are used to keep the wounds open in the first 72 hours. Intravenous antibiotics are continued for 7 to 10 days. After this, oral antibiotics are continued to complete a 4-week course of therapy.

If the clinical signs of infection are not improving in the first 24 to 36 hours, the patient is returned to the operating room for a repeat irrigation and débridement. Repeat cultures are obtained, and organism-specific intravenous therapy is continued. A low threshold for return to the operating room should be used in diabetics and immunocompromised patients.

Most pyogenic tenosynovitis, if treated promptly with adequate surgical débridement, appropriate antibiotics, and therapy will improve rapidly. Patients usually have an almost immediate sense of relief of the severe throbbing pain that was present before treatment. Wound healing of the volar incision occurs quickly as soon as the wicking is discontinued. The midlateral incision heals by secondary intention over the course of 10 to 20 days. When the swelling subsides, Steri-Strips can be used to bring the wound edges together, shortening the healing time. Despite healing by secondary intention, the midlateral scar is usually painless. Over time, the scar becomes soft and essentially unnoticeable. Reported range of motion after flexor tendon sheath infection varies. Ten to 20% of patients fail to recover full range of motion. A more rigorous analysis of motion by Schwendeman and Stern showed that only two thirds of normal motion was present at 6 weeks. This improved to 80% of normal motion at 30-month follow-up.[15]

The more severe the initial presentation, the more increased is the likelihood of complications and adverse outcome. Any infection of the flexor tendon sheath may cause scarring and adhesions within the sheath, limiting flexor tendon excursion and gliding. Tenolysis should not be considered until complete resolution of infection and failure to improve with occupational therapy. Passive motion should exceed active motion for a tenolysis alone to improve function. Stiffness of the PIP or DIP joints is not uncommon, particularly if early motion is not initiated or if the patient is noncompliant with therapy. Manipulation under anesthesia may be considered before open contracture release and/or tenolysis. Soft tissue necrosis occurs rarely. Local débridement should be done as needed. When the infection is controlled, healing by secondary intention will occur. If the flexor tendon is exposed, local flap coverage should be considered, especially in patients who have good tendon gliding. Late treatment or severe infection may result in tendon necrosis. This requires excision of the necrotic tendons from the level of the A1 pulley to its distal insertion. The flexor tendon sheath is left open. In our experience, staged reconstruction of the tendon sheath and tendon grafting is difficult and often has suboptimal outcome. In the index and small finger with tendon necrosis, amputation may be considered, because this is more likely to improve functional outcome and shorten the healing time. Severe flexor tendon sheath infections with tendon necrosis in conjunction with pyarthrosis of any digit except the thumb may best be treated by amputation.[19]

Radial and Ulnar Bursal Infections

Pertinent to the treatment of pyogenic flexor tenosynovitis are infections of the radial and ulnar bursae of the palm. Infections in these spaces occur rarely in isolation but are more commonly associated with flexor tendon sheath infections of the small finger or thumb.

Pertinent Anatomy

The radial bursa is a continuation of the tendon sheath of the FPL. The sheath begins at the base of the distal phalanx of the thumb. Technically, the sheath ends at the metacarpophalangeal (MP) joint. The radial bursa begins at this level and includes the length of the FPL tendon through the carpal canal. It ends 1 to 2 cm proximal to the proximal edge of the transverse carpal ligament. It is considered a separate bursal space from the FPL tendon sheath, even though in adults it was contiguous with the sheath in 95% of specimens.

The ulnar bursa begins at the proximal end of the small finger flexor tendon sheath. The bursa widens more proximally, overlapping the mid fourth metacarpal and the proximal base of the third and fourth metacarpals. The bursa lies ulnar to the flexor tendons, which are invaginated into the bursa but not surrounded by it. The relationship of the small finger flexor tendon sheath with the ulnar bursa is less consistent than the relationship between the flexor tendon sheath of the thumb and the radial bursa. Early studies showed direct continuity in only 50% of specimens. Other studies have demonstrated a higher rate of communication, often demonstrating an hourglass-type narrowing between the small finger tendon sheath and the ulnar bursa.[173]

Proximal to the transverse carpal ligament, the radial and ulnar bursa lie deep to the FDP tendons and above the fascia of the pronator quadratus. This plane between the FDP and the pronator quadratus fascia is the potential space of Parona. Communication between the radial and ulnar bursa can occur across this space.

Clinical Presentation and Preoperative Evaluation

Because radial and ulnar bursal infections rarely occur in isolation, the clinical presentations of these infections are similar to those of pyogenic flexor tenosynovitis of the thumb and small finger. In addition to the cardinal signs of Kanavel, there may be swelling and tenderness along the thenar or hypothenar eminence. The adjacent fingers assume a flexed posture, as does the wrist. Although the uninvolved fingers may not be swollen, passive extension is painful. Kanavel[93] believed that the most valuable sign of ulnar bursal infection was the presence of tenderness at the junction of the distal flexion crease of the wrist and the hypothenar eminence. Similarly for radial bursal infections was tenderness at the junction of the distal wrist flexion crease and the thenar eminence.

Extensive swelling may not be evident, because the bursae rapidly become necrotic. Accumulation of pus does not occur, because the bursae rupture and decompress into the surrounding space. The infection can track across the potential space of Parona, involving the opposite bursa. An ascending infection along the opposite border digit can then occur, forming the so-called horseshoe abscess. Anatomic variations in the interconnection of the tendon sheaths occur in approximately 15% of patients.[173] Therefore, clinical examination of any flexor tendon sheath infection should include examination of the palm, wrist, and all of the adjacent fingers.

Treatment

Ulnar and radial bursal infections rarely occur in isolation but are a part of pyogenic flexor tenosynovitis, most commonly of the thumb and small finger. There is no role for nonsurgical treatment of this condition. These infections can cause rapid destruction of the bursal sheath, swelling within the carpal tunnel causing acute median nerve symptoms,[122] and scarring and adhesions between the superficial and deep flexor tendons. Prompt surgical treatment is necessary. The septic flexor tenosynovitis must be treated in conjunction with the bursal infection. There is no general consensus regarding the surgical incision, use of drains, or open versus closed management with catheter irrigation. The following techniques have been described.

Open Treatment

Open treatment of ulnar bursal infections, as described by Boyes,[19] included two separate incisions The first incision is placed parallel to the proximal edge of the A1 pulley. It can be extended proximally along the radial margin of the hypothenar crease. The proximal end of the bursa in the forearm is exposed through a 3-inch incision, beginning just proximal to the wrist flexion crease. The incision parallels the volar edge of the distal ulna. The flexor carpi ulnaris and the dorsal sensory branch of the ulnar nerve are retracted volarward. By retracting these structures, the pronator quadratus muscle is exposed. The bulge of the ulnar bursa is easily visualized and opened. Cultures should be taken, and the wound is copiously irrigated from proximal to distal. Similarly, treatment of radial bursal infections is done through a distal incision placed at the level of the thumb MP joint. Boyes believed that the radial bursa could best be treated through the same proximal incision as the ulnar bursa, dissecting radially across the volar floor of the pronator quadratus to reach the radial bursa. He described a separate radial incision along the flexor carpi radialis; however, he believed this was superfluous when the ulnar incision was used. For advanced infections, Boyes advocated proximal extension of the palmar incision to include the decompression and drainage of the carpal tunnel. Drains are placed in the bursa and brought out through the skin; they are removed after 48 hours so that exercises can be started.[19]

Through-and-Through Closed Irrigation

In previous editions of this chapter, Neviaser described the method of through-and-through irrigation of bursal infections. The distal end of the bursa is exposed through a short extension of the zigzag incision used as the palmar approach to the tendon sheath of the small finger. The bursa is opened, and a 16-gauge polyethylene catheter is introduced into the wound and directed proximally into the bursa. Another incision, either straight or zigzag, is made in the volar ulnar surface of the wrist just radial to the flexor carpi ulnaris. The tendon and ulnar artery and nerve are retracted medially and the flexor superficialis and profundus retracted laterally to expose the bursa. The bursa is incised and saline flushed through it from the distal end. A rubber drain is brought out from the bursa through the skin in the proximal wound. The wounds are sutured around the implants. The irrigating system is managed the same as and in conjunction with the system in the finger as described earlier.[147,148]

With this method, a radial bursal infection is treated in a similar fashion. The palmar incision is made adjacent to the thumb flexion crease at the metacarpophalangeal joint. The proximal incision is placed just ulnar to the flexor carpi radialis. The respective ends of the bursa are opened, and the bursal sac is irrigated thoroughly.

Authors' Preferred Method of Treatment

We treat bursal infections by first addressing the flexor tendon sheath infection when present. The exposure of the distal bursa is the same as that described by Boyes and Neviaser. When a tendon sheath infection is present, the same incision used for exposure of the proximal tendon sheath is utilized for the distal exposure of the bursa. The proximal incision for ulnar bursal infections is a longitudinal incision beginning at the proximal wrist flexion crease. The incision is extended proximally for 5 cm, paralleling the radial margin of the flexor carpi ulnaris. The superficialis and profundus tendons are retracted radially. The flexor carpi ulnaris and ulnar neurovascular structures are retracted ulnarly. The bursa is exposed, opened, and drained. Cultures are taken. Proximal to distal irrigation with a 14- or 16-gauge angiocatheter or No. 5 pediatric feeding tube is performed with 600 to 800 mL of antibiotic-containing normal saline. The irrigation is continued until the distal effluent is clear. Radial bursal infections are treated in the same manner. Our incisions are the same as described under through-and-through treatment.

The incisions are left open. A ¼- to ½-inch Penrose drain is placed in the proximal incision site, placing the drain at the pronator fascia. Distally, a moist gauze wick is used to keep the incision open.

Postoperative Management and Expectations

The postoperative management of bursal infections is the same as that described for flexor tendon sheath infections. We remove the Penrose drain at 24 to 48 hours.

Outcomes after bursal infections are generally not as favorable as for isolated flexor tenosynovitis. Tendon adhe-sions, flexion contracture of the fingers and wrist, and restricted motion are more likely to occur. Tenolysis for recalcitrant adhesions may be necessary if therapy does not adequately restore function.

Deep Space Infections

The hand has three anatomically defined potential spaces and one forearm potential space. These septated spaces lie between muscle fascial planes (Fig. 3-8A). These spaces include the *thenar, midpalmar,* and *hypothenar spaces* in the hand and *Parona's space* in the forearm. There are three more superficial spaces in the hand: the *dorsal subcutaneous space, the dorsal subaponeurotic space,* and the *interdigital web space.* These infections are different from deep space abscesses, because they do not have well-defined anatomic borders. However, they have similar presentations as deep palmar space abscesses.

Palmar Space Infections
Clinical Presentation and Preoperative Evaluation
Both thenar and midpalmar space infections often present as swelling involving the entire hand, particularly on the dorsal side. The tight fascia on the palmar surface of the hand limits the amount of swelling. The more loosely arranged connective tissue dorsally allows greater expansion of the soft tissue in this area. This dorsal swelling should be distinguished from local dorsal abscess and dorsal cellulitis. All of the deep palmar space infections will have areas of palmar swelling and exquisite tenderness localized over the involved palmar space. Hypothenar infections generally have less dorsal swelling.

Preoperative evaluation includes a careful history of mechanism of injury and relevant comorbidities. Laboratory evaluation should include a complete blood cell count. Radiographs should be routinely obtained to evaluate for retained foreign body, underlying osteomyelitis, or fracture. Aspiration or ultrasound may be useful in identifying an abscess. However, if the clinical presentation strongly suggests deep infection, a negative aspirate should not negate surgical exploration.

Thenar Space. An infection of the thenar space may occur from a penetrating injury, from local spread from an adjacent flexor tendon sheath infection of the thumb, index, or long fingers, or from extension of infection from a subcutaneous abscess. It is the most common of the deep palmar space infections (see Fig. 3-8B).

On examination, the thenar region is quite swollen and exquisitely tender to palpation. The potential space becomes filled with purulent material and the cavity becomes engorged. The patient holds the thumb in a widely abducted position to minimize pressure in the abscess cavity. Any attempts to adduct or oppose the thumb cause severe pain. If the infection is not treated at this stage, the abscess usually spreads dorsally over the adductor pollicis and first dorsal interosseous muscles, resulting in a dumbbell or pantaloon abscess configuration. The injection studies by Kanavel[93] demonstrated that the abscess most likely tracks to the dorsum by destruction of the fascia of the adductor pollicis and extension of the abscess between its transverse and oblique heads, traveling into the space between the adductor pollicis and first dorsal interosseous muscle. From this location, it approaches the dorsal subcutaneous tissue on the lateral (radial) border of the first dorsal interosseous muscle. The clinical findings in this case may be more evident in the first dorsal web space. However, this should not be confused with a dorsal subcutaneous abscess.

Midpalmar Space. Midpalmar space infections are uncommon. They most commonly occur as a result of penetrating injury, although rupture of a tendon sheath infection of the long or ring finger into the midpalmar space can occur.

As with most hand infections, dorsal swelling is more evident. The palm is full, firm, and tender. The hallmark of the midpalmar space infection is loss of the normal palmar concavity. The palmar configuration becomes convex (see Fig. 3-8C). The fingers (most predominantly the middle and ring fingers) assume a semi-flexed posture. Although there may be pain with passive extension of the fingers, it is distinctly less than that associated with pyogenic tenosynovitis.

Hypothenar Space. Hypothenar space infections are extremely rare. These infections almost always result from penetrating injury. They may also occur from local spread of adjacent subcutaneous tissue abscesses. The boundaries of the hypothenar space are so separated from the other palmar spaces and bursae that spreading from or to adjacent palmar spaces almost never occurs.

The clinical signs of hypothenar space infection are localized tenderness and swelling of the hypothenar eminence. The absence of swelling in the palm and fingers and the lack of involvement of the flexor tendons help distinguish this infection.

Pertinent Anatomy

The thenar and midpalmar spaces of the hand are located dorsal to the flexor tendons and volar to the metacarpals and interosseous muscle fasciae. They are divided by the midpalmar (oblique) septum, which extends from the palmar fascia to the volar diaphyseal ridge of the third metacarpal.

Thenar Space. The thenar space occupies the area between the thenar eminence and the third metacarpal. The floor (dorsal boundary) of the thenar space is formed by the fascia covering the adductor pollicis muscle. The superficial (volar) boundary is the tendon sheath of the index finger and the palmar fascia. The radial border is defined by the confluence of the adductor pollicis tendon and fascia as they insert on the proximal phalanx of the thumb. The ulnar border is defined by the oblique (vertical midpalmar) septum, which extends from the palmar aspect of the third metacarpal shaft obliquely and radially toward the palmar fascia. The space is limited distally by the deep transverse fascia, one thumb's breadth proximal to the web. Proximally, it is limited by the base of the palm (see Fig. 3-8A).

Midpalmar Space. The midpalmar space occupies the mid palm between the thenar and hypothenar eminence. The floor (dorsal boundary) is formed by the fascia overlying the second and third volar interosseous muscles and the periosteum of the third, fourth, and fifth metacarpals. The superficial (volar) boundary is formed by flexor sheaths of the long, ring, and small fingers and the palmar aponeurosis. The radial border is formed by the oblique (vertical midpalmar) septum. The ulnar border is defined by the hypothenar septum, which extends from the volar ridge of the fifth metacarpal shaft to the palmar aponeurosis. The space is limited distally by vertical septa of the palmar aponeurosis, located approximately one thumb's breadth from the interdigital web spaces. Proximally, it is limited by the base of the palm (see Fig. 3-8A).

Hypothenar Space. The hypothenar space is a small potential area between the hypothenar septum and the hypothenar muscles. The floor (dorsal) boundary is formed by

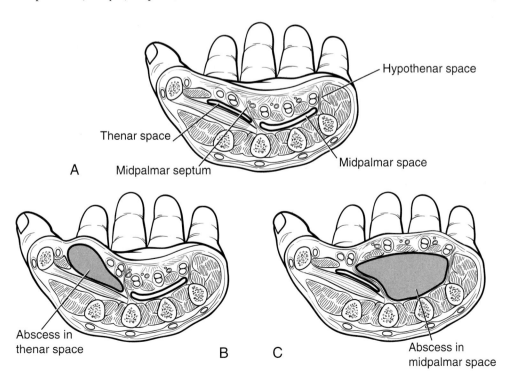

FIGURE 3-8. Deep palmar spaces. **A,** Potential spaces of the mid palm. **B,** Thenar space abscess. **C,** Midpalmar space abscess.

the periosteum of the fifth metacarpal and the fascia of the deep hypothenar muscles. The superficial (volar) boundary is formed by the palmar fascia and fascia of the superficial hypothenar muscles (see Fig. 3-8A).

Treatment

There is no role for nonsurgical management of deep space infections. These should be treated as surgical urgencies. Intravenous antibiotics are started preferably after obtaining a culture either from the site of a draining wound or from an aspirate of the affected palmar space. If the patient cannot be taken immediately to the operating room and cultures cannot be obtained from an aspiration, then antibiotic therapy with good staphylococcal coverage should be initiated.

Thenar Space.   Incisions to drain the thenar space should provide adequate exposure of the affected areas. It is also important to make incisions that will not lead to subsequent contracture. Access to the thenar space requires that an incision be placed near neurovascular structures, specifically, the recurrent motor branch of the median nerve, digital nerves to the thumb and radial side of the index finger, the princeps pollicis artery, and proper digital arteries. Careful dissection is necessary to avoid injury to these structures.

Drainage of the thenar space abscess has been described through dorsal incisions,[93] volar incisions,[13,115] or a combined volar and dorsal approach.[19,25,91,147,148] Kanavel described a dorsal transverse incision.[93] While he reported satisfactory access to both the dorsal and volar components of the thenar space abscess, the transverse scar can lead to contracture of the first web space. Burkhalter used a single incision to combine dorsal and volar approaches. This incision was carried across the first web space. Although providing excellent visualization, the scar across the web can be painful or cause contracture of the web space.[25]

Volar Approach (Thenar Crease).   An incision is made on the palmar surface of the hand just adjacent and parallel to the thenar crease (Fig. 3-9A). The incision begins approx-

imately 1 cm proximal to the web space and continues proximally for 3 to 4 cm. Blunt dissection through the palmar fascia is carried out toward the adductor pollicis muscle until abscess is encountered. In the proximal portion of the deep dissection, particular attention is necessary to protect the motor branch of the median nerve. After the area has been drained adequately, the dissection is extended over the distal edge of the adductor to decompress the first dorsal interosseous space.

Dorsal Transverse Approach.   An incision is made on the dorsum of the first web at the middle of a line between the distal ends of the metacarpals of the thumb and index finger (see Fig. 3-9B). Pus is usually encountered once the incision divides the skin. The approach is deepened between the first dorsal interosseous-adductor interval and volarly over the distal edge of the adductor (if necessary).

Dorsal Longitudinal Approach.   A straight or slightly curved longitudinal incision is made in the dorsum of the first web space, starting proximal to the web and extending perpendicular and proximal to the web, bisecting the interval between the first and second metacarpals (see Fig. 3-9C). The dissection is continued deeper into the interval between the first dorsal interosseous and the adductor pollicis, at which point pus should be encountered.

Combined Dorsal and Volar Approach.   Two incisions are made: one dorsally, which is the slightly curved longitudinal approach described earlier, and one volarly, which parallels the thenar crease. Each approach is used to drain the corresponding half of the space. A separate drain is used for each incision, but through-and-through drains are not used.

Closed Palmar Space Irrigation.   This method was described by Neviaser.[146a,147,148] He uses a combined volar and dorsal approach. A 16-gauge polyethylene catheter is sutured into the palmar wound and the wound closed around it; a drain is sutured into the dorsal wound, which in turn is

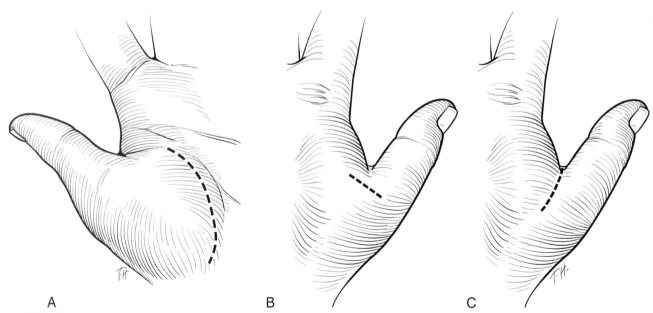

A   B   C

FIGURE 3-9. Incisions for drainage of the thenar space. **A,** Thenar crease approach. **B,** Dorsal transverse approach. **C,** Dorsal longitudinal approach.

nearly closed around it (some opening must be left around the drain to permit egress of the irrigating fluid). The hand is dressed in a compressive dressing with a plaster splint. The catheter is brought out of the dressing and connected to a bottle of sterile isotonic saline. The irrigating fluid runs continuously at the rate of 100 mL/hr for 48 hours. After 2 days the dressing is removed, and if the infection seems to have resolved clinically, the catheter and drain are removed. Active exercise is emphasized. Sutures are removed after 10 to 14 days. The advantages of this technique are the thorough mechanical lavage of the space and that the wound heals by primary intention. This technique requires careful nursing aftercare, and if the egress drain is not working well, there is a chance of developing increased pressure and swelling in the involved area.

Midpalmar Space

Transverse Incision in the Distal Crease. The midpalmar space is drained by a transverse skin incision in or parallel to the distal palmar crease overlying the third and fourth metacarpals (Fig. 3-10A). The nerves and arteries are protected. The flexor tendons of the ring finger are used as a guide to the midpalmar space. The deep dissection is continued longitudinally on either side of these tendons until the abscess is opened.

Combined Transverse and Longitudinal Approach. Boyes described a volar incision parallel to the distal palmar crease beginning at the long finger metacarpal and extending ulnarward and curving proximally along the radial margin of the hypothenar eminence (see Fig. 3-10B). The palmar fascia is divided, and the digital nerves and arteries, as well as the superficial palmar arch, are protected. The flexor tendons of the ring finger guide the deep dissection. Access to the midpalmar space is obtained by deep dissection on either side of these tendons.[19]

Curved Longitudinal Approach. A slightly curved incision is made in the mid palm, beginning just proximal to the distal palmar crease in line with the third ray (see Fig. 3-10C). This extends proximally and slightly ulnarward, parallel to the thenar crease. The palmar fascia is split, and the superficial palmar arch and the digital arteries and nerves are protected. The flexor tendons to the ring finger are identified. The midpalmar space is entered by dissecting on either side of these tendons. This approach was modified by Neviaser, who recommended primary wound closure with continuous catheter irrigation.[147,148] This is similar to the technique described earlier under treatment of thenar closed space irrigation method.

Distal Palmar Approach Through the Lumbrical Canal. This approach was described by Kanavel,[93] not as a routine approach to midpalmar space infection but as treatment for a special circumstance, when a midpalmar space infection involves the lumbrical canal. A longitudinal incision is made on the palmar surface of the third web space (between the middle and ring fingers). It extends from immediately proximal to the web and ends distal to the midpalmar crease. The incision should not cross the crease (see Fig. 3-10D). A

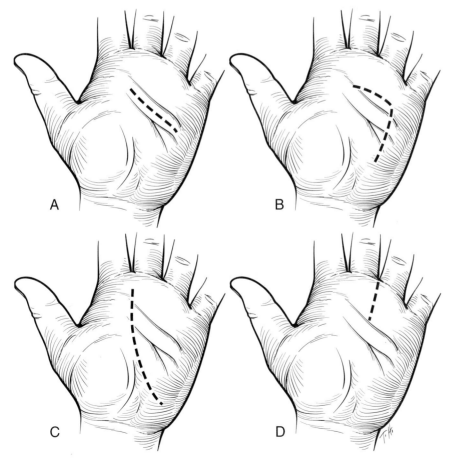

FIGURE 3-10. Incisions for drainage of the midpalmar space. **A,** Transverse incision in the distal crease. **B,** Combined transverse and longitudinal approach. **C,** Curved longitudinal approach. **D,** Distal palmar approach through the lumbrical canal.

clamp is inserted into the wound and directed proximally down the canal of the third lumbrical, dorsal to the flexor tendons, until the midpalmar space is entered and pus is encountered.

Dorsal Approach.   Mann described a dorsal approach to the midpalmar space. A longitudinal incision is made between the middle and ring, or between the ring and small, fingers. Blunt dissection is done above the periosteum on the ulnar side of the third metacarpal or along the radial or ulnar sides of the fourth metacarpal. Dissection is carried down between the metacarpal and interosseous muscles. Below the interosseous muscles lies the midpalmar space.

Hypothenar Space.   The hypothenar space is decompressed through an incision in line with the ulnar border of the ring finger, starting just proximal to the midpalmar crease and continued proximally to 3 cm distal to the wrist flexion crease (Fig. 3-11). The incision is deepened to the level of the hypothenar fascia. This layer is divided in the line of the incision. The abscess should be directly beneath it. After the purulence has been evacuated, a drain is placed in the wound.

Deep Subfascial Space Infections

The deep subfascial spaces include the dorsal subcutaneous space, the dorsal subaponeurotic space, and the interdigital web space. The dorsal subcutaneous space is an extensive area of loose connective tissue without distinct boundaries, in which pus can accumulate over the entire dorsum of the hand. The dorsal subaponeurotic space lies deep to the extensor tendons, above the periosteum of the metacarpals and fascia of the dorsal interosseous muscles. The interdigital web spaces are areas of loose connective tissue between the fingers. Infection in this area tracks both volarly and dorsally and is commonly called a collar-button abscess.

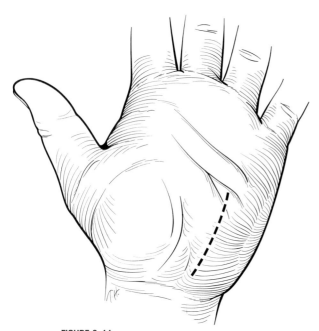

FIGURE 3-11. Approach to the hypothenar space.

Clinical Presentation and Evaluation

Dorsal Subcutaneous and Dorsal Subaponeurotic Space Abscess.   As with most infections of the hand, dorsal subcutaneous and dorsal subaponeurotic space infections typically result from penetrating injuries of the hand. The dorsal aspect of the hand is swollen, warm, and erythematous. The dorsal surface is tender to palpation. Fluctuance may be present. Finger extension may be difficult and is usually painful. Differentiating these infections from cellulitis or other hand infections can be difficult, because most hand infections present with dorsal swelling.

Web Space Abscess (Collar-Button Abscess).   The term *collar-button abscess* refers to the hourglass shape of the abscess and the resemblance to the collar buttons used for dress shirts in the early 1900s.[91] An infection in the web space (collar-button or collar-stud abscess) usually occurs through a fissure in the skin between the fingers, from a distal palmar callus, or from extension of an infection in the subcutaneous area of the proximal segment of a finger. The pain and swelling are localized to the web space and distal area of the palm. The adjacent fingers lie abducted from each other. The swelling may be more prominent on either the palmar or dorsal aspect, depending on the extent and location of the infection. Swelling is often greater on the dorsal side. However, one should not be misled into overlooking the more important volar component of this infection.

The position of finger abduction is helpful in differentiating a collar-button abscess from a dorsal subcutaneous infection. In the dorsal subcutaneous infection, the fingers are not abducted, because there is no purulence tracking between the base of the fingers or palmarly.

Pertinent Anatomy

The dorsal subaponeurotic space is limited on its dorsal surface by the dense aponeurosis of the extensor tendons. On its volar aspect, it is limited by the periosteum of the metacarpals and the dorsal fascia of the interossei. Medially and laterally, the aponeurotic sheet merges with the deep fascia overlying the dorsal interosseous muscles, the periosteum of the first through fifth metacarpals, and the capsules of the first through fifth MP joints. Kanavel described this space as a truncated cone, with the smaller end at the wrist and the larger end toward the MP joints.

The interdigital web spaces consist of the loose areolar connective tissue between the metacarpal heads and around the deep intermetacarpal ligament. The skin of the web space is densely attached to the palmar fascia. A web space infection most commonly begins on the volar surface. The strong attachments of the palmar fascia to the skin limit the volar extension of the abscess. Therefore, the infection track is along the path of least resistance to the dorsal surface.

Treatment

Dorsal Subcutaneous and Subaponeurotic Space Abscess. Exploration of the dorsal subcutaneous and subaponeurotic space can be performed through one or two dorsal longitudinal incisions. The first incision is placed over the longitudinal axis of the index metacarpal. The second incision is placed between the fourth and fifth metacarpals. These incisions allow exploration of the infection to determine if this is a superficial or deep infection. The subaponeurotic space can be opened by incising along the margin of the extensor tendon. Advanced infection often involves both the dorsal subcutaneous and the subaponeurotic space. The use of two incisions allows for good drainage of the abscess cavity, while maintaining soft tissue coverage over the extensor tendons.

Interdigital Web Space (Collar-Button Abscess). There are two important concepts to bear in mind when draining such abscesses. One is that the incision should not be placed across the web space because this will create a contracting scar that can restrict spreading of the fingers. The other is to be alert for the double-abscess configuration. Most authors agree with both dorsal and volar incisions for treatment of these abscesses. There is agreement on the use of a dorsal longitudinal incision. The most commonly described volar incisions are the curved longitudinal[24,25] and the zigzag[91] incision. Both provide access to the volar space.

Curved Longitudinal Incision. The volar incision is begun on the radial side of the affected web space. It is continued proximally and ulnarward, stopping just distal to the midpalmar crease overlying the metacarpal of the ulnar digit involved (see Fig. 3-12A). After the skin is divided, the subcutaneous tissue is spread with a clamp until pus is encountered. The opening in the abscess is enlarged longitudinally. Compression is applied to the dorsum of the web space by the surgeon while the wound is retracted. Increased drainage can be seen in the depth of the wound if there is a deep collar-button abscess.

A second incision is then made on the dorsum. It begins just proximal to the MP joints and lies between the metacarpal heads. It is extended distally in a straight line to end at the base of the involved web, a distance of 1 to 1.5 cm (Fig. 3-12D). The deep tissues are divided in a plane toward the palmar abscess. When the dorsal collection is entered,

the opening is enlarged in the direction of the wound. After the pus has been evacuated and the wound irrigated, gauze wicks are placed into both wounds.

One modification of this approach is a longitudinal volar incision between the metacarpals, but this provides less adequate exposure to the volar aspect of the abscess.

Volar Zigzag Approach. A zigzag incision is made on the palmar surface, starting just proximal to the web and stopping just distal to the midpalmar crease (see Fig. 3-12B). The flaps are reflected and the deep tissues dissected in the web while the digital arteries and nerves are retracted to either side. The superficial transverse metacarpal ligament and other fibers of the palmar fascia are divided to allow ample exposure of the volar and dorsal compartments of the dumbbell-shaped abscess. A 1.5-cm dorsal longitudinal incision is made between the bases of the proximal phalanges. Generous communication between the two incisions is established.

Neviaser used this method combined with primary wound closure and continuous catheter irrigation through a 16-gauge polyethylene catheter, allowing for fluid egress through a dorsally placed Penrose drain.[147,148]

Zigzag incisions provide excellent exposure for drainage of infection; but if they are left open, the flaps can retract and cause thick or tender scars. Therefore, if this incision is used, we recommend that the tips be tacked back into place with a single suture, leaving the remainder of the incision open.

Volar Transverse Approach. Kanavel described a volar transverse incision placed parallel with the distal flexion crease of the palm over the site of maximum swelling (see Fig. 3-12C). He believed this was generally adequate for drainage and did not require a second incision.[93] The deep dissection is as previously described. The dorsal approach

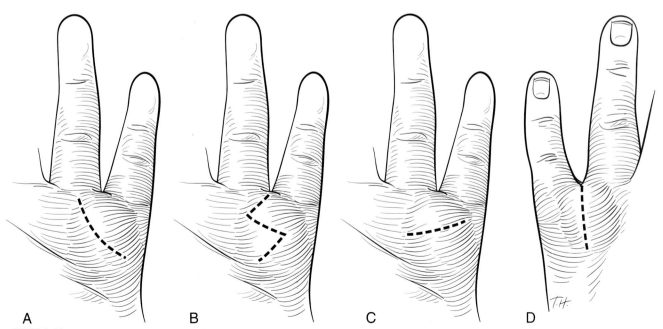

FIGURE 3-12. Incisions for web space abscesses (collar-button abscesses). **A,** Curved longitudinal incision. **B,** Volar zigzag approach. **C,** Volar transverse approach. **D,** Dorsal incision used in conjunction with any of the volar exposures.

may be needed as well. One potential disadvantage of this incision is placement of the transverse limb too far distally. If this part of the incision is inadvertently carried too close to the web, a web space contracture can result.

Parona's Space

Parona's space is a deep potential space in the distal volar forearm. It lies between the fascia of the pronator quadratus and the sheath of the FDP tendons. It is in continuity with the midpalmar space. Although infections of Parona's space most commonly result from extension of infection from either the radial or ulnar bursae, it is not in direct continuity with these bursae. Rupture of these bursae from infection lead to involvement of Parona's space. Isolated infection of Parona's space can occur after a penetrating injury.

Infections of Parona's space present as swelling, tenderness, and occasionally fluctuance in the distal volar forearm. Digital flexion is often difficult and painful. Surgical treatment is necessary for these infections. For isolated Parona space infections, we prefer the incision described for the treatment of the radial bursa. Only the proximal incision is necessary. In cases in which there is associated midpalmar infection, an extended carpal tunnel incision is necessary to drain both midpalmar and Parona spaces.

 ## Authors' Preferred Method of Treatment

Thenar Space. Our preferred method of treatment for the thenar space infections is through combined dorsal and volar approaches, as described earlier. We have found that a single volar incision is not adequate to address the dorsal abscess cavity between the adductor and first dorsal interosseous muscle. Similarly, a single dorsal incision, whether it is transverse or longitudinal, can provide access to the volar abscess, but it is more difficult and we have not been satisfied with our ability to adequately decompress and irrigate the involved space. We leave the wounds open, using a moist gauze wick. We occasionally use a Penrose drain on the volar side for large areas of abscess.

Midpalmar Space. Midpalmar space infections are treated as described earlier under the curved longitudinal approach. This method provides the best exposure of the midpalmar space. It is less likely to result in a severe scar contracture, because it lies adjacent to an anatomic crease. It is an extensile incision and can be used to simultaneously access the thenar space if necessary. We leave the incisions

---

CRITICAL POINTS: DEEP SPACE INFECTIONS

INDICATION

- Thenar, midpalmar, and collar-button abscesses

ETIOLOGY

- Penetrating injury is most common source of infection.

PREOPERATIVE EVALUATION

- Clinical examination is the hallmark of diagnosis.
- Aspiration is useful but can be misleading.
- Radiographs are necessary to evaluate for foreign body or fracture.
- MRI is rarely indicated but may help with early diagnosis of midpalmar space infection.

PEARLS

- Thenar space infections present as wide abduction of the thumb and difficulty with opposition.
- Midpalmar space infections result in loss of palmar concavity. Fingers are semi-flexed.
- Collar-button abscesses are distinguished by abduction of adjacent fingers.
- Urgent surgical treatment, especially in a patient with diabetes or immunocompromise, reduces the morbidity associated with this infection.

TECHNICAL POINTS

- Two incisions are required for thenar space infections. Use caution for the motor recurrent branch of median nerve.
- Single volar midpalmar incision. Use caution for superficial arch and digital nerves. Deep to the midpalmar space, pay attention to the deep palmar arch and motor branch of ulnar nerve.
- Two incisions are required for collar-button abscess. Do not incise across the web space.
- Use wick to keep incisions open.

PITFALLS

- Delayed surgical treatment
- Inadequate decompression
- Injury of the digital neurovascular structures

POSTOPERATIVE CARE

- Intravenous antibiotics
- Pain management to allow early range of motion
- First dressing change between 8 and 12 hours
- Soaks in dilute povidone-iodine solution three times per day
- Repeat débridement and irrigation in 48 hours if symptoms not improving

open using a moist gauze wick as described earlier. Healing by secondary intention occurs rapidly, provided the infection is well controlled and necrotic tissue has been removed.

Interdigital Web Space (Collar-Button Abscess).   We use both a dorsal and volar approach to treat these infections. Our preferred incision is the curved longitudinal incision. We find that this incision provides excellent exposure of the abscess, reduces the risk of skin edge necrosis, and provides easier access for wound management.

Postoperative Management and Expectations

We use the same general principles of management for all deep space infections. Postoperatively, the wounds are left open. A wet gauze sponge is placed into the wounds to allow continued drainage. A bulky dressing is applied. The hand is elevated, and the patient is continued on intravenous antibiotics. The first dressing change should be done at 12 to 24 hours. At this time the patient begins soaking in a dilute solution of povidone-iodine, as described earlier. Early motion is initiated. Therapist supervision may be necessary. Specific to dorsal subcutaneous and dorsal subaponeurotic space infections, we emphasize simultaneous three-joint digital flexion and wrist flexion. This is followed by active extension. This maintains the greatest excursion of the extensor tendons throughout healing. Moist gauze wicks are used to keep the wounds open in the first 72 hours. Splinting between dressing changes may be necessary for thenar and midpalmar space infections for up to 1 week. In general, we believe that active motion is necessary to allow tendons to glide and joints to move and thus reduce the problems of stiffness and contracture. Intravenous antibiotics are continued for 14 to 21 days. After this, oral antibiotics are continued to complete a 4-week course of therapy.

If the clinical signs of infection are not improving in the first 24 to 36 hours, the patient is returned to the operating room for a repeat irrigation and débridement. Repeat cultures are obtained, and organism-specific intravenous therapy is continued. Biopsy to diagnose fungal or atypical infections provides useful information more quickly than fungal and mycobacterial cultures. A low threshold for return to the operating room should be used in diabetics and immunocompromised patients.

Deep space infections are more likely to develop scarring and stiffness of the hand and fingers. With adequate treatment and rehabilitation, 70% to 80% of patients achieve full recovery. Most patients are able to return to their previous occupation.

Complications associated with deep space infections include stiffness and contracture. Extensor lag has been reported after dorsal subcutaneous and dorsal subaponeurotic space infections. Skin necrosis either dorsally or volarly can lead to exposed tendons or neurovascular structures. These problems may require secondary procedures for soft tissue coverage and contracture release. Tendon necrosis is less common with deep space infections but can occur, particularly on the extensor surface when there is significant soft tissue loss. Painful scar formation along the incision is reduced by proper placement of the incisions and postoperative management with desensitization, scar massage, and early motion.[120]

Nerve injury is uncommon but can occur during treatment. Infection causes soft tissue necrosis and distorts the local anatomy. This can lead to inadvertent placement of the surgical incision. It may be difficult to recognize a nerve or vessel within an ocean of pus and necrotic tissue.

Septic Arthritis

Septic arthritis is characterized by the presence of a purulent exudate within the closed confines of a joint. It is caused by the introduction and proliferation of pyogenic bacteria within the synovium in concentrations greater than 10^5 organisms/mL with subsequent production of a purulent exudate.[58] Inoculation of the joint usually occurs from penetrating trauma. *S. aureus* and streptococcal species are the most common organisms. Gram-negative, anaerobic, and mixed infections also occur, especially in the immunocompromised host. Expedient treatment is important to minimize articular destruction caused by infection.

Clinical Presentation and Patient Evaluation

Abscess within the joint cavity represents a cellular and immunogenic response within the synovium and reticuloendothelial system. Bacteria replicate within the joint cavity, producing toxins. This stimulates an immunogenic response. The responding leukocytes produce bactericidal enzymes that destroy the proteoglycan matrices and collagen of hyaline cartilage. Lymphocytes and related cells form immune complexes, which also can degrade articular surfaces. As the inflammatory response continues, there is increased pressure within the joint. This forces the joint into a position of maximum potential volume, producing pseudoparalysis. The increased volume within the joint further damages the articular cartilage through pressure necrosis. Untreated, pus under pressure may erode through the joint capsule and overlying skin. Alternatively, it may erode into the subchondral bone, resulting in osteomyelitis.[58,141,145]

Patients generally present with a history of penetrating trauma, which may occur from bites, splinters, thorns, hooks, needles, or any of a variety of penetrating injuries. The source of the injury is important in selecting empirical antibiotic therapy for the presumptive infecting organisms. Contiguous spread from an adjacent infection can occur. In the DIP joint other common mechanisms of occurrence are from infection or direct inoculation of a mucous cyst or from contiguous spread from a felon, paronychia, or purulent flexor tenosynovitis. In the PIP joint, contiguous spread is most commonly related to a purulent flexor tenosynovitis. At the MP joint, infection from a clenched fist injury is frequently encountered. Hematogenous spread, although uncommon, has been reported and is more common in immunocompromised patients.[145,152]

The clinical findings associated with a septic arthritis are swelling, redness, warmth, and pain around the affected joint. Both active and passive motion produce exquisite pain. Fluctuance within the joint may be demonstrated by ballottement. Systemic signs such as fever, chills, tachycardia, malaise, sweats, and rash may be present. The presence of systemic symptoms suggest hematogenous seeding and should alert the physician to look for a primary source of infection.[114,145,206]

Evaluation of the patient should address any history of penetrating trauma, insect, or animal bite, previous therapeutic joint injection or aspiration, or the possibility of retained foreign body. History of immunocompromising conditions or inflammatory conditions that may mimic joint sepsis should be obtained. Many inflammatory conditions can present as an acutely swollen and painful joint of the wrist and hand. These include gout, pseudogout, rheumatoid arthritis, systemic lupus erythematosus, psoriatic arthritis, acute rheumatic fever, sarcoidosis, and Reiter's syndrome. In the case of possible hematogenously spread infection, a careful review of systems may reveal the primary location.

Laboratory evaluation should include white blood cell (WBC) count, ESR, and CRP. The WBC count is elevated in less than half of patients. The ESR and CRP are consistently elevated in nonimmunocompromised patients. Blood cultures should be taken, particularly when systemic symptoms are present. History and clinical examination should direct culture of potential distant primary sources, such as urine, urethra, or oropharynx.

Aspiration of small joints may be difficult. Radiocarpal joint aspiration is more easily performed and can differentiate acute infection from other inflammatory processes, provided that the overlying skin is not cellulitic. The aspiration is performed through the dorsal skin, 1 cm distal to Lister's tubercle. An 18-gauge needle is introduced and directed proximally to accommodate the normal palmar tilt of the distal radius. If fluid is not easily obtained, 1 to 2 mL of sterile saline can be injected into the joint and then aspirated for analysis. The aspirate should be sent for Gram stain and aerobic and anaerobic culture. If adequate aspirate is available, cell count, fluid protein and glucose levels, and fungal and mycobacterial cultures should be obtained. The WBC count from the aspirate of more than 50,000/mm[3] suggests joint sepsis. A lower WBC count with a high percentage of polymorphonuclear cells (>90%) can indicate an early joint infection. A high WBC count (>90,000/mm[3]), regardless of the percentage of polymorphonuclear cells, should be treated as an acute infection. Synovial fluid glucose value of 40 mg/dL or less than the fasting blood glucose level also supports a septic process.[141]

Radiographs are useful to evaluate for retained foreign body, osteomyelitis, or gas within the joint or soft tissues indicating clostridial or other anaerobic infection. Initially, radiographs may show joint capsular distention and periarticular soft tissue swelling. Joint space narrowing on radiographs is seen as a late sequela of septic arthritis. Radioactive isotope bone scan is rarely necessary but may be helpful in localizing and diagnosing early cases.

Treatment

Septic arthritis of the hand is treated as a surgical emergency. Articular destruction from proteolytic enzymes and toxins that degrade glycosaminoglycans begins in the first 24 hours of infection. The principle of treatment for all septic joints is prompt surgical drainage. Serial aspiration has been proposed as a form of treatment for septic joint. In the hand and wrist, aspiration is useful diagnostically but therapeutically unpredictable.[58,141,145] Leslie and colleagues reported superior results with formal arthrotomy of the shoulder joint over serial aspiration. The same principle applies to the hand, where serial aspiration of small joints is more difficult and less reliable.[109]

Radiocarpal Joint

Arthrotomy of the radiocarpal joint is accomplished through the standard dorsal approach to the wrist joint. This is done through a longitudinal incision centered slightly ulnar to Lister's tubercle. The retinaculum between the third and fourth extensor compartments is opened. The extensor pollicis longus tendon is identified and retracted radially. The underlying joint capsule is exposed. The capsule can be opened longitudinally or with a "T" incision. Although the ligament sparing incision described by Berger and Bishop is an excellent approach to the wrist joint,[9] in the case of sepsis a longitudinal or "T-capsular" incision provides adequate exposure of the joint and can more easily be left open to allow continued drainage. Culture of the joint fluid is obtained. The joint is copiously irrigated with gravity irrigation or bulb syringe. Pulsed lavage is not used because this can cause additional soft tissue injury. The joint is taken through flexion and extension during the irrigation to maximize removal of purulent material. Articular surfaces are inspected for discoloration, areas of thinning, or softness. Necrotic tissue and inflammatory synovium are sharply removed. Synovial tissue should be sent for culture and histology. At the completion of irrigation, the joint capsule is left open. A gauze wick is placed down into the capsule to maintain a path for continuous drainage. Alternatively, the capsule may be closed over a drain. The skin incision is left open. One or two loosely placed sutures can be used to keep the skin edges from retracting. If the skin edges are markedly retracted, Steri-Strips can be placed to gently approximate the skin edges as the swelling decreases. A transverse skin incision can also be used to approach the joint, which results in a more cosmetic scar with less skin edge retraction. However, it is not extensile and may not provide adequate exposure in all circumstances.

Arthroscopic débridement and lavage of the infected radiocarpal joint may be a useful alternative to open débridement.[145] Viewing and working portals are established; usually the 3-4 portal is used for viewing and for fluid ingress. The working portal may be the 6R or the 4-5. An 18-gauge needle attached to intravenous tubing can be placed in the 6U portal for additional fluid egress. The efficacy of arthroscopic treatment of infection for larger joints such as the knee and shoulder has been shown. The efficacy of this method in the wrist has yet to be established. If the signs of infection are not improving in the first 24 hours, a formal open arthrotomy should be performed.

Metacarpophalangeal Joint

The MP joint can be opened through a dorsal longitudinal or dorsal curvilinear incision. If a wound is present, the incision is designed to incorporate the wound and to excise the wound margins. The skin flaps are elevated, and the extensor mechanism is defined. The joint capsule is exposed either through longitudinal splitting of the extensor tendon hood or through an incision in the sagittal band adjacent to the tendon. The MP joint capsule is often thin and inadvertently opened through the same incision. Once the joint is open, it is copiously irrigated with saline. Longitudinal traction opens the joint space and allows better access of the irrigant to the volar recesses of the joint. The joint should be carefully inspected for any articular surface damage or retained foreign body, especially in the scenario of MP joint infection resulting from a clenched fist injury, described later under human bite injuries. The joint capsule and wounds are left open and covered with a moist gauze dressing.

Proximal Interphalangeal Joint

Arthrotomy of the PIP joints is performed through a mid-axial incision. This incision avoids exposure of and injury to the central extensor tendon slip. The midaxial incision is placed from the distal margin of the interdigital web space and continued in the midaxial line to the level of the DIP joint. In the index finger, the incision is preferentially placed on the ulnar side of the finger. In the small finger, the incision is placed on the radial side. The central two digits can be accessed through either radial or ulnar incisions. If this approach is used for the thumb MP or interphalangeal (IP) joints, a radial incision is preferred. When the incision is correctly placed, the proper digital nerves lie protected in the volar skin flap (Fig. 3-13A). However, the dorsal sensory branch of the digital nerves can be jeopardized by this approach. The transverse retinacular ligament is incised, exposing the collateral ligament complex. The PIP joint is entered by excision of the accessory collateral ligament (see Fig. 3-13B), followed by capsulectomy. Alternatively, the joint may be exposed through subperiosteal elevation of the proximal origin of the collateral ligament. The joint is thoroughly débrided and irrigated. Inspection of the articular surfaces may be difficult through this incision, but a blunt probe or Freer elevator can be used to palpate the cartilage for areas of erosion or softening. The capsule and wounds are left open and covered with a moist gauze dressing.

Wittels and associates described a combined radial and ulnar midaxial incision for drainage. In conjunction with their functional rehabilitation, this provided very satisfactory results.[220] A dorsal arthrotomy is sometimes necessary, owing to the presence of a dorsal wound. In these cases, the central extensor slip and dorsal capsule are often injured or disrupted. This frequently leads to the development of a septic boutonnière deformity. When a septic PIP joint is encoun-

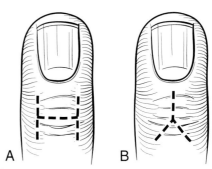

FIGURE 3-14. Dorsal approach to the DIP joint. **A,** "H" incision. **B,** Reverse "Y" or Mercedes incision.

tered in this setting, the wound is extended proximally and distally. The arthrotomy and capsulectomy are performed adjacent to the central slip, if it is intact.

Distal Interphalangeal Joint

The DIP joint is opened through a dorsal "H" incision or through a dorsal reverse "Y" or Mercedes incision (Fig. 3-14). Skin flaps are elevated over the terminal extensor tendon. The terminal tendon is retracted to the side, and a capsule is opened. It is important to protect the tendon insertion, because injury can result in a mallet finger deformity. Alternatively, the midaxial incision as described for PIP joint arthrotomy can be extended distally and used to expose the DIP joint. The collateral ligament is excised to gain access to the joint. This approach may be more useful when there is an associated flexor tendon sheath infection. The joint should be adequately débrided and irrigated. The wounds are left open.

Postoperative Management and Expectations

Surgical incisions are left open, with a gauze wick to maintain patency of the capsulotomy and allow for continued wound drainage. Moist gauze dressing changes three times per day prevent encrustation of the wound, which results in premature wound closure. Early range of motion is critical to postoperative treatment. This provides mechanical lavage of the joint and reduces the accumulation of pus within the joint.[120,218,220] We prefer that patients soak the affected hand in a dilute solution of povidone-iodine, as described previously. Active, active-assisted, and passive range of motion is done during the soaking period.

Empirical intravenous antibiotic therapy is started immediately after obtaining a culture from either an aspirate or surgical culture. Antibiotic selection is then tailored to treat the bacterial pathogen. There is some controversy regarding the duration of antibiotic therapy necessary for septic arthritis. Previous recommendations have included duration of therapy between 3 and 4 weeks. More recent recommendations use shorter courses of intravenous therapy, switching to oral antibiotics after 10 to 14 days. Oral antibiotics are continued to complete a 4- to 6-week course of therapy. We agree with others that intravenous antibiotic therapy should be continued through symptom resolution, followed by oral antibiotics for 4 to 6 weeks. Duration of antibiotic therapy should be based on surgical findings, pathogen virulence, and clinical response to treatment. If clinical improvement is not seen within the first 24 to 48 hours, repeat surgical irrigation and débridement should be considered. Amputation

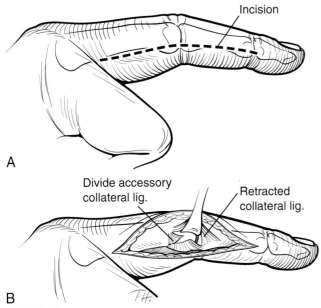

Incision

Divide accessory collateral lig.

Retracted collateral lig.

FIGURE 3-13. Lateral approach to the PIP joint. **A,** Skin incision. **B,** Arthrotomy is performed through the lateral ligamentous complex, dividing the accessory collateral ligament.

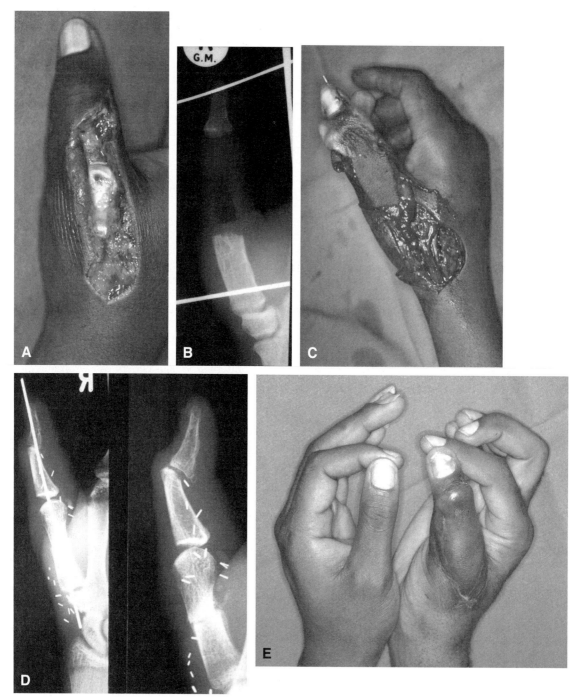

FIGURE 3-15. A 27-year-old man sustained a bite injury to his thumb during an assault. He developed a severe infection of the thumb MP joint, with subsequent spread to the metacarpal head and proximal phalanx. The volar soft tissue, flexor tendon, and neurovascular structures were intact. **A,** Open draining wound with exposed metacarpal head and necrotic proximal phalanx. **B,** Radiograph taken after resection of all necrotic bone. **C,** A free vascularized second toe transfer was used to reconstruct the bone defect, extensor pollicis longus tendon, and soft tissue defect. **D,** Radiographs immediately after surgery with Kirschner wire stabilization and at 1-year follow-up. **E,** Appearance and function of the reconstructed thumb at 1-year follow-up. There is no evidence of recurrent infection. (See also Color Figure 3-15A and C.)

may be necessary if an infection cannot be eradicated, or if an affected finger has a significant negative impact on overall hand function.[19,192] Every effort should be made to preserve the thumb, even if arthrodesis, shortening, or reconstruction is required (Fig. 3-15).

Symptom resolution and functional outcome after septic arthritis are correlated with the duration of symptoms before the initiation of treatment.[64,161] Some degree of joint stiffness is expected. In one study, only 13 of 33 infections of the PIP joint treated with early surgical decompression achieved full restoration of motion.[220] Early mobilization reduces the degree of postoperative stiffness but cannot reverse the changes that have occurred in the articular cartilage resulting from sepsis. Joint space narrowing is generally seen after completion of treatment. Joint arthrosis and ankylosis occur in cases in which the presentation or treatment has been delayed.

Complications associated with septic arthritis in the hand and wrist include stiffness of the affected and adjacent joints. Tendon adhesions associated with the swelling and inflammation caused by the infection or resulting from the surgical incision also occur and may require secondary surgery. Osteomyelitis of the adjacent bones may complicate or prolong the course of treatment. Additional surgical débridement, bone resection, resection arthroplasty, or amputation may be necessary. Late complications included arthrosis and arthritis. Salvage of the postinfectious arthritis may include arthrodesis, resection arthroplasty, or amputation. Implant arthroplasty in previously infected joints of the hand is very controversial. At the present time, most authors do not favor this treatment.

Septic Boutonnière Deformity

Unique complications of septic arthritis occur at the PIP and DIP joints. Septic boutonnière deformity is a complication of pyogenic arthritis of the PIP joint. It occurs in those cases in which a virulent organism has caused rapid tissue destruction or where there has been late presentation or treatment. The intra-articular collection of purulence has reached a volume that can no longer be retained within the joint. The path of least resistance for escape is dorsally. The joint is well supported palmarly by the volar plate, which blends with the accessory collateral ligaments, and by the collateral ligaments on the sides. All these structures are thick and unyielding; therefore, the pus escapes dorsally through the thin dorsal capsule. There, it can destroy the extensor mechanism over the dorsum of the joint. The central slip is attenuated or eroded, allowing the lateral bands to slip volarward. This results in a classic boutonnière deformity. Management of this problem is difficult. However, the first priority is eradication of the joint infection. Treatment of the boutonnière deformity is addressed *after* the infection is controlled.

If the boutonnière deformity is due to attenuation of the extensor mechanism, joint function is often salvageable. In these cases, the extensor tendon can be reefed or tightened to bring the lateral bands more dorsal. The PIP joint should be kept splinted in full extension for 6 weeks postoperatively. Compliance with full-time extension must be emphasized to the patient. Free motion is encouraged at the MP and DIP joints. If early joint motion is believed to be more critical to functional recovery, late boutonnière reconstruction can be done when the infection is resolved and the joint is supple.

If the PIP joint is significantly damaged, arthrodesis of the joint is the best treatment option. When the integrity of the joint has been maintained with good articular cartilage but there is a loss of the central slip, then late boutonnière reconstruction can be done after maximum passive joint mobility has been restored with appropriate hand therapy (see Chapter 6).

Mallet finger deformity can occur after DIP joint sepsis. The mechanism of injury is similar to that which occurs in the PIP joint. The terminal extensor tendon is attenuated or destroyed. DIP joint fusion is the most appropriate treatment.

Osteomyelitis

Osteomyelitis is an infection of the bone. Traditionally, it has been believed that once the bone has been infected, it remains infected: "Once an osteo, always an osteo." In the hand, it may be possible to eradicate infection, because amputation can remove the involved digit or portion of the digit. Additionally, with the introduction of microvascular reconstruction, adequate bone débridement can be undertaken with less risk of causing permanent structural and severe functional loss. In the hand, osteomyelitis is rare, likely owing to the hand's abundant vascular supply. It has been reported to represent between 1% and 6% of all hand infections.[58,82,134,163] When present, it is often related to adjacent soft tissue or joint infection. The most commonly involved bone is the distal phalanx.[5,58,163]

Osteomyelitis can occur after penetrating trauma, crush injuries, contiguous spread from adjacent soft tissue infections, and hematogenous seeding, and in the postsurgical setting. Penetrating trauma is the most common etiology for osteomyelitis.[5,114,163] Patients with immunocompromise, vascular impairment, and systemic illness are especially susceptible to develop osteomyelitis. Contributing factors to traumatic injuries that result in osteomyelitis include the environment in which the injury occurred and the resultant degree of contamination and the extent of soft tissue injury and devitalization.

Although most infections of bone are caused from penetrating trauma, hematogenous infections occur. Hematogenous spread of infection to the hand is rare. It is more likely to occur in children. In one study, only 1 of 62 cases of hematogenous osteomyelitis occurred in the hand. Reilly and colleagues reported a 13% incidence in their series. Of those patients, half were immunocompromised.[163] The susceptibility to infection in the long bones in children is believed to result from the vascular arrangement around the growth plate. The long capillary loops and venous sinusoids in the metaphysis adjacent to the growth plate have a tortuous course, leading to turbulent and sluggish blood flow. These capillary loops are actually terminal branches possessing gaps that allow blood cells and bacteria to pass into the extravascular space. Once in this space, the pathogen may proliferate, causing infection. Contributing to this process is the relative acellularity of this space, decreased oxygen tension, and suboptimal phagocytic activity.[5,58,85,211] Until the age of 1 year, there is vascular continuity between the metaphysis and epiphysis via the epiphyseal plate arteries. In infants, this can lead to the spread of infection from the metaphysis into the epiphysis and subsequently into the joint space. After the age of 1 year, the epiphyseal plate capillaries obliterate. This reduces the likelihood of contiguous spread of hematogenous osteomyelitis into the joint space.[5,85,205]

Acute infections after closed fractures are extremely rare,[80,200] but open fractures of the hand can result in deep infection. McLain and colleagues[134] reported an incidence of deep infection in 11% of patients. Factors associated with infection included grossly contaminated wounds and extensive soft tissue and skeletal injury. *S. aureus* was the dominant organism in only 30% of patients. Polymicrobial infections and enteric organisms were significant pathogens in more than 60% of cultures. Fixation of open or closed fractures with Kirschner wires can lead to a local osteomyelitis along the pin track. The incidence of pin track infection has been reported between 0.5% and 5%.[17,189]

The most common organisms responsible for osteomyelitis are *S. aureus* and other skin organisms. Coagulase-negative *Staphylococcus* is commonly associated with infections of implants, such as hardware used for internal fixation after a fracture. Many other organisms have been isolated and reported in the literature. Often the mechanism of injury and the environment in which the injury occurred may suggest a different infecting pathogen. For example, a penetrating injury from an animal bite would lead to empirical treatment for *Pasteurella multocida,* until definitive culture results are available.

Classification of osteomyelitis was refined by Cierny and Mader in 1985.[35,150] This classification applies to long bones and describes four anatomic sites of infection and three physiologic classes of host, defining 12 clinical types of osteomyelitis (anatomic site + physiologic class).

Anatomic Site

Type I: Medullary osteomyelitis. The infection is limited to the endosteum. Most commonly this is associated with hematogenous etiology. However, it can also be associated with intramedullary fracture fixation.

Type II: Superficial osteomyelitis. The infection involves the surface of the bone. The overlying soft tissue is deficient.

Type III: Localized infection. Both medullary and superficial characteristics are combined. Full-thickness sequestrum is present.

Type IV: Diffuse infection. The infection diffusely involves the bone. Instability of the bone is present either from the infection or the result of necessary débridement.

Physiologic Class (Host Characteristics)

A Host: Normal host with good immune system
B Host: Local or systemic compromise

C Host: Markedly compromised host. Treatment of the disease is worse than the disease itself.

Some of the factors that lead to a compromised host include systemic illnesses such as diabetes, liver or renal disease, malnutrition, malignancy, smoking, connective tissue disease, and peripheral vascular disease. Local compromise can occur from scarring, radiation, sensory compromise, lymphedema, and major vessel disease. All these factors can result in poor wound healing and difficulty in controlling infection.[5,35,150,206]

Clinical Presentation and Evaluation

Local clinical signs of infection often include redness, swelling, warmth, and tenderness. Fluctuance and/or drainage may be present. Findings depend in part on the etiology of the bone infection. When the osteomyelitis is resultant from contiguous spread of infection, it is frequently difficult to differentiate bone infection from soft tissue infection, as might be seen in a felon. Systemic clinical signs such as fever, chills, and malaise are more commonly seen in hematogenous osteomyelitis or in children. Waldvogel and colleagues reported that all patients with osteomyelitis of the hand had local signs of inflammation, but only one third of patients had fever and leukocytosis.[212] The presence of systemic symptoms should alert the examiner to the possibility of a remote source of infection. Failure of an apparent soft tissue infection to respond to appropriate treatment should suggest the diagnosis of an underlying osteomyelitis.[5,82]

Laboratory studies should include a WBC count, ESR, CRP, and blood culture. ESR and CRP are also useful in monitoring the response to treatment. CRP normalizes more rapidly than does ESR. Both levels increase in the first 48 hours after surgery.[154]

Radiographic findings are present in less than 5% of cases of acute osteomyelitis. Soft tissue swelling is one of the first radiographic findings. Metaphyseal rarefaction, osteopenia, osteosclerosis, and periosteal reaction are not noted until 2 to 3 weeks after the onset of infection[67] (Fig. 3-16). A not

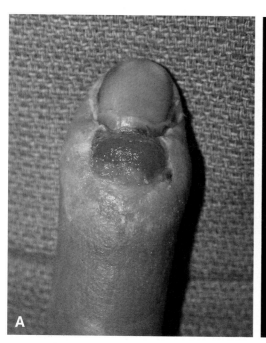

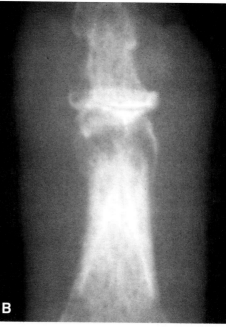

FIGURE 3-16. Osteomyelitis of the middle finger as a complication of pyarthrosis of the DIP joint. **A,** Granulation tissue overlying the DIP joint. **B,** Radiograph shows characteristic metaphyseal rarefaction and osteopenia. (See also Color Figure 3-16**A**.)

uncommon cause of osteomyelitis in the hand is the presence of dead bone. One should therefore always look on the radiograph for a fragment (often tiny) of bone with increased density.

Advanced imaging studies such as technetium-, gallium-, and indium-labeled WBC scans can be useful in identifying acute osteomyelitis. These studies are useful in the early stages of infection, when standard radiographs are normal.[45,67,213] Magnetic resonance imaging (MRI) can be a very useful study in the early presentation of osteomyelitis, owing to the contrast it generally provides between the abnormal and normal bone marrow. It should, however, be reserved for patients with inconclusive findings or as an aid in surgical planning. The sensitivity of MRI in the diagnosis of osteomyelitis has been reported between 82% and 100%.[18]

Aspiration may be useful diagnostically. Subperiosteal pus may be present, typically in the pediatric patient. If pus is not obtained adjacent to bone, metaphyseal aspiration can identify the offending pathogen and direct antibiotic therapy. A negative aspirate should not stop further investigation or suspicion of bone infection.

Treatment

Early diagnosis and treatment lead to an improved functional outcome. Both surgical and medical treatment are necessary. Adequate surgical débridement is critical to eradication of infection. Débridement of necrotic soft tissue and decompression and curettage of necrotic bone are mandatory. Repeat débridement and culture are necessary when clinical improvement is not seen in the first 72 hours. Wounds are left open, even though this may leave exposed bone, tendon, or implant. It is better to plan bone and soft tissue reconstruction once the infection is controlled than to inadequately débride the wound or to attempt a primary closure. Treatment of osteomyelitis of the distal phalanx or of a single finger, particularly osteomyelitis associated with septic arthritis, may be best managed with amputation.[5,19,58,163]

Osteomyelitis can occur in the setting of an acute fracture. This may be a pin track infection or a deep infection around hardware. Pin track infections can often be managed with oral antibiotics and local wound and pin care. However, if the infection cannot be controlled, removal of the pins may be necessary. Management of deep infections around implanted hardware depends on the stage of fracture healing, host factors, and the stability of fixation. In a healthy patient with stable fixation, it is usually preferable to control the infection with débridement and intravenous or oral antibiotics until the fracture is healed adequately to allow hardware removal. If this cannot be achieved, hardware removal and removal of all necrotic bone and tissue is necessary. Provisional stabilization with an external fixator or with an antibiotic impregnated methylmethacrylate spacer is used until the infection is controlled. Late reconstruction is planned based on the structural and functional deficits.

Prolonged intravenous antibiotic therapy is continued for 4 to 6 weeks and is based on the organism identified at surgical débridement and antibiotic sensitivity. Oral antibiotics that achieve therapeutic levels in bone can be used in conjunction with intravenous therapy. Resistant organisms are seen with increasing frequency. An infec-tious disease specialist is an invaluable resource in managing this problem.

Complications

Complications of acute osteomyelitis are common. Pain stiffness, deformity, and loss of strength frequently persist despite successful treatment and eradication of infection. Chronic pain and cold intolerance has also been described, particularly in patients with vascular insufficiency.[5] Fracture nonunion or malunion is not infrequent. Infection that requires amputation may result in a functional deficit. However, it is often less debilitating than preservation of a stiff and painful finger. Unresolved acute infection leads to chronic osteomyelitis and the complications associated with this process.

SPECIFIC TYPES OF INFECTIONS AND VECTORS

Animal Bites

Domestic animal bites by dogs and cats are common. Over 1 million dog bites are reported annually and represent 90% of all animal bites.[60,188,217] In more than 70% of cases, the dog is known to the victim.[60,68,69] Children younger than age 12 account for 50% of all dog bite injuries. Cat bites are less common and estimated at 5% of animal bite injuries. The remaining 5% include various domestic and wild animal bites.[68,69,186]

Of the multiple organisms cultured from the dog mouth, the more common pathogens include *S. aureus, Streptococcus viridans, Bacteroides,* and *Pasteurella multocida.* Similar flora is found in the cat mouth.[44,60,186,201] Cultures often show a polymicrobial infection.[44,60,69,77,186,201,217] Talan and associates cultured an average of five organisms per wound.[201] *P. multocida* is a frequent pathogen causing infection after dog and cat bites. It is particularly more prevalent in cat bite infections.[153] Cellulitis and serous or seropurulent drainage presenting in the first 12 to 24 hours after the bite injury is often caused by *P. multocida.*[2,68,186,188,215] Ulceroglandular tularemia has been reported after cat bites. The cat is thought to become a carrier of *Francisella tularensis* organisms in the mouth or claws through hunting and eating wild rodents or rabbits. The diagnosis of tularemia should be considered when patients with a history of cat bite present with pneumonia and have a soft tissue infection not responding to penicillin therapy.[30] Cat-scratch fever caused by infection with *Bartonella henselae* should also be kept in mind after feline contact.[186] *Capnocytophaga canimorsus* is a rare pathogen in dog bites. It is of particular interest because of the high fatality rate of 23% to 28% associated with this infection. History of splenectomy, alcoholism, and chronic pulmonary disease are significant risk factors for *C. canimorsus* infections.[60,142]

Although dog bites occur far more commonly than cat bites, they much less commonly become infected. In one report, cat bites were responsible for 76% of infected animal bites. Dog bites accounted for the remaining 24%.[60] Cat bites are produced by needle-sharp teeth, which produce a puncture wound. This allows bacteria to be injected deeply into the soft tissues. This soft tissue bed is a fertile medium for anaerobic and facultative anaerobic infections. The dog has blunt teeth and powerful masseter muscles that cause tearing of soft tissues, leaving large open wounds that are less susceptible to infection.

All animal bite wounds should be thoroughly irrigated. Necrotic tissue must be débrided. Any cat bite presenting as evolving pain requires incision of the puncture wound, irrigation, and débridement. All cat and dog bite wounds should be left open. However, large gaping wounds can be loosely closed after several débridements. Primary reconstruction of soft tissue defects can be considered if the tissue bed appears healthy with no evidence of necrotic tissue or sepsis after the first 48 to 72 hours.

Initial medical treatment includes an update of tetanus immunization if necessary. The rabies immunization status of the animal should be ascertained. Prompt and thorough wound irrigation with soap or povidone-iodine solution reduces the development of rabies by up to 90%.[52,60] Infected wounds should be cultured before irrigation and débridement. Aerobic and anaerobic cultures should be sent. Failure to culture for anaerobic organism will result in a significant number of missed pathogens and subsequent inadequate antibiotic coverage.[217] Antibiotic treatment depends on the severity of clinical signs and symptoms. Routine prophylactic treatment for an animal bite depends on the timing of presentation and the clinical signs and symptoms.

Other domestic and wild animal bites occur much less frequently. The organisms causing infection are similar to those involved in cat and dog bites.[127,188,209] Empirical antibiotic treatment should include coverage for gram-positive, gram-negative, and anaerobic organisms. The principles of surgical treatment remain the same. The wound should be opened to expose the depth of the bite. Necrotic or crushed tissue should be sharply débrided, and the wound should be thoroughly irrigated by gravity irrigation. The wounds should be left open and managed with dressing changes. Delayed primary wound closure may be considered when swelling and erythema have subsided and healthy wound base and tissue margins are present. Wound cultures taken 12 to 24 hours after débridement may be a useful diagnostic tool in determining whether a wound should be closed.[176]

Other animal bites and stings, caused by reptiles, arthropods, and marine animals, are associated with inflammation and tissue necrosis. The soft tissue injury results from the injection of toxin containing venom or from chemical inflammation, such as that seen with sea urchin spines. The swelling associated with these bite injuries can result in compartment syndrome. Secondary infection can occur and requires medical and surgical treatment.[121,188]

Marine Organisms

Multiple pathogens have been associated with an aquatic environment. Contact may occur through occupation or hobby. Infection has been reported from home aquariums. *Mycobacterium marinum,* although commonly associated with aquatic infections, generally presents as a chronic infection.[81] Organisms producing acute infections include species of *Staphylococcus, Streptococcus, Pseudomonas, Aeromonas,* and *Enterobacter.* Infection often occurs through contamination of a break in the skin or through an inadvertent penetrating injury by the bones or the spines of the fish. Rela-

tively minor wounds can be complicated by injection of venom, produced by glands on the dorsal and pectoral spines in some species, notably the catfish. When envenomation occurs, patients experience immediate severe throbbing pain. Pain may spread through the entire extremity. Muscles spasm and fasciculations may be noted. Over the first few hours, the site of injury may have local pallor that progresses to erythema and swelling. Occasionally, local skin necrosis and skin slough may occur. Swelling of the entire extremity may develop. Secondary infection can lead to death.[143]

The most serious aquatic infections are those caused by the non-*cholerae Vibrio* species, particularly *V. vulnificus* and *V. damsela. Vibrio* is a gram-negative, facultative anaerobic rod. Non-*cholerae Vibrio* infections are classified into two types. The more common primary septicemia type typically occurs in patients with underlying liver disease or other immunocompromising disorder.[92,146] The association with liver disease is thought to result from bypassing the hepatic reticuloendothelial system, as portal blood is shunted around the diseased liver. Also, high levels of serum iron associated with hepatic cirrhosis may increase the susceptibility to *V. vulnificus,* which requires iron for growth.[146] Primary septicemia is usually acquired through the gastrointestinal tract by the ingestion of raw seafood. Patients often present with rapidly developing extremity pain followed by skin lesions with bullae, purpura, and necrosis. The most common site of presentation is both lower extremities. It may also be seen in the upper extremity. The findings are similar to those of necrotizing fasciitis, but unlike necrotizing fasciitis, it is more commonly associated with an elevated serum creatine phosphokinase (CPK) level. In a report of eight patients with *Vibrio* septicemia, an elevated CPK level was found in seven. All patients with an elevated CPK level died. Even with aggressive medical and surgical management, these infections are associated with a very high mortality rate (67% to 88%).[146] The less common type of *Vibrio* infection, localized wound infection, occurs equally in immunocompetent and immunocompromised patients. The majority of these wounds are associated with a puncture wound from a fish spine or bone. Generally, these are self-limiting infections. However, development of necrotizing fasciitis has been reported. Aggressive surgical débridement, including amputation, and prolonged intravenous antibiotic therapy are necessary to treat these often fatal infections.[26,169,202,221]

Leeches

Iatrogenic animal bite infections have more recently been described with the re-introduction of medicinal leeches, *Hirudo medicinalis,* which are used for salvage of tissue with venous congestion.[41,43,170,216] The pseudomonad *Aeromonas hydrophila* is the organism most commonly associated with the medicinal leech. It has been frequently cultured from the intestinal flora of the leech. It can result in cellulitis, myonecrosis, abscess formation, endocarditis, and sepsis.[43,84] Lineaweaver and associates found that leeches that fed on antibiotic-containing blood had lower or absent intestinal cultures for *A. hydrophila.* Based on those findings, they recommended the use of broad-spectrum prophylactic antibiotics, which include coverage for *Aeromonas* species, before leech application.[12,84,112,113,119]

Human Bites

The overall incidence of human bite injuries to the hand is unknown. These injuries are often misdiagnosed or unreported. The patient frequently misreports the mechanism of injury to the hand. In one study, human bites ranked third in incidence below dog and cat bites.[68,70,130] Patzakis and colleagues reported on admissions to the orthopedic infection ward over a 5-year period: of 2288 admissions, 10% were due to human bites, specifically clenched-fist injuries.[151]

Four mechanisms of human bite injuries to the hand have been described.[49,123] The least frequent is inadvertent self-inflicted injury occurring from nail biting or secondary to sucking an open bleeding wound on the finger or thumb. The second mechanism is a traumatic amputation secondary to a bite injury. This usually occurs through the distal phalanx or the DIP joint. Full-thickness bite wounds into various parts of the hand represent the third mechanism of injury and inoculation. Although this is one of the more frequent modes of injury, it less commonly results in infection. When infection occurs, it is usually localized around the area of the penetration.[111] However, it has been reported to result in a rapidly spreading process continuing up to the forearm and arm, fitting a diagnosis of necrotizing fasciitis. Deaths associated with this condition were reported in the preantibiotic era.[123] The fourth mechanism of injury is a bite injury occurring when the hand strikes another person's mouth with a closed fist, more commonly known as a clenched-fist injury. The most commonly involved areas are adjacent to the third and fourth metacarpal heads of the dominant hand.[50,151,153] This type of bite injury is associated with the highest incidence of complications.

Clenched-fist injuries occur as the patient strikes the mouth of another person. The area around the MP joint may be impaled by a tooth, penetrating the skin and deeper structures. At the time of contact, the skin and extensor tendons are stretched tightly over the metacarpal head and a large surface area of the metacarpal head is exposed. Deep structures including tendon, joint capsule, and bone may be penetrated as well. The depth of penetration affects the location of spread of the infection. The dorsal subcutaneous space, the subtendinous space, the joint space, or all of these may be involved.[128] The site of the skin injury can be misleading in evaluating for injury to deeper structures. The position of the fingers at the time of impact affects the location of injury to the deeper structures. The more flexed position of the fingers results in more proximal injury to the tendon and joint capsule and a more distal injury to the metacarpal head (Fig. 3-17).

Patients often present with an innocuous-appearing wound on the dorsum of the hand around the MP joint. This presentation should be considered a human bite until proven otherwise. The patient may be reluctant to provide an accurate history regarding the method of injury and often presents to the emergency department either because of a functional loss, as might be caused by fracture or extensor tendon dysfunction, or because of infection. Pain, localized swelling, and erythema may be present. Drainage from the wound is frequently seen; however, fever, lymphadenopathy, and lymphangitis are rare.

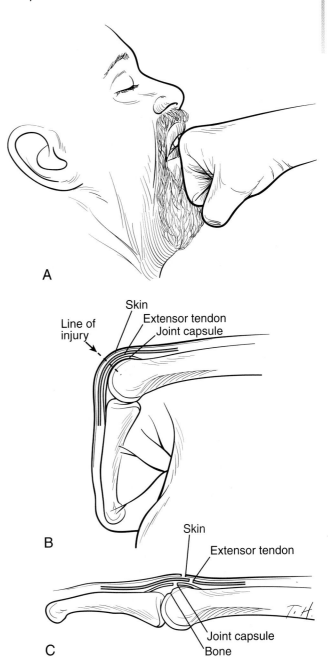

FIGURE 3-17. Clenched-fist injury of the MP joint. **A,** Mechanism of injury. **B,** Linear wound track with MP joint flexed. **C,** Position of injured structures in full extension.

A complete blood cell count, ESR, and CRP are obtained. Often these results are normal. Radiographs are used to evaluate for fracture or presence of a retained foreign body, such as a tooth.[135] These radiographs also provide a baseline for comparison to subsequent films used to evaluate for osteomyelitis. In cases of late presentation, osteomyelitis may already be evident.

The underlying injury to the hand is frequently more serious and extensive than the superficial wound and clinical presentation indicate. Patzakis and colleagues described the surgical findings in a group of 191 patients with clenched-fist injuries. Seventy-five percent had injury to the deep tissue layers, including tendon, capsule, and bone. Sixty-seven percent had a violation of the joint capsule. These findings emphasize the importance of surgical exploration and treatment of these injuries.[151] Wide exposure around the traumatic wound is required. The tendon, joint capsule, and bone are explored with the hand in a position of flexion. Small penetrations in the joint capsule may be inconspicuous or have sealed off. Therefore, even when the joint capsule appears intact, we prefer to open the capsule and inspect the articular surfaces. Cultures should be taken before irrigation. Necrotic tissue must be meticulously removed. Curettage of the affected portion of bone is performed. Softened areas of bone are débrided. Loose fragments of articular cartilage are removed. The wound is left open. No attempt is made to repair injuries to the extensor tendon or extensor mechanism. A moist gauze wick is placed in the wound, and a soft bulky dressing is applied. Dressing changes are started at 12 to 24 hours and combined with soaking in dilute povidone-iodine solution and early range of motion as described in previous sections. If clinical symptoms are not improving, repeat radiographs are obtained to evaluate for underlying osteomyelitis, and the patient should be returned to the operating room for repeat irrigation and débridement.

Intravenous antibiotic therapy should cover a broad spectrum of pathogens. *Eikenella corrodens* is the organism most associated with human bite infections. It is a gram-negative rod, which is a facultative anaerobe.[130] This is usually treated with high doses of penicillin. However, there are emerging strains of penicillin-resistant organisms. Empirical therapy should also cover *Staphylococcus* and *Streptococcus* species as well as gram-negative organisms.[50,70,183] Inpatient intravenous therapy should be continued until the clinical appearance is improving. Appropriate consideration of the patient's social situation and ability to comply with outpatient treatment is necessary.

Complications of infected bite wounds include septic flexor tenosynovitis, septic arthritis, osteomyelitis, stiffness, and pain. Toxic shock syndrome and deaths have been reported.[49,50] Amputations or resection arthroplasty may be necessary to eradicate infection and improve function. Complications may be minimized by recognizing the human bite wound as a serious injury and treating even small seemingly innocuous wounds with early and thorough débridement and appropriate antibiotic therapy.[137] Educating those physicians involved in the primary care of wounds to suspect human bite infections in the appropriate clinical setting can reduce the delay to treatment and subsequent complications associated with these injuries.[122,123]

Prosthetic Infections

Prosthetic joint replacements in the hand and wrist are more commonly performed in patients with rheumatoid arthritis. Although this patient population is generally immunocompromised, the infection rate around prosthetic implants is low, ranging from 0.5% to 3%.[6,51,61,139] When infection occurs, removal of the implant is necessary to control infection. Thorough débridement is done with removal of adjacent areas of necrotic bone. Treatment options include resection arthroplasty or fusion.[51,71,139] In the setting of severe infection or large dead space, temporary placement of an antibiotic-impregnated methylmethacrylate spacer can be

used until the infection is controlled. The choice of intravenous antibiotic is based on the offending organism. The duration of therapy should be the same as that for treatment of osteomyelitis. Rarely is there an indication for prosthetic reimplantation. If reimplantation is considered, the patient should have a normal WBC count, ESR, and CRP. At the time of surgery, Gram stain should be negative for bacteria; and a frozen section with less than five polymorphonuclear cells per high-power field suggests adequate eradication of infection. Infection around Silastic tendon rods can occur. Honner and associates reported an incidence of 2% in a series of 100 rods. Treatment included removal of the silicone rod, irrigation, débridement, and later reconstruction after all signs of infection were resolved and the skin and soft tissues were supple.[87]

Shooter's Abscesses: Infections Caused by Parenteral Drug Abuse

One of the most commonly encountered complications of intravenous drug abuse are infections of the skin and soft tissues. The hand and forearm provide easily accessible sites of venous access. Overall, abscesses of the upper extremity account for 40% to 80% of admissions for soft tissue infections.[74,83,174] Multiple sites of abscesses may be present. Many patients have underlying medical illnesses, poor medical care, and poor medical compliance. Bergstein and colleagues reported an incidence of hepatitis B seropositivity of 29%. The incidence of HIV in patients consenting to serologic testing ranged between 9% and 50%.[10,74,144,164,184] Recent studies have correlated the incidence of abscess formation with subcutaneous or intramuscular injection rather than intravenous injection. This may occur inadvertently when the vein is missed and the injected substance extravasates into the extravascular space. It may also occur volitionally. The repeated abuse of intravenous drugs leaves hardened sclerotic veins, which are no longer accessible for injection. Subcutaneous injection ("skin-popping) or intramuscular injections are used when venous access is difficult. The use of cocaine or of cocaine-heroin mixture (speedball) predisposes patients to abscess formation by inducing soft tissue ischemia.[144]

The organisms cultured from these abscesses are usually a mixed flora. Staphylococcal and streptococcal species predominate. Oral and enteric flora are also frequently present.[10,74,164,174,198] Summanen and coworkers isolated oral flora from 67% of abscesses caused by parenteral drug use. This compared with 25% in abscesses not associated with drug use. This is likely due to the use of sputum to clean either the injection site or the needle.[198] Schnall and colleagues found that gram-negative isolates were more common in patients older than the age of 40.[174]

The majority of these patients present to the emergency department with complaints of pain and swelling. Most patients do not have an elevated temperature and often do not have an elevated WBC count.[184] Examination may demonstrate fluctuance. Deep abscesses may be more difficult to identify. If abscess is suspected, aspiration with an 18-gauge needle in the area of suspicion may identify the presence of pus. Cultures should be sent from specimens obtained in the emergency department. Radiographs may demonstrate gas in the soft tissues or an underlying osteomyelitis.

Provisional drainage of any area of fluctuance should be performed in the emergency department. Once cultures are obtained, broad-spectrum antibiotics are given. Tetanus status is determined and updated as necessary. The patient should be admitted to the hospital. Expedient treatment with formal irrigation and débridement in the operating room can minimize the complications associated with these infections. A longitudinal extensile surgical incision is necessary to adequately drain the abscess cavity. Removal of all necrotic tissue and copious irrigation is performed. The wounds are left open and packed with gauze soaked with dilute povidone-iodine. Wounds may heal by secondary intention. Delayed primary wound closure can also be done and has been shown to reduce hospital stay.[176] Large wounds with associated skin loss or soft tissue fibrosis that precludes delayed primary wound closure can be skin-grafted when a healthy granulation tissue bed is present.

Large open wounds can also be managed with a vacuum-assisted wound closure device (V.A.C.). This technique can reduce the size of the wound, thereby requiring a smaller skin graft, or shorten the time needed for secondary wound healing.

Complications associated with soft tissue abscesses include spread of infection to adjacent potential spaces such as the flexor tendon sheath or adjacent joint space. Osteomyelitis can occur with long-standing infection. Bacteria and septicemia can spread infection to distant sites. Cardiac examination for murmur suggesting endocarditis should be performed on all patients. The most serious complication of soft tissue abscess is that of necrotizing fasciitis. Although this occurs rarely, it is a life-threatening infection that requires emergent surgical and medical treatment.

Many of these patients require prolonged hospitalization, often more owing to social concerns and medical compliance than because of medical necessity. Premature discharge to a situation in which the patient will not have a clean environment or be able to comply with antibiotic therapy and wound management may lead to more complications, greater morbidity, and higher social costs. The risk to the surgeon and health care team is considerable. Although universal precautions should be exercised with every patient, greater vigilance and attention is necessary to protect the health care providers in managing this patient population.

Herpetic Whitlow (Herpes Simplex Virus Infection of the Fingers)

Herpetic viral infections of the fingers are commonly misdiagnosed as bacterial infections, such as paronychia or felon. The inappropriate treatment of this condition as a bacterial process can result in severe complications. It is therefore important to be aware of the diagnosis and clinical presentation to avoid these adverse sequelae.[32,34,106]

The term *herpetic whitlow* is derived from the viral origin of the process and the middle English term *whitlow. Herpes* has a Greek origin, meaning "to creep," as this fits the general pattern of disease progression. Herpes simplex virus (HSV) types 1 and 2 are part of the alpha Herpes viridae. Humans are the only natural host. The term *whitlow* is believed to be a misnomer, because whitlow was generally used to describe a suppurative infection of the finger pulp, such as a felon. Other terms used to describe herpetic infection of the fingers include herpetic febrilis of the finger, herpetic paronychia,

and aseptic felon. The first reported case of herpetic infection of the finger in the English literature was reported by Adamson in 1909. Since Stern's publication in 1959, this infection has been commonly named herpetic whitlow.[88]

Herpetic infections are seen in both adults and children. In a child with herpetic gingivostomatitis, the thumb or finger can become inoculated by sucking. In adults, this infection has been reported as an occupational hazard, affecting those in the medical or dental profession who come into direct contact with saliva from patients who are actively shedding HSV. This is most often infection from HSV type 1. More recent studies emphasize the importance of autoinoculation or inoculation from a sexual partner infected with HSV type 2. HSV type 1 more commonly affects young children and the medical and dental professional in contact with saliva. HSV type 2 infections have been more common in adults.[4,62,117] Age and profession cannot be exclusively used to differentiate between HSV type 1 and HSV type 2 infections, and there is no difference in their clinical presentations.

Clinical Presentation and Diagnosis

The early symptoms of HSV infection of the hand mimic the presentation of herpetic lesions occurring in other locations. The incubation period of the virus ranges between 2 and 14 days, and a thorough history may provide clues to the diagnosis, possible vector, and viral type. Infection usually involves a single finger. Involvement of more than one finger may suggest another infection, such as coxsackievirus.[141]

The index finger and thumb are the most frequently infected digits. However, the infection may occur on any finger or any location on the hand or integument.[55] In the beginning of the infection the patient has intense throbbing and pain in the affected digit. Carter reported that one of the early symptoms may be tingling in the affected digit. In the early disease process, the patient's pain is disproportionately severe to the clinical findings.[34,223] Erythema and mild swelling are present; this is followed by the development of 1- to 2-mm clear vesicles. Over several days, these vesicles creep together and coalesce. The vesicle roof usually remains intact. As the vesicles coalesce, a large confluent bulla may form. The fluid within the vesicles is initially clear. It may rapidly become turbid and appear purulent, mimicking a bacterial hand infection. Lymphangitis and adenopathy may be present but are more commonly seen with bacterial superinfection.

Over the next 7 to 10 days, these signs and symptoms subside. Even though the symptoms are resolving, there is continued viral shedding over the next 12 to 14 days. It is during this time that the patient is most infective. The clinical course is generally self-limited and resolves over a 3-week period.

Early diagnosis depends on clinical suspicion. Distinguishing a viral infection from a bacterial infection is critical to the treatment. Suspicion of a viral infection depends on the patient history, quality and intensity of the pain, softness of the digital pulp, presence of vesicles, and a blood profile that does not fit a pattern of sepsis. Viral cultures definitively establish the diagnosis. However, the culture may take several days to become positive. The virus is sensitive to transport and cultures may be negative, even when transported in viral medium. Lesions that have crusted often do not produce positive cultures.

The Tzanck smear is performed on fresh vesicles. This microscopic examination will show multinucleated keratinocytes with steel-blue homogeneous karyoplasm. The base of the lesion is scraped vigorously with the edge of a scalpel blade. The material is touched to a glass slide and allowed to air dry. The Tzanck smear in all stages of the disease is less sensitive than viral culture. Immunofluorescent serum antibody titers, using type-specific monoclonal anti-HSV antibodies, can confirm the diagnosis and type. HSV blood testing for antibodies to the HSV type-specific G1 and G2 glycoproteins is now available and may provide a rapid diagnosis of HSV infection.[55,210]

Treatment of herpetic whitlow is essentially nonsurgical. The course of the disease is self-limiting. The main goal of treatment is to prevent autoinoculation or transmission of the infection. The digit should be kept covered with a dry dressing, and all contact with the lesion should be avoided. Unroofing of the vesicles may improve patient comfort. Intravenous, oral, or topical antiviral medication may be useful in shortening the natural course of the infection.[185] Partial nail excision may be indicated for a subungual herpetic lesion causing pressure below the nail plate.[158] Surgical débridement of bacterial superinfection must be done cautiously. Misdiagnosis of the viral infection as a paronychia or felon, which leads to surgical intervention, may result in disastrous complications. Viral encephalitis and death have been reported as a result of misdiagnosis and treatment of a herpetic infection as a felon.[4,32,34]

Once the disease resolves, the virus becomes latent in the nervous system. The responsible cell in the ganglia or the mechanism of latency is not completely understood. Twenty percent of patients will experience recurrence. The recurrent infection is usually less severe, except in immunocompromised patients in whom the recurrence rate and the infection severity is much higher.[55,185,210]

Upper Extremity Infections Associated With HIV Infection

Upper extremity infections in patients with HIV are more common in those patients with a concomitant history of intravenous drug abuse.[75] The clinical presentation of infection is similar to patients without HIV; however, the clinical course of the infection is often more severe. Gonzalez and coworkers reported on 28 patients with HIV infection. Eight of those patients had acquired immunodeficiency syndrome (AIDS), as defined by the Centers for Disease Control and Prevention guidelines. The most common presentation was that of soft tissue abscess. Patients with AIDS were more likely to present with a spontaneous infection,[75,129] and spontaneous septic arthritis should raise suspicion of underlying immunocompromise.[66,180] The organisms most frequently isolated were streptococcal and staphylococcal species. McAuliffe and Seltzer found *S. aureus* to be the most common pathogen in 74 patients infected with HIV.[129] Pyogenic infections responded well to aggressive débridement and antibiotic therapy. Herpetic viral infections were more commonly seen than in the general population.[66,75] The viral infections did not run a self-limited course and often became superinfected. Oral or intravenous antiviral therapy was necessary to resolve the infection. The incidence of necrotizing fasciitis was also disproportionately high in the patient group reported by Gonzalez and coworkers. Opportunistic infections of the hand have been reported, although less frequently than might be expected.[14,204]

Pyogenic infections respond well to early and aggressive surgical débridement and culture-directed antibiotic therapy. Viral infections have a prolonged course and do not resolve spontaneously. Intravenous antiviral therapy may be necessary to eradicate the infection. Amputation may be indicated for recalcitrant infection.

Diabetic Hand Infections

Approximately 7% of the adult population of the United States are diagnosed with diabetes mellitus.[28] It has been estimated that the prevalence of undiagnosed diabetes in the adult population older than the age of 50 is 10%. Among the many complications associated with diabetes is a susceptibility to infection, resulting in a high morbidity rate. Diabetics are known to have a higher rate of postsurgical infection, even after minor soft tissue procedures.[28,73] Infection may be the initial presenting complaint in patients previously undiagnosed with diabetes. Cohen and colleagues reported a 17% incidence of undiagnosed diabetes in patients treated for infections of the extremities.[37]

Several different mechanisms have been postulated for the increased susceptibility to infection in diabetics. Many studies have shown immune deficits, particularly lymphocyte dysfunction associated with elevated blood glucose levels. Deficits include decreased chemotaxis, decreased phagocytosis, decreased intracellular bactericidal activity, and decreased opsonic activity.[28,56,166] Overall, the leukocyte is less capable of performing its role of preventing infection and fighting sepsis. It has been further suggested that the local hyperglycemic environment may enhance bacterial proliferation, especially in staphylococcal infections.[56,166] Anatomic factors, notably peripheral neuropathies and diabetic angiopathy, contribute to poor wound healing and poor oxygen, leukocyte, and antibiotic delivery to the affected area. Wound healing activities including capillary ingrowth, fibroblast proliferation, and collagen synthesis have also been shown to be decreased in diabetics.[56]

Infections in diabetics have been separated into superficial and deep infections. The superficial infections include cellulitis and superficial localized abscess. These infections behave more like infections in nondiabetics and respond to broad-spectrum antibiotic therapy and local wound débridement.[79,157] Deep infections include involvement of bone, tendon sheath, or deep palmar spaces. Francel and colleagues[56] reported that 73% of patients in their series had deep infections. Gonzalez and coworkers reported that more than 50% of patients with deep infections required more than one surgical procedure.[73] The amputation rate in diabetics with deep infection ranges from 8% to 63%.[39,56,73,100,124,157] Necrotizing fasciitis occurs with greater frequency in diabetics and has been associated with a higher mortality rate.[57,65,187] Diabetics with associated renal failure represent a subgroup of patients with even higher morbidity and mortality rates. Francel and colleagues reported a 100% amputation rate in this patient group with upper extremity infections.[56] The most common pathogen remains *S. aureus*.

However, multiple organisms are present in most infections.[73,79,100,124] Gram-negative organisms were documented in up to 73% of positive cultures.[100]

Treatment includes broad-spectrum antibiotic therapy, careful monitoring and control of blood glucose level, and aggressive surgical management. Surgical incisions should extend past the area of erythema and should include the length of the areas of indurated skin and soft tissue. Wounds should be left open to heal by secondary intention. Secondary procedures for repeat débridement are common. When amputation is necessary, an open amputation is performed. The bone is shortened proximal to the level of skin resection. The wound will heal readily by secondary intention as long as the infection is controlled. Primary amputation may be the most appropriate procedure to control the infection, reduce disability, and improve functional outcome.

Necrotizing Soft Tissue Infections and Gas Gangrene

Necrotizing fasciitis is a rapidly advancing necrotizing infection affecting the skin, subcutaneous tissue, and fascia. It characteristically spares the underlying muscle. It is associated with high morbidity and mortality rates and severe systemic sepsis. Whereas necrotizing soft tissue infections were recognized in earlier literature, Meleney[136] is credited with the first detailed description of the disease process and first recognized the importance of early and extensive surgical débridement. Wilson first applied the term *necrotizing fasciitis,* recognizing that the constant feature of the infection was fascial necrosis.[219]

Two types of necrotizing infections have been described based on the bacteriology of the infection. Type 1 infections are mixed aerobic and anaerobic infections. Facultative anaerobic bacteria and non–group A streptococci are present. This is the most common type and is found in approximately 80% of cases. Type 2 infections are caused by group A *Streptococcus* species alone or in combination with staphylococcal species.[63,72,89,149]

The inciting event for the onset of infection may not be known. There may be a history of minor trauma or puncture wound. When seen in intravenous drug abusers, it is postulated that the contamination occurs through use of an unclean needle, use of saliva to clean the needle or injection site, or contamination of the street drug being injected. In the initial presentation, necrotizing fasciitis may resemble cellulitis. There is a swollen erythematous area of exquisite tenderness with an area of extensive cellulitis. Nonpitting edema is present and extends beyond the margins of the erythema, distinguishing this from cellulitis. Beyond the area of cellulitis, the skin may have an orange-peel appearance (peau d'orange skin). As the infection progresses, the skin changes from red and purple to a dusky blue-gray. The skin may be come hypoesthetic or anesthetic. By the fourth or fifth day, patchy areas of frank necrosis of the skin develop. The skin may slough, owing to thrombosis of the nutrient vessels that traverse the fascial layer and supply the overlying skin and subcutaneous tissue. Bullae form and are either clear or hemorrhagic (Fig. 3-18). Soft tissue crepitance is not common, although radiographs frequently demonstrate the presence of gas in the tissues.

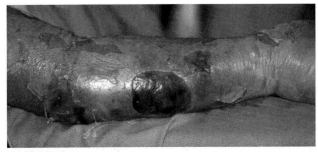

FIGURE 3-18. Characteristic appearance of necrotizing fasciitis. (See also Color Figure 3-18.)

Diagnosis begins with maintaining a high clinical suspicion in all patients, particularly with those patients with risk factors, including diabetics, immunocompromised patients, and intravenous drug abusers.[65,73] In the early stages the infection appears more like cellulitis. Marking the area of both cellulitis and edema followed by re-examination within an hour for signs of progression helps distinguish a necrotizing infection from cellulitis. Tenderness beyond the area of erythema is highly suggestive of necrotizing fasciitis. If an open wound is present, the wound can be explored. A probe or finger that dissects easily along the fascia below intact skin is a hallmark finding distinguishing this process from cellulitis.[98] When still in doubt regarding the diagnosis, an incisional biopsy can be performed at bedside. This is done proximal to the area of erythema and over the area of edema. The incision is carried down to the fascia. At least a 1-cm square section of fascia is obtained for frozen section.[190] Pus is not usually a component of these infections. A thin watery exudate may be encountered at the site of biopsy. Thrombosis obliterans of the perforating vessels and massive infiltration of polymorphonuclear cells confirm the diagnosis.[208]

Patients with necrotizing fasciitis often feel much worse than what would be expected from the initial presentation. They may experience a sense of impending doom. Fever and elevated WBC counts are not universally present. As the infection progresses, systemic signs of sepsis develop. Dehydration, electrolyte disturbance, and hypotension occur owing to the fluid shifts caused by the edema. Disseminated intravascular coagulopathy with rapidly progressing septic shock has been associated with necrotizing fasciitis.[89]

The infection can spread rapidly over hours, involving the entire upper extremity and continuing onto the chest wall. Surgical treatment and broad-spectrum intravenous antibiotic therapy covering gram-positive and gram-negative organisms as well as anaerobic organisms are mandatory. Careful monitoring and correction of fluid and electrolyte status should be done in the intensive care setting. Intubation may be necessary as systemic signs of sepsis progress. While the patient's medical condition should be optimized, surgical débridement should not be delayed, because this is the most important means of controlling the infection.

The surgical débridement should be extensive. Pus is rarely encountered, but a thin watery exudate, so-called dishwater pus, will be found. The infection dissects along the fascial planes, making easy finger dissection in this plane. The fascia appears gray or grayish green and may be liquefied. Areas of normal-appearing fascia may be seen. However, under microscopic examination, these areas may be involved.

Intraoperative frozen sections of the fascia can help guide the extent of débridement. Myonecrosis may be observed in cases of longer duration. In the hand, secondary thrombosis of the digital vessels results in necrotic fingers. Wide débridement of skin, subcutaneous tissue, fascia, and necrotic muscle, if present, is required. Amputation may be necessary, especially if muscle is involved or if the patient's condition is not improving despite aggressive débridement. The wounds should be left open and covered with moist gauze. Burn dressings should be used, and the patient is returned to the intensive care unit. Patient resuscitation should be the same as that used to resuscitate patients with extensive third-degree burns. These patients often require repeat débridement. However, it is the initial débridement that will most influence treatment outcome. It is mandatory to remove all necrotic tissue at the first surgery. The wound should be re-examined no more than 24 hours after the first surgery. If the patient's clinical course is deteriorating, an earlier re-examination and repeat débridement versus amputation is indicated. The use of hyperbaric oxygen as adjunctive treatment has been reported. In centers where this facility is readily available there may be some benefit.

When the infection is controlled and the patient is clinically stable, wound coverage with a split-thickness skin graft is necessary. Prolonged occupational therapy is often required for functional recovery. Despite aggressive management, these infections are associated with a high morbidity and mortality rate. Mortality rates range from 9% up to 75% when chest wall involvement is present.[57,72,76,89,133,172] Factors associated with increased mortality rate include age older than 50 years, diabetes mellitus, truncal involvement, and delay to diagnosis and treatment.[57,132,133,162,199] Early deaths, defined as within the first 10 days after initial débridement, were found consequent to sepsis syndrome, whereas late deaths were attributable to multiple organ system failure.[76,133]

Gas gangrene is an uncommon infection of the upper extremity. There are six types of *Clostridium* known to cause gas gangrene; however, *C. perfringens* is the most common. More than 60% of gas gangrene infections also involve nonclostridial species. Clostridial organisms are anaerobic gram-positive rods. They are spore forming, and the spores are highly resistant to environmental stresses. They survive for long periods and are ubiquitous in the soil. In the vegetative state, they produce toxins. It may be difficult to isolate clostridium from a wound culture. It must be grown in an anaerobic environment in a medium with a reducing agent such as sodium thioglycolate. Clostridia produce a number of toxins. Among these, alpha toxin is responsible for the myonecrosis, hemolysis, and myocardial depression through the inhibition of the calcium pump. Theta toxin is a hemolysin and is cardiotoxic. Kappa toxin destroys blood vessels through collagenase activity.[72,160,214]

Devitalized tissue provides an excellent environment for clostridial growth. Clinical signs occur within hours of inoculation. Endotoxin production quickly produces muscle, subcutaneous tissue, and fat necrosis. Thrombosis of local vessels further reduces the oxygen tension at the site of infection, continuing to promote a suitable environment for bacterial replication. Hydrogen sulfide and carbon dioxide gas are produced and dissect along the soft tissue planes, causing further tissue destruction. Local and systemic effects of the toxins are present as the infection continues, leading to severe hemolysis, hemoglobinuria, and, ultimately, renal failure. Death has been reported in as short a period as 12 hours after onset of infection.[160]

The clinical findings generally include a history of trauma, often with a crush component. Infections have also occurred in postsurgical wounds and as spontaneous infections. The principal signs of clostridial infection are pain, a closed wound, tachycardia out of proportion to fever or hydration status, and crepitus.

Treatment requires rapid recognition of the infection and emergent surgical débridement, removing all necrotic tissue. It is imperative to leave wounds widely open. Frequent dressing changes are initiated within 6 hours of the initial débridement. Intravenous antibiotic therapy, including high-dose penicillin therapy, is started immediately. Patient resuscitation in the intensive care unit must carefully manage fluid and electrolyte status. Hyperbaric oxygen is a valuable adjunct in the management of this devastating infection.

The principal differential diagnosis of clostridial myonecrosis includes necrotizing fasciitis and streptococcal gangrene, which also represent surgical emergencies. Gas gangrene progresses even more rapidly than necrotizing fasciitis, making early recognition imperative to patient survival. The mortality rate, despite aggressive management, remains high, approximating 25%.[167]

Cutaneous Anthrax Infections

Anthrax infection is caused by the gram-positive aerobic or facultative anaerobic bacterium *Bacillus anthracis*. The black eschar produced by the cutaneous disease gave rise to the name "anthrax" derived from the Greek word *anthrakos* meaning "coal." The bacillus exists in a vegetative or growing state and in a spore form. In the vegetative state it is very sensitive to environmental stress. Under these conditions, the cells undergo sporulation. The spore form is very resistant to environmental extremes, including temperature, pH, irradiation, disinfectants, sporicides, and many other stresses. The spore may remain viable in nature for up to 60 years (up to 200 years in one study).[104,203] Spores are present in the top 6 cm of soil and in animal products. Animals that die of anthrax release massive quantities of spores into the soil that may remain for decades before being ingested again. Burying animal carcasses is probably of little use in disrupting transmission because Pasteur showed that earthworms will carry spores back to the surface. Animal carcasses should be burned, not buried, to prevent long-term environmental contamination.

Anthrax infections have traditionally been transmitted through contaminated soil, animals, or animal products. With the growing threat of bioterrorism, it is important for clinicians to recognize the clinical manifestations of this disease. There are three main manifestations of anthrax. These are cutaneous, gastrointestinal, and inhalational. At present, the cutaneous form remains the most commonly seen, representing 95% of all reported cases worldwide. This form is also the most likely to be encountered by the hand surgeon.[207]

Clinical lesions of cutaneous anthrax usually appear within 2 to 7 days of handling sick animals or eating their meat; however, incubation periods of over 8 weeks have been reported. Cutaneous disease begins as a small, painless, red macule that progresses to a papule over 48 to 72 hours. The

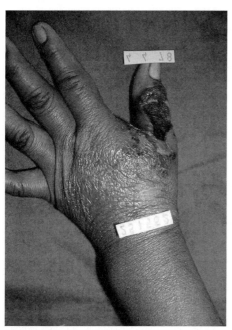

FIGURE 3-19. Cutaneous anthrax. (Courtesy of Dr. Eduardo Gotuzzo, Tropical Medicine Institute, Universidad Peruana Cayetano Heredia, Lima Peru.) (See also Color Figure 3-19.)

papule becomes vesicular and ruptures, ulcerates, and forms a 1- to 5-cm diameter brown or black eschar (Fig. 3-19). Even when the vesicle ruptures and ulcerates, the lesion remains painless. Weeping vesicles and open ulcers should be cultured. If the patient has not received antibiotic treatment, anthrax bacilli may be cultured from the fluid. Gram stain may reveal gram-positive rods. Polymerase chain reaction and immunohistochemical staining may help confirm the diagnosis. Lesions are not purulent or painful in the absence of superinfection. Satellite lesions and significant edema may surround the initial eschar.[104] Depending on the location and severity of disease, edema may be extensive and life threatening, especially if the lesions are close to the chest or neck. Tender regional lymphadenopathy, fever, malaise, and chills may accompany the skin lesion.

Even with prompt antibiotic therapy, cutaneous lesions progress through the eschar phase. Progression of the cutaneous lesion occurs despite antibiotic treatment, because the tissue necrosis and ulceration occur due to toxin, which is not neutralized by antibiotic therapy. Although antibiotics have no effect on the progression of the skin lesion, they do sterilize the ulcer. Several different antibiotics may be used, including penicillin, quinolones, or doxycycline. Intravenous therapy is used initially. Oral antibiotics are started as the patient shows clinical improvement. The duration of therapy is 60 days. Débridement of skin lesions is contraindicated because of the risk of spreading infection. Although 80% to 90% of lesions heal spontaneously, 10% to 20% of untreated cases may progress to malignant edema, septicemia, shock, renal failure, and death. Fatalities are uncommon with therapy.[104,207]

High-Pressure Injection Injuries

High-pressure injection injuries can result in extensive soft tissue damage, despite the often benign appearance of the entry wound. Material is injected through the skin at pressures up to 7000 psi. The nondominant index finger is the most frequently involved digit.[175,206] The extent of injury is related to the force of the injection and the type and amount of material injected. Mechanical and chemical injury results in local tissue necrosis and vascular occlusion. Oil-based paints and industrial solvents produce a greater degree of tissue necrosis than water-based paints and grease. Mirzayan and colleagues reported an amputation rate of 50% with oil-based paints. No amputations were required in water-based paint injections.[140]

Emergent surgical decompression and débridement is necessary. Despite wide and aggressive surgical management, it is usually impossible to remove all foreign material. Surgical delay more than 10 hours was found to result in higher rates of amputation.[191]

Infection is not frequently a component of these injuries unless treatment is delayed. These wounds are commonly contaminated with both gram-positive and gram-negative organisms.[140,156,178] The necrotic tissue resulting from the injury provides a good culture medium for the injected bacteria. Broad-spectrum antibiotic coverage is important in the treatment of these injuries.

Mimickers of Infection

A wide range of clinical conditions may mimic an infection of the hand. It is important to recognize these conditions to provide appropriate treatment and prevent unnecessary surgery. The following conditions do not represent an exhaustive list but include those that are more commonly encountered.[93,105,116] *Gout and pseudogout* represent the crystal arthropathies that may present as a pyarthrosis. Gouty tophi that erupt through the skin may have the appearance of infection with erythema of the skin and drainage. These lesions may also become secondarily infected and require surgical intervention. *Acute calcific tendinitis* presents as severe, well-localized pain overlying tendons or ligaments. Erythema and edema are often present. Other signs of infection such as fever, lymphadenopathy, or abnormal laboratory values are absent. Radiographs demonstrate characteristic calcific density in the area of tenderness. *Pyogenic granuloma* presents as a raised red friable lesion (Fig. 3-20). The friable tissue is sensitive to minor trauma and bleeds easily. In the hand it is usually on the volar surface of the palm or fingers. The etiology remains unclear, possibly related to repetitive irritation or minor trauma. *Pyoderma gangrenosum* is a very rare cutaneous lesion, seen principally in patients with a coexisting systemic disease, especially in patients with ulcerative colitis. The disease process begins with small papules that rapidly develop pustules. Central necrosis follows quickly, leaving a central ulcer. The border is raised and violaceous, and advances from the center at a rate of 1 to 2 cm/day. Treatment includes local wound care. Surgical excision is contraindicated and may exacerbate the disease, resulting in a larger area of necrosis. *Retained foreign bodies* may result in an inflammatory response that mimics an infection. Woody materials can be a significant irritant. Palm thorns are known to cause a chemical irritation of the soft tissues. Intra-articular thorns or thorns that pierce the tendon sheath can result in a chemical synovitis. Removal of the offending irritant is necessary for definitive treatment.[108]

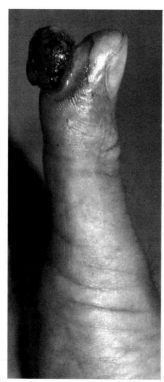

FIGURE 3-20. Pyogenic granuloma of the thumb. (See also Color Figure 3-20.)

Metastatic or primary tumors on the hand are rare. However, awareness of this possibility is important to prevent a misdiagnosis. Primary lesions include squamous cell carcinoma, basal cell carcinoma, melanoma, and keratoacanthoma (see Chapter 62). These are more likely to appear as a chronic infection.[118] Metastatic lesions to the hand are usually acral lesions, with more than 50% involving the distal phalanx. Radiographs may distinguish between tumor and infection. Primary lung tumors are the most common metastatic lesion to the hand.[1,168] Other sites of primary tumor include breast, kidney, colon, thyroid, and prostate.

ANNOTATED REFERENCES

7. Bednar M, Lane L: Eponychial marsupialization and nail removal for surgical treatment of chronic paronychia. J Hand Surg [Am] 16:314-317, 1991.

    Twenty-eight patients with chronic paronychia were treated with marsupialization or marsupialization in conjunction with nail removal. Patients with a nail deformity treated with marsupialization alone had a 28% recurrence rate. When no nail deformity was present, marsupialization alone was effective treatment.

16. Bolton H, Fowler P, Jepson R: Natural history and treatment of pulp space infection and osteomyelitis of the terminal phalanx. J Bone Joint Surg Br 31:499-504, 1949.

    This classic 1949 article outlines the pathophysiology of pulp space infections (felons) and describes surgical treatment and outcomes in 50 patients. Early surgical intervention with direct incision over the abscess site was recommended.

56. Francel T, Marshall K, Savage R: Hand infections in the diabetic and diabetic renal transplant recipient. Ann Plast Surg 24:304-309, 1990.

    This retrospective study reviewed the course of hand infections in diabetic patients and in diabetic patients who were renal transplant recipients. Severe infections were noted in diabetic patients with rapid progression to the involvement of deep spaces of the hand, bone, and tendon sheath. Sixty-three percent of diabetic patients progressed to amputation of the affected part. Diabetic patients who were renal transplant recipients had a 100% amputation rate, required an average of 7.3 surgical procedures, and had an average hospital stay of 41 days. This study emphasized the importance of early and aggressive management of diabetics with upper extremity infections.

62. Gill J, Arlette J, Buchan K: Herpes simplex virus infection of the hand. Am J Med 84:89-93, 1988.

    This article reported 79 patients with herpes simplex virus (HSV) of the hand. This large series contradicts previous reports in smaller series that this is predominantly a disease of health care workers, particularly those exposed to oral secretions, and was the first to assess the incidence of HSV infection of the hand in the general population. The incidence reported is 2.4 per 100,000. Only 8% of infections occurred among health care workers. The article reports the epidemiology and demographics of those infected, along with the breakdown of virology by age and gender.

70. Goldstein E, Barones M, Miller T: *Eikenella corrodens* in hand infections. J Hand Surg [Am] 8:563-567, 1983.

    A retrospective review of infections in the hand in which *Eikenella corrodens* was identified as a pathogen. Infections were associated with contamination by oral flora (e.g., in "fight bites"). The study emphasized the need for aerobic and anaerobic cultures of hand wounds and proper selection of antibiotic therapy when oral contamination of wounds is suspected.

93. Kanavel A: Infections of the Hand, 4th ed. Philadelphia, Lea & Febiger, 1921.

    Dr. Kanavel's classic text was the major pioneering work in the pathoanatomy and treatment of hand infections. Through his meticulous injection and anatomical studies, he defined the potential spaces of the hand and their anatomic predilection for infection.

117. Louis D, Silva J Jr: Herpetic whitlow: Herpetic infection of the digits. J Hand Surg [Am] 4:90-94, 1979.

    In this early report of 10 herpes simplex infections in the hand, all occurred in health care workers. It provides a detailed description of the clinical presentation and likely modes of exposure. The article raised the awareness for proper diagnosis and nonsurgical treatment of these infections.

118a. Lovette H (ed): Hand Clinics. Philadelphia, WB Saunders, 1998, vol 14.

    This volume of the *Hand Clinics* is focused on infections of the hand and is an excellent source of well-written and well-researched review articles on many topics related to hand infections.

128. Mason M, Koch S: Human bite infections of the hand. Surg Gynecol Obstet 51:591-625, 1930.

    Mason and Koch detailed the anatomy of the fascial spaces of the hand and the pathogenesis of infection following bite injuries. The authors, who were colleagues of Dr. Alan Kanavel, used his injection techniques to illustrate the pathways of infection.

129. McAuliffe J, Seltzer D, Hornicek F: Upper-extremity infections in patients seropositive for human immunodeficiency virus. J Hand Surg [Am] 22:1084-1090, 1997.

    The records of 74 HIV-positive patients treated for upper extremity infections were reviewed. Intravenous drug abuse was the most common risk factor for HIV infection in this group of patients. The disease course did not differ between HIV-positive patients and those patients who met criteria for AIDS. However, patients with AIDS were more likely to develop spontaneous infections.

134. McLain R, Steyers C, Stoddard M: Infections in open fractures of the hand. J Hand Surg [Am] 16:108-112, 1991.

An 11% incidence of infection was found in this review of 46 patients with open fractures. Infections occurred principally in injuries associated with a significant crush component, such as industrial injuries or farm-related injuries. *Staphylococcus aureus* was the most common pathogen isolated, but one third of the infections were polymicrobial. All polymicrobial infections occurred in wounds with extensive soft tissue injury, often in an agricultural environment. Overall, 47% of infected patients had enteric pathogens, polymicrobial infections, or both. These characteristics should be considered when initiating antibiotic therapy for open fractures.

139. Millender L, et al: Infection after silicone prosthetic arthroplasty in the hand. J Bone Joint Surg Am 57:825-829, 1975.

The incidence of infection in this study of 2105 silicone implant arthroplasties in 631 patients was found to be 0.48% (10 patients). The time from surgery to signs of infections averaged 17 days. Recommended treatment included removal of the implant when purulence or osteomyelitis was present.

140. Mirzayan R, et al: Culture results and amputation rates in high-pressure paint gun injuries of the hand. Orthopedics 24:587-589, 2001.

The importance of this study is that it provides the rationale for the use of prophylactic antibiotic therapy following high-pressure paint gun injuries. It further characterizes outcome of injury based on the type of injected material, noting a significantly higher amputation rate with oil-based paints (50%) compared with water-based paints (0%).

144. Murphy E, et al: Risk factors for skin and soft-tissue abscesses among injection drug users: A case-control study. Clin Infect Dis 33(July):35-40, 2001.

This case-control study was done to evaluate risk factors for the development of abscesses among IV drug abusers. The strongest risk factor identified for abscess formation was the injection of drug into the subcutaneous tissue or muscle ("skin-popping"). This was followed closely by the use of a dirty needle. In those patients who did not skin-pop, the technique of withdrawing blood into the syringe before injecting (so-called booting) was a risk factor. The substance injected was also identified as a risk factor. "Speedball," mixtures of heroin and cocaine, had a higher incidence of abscess, possibly by inducing soft tissue ischemia through the vasoconstrictive effect of the cocaine. HIV-positive status was not identified as a risk factor.

146. Nakafusa J, et al: The importance of serum creatine phosphokinase level in the early diagnosis, and as a prognostic factor, of *Vibrio vulnificus* infection. Br J Dermatol 145:280-284, 2001.

Vibrio vulnificus infections are uncommon infections. Importantly, this article describes an elevated serum CPK level as a feature of its presence, which helps to distinguish it from other soft tissue infections such as necrotizing fasciitis. An elevated serum CPK level was associated with a poor prognosis.

146a. Neviaser R: Closed tendon sheath irrigation for pyogenic flexor tenosynovitis. J Hand Surg [Am] 3:462-466, 1978.

The technique of closed tendon sheath irrigation with through-and-through irrigation for the treatment of pyogenic flexor tenosynovitis is described. The advantages of this technique in regaining range of motion are emphasized, with

18 of 20 patients regaining full motion by the end of the first postoperative week.

151. Patzakis M, Wilkins J, Bassett R: Surgical findings in clenched-fist injuries. Clin Orthop 220:237-240, 1987.

Patient demographics and surgical findings are presented for a group of 191 patients presenting in the emergency department with clenched-fist injuries. Seventy-five percent of patients were found to have injury to the tendon, joint capsule, cartilage, or bone. These findings support the importance of surgical exploration and débridement of dorsal hand wounds suggestive of clenched-fist injury mechanism.

161. Rashkoff E, Burkhalter W, Mann R: Septic arthritis of the wrist. J Bone Joint Surg Am 65: 824-828, 1983.

In 28 patients with septic arthritis of the wrist, *Staphylococcus aureus* was the most common organism, but an increased number of gram-negative organisms was seen compared with other series. Gram-negative organisms were believed to be correlated with a poorer outcome, but this could not be statistically confirmed. Those patients treated within 10 hours of presentation demonstrated better functional outcomes than those who were seen later. Idiopathic septic arthritis of the wrist was seen in patients older than age 60 and often associated with rheumatoid or osteoarthritis. Findings in this group were more subtle and often delayed surgical treatment.

186. Smith P, Meadowcroft A, May D: Treating mammalian bite wounds. J Clin Pharm Ther 25:85-99, 2000.

This article provides a comprehensive review of the literature on dog, cat, and human bites. Detailed analysis of pathogens and antimicrobial therapy is provided.

191. Stark H, Ashworth C, Boyes J: Paint-gun injuries of the hand. J Bone Joint Surg Am 49:637-647, 1967.

This was the first large series of patients with high-pressure injection injuries in the hand and fingers. Prior to this study, isolated case reports documented the severity of injury produced and the need for amputation. The role of wide decompression and débridement had not been defined. Risk factors associated with amputation included a delay in treatment and the use of a digital block anesthetic. Chemical inflammation was noted to be part of the disease process.

201. Talan D, et al: Bacteriologic analysis of infected dog and cat bites. N Engl J Med 340:85-92, 1999.

In a large series of patients with infections following dog or cat bites, 50% of dog bites and 63% of cat bites occurred on the hand. Most infections were polymicrobial. *Pasturella* was isolated from 50% of dog bites and 75% of cat bites. Antibiotic treatment recommendations were made based on pathogen isolates.

219. Wilson B: Necrotizing fasciitis. Am Surg 28:416-431, 1952.

The term *necrotizing fasciitis* was first used in this paper, because Wilson thought this term best described the consistent pathologic feature of fascial necrosis. Thoroughly describing the pathology and clinical course of the disease, Wilson recommended wide surgical incision and débridement. High fluid loss into the soft tissues (up to 3 L in an affected limb) was recognized, necessitating aggressive fluid and electrolyte replacement. The paper cited only an 8.7% mortality rate, lower than that seen in most current series.

220. Wittels N, Donley J, Burkhalter W: A functional treatment for interphalangeal pyogenic arthritis. J Hand Surg [Am] 9: 894-898, 1984.

The authors describe a midlateral approach to the PIP joint, with excision of the accessory collateral ligament. Early active range of motion in conjunction with dynamic splinting resulted in full range of motion in 39% of patients.

CHAPTER 4

Chronic Infections

Mukund R. Patel, G. N. Malaviya, and Alan M. Sugar

General Principles

Chronic infections of the hand and upper extremity are rare and are primarily a problem of diagnosis. They are often not considered in the differential diagnosis of hand lesions. Many surgeons encounter their first case by surprise unless an unusual diagnosis is considered in the presence of unusual symptoms and signs. One must consider infection in any chronic lesion of the hand. In an immunocompromised patient, infection must always be included in the differential diagnosis. *Biopsy and cultures must be considered as a part of a diagnostic work-up for atypical lesions. An infection that does not respond to antibiotics, drainage, or débridement is suspect.* Because infections are rare, diagnosis is often delayed unless a high index of suspicion is maintained. "Culture a tumor and biopsy an infection," is an adage to consider when an unusual lesion is encountered; otherwise, chronic and emerging infections will continue to elude us. With increasing numbers of jet travelers, we encounter old and exotic infections, and with more organ transplants and malignant lesions treated with chemotherapy, we encounter new and emerging infections. Recognition of these infections will save unnecessary surgery for medically treatable infections.

Chronic infections of the hand and upper extremity may be caused by a variety of agents: viruses, bacteria, mycobacteria, fungi, *Prototheca,* protozoa, and parasites (Table 4-1). The infection may be superficial and affect the skin or nails, or it may affect subcutaneous tissue; or it may be deep and affect the nerves, tenosynovium, joints, and bone. *Chronic lesions of the hand have a nonspecific presentation and need early biopsy and cultures for diagnosis. This is the best hope for early diagnosis and treatment.*

The most common chronic infection of the hand traditionally was tuberculosis. Nontuberculous mycobacterial infections (in past recognized as atypical or mycobacteria other than tuberculosis [MOTT]) of the hand are now more common than *Mycobacterium tuberculosis* infections.[8] Tenosynovial infections of both types are far more common than joint and bone infections. The most common fungal infection in North America is sporotrichosis. The most common chronic bacterial infection in North America is nocardiosis. The most common chronic infection affecting the hand in developing countries is Hansen's disease. Hansen's disease infects peripheral nerves, and the index of suspicion should be high when peripheral neuropathy of the ulnar nerve, with or without nerve enlargement, is seen in an immigrant. Chronic hand infections due to human immunodeficiency virus (HIV) have become increasingly common since 1981 in emergency departments and consultation rooms. Ten percent of patients with the acquired immunodeficiency syndrome (AIDS) are asymptomatic and can be diagnosed only with blood tests. HIV blood testing and counseling should be considered in acute and chronic infections of the hand. Hand surgeons should also use universal blood and body fluid precautions when dealing with any hand infection.[4,20] Chronic hand infections caused by protozoa, *Prototheca,* and parasites are sporadically encountered in Africa, Asia, and South America and are rare in North America.

Once a diagnosis is made, it is wise to arrange for consultation with an infectious disease specialist. Pharmacologic treatment of a chronic hand infection requires close monitoring for serious side effects and drug resistance. Recurrence of the infection due to drug resistance may occur from poor patient compliance or poor prescription practices.

DIAGNOSIS

A presumptive diagnosis of a chronic hand infection is made when one considers it as a possibility. Any chronic cutaneous, subcutaneous, tenosynovial, nerve, joint, or bone lesion (nodule, abscess, ulcer, sinus, fistula, or a nondescript mass) of the hand and upper extremity is suspect. The initial appearance of the lesion is nonspecific. A lesion suspected as an unusual tumor may be a chronic infection.[27] Immunocompromised states that may predispose a patient to a chronic hand infection include congenital hypogammaglobulinemia,[28] HIV infection,[10] corticosteroid therapy,[6] cytotoxic therapy,[6] organ transplantation,[14,26] hematologic malignancies,[9] pancytopenic anemia,[13] chronic renal

Table 4-1

ETIOLOGY, DIAGNOSIS, AND TREATMENT OF CHRONIC INFECTIONS OF THE HAND AND UPPER EXTREMITY

	Organism	Predilection	Diagnosis	Chemotherapy
Bacteria	*Actinomyces israelii*	S, SC, J, B	Actinomycosis	Penicillin
	Rochalimaea quintana	S	Bacillary angiomatosis/CSD	ERY
	Nocardia species	S, SC, B	Mycetoma (Actinomycetoma)	As per C&S
	Treponema pallidum	S, SC	Syphilis	Penicillin
	Bacillus anthracis	S	Anthrax	Doxycycline
Fungus	*Aspergillus*	S, SC	Aspergillosis	AB, fluconazole
	Blastomyces dermatitidis	TS, B	Blastomycosis	AB, KTC
	Candida albicans	S, TS	Candidiasis	AB
	Coccidioides immitis	TS, J	Coccidioidomycosis	AB, miconazole
	Cryptococcus neoformans	TS	Cryptococcosis	AB
	Exophiala jeanselmei	Deep abscess	Chromohyphomycosis	None
	Histoplasma capsulatum	TS, J	Histoplasmosis	AB, KTC
	Madurella mycetomatis	S, SC	Mycetoma (Eumycetoma)	As per C&S
	Rhizopus arrhizus	SC	Mucormycosis	AB
	Sporothrix schenckii	S, SC	Sporotrichosis	KTC, SSKI, AB
Mycobacterium leprae	*M. leprae*	N	Hansen's disease	D, RFM, CFZ, ETH
Tuberculous mycobacteria	*M. tuberculosis*	S, TS, J, B	Typical tuberculosis	INH, RFM, ETH, PZA
	M. bovis	TS	Typical tuberculosis	INH, RFM, ETH, PZA
Nontuberculous mycobacteria	*M. asiaticum*	TS	Atypical tuberculosis	TC, CLAR
	M. avium (MAC or MAI)	SC, TS, J, B	Atypical tuberculosis	AZI, CLAR, ETH, RFB
	M. chelonei	TS	Atypical tuberculosis	AMK, ERY
	M. fortuitum	Deep abscess	Atypical tuberculosis	INH, RFM, MIN
	M. haemophilum	J	Atypical tuberculosis	
	M. kansasii	S, TS, J, B	Atypical tuberculosis	INH, RFM
	M. marinum	S, TS, J, B	Atypical tuberculosis	RFM, TC, MIN, AMK
	M. malmoense	TS, J	Atypical tuberculosis	INH, RFM, ETH, PZA
	M. szulgai	TS, BU	Atypical tuberculosis	INH, RFM, ETH, PZA
	M. terrae	S, SC, T, J	Atypical tuberculosis	ETH, CYCLO
Parasites (worms)	*Gnathostoma spinigerum*	SC	Gnathostomiasis	None
	Onchocerca volvulus	TS	Onchocerciasis	None
Prototheca	*Prototheca wickerhamii*	S, TS	Protothecosis	AB, TC
Protozoa	*Leishmania*	S	Leishmaniasis	Antimony, AB
Virus	HIV	CD4 lymphocyte	AIDS	NRTI/PI
	Human papillomaviruses	S (epidermis)	Warts (verruca vulgaris)	Topical salicylic acid
	Paravaccinia virus	S	Human orf/milker's nodule	Cidofovir/idoxuridine

S, skin; SC, subcutaneous; TS, tenosynovium; J, joint; B, bone; N, nerve; BU, bursa; C&S, culture and sensitivity. CSD, cat-scratch disease; MAC, *Mycobacterium avium* complex; MAI, *Mycobacterium avium-intracellulare.*

Chemotherapeutic drugs are abbreviated as follows: AB, amphotericin B; AMK, amikacin; AZI, azithromycin; CFZ, clofazimine; CHL, Chloromycetin; CLAR, clarithromycin; CYCLO, cycloserine; D, dapsone; ERY, erythromycin; ETH, ethambutol; GNT, gentamicin, INH, isoniazid; KTC, ketoconazole; MIN, minocycline; NRTI, nucleoside reverse transcriptase inhibitor; PI, protease inhibitor; PZA, pyrazinamide; RFB, rifabutin (Mycobutin); RFM, rifampin (Rifadin); SSKI, supersaturated solution of potassium iodide; Sulfa, sulfonamides; TC, tetracycline.

failure,[21] systemic lupus erythematosus,[12] diabetes,[5,22,23] alcohol abuse,[19] extreme old age,[25] neutrophil count less than 500/mL,[15,18,24] or protein-calorie malnourishment (serum albumin level < 3.5 g/dL).[1,11] Vascular compromise (arterial injury, venous stasis, lymphangitis, severe scarring, radiation fibrosis) is always an added risk for infection. *The opposite is also true:* one must suspect immunodeficiency when a certain fungus—*Aspergillus, Candida, Cryptococcus, Pseudallescheria boydii,* or a zygomycete— is encountered in a culture from an infected wound.[17] An infective agent may live in balance with an immunocompromised host. Reactivation of a latent organism in the hand may occur when malnutrition sets in[1] or cytotoxic chemotherapy is administered to treat a malignancy.[15,18]

Diagnosis is delayed until tissue (drainage, aspirate, punch biopsy, needle biopsy, open biopsy) is sent for a smear and cultured for bacteria (aerobic and anaerobic), mycobacteria (typical and atypical), and fungus. Organisms in chronic infections are often sparse, and they grow slowly (*M. tuberculosis* divides approximately every 24 hours). Some organisms do not grow at all unless ideal growth medium is provided (*M. haemophilum* requires hemoglobin). *Improper collection and processing of specimens may result in delayed treatment.* There is no other area of clinical medicine in which specimen selection, collection, and transportation are so important and in which close communication with the pathologist, microbiologist, and infectious disease specialist is so imperative.

GUIDELINES FOR BIOPSY, SMEARS, CULTURES, AND ANTIMICROBIAL SENSITIVITY

The specimen must be kept moist and transported rapidly to the laboratory. If a delay is anticipated, the specimen should be refrigerated until prompt delivery can be ensured. A sterile container, securely covered, is adequate. Bacteriostatic saline or formalin should not be used for microbiology specimens. Sampled tissue is better as a specimen than swabs for routine anaerobic, mycobacterial, and fungal cultures. The suspected pathogen must always be specified if other than routine bacteria are suspected (e.g., *Nocardia,* actinomycetoma, *M. marinum, Sporothrix, Bartonella*). This facilitates the choice of the best culture medium and incubation temperature.

Swabs of superficial skin ulcers, from the skin surface of a sinus tract or from open abscesses, commonly yield a host of mixed bacterial flora and often do not reflect the organisms of true infectious significance. For these infections, every effort should be made to sample tissue from the deeper aspects of the lesion or from the margins where the organisms are actively spreading.

An adequate quantity of material should be obtained. Characteristically, chronic lesions contain few organisms. A swab is likely to obtain much serum but few organisms. To recover the most bacteria, mycobacteria, and fungi, a swab should never be submitted in lieu of curettings, biopsy material, or synovial fluid. Tissue biopsy is more likely to show the infecting organisms than pus or necrotic detritus. If a swab is used, the patient's interests are best served by vigorous rather than gentle application of the swab to the target tissue. Biopsy from the base or undermined edge of an ulcer is far superior to swab culture from the surface. Open biopsy is better than needle aspiration, punch biopsy, or superficial curettage of infected tissue. For meaningful culture results, laboratories prefer surgically obtained tissue samples, aspirates of closed abscesses, and a small amount of pus or fluid rather than swab samples. Organism concentrations in synovial fluids and pus may be low, so a minimum of several milliliters should be obtained whenever mycetoma or mycobacterial or fungal infection is a serious consideration. Specimens for smear and culture for mycobacteria should be collected and transported in closed, leak-proof, sterile containers.

The organisms are not uniformly distributed in the infected tissue. Several parts of the lesion should be sampled for smears and cultures to find the infecting organism. On tissue specimens, impression smears made by gently pressing a freshly cut surface of the tissue onto a slide should be requested in addition to routine ground tissue smears. Tissue impression smears are easier to read and interpret than those made from material that has been ground or macerated. Gram stains, Calcofluor white, or potassium hydroxide (KOH) stains for fungi and acid-fast stains for mycobacteria can be done on impression smears.

If results prove negative but signs and symptoms indicate otherwise, repetition of smears and cultures may be helpful. If antibiotic therapy has been initiated, direct smear may be the only available guide to the etiology because growth may be inhibited.

An "eight pack" tissue culture is sent to the microbiology laboratory for diagnosis (Table 4-2). The tissue specimen is immediately bisected: half of it is sent to the pathologist in formalin and the other half is sent promptly to the microbiologist *in sterile containers without formalin* for smears and cultures. *Formalin kills organisms, and they do not grow any more in the culture media. Tissue may be sent in formalin only to the pathologist for histopathology.* The first "three packs" are sent to the microbiology laboratory immediately for staining: Gram stain for bacteria, acid-fast stain for mycobacteria, and KOH stains for fungi (see Table 4-1). The next "five packs" are for cultures: two for aerobic and anaerobic bacteria, two for typical and atypical mycobacteria, and one for fungus. *M. marinum, M. haemophilum, M. ulcerans,* and *Sporothrix schenckii* grow best at 30°C. The rest of the mycobacteria grow best at 37°C. Only one, *M. xenopi,* grows best at 42°C. The

---

Table 4-2
THE "EIGHT PACK" TISSUE CULTURE FOR MICROBIOLOGY COVERS BACTERIA, MYCOBACTERIA, AND FUNGI

Biopsy Tissue	I	Histopathology 50% of tissue in formalin				
	II	Microbiology 50% of tissue *without* formalin	Smear and stain	(1) Gram stain	(2) Acid-fast bacillus stain (Ziehl-Neelsen or Kinyoun)	(3) Fungus stains (potassium hydroxide or Calcofluor white stain)
			Culture and sensitivity	(4) Aerobic (5) Anaerobic (Use transport medium, e.g.,"Portacul.")	(6) Tuberculous mycobacteria at 37°C (7)	(7) Nontuberculous mycobacteria at 30°C (*M. marinum*) and 42° (*M. xenopi*)	(8) Mycotic culture media Sabouraud's dextrose agar or brain heart infusion agar

The above smear and culture protocol is useful for bacteria, mycobacteria, and fungi from the biopsy specimen. The circulating nurse sends half of the biopsy specimen to the pathologist in formalin and the other half as an "eight pack" to the microbiologist in a sterile cup without formalin or saline. The specimen is delivered to the microbiologist immediately at the conclusion of surgery.

microbiologist must know that the specimen is from a chronic lesion so that it can be incubated at appropriate temperatures. The microbiologist also should get the tissue fluid (pus, synovial fluid, serosanguineous exudate), when available, for "eight pack" smears and cultures. The laboratory must know which antimicrobial agents, if any, the patient is taking. Whenever possible, the specimen is obtained before intraoperative antimicrobial agents are administered.

Tissue should be forwarded promptly to the laboratory. More often than not, I deliver the specimen to the microbiologist myself. This gives me an opportunity to communicate clinical history of the patient and tell the pathologist/microbiologist what organisms I am looking for. Fastidious organisms may not survive prolonged storage. Pus, fluid, and tissue should be placed into a transport vial in which anaerobes can survive for several hours, should the specimen not be delivered to the laboratory promptly.

Histoplasma capsulatum, Cryptococcus neoformans, M. bovis, M. avium, M. malmoense, Nocardia, and *Bartonella* may take more than 6 weeks to grow, and it is imperative to request the microbiology laboratory that the cultures not be discarded at the usual 4 weeks. I request the microbiologist not to discard the cultures for 10 weeks and to notify me promptly as soon as growth is positive. I seek help from an infectious disease specialist to closely follow the growth plates in the microbiology laboratory. In the care of immunocompromised patients or difficult diagnostic problems, numerous cultures or tests are often requested on a specimen, for which there may be inadequate quantity. The clinician should prioritize the test requests for the laboratory based on the highest clinical suspicions.

Three laboratory tests are used for identification of mycobacteria: stained smears, cultures in growth media, and, recently, nucleic acid (DNA and RNA) amplification techniques.

Staining

Two procedures are used for acid-fast staining, based on the ability of mycobacteria to retain certain dyes after washing with an acid-alcohol (hence "acid fast"). First, the Ziehl-Neelsen and Kinyoun stains are carbolfuchsin based and stain mycobacteria red. Second, fluorescent stains based on auramine dyes are more sensitive for the detection of mycobacteria in direct specimens. The organisms stain brightly and can be clearly distinguished from background material. Slides stained with a fluorescent dye can be examined reliably with an objective lens of lower magnification (25×) than the oil immersion lens (100×) required for carbolfuchsin-stained smears, and the reading of slides is faster and more reliable. This stain is preferred by the Centers for Disease Control and Prevention (CDC).

Nucleic Acid Amplification Techniques

Nucleic acid amplification techniques are recent advances in the early detection and diagnosis of mycobacterial disease. Two commercially available, Food and Drug Administration (FDA)–approved DNA probes are available for the detection of organisms in the *M. tuberculosis* complex. They are used with organisms grown in culture and, since September 1999,

directly on patient specimens.[30] The procedure can be performed and the organism identified within a matter of hours from the time an infection was suspected. Conventional cultures for tuberculosis generally take many weeks.

Cultures

Several quantitative studies have shown that a minimum of 10,000 bacilli per milliliter of specimen is necessary to detect bacteria in stained smears. When host immunity is high and bacterial virulence is low, infected tissue may have far fewer organisms per milliliter. In such cases, acid-fast staining may be negative. In contrast, fewer than 100 organisms are necessary to grow in culture. Three different types of traditional culture media are available for cultures: egg-based Löwenstein-Jensen, agar based, and liquid based. It is important that the clinician notify the laboratory if a pathogen with specific growth requirements is suspected so that special culturing media can be used. *M. haemophilum* grows best in the presence of hemoglobin, and *Bartonella* species are isolated best by using the Brenner's Isolator system.[7]

A major improvement in mycobacteriology has been the development of commercial broth systems for mycobacterial growth detection. Liquid systems allow for rapid growth and detection of mycobacteria within 1 to 3 weeks compared with solid media, where growth takes 3 to 8 weeks. Biochemical methods can distinguish mycobacterial species from cultures but are time consuming and laborious. Nucleic acid amplification technology and high-performance liquid chromatography have now gained widespread use because they provide rapid diagnosis. Polymerase chain reaction (PCR) analysis allows DNA sequence analysis and direct identification of *M. tuberculosis* in clinical specimens. PCR can detect fewer than 10 organisms/mL in a clinical specimen, compared with 100 for cultures and the 10,000 necessary for a positive smear. PCR analysis provides a useful method for instances when smear and culture are negative in the presence of a clinical presentation of tuberculosis. The test is generally accessible but is skill intensive and expensive, and is not yet considered the gold standard.[3,16] The potential for nucleic acid amplification testing (PCR) to enhance patient care is greatest when suspicion of tuberculosis is moderate to high and specimens are acid-fast bacillus (AFB) smear negative.[30] At least 2 g of tissue is necessary to do this test. The tissue should be set aside and preserved in 70% alcohol for later processing if all conventional smear and culture tests prove negative. The NAP (nitro-acetylamino-hydroxy propiophenone) test differentiates isolates of tuberculous mycobacteria with nearly 100% accuracy. High-performance liquid chromatography (HPLC) can identify virtually all mycobacteria that are clinically relevant to humans but is available only in public health and reference laboratories because the initial cost of equipment is high.[29]

Drug Susceptibility Tests

Drug susceptibility tests are performed on initial isolates from all patients to identify what should be an effective antituberculous regimen. To generate rapid testing and faster turnaround time for better patient management, the radiometric BACTEC system is used to test sensitivity of all primary antituberculous drugs: isoniazid, rifampin, pyrazinamide, and ethambutol.

Isolation of *Aspergillus* or *Nocardia* from a patient without a known immunodeficiency should trigger a work-up for an underlying host immune defect.[17] This work-up includes, at minimum, evaluation of B cell–mediated humoral immunity (serum immunoglobulins and isohemagglutinins) and T cell–mediated cellular immunity (absolute lymphocyte count which is part of a complete blood cell count and differential blood count, peripheral smear, platelet count, and erythrocyte sedimentation rate).[17] The most common cause of immunodeficiency today is acquired. AIDS and iatrogenic deficiencies that result from therapies that modulate the immune system (corticosteroids, post-transplant immunosuppression, and cytotoxic chemotherapy for malignancies) are leading causes of chronic infections. Primary (congenital) immunodeficiency syndrome associated with a hand infection is rare and has been documented in only one case.[28]

TREATMENT

In the war between man and microbe, the outcome depends on the dose and virulence of the infecting microbe and the immunity of the host. Antibiotics reduce the dose of the invading organisms, but final elimination of the infecting organism is determined by innate immunity (phagocytes, natural killer lymphocytes, plasma proteins of complement system) and two arms of acquired immunity: humoral immunity and cell-mediated immunity. *Humoral immunity* is conferred by B lymphocytes, which transform to plasma cells that produce immunoglobulin antibodies to eliminate extracellular organisms. *Cell-mediated immunity* is mediated by T lymphocyte helper cells [CD4+] and T lymphocyte cytolytic cells [CD8+], which eliminate intracellular

organisms in concert with neutrophils, monocytes, and macrophages. Eosinophils produce antibodies against multicellular parasites, and eosinophilia is a clue to a parasitic infection.[2] When humoral and cellular immunity are depressed, it is critical that three important components of treatment be implemented: antibiotics, surgical débridement of the infected tissue, and improved nutrition. Poor nutrition, whether from alcoholism, cancer, major trauma, or inadequate diet, predisposes the patient to infections that would otherwise be easily combated by healthy individuals. When a patient is therapeutically immunosuppressed and does not respond to adequate antibiotic therapy and surgical débridement, a reduction in immunosuppressive therapy and an improvement in nutrition may upgrade the host immunity to successfully combat the invading organisms.[26]

ANNOTATED REFERENCES

26. Sanger JR, Stampfl DA, Franson TR: Recurrent granulomatous synovitis due to *Mycobacterium kansasii* in a renal transplant recipient. J Hand Surg 12:436-441, 1987.

When host immunity exceeds mycobacterial virulence, antibiotics accelerate elimination of bacteria. When bacterial virulence exceeds host immunity, antibiotics and surgical excision of the infected tissue may be necessary. When host immunity is suppressed by chemotherapy and surgical excision is followed by recurrent infection, reduction of chemotherapeutic dose may help to elevate immunity and eliminate infection.

28. Tan ST, Blake GB, Chambers S: Recurrent orf in an immunocompromised host. Br J Plast Surg 44:465-467, 1991.

Infections that resolve naturally tend to perpetuate when host immunity is suppressed. The host may be immunocompromised from congenital lack of immunoglobulins as described by Tan or from acquired causes such as leukemia and lymphoma or chemotherapeutic suppression of immunity as in organ transplants and cancer.

Bacterial Infections

Actinomycosis, botryomycosis, brucellosis, mycetoma (actinomycetoma, eumycetoma), and syphilis are chronic bacterial infections that may affect the hand. They have been reported sporadically over many years. A newly emerging infection of the hand is *Actinobacillus* tenosynovitis. Pyoderma gangrenosum, although not infectious, is included here because it mimics a fulminating infection and must be included in the differential diagnosis. Treatment of this disease with surgery causes it to spread furiously and centrifugally (so-called pathergic reaction) and has even led to unnecessary amputations.[31,80]

Cutaneous anthrax has been classified by the CDC as a bioterrorism disorder since the September 11, 2001 attack and the subsequent bioterrorism incidents.[56] The CDC has categorized biologic agents with potential to be used as weapons based on ease of dissemination or transmission

potential for major public health impact, potential for public panic and social disruption, and the need for public health preparedness. Among the agents of the highest concern is *Bacillus anthracis* (anthrax).

ACTINOBACILLOCIS

Actinobacillosis is caused by *Actinobacillus actinomycetemcomitans,* a gram-negative bacillus that was originally described as a concomitant pathogen with actinomycosis in 1912. The organism is part of the endogenous flora of the mouth and can be recovered from about 20% of teenagers and adults. It is difficult to grow and identify. *Actinobacillus* infections are emerging only recently.

Diagnosis

Two cases of chronic tenosynovitis caused by *A. actinomycetemcomitans* affecting dorsal wrist tendons[45] and finger flexor tendons[49] have been reported.

Treatment

Tenosynovectomy and intravenous gentamicin in one case and oral tetracycline in the other rapidly resolved tenosynovitis without further recurrence.

ACTINOMYCOSIS

Actinomycosis is most commonly caused by *Actinomyces israelii*, a normal inhabitant of the oral cavity. Actinomycosis, by definition, is caused by intrinsic (endogenous) human flora; actinomycetoma is caused by exogenous pathogenic bacteria in soil. Two percent of actinomycosis cases occur in the upper extremity.[46] Most cases of hand actinomycosis have been reported sporadically in the literature between 1915 and 2001.*

Diagnosis

In the hand, a closed-fist injury is the most common cause of actinomycosis. Contents of oral flora may be implanted into the metacarpal head on impact.[39,50,60,112,113,131,142,148,150] Winner correctly called this type of injury "punch actinomycosis."[39,50,131,150] A dentist may contact it during examination of the mouth without gloves.[81] It may also occur in the subcutaneous tissues secondary to a human bite.[133] Clinical presentations are varied. Any suppurative inflammatory reaction that stubbornly resists treatment and tends to discharge continuously should lead one to suspect the possibility of actinomycosis, especially if it is at the site of a human bite wound.[133] It may start as an acute abscess,[39] or there may be a painless and persistent swelling of the hand after the acute inflammation from the initial trauma subsides. Subcutaneous tissue may become indurated and adherent to subjacent bone.[142] It may present as a hard mass,[66] or multiple sinuses may form that intermittently discharge purulent fluid. Once actinomycosis is established locally it spreads contiguously in a slow but progressive manner, ignoring tissue planes. Finally, contiguous invasion of bone occurs.[39,50,113,134] The identification of "yellow sulfur granules" of actinomycosis organisms from a draining sinus is diagnostic. Sulfur granules are a yellow conglomeration of microorganisms that form only in vivo and characteristically are identified in bandages that cover a draining sinus. Biopsy is necessary to obtain clinical material for diagnosis if a draining sinus is not present.

Treatment

Penicillin is the treatment of choice. Intravenous penicillin must be employed in high and prolonged doses followed by oral penicillin or amoxicillin[108] for 6 to 12 months. Short-term treatment with antibiotics may result in temporary cessation of drainage. When the therapy is discontinued,

*See references 39, 50, 60, 66, 81, 112-114, 117, 130, 133, 134, 142, 148, and 150.

however, drainage may recur. Without definitive treatment, the infection may persist for several decades and cause extensive deformities.[120] For penicillin-allergic patients, tetracycline, erythromycin, minocycline, and clindamycin are alternatives. If infection recurs, surgical débridement is an essential part of treatment.[120]

ANTHRAX

In the United States, the annual incidence of anthrax declined from 130 cases annually in the 1900s to a single case reported in 1992. It reappeared in the United States in this millennium as a bioterrorism disorder.[56] Ten cases of cutaneous anthrax and 10 cases of pulmonary anthrax (four fatal) were reported within a month after September 11, 2001. Of the numerous biologic agents that may be used as weapons, anthrax is one of the most serious.[82]

Anthrax is caused by *Bacillus anthracis,* a gram-positive, encapsulated, spore-forming bacillus. The name anthrax (Gk. *anthracis,* "coal") refers to the typical black eschar that is seen on affected areas. Ninety-five percent of patients with cutaneous anthrax are diagnosed when they have a relatively painless necrotic black ulcer.[36] Humans acquire the disease directly from contact with infected herbivores (agricultural anthrax), indirectly from contaminated meat, wool, hides, or leather from infected animals[36,145] (industrial anthrax), through accidental inoculation in the laboratory[151] (laboratory acquired anthrax), or unexpectedly from exposure to "weaponized" spores of bioterrorism (biocriminal anthrax).[82] The clinical forms include (1) cutaneous anthrax, which accounts for more than 95% of cases; (2) intestinal anthrax, from eating infected meat; and (3) pulmonary anthrax, from inhaling spore-laden dust. Cutaneous anthrax of the hand and upper extremity occurs in approximately one third of all cases[61] and may be seen primarily by a hand surgeon.

Diagnosis

Cutaneous anthrax occurs after the deposition of the organism into the skin at the site of a previous cut or abrasion. After an incubation period of 3 days (range, 1 to 12 days), the skin infection begins as an area of local edema that becomes a pruritic macule or papule. The papule progresses to a vesicle or vesicles, surrounded by erythema, in 1 to 2 days. The vesicle contains clear fluid that is dark blue (Fig. 4-1). Patients also may have fever, malaise, headache, and regional lymphadenopathy. The vesicle ruptures in 2 to 14 days and leaves behind a painless black eschar (Fig. 4-2). The eschar contracts into an ulcer, usually 1 to 3 cm in diameter, with small, 1- to 3-mm vesicles surrounding the ulcer. A characteristic black necrotic center develops by 4 weeks, often associated with extensive local edema.[145] Unless the disease becomes systemic, the eschar dries, loosens, and falls off in the next 1 to 2 weeks. A lesion on the finger heals and full mobility is restored.[151] Rarely, the black eschar on the hands may extend deeper than the dermis.[36,145] The common clinical description "malignant pustule" is actually a misnomer because the cutaneous lesion is not purulent. Anthrax is diagnosed by isolating *B. anthracis* from the vesicular fluid of skin lesions. Gram staining reveals bacilli in the subcutaneous tissue.

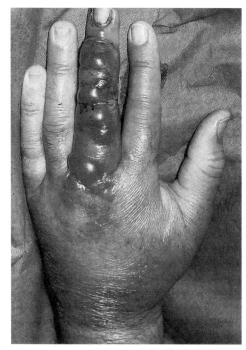

FIGURE 4-1. Initial lesion of cutaneous anthrax is a vesicle or vesicles surrounded by erythema. The vesicle contains clear fluid that is dark blue.

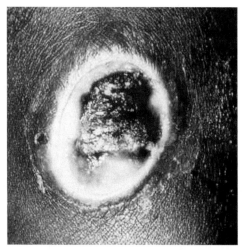

FIGURE 4-2. Vesicles rupture in 2 to 14 days and leave behind a black eschar that is characteristic of anthrax.

Treatment

About 20% of untreated cases of cutaneous anthrax become systemic and result in death. Antibiotic therapy does not appear to change the course of eschar formation and healing. It does decrease the likelihood of systemic disease and death. When treated with appropriate antibiotics, the death rate is less than 1% and lesions resolve without complications or scarring in 80% to 90% of cases. Rarely, the eschar extends deeper than the dermis, down to the muscle fascia. The eschar is then excised, and the defect is grafted using split-thickness skin grafts.[36,145] An eschar in

the forearm caused severe compression neuropathy of the ulnar nerve in one case.[145]

Duration of antibiotic treatment for animal-acquired and bioterrorism-acquired anthrax differs. Animal-acquired anthrax is treated with doxycycline (100 mg PO bid), ciprofloxacin (750 mg bid), or amoxicillin (500 mg tid) orally for 7 to 10 days. Lesions become sterile within 24 hours and resolve within weeks. Direct person-to-person spread of anthrax is extremely unlikely. There is no need therefore to treat contacts of infected individuals unless they were also exposed to the same primary source of infection. Bioterrorism-acquired anthrax is classified as anthrax exposure or anthrax infection. Both exposure and infection are treated for 60 days because aerosol inhalation anthrax is presumed in bioterrorism. A bioterrorist event should be reported to (770) 488-7100 or www.bt.cdc.gov, a website that also provides information about clinical diagnosis and management of all agents of bioterrorism.

In the United States, anthrax vaccine is recommended only for high-risk populations, including military combat personnel, persons who work directly with the organism in the laboratory, those who work with imported animal hides or furs, or those who handle potentially infected animal products in high-incidence areas.

BOTRYOMYCOSIS

Diagnosis

Chronic granulomatous infections of the hand in which grains of organisms are present in tissues are uncommon. Botryomycosis is a rare, chronic, granulomatous, suppurative, bacterial soft tissue infection that produces loose clumps of bacteria that resemble grains. Among more than 100 cases of botryomycosis reported in the literature, three cases affecting the hand have been identified.[51,67,70] The characteristic histologic finding of "granules" in clusters is the origin for the term *botryomycosis* (Gk. *botrys*, "bunch of grapes" in histology and *mycosis* for its clinical and histologic resemblance to fungal infection). The condition is, in fact, produced by bacteria and is truly a "granular bacteriosis." *Staphylococcus aureus,*[70] *Pseudomonas vesicularis,*[51] and *Moraxella nonliquifasciens*[67] have been reported to cause botryomycosis of the hand. Chronicity in botryomycosis may be a state of "equilibrium" between the host and the microorganism. It is not clear if this results from low pathogenicity of the organism or from some peculiar immunologic characteristic of the host. *Moraxella nonliquifasciens,*[67] an organism of low virulence, caused hand botryomycosis as reported by Feldman and coworkers.[67] A staphylococcal botryomycosis of the hand and arm occurred in a patient with decreased resistance due to systemic lupus erythematosus, nephritis, and corticosteroid and azathioprine therapy.[70]

Treatment

Clinically, histologically, and therapeutically this bacterial infection resembles a fungal infection. The condition may respond rapidly to oral antibiotics,[70] or it may be resistant to antibiotic therapy and may need complete excision and skin grafting to eradicate the infection.[67]

BRUCELLOSIS

Brucellae are gram-negative coccobacilli that chronically infect animals. Virtually all human infections derive from direct or indirect contact with cattle *(B. abortus)* or goats and sheep *(B. melitensis)*. Routes of transmission to humans include cuts in the skin, inhalation of infected aerosols, and ingestion of unpasteurized milk. Brucellosis is endemic in the Middle East, South America, and the Mediterranean area. In Texas and California, the epidemiology of brucellosis has changed from a disease associated with exposure to cattle to one linked to ingestion of unpasteurized goat milk products imported from Mexico.

Diagnosis

The musculoskeletal system is affected in approximately one third of the cases.[119] Osteomyelitis and septic arthritis may occur in the upper extremity.[74,119,123] Septic arthritis occurred in the sternoclavicular joint in three cases (1.8%), shoulders in eight (5%), elbows in nine (5.3%), and wrists in six (3.5%). Osteomyelitis occurred in four (2.4%), and tendinitis was noted in one (1.2%).[119] Dactylitis due to osteoarticular brucellosis was described by Ozgocmen and coworkers[124] and by Howard and associates.[79] Diagnosis was made when blood culture[124] or bone needle aspiration culture[79] grew *B. melitensis.* Gonzalez-Alvero,[74] Mousa,[119] and Colmenero[59] and their colleagues have described chronic brucellar olecranon bursitis in which synovial fluid and serum were positive for serologic tests and *B. melitensis* grew on chocolate agar.

Treatment

Repeated 4- to 6-week courses of rifampin and tetracycline may cure the patient without a relapse.[119]

MYCETOMA (ACTINOMYCETOMA AND EUMYCETOMA)

Mycetoma is a disease complex caused either by bacteria (actinomycetoma) or by fungi (eumycetoma, Madura foot, maduromycosis). Eumycetoma is so called because it is caused by the Eumycetes group of fungi.[111] The term *mycetoma* (fungus tumor) was coined in Madura, India, in 1860.[53-55] The infection is characterized by a slowly evolving, often painless, cutaneous and subcutaneous destructive inflammatory granuloma, riddled with abscesses, sinuses with interconnecting channels, and fistulas that drain characteristic colonies of the infecting organisms in the form of granules. *The granules are the defining characteristic of this infection.*[44,54,55,111] These granules are colonies of the organism.[104] Only 2% to 10% of all mycetomas involve the hands,[41,77,78,93,94,100,118,139] whereas the majority occur in the feet.[53] Twenty-one cases of the hand and arm were reviewed by Moore in 1954,[118] and since then several more cases have been reported.* In only three recent cases was the disease diagnosed early at a nodular or abscess stage.[34,92,129] In all other cases, diagnosis was delayed until it was in the sinusoidal or musculoskeletal stage and treatment was difficult.

A mycetoma caused by aerobic bacteria, actinomycetes, is referred to as actinomycetoma.[127] Actinomycetes are

"higher" bacteria with morphologic characteristics between bacteria and fungi. The majority of actinomycetomas in North America are caused by *Pseudallescheria boydii*[75,98] (its asexual anamorph is *Scedosporium apiospermum*[43,90]; previous other names: *Allescheria*[98] and *Monosporium*) and *Nocardia* species.[52,73,75,109,116,129,146] The spectrum of chronic nocardiosis of the hand varies from a nondraining skin plaque[139] to a draining abscess or multiple discharging sinuses, to typical stage 1, 2, and 3 actinomycetoma.[52,116,129]

A mycetoma caused by true fungi is referred to as eumycetoma, true mycetoma,[127] or maduromycosis.[57,58] More than 30 fungi are known to cause eumycetoma.[44] Distinguishing mycetomas caused by actinomycetes bacteria (actinomycetoma) and fungi (eumycetoma) is extremely important because the treatment and prognosis of the two are distinctly different. In contemporary medical mycology, actinomycosis is not classified as an actinomycetoma because the etiologic agents of actinomycosis are anaerobic and components of the endogenous oral flora. Rippon has stipulated that only infections caused by aerobic exogenous pathogenic bacteria and fungi are included in mycetoma.[132] This clearly differentiates actinomycosis from actinomycetoma.

Microbiology

Major actinomycetes bacteria and fungi causing mycetoma are found all over the world and are associated with woody plants and soil.[110] The largest number of infected patients live in the tropics.[110] In the United States, several cases of hand mycetoma have been reported, and they are almost equally divided between actinomycetoma and eumycetoma.†

Agents of mycetoma differ in different parts of the world. The most common cause of mycetoma in the United States is *Pseudallescheria boydii* (asexual anamorph, *Scedosporium apiospermum*; older names: *Allescheria, Monosporium, Petriellidium*)[98] and *Nocardia.*[37,52,76,92,109] *Madurella mycetomatis, Actinomadura madurae,* and *Nocardia brasiliensis* predominate in India,[88] and *N. brasiliensis* and *A. madurae* are the most common causes of mycetoma in Mexico and Central and South America. *Streptomyces somaliensis* and *Actinomadura pelletieri* are seen in Africa. *N. asteroides* and *Scedosporium apiospermum*[95] are reported to predominate in Japan. A case of *Arthrographis kalrae* hand eumycetoma successfully treated with itraconazole was reported from France,[63] and a case of *S. somaliensis* hand actinomycetoma sensitive to cotrimoxazole and streptomycin was reported from the United Kingdom.[77] *Phialophora jeanselmei (Torula jeanselmei)* hand eumycetoma was reported from Thailand.[153] At times, granules are identified in the lesion but fail to grow organisms and challenge diagnosis and treatment.[34,77,84]

Diagnosis

A mycetoma is defined by the characteristic triad of signs—tumor, sinus, and grains—in the distal aspect of a limb.

---

*See references 33, 34, 37, 64, 72, 76, 84, 92, 98, 109, 115, 118, 129, and 144.

†See references 34, 37, 52, 64, 72, 75, 76, 84, 109, 115, 118, 129, and 144.

Swelling is woody and indurated, and multiple sinus tracts drain grain-filled pus. Characteristic grains in draining sinuses are 0.2 to 3.0 mm in diameter and may be black, white, yellow, pink, or red, depending on the causal organism. Grains may be difficult to locate in histopathologic sections and require multiple cuts through the paraffin-embedded tissue. Hematoxylin and eosin stain is adequate to detect the grains. Tissue Gram staining detects fine, branching hyphae within the actinomycetoma grain, and Gomori's methenamine silver or periodic acid–Schiff stain detects the larger hyphae of eumycetoma. Species of the agent can often be recognized by the color, size, compaction, and hematoxylin-staining character of the grain when organisms fail to grow.

Mycetoma, regardless of fungal or bacterial origin, has a similar clinical presentation. The majority of the patients are males and between 30 and 60 years old. The male-to-female ratio is 5:1. The disease begins following the traumatic implantation of the etiologic agent from the soil, thorn, or wood splinter into a bare hand of a healthy person.[110] The lesions may be restricted to a finger[92,94,101,136,153] (Fig. 4-3A), hand[42,84,97,115,144] (see Fig. 4-3B), wrist,[94] or forearm[109,116] or may extend to the axilla and the chest wall.[65]

The infection begins in the skin and subcutaneous tissues. Mycetoma tends to follow fascial planes as it spreads proximally, laterally, and with increasing depth it progressively infects and destroys all connective tissues and bone. I have graded mycetoma of the hand into four stages. Initially, the lesion is a small, firm, painless subcutaneous nodule or nodules under the skin (duration, 2 to 3 months)[84,85,100] or the nodules may grow to a large size[72,84] (nodular stage) (see Fig. 4-3A). Nodules become abscesses and drain granules through sinuses to the surface of the skin or to the surface of an ulcerated nodule (duration, 4 to 12 months)[77,100,110] (sinusoidal stage). Sinuses may close after pus and granules have been discharged. Old sinuses heal and new ones crop up. If left untreated, the infection progresses to osteomyelitis and limb deformity over the course of a year or more[94,100,109] (skeletal stage). A network of connected sinuses is present in the soft tissues from the bone to skin. Hand mycetoma has been reported to extend through the lymphatics to the chest wall after many years (metastatic stage).[135]

Constitutional symptoms are absent. Pain is not a predominant symptom. The patient, usually an immigrant, a rural farmer, or a laborer of lower socioeconomic status, postpones seeking medical care until the second or third stage is reached. Granules, which are aggregates of the organism, are discharged through these sinuses. Eventually the hand and forearm become grossly enlarged, nodular,

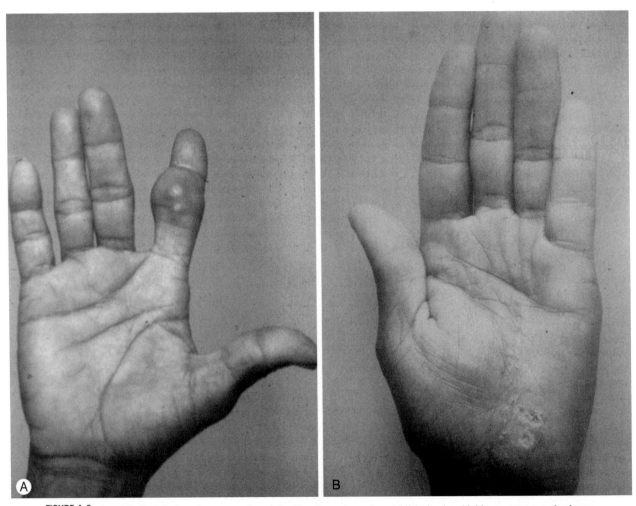

FIGURE 4-3. **A** and **B,** Early lesion of mycetoma is nodular. The diagnosis can be established only with biopsy, smears, and cultures.

discolored, indurated, and deformed, although there may be little pain or tenderness experienced by the patient. The progression of the disease is marked by remissions and exacerbations. The period necessary for the development of the deformity varies from several months to several years. The extent of soft tissue invasion (staging) is best appreciated on magnetic resonance imaging. A more exact species diagnosis depends on the culture of the grain and isolation of the organism. The grain obtained for culture must be as free as possible from bacterial and fungal contamination. A deep-tissue, wedge-shaped biopsy provides a good specimen for both histologic and microbiologic diagnosis. Fungi that cause eumycotic mycetoma can be difficult to grow.[34] Optimizing growth of a eumycotic mycetoma involves an important step. Before being inoculated onto culture media, the grains should be rinsed quickly in 70% alcohol and washed several times in sterile saline. Biopsy specimens are preferred over discharged grains, because such grains may be contaminated with surface organisms or may already be dead. For primary isolation, actinomycetoma grains are grown on Löwenstein-Jensen medium and fungal grains on blood agar. Sabouraud agar (2% glucose, 1% peptone agar) without antibacterial antibiotics is satisfactory for subcultures.

Two sets of cultures are prepared: one is inoculated at 37°C and the other at 26°C. Characteristic colonies are expected to develop within 10 days. Apart from *M. mycetomatis,* which secretes a brown pigment in the medium, all other organisms, both bacteria and fungi, tend to maintain the color of the original grain. Bacterial colonies are usually granular or cerebriform, whereas fungal colonies are either velvety or fluffy. Further identification is made by microscopic examination of fungi in lactophenol blue preparation and of bacteria in Gram and modified Ziehl-Neelsen stains.

Actinomycotic granules may be white *(Actinomadura madurae),* pink or red *(A. pelletieri),* yellow *(Nocardia asteroides, Streptomyces somaliensis[109]),* or orange *(N. asteroides).* Black granules are always eumycotic *(Leptosphaeria senegalensis, Exophilia jeanselmei, Madurella grisea, M. mycetomatis),* but eumycotic granules may also be pale *(Pseudallescheria boydii).*[103]

In histologic sections stained with hematoxylin and eosin, involved tissue reveals a suppurative granuloma. Grains are seen embedded in an abscess composed of neutrophils accompanied by an outer epithelioid cell, plasma cell, and multinucleated giant cell reaction intermingled with areas of fibrosis. The size of various grains in sections is so characteristic that it allows specific diagnosis of the causative organism. Eumycetic hyphae within the grain are easy to see at 400× magnification, whereas those of actinomycetes are difficult to visualize even at 800×.[104] In electron micrographs, concentric rings of cell wall thickening and coarse cell wall fibrils around cells are seen within eumycetic grains. Persons afflicted with mycetoma generally have deficient cell-mediated immunity. This is evidenced by their inability to react to tuberculin.[89]

Differential Diagnosis

Tentative diagnosis is made in the presence of a chronic cutaneous and subcutaneous lesion that is swollen, indurated, and riddled with nodules, abscesses, sinuses, and fistulas that discharge granules. Tuberculosis, syphilis, sporotrichosis, blastomycosis, botryomycosis,[51,67,70] and coccidioidomycosis should all be considered in the differential diagnosis. In only one case, *Aspergillus nidulans* was reported to cause eumycetoma of the forearm.[128]

Treatment

The success of treatment depends not only on the differentiation between actinomycetoma and eumycetoma but also on a definitive identification of the causal organism. The correct approach for initial treatment of actinomycetoma is medical.[102] The correct approach for the initial treatment of eumycetoma is a wide surgical débridement of acute and necrotic tissues[78,110] followed by chemotherapy.

Actinomycetoma

In all cases of actinomycetoma, a combination of two drugs has been used for the past 25 years. One of these is always streptomycin sulfate[104] (14 mg/kg daily for the first month and on alternate days thereafter). In patients with *A. madurae* mycetoma, dapsone is given orally (1.5 mg/kg in the morning and evening). Similarly, *S. somaliensis* mycetoma is treated by dapsone first, but if no response appears after 1 month, treatment is changed to trimethoprim-sulfamethoxazole tablets (23 mg/kg/day of sulfamethoxazole and 4.6 mg/kg/day of trimethoprim in two divided doses). *A. pelletieri* mycetoma responds better to streptomycin and trimethoprim-sulfamethoxazole; this was also the experience with *N. brasiliensis* in Sudan. However, such mycetomas caused by *Nocardia* in the Americas are treated with trimethoprim-sulfamethoxazole and dapsone or trimethoprim-sulfamethoxazole and amikacin. Because amikacin could have deleterious side effects in patients with renal disease (and because of its high cost in developing countries), it is kept as a second-line treatment when first-line treatment that includes dapsone fails. Treatment is given in cycles of simultaneous administration of two divided doses of amikacin (15 mg/kg/day) for 3 weeks and trimethoprim-sulfamethoxazole (35 mg/kg/day) for 5 weeks. The cycle is repeated for a second and, rarely, a third time as the need arises.[104]

Eumycetoma

Combined surgical and medical management is the currently recommended approach.[110] Early resection with a wide margin of uninfected tissue results in the most successful outcomes. Surgery is used as a means to remove bulk of the lesion, and treatment is then supplemented with antifungal drugs. Ketoconazole,[77] itraconazole,[78] and fluconazole are drugs of choice for fungi that cause eumycetoma.[110,149] Eumycetoma caused by *M. mycetomatis* often responds to ketoconazole, 200 mg twice daily, and debulking of the lesion. Miconazole is an option to manage mycetoma caused by *P. boydii.*[149] Rare cases of mycetoma caused by *Acremonium falciforme, Aspergillus flavus,* or *Fusarium* have responded well to itraconazole in a dose of 200 mg twice daily. Ketoconazole, given preoperatively, permits less radical excision of the infected tissues.[42,105] Altman and associates successfully used oral fluconazole for 6 months to treat a eumycotic hand infection.[34] In all cases of medical management, treatment is given for at least 6 to 12 months and has been required for up to 3 years in some cases.[104] The cure rate is approximately 70%.[78] Although side effects are few, patients are regularly monitored to assess hematologic, kidney, or liver function, depending on the medication used. Surgical management should include excision to uninfected margins; otherwise, the recurrence rate is as high as 80%. For further reading, Mahgoub,[78,101,103-105] Mariat,[107] and McGinnis[110,111] and their colleagues have detailed discourses on this difficult infection.

SYPHILIS

Diagnosis

Syphilitic lesions of the hand may be congenital, primary, secondary, or tertiary. The primary syphilitic lesion in the hand usually occurs on the tip of a finger because infection is acquired from the mouth,[81] teeth,[140] or genitals[35,143] of an infected person through direct contact. The lesion may present at the tip of a finger as an ulcer[35,81,143,147] or an ulcerative paronychia.[81,91,143] Paronychia may present as a "discharging horseshoe ulcer" around the nail fold or as inflammatory periungual and subungual papules.[32] Lesions on multiple fingers may occur.[62,91] The chancre appears on a finger approximately 3 weeks after exposure. The ulcer is indolent and has a firm granulomatous base, raised margins, and serous discharge.[147] A concurrent lesion on the genitalia may or may not be present.[143] Epitrochlear and axillary lymph glands are enlarged.

Lesions of secondary syphilis in the hand consist of syphilitic dactylitis.[143] Tertiary lesions of syphilis in the hand are called *gummas*. A gumma is a chronic granulomatous lesion that involves tissues from skin to bone. Congenital syphilis may present as bilateral metacarpal and phalangeal dactylitis in a newborn.[40,69] Syphilitic dactylitis may present as edema of the hands and fusiform swelling of digits.[40] Metacarpals and phalanges show bone formation (reactive sclerosis), bone destruction (patchy rarefaction), and periosteal new bone formation.[40] Syphilitic dactylitis in the infant may resemble spina ventosa that is typical of tuberculosis.[71] Pathologic fractures of the metaphysis may masquerade as pseudoparalysis.[69] Syphilis should be remembered in the differential diagnosis of infantile osteomyelitis.

A presumptive diagnosis of syphilis is made by using two types of serologic tests: treponemal tests (e.g., fluorescent treponemal antibody absorbption test [FTA-ABS]) and nontreponemal tests (e.g., Venereal Disease Research Laboratory test [VDRL]; or the rapid plasma reagin test [RPR]). Diagnosis is confirmed by darkfield examination of the exudate from the lesion for *Treponema pallidum*.

Treatment

Congenital Syphilitic Hand Lesions. Pathologic fractures and dactylitis are treated with protective splints in addition to an appropriate dose of penicillin.

Primary Syphilitic Hand Lesion. Treatment is with one dose of 2.4 million units of intramuscular benzathine penicillin G. The regimen for penicillin-allergic patients is doxycycline, 100 mg, orally two times daily for 2 weeks.

Secondary and Tertiary Syphilitic Hand Lesions. Secondary and tertiary syphilis are treated with benzathine penicillin G, 2.4 million units intramuscularly, given 1 week apart for 3 consecutive weeks.

PYODERMA GANGRENOSUM (GANGRENOUS PYODERMA)

Pyoderma gangrenosum can mimic an acute or chronic infection. It is a progressive necrotizing and ulcerative disease of the skin (Fig. 4-4A), and there may be a predisposition in hosts with immunologic compromise. The condition is characterized by prompt deterioration with surgical excision and/or grafting and a relatively rapid resolution with oral prednisone. Pyoderma gangrenosum is well known to dermatologists but may be misdiagnosed as a "fulminating" infection. Diagnosis of pyoderma gangrenosum often requires consultation by multiple specialists. Misdiagnosis results in inappropriate initial medical treatment (antibiotics[38,68,80,83,86,96,125,152]), unnecessary incision and drainage,[38,68,86,96] multiple débridements,[38,86] unnecessary skin grafts,[80] digital necrosis,[87] and even amputation.[31,80]

Pyoderma gangrenosum was first described at the Mayo Clinic in 1930 as a fulminant streptococcal infection.[48] Although this was subsequently disproved by bacteriologic and histologic studies, the name "pyoderma gangrenosum" persisted because of the original assumed etiology. It is most common in the lower limbs and trunk and rare in the hands and upper extremity.[80] Only 20 cases in the hand and upper extremity were reported in the English literature between 1983 and 2001, and all were misdiagnosed initially as infection.*

Diagnosis

Pyoderma gangrenosum characteristically affects the dorsal surface of a finger,[80,106,122] hand,[31,38,47,68,80,83,86,125,152] wrist, forearm,[86] or elbow.[80] Patients are most often in their third and fourth decades. A centrifugally creeping and weeping ulcer is surrounded with a rough, serpentine, undermining, burrowing, black-blue rim, which is further encircled with a 5- to 10-mm rim of raised purplish erythema and covered by a thin, translucent graying epidermis (see Fig. 4-4A). It spreads 1 to 2 cm per day in a centrifugal pattern. Pain is a significant symptom in 75% of cases. The central portion undergoes wet gangrenous necrosis, oozes, and impersonates infection.[87,99] Pyoderma gangrenosum does not respond to traditional antibiotics, local wound débridement, or skin grafting. Wound débridement consistently leads to deterioration of the condition; this so-called pathergic response is a hallmark of this disease.[80,137] In a review of 13 cases in the literature and 7 cases added by Huish and colleagues, every patient initially had a misdiagnosis of infection. Thirteen misdiagnoses resulted in 16 unnecessary surgeries, including four amputations and two failed skin grafts. No surgical procedure resulted in clinical improvement. All surgical

---

*See references 31, 38, 47, 68, 80, 83, 86, 96, 106, 122, 125, and 152.

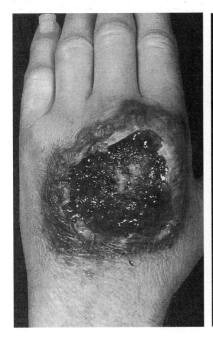
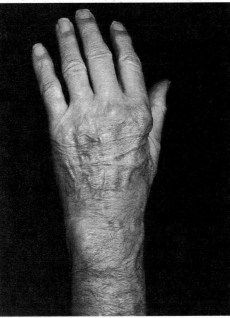

FIGURE 4-4. **A** and **B,** Pyoderma gangrenosum ulcer is a centrifugally creeping ulcer surrounded by a rough, serpentine, undermining black-blue rim, which is further encircled with a 5- to 10-mm rim of raised purplish erythema covered by a thin, translucent, graying epidermis. The central portion undergoes wet gangrenous necrosis, oozes, and impersonates infection.

procedures were followed by unrelenting extension of the ulcer. All cultures were negative. Five physicians on an average examined each patient before the final diagnosis of pyoderma gangrenosum was made by or in conjunction with a dermatologist. Clinical improvement after correct medical treatment with oral prednisone, azathioprine, or dapsone was dramatic and occurred within 1 week.[80]

More than 50% of the hand patients had ulcerative colitis,[31,68,80] Crohn's disease,[38] myelodysplastic syndrome,[80,86,152] or an accompanying immunologic disorder. Twenty-five percent of patients had no known underlying medical condition.[38,83,96,122,125,152] The prevalence of pyoderma gangrenosum in ulcerative colitis is about 5%; and in Crohn's disease it is about 2%. Pyoderma gangrenosum is a clinical diagnosis, and a high clinical suspicion aids in its correct diagnosis and treatment. Biopsy is of little diagnostic value, and no laboratory test is confirmatory.

Treatment

Management includes oral administration of corticosteroids (prednisone, 100 mg/day), treatment of associated medical conditions, and avoidance of surgical intervention. The administration of corticosteroids is tapered when the ulcers show signs of healing. Within 6 weeks, the lesion is completely epithelialized because the deeper layers of the dermis, sweat glands, and hair follicles remain intact (see Fig. 4-4B).[86] It responds to oral dapsone[47] or azathioprine[31] or intralesional steroid injections[83] when oral corticosteroids are contraindicated. Before the advent of these drugs, the skin lesions healed with an atrophic scar when the underlying disease, such as ulcerative colitis, was controlled.[48]

ANNOTATED REFERENCES

36. Aslan G, Terzioglu A: Surgical management of cutaneous anthrax. Ann Plast Surg 41:468-470, 1998.

145. Terzioglu A, Aslan G: Ulnar nerve lesion due to cutaneous anthrax. Ann Plast Surg 43:644-645, 1999.

Black eschar of anthrax rarely transcends the dermis and subcutaneous tissue. When the eschar is thick and causes pressure on the subjacent nerve, it may need early excision and coverage of the nerve with a skin graft, as shown above by Terzioglu and Aslan.

80. Huish SB, de La Paz EM, Ellis PR III, Stern PJ: Pyoderma gangrenosum of the hand: A case series and review of the literature. J Hand Surg [Am] 26:679-685, 2001.

This article is a worthwhile reading for every hand surgeon who wants to avoid an embarrassing encounter with this rare acute fulminating disease. It summarizes personal experience and review of literature on cases affecting the upper extremity. It shows how rapidly the condition resolves when treated with prednisone and how rapidly it deteriorates when treated with surgery.

99. Louis DS, Jebson PJ: Mimickers of hand infections. Hand Clin 14:519-529, 1998.

This article is a good collection of hand conditions that mimic hand infections. The examples are well illustrated and rare and serves both the novice and well experienced.

101. Mahgoub ES: Treatment of actinomycetoma with sulfamethoxazole plus trimethoprim. Am J Trop Med Hyg 21:332-335, 1972.

102. Mahgoub ES: Medical management of mycetoma. Bull WHO 54:303-310, 1976.

103. Mahgoub ES: Mycetoma. Semin Dermatol 4:230-236, 1985.

104. Mahgoub ES: Agents of mycetoma. *In* Mandell GL, Bennett C, Dolin R (eds): Principles and Practice of Infectious Diseases, 5th ed. New York, Churchill Livingstone, 2000, pp 2702-2706.

105. Mahgoub ES, Gumaa SA: Ketoconazole in the treatment of eumycetoma due to *Madurella mycetomii*. Trans R Soc Trop Med Hyg 78:369-376, 1984.

Mahgoub has the largest experience in epidemiology, bacteriology, diagnosis, treatment, and prognosis of actinomycetoma and eumycetoma. This rare disease has been reported in the Western Hemisphere with regularity in every decade since it was first described. It serves to keep this disease in the differential diagnosis of any chronic infection of the hand and upper extremity. If a hand surgeon encounters a case of mycetoma, Mahgoub will provide the most comprehensive update on the subject.

Fungal Infections

CLASSIFICATION

Fungal (*L. fungosus*, "mushroom") infections of the hand can be divided into three anatomic categories: cutaneous, subcutaneous, and deep.[158,215] The most common fungal infections of the hand are cutaneous infections (skin and nail), and these are commonly treated by dermatologists and primary care physicians. Subcutaneous (phaeomycotic cysts) and deep infections (tendon, bone, joint) are rare and are likely to be seen by hand surgeons after patients are treated for variable durations by other physicians and surgeons.[157] Fungi can appear microscopically as either yeasts or molds. Yeasts are unicellular, typically round or oval, and usually reproduce by budding. Molds have multinucleate, long, filamentous structures called hyphae that grow by branching and longitudinal extension. The fungi are somewhat artificially divided into nonopportunistic and opportunistic fungi. Nonopportunistic fungal infections (such as those causing the endemic mycoses) of the hand are common, affect healthy subjects, and grow in the host at body temperature (37°C) as yeastlike forms. They grow in nature at room temperature (27°C) as molds, and their growth is thus facilitated when incubated in the laboratory at ambient temperature. The endemic fungi known to infect the hand include the agents of blastomycosis, coccidioidomycosis, histoplasmosis, and sporotrichosis.[158] In contrast, opportunistic fungi infect immunocompromised patients, and the fungi are ubiquitous in the environment. These infections are rare and usually present as deep infections. Any yeast or mold recovered from an immunocompromised patient should not be dismissed as a "contaminant" or colonizer without first ruling out its role in the patient's disease.[282] Fungi commonly associated with immunodeficiencies are shown in Table 4-3.

Table 4-3
RISK FACTORS AND COMMONLY ASSOCIATED FUNGI

Predisposing Host Risk Factors	Fungi/Infection
Neutropenia (hematogenous malignancies)	*Aspergillus*, mucormycosis
Cell-mediated immune defects including AIDS	*Cryptococcus*
Malnutrition	*Aspergillus*, mucormycosis
Diabetes	Mucormycosis
Corticosteroids	*Cryptococcus, Pseudallescheria boydii (Allescheria boydii, Petriellidium boydii)* (Bower), mucormycosis
Cytotoxic chemotherapy	*Aspergillus*

DIAGNOSIS AND TREATMENT: GENERAL PRINCIPLES

Although most commonly diagnosed in patients with immunodeficiency, a high index of suspicion is necessary to avoid misdiagnosis. Fungal infections have been reported in patients with AIDS,[200,290] with hematologic malignancies,[155,203,219,221,238,255,300] on cancer chemotherapy, and on corticosteroid therapy[205,288,298]; in recipients of bone marrow and organ transplants[155]; in patients with prosthetic joint implants[185]; in patients with prosthetic arteriovenous shunts[287] and distal steal phenomena[229]; in patients with chronic renal failure[155]; in diabetics[155,179,188,275,298]; and in alcoholics.[157] Similarly, one must suspect immunodeficiency when certain fungi, such as *Aspergillus, Candida, Cryptococcus, Pseudallescheria boydii*, or the Zygomycetes are encountered in a culture from an infected patient.[216] An appropriate work-up to identify the immunodeficiency is then warranted. When a soft tissue, joint, or bone infection presents as a chronic draining sinus that has not responded to usual antibiotics, deep fungal infection should be considered. Nondiagnostic surgical wound cultures also raise the possibility of a fungal infection. The main role of the surgeon is to perform an adequate biopsy and request smears and cultures for fungi. Fungi can often be identified in biopsy tissue, even when they do not grow in culture. A 10% KOH solution or a preparation stained with Calcofluor white may be requested to prepare wet tissue mounts. Calcofluor white stains the fungal elements so that they are relatively more visible, but a fluorescence microscope is needed. The histologic features of a biopsy specimen can be more rapidly diagnostic than culture when the mycosis is caused by a slow-growing fungus, which can take weeks to a month or more to grow in the laboratory and may require special growth media.

Finally, biopsy may provide proof that the fungus is invading tissue and is not just a contaminant (e.g., a saprophyte growing on a skin ulcer). It is important to transport the specimen rapidly to the microbiology laboratory to minimize overgrowth of contaminating bacteria. Most fungi grow within 4 weeks but occasionally will take 8 weeks to grow (as is the case with *Sporothrix schenkii* and some of the filamentous fungi), and it is wise to request the microbiology laboratory not to discard the cultures at their usual 4 weeks when fungi are suspected.[184] Testing for the presence of antibody has been used for diagnosis of coccidioidomycosis and histoplasmosis but has not proved to be very useful in cases of blastomycosis and sporotrichosis.

Correlation of clinical and microbiologic results is always necessary.[282] Some fungi (*Blastomyces dermatitidis, Coccidioides immitis, Histoplasma capsulatum*) usually infect immunocompetent hosts while other fungi (*Aspergillus, Rhizopus, Cryptococcus*, and *Pseudallescheria*) infect immunocompromised hosts. However, the endemic fungi are important causes of infection in seriously immunocompro-

Table 4-4

SPECTRUM OF ACTIVITY OF ANTIFUNGAL AGENTS AND PREFERRED AGENT(S)* FOR MOST CLINICAL INFECTIONS

	Amphotericin B	Flucytosine	Ketoconazole	Fluconazole	Itraconazole
Aspergillus	+*	+	–	–	+
Blastomyces +*		+	+	+*	
Candida albicans	+*	+	+	+*	+
Chromomycosis		+*	+		+
Cryptococcus	+*	+*	+	+	+
Coccidioides	+*	–	+	+	+*
Histoplasma	+*	–	+	+	+*
Mucormycosis	+	–	–	–	–
Pseudallescheria			+		+*
Sporothrix	+	–	+	+	+*

In general, acutely ill patients with life-threatening mycosis should be treated with amphotericin B. Azole therapy can follow once the patient's condition is stabilized.

mised hosts such as those with AIDS or heart transplants. The major principle is to suspect fungal infection when any fungus is recovered from an immunocompromised host, rather than dismiss the isolate as a contaminant. Recovery of *Aspergillus* or *Candida* from an otherwise normal host may not be indicative of invasive disease, but the burden is to consider these seriously before ruling out infection. Many risk factors are specific to certain fungal infections. The differential diagnosis can often be narrowed on the basis of the specific immune defect present (Table 4-4).

The diagnostic laboratory should be alerted when specimens from patients suspected of having coccidioidomycosis or histoplasmosis are sent for culture. The yeastlike forms present in tissue will convert to the mycelial form at room temperature and can be easily aerosolized if the cultures are not maintained in a biohazard hood. Infection of the laboratory with *H. capsulatum* or *C. immitis* is a well-appreciated occurrence and can lead to considerable morbidity and even mortality in the infected laboratory worker.

Surgical débridement of infected tissue is the keystone of treatment in aspergillosis[174,203,221,238,255] and mucormycosis,[155] irrespective of the host's immunocompetence. Secondary to their angioinvasive nature, these two fungi cause severe and often progressive tissue infarction and necrosis. Removal of nonviable tissue is critical to the success of treatment. If possible, reversal of the underlying immunocompromising predisposition should be vigorously attempted.

Amphotericin B (Fungizone) was the treatment of choice for patients with fungal diseases from the time of its introduction in 1958 and by default became the gold standard for antifungal therapy of invasive mycoses.[282] It is given intravenously and has serious toxic effects on kidney, liver, and blood. The availability of lipid formulations of amphotericin B, such as Abelcet and AmBisome, has resulted in the ability to administer higher doses of amphotericin B with significantly fewer side effects. Currently, there is some controversy concerning whether the lipid formulations should replace Fungizone for most indications. Because these lipid formulations of amphotericin B are rather expensive, many are loathe to prescribe them, when the much less expensive conventional amphotericin B can be used. Consultation with experts in the treatment of invasive fungal diseases is encouraged, so that the most effective and least toxic regimen can be recommended.

Use of effective oral antifungal therapy for the treatment of invasive mycoses is a relatively recent development. Since the FDA approval of ketoconazole (Nizoral) in 1983,

CRITICAL POINTS: HIGH SUSPICION FOR FUNGAL INFECTION

- Any infection in an immunocompromised patient
- An infection that does not respond to antibiotics, drainage, and débridement
- Sterile or nondiagnostic cultures of the surgical wound

CRITICAL POINTS: TREATMENT OF FUNGAL INFECTIONS

- Fungal infections require a high index of suspicion, long incubation periods, and special growth media.
- Tissue biopsy is often necessary to differentiate true infection from a culture contaminant.
- Surgical débridement of infected tissue is the keystone of treatment in aspergillosis[174,203,221,238,255] and mucormycosis,[155] irrespective of a host's immunocompetence.
- Side effects of antifungal antibiotics and emerging resistant strains necessitate a consultation with an infectious disease specialist.

fluconazole (Diflucan) in 1990, and itraconazole (Sporanox) in 1994, these synthetic oral antifungal azoles have been increasingly used as therapy for various systemic mycoses. In certain circumstances they have equivalent efficacy and improved safety and ease of administration when compared with amphotericin B. Itraconazole has emerged as a possible alternative to amphotericin B in treating several fungal infections, including aspergillosis, blastomycosis, coccidioidomycosis, histoplasmosis, pseudallescheriasis, and sporotrichosis. Antifungal agents in current use are shown in Table 4-4. Because of the infrequency of these infections, potential side effects of medications and the emergence of resistant strains, an infectious disease consultation is advisable. Some drugs, such as itraconazole capsules, are erratically absorbed and have multiple drug interactions. When antifungal agents are used for chronic therapy, serum blood concentrations should be obtained and doses adjusted as necessary.

CUTANEOUS FUNGAL INFECTIONS

Cutaneous (superficial) infections are caused by fungi that metabolize keratin. Because these organisms depend on keratin for nutrition, they do not invade beneath the skin. Most of the clinical manifestations of skin infection are a consequence of host reaction to fungal metabolic products.[158] Patients with skin and nail infections usually seek medical care from dermatologists. Most of these fungi are easily identified on wet KOH preparations. They grow hyphae (Gk. *hyphos,* "a web") readily on Sabouraud's medium. Skin or nail scrapings from the suspected area are placed in 10% KOH on a glass slide. The slide can be heated over an alcohol lamp until bubbles are seen. Spores or branching mycelia under the microscope confirm the presence of fungus. *Candida albicans* and dermatophytes (*Trichophyton, Microsporum,* and *Epidermophyton)* cause the majority of chronic cutaneous and nail infections.

Etiology

Chronic cutaneous *C. albicans* infection occurs in the moist palms and webs of a "clenched fist" in patients with spasticity. Trichophytosis ("ringworm") is the most common cutaneous (and nail) infection. It is more often treated by a family physician or dermatologist, although hand surgeons are now consulted by the patients directly and often. The skin diseases associated with *Trichophyton* are also commonly referred to as "tinea." Other fungi that infect the skin are *Epidermophyton* and *Microsporum.* "Wristwatch ringworm" occurs in moist skin under a watch or its strap.[160] Tinea nigra palmaris has been reported to be misdiagnosed as malignant melanoma.[269,299]

Diagnosis

Definitive diagnosis requires fungal cultures, because the infections caused by *Trichophyton* and *C. albicans* may not be clinically distinguishable and they respond to different antifungal agents.

Treatment

In the cerebral palsy patient with a clenched fist, tendon or fascial lengthening (see Chapter 34) may be necessary to prevent recurrent infections if routine hand hygiene fails to keep the skin dry.

Uncomplicated cases of tinea are easily treated with cream or lotion of tolnaftate (Tinactin),[270] miconazole (Monistat),[180] or ciclopirox (Loprox).[270] Widespread lesions require treatment with oral griseofulvin, ketoconazole, fluconazole, or itraconazole. It is probably not necessary to use the newer broad-spectrum triazole derivatives, such as voriconazole, for the treatment of these infections.

SUBCUTANEOUS FUNGAL INFECTIONS

There are three major subcutaneous fungal infections of the hand: chronic paronychia, sporotrichosis, and phaeomycotic cysts. Chronic paronychia is easy to diagnose but is usually initially misdiagnosed as a bacterial infection. Lack of response to repeated courses of the usual antibiotics is an important clue to the fungal etiology of this infection. Drainage and débridement may be needed if medical management fails. Sporotrichosis is rare and responds readily to medical treatment. Phaeomycotic cyst is a deep dermal or subcutaneous infection that results from the traumatic implantation of a dematiaceous (brown) fungus such as *Exophiala* or *Phialophora.*

Chronic Paronychia

Chronic paronychia is characterized by a relatively well-localized area of skin inflammation proximal to the cuticle. The skin becomes warm, glistening, and tense and extends to the cuticle. The cuticle is chronically indurated, retracted, and rounded at the base of the nail. It usually affects a female patient who frequently soaks her hands in water, as required either by her job or her domestic duties. Mechanical trauma that damages the cuticle is responsible for fungal invasion of the nail fold. Patients with chronic paronychia have a higher incidence of colonization of the mouth, bowel, and vagina than controls.[197,198] Patients do not routinely give a history of acute paronychia, and surgical exploration does not identify pus deep to the nail plate. Unless the disease process is stopped, secondary thickening, ridging, and discoloration of the nail may occur, and eventually nail loss may result. Specific diagnosis is made by biopsy, Gram stain, or KOH preparation and culture.

Etiology

C. albicans is responsible for the majority (70%[194] to 97%[236]) of cases of chronic paronychia. *C. albicans* is part of the normal resident flora of human skin and nails.[237] Stone and Mullins first reproduced this entity in 1964 by soaking fingers in water until the skin macerated and inoculated either viable or nonviable *Candida* into the cul-de-sac between the base of the nail and eponychium.[275-277] Inflammatory reaction in the presence of dead *C. albicans* indicated that the exogenous byproducts of fungal organisms caused local chronic inflammation. Chronic maceration of the fingers is accompanied by separation of the cuticle from the nail, so that a pocket of water develops under the proximal nail fold. Once this pocket is formed, capillary action retains water in it and transient flora such as *C. albicans* and gram-negative rods thrive in it. As Stone calls it, the process forms a "dermatologic cesspool" and cultures yield *C. albicans* and mixed bacterial flora, including *Proteus,* streptococci, and gram-negative rods (usually *Escherichia coli* and *Pseudomonas*).[274,278] The condition has been reported in up to 9% of diabetic and in 3% of nondiabetic women older than the age of 20 years.[275] Thumb sucking is the usual etiology of chronic paronychia in children.[278] In men the condition is always occupational.[272,275] In a barber, chronic paronychia may occur when hair is embedded in the paronychium.[272]

Diagnosis

Chronic paronychia is entirely a clinical diagnosis, but the picture presented is so characteristic as to present no diagnostic difficulties.[275] Ninety-two percent of patients are women.[194] Of the affected men, 25% are chefs, barmen, or fishmongers. A chronically indurated, retracted, and rounded hyponychium is the hallmark of the chronic paronychia. Recurrent episodes cause inflammation and drainage, followed by thickening and transverse grooving of the nail plate.[161,194,212] Patients with chronic paronychia complain of a long history of annoying and disfigured thickening of the eponychial skin.[161,225,273]

Usually the lateral nail fold shows the first signs of chronic swelling, with a separation of this fold from the lateral margin of the nail. After weeks or months, the process progresses to the posterior nail fold, the eponychium. The cuticle separates from the nail plate and allows moisture and *C. albicans* to harbor in the subeponychial cul-de-sac. Germinal matrix in the eponychial area is eventually invaded and causes irregularities of the dorsum of the nail plate, usually grooving. In 30% of the cases, the nail plate becomes greenish owing to secondary colonization by *Pseudomonas aeruginosa,* which are normal colonizers of the hyponychial space between the skin and free edge of the nail.[237,258] Subacute intermittent flare-ups by secondary bacterial infection may require treatment with oral antibiotics but do not cure the underlying chronic hyponychial candidiasis. Smears of skin and nail scrapings may be negative for *C. albicans,* and diagnosis must be established with a culture. Other causes of paronychia include syphilis,[228] blastomycosis,[244] tuberculosis,[248] and herpetic paronychia.[262] Squamous cell carcinoma,[167,192] subungual keratoacanthoma,[232] leukemia cutis,[214] amyloidosis,[156] and pilonidal sinus[272] have been reported to mimic chronic paronychia.

Treatment

Keeping the area as dry as possible and prolonged application of a topical azole antifungal agent such as clotrimazole (Lotrimin, Mycelex) or econazole[297] may adequately treat a *C. albicans* infection. Oral therapy with fluconazole, 200 to 400 mg/day, is a more effective alternative, but long-term prognosis of either topical or oral therapy remains unsatisfactory. Approximately 40% of patients remain free of paronychia, 40% heal periodically, and 20% have continuous disease after 1 year.[196] When medical management does not succeed, eponychial marsupialization should be considered.[224,225] In this operation, the fibrotic cutaneous and subcutaneous tissue of the eponychium is excised to permit unrestricted drainage of the fungi and their exogenous byproducts so that the infectious and inflammatory processes are reversed.

Technique of Marsupialization. Under digital or wrist block, with tourniquet hemostasis, a symmetrical 2- to 3-mm wide crescent-shaped piece of skin and subcutaneous tissue is excised approximately 2 mm proximal to the nail fold of the affected digit (Fig. 4-5).[225] The excision extends to the lateral nail plate margin on both sides. Asymmetrical excision produces an asymmetrical nail margin when it is healed. Nail removal should be done when concurrent nail irregularities are seen. Nail irregularities may indicate that the infection is deeper under the nail; and if the nail is not removed, infection tends to recur.[165] The tourniquet is removed, and hemostasis is obtained by several minutes of direct compression. This is dressed initially with a nonadherent dressing that is removed on the first postoperative day, and warm soaks are initiated. The wound is redressed. The patient then soaks the wound in hydrogen peroxide periodically and keeps it covered. Epithelialization occurs in 2 weeks, and in most cases this will be curative. Full-length improvement of the nail plate may take 9 to 12 months. In one study, normal cuticular contour and nail growth resulted in 28 of 31 digits. Keeping the fingers dry and basic hygiene are essential to prevent recurrence. Mouth, anus, and vagina may provide a reservoir of *C. albicans* from which the nail fold may be reinfected.[236]

CRITICAL POINTS: MARSUPIALIZATION OF CHRONIC PARONYCHIA

- Do not injure the free margin of the eponychium.
- Excise a crescent-shaped segment of the skin symmetrically.
- Let the patient soak the finger in warm water once daily and redress the wound.

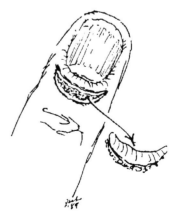

FIGURE 4-5. Technique of marsupialization.[224,225] A symmetrical, crescent-shaped segment of skin is excised from the dorsum of the distal phalanx, leaving an adequate bridge of skin and cuticle (hyponychium). (From Keyser JJ, Littler JW, Eaton RG: Surgical treatment of infections and lesions of the perionychium. Hand Clin 6:137-153, 1990.)

Sporotrichosis (Rose Thorn Disease)

Etiology

Sporotrichosis is the most common cutaneous and subcutaneous (lymphocutaneous) fungal infection in North America.[158] If sporotrichosis is promptly diagnosed, it can usually be cured with medical treatment. If unrecognized, the disease can result in progressive disability.[186]

Sporotrichosis was first diagnosed by Schenk in 1898 at Johns Hopkins Hospital in a patient with a primary lesion in his finger and secondary lymphatic lesions in the forearm.[265] The infecting organism was a dimorphic fungus and was termed *Sporothrix (Sporotrichum) schenckii.* In the United States, the infection in humans is an occupational hazard of rose growers, gardeners,[222] and florists, as well as farmers, horticulturists, and nurserymen.[199] The organism is ubiquitous in soil and frequently inoculated into the skin and subcutaneous tissues by a rose thorn. The majority of cases are reported around the Missouri and Mississippi rivers, but the disease occurs worldwide. The fungus has been recovered from nails of cats, and sporotrichosis has followed cat scratches.

Diagnosis

Lymphocutaneous infection accounts for 80% of cases of sporotrichosis, and 80% of infections occur in the upper extremity.[171] Localized cutaneous infections are less frequent. The infection is nonopportunistic and affects healthy subjects. Alcoholism has been reported to be a predisposing factor.[159,222] The disease occurs rarely in childhood.[231]

Infection begins when the fungus is inoculated into a site of skin injury on the exposed part of hand or forearm. It produces an erythematous, ulcerated, or verrucous nodule. The ulcers develop raised borders. The ulcer closely resembles a chancre. The infection is characterized by linear marching nodules on the forearm and arm, which represent spread through local lymphatic channels. Regional lymph nodes become enlarged, and seropurulent drainage may occur from both the primary lesion and the involved nodes. The lymphocutaneous lesions are typically painless, and a chronic cyclical process of spontaneous healing, nodule formation, ulceration, and drainage may continue for years. Sporotrichosis should be included in the differential diagnosis of a chronic ulcerated skin lesion.[263]

Among the differential diagnosis of the nodular lymphangitis pattern of lymphocutaneous sporotrichosis is nocardiosis,[208] leishmaniasis, tularemia, and atypical mycobacterial infections, especially *M. marinum.* The ulceroglandular form of tularemia is usually accompanied by systemic symptoms. Much less often, botryomycosis,[172,190,193] *Blastomyces dermatitidis, Coccidioides immitis, Cryptococcus neoformans, Histoplasma capsulatum, Mycobacterium kansasii, Staphylococcus aureus, Streptococcus pyogenes, Burkholderia pseudomallei, Bacillus anthracis,* and vaccinia virus may also be characterized by nodular lymphangitis.[260]

Diagnosis may be missed owing to the relative rarity of the disease. Only 36 cases were treated in 29 years at the Mayo Clinic between 1957 and 1986.[186,263] The average delay in diagnosis was 4 months. The standard histologic stains may not show the organism. The organism may sometimes be identified in biopsy specimens using specific fluorescent antibody staining, but this is not a routine test.[178] Periodic acid–Schiff or silver staining will highlight the fungus as red or black, respectively. Examination of biopsy specimens reveals a pyogranulomatous response and is diagnostic if characteristic cigar-shaped yeast forms are seen. Unfortunately, the yeast may be difficult to detect unless multiple sections are examined, because there are characteristically very few organisms in the infected tissue. The diagnosis is best made by culture of the affected site, although repeated attempts at culture may have to be made.[260] Aspirates or deep cultures are preferable to swabbed specimens because the organisms are sparse. Cultures become positive in a few days to a month. Cultures must be incubated at 30°C or room temperature in modified Sabouraud's agar fungal media. False-negative cultures may result if the specimens are cultured at 37°C.

Treatment

Itraconazole is now the drug of choice for lymphocutaneous sporotrichosis.[259,267] Treatment with 100 to 200 mg/day for 3 to 6 months results in complete resolution in most patients. The drug should be administered with a fatty meal or carbonated beverage to enhance absorption. Heat is considered a useful adjunct to medical therapy as the organism grows at temperatures below 37°C.[195] Cutaneous sporotrichosis was treated in the past with a saturated solution of potassium iodide (SSKI, 1 g/mL) and may still be considered if itraconazole causes hepatotoxic side effects. SSKI may not be convenient because it causes bitter taste and gastrointestinal upset. Oral terbinafine (125 mg/day) has been shown to be effective against sporotrichosis in Japan.[242] Fluconazole, 400 to 800 mg/day, can also be used. The role of voriconazole and the newer triazole antifungal agents is not known, but they are expected to be highly efficacious. Isolated cutaneous sporotrichosis responds well to medication and has an excellent prognosis. Rarely, sporotrichosis can present as a deep fungal infection in immunocompromised hosts.

Phaeomycotic Cysts

A phaeomycotic cyst is a rare deep dermal and subcutaneous infection due to a darkly pigmented fungus such as *Exophiala, Phialophora,* or *Bantalis.* It most commonly results from the traumatic implantation of a wood splinter, but it may be nosocomially acquired at the site of an intravenous catheter in an immunocompromised patient.[189,281]

In a review of phaeomycotic cysts from the Armed Forces Institute of Pathology, 25 cases were seen over 19 years.[302] Eleven were on the upper extremity, 12 on the lower extremity, and 2 on the face. The standard of care for this infection is surgical removal. It is not clear whether antifungal therapy alone may be successful.

DEEP FUNGAL INFECTIONS

Deep fungal infections are serious clinical problems that often result in significant morbidity and even mortality. Several of the organisms described in the following section can also present as cutaneous or superficial infections. Fortunately, deep infections are rare in the hand and upper extremity. Deep fungal infections may affect the tenosynovium, joints, or bone. The only way to make a diagnosis of fungal infection of the hand or upper extremity is to include fungal stains and cultures in the biopsy of every chronic tenosynovitis, arthritis, or osteomyelitis. Infectious disease consultation is recommended for diagnosis and treatment of deep fungal infections. These infections may be difficult to treat because drug therapy requires prolonged therapy and recurrences are common in both immunocompetent and immunocompromised patients.

Aspergillosis

Diagnosis

Aspergillus infection of the hand has only occasionally been encountered in a healthy person.[246] It has been reported as an opportunistic pathogen in an immunocompromised adult with diabetes[188] and in immunocompromised children with acute leukemia.[203,221,238,255,300] *A. fumigatus* is the most common species recovered from patients with aspergillosis. Granulocytopenia (<500 polymorphonuclear leukocytes/mL) that results from cytotoxic chemotherapy predisposes children to invasion by *Aspergillus*. A hemorrhagic vesicle, bleb, or necrotic ulcer on the finger,[255] hand,[203,221,300] forearm, or arm[255] of a child who is undergoing chemotherapy for acute leukemia should alert the hand surgeon to aspergillosis. Puncture wounds after intravenous infusion are common sites of infection. Biopsy of the necrotic lesions shows numerous fungal hyphae on a wet KOH preparation. Biopsy is essential in establishing diagnosis, because blood cultures fail to reveal the diagnosis. *Aspergillus* species are common contaminants in the bacteriology laboratory but should not be dismissed when the culture is obtained from an immunosuppressed patient. Definitive diagnosis of *Aspergillus* infection is dependent on identification of the organism in cultures of the infected biopsy tissue.

Treatment

Radical surgical débridement and intravenous amphotericin B therapy are the mainstays of treatment. Itraconazole has been successful in the treatment of localized cutaneous *Aspergillus* infection of the hand.[188] Metastasis to different sites occurs rapidly and generally proves fatal. Necrosis of tendons, joints, and neurovascular bundles occurs and necessitates ray amputation. Consultation with an infectious disease specialist is advised because high-dose therapy with amphotericin B is usually required in the immunocompromised host. Various newer azoles might be indicated for prolonged treatment.

Blastomycosis

Blastomycosis is caused by *Blastomyces dermatitidis*. It is reported mostly in North America, in the Ohio and Mississippi River valleys, and has a similar distribution as histoplasmosis. It is a primary pathogen and infects an immunocompetent host who works in contact with soil. The fungus is inhaled and causes a clinical or subclinical lung infection. Cutaneous blastomycosis can be caused by direct implantation into the skin or by dissemination of the fungus from the lungs. Hand infections are sporadically reported.[164,166,201,206,233,241,244,247,251] Traumatic implantation of *B. dermatitidis* has been reported in the hand

of a veterinarian who handled an infected necropsy specimen.[206]

Diagnosis

Skin lesions can be solitary or multiple and may appear concurrently in separate regions of the body. Ulcerations of the hand and forearm are most frequently located on the dorsal surfaces.[166] Subcutaneous nodules develop into abscesses and progress to draining fistulas. Contiguous spread to bone may occur. Lesions may be exudative, suppurative, or granulomatous. Lymphangitis and lymphadenitis may occur.[206] Histopathologic diagnosis of biopsy tissue may require special stains, including periodic acid–Schiff or silver stain. The fungus has a characteristic histologic appearance with a double refractile cell wall and broad-based buds between the mother/daughter cells. Hyphae are not seen in the tissues.

Osteoarticular Lesions

Osteoarticular lesions occur in 60% of patients who have systemic blastomycosis[233] and may include septic arthritis and osteomyelitis in the hand[166,201,244] and elbow. A localized osteomyelitis of the distal radius that simulated a sarcoma was reported in an otherwise asymptomatic patient.[241]

Treatment

Amphotericin B, ketoconazole, and itraconazole are highly effective against *B. dermatitidis*. Fluconazole has not been as effective but may be used at a dose in excess of 400 mg/day if alternatives are not available for use. Surgery is necessary only for diagnostic biopsy. The value of surgical debulking is questioned.

Candidiasis

The increasing incidence of HIV infection and the implantation of prosthetic devices are important in the increasing incidence of systemic candidiasis. The most common species recovered from clinical specimens include *C. albicans*, *C. tropicalis*, *C. glabrata*, and *C. parapsilosis*. Many other less common species have also been described. Flexor and extensor tenosynovitis of the hand has been reported in a newborn[301] and in AIDS.[286] Septic arthritis of the wrist with *C. parapsilosis* has been reported.[183] Silicone arthroplasty of the metacarpophalangeal joint may become infected by *C. albicans*.[185] Fluconazole and amphotericin B are the drugs of choice for use in patients with candidiasis. Specific drugs and doses should be selected in conjunction with an infectious diseases specialist. Combinations of amphotericin B and fluconazole may be effective but have not been specifically studied in this type of *Candida* infection. For periprosthetic infection, radical tenosynovectomy and removal of the implant are necessary in addition to combined chemotherapy with amphotericin B and 5-fluorouracil.[301]

Coccidioidomycosis

Diagnosis

Coccidioides immitis is a highly infectious fungus that is found only in hot and arid regions of the San Joaquin Valley in California and the deserts of the southwest of the United

States,[182,207,218] where the infection is endemic. This fungus has a predilection for synovium, and 10% of coccidioidal infections occur in the wrist and hand (Fig. 4-6).[162] Cases of tenosynovitis,[182,207,218,293] joint infection,[181,296] and osteomyelitis[168,181,217,284] of the hand have been reported. Coccidioidal osteomyelitis of a metacarpal may mimic an enchondroma.[217] Patients with tenosynovitis present with chronic diffuse swelling over the dorsal[182] or volar[207] side of the wrist or palm.[218] If untreated, septic tenosynovitis may lead to extensor tendon rupture and may mimic rheumatoid arthritis.[283] Clinical, gross histopathologic (rice bodies and melon seed bodies[293]) and microhistopathologic similarities (noncaseating granulomas) between coccidioidal, other fungal, and tuberculous infection are well recognized. Diagnosis is made from positive complement fixation titer,[207,218,293] presence of chronic granuloma, microabscesses in the synovial biopsy, and identification of *C. immitis* in synovial stains and cultures. The organism has a characteristic appearance in tissue and can be identified in many cases under the microscope. Rarely, concurrent pulmonary coccidioidomycosis will be diagnosed.[207] Coccidioidomycosis of the hand may occur as a part of disseminated coccidioidomycosis or after traumatic implantation of the fungus.

Histopathology of excised synovium shows the characteristic *C. immitis* spherules in synovium, and the dimorphic fungus grows in synovium culture. The laboratory should be alerted to the presumed diagnosis so that it can handle the specimens and cultures in an appropriate biohazard hood to prevent airborne dissemination. The fungus in its hyphal form is highly infectious.

Treatment

Coccidioidomycosis is one of the most difficult to treat of the invasive mycoses. Nonpulmonary infection often requires years to cure, and life-long suppressive therapy may be needed. The infection resists aggressive treatment with synovectomy, tenosynovectomy, and high doses of amphotericin B. Patients may have multiple recurrences of tenosynovitis, even when they are treated with adequate tenosynovectomy and intravenous amphotericin B. The

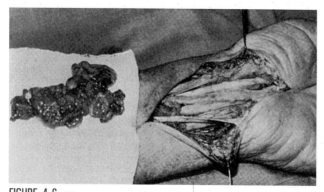

FIGURE 4-6. Flexor tenosynovitis caused by *Coccidioides immitis* of 3 years' duration in a patient with acute lymphoblastic leukemia. It flared up when chemotherapy was started. A combination of tenosynovectomy and intravenous amphotericin B is essential in immunosuppressed patients. (From Gropper PT, Pisesky WA, Bowen V, Clement PB: Flexor tenosynovitis caused by *Coccidioides immitis*. J Hand Surg [Am] 8:344-347, 1983.)

infection flares up during periods of immunosuppression or lowered host resistance. Patients with dormant tenosynovitis and leukemia may suffer flare-up of preexisting infection during cancer chemotherapy. Complement fixation titers correlate closely with clinical response to therapy and are useful in detecting subclinical recurrences.[168]

Therapy with fluconazole, itraconazole, or amphotericin B may be indicated depending on the patient's condition. The azoles are particularly useful for long-term therapy and have provided many patients with chronic suppression of otherwise relapsing manifestations of disease. Consultation with a knowledgeable infectious disease consultant is highly recommended, because a long-term commitment to therapy with its attendant side effects, drug interactions, and possibly disease flares are frequently necessary.

Cryptococcosis

Diagnosis

Cryptococcosis (European blastomycosis, torulosis) is an infection caused by the opportunistic fungus *Cryptococcus neoformans*. It is usually associated with avian habitats, and in particular with pigeons.[205,239] *C. neoformans* is a saprophytic fungus present in the environment. There are two varieties: var. *neoformans,* which is a true opportunistic fungus, and var. *gatti,* which behaves more like a primary pathogen, similar to *C. immitis, B. dermatitidis,* and *H. capsulatum. C. neoformans* var. *gatti* has been associated with the flowering of certain eucalyptus trees.

Cryptococcus species may rarely cause disease of the hand in immunocompetent patients.[239] Opportunistic cryptococcal infection of the hand has been reported in patients with AIDS,[200,268,290] renal failure,[170,229,287] and end-stage renal disease[229,287]; in renal allograft recipients[154]; in patients receiving long-term corticosteroids[205,229,288,298]; and in diabetics.[229,298]

Cryptococcal infections of the hand may occur in the skin,[175,200,205,268,298] tenosynovium,[191] or joint.[256] Cutaneous cryptococcosis can present in a variety of ways, including papules,[175] pustules, plaques,[205] cellulitis, abscesses, nodules,[268] sinuses, and ulcers,[200,268] all of which may present diagnostic problems for the hand surgeon. Thick and tenacious purulent fluid in the wound should arouse suspicion of cryptococcal infection and, typically, thorough surgical débridement fails to clear the infection. Diagnosis is confirmed by a high cryptococcal antigen titer and growth of the fungus from biopsy specimens. Worland reported an extensive suppurative wound of the hand in an immunosuppressed patient with diabetes and chronic obstructive lung disease on prednisone.[298] Tsai and colleagues and Braun and associates separately described the same patient with diabetes, end-stage renal failure, and uremia who developed infection of the hand with ipsilateral synthetic arteriovenous fistula. The infection did not resolve with amphotericin B, 5-flucytosine, and repeated surgical drainages until the graft was removed.[170,287] Casadevall and coworkers[175] reported four skin-puncture accidents of fingers and hand with needles that were heavily contaminated with *C. neoformans*. In one of these accidents, delayed administration of antifungal drugs resulted in a granuloma of the finger. In the other three accidents, immediate prophylaxis with oral fluconazole prevented skin infection. Their experience suggests that early therapy with fluconazole is a reasonable means of managing skin injuries caused by instruments contaminated with viable *C. neoformans.*[175]

Treatment

Fluconazole,[154,175,191,200,205,268,288,290] itraconazole,[239] and flucytosine[288] are all effective in eradicating the infection. Treatment of hand infections with a minimum of 12 weeks of therapy with fluconazole, 400 mg/day, or more should control most of these infections. Alternatives include amphotericin B with or without flucytosine, itraconazole, or the newer azoles such as voriconazole. If significant immunosuppression is present, long-term suppressive therapy is recommended.

Histoplasmosis

Diagnosis

Histoplasma capsulatum is a highly infectious fungus, endemic in the Mississippi and Ohio river valleys. The diagnosis of histoplasmosis is difficult because the clinical syndrome is nonspecific. It may be difficult to isolate *H. capsulatum* from clinical specimens.

Histoplasmosis may present as cutaneous infection,[261] tenosynovitis,[253,254,264] tendon ruptures,[264] carpal tunnel syndrome,[187,253,257,280] arthritis,[249,264] or fatal necrotizing myofascitis[291] in the upper extremity. A case of recurrent osteomyelitis of capitate bone with a 10-year latency between initial inadequate curettage and clinical recurrence was reported.[173] Infected synovial tissue is red brown, contains many rice bodies, and undergoes active caseous granulomatous inflammation.[264] *H. capsulatum* is demonstrated in the biopsy tissue if Grocott silver stain is specified.[294] *H. capsulatum* may take several weeks and be difficult to grow. Close collaboration between surgeon, rheumatologist, infectious disease specialist, pathologist, and microbiologist is paramount in the diagnosis and treatment of these cases.[264]

Since the late 1940s, serology has been important in the diagnosis of infection with *H. capsulatum.* Complement-fixing (CF) antibodies and precipitin bands have been most commonly used in the clinical laboratory. For CF antibodies, a titer of 1:8 is considered presumptive and a titer of more than 1:32 is strongly suggestive of active infection.[234,294] The histoplasmin skin test becomes positive in 2 to 4 weeks after the onset of infection and remains positive for life in 90% of patients.[294] Skin testing is not recommended in the clinical setting and is primarily an epidemiologic tool. Sensitivity of antibody tests may be lower in immunocompromised hosts. A polysaccharide antigen test is available commercially and can help in diagnosis of histoplasmosis, as well as to gauge the efficacy of antifungal therapy.

Treatment

Combined medical and surgical treatment is critical to prevent recurrence. A combination of complete tenosynovectomy, bone débridement,[173] and prolonged systemic antifungal therapy, such as oral ketoconazole[247] or itraconazole or intravenous amphotericin B,[264] is utilized. The drug of choice for long-term therapy is itraconazole, 200 mg twice daily. Fluconazole, 400 to 800 mg/day can serve as an alternative. The histoplasmosis reference laboratory in Indianapolis, Indiana (317-630-2515, histodgn@indyunix. lupui.edu) provides services in histoplasmosis antigen testing and itraconazole serum levels.

Mucormycosis

Mucormycosis is the common name given to several different diseases caused by fungi of the order Mucorales. *Rhizopus* species are the most commonly isolated agents of mucormycosis, followed by *Rhizomucor.* They are opportunistic fungi known to invade blood vessels. Mucormycosis is an acute and chronic fungal infection characterized by vascular infection, thrombosis, and gangrenous tissue necrosis. These infections are among the most aggressive and destructive of the fungal infections and are fortunately rare.[282] Rapid diagnosis and radical débridement are essential to preserve tissue devastation. Cutaneous mucormycosis predominantly involves the epidermis and dermis, and necrosis develops secondary to vascular invasion. The most important association to remember that may point to mucormycosis is a triad of diabetes, blood vessel thrombosis, and rapid, cutaneous and subcutaneous gangrenous destruction.

A nationwide epidemic that was caused by contaminated elastic bandages in the 1970s focused attention on primary cutaneous mucormycosis as a distinct entity. Patients presented with cellulitis under areas covered by the bandages, which presumably was caused by direct inoculation of fungi into skin occluded by the adhesive. Failure to recognize the mycotic nature of the infection or failure to remove the bandages resulted in penetration of hyphae into the skin and areas below the skin. Use of sterilized bandages and dressings eliminated this form of mucormycosis.

Diagnosis

Rhizopus and *Mucor* infection of the hand is usually cutaneous and subcutaneous. The upper extremity is involved in 24% of all cutaneous cases.[155] Fifty percent of cases of primary cutaneous mucormycosis occur in patients with severe trauma where the wound is contaminated by soil or water. Of the other 50%, most of the patients have diabetes (20%), leukemia (9%), chronic kidney failure (5%), or organ transplantation (4%).[155]

Cutaneous and subcutaneous infections present as progressive gangrenous cellulitis and progressive necrosis of the wound margin. Black eschars and black pus indicate advanced disease and should lead one to consideration of mucormycosis, especially in an immunocompromised host. Cutaneous and subcutaneous mucormycosis is more localized than other types of mucormycosis and has much better prognosis (mortality, 15%) than deep-seated infections (mortality, 32%).

An infection of the forearm may occur at an intravenous infusion site[155] or follow an intramuscular injection in an immunocompromised patient.[219] Contamination of devitalized tissue after major trauma[155,179,250] or minor trauma[179] can result in mucormycosis. The disease has been reported in patients whose burn wounds have been dressed with contaminated elasticized tape.[230] *Mucor hiemalis,* a common soil inhabitant, was recovered from a diabetic gardener with a localized subcutaneous infection of a finger.[179]

Whereas some mild and localized cases have been described in the hand,[179,289] the disease more often results in devastating tissue necrosis. In older patients, tissue necrosis may be so extensive that major débridement and multiple skin grafts are necessary.[213] It may behave like necrotizing fasciitis with rapid necrosis of subcutaneous tissue. Progressive gangrene has prompted finger, hand, or below-elbow amputation.[223]

Mucormycosis is notorious for its tendency to invade deep tissues, although mucormycosis osteomyelitis in the hand is rare.[271] Extension of pathology across tissue planes strongly suggests a fungal etiology and urgent need for a biopsy. The diagnosis is typically made histologically, but yield on superficial swab cultures is low. The diagnosis of mucormycosis requires that tissue be examined for presence of the characteristic irregular, broad, nonseptate, right-angle branching hyphae. The organisms are scattered within a large area of necrosis. Biopsy and smears often reveal the organisms when cultures are negative. Cultures from an excised ulcer may grow *Rhizopus, Mucor,* or *Absidia,* as well as other Mucorales, such as *Cunninghamella* and *Apophysomyces.* They grow abundantly in 1 to 3 days on routine fungal media when the biopsy material is sampled from deep tissue. For histopathologic examination, the laboratory must be alerted as to the nature of the lesion because certain fungal media contain cycloheximide, which suppresses growth of Mucorales species.

Treatment

The standard therapy for mucormycosis is prompt and aggressive surgical débridement of necrotic tissue, skin grafting, and amphotericin B. Reversal of any underlying predisposing systemic factors is a critical first step, and diabetes should be aggressively managed. The dose of immunosuppressive medications should be reduced if possible. Intravenous amphotericin B remains the drug of choice for the treatment of mucormycosis and should be given in full dose without the delay of increasing dose titration. The lipid formulations of amphotericin B such as Abelcet and AmBisome can probably be used. High doses of these agents are necessary in patients who are at risk of dying of this infection, despite their known toxicity.

Extracutaneous Sporotrichosis

Diagnosis

Extracutaneous sporotrichosis is rare and usually occurs within the musculoskeletal system of an immunocompromised host. The organism usually enters the body through the lungs, and a concomitant pneumonia is often present. Deep sporotrichosis infection may localize to the bones, joints, or tenosynovium in the hand. Sporotrichal osteomyelitis may present as multifocal subchondral and periarticular erosions of the bones of the hand.[177,202] Among articular lesions, wrist[210,220,235] and hand joints[163,235,295] are the most frequently involved. A joint infection with a sinus should arouse suspicion.[235] Tenosynovial lesions may occur on the dorsal wrist tendons.[184,209,211,222] Extensor tenosynovitis may cause rupture of an extensor tendon.[279] Sporotrichal flexor tenosynovitis may result in carpal tunnel syndrome[159,209,279] or ulnar nerve entrapment.[159] Bursal sporotri-

chosis has been reported in the olecranon bursa.[177] Sporotrichal myositis of the biceps muscle has been reported without skin or lymphatic involvement.[210]

A high index of suspicion is needed to make the diagnosis of sporotrichal arthritis, osteomyelitis, and tenosynovitis. The diagnosis of sporotrichal arthritis is often delayed for two reasons. First, *Sporothrix schenckii* is an uncommon cause of arthritis and, second, sporotrichal arthritis often occurs in the absence of the clinically familiar cutaneous lesions. Eighty-four percent of sporotrichal joint infections presented as monoarthritis.[163] Sporotrichosis should be considered in the differential diagnosis when granulomatous synovitis is recognized by histologic examination.[220] Sporotrichal osteomyelitis is equally rare. Infected patients have localized swelling, local sinus tract formation, and concomitant arthritis. Roentgenographic findings in osseous sporotrichosis are nonspecific and include destruction of bone without reactive sclerosis or periosteal reaction. Tenosynovial swelling of sporotrichosis is clinically similar to rheumatoid tenosynovitis (Fig. 4-7A); and on gross and histologic examination, proliferative tenosynovium is similar to rheumatoid tenosynovium (see Fig. 4-7B and C). Rice bodies may be found in the inflamed tenosynovium, as is common in tenosynovitis due to rheumatoid arthritis, tuberculosis, and many other causes.[222,279] Olecranon bursal sporotrichosis has been reported.[295] Even when biopsy is done expeditiously, diagnosis may be missed on histopathologic examination[220] unless multiple sections are diligently examined.[171] S. schenckii may grow from aspirated pus or from tenosynovium[209] or not grow on repeated cultures.[184] Delay in diagnosis can range from 2 to 12 months.[184,220] Repeated synovial fluid cultures and synovium biopsies may be necessary before a diagnosis is made.[184,279] Cultures usually grow in 4 weeks, but growth may be delayed up to 8 weeks.[184] Histologic examination typically reveals a nonspecific pyogranulomatous response or a noncaseating granuloma. It is diagnostic only when characteristic cigar-shaped yeasts are seen and *Sporothrix schenckii* grow on culture.

Treatment

Aggressive chemotherapy in combination with surgical débridement is necessary to cure deep sporotrichosis (see Fig. 4-7B). For bone, joint, and tenosynovial sporotrichosis, SSKI is not adequate as it is in the treatment of cutaneous and lymphocutaneous sporotrichosis.[184,202] Amphotericin B is the drug of choice.[184,209,220,279] 2-Hydroxystilbamidine,[209] ketoconazole,[211] itraconazole,[267] and fluconazole[176] have all been successfully used. If surgical débridement in conjunction with chemotherapy does not eradicate the infection, arthrodesis or amputation may be necessary.[263] Appropriate use of antifungal agents, however, should make such radical surgery less likely. Osteoarticular sporotrichosis may require prolonged therapy but is not life threatening.

NEWLY EMERGING HAND FUNGAL INFECTIONS

In recent years, a number of emerging infections have become apparent. This category includes infections due to resurgent organisms that had previously declined in

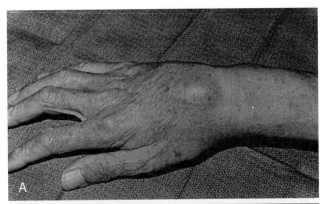

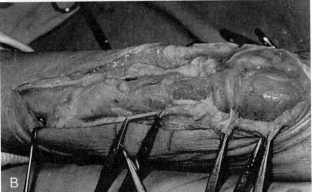

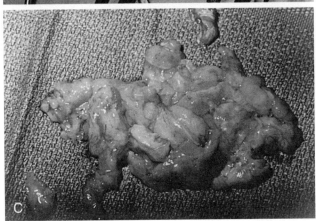

FIGURE 4-7. Sporotrichosis tenosynovitis. **A,** Swelling on the dorsum of the hand resembles that of rheumatoid tenosynovitis. **B,** The synovial proliferation involves all the extensor tendons. **C,** The resected tenosynovium is thick, extensive, and proliferative. (From Hay EL, Collawn SS, Middletown FG: *Sporothrix schenckii* tenosynovitis: A case report. J Hand Surg 11:431-434, 1986.)

prevalence, as well as newly identified pathogens. These are generally rare fungal infections that are often low grade, encapsulated, and localized to subcutaneous tissue. *Exophiala (Phialophora) jeanselmei*,[226,240,243] *Geotrichum candidum*,[204] *Phialophora richardsiae*,[266,285] and *Cladophialophora bantiana*[252] invoke minimal inflammation and result in formation of a thick capsule. *Exophiala, Phialophora,* and *C. bantiana*[252] colonies are darkly pigmented on Sabouraud's dextrose agar (the so-called dematiaceous fungi), giving them the name of chromomycosis,[292] chromohyphomycosis,[240] and phaeohyphomycosis.[226]

No antibiotics are necessary if the entire encapsulated mass of fungus is excised. If a cyst filled with yellow creamy material is opened, it is important to irrigate the wound before the tourniquet is released to prevent hematogenous dissemination of live fungi. Itraconazole may be given orally. Because of nodular tumefaction, these infections may be considered as a grade 1 eumycetoma. *P. richardsiae* is a rare fungus found in wood pulp that has caused two infections in the upper extremity, one in the hand[266] and one of the elbow in the olecranon bursa.[285] The infectious granuloma is safely encapsulated by the host and surgical excision is adequate. No antibiotic is necessary if the capsule is left intact during excision.

Torulopsis holmii[245] is generally considered a saprophyte of the gastrointestinal and urogenital tracts of humans and is also found in animals and soil. Unnecessary digital amputations can be avoided by maintenance of a high level of vigilance for these organisms in immunocompromised patients with penetrating hand trauma. *Scedosporium (Monosporium) apiospermum* (anamorph synonyms: *Pseudallescheria boydii* [the currently approved name], *Allescheria boydii, Petriellidium boydii*) may cause infection of hand,[227] wrist joint, tendons,[169] and soft tissues of the forearm[227] in immunocompromised patients. *Scedosporium* infections respond to itraconazole,[169,227] although surgical excision is an important adjunct in treatment of this infection. These fungi are inherently resistant to amphotericin B and may be less sensitive to azoles as well. Treatment with voriconazole, high-dose fluconazole, or itraconazole is the preferred strategy. Long-term therapy (>3 months) is likely to be necessary.

Interaction with CDC, Mycotic Disease Branch, Atlanta, Georgia 30333 (www.cdc.gov) or Fungus Testing Laboratory, University of Texas, Health Sciences Center, San Antonio, TX 78284 (210-567-4132, rinaldi@uthscsa.edu) may help with choosing the latest diagnostic and therapeutic laboratory tests and treatment.

ANNOTATED REFERENCES

186. Duran RJ, Coventry MB, Weed LA: Sporotrichosis: A report of 23 cases in the upper extremity. J Bone Joint Surg Am 39:1330-1957, 1957.

     This is as good a description of this rare fungal infection as anywhere. The reader will make diagnosis of sporotrichosis easily after reading this article written more than 40 years ago.

224. Keyser JJ, Eaton RG: Surgical cure of chronic paronychia by eponychial marsupialization. Plast Reconstr Surg 58:66-69, 1976.

225. Keyser JJ, Littler JW, Eaton RG: Surgical treatment of infections and lesions of the perionychium. Hand Clin 6:137-153, 1990.

     The above two articles describe in detail surgical treatment of chronic paronychia that resists medical treatment. The surgical technique is illustrated well and is the one that I have followed with gratifying results. The technique of excising a crescent of skin preserves the eponychium and drains the infection adequately.

278. Stone OJ, Mullins JF: Chronic paronychia in children. Clin Pediatr 7:104, 1968.

Stone and Mullins provide experimental proof that *Candida* infection causes chronic paronychia. They describe the natural course of the disease in children—it is self curing in the majority, unless the patient is immunocompromised.

282. Sugar AM, Lyman CA: A Practical Guide to Medically Important Fungi and the Diseases They Cause. Philadelphia, Lippincott-Raven, 1997, pp 3-146.

This is a short and practical reading that clarifies common fungal infections. It covers salient features of all fungal infections that are included in this chapter. There are references to specialized laboratories for rare tests for fungal infections. Sugar has edited this chapter and brought it up to date.

Hansen's Disease (Leprosy)

Leprosy is now officially called Hansen's disease (HD) to help get rid of the stigma of the words "leper" and "leprosy," which since Biblical times have been surrounded by revulsion and horror.[512] HD is a chronic infection of the peripheral nerves and skin caused by *Mycobacterium leprae.* It is both a neurologic and an immunologic disease. Ulnar, median, and radial nerves, usually in that order, are affected in the upper extremity in 70% of active and relapsing cases of leprosy.[475] The nerves suffer a triple blow from *M. leprae:* infective neuropathy, immunologic neuropathy, and compressive neuropathy (intraneural and extraneural compression). Peripheral neuropathy (motor, sensory, and autonomic) ultimately causes the deformities of HD. Motor damage causes imbalance, leading to flexible and subsequently fixed deformities; sensory damage and sensory loss lead to autoamputation of fingers from recurrent injury and infection; and autonomic damage causes loss of protective sudomotor and vasomotor functions. HD is curable with outpatient oral chemotherapy. Dapsone renders the patient noncontagious in less than 6 weeks, and rifampin is effective in 2 days.[326] Treated early, it is cured; treated late, infection is cured but the nerve damage lingers.[549] The care of HD patients is now firmly integrated into general outpatient health care services. Fear of the disease is no longer justified by the lay public or the medical profession.

MICROBIOLOGIC CHARACTERISTICS

Gerhard Armauer Hansen from Norway identified the AFB *M. leprae* in 1873,[379] 10 years before Robert Koch, his contemporary, described *M. tuberculosis. M. leprae* was the first bacterium to be implicated as a cause of a human infection. It has not yet been grown in conventional media, but Shepard first demonstrated that it grows in the mouse foot pad.[524] In mice and humans it divides every 13 days. *M. leprae* grows best at temperatures below 37°C.[321] In humans, the bacteria infect nerves in the cooler parts of the body: the fine terminal dermal nerves, small subcutaneous nerves, and the superficially located large nerve trunks.[398] Sensory loss always precedes motor loss because superficial dermal nerve damage precedes deeper nerve trunk damage and nonmyelinated fibers are affected before myelinated fibers. Kirchheimer (1913-2001) first showed that *M. leprae*

grows luxuriously in cold-blooded, nine-banded armadillos,[412] a mammal found exclusively in Texas and Louisiana.

EPIDEMIOLOGY

The highest incidence of the disease is seen in Asia and Africa, with smaller numbers in South and Central America, the Pacific, and Caribbean islands. In the United States, in 1993 there were about 7000 patients, mostly immigrants from Mexico,[384] the Caribbean,[384] India,[374] Southeast Asia,[413] and Philippines.[384] The annual incidence of newly diagnosed patients in 1997 in the world was 566,000,[579] and in the United States it was 122 patients.[458] Most of the patients (80%) are located in California, Florida, Louisiana, New York, and Texas,[384] major sites of immigration. The island populations in Hawaii and Puerto Rico have the highest incidence and prevalence of HD in the United States.

In terms of reservoirs, most consider that HD is uniquely a human disease. In Texas and Louisiana, 15% of wild armadillos are infected with *M. leprae.*[535] It has been suggested that contact with infected armadillos can result in HD.[421] The most commonly held view of transmission of HD is that it is spread from human to human, primarily as a nasal droplet infection. Skin-to-skin contact is unproven. Incidence rates rise to a peak between 10 and 20 years of age and then decline. Sixty percent of HD patients develop the disease as children or young adults.[403]

CLINICAL PATHOLOGY

HD is essentially an infection of the peripheral nerves, and it is the only bacillary infection of the nerves. The peripheral nerve is an immunologically protected site where *M. leprae* preferentially thrive. *M. leprae* proliferate preferentially in the Schwann cells.[528] Some patients develop peripheral neuropathy before the diagnosis of the disease (pure or primary neuritic leprosy [PNL]), some develop it after starting therapy (infectious and immunologic neuritis), and yet others continue to develop neuropathies well after the therapy is stopped (immunologic neuritis or relapse). HD causes mononeuritis or mononeuritis multiplex. There is always nerve damage in HD.[381,408] Initially, Fite[363] taught that "all leprosy is neural leprosy" and Dastur,[345] that "there is no such thing as nonneural leprosy." From the onset, the cutaneous nerves[411] and fine intradermal nerve fibers[326] are involved in all forms of HD, and sensory loss is the first and most devastating casualty of HD.[345] Skin lesions and sensory loss develop simultaneously[564]; when skin lesions are present, the underlying dermal nerves are always infected.[395] Although it is the skin lesions that bring the patient to the doctor, it is the nerve lesions that cripple the patient. About 30% of sensory fibers must be destroyed before evidence of sensory impairment can be detected.[484] Thus by the time an anesthetic skin patch is detected, the nerve infection is well advanced. If a skin lesion is found to be insensitive, or an adjacent subcutaneous nerve is visible or palpable, HD can confidently be suspected.[403]

The bacillary load in the nerves is always higher than that observed in the skin in all stages and all types of HD.[410,528,545] The earliest change observed in lepromatous (LL) HD is the presence of *M. leprae* inside the Schwann cells.[394] The bacilli are found in 70% of the nerves in tuberculoid HD when they are hardly found in the skin.[527] At the time of diagnosis of HD, 50% of patients have nerve impairment or disability, motor and/or sensory.[501,536] An additional 10% to 20% develop a nerve impairment during and after completion of treatment.[536,542] Of 310 patients who had no nerve disability at diagnosis, 10% developed it within 2 years of treatment.[501]

Nerve lesions are due to infection of the nerve and are compounded by the immune reactions that continue in the nerves long after the patient is rendered free of living bacteria. Dead bacterial remnants persist in the nerves after a full course of antibiotic treatment.[399] The presence of these antigens may cause intraneural inflammation and fibrosis indefinitely.[399] The maximum concentrations of bacilli, and hence the greatest damage, are found in the fine dermal nerves, subcutaneous nerves, and the superficially located nerve trunks. In all types of HD the infected nerve is ultimately replaced by hyalinized fibrous tissue.[395] *M. leprae* conveniently hide in the fibrous tissue and are not reached by drugs. There is the possibility of relapse of the disease from persistent *M. leprae* in the fibrosed nerves.[395] Profound loss of sensation allows uncontrolled and progressive tissue damage from unrecognized injury and infection.[358] With repeated tissue necrosis and self-débridement, the fingers and toes may shorten to form mitten hands and feet. Antia has described three patterns of sensory loss in HD: (1) anesthetic patch from infection of a dermal or subcutaneous nerve; (2) regional loss from infection of a nerve trunk in tuberculoid disease; and (3) a glove-and-stocking pattern due to confluent involvement of sensory nerves in lepromatous disease.[305]

The incubation period of HD is not accurately known. Two to 7 years is considered usual. Ninety percent of the people who are exposed to *M. leprae* infection are naturally immune to the infection. Most people who are infected with *M. leprae* develop a subclinical infection and recover naturally without having symptoms or signs of disease.[326] In the remainder, HD progresses slowly over months and years. Most of the serious sequelae are the result of infection of the peripheral nerves. Bacterial multiplication occurs within Schwann cells, and they spread intraneurally to adjacent

Schwann cells. A stage is reached when intraneural infection is "recognized" by the host immune system and the nerve is invaded by lymphocytes and macrophages. A granuloma forms and fibrosis occurs within the epineurium, perineurium, and endoneurium.[509] Enlargement of peripheral nerves results not from initial infection but instead from subsequent immunologic reaction and caseation.[557] Enlarged nerves are pathognomonic of HD.[326,349] They are present in 25% of newly diagnosed cases.[542] Neurologic deficit is present in 95% of enlarged nerves.[542] In addition to the peripheral nerves, pathology of HD is largely confined to the skin, eyes, upper respiratory tract, and testes.

CLASSIFICATION

The clinical manifestations of HD vary, depending on the host's resistance or immunity. At one end of the spectrum, a patient may have high cell-mediated immunity and ability to resist, fight, and contain bacteria. At the other end of the spectrum, a patient may have complete tolerance to *M. leprae,* because the patient is without any detectable cell-mediated immunity against the microbe. These patients are actually teeming with bacteria; the host becomes a perfect culture medium for them. Between these two ends of the spectrum, the borderline group is found, encompassing most of the patients. The three main clinical types of HD are tuberculoid (TT, high immunity), lepromatous (LL, low immunity), and borderline (BB, unstable and intermediate immunity) according to the Madrid classification.[350] In tuberculoid HD, a cell-mediated immune response to *M. leprae* destroys both the bacillus and the Schwann cell in which it resides. This process leads to early caseous necrosis with total destruction of the nerve. In lepromatous HD, on the other hand, there is very little immune response to the bacillus. *M. leprae* multiply freely in the Schwann cells, producing a slow fibrosis over many years. Histoid and Lucio leprosy are variants of lepromatous leprosy. For research purposes, Ridley and Jopling[508] and Leiker[417] coincidentally and independently in 1966 divided the borderline cases into three subsets: BL, BB, and BT (Table 4-5). Ridley further divided TT and LL into polar (LLp, TTp) and subpolar (LLs, TTs) groups.[507] In 1982, the World Health Organization (WHO) recommended operational classification of HD into paucibacillary and multibacillary for treatment purposes based on the result of slit-skin smears. When a skin smear is positive, the disease is classified as multibacillary (MB). Under this classification most of indeterminate (I), TT, and BT cases are paucibacillary but any of them showing smear positivity is classified as multibacillary for purpose of drug therapy. The smears are positive in LL, BL, and BB cases and are classified as multibacillary. The number of drugs and length of therapy are higher for multibacillary than paucibacillary disease.

When a slit smear is not possible, a patient can be classified clinically. A patient with six or more lesions is classified as multibacillary (MB), and one with fewer than six lesions as paucibacillary (PB), with a reasonable balance between sensitivity and specificity.[342] PB patients are further classified into those with a single lesion and those with two to six lesions because the treatment of the two differs in drugs

Table 4-5
CLINICAL, BACTERIOLOGIC, HISTOLOGIC, AND IMMUNOLOGIC FEATURES OF HANSEN'S DISEASE

Lesions and Tests	Type of Hansen's Disease				
	TT	BT	BB	BL	LL
Number of skin lesions	Usually single	Single or few, may be distant	Several	Many	Very many
Size of skin lesions	Variable	Variable	Variable, mixed large and small lesions	Variable	Small
Surface of skin lesions	Very dry, sometimes scaly	Dry	Slightly shiny	Shiny	Shiny
Sensation in skin lesions	Absent	Moderately to markedly diminished	Slightly/moderately diminished in large lesions	Slightly diminished in large lesions	Not affected
Loss of hair and sweating in skin lesions	Absent	Markedly diminished	Moderately diminished	Slightly diminished	Not affected
AFB in skin lesions	Nil	Nil or scanty	Moderate numbers	Many	Very many (plus globi)
AFB in nasal scrapings or nose blows	Nil	Nil	Nil	Usually nil	Very many (plus globi)
Nerve lesions	Nerve may be thickened (one or two nerves only)	Thickening of several nerves	Thickening of several nerves	Thickening of several nerves, bilateral	Nerve thickening mild, may not be obvious till late stages
Histology	Dermal nerves are destroyed and cannot be recognized. AFB not seen. Foci of lymphocytes, epithelioid cells and giant cells invading skin indicating host cell-mediated immunity. Cutaneous nerves are greatly swollen due to epithelioid cell granuloma; they may caseate or are destroyed. Nerve abscess more common.	In BT there is a tuberculoid reaction more diffuse than in TT. AFB may or may not be seen.	In BB there is a diffuse epithelioid cell granuloma with occasional foam cells. AFB in small numbers.	In BL there is a granuloma composed of macrophages with lymphocytes in clumps or sheets. AFB present.	Diffuse leproma of foamy macrophages with few lymphocytes and plasma cells indicating poor cell-mediated immunity. Cutaneous nerves may show slight cellular infiltrate with foam cells. AFB seen in clumps. Nerve abscess less common.
Lepromin test	Strongly positive (+++)	Moderately or weakly positive (++ or +)	Negative	Negative	Negative

TT, tuberculoid; BT, borderline tuberculoid; BB, borderline; BL, borderline lepromatous; LL, lepromatous; AFB, acid-fast bacillus.

used. The limitation of using a purely clinical classification is that a single-lesion or paucilesional smear–positive case is falsely classified as PB and will receive inadequate chemotherapy, with the a risk of relapse and resistance, because approximately 3% of single-lesion patients[338] and 1% of paucilesional smear–positive cases[342] are multibacillary.

All the just-described classifications are based on host resistance or immunity. Clinical characteristics, skin and nerve lesions, bacteriology, histology, and immunology of HD in its spectrum are summarized in Table 4-5. It remains unknown why certain individuals develop HD and others do not.

EARLY DIAGNOSIS

Early diagnosis of HD can usually be made by clinical examination[446] supported by slit-skin smear.[326,474] Early diagnosis is conducive to cure and normal life.

Cardinal Signs

WHO has emphasized three cardinal signs for clinical diagnosis of HD: an anesthetic skin patch, nerve thickening, and a hypopigmented skin lesion. It must be confirmed by bacteriologic examination. A skin smear positive for HD bacilli confirms the diagnosis. At least two of the first three cardinal signs, or the fourth, should be present for the diagnosis of HD to be made.[578] To this Saunderson and Groenen have added unexplained loss of sensation in hand or foot *without a skin lesion*, and this ensures inclusion of pure (primary) neuritic cases of HD.[520]

Anesthesia
There are numerous diseases that produce anesthetic patches on the skin, and there are varied neurologic conditions that cause sensory loss. *Demonstrable loss of sensation restricted to a patch is not only unique but also pathognomonic of HD* and often requires no further tests for diagnosis. The tests (slit-skin smears) help further in classification and treatment of the disease.[564] Anesthesia is found on careful physical examination. Patients seldom complain of numbness because they adapt to gradual loss of sensation. Anesthesia may be patchy in the distribution of the dermal and cutaneous nerves, regional in the distribution of the peripheral nerve trunks, or in a diffuse glove-and-stocking pattern when damage has occurred to the dermal, subcutaneous, and the main nerve trunk as seen in lepromatous HD. The first tests to show and quantitate sensory nerve function impairment are moving two-point discrimination and Semmes-Weinstein monofilament testing.[568] In lepromatous HD, a period of formication or pruritus may precede all other symptoms, very early in the course of the disease.[407] A painless burn may be the presenting symptom or sign of HD.[407]

Thickened Nerves
Thickened nerves at the site of predilection are pathognomonic of HD (Fig. 4-8).[326,349] The ulnar nerve is always the first nerve trunk to be involved in the upper extremity and is the most commonly affected nerve with or without skin

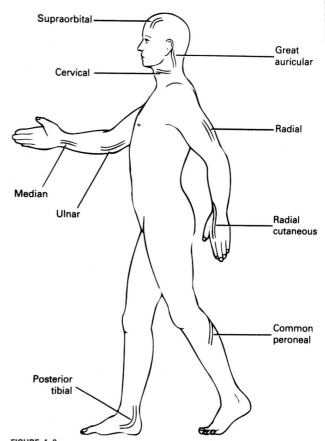

FIGURE 4-8. Hansen's disease. The common sites of nerve involvement in the upper extremity are the ulnar nerve at the elbow and the median nerve and the sensory branch of the radial nerve at the wrist. Radial nerve involvement in the upper arm is rare. (From Hastings RC: Leprosy, 2nd ed. New York, Churchill Livingstone, 1994.)

lesions. In an immigrant from an endemic region of the world who presents with an ulnar nerve entrapment or carpal tunnel syndrome[413] or an unexplained neuropathy, with or without a skin lesion (pure neuritic HD), consider HD as an etiologic basis for the diagnosis.[420,457,464] There are four clinical stages of nerve infection in HD:

I. *Parasitization:* Bacteria invade the Schwann cells; clinically the nerve is normal, but 50% of the patients have neurologic deficit.[542]
II. *Inflammation:* Adhesion of the nerve to the perineurium is noted with inability to roll the nerve during palpation.[304]
III. *Enlargement:* The nerve is palpably enlarged (with caseation and without or with an abscess). Ninety-five percent of these patients have a neurologic deficit.
IV. *Destruction:* The nerve is irreversibly damaged and converted to a cord of scar tissue.

Twenty-five percent of newly identified cases have one or more enlarged nerves. The enlarged nerves may be palpable but not visible, palpable and visible, or palpable and fluctuant. The nerve may be soft (parasitization), firm (caseation), or hard (fibrosed). Thickening of nerve trunks occurs most often in the borderline, lepromatous, and pure neuritic types of HD. Fifty-one percent of patients without enlarged nerves also have some nerve deficit on careful clinical examination. Pain in one or several nerves may be the presenting symptom in tuberculoid or borderline tuberculoid HD even before the skin lesions have appeared. In the beginning, the nerve may be normal in size but may be tender. As granuloma, edema, and fibrosis occur in the nerves, they become enlarged and firm. Enlarged nerves may or may not be tender.[515,560] Caseation may follow and progress to a solitary tuberculoid lesion of the nerve or a cold nerve abscess without sinus formation[316,378,419,435,514,519,530,553] or with sinus formation.[377] Finally, the nerve is calcified.*

If the body's cellular immunity anchors the infection within one or more nerves, the patient may present initially with clinical nerve deficit but no skin lesions and negative slit-skin smears.[445,446] This is called "pure neuritic" or "primary neuritic" HD.[353,380,404,445,461,552,561] Mean prevalence rate of pure neuritic HD varies from 0.8% to 18%.[461,564] In pure neuritic HD, commonly one nerve is involved, typically the ulnar nerve at the elbow, or the patient may have polyneuropathy. The most common clinical presentation is with numbness or weakness; wasting, deformity, and pain/tingling may also be presenting symptoms in a small minority.[552] The nerve is palpable or visible in 80% of patients with pure neuritic HD. An early and accurate diagnosis of pure neuritic HD is essential to avoid mismanagement and should be suspected in an immigrant from an endemic region.[374,413] In absence of anesthetic skin patches or absence of AFB in slit-skin smears, fine-needle nerve aspiration[393,569] or an open nerve biopsy[335,361,374,413,443,482] may establish diagnosis. Histopathology of pure neuritic lesions reveals a spectrum from paucibacillary (tuberculoid) to multibacillary (lepromatous) type.[569] When it is not possible

*See references 312, 330, 333, 337, 356, 364, 368, 434, 460, 477, 495, 498, 519, and 556.

to biopsy a nerve in pure neuritic HD, three factors help to decide the classification and choice of treatment regimen.[309,565] First, a pure mononeuritic case generally responds well to paucibacillary regimen but it is reasonable to consider HD involving multiple nerves on both sides of the body (mononeuritis multiplex) as multibacillary. Second, a clinically mononeuritic case may show multiple nerve involvement on electrophysiologic studies, indicating a more widespread involvement and need for a multibacillary regimen. Third, the lepromin reaction is helpful in both mononeuritis and mononeuritis multiplex in determining the patient's position on the immunologic spectrum.

Skin Lesions

Skin lesions may became visible at any time during the course of primary neuritic HD.[388,493] The body of the patient should be examined for pigmented or hypopigmented patches and nodules in light that should preferentially fall on the patient from behind the shoulders of the examiner. Classically, the first lesion is a symptomless, ill-defined, slightly hypopigmented macule that is commonly seen on the face, trunk, or limbs. Sensation is only slightly impaired or normal. Bacilli are difficult to find, and diagnosis depends on careful, continuing observation. This lesion is called "indeterminate"; it may heal or progress to one of the three determinate types: tuberculoid, borderline, or lepromatous HD.[522] An indeterminate lesion most often heals spontaneously, but about 30% progress to a determinate type (Fig. 4-9).[403]

The most common clinical manifestation in HD is a hypopigmented, numb patch of the skin. Discolored skin lesions occur in many diseases and numbness of skin occurs in many nerve disorders but *a skin lesion that is anesthetic occurs only in HD*. When such a lesion is encountered, diagnosis of HD is clinically confirmed. Increasing anesthesia and elevation of the margins of the skin lesion

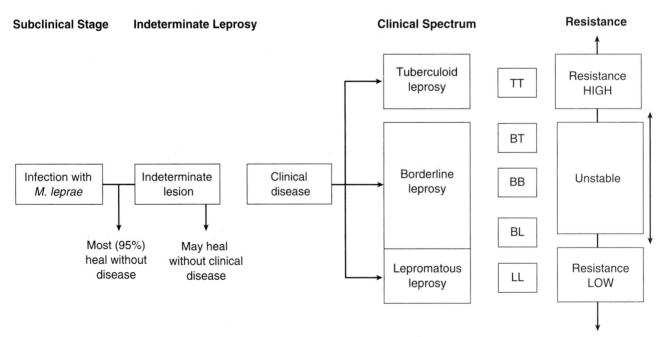

FIGURE 4-9. The course of leprosy after infection with *Mycobacterium leprae*.

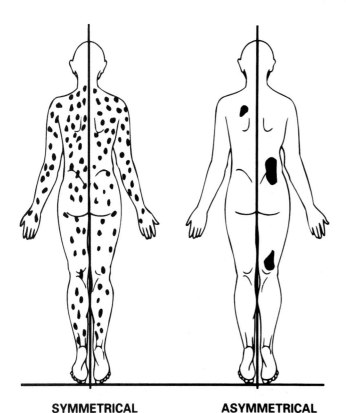

SYMMETRICAL   **ASYMMETRICAL**

FIGURE 4-10. The lesions of multibacillary Hansen's disease are symmetrical, and those of paucibacillary Hansen's disease are asymmetrical. (From Hastings RC: Leprosy, 2nd ed. New York, Churchill Livingstone, 1994.)

indicate movement toward the tuberculoid pole. An increase in the number of the lesions and central elevation of the skin lesion indicate movement toward the lepromatous pole. On light skin, the lesions are copper colored; and on dark skin, they are hypopigmented. Clinically, a patient with six or more lesions is classified as multibacillary and one with fewer than six lesions as paucibacillary, and there is a reasonable balance between sensitivity and specificity of this method (Fig. 4-10).[342] A hyperpigmented palmar lesion is a rare presentation of HD and is seen in borderline tuberculoid.[375]

The diagnosis of HD may occasionally be difficult, as in the following three situations: (1) there is a skin lesion without sensory loss, (2) there is a sensory loss without a skin lesion, and (3) there is an enlarged nerve without motor or sensory loss and a skin lesion is absent (primary neuritic HD).

Diagnostic Tests

Lepromin Skin Test (Mitsuda Reaction)

Mitsuda, a Japanese leprologist, described in 1919 the value of skin reaction to a suspension of leprosy nodules, the reaction that is named after him.[447] Dharmendra purified leprosy antigen (Dharmendra antigen) and unequivocally established the prognostic value of lepromin testing in 1955.[351] This led to classifications of HD spectrum on an immunologic basis.[417,508] A majority of individuals exposed

---

CRITICAL POINTS: LEPROMIN TESTING

- The lepromin test is not to make a diagnosis of leprosy.
- The lepromin test helps to classify leprosy.
- In pure neuritic leprosy, the lepromin test may help in deciding whether the patient should be treated with a paucibacillary regimen (lepromin test 1+ to 3+) or a multibacillary regimen (lepromin test negative).

---

to *M. leprae* get infected; only a small percentage of these go on to develop the disease. The lepromin test is positive in people who develop subclinical infection, because their inherent resistance is high. It is thus positive in the majority of healthy individuals in endemic areas. It is thus not a diagnostic test for HD. *It is of great value in classifying a case of HD, once the diagnosis has been made.* It essentially indicates the resistance of the patient. The patients on the tuberculoid side of the spectrum have higher resistance and show a positive reaction, whereas those on the lepromatous side have lower resistance and show a negative reaction.

Slit-Skin Smears

Slit-skin smear is the gold standard for diagnosis of HD. This is the simplest and yet the most important investigation that helps not only in diagnosing HD but also in classifying the disease.[403] *Presence of AFB in slit-skin smears confirms the diagnosis of HD.*[403] A negative result, of course, does not rule out the diagnosis of HD. In pure (primary) neuritic HD, skin lesions are absent and nerve aspiration or open nerve biopsy may be considered if the clinical diagnosis of HD is not certain.*

Slit-skin smears are made from a suspect lesion, as well as from sites commonly affected in lepromatous HD. These sites include skin from the dorsum of proximal phalanges of fingers and extensor surfaces of the forearms. In lepromatous patients, nodules are the preferred sites for slit-skin smears but these may also be obtained from the trunk, buttocks, or the ear lobes. In tuberculoid patients, rims of skin lesions should be sampled.

Technique. The skin lesion is cleansed with isopropyl alcohol or ether, and a portion of it is pinched between the thumb and index finger of the left hand to squeeze out the blood off the skin fold. With a No. 15 scalpel, the skin is slit between the thumb and finger, about 5 mm long, and deep enough (about 3 mm) to get well into, but not through, the infiltrated layer of the dermis. The blade is then used to scrape the cut edges of dermis several times so that tissue fluid and dermal pulp (not blood) collects on one side of the blade; this is gently smeared onto a glass slide. The smear is fixed over a flame before being sent for staining. A total of six or eight smears should be made.

---

*See references 388, 391, 404, 415, 422, 454, 481, 493, 561, and 565.

CRITICAL POINTS: SLIT-SKIN SMEARS

- Slit-skin smear confirms diagnosis of HD, when it is positive.
- It classifies the patient as multibacillary for chemotherapy.
- Do not allow the skin to bleed. Bloody smears are useless.
- Cut through part of the dermis but not through the dermis.

Skin Biopsy

When a slit-skin smear is negative, a skin biopsy may be considered, if the clinical diagnosis is in doubt. The probability of finding bacilli in an HD patient is greater in skin biopsy than slit-skin smears.[492] A biopsy in HD must include the full depth of the dermis together with a portion of subcutaneous fat to include a dermal nerve. It is difficult to opine on a section that fails to show a dermal nerve.

Technique. A deep skin biopsy at the active edge of a lesion is done that includes large deep dermal nerves entering the deep surface of the dermis and nerve fibers in the subcutaneous tissue. The biopsy can be preserved in a suitable preservative such as 10% formaldehyde for further processing. A portion of the skin may be saved in 70% ethyl alcohol so that PCR may be done if bacilli are not found in the skin. PCR can detect in a skin sample as few as 10 to 100 bacilli in an early or TT lesion.[400] When a biopsy is being sent for a mouse foot pad test, it should be placed in a small sterile bottle without any additive and kept at 4°C in a flask containing ice.

Viable *M. leprae* are solid, are nonfragmented, and stain uniformly, whereas dead bacilli are fragmented and stain irregularly. The percentage of solidly staining bacilli, termed the *morphologic index* (MI),[505] is useful for assessing viability of the bacilli in skin and tissue sections. It tells if the patient is still infective and if the disease is still active, gives valuable information as to response to treatment, and provides an early indication of bacterial resistance to treatment or of noncompliance with chemotherapy. The total number of bacilli in the dermis, the *bacteriologic index* (BI),[403,505] includes both live (solid) and dead (fragmented) bacteria. The BI is useful in assessing the number of live bacteria at

CRITICAL POINTS: SKIN BIOPSY

- Always include subcutaneous tissue with a subcutaneous nerve.
- Do not place skin in preservative if growth of mycobacteria in mouse foot pad is contemplated.
- Save a portion of skin in 70% alcohol if PCR test is planned.

Table 4-6

METHOD OF GRADING BACTERIOLOGIC INDEX IN SLIT-SKIN SMEAR OR SKIN BIOPSY OR NERVE BIOPSY SPECIMEN

Bacterial Index	Average No. of Bacilli per (100×) Field	WHO Classification
0	0 in 100 fields	Paucibacillary
1	1-10 in 100 fields	Multibacillary
2	1-10 in 10 fields	Multibacillary
3	1-10 per field	Multibacillary
4	10-100 per field	Multibacillary
5	100-1000 per field	Multibacillary
6	>1000 per field	Multibacillary

Classification of patients into paucibacillary (BI = 0) and multibacillary (BI > 0) for treatment purpose makes detailed computing unimportant in diagnosis. The index is nevertheless useful in following the improvement or deterioration of the disease (drug compliance and drug resistance). Morphologic index calls for consistently high standards of staining, fixation, and microscopy, which are rarely available outside research and scientific units.[1]

the onset of diagnosis (Table 4-6). It assesses the natural host resistance to *M. leprae* and classifies the patient into paucibacillary or multibacillary disease, which determines their respective treatment regimens. Using the WHO definition, paucibacillary refers to patients with a BI of 0 on the Ridley scale at all skin smear sites and multibacillary refers to patients with a BI of 1+ or more at any site.

Nerve Biopsy

Neuritic pain with an enlarged nerve and without a skin lesion may be the first symptom/sign of HD. In this type of nerve lesion, called pure or primary neuritic HD, in the absence of skin lesions, fine-needle nerve aspiration cytology[348,393,533] or open biopsy[403,443,564] may be the only way to confirm the diagnosis of HD. Nerve aspiration cytology is simple and rapid; material obtained is abundant, absence of trauma and scarring are appreciated by the patient, and an operating room visit for nerve biopsy is avoided. A thickened pure sensory nerve with minimal functional deficit (sural, radial sensory, supraclavicular) is suitable. When *M. leprae* is not visible on microscopy in the nerve as in pure neuritic HD or TT disease, PCR, which is positive in 80% of cases, is the last resort to find *M. leprae* in the nerve[334] or the skin.[400]

Technique of Fine-Needle Nerve Aspiration. The nerve is palpated and the most prominent site is noted. Skin is anesthetized 1 cm proximal to the site of aspiration. A 22-gauge 4-cm needle fixed to a 10-mL disposable syringe is used, and aspiration is performed using a single puncture. The direction of the needle is always kept parallel to the length of the nerve. The material aspirated is smeared on glass slides. Hematoxylin and eosin and acid-fast stains are done. Sixty-six percent of the aspirated nerves showed inflammatory cells, 25% showed granulomas consistent with the diagnosis of HD, and 24% showed AFB.[569] No neurologic deficit has occurred at 1-year follow-up.[348,569]

Technique of Open Nerve Biopsy.   Pearson recommends biopsy of one or two fascicles of a branch of the radial sensory nerve.[482] If the nerve is severely damaged and fascicles are obliterated, a small longitudinal wedge of nerve can be removed. A 2-cm nerve biopsy provides enough length for histology and electron microscopy.[306] It is important to identify proximal and distal ends of the nerve for the pathologist. The excised portion is immediately immersed in a fixative (10% buffered formalin or alcohol).

Electrophysiologic Studies

Nerve conduction studies and electromyography are not specific in the diagnosis of HD.[564] They are useful before surgery in confirming the site of compression neuropathy and assessing the extent of nerve damage in early stages of leprosy.

TREATMENT

The patient is classified on the immunologic spectrum of HD based on the lepromin test, skin smears, skin biopsy, or nerve biopsy. Based on this, chemotherapeutic agents and duration of treatment are decided. The primary aim in managing patients with HD is to prevent deformities in those who do not have them and to reduce disabilities in those who have them. If treated early, the disease leaves no residual marks. The diagnosis should not be made by exclusion or by therapeutic trial. *No one should be treated for HD unless the diagnosis is established. A mistaken diagnosis may cause severe social complications.*

Six objectives of treatment of HD include:

1. Elimination of infecting bacteria (multidrug therapy)
2. Relief of pain (anti-inflammatory medications and nerve decompression)
3. Preservation of sensation (corticosteroids, thalidomide, and nerve decompression)
4. Restoration of sensation (innervated skin flaps, nerve transfer, nerve decompression, sensory re-education)
5. Treatment of deformities: flexible and fixed (hand therapy and reconstructive surgery) (see Chapter 41)
6. Rehabilitation (psychological, social, vocational, and avocational)

Elimination of Infecting Bacteria (Multidrug Therapy)

Drug therapy renders the patient noninfective very quickly. In the 1940s, dapsone was shown to cure patients with HD and was the first landmark in the treatment of HD.[362] Monotherapy with dapsone led to drug resistance.[483] In 1982, WHO recommended multidrug therapy (MDT) to reduce drug resistance.[581] Dapsone, which is bacteriostatic, makes the patient noninfective in 6 weeks, and rifampin, which is bactericidal for *M. leprae,* makes the patient noninfective in 2 days.[326] Since the mid 1980s, bactericidal activities of ofloxacin, minocycline, and clarithromycin have provided treatment for rifampin-resistant *M. leprae.* Mouse foot pad antibiotic sensitivity testing should be routinely done on all multibacillary patients when possible.[418] Treatment for paucibacillary and multibacillary HD is different in the number of drugs and their duration.

Paucibacillary HD

Paucibacillary HD is treated with two drugs: dapsone, 100 mg once daily, orally, unsupervised; and rifampin, 600 mg once monthly, orally, supervised.

The drugs are given orally on an ambulatory basis. WHO recommends treatment for 6 months. In developing countries, rifampin is given once a month because it is very expensive. American recommendations include rifampin in a "full" dosage of 600 mg daily. A *single dose* of a three-drug bactericidal combination of rifampin, 600 mg, plus ofloxacin, 400 mg, plus minocycline, 100 mg (ROM) is shown to kill 99% of viable *M. leprae.*[534] In 1997, WHO endorsed the use of single-dose ROM for the treatment of patients with single-lesion paucibacillary HD.

Multibacillary HD

Multibacillary HD is treated with three drugs: dapsone, 100 mg daily, orally, unsupervised; rifampin, 600 mg once monthly, orally, supervised; and clofazimine, 300 mg once monthly, orally, supervised, and 50 mg daily, orally, unsupervised.

WHO recommends treatment for 12 months.[580] If the skin smears remain positive, the treatment is continued until the smears become negative. Patients in the urban United States often refuse to take clofazimine because it discolors the skin. Rifampin is hepatotoxic, and its use must be monitored with periodic bilirubin determinations. An elevation of serum bilirubin is an indication to stop rifampin. It should not be prescribed in the first 3 months of pregnancy.[326]

With this treatment, the number of patients worldwide requiring treatment decreased from 12 million in 1982[462] to 0.8 million in 1999. Still, more than 500,000 new cases are detected each year worldwide. WHO's goal is to eliminate HD as a public health problem by reducing its prevalence to less than 1 case per 10,000 population worldwide. However, drug resistance,[483] persistence of viable *M. leprae* in the tissues for many years after effective therapy (persisters),[307,361,390,486,529] and relapses after release from treatment[313,376,555] make eradication of HD difficult. Persisters relapse when their immunity falls for any reason. Relapse rate after dapsone monotherapy was 10% after 5 years, and after MDT it was 0.6% after 5 years. Relapses are more often in multibacillary than paucibacillary patients after both monodrug therapy and MDT. Relapses in multibacillary patients occur more often in patients who have a higher bacillary load (BI > 4 before MDT).[392]

Relief of Pain

Neuritic pain in HD occurs secondary to nerve infection, nerve reactions due to immunologic defense mechanisms,[452,491,506] nerve compression,[543] and nerve abscess.[303,344,416,516,518,530] Non-neuritic pain in HD may arise from dermatitis, tenosynovitis,[437,489] arthritis,[372,409,532] and myositis (Fig. 4-11).[401]

Reactions

The term *reaction* is used to describe the sudden exacerbations in the manifestations of the HD that may occur before, during, or after the course of MDT. Reactional episodes are said to be brought about by alterations in immunologic balance. They are antigen-antibody reactions

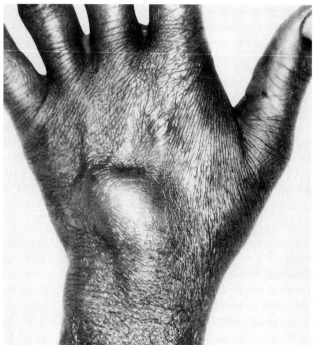

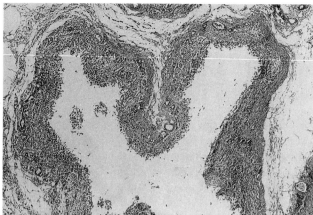

FIGURE 4-11. **A** and **B,** A rare initial presentation in Hansen's disease is tenosynovitis. Clinically it presents as a moderately painful swelling on the dorsum of one or both wrists, hands, and fingers.

to *M. leprae* polysaccharides and proteins. In the upper extremity, they manifest with acute inflammation in the skin, nerves, tenosynovium, and joint. The patient suffers pain from tender nerves, tender skin, tender tenosynovitis, and tender and swollen joints. Swelling of the joints is symmetric and occurs mainly in the wrist, metacarpophalangeal joints, and proximal interphalangeal joints and resembles rheumatoid arthritis.[372,409,532] All are precursors to edema. The shoulder-hand-finger syndrome can develop in the reactive phases of HD[367] as an edematous, painful, stiff upper extremity. Furness and colleagues call this the "stasis hand" of leprosy.[367]

Much of the nerve damage in HD takes place during the reactive phase. The reactive phase in HD produces intraneural caseous necrosis in tuberculoid disease and microabscesses in lepromatous disease.[395] Lepra reaction neuritis is a medical emergency. Unless it is treated immediately, sensory loss may become devastating and irreversible.[438] *A reaction may be the initial manifestation of HD.* Reactions plague the patient before treatment, during treatment, and long after MDT has practically eliminated all viable organisms from the body. New deformity or disability occurs in 5% of multibacillary patients during therapy and 2.5% during surveillance period as a result of lepra reactions.[570] They continue to disable and deform the patient for life. HD is thus truly an immunologic disease.

Three types of reactions occur in HD: reversal reaction (type 1), erythema nodosum leprosum (type 2), and Lucio's reaction.[373]

Reversal Reactions (RR) (Lepra Type 1)

There is rapid increase in cell-mediated immunity when a patient is under adequate and regular treatment. This results in an improvement of immunologic resistance that is associated with a reaction that is characterized as an "upgrading reaction" or "reversal reaction." These type 1 reactions are most common in borderline and tuberculoid patients. Clinically, reaction is manifested in the skin, nerves, and tendons. The reaction may be mild and manifested by dull pain or with severe neuritic pain and skin lesions and tenosynovitis.[326]

Erythema Nodosum Leprosum (ENL) (Lepra Type 2 Reaction)

Lepra type-2 reactions affect mainly the lepromatous (LL > BL[440]) patients. In contrast to a reversal reaction, erythema nodosum leprosum is a generalized process, involving several organ systems, concurrently or sequentially. The patient is often ill, with fever and granulocytosis. The process takes its name from crops of painful, red, cutaneous and subcutaneous nodules that develop all over the face, limbs, and trunk. Joints may become swollen and tender. Neuritis occurs in 20% of cases owing to formation of microabscesses. Periostitis, tendinitis, and myositis are sometimes observed. It has been hypothesized that a high bacterial antigen load leads to an immune reaction in which immune complexes cause vasculitis, which is the histologic hallmark of ENL (Table 4-7).

Lucio's Reaction

In 1852, Lucio and Alvarado described a necrotizing skin reaction associated with non-nodular diffuse LL HD.[451] Lucio's reaction is common in Mexico and Central America.[403] Large recurrent, sloughing cutaneous ulcerations occur that heal poorly. It may present as intense hand (and foot) edema. Necrosis, ulceration, and purulent exudate are superimposed on purpuric cutaneous plaques on hands and feet.[537] There may be rapid and profound deterioration of health, with delay in diagnosis and high morbidity and mortality.[537] This is considered to be a type of HD reaction associated with necrosis of arterioles, whose endothelium is massively invaded by *M. leprae* (see Table 4-7).[451]

Table 4-7
CLASSIFICATION OF LEPRA REACTION (REACTION IN LEPROSY)

Type of Reaction	Types of Leprosy Involved	Main Clinical Features	Main Histologic Features	Main Hematologic Findings
Type 1 reaction Reversal reaction (RR reaction) Increased hypersensitivity to *M. leprae*	1. Borderline (BT < BB < BL)	Erythema and swelling of some or all leprosy skin lesions. New lesions may appear. Edema of extremities. Neuritis.	In upgrading reaction there is edema, reduced bacilli, and increased defensive cells, such as lymphocytes, epithelioid cells, and giant cells. In downgrading reaction there is increase in bacilli and defensive cells are replaced by macrophages.	Nil
Type 2 reaction Erythema nodosum leprosum (ENL reaction) Immune complex formation	1. LL 2. BL	Fever, skin eruptions, ENL, with any of the following, singly or in various combinations: *Hand:* neuritis, bone pain, joint pain, dactylitis, tenosynovitis, lymphadenitis. *Systemic:* fever, malaise, rhinitis, epistaxis, iritis, epididymo-orchitis, proteinuria. In severe cases (erythema necroticans), skin lesions may become vesicular or bullous and break down.	In ENL lesions there is edema, neutrophil infiltration, and vasculitis (veins and arterioles). In erythema necroticans there is obliterative angiitis and endarteritis. Bacilli are fragmented and granular.	Polymorphonuclear leukocytosis Raised ESR Thrombocytosis Raised IgG, IgM, complement 2 and complement 3 Normocytic normochromic anemia
Lucio's reaction	Lucio's leprosy (in Mexico and South America)	Small pink lesions on skin become large, develop bullae, become necrotic, and cause large painful ulcers.	Necrosis of superficial blood vessels. Deposits of immunoglobulin and complement in vessel walls. Abundant AFBs.	High titers of circulating immune complexes and cryoglobulins

LL, lepromatous; BL, borderline lepromatous; ENL, erythema nodosum leprosum; ESR, erythrocyte sedimentation rate; AFB, acid-fast bacilli.

Treatment of Reactions (Table 4-8)

Leprosy is cured but nerves die,[549] unless reactions are prevented or treated early.[339,341] Mild reactions are accompanied by nagging pain without neurologic deficit. Aspirin is adequate for pain relief and is the drug of choice. More severe reactions are best managed by resting the nerve (splinting the affected joint) and oral corticosteroid therapy.[339-341] Prednisone reduces edema virtually overnight and decreases the postinflammatory scarring.[452] In reversal reaction, corticosteroids may be needed for 6 months or longer to prevent relapses[452] and use for up to 5 years has shown very beneficial results.[549] In ENL, clofazimine[488] and thalidomide[479,575] help to reduce the corticosteroid dose once the acute pain subsides. Acute tenosynovitis is treated with oral cortisone, hand elevation, and a balanced combination of splinting and mobilization of the joints.

In Lucio's reaction, débridement of sloughing skin and skin grafting are indicated early, particularly when joints are exposed. It is also necessary to provide immunosuppressive drug therapy and MDT. Naafs has reviewed current views on reactions in HD and is a valuable reading.[452] Hands affected by reactive phases of HD do well if occupational and physical hand therapists prevent "frozen hands" and "frozen shoulders."[366]

Compression Neuropathy

There may be internal compression of the nerves where the nerve fibers are strangulated by the thickened epineurium because of intraneural edema ("acute nerve compartment syndrome") or intraneural granuloma formation and caseation ("chronic nerve compartment syndrome"). Surgical decompression is complementary to, and not a substitute for, medical treatment of acute neuritis.[407] Nerve compression is surgically decompressed when (1) nerve pain is severe even though nerve function may have been lost for months or years[365] and (2) when there is recent and/or progressive loss of nerve function (motor or sensory) after adequate cortisone treatment from 3 days[305] to 3 weeks.[365,381] Those with extensive surgical experience in HD, including Brand and Fritschi,[322,365] Antia,[304] Callaway and colleagues,[327] Enna

Table 4-8

TREATMENT OF LEPRA REACTION

Type of Reaction	Corticosteroids	Clofazimine	Thalidomide
Type 1 reaction	At least 60 to 80 mg prednisone daily. Initially attempt to taper over 2 to 3 months. For chronic reactions try to taper to an every-other-day schedule.	300 mg daily until controlled off corticosteroids; then taper to 100 mg daily. Increase as needed if reaction recurs.	Ineffective
Type 2 reaction	Usually 60 mg of prednisone daily. Initially attempt to taper over 2 to 3 months. For chronic reactions try to taper to an every-other-day schedule.	300 mg daily until controlled off corticosteroids; then taper to 100 mg daily. Increase as needed if reaction recurs.	100 mg four times daily tapered after reaction controlled. For chronic reaction, maintenance level of 100 mg every other day to 100 mg twice daily. Try to discontinue after 6 months.
Lucio's reaction	At least 60 mg of prednisone daily. Initially attempt to taper over several weeks. For chronic reactions try to taper to an every-other-day schedule.	Value questionable except as antileprosy therapy	Ineffective

and Delgado[360] Palande,[470,471,473] Srinivasan,[540,541,544] and others,[387,436,476,478,571] found that when unrelenting pain was the patient's main problem, ulnar nerve decompression was a gratifying operation for the patient and the surgeon (Fig. 4-12). Varying grades of motor and sensory recovery were additional benefits in 50% of the patients when surgery was done early.[327,468,478]

Results of carpal tunnel release are mixed. Husain and colleagues,[386] Antia,[305] and Parikh[478] have observed that the decompression of median nerve was beneficial. Pain relief was dramatic, sensory recovery was seen in 90% of cases, and in 45% of cases muscle strength improved.[386] Palande observed motor recovery in 75% of patients with median nerve palsy if operated on within 2 months of paralysis.[470] Fritschi observed that after carpal tunnel release, recovery of any measurable motor or sensory function was rare.[365]

Results of radial nerve release in the radial nerve groove of humerus are equivocal.[365] The number of cases requiring nerve decompression has been significantly reduced after

CRITICAL POINTS: ULNAR NERVE DECOMPRESSION

- Release of fibro-osseous canal relieves extraepineurial pressures.
- Longitudinal epineurotomy relieves intraepineurial pressure.
- Vascular supply of the nerve should not be disturbed. Let the nerve rest in its bed.
- Caseated material within the nerve should be débrided gently and irrigated thoroughly.
- When a nerve has been destroyed by the process, total excision of the involved nerve results in complete relief of pain.

using cortisone,[339,341] clofazimine,[488] and thalidomide[575] to control acute leprous reactions.

Nerve Abscess

Nerve abscess may be the initial presenting problem in HD,[449,553] may be seen during therapy,[530] and may appear during post-MDT surveillance.[303,344] A nerve abscess may appear as a single swelling (Fig. 4-13), multiple swellings on a single nerve,[377,496] or multiple swellings on different nerves.[516] Salafia and Chauhan reported that children and teenagers accounted for 47% of 145 nerve abscesses.[516] Nerve abscess occurs across the entire spectrum of HD. The abscess may be fluctuant, nonfluctuant, subcutaneous, deep, painless, painful, collar-stud,[304] moderate in size, giant in size,[378] without a sinus, with an impending sinus (Fig. 4-14), with a draining sinus, with a dry sinus, without calcification, or with calcification (Fig. 4-15).* It is most commonly seen in the ulnar nerve (58%)[316,530] and rarely in the median (7%)[369] or the radial nerve[312] and may be unilateral or bilateral (Fig. 4-16).[370,490,516]

Treatment

A painless abscess may subside with oral corticosteroid therapy.[303] If a painful and fluctuating abscess does not respond to oral corticosteroid therapy, it is drained to debulk the caseous granulation tissue and to decompress the surviving nerve fascicles. This relieves pain and may prevent further deterioration of nerve function.[316,378,419,435,514,519,530,553]

Technique of Nerve Abscess Drainage. A painless and fluctuating abscess without progressive nerve deficit may simply be aspirated under sonography.[553] An abscess with progressive neurologic deficit is drained with a single longitudinal epineurotomy. Drainage may yield caseous material. No nerve fascicles are disturbed. The epineurium is not

---

*See references 312, 330, 333, 337, 356, 364, 368, 434, 460, 477, 495, 498, 519, and 556.

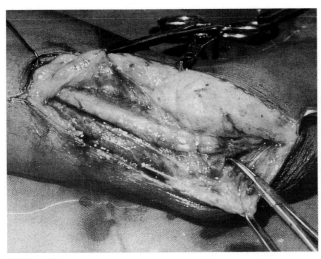

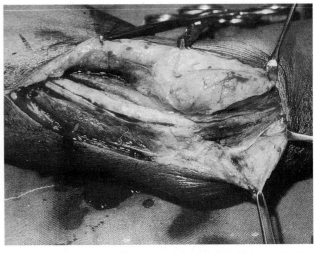

FIGURE 4-12. **A,** An incision is made in the upper arm, over the palpable nerve, or at least 10 cm proximal to the medial epicondyle, and carried behind the medial epicondyle and distal to the elbow. Extraepineurial pressure in the fibro-osseous tunnel containing the enlarged nerve is decompressed. **B,** Longitudinal epineurotomy is then done along the length of the enlarged nerve proximal and distal to the medial epicondyle to decompress intraepineurial pressure.

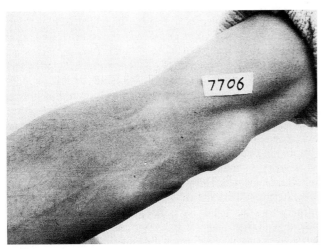

FIGURE 4-13. Clinical features of a nerve abscess are many and varied. A single swelling is the most common surgical presentation.

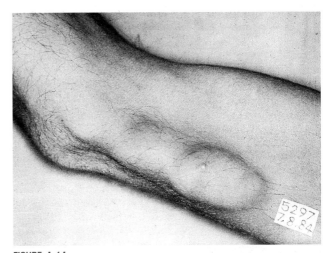

FIGURE 4-14. A nerve abscess with an impending sinus may need early incision and drainage to prevent formation of a chronic sinus and more perineurial fibrosis.

closed. The skin can be primarily closed over a drain that is removed 24 to 48 hours after surgery. A chronic sinus secondary to a discharged nerve abscess can be treated by excision of the sinus tract along with necrotic nerve tissue. In cases of complete nerve trunk palsy, a course of rifampin and isoniazid can heal the sinus in about 6 months.[385]

Preservation of Sensation

Infection of the peripheral nerve in HD impairs pain perception. Loss of pain allows the patient to injure himself or herself. Fingertips undergo "terminal absorption"[358] due to recurrent trauma and infection.[319] Shortening of the fingers can result in "mitten" hands.

Sensory loss occurs in HD from several causes, but the basic pathology is a varying mixture of segmental demyelination and axonal degeneration. Swelling of the endothelium in leprous vasculitis causes narrowing of lumina and ischemia.[395] Progressive nerve fibrosis converts the nerve

into a fibrous cord. Complete and early elimination of bacteria by MDT may cure the patient. Reactions are treated by prompt administration of corticosteroids. In patients with recent loss of sensation who do not respond to corticosteroids, surgical decompression of the involved nerve is indicated.[563] Surgery done no later than 3 months after the onset of nerve damage has been shown to be beneficial.[452]

Silent Neuritis. Silent neuritis occurs with neurologic loss (sensory and motor) but without neuropathic pain or tenderness and in absence of a leprae reaction (types 1, 2, or Lucio) in a large population of HD. In 67% to 75% of those who developed deformities, patients gave no history of reactions; 95% of those with pure neuritic HD did not give history of neuritic pain. Srinivasan and associates[544] and van Brakel and Khawas[567] have postulated that the nerves have been silently damaged by Schwann cell destruction and segmental demyelination during continuous or recurrent

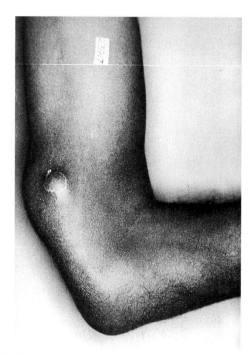

FIGURE 4-15. A nerve abscess may eventually become calcified and seen on radiographs as a longitudinal opacity corresponding to the location of the nerve.

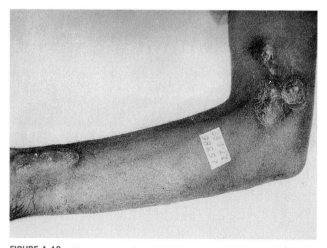

FIGURE 4-16. Abscesses may be seen along one or more cutaneous nerves of the arm or forearm. The median cutaneous nerve of the arm and median cutaneous nerve of the forearm account for 35% of abscesses.

subclinical type 1 and 2 reactions. In silent neuritis, corticosteroids are beneficial in reversing motor weakness,[546] but their benefit in impaired sensibility is not known.[407]

Restoration of Sensibility

Antia reported that 20% to 30% of patients develop irreversible nerve damage in HD.[308] Restoring sensibility in anesthetic extremities of HD patients[426] is the next surgical frontier.[503] The minimum desirable level of sensibility in Hansen's disease is protective sensibility. This prevents self-mutilation of the hand. Surgery is successful if the patient can resume "injury-free" hand activities. The recovery of sensory abilities therefore will help in "normalization" of the activities of the patients.[426] Procedures to restore sensibility should be delayed until all indicated tendon transfers have been done and the patient has supple tissues with an established range of motion. The following possibilities have currently been used in HD with varying success.

Sensory Nerve Transfers

The radial digital nerve of the middle finger has been transferred to the ulnar digital nerve of the little finger to restore sensibility on the ulnar side of the hand.[314] Similarly, the radial digital nerve of the ring finger has been used to restore sensibility to the ulnar side of the thumb.[442] Based on this principle, Ozkan and associates have described restoration of sensibility in leprotic hands by transferring a sensory branch of the radial nerve to appropriate median or ulnar nerve branches.[466,467]

Frozen skeletal muscle bridge grafts have been used to replace damaged nerve segments. After freezing, muscle fibers degenerate and leave their sarcolemmal tubes intact. These tubes act as a framework, along and through which the regenerating axon sprouts can migrate distally toward the receptors.[487] Muscles like sartorius and gracilis, which have parallel arrangement of fibers, are preferred as grafts. Narayankumar and coworkers[455] and Pereira and colleagues[485,487] have reported an autogenous muscle graft technique for restoration of sensibility in hands of HD patients with complete and irreversible loss of sensation. Postoperatively, six of nine patients who were followed reported that they felt pressure, joint movements, and temperature difference. Ability to sweat in the affected area was also restored in one of nine hands.[485]

Sensory re-education introduced by Dellon[347] is useful for all patients with HD with sensory loss, with[467] or without surgery. Some patients who have undergone reconstructive surgery of the hand have been observed to get some "feeling" in their hands 2 to 3 years after surgery, especially when the hand has been put to considerable use.[426]

Treatment of Deformities

The horror and stigma of the disease are rooted in the deformity. The normal appearing but infected HD patient moves about freely in the society. The deformed but noncontagious patient is an outcast. To the deformed patient, appearance means the difference between being an outcast and a normal life.[473] In HD, *the appearance of the hand is as important as its function.* The correction of deformity is often indicated even if it does not substantially restore hand function because it restores a patient's dignity.

The ulnar nerve damage is responsible for 50% of the primary deformities of the hand. The ulnar claw hand is the most common paralytic deformity in HD. The second most common deformity of the hand is due to a combined ulnar and median nerve paralysis, the complete claw hand, with simian deformity. Deformities due to radial nerve paralysis are rare, occurring only in 1% to 2% of the deformed cases. Radial nerve palsy is usually a part of a "triple nerve paralysis." Pure median and radial nerve involvement is rarely encountered in HD. Surgical treatment of hand deformities in HD is reviewed extensively in Chapter 41.

Rehabilitation

Psychiatric morbidity is common in HD patients.[499] One must therefore evaluate the deformity that the patient has as well as the patient as a whole. For patients to make a decision, it is important that they know what surgery has to offer and what is expected of them in the postoperative period. Patients with HD have to face three different sets of problems—overuse, misuse, and protected use. The entire process of rehabilitation depends on the patient's understanding of the three problems, acceptance of residual disability, and desire to adapt to new situations. Among these acceptance of disability is the most important and most difficult.[430] It is the patient who needs rehabilitation, not the hand alone.

It is important that the surgeon assemble a multidisciplinary team to follow the patient, including an infectious disease specialist, a physical and occupational therapist, and a social worker. Rehabilitation of the patient's psychological, social, vocational, and avocational life restores his or her self-esteem. These are the final and most important chapters in restoring social acceptability[332] and dignity[318] to the dejected and stigmatized HD patient. In his enthusiasm for surgery and research, Brand never forgot the person behind the disease (cited in Nash[456]).

RESOURCE MATERIALS

For the latest guidelines on diagnosis and treatment of HD, National Hansen's Disease Programs (in Baton Rouge, LA, 70816) maintains a referral service to several federally funded ambulatory HD centers in Boston, Los Angeles, Martinez, San Diego, Chicago, Miami, New York, Phoenix, Puerto Rico, Seattle, Dallas, Houston, Harlington, and San Antonio (Phone: 1-800-642-2477, Fax: 225-756-3760) (http://bphc.hrsa.gov/nhdp/default.htm). Several texts on medical and surgical treatment have been published by physicians[326,381,403,407,414] and surgeons[305,309,365,544] experienced in HD. Five journals are dedicated to basic and clinical research on HD.[306,349,361,402,424] The International Congress of Leprosy first met in 1897, convenes every fifth year, under the auspices of the International Leprosy Association, to update research and clinical information, and last met in 2002, in Brazil.

ANNOTATED REFERENCES

306. Antia NH, Mehta LN, Shetty VP, Irani PF: Clinical, electrophysiological, quantitative, histological and ultrastructural studies of the index branch of the radial cutaneous nerve in leprosy. Int J Lepr 43:106-113, 1975.

   Antia and colleagues have done extensive clinical and laboratory studies on nerve involvement in HD. This article describes observations on the index branch of radial nerve where it is easily available and safe to biopsy. Even though it is not palpably thickened, it shows histologic and conduction velocity changes, suggesting that in HD, neural involvement is widespread.

309. Antia NH, Shetty VP: The Peripheral Nerve in Leprosy and Other Neuropathies. New Delhi, Oxford University Press, 1997.

   This monograph is recommended for all those who are keen to know more about nerve damage in HD.

317. Birke JA, Brandsma JW, Schreuders TA, Piefer A: Sensory testing with monofilaments in Hansen's disease and normal control subjects. Int J Lepr Other Mycobact Dis 68:291-298, 2000.

   This article gives an opportunity to compare sensory thresholds for monofilament nylons in the hands of normal subjects and those affected by HD. The levels of protective sensations have been defined and the reproducibility of the observations in HD-affected hands has been examined.

320. Brand PW: Paralytic claw hand. J Bone Joint Surg Br 40:618-632, 1958.

   Reconstruction in HD was initiated by Brand. In this landmark article the surgical procedure for correction of claw hand with special reference to HD is discussed. A new method to make tendon junctures is described.

321. Brand PW: Temperature variation and leprosy deformity. Int J Lepr 27:1-7, 1959.

   The paralysis in HD has more or less a set pattern, like ulnar nerve involvement in cubital tunnel syndrome, median nerve involvement in carpal tunnel syndrome, and so on. The cause of this peculiar presentation to some extent depends on the selective localization of *M. leprae* in these superficial nerve trunks. This study showed that the tissues have lower temperature at these sites—a condition that favors the growth of the invading germ.

333. Chauhan SL, Girdhar A, Mishra B, et al: Calcification of peripheral nerves in leprosy. Acta Leprol 10:51-56, 1996.

   This article has some typical pictures of calcified nerves in HD, and the mechanism of calcification in nerve abscess is discussed. Calcification of only common peroneal and ulnar nerves has been observed.

347. Dellon AL: Functional sensation and its re-education. Clin Plast Surg 11:95-99, 1984.

   The sensory recovery is important for the efficient use of the hand. Sensory evaluation in terms of monofilament nylons or 2-PD (two-point discrimination) may be academically sound, but actual tests of sensory function involve activities of day-to-day use of the hands that depend on sensory feedback. This article has highlighted the significance of this concept and describes how to retrain sensation to numb hand.

360. Enna CD, Delgado DD: The surgical management of Hansen's disease: A survey updated. Plast Reconstr Surg 67:79-93, 1981.

   This is a review article on surgical correction of deformities in HD. Various deformities are described and their surgical management is discussed in a comprehensive manner.

365. Fritchi EP: Surgical Reconstruction and Rehabilitation in Leprosy, 2nd ed. New Delhi, The Leprosy Mission, 1984.

   This book is a primer on reconstructive surgery in HD written by a person who spent his life analyzing and managing the surgical problems of HD-affected persons. The book describes in very clear and simple language the deformities in HD and the procedures to correct it. Details of the operative procedures are described. It is recommended for those who want to take up reconstructive surgery for HD.

381. Hastings RC: Leprosy, 2nd ed. New York, Churchill Livingstone, 1994.

   This title gives a comprehensive account of HD—its clinical course, diagnosis, and treatment, including complications. The immunology of HD is described in a very clear and concise manner.

393. Jayaseelan E, Shariff S, Rout P: Cytodiagnosis of primary neuritic leprosy. Int J Lepr Other Mycobact Dis 67:429-434, 1999.

This article describes diagnosis of neuritic leprosy by cytologic studies of the material obtained by nerve aspiration. The technique is likely to be very useful in situations in which HD is less frequently seen and also for diagnosis of early cases. A positive aspirate confirms the diagnosis, but a negative aspirate has to be examined by open biopsy and more sophisticated methods (viz., PCR and immunohistologic techniques) before HD can be ruled out.

395. Job CK: Pathology and pathogenesis of leprous neuritis, a preventable and treatable complication. Int J Lepr Other Mycobact Dis 69:19-29, 2001.

C. K. Job, an eminent pathologist dedicated to leprosy, has carried out studies on various aspects of gross and microscopic pathology of leprosy. The present article deals with the current concepts about leprous neuritis and is recommended for all those who would like to have a better understanding of the disease.

403. Jopling WH, McDougall AC : Handbook of Leprosy, 5th ed. New Delhi, CBS Publishers, 1996.

This short concise pocket book written by an experienced leprologist gives all relevant details about HD in a simple, clear language.

425. Malaviya GN: Correction of claw fingers in leprosy—current status. Acta Leprol 7:239-245, 1991.

This article reviews various surgical options available for correction of claw finger deformity. An attempt has been made to define the indications for each procedure, based on their relative merits and demerits in the context of leprosy.

426. Malaviya GN: Towards restoring sensibility in anesthetic extremities of leprosy patients. Acta Leprol 9:111-115, 1995.

Various possibilities of restoring sensation to the anesthetic hands and feet of HD-affected persons are explored in this article. Different possible options that have been used in the past are analyzed. It has been suggested that multiple approaches be tried with an objective to restore at least protective sensation so that these patients can live an injury and ulcer-free life.

427. Malaviya GN: Unfavourable results after surgical correction of claw fingers in leprosy. Indian J Lepr 69:42-52, 1997.

In this article various unfavorable outcomes seen after correction of claw fingers in leprosy affected hands are described. Even though the article fails to give the true prevalence of each problem, it enumerates most of them, many of them in the author's own hands. It is valuable reading for those who undertake reconstructive surgery and is mandatory for those who occasionally operate on an HD-affected hand.

446. Mishra B, Mukherjee A, Girdhar A, et al: Evolution of early lesions in leprosy. Lepr Rev 64:259-266, 1993.

This is an interesting article through which the evolution and progression of leprosy lesions are traced. It highlights that the initial symptom is some sort of paresthesia that many times is ignored by the patient. Later on either a nerve thickening appears at these sites or a hypopigmented skin lesion develops. Some of the patients who developed nerve thickening first were found to develop a skin lesion in the innervated area of that nerve. This progression is rather slow but definite.

452. Naafs B: Current views on reactions in leprosy. Indian J Lepr 72:99-122, 2000.

This very experienced leprologist tells the newer concepts about lepra reactions. The mechanism of type-1 and ENL reactions is discussed. The article is comprehensive in clinical diagnosis, treatment, and prognosis of reactions in leprosy that damage peripheral nerves before, during, and after *M. leprae* and are more or less eliminated by MDT.

471. Palande DD: Surgery of ulnar nerve in leprosy. Lepr India 52:74-88, 1980.

Palande has been actively involved in the surgical problems affecting leprosy patients. Having more than three decades of work experience to his credit, he has written several important articles on the topics of current interest. In these articles he discusses the issue of nerve trunk decompression in leprosy in general and decompression of the ulnar nerve in particular, which is more frequently affected. The clinical signs of nerve compression and indications for surgery are discussed.

473. Palande DD: The promise of surgery, its scope and limitations in leprosy. Lepr Rev 69:168-172, 1998.

This article deals with issues involved with the outcome of corrective surgery. The benefit of surgery and its limitations are discussed. The person who undergoes corrective surgery will come to understand that surgery is some sort of palliation and that one should not expect that normalcy will be restored.

485. Pereira JH, Bowden TS, Narayankumar TS, Gschmeissner SE: Peripheral nerve reconstruction using denatured muscle autografts restoring protective sensation in hands and feet of leprosy patients. Int J Lepr 68:83-91, 1996.

The authors have reported their results in a series of patients in which a swollen segment of the nerve trunk (at classic sites of nerve thickening, namely, carpal tunnel and tarsal tunnel) was excised and continuity was restored by replacing the excised segment with a cold denatured muscle graft. The details of the technique and its limitations are discussed. Even though limit of length for the graft exists, the procedure might have potential use. The authors provide more detailed understanding of nerve regeneration.

508. Ridley DS, Jopling WH: Classification of leprosy according to immunity, a five group system. Int J Lepr 34:255-273, 1966.

This article was written by experienced pathologists when there was not much information available on the immunologic aspects of leprosy. Their classification of leprosy into different groups, based on the immunologic responses of the host, remains valid and is used to classify patients in research studies.

516. Salafia A, Chauhan G: Nerve abscess in children and adult leprosy patients: Analysis of 145 cases and review of literature. Acta Leprol 10:45-50, 1996.

This is a large series of nerve abscesses in leprosy patients. Nerve abscesses in superficially placed cutaneous nerves and deeply located nerve trunks are described, and the authors share their experience in treating them.

524. Shepard CC: Multiplication of *M. leprae* in the foot pad of mice. Int J Lepr 30:291-306, 1960.

Shepard, an eminent American researcher at Carville Hansen Center, Louisiana, was first to show that *M. leprae* can grow manyfold if injected into the foot pad of laboratory mice. This opened the doors for further research on *M. leprae,* leading to the development of newer drugs effective against the germ and the detection of drug-resistant organisms.

540. Srinivasan H: Surgical decompression of the ulnar nerve. Indian J Lepr 56:520-531, 1984.

Srinivasan has been active as a full-time surgeon doing reconstructive surgery of the hand and foot for nearly four decades. In this review article, written in 1984, he has analyzed the results of various series of ulnar nerve decompression in HD. The most certain benefit of nerve trunk decompression was relief from intractable nerve pain. He concludes that a combined approach (i.e., corticosteroid therapy and nerve decompression) is more rewarding than either alone. The most controversial issue about nerve decompression is still the timing of surgery.

545. Srinivasan H, Rao KS, Iyer CG: Discrepancy in the histological features of leprosy lesions in the skin and peripheral nerve: Report of a preliminary study. Lepr India 54:275-282, 1982.

This article tells us that skin and nerve involvement in HD is not parallel. The lesions in the nerve may be more advanced than what is manifested in the skin and vice versa. It is possible that the lesions may be in the different stages of progression in the skin and nerve.

546. Srinivasan H, Rao KS, Shanmugam N: Steroid therapy in recent "quiet nerve paralysis" in leprosy: Report of a study of twenty-five patients. Lepr India 54:412-419, 1982.

This widely quoted article on painless nerve damage in HD is a classic. This slowly progressive nerve damage has been called "quiet nerve damage." Because nerve function deterioration is not punctuated with pain, the patients report for treatment when the nerve damage is fairly advanced. Corticosteroids are the only available option for this type of case when early diagnosis is made. Prognosis is relatively poor.

550. Sunderland S: The internal anatomy of nerve trunks in relation to neural lesions in leprosy: Observations on pathology, symptomatology and treatment. Brain 96:865-888, 1973.

Sunderland made extensive dissections of the nerve trunks and described the neural topography in great detail. His monumental work still remains to be reproduced. In this beautifully documented article he attempts to explain the intraneural spread of infection from one funiculus to another in a nerve trunk. It describes very clearly how the whole nerve trunk gets involved in HD even though it may not clinically manifest the damage. It gives a clear understanding about the neural affections in HD and explains why nerve grafting may not be a good option to restore sensibility in anesthetic hands of HD-affected persons.

Mycobacterial Infections (Tuberculous and Nontuberulous Mycobacteria)

Tubercle bacillus was identified, isolated, and grown in 1872 by Robert Koch, for which he received a Nobel prize in 1905. More than 100 years after Koch, *M. tuberculosis* continues to affect a third of the world's population. In the United States there is an increased prevalence among immigrants, accounting for 40% of all reported cases in 2000. Understandably, the most common chronic infection of the hand is tuberculosis.

Tuberculous tenosynovitis, arthritis, and bursitis simulate rheumatoid synovitis but are localized to a few tendons, a joint, or a bursa. Absence of generalized findings of rheumatoid arthritis should alert the clinician to the possibility of tuberculosis.

Biopsy for histopathology and microbiology is always necessary for definitive diagnosis. The sine qua non histologic hallmark of a tuberculous infection is the granuloma (tubercle). A granuloma is a minute aggregation of activated T lymphocytes, macrophages, epithelioid cells, and Langhans' giant cells that limits the multiplication and spread of the tubercle bacillus. The tuberculosis granuloma can be distinguished from those of atypical mycobacteria by its characteristic central necrosis or caseating granuloma.[606,646] If an initial biopsy does not confirm the diagnosis, a repeat biopsy may help to establish a diagnosis, because the organisms are often sparse and grow with difficulty.

All mycobacterial infections reported before 1960 were attributed to *M. tuberculosis.** Only a few authors reported more than 20 cases.[584,614,626,809,839,881] Runyon described four new classes of mycobacteria (atypical mycobacteria or

mycobacteria other than tuberculosis [MOTT]) in the 1950s[857,893] (Table 4-9), and, since then, at least 16 species have been identified. Runyon's classification is now superceded by grouping atypical mycobacteria within the laboratory on their growth rates as slow or rapidly growing mycobacteria (Table 4-10).[623] *M. marinum* is the most common cutaneous tuberculosis in the West. Most common AIDS-related mycobacterial infections are caused by *M. avium* and *M. haemophilum.*

The clinical presentation of the tuberculous and atypical mycobacterial infection is indistinguishable. Mycobacterial identification is paramount because the virulence, growth requirements, drug sensitivity, and treatment of the various species differ vastly. The constitutional symptoms usually present in tuberculosis involving other parts of the body are notoriously lacking.[614] The erythrocyte sedimentation rate (ESR) may be slightly elevated in infection with *M. tuberculosis* but is almost invariably normal in immunocompetent patients with infections caused by atypical mycobacteria. A higher ESR indicates lower immunity and a more severe infection. It may necessitate diagnostic work-up for a primary focus and multicentric tuberculosis.[605,649] Regional lymphadenopathy is usually absent. A positive tuberculin skin test is not indicative of a currently active infection, is

---

*See references 614, 629, 632, 652, 655, 669, 684, 686, 702-704, 708, 712, 723, 727, 728, 733, 734, 754, 763, 809, 814, 815, 821, 822, 825, 839, 850, 874, 876, 881, 884, and 901.

Table 4-9
RUNYON'S CLASSIFICATION OF ATYPICAL MYCOBACTERIA

Runyon Group	Pigment of Colonies on Characteristics	Exposure to Sunlight	Organisms	Natural Habitat
I	Photochromogens	Yellow colonies	M. marinum	Water, fish
			M. kansasii	Water
			M. asiaticum	
II	Scotochromogens	Orange colonies	M. gordonae	Water
			M. szulgai	Unknown
			M. scrofulaceum	
III	Nonchromogens	None	M. avium	Ubiquitous
			M. terrae	Water, soil
			M. malmoense	Unknown
			M. haemophilum	? Unknown
			M. ulcerans	
IV	Rapid growing	Variable	M. chelonae	Water, soil
			M. fortuitum	Water, soil, animals
			M. smegmatis	

Atypical mycobacteria that have caused chronic infections of the hand are arranged by Runyon's classification. There are more atypical mycobacteria, but they have not yet been found to cause hand infections.

Table 4-10
GROWTH RATES OF MYCOBACTERIA

Slowly Growing	Intermediately Growing	Rapidly Growing < 7 Days
M. avium complex (M. avium and M. intracellulare) M. kansasii M. xenopi M. szulgai M. scrofulaceum M. malmoense M. terrae M. haemophilum M. asiaticum	M. marinum M. gordonae	M. fortuitum M. chelonae M. smegmatis M. abscessus

Growth rates have become a practical means of grouping the species within the laboratories.

negative in anergic patients, and is not useful in diagnosis.[700] Pulmonary disease does not generally accompany mycobacterial infection of the hand.[608,763]

Surgical findings of tuberculosis and atypical mycobacterial infection may also be indistinguishable. AFB smears of sampled granuloma may not show any organisms or reveal only sparse bacilli after painstaking scrutiny.[641] The purulent aspirate from an infected joint often shows the organisms on a smear.[651] Cultures most often grow the organism in 7 to 70 days on Löwenstein-Jensen media. M. marinum, M. haemophilum, and M. ulcerans grow at 25°C to 30°C (room temperature), whereas M. tuberculosis and other atypical mycobacteria grow at 37°C (body temperature). M. xenopi grows best at 42°C. It is critical to request incubation at three temperatures because many laboratories do not routinely incubate mycobacterial cultures at 30°C and 42°C. The tuberculous and atypical infections differ in their prognosis, and their sensitivity to antimicrobial drugs varies widely. The clinical course of atypical infections varies from self-healing cutaneous lesions to highly resistant deep lesions, resistant both to surgical débridement and chemotherapy. M. avium, M. chelonei, and M. malmoense infections are tenacious, resistant, and recurrent, often requiring amputation. Some grow readily on cultures, and others like M. avium, M. chelonae, and M. malmoense do not. Some grow quickly (fast-growing mycobacteria), and others take 8 to 10 weeks (M. avium, M. malmoense).

There are six locations of tuberculous and atypical mycobacterial infections in the upper extremity: the skin, subcutaneous tissues, tenosynovium, bursa, joints, and bone. A combination of the above may be seen in immunocompromised patients.[605,649,680] The three most common M. tuberculosis infections of the hand are flexor tenosynovitis, wrist joint infection, and phalangeal osteomyelitis (dactylitis).[718] Rarely, mycobacterial infections cause a midpalmar space abscess,[653] fasciitis,[781,833] compartment syndrome in the forearm,[683] or a cold abscess in a muscle.[583,597] Infection of an olecranon bursa is rare and is usually caused by atypical mycobacteria.[600,696,803]

CUTANEOUS TUBERCULOSIS

The most common tuberculous infection of the hand involves the skin. Eighty percent of cutaneous tuberculosis affects the hand and the upper extremity.[612,759] Tuberculosis may be acquired in one of the following ways: by inoculation from an exogenous source through a breach in the skin,* by contiguous spread from bone to skin (scrofulo-

---

*See references 594, 630, 706, 712, 734, 738, 754, 777, 789, 807, 825, 827, 859, 861, 884, and 906.

derma[664,733]), or by hematogenous spread to skin from a pulmonary or extrapulmonary focus (lupus vulgaris).[612] *M. marinum (M. balnei)* is the most commonly reported mycobacterial skin infection of the hand in the West[670,745,759,837] and *M. tuberculosis* in the East.[870] An underlying disease that compromises host immunity may be found in up to 30% of cases.[612] Cutaneous tuberculosis of the hand in AIDS is rare.[639]

Skin infections can be caused by primary inoculation in medical personnel with a needle withdrawn from an infected patient,[777] accidental injection of infected fluid in the laboratory,[699] or mycobacterial infection from autopsy material.[630,706,738,807,818] Tuberculous paronychia has been reported in a nurse caring for a patient with active pulmonary tuberculosis.[824] The disease is usually self-limited if host immunity is high, but chemotherapy expedites cure and reduces morbidity. Surgical excision of the lesion is clearly indicated in a lesion caused by accidental inoculation by a known drug-resistant organism.[861] The cutaneous infections by *M. kansasii* heal spontaneously over a period of time, and chemotherapy is given to expedite the healing and prevent scarring. A tuberculous skin gumma can occur on the hand after a contaminated skin venipuncture.[906] *M. bovis* skin infection may occur occupationally in butchers (butcher's wart).[918]

Diagnosis

The most common presentation is a nodular and/or pustular lesion on the finger, hand, or forearm (Fig. 4-17). A nontender nodule gradually progresses to single or multiple abscesses that drain clear liquid. Nodules do not heal with antibiotics and soaks. Less common presentations include erythema, swelling, cellulitis,[841] crusting, verrucous plaque,[730,797,853] verrucous nodule,[628] sporotrichoid lesion,[762] and ulceration. Cortisone exacerbates the disease.[582] Signs of lymphatic spread are evident in 70% of cases. Multiple, marching, linear lesions may be seen along the lymphatics on the forearm simulating a sporotrichoid (*Sporothrix schenckii*) skin infection.[582,585,662,731,828,846] Most patients have lesions for 2 months or more before they are seen, and there is usually a substantial delay between initial consultation

and correct diagnosis,[625] because of the rarity of the condition. Patients infected with *M. marinum* give a history of a puncture wound involving fish[644,689,816] or fish tank* in more than half the cases,[670] and the lesion is known as "fish tank granuloma,"[616,714,800] "swimming pool granuloma,"[689,759,892] or "fish fancier's finger."[744,790,795]

M. tuberculosis infections of the hand are characterized by a pustular or nodular phase that subsequently ulcerates to form a "tuberculous chancre."[594] Regional lymphadenopathy develops in 3 to 4 weeks after the primary skin lesion is noted. The tuberculous chancre and affected regional lymph nodes constitute the "tuberculous primary complex" of the skin, akin to classic Ghon's lesion. Organisms may not be seen on AFB staining. Cultures may not grow mycobacteria. Under these circumstances, the detection of mycobacteria by PCR to analyze nucleic acid sequences is recommended because it is rapid and accessible in most hospitals.[796] Prompt chemotherapy is curative.

Differential Diagnosis

The linear, marching lymphangitis typical of *Sporothrix* infection can also be seen with infections caused by *M. marinum, M. kansasii,*[828] *Leishmania,*[682] *Coccidioides, Cryptococcus,* and *Nocardia,* lupus vulgaris,[773] and tularemia.[731] Tuberculous cutaneous infection of the hand may also be confused with infection by blastomycosis, histoplasmosis, syphilis, and yaws. Final diagnosis of tuberculous infection requires skin biopsy with mycobacterial culture.

Treatment

Selman Waksman was awarded a Nobel Prize in 1952 for his discovery of streptomycin, the first antibiotic demonstrated to be effective against tuberculosis. Monotherapy with streptomycin, however, led to the development of resistant strains. To avoid resistance, *M. tuberculosis* skin infection is treated with a combination of bactericidal drugs, including isoniazid and rifampin, taken daily for at least 6 months, as well as ethambutol for the first 2 months.[870]

Treatment of atypical mycobacterial infection differs from treatment of tuberculosis. Optimal treatment of cutaneous *M. marinum* infection is not well established. Mild infection resolves spontaneously but complete resolution may take up to 2 years. A variety of antibiotic regimens have been used successfully, including tetracycline,[670] minocycline,[670] doxycyline,[670] sulfamethoxazole-trimethoprim,[670,744,778] and amikacin and ethambutol-rifampin combination.[670,745] Resistance to tetracycline, minocycline, doxycycline, rifampin, and cotrimoxazole[654] is emerging. Thus, results of antimicrobial sensitivity tests are helpful in guiding chemotherapy. Treatment of *M. kansasii* cutaneous infection is usually effective with the standard antituberculous drugs erythromycin and cotrimoxazole. Drug sensitivity testing against *M. kansasii* is recommended because resistance to rifampin is emerging.[913]

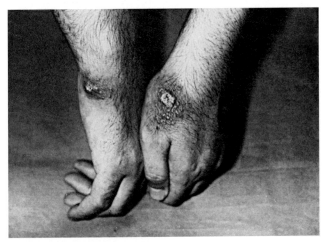

FIGURE 4-17. Tuberculosis of the skin showing pustular, nodular, and ulcerative lesions in both hands.

*See references 604, 615, 678, 714, 744, 745, 771, 780, 800, 804, and 891.

Large series of *M. marinum* and *M. kansasii* skin infections of the hand have been reported by Huminer and associates,[745] Johnston and Izumi,[759] Kullavanijaya and coworkers,[778] Breathnach and colleagues,[622] and Edelstein.[670] Current concepts of cutaneous *M. tuberculosis* treatment have been reviewed by Sehgal.[870] When the infection is caused inadvertently by inoculation of drug-resistant *M. tuberculosis,* surgical excision of the lesion is important.[861]

SUBCUTANEOUS TUBERCULOSIS

Subcutaneous infection by *M. tuberculosis* is rare. Hurst described six cases of subcutaneous granulomas from *M. marinum.*[747] Christensson[642] and Love[798] and their colleagues described one case each of subcutaneous granuloma caused by *M. terrae.* Parker and Irwin described a subcutaneous granuloma on the dorsum of a finger caused by *M. kansasii.*[829] Baack and coworkers described a case of subcutaneous infection caused by *M. chelonei* on the radial side of the wrist after a cortisone injection.[601] Sahn and Pierson described a subcutaneous nodule in the thumb pulp from accidental injection of tuberculous organisms while performing guinea pig inoculation.[861] By far the most common cause of subcutaneous infection is *M. ulcerans* (Buruli ulcer). Buruli ulcer is diagnosed in immigrants from endemic countries,[776,792] and it is the third most common tuberculous disease in the world after *M. tuberculosis* and *M. leprae.*[903]

Diagnosis

Buruli ulcer was first described in 1948 by MacCallum and coworkers in six Australian patients, who each had a single ulcerative lesion on an arm or leg.[799] In the 1960s, many patients in the Buruli district of Uganda, near the Nile River, had ulcers that were caused by *M. ulcerans.*[643] The disease has since become known as Buruli ulcer (BU). BU is an emerging infectious disease in Africa, Asia, Australia, and South America.[883] The first case in the United States was reported in 1974[792] in an immigrant physician from Nigeria who developed a chronic ulcer around the elbow.

Necrosis of subcutaneous fat is the pathologic hallmark of BU. Inoculation into subcutaneous tissue usually occurs through penetrating skin trauma. Secretions of toxins by the organisms (mycolactone, phospholipase C) cause extensive subcutaneous fatty tissue necrosis, resulting in extensive fibrosis. The disease progresses in four stages: subcutaneous nodule, cellulitis, ulceration, and scar formation with deformity.[820] The lesion is a painless ulcer that has undermined edges and a necrotic center with hyperpigmented and shiny surrounding skin. If untreated, the infection may invade underlying bones. Hofer and Hirschel[736] and Hu[742] described a case in which the infection invaded ulna, metacarpal, and thumb phalanges. Aquilar described a case of *M. ulcerans* of the hand in a Mexican farmer.[593] AFB are usually found in the base, not in the ulcer edges. *M. ulcerans* grows at 30°C. It is difficult to grow, and attempts to culture the microorganism from clinical specimens fail in over half of all cases. Up to 3 months of incubation are required, and the laboratory should be alerted not to discard the media prematurely.

Treatment

At present, antimycobacterial drug treatment is ineffective and treatment is surgical. Early excision of a pre-ulcerative papule or nodule is curative. A necrotic ulcer should be excised to normal healthy tissue, so as to prevent persistent infection from residual bacilli. The underlying defect may be skin grafted. In stage IV disease with extensive contractures and ankylosis, reconstructive surgery may be necessary. Van der Werf and associates summarized a seminar on this important, emerging, and elusive infection in 1999.[903] Similarities between *M. ulcerans, M. marinum,* and *M. haemophilum* are striking in that they all grow at lower than body temperature at 30°C.

MYCOBACTERIAL TENOSYNOVITIS

Mycobacteria have a predilection for tenosynovium. Flexor tendons of the fingers (Fig. 4-18A),[595,609,834,839] palm,[652] wrist,[770] and forearm* (see Fig. 4-18C) are affected more often than extensor tendons (see Fig. 4-18B).[595,600,627] The physician may feel rice bodies glide beneath the examining fingers.[692] Flexor tenosynovitis of the digit produces a characteristic "sausage finger."[748] Tuberculous tenosynovitis involving the first dorsal compartment at the wrist may mimic de Quervain's disease.[636] Over half of the reported hand tenosynovial infections are due to *M. marinum.*[†] The second most common infecting organism is *M. kansasii,*[663,667,716,764,785,829] and the third most common infecting organism is *M. avium-intracellulare complex.*[658,672,769,770,805,880] Reports of *M. tuberculosis* tenosynovitis since 1960 have been sporadic[587,619,674,889,908] compared with larger series in prior years.[‡] The patient is generally healthy, and constitutional symptoms are lacking. Inflammatory signs (erythema, warmth, and tenderness) are absent (cold abscess). Coexistent pulmonary or extrapulmonary tuberculosis is rare.[§] Wrist and hand radiographs are almost always normal. Late in the disease the infection may spread to adjacent joints or bone.[794] The ESR may be elevated in *M. tuberculosis* infection but is almost always normal in atypical infections.[890] The delay between the onset of symptoms and diagnosis is lengthy.[587,627,686,716-718,763,809] In 1923, Kanavel emphasized the necessity for early diagnosis because tendon rupture, wrist infection, or secondary osteomyelitis can occur.[763] Treatment with steroid injection for presumed aseptic tenosynovitis is harmful.[658]

Diagnosis

Delay in diagnosis occurs for several reasons. Clinically, the disease pattern is nonspecific. It starts insidiously and becomes indolent. Other than the hand lesion, the patient is healthy. Pain is conspicuously absent until late in the disease. The diagnosis is not suspected because the tenosyn-

---

*See references 584, 586, 587, 621, 681, 683, 686, 716, 718, 763, 775, 809, 839, 847, 881, and 908.

†See references 590, 606, 640, 641, 644, 717, 718, 747, 779, 909, and 919.

‡See references 584, 632, 652, 655, 686, 692, 704, 763, 809, 815, and 881.

§See references 584, 615, 619, 640, 641, 729, 747, 763, 809, and 839.

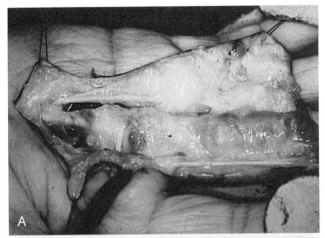

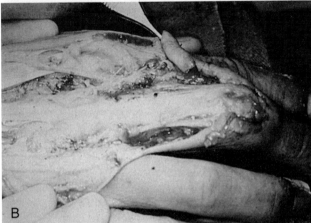

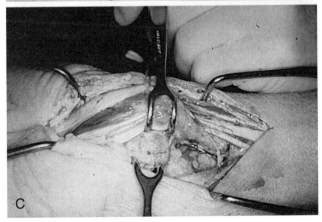

FIGURE 4-18. *Mycobacterium marinum* tenosynovitis may involve flexor tendons in the finger (**A**), extensor tendons in the finger (**B**), or flexor tendons in the palm, wrist, and forearm (**C**). (Courtesy of S. P. Chow, Hong Kong.)

ovitis resembles nonspecific or rheumatoid tenosynovitis. Carpal tunnel syndrome can be an initial manifestation of tuberculosis.* Smears of fluid aspirated from the lesion may provide the first clue to diagnosis,[631,659] but this is often not done.[663] Synovial biopsy is often not done at the time of tenosynovectomy or carpal tunnel release. When biopsy is done, tissue is sent for histopathology but may not be sent for microbiology.[844] Histopathology shows poorly or noncaseating granuloma[641] and may be interpreted as sarcoidosis.[663] When biopsy tissue is sent for culture, it may be mistakenly sent in formalin.[672] Even when properly

done, histopathology studies reveal only scanty bacilli after painstaking scrutiny.[641] Cultures may not be requested for or not done at 30°C for *M. marinum* at some hospitals. Two patients underwent finger amputations for a missed diagnosis of *M. marinum* infection.[743]

The disease may present in one of four stages depending on the duration of the infection and host immunity. In the first stage, a serous exudate alone is present. In the second stage (up to 2 years), granulation tissue, tenosynovial proliferation, and rice bodies appear. In the third stage, infection invades the tendon; the tendons may be frayed, infiltrated,[655] ruptured, or caseated into a fungoid mass.[809] Fraying of the tendons occurs at an average of 3 years and rupture of the tendons occurs at an average of 4 years from the onset of tenosynovitis.[809] In the fourth stage, and only very late, the infection spreads to the adjacent joints,[587,627,763,809,839,851] or bone[763,809] and a sinus with or without superimposed pyogenic infection may be present.

Histologic sections are first examined with the hematoxylin and eosin stain. This is best done as rapid intraoperative biopsy (frozen section). If granulomas are observed, even if poorly formed,[718] additional stained specimens with Ziehl-Neelsen stain (for AFB) and Gomori's methenamine silver stain (for fungi) are examined. Failure to demonstrate AFB by staining the synovium does not rule out tuberculosis[587] because cultures may be positive when smears are negative. A definitive diagnosis is made by culturing infected synovium or rice bodies.[889] Rice bodies contain live mycobacteria that grow on culture.[587,763,839] A bacteriologic diagnosis can often be made by smearing and culturing drainage from a sinus. Aspirated synovial fluid from a fluctuating bursa may grow mycobacteria.[659]

Treatment

Multidrug therapy with antituberculous antibiotics remains the cornerstone of treatment. Before the development of effective antituberculous therapy, fewer than one half of patients with tuberculous tenosynovitis were cured by complete surgical extirpation of all infected synovium.[584,809] Synovectomy of the tendons or a joint is often carried out by the surgeon at the time of exploration because the diagnosis is not known and removal of the pathologic tissue is logical. If the synovectomy is thorough and the host resistance is exceptionally high, the patient may be cured.[592,814] Otherwise, the patient temporarily improves, tenosynovitis recurs, a sinus forms, or the wound breaks down.[718] There is a small window of time before these wound complications occur, during which one awaits the results of culture and sensitivity testing.[674] It is reasonable to start chemotherapy based on smear staining or histopathology and revise chemotherapy when results of sensitivity testing become available.

The role of synovectomy in an immunocompetent patient is controversial. Gunther and Levy recommend a combination of surgical synovectomy and chemotherapy.[718] Chow and colleagues[640] and Skoll and Hudson[875] recommend a "minimal" biopsy to make a diagnosis with removal of enough synovium for histopathology, smears, and cultures. If the diagnosis is established through a "minimal" biopsy,

---

*See references 600, 619, 627, 663, 665, 667, 711, 716-718, 756, 760, 763, 764, 775, 779, 785, 786, 803, 811, 843, 845, 886, and 889.

or through culture of drainage material, the patient receives chemotherapy without synovectomy.[640] The danger of this approach is that fibrosis may reduce vascular supply of infected tissues and reduce local antibiotic perfusion, necessitating later synovectomy and prolonging treatment. Thorough synovectomy and concomitant antituberculous medication seems logical.[640]

When mycobacteria are sensitive to chemotherapy, but the host is immunocompromised, "aggressive synovectomy" helps to reduce the mycobacterial load to chemotherapy.[658] When the patient is on immunosuppressive therapy, in addition to chemotherapy and thorough synovectomy, the physician may be forced to decrease the dose of immunosuppressive drugs to control the infection.[864] When the mycobacteria are partially or completely resistant to one or more first-line drugs,[659,882] or the organism is known to be pernicious (e.g., *M. avium,*[672] *M. malmoense, M. terrae*) "thorough" synovectomy and chemotherapy are clearly indicated regardless of immune status. Synovectomy alone in such circumstances is inevitably followed by recurrence[729] and may even necessitate amputation.[882]

Tuberculous tenosynovitis in the finger and wrist eventually leads to painless tendon attrition and rupture.[809] Flexor tendon grafting restores finger flexion, if the infection is contained within the flexor tendon sheath and the sheath and underlying joints are spared. When a tendon ruptures in the palm or wrist, the ruptured distal end can be "piggy backed" to an adjacent functional tendon. When infection spreads from a tendon sheath in a finger to adjacent joint and bone, chemotherapy controls the infection but mobility is lost.

Reactivation of a dormant tuberculous infection of the hand may recur many years after it is successfully treated with tenosynovectomy and MDT.[760]

TUBERCULOUS ARTHRITIS

Osteoarticular tuberculosis of the extremities is second only to the spine in frequency and affects the lower extremities more frequently than the upper extremity. The wrist is the upper extremity joint most commonly infected by *M. tuberculosis.** Tuberculous infection of the wrist can be seeded by a blood-borne infection or may spread from untreated flexor tenosynovitis.[675,718,735,763,809] The infection has been demonstrated to spread from flexor tendons across the wrist joint to the dorsal tenosynovium and result in a swelling on both sides of the wrist.[627,718] The elbow[638,769, 808,930] and interphalangeal joints[587,589,608,674,717,724,761] are less commonly infected. Elbow infections commonly start from the olecranon or the lower end of the humerus and spread to the elbow joint.[898]

Diagnosis

In contrast to mycobacterial tenosynovitis, the earliest manifestation of tuberculous arthritis is pain. Tuberculous joint infection may present in one of three stages. The first stage involves infection of the joint synovium and is marked by pain, swelling, and limitation of joint motion. The joint may be held in flexion. Roentgenographic hallmarks of early joint infection are soft tissue swelling, periarticular

osteoporosis, and absence of a subchondral plate. In the second stage, infected synovium invades subchondral bone and causes cystic changes (Fig. 4-19A). The hyaline cartilage is invaded, and joint space is reduced or lost (see Fig. 4-19B). A draining sinus may form and may be the presenting clinical feature.[621] A triad of radiographic findings—juxta-articular osteoporosis, subchondral cysts, and gradual narrowing of the cartilage space (Phemister's triad)—is characteristic of tuberculous arthritis. Subchondral cysts characteristically form on both sides of the infected joint. In the third stage, the joint is deformed, dislocated, or partially ankylosed, with or without pain (see Fig. 4-19C). Tuberculous arthritis may be suspected when drainage persists from an infected elbow, wrist, or finger joint, despite multiple courses of antibiotics and multiple drainage procedures.[587] Most joint infections are monoarticular and may strongly resemble a case of monoarticular rheumatoid arthritis. Concurrent pulmonary or extrapulmonary tuberculosis is uncommon.[611]

In the absence of coexistent extra-articular tuberculosis, diagnosis of *M. tuberculosis* infection almost always requires arthrocentesis or biopsy.[611,621] Synovial fluid aspirate may show AFB on smear, and cultures are generally positive. Granulomas with caseation are present in three fourths of the biopsy specimens.[611] Clinical confusion occurs when *M. tuberculosis* infects joints previously involved with rheumatoid arthritis[661] or gouty arthritis.[739]

There are some differences between joint infections with *M. tuberculosis* and *M. marinum*.[589,603,640,641,651,707,724,916,919] *M. marinum* infections are associated with traumatic exposure to salt water[644,743,790,795,816,856,872,909] or a fish tank[†] in vocational[644,689,690,816,872,909] or avocational[585,620,707,774,778] activities. Diagnosis is made with biopsy and culture. Cultures are positive between 2 and 6 weeks of incubation at 30°C on Löwenstein-Jensen media.[670]

Unlike *M. tuberculosis,* in *M. marinum* infections a finger joint is infected in three fourths of the cases and the wrist is infected in the rest. Infections are typically monoarticular. Symptoms usually begin within 1 to 2 weeks after the initial trauma. The mean time from onset of symptoms to bacteriologic diagnosis is 8 months (range, 3 months to 3 years). The pain is mild, but swelling of the involved joint is marked and boggy. Organisms may be stained from draining joint fluid,[724] aspirated joint fluid,[603] or synovial biopsy in 75% of cases. Mycobacterial cultures are positive in almost all (95%) of synovial fluid and synovial biopsy specimens.[610] A severely immunocompromised patient (chemotherapy, corticosteroids, systemic lupus[705]) may develop a multicentric *M. marinum* mycobacteriosis that may include bones, joints, tendons, and skin.[605,680,705] Rarely, early amputation may be necessary.[916]

Brashear and Winfield have reviewed *M. tuberculosis* infections of the wrist joint.[621] The largest number of cases of *M. marinum* joint infections of the hand have been reviewed by Harth and associates[724] and Alloway and colleagues.[589] *M. kansasii* joint infections have been reviewed

---

*See references 608, 611, 621, 627, 633, 674, 675, 735, 758, 840, 851, 871, and 908.

†See references 585, 596, 604, 605, 615, 616, 620, 678, 714, 744, 771, 800, and 858.

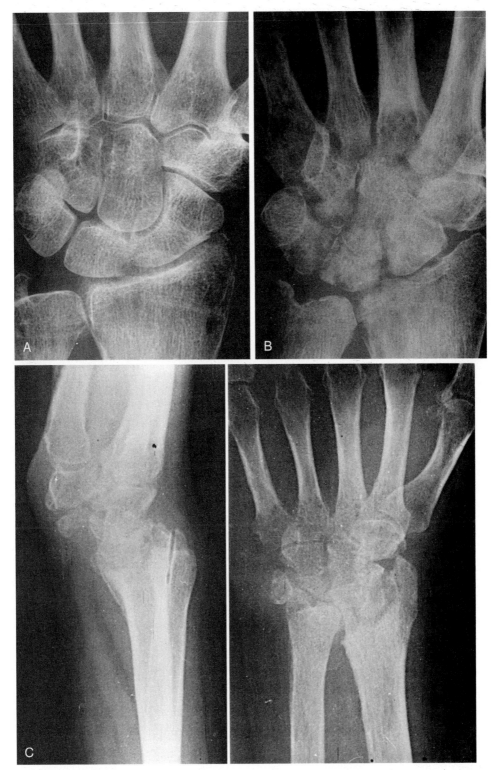

FIGURE 4-19. A, Tuberculosis of the wrist may start in the synovium and cause subchondral erosions in the carpal bones. **B,** Gradually the hyaline cartilage is destroyed, the joint space is reduced, and the bones become osteopenic. **C,** Finally there is destruction and volar subluxation of the radiocarpal joint. (Courtesy of S. M. Tuli, New Delhi, India.)

by Bernard and associates,[610] DeMerieux and coworkers,[661] Dillon and colleagues,[663] and Gunther and Levy.[718]

Treatment

Treatment of *M. tuberculosis* septic arthritis consists of chemotherapy and prevention of deformity by splinting during the first and second stages.[897-899] Intermittent active exercises for the elbow, forearm, wrist, and finger joints should be encouraged as pain permits. Although total or subtotal synovectomy has been performed at the time of biopsy, the value of synovectomy is controversial. Gunther and coworkers[717] favor chemotherapy and surgical débridement once diagnosis is confirmed. Benkeddache and Gettesman[608] recommend biopsy for diagnosis and chemotherapy for treatment. In its earliest stage almost all infected joints recover fully with chemotherapy and without surgical débridement. In the second stage, painful joints are fused.[608] If the source of pain can be localized to the distal radioulnar joint, resection of the distal end of the ulna may be all that is required.[898] In patients with unfavorable response in 3 months, or with recurrence of infection, Tuli[898] recommends surgical débridement. Unfavorable therapeutic response may occur if the organism is marginally sensitive to drugs or if the host resistance is low due to malnutrition, drug immunosuppression, or an underlying immune deficiency disease. In the third stage, a painful, dislocated, unstable, ankylosed, or deformed joint requires fusion, excisional arthroplasty, or corrective osteotomy. Fusion is delayed until progressive bone destruction is halted and bone is sufficiently vascularized after chemotherapy. Chemotherapy is given for 9 months.[587] Successful outcome with this method (biopsy for diagnosis and chemotherapy for treatment) has been confirmed by Martini and Gottesman in the elbow[808] and by Tuli in the wrist.[898]

M. marinum arthritis does not have as favorable a therapeutic response to chemotherapy as *M. marinum* tenosynovitis. A combination of chemotherapy and synovectomy is preferred in the treatment of *M. marinum* arthritis. Patients with involvement for longer than 6 months had worse results. *M. marinum* strains are uniformly resistant to isoniazid. They are sensitive to rifampin, ethambutol, and ciprofloxacin. Monotherapy with minocycline and trimethoprim-sulfamethoxazole has been effective for superficial infections, but combination chemotherapy is recommended for *M. marinum* arthritis to prevent resistance. Rifampin-ethambutol combination is the most successful in past reports. Chemotherapy for a minimum of 6 months or for at least 2 months after complete resolution of joint infection is recommended for all atypical mycobacterial joint infections.[589]

The largest numbers of deep atypical infections of the hand are reported and reviewed by Kelly[769] (1967), Cortez[651] (1973), Sutker[890] (1979), Hurst[747] (1987), Chow[640] (1987), Gunther[716-718] (1976-1989), Kozin[776] (1994), Hellinger[729] (1995), and Alloway[589] (1995) and their colleagues.

TUBERCULOUS OSTEOMYELITIS

It is estimated that 10% of tuberculosis is extrapulmonary and that 10% of extrapulmonary tuberculosis is skeletal and

that approximately 10% of skeletal tuberculosis affects the hand, wrist, and elbow.[608,851] Tuberculosis of the bones of the hand is less common than the joints. It typically occurs in the phalanges (tuberculous dactylitis[685,723,733,757,822,867,901,924] and metacarpals[736,831,851,910]). Twenty-five percent of children who have tuberculous dactylitis have multiple foci.[723,733,867] It is rare in carpal bones,[817] radius,[736,742,898] and ulna.[898]

Diagnosis

Clinical presentation of skeletal tuberculosis of the hand in children and adults is different and has changed in character over the years.

Tuberculous Osteomyelitis of the Hand in Children

The highest incidence of skeletal tuberculosis of the hand before the era of antitubercular therapy was in infants[733] and children.[702,723] In children, two thirds of the patients are age 2 or younger[723,733]; it is uncommon after age 5 and scarce after 10 years.[733] The natural course of the disease was often self-limiting[723] but was accompanied by residual deformity.[851] *M. bovis* was then the infecting organism, and with pasteurization of milk it is rarely reported in children today. Adult cases are more often reported today and are caused by *M. tuberculosis*[629,898,900] or atypical mycobacteria.[608,685] Concurrent pulmonary infection was common in the past[737] but is rare today both in children and adults.[608,685]

Tubercular dactylitis is the most common form of skeletal tuberculosis in infants and children, and the proximal phalanx of the second and third fingers is the most frequent site.[849] From a clinical viewpoint, there are two types of dactylitis. One group consists of those individuals who have generalized tuberculous infection and tuberculous dactylitis is a minor manifestation of the whole.[723] The second group consists of patients whose dactylitis is the presenting symptom and who have a relatively mild or no generalized tuberculous infection. In either case, symptoms begin with a painless, nonsuppurative, and insidious swelling on the hand or fingers. Often, multiple fingers are affected.[851] On examination, there is a typical fusiform swelling of a finger or a diffuse swelling on the dorsum of the hand. There is practically no tenderness or local heat, but the part may appear taut and shiny. It is not easily diagnosed at this early stage because the presentation is nonspecific and may simulate a tumor.[757] The swelling often reaches considerable size, doubling the digital girth. In late cases, an abscess may form, with skin discoloration and fluctuation. The abscess may burst and leave a sinus that drains a cheesy, yellowish exudate. Where secondary infection of a sinus occurs, the condition closely resembles a subacute osteomyelitis of pyogenic origin.[733]

Radiographs are characterized by endosteal resorption of bone and progressive subperiosteal hyperplasia. During infancy and childhood, the short tubular bones have a lavish blood supply through a large nutrient artery entering in the middle of the bone. The agent lodges in the center of the marrow cavity, and the interior of the short tubular bone is converted into a virtual granuloma. This leads to a spindle-shaped expansion and inflated shape of the bone. Endosteal resorption of bone and progressive subperiosteal hyperplasia is recorded as "spina ventosa" in the literature[849,876,905] (L. *spina*, "spine"; *ventosa*, "distended with air"). Syphilitic dactylitis has a similar radiographic appearance,[617,698] but serology distinguishes the two clinically. Early in the course of tuberculous infection, the epiphysis is spared because of its rich blood supply,[702] but in late cases it is invaded and causes shortening or deformity of the digit. Radiographic findings of tuberculosis in children include joint effusion, periarticular osteopenia, joint space narrowing, cortical irregularity, lytic lesions, periosteal new bone formation, and advanced epiphyseal maturity.[726] Diagnosis cannot be made without a biopsy. If the biopsy shows granulomatous inflammation on frozen section, AFB staining of the tissue should be requested because it may show tubercle bacilli. A high index of suspicion for tuberculosis in a chronic bone lesion and an "eight pack" culture at the time of biopsy expedite the diagnosis.

Tuberculous Osteomyelitis of the Hand in Adults

Tuberculosis osteomyelitis in the adult occurs most commonly in a phalanx[587,608,728,901] or a metacarpal.[608] In the distal phalanx, it is very rare. Tuberculosis osteomyelitis of carpal bones is also rare.[817] A single bone lesion that appears to be a bone tumor may be tuberculosis.[915] Multicentric tuberculosis may be mistaken for a malignant metastatic disease.[896] Local discomfort and swelling are the usual presenting findings. A pathologic fracture of a metacarpal or a phalanx may occur.[901] A draining fistula forms in untreated cases. Radiographic criteria for diagnosis of skeletal tuberculosis in the adult hand and wrist include bone destruction with honeycombing, diffuse bone loss or cystic lesions, metaphyseal osteoporosis, and preservation of articular cartilage (Fig. 4-20).[685] Increased bone density and sequestra may be seen if staphylococcal osteomyelitis is superimposed. Osteomyelitis due to *M. marinum*[644,919] and *M. kansasii*[782] is clinically similar.

Treatment

Tuli's approach of "do not operate when antibiotics can do the job and operate when you must" is based on experience of thousands of cases of musculoskeletal tuberculosis treated over 3 decades.[897-899] MDT is the keystone of treatment of tuberculosis.[645,822,897,899] Curettage is chosen by the treating surgeon at the time of biopsy, because it is easy, it removes pathologic tissue, and it reduces the bacterial dose. Because of the efficacy of available chemotherapy today, it is not essential. On the other hand, if the organism is resistant, or if the host is immunosuppressed or there is evidence of bone sequestrum, surgical débridement of infected bone is essential. Histologic findings compatible with tuberculosis (chronic granuloma, with or without caseation) in the presence of negative fungal cultures warrant MDT. Before the advent of chemotherapy, many infants and children with localized tuberculous dactylitis without generalized active tuberculosis recovered without surgical débridement in 1 to 3 years.[737] When tuberculous dactylitis occurs in an infant or a child as a part of a severe generalized tuberculosis, it does not resolve spontaneously.[702,723] When it occurs in an adult patient, untreated, it progresses slowly and may necessitate amputation.[685] Pearlman and Warren advised protection of the weakened bone to prevent fracture during chemotherapy. They reported arrest of the tuberculous process where cast and chemotherapy alone were used.[831] Benkeddache and Gettesman treated all their skeletal cases with surgical biopsy for diagnosis and antimyco-bacterial drugs for treatment without further surgical débridement.[608] In early stages, treatment with chemotherapy results in complete resolution. The immune status of the host is an overwhelming predictor of eventual outcome.[776] In the immunocompromised patient population, only 4 of 10

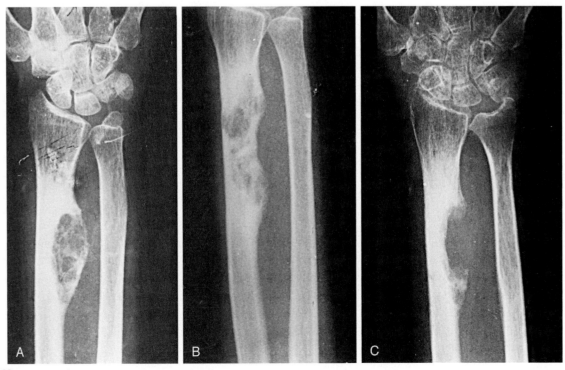

FIGURE 4-20. Tuberculous osteomyelitis of the shaft of the radius resembled a "tumorous lesion" of the bone. **A,** Cultures grew *Mycobacterium tuberculosis.* **B** and **C,** The lesion healed in response to oral antituberculous chemotherapy. (Courtesy of S. M. Tuli, New Delhi, India.)

patients had resolution of deep infection at final follow-up evaluation.[776]

ANTITUBERCULOUS DRUGS AND MULTIDRUG THERAPY REGIMENS

The modern era of tuberculosis began in 1944 with the demonstration of the efficacy of streptomycin in humans. In 1952, the much more effective bactericidal drug isoniazid (INH) became available, making tuberculosis curable in the great majority of patients. In 1970, the bactericidal drug rifampin (RMP) attained equal status to INH. The duration of chemotherapy progressively decreased from approximately 2 years before the availability of RMP, to 9 months with INH and RMP given together, and to 6 months using MDT including INH, RMP, and the bacteriostatic pyrazinamide (PZA) and/or ethambutol (EMB).[719]

INH is bactericidal and is the cornerstone of therapy. It is included in all regimens until resistance is established on cultures. It can cause hepatitis and peripheral neuropathy. Pyridoxine (50 mg PO daily) is given conjointly with INH to minimize peripheral neuropathy. RMP is also bactericidal and is the second major antituberculous agent. The most important complication of RMP is hepatitis. Rifabutin (RFB) is a semi-synthetic derivative of rifamycin that shows good activity against about one third of rifampin-resistant strains of *M. tuberculosis*. PZA is an essential component of three- or four-drug regimens. It is bacteriostatic and its beneficial effect is mostly limited to the first 2 to 3 months of treatment. EMB is bacteriostatic and is an initial component of most regimens. The most important complication of EMB is optic nerve toxicity that may require its removal from the regimen. Blurring and acuity of vision are closely supervised. Tuberculosis should be treated in collaboration with an infectious disease specialist. Second-line agents are less efficacious and more toxic than the first-line drugs. Drug resistance to one or more antituberculous drugs has developed and remains a challenge. Nationwide survey of resistance of new cases in 1997 was 8% for INH, 2.3% for RMP, 2.3% for PZA, 2.2% for EMB, and 3% simultaneously for both INH and RMP (multiple drug–resistant tubercle bacilli).[819] Multiple drug–resistant strains of tuberculosis both to RMP and INH have occurred in AIDS and require directly observed therapy.

Indications

Histologic findings compatible with tuberculosis (granulomatous synovitis, with or without caseation) warrant chemotherapy, although other chronic infections can cause an identical clinical and histologic picture. This is best established on frozen section of biopsy material. The differential diagnosis of granulomatous synovitis includes tuberculous[655,683,703,708,758,906] and atypical[886] mycobacterial infections, fungus,[885] foreign bodies,[710] brucellosis, sarcoidosis,[813] and Crohn's disease,[695] among others. In the presence of negative fungal smears and cultures, a diagnosis of tuberculosis is presumed. Once sensitivity results are reported by the laboratory, chemotherapy is revised to appropriate drugs. In early stages, treatment with chemotherapy will result in complete resolution.

Regimens

Modern tuberculosis therapy guidelines by the CDC and the American Thoracic Society are summarized in Table 4-11. The basic principles that underlie the treatment of pulmonary tuberculosis apply to extrapulmonary forms of the disease. Although relatively few studies have examined treatment of extrapulmonary tuberculosis, increasing evidence suggests that 6- to 9-month regimens that include INH and RMP are effective. In bone and joint disease, 9 months of cumulative chemotherapy is advised.[650] The first 2 months include a four-drug regimen of INH, RMP, PZA, and EMB.[634] After the initial four-drug regimen, a two-drug regimen (INH and RMP) may be resumed if the bacillus is sensitive to both. Patients with initial resistance to RMP or INH are treated with a four-drug regimen plus three second-line drugs to which the organism is sensitive (e.g., amikacin, cycloserine, ciprofloxacin, capreomycin, clofazimine, ethionamide, kanamycin). All patients with organisms resistant to either INH or RMP should receive directly observed therapy. The four-drug regimen can be administered three times a week for 6 months if the therapy is directly observed. Concurrent pulmonary tuberculosis with chronic tuberculous hand infection is rare but must be ruled out in every case because cases with positive sputum smears or positive sputum cultures are highly infectious. Every patient who has hand tuberculosis must have chest radiography. Patients receiving chemotherapy become noninfectious within 2 weeks. If the chest radiograph and sputum are positive, isolation for the first 2 weeks of treatment is recommended to control the spread of tuberculosis. No isolation is necessary for extrapulmonary tuberculosis without active pulmonary tuberculosis.

SPECIAL FEATURES AND TREATMENT OF ATYPICAL MYCOBACTERIA

Of 50 species of atypical mycobacteria that are currently considered to be potential sources of disease, only 16 have been reported to cause infection of the hand and upper extremity. There is a wide range of virulence among atypical species and the very indolent diseases that they are capable of producing.[623] These are described to raise awareness for early biopsy and cultures that will help to identify them in clinical practice. Atypical mycobacterial infection occurs both in immunocompetent and in immunodeficient patients. When atypical mycobacterial infection is encountered, a cause for underlying immunodeficiency should be sought. Chemotherapy and treatment of atypical mycobacteria differs from that of *M. tuberculosis*. The year the bacillus was discovered is placed in parentheses after the bacillus name below.)

Mycobacterium abscessus
M. abscessus causes digital tenosynovitis that grows in culture in approximately 6 weeks. It is cured with clarithromycin and ciprofloxacin.[928,929]

Mycobacterium asiaticum (1965)
M. asiaticum is an emerging chronic mycobacterial hand infection. In a case of *M. asiaticum* flexor tenosynovitis,

Table 4-11

ANTITUBERCULOUS DRUGS USED IN THE UNITED STATES (JUNE 2003)

Drug	Adult Daily Dosage	Pediatric Daily Dosage	Main Drug Toxicity
First-Line Drugs			
Isoniazid (INH)*†	300 mg PO, IM	10-20 mg/kg (max. 300 mg)	Hepatic toxicity, peripheral neuropathy
Rifampin*‡ (Rifadin, Rifocin, Rimactane) or rifapentine	600 mg PO, IV	10-20 mg/kg (max. 600 mg)	Hepatic toxicity, flu-like syndrome
Pyrazinamide§	1.5-2.5 g PO	15-30 mg/kg (max. 2 g)	Arthralgias, hepatic toxicity, hyperuricemia
Ethambutol‖ (Myambutol)	15-25 mg/kg PO	15-25 mg/kg PO	Optic neuritis
Second-Line Drugs (in alphabetical order)			
Capreomycin (Capastat)	15 mg/kg IM	15-30 mg/kg	Auditory, vestibular, and renal toxicity
Cycloserine** (Seromycin)	250-500 mg bid PO or 1 g single dose	10-20 mg/kg	Psychiatric symptoms, seizures
Ethionamide/prothionamide (Trecator-SC)	250-500 mg bid PO or 1 g single dose	15-20 mg/kg	Gastrointestinal and hepatic toxicity
Gatifloxacin			
Kanamycin (Kantrex)	15 mg/kg IM, IV (max. 1 g/day)	15-30 mg/kg	Auditory and renal toxicity
Levofloxacin			
Moxifloxacin			
Para-aminosalicylic acid (PAS)	4-6 g bid PO or 12-g single dose	75 mg/kg bid	Gastrointestinal disturbance
Streptomycin	15 mg/kg IM	20-30 mg/kg	Vestibular toxicity, renal toxicity

*Intravenous preparations of isoniazid and rifampin are available.

†Pyridoxine, 10 to 25 mg, should be given to prevent neuropathy in malnourished or pregnant patients and in those with HIV infection, alcoholism, or diabetes. For intermittent use after initial daily therapy of a few months, dosage is 15 mg/kg (max. 900 mg) twice a week for adults.

‡For intermittent use after a few months of daily therapy; dosage is 600 mg twice a week.

§For intermittent use after first 8 weeks of daily therapy; dosage is 2.5 to 3.5 g twice a week.

‖Usually not recommended for children younger than 6 years old because visual acuity cannot be monitored. May use 25 mg/kg/day during first 1 or 2 months or longer if organism is isoniazid resistant. Decrease dosage if renal function is diminished. For intermittent use after a few weeks to months of daily therapy; dosage is 50 mg/kg twice a week.

¶May recommend pyridoxine 50 mg for every 250 mg of cycloserine to decrease the incidence of adverse neurologic effects.

**Rifabutin is effective against 30% of rifampin-resistant *M. tuberculosis*. It is the drug of choice against *M. avium* infections.

successful management included radical flexor tenosynovectomy, oral minocycline, and clarithromycin.[694]

Mycobacterium avium-intracellulare complex (MAC) (1943)

MAC is the most resistant,[920] tenacious, and troublesome organism that infects the hand. Hellinger and associates[729] have reported and reviewed several cases.[672,769,805,844,880] It most commonly causes tenosynovitis of the finger, palm, or wrist and carpal tunnel syndrome.[672,787] Tenosynovial biopsy fails to show the organism on smears, and the growth on cultures takes 2 months. It is resistant to drugs commonly used for the treatment of tuberculosis. The current antibiotics recommended against MAC are a combination of clarithromycin, rifabutin, and ethambutol.[729] Rifabutin shows better activity against the MAC complex of organisms than rifampin. A combination of thorough surgical

débridement and multidrug chemotherapy is recommended for treatment. Extensive exposure of the tendons from the musculotendinous junctions to their terminal insertion in the affected digits is recommended for "aggressive" tenosynovectomy followed by aggressive hand therapy as soon as wound healing allows.[729]

Mycobacterium chelonae

M. chelonae grows rapidly when compared with other mycobacteria. They grow in 1 week,[592] but multiple cultures may be needed. The infection presents as a chronic nodule or tenosynovitis in a finger.[592,783,882,926] Due to difficulty in isolation, diagnosis was delayed in all reported cases, resulting in ray amputation in three of five cases.[592] Some organisms are susceptible to erythromycin, doxycycline, and kanamycin.[592] Clarithromycin is the drug of choice for localized disease.

Mycobacterium fortuitum (1972)

M. fortuitum is mainly associated with traumatic wound abscess[653] or tenosynovitis.[595,749,845] The infection responds well to surgical excision alone[845] or antituberculous drugs.

Mycobacterium gordonae

M. gordonae causes tenosynovitis, and biopsy and culture are necessary for a timely diagnosis.[609]

Mycobacterium haemophilum (1978)

Since the initial recognition of *M. haemophilum* in 1978,[878] several hand and upper extremity infections have been reported in immunocompromised patients. *M. haemophilum* is an emerging opportunistic pathogen that grows in a medium that is obligatorily supplemented with hemoglobin and incubated at 30°C. Approximately 50% of cases in AIDS, renal transplant, bone marrow transplant, and lymphoma patients have *M. haemophilum* skin or joint lesions in the upper extremity. Infections may occur in the arm,[887] wrist,[802,852] hand,[887] and finger.[852] It is a fastidious, slow-growing, non-pigmented mycobacterium, but diagnosis is relatively easy if the culture is requested in a hemoglobin-containing medium at 30°C. It may grow from tissue biopsy or aspirated synovial fluid.[802,852] Its prognosis is poor because of the underlying host immune deficiency[852] and lack of drugs that inhibit its growth.[802] Lesions may heal slowly over months to years and may occur owing to improved immune function from antiretroviral HIV treatment. Saubolle and coworkers[865] and Straus and colleagues[887] have reviewed cases in the upper extremity of this troublesome, emerging infection.

Mycobacterium kansasii (1953)

The natural reservoir of *M. kansasii* may be water.[679] *M. kansasii* hand infections are generally low grade. Diagnosis is established by easy growth of AFB in the aspirated synovial fluid from a synovial bursa,[665] joint,[930] excised rice bodies, or synovium. Once the bacteriologic diagnosis is confirmed, further surgical débridement of the infected tissue is unnecessary. Chemotherapy with rifampin, isoniazid, and ethambutol[829] and erythromycin is predictably successful. When flexor tenosynovitis recurs in an immunosuppressed patient, such as a renal transplant recipient, recovery occurs after thorough synovectomy, prolonged chemotherapy, and reduction of immunosuppressive therapy.[864] Resistant strains of *M. kansasii* to rifampin[913] and isoniazid[663] have emerged.

Mycobacterium malmoense (1977)

M. malmoense infection is difficult to diagnose because the organism takes 12 weeks to grow[676] and microbiology laboratories often discard their cultures prematurely.[741] It may cause an abscess with a draining sinus, carpal tunnel syndrome,[927-929] and tenosynovitis,[697,927] followed by fraying and rupture of the flexor tendons.[843] Treatment is with standard antituberculous drugs: isoniazid, rifampin, ethambutol, and pyrazinamide.[843]

Mycobacterium marinum (1926)

M. marinum infection is described in the earlier sections dealing with tenosynovial and joint infections. It is sensitive to and responds well to ethambutol and rifampin[778] and to

sulfamethoxazole-trimethoprim.[744] It also responds well to monotherapy with clarithromycin.[863] Clarithromycin has been used increasingly because of good clinical efficacy and minimal side effects. Isoniazid is contraindicated because of high resistance.[745] Single and multiple drug resistance is emerging.[641] Most infections may be successfully treated with chemotherapy alone.[640,707]

Mycobacterium scrofulaceum (1956)

A 66-year-old man in Singapore who suffered from diabetes mellitus presented with osteomyelitis of the right wrist and extensive synovial swellings of the flexor tendons.[838] The clinical features, radiologic appearances, and histology suggested a tuberculous infection, but subsequent culture grew an atypical *M. scrofulaceum*. This case illustrates the need to be aware of the possibility of atypical mycobacterial infection in cases of suspected skeletal tuberculosis.

Mycobacterium smegmatis (M. goodii)

The first case of olecranon bursitis due to *M. goodii* was reported in 2001. This case illustrates that previously unrecognized members of the *M. smegmatis* group of mycobacteria have pathogenic potential.[696]

Mycobacterium terrae complex (1950)

First identified in 1950, *M. terrae*, *M. nonchromogenicum*,[848] *M. triviale*, and radish bacillus[748] are commonly referred to as *M. terrae complex*. In the hand, it is reported to infect subcutaneous tissue,[642] tenosynovium,* joints,[855] and bone.[671,855] *M. terrae* arthritis may occur in immunocompromised patients.[671]

Mycobacterium ulcerans (Buruli ulcer) (1930)

Buruli ulcer is described in detail under subcutaneous tuberculosis.

Mycobacterium xenopi (1957)

The first hand infection due to this organism is a case of wrist tenosynovitis in an immunocompetent male patient, described in 1996.[648] It grows best at 42°C, unlike the rest of atypical mycobacteria.

Mycobacterium szulgai (1972)

Since identified in 1972, olecranon bursitis and carpal tunnel syndrome are reported to be caused by this emerging mycobacterium.[803,806,886] *M. szulgai* is susceptible to first-line antimycobacterial agents.

Author's Preferred Treatment: Diagnosis and Treatment of Mycobacterial Hand Infections

Diagnosis

The most common manifestation of tuberculosis and mycosis in the hand is chronic tenosynovitis. When chronic

---

*See references 659, 671, 721, 748, 766, 798, 810, 812, 834, and 848.

tenosynovitis is nonspecific (there is no indication of rheumatoid arthritis), worsened by cortisone injection, recurrent after tenosynovectomy, or accompanied by sinus formation, I would consider tuberculosis or fungal infection as a cause of the disease. I always sample the synovium in cases of chronic monoarticular arthritis. As soon as I get enough biopsy material, I bisect it and save one specimen without formalin for the microbiology laboratory; the other is sent to the histopathology laboratory in formalin. The pathologist is asked to look at the frozen section for a granuloma in multiple sections. If a granuloma is reported on frozen section, the need for multiple smears and cultures is reinforced.

In addition to biopsy, I send the fluids (e.g., pus, synovial fluid, exudates) for smears and cultures. I request three smears (Gram, AFB, and KOH fungus) on the biopsy tissue as well as the fluid. I request five cultures (aerobic and anaerobic bacteria, tuberculous and atypical mycobacteria, and fungi) on the tissue specimen as well as fluids. I request the mycobacterial cultures at 30°C for *M. marinum, M. haemophilum, M. ulcerans,* and *Sporothrix* and at 36° ± 1°C for the rest of the mycobacteria and 42°C for *M. xenopi.* More often than not, I personally take the specimen to the microbiology laboratory and I urge the microbiologist not to discard the cultures for 12 weeks because that covers the slowest-growing *M. ulcerans* species. I alert the microbiologist and the pathologist of the rarity of the possible chronic infection. I request the infectious disease specialist to supervise the smears and cultures. This partnership improves the chances of laboratory diagnosis of these rare, unexpected, and newly emerging infections.

Treatment

If there is histopathologic evidence of granuloma, caseating or noncaseating, I start treatment for tuberculosis with four drugs (isoniazid, rifampin, pyrazinamide, ethambutol) until the cultures and sensitivities become available. Histologic findings compatible with tuberculosis warrant MDT, although other chronic infections (fungi and atypical mycobacteria) can cause identical clinical and histologic pictures. It may be difficult to distinguish between granuloma of various mycobacteria and fungi, and it is reasonable to treat for *M. tuberculosis* because this is the most common granulomatous infection of the hand. Cultures may take 1 to 12 weeks depending on the organism. Once the sensitivity of the organism is determined, I revise the chemotherapy. Wounds generally heal without complications before mycobacteria are cultured. I seek the help of an infectious disease specialist because the drugs are toxic to liver and kidneys among other tissues, and drug resistance may develop at any time owing to inadequate drug compliance. I monitor therapy with monthly examinations. Bone and joint lesions on chemotherapy are monitored with radiographs every 3 months for improvement or deterioration. If improvement is not seen, surgical débridement is considered, especially in immunocompromised patients. Resistance to drugs is a problem. This is the real challenge of this millennium.[709]

SOURCES OF MOST RECENT POLICIES AND RECOMMENDATIONS ON TREATMENT OF TUBERCULOSIS

Centers for Disease Control and Prevention, Division of Tuberculosis Elimination (404) 639-3311, www.cdc.gov/ or www.hopkins-id.edu.
For management of drug-resistant tuberculosis, call (212) 491-8403 or (415) 502-4700.

ANNOTATED REFERENCES

Most annotated references are some of the largest series of tuberculosis of the hand. Some other references have been included because they describe unique observations on diagnosis or treatment.
584. Adams R, Jones G, Marble HC: Tuberculous tenosynovitis. N Engl J Med 233:706-708, 1940.
809. Mason ML: Tuberculous tenosynovitis of the hand: A study of 33 cases of chronic tenosynovitis of the hand. Surg Gynecol Obstet 59:363-396, 1934.
839. Pimm LH, Waugh W: Tuberculous tenosynovitis. J Bone Joint Surg Br 39(1):91-101, 1957.

Mason, Adams and colleagues, and Pimm each reported more than 20 cases of tuberculosis of the hand before the use of streptomycin. They provide a description of the natural course of the disease and a useful historical control for the treatment and results of synovectomy without antibiotic intervention. Mason, working with Kanavel and Koch in Chicago, reported on 18 cases after tenosynovectomy done between 1914 and 1934; 13 (over 72%) remained free of recurrence between 2 months and 12 years after operation and 6 of them required two or more operations before the process could be eradicated. Adams from Massachusetts General Hospital recorded over 45 years and noted that 7 of 17 patients treated with tenosynovectomy were cured and an additional 7 improved. Pimm, of Oxford, in a study of 42 patients after tenosynovectomy without antibiotics followed between 2 and 27 years, noted that 20 had no recurrence and the remaining 22 had a recurrence, most within 1 year.
589. Alloway JA, Evangelisti SM, Sartin JS: *Mycobacterium marinum* arthritis. Semin Arthritis Rheum 24:382-390, 1995.
724. Harth M, Ralph ED, Faraawi R: Septic arthritis due to *Mycobacterium marinum.* J Rheumatol 21:957-960, 1994.

Both of these articles are important because they point out that septic monoarthritis (wrist, metacarpophalangeal joint, proximal interphalangeal joint) in a patient with a history of vocational or avocational contact with aquatic activities or fish may be caused by *M. marinum* and intra-articular steroid injection will aggravate the condition. They showed that joint aspiration has a high yield for positive staining and cultures. This opens a window for initial treatment with antibiotics only. Treatment with minocycline or trimethoprim-sulfamethoxazole can be initiated until sensitivity results become available.
606. Beckman EN, Pankey GA, McFarland GB: The histopathology of *Mycobacterium marinum* synovitis. Am J Clin Pathol 83:457-462, 1985.
646. Collins RJ, Chow SP, Ip FK, Leung YK: Synovial involvement by *Mycobacterium marinum:* A histopathological study of 25 culture-proven cases. Pathology 20:340-345, 1988.

The above two articles are important because they contrast the age-old axiom that caseating granuloma is an essential part of the histopathologic diagnosis of tuberculosis. Beckman first reported that *M. marinum* may cause a noncaseating granuloma. Collins and Chow showed that caseating granuloma was present in only 33% of the *M. marinum* tenosynovitis, and mycobacteria were seen in a stained specimen in only 60% of the cases. Pathologists often rule out tuberculosis if bacilli are not seen on stained sections or caseating granulomas are not seen in histopathology. Beckman and Chow have taught us that *M. marinum* can and should be considered in the absence of caseating granulomas. It is here that cultures at 30°C are essential to grow *M. marinum*.

614. Bickel WH, Kimbrough RF, Dahlin DC: Tuberculous tenosynovitis. JAMA 151:31-35, 1953.

Bickel reported on 40 cases after the advent of streptomycin. Bickel's report from the Mayo Clinic is important; his results of tenosynovectomy are analyzed without and with the use of streptomycin. Fifteen of 30 patients who had tenosynovectomy only had recurrence. Eight of his 10 patients treated with tenosynovectomy and streptomycin did not have a recurrence. One outcome is clear: in war between man and microbe, once the dose of the microbe is reduced by tenosynovectomy, the man can handle the microbe with his host immunity, at least in 50% of cases Bickel and colleagues studied. This is good fortune on the part of the patient today when synovectomy is carefully done and the surgeon fails to request microbiology testing or the laboratory fails to reveal the underlying microbe or because the microbe is scarce or grows with difficulty because it is seeded on media without special ingredients *(M. haemophilum)* or at unfavorable temperature *(M. marinum)*. The outcome of combined medical and surgical treatment is clear: it is far superior to surgery only.

622. Breathnach A, Levell N, Munro C, et al: Cutaneous *Mycobacterium kansasii* infection: Case report and review. Clin Infect Dis 20:812-817, 1995.

This is an important contribution because the authors have reviewed 29 cases of cutaneous tuberculous infection caused by *M. kansasii*. This is the largest review on this disorder, which is much rarer than *M. marinum* cutaneous infection.

623. Brown B, Wallace R: Infections due to nontuberculous mycobacteria. *In* Mandell GL, Bennett JE, Dolin R (eds): Principles and Practice of Infectious Diseases, 5th ed. New York, Churchill Livingstone, 2000, pp 2630-2636.

Brown's classification of nontuberculous mycobacteria (NTM) supersedes that of Runyon by grouping nontuberculous mycobacteria within the laboratory on their growth rates as rapidly or slowly growing mycobacteria. It is important to warn the microbiology laboratory not to discard cultures until all slowly growing mycobacteria are ruled out.

640. Chow SP, Ip FK, Lau JH, et al: *Mycobacterium marinum* infection of the hand and wrist: Results of conservative treatment in twenty-four cases. J Bone Joint Surg Am 69:1161-1168, 1987.

641. Chow SP, Stroebel AB, Lau JH, Collins RJ: *Mycobacterium marinum* infection of the hand involving deep structures. J Hand Surg [Am] 8:568-573, 1983.

Chow made a significant contribution to surgery by suggesting that diagnosis of tuberculosis can be made by synovial biopsy through a small incision and that conservative treatment of tuberculosis of the hand is effective and safe in immunocompetent patients when tenosynovitis is painless, there are no sinuses, and the patient has not received cortisone injections. Fourteen of 24 patients (60%) were cured with antibiotic treatment (rifampin and ethambutol for 8 to 15 months) without radical tenosynovectomy. When a patient has painful tenosynovitis, has a sinus, or previously has had cortisone injection, radical synovectomy and antibiotic treatment are obligatory.

672. Eggelmeijer F, Kroon FP, Zeeman RJ, et al: Tenosynovitis due to *Mycobacterium avium-intracellulare:* Case report and a review of the literature. Clin Exp Rheumatol 10:169-171, 1992.

658. Darrow M, Foulkes GD, Richmann PN, et al: *Mycobacterium avium intracellulare* infection of the hand: Two case reports. Am J Orthop 24:914-917, 1995.

729. Hellinger WC, Smilack JD, Greider JL Jr, et al: Localized soft-tissue infections with *Mycobacterium avium/Mycobacterium intracellulare* complex in immunocompetent patients: Granulomatous tenosynovitis of the hand or wrist. Clin Infect Dis 21:65-69, 1995.

These articles have shown that MAC is the most resistant, tenacious, and troublesome of the mycobacteria that infect the hand. Hellinger and colleagues from the Mayo Clinic have reported on 6 cases and reviewed 11 previously reported cases up until 1995. This is an in-depth review of this rare infliction. They pointed out that combination of antibiotics and thorough tenosynovectomy is essential to get a cure and that surgical exposure extends from musculotendinous junction to the terminal insertion of the tendon in the distal digital phalanx. Multiple débridements may be necessary. Antibiotic coverage with clarithromycin and ethambutol is provided until culture and sensitivity results are available.

663. Dillon J, Millson C, Morris I: *Mycobacterium kansasii* infection in the wrist and hand. Br J Rheumatol 29:150-153, 1990.

Dillon reported 3 new cases and reviewed 24 cases of tenosynovitis due to *M. kansasii*. *M. kansasii,* similar to *M. marinum,* was found to be resistant to para-amino salicylic acid and isoniazid and sensitive to rifampin and ethambutol.

686. Fellander M: Tuberculous tenosynovitis of the hand treated by combined surgery and chemotherapy. Acta Chir Scand 11:142-150, 1956.

Fellander, of Sweden, confirmed the findings of Bickel from the United States that addition of antibiotics to synovectomy improved the results from 50% success to almost 100%. Thirteen of his 14 patients did not have recurrence after combination treatment. This experience is a precursor to Chow's attempt 30 years later to treat tuberculosis with biopsy diagnosis and antibiotics only.

716. Gunther SF, Elliott RC: *Mycobacterium kansasii* infection in the deep structures of the hand: Report of two cases. J Bone Joint Surg Am 58:140-142, 1976.

717. Gunther SF, Elliott RC, Brand RL, Adams JP: Experience with atypical mycobacterial infection in the deep structures of the hand. J Hand Surg [Am] 2:90-96, 1977.

718. Gunther SF, Levy CS: Mycobacterial infections. Hand Clin 5:591-599, 1989.

Gunther continued to remind us of nontuberculous mycobacterial infections of the hand in the 1970s and 1980s. His personal experience of cases in Washington, DC, and review of the literature can bring a wealth of information to the reader. His description includes *M. marinum, M. kansasii,* and *M. avium* infections of the skin, tenosynovium, joint, and bone.

745. Huminer D, Pitlik SD, Block C, et al: Aquarium-borne *Mycobacterium marinum* skin infection: Report of a case and review of the literature. Arch Dermatol 122:698-703, 1986.

759. Johnston JM, Izumi AK: Cutaneous *Mycobacterium marinum* infection (swimming pool granuloma). Clin Dermatol 5:68-75, 1987.

These two articles are comprehensive review articles about cutaneous *M. marinum* infection. The authors review 500 cases reported in literature between 1963 and 1986. They clarify clinical diagnosis, differential diagnosis, laboratory diagnosis, and medical treatment. Huminer and colleagues have detailed drug sensitivity studies, and Johnston and Izumi have emphasized minocycline, 100 mg twice a day for up to 4 months. Both authors point out that the organism is resistant to isoniazid and para-amino salicylic acid.

748. Huskisson EC, Doyle DV, Fowler EF, Shaw EJ: Sausage digit due to radish bacillus. Ann Rheum Dis 40:90, 1981.

Flexor tenosynovitis limited within a finger may produce a characteristic "sausage finger" in tuberculosis.

763. Kanavel AB: Tuberculosis tenosynovitis of the hand: A report of 14 cases of tuberculosis tenosynovitis. Surg Gynecol Obstet 37:635-647, 1923.

No review of tuberculous tenosynovitis is complete without studying the clinical and operative observation of Kanavel of Chicago. Mason's compliment, "The report of Dr. Kanavel in 1923 has described the condition so well that additions are superfluous and deletion impossible" is still true today. In a study of 14 cases, he staged the disease into exudative, granulation, locally necrotic, and finally metastatic phases into adjacent joints and bone. He recommended careful and complete tenosynovectomy and achieved excellent results when additional extrapulmonary lesions were absent, indicating better host immunity.

769. Kelly PJ, Karlson AG, Weed LA, Lipscomb PR: Infection of synovial tissue by mycobacteria other than *Mycobacterium tuberculosis.* J Bone Joint Surg Am 49:1521-1530, 1967.

770. Kelly PJ, Weed LA, Lipscomb PR: Infection of tendon sheaths, bursae, joints, and soft tissues by acid-fast bacilli other than tubercle bacilli. J Bone Joint Surg Am 45:327-336, 1963.

Kelly and colleagues from the Mayo Clinic reported on infections of the hand caused by mycobacteria other than tuberculosis soon after Runyon had just classified them in 1959. These were some of the earliest nontuberculous mycobacterial infections of the hand that were treated with a combination of surgery and antituberculous antibiotics. In three cases so treated, none recurred. The era of medical treatment had just begun.

857. Runyon EH: Anonymous mycobacteria in pulmonary disease. Med Clin North Am 43:273-290, 1959.

893. Timpe A, Runyon EH: Relationship of "atypical" acid-fast bacilli to human disease: Preliminary report. J Lab Clin Med 44:202-209, 1954.

Runyon and Timpe classified mycobacteria other than tuberculosis (MOTT) or atypical mycobacteria into four classes in 1950s. This was a milestone in the identity of mycobacteria, the classification of which was in a chaotic state. After their description, more cases of what are now called nontuberculous mycobacteria (NTM) are reported than those caused by tuberculous mycobacteria.

870. Sehgal VN: Cutaneous tuberculosis: Current concepts. Int J Dermatol 29:237-247, 1990.

One of the most thorough reviews of cutaneous tuberculosis of *M. tuberculosis origin* is by Sehgal. This is a dissertation of his personal experience of many years. He explains the routes of infection, clinical presentations, diagnosis, and treatment in enjoyable detail.

Occupational Infections

Barber's interdigital pilonidal sinus, shearer's disease, milker's interdigital granuloma and slaughterer's interdigital granuloma are foreign-body occupational infections of the hand caused by penetration of human or animal hair into skin. Anthrax,[962] *M. marinum*,[936] tuberculous paronychia,[951] herpetic paronychia,[956] prosector's wart,[946,949] milker's nodule,[938] human orf,[935] and viral warts[941] are also infectious occupational diseases of the hand and are described in detail in the bacterial, tuberculous, and viral sections.

BARBER'S INTERDIGITAL PILONIDAL SINUS

Barber's interdigital pilonidal sinus of the hand is a foreign-body hair granuloma.[952] The term *pilonidal* is derived from the Latin terms *pilos,* which means "hair," and *nidus,* which means "nest." Interdigital pilonidal sinus in barbers was first described in 1942 as a foreign-body reaction or a granuloma of the customer's hair implanted in the interdigital skin of the barber.[958] Since then cases have been described as hair-bearing sinus,[934] barber's interdigital pilonidal sinus,[933,940,942,944,952,953,955,961] barber's disease,[960] and interdigital sinus.[932,939] Interdigital pilonidal sinus is a disease of only male barbers and hairdressers. It has never been reported in female

hairdressers. The reason for this is not clear. It may rarely affect the pulp of a finger.[937] The condition is not a congenital cyst because hair roots are not seen in the sinus or the cyst, and the hairs are not immature, curly, or fine like those found in a congenital pilonidal cyst.

Diagnosis

Clinically, a pit or sinus develops in the interdigital web space dorsally. The sharp snipped hair ends enter the soft skin of the digital webs when barbers use their fingers to comb the customer's hair. Constant rubbing of the fingers against each other exacerbates the problem. Once inside the web space the hairs cause a foreign-body reaction and sinus formation. As more hairs enter into the web space through the sinus, a cyst may form. In due time the sinus or the cyst becomes infected and an abscess forms that intermittently discharges purulent fluid with pieces of hair. Histologically, the lesion reproduces the features of a nonspecific inflammatory granuloma.[952,958]

Several loose and easily removable hairs, of different lengths, color, and texture, generally protrude from the sinus. They have sharp, pointed ends and are consistently thick, stiff, and straight, essentially the male type. This may explain why the condition occurs in men's hairdressers. Women's hair is generally soft and thin, and the ends are more likely to bend rather than penetrate. Rarely is more than one interdigital web space affected.[958] The order of predilection is the third web space followed by the second and fourth. The first web space has been reported to be involved only once.

Treatment

Excision of the lesion and primary wound closure results in a less obvious scar than incision and drainage.[933,934, 943,945,952,953,958]

SHEARER'S DISEASE

A similar and related condition to barber's interdigital sinus occurs in the interdigital spaces of sheep shearers and is caused by wool. Small tufts of wool may protrude from the sinus. Symptoms are worse after shearing lambs, because newer, finer wool passes into the sinus more easily.[947,954] A recurrent subungual pilonidal sinus of the thumb in a dog groomer caused chronic osteomyelitis of the terminal phalanx. The foreign-body hair granuloma is a well-recognized occupational hazard in dog groomers in the United Kingdom.[950]

MILKER'S INTERDIGITAL GRANULOMA

The hairs of cattle, barbed at an angle, may penetrate skin of milker's hands and migrate slowly and deeply under the skin and cause a foreign-body reaction. Milker's interdigital granuloma is a painful, red, granulating, discharging, vege-tating lesion found in the hands of milkers. It may vary from pea size to nut size. The surface may be irregular and riddled with sinuses. The second and third interdigital spaces of the dominant hand are the usual location. Treatment is removal of the hair and control of the inflammatory process. A persistent granuloma should be excised.[948]

SLAUGHTERMAN'S INTERDIGITAL GRANULOMA

Slaughterhouse employees may develop a pilonidal sinus in the interdigital space from hair of the animals they slaughter.[957] The lesion persists with conservative treatment until it is completely excised.

ANNOTATED REFERENCES

948. Meneghini CL, Gionitti F: Granulomatosis fistulosa interdigitalis of milker's hands. Dermatologica 129:38-50, 1964.
950. Mohanna P, Al Sam SZ, Flemming AFS: Subungual pilonidal sinus of the hand in a dog groomer. Br J Plast Surg 54:176-178, 2001.
952. Patel MR, Bassini L, Nashad R, Anselmo MT: Barber's interdigital pilonidal sinus of the hand: A foreign body hair granuloma. J Hand Surg [Am] 15:652-655, 1990.
954. Philips PJ: Web space sinus in a shearer. Med J Aust 2:1152-1153, 1966.
957. Sloan JP, Brenchley J: An unusual cause of pilonidal sinus. J Accid Emerg Med 17:232, 2000.

In each of these articles, interdigital sinus has been caused by hair in a milker, dog groomer, barber, cattle shearer, and slaughterhouse worker. The sinus does not respond to antibiotics. Surgical excision cures it.

Protothecal, Protozoal, and Parasitic Infections

PROTOTHECOSIS (ALGAE INFECTIONS)

Protothecosis is a rare infection that is caused by microscopic, unicellular, colorless algae of the genus *Prototheca*, also classified sometimes as a fungus.[1007] *P. wickerhamii* is the most frequent alga infection in the upper extremity.[1006] In the United States, it is common in the southeastern states.[1013]

Diagnosis

The most common presentation of protothecosis in the upper extremity is a single lesion of the skin or subcutaneous tissue or olecranon bursitis. The typical skin lesion is a painless, slowly progressive, well-circumscribed plaque or papulonodular lesion that may become ulcerated. The skin and soft tissue lesions typically enlarge over a period of weeks to months, with no tendency for self-healing. *P. wickerhamii* favors the olecranon bursa, and recurrent olecranon bursal infection can occur after open trauma.[963,977, 995,1009,1013] The infection follows minor trauma, corticosteroid injection, or wounds exposed to soil or water. Protothecal infection may also occur on the forearm,[1015] dorsum of the hand,[997,1003,1009] palm,[982,986] or digit.[976] It may mimic a neoplasm if a nodule recurs several times.[1003] Incision and drainage of an infected abscess will generally be complicated by recurrence.[1003] Diagnosis can only be made by open biopsy.

Protothecosis is best diagnosed by biopsy for histologic study and culture. Excised olecranon bursa or abscess wall shows foci of chronic granulomatous inflammation and small, refractile, oval objects in epithelioid cells consistent with *Prototheca*. The inflammatory response shows both microabscesses and granulomas with multinucleated giant cells. *Prototheca* cells usually range from 8 to 20 mm in diameter, stain well with Gomori's methenamine silver or periodic acid–Schiff, and often contain two to eight tightly packed endospores in each cell or sporangium. Cultures for *Prototheca* are rarely positive.[982,1003] When the organisms grow, white opaque colonies appear in a few days on Sabouraud's agar. Identification is by gross and microscopic appearance plus biochemical tests.

Treatment

Protothecosis has little, if any, tendency toward self-healing. Organisms are sensitive to tetracycline and amphotericin B.[986] Surgical excision of lesions and intravenous therapy with amphotericin B and tetracycline have been used successfully. Prolonged therapy with ketoconazole, itraconazole, or fluconazole has been reported to benefit some patients with skin lesions.[989] Complete excision of the infected tissue is necessary for cure.

PROTOZOAL INFECTIONS

Leishmaniasis is an intracellular infection caused by the protozoa *Leishmania*. Rodents and canines are the normal reservoirs, humans are the hosts, and the vector is the sandfly. Humans can also act as reservoirs when actively infected. The parasite multiplies in the cytoplasm of macrophages, which then rupture and release the *Leishmania* organisms into the bloodstream. Three clinical entities caused by leishmaniasis have been described: cutaneous, mucocutaneous and visceral. Cutaneous leishmaniasis (Baghdad boil, Delhi boil,[1017] tropical sore, oriental sore, Chiclero's ulcer[1011]) is the most common form. The initial lesion is a red-brown papule at the bite site. It gradually enlarges to a 2- to 4-cm painless, chronic ulcer within 6 months. The ulcer has a necrotic base and indurated margin and is covered by a firmly adherent crust. It develops a "pizza-like" appearance with a raised outer margin. Lymphadenopathy is absent. A solitary lesion occurs in 76% of cases, two lesions in 15%, three lesions in 6%, and four lesions in 1%.[1010] Multiple ulcers occur in immunocompromised patients.[964] Eighty percent of the lesions are located on exposed body sites (face, upper extremity,[964,988,990,999,1001,1005,1014] and lower extremity). The ulcer usually heals without treatment over the course of a year, leaving a characteristic cribriform scar.[983] Basal cell carcinoma[992,1008] or epidermoid carcinoma[984] may develop in a leishmaniasis scar.

Leishmaniasis is endemic in 88 countries with an estimated yearly incidence of 1 to 1.5 million cases of the cutaneous variety and 500,000 cases of visceral leishmaniasis (kala-azar).[971,972] Cutaneous leishmaniasis occurs widely throughout South America, Africa, Mediterranean, the Middle East,[985] and Asia. More than 80% of the total of 12 million infected patients live in Brazil (New World leishmaniasis), Tunisia,[972] Syria,[972] Iran,[1018] and Afghanistan,[972,1012] (Old World leishmaniasis). The disease is endemic in southern Texas,[978,988] because of its proximity to Mexico. Holiday visitors to Costa Rica[1014] and Central America[979] are the most common importers of leishmanial ulcer to the United States. It should be included in the differential diagnosis of skin lesions in personnel returning from the military.[981,983,994,1004]

Diagnosis

A chronic nonhealing ulcer in the exposed part of the upper extremity in a traveler from an endemic country,[979,980,1014] in a recent immigrant from those countries, or in military[983,994,1016] personnel should arouse suspicion of a leishmanial ulcer. A nonhealing nodular ulcer is an indication for a smear, culture, or biopsy. Final diagnosis is usually delayed unless the index of suspicion is high. In a series of 28 patients, the diagnosis of leishmaniasis was delayed an average of 125 days, despite an average of three physicians' examinations.[1005] Diagnosis is made by identification of the parasite from smear, fine-needle aspiration cytology,[987] or biopsy specimen. The first smear may be positive in 80% of cases, and a second smear may be positive in an additional 10% of cases.[1010] Smears taken from the center of the ulcer have a greater sensitivity than those from the edge of the ulcer.[1000] A positive culture may take a month to grow. Before a biopsy sample is immersed in formaldehyde, an impression smear of tissue should be taken and a prolonged Giemsa stain (45 minutes) should be performed on the smear. The microorganism has to be cultivated from biopsy material on special medium (Novy-McNeal-Nicole medium). PCR is the most accurate test identification of *Leishmania* species but is limited to specialized laboratories.[974,991,1012]

Treatment

Treatment minimizes the scar and may ultimately avert formation of carcinoma.[984,992,993,1008] Topical therapy with paromomycin and methylbenzethonium chloride has been used successfully for the treatment of Old World leishmaniasis.[968,973] Intralesional injection of antimony compounds was successful in 76% of cases by Uzun.[1010] Therapy was carried out using intralesional injection of 1 mL/cm^2 of meglumine antimonite or sodium stibogluconate, once a week. The average number of injections was 11.[1010] The recommended dose of sodium stibogluconate is 20 mg/kg/day, and the duration of therapy varies from 10[1016] to 28[989] days. Liposomal amphotericin B may be used as an alternative.[989]

As a preventive measure, the CDC recommends application of repellent with DEET (diethyltoluamide) to exposed skin and edges of clothing to prevent sandflies from biting.[970]

PARASITIC WORM (NEMATODE, FILARIAL) INFECTIONS

Parasitic worm (nematode) infections of the upper extremity have been reported due to two roundworms, *Gnathostoma spinigerum* and *Onchocerca volvulus,* and a tapeworm, *Taenia soleum.*

Gnathostomiasis

Gnathostomiasis is a subcutaneous infection caused by a roundworm (nematode), *Gnathostoma spinigerum.* It is a chronic, cutaneous "migrating" larval infection. It is common in Thailand, Southeast Asia, and Japan, where people eat uncooked fish or raw pork. In the United States, the patient is likely to be an immigrant.[998] Multiple migrating episodes of swelling and pain occur in the hand, foot, shoulder, and face over several years as larva migrate subcutaneously. Eosinophilic count is typically high, because eosinophils are specifically effective against helminthic parasites. A skin test and a serum precipitin test are useful in confirming the clinical diagnosis.[975]

Exploration, recognition, and removal of the larva (1 cm by 1 mm) from the infected part of the hand is curative.

Onchocerciasis (Onchocercosis, Filarial Infection)

Onchocerciasis is a rare parasitic infection of the soft tissues caused by a roundworm (nematode), *Onchocerca volvulus.* Onchocerciasis of the flexor tendons of finger,[1002] wrist,[965,966,1002] carpal tunnel, and forearm[969,1002] have been reported in North America.[965,969,1002] Eosinophilia is pathognomonic of parasitic infestations and has been reported as high as 16% in one case.[1002]

Synovectomy is curative. Drug therapy is not necessary if all the parasites are removed with the infected tissue.

TAPEWORM INFECTION (CYSTICERCOSIS)

The tapeworm (*Taenia soleum*) may infect a muscle and present as a mass that can be mistaken clinically for malignant sarcoma. Tapeworm infections of the upper extremity have been reported in the triceps muscle[996] and flexor digitorum profundus muscle.[967] Tapeworm infection is acquired by ingestion of inadequately cooked and infected pork. The differential diagnosis of a muscle mass should include cysticercosis. The diagnosis is made by fine-needle aspiration of the cyst.

Simple surgical excision cures the condition.

ANNOTATED REFERENCES

963. Ahbel DE, Alexander AH, Kleine ML, Lightman DM: Prothecal olecranon bursitis: A case report and review of the literature. J Bone Joint Surg Am 62:835-836, 1980.

The authors report a case and review the literature of 26 cases, with 7 involving the olecranon bursa and 3, the hand. Eight of 10 cases were indigenous to the United States. It is useful to keep this diagnosis in mind when a bursa recurs after multiple aspirations. Fluid does not yield positive cultures. Diagnosis is easily and usually made on routine biopsy sections stained with hematoxylin and eosin. Among giant cells and histiocytes are seen small, clear, refractile, oval objects consistent with *Prototheca* species.

977. Grocott, RG, Huffaker AK, White CB: Prothecal bursitis: A case from Panama. Lab Med 10:89-96, 1979.

The authors report a case and review 15 cases in the literature. Half of them affected the upper extremity, with six involving the olecranon bursa and two, the hand. This is consistent with others who report that it mainly affects the extremities.

988. Maloney DM, Maloney JE, Dotson D, et al: Cutaneous leishmaniasis: Texas case diagnosed by electron microscopy. J Am Acad Dermatol 47:614-616, 2002.

Maloney reported 1 case in the forearm and reviewed 29 other cases of cutaneous leishmaniasis in southern Texas. He emphasized the endemic nature of this condition in Texas. Electron microscopy is useful if histopathology does not confirm the disease.

996. Ogilvie CM, Kasten P, Rovinsky D, et al: Cysticercosis of the triceps—an unusual pseudotumor. Clin Orthop Rel Res 382:217-221, 2001.

Ogilvie and colleagues have given us a concise description, diagnosis, and misdiagnosis of tapeworm infection of a muscle: ingestion of inadequately cooked infected pork, development of adult worm in the intestine, release of eggs in the intestine, re-ingestion of eggs in the contaminated food, hematogenous spread, destination in a muscle, encystation of larva, their demise, painful granulomatous mass, misdiagnosis of malignant sarcoma, operative plan for wide resection of muscle, correct diagnosis on histopathology. Beware of an isolated muscle mass.

998. Raturi U, Burkhalter W: Gnathostomiasis externa: A case report. J Hand Surg [Am] 11:751-753, 1986.

Raturi and Burkhalter remind us that immigrants from Japan and Thailand who relish raw fish (sashimi and somfuk) may harbor worms of gnathostomiasis species. The worm wanders around (1 cm/hr) in the subcutaneous tissue and causes pain and swelling as it secretes its toxin. There are two clinical markers of the disease: migrating subcutaneous pain and eosinophilia.

1002. Simmons EH, Van Peteghem K, Trammell TR: Onchocerciasis of the flexor compartment of the forearm: A case report. J Hand Surg [Am] 5:502-504, 1980.

Flexor tenosynovitis, carpal tunnel syndrome, and eosinophilia do not occur in rheumatoid, tuberculous, or fungal disease. The authors remind us that eosinophilia is a clinical marker for worm infections. Pathologic analysis shows a filarial worm in the tissue. That incites eosinophilia.

1003. Sirikulchayanonta V, Visuthikosol V, Tanphaichitra D, Prajaktham R: Protothecosis following hand injury. J Hand Surg [Br] 14:88-90, 1989.

The authors remind us that it is wise for surgeons to be aware of this condition if they find patients having recurrent nodule formation after a penetrating hand injury. They recommend surgery and tetracycline for treatment.

1005. Sotiropoulos G, Wilbur B: Two cases of cutaneous leishmaniasis presenting to the emergency department as chronic ulcers. J Emerg Med 20:353-356, 2001.

The authors describe a case of forearm painless ulcer in a man who returned after a 2-month missionary trip to Costa Rica. Biopsy proved negative, but the CDC was able to help with diagnosis by growing the *Leishmania* on culture.

1010. Uzun S, Uslular C, Yucel A, et al: Cutaneous leishmaniasis: Evaluation of 3,074 cases in the Cukurova region of Turkey. Br J Dermatol 140:347-350, 1999.

This recent article is about Old World leishmaniasis. It shows how common leishmaniasis is in Turkey. Other two countries with high incidence and prevalence are Tunisia and Syria. Eighty percent of the lesions were located on exposed body sites. Diagnosis was made in 90% of cases by the smear method. Overall healing rate was 90% when the lesion was injected with antimony compounds locally.

1014. Wilson ME, Lucchina LC: Photo quiz: Healthy student with a papule. New World cutaneous leishmaniasis. Clin Infect Dis 33:816, 899-900, 2001.

In 1998 and 1999, Costa Rica was the place of exposure for 30 of the 81 cases of American cutaneous leishmaniasis for which sodium stibogluconate was requested from the CDC. Healthy students spending holidays in Costa Rica may return with an ulcer on the exposed part of the upper extremity.

Viral Infections

Chronic viral infections of the hand include AIDS, human orf, milker's nodules, and warts. AIDS presents as infections and tumors of the hand that are secondary to suppressed immunity. Orf in an immunodeficient patient attains "giant" size and can be misdiagnosed and mistreated as a malignancy. Warts are often seen by hand surgeons, and most are managed conservatively.

WARTS

A wart is a cauliflower-like, raised, demarcated, grayish mass with an irregular surface traversed by many projections. Ciuffo, in 1907, first provoked warts in the skin of volunteers by injection of appropriately filtered wart tissue and suggested that it is a viral infection.[1043] Strauss and colleagues, in 1950, demonstrated the virus under electron microscope,[1143] which has subsequently been included in the group of human papillomaviruses (HPVs).

Classification

Two types of cutaneous warts are widespread in hands. Common warts, verruca vulgaris (L. *verruca,* "a little hill"), represent 95% of cutaneous warts in the hands. The second most common are flat or plane warts (verruca plana) (5%). Both types are seen predominantly in children[1126] but also affect adolescents and young adults. Adults at high risk for the development of warts are veterinary surgeons,[1046] butchers,[1046] meat packers,[1078] fowl handlers, poultry processors,[1140] and fish handlers,[1129] all occupations in which hands are frequently exposed to moisture.

Pathogenesis of Human Papillomavirus

The incubation period of HPV disease is 1 to 3 months.[1126] The virus infects only the epidermis. Warts have a characteristic histologic appearance, showing acanthosis, papillomatosis, hyperkeratosis, and parakeratosis.

Diagnosis

Common Verrucated Wart

The clinical appearance of a common verrucated wart is quite characteristic and usually consists of a single lesion on the dorsum of the hand, fingers, or around the nail. It may occur in the palm of the hand. It is a cauliflower-like, raised, demarcated, and grayish mass, with an irregular surface traversed by many projections. It is often painless, and the adjacent skin is healthy. Warts in the palm may be painful because of pressure during grip. If untreated, the common wart may multiply and infect the surrounding skin or the opposite hand. When multiple, there may be several dozen "seed lesions" surrounding a larger and older "mother wart." A cluster of closely spaced papules may coalesce into a large "mosaic wart." "Kissing warts" are seen in areas of skin contact (web spaces) and appear to represent direct inoculation. Filiform warts are slender, finger-like papules. Periungual warts may extend into the nail bed under the nail plate (subungual warts) and may persist for many years in spite of treatment.

Flat (Plane) Warts

Flat (plane) warts are minimally elevated papules that are 2 to 5 mm in diameter. They appear as multiple lesions with a smooth surface. Flat warts have an enhanced likelihood of spontaneous involution.[1101,1122,1144] Flat warts in adults are more common in women.

Multiple Warts

Common warts rarely if ever transform into squamous cell carcinoma.[1064,1068] Immunosuppressed patients with an inherited defect such as epidermodysplasia verruciformis,[1095] acquired defects in immunity (renal transplant recipients),[1031] lymphoproliferative disorders, or those on chemotherapeutic drugs may develop multiple warts. These warts may transform into squamous cell carcinoma. Biopsy is indicated when the diagnosis is doubtful.

Treatment

No antiviral chemotherapy is available for HPV warts. They are a cosmetic nuisance in most cases and often disappear spontaneously. Spontaneous resolution appears to occur in children,[1102,1085,1098,1151] in 50% within 1 year[1098] and 90% within 5 years.[1151] Fluctuations in immunity to human papillomavirus may be responsible for spontaneous regression or resurgence of preexisting warts.[1122] However, if left untreated, they may persist for many years and attain large size. Gardner and Acker reported a case of bone destruction of a distal phalanx caused by a periungual wart.[1060] Rarely, a wart transforms into a carcinoma.[1064,1068] These rare instances require aggressive surgical treatment, but conservative treatment remains the hallmark for management of common warts.

Multiplicity of treatments for warts attests to the lack of any single satisfactory method of therapy. Simple topical treatment is just as successful as more invasive methods.[1033,][1034,1036] Cooperation of the patient and experience of the physician determine the appropriate treatment modality. Most therapeutic modalities consist of chemical or physical destruction of the warts or excision of large lesions. Salicylic acid is the most commonly used ingredient in the chemical destruction of the lesion and the virus it harbors. Less aggressive therapy of common warts in childhood is preferred because of the increased likelihood of spontaneous resolution[1098,1151] and lack of tolerance for painful ablative treatments. In contrast, warts in immunosuppressed adults are likely to be progressive, recalcitrant, recurrent, unresponsive to all but the most aggressive therapy,[1104] and more likely to become malignant.[1031] Infectious disease and dermatology specialists should be consulted for treatment recommendations.

Patients with verrucated warts usually seek treatment for cosmetic reasons. Patients with flat warts usually do not seek treatment. Keratolytic therapy is simple, inexpensive, painless, and preferred because it is as effective as cryotherapy, with a success rate of approximately 70% and a minimal recurrence rate of 4%.

Keratolytic Therapy

Local applications of keratolytic agents result in chemical débridement of the infected epidermal cells. The most used method is a self-applied paint of 16% salicylic acid with lactic acid in collodion (1:1:4). A drop of the solution (Duofilm, Occlusal, Paplex) is placed over the wart and left in place for a few minutes. It is then soaked in warm water, and white sloughing keratin is mechanically débrided gently with a cloth. This is repeated daily. It takes a few days to a few weeks to "melt" a wart. Seventy percent cure in 12 weeks was reported in a randomized trial by Bunney, and the treatment was as effective as cryotherapy.[1034-1036] Compliance is a major limitation. A high-potency 26% salicylic acid reduces the treatment period to 2 weeks.[1110] Forty percent salicylic acid is available as a thin layer applied on a tape and is an excellent alternative (Mediplast). A small piece of the tape is cut that is a little larger than the wart. Protective plastic that covers the salicylic acid on the tape is peeled off. The tape firmly adheres to the wart (Fig. 4-21A and B). On a finger, it may be reinforced with waterproof 3M tape (see Fig. 4-21C). It is left in place for a day or two. At the time of shower, it is removed, the sloughed epidermis is scrubbed off with a brush, and a new tape is applied over dry skin. Slow tissue necrosis removes the infected epidermis over a few days to few weeks. Adverse reactions include occasional irritation of normal tissue surrounding the wart. This treatment is painless, convenient, and safe. Patient compliance is good and self-treatment is inexpensive.

Taping for Periungual Warts

Periungual warts are difficult to treat when they extend under the nail plate. Litt[1092] has recommended application of plain adhesive tape to the entire finger distal to the proximal interphalangeal joint. The patient is instructed to remove the tape in 6.5 days, scrub off the necrotic skin, and reapply the tape in 12 hours. The process is repeated for 6 to 9 weeks. Additional fingers may be taped similarly. He claims excellent results. He does not offer any reason why the method works.

Cryotherapy

Liquid nitrogen or carbon dioxide,[1034,1036] without local anesthesia, is preferred for the management of refractory periungual warts. Burning pain associated with cryotherapy

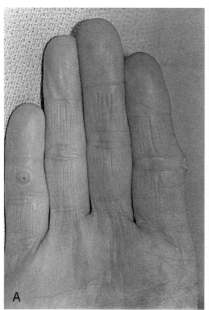
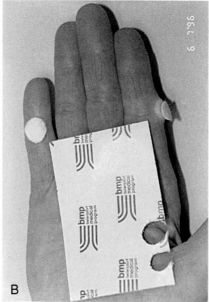
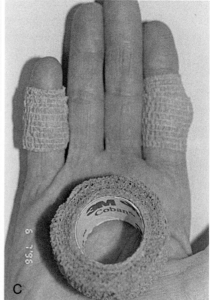

FIGURE 4-21. **A,** Typical warts in the hand of a cafeteria worker whose hands are frequently immersed in water. **B** and **C,** A piece of medicated adhesive tape (Mediplast) slightly larger than the wart is applied over the lesions secured in place with (Coban) waterproof 3M tape.

is well tolerated by adults but not children.[1110] Adverse reactions in children have included premature closure of the distal phalangeal physis and angular deviation of the distal interphalangeal joint[1055] and destruction of the proximal interphalangeal joint.[1101]

Intralesional Injection of Bleomycin

Intralesional injection of bleomycin (0.1 to 0.2 mL of 1 unit/mL) is indicated in the treatment of recalcitrant warts[1020,1035,1138] and is successful in 88%.[1035] Raynaud's phenomenon is reported in digits injected with bleomycin.[1052]

Electrosurgery

Electrosurgery includes electrocautery, electrocoagulation, electrodesiccation, and laser ablation. Ablation of the wart may be done by a diathermy knife under local anesthesia or under general anesthesia for multiple lesions. There is risk of recurrence of warts in and around the site of treatment. Electrodesiccation is useful for filiform warts. Concerns about laser therapy include risk to the operator and paramedics from the dispersion of virus in the plume of vapor generated by the laser.[1052,1059,1133]

Curettage and Surgical Excision

A wart can be curetted out with a small curet. No controlled studies have been published, but gratifying results have been reported.[1034,1116] To prevent recurrence, it is safe to apply a tape with a keratolytic agent (e.g., Mediplast) to débride the curetted margins of the wart. Simple surgical excision has not been prospectively studied. I have had success with it and have not had recurrences. It is important to excise the wart through a wide margin to prevent recurrence. The size of the margin I use is at least 1 mm. If the excision is not complete, there may be a risk of recurrence in the suture tracts.

Outcome

Prognosis in general depends in part on the age and immunity of the patient, as well as on the type, number, and chronicity of warts. Warts in children respond to treatment more readily than adults. Immunodeficiency inhibits the response to treatment. Mosaic and plane warts are more resistant to treatment. Single warts disappear more rapidly than multiple warts, and chronic warts tend to be more recalcitrant to treatment.[1034] Warts frequently recur, and they should not be considered cured until a 6-month period has elapsed.

Author's Preferred Method of Treatment

I use 40% acetylsalicylic acid keratolytic therapy with Mediplast as my first choice for treatment. The treatment is acceptable to patients, is simple to execute, and is effective in a large percentage. When a patient does not want to undertake prolonged treatment and the wart is large, I surgically excise it with a 1- to 2-mm margin. I excise the infeced nailbed after removal of nail plate in cases of periungual and subungual warts.

ACQUIRED IMMUNODEFICIENCY SYNDROME (AIDS)

Etiology and Epidemiology

AIDS was first recognized in mid 1981. In 1982, the CDC developed a case definition based on the opportunistic infections and tumors that developed secondary to a failure of host immunology and coined the term *acquired immunodeficiency syndrome.* In 1983, a cytopathic retrovirus (HIV) was isolated from persons infected with AIDS. By 1985, serologic tests to detect HIV were developed and a diagnosis of AIDS could be confirmed in the laboratory. As of 1998, it was estimated that, worldwide, more than 33 million adults and children were living with HIV infection/AIDS, from a cumulative total of well over 47 million persons infected since the beginning of the epidemic. These figures keep increasing, with approximately 16,000 new infections per day. Half of all new infections occur in young people between 10 and 24 years of age. In 1993, HIV infection became the most common cause of death among persons aged 25 to 44 years. As of December 31, 2002, in the United States, a total of 886,575 persons were reported to be infected with AIDS, 501,699 of these persons had died, and the number of persons living with AIDS (384,876) was the highest ever reported. Approximately one third of persons in the United States infected with HIV may not know they are infected. Globally, 38 million people were infected with HIV by the end of 2003.

AIDS is a sexually transmitted disease of homosexual and bisexual men and of heterosexual intravenous drug abusers that is transmitted through pooled contaminated needles. Before serologic testing for HIV was begun in 1985, AIDS was common in hemophiliacs who received infected blood transfusions. Percutaneous, mucous membrane, and cutaneous exposure to blood-contaminated body fluids can occur frequently in the health care setting. Such exposure has infrequently resulted in occupationally acquired HIV infection in health care workers. The average risk of seroconversion after a needlestick injury with HIV-infected blood is 0.33%. Transmission of HIV has also been reported after mucous membrane and cutaneous exposure to blood. As of December 2001, a total of 57 health care workers have been reported to the CDC with documented HIV seroconversion after occupational exposure. Of these 57 persons, 50 had a percutaneous exposure, 5 had a mucocutaneous exposure, and 2 had both percutaneous and mucocutaneous exposure. Three major occupations were nurses (22), laboratory technicians (19), and physicians (6). To date there are no confirmed seroconversions in surgeons with exposure to a suture needle. Transmission of HIV from a health care worker to patients has been documented in two instances: one in a dental practice and one from an orthopedic surgeon in France.[1114]

HIV subverts the cell-mediated immune system by infecting T lymphocytes, specifically the subset CD4+ lymphocytes that normally orchestrate immune responses responsible for phagocytosis of infecting organisms.[1019]

Clusters of T lymphocytes are differentiated by a specific protein molecule on the cell surface. Depletion of CD4+ T lymphocytes (<500/mL) is the hallmark of HIV disease. The opportunistic infections and tumors are primarily due to fall in T-cell number and failure of immune surveillance. *Death in AIDS ultimately results from infection or malignancy.* AIDS patients acquire chronic infections from bacteria,[1024,1066] fungi,[1136] and viruses[1118] that ultimately prove fatal. Tuberculosis[1057] and Hansen's disease[1103,1115] may relapse once host resistance is reduced with HIV infection.

Clinical Manifestations and Stages of HIV Infection

The spectrum of HIV infection ranges from asymptomatic to severe immunodeficiency associated with serious secondary infections, neoplasms, and other conditions. AIDS is the most advanced stage of this illness, in which the infected host can no longer control opportunistic organisms or malignancies that rarely cause illness in immunocompetent individuals. Without therapy, AIDS develops in approximately 5% of HIV-infected adults within 2 years of infection, in approximately 25% within 6 years of infection, and in 50% within 10 years. Approximately 10% of HIV-infected individuals remain clinically asymptomatic with normal CD4 T-lymphocyte counts for 10 years after infection. After 11 years, however, more than 75% of HIV-infected patients develop AIDS or die.[1097]

The clinical spectrum of HIV infection includes (1) primary infection (the acute retroviral syndrome), (2) asymptomatic latent infection for several years, (3) resurgence of early symptomatic infection with persistent generalized lymphadenopathy (PGL), and (4) advanced immunodeficiency (AIDS) with opportunistic infections and malignant tumors.

The primary infection is accompanied by decline in CD4+ cell count. High levels of viremia and high plasma concentrations of HIV RNA persist for 1 to 3 weeks. During the second latent asymptomatic period, virus load increases by 10^{10}/day and the CD4+ cell count declines by 50/mL/yr. In the third phase, PGL is related to the rapid infection of CD4+ cells in lymph nodes by HIV. PGL is defined as the presence of two or more extrainguinal sites of lymphadenopathy for a minimum of 3 to 6 months. Fifty to 70 percent of HIV-infected individuals develop PGL. In the final and fourth overt phase, plasma viremia rapidly increases, accompanied by a more rapid decline in CD4+ count before the onset of symptoms. As the viral load rises and CD4+ cell count falls, the risk of opportunistic infections, malignancies, wasting, and death increases. During each phase, viral load (viremia) is monitored by measurement of HIV RNA in plasma, and immunologic status is measured by absolute number of CD4+ lymphocytes. Certain diseases are more common in persons infected with AIDS than in the uninfected population and are considered suggestive of HIV infection. Among the conditions included in the 1993 AIDS Surveillance Case Definition by the CDC, those of particular importance to a hand surgeon are listed in Table 4-12. Clinical staging of the disease based on clinical findings and CD4+ T-lymphocyte count is shown in Table 4-13.

Table 4-12
AIDS INDICATOR CONDITIONS

Bacterial infections, multiple or recurrent

Coccidioidomycosis, extrapulmonary

Cryptococcosis, extrapulmonary

Herpes simplex

Histoplasmosis, extrapulmonary

Kaposi's sarcoma

Mycobacterium avium-intracellulare complex or *Mycobacterium kansasii,* extrapulmonary

Mycobacterium tuberculosis, any site (pulmonary or extrapulmonary)

Mycobacterium, other species or unidentified species, extrapulmonary

Wasting syndrome of HIV infection

From the 1993 AIDS Surveillance Case Definition.

Clinical Manifestations of AIDS Infection in the Hands

Glickel,[1063] Seltzer and associates,[1136] Ching and coworkers,[1042] McAuliffe and colleagues,[1099] and Gonzalez and coworkers[1066] described hand infections in patients with HIV disease. Approximately 10% of the patients who present with hand infections in metropolitan hospital emergency departments have HIV infection. Eighty percent of intravenous drug abusers who present with hand and upper extremity infections have HIV infection. Glickel suggests that diagnosis of AIDS should be considered in any unusual hand infection.[1063] It should be considered in any patient who needs a repeat drainage or débridement procedure.[1042,1066,1099] Fingers in AIDS may be red with painless erythema and periungual telangiectasia.[1111] Nails may be blue[1026] or show clubbing.[1026,1030] Ching noted that among 14 AIDS patients with hand infections, almost one third needed multiple débridements and resulted in an amputation of a finger or hand.[1042] McAuliffe,[1099] in a review of 74 HIV-seropositive patients who were treated for upper extremity infections, found that intravenous drug use was the most common risk factor for HIV infection as well as the most common cause of the infection necessitating admission. These patients were admitted a total of 97 times for the treatment of 89 different infections and underwent 120 surgical procedures. Twenty-six (29%) infections required more than 1 operation, and 11 (12%) resulted in amputation. Patients with AIDS were significantly more likely to present with spontaneous onset of infection than were those who were HIV seropositive. The infections may be seen early in the course of the disease, and in one half of the patients they preceded the diagnosis of AIDS.[1025] Gonzalez, in a study of 28 patients, found five patients who had necrotizing fasciitis; all needed more than one débridement, and one required forequarter amputation.[1066]

Herpes simplex virus (HSV 1 and 2) infection of the hand is clinically diagnosed when characteristic multiple vesicu-

Table 4-13

CLINICAL GRADING OF AIDS BASED ON CLINICAL CONDITIONS AND CD4⁺ LYMPHOCYTE COUNT

CD4⁺ T-Cell Count	Clinical Categories		
	A Asymptomatic Acute (Primary) HIV or PGL	B Symptomatic, Not A or C Conditions	C AIDS Indicator Conditions*
1. 500/mL	A1	B1	C1
2. 200–499/mL	A2	B2	C2
3. <200/mL	A3	B3	C3

Shading indicates revised conditions included in the 1993 Revised Classification System for HIV Infection and Expanded AIDS Surveillance Case Definition for Adolescents and Adults, which included CD4⁺ counts because low counts can occur without clinical signs and symptoms of indicator conditions.

*Clinical conditions in category C are listed in Table 4-12.

PGL, Persistent generalized lymphadenopathy.

lar lesions on an erythematous base are present. It generally resolves within 3 weeks. When it lasts longer than 3 weeks, an index of suspicion for immunosuppression or AIDS should be raised. In an occult[1048] or overt[1066] HIV infection, herpes simplex may present as a chronic granulating infection in the hand that does not respond to routine antibiotics and may progress to finger necrosis[1023,1118] or gangrene.[1153] Staining of scrapings from the base of the lesions with Wright's, Giemsa's (Tzanck preparation), or Papanicolaou's stain demonstrates characteristic giant cells or intranuclear inclusions of HSV infection. These cytologic techniques are often useful as quick office procedures to confirm the diagnosis. Direct immunofluorescent antibody and indirect immunoperoxidase staining are equally sensitive and specific for the detection of HSV antigen.[1134] In the eyes of most virologists, viral cultures remain the gold standard by which other methods of diagnosis of HSV are judged.[1055] Laboratories that do viral cultures provide transport media for clinical specimens. For cutaneous HSV infections, acyclovir and its related compounds, famciclovir and valacyclovir, have been the mainstay of therapy. Treatment with intravenous acyclovir is followed by oral acyclovir (200 mg q 4-5h)[1118] to prevent recurrences. Famciclovir and valacyclovir have more convenient dosing schedules (three times daily) compared with acyclovir (five times daily). Necrotic and gangrenous parts of the hand are excised. Acyclovir-resistant strains of HSV are being identified with increasing frequency, especially in HIV-infected persons. Isolation of HSV from persisting lesions despite adequate dosages of acyclovir should raise the suspicion of acyclovir resistance.[1139] Therapy with the intravenous foscarnet (Foscavir)[1130] and topical cidofovir gel (Forvade),[1100] trifluorothymidine ointment,[1083] and vidarabine[1107] speed healing of acyclovir-resistant herpes. Herpetic infections of the pulp should not be mistaken for felons or paronychia and should not be violated with incision and drainage. If inappropriately treated with surgery, patients may develop local secondary bacterial bone lysis or metastatic viral encephalitis.[1093]

Other Opportunistic Hand Infections

M. haemophilum may cause a skin infection,[1142] joint infection,[1121,1142] or tenosynovitis[1096] in the hand in an AIDS patient. It is a fastidious, slow-growing, atypical *Mycobacterium* that optimally grows at 30°C in 10% CO_2 and hemoglobin. *M. avium* has been demonstrated to cause chronic tenosynovitis in an AIDS patient.[1090] Any chronic infection of the hand in AIDS should be sampled for tuberculous mycobacteria, nontuberculous mycobacteria, and fungi.

Bacillary angiomatosis was first described by Stoler in 1983[1141] and is an infectious, cutaneous, vascular, tumor-like disorder found almost exclusively in HIV-positive individuals.[1024,1044,1045] The lesion resembles a benign pyogenic granuloma[1024] or a Kaposi sarcoma. A previously unidentified, pathogenic species of *Bartonella* (formerly *Rochalimaea*), *B. henselae*, has been identified as an emerging opportunisitic gram-negative bacillary infection.[1045] The lesion may be pea sized when first recognized. It may be pedunculated and friable. There may be ulceration with crusting. The lesions may be solitary or multiple. When punctured by a needle or scalpel, the lesion may bleed profusely. Clinical differential diagnoses include pyogenic granuloma, hemangioma, and Kaposi's sarcoma. The diagnosis of bacillary angiomatosis is best made by fine-needle aspiration biopsy.[1131] Hematoxylin and eosin stains of biopsy specimens from skin lesions show proliferation of small blood vessels in the dermis, enlarged endothelial cells with abundant cytoplasm, and necrotic and granulomatous changes. Warthin-Starry stains show perivascular accumulations of bacilli; these findings may be confirmed by electron microscopy, although this is not usually necessary. The diagnosis can also be established by culture of the organism in several special media or by detection of *Bartonella* DNA by polymerase chain reaction. Serologic assays for anti-*Bartonella* antibodies are available through the Special Pathogens Branch of the CDC. If left untreated, bacillary angiomatosis follows a progressive and potentially a fatal course. Once it is properly identified, treatment of bacillary angiomatosis consists of prolonged therapy with erythromycin or doxycycline. Fluoroquinolones, other macrolides, and trimethoprim-sulfamethoxazole also have activity against *Bartonella*.[1023,1044]

Kaposi's sarcoma (KS) may occur in the hand[1025,1054,1072,1081,1109,1117] and may need punch or open biopsy or excision. Moritz Kaposi first described the entity Kaposi's sarcoma in 1872.[1080] In 1994, Chang and coworkers discovered a new herpesvirus, human herpesvirus type 8 (HHV-8) or KS herpesvirus. It was identified both in AIDS-related KS as well as in non–AIDS-related KS (classic Mediterranean KS; African or endemic KS; renal, cardiac, and hepatic transplant-recipient KS). The virus is also found in peripheral blood mononuclear cells in patients with KS, and this frequently precedes the development of KS in AIDS patients. Human herpesvirus type 8 is transmitted sexually and proliferates in an immunosuppressed AIDS environment.

KS is the most common neoplasm affecting HIV-infected individuals. It is a vascular neoplastic disorder that in the United States is seen predominantly in HIV-infected homosexual men. KS is staged as (I) cutaneous, locally indolent; (II) cutaneous, locally aggressive ± regional lymph nodes; (III) generalized mucocutaneous ± regional lymph nodes; and (IV) visceral.[1086] KS in an AIDS patient is a more aggressive tumor than that identified in non-AIDS patients.

The characteristic finding in stage I is a cutaneous red-purple nodule or plaque. The skin is the most common first site of presentation. The lesions are generally painless and nonpruritic and appear as firm, slightly raised or nodular tumors. Cutaneous nodules ranging from 0.5 to 2.0 cm in diameter are frequently observed. Cutaneous KS does not cause the death of patients with HIV infection. Despite the relative lack of mortality associated with KS, morbidity associated with more advanced disease can be considerable. Bulky cutaneous lesions may become painful. Large, plaque-like lesions may coalesce and restrict joint movement. Lesions of KS are often difficult to distinguish from those of bacillary angiomatosis; biopsy is required for diagnosis. For cutaneous lesions, a small punch biopsy (2 to 4 mm) is usually adequate. Tumor registry data from San Francisco General Hospital demonstrated a decline in the number of newly diagnosed cases of KS from 103 in 1995 to 62 in 1996 to 36 in 1997. This corresponds to the more widespread use of highly active antiretroviral therapy. The social problems associated with this disfiguring neoplasm in an already socially stigmatizing disease cannot be overemphasized, and KS may need excision for social and cosmetic reasons.[1114]

Vascular lesions other than KS occur as serious complications of the hand in HIV infection. HIV-infected patients develop symptoms of Raynaud's phenomenon when treated with bleomycin and vincristine.[1052,1112,1117,1149] *Digital gangrene* may occur from vasculitis,[1023,1051,1123] obliteration of digital arteries,[1051] and vascular injury resulting from chemotherapy.[1054,1072,1091,1112,1117,1148] HIV-induced thrombocytopenia may cause compartment syndrome of the forearm.[1047,1054,1081,1109]

Tumors of smooth muscle origin (leiomyomas and leiomyosarcomas) have nonrandom relationship with HIV infection in children,[1038] and leiomyoma of the hand has been reported in a child with AIDS.[1152]

Laboratory Diagnosis

There are two laboratory tests for the diagnosis of HIV infection: serologic tests that detect antibodies to human immunodeficiency virus and plasma HIV-1 RNA concentration that determines the HIV viral load in the blood.

Serologic tests becomes positive within 2 to 8 weeks of infection. In adults, testing for HIV antibodies is considered positive when a repeatedly reactive enzyme-linked immunosorbent assay (ELISA) is confirmed by a more specific assay, such as a Western blot. This combination of findings should generally be considered to indicate a current infection with HIV. The sensitivity of ELISAs ranges from 93% to 100%. The specificity of a repeatedly reactive ELISA is approximately 99%. A rapid ELISA to detect HIV antibodies within 1 hour is commercially available in the United States and is useful when postexposure prophylaxis is imminent in a health care setting. The assay most commonly used to confirm ELISA reactivity is the Western blot. This test involves incubation of the patient's serum with HIV proteins. A negative result rules out AIDS.

Monitoring HIV-1 ribonucleic acid levels (also known as HIV viral load) has become the standard of care for monitoring response to therapy in HIV-infected patients. Because patients with primary HIV infection may not yet have mounted an antibody response, ELISA and Western blot assays may be negative or indeterminate. Detection of plasma HIV RNA is used to detect the presence of HIV infection in patients with acute HIV infection and in those who have reactive ELISAs but indeterminate Western blots. Patients with primary HIV infection have high levels of viremia (usually 10^5 to 10^6 copies per milliliter of plasma). All patients with suspected primary HIV infection should have follow-up studies to confirm seroconversion; this occurs in the majority of patients within 3 to 6 months of presentation. The diagnosis of established HIV infection in adults is relatively straightforward and can be made serologically. A reactive ELISA that is confirmed with a Western blot is generally diagnostic for HIV infection. A negative ELISA should be repeated in 3 to 6 months for someone at risk for acquiring HIV infection, because false-negative ELISAs can occur during the seronegative window of primary HIV infection. In someone with a clinical picture strongly suggestive of AIDS and a negative ELISA, consideration should be given to pursuing the diagnosis of infection with unusual subtypes of HIV-1 or HIV-2, which may not be detected in the serologic assays used. The ultimate diagnosis of HIV infection requires the demonstration of serologic conversion.

CD4+ count is helpful in prognosis, prevention, and treatment and is one of the most important tests for HIV infection. CD4+ count of less than 500/mL is used for AIDS surveillance but is not diagnostic of HIV infection. Reduced counts at this level occur in disease situations without AIDS, and a false-positive result is detrimental for both the patient and the treating physician.

Prognosis

Prognosis is based largely on CD4+ lymphocyte counts and plasma viral load assays. There is risk of opportunistic complications among individuals with CD4+ cell counts below 200/mL. The median time to an AIDS-defining condition after reaching 200/mL is 18 to 24 months; the median survival after a CD4+ count of 200/mL is 3 years, and survival after developing an AIDS-defining complication is 1 year without antiretroviral therapy. Those with CD4+ counts below 50/mL are considered to have advanced HIV disease and are at much higher risk for development of opportunistic infections such as *Mycobacterium avium* infection. Taken together, the CD4+ lymphocyte count and plasma viral load are the best prognostic markers for subsequent disease course in an HIV-infected individual. The CD4+ lymphocyte count, a specific test for cellular immunocompetence, is a sensitive predictor of the development of symptomatic HIV infection and AIDS in the near term. Conversely, the plasma viral load (HIV-1 RNA) is an extremely useful predictor of disease course over a more extended period of time. Plasma HIV RNA of 10^3/mL is predictive of slow progress and that of 10^5/mL is predictive of rapid progress. The more rapid the decline in CD4+ count, the faster is the clinical progression of the disease. A popular analogy of this situation proposed by Coffin likens AIDS to an impending train wreck, with the viral load reflecting the speed of the train and the CD4+ count reflecting the distance to the disaster.

In the absence of treatment, survival is short after the diagnosis of clinically defined AIDS. Before the availability of combination antiretroviral therapy, median survival after the diagnosis of AIDS was estimated to be between 12 and 18 months. Patients diagnosed with an opportunistic infection had the most rapid mortality. Most of these patients had CD4+ counts less than 100/mL.

Prevention

In surgery of the hand in a known AIDS patient, the hand surgeon has a special responsibility in protecting the entire operating room personnel[1029] from accidental spread of infection. Universal blood and body fluid precautions should be observed during surgery.[1029,1037] This includes attention to barrier techniques (double gloves, goggles, or masks with plastic eye guards) and measures designed to prevent injury (indirect transfer of sharp instruments between the surgeon and the scrub nurse via an instrument receptacle and self-sheathing needles). Bare needles should be recapped without using two hands by introducing the needle into the cap placed on the table. These precautions should always be used in areas where AIDS prevalence is high.

In 1990 the CDC recommended the use of zidovudine for postexposure prophylaxis after occupational exposure to HIV among health care workers. HIV seroconversion after occupational exposure was decreased by approximately 81% with the use of zidovudine. This has led to subsequent recommendations that incorporate the newer antiretroviral drugs based on quantity of source material (viral load) and the HIV status of the source person (virulence). Zidovudine, lamivudine, and indinavir are now recommended for 4 weeks for postexposure prophylaxis.

Treatment

Medical treatment cannot cure HIV disease but has improved the quality and length of life for HIV-infected persons. Treatment of AIDS consists of (1) eradication of the HIV viremia with antiretroviral drugs, (2) treatment of opportunistic infections (bacterial,[1024,1042,1066] mycobacterial,[1041,1058,1096,1103] fungal,[1136,1147] and viral,[1048,1063,1066,1107,1118]) with specific antibiotics and surgical drainage, débridement, and excision of the infected tissues or amputation of the necrotic or gangrenous part of the hand, and (3) treatment of malignancies.

The use of combination antiretroviral therapy with nucleoside reverse transcriptase inhibitors (NRTI) and protease inhibitors (PI) in 1995 led to a dramatic decrease in drug resistance and dramatic improvement in the natural history of treated HIV disease. In the United States, deaths attributed to AIDS decreased by 23% in 1996 and by 44% in 1997. Multidrug antiviral therapy with two NRTI drugs (abacavir, didanosine, stavudine, lamivudine, zalcitabine, zidovudine) plus a PI drug (efavirenz, indinavir, nelfinavir, ritonavir, saquinavir) appears to be the most potent antiretroviral regimen available in preventing disease progression (maintaining or increasing CD4+ cell counts), and preventing drug resistance. Strongly recommended regimens include either indinavir, nelfinavir, ritonavir + saquinavir, ritonavir + indinavir, ritonavir + lopinavir, or efavirenz in combination with one of several two-drug NRTI combinations. Clinical outcome data support the use of a PI in combination with two NRTIs. Zidovudine monotherapy is no longer acceptable for patients with HIV infection. Monotherapy, as in tuberculosis, leads to drug resistance.

HUMAN ORF (ECTHYMA CONTAGIOSUM, CONTAGIOUS PUSTULAR DERMATITIS, FARMYARD POX, MILKER'S NODULE)

Human orf infection is important to a hand surgeon because it causes a large tumor-like lesion in immunodeficient hosts that resolves with medical treatment. Misdiagnosis has led to an unnecessary excision,[1040] sometimes multiple excisions,[1145] and even amputations.[1039,1079]

The word "orf" is an old Anglo-Saxon name for cattle, and the disease is endemic in sheep and goats. It is a large paravaccinia DNA virus that belongs in the subgroup of poxviruses. It is common in humans who have direct contact with infected sheep and goats or with products or objects that come in contact with sheep and goats. The virus can persist for long periods on such objects as fences, barn doors, and feeding troughs from which the disease is indirectly transmitted to a susceptible host. In 1 year, 1.4% of 16,484 sheep and goat handlers in New Zealand were infected.[1119] The risk was highest (4%) in mutton slaughterers. It occurs on the exposed parts of the body, especially the hands.[1021,1022,1065,1071,1108,1132,1150] Human orf is an occupational disease[1053] in "risk populations" such as shepherds,[1094] sheep shearers,[1084] butchers,[1119] and veterinary surgeons.[1039,1127,1137] There is a yearly outbreak of orf infection of the hand in Saudi Arabia.[1071] Two million people visit Saudi Arabia for "Hajj" every year, and hundreds of thousands of sheep are slaughtered by nongloved hands at the end of the ceremony. Inoculation occurs in preexisting or incidental new injuries of the hand from the infected animals.[1071] Outbreaks in Turkey[1069] and Belgium[1062] occur 2 to 3 weeks after Islamic *"Feast of Sacrifice"* (Aid el Kabir or Aid el Adha) in men who bleed the sheep and in women who handle their skin and meat. The epidemic is predictable 9 weeks after the end of Ramadan every year, and 75% of patients are Islamic.

Diagnosis

Ninety-five percent of the lesions are on the finger,[1021,1061,1075,1094,1108,1119,1124] hand,[1105] wrist, or forearm.[1074,1128] The lesion is usually unilateral, rarely bilateral.[1105] There is a history of exposure to sheep or goats, a goat/sheep bite, or handling of goat/sheep for "sacrifice." After an incubation period of 3 to 7 days,[1127] the infected skin lesion erupts clinically. In humans, orf is commonly known as ecthyma contagiosum[1056,1076,1108,1119,1127] or contagious purulent dermatitis (CPD), but this is in part a misnomer because pustules are not purulent (ecthyma = purulent pustules) in human orf.

Leavell has described the lesion in six clinical stages in a study of 19 cases of human orf.[1087] Each stage lasts approximately 1 week, and the disease resolves without treatment in approximately 6 weeks (range, 14 to 72 days). The first stage is characterized by an erythematous macule or papule. In the second (target) stage the lesion turns into a nodule with a central red center, a middle white ring, and peripheral erythematous halo.[1074] The third, or the weeping, stage is characterized by a weeping surface on a nodule. The fourth stage consists of a thin yellow crust with underlying black dots over the nodule. The fifth (papillomatous) stage consists of small surface papillomas and finger-like projections of the epidermis. The sixth and final stage is characterized by reduction in the size of the lesion and formation of a thick crust that looks like an ulcer[1124] before final healing. Lesions do not always correspond to these stages and may present as an erythematous nodule,[1108] a tense bullous lesion,[1021,1094] a giant lesion,[1120] or a felon.[1022] In orf felon there is absence of local pain and drops of clear fluid exude from the lesion.[1022] The lesions may be single or multiple.

Diagnosis is confirmed by electron microscopy of negatively stained suspensions from lesions and is found to be simple and the most useful and rapid laboratory method available. Provisional diagnosis can be made in an hour, compared with several weeks when tissue culture techniques are used. The virus survives without preservatives in crusts, vesicular fluid, or biopsy of suspected lesions for as long as 30 days and can be safely saved and mailed to a distant electron microscopic facility for identification.[1045] A scab from the surface of the lesion is usually sufficient to establish the diagnosis because these contain large amounts of orf virus. Up to 1.6×10^{11} virus particles can be recovered from 1 g of the scab material.[1119] Characteristic large multiple oval viral particles may be seen within the keratinocytes under an electron microscope. In most cases, however, the clinical appearance of the lesion on a finger, hand, wrist, or forearm and a history of contact with sheep or goats are sufficient to make diagnosis of human orf.

In an immunocompromised patient, the lesion may attain a large size. Immunosuppressed patients with chronic lymphatic leukemia,[1077] patients on immunosuppressive medication for a lymphoma,[1132] and renal transplant patients[1061,1127] have been reported with "giant" orf lesions on their fingers or palms. The lesion may recur several times after thorough excision and skin grafting in a patient with severe congenital impairment of cellular and humoral immunity (Nezelof's syndrome).[1145] It may assume giant proportions in atopic dermatitis.[1050] Giant orf in a normal individual is rare,[1113] and immunologic work-up is in order.[1073] It has been erroneously stated that infection with the orf virus confers lifelong immunity.[1087,1108] Eighteen cases of re-infection in immunocompetent patients were reported by Robinson and Peterson.[1119] Person-to-person transmission is rare.

Differential Diagnosis

Orf and milker's nodule are essentially identical on clinical, histologic, and virologic examination.[1049,1067,1106] Orf is diagnosed if the patient has been in contact with sheep or goats, whereas milker's nodules are suspected if the patient has been manually milking cows[1088] or buffaloes.[1102] Often the patient can remember seeing a scabby mouth lesion on a sheep or a crusting pseudo-cowpox lesion on an udder. In the absence of such history, diagnosis of "farmyard pox"[1137] or parapox infection[1120] affords the clinician a diagnosis based on common clinical and electron microscopic findings. Lesions in immunosuppressed patients progress to giant epithelioma-like tumors and have led on occasion to unnecessary amputation.[1065,1079,1132]

Treatment

If untreated, spontaneous resolution of the lesion occurs within 6 weeks in immunocompetent hosts. The lesion may persist or continue to grow in immunocompromised hosts and may recur even after multiple and radical excisions and skin grafts.[1071,1127,1145] Two antiviral agents have been successfully used in isolated cases since 1986: topical idoxuridine (40%) in dimethylsulfoxide[1077] and cidofovir cream (1%).[1061] Tan described one case of congenital impairment of immunity (Nezelof's syndrome) that defied treatment with multiple radical excisions, skin grafts, topical idoxuridine, and intralesional injections of interferon alfa. It finally healed when the lesion was liberally irrigated with hypochlorite solution before, during, and after surgical excision.[1145] Hypochlorite solution is virucidal against poxviruses. To date, topical cidofovir appears to be the drug of choice for the treatment of human orf.

Latest updates on diagnosis and treatment of AIDS are available from the website of the AIDS Treatment Information Service (ATIS) at http://www.hivatis.org, or from ATIS (telephone: 800-448-0440 or www.hopkins-aids.edu).

MILKERS' NODULE (Paravaccinia Virus, Pseudo-Cowpox)

Diagnosis

Edward Jenner, in his "Inquiry into the Causes and Effects of the Variolae Vaccinae" in 1798, was the first to observe that pustular material from the lesions of cowpox, when inoculated into humans, protected them from infection with smallpox. A related bovine disease is termed *pseudo-cowpox* because the disease demonstrates similar symptoms in cows but fails to protect humans from smallpox. Pseudo-cowpox is caused by the paravaccinia virus. In humans, this virus causes milker's nodule of the hand. Milkers usually acquire hand infection from the cow's infected udder through direct contact or indirectly through contaminated objects.[1135] Milkers' nodule is usually regarded as an occupational disease of dairy farm workers.[1070] The initial lesion is on the exposed part of the hand and upper extremity in more than 50% of cases.[1067] The incidence of milkers' nodule has fallen since the majority of cows are now milked by machine.

The bovine virus is morphologically indistinguishable from the ovine orf virus.[1106] When the animal source is unknown, or in doubt, it is not possible to clinically differentiate between ovine and bovine nodular lesions on the exposed hand and upper extremity and under the electron microscope. Diagnosis of the disease is based largely on knowledge of the animal source.[1106] Shelley has thus proposed a collective term *farmyard pox*[1137] when the source is unknown.[1067]

Treatment

Orf and milkers' nodule are easily recognized by those working with sheep and cows. The understanding that the disease spontaneously resolves in 6 weeks inclines many patients not to seek medical attention. When a physician who is unaware of such a lesion encounters one, misdiagnosis and mistreatment may occur.

SOURCES FOR UPDATES ON DIAGNOSIS AND TREATMENT OF AIDS

Contact the AIDS Treatment Information Service (ATIS) at http://www.hivatis.org or ATIS (telephone 800-448-0440) or the Centers for Disease Control and Prevention, 1600 Clifton Rd., Atlanta, GA 30333 (telephone 404-639-3534 or 800-311-3435 or http://www.cdc.gov/ or www.hopkins-aids.edu) for additional information.

ANNOTATED REFERENCES

1036. Bunney MH, Nolan MH, Williams DM: An assessment of methods of treating viral warts by comparative treatment trials based on a standard design. Br J Dermatol 94:667-677, 1976.

This study is valuable because it is statistically well designed. It has a large random sample (n = 1800) and a minimum follow-up of 12 weeks. The study was prospectively done by a dermatologist and a statistician from Edinburgh University with comparison of results from two centers. They found no statistically significant difference between the percentage of patients cured with hand warts treated with liquid nitrogen (69%) and those who applied a paint containing salicylic acid and lactic acid (67%) at 3-month follow-up. Liquid nitrogen freezing is painful, and patients prefer salicylic acid paint.

1042. Ching V, Ritz M, Song C, et al: Human immunodeficiency virus infection in an emergency hand service. J Hand Surg [Am] 21:696-700, 1996.

This article highlights the severity of hand infections in AIDS. Five of fourteen AIDS patients with upper extremity infections required multiple débridements. Finally the sepsis could be controlled with amputation of a finger in four and the forearm in one. Patients with low CD4+ counts (<500/mL) required more aggressive management and more operations.

1061. Geerinck K, Lukito G, Snoeck R, et al: A case of human orf in an immunocompromised patient treated successfully with cidofovir cream. J Med Virol 64:543-549, 2001.

1076. Hunskaar S: A case of erythema contagiosum (human orf) treated with idoxuridine. Dermatologica 168:207, 1984.

1127. Roy-Boulos AM, Akhtar M, Bendl B: Human orf (ecthyma contagiosum): A report of two cases from Saudi Arabia. Ann Saudi Med 6:49-52, 1996.

These three articles are a reminder that orf normally resolves in 6 weeks in immunocompetent subjects but manifests as a vigorously proliferative giant lesion in an immunocompromised patient. The lesion may be misdiagnosed as a malignant tumor and mistakenly treated with amputation. The lesion is curable with application of topical antiviral agents.

1063. Glickel SZ: Hand infections in patients with acquired immunodeficiency syndrome. J Hand Surg [Am] 13:770, 1988.

This article marks the identification of hand infections in AIDS by an author who was in the midst of the AIDS epidemic in New York City. His message is clear: Beware of AIDS when unusual infections are caused by usual organisms, and beware that unusual hand infections may precede the diagnosis of overt AIDS because a majority of patients harboring HIV infection are unaware that they have HIV disease.

1066. Gonzalez MH, Nikoleit J, Weinzweig N, Pulvirenti J: Upper extremity infections in patients with the human immunodeficiency virus. J Hand Surg [Am] 23:348-352, 1998.

In this article, the authors have three messages. First, the duration of herpetic lesions of digits was longer than 6 months and did not respond to intravenous acyclovir but responded to intravenous foscarnet. Second, necrotizing fasciitis required two to seven débridements in five patients and one patient required forequarter amputation to control the infection. Finally, all intravenous drug abusers tested positive for hepatitis B and C.

1087. Leavell UW, McNamara MJ, Muelling R: Orf: Report of 19 human cases with clinical and pathological observations. JAMA 203:657-664, 1968.

This article traces the natural history of orf in humans with normal immunity. The authors divide the lesions into six stages, with natural healing in an average of 36 days without a scar. Electron microscopy confirmed the presence of poxvirus in the lesion.

1089. LeBoit PE, Berger TG, Egbert BM: Bacillary angiomatosis. Am J Surg Pathol 13:909, 1989.

This is a landmark article on cutaneous vascular proliferation that clinically and pathologically resembles Kaposi's sarcoma, pyogenic granuloma, or histiocytoid (epithelioid) hemangioma in an AIDS patient. It was so named at the height of AIDS epidemic from San Francisco. It is clinically very important because these lesions are easily treatable with antibiotic therapy, including erythromycin. The infecting organism was later identified as *Bartonella henselae.*

1098. Massing AM, Epstein WL: Natural history of warts: A two year study. Arch Dermatol 87:306-310, 1963.

This rarely quoted article is worthwhile for those who treat warts. In this study, 50% of warts completely resolved in 1 year and 67% in 2 years without any treatment in a follow-up study of 1000 institutionalized, mentally defective children, ranging in age from 4 to 20. The children were examined three times a year for 2 years.

1099. McAuliffe JA, Seltzer DG, Hornicek FJ: Upper-extremity infections in patients seropositive for human immunodeficiency virus. J Hand Surg [Am] 22:1084-1090, 1997.

This paper presents one of the largest experiences in hand infections in AIDS patients. Seventy four patients were admitted a total of 97 times for the treatment of 89 different infections and underwent 120 surgical procedures. One third of the patients (26) required more than one operation and 11 (12%) required amputation.

1110. Parish LC, Monroe E: Treatment of common warts with high potency salicylic acid. Clin Ther 10:462-466, 1988.

This is one of many ways to control an ugly looking lesion on the hand. In this study 50% of the lesions were cured or improved in a week and 80% of the patients were cured in 2 weeks. The polyacrylic vehicle that carries salicylic acid (Occlusal HP) eliminates the need for bandaging the treated areas, unlike collodion-based products. Good compliance is the key to success in treating warts with keratolytic agents, and with rapid resolution and no need for bandaging improves compliance with this method.

1137. Shelley WB, Shelley ED: Farmyard pox: Parapox virus infection in man. Br J Dermatol 108:725-727, 1983.

This is an important article because it emphasized that orf and milker's nodule are the same disease caused by the same virus; the former is caused by contact with sheep or goats and the latter is caused by milking cows. The term *farmyard pox* is thus an appropriate one for this parapox virus infection, also known as pseudo-cowpox.

1151. Williams HC, Pottier A, Strachan D: The descriptive epidemiology of warts in British schoolchildren. Br J Dermatol 128:504-511, 1993.

This is a study of the natural course of warts in British schoolchildren. Of the 364 children noted to have warts at the age of 11, 93% no longer had warts at 16. This is a solace for parents whose children have anxiety about their warts.

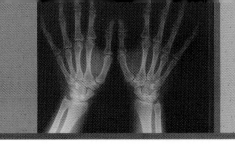

CHAPTER 5

Dupuytren's Contracture

D. A. McGrouther

The application of new science has given us a much better understanding of the biologic processes in Dupuytren's disease (DD), leading to a more logical approach to treatment; surgery remains the mainstay of management of the contracture, although some minimally invasive approaches have been introduced for selected cases.

An enormous number of different operative techniques are in use, extending from simple division of contracted tissue (fasciotomy) to limited or more radical excision (various types of fasciectomy). The fact that these very different approaches can be equally effective means that there must be some common influence on the disease process over and above that of simply cutting it out.

From the patient's point of view, as the disease develops, flexion contracture results in a progressive loss of hand function. For the hand surgeon, the disease presents a fascinating technical challenge that requires careful dissection amid the complex anatomy of the hand. Many factors will contribute to treatment outcome: the rate of onset and stage of the disease, technical performance of the operation, the therapy program, and patient "motivation." The preoperative consultation will set the course for the entire episode, and it is important for the surgeon to have the appropriate background to enable questions to be answered and proper informed consent to be given. In this chapter I will review what is known about the biology of the condition and try to rationalize surgical treatment.

THE NATURE OF DUPUYTREN'S DISEASE

Biologic Behavior

Although first reported by Henry Cline and Astley Cooper of London, just credit is given to Baron Guillaume Dupuytren, who described the treatment of this malady by operative demonstration of contracture release before a class of medical students.[41, 44] The patient was operated on in a seated position with the hand elevated. No tourniquet was used, and no anesthetic, as we now understand it, was available.

Dupuytren stood behind the patient because in this position it is less easy for the patient to withdraw the arm, and he performed a simple release of the contracted fascia, which was probably all that was possible under the circumstances. (Following the procedure the patient was described as *très faible*.) Perhaps the major lesson of history is the controversy set up by Dupuytren, who advocated simple *division* of cords (*fasciotomy*), whereas Goyrand[55] advised *removal* of palmar fascia (*fasciectomy*). This disagreement still exists despite all the sophistication of modern technique,[98] but it points the way to our understanding of the nature of the condition.

Dupuytren's disease is a condition of the hand characterized by the development of new tissue in the form of nodules and cords.[89] This new tissue is of great biologic interest inasmuch as it seems to have some features in common with benign neoplastic fibromatosis[97,133] and yet undergoes an evolution, through contraction and maturation, similar to wound-healing tissue. It is now appreciated that digital contracture may be preceded by the appearance of nodules and cords in the palm and fingers, and the description *Dupuytren's disease* is fashionable, but it is not clear whether there is a single entity or a number of diseases resulting in the same pathologic features. The disease has certainly acquired a nomenclature all its own; the tendency to get it has been termed a *diathesis*,[65] the new cellular masses are often called *Dupuytren's tissue,* and even the terms *fascia, fasciotomy,* and *fasciectomy* are time-honored rather than specific descriptions.

The *site* of onset is the fibrofatty layer between the skin and deep structures of the palmar surface of the hand, which has a precisely ordered system of subcutaneous ligamentous fibers. The abnormal fibromatous Dupuytren's tissue seems to develop within or around certain of the ligamentous strands that have a predominantly longitudinal orientation.

The description of Luck[89,135] remains a useful starting point for histopathologic understanding; the nodule was seen as the fundamental lesion. The term *nodule* has become confused and is used both in the *clinical* sense of a palpable subcutaneous lump and in the *histologic* sense of a collection of cells in a whorled pattern (a much smaller focus than

The author would like to acknowledge **Robert M. McFarlane**, not only for his superbly written chapters in the first three editions of this book, but also for his major contributions to our understanding of Dupuytren's contracture.

the clinical nodule and not palpable). Even the clinical nodule is not a homogeneous entity. Some nodules appear to arise principally from longitudinal contraction of the underlying fascia, which bunches up the skin to form a nodule.[46,104] Others seem to be due more to a space-occupying lesion pushing upward on the skin, and the major components of such a nodule are cell proliferation and connective tissue matrix. Nodules do not occur randomly but at precise positions, generally in the lines of the digital rays in the palm or digit; *Dupuytren's disease seems to follow certain anatomic pathways determined by longitudinal tension lines.* Luck viewed the nodule as the "powerhouse" of the contracture and an evolutionary lesion of the disease that later matures to form a *cord.* This may account for some cord formation, but an alternative explanation is that normal bands (the convention is to use the term *band* for a normal palmar fascial structure and *cord* for a diseased band) hypertrophy and thicken in response to increased tension. McFarlane,[95] in a key article, showed the way in which Dupuytren's disease propagates from one anatomic structure to another to form a longitudinal contracted cord.

Cell and Molecular Mechanisms

Luck's classification[89] of the disease into three phases has been widely accepted: *proliferative* phase characterized by cell proliferation "with no purposeful arrangement," *involutional* phase in which fibroblasts show alignment along tension lines, and *residual* phase in which tissue is largely acellular and tendon-like. To fit Dupuytren's disease into the current knowledge of pathogenetic mechanisms it is possible to reduce Luck's plan to two separate but overlapping processes: proliferation and mechanotransduction. There is clearly a *proliferative process* characterized by immature fibroblasts, many of which are myofibroblasts,[50, 129,133] in a characteristic whorl pattern. Myofibroblasts produce an extracellular matrix with predominantly type I collagen and fibronectin, laminin, type IV collagen, and tenascin as constituents.[17] Moreover, the myofibroblast phenotype and growth factors are mainly localized to the active proliferative nodules[18,38,63] and myofibroblast cytoskeletal characteristics persist in culture. The cell of origin for the masses of proliferation is unknown, but the vascular pericyte has been suggested.[78] Other cell types have been recognized in Dupuytren's tissue: Langerhans cells[123] and T and B lymphocytes.[56] Evidence is certainly accumulating for raised levels in Dupuytren's tissue of growth factors known to stimulate fibroblasts[5,10,69,80,145]; interleukin-1, basic fibroblast growth factor, transforming growth factor (TGF)-β_1, TGF-β_2, epidermal growth factor (EGF), platelet-derived growth factor (PDGF), and connective tissue growth factor (CTGF) have been suggested to have a role. At the present time there is no clear knowledge of what starts the proliferation phase, although speculation includes rupture of fascial fibers[45,136] and an inflammatory process with adhesions between ligamentous structures.[2,104] A different glycosaminoglycan profile, in uninvolved fascia from patients with Dupuytren's disease, suggests some sort of predisposition in certain individuals.[151] Genetic susceptibility to Dupuytren's disease has been associated with a *ZF9* gene polymorphism.[13] This transcription factor increases TGF-β_1 expression, a known fibrogenic growth factor, although polymorphisms of TGF-$\beta1$[12] or TGF-β_2[11] were not found. This illustrates the complexity

in understanding a genetic component in this condition, and it seems likely that multiple genes are involved.

The understanding that there is a proliferative component to the pathogenesis has resulted in trials of antiproliferatve drugs such as 5-fluorouracil[71] and radiotherapy.[134]

The second *mechanical process* demonstrates the phenomenon of mechanical transduction whereby the cellular tissue once formed responds to the mechanical environment, a process by which physical forces (tension or compression) and cellular events (gene expression) are linked. As a result, cell motility, shape, and differentiation and the production of matrix and other proteins are influenced by the forces acting on the cell. In a series of elegant experiments on tendons, Flint[45] showed that connective tissues respond to tensile and compressive loads. Lateral force on a tendon where it passes around a bony prominence results in differentiation toward cartilage, whereas allowing the tendon to bowstring by cutting retinacular structures restores longitudinal uniaxial load with a return to tensile tendinous structure.

Cell culture experiments provide some clues about what is happening. Fibroblasts respond not only to chemical signals,[4] growth factors, and cytokines but also to physical mechanical stimulation.[125] In fact, they appear to perceive strain and try to "hide" from it by aligning along isostrain lines when grown in collagen gel.[42] Curiously, in general not only do fibroblasts respond to force but they also generate it as though there is an optimum level of strain that they enjoy, and they will influence their microenvironment to bring this about; fibroblasts exhibit tensional homeostasis.[26] Collagen lattice contraction studies have shown a correlation between the expression of α smooth muscle actin, that is, the myofibroblast phenotype, and the generation of contractile force,[147] but we remain uncertain about exactly how contraction occurs.

Tension in Dupuytren's disease seems to be important: it acts intermittently on Dupuytren's tissue as the digits are actively extended against the passive restraint of the tethered palmar fascial ligaments. This degree of "tension" seems in some way to "perpetuate" the disease process. Tomasek and colleagues[148] have shown that TGF-β_1 combined with mechanical stress can promote differentiation of fibroblasts into myofibroblasts. The work of Messina[111] is biologically important inasmuch as it has shown that greatly increasing tension by an external fixator can result in remodeling of contractile tissue, with subsequent lengthening of fascia and extension of the digit. The biochemical mechanism seems to be an increase in the level of degradative enzymes, neutral metalloproteinases, and acid cathepsins and an increase in newly synthesized collagen to allow extension.[9,144] This is what surgeons would call "remodeling."

By contrast, fasciotomy releases tension and causes softening of the residual nodules. We therefore have the seeming paradox that an increase in tension causes lengthening of contracted tissues whereas reducing tension in the fascia causes resolution of nodules. Much more needs to be done, but there is enough fundamental knowledge now to indicate that *the aim of treatment is not simply radical excision.*

There will be further development of our understanding of these pathogenetic mechanisms pointing the way toward new treatment strategies. Early in-vitro and clinical studies of collagenase injection show promise.[7,142] Meanwhile, the standard management is to relieve contracture by surgery.

The Questions Patients Will Ask

Is There a Cause-and-Effect Relationship?

A simple cause-and-effect relationship has long been sought, and Dupuytren's disease has been linked in often anecdotal literature to almost every fashionable etiologic concept, including neurosyphilis,[136] pulmonary tuberculosis, and, more recently, free radicals[88] and human immunodeficiency virus (HIV) infection,[22] but the vast majority of patients with Dupuytren's disease do not suffer from any of these conditions. Essentially it remains an idiopathic disorder. A link to diabetes is accepted,[3] but this type of Dupuytren's disease has a slightly different form, seemingly more widespread, especially on the radial digits, and often less progressive. Alcohol is forever linked with Dupuytren's disease in the minds of medical students; this remains a controversial association,[29,59,68] as does tobacco consumption. The increased incidence in patients with epilepsy may be due to the drugs rather than to the disease.[68] The significance of these studies to the surgeon is that there is no mandatory requirement to order batteries of laboratory tests for patients with Dupuytren's disease unless otherwise indicated by the history and general medical examination. There is also no evidence of benefit to the hand by treating disease or altering alcohol or tobacco consumption.

Occupation or Injury?

Because Dupuytren's disease affects the hand, occupational use is an obvious target for association. Dupuytren himself related contracture to heavy use in one patient, a coachman, and to trauma in another, a wine merchant who felt a cracking on lifting a barrel many years before. Neither of these suggestions of occupational use[39,109] or trauma[75] have withstood scientific scrutiny. Vibration is often suggested, but the contribution is uncertain.[86] The fact remains, however, that even if we attribute the disease to genes, it is necessary to explain why it should start at a particular age or even at different times in the two hands. Two sets of identical twins have been reported, only one partner of each having Dupuytren's disease.[90] A single injury may seem to start it off in some patients,[74,81] and this can be of considerable medicolegal importance. McFarlane and Shum[101] have defined criteria for judging whether an injury is significant for this purpose. There is no clear evidence that a patient should change his or her lifestyle or occupational use after a Dupuytren's operation, although common sense may be more appropriate than science here.

Is Dupuytren's Disease Genetically Determined?

What epidemiologic studies are available have suggested that it is a condition common in populations of Northern European extraction. In an extensive survey of the population of Iceland the prevalence of Dupuytren's disease has been reported as 7.2% at age 45 to 49, rising to 39.5% at age 70 to 74.[58] In one study a reported incidence in relatives of 16% rose to 68% when the relatives were examined.[85] Autosomal dominant inheritance is seen in some pedigrees, but other modes of inheritance occur and there are many sporadic cases.[30] It is rare in children.[153]

The racial distribution in Veterans Administration patients[139] is reported as a prevalence of 130/100,000 in blacks, 734/100,000 in whites, 237/100,000 in Hispanics, 144/100,000 in Native Americans, and 67/100,000 in Asians. McFarlane[102] has cast doubt on the often-quoted hypothesis that the disease is linked to Viking migrations of the 9th to 13th centuries and that it existed in Europe before then. Surgeons in Africa, India, and Asia rarely see it, although Indian patients living in Birmingham, England, are now contracting the disease,[140] which raises the intriguing possibility that there is an environmental influence acting over a long term. It is not at all clear whether the outcome of surgery is different in different population groups. Certainly, formal studies of postoperative results in the long term suggest a very high incidence of recurrence and progression in all continents. Recent epidemiologic data[60,112,157] suggest that patients with Dupuytren's contracture followed over a 15-year time cycle show an increased mortality from a range of cancers. This finding needs much further corroboration to see if there are common genetic mechanisms, such as progressive mutations.

Good news for patients is that there is a negative association with joint complaints.[57]

Surgical Anatomy of the Palmar Fascia

Palmar fascia is not fascia, nor is it just palmar! What the hand possesses is a three-dimensional system of fine ligamentous structures, each with a precise origin and insertion and all together constituting a fibrous tissue continuum[20,73,104,113,141] (Fig. 5-1). This can be regarded as a fibrous skeleton or framework providing guide channels and retinacular restraint for longitudinally running structures and also as a system that anchors the skin while still allowing it to flex and extend. Altogether, it is like a chassis or airframe. For convenience and understanding, parts of this continuum are named separately, although there is considerable merging and convergence.

The lesions of Dupuytren's disease do not occur in a random pattern, but the pathologic process seems to follow certain well-defined anatomic pathways through the fibrous tissue continuum of the hand, as determined by longitudinal lines of tension. The principal longitudinal pathway comprises the fibers of insertion of the palmaris longus or, when this is absent, the longitudinal fibers of the palmar fascia merge with the deep fascia of the forearm or the anterior surface of the flexor retinaculum. Following the longitudinal fibers in a proximal-to-distal direction, the anatomic arrangement in a normal hand is such that in the mid palm (just distal to the distal palmar crease) the longitudinal fibers pass distally in three layers (the individual structures are reviewed in detail by McFarlane[96] and McGrouther[106]):

Layer 1: The most superficial fibers insert into the skin of the distal palm (midway between the distal palmar crease and the proximal digital crease [see Fig. 5-1A]; Zancolli[159] described fibers that pass distally in the palmar midline of the digit). The insertion into skin is progressively more proximal on passing from the ulnar to the radial side of

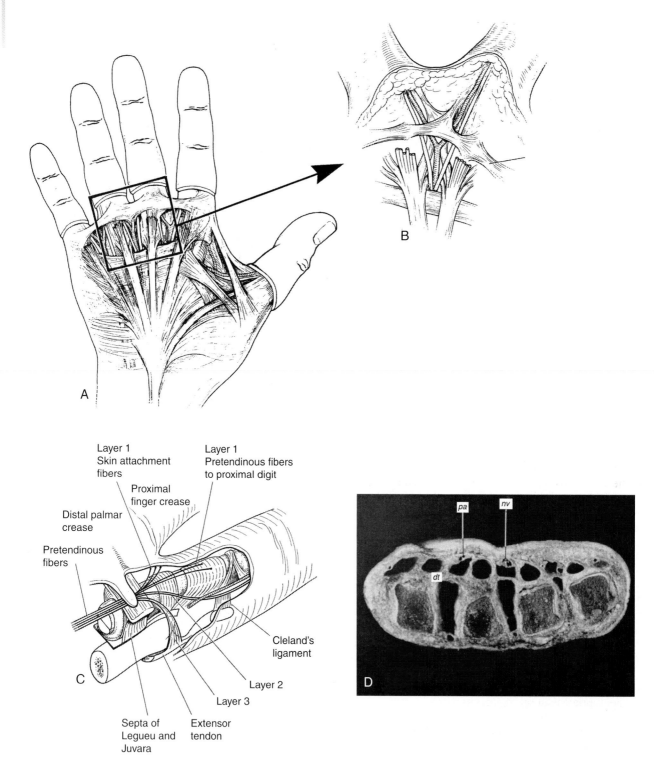

FIGURE 5-1. The components of the palmar fascia (**A**) with a magnified view of the structures in an interdigital web (**B**). The longitudinal pretendinous fibers are shown passing anterior to the transverse fibers of the palmar fascia and then dividing into three layers. The most anterior layer inserts into the distal palm, the second layer passes distally as the spiral band of Gosset to reach the lateral digital sheet. Layer 3 passes on either side of the MP joints to deeper planes. These structures are represented diagrammatically (**C**). **D,** Cross section of the hand at the level of the metacarpal heads, showing the palmar fascial continuum, contributed to by the above fibers and retaining all structures in place. The subdivision of the distal part of the central compartment into eight narrow compartments is demonstrated. The interdigital nerves and vessels (nv) have been left to show their relation to the lumbrical compartments. dt, deep transverse metacarpal ligament; pa, palmar aponeurosis. (**A-C,** From McGrouther DA: The palm. *In* McFarlane RM, McGrouther DA, Flint MH [eds]: Dupuytren's Disease. Biology and Treatment, Vol. 5. The Hand and Upper Limb Series. Edinburgh, Churchill Livingstone, 1990, pp 127-135. **D,** from Bojsen-Moller F, Schmidt L: The palmar aponeurosis and the central spaces of the hand. J Anat 117:55-68, 1974, with permission.)

the hand, which may be one of many reasons why contracture is more common in the ulnar fingers.

Layer 2: The spiral fibers pass on either side of the flexor tendon deep to the neurovascular bundle to reach the lateral digital sheet (see Fig. 5-1B). In their course these fibers therefore pass through several structures, which form a continuum, but our understanding is improved by considering them as separate entities; in a proximal-to-distal direction they are the longitudinal fibers of the palmar fascia, the spiral fibers of Gosset,[54] which in the normal hand may be a very flimsy sheet, and the lateral fascia in the digit, which has been variously described as a retrovascular band or a lateral digital sheet. This receives fibers from the natatory ligaments (which arch around the skin webs) and gives fibers to Cleland's ligaments (which anchor the digital skin to the proximal interphalangeal [PIP] and distal interphalangeal [DIP] joints) posterior to the neurovascular bundles and Grayson's ligaments anterior to the neurovascular bundles.

Layer 3: The deepest longitudinal fibers of the palmar fascia pass deeply on either side of the flexor tendons and on either side of the metacarpophalangeal (MP) joints (see Fig. 5-1C). Zancolli[159] has described the deep course of these fibers.

The importance for the surgeon of this anatomic arrangement is that the different layers of a Dupuytren contracture can be followed distally as separate layers 1, 2, and 3, thus presenting a more logical approach to excision than simply preserving neurovascular bundles and excising all else.

There are safe surgical landmarks. Skoog[138] has shown that the contracture can be dissected from the anterior surface of the transverse fibers of the palmar aponeurosis (Fig. 5-2) (which extend as far distally as the distal palmar crease and are now often termed the *palmar aponeurosis pulley of Manske*[92]), with these fibers left intact and thus ensuring that at this level in the distal palm the neurovascular bundles are safe in their tunnels deep to these fibers. Following the contracture distally it is possible by gentle blunt dissection to recognize the three layers of the longitudinal fibers. Layer 2 (the spiral cord) is the one that, as it contracts, characteristically displaces the neurovascular bundle in the manner described by McFarlane.[95] Within the digit the normal fascial structures lie laterally. McFarlane has shown the way in which contracture runs through the anatomic pathways (Figs. 5-3 and 5-4) to form different patterns of cord contraction as follows:

The *central cord* (Figs. 5-4 and 5-5) essentially follows layer 1 but passes farther distally, following the longitudinal pretendinous fibers in the palm and passing to the digit either through the midline fibers described by Zancolli[159] or through the deep dermis and resulting in skin involvement.[104] This cord attaches to the base of the middle phalanx, usually on one or the other side and often the tendon sheath.

The *lateral cord* runs from the natatory ligament (anterior to the neurovascular bundle) to the lateral digital sheet. It does not usually cause PIP joint contracture, but on the ulnar side of the little finger it attaches to an abductor cord overlying the abductor digiti minimi and can cause severe PIP joint flexion. White[156] has described the fascial structures on the ulnar side of the palm in detail.

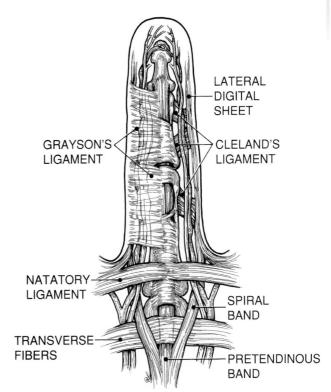

FIGURE 5-2. Parts of the normal digital fascia that become diseased. Grayson's ligament is shown on the left. It is an almost continuous sheet of thin fascia and is in the same plane as the natatory ligament. Cleland's ligament is shown on the right. It does not become diseased. The lateral digital sheet receives fibers from the natatory ligament as well as the spiral band. The spiral bands pass on either side of the MP joint, deep to the neurovascular bundles, to reach the side of the finger. (From McFarlane RM: Patterns of the diseased fascia in the fingers in Dupuytren's contracture. Plast Reconstr Surg 54:31-44, 1974, with permission.)

The *spiral cord* (see Figs. 5-4 and 5-6) arises from the longitudinal pretendinous fibers and follows layer 2 through the spiral cord (Gosset[54]) to the lateral digital sheet. From there it gains attachment to the middle phalanx by Grayson's ligament. Strickland and Bassett[143] have demonstrated that a deep digital cord may arise from the base of the proximal phalanx or the intrinsic tendons and therefore not be obvious in the palm.

In the first web space the structures generally involved[62] are the natatory ligament in the free edge of the web (also known as the distal commissural ligament) or the proximal commissural ligament, which lies parallel and proximal to the natatory ligament in continuity with the transverse fibers of the palmar aponeurosis. In addition to these essentially transverse structures there are longitudinal fibers, but because these largely insert on the radial side of the thumb, flexion of the thumb joints is uncommon. There are individual variations in the arrangement of all of these structures.

The major anatomic hazard for the surgeon is displacement of the neurovascular bundle, which can occur at any point between its proximal fixed position in the mid palm (under the transverse fibers of the palmar aponeurosis) and a second fixed position at the base of the middle phalanx, where the nerve is held laterally by Grayson's ligament (Fig. 5-7). Between these two fixed points the nerve bundle can be markedly displaced to or across the digital midline

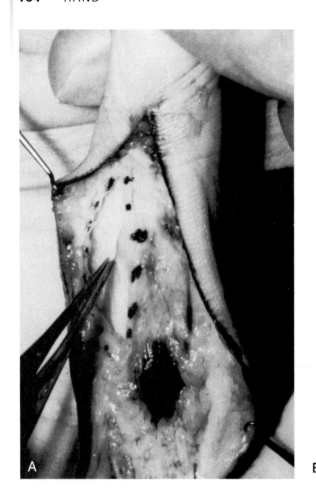

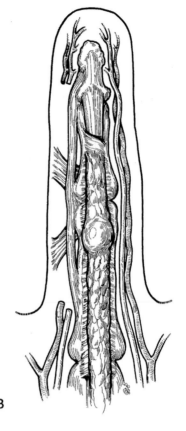

FIGURE 5-3. **A,** An unusually prominent retrovascular cord lies deep to
the neurovascular bundle, which is
marked with dots. **B,** The cord arises
from the periosteum on the side of the
proximal phalanx, courses very close
to the capsule of the PIP joint, and
attaches to the side of the distal phalanx. It is an occasional cause of
flexion contracture at the PIP joint
and the usual cause of DIP joint contracture. (Courtesy of Dr. R. M.
McFarlane.)

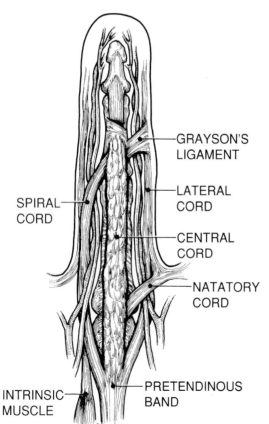

FIGURE 5-4. The change in the normal fascia bands to diseased cords. The
pretendinous cord causes MP joint contracture, and the others cause PIP
joint contracture. When the natatory cord is diseased, it becomes adherent
to the pretendinous cord. As it is drawn proximally, it appears to bifurcate
from the pretendinous cord. Grayson's ligament is diseased in two ways.
On the right it is shown simply thickened. On the left it has contributed to
the attachment of the spiral cord onto the flexor tendon sheath. (Courtesy
of Dr. R. M. McFarlane.)

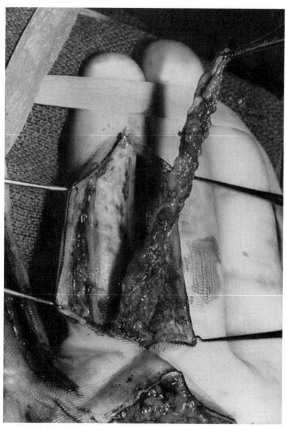

FIGURE 5-5. There is a variable amount of fibrofatty tissue between the neurovascular bundles in the finger that becomes the central cord when diseased. (Courtesy of Dr. R. M. McFarlane.)

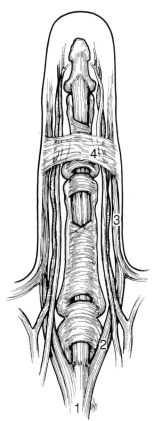

FIGURE 5-6. The parts of the normal fascia that compose the spiral cord: (1) pretendinous band, (2) spiral band, (3) lateral digital sheet, (4) Grayson's ligament. (From McFarlane RM: Patterns of the diseased fascia in the fingers in Dupuytren's contracture. Plast Reconstr Surg 54:31-44, 1974, with permission.)

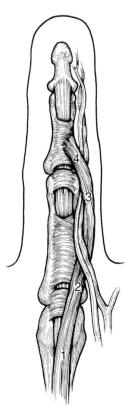

FIGURE 5-7. With contraction, the spiral cord straightens and the neurovascular bundle spirals around it and is displaced toward the midline. 1, pretendinous band; 2, spiral band; 3, lateral digital sheet; 4, Grayson's ligament. (From McFarlane RM: Patterns of the diseased fascia in the fingers in Dupuytren's contracture. Plast Reconstr Surg 54:31-44, 1974, with permission.)

(Fig. 5-8). Although there is difficulty in predicting the position in individual cases, displacement is particularly likely in a severely flexed digit.[154] As the fascia is progressively excised, the surgeon must be certain that the neurovascular bundle is preserved (Fig. 5-9). Different surgeons vary in the amount of exposure they use to achieve this end.

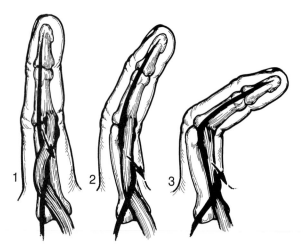

FIGURE 5-8. The neurovascular bundle is displaced in three directions with increasing PIP joint contracture: (1) toward the midline; (2) proximally; (3) superficially. (Courtesy of Dr. R. M. McFarlane.)

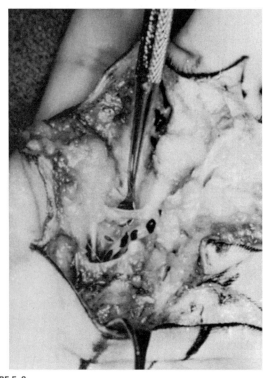

FIGURE 5-9. Displacement of the neurovascular bundle almost at the distal crease of the palm due to a spiral cord contracture. The MP joint was flexed 70 degrees and the PIP joint was flexed 90 degrees. The nerve is dotted and the artery is supported by the instrument. Both are immediately subcutaneous and thus in danger of being cut when the skin is incised. (Courtesy of Dr. R. M. McFarlane.)

SURGICAL MANAGEMENT OF DUPUYTREN'S DISEASE

There is no perfect operation for Dupuytren's disease or even one approach that is clearly better than another, at least not in the published literature. Much emphasis has been placed on surgical technique, but the outcome of treatment depends not so much on the knife alone as on an integrated treatment plan taking into account case selection, timing of surgery, the patient's expectations modified by the informed consent process, the actual operation, and the postoperative rehabilitation program, including splinting.

Aims of Treatment

There is currently strong evidence that Dupuytren's disease is a genetic disease. The genes cannot be surgically removed! It is therefore wrong to contemplate a lasting cure. The patient can potentially be helped by surgery, but equally there is a potential to make the patient worse, so a careful decision is advised before embarking on operative treatment. An operation is not merely excision of a lump or mass of pathologic tissue. It is impossible to define where the lesion stops. A margin of clearance is not possible, and in any case the residual tissues seem to be capable of mounting the same response of nodules, cords, and contracture. The fascination of Dupuytren's surgery is that the curious biologic behavior does not require the wide resection that would be appropriate in oncology; such an approach would not in any event be possible. The key aim is to achieve an alteration in the biomechanics of the hand to shield any residual DD tissue from tensile forces, and this seems to be the common principle of all surgery. Simply *cutting* a cord may achieve this successfully in a hand with otherwise well-preserved anatomy inasmuch as the divided cord will retract into fat, the ends will be separated, and force transmission will be prevented. When the tissues of the hand are rigid and infiltrated, *resection* will be necessary to separate the divided ends of the palmar fascial ligamentous structures. When skin is heavily involved, it will need to be replaced or separated by a firebreak to interpose a segment of healthy uninvolved tissue that will break up lines of longitudinal tension through Dupuytren's tissue. In fact, the surgeon is challenged to reconstruct the hand in such a way to avoid any of the wound-healing tissues or residual Dupuytren's cells being subjected to tractional forces. This is analogous to the challenge of release of a post-burn contracture of the hand. All wound and scar lines and graft edges should be zigzagged or placed in the neutral lateral skin lines to limit tensional forces on the wound-healing (and Dupuytren's) fibroblasts.

An operation has a *potential to do good* through release of joint contractures, possibly through the actual removal of Dupuytren's tissue and possibly by interposing healthy tissue between the ends of cords and nodules to prevent them from linking up again.

However, surgery has a significant *potential to do harm* through inadvertent division of digital nerves or vessels, creation of PIP joint hyperextension, and problems in wound healing with the triad of hematoma, skin necrosis, and infection. In addition, treatment may be followed by stiffness

CRITICAL POINTS: INDICATIONS AND TIMING OF OPERATIVE TREATMENT

INDICATIONS

- Definite progression of contracture
- Functional disability

PREOPERATIVE EVALUATION

- Consider the condition of the hand tissues, the rate and extent of the contracture, and the likely compliance of the patient.
- Select, advise, and warn!

PEARLS

- Understand the three anatomic layers of palmar fascial ligaments: the contracture follows anatomic structures.
- Surgery can release the contracture, but it cannot remove the genes. Expect recurrence.
- The aim of surgery is release: Dupuytren's tissue cannot be totally excised.

TECHNICAL POINTS

- For MP joint contracture
  - Release in mid palm.
  - Preserve transverse fibers of palmar aponeurosis.
  - Excise contracted longitudinal cords.
  - Limited dissection of 1 to 2 cm is effective; there is no evidence that more extensive surgery reduces recurrence.
  - Use loose wound closure; avoid hematoma.
- For PIP joint contracture
  - Excise fascia in proximal digit using non-straight-line incision.
  - Or dermofasciectomy excising skin fat and fascia.
  - Identify the neurovascular bundles (likely to be displaced) proximally.
- Dissect and preserve neurovascular bundles by blunt and sharp dissection.
- Close skin with Z plasties (or similar) or replace with full-thickness graft from upper arm as a fire-break.
- Identify neurovascular bundles by initial transverse incision at proximal digital crease.
- Dissect and preserve neurovascular bundles by blunt and sharp dissection.
- Use full-thickness graft from upper arm.
- Fixed joint contracture despite fasciectomy
  - Less than 40 degrees: persistent contracture—accept
  - More than 40 degrees: salvage procedure—possible arthrodesis

PITFALLS

- Nerve division: the neurovascular bundles can be displaced to or across the midline.
- Artery division: critical ischemia may occur if both digital arteries are damaged.
- The surgery is more difficult, recovery longer, and recurrence more common than the patient imagines!

POSTOPERATIVE CARE

- The amount of rehabilitation required is very variable.
- Spot the patient whose hand is becoming stiff and intervene with therapy and night splintage.

FUNCTIONAL USE

- The patient is advised to do no heavy work or sports requiring gripping for 6 to 12 weeks.

---

with or without reflex sympathetic dystrophy and increasing stiffness elsewhere in the hand.

For the hand surgeon it is important to have a concept of the nature of the disease and to then derive a plan of management appropriate to the surgeon's own practice and rehabilitation facilities. As a general rule, patients and surgeons underestimate what is involved in recovery from Dupuytren's surgery and may overestimate the benefits to be derived from surgery.

Clinical Findings

The disease may be diagnosed when the patient appreciates that there is a *nodule* in the palm of the hand, or the condition may have been noted as an incidental finding on general physical examination for other purposes and the patient may have very little awareness and few symptoms. The general physician may send the patient along to "have his hand fixed." Frequently the patient will have been given a mistaken view about causation and treatment. A solitary nodule may remain unchanged for years and requires no action except perhaps occasional review. When a nodule is painful, corticosteroid injection can be tried.[76] Rarely, excision of a very tender solitary nodule is indicated when grip is inhibited. Corticosteroid injection may also be used for knuckle pads, and it is my policy to avoid operating on these lesions; they may regress spontaneously and do not cause functional problems.

Operative Indications

An operation for Dupuytren's contracture is not necessarily indicated immediately on diagnosis. It is important to demonstrate *loss of function* or *progression of disease* before submitting the patient to the time off work, inconvenience, cost, and discomfort of a procedure without a guaranteed long-term outcome.

Loss of Function

The patient may complain of flexion contracture, particularly when progression has been relatively rapid. The contracture may cause difficulty with manipulative tasks or putting the hand into a pocket, problems with washing, or loss of function at work or recreational use. In addition, there may be embarrassment about the hand's role in communication, its appearance, or the shape of the hand in handshaking.

It is better to rely on functional difficulty and the rate of progression when deciding on surgery rather than choosing a set amount of joint contracture. McFarlane and Botz[99] have shown in a large patient survey that when the PIP joint contracture was less than 30 degrees the patient was more often made worse than better. Certainly, MP joint contracture can be corrected no matter how long lasting. By contrast, PIP joint flexion may not be correctable, and there is an impression that longer-lasting contractures are more difficult to release. However, this is not necessarily an argument for early aggressive surgery.

Rate of Progression

During consultation with the patient it is wise to try to establish a mental picture of the time course of progress in that particular hand. When did it start? Has it changed much in the past year? When was it last possible to place the hand flat on a tabletop? When there is no clear indication of recent progression in that hand, it is useful to chart the state of the deformity and review the patient after an interval, the timing of which can be judged from the history, but usually up to 6 months. If progress is then demonstrated by measurement, both parties will be in agreement about the need for intervention. If there is no significant progress, further review is indicated and serves to build the doctor-patient relationship, which is so important in this condition.

Patient Considerations

It is unwise to operate until the patient appreciates the full picture of the possible outcomes. Left alone, the natural history of the condition is probably deterioration in function because of progressive loss of finger extension. This is, however, by no means inevitable inasmuch as palmar nodules may remain relatively static over several years. The patient must appreciate that the condition is progressive and recurrent and that surgery can produce improvement that may be long lasting in some cases but may be quite short lasting in others (see the section on recurrence).

It is necessary to consider the patient, the hand, and the disease.

The Patient

For the *patient,* the prognosis for the disease is worse for the young, but although early radical surgery has often been advocated, there is no clear evidence that this is the best way to proceed. It is best to be steered by the rate of progression, and it is my own view to not vary operative procedure for age.

It is usual to ask about family history, not so much because it will affect treatment decisions as because it will condition the patient's expectation of outcome. "My brother had a simple operation and he was OK!"

Some patients should not have surgery for a variety of different reasons. The patient may be too frail or may have intercurrent pathology such as parkinsonism or a stroke, which limits possible rehabilitation. The patient may have unrealistic expectations or be unwilling to make the rehabilitation effort; beware of the patient who criticizes the last surgeon! The surgeon must consider how the patient is reacting to the disease. Is the digit being voluntarily flexed out of the way to allow function?

The Hand

For the *hand,* the surgeon must balance its severity of contraction and its importance to this patient: musicians, artists, or laborers will almost always be more motivated to rehabilitate the dominant hand. Douglas Lamb (personal communication, 1980) used to lecture "Beware of the sweating hand, it is likely to become stiff postoperatively," and beware of the warnings of a wise and experienced surgeon!

The Disease

How aggressive is the *disease* in this patient (i.e., is there a strong diathesis)? The age, duration, and speed of the contracting process can be assessed from the history, but the rate seems to be quite different in different patients. Intercurrent disease must be assessed; diabetes may suggest a milder course, and alcoholism may indicate difficulty in compliance with postoperative rehabilitation. The presence of the disease in other sites, knuckle pads, palmar fibromatosis, and Peyronie's disease suggests a more aggressive course.

Taking all of these factors into account, a decision will be made to operate or alternatively to keep the situation under review and consider an operation at a later stage if the situation deteriorates. It is wise to try to organize treatment at a time of the year when work and recreational demands are least disturbed.

Preoperative Information

It is advisable to tell the patient the following in general terms:

1. The condition is of unknown cause, it is possibly genetic, and the underlying disease tendency cannot be treated. The patient can be reassured, however, that the disease per se is not sinister, that is, it is not cancer, not malignant.
2. The purpose of the operation is to straighten the hand. Different surgeons vary in their approach regarding whether tissue is divided or excised. If palpable tissue is to be left behind, the patient should be informed.
3. The operation will result in scars.
4. The healing time is surprisingly long (surgeons are eternal optimists) and likely to require dressings for a minimum of 3 to 4 weeks or up to 6 weeks with a skin graft. A skin graft will leave a donor site scar. Full recovery takes *at least* 3 months.
5. There will be temporary loss of function and a need to be referred to a hand therapist.
6. There are possible complications. A nerve may be cut (1% to 3% in most series) despite the best efforts to avoid

this. Should this occur, there will be sensory loss and tingling. There is a definite risk of stiffness (with or without reflex dystrophy, which is a difficult condition to explain to a patient until it develops). In recurrent cases it is wise to mention the rare possibility that there may be damage to digital arteries resulting in a need to revascularize a digit [72] or even leading to loss of that digit.

7. The correction of flexion contracture may be incomplete.
8. The possibility of recurrence depends not only on the operation but also on the rehabilitation program and the patient's own diathesis.
9. The possibility of recurrence and extension is high—on the order of 50% after 5 to 10 years in most published series.

Operative Techniques

It is desirable to have a surgical plan that will be effective and yet as safe as possible. It must be recognized that a desire for wide exposure of vital structures to avoid damage will conflict with the aim of limiting tissue trauma and its subsequent inflammatory response in the hope of minimizing pain, stiffness, swelling, and scarring.

The surgeon must have a clear plan for each of the tissue layers that will be encountered, even though the operation will be an integrated intervention tackling all layers. It is necessary to consider three aspects of the surgical plan: (1) management of the skin, (2) management of the fascia, and (3) management of the joints, especially the PIP joint.

General Preparations for Surgery

As in all hand operations, preoperative preparation consists of adequate cleansing of skin and nails, which may be difficult in a chronically flexed digit. Skin intertrigo should be treated by antifungal medication. Many cases are now performed as outpatient cases,[91] although in an extensive operation it is better to elevate the hand overnight; and, when circulation is in doubt, it is mandatory to observe skin color for at least 24 hours. In my view, patients having operations for recurrent Dupuytren's disease are best admitted overnight. The choice of anesthetic will depend on the individual surgeon's preferences and practice, but general anesthesia and supraclavicular or axillary blocks are all in common use. For a localized procedure confined to one or two digital rays, a midpalmar block is possible by insinuating a needle beneath the ulnar side of the palmar longitudinal fascial fibers. An arm tourniquet should be used but will only be tolerated for 20 minutes if the tourniquet area is not anesthetized. When it seems likely that a more prolonged procedure will be necessary to identify vital structures or when the surgeon has limited experience, it is necessary to use one of the methods of anesthesia that ensures that tourniquet discomfort does not hasten the operative dissection (see Chapter 2). For a local block the tourniquet should not be inflated until after skin preparation, and this should be reserved for straightforward cases.

After skin preparation and draping, the hand is placed on the hand table supine and immobilized by a lead hand or other retraction system to apply an extension force to the flexed digits. Loupe magnification will facilitate the dissection.

Management of the Skin

Choices in management of the skin are *skin incision,* in which the skin is incised for exposure and then repositioned, and *skin excision.* If the decision is to excise and replace the skin cover, this will probably be done en bloc with the fascia as a dermofasciectomy, and the first choice for replacement skin cover is usually a skin graft, rarely a skin flap. The judgment about whether skin requires removal and replacement is an individual one. Some would do this at the first operation routinely, when there is a strong diathesis, or in recurrence, in rising order of general acceptance.

Skin Incision

In choosing a skin incision, of which there are many (Fig. 5-10), longitudinal incisions have the advantage of progressive extensile exposure whereas transverse incisions are less likely to be a pathway for subsequent scar contracture.

Longitudinal Incisions. Of the many patterns of *longitudinal* exposure, there are common principles of design.

1. The scar should not cross concavities; for example, a palmar midline incision is not satisfactory unless broken up by "Z"-plasties.
2. A zigzag scar can allow better exposure by creating flaps that can be elevated and retracted.
3. Shortened skin can be lengthened either by "Z"-plasty or by multiple "Y-V" advancement. This is generally done at the end of the dissection,[80] when areas of poor vascularity can be identified.

Popular incision patterns for a *single digital ray* include the following.

Straight Line Incision Subsequently Broken up by "Z"-Plasties. This is perhaps the most popular technique in general use today.[64,98] It has the advantage of allowing exposure of neurovascular structures progressively but the disadvantage of creating a longitudinal deep wound as a pathway for later recurrence. After incision of the skin, the margins are retracted; it is better in the palm to keep all the fat on the skin flaps rather than dissecting in the plane between dermis and fat. The latter is more likely to result in skin necrosis because skin vascularity must now rely on horizontal circulation through the dermis itself and this is unreliable when the dermis is involved in the Dupuytren process. Great care must be taken at the palmodigital junction to not cut down onto cords of contracted fascia until the neurovascular bundles have been identified because the nerve may be spiraling over the cord and can be inadvertently divided. For this reason it is usual to commence dissection of the fascia proximally[64] or, alternatively, distally[98] when the nerves can be identified in their normal location.

At the end of the fascial dissection, "Z"-plasties are designed and fashioned by taking into account any areas where the dermis is thinned, involved, or even buttonholed by the previous dissection. Opinions vary about whether the "Z"-plasties should be centered on the flexion creases or midway between, and it is not possible to give a scientific answer on this question. For a "Z"-plasty to transfer, the tissue must be capable of shortening transversely to allow

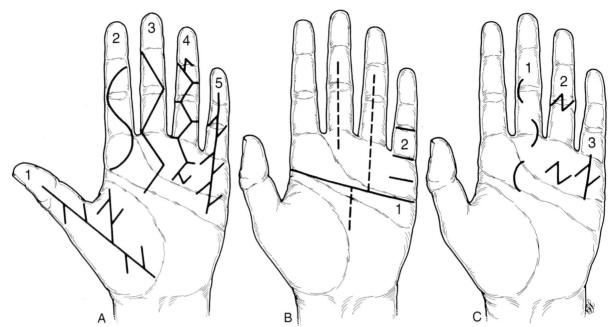

FIGURE 5-10. Basic incisions. **A,** Longitudinal incisions: 1, A "T"-shaped incision exposes all three cords that contract the thumb and first web space. The incisions are closed with "Z"-plasties. 2, A lazy-"S" incision is not recommended in the palm or the finger because it becomes straight and contracts. 3, The Bruner incision[20] is preferred to the lazy-"S" because sharp angles remain and prevent scar contracture. 4, A multiple "Y-V" incision with a "Z"-plasty at either end provides good exposure and corrects relative skin shortage.[8,54] 5, A midline longitudinal incision, closed with Z-plasties. **B,** Transverse incisions. 1, Most of the palmar aponeurosis can be removed through an incision that begins in the distal palmar crease on the ulnar side and ends in the proximal crease on the radial side of the hand.[81] A proximal extension is unnecessary but is used by many surgeons. A variety of distal incisions, separate or in continuity, can be added to remove digital disease. 2, Multiple, short, transverse incisions are used by some surgeons.[14,22] The transverse incision can be sutured, skin grafted, or left open. **C,** Minimal exposure. 1, Moermans' short curved incisions used for segmental fasciectomy.[86] The incisions for fasciotomy (2) and limited fasciectomy (3). (Courtesy of Dr. R. M. McFarlane.)

longitudinal lengthening. It can be argued that there is more skin available in the mid segment of the digit and also that there is more subdermal tissue and possibly more blood vessels here. By contrast, placement of the "Z"-plasties at the crease lines places the transverse limb of the "Z" in the crease line. A "Z"-plasty using large flaps at this point can result in a constriction ring. The real point to note, however, is that the skin on the palmar surfaces of the palm and digits has material properties all its own and is surprisingly weak. This skin tears readily and stitches cut out all too easily. This natural situation is often apparently worse in a flexed Dupuytren digit, where the skin can appear quite atrophic in areas and thickened in others. The palmar skin is stiff and does not easily tolerate tension or rotation such that small flaps often appear blanched after transfer and there is a significant necrosis rate.

Bruner-Type Zigzag Incision. This incision is also popular in Dupuytren's disease but has the disadvantages that it does not allow lengthening, and the tips of the flaps may be ischemic if the contracture runs longitudinally through the skin.[27] As in all situations, care must be exercised in elevating the tips of the flaps because the neurovascular bundles may be very superficial at this point and can be "nicked."

Multiple "Y-V" Advancement Flaps. This incision has numerous advantages. It can be raised as a zigzag incision initially and the lateral limbs added later. In some cases the lateral limbs may not be necessary if lengthening is not required, and therefore the design does have considerable

flexibility. Popularized by Deming[40] and Watson,[77] this incision was, in fact, a popular incision in the French literature throughout the early 20th century.[120] Lengthening is achieved by each lateral extension forming the stem of a "Y", which can be advanced as a small advancement flap to become a "V".[14] An interdigitation of several flaps achieves overall digital lengthening. The flaps are very safe, provided that both neurovascular bundles are intact, because they are not required to rotate as in a "Z"-plasty.

Moermans' Small Curved Incisions. These incisions are made along the cord but with the aim of excising intermittent lengths of the cord and leaving alternate lengths of fascia intact in situ. Moermans described this as segmental aponeurectomy.[116,117] In each wound a short excision of the cord is performed, with care taken to not damage nerves. Particular care must be exercised when a spiral cord is suspected at the base of the finger. Moermans has shown an incidence of nerve damage similar to that of other operative techniques.

Transverse Skin Incisions. Dupuytren[41] used a transverse incision dividing the "aponeurosis" and leaving the wound open, followed by splintage during the healing period. McCash[94] revised this approach, and the controversy that followed the presentation of his work rages on. It is doubtful whether anybody today does a true McCash operation, which in addition to leaving wounds open had several other features: radical skin undermining to allow extensive fascial dissection; tunneling from a transverse palmar wound to transverse digital wounds; advancement of skin distally to allow digital closure, with the palm left open; and prolonged night splintage. It would now be best to avoid the inflammatory McCash eponym and use the term *open palm technique*[31,131,132] when the skin is not closed, inasmuch as this may accompany a wide range of different deeper procedures. The open palm technique is not therefore a technique of releasing Dupuytren's contracture, merely a technique of wound management that avoids postoperative hematoma.[88]

Transverse incision may be accompanied by skin grafting (split skin or full thickness). McGregor[103] described an operation of fasciotomy and grafting in which the palm is divided across transversely so that all fascial cords are divided and the fascial ends can retract. A split-skin graft was then inserted. This is a large operation for primary palmar disease, although it has a very useful place in managing recurrence associated with much shortening and induration of the palm.

Gonzales[51,52] performed a transverse release at the proximal digital crease as a means of releasing PIP joint contracture and filled in the defect with a full-thickness graft. Transverse incisions at the PIP skin crease are of much less value in giving adequate exposure for dissection. Borden[21] and Beltran and colleagues[15] have, however, performed open digital incisions.

For two adjacent rays it is usual to combine longitudinal and transverse elements to give adequate exposure while helping to eliminate the straight line of the incision. A popular approach is to make an incision along the distal palmar crease with a proximal extension and then make distal longitudinal incisions for each involved digit, offset from the proximal one, in one of the patterns described earlier (see Fig. 5-10B).

Skin Excision: Dermofasciectomy

Skin replacement in patients with DD is not a new idea and was advocated by Busch[32] in 1882 and Lexer[84] in 1931; these surgeons performed wide excisions of involved palmar and digital skin combined with skin grafting. Hueston[66,67] popularized the use of skin grafts for three separate logical reasons: to replace a skin shortage, to produce a firebreak (and this is biologically a concept now gaining much support), or to replace dermis infiltrated with myofibroblasts.[93] In dermofasciectomy, Hueston achieved all these aims; initially he advised this operation for recurrence, but later he advocated it for primary surgery in young patients. The use of this operation for primary treatment has become more popular (Logan, personal communication, 1992), and there are suggestions of a lower recurrence rate,[25,61,75] although a skin graft does not guarantee freedom from further contraction.[127]

Management of the Fascia

It is artificial to describe the skin incision in isolation, and a decision on how much fascia to remove must be made in conjunction with the skin plan. Currently, on the international scene there are three approaches:

1. Limited fasciectomy popularized by Hueston[64] or one of its many variants (Fig. 5-11). The underlying principle is to remove all the involved fascia in that ray by progressive longitudinal dissection proceeding usually in a proximal-to-distal direction. The term *limited* is used in

comparison with the operations that preceded it in a historical sense.[107] It is, in fact, a big operation, and a traumatic wound of this extent would be expected to have a prolonged course of recovery.

2. Resection greater than in the first approach in which uninvolved fascia is removed in the hope of preventing recurrence. Radical fasciectomy in the palm is popular in central Europe,[114] and a radical approach to the digit has been advocated by McFarlane.[98]

3. A more limited approach than Hueston's technique in which the aim is to produce a release of tension in the palmar fascia without necessarily removing all the fascia in that digital ray. Fasciotomy has been performed in selected cases in many published series, but Moermans[116,117] has shown that discontinuous removal (i.e., segmental aponeurectomy) can be effective as a general plan of management.

Standard Limited Fasciectomy

Through a longitudinally oriented incision extending from the palm to the digit, the skin is carefully reflected with small skin-perforating vessels preserved as much as possible and bipolar hemostasis secured when vessels need to be divided. Fat is preserved on the skin, the plane of dissection being between fat and fascia, to ensure the best chance of retaining skin vascularity.

The longitudinal fibers of the palmar fascia are dissected free as far proximally as the proximal palmar crease. There are considerable variations in the proximal extent of this dissection; some surgeons continue as far as the proximal end of the nodules or cords, whereas others simply excise a set distance proximal to this crease.

The longitudinal cord is divided by pressure with a sharp scalpel and elevated in a proximal-to-distal direction. Some of the fibers pass deeply into the septa (of Legueu and Juvara,[20,82] see Fig. 5-1C) under the transverse fibers of the palmar aponeurosis. Many surgeons excise the transverse fibers together with the involved underlying septa, but Skoog[138] advocated preserving these transverse fibers intact because they are never contracted. Certainly their preservation permits a much more superficial dissection, with the neurovascular bundles kept safe deep to them, but only in the mid palm proximal to the distal palmar crease. At this point the transverse fibers cease, and distally the longitudinal cords may pass more deeply and the neurovascular bundles are at risk of being injured. The surgeon must identify these and know where they are. In the standard limited fasciectomy, Hueston advised wide exposure of the neurovascular bundles.[64,65] Skoog advocated a more selective resection, merely uncovering bundles at intervals to ensure that they are safe.

Whatever approach is followed, the dissection then proceeds distally and a knowledge of the three layers of the fascia will facilitate dissection. Care must be taken to not damage displaced neurovascular bundles. It is important to identify not just the nerves but also the digital arteries; they tend to be displaced together, although in some cases there may be some fascia or space between.

In the digit, Hueston's approach[64] was to remove involved fascial cords rather than perform a prophylactic fasciectomy. Most surgeons seem content to isolate the contracted cords and nodules and follow them to their distal attachments. If

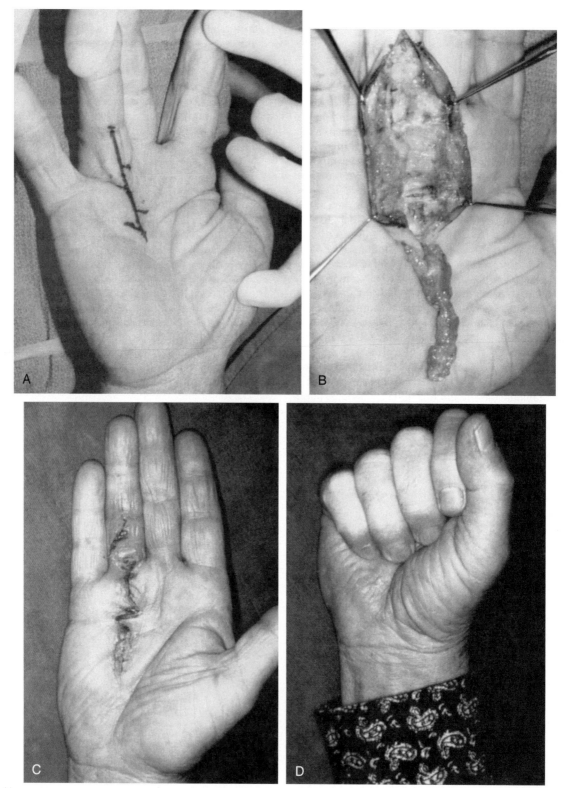

FIGURE 5-11. This 71-year-old retired trucker had noted thickening in the right palm for 1 year. The left hand was clear. **A,** He had disease in the ring finger ray only, with 30 degrees of MP joint contracture. He was a good candidate for a limited fasciectomy because his disease was mild, appeared late, and progressed slowly. **B,** He was operated on as an outpatient under local anesthesia. The exposure and amount of excised fascia are shown. **C** and **D,** Appearance of the hand 10 days after operation. The wound was closed with two "Z"-plasties. He had full flexion and extension. One year later he had full movement and no evidence of recurrence or extension of disease. (Courtesy of Dr. R. M. McFarlane.)

division of Dupuytren's tissue results in release of the joint contracture, the tissue is removed and the dissection is discontinued. If despite removal of cords the contracture persists, the surgeon must look for additional cords and then consider joint release.

Radical Fasciectomy

The term *radical fasciectomy* has usually been applied to extensive removal of fascia in the palm, with extension into the involved fingers only. The aim in the palm has been to remove all the longitudinal fibers to the four digital rays. A variety of incisions have been used, but the Mercedes-Benz three-pronged star-shaped incision is popular (Millesi[114]). Whatever skin incision is used, it is necessary to form quite large skin flaps to gain access to the entire palmar area, and there is therefore a risk of skin necrosis, so great care must be exercised to preserve small perforating blood vessels. This more extensive procedure would seem likely to carry an increased risk of wound-healing complications and postoperative stiffness. Perhaps the greatest argument against it is that most of the later problems of recurrence are in the PIP joint or in the digit.[33] For this reason, extensive palmar dissection is less popular than it was 50 years ago.[108] There is certainly no clear evidence that the more extensive palmar procedures give a longer disease-free interval. McFarlane[98] has advocated a radical approach in the individual involved digit in the hope of reducing the incidence of recurrence. He commenced his dissection distally because the neurovascular bundles are readily found near the distal crease of the finger, and by following the bundles in a distal-to-proximal direction they can be preserved. All the fascia between the bundles is removed in a block, thus ensuring that all contracted cords and potentially contracted fascia are removed. A separate search behind the cords is made for a retrovascular band of Thomine.[146]

Fasciotomy

Many published series describe a limited role for fasciotomy in selected cases. It has been suggested for elderly patients in whom anesthesia is best avoided. This patient group, however, may not benefit from rehabilitation and perhaps should be left alone. It is perhaps more appropriate to consider the type of lesion that may be treated by fasciotomy.[128] Colville[35] has designed a knife for closed division of cords. All closed procedures carry a risk of neurovascular injury, although this is lowest in palms with a mature cord bowstringing across a concavity and highest in digits in which the position of the neurovascular bundles cannot be ascertained with any certainty. Moermans[116,117] has developed a different approach to fasciectomy by not attempting to remove all the longitudinal fascia in an individual ray; instead he performs a discontinuous removal through a series of short curved incisions and leaves intermediate sections of fascia undisturbed (Fig. 5-12). This procedure, segmental fasciectomy, is intermediate between fasciotomy and limited fasciectomy and offers the advantage of less disturbance of the physiology of the hand.

Nonoperative Treatments

Closed needle fasciotomy has become popular in rheumatologic practice in France, with a corticosteroid being inject-

ed after needle division of the cords.[8,49] There is an obvious risk of damage to nerves and tendons. Ketchum and Donahue[76] have treated Dupuytren's nodules with a series of injections of triamcinolone acetonide directly into the lesion. Although some patients had complete resolution of the nodules, 50% experienced reactivation 1 to 3 years later.

Study of Dupuytren's nodules that had been injected preoperatively with corticosteroid has found that these agents reduced the rate of fibroblast proliferation and increased the rate of apoptosis of both fibroblasts and inflammatory cells.[110]

Badalamente, Hurst, and coworkers[6,7] have raised enormous interest among colleagues and patients (judging by Internet patient websites) in the possibility of nonoperative intervention by injecting enzyme (clostridial collagenase) to lyse and rupture Dupuytren's cords. They are proceeding in a careful manner, and the results of phase 3 efficacy trials are awaited. Other nonoperative treatments such as ultrasound, massage, radiotherapy, and splintage lack evidence of benefit.

Management of Joint Contracture

The MP joint is rarely a problem in that it can almost always be released by a simple fascial procedure. The basic rule is that the MP joint will tolerate prolonged immobilization in flexion whereas the PIP joint will not. For a variety of anatomic reasons this seems to be related to the joint itself rather than being a feature of Dupuytren's disease alone.

For this reason, MP flexion is not an urgent indication for surgery. The difficulty comes in knowing what to advise for PIP joint contracture (Fig. 5-13). Certainly, prolonged flexion seems to make release more difficult, although there is always some unpredictability about this. It is almost impossible to predict with any degree of certainty on clinical examination whether a joint will be released by fascial surgery or not; on occasion the joint is released by fascial excision quite far proximally. However, it is also possible that even after all fascia has been excised the joint may remain flexed. It is always *possible* to release a PIP joint provided that enough structures have been released. The real question is whether this is wise because the more extensive the surgery, the more likely there will be postoperative joint stiffness.

The flexor tendon sheath or what appear to be additional cruciform fibers may be inextensible and overlie the neck of the proximal phalanx distal to the distal edge of the A2 pulley. It may be possible to release all the oblique strands in this area without opening the synovial membrane, and this is desirable. Farther laterally there may be involvement of fibers of Grayson's or Cleland's ligaments. In this sort of advanced Dupuytren's disease it is often difficult to identify specific lateral structures, but there may be a tight amorphous sheet.

A number of structures may be examined and released sequentially, but all have in common the feature that their release will require opening the flexor tendon sheath or PIP joint capsule because the structures that we are now about to consider are components of this sheath. If the PIP joint remains in fixed flexion, the checkrein ligaments[154] are examined next. These are two ligamentous cords lying anterolaterally and running from the proximal swallowtail extensions of the volar plate to the neck of the proximal phalanx. If these structures are studied from video magnetic resonance imaging (MRI) recordings, the checkrein ligaments

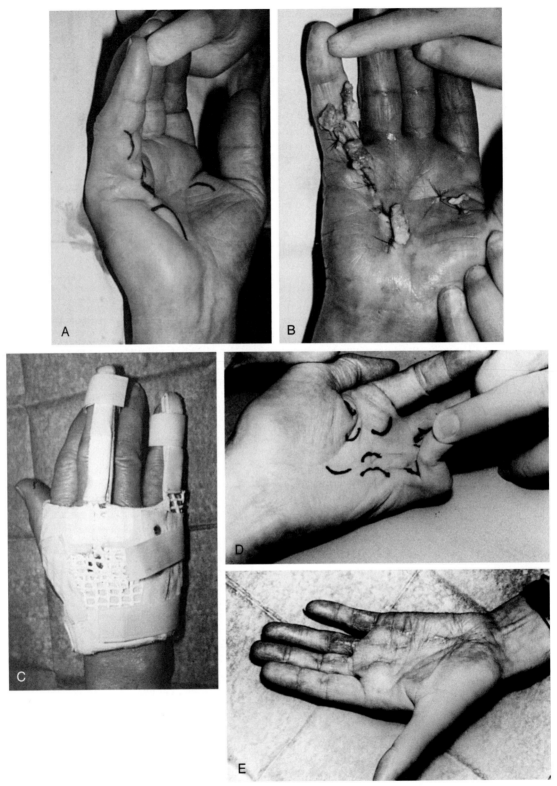

FIGURE 5-12. The segmental aponeurectomy technique of Moermans. **A,** Staged curved skin incisions. **B,** Segmental aponeurectomy. **C,** Custom-made extension splint. **D,** A patient with involvement of all digital rays. **E,** The correction achieved 6 weeks after operation. (From Moermans JP: Various views and techniques: Segmental aponeurectomy. *In* McFarlane RM, McGrouther DA, Flint MH [eds]: Dupuytren's Disease. Biology and Treatment, Vol 5, The Hand and Upper Limb Series. Edinburgh, Churchill Livingstone, 1990.)

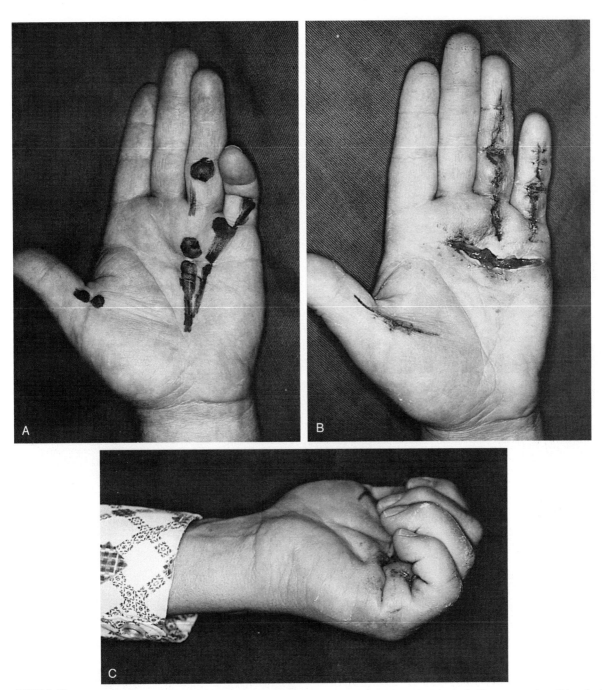

FIGURE 5-13. This 49-year-old locomotive engineer had progressive bilateral contracture for several years. **A,** He was a good candidate for the open palm technique, not only because two rays were involved but also because his endomorphic build suggested that his hand would swell postoperatively and result in prolonged joint stiffness (**B** and **C**). *Continued*

seem to coil up proximally on the neck of the proximal phalanx. They therefore need to be slack in flexion, but if infiltrated by fibroblastic tissue they become inextensible. They can be approached from the palmar fasciectomy approach by dissecting around the lateral borders of the neck of the proximal phalanx.

The next structure to release is the accessory collateral ligament running from the condyle on the head of the proximal phalanx to the lateral edges of the volar plate.[37] Finally, *gentle* manipulation may be necessary; this is often followed by a cracking sound, which may be due to separation of the vincula. The problem is that every structure is

shortened and contracted. Only the most determined hand therapy and patient compliance will maintain the gain of such a procedure, and the tendency to relapse will persist for months because of immature scar tissue replacing the divided structures. The outcome of PIP joint release is uncertain; in one series,[16] an average preoperative contracture of 65 degrees was improved to 35 degrees. However, there seems to be general agreement that when fasciectomy accompanied by capsuloligamentous (joint) release is compared with fasciectomy alone[36,155] there is no clear benefit and management of PIP joint contracture remains controversial. The possibility of using an orthotic preoperative soft tissue

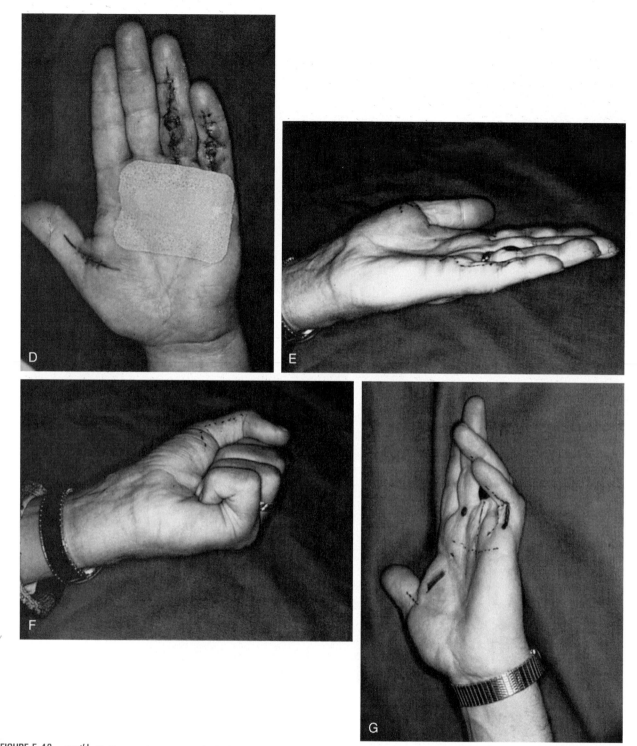

FIGURE 5-13—cont'd. **D,** Two weeks postoperatively there was no swelling of the hand. The palmar wound was covered by granulation tissue and was contracting. He had good flexion and extension. A light dressing was sufficient and facilitated the wearing of a splint. He returned to work in 3 weeks with the wound healed. **E** and **F,** At 1 year, he had full flexion and extension. **G,** At 2 years, he had recurrent PIP joint contracture of the little and ring fingers. (Courtesy of Dr. R. M. McFarlane.)

distraction device[19,121] or a Pennig external fixator[158] may improve results. Alternatively a two-stage operation has been suggested with fasciotomy and accessory collateral ligament release and S-Quattro distraction followed by a later fasciectomy.[124]

Total anterior tenoarthrolysis[130] may be considered for the patient determined to seek improvement.

Author's Preferred Method of Treatment

After experiencing many different approaches and having the opportunity to see the problems inherent in each, I have settled on relief of the joint contracture as my guiding principle of surgery and do not attempt to completely excise Dupuytren's tissue. It is necessary, however, to ensure that the contracture does not simply join up again, and I do this by using the concept of a "firebreak" of healthy tissue between separated fascial ends. I prefer to consider each joint contracture separately and devise a plan for each. For MP joint contracture, the longitudinal fibers of the palmar fascial ligaments are released in the mid palm. This operation has become more and more limited and anatomically precise over the years. For PIP joint contracture, a number of different approaches have been tried: initially a limited approach via a "Z"-plasty incision, then a transverse incision (sometimes left open), and then a short skin graft of the Gonzales type,[51,52] and currently for the past 15 years I have preferred dermofasciectomy. This approach seems to give the lowest chance of requiring further surgery in that digit, although this is an impression that cannot be proved by comparative trial. I would prefer to think that my technique has evolved like an aircraft design by finding the faults and designing them out. No procedure seems to guarantee long-term cure, and it is important to disturb the anatomy and physiology of the hand as little as possible. I would argue that preserving the original anatomy of the hand as much as possible will make the next operation much simpler, should it be required.

For MP joint contracture, a very superficial incision is made along the distal palmar crease, and the proximal skin edge is elevated along with fat, but all fascial structures are left in the bed of the wound. By dissecting under vision on either side of the contracted longitudinal cord, the transverse fibers of the palmar aponeurosis are identified and preserved. The neurovascular bundles lie beneath these fibers (which terminate in a free border at the distal palmar crease) and are generally safe and do not need to be visualized. I do, however, identify the ulnar digital nerve in the case of the little finger because the transverse fibers are poorly developed in this area. It is possible to separate the involved longitudinal cord from the underlying intact and uninvolved transverse fibers and remove a short length of the longitudinal cord by transecting it 1 to 1.5 cm proximal to the distal palmar crease. I do not dissect any farther proximal than this because it does not seem to affect the outcome. More proximal fascia cannot cause joint contracture, and residual nodules and cords generally soften and regress once tension is released.[1] The divided cord is lifted off the transverse fibers, and it will usually be found that the MP joint contracture has been relieved by this limited and specific dissection. This technique at this level has much in common with that of Moermans,[116] but I try to rely on visualization of the transverse fibers to preserve the nerves. Preserving the transverse fibers may seem an unnecessary sophistication of technique, but it can be argued that by this limited dissection there is more rapid recovery, a lesser chance of hematoma, and less disturbance in anatomy should further surgery be necessary. In my own case I have had to re-explore only two palms in which this limited procedure has been done, and in both cases it was possible to re-excise contracted longitudinal fibers and still keep the transverse fibers intact on this second occasion.

Passing just distal to the free border of the transverse fibers at the distal palmar crease is the point where knowledge of the three layers of insertion of the longitudinal fibers will be useful. The proximal end of the cords developing in each of these layers can be identified. It is not my practice to chase the cords for any considerable distance because to do so necessitates either undermining of the skin or a longitudinal incision, both of which are better avoided. The aim of the dissection at this point in the mid palm is principally to release the MP joint, which in most cases will already have been achieved by proximal division of the longitudinal fibers. In a few cases there will be an additional cord in layer 3 that requires division to release the MP joint contracture. Under these circumstances the neurovascular bundle should be exposed in the proximal web fat just distal to the transverse fibers and protected as a short length of the cord is removed. Occasionally there is a large subcutaneous nodule (layer 1) just distal to the distal palmar crease, and this is removed in continuity with the cord. Otherwise, no further dissection is performed at this point. The total length of the longitudinal tissues removed in the mid palm is on the order of 1 to 2 cm. The cords under the distal palm, between distal palmar crease and the proximal digital crease, are left in situ and not dissected. This avoids a longitudinal scar and longitudinal wound bed, potentially a site of recurrence.

The flexed PIP joint is then tackled as a separate problem. The critical area is the front of the proximal segment of the digit. Again, it is my practice to excise only sufficient contracted fascia to allow release and prevent immediate reestablishment of a contracture line through the wound-healing process. Although fascia can be satisfactorily released through any of a variety of skin incisions, retention of the original digital skin increases the likelihood of recurrence, and management of digital recurrence is the greatest challenge in Dupuytren's disease. For this reason I have now almost universally adopted the procedure of insertion of a skin graft (Fig. 5-14). Digital dermofasciectomy is performed in which the entire skin of the proximal segment of the digit is excised from one neutral lateral line to the other together with all of the underlying fascia. The proximal transverse incision is generally made first in the proximal digital crease, and the lateral corners of the skin are elevated to locate the neurovascular bundles, which are preserved by gentle retraction while the fascial dissection proceeds in a proximal-to-distal direction. Bipolar coagulation is used throughout for hemostasis. The skin is excised together with all the underlying fascia and fat (because this is the layer in which the disease would recur), but the digital flexor tendon sheath is left intact and both neurovascular bundles are preserved.

I have had considerable hesitation about advocating this method, which seems so radically different from that of Dr. Robert McFarlane, who wrote previous editions of this chapter. It is curious, however, how many of the key elements coincide. I certainly differ from Dr. McFarlane in not removing fascia from end to end in the involved ray, but we both support the concept of complete removal of fascia in the proximal segment of the digit. Dr. McFarlane replaced the original skin whereas I prefer a graft. Perhaps the lowest common denominator is the creation of a definite area of discontinuity in the fascia in the proximal segment of the digit.

In recurrent or severely involved cases in which it is anticipated that the flexor tendon sheath may be involved, it is possible to lift the proximal skin of the digit as a distally based flap by cutting it transversely at the proximal digital crease and then making two midlateral incisions distally from this point. This flap will then "retreat" distally as the finger is extended and will provide cover for any windows made in the synovial sheath. On occasion when making the proximal transverse incision alone, there will be complete release of the PIP joint; under these circumstances a simple ellipse of skin may be inserted as a firebreak[52,67] without the need to remove all the skin of the proximal segment.

An important principle of surgery for Dupuytren's disease is to *avoid hematoma,* and there are many ways of achieving this. My own approach is to use a bipolar coagulator throughout, release the tourniquet at the end of the dissection, elevate and hold the hand in a swab to wait for reactive hyperemia to wear off, and then secure further hemostasis with the bipolar coagulator. Wounds may be left completely or partly open and drains inserted. Gaps may be left at the margins of skin grafts; it is my practice to carefully suture

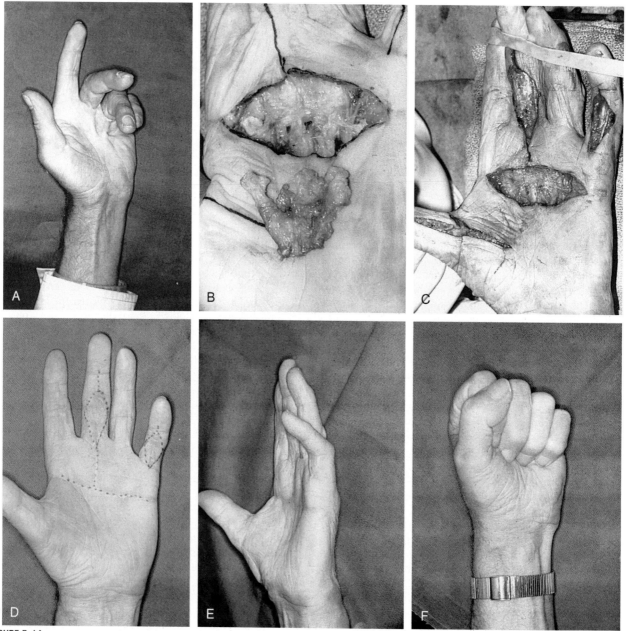

FIGURE 5-14. This 66-year-old painter had severe bilateral disease of at least 10 years' duration. His father had Dupuytren's disease, but his sons (44 and 36 years old) did not. He had no knuckle pads or foot involvement. **A,** The MP joints of the little, ring, and long fingers were flexed about 60 degrees, and the PIP joints of the little and long fingers were flexed 50 and 40 degrees. The index finger was not involved, but the MP joint of the thumb was flexed by a pretendinous cord and the web space reduced to 60 degrees. **B,** The palmar aponeurosis was removed through a transverse incision. **C,** At the completion of the dissection and release of the tourniquet, the width of the palmar wound is shown. Skin was excised over the PIP joints of the little and long fingers and replaced with full-thickness skin grafts. **D,** At 1 year postoperatively the palmar wound had been left open and healed in 4 weeks. The skin grafts on the little and long fingers are outlined. The thumb wound was closed with "Z"-plasties. **E and F,** He gained full extension of the PIP joint of the long finger but had 30-degree residual contracture of the PIP joint of the little finger. The residual contracture might have been less with better compliance with postoperative splinting. He regained full flexion within 3 months of operation. (Courtesy of Dr. R. M. McFarlane.)

the midlateral lines but leave the transverse edges unsutured because these will heal spontaneously to linear scars. Skin grafts can be positioned with tie-over sutures to apply gentle pressure. Pressure dressings are going out of fashion inasmuch as they are uncomfortable and hardly necessary with modern hemostasis. Postoperative elevation overnight is desirable but difficult to achieve with day surgery; the patient should be advised to elevate the hand on pillows overnight. The precise method will depend on the surgeon's experience, the logistics of the practice, and the last-remembered complication! There is no right way or wrong way to avoid hematoma, but every effort must be made to do so.

If despite all a hematoma should develop, the level of postoperative pain will rise and under such circumstances the patient must be advised to report back to the surgeon.

POSTOPERATIVE REHABILITATION

The treatment plan must take into account the wide range of reactions to surgery such that some patients will heal and recover with minimal attention whereas others will require constant and prolonged supervision by a hand therapist to regain motion and function. For this reason, the management plan must be flexible, more so than in most areas of hand surgery. The hand therapist should see all patients initially on removal of the operative dressing and provide advice on a program of active mobilization. Thereafter, patients should be seen routinely at weekly intervals to ensure that recovery of motion is progressing. If there is prolonged stiffness, a more active regimen will be required with more frequent attendance to ensure patient compliance with therapy advice. A much improved postoperative range of joint motion has been reported in patients who comply with splintage.[126]

In the immediate postoperative period there seem to be two views about the best position in which to splint the hand. One school of thought believes that the hand should be splinted with the MP joints flexed and the PIP joints extended, this being the most favorable position in which to immobilize the hand regardless of pathology. Alternatively, the hand can be immobilized with the MP and PIP joints extended to allow maximal elongation of the wound bed. The latter is easier to achieve. The period of immobilization should be principally for comfort and for a limited period only of 2 or 3 days. The optimum time to begin active mobilization is approximately 3 days postoperatively, but more prolonged splintage will be necessary when a skin graft has been used: 10 days' immobilization followed by protection from abrasion for 1 month. When active mobilization is commenced, splintage should be used between periods of exercise and at night (Fig. 5-15). Stiffness can be a problem, and it is difficult to know whether some patients have a greater physiologic tendency toward stiffness or whether they just do not move enough. Relapse into a position of flexion is likely to occur for many weeks after surgery. Static night splintage may be beneficial for months. When PIP joint correction has been incomplete, a program of dynamic splintage may improve slightly on the postoperative correction or at least prevent relapse (Fig. 5-16). A custom-made thermoplastic splint with an elastic outrigger is a

possibility. Spring-loaded splints exerting a constant strong pull are poorly tolerated. When good correction is achieved at surgery but followed by relapse, a Joint Jack or similar static splint may be beneficial.

Return to everyday and occupational activities is to be encouraged at the earliest opportunity. It is a mistake to rest the hand until the wounds have healed. After the open palm technique the patient should be encouraged to use the hand in a dressing for as many activities as possible.

POSTOPERATIVE COMPLICATIONS

The rate of complications is high, having been reported at 17% overall,[73,122] and published outcomes of surgical procedures often underestimate the complete picture. Complications can be due to damage to structures at surgery or problems in wound healing in the short or long term.

Damage to the digital nerves and vessels is possible. Division of a nerve is a rare event (1.5%[99]), so rare that at the end of a career the surgeon should be able to remember the names of each patient! When it happens, it is because the neurovascular bundles are out of position; and even though surgeons must be armed with this knowledge, they may mistakenly believe that a strand of fascia is the nerve and while preserving this false nerve the true one can be injured. Alternatively, the dorsal branch may be quite large and be

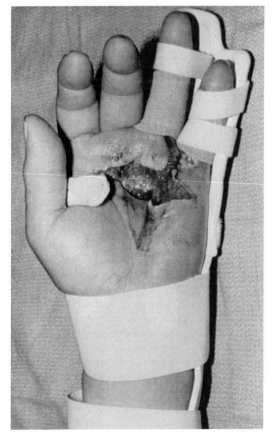

FIGURE 5-15. A static dorsal splint, firmly supported on the forearm, which holds the operated digits in maximum extension. The purpose of the splint is to maintain the correction gained at operation, but occasionally a residual flexion contracture is improved. (Courtesy of Dr. R. M. McFarlane.)

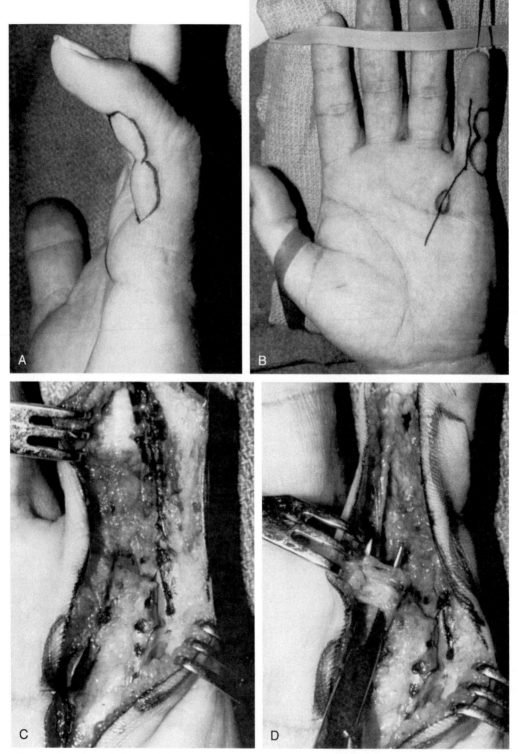

FIGURE 5-16. This 51-year-old appliance dealer noted thickening in the left little finger and gradual contraction over 20 years. His right hand was clear. His father and brother had Dupuytren's contracture. He was taking medication for gout. **A,** The disease was confined mainly to the ulnar side of the little finger with 45 degrees of PIP joint contracture. **B,** A midline longitudinal incision is shown that began in the mid palm and extended to the distal crease of the finger. **C,** The ulnar neurovascular bundle was exposed as well as the fascia that originated at the insertion of the abductor digiti minimi tendon. **D,** The radial neurovascular bundle was exposed. A natatory cord is shown just before it was cut.   *Continued*

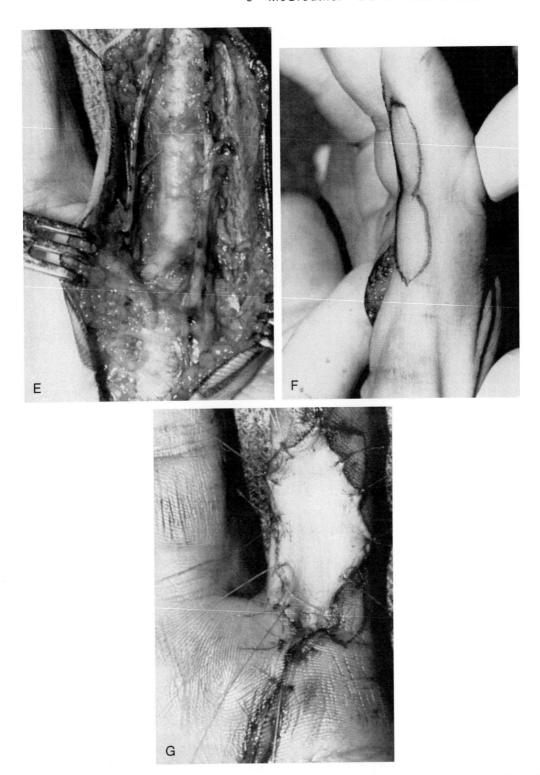

FIGURE 5-16—cont'd. E, The disease between the neurovascular bundles, including the pretendinous cord in the palm, and the disease lateral to each neurovascular bundle were removed. **F,** With excision of all diseased fascia, the PIP joint could not be fully extended. A soft tissue release of the joint was not performed. **G,** The skin over the PIP joint was excised and replaced by a full-thickness skin graft. Splinting was used postoperatively to maintain extension.

Continued

mistaken for the proper digital nerve. There is little published information on why nerves get cut! The consequence is that the patient will suffer numbness, which may be tolerable, and pain and paresthesia, which may not be.

Division of an artery is almost certainly much more frequent and often goes unnoticed (or unrecorded). In my expe-rience it is frequent to see patients with a recurrence and only one digital artery. In the rare cases in which vessel injury is found to have occurred during surgery, the key step is to release the tourniquet at the end of dissection and ensure that the fingertip and all the skin flaps are viable; if not, arte-rial reconstruction is necessary. Loss of one digital artery may

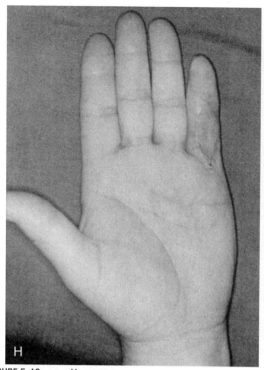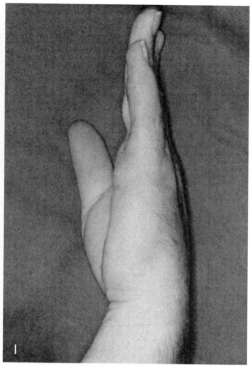

FIGURE 5-16—cont'd. **H** and **I**, At 3 months, he had full flexion and almost full extension. (Courtesy of Dr. R. M. McFarlane.)

endanger the skin flaps or the viability of the wound edge despite seemingly adequate perfusion of the digit overall.

Another surgical injury is buttonholing of the skin during the dissection. Depending on the location of the buttonhole, this may lead to inadequate circulation to a skin flap.

Tendon sheath opening and exposure of the flexor tendons should be avoided, and when a contracted sheath requiring excision is anticipated, it is wise to retain skin flaps sufficient to cover these.

Early difficulties in wound healing center around the triad of hematoma, skin ischemia, and infection. *Hematoma,* a fluid collection of blood, is due to insufficient hemostasis and/or drainage. A hematoma creates a dead space in the tissues that must resolve either by drainage in due course or by fibrosis. The presence of blood seems to aggravate inflammatory mechanisms and result in swelling, and it seems that this and possibly other mechanisms (division of a digital artery, poor flap design, failure to preserve skin vascularity) cause skin ischemia. Finally, the pool of blood is a nidus for infection, which spreads in ischemic tissue.

Later problems in wound healing comprise all the features of reflex dystrophy: pain, swelling, stiffness, and associated vasomotor disorders. It is important to maintain joint motion by active and passive exercises until the condition resolves (see Chapter 57).

RECURRENT DUPUYTREN'S DISEASE

Recurrent Dupuytren's disease may look much like the original condition, but it is a *completely different management problem* that must be approached with extreme caution. The surgeon should have a surge of adrenaline on looking at the hand. Gordon[53] distinguished between recurrence (Dupuytren's disease in the same area) and extension (nodules and cords in other areas). This seems straightforward, although in practice distinction can be difficult. The key factor is whether the operative field has been dissected before.

Recurrent contracture has many causes, and patients have a variety of different pathologies. There is no clear evidence that recurrence is due to failure to adequately excise Dupuytren's tissue at the first operation. Postmortem examinations of hands with Dupuytren's disease by the author have shown much wider involvement than suggested by clinical examination of cords and nodules, and complete excision is not possible. It is better to consider that any residual Dupuytren's tissue was not protected from tension. Some recurrences are due to regrowth or new growth of Dupuytren's tissue, although clinically and histologically this growth is indistinguishable from scar. However, failings during the first operation almost certainly make recurrence more likely. Ischemia, hematoma, skin loss, and infection increase scarring.

Recurrent contracture often shows flexion at both the PIP and DIP joints, the latter being uncommon in primary disease, and some of these digits are flexed in an intrinsic-minus posture. This situation is due to adherent scarring of the intrinsic tendons, which normally have a very small excursion, following extensive palmar dissection. Alternatively, there may be adhesions of the extensor apparatus to the proximal phalanx after extensive digital exposure. Failure to mobilize the digit adequately in the postoperative period may be due to a limited therapy program or to poor patient compliance, and this will contribute significantly to recurrent contraction. The published incidences of recurrence vary widely in different series, largely because of the criteria for defining recurrence and the time of follow-up rather than true differences in surgical outcome. In a personal study of 100 patients at up to 20 years' follow-up, no hand was free from Dupuytren's disease after 10 years. Typical series suggest a rising recurrence rate with time[47] to approximately 50% at 5 years: Hueston[64] reported a 40% recurrence with 40% extension; Tonkin and associates[149] showed 54% recurrence with limited fasciectomy, 33% with dermofasciectomy; and Foucher[48] listed a 41% recurrence, 23% of which was severe. Moermans' segmental fasciectomy[117] has shown a similar pattern of recurrence, thus suggesting that it is the disease process rather than the operation that determines the recurrence rate. This suggestion is supported by Bryan and Ghorbal,[28] who noted that 55% of fasciotomy patients maintained correction for 5 years. However, there is some evidence that the recurrence rate after dermofasciectomy may be lower[75]: Tonkin,[149] 33%; Hall and associates,[61] 8% at 24 to 100 months; and Brotherston and coworkers,[25] no contracture exceeding 15 degrees in 34 patients at 80 to 120 months.

In operating on a recurrent contracture it is critical to appreciate several important points:

1. "Standard" anatomy cannot be relied on—the nerves and vessels can be anywhere.
2. Dissection will be much more difficult and time consuming—all structures are likely to be encased in hard scar tissue. Unlike a primary case, there may be no definable adventitial layer around nerves and vessels; and in the worst cases, which may look quite simple from the skin surface, it can be almost impossible to dissect out the neurovascular structures. The patient must be warned of potential damage.
3. Nerves and vessels may have been damaged the first time round. Clinical examination may need to be supplemented by Doppler examination and angiography.
4. The PIP joint may be fixed in flexion by extensive fibrosis, and a salvage procedure may be necessary.
5. When there has been an extended period of remission after the first operation, the patient will expect the same result or better. This is unlikely.
6. When there has been a short period of release after the first procedure, the patient may not have cooperated adequately with the postoperative therapy plan but relied on the surgeon to straighten the digit. It is important to ascertain when the recurrence developed and whether any identifiable factors contributed to it.
7. The risk of all complications is higher on the second and each subsequent occasion.
8. It is important to have a sense of realism about the goals of surgery in recurrence. If a PIP joint release has had a short-lasting benefit, it may be better to proceed to an arthrodesis rather than attempt another release.
9. Dermofasciectomy is preferable to retaining scarred skin.
10. There is likely to be a greater inflammatory reaction with swelling, and it is preferable to admit the patient overnight for elevation of the hand and observation of the circulation.

Translating these points into practical advice, the operation should proceed with an anesthetic technique providing prolonged anesthesia in the tourniquet area. The dissection may have to follow the important principle of finding the neurovascular bundles in a safe area and preserving these as the area of recurrent disease is approached. Dissection usually proceeds in a proximal-to-distal direction, and it may be possible to release the MP joint with a limited dissection in the mid palm as in a primary case. The major problem is the difficulty in releasing the PIP joint, which may be held by numerous cords, scar contracture, and checkrein ligament contracture. It is my practice to discuss options with the patient preoperatively. If the PIP joint can be straightened to 35 degrees or better, this is accepted and postoperative splintage instituted to try to improve on or at least hold this range. If the correction is 40 degrees or worse, a salvage procedure is required for the PIP joint. I have had disappointing results in the long term with checkrein ligament release, and I would generally advocate PIP joint arthrodesis as the best means of keeping the patient out of the operating theater in the future. A stiff finger is well tolerated by patients with DD, who are not strangers to stiffness. Amputation is rarely indicated and only on specific request by the patient (I have done this only twice). Arthrodesis is performed through a dorsal incision with the use of a single longitudinal Kirschner wire and an interosseous wire loop. Alternatives are PIP joint replacement arthroplasty (Fig. 5-17) or osteotomy of the neck of the proximal phalanx, but published results of outcome are limited. I have a series of 20

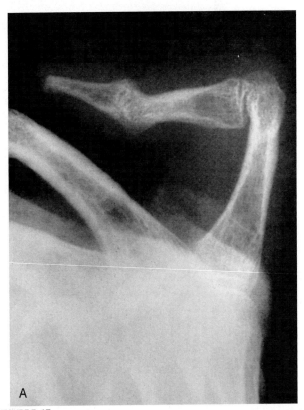

A

FIGURE 5-17. This 70-year-old housewife noted contracture of her left little finger for about 4 years. She had an operation 2 years previously that did not correct the contracture. She came seeking amputation because the finger was in the way. **A,** A preoperative radiograph shows that the DIP joint was fused at the first operation. The range of movement of the PIP joint was from 90 to 110 degrees. At operation, the finger was opened through the palmar scars and the residual disease excised. This did not correct the PIP joint contracture, so the joint was opened by reflecting the palmar plate. One centimeter of proximal phalanx was removed and a size 0 Swanson implant was inserted. The palmar plate and collateral ligaments were reattached to the proximal phalanx, and the flexor tendon sheath closed. The skin could not be closed, so a full-thickness skin graft was applied.   *Continued*

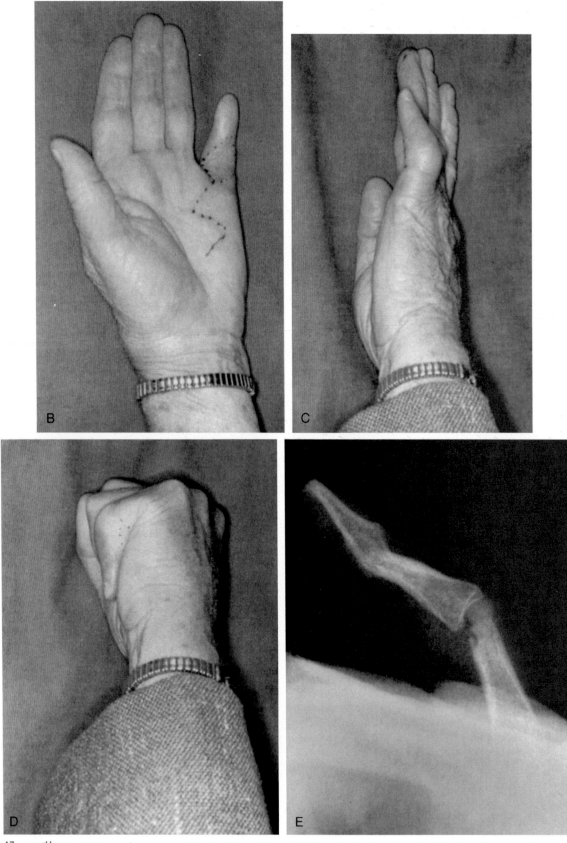

FIGURE 5-17—cont'd. **B** to **D,** Six months postoperatively the skin graft has settled. Note that the finger is noticeably short. The range of movement at the PIP joint was from 30 to 90 degrees. **E,** A radiograph shows the implant in place. (Courtesy of Dr. R. M. McFarlane.)

patients with recurrence of up to 90 degrees of contracture straightened by an external fixation device—mini Pennig fixator pins and blocks are placed in the dorsal midline and rubber bands are used to apply an extension force.

CONCLUSION

None of the arguments in Dupuytren's disease are new. Although new biologic knowledge is providing a better understanding of how surgery may work, there are as yet no fundamentally new treatments. Comparative clinical trials have made little contribution to surgical practice, probably because of the heterogeneous nature of the contractures and the patients. Much more could be achieved by an analysis of the factors leading to success or failure in the individual case to provide a more rational approach to case selection and the choice of operation.

ANNOTATED REFERENCES

7. Badalamente MA, Hurst LC, Hentz VR: Collagen as a clinical target: Nonoperative treatment of Dupuytren's disease. J Hand Surg [Am] 27:788-798, 2002.

   The team of Marie Badalamente and Larry Hurst has produced many good publications on the science and treatment of Dupuytren's disease. They have been conducting a careful clinical trial to evaluate the use of clostridial collagenase injections to release Dupuytren's cords in selected patients; in those with a well-defined cord it is released away from the location of digital nerves. This study is likely to be the forerunner of future injection therapies, perhaps combining imaging with active biologic agents.

44. Elliot D: The early history of contracture of the palmar fascia. *In* McFarlane RM, McGrouther DA, Flint MH (eds): Dupuytren's Disease: Biology and Treatment, Vol 5, Hand and Upper Limb Series. Edinburgh, Churchill Livingstone, 1990, pp 1-10.

   Much that has been written about Dupuytren's disease is wrong, and errors have been handed down from article to article. Elliot is the most reliable source because he spent weeks in dusty libraries in Paris and elsewhere tracking every original document and article from the entire 19th century. He obtained new translations and applied the intellectual rigor and uncompromising thoroughness for which he is renowned to this scholarly work, which will never be bettered. For history, this is the reference source.

64. Hueston JT: Limited fasciectomy for Dupuytren's contracture. Plast Reconstr Surg 27:569-585, 1961.

   This paper led a move away from the previous radical operations toward a more limited approach whereby only the fascia in the involved digital rays is dissected out. Hueston also popularized incorporation of the "Z"-plasty in wound closure. It remains a popular approach but is still a fairly extensive dissection in which the digital nerves are widely exposed, thus making dissection of recurrence more difficult.

66. Hueston JT: Dermofasciectomy for Dupuytren's disease. Bull Hosp Jt Dis 44:224-232, 1984.

   Although Lexer[84] used extensive skin grafting, Hueston introduced a more limited skin replacement for recurrent cases, which he later called a "firebreak." Hueston believed that the dermis had some sort of etiologic role in the condition. McFarlane has said that the irritating thing about Hueston is that he introduced innovations "on a hunch" that years later, after scientific assessment, were often found to be correct. The jury is out on the role of the dermis.

95. McFarlane RM: Patterns of the diseased fascia in the fingers in Dupuytren's contracture. Plast Reconstr Surg 54:31-44, 1974.

   Robert McFarlane changed our perception of Dupuytren's disease by identifying the individual anatomic ligamentous bands along which Dupuytren's disease propagated. McFarlane deserves credit for pointing out that Dupuytren's disease was not an amorphous fibromatosis but followed anatomic structures in a longitudinal orientation through the palm. McFarlane went on to stimulate basic scientists to work on all aspects of the biology of this curious disease and much subsequent literature has been stimulated by his efforts.

107. McGrouther DA: An overview of operative treatment. *In* McFarlane RM, McGrouther DA, Flint MH (eds): Dupuytren's Disease: Biology and Treatment, Vol 5, The Hand and Upper Limb Series. Edinburgh, Churchill Livingstone, 1990, pp 295-310.

   My excuse for citing one of my own book chapters is that it categorizes all of the published operative techniques of other authors in terms of their separate approaches to the skin, the fascia, and the joint. The aim was to derive logical principles that would unite the widely different operative approaches.

117. Moermans JP: Long-term results after segmental aponeurectomy for Dupuytren's disease. J Hand Surg [Br] 21:797-800, 1996.

   Although the concept was published as long ago as 1878 by Adams (Adams W: Contraction of the fingers [Dupuytren's contraction] and its successful treatment by subcutaneous divisions of the palmar fascia and immediate extension. BMJ 1:928-932, 1878), Moermans has shown more recently that contracted fascia divided but not excised will soften (involute). Moermans removes intermittent lengths of the contracted fascia, using discontinuous short curved incisions. His series is remarkable for the length of detailed follow-up, and nerve damage was no different from other techniques

137. Skoog T: The transverse elements of the palmar aponeurosis in Dupuytren's contracture. Scand J Plast Surg 1:51-63, 1967.

   Tor Skoog was a perfectionist who published a doctoral thesis on Dupuytren's contraction (Skoog T: Dupuytren's contraction with special reference to aetiology and improved surgical treatment, its occurrence in epileptics. Notes on knuckle pads. Acta Chir Scand 96[Suppl]:139, 1948) in which he apparently reviewed every publication in English, German, the Scandinavian languages and many in French and Russian since the time of Dupuytren. He went on to describe a selective operation (these names are confusing and differently interpreted by many surgeons). He wished the essential elements to be remembered as preservation of the transverse fibers of the palmar fascia (thus limiting the dissection in the mid palm) and limited exposure of the neurovascular bundles, just enough to ensure they are safe—a truly minimally invasive procedure!

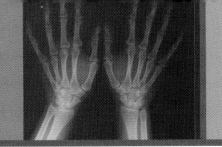

CHAPTER 6

Extensor Tendon Injuries

**Mark E. Baratz, Christopher C. Schmidt,
and Thomas B. Hughes**

Extensor tendon injuries are frequently underestimated. Although few surgeons without hand surgery training will attempt repair of an injured flexor tendon, many will tackle the lacerated extensor tendon. Extensor tendons are easy to expose and seem easy to repair. The postoperative care for extensor tendon injuries does not carry the mystique surrounding flexor tendon injuries. The consequences of extensor tendon repair vary with the severity of the injury, the location of the laceration, the technique used for repair, and the care that follows. A laceration of the extensor over the proximal phalanx involving 40% of tendon in which the patient can extend the finger against resistance will do well with or without repair. A similar laceration over the proximal interphalangeal (PIP) joint with a loss of active extension may result in poor finger function regardless of treatment. Reconstruction of extensor injuries presents a greater challenge than treatment of acute extensor tendon laceration. Success is predicated on the preoperative evaluation. Is the skin supple? Is there an associated joint contracture or arthritis? Does the solution require tenolysis, tendon graft, or tendon transfer? Can expectations ever match predicted outcome?

In this chapter there is a review of anatomy, treatment, and expected outcome for acute and chronic extensor tendon injuries. The injuries are considered starting with mallet injuries and progressing proximal into the forearm.

Anatomy

Normal Anatomy

Wrist extension is possible by virtue of the extensor carpi radialis brevis (ECRB), extensor carpi radialis longus (ECRL), and the extensor carpi ulnaris (ECU). These muscles originate on the lateral condylar ridge and lateral epicondyle of the distal humerus. The finger and thumb extensors (abductor pollicis longus [APL], extensor pollicis brevis [EPB], extensor pollicis longus [EPL], extensor digitorum communis [EDC], extensor indicis proprius [EIP], and extensor digiti minimi [EDM]) have a broad origin, including the lateral epicondyle, proximal radius, proximal ulna, and the interosseous membrane. Muscle fibers give rise to tendon 3 to 4 cm proximal to the wrist joint. The EIP muscle is an exception in that it has muscle fibers that extend to or beyond the level of the wrist joint. The fascia of the extensor muscles condenses at the level of the wrist to form the extensor retinaculum. Vertical septa divide the space beneath the retinaculum into six extensor compartments, as depicted in Figure 6-1. The multiple slips of the APL exit the first compartment and insert into the fascia of the thenar muscle and the base of the thumb metacarpal. The tendon of the EPB blends with fibers of the extensor hood over the metacarpophalangeal (MP) joint before inserting into the base of the thumb proximal phalanx. The radial wrist extensors (ECRL and ECRB) exit the second compartment before inserting onto the index and middle metacarpals, respectively. The ECRL tendon inserts on the radial aspect of the index metacarpal. The ECRL applies a radial deviation moment to the wrist. The ECU tendon that inserts on the ulnar aspect of the fifth metacarpal after passing through the sixth extensor compartment neutralizes the radial deviation moment applied by the ECRL. The ECRB tendon inserts on the base of the third metacarpal and provides a pure extension moment to the wrist. The balance of the three wrist extensors is lost when the ECU is paralyzed as a result of posterior interosseous nerve palsy. In this situation the ECRL and ECRB are capable of extending the wrist, but with obvious radial deviation. The EPL wraps around Lister's tubercle as it passes through the third compartment. The tendon passes ulnar to the EPB at the MP joint, connected to the EPB by fibers of the extensor hood. The EPL tendon flattens as it continues toward its insertion into the base of the distal phalanx. The fourth compartment supports

The authors would like to acknowledge the important contributions to the understanding of acute and chronic extensor tendon injuries by **Dr. James R. Doyle, Dr. Richard I. Burton,** and **Dr. Julie A. Melchior** in previous editions of this book. Some of their material, including illustrations, has been incorporated into this newly combined chapter.

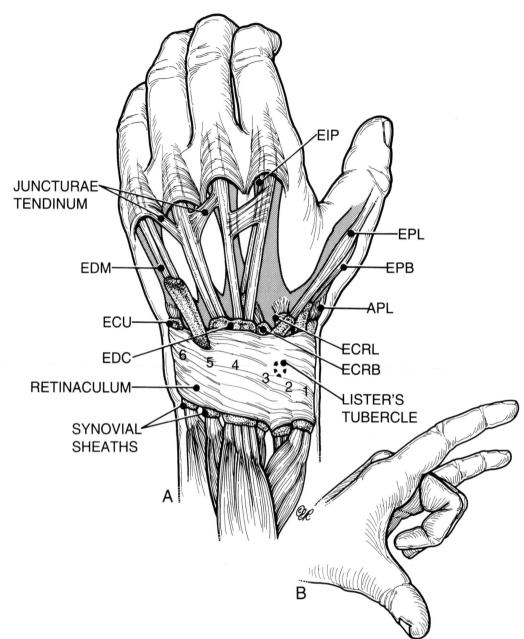

FIGURE 6-1. **A,** The extensor tendons gain entrance to the hand from the forearm through a series of six canals, five fibro-osseous and one fibrous (the fifth dorsal compartment, which contains the extensor digiti minimi [EDM]). The first compartment contains the abductor pollicis longus (APL) and extensor pollicis brevis (EPB); the second, the radial wrist extensors; the third, the extensor pollicis longus (EPL), which angles around Lister's tubercle; the fourth, the extensor digitorum communis (EDC) to the fingers, as well as the extensor indicis proprius (EIP); the fifth, the EDM; and the sixth, the extensor carpi ulnaris (ECU). The communis tendons are joined distally near the MP joints by fibrous interconnections called juncturae tendinum. These juncturae are found only between the communis tendons and may aid in surgical recognition of the proprius tendon of the index finger. The proprius tendons are usually positioned to the ulnar side of the adjacent communis tendons, but variations may be present that alter this arrangement (see text). Beneath the retinaculum, the extensor tendons are covered with a synovial sheath. **B,** The proprius tendons to the index and little fingers are capable of independent extension, and their function may be evaluated as depicted. With the middle and ring fingers flexed into the palm, the proprius tendons can extend the ring and little fingers. Independent extension of the index finger, however, is not always lost after transfer of the indicis proprius[110] and is less likely to be lost if the extensor hood is not injured[117] and is probably never lost if the hood is preserved and the juncturae tendinum between the index and middle fingers is excised (see text).[84] This figure represents the usual anatomic arrangement found over the wrist and hand, but variations are common, and the reader is referred to the section on Anatomic Variations. ECRB, extensor carpi radialis brevis; ECRL, extensor carpi radialis longus.

the tendons of the EIP and EDC. The EIP tendon melds with fibers of the extensor hood over the MP joint as it passes ulnar to the EDC tendon to the index finger.

Hirai and colleagues studied the intertendinous connections of the hand. The connections were classified as filamentous, fibrous, or tendinous and noted to be either "r"-shaped or "y"-shaped. An "r"-shaped filamentous band was commonly seen in the second intermetacarpal space. An "r"-shaped tendinous band typically joined the tendons of the third intermetacarpal space. A "y"-shaped tendinous band was the most frequent type of intertendinous connection between tendons of the fourth intermetacarpal space.[73]

MP joint extension is accomplished via fibers of the sagittal band that extend from the extensor hood to the palmar plate. Young and Rayan studied the anatomy and biomechanics of the sagittal band in cadaver fingers, finding that Swan-Ganz catheter measurements deep to the sagittal band were highest when the MP joint was fully flexed and least with 45 degrees of MP joint flexion. No instability of the extensor was seen with sectioning of the ulnar sagittal band. Instability of the tendon was seen with partial proximal sectioning of the radial sagittal band. Complete sectioning of the radial sagittal band resulted in tendon dislocation. Tendon instability after section of the radial sagittal band was amplified by wrist flexion.[180]

Fibers of the common extensor blend with fibers of the lateral band to form the central slip of the extensor tendon. The central slip inserts on the base of the middle phalanx to effect PIP joint extension. The central slip is maintained in its dorsal position by virtue of the medial and lateral fibers of the transverse retinacular ligament. These fibers originate on the flexor sheath and lateral margin of the middle phalanx. Portions of the common extensor and lateral bands combine to form the terminal tendon. These slips of the extensor are held dorsal to the axis of the PIP joint by the fibers of the triangular ligament.' The terminal tendon is responsible for distal joint extension. Extension of the fingers is primarily an active event powered by the extensor muscles. Some authors believe that the spiral oblique retinacular ligament (SORL) provides a passive assist to extension of the distal interphalangeal (DIP) joint.[51,67,94,181] Other authors have ascribed a static, support role to this ligament,[70,83,140] a ligament that Shrewsbury and Johnson[144] found in about 50% of fingers, with the exception of the ulnar side of the ring finger, where it could be identified in 93% of the specimens examined. Fibers of the SORL originate on the palmer plate and flexor sheath beneath the PIP joint. These fibers

move dorsally to insert in the terminal tendon. With PIP extension, fibers of the SORL tighten to assist DIP extension (Fig. 6-2).

Anatomic Variations

Second Compartment

A third radial wrist extensor, the extensor carpi radialis intermedius (ECRI), was identified by Wood[179] in 12% of specimens and by Albright[2] in 24%. This tendon was substantial enough, in most cases, to function as a tendon transfer. In fact, Albright included in his report two cases in which the ECRI was used as a transfer to restore thumb function in paralytic disorders. The origin and insertion of the ECRI varied among specimens.[2]

Third and Fourth Compartments

McMurtry and Jochims[114] described hypoplasia of the thumb and finger extensors transmitted over four generations of a family with an autosomal dominant pattern of inheritance.

Gonzalez and colleagues[63] identified variations of the EIP in 19% of specimens. They noted duplicate slips of the EIP in 10 hands and duplicate slips of the EDC in two specimens. The EIP was either palmar or radial to the EDC at the level of the metacarpal head in two specimens.

Gonzalez and colleagues,[61] in a separate study, found a slip of the EDC to the small finger in 35 of 50 specimens. Twelve of 50 had only a junctura to the small finger, and the remaining three small fingers relied on the EDM for MP joint extension.

Ogura and associates[123] found the extensor digitorum brevis manus (EDBM) muscle in 3% of 559 cadaver hands. The muscle typically originated from the dorsal lip of the distal radius and inserted on the index extensor with the EIP. The authors believed that the EDBM muscle was a variant of the EIP muscle because the two were frequently connected and shared the same nerve and arterial supply.

Zones of Injury

Klienert and Verdan[92] proposed a system of classifying extensor tendon lacerations according to eight zones in the hand, wrist, and forearm. Doyle suggested adding a ninth zone to characterize injuries to the extensor muscles of the mid and proximal forearm.[39] A written description of the zones is listed in Table 6-1, and the zones are illustrated in Figure 6-3.

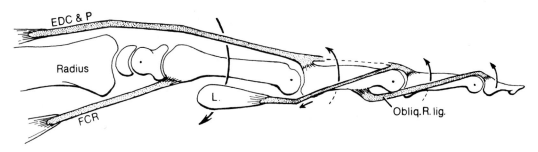

FIGURE 6-2. Schematic representation of the spiral oblique retinacular ligament (Obliq. R. lig.) and its contribution to DIP joint extension.

Table 6-1
ZONES OF INJURY

Zone	Finger	Thumb
I	Distal interphalangeal joint	Interphalangeal joint
II	Middle phalanx	Proximal phalanx
III	Proximal interphalangeal joint	Metacarpophalangeal joint
IV	Proximal phalanx	Metacarpal
V	MP joint	Carpometacarpal joint/radial styloid
VI	Metacarpal	
VII	Dorsal retinaculum	
VIII	Distal forearm	
IX	Mid and proximal forearm	

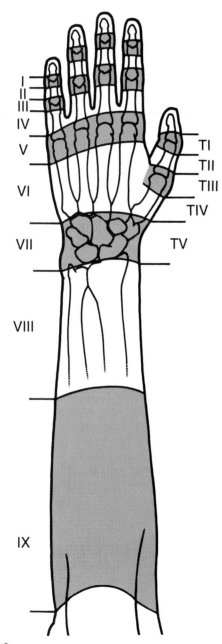

FIGURE 6-3. Extensor tendon zones of injury as described by Klienert and Verdan and by Doyle.

TREATMENT

Suture Techniques

Extensor tendon repair must be performed with two goals in mind: maximize strength and minimize shortening of the tendon. The technique used to repair extensor tendons will vary according to the thickness of the extensor. Doyle[39] found that the thickness ranged from 0.55 mm in zone II to 1.7 mm in zone VI. In the more distal portions of the thumb and finger, the tendon is flat and is best repaired with a simple, running, mattress, or cross stitch suture. Doyle recommended a running stitch that included the skin for repairs at the DIP joint (Fig. 6-4) and also advocated a running suture oversewn with a cross stitch for repairs done over the mid and proximal phalanges (Fig. 6-5).[39] Extensor tendon repairs for central slip lacerations and injuries at or proximal to the level of the MP joint can be repaired using core sutures, with or without an epitendinous stitch. Howard and coworkers[75] found that the Becker (MGH) version of a four-strand repair in zone VI was more resistant to gap formation than the modified Bunnell and modified Krackow-Thomas repairs (Fig. 6-6).

Principles of Rehabilitation

After tendon repair or reconstruction, finger mobilization depends on the quality of the tendon repair and associated bone or soft tissue damage. The surgeon directing the postoperative care should take into consideration the existing literature on rehabilitation of extensor tendon injuries.

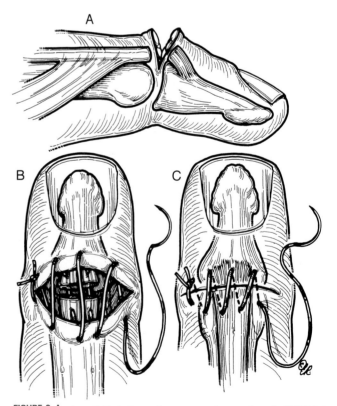

FIGURE 6-4. A to C, Technique of extensor tendon repair at the DIP joint as described by Doyle, in which the skin and tendon are simultaneously approximated.

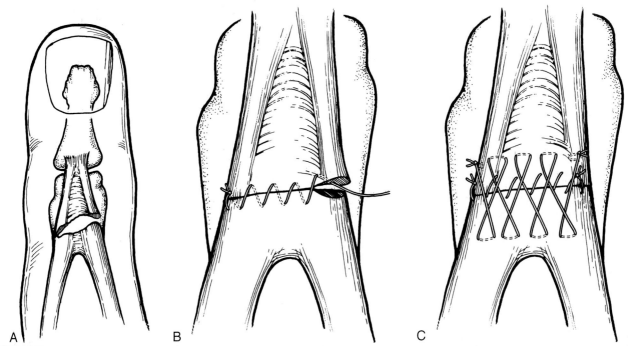

FIGURE 6-5. The relatively thin extensor tendon just proximal to the DIP joint can be repaired with this technique. **A,** Sharp laceration in zone II of the extensor tendon. **B,** Laceration repaired with a running suture and (**C**) oversewn with a Silfverskiöld cross stitch.

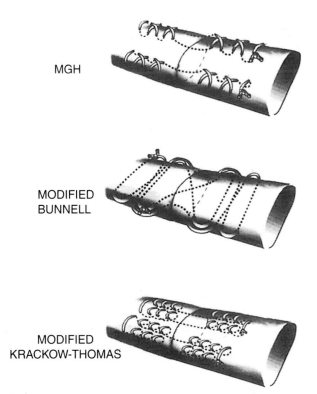

MGH

MODIFIED BUNNELL

MODIFIED KRACKOW-THOMAS

FIGURE 6-6. Schematic representation of the four-strand MGH, the modified Bunnell, and the modified Krackow-Thomas repairs. (Reprinted from Howard RF, et al: Biomechanical analysis of four-strand extensor tendon repair techniques. J Hand Surg [Am] 22:838-842, 1997. With permission from The American Society for Surgery of the Hand.)

Evans and Burkhalter[50] examined extensor tendon excursion for the fingers in zones IV to VII (MP joint through wrist) and the EPL tendon in zones IV and V. They compared intraoperative measurements of tendon excursion with values measured by Bunnell in cadaver specimens.[13] Their measurements were also compared with values calculated using the relationship between tendon excursion and angular motion at the MP joint as proposed by Brand.[15] While tendon excursion varies from finger to finger, Evans and Burkhalter[50] estimated that 30 degrees of MP flexion in the fingers results in 5 mm of extensor tendon glide. Based solely on intraoperative findings they estimated that 60 degrees of motion at the interphalangeal (IP) joint produced 5 mm of EPL glide at Lister's tubercle. Motion producing 5 mm of tendon glide was thought to be critical, because Duran and Houser[42] had previously found that 3 to 5 mm of passive tendon glide is necessary to prevent tendon adhesions at the site of tendon repair. Evans and Burkhalter applied their findings to a series of 66 patients with extensor tendon injuries in zones V to VII.[50] Dynamic splinting was begun at day 3 with the wrist in 45 degrees of extension and the MP and IP joints supported by traction slings in 0 degrees of flexion. A flexion block limited MP flexion to approximately 30 degrees. EPL lacerations were treated with the wrist, carpometacarpophalangeal (CMC), and MP joints splinted in extension. The dynamic traction placed the thumb at 0 degrees and permitted active flexion to 60 degrees. Active flexion and passive extension were performed 10 times an hour for 3 to 4 weeks. Active motion was initiated at week 4, and passive flexion and resisted extension were begun at 7 weeks after tendon repair.[50] The efficacy of this technique for managing extensor lacerations at or proximal to the MP joint has been supported by other authors.[16,32]

Expected Outcome

There are relatively few articles describing the outcome of extensor tendon repair and reconstruction. In 1942, Miller[116] suggested criteria for assessing the results of extensor tendon repair (Table 6-2).

Newport and colleagues[118] reviewed finger motion after extensor tendon repair in 101 fingers. Sixty percent of tendon injuries had an associated injury such as fracture, dislocation, or flexor tendon injury. Approximately 60% of tendon injuries were in zones V to VIII (MP joint to distal forearm). Fingers were splinted for 3 to 4 weeks after repair, followed by 2 weeks of active motion. Passive motion was initiated at approximately 6 weeks post repair. Good or excellent results with total active motion (TAM) averaging 230 degrees were achieved in 64% of patients without an associated injury. Forty-five percent of patients with an associated injury had good or excellent results with an average TAM of 212 degrees. Extensor injuries over the fingers (zones I to IV) had less motion at follow-up than extensor tendon injuries over the metacarpals, wrist, and distal forearm (zones V to VIII).[118]

Crosby and Wehbe[32] treated 50 repaired extensor tendons with dynamic splinting and tendon mobilization. Full range of motion was achieved in 45 of 50 digits after an average of 9 weeks. Five digits had an extension lag of 10 degrees or less. All patients achieved at least 93% of their predicted strength by 12 weeks. Return to their preinjury activities took an average of 10 weeks.

Chester and coworkers[28] suggested that total active motion at 4 weeks was superior in those patients treated with dynamic splinting of extensor tendon injuries in zones IV to VIII compared with patients who were instructed to perform immediate active extension while wearing a palmar splint. At final follow-up, there were no ruptures and the differences in finger motion between the two groups were not significant.

Complications

The most common complication after tendon repair is the formation of adhesions between the repair site, adjacent skin, and bone. These adhesions can restrict joint flexion as well as extension. Therapy is designed to improve tendon gliding. If loss of motion persists 4 to 6 months after repair, an extensor tendon tenolysis may improve motion. Tenolysis is not considered until progress in therapy has reached a

plateau and the skin over the repair site is supple. Swollen, densely scarred skin will restrict digit motion post tenolysis even if full motion is achieved intraoperatively. Depending on the injury and subsequent scarring, the patient may require a tenolysis and capsulotomy, collateral ligament release, and flexor tenolysis.[169] The need for releases in addition to an extensor tenolysis can be assessed if the procedure is done with a local anesthetic and sedation (see Neurolept Anesthesia in Chapter 2). The adhesions are released between the skin and tendon and between tendon and bone using a combination of sharp dissection and a thin, blunt-edged elevator. An intrinsic release, resection of a triangular portion of the lateral bands, will improve PIP motion in those patients with intrinsic tightness. If passive motion is not restored, then a joint release is performed.[169] The dorsal capsule is incised along with the dorsal half of the collateral ligaments. This should permit full, passive PIP flexion. The tourniquet is then released, and the patient is asked to make a full fist. A discrepancy between active and passive flexion suggests flexor tendon adhesions, a finding common when the patient has sustained a phalangeal fracture in association with the extensor tendon laceration. If active flexion is not restored, a flexor tenolysis is performed. Creighton and Steichen[31] reported the results of tenolysis after fracture with tendon repair and showed a 31% improvement in total active range of motion. They found 50% improvement in active extensor lag when only an extensor tenolysis was required. Improvement in motion decreased when a dorsal capsulotomy was needed: 21% improvement in total active range of motion and 0% improvement in active extensor lag.

Zone I Injuries (DIP level)

Mallet Finger
Acute Injuries

Loss of active extension at the DIP joint is the hallmark of a mallet injury. Loss of passive extension suggests that the injury is chronic. Hyperextension of the injured PIP joint in a mallet injury is described as a "compensatory" swan neck deformity (Fig. 6-7).[99] Hyperextension of the adjacent PIP joints suggests a propensity to develop a swan neck deformity even if the deformity is not apparent on the initial examination (Fig. 6-8).

Most mallet injuries are treated with immobilization of the DIP joint in extension. Cast immobilization of both the DIP and PIP joints was an established treatment in the past but has limited indications at this time.[17,64,146,157,173,177] Extension splinting of just the DIP joint has become the standard of care for most mallet injuries.* Katzman and colleagues used cadaver specimens to show that PIP joint motion and intrinsic tendon retraction did not create a tendon gap in fingers with a terminal tendon laceration.[84] Most authors recommend full-time splinting with the DIP joint in extension for 6 weeks, followed by 2 to 6 weeks of splinting at night and during strenuous activities.[82] By using a residual extension lag of 10 degrees or less as the measure of successful treatment with splinting, most authors have reported a success rate of about 80%.[1,30,58]

Table 6-2

MILLER'S[116] CRITERIA FOR ASSESSING EXTENSOR TENDON FUNCTION

Result	Total Extension Lag (degrees)	Total Flexion Loss (degrees)
Excellent	0	0
Good	≤ 10	≤ 20
Fair	11-45	21-45
Poor	≥ 45	≥ 45

---

*See references 45, 64, 77, 90, 96, 142, 152, 155, 171, and 172.

There are conflicting views on the management for fractures with subluxation of the distal phalanx. Wehbe and Schneider[175] suggested nonoperative treatment for all mallet fractures, including those with palmar subluxation of the distal phalanx. Many authors have recommended operative treatment for mallet fractures with a large dorsal fragment and palmar subluxation of the distal phalanx.[30,64,68,156] Doyle described the use of a pull-out suture for the fracture fragment and longitudinal pinning of the DIP joint (Fig. 6-9).[39] Damron and Engber reviewed 19 patients treated for irreducible fracture-subluxations using a tension band technique. At an average follow-up of 8 years DIP joint motion ranged from 1 to 69 degrees.[34]

Several authors have described the use of closed reduction of mallet fractures with extension block pinning of the DIP joint,[126,164] including Mazurek and coworkers.[110] The distal phalanx is maximally flexed, and a 0.045-inch Kirschner wire is introduced into the head of the middle phalanx at a 45-degree angle (Fig. 6-10A-C).[110] The wire creates an extension block for the bony fragment. Occasionally, manipulation of the distal phalanx against the wire is required to achieve an anatomic reduction (see Fig. 6-10D). Once the fragment is reduced, a second wire is placed longitudinally from distal to proximal across the DIP joint to maintain extension and reduction (see Fig. 6-10E and F). If the fracture fragment is large enough, a smaller wire may be placed through the fragment perpendicular to the fracture line from dorsal to palmar. The wires are cut short, and a splint is applied. The digit is kept dry. Pins are cleaned and treated with antibiotic ointment twice a day. Bridging trabeculae are usually apparent at 4 weeks, at which time the pins are removed and motion is begun.

Tetik and Gudemez[164] documented their experience with a modification of extension block pinning for fractures involving more than 33% of the articular surface and those fractures with subluxation of the distal phalanx. At an average follow-up of 27 months, all fractures healed and a congruent joint was achieved in 17 of 18 patients. One patient had

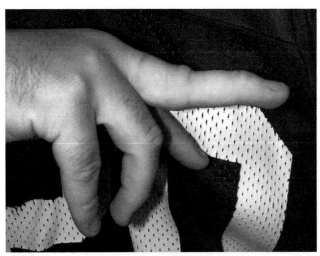

FIGURE 6-7. Mallet deformity with a mild compensatory swan neck deformity.

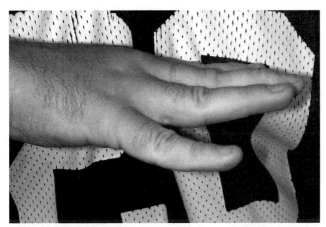

FIGURE 6-8. Ligamentous laxity as evidenced by hyperextension of the PIP joints in all fingers.

The indications for operative treatment are controversial, although only a few authors recommend surgery for both soft tissue and bony mallet injuries.[80] Three situations are consistently cited as indications for surgery: open injuries; closed injury in a person who would be unable to work with a splint (e.g., health care worker); and a large dorsal fragment with palmar subluxation of the distal phalanx. Authors agree on operative treatment for open injuries. Mattress sutures, pull-out wires, and running sutures or wires have been recommended for repair of open mallet lacerations.[44,121,157] Doyle recommended repair with a synthetic monofilament suture that concurrently approximates skin and tendon (see Fig. 6-4).[39]

Kirschner wire fixation of the DIP joint has been described as an adjunct to tendon repair and as the sole treatment for a mallet injury.[25,26,46,52,128,174] Doyle proposed Kirschner wire fixation of the DIP joint for 6 weeks, followed by night splinting for 2 weeks.[39] Tubiana suggested that the wire be inserted to one side of the fingertip and advanced obliquely across the DIP joint to avoid scarring on the apex of the pulp.[168]

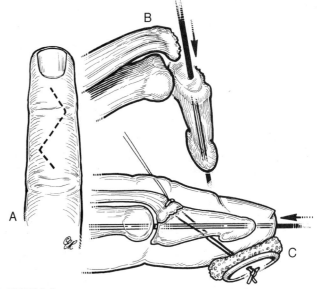

FIGURE 6-9. **A** to **C,** Doyle's technique of open repair of a mallet fracture with a pull-out suture and pinning of the DIP joint.

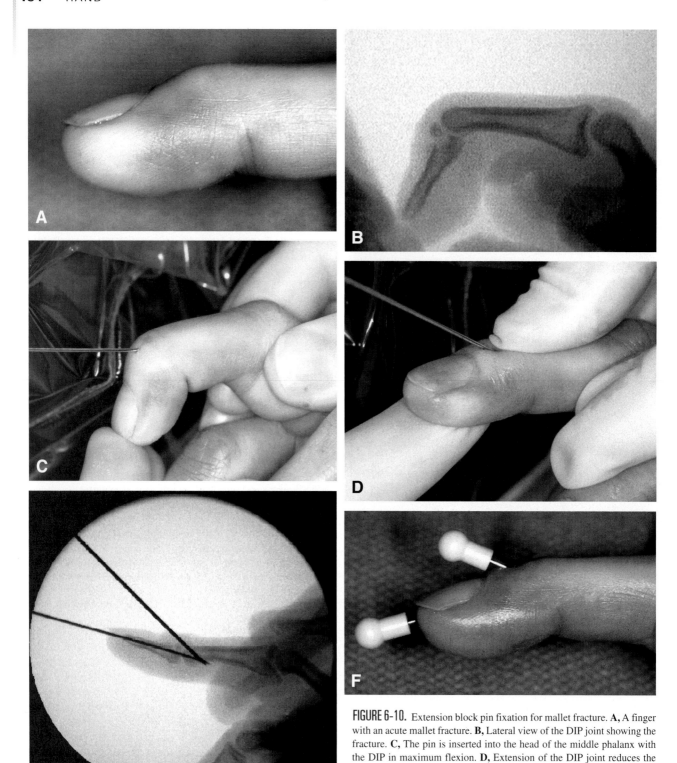

FIGURE 6-10. Extension block pin fixation for mallet fracture. **A,** A finger with an acute mallet fracture. **B,** Lateral view of the DIP joint showing the fracture. **C,** The pin is inserted into the head of the middle phalanx with the DIP in maximum flexion. **D,** Extension of the DIP joint reduces the mallet fracture fragment against the extension block pin. **E,** A second pin is then passed across the DIP joint. **F,** The pins are left protruding and are capped. (All images courtesy of Alex Shin, MD.)

minimal pain. Motion at the DIP joint averaged 80 degrees with an average lag of less than 2 degrees.[164]

Chronic Injuries

Three points are important in evaluating mallet deformities seen at some point remote from the injury: prior treatment, passive motion of the DIP joint, and position of the PIP joint. The passage of up to several months does not preclude successful splinting of a mallet finger.[58,83,101] Fingers that have been splinted appropriately for 6 to 8 weeks may improve with a continued trial of splinting. Previous splinting with inadequate DIP extension is easily corrected. A chronic mallet deformity with a flexion contracture of the DIP joint needs to be evaluated with a lateral radiograph.

Arthritis of the DIP joint or chronic palmar subluxation of the distal phalanx may preclude further nonoperative treatment. If the joint space is preserved, passive extension can be restored with therapy and dynamic splinting or with serial casts.

Several authors have advocated operative treatment for chronic mallet deformities.[44,80,97] Most describe removing several millimeters of attenuated tendon followed by repair of the tendon and pinning of the DIP joint. Burton and Melchior suggested that the DIP joint should be pinned for 4 to 6 weeks and splinted for 6 to 8 weeks. They recommended gradual weaning of the splint to prevent recurrence of the mallet deformity.[22] Kaleli and colleagues[80] reported excellent results using a miniature external fixator after resecting and repairing the injured portion of extensor tendon along with an elliptical wedge of dorsal skin. Burton and Melchior[22] stated that reconstruction of the extensor tendon in chronic mallet injuries is often successful, except in those instances in which there is a nonunion of a large dorsal fragment with palmar subluxation of the distal fragment.

A tenotomy of the central slip has been used to treat chronic mallet deformities with and without a compensatory swan neck deformity.[11,66,74,104] Grundberg and Reagan treated 20 patients with an average extension lag of 37 degrees at the DIP joint and an average hyperextension deformity of 10 degrees. Three patients had a palmar capsulotomy performed concurrently to treat a flexion contracture of the DIP joint. At an average follow-up of 29 months, the average lag at the DIP joint was reduced to 9 degrees with an average extension deficit at the PIP joint of less than 2 degrees.[66] However, Grundberg and Reagan had 6 of 20 patients with a residual DIP lag of 20 degrees or more. They noted that

Bowers and Hurst had splinted the IP joints for 2 weeks postoperatively and had achieved an average correction of 59 degrees in a series of five patients,[11] compared to the 28-degree average correction in the series published by Grunberg and Reagan.[66]

In 1978, Thompson and coworkers[165] published their experience with reconstruction of the SORL. A palmaris longus graft is sutured to the terminal tendon and passed between the flexor tendon and the palmar plate of the PIP joint. The graft is then passed into a bone tunnel in the diaphysis of the proximal phalanx. The graft is held in place with a pull-out suture that exits the opposite side of the finger and is tied over a button (Fig. 6-11). Girot and associates[59] published a series of SORL reconstructions with satisfactory results. Kinoshita and coworkers[91] reported the use of a SORL reconstruction to correct a swan neck deformity after a free vascularized PIP joint transfer.

Authors' Preferred Method of Treatment of Mallet Fingers

We prefer to treat most mallet injuries with splints. The finger is examined with attention to the degree of flexion at the DIP joint, the passive motion of the DIP joint, and the position of the PIP joint of both the injured finger and the adjacent fingers. A finger with loss of active DIP extension, full passive extension, and no swan neck deformity is treated

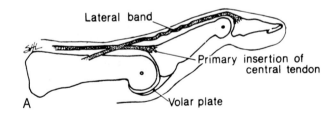

A

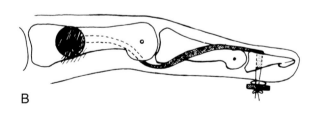

B

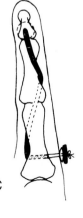

C

FIGURE 6-11. SORL reconstruction. **A,** Schematic representation of the mallet deformity with compensatory swan neck deformity. **B** and **C,** The tendon graft is fixed to the distal phalanx with a pull-out suture. The graft is passed between the flexor tendon sheath and the neurovascular bundles palmar to the PIP joint. The graft is tensioned and anchored into the shaft of the proximal phalanx.

with a dorsal splint over the DIP joint. This protocol is followed for mallet injuries with and without an associated fracture of the distal phalanx. A large dorsal fragment with or without palmar subluxation of the distal phalanx has not been a contraindication to splinting in our practice (Fig. 6-12). Although we have no experience with the technique, we are intrigued by the reports of closed reduction and extension block splinting.

Several types of splint can be used: foam-padded aluminum splints, molded plastic splints, and custom thermoplastic splints. Splints are chosen based on comfort, fit, and patient preference. Splints should maintain the DIP joint in extension. Hyperextension of the DIP joint may contribute to breakdown of the dorsal skin,[130] reported with an incidence as high as 38%.[158] Splinting is initiated for 6 weeks on a full-time basis. Patients are instructed to maintain DIP extension when the splint is removed, such as when cleaning the finger. If extension is restored after 6 weeks of full-time splinting, the finger is splinted at night for 6 weeks and during the day while performing heavy tasks. The duration of splinting may be shortened in patients with stiff joints, such as elderly patients and laborers. Splinting duration may need to be extended in patients with supple joints. Fingers with a mallet deformity and compensatory swan neck deformity are treated with a custom splint that maintains DIP joint extension and the PIP joint in slightly flexed position (Fig. 6-13). The adequacy of joint positioning in the splint can be confirmed with a lateral radiograph of the digit (Fig. 6-14). In health care workers, we have had good success with a small thermoplastic splint that can be covered

with a glove or a clear, sterile adhesive wrap. We have not performed percutaneous pinning of the DIP joint.

Open mallet injuries are repaired with an interrupted or running 5-0 nylon suture. If the repair is tenuous, the DIP joint is pinned with a 0.045-inch Kirschner wire for 6 weeks, followed by 6 weeks of night splinting. Open mallet fractures are treated using the method described by Doyle, as illustrated in Figure 6-9.[39] With a segmental defect in the tendon, a "turndown" slip of the lateral band is used to restore tendon continuity with normal tendon tension (Fig. 6-15). Soft tissue defects are concurrently managed with local flaps, such as the reversed cross finger flap (see Chapter 47).

Chronic mallet deformities are all given an additional trial of splinting if there is any question regarding the adequacy of the initial treatment. We have never been confronted with a patient in whom it was not possible to at least partially improve the extensor lag with additional splinting. We have no personal experience with either central tendon tenotomy or resection and repair of attenuated tendon in chronic mallet deformities. Chronic mallet deformities with compensatory swan neck deformities are reconstructed with the SORL reconstruction technique as described earlier and illustrated in Figure 6-11. Chronic mallet deformities that are painful, arthritic, and interfere with hand function are treated with DIP fusion.

Mallet Thumb

Both operative and nonoperative treatment have been recommended for closed mallet injuries involving the thumb.[1,37,125,129] De Monaco and colleagues[35] described good

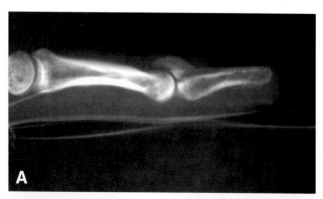

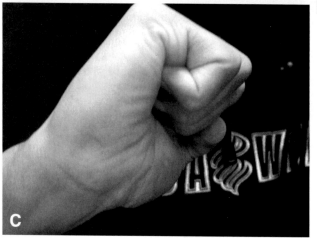

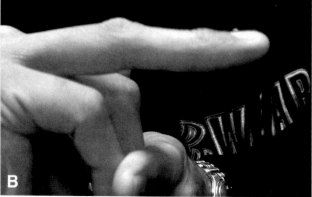

FIGURE 6-12. A, A mallet fracture treated with splinting in extension. This treatment resulted in a painless, fibrous union with full extension (**B**) and excellent flexion (**C**).

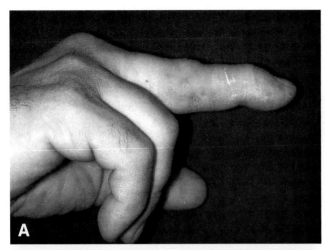

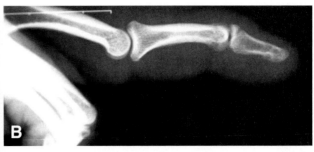

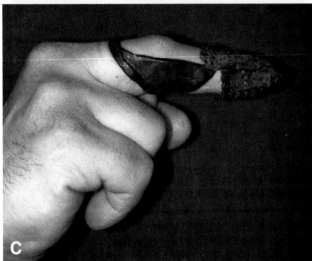

FIGURE 6-13. **A,** A mallet finger with compensatory swan neck deformity. **B,** Lateral radiograph with no fracture and obvious swan neck deformity. **C,** The distal static splint holds DIP joint in full extension. A figure-of-eight splint blocks PIP extension and permits PIP flexion.

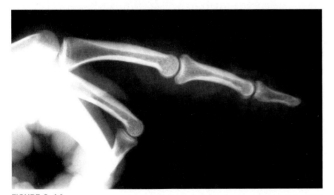

FIGURE 6-14. Lateral radiograph confirms appropriate position of the PIP and DIP joints in splint used in Figure 6-13 to treat a mallet deformity with a compensatory swan neck deformity.

CRITICAL POINTS: TREATMENT PRINCIPLES FOR EXTENSOR TENDON INJURIES

- Suture technique should be chosen to maximize strength and minimize shortening of the tendon.
- Success of rehabilitation depends on associated bone and soft tissue damage and the quality of the initial tendon repair.
- Injuries over zones I to IV typically result in less motion on follow-up than for zones V to VIII.
- The most common complication is adhesions between the repair site and adjacent tissue.
- Adhesions may require tenolysis and capsulotomy, collateral ligament release, or flexion tenolysis, or a combination of these methods.

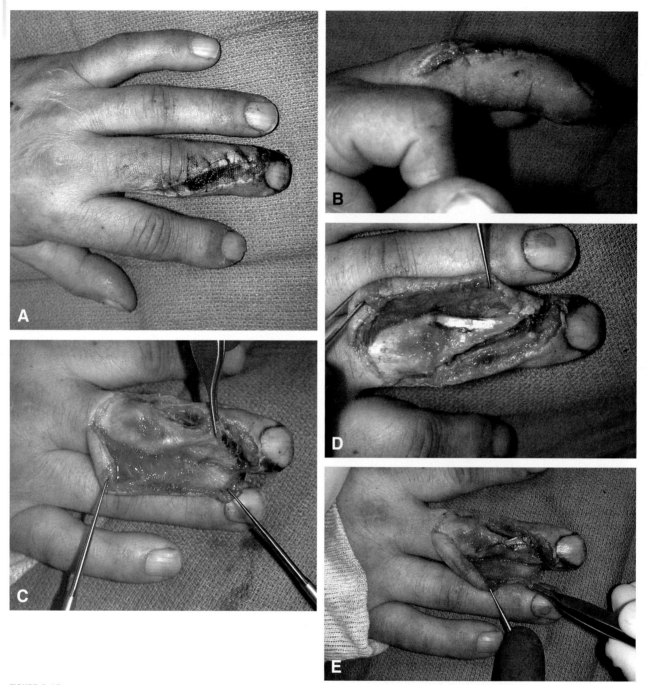

FIGURE 6-15. A, Saw injury to the dorsal aspect of the middle phalanx and DIP joint. **B,** Damage to the terminal tendon results in a mallet deformity. **C,** The kerf of the saw blade has created a segmental defect in the extensor tendon that cannot be directly repaired without excessive tension. **D,** A segment of the lateral band is marked to design a turndown flap of tendon to reconstruct the extensor tendon. **E,** The tendon flap has been sutured distally, restoring tendon continuity without undue tension.

restoration of function with transosseous repair of the tendon and early motion. Patel and coworkers and Primiano and associates reported similarly good results with nonsurgical treatment.[125,129]

Authors' Preferred Method of Treatment of Mallet Thumb

We treat mallet thumb injuries in the same manner as mallet fingers. Closed injuries are splinted for 6 weeks full time and at night for an additional 6 weeks. Open injuries are treated with direct repair.

Zone II (Middle Phalanx Level)

Extensor tendon injuries over the middle phalanx are typically seen in conjunction with sharp lacerations, saw injuries, and crushing injuries. Doyle recommended a running stitch oversewn with a Silfverskiöld cross stitch see (see Fig. 6-5).[39,145] Lacerations with a crush component can injure the periosteum and incite bone formation on the dorsal surface of the bone. This mass, described as a turret exostosis, can limit DIP flexion.[178] Once the mass is mature, as evidenced by a sclerotic border on plain radiographs, the bone can be resected to improve DIP motion.

Authors' Preferred Method of Treatment of Zone II Injuries

Acute lacerations are evaluated by having the patient extend the DIP joint. An extensor lag is treated with exploration and repair. Active extension with weakness against resistance is treated with the DIP joint splinted in extension for 3 to 4 weeks. Active extension with normal strength against resistance is treated with gentle active motion followed by re-evaluation in 1 week to ensure an extension lag has not developed. Lacerations with a segmental defect are treated with a lateral band turndown, as illustrated in Figure 6-15. Chronic zone II injuries that create a swan neck deformity can be managed with a SORL reconstruction, as described earlier and illustrated in Figure 6-11.

Zone III (PIP Joint)

Disruption of the extensor apparatus at or just proximal to the PIP joint results in a loss of extensor power at the PIP joint. Forced flexion of the PIP joint can damage the central slip of the extensor tendon. Injuries to the central slip range from a sprain with attenuation of the central slip to complete disruption of the central slip resulting from palmar dislocation of the PIP joint.[150,151,153,159,160] Avulsion injuries may

include only soft tissue or a fragment of bone. Lacerations can include part or all of the central slip and the adjacent lateral bands. If the injury results in palmar subluxation of the lateral bands, the DIP joint will be drawn into hyperextension, creating a boutonnière deformity.[70,115,139,181] This deformity often evolves within a week of the initial injury. McCue and Bowers discussed the pseudo-boutonnière deformity, which is a deformity resulting from a hyperextension injury in which contractures of the soft tissues palmar to the PIP joint simulate a disruption of the central slip.[10,12,112]

An extension lag at the PIP joint, weak extension against resistance, loss of extension at the DIP, and intra-articular injection of a contrast dye have all been recommended as means to diagnose the boutonnière injury.[14,103]

Acute Closed Boutonnière Injuries

Extension splinting of the PIP joint can restore continuity of the central slip without operative intervention. The PIP joint can be maintained in an extended position with a variety of splints or a transarticular pin.[44,113,136] Flexion of the DIP joint draws the extensor distally and facilitates dorsal translation of the lateral bands. Stewart recommended casting the DIP joint in flexion and the PIP joint in extension for 6 weeks.[159,160] McFarlane and Hampole thought it was easier to achieve PIP extension without tension by immobilizing the MP and wrist joint.[113] They also advocated pinning the PIP joint in extension. The pin was removed after 3 weeks and the splint after 4 weeks. Tubiana recommended a similar treatment without pinning of the PIP joint.[168] Boyes,[14] King,[89] and Doyle[39] described extension splinting of the PIP joint alone to restore and maintain PIP extension (Fig. 6-16). Active DIP flexion was encouraged. The treatment was terminated

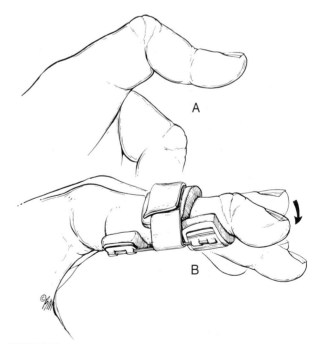

FIGURE 6-16. A, Schematic representation of a boutonnière deformity. **B,** A Bunnell splint is applied to maintain extension at the PIP joint. The strap over the PIP joint is progressively tightened until the PIP joint is fully extended. The patient is encouraged to actively and passively flex the DIP joint. The splint is worn until the patient can maintain active extension of the PIP joint.

when full DIP flexion was restored and PIP extension maximized. Elliott[44] and Sakellarides[136] both reported a preference for pinning the PIP joint in extension for 5 to 6 weeks, while allowing active DIP flexion.

Open treatment for acute, closed boutonnière injuries has been recommended for central slip ruptures with an avulsed bone fragment.[14,168] Small fragments are excised with repair of the central slip to bone; large fragments are reduced and pinned. Spinner and Choi[153] suggested operative treatment for closed anterior dislocations of the PIP joint with rupture of the central slip and a collateral ligament.

Authors' Preferred Method of Treatment of Acute Closed Boutonnière Injuries

Boutonnière deformities that have full passive extension of the PIP joint and full passive flexion of the DIP joint are treated with a dorsal or palmar thermoplastic splint for the PIP joint that permits active MP and DIP motion. The splint immobilizes the PIP joint in full extension and is worn full time for 6 weeks and at night for 6 weeks. Concomitant active and passive flexion of the DIP joint must be done as well. Splinting is shortened for older patients and extended for young patients if the initial 6-week trial is unsuccessful or if the lag recurs once PIP flexion is initiated.[49] Patients with a loss of passive extension at the PIP joint and flexion at the DIP joint are warned that, despite treatment, restoration of a normal finger is very difficult. Contractures of the PIP joint that are 30 degrees or less are treated with a dynamic extension splint. Contractures that are 30 degrees or more are treated with serial casting. We have not offered surgical treatment for closed anterior dislocations of the PIP joint with a ruptured collateral ligament unless the dislocation is irreducible. Central slip ruptures with a small fleck of bone are treated with splinting of the PIP joint. Larger fragments that are too small to pin are excised (Fig. 6-17A to C). The central slip is repaired with a suture anchor (see Fig. 6-17D and E). Care must be taken to avoid advancing the central slip because this will disrupt the balance of the extensor apparatus. In the example shown in Figure 6-17, the balance was tested by flexing the PIP and DIP joint. The defect distal to the repaired central slip was reconstructed by rotating and suturing in a slip of the lateral band. The entire digit is splinted for 5 to 7 days, followed by continuous splinting of the PIP joint for 5 weeks and night splinting for 6 weeks.

The most common complication encountered in treating acute closed boutonnière injuries is incomplete correction of the deformity, but full flexion of the PIP joint and DIP joint with an extension lag of 20 degrees or less usually produces a finger that has few functional limitations.

Acute Open Boutonnière Injuries: Zone III Lacerations

Lacerations over the extensor surface of the PIP joint should be carefully managed to prevent joint infection and loss of extension. Primary repair is advocated; the method varies,

particularly when there is loss of tendon substance.[7,39,44,136,137] Doyle described the use of a core stitch to repair the central slip passed tendon to tendon or tendon to bone. The tendon is then oversewn using a Silfverskiöld cross stitch (Fig. 6-18). With loss of tendon substance, Snow[148] performed a turndown of the central slip (Fig. 6-19) whereas Aiche and coworkers[3] chose to split and centralize the lateral bands (Fig. 6-20). Doyle noted that an adequate repair was measured by the ability to flex the PIP joint without gapping at the repair site. His preferred postoperative regimen consisted of short arc flexion under the supervision of a therapist, as described by Evans.[48]

Lacerations over the MP joint of the thumb may injure the joint capsule, the EPB tendon, and the EPL tendon. Doyle recommended repairing the capsule with interrupted sutures and repairing the tendons with a 4-0 core suture and a 5-0 Silfverskiöld cross stitch. He and others suggested a postoperative protocol using dynamic extension.[40,47,48,50] The wrist is held in 40 degrees of extension, the CMC in neutral, and the MP and IP joints in 0 degrees. Flexion up to 60 degrees is permitted at the IP joint. Hung and associates began MP motion 3 weeks after surgery.[76]

Authors' Preferred Method of Treatment of Zone III Lacerations

Patients with lacerations over the PIP joint in a finger that has full, active extension against resistance are permitted immediate active motion with re-examination in 1 week. If the digit has full, active extension but is weak with resisted extension, the PIP joint is splinted in extension for 3 to 4 weeks and re-examined. If extension against resistance is restored, the PIP joint is splinted at night and with strenuous activities for 4 to 6 weeks. If there is an extensor lag in association with a laceration over the PIP joint, repair is recommended. The repair is completed with 3-0 braided synthetic suture on a tapered needle. If the central slip is lacerated at its insertion, the repair is performed using a microsuture anchor. When possible, the repair is oversewn with a 5-0 nylon suture using the Silfverskiöld cross stitch, as illustrated in Figure 6-18. The repair is evaluated intraoperatively. Both the PIP and DIP joints should be able to flex 60 degrees without gapping. In cases of extensor tendon deficiency, a turndown of the central slip and/or the lateral band is performed, as described by Snow[148] and illustrated in Figure 6-19. The PIP joint is splinted in extension for 3 to 4 weeks, allowing MP and DIP flexion and extension. Progressive PIP flexion is then begun under the supervision of a therapist, with continued splinting in extension at night. If an extensor lag recurs, part-time splinting is resumed during the day. Gentle static flexion is begun at 8 weeks. The digit is protected from impact for 12 weeks from the date of the repair. Tenolysis and joint releases are not considered until 6 months from the time of surgery.

Zone III lacerations over the thumb MP joint are repaired with a modified Kessler core stitch using braided 3-0 syn-

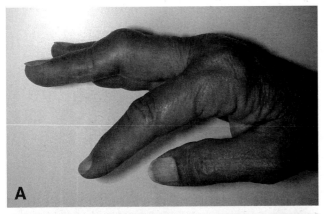

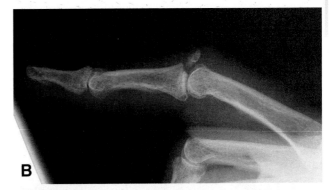

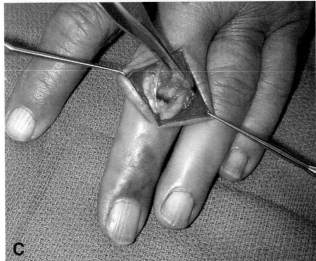

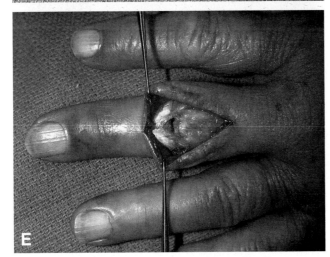

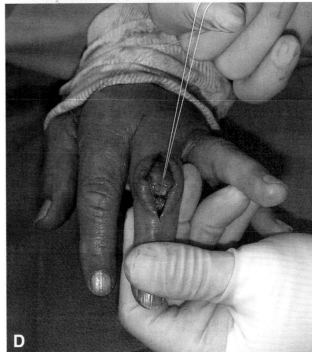

FIGURE 6-17. **A,** An acute boutonnière deformity. **B,** An avulsed bone fragment at the insertion of the central slip. **C,** The avulsed bone fragment usually is larger than anticipated based on plain radiographs. **D,** The bone fragment has been excised, and a suture anchor has been inserted into the base of the middle phalanx. **E,** The central slip has been reattached to the base of the middle phalanx using the suture anchor.

thetic suture on a taper needle. The repair is reinforced with an epitendinous repair, using 5-0 nylon and a Silfverskiöld cross stitch. Before skin closure, the MP joint is held in 20 degrees of flexion. The IP joint is flexed until there is tension on the repair. The thumb is supported in a thumb spica splint with the wrist in 20 degrees of extension, the thumb MP joint in 20 degrees of flexion, and the IP joint free. The patient is permitted gentle, active IP motion using the limits defined intraoperatively. After 4 weeks, the splint is removed and active thumb MP motion is initiated.

Chronic Boutonnière Deformity

The central slip may be disrupted by traumatic injury or through attenuation secondary to inflammatory arthritis or osteoarthritis.[6,72,127] As previously described, disruption of the central slip is accompanied by disruption of the triangular ligament. The loss of these transverse fibers allows the lateral bands to drift palmar to the axis of the PIP joint. Palmar subluxation of the lateral bands accentuates flexion of the PIP joint and creates hyperextension at the DIP joint. If treatment is unsuccessful, the transverse retinacular liga-

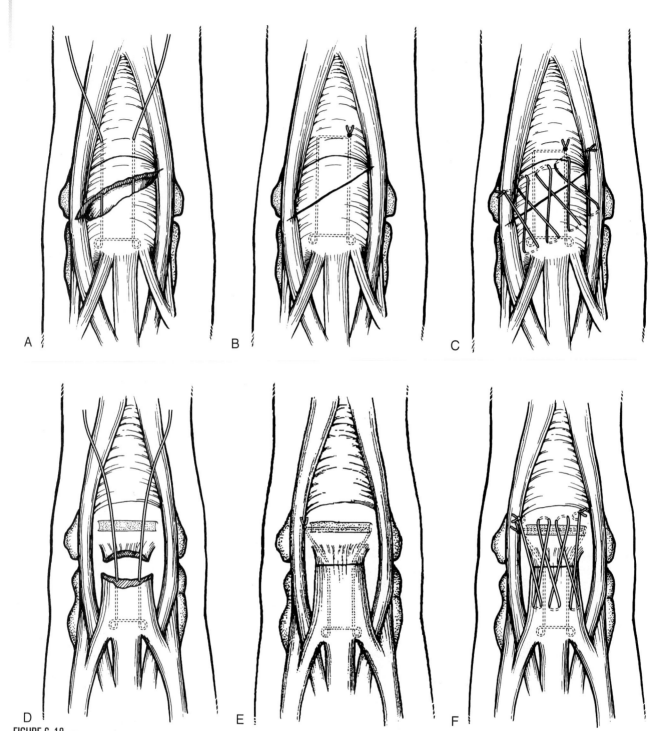

FIGURE 6-18. Doyle's preferred technique for repair of zone III lacerations. **A** to **C,** Central slip laceration with sufficient tendon to repair with core suture and oversew with Silfverskiöld epitendinous stitch. **D** to **F,** The core stitch can be passed through a trough in the base of the middle phalanx when the tendon laceration is distal, leaving a small stump of central slip.

ment shortens and holds the lateral bands palmar to the axis of the PIP joint. In time, the PIP joint can develop a fixed flexion contracture and the DIP joint can develop a fixed extension contracture (Fig. 6-21).[19-21,100,102,105,138,154]

Burton and Melchior[22] classified chronic boutonnière deformity into three stages:

Stage 1: Supple, passively correctable deformity
Stage 2: Fixed contracture: contracted lateral bands

Stage 3: Fixed contracture: joint fibrosis, collateral ligament and palmar plate contractures

They recommended that a therapy regimen of active-assisted extension of the PIP joint combined with passive flexion of the DIP joint be attempted in any stage 1 or 2 deformity. They further recommended that the exercises should be supplemented by a combination of static and dynamic extension splinting during the day and static splinting at

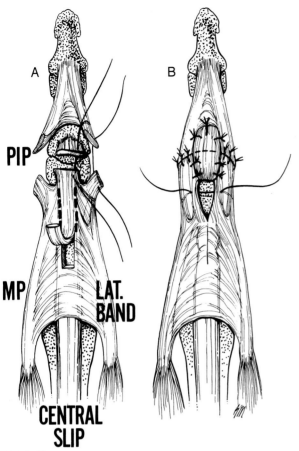

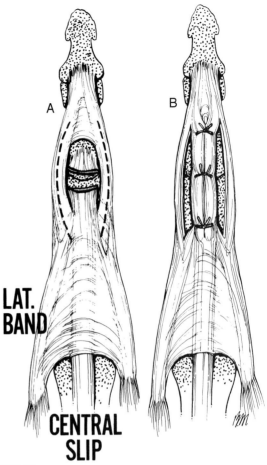

FIGURE 6-19. Snow's technique of central slip reconstruction. **A,** A distally based flap of extensor tendon is raised to span a defect in the central slip. **B,** The flap is sutured to any distal tissue and to the lateral bands. This must allow PIP flexion to at least 60 degrees without excessive tension.

FIGURE 6-20. Aiche's technique of central slip reconstruction. **A,** A segmental defect in the central slip is managed by designing a tendon flap using the central half of the lateral bands. **B,** The lateral bands are mobilized and sutured to each other using a 5-0 nonabsorbable suture.

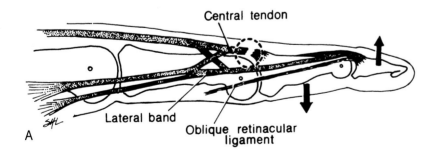

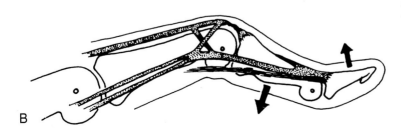

FIGURE 6-21. Pathomechanics of the boutonnière deformity. **A,** Attenuation of the central slip results in unopposed flexion at the PIP joint. **B,** With PIP joint flexion the lateral bands drift palmar to the axis of rotation at the PIP joint. The lateral bands stay in this palmar position due to loss of dorsal support from the attenuated triangular ligament and to contracture of the transverse retinacular ligament.

night.[22] For those patients who fail nonoperative treatment, Burton and Melchior listed several points for surgeons to consider before embarking on surgical correction of a boutonnière deformity. To paraphrase:

1. Splinting is an important component of postoperative care; it may be necessary for several months after surgery.
2. Boutonnière reconstructions are most successful on supple joints. If necessary, a joint release can be performed as a first stage.[95] If the release is followed by an intensive exercise and splinting program, the second stage may be avoided.
3. An arthritic joint usually precludes soft tissue reconstruction. The surgeon should consider either a PIP joint fusion or arthroplasty with extensor tendon reconstruction.
4. Boutonnière deformities rarely compromise PIP flexion and grip strength. Do not trade extension at the PIP joint for a stiff finger and a weak hand.

5. The goal of boutonnière reconstruction is to rebalance the extensor system by reducing extensor tone at the DIP joint and increasing tone at the PIP joint.[135,139]

Reconstructive procedures for chronic boutonnière deformities can be divided into three categories: tenotomy, tendon grafting, and tendon relocation.

Tenotomy

Transection of the extensor mechanism over the middle phalanx has been described by a number of authors.[38,43,53-55,117] It is often referred to in the literature as the Dolphin or Fowler procedure. This procedure is recommended for supple boutonnière deformities where there is full passive extension at the PIP joint and full passive flexion at the DIP joint. The tendon is divided just distal to the central slip and dorsal transverse retinacular fibers (Fig. 6-22). The SORL is preserved to maintain DIP joint extension. Burton and

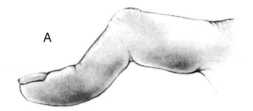

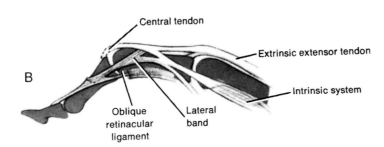

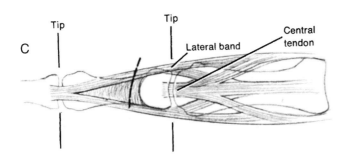

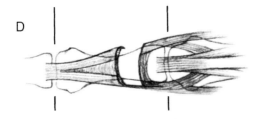

FIGURE 6-22. Extensor tenotomy for supple boutonnière deformity. **A** and **B,** Deformity characteristic of the chronic boutonnière deformity. **C** and **D,** The lateral bands are released distal to the insertion of the central slips. The lateral resulting proximal migration of the extensor mechanism reduces tension at the DIP joint and increases extensor tension at the PIP joint.

Melchior recommended a postoperative protocol in which the PIP joint is splinted in extension for 6 to 8 weeks.[22] The splint is removed to allow active motion of the DIP and PIP joints.

Tendon Grafting

Tendon grafts have been used in chronic boutonnière deformities where there is full passive extension of the PIP joint and insufficient extensor to perform a reconstruction with local tendon.[55,99,137] Littler illustrated this technique using a thin tendon graft with a figure-of-eight weave through the base of the middle phalanx and the lateral bands (Fig. 6-23). An obliquely oriented pin is used to maintain the PIP joint in extension for 3 weeks. The pin is removed, and the PIP joint is splinted in extension on a part-time basis for 2 to 3 months.

Tendon Relocation

Mobilization and relocation of adjacent extensor tendon tissue has been described in various forms for the treatment of chronic boutonnière deformities.* Many authors have reported their experience with resection of the attenuated central slip and direct repair of the central tendon and lateral bands.[33,44,65,81,88,124,141,150] Transfer of the lateral bands is recommended in those instances in which the lateral bands are fixed palmar to the axis of the PIP joint. Many variations on this technique have been described. In each, the lateral bands are mobilized by releasing the contracted fibers of the transverse retinacular ligament. Littler described dividing the lateral bands over the middle phalanx, rolling the bands dorsally and suturing them to the insertion of the central slip (Fig. 6-24).[99,102] Burton and Melchior[22] noted that this technique is not an option when the central tendon is too attenuated to hold sutures. Littler proposed an alternative; the ulnar lateral band can be detached distally, transferred through the radial lateral band and inserted through drill holes into the base of the middle phalanx.[98]

Matev's variation on this procedure involved distal detachment of the ulnar lateral band at the DIP joint and more proximal detachment of the radial lateral band at the midportion of the middle phalanx.[108,109] The ulnar lateral band is sewn to the distal stump of the radial lateral band, effectively creating a lengthened terminal tendon. The proximal limb of the radial lateral band is woven into what remains of the central slip and sutured to the periosteum over the base of the middle phalanx. Matev's version of reducing tension in the extensor at the DIP joint and increasing extensor tone at the PIP joint was reviewed in a series by Terrill and Groves.[163] Fourteen of 20 patients with supple deformities improved their extension lag at the PIP joint from 59 to 14 degrees with only a modest loss of PIP flexion. DIP flexion improved, on average 57 degrees. Six patients had a PIP flexion contracture and were treated with a palmar plate release and extensor tendon reconstruction, concurrently. The results in this group were less predictable, spurring the authors to recommend a staged procedure in which the Matev procedure is performed 3 months after the palmar plate release.

*See references 23, 43, 44, 65, 81, 88, 98, 99, 102, 107-109, 141, 148-151, and 174.

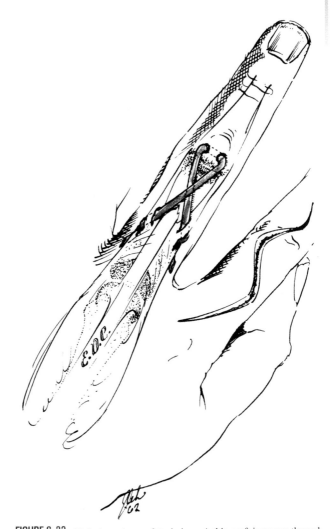

FIGURE 6-23. Littler's tendon graft technique. A thin graft is woven through the base of the middle phalanx and through the extensor tendon to restore extensor tone to the PIP joint.

Zone IV injuries: Finger Proximal Phalanx and Thumb Metacarpal

A partial zone IV tendon injury is more commonly seen than a complete laceration, because the extensor mechanism is flat and it curves around the proximal phalanx.[147] Failure to extend the PIP joint alerts the examiner that a complete tendon injury exists. The diagnosis of a partial tendon laceration is based on a skin laceration over the proximal phalanx and a weakness with resisted extension. The extent of the tendon injury can be determined only by surgical inspection.[39] Even with a complete tendon laceration, the proximal end of the tendon does not migrate proximally from the open wound because the sagittal band tethers the severed end.

Zone IV extensor tendon injuries are often associated with a proximal phalanx fracture.[118] These fractures should be operatively stabilized to allow for tendon rehabilitation.

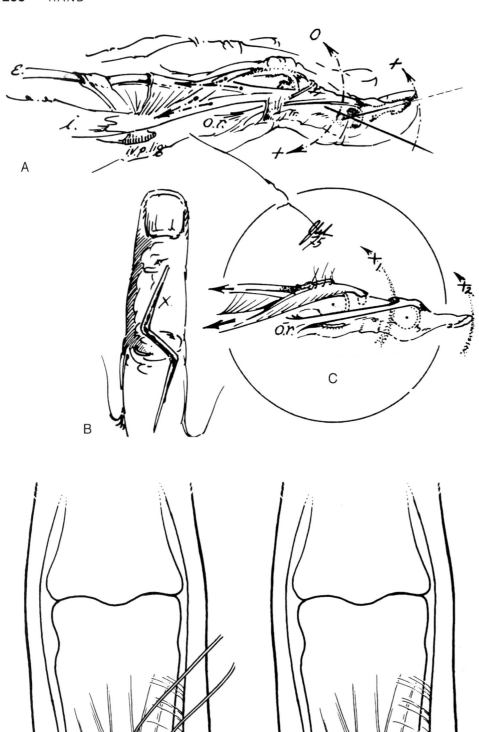

A

B

C

FIGURE 6-24. Littler's illustration of his technique for management of the chronic boutonnière deformity: transection of the lateral bands and repair dorsal to the base of the middle phalanx.

A

B

FIGURE 6-25. Lacerations in zone IV are repaired with a modified Kessler suture and epitendinous cross stitch.

Authors' Preferred Method of Treatment of Zone IV Injuries

To see the injured tendon, the laceration site should be longitudinally extended. Partial lacerations greater than 50% and complete lacerations are repaired with a modified Kessler suture using 4-0-braided polyester (Fig. 6-25). In a biomechanical study, Newport and coworkers[119] showed that a modified Kessler suture in zone IV would not shorten the tendon or limit PIP or DIP joint flexion. In addition, the repair did not gap when active motion was simulated, creating 30 degrees of PIP joint flexion.

Within the first week after tendon repair, the injured finger is started on a passive extension and active flexion protocol combined with a tendon mobilization program.[32] The hand therapist makes a dynamic extension splint in which a rubber band supplies the extension force (Fig. 6-26). Flexion blocks can be added to the splint by placing a washer on the outrigger line. The need for the flexion blocks is based on observed tension at the repair site intraoperatively; the goal of the flexion block is to allow early tendon motion without tension at the repair site. The patient wears the splint 24 hours per day for 4 to 6 weeks. During that time, he or she is instructed to flex the finger 10 times per hour while awake. The therapist starts the tendon mobilization program within the first week after repair; the program involves passive range of motion of either the MP or the PIP joints while the wrist and/or digit is in maximal extension (Fig. 6-27).[32]

In zone IV, over the thumb metacarpal, the EPB and EPL tendons are oval. Both can often be repaired with a core type suture such as a Kessler-Tajima.[161] The rehabilitation is the same for zone III injuries in the thumb, as described earlier in this chapter.

Zone V injuries (Finger MP)

Human Bite Injuries

Partial extensor tendon injuries over the MP joint are often caused by a punch to an opponent's mouth, so-called clench fist injury or fight bites. A small skin laceration is present over the MP joint, and the joint often becomes contaminated with oral flora. An inoculum of saliva contains over 42 different bacterial species and 100 million organisms per milliliter.[143] Because these injuries appear innocuous, the patient often does not recognize the severity of the injury until the joint becomes infected.[27,62,106,167] This delay has a deleterious effect.[41] Septic joints create pain, swelling, erythema, and loss of joint motion. The dominant long finger MP joint is most often involved.[167] Radiographs may be normal but can show a retained tooth, defect in the metacarpal head, or osteomyelitis.[106,167]

Bacterial cultures grow gram-positive and gram-negative organisms with *Streptococcus* species and *Staphylococcus* species being the most frequently cultured organisms.[41,106] Anaerobic bacteria such as *Bacteroides, Peptococcus, Peptostreptococcus, Clostridium,* and *Fusobacterium* have also been isolated.[18,167] *Eikenella corrodens,* an anaerobic gram-negative rod, was cultured in 6% to 30% of patients.[5,60] Rayan and coworkers showed that *Eikenella* is not universally susceptible to penicillin but was 100% susceptible to a second- or third-generation cephalosporin.[132] Streptococci and staphylococci consume oxygen, creating an ideal environment for *Eikenella* growth. There is no evidence to suggest that the presence of *Eikenella* adversely affects the outcome.[18]

Treatment consists of prompt surgical exploration of the wound. The tendon injury is proximal to the skin laceration, because the MP joint is flexed at the time of injury. The extensor tendon should be split longitudinally and the MP joint opened, cultured, and irrigated with antibiotic solution.[41] The metacarpal head should be inspected for a retained

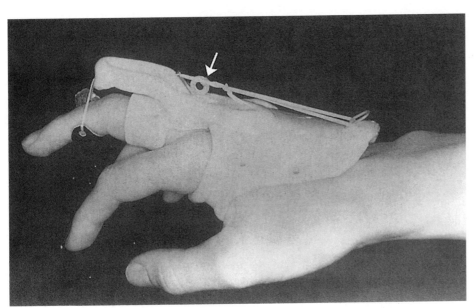

FIGURE 6-26. A hand-based dynamic splint for extensor tendon repairs distal to the MP joint. PIP flexion is limited by the blocking washer *(arrow)*. (From Crosby CA, Wehbe MA: Early protected motion after extensor tendon repair. J Hand Surg [Am] 24:1064, 1999, with permission from The American Society for Surgery of the Hand.)

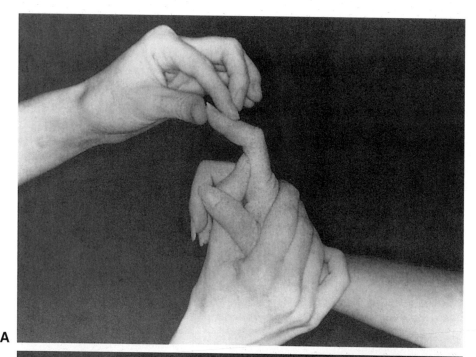

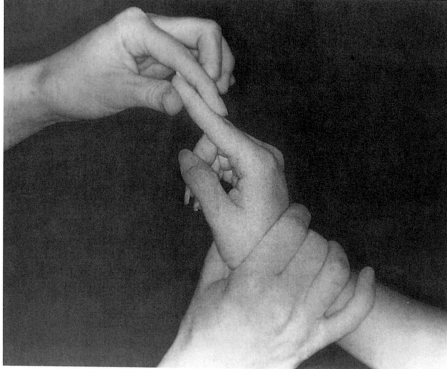

FIGURE 6-27. The tendon mobilization program for extensor tendons. **A,** The PIP joint is ranged with both the wrist and MP joints in extension. **B,** The MP joint is ranged with the wrist, PIP, and DIP joints in extension. (From Crosby CA, Wehbe MA: Early protected motion after extensor tendon repair. J Hand Surg [Am] 24:1065, 1999, with permission from The American Society for Surgery of the Hand.)

CRITICAL POINTS: CLENCH FIST INJURIES

- First priority is prevention of infection.
- Extensor tendon repair can be delayed 7 to 10 days until absence of infection is ensured.
- Treat infection empirically with IV antibiotics for 48 hours, then adjust regimen based on intraoperative culture results.

tooth or articular damage. Partial tendon lacerations usually require no suturing. Repair of complete lacerations is deferred until the infection has cleared.

The results of treatment depend on the severity of the infection. Chadaev and colleagues[27] reported that when the MP joint was septic, 6 of 48 joints lost more than 30% range of motion, and the hand lost more than 25% power pinch and 30% grip strength. The same authors reported that when there was destruction of cartilage or bone, 27 of 41 joints lost more than 30% of motion and the hand lost more than 25% power pinch and 30% grip strength.[27] Amputations or joint resections were necessary in 37 of 41 of these cases.[27] Poor prognostic factors for the development of osteomyelitis include delayed initial treatment, inadequate initial débridement, and closure of the wound at the time of injury.[62]

Authors' Preferred Method of Treatment of Zone V Injuries

In the case of a human bite, the extensor tendon injury is usually a transverse, partial laceration that does not need to be repaired. If the extensor injury is complete, the repair is delayed for 7 to 10 days until absence of infection is ensured. The portion of the wound created by the bite is not closed. The hand is splinted in a "safe position," with the wrist in 30 degrees of extension, the MP joints in 60 degrees of flexion, and the PIP joints in extension. The next day the infected hand is cleansed in a chlorazone whirlpool bath twice daily followed by resumption of splinting. Active motion exercises are initiated once the infection has started to clear. Intravenous antibiotics (ampicillin/sulbactam) are used for at least 48 hours. Patients with a significant allergic reaction to penicillin are treated with clindamycin and gentamicin.[106] When the intraoperative culture results are known, the antibiotic regimen is adjusted to an appropriate oral agent. The duration of antibiotic coverage depends on the operative findings, comorbidities, organisms, and response to treatment.

For complete, clean lacerations a core stitch of 3-0 braided polyester is used with a 5-0 nylon epitendinous stitch using the Silfverskiöld technique (Fig. 6-28).

Open Sagittal Band Injuries

Complete lacerations of either the radial or ulnar sagittal band are rare. The laceration usually causes extensor tendon subluxation or dislocation opposite the side of the injury, as well as loss of MP joint extension.[39] Partial sagittal band lacerations may or may not create tendon instability or extension loss. Koniuch and colleagues[93] demonstrated extensor tendon instability after a laceration involving two thirds of the proximal sagittal band. These injuries should be explored with the use of local anesthesia by extending the skin lacera-

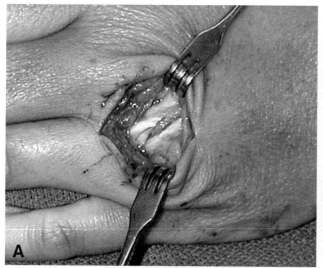

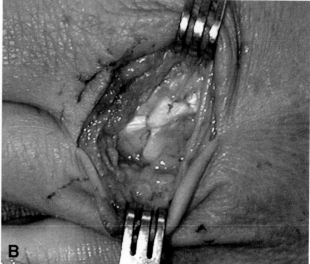

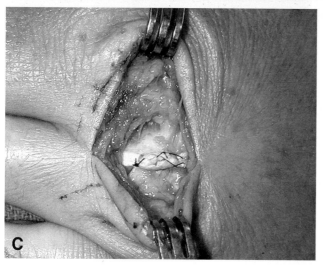

Figure 6-28. **A,** Complete laceration of the extensor tendon over the MP joint. **B,** The tendon has been approximated with a core stitch using a 3-0 braided, polyester suture. **C,** The repair is oversewn with a 5-0 nylon suture using a Silfverskiöld epitendinous repair.

tion and visualizing the extensor tendon during active flexion. If the laceration involves more than two thirds of the sagittal band or the extensor tendon becomes unstable with motion, it should be repaired.

Closed Sagittal Band Injury (Extensor Tendon Subluxation)

Closed injuries to the sagittal band are more common than open lacerations and can result from a direct blow, from forced MP joint flexion, or even from mundane daily activities such as flicking the finger or crumbling paper.[69,79] Symptoms range from pain and loss of MP joint motion to extensor tendon snapping or catching during finger flexion. Snapping from a sagittal band injury can be confused with a trigger finger. There have been a few reported cases of radial extensor tendon subluxation[4,69,134] secondary to ulnar-sided tears. The more common partial or a complete radial-sided tear commonly results in ulnar extensor tendon subluxation during finger flexion. The extensor tendon may even dislocate and cause ulnar deviation of the injured finger (Fig. 6-29). A small finger dislocated extensor tendon can cause the finger to lock in a 15- to 30-degree abduction deformity.[131] The long finger extensor tendon is prone to ulnar subluxation after injury because it tends to be loosely anchored to the sagittal band and the tendon blends into the extensor hood at a more distal level.[4,86]

Ishizuki demonstrated that the sagittal band has a thin superficial layer that runs over the extensor tendon and a thick deep layer, which lies beneath the extensor tendon. The superficial layer fuses with the deep layer on each side of the extensor tendon (Fig. 6-30).[79] Ishizuki hypothesized that spontaneous ulnar subluxation was the result of disruption of the superficial layer, whereas traumatic ulnar subluxation was caused by a tear in both layers of the sagittal band radial to the extensor tendon (Fig. 6-31).[79] The sagittal band of both the index and small fingers can be disrupted between the communis and proprius tendons.[78] This sagittal band

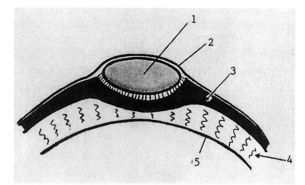

FIGURE 6-30. Ishizuki's diagrammatic representation of a transverse section of the sagittal band at the level of the MP joint: (1) The EDC tendon; (2) superficial layer of the sagittal band; (3) deep layer of the sagittal band; (4) connective tissue between the sagittal band and dorsal MP joint capsule; (5) MP joint capsule. (From Ishizuki M: Traumatic and spontaneous dislocation of extensor tendon of the long finger. J Hand Surg [Am] 15:967, 1990, with permission from The American Society for Surgery of the Hand.)

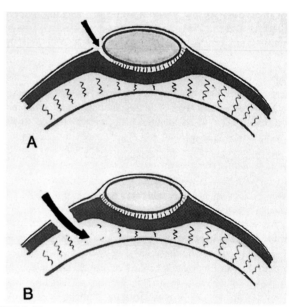

FIGURE 6-31. A, Ishizuki's interpretation of a spontaneous dislocation, in which the superficial layer of the sagittal band is disrupted. **B,** A traumatic dislocation is shown in which both the superficial and deep layers are torn. (From Ishizuki M: Traumatic and spontaneous dislocation of extensor tendon of the long finger. J Hand Surg [Am] 15:969, 1990, with permission from The American Society for Surgery of the Hand.)

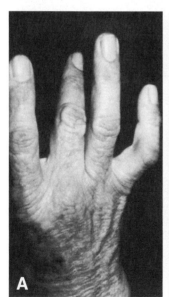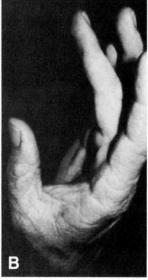

FIGURE 6-29. A and **B,** The dislocated EDC tendon is causing ulnar deviation and flexion of the long finger.

injury results in ulnar subluxation of the index or small finger EDC tendon and radial subluxation of the index or small finger proprius tendon during digital flexion.

Sagittal band injuries that do not result in symptomatic extensor tendon subluxation can be treated with buddy-taping the finger to an adjacent digit. It is imperative to rule out a collateral ligament injury by stressing the finger in flexion and obtaining radiographs to detect an avulsion fracture.[40,131] In most patients the acute symptoms resolve within 3 weeks, but it may take up to 9 months for the pain to dissipate fully.[131] If pain and loss of MP motion persist for 3 months after direct MP trauma, the patient should be given

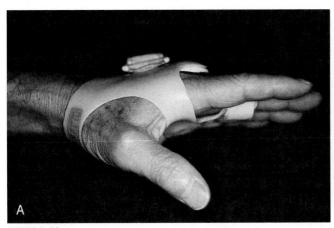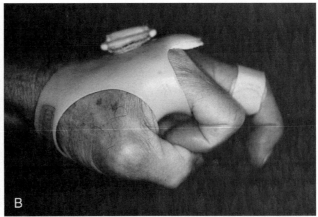

FIGURE 6-32. **A,** The splint maintains the injured finger in extension and neutral abduction-adduction. **B,** The splint permits only 10 to 20 degrees of active MP joint flexion.

the option to have the sagittal band and MP joint surgically explored. Koniuch and colleauges[93] reported on nine patients who underwent surgical exploration of the sagittal band and MP joint because of persistent pain and swelling without extensor tendon subluxation and found a partial tear of the ulnar sagittal band in seven and radial sagittal band in four. The MP joint was inspected and lavaged, and 25% of the patients had joint pathology. The MP capsule and sagittal band were repaired in separate layers with nonabsorbable mattress sutures. Within 5 postoperative days, all patients were started on a 3-week course of dynamic passive extension and active flexion splinting. Eight of the nine patients returned to full activities, and no patient experienced tendon subluxation, pain, or swelling.

Acute injuries that are 2 to 3 weeks old can be treated with extension splinting of the MP joint.[4,24,78,131,134] Inoue and Tamura[78] reported on six patients seen within 2 weeks after injury who suffered either a traumatic or a spontaneous dislocation. A splint was used for 6 weeks that blocked MP joint flexion and allowed active motion of the IP joints (Fig. 6-32). At a minimum of 8-month follow-up, all of the patients had full range of motion without recurrent tendon dislocations.[78] Despite reporting successful results with acute subluxations or dislocations treated with MP blocking splints, Rayan and Murray noted persistent pain-free tendon subluxation in four of the nine patients.[131]

Patients who fail splint treatment or who have an injury more than 3 weeks old should be treated with direct repair of the radial sagittal band and, if necessary, release of the ulnar sagittal band (Fig. 6-33).[79,86] The goal is to restore alignment of the extensor tendon by repairing the defect in the radial sagittal band. If the defect is through both the superficial and deep layers, a 4-0 nonabsorbable cross stitch is placed. If the deep layer is intact, the tendon is centered in its groove with a few simple sutures and the superficial layer is secured with a cross stitch. Local anesthesia with a distal forearm tourniquet is used to ensure that the tendon, after suture, remains centered during full active finger flexion. A contracted ulnar sagittal band may have to be released to aid in centralizing the extensor tendon. After repair, the MP joint is immobilized in slight flexion with the IP joints free

for 4 weeks. Protected range of motion exercises are continued for another 6 weeks. In a series of 13 patients, Ishizuki reported no recurrence of the tendon instability after direct repair.[79]

In some cases, a direct repair of the radial sagittal band is not possible because of scarring and deficient tissue. A number of surgeons have described operative techniques that use local tissue to reconstruct the radial sagittal band (see Fig. 6-33).[24,111,176] Wheeldon reported using the junctura tendinum between the long and ring fingers to reconstruct the radial sagittal band of the long finger.[176] With the damaged digit in flexion, the ulnar junctura tendinum is released from the adjacent tendon and transferred across and sutured to the palmar radial sagittal band remnant of the deep intermetacarpal ligament. It may not be possible to use the junctura tendinum because of its irregular location, inadequate length, or absence.[111] McCoy and Winsky described a sagittal band reconstruction that uses a distal slip of the extensor tendon. The distal extensor tendon is split on the radial side, and the tendon is wrapped around the lumbrical muscle to reconstruct the radial sagittal band.[111] In contrast to McCoy and Winsky, Carroll and coworkers[24] described using a proximal ulnar slip of the EDC to reconstruct the sagittal band. This operation using the ulnar slip of the EDC is performed under local anesthesia to allow for assessment of tendon stability and active range of motion of the finger joints. A longitudinal skin incision is made over the dorsal MP joint. The sagittal band is examined to determine if a primary repair is possible. If insufficient tissue remains that can adequately hold sutures, then the EDC tendon is centralized by releasing the ulnar sagittal band and a distally based slip of the EDC is created on the ulnar side of the damaged digit. The slip is routed deep to the EDC tendon, looped around the radial collateral ligament, tensioned to allow full flexion, and sutured back on the EDC tendon. The MP joint is splinted in extension for 6 weeks, and IP joint motion is started after 2 weeks. At 6 weeks, MP joint motion is initiated to regain full MP flexion. Carroll and coworkers[24] reported the results from five sagittal band reconstructions in three patients. At follow-up all five reconstructions produced a painless, 90-degree arc of MP joint motion without residual tendon subluxation.

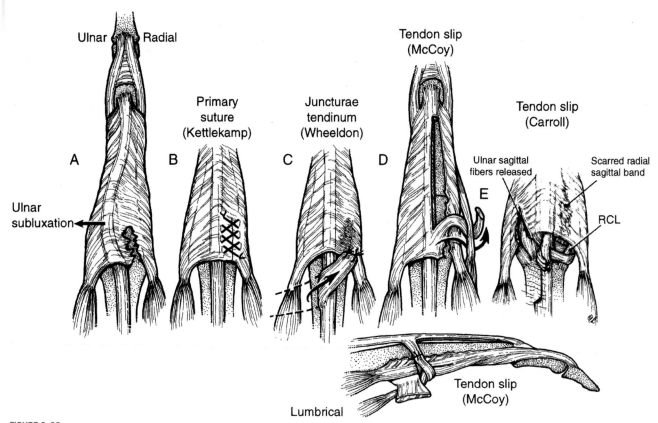

FIGURE 6-33. Methods of extensor hood reconstruction. **A,** Ulnar subluxation of the EDC tendon caused by a torn radial sagittal band. **B,** Primary suture of the radial sagittal band centering the EDC tendon. **C,** The ulnar junctura tendinum is released from the adjacent tendon and sutured to the palmar radial sagittal band remnant of the deep intermetacarpal ligament. **D,** The distal tendon is splinted on the radial side and wrapped around the lumbrical muscle. **E,** An ulnar, distally based slip of the EDC is looped around the radial collateral ligament.

Authors' Preferred Method of Treatment of Extensor Tendon Subluxation

Lacerations of the sagittal band that involve more than two thirds of the band substance or that result in tendon subluxation or loss of MP joint extension are repaired. We recommend repair of the tendon with a 4-0 braided polyester Kessler suture and a 4-0 locked running nylon suture.

Sagittal band ruptures that cause extensor tendon subluxation, if diagnosed within 3 weeks of injury, are treated with a hand-based MP extension splint. Patients with symptomatic ulnar subluxating EDC tendons diagnosed more than 3 weeks earlier and those who fail splint treatment should undergo surgical exploration under local anesthesia and primary repair of the radial sagittal band. The surgeon may have to release the ulnar sagittal band to centralize the EDC tendon. If the radial sagittal band is deficient to prohibit repair, then a sagittal band reconstruction, as described by Carroll and coworkers,[24] is performed.

Thumb CMC Joint

Lacerations over the thumb CMC usually involve the EPB and APL tendons. Patients present with limited MP joint extension and/or CMC joint abduction. Care should be taken to rule

out an injury to the sensory branch of the radial nerve and/or the radial artery. The EPB and APL are sizeable tendons and can be repaired with a 3-0 polyester modified Kessler-Tajima suture.[161] Within 2 to 5 days after repair, tendon gliding is initiated by using a dynamic splint program.[32] The rubber band on the splint holds the MP in neutral and allows full active MP joint flexion across the palm (Fig. 6-34).

Zone VI injuries (Finger Metacarpal)

Acute Injuries

As noted by Doyle, zone VI injuries tend to have a better prognosis than distal injuries because "zone VI injuries are unlikely to have associated joint injuries, decreased tendon surface area in zone VI lessens the potential for adhesion formation, increased subcutaneous tissue lessens the potential for adhesions, there is greater tendon excursion in zone VI, and complex tendon imbalances are less likely to occur."[39]

The function of the EDC tendon in zone VI is to extend the MP joint. Even with a complete laceration of the EDC tendon, a patient may still be able to extend the MP joint with the aid of either the EIP, extensor digiti quinti, or juncturae tendinum. The integrity of the proprius tendons to the index and small fingers can be tested by having the patient flex the long and ring fingers while extending the index and small fingers. Failure to extend the index or small

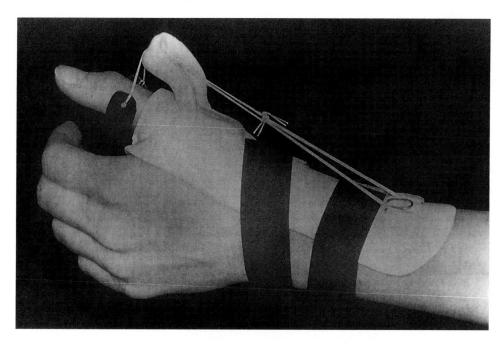

FIGURE 6-34. This forearm based dynamic splint permits active MP and IP flexion. (From Crosby CA, Wehbe MA: Early protected motion after extensor tendon repair. J Hand Surg [Am] 24:1064, 1999, with permission from The American Society for Surgery of the Hand.)

finger indicates a laceration to the respective proprius tendon.[56] The juncturae tendinum interconnect the extensor tendons of the long, ring, and small fingers. In the case of a complete laceration of the EDC tendon proximal to the juncturae, the patient may still be able to extend the MP joint through the pull of the adjacent tendons. Wounds should be explored in patients with loss of hyperextension of the MP joint or weakness with resisted extension to rule out the possibility of a significant partial or complete extensor tendon laceration.

The extensor tendons in zone VI have a sufficient diameter to allow placement of a 2-0 braided, polyester core suture.

Newport and Williams[120] compared the biomechanical properties of zone VI tendon suture using either a mattress, figure-of-eight, modified Bunnell, or modified Kessler suture; the results showed the modified Bunnell suture to have the greatest repair strength with the least loss of MP and PIP joint motion (Fig. 6-35). The skin laceration should be extended to allow enough visualization to place a modified Bunnell suture. At least 1 cm of tendon proximal and distal to the laceration should be grasped with the suture.

A dynamic splint and tendon mobilization program as described by Crosby and Wehbe is recommended.[32] A dynamic forearm-based splint is made with the wrist in

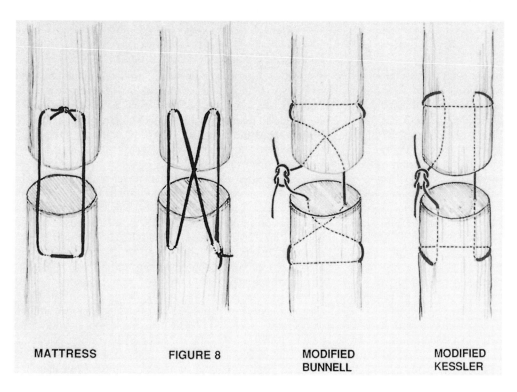

MATTRESS   FIGURE 8   MODIFIED BUNNELL   MODIFIED KESSLER

FIGURE 6-35. The modified Bunnell suture was the strongest suture with the least loss of MP or PIP joint motion. (From Newport ML, Williams CD: Biomechanical characteristics of extensor tendon suture techniques. J Hand Surg [Am] 17:1119, 1992, with permission from The American Society for Surgery of the Hand.)

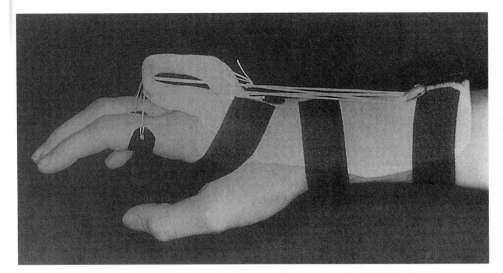

FIGURE 6-36. A dynamic extensor splint is used for repairs proximal to the MP joints. (From Crosby CA, Wehbe MA: Early protected motion after extensor tendon repair. J Hand Surg [Am] 24:1063, 1999, with permission from The American Society for Surgery of the Hand.)

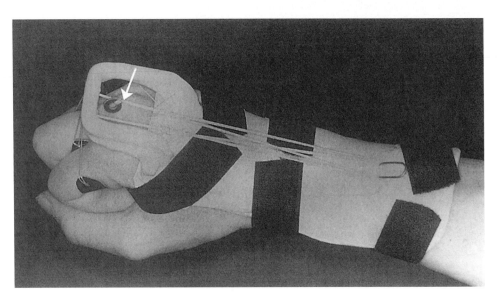

FIGURE 6-37. The washer (arrow) blocks active flexion to protect the repair site. (From Crosby CA, Wehbe MA: Early protected motion after extensor tendon repair. J Hand Surg [Am] 24:1063, 1999, with permission from The American Society for Surgery of the Hand.)

30 degrees of extension; the rubber-band traction produces MP extension and allows active MP flexion (Fig. 6-36). A blocking washer can be applied to the splint to limit active flexion (Fig. 6-37). The level of the flexion block (i.e., how much MP flexion can be allowed) should be determined at the time of surgery. The goal is to allow tendon gliding to limit adhesion formation and decrease tension on the repair to prevent gap formation. Patients are instructed to actively flex the injured finger 10 times per hour in the splint that is worn 24 hours per day for 4 to 6 weeks. Tendon mobilization program is also started within the first week as described earlier in the discussion on zone IV repairs. The patients are weaned from the dynamic splint 4 to 6 weeks after surgery, and during that time active range of motion and tendon gliding exercises are started. The patients are allowed full, unrestricted activity 8 to 12 weeks after surgery.

Crosby and Wehbe reported on six tendons with zone VI repairs using the just-described dynamic traction and tendon mobilization program. Their findings showed a total active motion of 265 degrees (normal 260 degrees), pinch strength of 95%, and grip strength of 92%.[32] Both pinch and grip strength were compared with that of the uninjured hand. Other investigators have reported good and excellent results after zone VI tendon repairs using dynamic extension, active flexion tendon protocols.[16,29,76,85] In contrast to the good results reported after early passive motion protocols, Newport and associates reported 10 of 29 patients having a fair or poor result after zone VI tendon repair followed by 3 to 4 weeks tendon immobilization before active range of motion was allowed.[118] Khandwala and colleagues compared two groups of 50 patients with zone V and VI extensor tendon injuries and found no statistically significant difference between postoperative rehabilitation with either a dynamic outrigger splint or a palmar blocking splint.[87]

Complications after zone VI tendon repair include loss of flexion, loss of extension, and tendon rupture.[16,29,32,76,85,118] Loss of finger flexion has been reported to be more common than loss of extension.[118] This loss of flexion is believed to be due to shortening of the extensor tendon during the repair. In a biomechanical study, the investigators reported that 8 mm of extensor tendon shortening in zone VI resulted in a decrease of 23 degrees for MP flexion and 22 degrees for PIP flexion.[120] Avoiding shortening the tendon during repair can prevent this extrinsic extensor tightness. In Crosby's series, tendon ruptures were a result of patients removing their dynamic splints within the first 3 weeks of surgery.[32] If tendon rupture occurs, the tendon should be explored and sutured again as soon as possible.

Authors' Preferred Method of Treatment of Zone VI Injuries

Extensor tendon lacerations over the metacarpal are repaired using a core suture of 3-0 braided, synthetic suture. A modified Kessler stitch for the core stitch is supplemented by a Silfverskiöld epidendinous stitch. Our experience has been similar to that of Khandwala and colleagues[87] in that equal success can be achieved with either dynamic extension splinting or a palmar splint. When using a palmar splint, splint position is determined based on the tension observed after tendon repair. In general, we place the wrist in 20 degrees of extension and the MP joints in 30 degrees of flexion and leave the IP joints free.

Chronic Injuries

Tethered by the juncturae, lacerated extensors over the metacarpal frequently remain close to the site of injury, permitting delayed repair. The juncturae can be used to bridge short segmental defects resulting from muscle shortening or débridement of the tendon ends. Intercalary tendon grafts or tendon transfers can be used for long-standing injuries. A two-stage reconstruction with silicone rods should be considered when the dorsal skin adheres to the underlying metacarpals. Tomaino and Plakseychuk[166] described a two-stage extensor tendon reconstruction with free-tissue transfer in a patient with chronic osteomyelitis after a severe burn.

Zone VII Injuries

Acute Injuries

Acute extensor tendon injuries in zone VII are usually the result of penetrating trauma. As a result, there is almost always an associated injury to the extensor retinaculum. Zone VII tendons have a diameter close to that of a flexor tendon. Consequently, it is easier to place core sutures and circumferential epidendinous stitches.

There has been considerable debate concerning the appropriate management of the extensor retinaculum. Some surgeons advocate excising the retinaculum overlying the repaired tendon to prevent adhesions forming between these two structures. Excision of the retinaculum can also improve exposure and prevent friction between bulky repairs and the overlying retinaculum. Other surgeons have noted no difference in results in zone VII when the retinaculum is repaired overlying tendon repairs. If at all possible, some portion of the retinaculum should be maintained, repaired, or recon-

structed to prevent bowstringing or subluxation of the extensor tendons.

Primary repair of lacerated tendons is performed using 3-0 or 4-0 nonabsorbable suture and a grasping or locking stitch. In zone VII injuries, there are frequently multiple lacerated tendons and dissection into areas of normal anatomy may be required to correctly identify the cut tendon ends. Typically, the tendons will retract into the forearm, and correct anatomic identification can be more challenging. A thorough understanding of the normal anatomy can prove invaluable in these cases. The technique of Botte and coworkers[8] helps keep multiple tendon ends organized. Once a tendon is identified based on the proximal and distal anatomy, a suture is placed and a hemostat clamped on the suture material. A sterile tape is used to label the hemostat with the name of the identified tendon.

Chronic Injuries

The management of chronic injuries in zone VII is difficult for several reasons. There is no paratenon in this intra-synovial portion of the tendon. As a result, the proximal tendon tends to retract. Over time, the ability to reapproximate the tendon ends is limited by this retraction. Attempts to repair tendons after muscle contracture leads to extrinsic tightness and limited flexion. Additionally, the fibro-osseous compartments through which the tendons pass tend to scar.

Chronic injuries can be a result of a delay in diagnosis, poor patient compliance, or concomitant trauma that delays surgical care. The most common cause of chronic tendon injuries is attritional rupture, such as rupture of the EPL tendon after a distal radius fracture. The etiology of this rupture remains uncertain. Some propose that it is related to the disruption of the tendon's blood supply or wear of the tendon on a malreduced fracture fragment. However, this does not explain why EPL ruptures are more common in nondisplaced fractures. Denman proposed that the mechanism of a distal radius fracture directly injures the EPL tendon, whereas Helal and coworkers suggested that the failure of the third compartment retinaculum to tear after nondisplaced fractures constricted the EPL, leading to delayed attritional ruptures.[36,71] EPL longus ruptures usually occur from 3 weeks to 3 months after a distal radius fracture. The tendon ruptures at the distal edge of the extensor retinaculum near Lister's tubercle. Patients note a sudden loss of thumb extension.

Chronic tendon injuries can be managed with an intercalary graft or a tendon transfer. Tendon grafting can be performed with a palmaris longus or toe extensor. This gives the original muscle control of finger function, obviating the need for retraining. Before grafting, the muscle should be tested for excursion. A muscle that is shortened or scarred will not be an effective motor. Tendon transfers using the EIP can provide independent extension with sufficient length to reach the thumb and all four fingers. The EIP can be identified preoperatively by having the patient hyperextend the index finger MP joint. Surgeons should remember that Gonzales and coworkers noted variations of the EIP in 19% of cadaver specimens examined.[63]

Rupture of multiple tendons can be challenging and is seen predominantly in patients with rheumatoid arthritis (see Chapter 59).

Authors' Preferred Method of Teatment of Zone VII Injuries

We use the EIP to EPL tendon transfer in cases of EPL rupture. The EIP has a similar amplitude and line of pull to the EPL muscle-tendon unit. There is little re-education necessary, and there is only one tendon junction. Patients must confirm independent EIP function by extending the index finger while fully flexing the remainder of the digits. Three small incisions are used to perform the transfer. First a 1-cm, transverse incision is made over the index finger MP joint and the ulnarmost tendon is isolated. A second transverse incision is made just proximal to the extensor retinaculum. Through this proximal incision the EIP tendon is identified in the radial aspect of the fourth extensor compartment. The EIP is usually the only tendon to have muscle fibers as far distal as the extensor retinaculum. Through the incision over the MP joint the EIP tendon is separated from interconnections to the EDC and transected. The EIP tendon is then brought through the proximal incision. A third incision is centered over the scaphotrapezial trapezoid joint, the usual location of the distal stump of the ruptured EPL tendon. A subcutaneous tunnel is created to connect the incision in the distal forearm and the incision near the base of the thumb. The EIP tendon is passed through the tunnel and attached distally to the distal stump of the EPL with a Pulvertaft weave. The tension on the transfer should be set so that when the wrist is extended the IP joint flexes, allowing the tip of the thumb to touch the tip of the index finger. The thumb IP joint should fully extend when the wrist is flexed. The thumb is immobilized with the wrist extended 20 degrees and the thumb IP joint at 0 degrees for 4 weeks. Active motion is permitted at 4 weeks. The transfer is protected from heavy resistance for 12 weeks.

Zone VIII: Distal Forearm

Injuries in zone VIII include ruptures of the musculotendinous junction and muscle belly lacerations. Repair of these injuries is complicated by the difficulty of placing sutures in the thin fascia overlying the muscle. Occasionally, an adequate repair can be obtained by placing sutures in the muscle fascia distally, where it is thickening to form the tendon. When repair is not feasible, a side-to-side tendon transfer may provide the best means to restore tendon function.

Ruptures at the musculotendinous junction are rare. Takami and associates[162] reported 10 cases, usually resulting from violent, resisted wrist or finger extension. Five injuries were sports related and five resulted from industrial accidents. The EDCs to the long and ring fingers were the tendons most frequently injured. Two ruptures were partial. The remaining eight ruptures were explored and managed with a side-to-side repair to an adjacent extensor tendon. Good or excellent results were obtained in seven of the eight patients.

Zone IX: Proximal Forearm

Zone IX is defined as the proximal half of the forearm and is composed of the muscle bellies of the extensor tendons.

Penetrating trauma in this region can be accompanied by nerve injuries that can make proper assessment difficult. As is true distally, small skin lacerations can cover extensive muscle disruption, and careful examination is required. In some cases, disruption of muscle tissue in the forearm may not impair wrist or finger function.

Surgeons should attempt to repair injuries that involve complete disruption of a muscle belly. A thorough exploration should be performed to identify associated nerve or arterial injuries. Débridement of devitalized tissue may make repair more difficult but is necessary to prevent infection. Multiple, interrupted absorbable sutures are used to repair the epimysium and fibrous intramuscular septa.

Botte and colleagues[9] described a technique for tendon grafting muscle lacerations in the proximal forearm that involved 50% or more of at least two muscle bellies. A palmaris or toe extensor graft is harvested and passed through the superficial and deep epimysium on each side of the laceration. The ends of the tendon are sewn to themselves in a Pulvertaft fashion. This loop of tendon helps to reinforce the epimysial repair. In 58 patients, 54% achieved grade 4 or 5 muscle strength after these repairs.

ANNOTATED REFERENCES

3. Aiche A, Barsky AJ, Weiner DL: Prevention of the boutonnière deformity. Plast Reconstr Surg 46:164-167, 1970.

    Describes a procedure using 50% of the lateral band to reconstruct the central slip in cases of acute central slip loss, but the authors do not report their results.

38. Dolphin JA: Extensor tenotomy for chronic boutonniere deformity of the fingers: Report of two cases. J Bone Joint Surg Am 47:161-164, 1965.

    Although Dolphin reported only two cases, this is the classic description of terminal extensor tendon division distal to the triangular ligament for treatment of chronic boutonnière deformities. The division is performed distal to the triangular ligament, and neither patient developed an extensor lag at the DIP joint level.

57. Gama C: Results of the Matev operation for correction of boutonnière deformity. Plast Reconstr Surg 64:319-324, 1979.

    A report of 41 patients treated using the Matev extensor tendon reconstruction in patients who had boutonnière deformity for less than 6 months. Postoperatively, all patients had a slight PIP extensor lag and the majority had full composite finger flexion. The author recommended immobilization for only 3 weeks postoperatively in 40 degrees of flexion at the PIP joint level.

88. Kilgore ES, Graham WP: Operative treatment of boutonnière deformity. Surgery 64:999-1000, 1968.

    Describing the pathology of boutonnière deformity, these authors recommended a "V" incision in the central slip with excision of redundant scar and advancement of the proximal tendon. This is purely a description of technique and no report of results.

102. Littler JW, Eaton RG: Redistribution of forces in the correction of the boutonnière deformity. J Bone Joint Surg Am 49:1267-1274, 1967.

    Littler and Eaton described the pathology of the boutonnière deformity and a method of repair using the lateral bands, which are detached from the oblique retinacular ligament. The lateral bands are detached from the terminal tendon, flipped over, and repaired to the central slip insertion site. The lateral bands then function to simply extend the PIP joint. This reconstruction is used for chronic boutonnière deformities, and the article reported good results in eight cases.

108. Matev I: Transposition of the lateral slips of the aponeurosis in treatment of long-standing "boutonnière deformity" of the fingers. Br J Plast Surg 17:281-286, 1964.

    The original description of a procedure that involves using one of the lateral bands to reconstruct the central slip and lengthening of the terminal extensor tendon with the other. The author reported results of nine cases.

122. Nichols HM: Repair of extensor-tendon insertions in the fingers. J Bone Joint Surg Am 33:836-841, 1951.

    By using palmaris longus tendon grafts for repair of late mallet and boutonnière deformities, Nichols reported a successful outcome in 11 of 12 cases.

133. Rico AA, Holguin PH, Vecilla LR, del Rio JL: Tendon reconstruction of postburn boutonnière deformity. J Hand Surg [Am] 17:862-867, 1992.

    A tendon graft is used to keep the lateral bands dorsal to the axis of rotation of the PIP joint, allowing them to act as the primary extensor of the PIP joint. The authors employed this technique in 22 fingers with satisfactory results.

150. Souter WA: The boutonnière deformity: A review of 101 patients with division of the central slip of the extensor expansion of the fingers. J Bone Joint Surg Br 49:710-721, 1967.

    The classic article that showed better results with nonoperative treatment as compared with surgery. A series of 106 central slip injuries without fixed flexion contracture of the finger were treated within the first 6 weeks.

151. Souter WA: The problem of boutonnière deformity. Clin Orthop 104:116-133, 1974.

    An excellent overall description of the deformity, which also describes the treatment, both conservative and operative, and lists the multiple late reconstructive options when there is not adequate central slip tissue available for repair.

163. Terrill RQ, Groves RJ: Correction of the severe nonrheumatoid chronic boutonnière deformity with a modified Matev procedure. J Hand Surg [Am] 17:874-880, 1992.

    A retrospective review of 20 patients treated for chronic boutonnière deformity with the Matev procedure, with a good description of the procedure and postoperative protocol. There was an 85% satisfactory outcome in the group without preoperative fixed flexion contracture and 67% good or satisfactory outcome in the group with a preoperative fixed flexion contracture. The release of the fixed flexion contracture and extensor reconstruction was performed simultaneously. Based on these results, the authors recommended staged reconstruction with initial fixed flexion contracture release followed by second-stage extensor reconstruction.

170. Urbaniak JR, Hayes MG: Chronic boutonnière deformity—an anatomic reconstruction. J Hand Surg [Am] 6:379-383, 1981.

    A description of a technique for chronic boutonnière deformities that involves release of the transverse retinacular ligament and reconstruction of the central slip using a flap of capsule attached to the base of the middle phalanx. A prerequisite for the procedure was full passive range of motion. Twelve of 13 patients had satisfactory results.

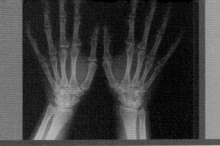

CHAPTER 7

Flexor Tendon Injury

Acute Injuries

Martin I. Boyer

Major advances in the understanding of intrasynovial flexor tendon biology, repair, and rehabilitation have been made since the 1960s, when reports first demonstrated that flexor tendon lacerations within the confines of the fibro-osseous flexor digital sheath could be repaired primarily and that rehabilitation could be carried out successfully without excision of the lacerated tendons followed by primary tendon grafting.* The concept of adhesion-free tendon healing has been validated both in experimental and in clinical studies since that time,† lending support to efforts attempting to achieve a reliable technique of primary flexor tendon repair and digital rehabilitation without the inevitable need for later tenolysis.‡ Although investigators have focused recently on restoration of the gliding surface of the visceral and parietal paratenon, on in-vitro and in-vivo repair site biomechanics, and on understanding the molecular processes operant during flexor healing, the goals of the surgical treatment of the lacerated intrasynovial flexor tendon have remained constant: the achievement of a primary tendon repair of tensile strength sufficient to allow the application of a postoperative motion rehabilitation protocol that inhibits the formation of intrasynovial adhesions, stimulates restoration of the gliding surface, and facilitates healing of the repair site.

---

*See references 49, 69, 137, 186, 237, 290, 359, 449, 459, 463, 473, and 474.

†See references 117, 121-123, 127-130, 241, 244, 245, 248-250, 259, 262, 263, 267, and 271.

‡See references 109, 173, 177, 252, 289, 384, 420, 428, 433, 461, 472, and 485.

PREOPERATIVE EVALUATION

The preoperative clinical examination of the traumatized hand is done before the administration of local anesthesia or sedation so that neurologic or vascular injury can be documented and the appropriate operating room supplies requested should microsurgical repair be required. After completion of the clinical examination, a median and/or ulnar nerve block can be performed for analgesia if required.

The integrity of the skin on both the volar and dorsal aspects of the injured digit(s) is examined to ascertain the presence or absence of additional injuries. Obvious angular or rotational deformity of the digit signifies either a metacarpal or a phalangeal fracture or a dislocation of the metacarpophalangeal (MCP), proximal interphalangeal (PIP), or distal interphalangeal (DIP) joints. Realignment of a fracture or reduction of the dislocation may be required before the evaluation of flexor tendon integrity or the presence of digital neurovascular injury. If the flexor tendons are lacerated in the absence of any underlying skeletal injury (as is usually the case), the digit assumes an extended posture at the PIP and DIP joints even on the application of a passive moment of wrist extension, which would effect a tenodesis force in the presence of intact tendons.

Examination for continuity of the flexor digitorum superficialis (FDS) tendon, as distinct from the flexor digitorum profundus (FDP) tendon, is performed (Fig. 7-1). To isolate the FDS tendon, the adjacent digits are held in full extension or in mild hyperextension by the examiner at the MCP, PIP, and DIP joints. Active flexion of the PIP joint is evaluated for each digit separately and, if present, indicates intact fibers of the FDS inserting into the middle phalanx. It does not, however, rule out partial FDS injury.

Evaluation for continuity of the FDP tendon is done by asking the patient to flex the DIP joint actively while the

The authors acknowledge the work of **Drs. James Strickland** and **Lawrence Schneider,** whose outstanding chapters in previous editions have been modified, combined, and updated. Their contributions to our understanding of repair and reconstruction of the damaged flexor tendon system have greatly advanced our ability to care for these injuries.

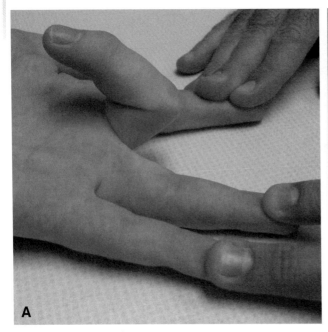

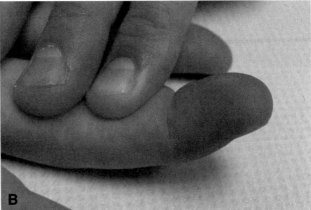

FIGURE 7-1. **A,** Continuity of the FDS tendon is evaluated by asking the patient to flex the finger actively while holding the MCP joints of the uninvolved fingers in hyperextension and the PIP and DIP joints of the uninvolved fingers in full extension. This effectively eliminates the profundus and allows the superficialis action to be evaluated. **B,** The middle phalanx is held firmly, and active flexion at the DIP joint is carried out. This demonstrates continuity of the FDP tendon.

examiner grasps the middle phalanx. Active flexion of the digit against resistance in an attempt to elicit pain to diagnose partial tendon laceration is to be condemned.

The digital neurovascular status is examined. Both the radial and the ulnar digital nerves are tested by means of static two-point discrimination, and the capillary refill of both the volar digital pulp and the nail bed are recorded. Slowing of the capillary refill of the involved digit may imply digital artery laceration, and microvascular repair should be anticipated.

Although a complete evaluation of the skin, digital nerves, blood supply, and skin cover enables the surgeon to prepare for most of the operative findings that will be encountered, some elements of the injury will by necessity be appreciated fully only on surgical exploration. These include damage to the vincula, the deep layer of the parietal paratenon (overlying the phalangeal periosteum layer), the fibrous pulley system (most notably the A2 and the A4 pulleys), and the volar plates overlying the MCP and interphalangeal (IP) joints. Failure to address these injured structures could lead to complications in the immediate, early, and late periods postoperatively.

Plain radiographs are taken while the patient is in the emergency department, because fluoroscopic images taken intraoperatively can lack the necessary resolution and detail required to diagnose subtle bony injury. In addition, indirect injury to the flexor mechanism such as occurs in avulsions of the FDP from its insertion into the proximal aspect of the distal phalanx may be accompanied by bony injury. On occasion, a small fleck of bone indicates the extent of proximal tendon stump retraction and will minimize proximal dissection that would be unnecessary. Surgical supplies necessary for the fixation of small fragments of bone may be required and should be available.

Remote injuries of the skeleton are diagnosed radiographically, and their presence may affect the results expected from tendon repair. Occasionally, additional imaging studies may be requested to delineate precisely the location of the proximal tendon stump after a delay in presentation. High-resolution ultrasound examination of the digit has been shown to be effective, and magnetic resonance imaging (MRI) has also been reported to achieve good results in determining the location of the proximal stump. A blinded clinical study evaluating whether localization of the proximal stump by clinical examination of a tender nodule along the course of the flexor tendon is less accurate than either ultrasound or MRI has not been performed.

Anatomy

The FDS muscle belly has two heads of origin: the ulnar head arises from the anterior aspect of the medial epicondyle, the ulnar collateral ligament of the elbow, the medial aspect of the coronoid process, and the proximal ulna; and the radial head arises from the proximal radius immediately distal to the insertion of the supinator muscle. It lies deep to the pronator teres, flexor carpi radialis, palmaris longus, and flexor carpi ulnaris muscles and superficial to the FDP and the flexor pollicis longus muscle bellies. The median nerve is loosely adherent to the deep surface of the FDS muscle. At the level of the mid forearm, the FDS muscle divides into superficial and deep layers, which send tendons to the middle and ring fingers (superficial) and the index and small fingers (deep). The FDS tendon to the small finger may be hypoplastic or absent in some individuals. The innervation of the FDS muscle is from the median nerve, which enters the muscle belly in the proximal forearm. The blood supply is from both the radial and the ulnar arteries.

The FDP muscle belly arises from the volar and medial aspects of the proximal three fourths of the ulna immediately distal to the insertion of the brachialis muscle and from the medial half of the volar aspect of the interosseous membrane. It lies deep to the FDS muscle belly and is adjacent to the flexor pollicis longus muscle belly in the forearm. The ulnar nerve travels distally in the forearm loosely adherent to the FDP muscle belly, supplying innervation to the muscle-tendon units of the ring and small fingers. The anterior interosseous branch of the median nerve innervates the FDP muscle tendon units of the index and middle fingers. The tendons of the FDP usually arise from a common muscle belly, although the FDP tendon of the index finger exhibits a greater independence because it frequently arises from a separate muscle belly. The blood supply of the FDP muscle is from the ulnar artery predominantly.

The flexor pollicis longus (FPL) tendon arises from the volar aspect of the middle third of the radial shaft and from the lateral aspect of the interosseous membrane. It is located deep to the tendon of the flexor carpi radialis muscle and the radial artery at the level of the proximal wrist flexion crease. The anterior interosseous branch innervates the FPL muscle belly in the proximal or mid forearm. The blood supply of the FDP muscle is predominantly from the radial artery.

The tendons of the nine digital flexors enter the proximal aspect of the carpal tunnel in a fairly constant relationship: the four FDP tendons are deep to the FDS tendons of the index and small digits, and the FDS tendons to the ring and middle digits lie superficially immediately ulnar or subjacent to the median nerve. The tendon of the FPL lies deep and radial within the carpal tunnel, adjacent to the scaphoid and the trapezium.

The FDP tendon is divided into five anatomic zones (Fig. 7-2). Zone V extends from the muscle-tendon junction to the proximal aspect of the carpal tunnel, and zone IV describes the flexor tendons within the carpal tunnel. Distal to the transverse carpal ligament at approximately the level of the superficial palmar vascular arch, the lumbrical tendons take their origin from the FDP tendons. Zone III denotes the origin of the lumbricals from the FDP tendon. A reflection of synovial tissue covers the distal aspect of zone III of the flexor tendon, and the proximal aspect of the A1 pulley is the entrance to the fibro-osseous flexor sheath: zone II of the flexor tendon. Zone I lies distal to the insertion of the FDS tendon and includes the C3 and A5 pulleys. A laceration in zone I, by definition, injures only the tendon of the FDP.

As the FDS tendon enters the A1 pulley it divides into two equal halves that rotate laterally and then dorsally around the FDP tendon (Fig. 7-3). The two slips rejoin deep to the FDP tendon over the distal aspect of the proximal phalanx and the palmar plate of the PIP joint at Camper's chiasm and then insert as two separate slips on the volar aspect of the middle phalanx.

The fibro-osseous digital sheath defines zones I and II of the FDS and FDP tendons (Fig. 7-4). Within this sheath, the flexor tendons are covered by a thin layer of visceral paratenon, and the internal aspect of the sheath and the pulley system is covered by a continuous layer of parietal paratenon. These two layers of paratenon comprise the so-called gliding surface of the flexor tendons within the digital sheath, the restoration of which is critical to the unimpeded function of the digit after flexor tendon repair.

The pulley mechanism of the flexor sheath consists of (1) annular pulleys, which serve to keep the tendon applied

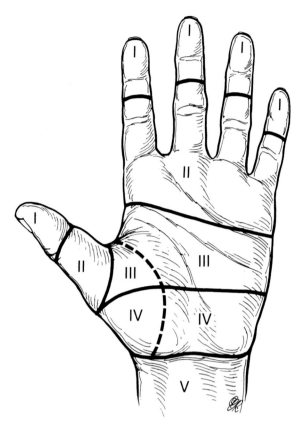

FIGURE 7-2. The flexor system has been divided into five zones or levels for the purposes of discussion and treatment. Zone II, which lies within the fibro-osseous sheath, has been called "no man's land" because it was once believed that primary repair should not be done in this zone (see p. 241).

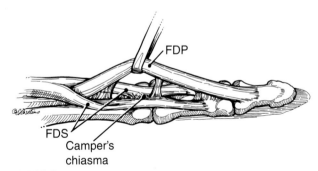

FIGURE 7-3. In the proximal part of the flexor sheath the FDS tendon divides into two slips, which then encircle the FDP tendon first volar, then radial and ulnar, and then finally dorsal. The two portions of the FDS tendon reunite at Camper's chiasm and then re-divide before inserting onto the middle three fifths of the volar aspect of the middle phalanx, forming the floor of the flexor sheath in this area.

closely to the underlying bone and thus improve the mechanical efficiency of joint rotation, and (2) cruciform pulleys, which are compressible and allow for digital flexion to occur without undue deformation of the annular pulley system (see Fig. 7-4). The A1, A3, and A5 pulleys take origin from the palmar plates of the MCP, PIP, and DIP joints, and the A2 and A4 pulleys take origin from the middle halves of the proximal and middle phalanges, respectively. The cruciform pulleys are located proximal and distal to the PIP joint between the A2 and A3 pulleys (C1)

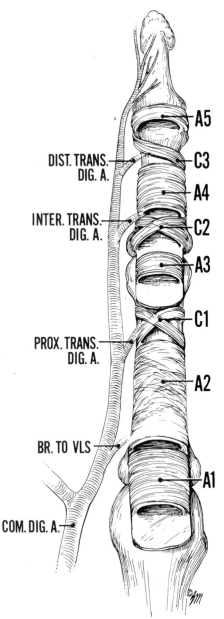

A5
DIST. TRANS. — C3
DIG. A.
A4
INTER. TRANS. — C2
DIG. A.
A3
C1
PROX. TRANS. —
DIG. A.
A2
BR. TO VLS —
A1
COM. DIG. A. —

FIGURE 7-4. The fibrous retinacular sheath starts at the neck of the metacarpal and ends at the distal phalanx. Condensations of the sheath form the flexor pulleys, which can be identified as five heavier annular bands and three filmy cruciform ligaments (see text). Dist. Trans. Dig. A., distal transverse digital artery; Inter. Trans. Dig. A., intermediate transverse digital artery; Prox. Trans. Dig. A., proximal transverse digital artery; Br. to VLS, branch to vinculum longum; Com. Dig. A., common digital artery.

and between the A3 and A4 pulleys (C2), and the C3 pulley is located proximal to the DIP joint between the A4 and A5 pulleys.

The nutritional supply of the FDS and FDP tendons is twofold (Fig. 7-5).* The parietal paratenon[86,94] allows for passive nutrient delivery to, and waste removal from, the flexor tendon within the flexor sheath by means of diffusion. In addition, a direct arterial supply to the flexor tendons

*See references 73, 80, 93, 115, 120, 171, 225, 243, 246-248, 261, 266, 270, 283, 284, 314, 326, 382, and 467.

through the vincular system as well as the bone of both the middle (FDS) and distal (FDP) phalanges allows for the active delivery of nutrients and the removal of wastes.[24,36,171,172,224,314,333] The vinculum longum superficialis (VLS) arises from a ladder branch of the digital arterial system over the proximal metaphysis of the proximal phalanx, and the vinculum brevis superficialis (VBS) arises from an arterial ladder branch at the level of the origin of the volar plate of the PIP joint. The vinculum longum profundus (VLP) arises from the same source as the VBS and is related intimately to it. The vinculum brevis profundus (VBP) arises from the digital arteries at the level of the distal metaphysis of the middle phalanx. The avascular zone of the FDS tendon lies between the VLS and the VBS. The avascular zones of the FDP tendon lie proximal to the VLP and between the VLP and the VBP. Flexor tendon nutrition in these avascular zones is effected by diffusion only. In the flexor tendon segments supplied directly by the digital vincular system, the predominance of the blood supply is to the dorsal (deep) aspect of the flexor tendon.

HISTORICAL REVIEW

An historical catalogue of the main contributors to the current state of the art and science of intrasynovial flexor tendon repair and rehabilitation is presented in Table 7-1. The annotated references listed at the end of this subchapter summarize the "classic" articles on the basic and clinical science of flexor tendon injuries and their treatment.

SURGICAL TREATMENT

Preoperative Considerations

Whether to proceed with primary repair of a lacerated intrasynovial tendon depends on several factors related to the extent and the timing of the injury and to the state of the soft tissues of the digit. In combined injuries of the hand (those that involve substantial injury of two or more of the following elements: skin, nerve, arterial supply, venous drainage, flexor tendon(s), extensor mechanism, bone, or joint) wherein the traumatized tissues cannot be repaired adequately to allow for postoperative rehabilitation to proceed or if extensive contamination or deficiency of the overlying soft tissues is present, then primary repair of the flexor tendon may not be indicated. In the setting of a neglected palmar or digital laceration with both purulent infection and tendon laceration present, primary tendon suture may also be contraindicated.

Usually it is preferable to perform tendon repair early rather than delay and allow for myostatic shortening of the proximal muscle-tendon unit to occur.[51,125,447] The upper limit of time past which proximal stump contracture is more likely than not to cause technical difficulty is variable, although 3 weeks is a commonly cited interval after which primary tendon repair would probably be unsuccessful.

In the setting of a delayed presentation and an unreliable history, the interval between injury and diagnosis is not known. The likelihood of proximal myostatic muscle-tendon retraction and the resultant inability to bring the

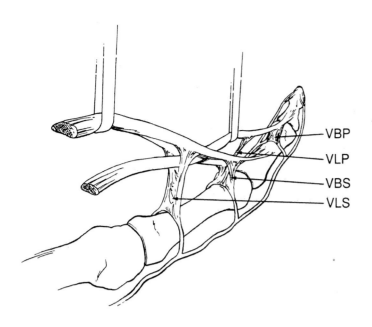

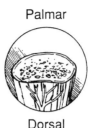

Palmar

Dorsal

FIGURE 7-5. Blood supply to the flexor tendons within the digital sheath. The segmental vascular supply to the flexor tendons is by means of long and short vincular connections. The vinculum brevis superficialis (VBS) and the vinculum brevis profundus (VBP) consist of small triangular mesenteries near the insertion of the FDS and FDP tendons, respectively. The vinculum longum to the superficialis tendon (VLS) arises from the floor of the digital sheath of the proximal phalanx. The vinculum longum to the profundus tendon (VLP) arises from the superficialis at the level of the PIP joint. The cutaway view depicts the relative avascularity of the palmar side of the flexor tendons in zones I and II as compared with the richer blood supply on the dorsal side, which connects with the vincula.

Table 7-1

HISTORICAL CONTRIBUTIONS TO FLEXOR TENDON REPAIR

Author(s)	Publication Activity	Main Area of Contribution	Significance	References
Bunnell	1918-1951	Surgical technique of tendon repair, grafting	Stressed the importance of gentle and precise surgical technique as having a direct effect on results	63-68
Mason, et al.	1932-1959	Animal model study of repair site healing	Classic in-vivo study of repair site healing and accrual of strength	37, 274-277
Boyes, et al.	1947-1989	Surgical technique of tendon repair, grafting	Detailed techniques and results of intrasynovial flexor tendon grafts	49-54, 412, 413
Peacock, et al.	1957-1987	Tendon biology, healing	Stressed the contribution of surrounding sheath to tendon repair site healing	87, 254, 321-329, 469
Verdan, et al.	1960-1987	Primary tendon repair	First report of successful primary tendon repair within the digital sheath	77, 207, 388, 454-463
Potenza, et al.	1962-1986	Tendon biology, healing	Stressed the contribution of surrounding sheath to repair site healing	344-354
Kleinert, et al.	1967-present	Early motion rehabilitation	Reported technique of reliable and reproducible postoperative "rubber-band" rehabilitation. Also the first valid report in the United States of primary zone II repair	195-207, 236,. 383, 471
Bruner	1967-1975	Skin incisions	Zigzag volar approach to the digital sheath	58-60
Kessler, et al.	1969-1987	Primary tendon repair	Core suture technique	182-186
Ketchum, et al.	1971-1985	Biology and biomechanics of tendon repair	Experimental study of tendon repair and healing	187-191

Continued

Table 7-1

HISTORICAL CONTRIBUTIONS TO FLEXOR TENDON REPAIR—cont'd

Author(s)	Publication Activity	Main Area of Contribution	Significance	References
Lundborg, et al.	1975-present	Tendon healing, vascularity, nutrition	Advocated the concept of "intrinsic" tendon healing, detailed the vascularity of flexor tendon	5-9, 102, 103, 122, 127, 154, 155, 241-250, 362, 371, 478, 479
Duran, et al.	1975-1990	Early motion rehabilitation	Passive motion rehabilitation protocol	100, 101
Manske, et al.	1977-present	Tendon biology, biomechanics	Classic studies of tendon nutrition, repair site biology and biomechanics	17-22, 48, 99, 121-123, 128, 132, 150, 159-161, 169, 178, 179, 210, 211, 239, 240, 256-272, 289, 336-340, 356-358, 373-375, 475, 476
Leddy, et al.	1977-1993	FDP avulsion injuries	Classification of FDP avulsions	219-222
Lister, et al.	1977-1986	Rehabilitation, pulley reconstruction	Clinical studies of pulley reconstruction and handling of the digital sheath	232-236, 383
Gelberman, et al.	1980-present	Tendon biology, biomechanics, rehabilitation	Classic experimental and clinical studies of tendon repair site biology, biomechanics, vascularity and rehabilitation	3, 14-16, 23, 39, 40, 43-46, 48, 92, 93, 97, 98, 115-130, 133, 134, 157, 158, 163, 168, 225-228, 262, 263, 271, 308, 309, 372, 397-401, 439, 481-484
Strickland, et al.	1982-present	Tendon repair, rehabilitation	Classic clinical and experimental studies of flexor tendon repair and rehabilitation	72, 218, 418, 421, 431, 433-436, 472
Silfverskiöld, et al.	1983-1994	Tendon repair, rehabilitation	Clinical and experimental study of repair site gap formation and rehabilitation	285-287, 390-396
Amadio, et al.	1984-present	Tendon and pulley biology, biomechanics, rehabilitation	Classic experimental studies of tendon repair site biology, biomechanics, and rehabilitation	13, 85, 229-231, 297-300, 304, 306, 307, 318, 450-452, 491-498, 500, 501
Hitchcock, et al.	1987	Tendon biology, rehabilitation	Experimental study of the biological effect of passive motion rehabilitation	166
Doyle	1988	Flexor pulley system	Relative importance of each pulley	94
Mass, et al.	1989-present	Tendon biomechanics	Experimental study of in-vitro repair site biomechanics	56, 61, 82, 139, 140, 152, 209, 278-281, 295, 305, 341, 342, 369, 376, 414
Abrahamsson, et al.	1989-present	Growth factors in tendon healing	In-vitro studies of growth factor synthesis during repair site healing and their effects	2-9, 15, 23, 153, 367, 477-480
Schuind, et al.	1992-present	In-vivo flexor tendon forces	Classic study documenting in-vivo flexor forces during digital motion	385
Diao, et al.	1996-present	Core and epitendinous suture techniques	Experimental study of the role of epitendinous suture in time-zero repair site strength	90, 91, 162, 238, 409
Sandow and McMahon	1996-present	Core suture technique	Improved time-zero core suture technique	381

Table 7-1

HISTORICAL CONTRIBUTIONS TO FLEXOR TENDON REPAIR—cont'd

Author(s)	Publication Activity	Main Area of Contribution	Significance	References
Boyer, et al.	1997-present	Tendon biology, biomechanics, rehabilitation	Experimental studies of tendon repair site biology, biomechanics, vascularity, and rehabilitation	39, 43-48, 92, 93, 119, 133, 134, 225, 397-401
Wolfe, et al.	1999-present	Core suture technique	Core suture technique	28-30, 292, 293, 404
Taras	1999-present	Core suture technique	Core suture technique	31, 443, 444
Leversedge	2000-present	Tendon vascularity and neovascularization after repair	Experimental studies of tendon repair site and insertion site vascularity	43, 47, 93, 225, 226

proximal and distal stumps together without substantial digital flexion or tension within the muscle-tendon unit is anticipated. In such cases, the appropriate surgical supplies for reconstruction (primary tendon graft, artificial tendon rod, or pulley reconstruction) rather than primary repair are made available (see the subchapter for reconstructive techniques in flexor tendon surgery on p. 241).

In general, the repair of flexor tendon lacerations need not be performed on an emergent basis unless division of both digital arteries is suspected. If digital perfusion is compromised or if the mechanism of injury is such that both arteries are likely to be divided (as is the case if both digital nerves are lacerated and the patient is unable to discriminate a static two-point stimulus on both radial and ulnar aspects of the digital pulp), then urgent exploration and repair is indicated.

If the tendon stumps are either unclean or ragged, excision of the FDS tendon and repair of the FDP tendon only may be indicated.[468] Whereas this repair protocol has the potential benefit of lessening adhesion formation in a severely traumatized soft tissue bed, the risks of excising primarily the FDS tendon are substantial, because creation of a "one-tendon" finger limits reconstructive options if significant FDP repair site elongation or rupture occurs. In these cases, the straightforward option of DIP joint arthrodesis with preservation of the FDS alone is unavailable. The previously held notion that only the FDP be repaired (and the FDS tendon be left alone or excised) for an otherwise clean laceration with an intact soft tissue bed has been invalidated experimentally.[318]

Repair of Zone I Lacerations or Avulsions

Recent in-vivo experiments on the canine FDP-bone repair site have led to several new concepts of flexor tendon repair to bone.[43,45,47,397] First, the tendon-bone repair site does not appear to accrue strength during the 3 to 6 week period postoperatively.[397] Second, even at 6 weeks postoperatively (the time at which the grasping suture and dorsal button are usually removed) there is substantial inflammatory tissue still present at the repair site, signifying a potential biologic "immaturity" of the repair site.[45] In addition, there is a substantial tendency for the repair site to elongate during the immediate postoperative period, which may not be apparent

clinically. These findings suggest that tendon-bone healing does not follow the same time course as the healing of intrasynovial flexor tendon repairs.

Laceration of the FDP tendon distal to the insertion of the FDS tendon or avulsion from its insertion at the base of the proximal aspect of the distal phalanx is by definition an injury in zone I of the flexor sheath. If the tendon is lacerated and the distal tendon stump is less than 1 cm long, FDP tendon advancement and primary repair to bone are indicated. If more than 1 cm of FDP stump is available for suture, then primary tenorrhaphy is indicated because shortening of the FDP tendon by greater than 1 cm may result in a quadriga effect on attempted composite flexion of the digits.[458] In this clinical situation, the laceration may lie near or beneath the A4 pulley, making the repair technically difficult.

Tendon to Bone Repair

Many techniques of core suture placement have been advocated for affixing the FDP tendon stump to bone. Theoretically, most of the techniques employed for tendon-tendon repair can be utilized for tendon-bone repair; however, several of these have been accepted more widely since removal of the dorsal button and transfixing suture at 6 weeks postoperatively has been advocated generally. The utilization of suture material of high tensile strength that is absorbed after months rather than weeks has led to increased advocacy of core suture techniques that need not be placed in the proximal stump with an intention toward their eventual removal.[43,47,397] In addition, the increased utilization of intraosseous anchors in hand surgery has led some investigators to advocate their utilization in this clinical setting.[61,62,151,365,403] If bone quality is good and experimental data are supported with clinical efficacy, their use could become more widespread.

The classic technique for repair of FDP tendon to bone involves passage of the suture strands utilized to grasp the tendon stump through the distal phalanx by means of straight needles and tying them over a button placed dorsally on the nail plate distal to the lunula. Ex-vivo studies have suggested superiority of the multistrand Becker (or MGH) technique in terms of improvements in time-zero biomechanical indices (Fig. 7-6).[43] This core suture technique is also useful if intraosseous anchors are used.[294] Several

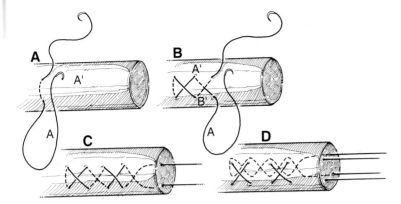

FIGURE 7-6. **A** to **D,** The four-strand modified Becker repair (see text).

authors have suggested modifications of these techniques wherein both the sutures and knot are placed subcutaneously and a dorsal button is not utilized.[180,386] These techniques have not been studied experimentally. Whichever technique is employed, apposition of the FDP stump to the bone should be confirmed visually before tensioning and tying the suture knot.

Specific techniques for retrieval of the proximal tendon stump[1,165,193,332,368,410,423,430,446] and for difficulties that might be encountered while attempting to pass the tendon stump through the pulley system (most notably the A4 pulley)[104,214,296] are discussed next.

FDP Avulsion

Leddy and Packer classified FDP avulsions into three types (Fig. 7-7).[221,222] In type I avulsions, the FDP tendon retracts into the palm. By definition, the vincular blood supply of the tendon has been disrupted. The sheath may, after a few days, be noncompliant and not permit passage of the FDP tendon through it in an attempt to repair the stump to bone. Additionally, proximal muscle contracture may prevent tendon stump advancement. In type II avulsions, the tendon stump retracts to the level of the PIP joint. The sheath is not

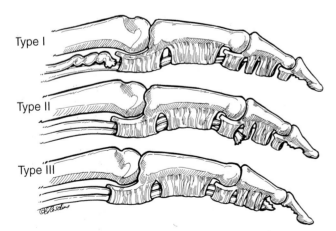

FIGURE 7-7. Profundus avulsion classification of Leddy and Packer. Type I: FDP is avulsed from its insertion and retracts into the palm. Type II: the profundus tendon is avulsed from it insertion but the stump remains within the digital sheath, implying that the vinculum longum profundus is still intact. Type III: a bony fragment is attached to the tendon stump, which remains within the flexor sheath. Further proximal retraction is prevented at the distal end of the A4 pulley.

compromised, and proximal muscle-tendon contracture does not develop substantially. Attempts to advance the tendon stump through the sheath, especially the A4 pulley, may require gentle pulley dilation as well. Repair may be attempted for 6 weeks, or longer, after injury. A large bone fragment is attached to the stump of the FDP tendon in type III injuries. This fragment usually prevents tendon retraction proximal to the distal edge of the A4 pulley. Bony repair using Kirschner wire or screw fixation is often all that is required. A type III injury may be deceptive preoperatively after clinical and radiographic examination because, on occasion, the FDP stump itself is avulsed from the bony fragment (a so-called type IV injury, not initially classified by Leddy and Packer).[222] The stump may be located either within the tendon sheath or within the palm. Repair of the fracture is done first, after which the tendon is advanced and affixed to the distal phalanx. Immobilization of the DIP joint is required, and the range of motion that may be expected after repair is substantially less.

Repair of Zone II Lacerations

Attempts to improve the time-zero early postoperative strength of the repair construct have focused on attempts to vary the configuration of the core suture, to alter the number of suture strands passing across the repair site, to use core sutures of different caliber and materials, and to vary the pattern and depth of placement of the circumferential epitenon suture. While clinical application of repair site augmentations such as onlay tendon grafts, patches, or synthetic materials has been disappointing owing to both increased repair site bulk and poor ability to restore the gliding surface, recent ex-vivo results suggest that these techniques might warrant further investigation.

Core Sutures

Ex-vivo and in-vivo investigations in linear, in situ, and other models have suggested that core suture configurations with the greatest tensile strength are those in which there are multiple sites of tendon suture interaction.* Although the Kessler or modified Kessler techniques still enjoy widespread acceptance, newer techniques such as Tajima,†

---

*See references 38, 44, 159, 169, 209, 357, 363, 379, 387, 389, 408, 409, 431, 442, 445, 465, 481, 482, 496, and 501.

†See references 42, 135, 175, 215, 309, 311, 377-379, 431, 434, 438, 466, and 482.

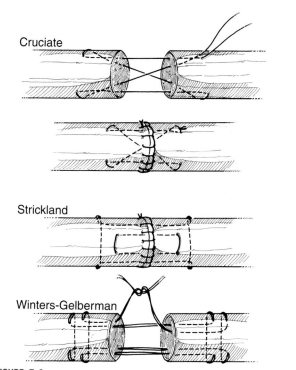

FIGURE 7-8. Commonly used techniques for end-to-end flexor tendon repair.

Strickland,[82,175,292,414,431,434] cruciate,[292] Becker,[*] and Savage[†] configurations all offer greater suture hold on the tendon that is independent of the suture knot (Fig. 7-8). These modern methods of core suture technique have not only been shown to offer greater time-zero repair site tensile strength but also to improve strength up to and including 6 weeks postoperatively. A significant relationship between tendon cross-sectional dimension and suture "hold" on the tendon stump, however, has not been proven.[46]

It is well accepted that core suture strength is directly related to the number of suture strands crossing the repair site between proximal and distal tendon: all else being equal, more strands mean a stronger repair.[‡] This fact holds true in both ex-vivo time-zero studies as well as in-vivo studies for up to 6 weeks postoperatively. The results of numerous studies employing commonly used core suture techniques have demonstrated the superiority of the four-strand core suture over the two-strand core suture and the greater strengths achieved with both six- and eight-strand core suture techniques.[119,381,481,482] The limiting factor to more widespread use of modern multi-strand suture techniques remains the surgeon's ability to perform the repair using atraumatic technique such that further damage to the tendon stumps and the circumferential visceral epitenon is

---

*See references 20, 21, 43, 82, 141, 142, 170, 294, 299, 318, 355, 414, 493, 498-500, and 501.

†See references 17-21, 30, 292, 309, 311, 356, 377-379, 389, 404, 466, 482, 496, 497, and 501.

‡See references 28-30, 44, 92, 215, 292, 299, 313, 356, 379, 389, 398, 445, 466, 482, 490, and 501.

minimized. While several investigators have evaluated the effect of different suture materials (both the caliber and composition of the core suture itself), most surgeons use semi-resorbable suture of 4-0 or higher caliber.

Other variables relevant to core suture placement shown to have a positive effect on time-zero core suture tensile strength include the dorsovolar location of the core suture,[19,409] the cross-sectional area of tendon grasped or locked by the redirecting loop of suture,[159,161,169] and the total number of times that the tendon has been grasped by the suture. Studies in an ex-vivo in-situ human model have shown that greater time-zero strength is achieved with a more dorsal placement of the core suture within the tendon stumps.

The effect on intrasynovial flexor tendon vascularity with a more dorsal suture placement, especially in the areas where the vinculum enters the tendon, is not known. Ex-vivo studies have suggested that the redirecting loop of the core suture that is positioned to "lock" rather than "grasp" the tendon stumps show greater time-zero. In addition,[159,161,169] increasing the number of locks or grasps increases the time-zero tensile strength of the flexor tendon repair site (Fig. 7-9). The placement of the suture knot either within or away from the repair site has not been shown conclusively to have an effect on core suture tensile strength.[298,356] Greater quantity of suture within the repair site may increase repair site bulk and decrease tendon glide, whereas knot placement away from the repair site may also affect tendon gliding detrimentally owing to increased friction between tendon and sheath proximal or distal to the repair site. Techniques of intrasynovial core suture placement that do not require the tying of sutures have not gained acceptance.

Epitendinous Suture

Additional technique by which hand surgeons have attempted to augment repair site strength is by alteration of the configuration of circumferential epitendinous suture.[238,273] Several studies have suggested that a clinically and statistically significant component of time-zero repair site strength is provided by a circumferential epitendinous suture passed

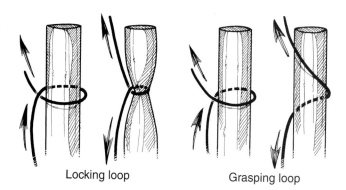

FIGURE 7-9. The relationship between the longitudinal and transverse intratendinous components of the core suture defines whether the suture is "locking" or "grasping." When the transverse component passes within the tendon superficial to the longitudinal component, the suture "locks" a bundle of tendon fibers. When the transverse component passes deep to the longitudinal component, however, the suture does not "lock" a bundle of tendon fibers but pulls through the tendon.

multiple times across the repair site,* most investigations suggest that while the epitendinous suture does increase time-zero and early postoperative strength of the repair site, it cannot be relied on to solely provide the majority of repair site tensile strength. It has been shown, however, that the role of the epitendinous suture regardless of its configuration is twofold: first to decrease repair site bulk by smoothing out the tendon stump surface and, second, to increase tensile strength of the repair site. Based on studies of core suture biomechanics and in-vivo clinical and experimental studies of tendon force in both canines and humans, four-strand (or higher) core suture techniques supplemented by a running epitendinous suture are recommended to achieve sufficient repair site tensile strength to allow for postoperative passive motion rehabilitation to proceed without significant risk of gap formation at the repair site.

Gap Formation

Whereas greater degrees of strength have been achieved with modern core and epitendinous suture techniques, the effect of small degrees of early repair site dehiscence and repair site gap formation on tendon healing and accrual of repair site strength has been appreciated only recently.[27,29,33,92,119,361,390,392,395] Previous investigators have assumed that the presence of repair site gaps was accompanied uniformly by the presence of intrasynovial flexor tendon adhesions, decreased tendon glide, and digital stiffness.[27,29,33,92,119,361,390,392,395] A recent in-vivo canine study has refuted this assumption and has demonstrated that the presence of a repair site gap, even greater than 3 mm, is not correlated with the presence of intrasynovial adhesions or with decreased digital arc of motion.[119] Whereas large gaps did not seem to affect tendon function, that is, excursion, large repair site gaps that occurred during the first 21 days postoperatively were observed to have a significant negative effect on tendon structure, that is, the accrual of tendon repair site tensile strength. In tendons without gaps or with gaps less than 3 mm in length, a significant increase in repair site tensile strength was seen between 3 and 6 weeks postoperatively, whereas in tendons with a repair site gap greater than 3 mm, significant accrual of repair site strength did not occur. Although the biologic processes at work within the larger repair site gaps remain open to further investigation, large repair site gaps seen early in the postoperative period pose a greater risk of rupture as motion rehabilitation progresses after 3 weeks (Fig. 7-10). Evaluation of imaging modalities such as ultrasound,[192,223] MRI,[96,282] and plain radiographs to determine precisely the extent of repair site gap has yielded inconsistent results that are not yet applicable to the clinical situation.

Biologic Considerations

Important strides have been made in the investigation of the biologic processes taking place at the repair site during the early postoperative period. Increased synthesis of type I collagen mRNA and protein has been demonstrated within repair site cells and cells within the adjacent epitenon early in the postoperative period.† However, in one study it was shown that neither the total amount nor the maturity of the collagen at the repair site increased significantly during the first 6 weeks postoperatively.[133] The accrual of repair site tensile strength demonstrated between 3 and 6 weeks

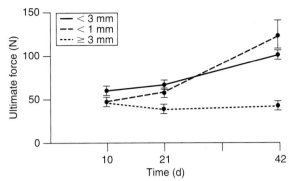

FIGURE 7-10. Ultimate tensile strength is plotted as a function of time. Tendons with repair site gaps less than 3 mm accrue strength during the fourth to sixth week postoperatively, whereas tendons with repair site gaps greater than 3 mm show no significant increase in ultimate tensile strength during the early postoperative period. (Redrawn from Gelberman RH, Boyer MI, Brodt MD, et al: The effect of gap formation at the repair site on the strength and excursion of intrasynovial flexor tendons: An experimental study on the early stages of tendon-healing in dogs. J Bone Joint Surg Am 81:965-982, 1999.)

postoperatively in tendons with repair site gap of less than 3 mm must be due to mechanisms other than increased synthesis or more rapid maturation of collagen at the repair site. Fibronectin, an abundant extracellular matrix protein involved in cell-matrix communication,[14,25,55] as well as $\alpha_5\beta_1$ and $\alpha_v\beta_3$ integrins, cell-surface compounds involved in the binding of fibroblasts to extracellular matrix,[157,158] are likewise up-regulated during the early postoperative period. Fibroblasts grown in culture have demonstrated responsiveness to externally applied stress both on a cellular and molecular level[26,55,189]; however, the exact relationship between synthesis of collagen and integrins and the accrual of tensile strength at tendon repair site remains unknown. Up-regulation of the synthesis of mRNA of angiogenic mediators has been demonstrated both within the flexor tendon repair site and in surrounding epitenon[39,48] and has been shown to precede temporally and be distinct spatially from longitudinal blood vessel growth both on the tendon surface and within the flexor tendon substance.[120] The cellular origin of these angiogenic mediators and their role in blood vessel ingrowth through the avascular region of the flexor tendon remain unknown. The identification of fibroblast responsiveness in culture to growth factors such as transforming growth factor-β and insulin-like growth factor merits further investigation into their role in early tendon healing.

The Role of Postoperative Passive Motion Rehabilitation

Despite advances made in the improvement of repair site strength and in the understanding of repair site biology, formation of adhesions between the tendon and the surrounding fibro-osseous sheath and the resultant digital stiffness and range of motion remain frequently encountered

---

*See references 27, 85, 135, 215, 319, 379, 380, 387, 389, 391, 402, and 490.

†See references 88, 112, 114, 116, 133, 194, 213, 255, 302, 303, 370, 375, 448, and 499.

complications after intrasynovial flexor tendon repair and rehabilitation. Recent in-vivo studies have suggested that the formation of these restrictive intrasynovial adhesions both at the repair site as well as at remote sites between tendon and sheath may be obviated if a sufficient amplitude of intrasynovial tendon excursion is achieved during passive motion rehabilitation.[41,119,228,399,481,482,494,498] Recent canine studies have suggested that the extent to which intrasynovial tendon repair sites must be moved passively during postoperative rehabilitation to obviate clinically relevant adhesion formation may be as low as 1.6 mm.[227,228] Despite the experimental success of increased levels of applied intrasynovial repair site excursion during passive motion rehabilitation, mechanical and pharmacologic methods to decrease intrasynovial adhesions have been attempted.* Although both in-vivo and in-vitro studies have demonstrated beneficial effects of locally applied compounds such as 5-fluorouracil (a mitotic inhibitor)[11,76,301] and hyaluronic acid (a lubricant)[16,25,147-149,297,376,411,451,477] on tendon gliding (both have been shown to increase tendon glide, decrease adhesion formation, and decrease work of digital flexion), they have not enjoyed widespread clinical application owing to expense, potential side effects, and the difficulty in obtaining and maintaining a high concentration of the substance. Mechanical barriers placed between tendon and sheath after the primary repair of intrasynovial flexor tendon lacerations have not gained acceptance.

In an effort to improve the strength of the intrasynovial flexor tendon repair site, investigators have advocated rehabilitation methods that generate increased levels of applied in-vivo force across the repair. My colleagues and I have demonstrated that increasing levels of clinically relevant applied force during postoperative rehabilitation from 5 to 17 N did not accelerate the accrual of repair site strength.[44] Although more vigorous rehabilitation protocols may help to improve hand function, we found no evidence that it enhances repair site strength in the context of multi-strand repair technique.

FPL Lacerations

Intrasynovial lacerations of the FPL tendon may pose a unique difficulty in that the proximal tendon stump frequently retracts deep to the thenar musculature, and retrieval by direct exposure of the proximal stump is not possible.[†] Similar to techniques recommended for FDS and FDP tendon location and retrieval, blind passage of grasping instruments into the flexor sheath is to be condemned. If the proximal stump has retracted proximal to the distal edge of the thenar musculature, it is localized through a separate incision in the distal forearm. The stump of the FPL lies deep to the flexor carpi radialis tendon and the radial artery. A small hematoma can be seen often within the synovial tissue surrounding the tendon and can help locate the proximal stump without undue dissection. Delivery of the proximal tendon stump into the distal wound can be accomplished by any one of the techniques just described.

---

*See references 11, 16, 32, 35, 76, 78, 89, 106, 107, 111, 119, 121, 136, 138, 147, 148, 162, 176, 183, 212, 216, 217, 241, 245, 253, 301, 312, 316, 317, 343, 372, 392, 395, 396, 437, 440, 441, 464, 478, 494, 495, and 501.
†See references 57, 105, 145, 243, 310, 334, 360, 402, and 453.

Repair of Zone III, IV, and V Lacerations

The exploration and repair of flexor tendon injuries proximal to the A1 pulley are carried out in a fashion similar to the more common distal lacerations. Important differences between the more proximal lacerations and those within the fibro-osseous flexor sheath are that restrictive adhesions are less likely to impede motion of the more proximally lacerated and repaired tendons, since the narrow confines of the fibro-osseous digital sheath have not been breached. In addition, apparently small lacerations frequently involve multiple tendons and often damage major neurovascular structures (median or ulnar nerves or radial or ulnar arteries) as well. Preoperative preparation for tendon repair in these injuries should consider these possible eventualities, and microsurgical instrumentation as well as an operating microscope should be available. Techniques and considerations for the placement of the core and epitendinous sutures and the postoperative rehabilitation are the same as those described for zone II injuries.

Partial Tendon Lacerations

There has been considerable debate about the appropriate management of partial tendon lacerations.[41,143,144,288,383,495,498,501] Despite several in-vivo studies evaluating tendon gliding as well as biomechanical properties, current recommendations are evolving. Presently, repair of lacerations of greater than 60% of the tendon cross-sectional area is recommended by some authors, utilizing a technique similar to that recommended for complete lacerations. If the cross-sectional area lacerated is less than 60%, the tendon is neither repaired nor débrided unless complete or partial entrapment (i.e., triggering) of the tendon under the fibrous pulley system is observed.

 ## Author's Preferred Method: Zone I (Fig. 7-11)

Before definitive surgical treatment in a well-lit operating room, either a general anesthetic or an interscalene or axillary block is administered. Local anesthesia in the form of peripheral nerve blocks or digital ring blocks, and intravenous anesthesia administered after inflation of a brachial tourniquet, is not recommended. The patient is supine on the operating table, and the arm lies at a right angle to the long axis of the body. A high brachial tourniquet is placed over the biceps muscle belly and is set at greater than 100 mm Hg above systolic blood pressure. The limb is exsanguinated by an elastic bandage or by passive elevation, and the tourniquet is inflated after preparation of the exposed skin surfaces with povidone-iodine scrub and paint.

A midlateral incision is utilized to expose the volar insertion site of the FDP at the base of the distal phalanx, as well as the proximal and distal end of the A4 pulley and both neurovascular bundles. If a large bony fragment has arrested tendon retraction at the distal end of A4 pulley, the FDP tendon insertion into the fragment is confirmed by direct

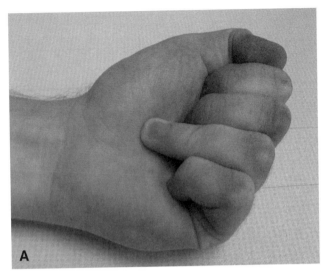

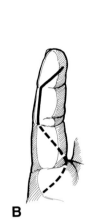

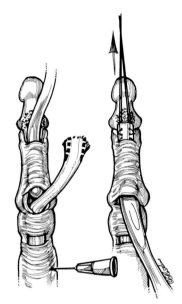

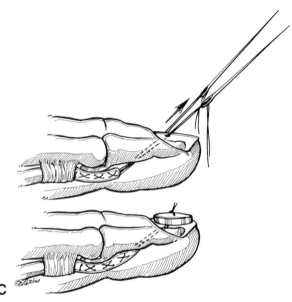

FIGURE 7-11. Author's preferred technique for FDP tendon reattachment to bone. **A,** Clinical photograph of a patient without active DIP flexion. **B,** Midlateral exposure over the middle phalanx is preferred. This incision may be extended diagonally over the pulp of the finger distally and into a Bruner incision proximally. Sourmelis-McGrouther technique of proximal stump retrieval is preferred (see p. 233). The stump of the profundus tendon may be delivered under the A4 pulley after sequential dilatation of the pulley with pediatric cervical sounds of increasing diameter. A modified Becker grasping stitch core suture is placed within the tendon stump. **C,** Straight Keith needles are drilled from the volar proximal base of the distal phalanx in a distal dorsal direction to exist the nail plate through the sterile matrix (distal to the lunula and eponychial fold). The individual grasping core sutures are delivered to the dorsum of the finger after placement of the needles through the holes in the button. The sutures are tied while holding the tendon directly to bone using forceps.

identification and longitudinal traction of the fragment distalward. Occasionally, only the volar plate of the DIP joint will have remained attached to the fragment and the FDP will have avulsed off and retracted further proximally. The tendon stump is then located proximally and is retrieved into the distal wound by any of the techniques described for zone II injuries below. The tendon is then transfixed with a 25-gauge needle.

It is often difficult to deliver the flared-out stump of the FDP tendon through the A4 pulley after it has avulsed from the distal phalanx and retracted proximally. There are several techniques available for this difficult situation. First, sequential dilation of the A4 pulley using pediatric cervical sounds or dilators should be carried out. The A4 pulley itself is fairly noncompliant, and sequential dilation will facilitate tendon delivery beneath the pulley. Second, the edges of the stump are trimmed so that the width of the stump does not exceed that of the tendon. Care is taken to not excise the stump entirely, because recent investigation has shown that this stump may play an active role in the healing of

the tendon stump to bone. After sequential dilatation of the pulley, the core suture is placed in the stump and the suture strands are delivered in a proximal to distal direction through the pulley. Gentle traction on the suture ends while "guiding" the tendon stump beneath the A4 pulley using a Freer elevator is done. Partial or complete resection of the A4 pulley to facilitate tendon stump delivery is discouraged.

The bone at the volar base of the distal phalanx need not be roughened to expose bleeding medullary bone. A modified Becker repair is carried out, utilizing a 3-0 braided caprolactam suture (Supramid) with small, tapered needles affixed to both ends. The suture is first passed through the tendon in a plane parallel to the volar-dorsal axis of the tendon, midway between the central axis of the tendon and its radial or ulnar edge. Thus, the suture exits the tendon both at the volar and the dorsal aspects of the tendon. Subsequently, the segment of suture that exits volarly is passed in a dorsal-to-volar direction entering the tendon 3 mm distal to the point of exit from the tendon of the other suture strand. Similarly, the suture segment that exits from

CRITICAL POINTS: ZONE I REPAIR

SURGICAL TIMING

- Leddy type I injuries require early (within 3 weeks) diagnosis and treatment.
- Leddy type II and III injuries potentially may be repaired even after 6 weeks.

PEARLS

- Ultrasound or MRI may be helpful in locating the proximal stump.
- Microsuture anchors or dorsal button constructs may be used.
- Observe the tendon-bone site directly before final knot-tying.

PITFALLS

- A tendon advanced and inserted too tight will lead to quadrigia.
- Two-strand repair techniques may be insufficient.

TECHNICAL POINTS

- Make a midlateral exposure over the middle phalanx with an oblique extension over the pulp.
- Expose the trifurcation of the digital nerve.
- Identify and prepare the bony insertion site (creating a trough is unnecessary).
- Retrieve proximal stump: skin hooks, reverse Esmarch, Sourmelis, direct exposure.
- Use modified Becker four-strand (3-0 or 4-0) core sutures placed proximally, and deliver stump beneath A4.

- Realize that pulley dilatation may be necessary with sounds/dilators.
- Drill Keith needles to exit the nail plate distal to the lunula.
- Place each suture (two strands) through each eyelet.
- Place needles through button and padding before tendon sutures are delivered dorsally.
- Hold tendon down at repair site while tying knot.
- Use additional peripheral sutures to periosteum if possible (6-0 Prolene is sufficient).
- Place frequent skin sutures to prevent wound dehiscence during motion.

POSTOPERATIVE CARE

- Apply dorsal splint with wrist and MCPs flexed and PIPs and DIPs extended.
- Use a graded rehabilitation protocol under supervision of a qualified therapist.
- Know that synergistic wrist motion is helpful to lessen force and increase excursion.
- Know that edema control is critical to success (avoid corticosteroids).

RETURN TO ACTIVITIES

- May return to full activity at 4 to 6 months after surgery.

---

the dorsal aspect of the tendon is passed in a volar-to-dorsal direction, entering the tendon 3 mm distal from where the first strand exits the tendon. The suture strands cross the tendon on both its external and internal surfaces and, after repeated passes, grasp the tendon along its radial and ulnar aspects at multiple points. The suture segments are delivered through the cut ends of the tendon stumps. The second suture is passed on the ulnar side of the tendon in an orientation similar to the first, completing the four-strand grasping suture. The sutures are then passed through the distal phalanges using straight Keith needles that are drilled through exposed bone at the base of the distal phalanx using a small hand-held drill and are tied over a button placed on the nail plate dorsally. It is preferable to have the needles exit the nail plate beyond the lunula (and therefore beyond the germinal matrix) to avoid nail deformity or eponychial injury. The button is left in place for 6 weeks and is then removed by cutting the suture flush with the nail plate after the application of gentle traction to the button.

In general, the rehabilitation protocol follows the same progression as that described for zone II injuries.

Author's Preferred Method: Zone II (Fig. 7-12)

After the initial administration of intravenous antibiotics and tetanus toxoid as appropriate, the wound is irrigated in the emergency department and is closed loosely so as to prevent desiccation of the underlying tendons, sheath, and neurovascular structures. A dorsal splint that includes all digits is applied. Before definitive surgical treatment in a well-lit operating room, either a general anesthetic or an interscalene or axillary block is administered. Use of local anesthesia in the form of peripheral nerve blocks, digital ring blocks, or intravenous anesthesia administered after inflation of a brachial tourniquet is not recommended. The patient is supine on the operating table, and the arm lies at a right angle to the long axis of the body. A high brachial tourniquet is placed over the biceps muscle belly and is set at greater than 100 mm Hg above systolic blood pressure. The limb is exsanguinated by an elastic bandage or by passive elevation, and the tourniquet is inflated after

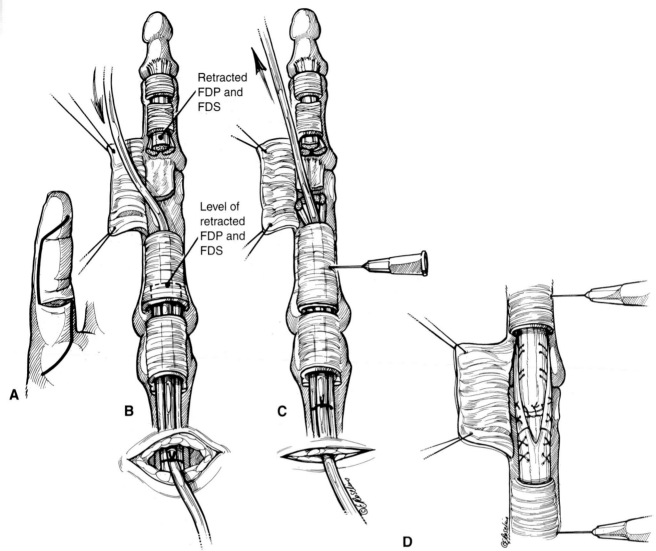

FIGURE 7-12. Author's technique of flexor tendon repair in zone II. **A,** Knife laceration through zone II with the digit in full flexion. The distal stumps retract distal to the skin incision with digital extension. **B,** Radial and ulnar extending incisions are used to allow wide exposure of the flexor tendon system. Note appearance of the flexor tendon system of the involved fingers after the reflection of skin flaps. The laceration occurred through the C1 cruciate area. Note the proximal and distal position of the flexor tendon stumps. Reflection of small flaps ("windows") in the cruciate-synovial sheath allows the distal flexor tendon stumps to be delivered into the wound by passive flexion of the DIP joint. The profundus and superficialis stumps are retrieved proximal to the wound by passive flexion of the DIP joint. The profundus and superficialis stumps are retrieved proximal to the sheath by the use of a small catheter or infant feeding gastrostomy tube. **C,** The proximal flexor tendon stumps are maintained at the repair site by means of a transversely placed small-gauge hypodermic needle, allowing repair of the FDS slips without tension. **D,** Completed repair of both the FDS and FDP tendons is shown with the DIP joint in full flexion. Extension of the DIP joint delivers the repair under the intact distal flexor tendon sheath. Wound repair is done at the conclusion of the procedure.

preparation of the exposed skin surfaces with povidone-iodine scrub and paint. The sutures utilized to close the initial wound are not removed until this time.

A midlateral incision is preferred irrespective of the site of the skin laceration, because it affords a wide exposure, places intact skin and subcutaneous fat directly over the flexor sheath and the neurovascular bundles, and can minimize the creation of small distally based skin flaps whose perfusion might become compromised and be at a higher risk of flap necrosis (Fig. 7-13).

Exposure of the neurovascular bundle on the side of the skin incision is performed by dividing Grayson's ligament. The skin and subcutaneous fat are raised off of the fibro-

osseous sheath as a single layer. Separation of these tissues is to be avoided because skin perfusion is by random vascular supply, and unnecessary thinning of the skin flap can cause decreased perfusion at the tip of the flap.

The laceration of the sheath is identified and a limited débridement of the hemorrhagic ends of the sheath is performed. Sheath resection is rarely necessary, especially if the laceration was sharp and the overlying skin edges are clean and viable. Exposure of the contents of the sheath is done by reflecting a radial- or an ulnar-based flap of sheath located between the distal edge of the A2 pulley and the proximal edge of the A4 pulley. The distal stump may be delivered by passive flexion of the DIP and the PIP joints. It

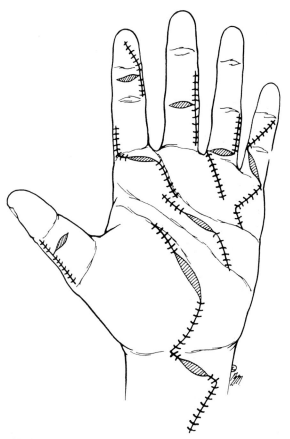

FIGURE 7-13. Incision options for wound extension during flexor tendon repair.

is then transfixed to tissue deep to the neurovascular bundle by a 25-gauge needle.

If the digit was in a position of maximal or submaximal flexion at the time of injury, the distal stump will usually lie quite distal to the skin laceration and may come to rest beneath or distal to the A4 pulley after digital extension. Gentle sequential dilation of the A4 pulley with pediatric cervical sounds or dilators is of benefit so that the tendon stump can be passed through the narrow A4 pulley more easily. Partial pulley resection or oblique incision with subsequent repair of the A4 pulley is to be avoided if at all possible.

If the proximal stump of tendon is visible within the fibro-osseous sheath, it may be retrieved by means of a gentle proximal to distal milking of the tendon stump along its course. The tendon is grasped directly on its cut end with nontoothed forceps and is held in a position to be sutured by a 25-gauge needle. If the proximal tendon stump is not visible, repeated blind passes into the digital sheath using a hemostat or similar device in an attempt to grasp the tendon end should not be done. Several techniques have been described to find and deliver the proximal stump in this situation.

The method advocated by Sourmelis and McGrouther[410] is reliable. A small pediatric feeding tube is passed from the wound into the palm beneath the annular pulley system. The flexor tendons are left in situ in the sheath, and, through a midpalmar incision, the catheter is sutured to both tendons several centimeters proximal to the A1 pulley. The catheter

is pulled distally, delivering the tendon stumps into the distal repair site easily. A 25-gauge needle is utilized to secure the tendons in situ. In situations in which the tendons have retracted proximally into the palm, an incision is made just distal to the transverse carpal ligament to isolate the tendon stump. The superficial palmar arch is identified, as well as the common metacarpal arteries and common digital nerves. The proximal stump(s) are then delivered distally by a catheter method as described or by direct identification, grasping, and distal traction at the cut end directly. Dilation of the A1 and A2 pulleys as described for the A4 pulley is required infrequently. It is important, however, to reestablish the proper anatomic relationship of the FDS and FDP tendons proximally and at the decussation of the FDS slips and the chiasm of Camper, as well as within the fibro-osseous pulley system before repair.

The FDS tendon is repaired first. If the tendon is lacerated proximal to the decussation, an eight-strand core suture as described by Winters and Gelberman is used (see Fig. 7-8).[481,482] The identical technique as described is used for core suture placement in FDP tendon lacerations. The technique utilizes a 3-0 or 4-0 braided caprolactam (Supramid) looped suture affixed to a tapered needle end. This multistrand core suture technique offers a substantial improvement in time-zero repair site tensile strength and stiffness over conventional core suture techniques that utilize two, four, or six strands of suture across the repair site.

Two continuous modified four-strand Kessler sutures serve as the basis of the construct. Both sutures are placed with their transverse limbs oriented along the long axis of the tendon cross section. The second limb of the core suture is placed with the transverse loop of suture at a slightly greater distance from the repair site; either one or two sutures can be utilized, thus resulting in either one or two knots located within the repair site at completion of the core. In general, the transverse limbs of the core sutures should be 1 cm from the repair site. Locking loops of suture are not utilized. When using one suture, the core suture is tensioned to bring the stumps together before beginning the second modified Kessler component of the core oriented parallel to the first. A running epitendinous suture is then placed circumferentially around the tendon after completion of the core suture; the "tail" of the suture after the first knot is tied is left long to assist in tendon inversion to facilitate placement of the posterior aspect of the epitendinous suture. A 6-0 Prolene suture is utilized; the suture takes deep bites into the substance of the tendon to improve strength and need not be locked after each suture pass (Fig. 7-14).

If the FDS tendon has divided proximal to the site of laceration, the repair is made difficult by the thin, flat shape of the tendon slips as they wrap around the FDP tendon. Use of a large needle and 3-0 or 4-0 suture as described for the entire FDS or FDP tendon can cause undue trauma to the FDS slips and may lead to excessive repair site bulk that impairs gliding beneath the A2 pulley. In addition, multistrand repair techniques may not be possible owing to the size and orientation of the tendon slips. It is preferable, therefore, to use a smaller needle along with a smaller-caliber suture so as to minimize tissue trauma. A 4-0 or 5-0 Ethibond suture affixed to a small, tapered needle at each end is used currently. Recent ex-vivo investigation has suggested the superiority of the Becker suture for such

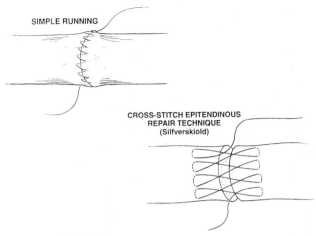

SIMPLE RUNNING

CROSS-STITCH EPITENDINOUS
REPAIR TECHNIQUE
(Silfverskiöld)

FIGURE 7-14. Epitendinous suture techniques.

repairs.[294] This method of core suture placement is recommended. A circumferential epitendinous suture is placed if possible. The FDP tendon is then repaired with the Winters and Gelberman technique.[481,482]

After completion of the epitendinous suture, it is mandatory to confirm that the repair site itself glides beneath the A2 and the A4 pulleys with passive digital flexion and extension. Failure to evaluate tendon glide after repair may lead to substantially decreased digital range of motion. If the repair is "trapped" proximal to the A4 pulley, a DIP flexion deformity may result. Similarly, if the repair site does not glide under the A2 pulley during attempted flexion, significant loss of PIP flexion may be expected. It may be helpful, before skin closure, to place the repair site within either the A2 or the A4 pulleys, so as to allow for gradual pulley dilatation during the immediate period postoperatively. Gentle pulley dilation using a Freer elevator or pediatric cervical sounds or dilators may be required.

Repair of lacerations to the digital arteries or nerves is done before flexor tendon suture, because the flexed posture of the finger after completion of the tendon repair leads to technical difficulty in performing the microsurgical vessel and nerve repairs.

After tourniquet deflation, bleeding points are controlled using bipolar cautery and by gentle manual pressure. The skin is closed using multiple sutures of 4-0 nylon placed in horizontal mattress configurations. A passive drain may be left subcutaneously overlying the tendon sheath and is removed the following day. A well-padded compressive nonconstrictive dressing with a dorsal plaster slab is applied from the fingertips to the proximal forearm to hold the wrist, MCP, PIP, and DIP joints in slight flexion so as to minimize passive myostatic tension on the repair site. All digits are included in the postoperative dressing. If the FPL tendon is repaired, the plaster splint overlies the dorsal aspect of the thumb to hold the carpometacarpal, MCP, and IP joints in slight flexion.

CRITICAL POINTS: ZONE II REPAIR

SURGICAL TIMING

- This is an emergency if both digital nerves and arteries are lacerated.
- For an injury less than 3 weeks old nonemergent repair is indicated unless there is active purulent infection.
- An injury greater than 6 weeks old is a relative contraindication to attempt primary repair.

PEARLS

- Multi-strand core suture technique with a running circumferential epitendinous suture is used.
- Urethral/cervical dilators should be ready for pulley dilatation, especially A4.
- A pediatric No. 8 feeding tube should be ready if retrieval is required (Sourmelis).
- Goal of repair and rehabilitation is a strong repair site that will not elongate beyond 3 mm with gentle passive range-of-motion therapy designed to prevent adhesion formation.

PITFALLS

- If less than 1 cm of FDP stump is remaining, FDP advancement and repair to bone should be considered.

- Lacerations of the slips of the FDS require different sutures, techniques, and needles than do FDP lacerations.
- "Active" range of motion after surgery has not been shown to be of benefit.
- Frayed tendon end may require judicious débridement to lessen repair site bulk.

TECHNICAL POINTS

- Use a midlateral exposure if possible.
- Enter sheath between distal A2 and proximal A4.
- Retrieve proximal stump: skin hooks, reverse Esmarch, Sourmelis, direct exposure.
- Deliver distal stump by passive DIP hyperflexion.
- Know that the A4 pulley may require dilatation before distal stump can be passed beneath it.
- Transfix tendons, once delivered through pulleys, with 25-gauge needle.
- Repair distal lacerations distal to A4 if difficult to deliver distal stump through A4.
- Use a minimum of a four-strand core suture technique (3-0 or 4-0 suture) with a running 6-0 Prolene epitendinous suture (nonlocked, deep bites into tendon).

CRITICAL POINTS: ZONE II REPAIR—cont'd

- Immobilize the digit with the repair site under a pulley if possible.
- Sheath repair is recommended but not required.
- Place frequent skin sutures to prevent wound dehiscence during motion.

POSTOPERATIVE CARE

- Apply dorsal splint with wrist and MCPs flexed and PIPs and DIPs extended.
- Use graded rehabilitation protocol under supervision of a qualified therapist.

- Use synergistic wrist motion to lessen force and increase excursion.
- Know that edema control is critical to success (avoid corticosteroids).

RETURN TO ACTIVITIES

- May return to activity at 4 to 6 months after surgery.

POSTOPERATIVE MANAGEMENT: REHABILITATION

Young and Harmon first described the concept of passive motion utilizing elastic band traction in 1960.[489] This technique became popular after some initial skepticism, following publication of the Louisville experience in 1977 in which the results of 156 flexor tendon lacerations repaired in 68 patients were reported.[236] A controlled motion rehabilitation protocol was utilized. An extension block splint was fabricated to keep the wrist flexed, MCP joints flexed slightly, and the IP joints in full extension. Active digital extension is done, and digital flexion is achieved passively by rubber bands secured at the wrist and attached to the injured digit at the nail plate. Eighty percent of these patients had good or excellent results, a substantial improvement over reports published previously. These data were instrumental in demonstrating that the gliding surface of the flexor tendon sheath could be restored after primary repair and rehabilitation of intrasynovial flexor tendons and that satisfactory functional results could be achieved. Modifications to this "rubber band traction" system also showed substantial promise.

The Louisville protocol was modified further by the placement of a bar or pulley at the midpalmar level to improve the vector of pull; biomechanical studies demonstrated that this change created greater flexion at both the DIP and PIP joints than the original Louisville splint and rehabilitation protocol and that flexion contractures of the digits could be obviated. Further splint refinement over the past decade has led to the creation of a splint with a mobile joint at the wrist (a synergistic wrist splint) allowing for greater degrees of intrasynovial tendon excursion to be achieved owing to the tenodesis effect of wrist position on flexor tendon motion.*

Although Duran and Houser determined that 3 to 5 mm of intrasynovial repair site excursion was necessary to obviate the development of intrasynovial adhesions,[100,101] recent canine studies have suggested that the extent to which intrasynovial tendon repair sites must be moved passively during postoperative rehabilitation to obviate clinically relevant adhesion formation may be as low as 1.6 mm.[399] The degree of intrasynovial repair site excursion was achieved by Duran through a passive digital range-of-motion protocol taught to the patients. This passive motion rehabilitation technique decreased the frequency of PIP joint flexion contractures often seen with rubber band protocols. Strickland improved on this protocol by utilizing a dorsal blocking splint with the wrist in 20 degrees of flexion, the MCP joints in 50 degrees of flexion, and the IP joints in full extension. For the first 3.5 weeks postoperatively the patient flexed and extended the PIP joint, DIP joint, and entire digit 25 times daily within the confines of the dorsal block splint. At 3.5 weeks postoperatively active digital flexion and extension is initiated again within the confines of the dorsal blocking splint. Active range-of-motion exercises outside the splint are initiated 1 week later, and the splint is worn until 5.5 weeks postoperatively. Blocking exercises for both the DIP and PIP joints are initiated at that time.

Although a variety of early motion protocols that advocate "place and hold," "light active," or "active" components have been described, there are conflicting reports regarding their success. Repair site rupture rates have been reported to be as high as 46%[330] with some early motion protocols.

In an effort to improve the strength of the intrasynovial flexor tendon repair site, investigators have also advocated rehabilitation methods that generate increased levels of applied in-vivo force across the repair.[44] An experimental study in canines in which 214 FDP tendons were transected, repaired, and assigned to either low-force (5 N) or high-force (17 N) passive range-of-motion rehabilitation regimens demonstrated that increasing the level of clinically relevant applied force during postoperative rehabilitation did not accelerate the accrual of repair site strength (Fig. 7-15). These findings suggested that there be a reexamination of the concept of increases in force produced by more vigorous mobilization protocols and whether they are beneficial to tendon healing.

Presently available experimental and clinical data suggest therefore that repair of an intrasynovial flexor tendon laceration be performed within 10 to 14 days of injury using

---

*See references 34, 83, 108, 131, 164, 208, 334, 366, 405-407, 417, and 471.

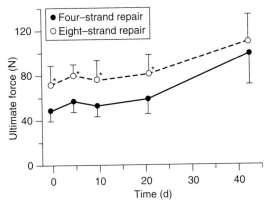

FIGURE 7-15. Comparison of ultimate force versus time between suture techniques from 0 to 21 days. The repairs with the eight-strand technique were significantly stronger than those that used the four-strand technique. *Asterisks* denote a significant difference between the eight- and four-strand techniques at $P < .05$. (Redrawn from Boyer MI, Gelberman RH, Burns ME, et al: Intrasynovial flexor tendon repair: An experimental study comparing low and high levels of in vivo force during rehabilitation in canines. J Bone Joint Surg Am 83:891-899, 2001.)

a core and epitendinous suture technique able to withstand repair site gap formation of 3 mm during the first 3 weeks postoperatively. A passive motion rehabilitation protocol that strives to emphasize intrasynovial repair site excursion, rather than increased application of musculotendinous force across the repair site, should be utilized.

Author's Preferred Method: Postoperative Rehabilitation of Zone I and Zone II Repairs (Figs. 7-16 to 7-18)*

Within 1 week after tendon repair, a synergistic wrist splint is fabricated so that passive digital flexion may be combined with active and passive wrist extension, and active digital extension may be combined with active or passive wrist flexion. In the resting position, the wrist is blocked at 30 degrees of flexion with a removable dorsal foam block; the splint permits up to 30 degrees of wrist extension without resistance when the block is removed. The MCP joints are blocked dorsally at 60 degrees of flexion, and the PIP and DIP joints are in full extension. A home exercise program is taught to the patient. Hourly performance of a passive range-of-motion protocol for the MCP, PIP, and DIP joints is done within the confines of the splint. Synergistic wrist extension within the splint is done to increase tendon excursion intrasynovially. In addition, gentle "place and hold" synergistic digital flexion combined with wrist extension may allow for greater degrees of intrasynovial repair site excursion. The goal is not the application of tension to the

*This section was written with the assistance of Rebecca von der Heyde, OT.

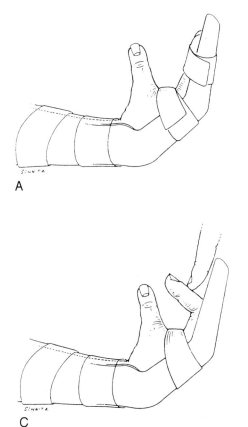

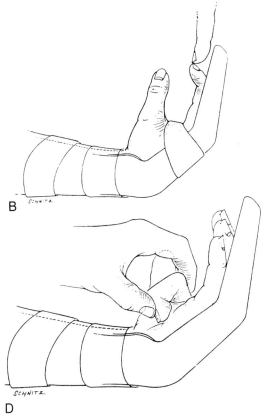

FIGURE 7-16. Controlled passive motion method. **A,** An Orthoplast dorsal blocking splint is used to hold the wrist in mild flexion, the MCP joints in about 45 degrees, and the PIP and DIP joints in nearly full extension. **B,** Full isolated passive flexion of the DIP joint. **C,** Full isolated passive flexion of the PIP joint. **D,** Full passive flexion of the MCP, PIP, and DIP joints.

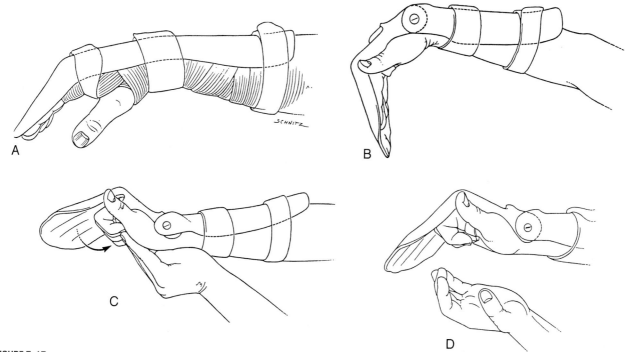

FIGURE 7-17. Controlled "place-and-hold" motion after flexor tendon repair protocol. **A,** After removal of the surgical bandage, a traditional dorsal blocking splint that positions the wrist in 20 degrees of palmar flexion, the MCP joints in 50 degrees of flexion, and the IP joints in extension is applied. **B,** A tenodesis splint with a wrist hinge is fabricated to allow for full wrist flexion, wrist extension of 30 degrees, and maintenance of MCP flexion of at least 60 degrees. **C,** After composite passive digital flexion, the wrist is extended and passive flexion is maintained. **D,** The patient actively maintains digital flexion and holds that position for about 5 seconds. Patients are instructed to use the lightest muscle power necessary to maintain digital flexion.

repair site but the encouragement of tendon excursion with the goal of restoration of the gliding surface. Edema is controlled at each visit with compressive digital wraps. Objective measurement of active place-and-hold range of motion is recorded at each visit.

Beginning at 1 week postoperatively, gradual progression of a home exercise program is initiated based on gentle place-and-hold measurements. Between 1 and 3 weeks, the passive digital range of motion within the confines of the dorsal block splint are continued, as are the gentle place-and-hold exercises. At 4 weeks, differential tendon gliding exercises are begun. These consist of MCP flexion with PIP and DIP extension (flat fist) and MCP extension with PIP and DIP flexion (hook fist), both with synergistic wrist extension within the splint. At 5 weeks, composite wrist flexion and full digital extension are begun along with composite wrist extension and digital flexion within the confines of the splint. At 6 weeks postoperatively the splint is discontinued, and isolated FDS and FDP gliding exercises are begun.

An increased range of motion of between 5% and 10% is expected each week. After discontinuation of the splint, resisted composite fist exercises are begun (gentle putty) and are followed by gentle resisted differential tendon gliding (hook fist, flat fist) and then by blocking of the PIP and DIP joints to isolate FDS and FDP, respectively. Resisted "strengthening" exercises are not performed until 3 months postoperatively. Progression for patients with decreased tendon glide, and therefore decreased range of digital motion, is made after consultation with the treating surgeon (e.g., adding active range of motion by the fourth

week or discontinuing the splint before the sixth week postoperatively).

COMPLICATIONS

Despite continued refinements made to the surgical care and rehabilitation of flexor tendon lacerations and avulsions, complications can be frequent and can have devastating effects. The greatest protection against the most dreaded of complications, namely, rupture,* is a well-done core suture and running epitendinous time-zero repair, along with a well-educated patient. It has been shown experimentally that digital extension at the MCP, PIP, and DIP joints, when combined with wrist extension, leads to forces on the flexor tendon repair site that can lead to excessive repair site gap formation and rupture.[44,227,228] The patient is educated by both the therapist and the surgeon that combined digital and wrist extension is to be avoided and that any digital extension must be combined with synergistic wrist flexion. Likewise, any motion of the wrist into extension beyond neutral is accompanied by passive placement of the digits into the flexed posture at the MCP, PIP, and DIP joints. It remains difficult despite the availability of new imaging techniques to determine whether repair site elongation

---

*See references 10, 12, 17, 20, 71, 74, 75, 84, 95, 96, 105, 110, 113, 156, 167, 174, 181, 190, 282, 288, 291, 320, 330, 331, 335, 378, 383, 402, 412, 436, and 485-488.

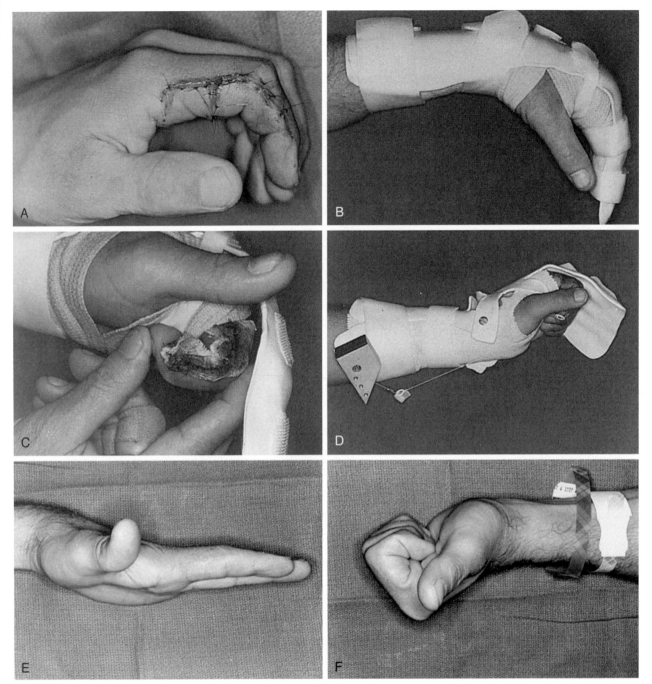

FIGURE 7-18. Clinical examples of the author's post–flexor tendon repair program. **A,** Index finger after a four-strand repair of the FDS and FDP. **B,** Resting splint with the wrist and MCP joints flexed and the IP joints extended. **C,** The finger is passively flexed with the wrist in flexion. **D,** The wrist is extended while maintaining passive digital flexion. The patient then holds this position with light active flexion. **E,** Extension at 3 years. **F,** Flexion at 3 years. (Courtesy of James W. Strickland, MD.)

beyond 3 mm has occurred. It is therefore imperative for repair site strength accrual to occur beginning at 3 weeks postoperatively so that the potential for gap formation be minimized up to that time.

Should rupture or substantial elongation occur up to 3 weeks postoperatively, or, in the case of zone I repairs if the dorsal button becomes loose, surgical exploration and re-repair is advocated. At time periods longer than 3 weeks postoperatively, the chances of a successful repair may

diminish. An attempt should be made, however, to explore the sheath and proceed with repair or reconstruction (as described in the next subchapter) should catastrophic sudden loss of digital motion occur during the postoperative time period.

On occasion, the tendons may become adherent and fail to glide sufficiently to restore unimpeded digital function. The decision to proceed with tenolysis is made after serial joint measurements fail to demonstrate improved active digital motion despite continued therapy. A prerequisite for successful tenolysis is that full or nearly full passive digital flexion has been achieved.[420,425,428] In this case, dorsal impedance to passive and therefore active motion of the digit does not occur.

After a flexor tendon injury or avulsion that has not been treated, attempts to advance the proximal stump and repair the tendon in a relatively shortened position can occur. If this occurs in the middle, long, or small finger, the syndrome of quadrigia may result (see p. 273). If the FPL or the index FDP is advanced and repaired beyond the point of musculotendinous compliance, digital flexion contracture rather than incomplete flexion in adjacent uninvolved digits may ensue. The most efficacious treatment is prevention: for the surgeon to recognize that a repair is too tight and for secondary reconstructive options to be utilized.

If PIP or DIP flexion contractures occur as was the case in patients treated with the passive rubber-band rehabilitation modalities, gentle passive stretch and splinting techniques can be employed. The danger in too-aggressive attempts to correct flexion deformities is that subjacent tendon rupture can occur.

ANNOTATED REFERENCES

44. Boyer MI, Gelberman RH, Burns ME, et al: Intrasynovial flexor tendon repair: An experimental study comparing low and high levels of in vivo force during rehabilitation in canines. J Bone Joint Surg Am 83:891-899, 2001.

    Increasing the level of force applied during postoperative rehabilitation did not accelerate the time-dependent accrual of repair site stiffness or strength. Suture technique (the number of core suture strands) was of primary importance in providing a stiff and strong repair throughout the first 6 weeks postoperatively. This manuscript suggests that there be should be a re-examination of the concept that increases in force produced by more vigorous mobilization protocols are beneficial to healing of tendons. Although more vigorous rehabilitation may help to improve hand function, no evidence was found that it enhances tissue healing or strength in the context of a multi-strand modern suture repair.

47. Boyer MI, Strickland JW, Engles D, et al: Flexor tendon repair and rehabilitation: State of the art in 2002. Instr Course Lect 52:137-161, 2003.

425. Strickland JW: Development of flexor tendon surgery: Twenty-five years of progress. J Hand Surg 25:214-235, 2000.

    These review articles outline the basic science and clinical investigations that have advanced significantly the treatment and outcome after intrasynovial flexor tendon repair, reconstruction, and rehabilitation over the past three decades. The application of modern multi-strand suture repair techniques as well as postoperative rehabilitation protocols emphasizing the application of intrasynovial repair site excursion have led to protocols for treatment of intrasynovial flexor tendon lacerations that include a strong initial repair followed by the application of postoperative passive motion rehabilitation. Currently accepted treatment protocols after flexor tendon repair and reconstruction are based on current clinical and scientific data.

119. Gelberman RH, Boyer MI, Brodt MD, et al: The effect of gap formation at the repair site on the strength and excursion of intrasynovial flexor tendons: An experimental study on the early stages of tendon-healing in dogs. J Bone Joint Surg Am 81:975-982, 1999.

    Elongation at the repair site had been thought to result in the formation of adhesions and a poor functional outcome after repair of flexor tendons. In a clinically relevant canine model it was shown that after sharp transection followed by repair, a gap at the repair site of more than 3 mm does not increase the prevalence of adhesions or impair the range of motion but does prevent the accrual of strength and stiffness that normally occurs with time. Suture repair techniques therefore should be directed toward the prevention of repair site gap formation during the critical first 3 weeks postoperatively.

122. Gelberman RH, Manske PR, Akeson WH, et al: Flexor tendon repair. J Orthop Res 4:119-128, 1986.

    Healing canine flexor tendons treated with either total immobilization, delayed protected mobilization, or early protected mobilization were studied by biomechanical, microangiographic, biochemical, and histologic techniques at intervals through 12 weeks. Although adhesions obliterated the space between the tendon surface and the tendon sheath of the immobilized repairs, mobilized tendons demonstrated coverage of the repair site by cells from the epitenon by 10 days and a smooth, gliding surface that was maintained free of adhesions through 42 days. This in-vivo canine study demonstrated convincingly that adhesion-free healing could occur for lacerations of the flexor tendons within the confines of the fibro-osseous digital sheath.

125. Gelberman RH, Siegel DB, Woo SL, et al: Healing of digital flexor tendons: Importance of the interval from injury to repair: A biomechanical, biochemical, and morphological study in dogs. J Bone Joint Surg Am 73:66-75, 1991.

    In an in-vivo canine model, intrasynovial flexor tendons were repaired either immediately or after a delay of 7 or 21 days. For both biochemical and biomechanical indices, immediate repair demonstrated superiority to those tendons repaired after a delay of 7 or 21 days.

127. Gelberman RH, Vande Berg JS, Lundborg GN, Akeson WH: Flexor tendon healing and restoration of the gliding surface: An ultrastructural study in dogs. J Bone Joint Surg Am 65:70-80, 1983.

    Healing canine flexor tendons were treated with either total immobilization or by early mobilization. Immobilized tendons healed by ingrowth of connective tissue from the digital sheath and cellular proliferation of the endotenon. In contrast, the mobilized tendons healed by proliferation and migration of cells from the epitenon. Ingrowth of reparative tissue from the tendon sheath was notably lacking in this group. The epitenon cells exhibited greater cellular activity and collagen production at each interval compared with cells of the immobilized repairs. This manuscript demonstrated that the intrasynovial gliding surface could indeed be restored and that early mobilization after flexor tendon laceration and repair in zone II could achieve good results.

186. Kessler I, Nissim F: Primary repair without immobilization of flexor tendon division within the digital sheath: An experimental and clinical study. Acta Orthop Scand 40:587-601, 1969.

    This article described Kessler's eponymous core suture technique, as demonstrated in an experiment performed on chickens. Seven clinical cases are summarized as well. The two-strand core suture technique is illustrated and demonstrated radiographically. The authors' goal was to "examine and demonstrate the condition of an injured flexor tendon after primary end-to-end suture without immobilization." In the manuscript, they showed that "early motion may change the nature of the adhesions and preserve good physiological range of excursion." The subsequent two decades would see the rise in popularity of the concept of primary tendon healing and the application of early motion protocols to the armamentarium of hand surgeons for the treatment of flexor tendon lacerations.

236. Lister GD, Kleinert HE, Kutz JE, Atasoy E: Primary flexor tendon repair followed by immediate controlled mobilization. J Hand Surg [Am] 2:441-451, 1977.

The results of immediate repair and controlled mobilization in 156 severed flexor tendons in 68 patients over an 18-month period were reported in this classic manuscript. Seventy-nine (56%) of the injuries occurred in zone II; of these, 75% of patients were rated as "excellent" or "good." In one fourth of the cases the FDS was excised. This report was the first large series in the United States advocating what has become the accepted method of treatment: primary repair of intrasynovial flexor tendon lacerations within the digital sheath.

246. Lundborg G, Holm S, Myrhage R: The role of the synovial fluid and tendon sheath for flexor tendon nutrition: An experimental tracer study on diffusional pathways in dogs. Scand J Plast Reconstr Surg 14:99-107, 1980.

This is the "classic" article describing the vascular supply to the intrasynovial flexor tendon. Angiographic and histologic studies on the FDP tendons of fresh amputation specimens demonstrated three separate vascular systems of various origin, with little communication between each; in the FDS tendon, two systems were observed. It was postulated that the synovial fluid is of importance for the nutrition of the tendons in these avascular zones and that the synovial sheath should be preserved if possible.

263. Manske PR, Gelberman RH, Vande Berg JS, Lesker PA: Intrinsic flexor-tendon repair: A morphological study in vitro. J Bone Joint Surg Am 66:385-396, 1984.

Advocates of the intrasynovial flexor tendon's ability to heal in the absence of the ingrowth of fibrous adhesions from the surrounding sheath, Manske and colleagues cultured flexor tendon explants in a cell-free medium for 6 weeks. It was concluded that flexor tendons have the intrinsic capacity to participate in the repair process, because "capping" was observed of the free tendon end. This phenomenon occurred by proliferation and migration of cells from either the epitenon or endotenon cell layer.

266. Manske PR, Lesker PA: Flexor tendon nutrition. Hand Clin 1:13-24, 1985.

The concepts regarding nutrient pathways to flexor tendons within the digital sheath are reviewed in this paper, which supports both diffusion and perfusion as modes of nutritional supply to the intrasynovial flexor tendon.

268. Manske PR, Lesker PA: Nutrient pathways of flexor tendons in primates. J Hand Surg [Am] 7:436-444, 1982.

The perfusion and diffusion pathways to the FDP tendons of 40 monkeys were investigated by measuring the uptake of tritiated proline by various tendon segments. This classic article demonstrated the importance of both perfusion and diffusion in the delivery of nutrients to the various segments of the FDP tendon. In the areas supplied by vincula, the perfusion was relatively greater, whereas in the avascular areas, diffusion served a greater role.

320a. Parkes A: The "lumbrical plus" finger. J Bone Joint Surg Br 53:236-239, 1971.

458. Verdan C: Syndrome of quadrigia. Surg Clin North Am 40:425-426, 1960.

Two short classic articles on complications after DIP level disarticulations, too-tight and too-loose tendon repairs, reattachments, and grafts. Weak flexion of unaffected digits (quadrigia) and paradoxical extension of affected digits can cause difficulties in rehabilitation after flexor tendon repair and reconstruction.

385. Schuind F, Garcia-Elias M, Cooney WP 3rd, An KN: Flexor tendon forces: In vivo measurements. J Hand Surg [Am] 17:291-298, 1992.

"S"-shaped force transducers were developed for measurement of in-vivo forces along intact tendons. Basic numerical data on the intratendinous forces realized during various types of pinch and grasp were recorded.

397. Silva MJ, Boyer MI, Ditsios K, et al: The insertion site of the canine flexor digitorum profundus tendon heals slowly following injury and suture repair. J Orthop Res 20:447-453, 2002.

In a clinically relevant canine model, the results of this study indicate that the canine FDP tendon heals slowly after it is injured at its insertion site and sutured onto the distal phalanx. While these findings may be limited to the particular repair method used, they demonstrate a need for devising new treatment strategies to improve healing of flexor tendon insertion site injuries (Leddy type II and III avulsions).

436. Strickland JW, Glogovac SV: Digital function following flexor tendon repair in zone II: A comparison of immobilization and controlled passive motion techniques. J Hand Surg 5:537-543, 1980.

In one of the two classic articles on the clinical outcome after zone II flexor tendon repair and rehabilitation, the other being the Louisville experience, two groups (mobilization vs. immobilization) were compared. The immobilization group demonstrated a higher number of ruptures, and no results were graded as excellent. Early passive motion appeared to be an effective technique to improve the results of flexor tendon repairs in zone II.

455. Verdan C: Primary repair of flexor tendons. J Bone Joint Surg Am 42:647-657, 1960.

This "classic" article described Claude Verdan's technique for the primary repair of intrasynovial flexor tendon lacerations after a "fresh, cleanly cut wound." He used four 6-0 silk sutures placed at 90 degrees to each other in the epitendinous layer of the FDP, and he stressed precise approximation of the tendon ends. The FDS and the surrounding sheath were both excised; a core suture was not described. Active range-of-motion exercises began at 3 weeks after removal of "blocking" pins. This article showed, in Verdan's own words, that "primary repair of flexor tendons in no man's land, performed according to certain technical rules, is a valid operation."

494. Zhao C, Amadio PC, Momose T, et al: Effect of synergistic wrist motion on adhesion formation after repair of partial flexor digitorum profundus tendon lacerations in a canine model in vivo. J Bone Joint Surg Am 84:78-84, 2002.

In a canine study of synergistic wrist and finger motion, these Mayo Clinic surgeons demonstrated a positive effect of passive digital motion, performed with either wrist fixation or synergistic wrist motion, on adhesion and gap formation after flexor tendon repair. These data support the use of synergistic wrist and digital rehabilitation techniques in the rehabilitation of intrasynovial flexor tendon partial lacerations, and, by extension, total lacerations after repair.

Flexor Tendon Reconstruction

John S. Taras and Robert A. Kaufmann

Restoring satisfactory digital function after an unrepaired flexor tendon laceration or a failed repair remains one of the most difficult challenges in hand surgery. Flexor tendon reconstruction was commonly performed before 1960 for treatment of both acute and chronic zone II lacerations. This region was termed "no man's land" (see Fig. 7-2) because primary repair was believed to result in a poorly functioning digit. A post-injury delay of 3 weeks or longer was recommended before tendon grafting. Today, successful results with primary repair of flexor tendon lacerations are commonly obtained, but "no man's land" remains an anatomic region in which it is very difficult to reestablish flexor tendon function.[384a] Successful surgical management of the acute or chronically injured flexor tendon system presupposes a thorough understanding of flexor tendon anatomy,[*] pertinent biomechanics,[109,193,498] and indications for appropriate intervention.[†]

In this section I review indications and techniques for tenolysis, primary tendon grafting, staged tendon grafting, select tendon transfers, and pulley reconstruction. The hand surgeon must be skilled in all of these management options because the intraoperative findings may necessitate a departure from the planned procedure. A flexor tendon tenolysis may need to be changed to a primary or multistage grafting procedure if poor tendon integrity or excessive scarring is present. Knowledge of appropriate management algorithms is essential not only to guide intraoperative decision making but also to discuss the possibility or eventuality of each to the patient. The latter is of utmost importance in today's health care environment that demands thorough preoperative communication between the surgeon and patient.

Before embarking on what may result in a lengthy multiprocedure voyage, the question of whether tendon reconstruction is indicated needs to be asked. Doing no operation, performing an arthrodesis, or amputating the digit may be a more prudent intervention than subjecting the patient to what may ultimately restore little functional improvement. Proper patient selection is, therefore, essential for the success of flexor tendon reconstruction. Before proceeding with surgery, the rigors of postoperative therapy need to be explained. The patient must agree to strict adherence to protocol or risk a compromised outcome. Additionally, the drawback of not undergoing flexor tendon reconstruction must be weighed against the risks of surgery. Age, functional status, occupational needs, and the patient's individ-

ual desires must all be considered. An elderly person with few functional demands may be content with a total arc of motion that is 50% of normal. Careful attention must also be placed on the preoperative sensory and circulatory status of the finger. Flexor tendon reconstruction will invariably add an additional neurovascular insult and may result in a cold and atrophic finger, not to mention an unhappy patient, even when satisfactory range of motion has been attained.

Reconstruction of the flexor tendon system can be viewed as a management ladder with each step representing a need to address greater impairment (Fig. 7-19). Once the decision for surgery has been made this ladder is used as a guide for operative intervention. Initial consideration is given to adhesions that may be present. A tenolysis to restore tendon gliding is performed if tendon and pulley integrity is found to be satisfactory; if it is not, then a suitable replacement is required. In certain circumstances a tendon transfer can more predictably achieve restoration of finger function. When a tendon transfer is not appropriate, a tendon graft should be considered. A primary tendon graft can be carried from palm to fingertip when the palm is uninjured and there is minimal scarring. If extensive scarring is present, a tenolysis, tendon transfer, or primary graft may not be adequate. In this scenario, scarring around an area that received significant trauma may require a joint contracture release and possibly pulley reconstruction. A temporary silicone spacer is needed to develop a smooth gliding bed around the implant before placing a tendon graft in a staged manner. When the palm is relatively scar free, the graft may be placed from the palm to the fingertip. If the palm is also scarred, then this graft is best extended from the fingertip to the distal forearm.

Ensuring smooth tendon gliding is of paramount concern during flexor tendon reconstruction, but each surgical intervention evokes its own scar response from the adjacent tissues. Postoperative healing may result in the formation

---

[*]See references 7, 114, 154, 155, 164, 208, 232, 233, 260, 384, 516, and 517.

[†]See references 38, 58, 59, 62, 112, 119, 177, 191, 198, 203, 229, 234, 279, 300, 302, 304, 305, 309, 325-327, 334, 335, 341, 352, 353, 359, 372, 403, 442, 443, 445, 466, 472, 474-477, 504, 511, and 520a.

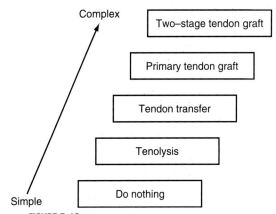

FIGURE 7-19. Ladder of tendon reconstruction options.

of adhesions between the tendon and its surrounding structures.[95,286-291] Factors that need to be considered are as follows*:

1. *Age of the patient.* Younger patients do better than the elderly, except in the very young when technical difficulties may compromise the end result.
2. *Mechanism and extent of trauma.* Crushing injuries, fractures, joint disruption, nerve and artery damage, skin loss, or infection contribute to a worse prognosis than after surgery to reconstruct tendons that were cleanly lacerated.
3. *Level of tendon laceration.* As a rule, tendons injured outside the flexor sheath yield better results than do those injured within the fibro-osseous sheath.
4. *Healing response of the patient.* Assuming that the reconstruction is performed by a well-trained and experienced surgeon, the patient's innate healing response to injury will likely influence the end result more than the actual technique of suturing, the type of suture material chosen, or the timing of the procedure.

FLEXOR TENOLYSIS

Preoperative Evaluation

Active finger motion is predicated on the flexor tendon gliding smoothly in its sheath and is adversely affected by adhesions. Tendon adhesions occur whenever the surface of a tendon has been violated either through the injury itself or from surgical manipulation.[145,248,280,286,287,488] Failed primary tendon repairs, crush injuries, fractures, and infections can individually or in combination cause peritendinous adhesions to adjacent soft tissues or fracture callus. Additionally, adhesions may form at the juncture between the graft and native tendon after a grafting procedure. If the adhesions are mild, a conscientious therapy program will usually restore full gliding. Once a patient's progress has plateaued and a significant difference between passive and active range of digital motion exists, then a tenolysis may be considered. Surgical release of restrictive adhesions has been shown to be an excellent salvage procedure when tendon and pulley integrity are maintained and the involved joints are supple.†

Flexor tenolysis is often more technically demanding than tendon repair itself. If unsuccessful, the patient's hand function may be even worse than before surgery. The best candidate for tenolysis is a patient whose repaired tendon has localized adhesions that limit gliding (Fig. 7-20). Once surgical release of this region has been successfully accomplished, a full range of motion is usually regained. More frequently, however, the adhesions involve a long segment of the involved tendon and require extensive exposure for release (Fig. 7-21).

---

*See references 30, 68, 127, 128, 153, 244, 264, 265, 277, 294, 317, 420, and 455.

†See references 12, 33, 118, 129, 192, 202, 395, 396, 399, 405, 406, 439, 440, 443, 479, 480, and 503.

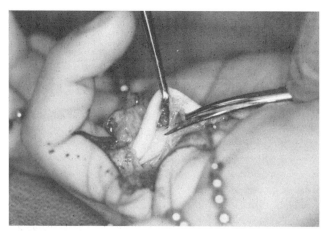

FIGURE 7-20. Localized area of tendon adhesion permits simple tenolysis to restore full tendon gliding.

Successful tenolysis demands immediate mobilization and, therefore, any concomitant surgery that requires immobilization or protection in the postoperative period will tend to compromise the procedure. Joint contracture is frequently seen in patients requiring tenolysis. These patients may also require a capsulectomy, which further complicates the problem and results in a lesser degree of recovery.[479] Any additional procedures that require postoperative immobilization, such as tendon lengthening or shortening, free skin grafts, or osteotomies, will all negatively affect the outcome[479] and may be a contraindication to doing the tenolysis concomitantly. Additional negative prognostic indicators are age older than 40 years, nerve suture, late tenolysis (more than 1 year postoperatively), and tenolysis requiring a prolonged operative time.[479,480] Some hand surgeons have rebuilt pulleys at the time of flexor tenolysis,[131a,250,439] but I believe the need for pulley reconstruction is a strong indication for staged tendon grafting.

There is some disagreement about the exact timing of tenolysis. Certainly all surgeons would agree that a reasonable period of time should be allowed for softening of the wound and spontaneous remodeling of adhesions and

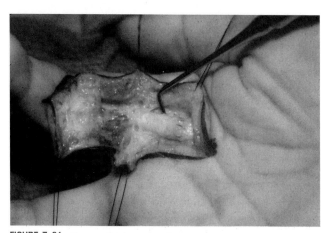

FIGURE 7-21. Dense adhesions completely restrict tendon gliding, which requires difficult and meticulous tenolysis to restore tendon function.

scar tissue. Only after the compliant patient, trying to regain gliding movement through hand therapy measures, has reached a plateau should tenolysis be considered. Fetrow,[118] after reviewing Pulvertaft's cases, stated that 6 months should be allowed after a free tendon graft to lessen the risk of graft rupture. He also suggested that a minimum of 3 months of healing be allowed after tendon repair to prepare the tissues for tenolysis. Rank and Wakefield[363] originally waited 3 months but later advocated a delay of 6 to 9 months before considering tenolysis.[364] Weeks and Wray[492] showed that most of the active function obtained after a tendon graft was achieved by 22 weeks postoperatively, which suggests that this point is a good time to perform tenolysis when indicated. The surgeon's judgment should prevail,[123] and I do not perform tenolysis earlier than 3 months in cases of either direct repair or grafting. A tenolysis invariably strips the tendon of soft tissue connections and thereby endangers tendon nutrition, increasing the likelihood of rupture. Delay is believed, although surely not guaranteed, to reduce the incidence of this complication. The effect of patient age at the time of tenolysis on functional improvement was investigated in a report by Birnie and Idler.[33] These authors noted that tenolysis in children younger than age 11 years resulted in only minimal gains, whereas older children benefited from tenolysis even when it was carried out more than 1 year after their original operation.

Several investigators have researched the use of agents to block the formation of restrictive adhesions after tenolysis or tendon repair.* Steroid preparations have been locally instilled to alter the wound healing in the belief that adhesion formation would be less robust.[216] Whitaker and colleagues,[503] James,[201] Carstam,[69,70] Rank and associates,[364] and Wrenn and coworkers[520] suggested locally administered steroids to be of some value, whereas Verdan,[479] Brooks,[53] and Fetrow[118] concluded that steroids do not improve the results of tenolysis. Bora and colleagues[36] found that the use of many of these materials promoted additional scarring. My colleagues and I use a technique that stresses immediate and continued active range of motion in a vigorous postoperative hand therapy program that has obviated the need for these materials. Formal hand therapy should begin 2 to 3 days after surgery and should continue until range of motion has plateaued and adhesions have stabilized.[82] An aggressive active and passive range-of-motion program is carried out daily for 2 to 4 weeks and is then reduced in frequency. Static and dynamic splinting techniques are often used to augment the rehabilitation program.

Technique

Schneider[400,405] and Hunter[183,185] and their coworkers advocated the use of local anesthesia complemented by intravenous sedation to allow active participation of the patient during tenolysis (see the section on neuroleptanalgesia in Chapter 2). Easily awakened, the patient cooperates dynamically during the surgical procedure. The surgeon can be

certain that the tendon has been completely freed and that the tendon motor can actively pull the finger into full flexion. Although Schneider and Hunter and their coworkers favored 1% or 2% lidocaine,[183,185] my colleagues and I prefer the longer-acting agent 0.5% bupivacaine (without epinephrine) infiltrated locally in the skin or as digital nerve blocks at the metacarpal level. Wrist blocks can also be useful but will invariably result in altered metacarpophalangeal (MCP) joint motion from intrinsic muscle paralysis.

Although the use of neuroleptanalgesia is strongly recommended for tenolysis, sometimes it is not feasible. General anesthesia is recommended for those patients with extensive scarring when the tourniquet time will likely exceed 1 hour. Additionally, some patients may not be ideal candidates for neuroleptanalgesia. When a patient is under general anesthesia the surgeon must be certain to extend the tenolysis proximal and distal to the zone of injury to ensure that all adhesions are lysed. Whitaker and colleagues[503] recommend a "traction flexor check" by pulling on the involved tendon through a separate incision at the wrist. This gives an estimate of the potential range of motion and has the additional benefit of breaking up any adhesions that may have been missed.

The involved flexor system is preferably approached through an ample zigzag incision[55,56] sufficiently long to uncover the entire length of the flexor tendon if necessary. Flexibility of the surgical approach may be required to utilize previous surgical scars. All limiting adhesions are methodically excised,[411] and care is taken to define the tendon border, a task that is not simple in dense scar tissue. Specialized tenolysis knives designed by Meals are particularly useful to cleave tendon adhesions (Fig. 7-22). It is absolutely imperative to preserve the pulley system, especially the critical A2 and A4 pulleys. If this is not possible, new pulleys can be constructed at the time of tenolysis,[131a,250,439] but I believe this practice greatly reduces the probability of success. A staged tendon implant should be considered when an adequate pulley system cannot be preserved at the time of tenolysis. Often a poor quality tendon will rupture during a tenolysis, forcing the surgeon onto the reconstructive ladder of options (see Fig. 7-19). The next step would then be tendon grafting or transfer. In cases

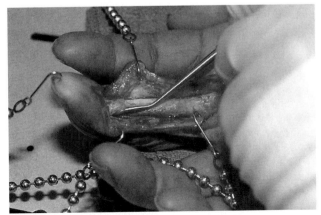

FIGURE 7-22. Knives specifically designed by Meals for tenolysis are invaluable in cleaving dense tendon adhesions.

---

*See references 10, 17-19, 22, 29, 64, 70, 90, 117, 134, 141, 143a, 190, 201, 202, 220, 315, 340, 373, 431, 446, 451, 491, 501, 510, and 520.

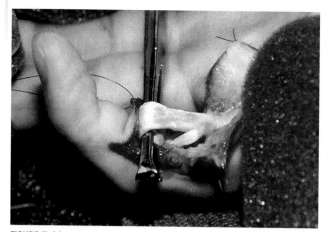

FIGURE 7-23. By gently twisting the tendons with an Allis clamp, tendon excursion can be confirmed during tenolysis.

in which the tenolysis results in considerable trauma to the tendon sheath and significant scarring is encountered, staged reconstruction (including pulley reconstruction) with a temporary silicone implant is indicated.

During tenolysis the patient's active motion is reevaluated frequently as each area of scar is lysed. An Allis clamp is placed around the tendons. By twisting the clamp, the excursion of the tendon is periodically checked during the procedure to complement the active motion testing (Fig. 7-23). Tourniquet paralysis intervenes between 20 and 30 minutes in most patients; and if the procedure is prolonged, the tourniquet can be continued without the patient's activity for more than 1 hour. The tourniquet is then released, bleeding is controlled, and after a few minutes the patient is able to actively flex the digits again. If necessary, the tourniquet can be reinflated, but this is rarely needed. When performing a tenolysis in cases complicated by a prior crush injury or fracture, it may be necessary to evaluate the extensor system also to ensure that both tendon systems are free of adhesions.

Postoperative Care

After closure, a nonconstricting dressing is placed so that immediate flexion can be performed within the bandage to maintain the gliding obtained through tenolysis.[129,131] Active motion is begun under the supervision of a hand therapist 2 to 3 days postoperatively. Most authors find that if the patient shows improving motion in the first week and maintains this gain for the next 2 to 3 weeks, useful motion will be maintained.[122] To help the patient get through the difficult and often painful first week after tenolysis, an indwelling polyethylene catheter can be left in the involved area at the time of surgery.[185,407] Small amounts of local anesthetic are instilled during exercise periods when discomfort is greatest. This catheter is left in place for 5 days.

Continuous passive motion (CPM) devices can be useful when joint contracture releases are performed concomitantly after tenolysis,[219,297] but it is clear that they will not substitute for immediate active pull-through of the lysed tendon system. Active range-of-motion exercises must be the primary therapeutic modality after tenolysis.[117a,122] CPM devices may in fact impart a false impression of success if

CRITICAL POINTS: TENOLYSIS

INDICATION

- Tendon adhesions

PREOPERATIVE EVALUATION

- Discrepancy exists between passive (full) and active (limited) range of motion after hand therapy has plateaued.

PEARLS

- Do not operate earlier than 3 months status post repair or grafting.

TECHNICAL POINTS

- Use neuroleptanesthesia if possible. Otherwise "traction check" through additional wrist incision.
- Use zigzag incisions.
- Use tenolysis knives.

PITFALL

- Worse prognosis: concurrent capsulectomy, concurrent osteotomy, age older than 40, 1-year delay

POSTOPERATIVE CARE

- Immediately begin active range-of-motion exercises.

they are used without active-assisted exercises, and I rarely use CPM after tenolysis.

SINGLE-STAGE FLEXOR TENDON GRAFTING: FDP, FDS DISRUPTED

Indications

Despite the rightful popularity of direct early repair,[380,404,415,416] there still exists a group of patients in whom a free tendon graft is indicated as the initial procedure.[84,281,282,357,360,361,397] The indications have been well established and include the following[2,3,42-47,147,269,484,486]:

1. Injuries resulting in segmental tendon loss
2. Delay in definitive repair making it impossible to do an end-to-end repair. The delay can be caused by late referral, as well as cases in which the flexor tendon injury was not appreciated at the time of injury. Lacerations that have been neglected for over 3 to 6 weeks will have evidence of degeneration of the tendon end with scar tissue filling the tendon sheath.
3. Patients in whom the surgeon believes delayed grafting is the better treatment alternative for a zone II injury

4. Delayed presentation of *some* flexor digitorum profundus (FDP) avulsion injuries

Single-stage free-tendon grafting after flexor division in a digit remains one of the most elegant (and difficult) procedures in the hand surgeon's armamentarium. The injured tendons are excised and replaced with a suitable tendon graft secured to the base of the distal phalanx at the FDP insertion and joined to a proximal motor in the palm or distal forearm. The palm-to-fingertip tendon graft (Fig. 7-24) is usually performed in those fingers that have had both flexor tendons severed in zone II.[465] Surgical principles to be followed include placement of only one graft in one finger, never sacrificing an intact FDS, ensuring that the graft is of small caliber with its ends fixed away from the tendon sheath, and ensuring adequate graft tension.[459a]

Before surgery, the wound should be well healed and the joints without contracture and demonstrating maximum passive motion (Boyes' grade 1) (Table 7-2).[39,40,71] Pulvertaft[360] emphasized that, "The hand is in good overall condition. There is no extensive scarring. Passive movements are full or nearly full. The circulation is satisfactory. At least one digital nerve in the affected digit is intact." Patients presenting with joint contracture should undergo a hand therapy regimen to regain as much passive digital motion as possible before tendon grafting. The patient should be instructed preoperatively that alternative measures

may need to be performed. In cases in which there is extensive scarring, pulley incompetence or joint contracture single-stage tendon grafting is not advocated. In these patients two-stage tendon graft procedures are performed. Single-stage grafting is contraindicated for insensate or poorly vascularized digits, in children younger than the age of 3 years, and in elderly patients.[514]

The Distal Juncture

No gliding motion takes place at the distal juncture, making it of paramount concern to ensure a durable[274] and firm union between the tendon and the FDP stump or volar base of the distal phalanx.[120,211,222,272,469,502] When the distal juncture is created first, the finger can be more easily closed in the extended position and the appropriate graft length determined in the palm. The proximal juncture is then accomplished after the distal juncture has been completed. Uniform agreement does not exist on this sequence, however. Creating the proximal juncture initially with subsequent length adjustment at the fingertip has been advocated,[358,426,433,497,514] but I find this technique to be less reliable for judging the proper tension required to restore the natural digital cascade. There are a number of techniques for attaching the tendon graft to the distal phalanx, and these are based primarily on the length and condition of the distal FDP stump (see p. 248).

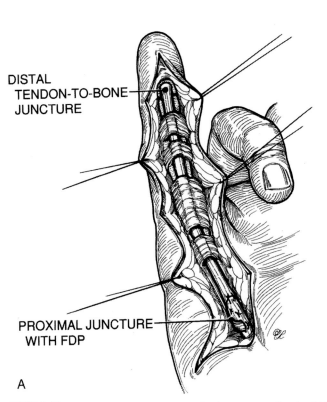

DISTAL TENDON-TO-BONE JUNCTURE

PROXIMAL JUNCTURE WITH FDP

A

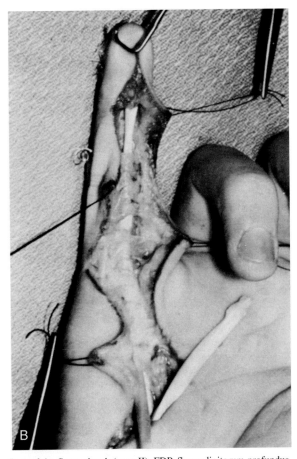

B

FIGURE 7-24. A, Flexor tendon graft. The tendon junctures are placed outside the confines of the flexor sheath (zone II). FDP, flexor digitorum profundus. **B,** In this clinical case the graft has been fixed into the distal phalanx and the proximal juncture will be completed in the palm by using the FDP as the motor.

Table 7-2
BOYES' PREOPERATIVE CLASSIFICATION

Grade	Preoperative Condition
1	Good. Minimal scar with mobile joints and no trophic changes.
2	Cicatrix. Heavy skin scarring due to injury or prior surgery. Deep scarring due to failed primary repair or infection.
3	Joint damage. Injury to the joint with restricted range of motion.
4	Nerve damage. Injury to the digital nerves resulting in trophic changes in the finger.
5	Multiple damage. Involvement of multiple fingers with a combination of the above problems.

From Boyes JH: Flexor tendon grafts in the fingers and thumb: An evaluation of end results. J Bone Joint Surg Am 32:489-499, 1950, with permission.

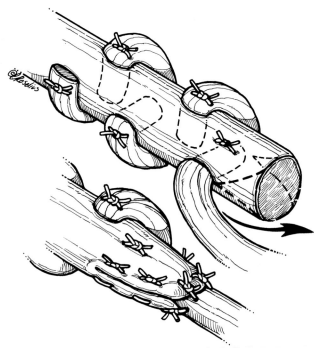

FIGURE 7-25. The modified Pulvertaft end weave technique. The graft is secured to the proximal motor tendon via multiple weaves through the motor tendon held in place with 3-0 polyester sutures.

The Proximal Juncture

It is desirable to create a proximal juncture that can withstand muscle pull in the early healing period and prevent gap formation. A gap will lengthen the repair, make the graft too long, and create an area of potential rupture.[218,220,249,463] The tendon weave is my preferred method of proximal tendon graft juncture in any area outside the flexor sheath, where it would be too bulky. This type of juncture is stronger than the end-to-end suture techniques,[88,93,463] and it has the advantage of being very strong[88,463] and allowing careful adjustment of graft tension[354-358,449c] (Fig. 7-25). An in-vitro analysis of this technique by Gabuzda and coworkers[125] in human cadaver tendons confirmed its strength. They found that the strength of the repair increased significantly with additional weaves and recommended using as many as four or five. I use at least three weaves to create a strong juncture. End-to-end suture techniques have also been used in tendon grafting by various authors,* but these methods leave little margin for error as far as tension adjustment is concerned and the graft is often a different size than the motor tendon.

Single-Stage Grafting Technique

All flexor tendon surgery should be carried out under tourniquet control. I favor a Bruner-type incision to expose the tendon system (Fig. 7-26),[398] but the midlateral approach can be used as well and is favored by some surgeons.[143,306,363,364,441] The neurovascular bundles are protected throughout the dissection. The area of injury to the sheath is noted, and the damaged sheath is minimally resected. As much of the uninjured flexor sheath is preserved as possible.[487] This is in contradistinction to the older teachings of many leading tendon surgeons,[40,41,61,231,348,355,363,364] who believed that all the sheath, except for critical narrow bands

of pulley, should be removed. Handling, pinching, or probing of the tissues must be minimized because of the risk of increasing the number and density of adhesions. Approximately 1 cm of the FDP stump is preserved distally. The remainder of the injured FDP is sharply excised proximally to the lumbrical origin in the palm. The FDP is used for the motor, unless it is of poor quality, in which case the flexor digitorum superficialis (FDS) can be used.

In the majority of cases both digital flexor tendons are not functioning. When this is true, the proximal stump of the FDS is pulled distally and the tendon transected, allowing the remaining stump to retract proximally. The distal FDS is excised sharply, but 1 to 2 cm of its insertion is left undisturbed because this provides a more favorable posterior bed for the graft than does a surgically invaded, freshly granulating area. The FDS tail may, by virtue of adhesion to the flexor canal floor, provide stability at the proximal interphalangeal (PIP) joint, thereby helping to prevent hyperextension deformity, a problem occasionally seen in fingers without an FDS tendon.[320,462]

Obtaining the Graft

At this point the wound is covered with a moist dressing and attention is directed at obtaining the appropriate graft. If it is necessary to harvest from the lower extremity, the tourniquet is released. The technique of obtaining a flexor graft is discussed in detail on page 263.

Placement of the Graft

After hemostasis is achieved, the extremity is once again exsanguinated and the tourniquet reinflated. A holding suture is placed to secure the distal end of the graft, and the graft is threaded under the pulleys. Various techniques can

*See references 26, 27, 93, 214, 215, 217, 220, 242, 278, 371, 382, 456-459, 463, 470, 482, 490, and 519.

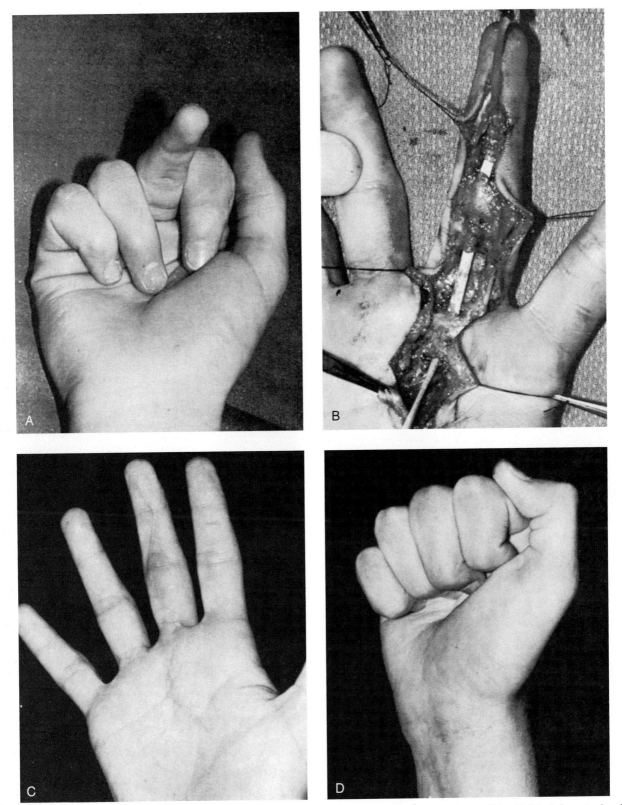

FIGURE 7-26. Example of a flexor tendon graft. **A,** A 16-year-old boy presented with a 3-month-old laceration in zone II in which both flexor tendons had been severed. The patient maintained supple joints and had minimal scarring. **B,** As much uninjured flexor sheath was preserved as possible. The tendon graft (palmaris longus) has been threaded into the retinacular system in preparation for distal and proximal junctures. Note preservation of the pulleys. **C** and **D,** Extension and flexion at 6 months postoperatively.

be used to pass the graft, but my preferred method is with the Swanson disposable suture passer (Smith and Nephew, Memphis, TN). It is directed beneath the pulleys in a distal to proximal direction. The holding suture attached to the grafted tendon is placed through the wire loop and then pulled distally. A flexible silicone tendon implant to which the graft is sutured can also be used as a tendon passer. Leddy[236] and Sourmelis and McGrouther[428] have used a flexible rubber catheter as a passer, but regardless of which method is used, care must be taken to minimize trauma to the intact sheath. A clamp is placed at the proximal end of the graft to prevent inadvertent withdrawal.

Distal Juncture Technique

If the distal profundus stump has been preserved, it is reflected to its insertion on the volar lip of the distal phalanx. The graft is initially secured by utilizing a 3-0 Prolene suture placed in the end of the graft and crisscrossed twice in the method of Bunnell. The needle is cut off. A tendon braider is then used to pass the graft through the FDP stump. The ends of the suture are threaded onto a Keith needle. Regardless of whether the FDP stump is present, I fasten the sutures using an "around the bone" technique. With the use of a needle holder, the Keith needles are passed around both sides of the distal phalanx to emerge through the middle third nail plate (Fig. 7-27). An effort should be made to avoid the germinal nail matrix; the ideal point of exit through the nail plate should be 3 to 4 mm distal to the lunula and approximately 2 mm from the midline. The tails of the suture are then tied directly over the nail plate (see Fig. 7-27C). At least two 3-0 braided polyester sutures are used then to reinforce the FDP graft juncture (Fig. 7-28).

When the distal FDP stump is insufficient to allow braiding, it may be split longitudinally and the graft laid within the split (Fig. 7-29). The graft is then drawn through

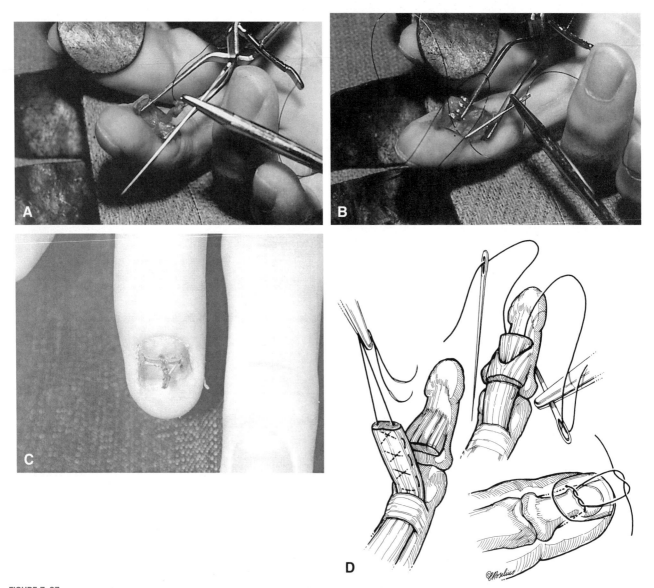

FIGURE 7-27. **A** and **B,** The pullout suture for the distal juncture of securing a tendon graft is passed around the sides of the distal phalanx with the aid of Keith needles. **C,** The pullout suture is then tied directly over the middle third of the nail plate. **D,** Diagram of technique.

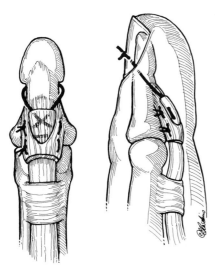

FIGURE 7-28. The distal juncture. The tendon graft is woven through the distal stump of the profundus. The pullout suture is then passed around the sides of the distal phalanx through the nail bed and tied over the nail plate.

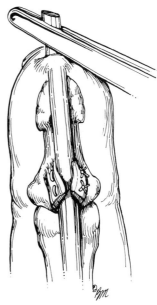

FIGURE 7-30. Distal juncture technique. The graft itself is drawn through the pulp and, after tension adjustments are made, is sutured to the profundus stump.

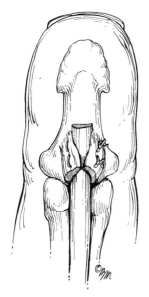

FIGURE 7-29. Distal juncture technique. In this tendon-to-tendon technique an interweave suture is used to fix the graft to the stump of the FDP.

the pulp with a large needle and the projecting graft temporarily clamped at the fingertip,[358] (Fig. 7-30) allowing for precise tension adjustment. Additional sutures are placed between the graft and the FDP stump through which it was passed. I prefer this technique in children with open growth plates but do not hesitate to augment the distal juncture with a standard pullout suture in the skeletally mature. Similar techniques have been described.[385,427,433,497,514]

Another acceptable method is a modification of the classic Bunnell tendon-to-bone pull-out technique (Fig. 7-31).[41,257,358,436,459,487] A drill hole is made in the volar cortex of the distal phalanx into which Keith needles are passed through the nail plate. Although passing the suture through the bone, nail matrix, and plate provides a strong bone-to-graft junction when healed,[204,370] I find it more cumbersome

and have not encountered distal ruptures using the aforementioned "around the bone" technique. Many surgeons employ a sterile button tied over a stent on top of the nail plate for securing the pullout suture. I believe this to be unnecessary, and my concerns with button use have grown after encountering permanent nail deformities secondary to pressure-related eponychial necrosis.

Another alternative places a transverse drill hole across the base of the distal phalanx with the graft threaded through and sutured to itself[227,304a,354,358] (Fig. 7-32). This technique allows for easy graft tension judgment, but the graft must be thin to pass through the bony tunnel.[354,358]

Proximal Juncture Technique

In the palm-to-tip graft the proximal juncture is made into the FDP tendon just distal to the lumbrical origin. The lumbrical muscle itself is left undisturbed unless it is involved in scarring, in which case the scar tissue is excised. Abundant scar is an indication for two-staged tendon reconstruction. The motor tendon is slit at its end with a fine blade, or preferably a Brand tendon braider is used, and the graft is threaded into the slit. The graft is then threaded transversely in a different plane. Buried 3-0 polyester sutures are used to join the tendons at the interweaves, and the "fish mouth" created is closed to embrace the graft (see Fig. 7-25).

Most surgeons agree that graft length is estimated in an anesthetized patient by the relaxed position of the fingers with the wrist in neutral position.[41,254,434,437,487] Each finger should fall into semiflexion, slightly less flexed than its ulnar neighbor or more flexed than its adjacent radial finger (Fig. 7-33). The interweave technique[354,487] is especially amenable to adjusting tension; if the posture of the hand is satisfactory with one suture in place, the juncture is completed by adding additional sutures.

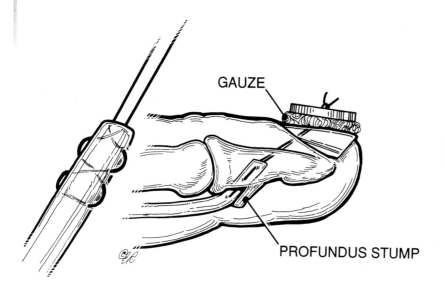

FIGURE 7-31. Modified Bunnell distal juncture technique.

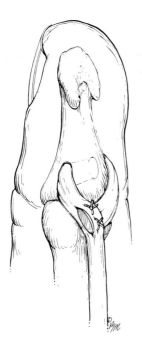

FIGURE 7-32. Distal juncture technique. The tendon graft, which must be thin, is passed through a transverse drill hole in the distal phalanx.

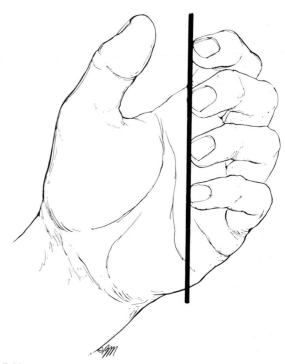

FIGURE 7-33. Determining tension in a reconstructed flexor system at the time of suturing the proximal juncture. With the wrist in neutral position, each finger falls into slightly less flexion than its ulnar neighbor.

Postoperative Care of Tendon Grafts

Postoperative care of tendon grafts has undergone a significant transformation favoring newer early motion protocols over immobilization. Traditional treatment called for 3 weeks of immobilization in which a posterior plaster splint was applied from the fingertips to below the elbow with the wrist flexed approximately 35 degrees, the MCP joints maintained at 60 to 70 degrees, and the interphalangeal (IP) joints at rest in extension.[63] The dressings were changed at 10 days when the skin sutures were removed. The splint was replaced and worn full time for 21 days, at which point an active exercise program was instituted.[460] The patient wore the splint in between exercise periods for 1 or 2 additional weeks. When the distal pullout suture was removed at 6 weeks more vigorous exercises could be started.

As early motion exercises have been utilized after primary flexor tendon repairs,[78,101,224,225,253,283,432a,449b,500] so, too, have these techniques been applied to flexor tendon grafting.[23,454] Our early motion protocol, directed by an experienced hand therapist, greatly benefits the compliant patient. It should be utilized only when the surgeon is confident that the graft junctures are strong enough to withstand the additional tensile stresses of this regimen. The postoperative splint utilized in this early motion scenario is a static dorsal blocking splint with the wrist positioned in

CRITICAL POINTS: SINGLE-STAGE TENDON GRAFTING: FDP, FDS DISRUPTED

INDICATION

- Definitive repair is delayed, making it impossible to do an end-to-end repair.

PREOPERATIVE EVALUATION

- Joint contractures need aggressive therapy before grafting.

PEARLS

- Interweave technique allows easy graft tensioning when creating the proximal juncture.
- Graft length is correct when, with the wrist in neutral, each finger is slightly less flexed than its ulnar neighbor or more flexed than the adjacent radial finger.

TECHNICAL POINTS

- Use a Bruner-type incision.
- Preserve 1 cm of FDP stump distally.
- Excise the distal FDS sharply leaving 1 to 2 cm of its insertion undisturbed.
- Use the FDP for the motor.
- Use a tendon weave for proximal tendon graft (if outside flexor sheath).
- Obtain a flexor graft.

- Place a holding suture through the distal end of the graft.
- Thread the graft under the pulleys with a disposable suture passer.
- Create a distal juncture with an "around the bone" technique.
- Make a proximal juncture into FDP just distal to the lumbrical origin.
- Use three or more interweaves.

PITFALLS

- Two-stage tendon graft is needed if the surgeon finds extensive scarring, pulley incompetence, or joint contracture.
- Careless handling, pinching, or probing of graft will increase the number and density of adhesions.

POSTOPERATIVE CARE

- Use an early range-of-motion protocol if graft junctures are strong.
- Apply a static dorsal blocking splint (4 to 6 weeks) with wrist neutral, MCP joints at 45 degrees, and IP joints neutral.
- Treat flexion contractures with passive stretching and splinting (6 to 8 weeks).

---

neutral, the MCP joints in 45 degrees of flexion, and the IP joints in neutral. This splint is worn for protection until 6 weeks after surgery. Therapist-guided protected passive range-of-motion exercise can be instituted at the first postoperative visit 2 to 3 days after surgery. At 2 weeks after surgery, gentle place-and-hold flexion exercises along with active short-arc digital flexion and extension exercises are added to the therapy program. Blocked flexion exercises involve blocking flexion at the MCP or PIP joint while attempting active flexion at the distal joints and will put additional stress on the junctures. Despite this tensile stress, the blocked flexion exercise method optimizes tendon gliding[494,495] and is instituted actively at 4 weeks and with resistance at 6 weeks. Other experienced therapists prefer to be more cautious with their protocol and defer resisted exercises, including blocking, until after 8 weeks. Flexion contractures are treated with protected passive stretching and specific splinting techniques. Patient education is of utmost importance, and judgment must be used in guiding the more active patient and prodding the reluctant one.

Long-Term Graft Integrity

If a grafted tendon is explored after a period of 6 or more months, it is often identified to be of normal appearance and is indeed a histologic replica of the original tendon. Whether the tendon is in reality the original graft or a new creation brought about by fibroblasts from the host building on a scaffold provided by the graft is a question pondered by many writers.[31,142,245,336,346] The answer, according to Lindsay and McDougall,[247] is that the graft as a whole survives and is reconstructed by a repair process manifested by an increase in the number of mature fibroblasts, revascularization of the graft, and gradual reconstruction of the original collagen. This concept was confirmed in a later study by the same group.[32] It is likely that the graft is nourished by local synovial fluid before revascularization of its tissue. Blood supply is then carried in by local granulation tissue in the form of adhesions.

SINGLE-STAGE FLEXOR TENDON GRAFTING: FDP DISRUPTED, FDS INTACT

Indications

In patients with an injury to the FDP but an intact FDS, early direct repair is indicated, provided that the lesion is recognized and referred within an appropriate time frame.[236] It is unusual that direct repair can be performed after 3 to 4 weeks have elapsed unless the short vinculum to the FDP has remained intact and maintained the tendon in a distal location. This may not be apparent until exploration, although it can usually be determined with magnetic resonance imaging (MRI) preoperatively. When more than 4 weeks have elapsed from the time of injury and the FDS is

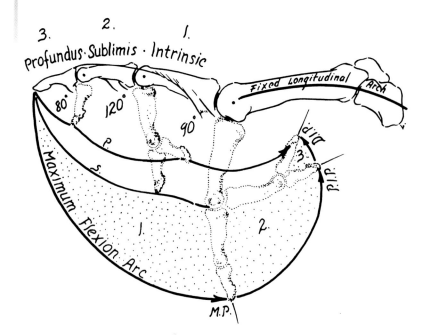

FIGURE 7-34. The flexion arc. In isolated injuries to the FDP when the FDS is fully functional, the greatest part of the flexion arc is maintained *(stippled areas 1 and 2)*. Restoration of active profundus function provides only that portion of the arc denoted by the small stippled 3. PIP, proximal interphalangeal; DIP, distal interphalangeal; MCP, metacarpophalangeal. (From Littler JW: The physiology and dynamic function of the hand. Surg Clin North Am 40:259, 1960.)

fully functional, caution must be exercised in offering a free tendon graft to restore distal joint function.[397] Realizing that most of the useful motion has been maintained when the FDS is fully functional (Fig. 7-34),[256] patients with a severed FDP but who still have an intact FDS may adapt nicely and require no treatment. This is especially true in patients in whom the distal joint does not hyperextend. Appropriate

preoperative explanation of the considerable risk to this function is mandatory. The patient must understand that while passing the tendon graft through or around the FDS, injury may occur that ultimately results in the formation of adhesions and an overall loss of function (i.e., loss of PIP motion). The patient's hand function may, therefore, be significantly impaired by attempts to restore active DIP

CRITICAL POINTS: SINGLE-STAGE TENDON GRAFTING: FDP DISRUPTED, FDS INTACT

INDICATIONS

- Young people with supple joints and a reasonable need for active DIP joint function
- Better justified on ulnar side of hand for power grip
- When FDS is not pulling through completely
- Hyperextension of DIP, but joint supple

PREOPERATIVE EVALUATION

- Early direct repair is indicated until 3 to 4 weeks after injury.
- Later repair is possible if a short vinculum to FDP maintains tendon in distal location.
- MRI may be used to determine location of the proximal stump.

PEARLS

- Never remove an intact, fully functioning FDS tendon in an effort to place a graft.

TECHNICAL POINTS

- Use similar technique as in free tendon grafting.
- Know that a thinner graft is easier to pass (plantaris).

- Pass graft through FDS decussation.
- If area is tight, pass graft around FDS.
- Can remove one FDS tail for tendon graft passage.
- Can be done in two stages.

PITFALLS

- Caution must be exercised with patient selection.
- Patients with intact FDS may adapt nicely and require no treatment.
- During the procedure, injury may occur, resulting in adhesions and overall loss of function.
- In patients with DIP hyperextension, tenodesis or arthrodesis can be offered.

POSTOPERATIVE CARE

- Use early motion protocol if graft juncture is strong.
- Apply static dorsal blocking splint (4 to 6 weeks) with wrist neutral, MCP joints at 45 degrees, and IP joints neutral.
- Treat flexion contractures with passive stretching and splinting (6 to 8 weeks).

flexion, leading many surgeons to implore conservatism, especially in the aged and heavy laborers.[156,313,316,366,371,483] In those patients troubled by instability at the tip or by the lack of involvement of the distal portion of the finger in grip, stabilization of the distal interphalangeal (DIP) joint by tenodesis[205] or arthrodesis can be offered. Despite the difficulties and not inconsiderable risks, outstanding results with FDP grafting in carefully selected patients have been reported.[35,88a,132,195,200,298,356,377,432] I believe that much of the

variability in patient results can be attributed to the different methods of patient evaluation.[139,319,391,397] The procedure should be restricted to young people with supple joints and a reasonable need for active DIP joint function. The graft is probably more frequently justified on the ulnar side of the hand (i.e., in the ring and little fingers for power grip) than on the radial side of the hand (Fig. 7-35). The indications of this operation are greater when the FDS is not pulling through completely and there is limited active PIP flexion.

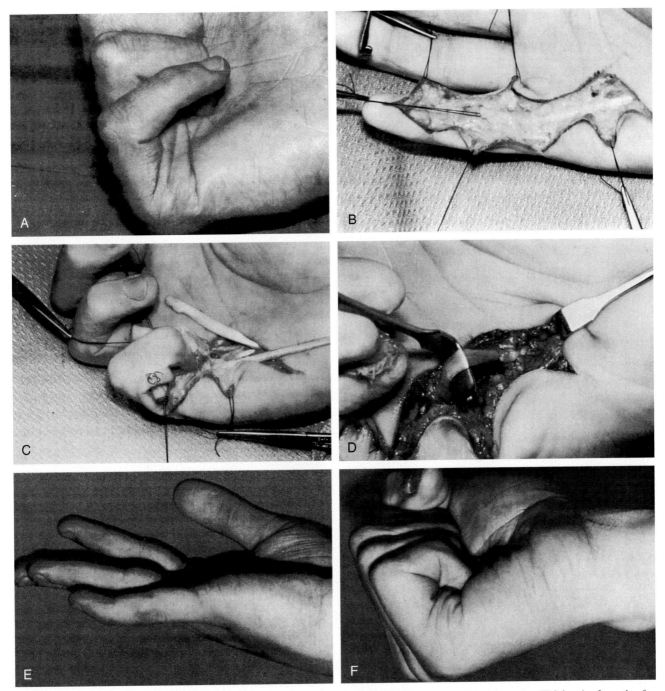

FIGURE 7-35. Tendon graft through an intact FDS. **A,** This 17-year-old boy had ruptured the FDP and demonstrated incomplete FDS function 3 months after injury. **B,** The FDP was retrieved and mobilized, but it was not possible to advance it to the insertion. A tendon graft was then placed. **C,** The graft in place. The finger will be closed before completing the proximal juncture. **D,** An interlace juncture in the palm using the FDP as the motor. **E** and **F,** End result at 1 year. There is a flexion deformity at the tip, but a total of 50 degrees of strong flexion has been gained at the DIP joint.

Single-Stage Grafting Technique With an Intact FDS (Zone I Injuries)

The technique is similar to that for free tendon grafting in the previous section. A thinner graft is easier to pass, and the plantaris should be useful here. The graft is passed through the FDS decussation, but if this area appears tight, the graft may be passed around the FDS. Under no conditions is it ever justified to remove an intact, fully functioning FDS tendon, although Harrison did suggest removal of one tail of the tendon for graft passage.[146] On occasion the procedure has been done in two stages,[88a,156,481,515] with a tendon implant placed at the first stage, particularly if there has been some element of injury to the FDS or the flexor tendon bed or pulley system. Use of the staged tendon graft has been gratifying when appropriately utilized in fingers with a poor sheath.[88a,444]

Postoperative Care of Tendon Grafts With an Intact FDS (Zone I Injuries)

I favor early active range-of-motion protocols to maintain normal FDS function, particularly after Schneider noted that, despite careful preoperative patient selection, a considerable number required subsequent tenolysis.[397] To avoid adherent scarring, short-arc active extension and flexion exercise can be instituted within the first postoperative week along with gentle place-and-hold and straight-fist flexion exercises.

TWO-STAGE FLEXOR TENDON RECONSTRUCTION

Indications

The past four decades have witnessed significant advances in the ability to restore flexor tendon function to badly scarred digits. Staged reconstruction uses passive or active tendon implants, followed secondarily by a replacement graft. A significant number of patients afflicted with flexor tendon injury will not benefit from reconstruction by conventional one-stage tendon grafting techniques. The reasons for this are numerous and include the severity of the original trauma, that is, crushing injuries associated with underlying fracture or overlying skin damage, and failure of previous operations with excessive scarring of the tendon bed.[343-345,347-349] Occasionally, the retinacular pulley system may have been damaged either at the time of injury or through prior surgery. Joints restricted by contracture that are not responsive to therapy measures and injury to both digital nerves are also poor prognostic factors in flexor tendon reconstruction.[390] Patients with all or some of the problems just described, in whom conventional tendon grafting is not advocated, may undergo staged tendon reconstruction as an alternative method in an attempt to salvage useful finger function.

Many factors must be considered when determining the feasibility of two-stage tendon reconstruction. The patient should be helped to understand the complexity of the problem and be willing to undertake an arduous postoperative therapy program. The surgeon should decide whether it is justifiable to subject a severely damaged finger to two additional surgical procedures, and possibly a third (some of these patients will require tenolysis after the second stage). In some instances, arthrodesis or amputation may be a better alternative. It is wise to start the patient on a range-of-motion and scar-softening therapy program[266-268] to attain maximum preoperative passive range of motion. The surgeon is then afforded the opportunity to better evaluate the patient's willingness to actively participate in postoperative therapy. It is probable that patients with severe neurovascular impairment will at best make limited gains and should be rejected as candidates for staged reconstruction.[182,194]

Historical Review

In 1965, Hunter[161] first published his personal experience with tendon implants and, in 1971, with Salisbury[180] presented more than 10 years' experience with this technique in which severely damaged flexor tendons were excised and the system rebuilt around a silicone/Dacron–reinforced implant. This work was based on earlier studies of artificial tendon and tendon implants by Bassett and Carroll.[25] With Hunter's technique the implant was attached only at its distal end and left free proximally in the distal forearm. The proximal end of the implant was placed in the distal end of the forearm because of the many patients having severe scarring involving the palm as well as the digit. The proximal juncture thereby bypasses the scarred palm and is placed in an area relatively favorable for tendon juncture. During wound healing, a passive exercise program was used to mobilize the finger before the second stage proceeded. In response to the implant, a smooth, well-organized pseudo-sheath was formed, creating order in what was previously a chaotic tendon bed.

The second stage is usually performed approximately 3 months after the first when the implant is replaced with a long tendon graft. Of paramount concern in this second operation is to disturb the newly formed sheath as little as possible. Many authors have written about their tendon reconstruction experience in which a silicone rubber implant is placed at the first stage.*

Other researchers have investigated alternate techniques to reconstructing the damaged flexor tendon system.† An interesting approach to the problem of severe tendon injuries was published by Paneva-Holevich in 1969.[330] In this staged technique, the proximal cut end of the FDS is sutured to the proximal cut end of the FDP tendon in the palm. This will become the proximal juncture. At the second stage the FDS is used as a pedicle graft by severing it as far proximal as possible and bringing this end out to be inserted at the distal phalanx. This technique has been combined with implantation of a silicone prosthesis during the first stage to prepare a bed for the subsequent distal pedicle transfer.[5,54,77,79,212,312a]

---

*See references 4, 9, 34, 48, 65, 74, 123a, 126, 149, 157, 162, 163, 165, 168, 181, 235, 238, 318, 376, 378, 386, 388-390, 402, 467, 492, 496, and 499.

†See references 196, 197, 258, 259, 310, 350, 417, 421, 489, and 521a.

One elegant technique devised was the use of a homograft consisting of the entire flexor system, tendon, and supportive structures transplanted into a damaged finger. This procedure, published by Peacock,[332] showed that such grafts were well tolerated. Hueston and colleagues[159] also presented an encouraging series of cases using homografts, but because of difficulty in obtaining these grafts, widespread use of this technique did not follow. In 1974 Chacha[72] used autologous composite grafts from the toe to the flexor system of the hand with only modest results. More recently, Asencio and associates[16] implanted human composite flexor tendon allografts into two fingers with irreparable injuries of the flexor tendon system.

Permanent (active) tendon implants varying in size, shape, material, as well as the type of end device for distal and proximal fixation have been reported in the literature.[161] Rigid, permanent bonding between the tendon implant distally to bone and proximally to native tendon has not been reliably achieved. At the present time, although the search for a permanent active tendon implant continues, it cannot be recommended.*

Technique: Stage I

The flexor system of the involved finger is exposed through the volar zigzag approach and continued to the lumbrical origin level in the palm. Previous scars can be partially used, when feasible, by combining them with the modified Bruner[55] incision. If a midlateral incision was previously used, it can be revisited or ignored and the volar approach utilized. All potential pulley material, injured or uninjured, is preserved. The flexor tendons are then excised, with a 1-cm length stump of FDP left attached to the distal phalanx. If an FDS tail can be preserved, it is left attached to the middle phalanx. Excised tendon material is set aside in moist sponges for possible use in pulley reconstruction. The proximal FDP is transected at the lumbrical origin level; and if the lumbrical is scarred, it is also excised. As much as possible of the original flexor retinaculum is preserved. If joint flexion deformities are not corrected by excision of the injured tendons, volar plate and accessory collateral ligament release are performed at this time. A second curvilinear incision is made proximal to the wrist crease in the ulnar half of the volar aspect of the forearm. The involved FDS tendon is identified, drawn into the wound, and transected near the musculotendinous junction.

A trial set of silicone tendon implants is useful here to determine the appropriate size needed. The adult man generally can accommodate a 5- or 6-mm tendon implant, but I usually use a smaller 4-mm implant. This is closer in size to the expected tendon graft and will hopefully create a more snugly fitting tendon sheath. The implant, once threaded into the pulley system, should glide freely. At this point the integrity of the pulley system is assessed. A minimal requirement is the presence of A2 and A4 pulleys at the proximal and middle phalangeal levels, respectively. However, some evidence suggests superiority of a four-pulley system. The pulleys must be strong[37] and snug but not binding so that

*See references 21, 89, 138, 161, 162, 166-168, 172-175, 181, 186-188, 199, 213, 351, 379, and 381.

passive gliding of the implant is possible. Pulley reconstruction options are discussed on page 269.

The implant is removed from its sterile package, and care is taken only to handle the implant with smooth forceps so as not to damage the surface. Handling with gloves will lead to talc adhering to the implant and increase the likelihood of an inflammatory reaction. The implant is passed with a tendon passer from the proximal region of the palm to the distal end of the forearm in the plane between the FDP and FDS.[236,414,428] A finger placed in the distal forearm wound, proximally in the muscle plane, ensures a space for migration of the proximal end of the implant during passive exercise after stage I. The distal juncture is now carried out.[162,180] A 3-0 polyester suture is used in a figure-of-eight stitch, and the implant is fixed beneath the FDP stump (Fig. 7-36). Two sutures that go through the stump, local periosteum, and the implant reinforce this construct. The surgeon must be certain that these added sutures catch the Dacron tape within the silicone rubber because the sutures will have little holding power in the rubber alone.

Traction is then exerted on the proximal end of the implant to ensure free passage under the pulleys and to observe the potential range of motion (Fig. 7-37). If the tendon bowstrings such that lost range of motion is observable, tighter or additional pulleys must be constructed at this time (Fig. 7-38). If any portion of the salvaged retinacular system is too tight, it is gently stretched with a curved hemostat or removed and this area reconstructed. The implant must glide freely without buckling when the finger is flexed passively. Tendon implant length is determined so that in an extended hand position the proximal end lies in the distal forearm and does not buckle with passive finger flexion. This usually requires trimming 3 to 5 cm of the implant. The proximal implant is left free to glide and is never sutured to surrounding tissue.

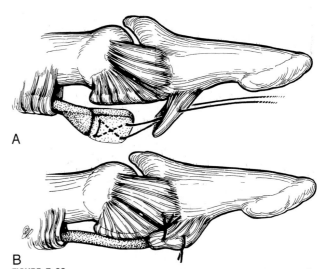

FIGURE 7-36. Stage I flexor reconstruction. In the distal juncture wire suture technique a figure-of-eight suture of 3-0 Prolene is placed in the implant and sutured to the profundus stump. Additional sutures are placed on each side of the implant. (After Hunter JM, Salisbury RE: Use of gliding artificial implants to produce tendon sheaths: Techniques and results in children. Plast Reconstr Surg 45:564-572, 1970.)

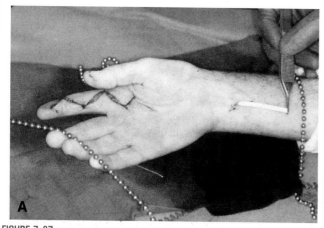 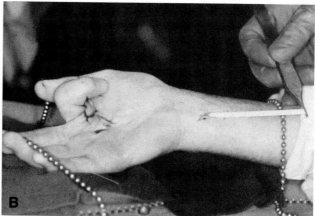

FIGURE 7-37. **A** and **B,** The potential of the planned graft is tested by pulling the implant proximally. Bowstringing of the implant indicates the need for pulley reconstruction.

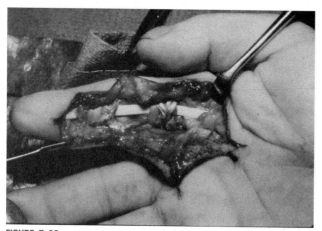

FIGURE 7-38. At the time of the implant placement deficiencies in the pulley system are addressed by reconstruction of the A2 and A4 pulleys.

Postoperative Care: Stage I

After wound closure, a bulky dressing is applied with a posterior plaster splint maintaining the wrist in about 35 degrees of flexion. This ensures more proximal placement of the implant, which in turn creates a longer proximal extension of the sheath, giving the implant more room to move without buckling during the passive range-of-motion program between stages I and II. The splint should extend past the fingertips with the MCP joints kept in 60 to 70 degrees of flexion and the IP joints relaxed in the extended position.

Passive motion is started on the first postoperative visit 2 to 3 days after surgery.[66] Patients are taught passive range-of-motion exercises, including the use of trapping with adjacent normal fingers to regain mobilization in the operated finger. Concomitant nerve repair at stage I may delay the onset of mobilization.[268] Patients having contracture releases may benefit from the addition of dynamic splinting.

Time Interval Between Stage I and Stage II

The appropriate interval between stages I and II is the time needed for wound healing and the development of a gliding sheath formed in response to the implant. The joints are mobilized in an effort to regain full passive mobility. Lateral flexion and extension radiographs will demonstrate the implant excursion after passive range of motion is restored and reveal whether buckling, which is associated with synovitis, impedes smooth implant movement. The time interval allowed is generally 3 months. Occasionally, conditions allow or demand an earlier stage II and treatment of each patient is individualized after assessing the condition of the hand. Generally, at 3 months the hand is soft, the joints are well mobilized, and the patient is ready for stage II. A case report details a successful stage II procedure done 18 years after stage I.[521]

CRITICAL POINTS: TWO-STAGE FLEXOR TENDON RECONSTRUCTION: STAGE I

INDICATIONS

- Crushing injuries associated with underlying fracture or overlying skin damage
- Failure of previous operations
- Excessive scarring of the tendon bed
- Damaged pulley system
- Contracted joints

PREOPERATIVE EVALUATION

- Patient must understand necessity of arduous postoperative therapy program.
- Arthrodesis or amputation may be a better alternative.

PEARLS

- A range-of-motion and scar-softening therapy program is important to attain maximum preoperative passive range of motion and to evaluate willingness to participate in postoperative therapy.

CRITICAL POINTS: TWO-STAGE FLEXOR TENDON RECONSTRUCTION: STAGE I— cont'd

TECHNICAL POINTS

- Preserve potential pulley material, injured or uninjured.
- Excise flexor tendons leaving 1-cm FDP stump.
- Transect the proximal FDP at the level of the lumbrical origin.
- Correct joint flexion deformities.
- Make second incision in the distal forearm.
- Identify the involved FDS tendon, draw it into the wound, and transect it near the musculotendinous junction.
- Determine the appropriate size of silicone implant.
- Assess the integrity of pulley system. Need at least A2 and A4 pulleys.
- Pass the implant from the proximal palm to the distal forearm between FDP and FDS.
- Fix the implant beneath the FDP stump.
- Exert traction on the proximal end of implant to observe potential range of motion.
- If implant bowstrings, then reconstruct needed pulleys.

PITFALLS

- Ensure that tendon implant does not buckle with passive flexion.
- Severe neurovascular impairment will limit result; these patients are poor candidates.

POSTOPERATIVE CARE

- Apply splint with wrist in 35 degrees of flexion, MCP joints at 60 to 70 degrees of flexion, and IP joints extended.
- Start passive motion on first postoperative visit.
- Remember that contracture releases may benefit from dynamic splinting (6 to 8 weeks).

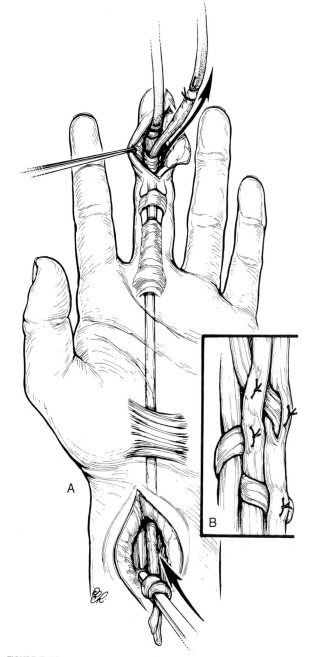

FIGURE 7-39. Stage II flexor reconstruction. **A,** The distal portion of the finger wound and the distal forearm wound are opened, and both ends of the implant are located. The tendon graft is now sutured to the proximal end of the implant and drawn into the newly created sheath. **B,** The proximal juncture is either an interweave of the graft into the adjacent FDP motor in the case of the long, ring, and little fingers or an interlace into the FDP of the index finger. (See Fig. 7-25 for the Pulvertaft end weave technique.) (After Hunter JM, Salisbury RE: Use of gliding artificial implants to produce tendon sheaths: Techniques and results in children. Plast Reconstr Surg 45:564-572, 1970.)

Technique: Stage II

The distal portion of the finger incision is opened to about the middle of the middle phalanx (Fig. 7-39). The implant is located at its attachment to the FDP stump. Care is taken to not injure the most distal pulley over the middle phalanx. The proximal incision is then reopened in the distal end of the forearm. The forearm fascia is excised to visualize the sheath, which is ideally soft, thin, and translucent. The sheath is incised, and the proximal implant is exposed. The motor is selected, most commonly the profundus mass to the long, ring, and little fingers. For index finger reconstruction, the FDP to the index finger is chosen. The superficialis muscle can be used if the FDP is unsuitable.[389] The wounds are then packed and the tourniquet is deflated while a tendon graft is obtained (see page 263). If the proximal juncture is to be in the forearm, the palmaris longus is not long enough and either the plantaris or a toe extensor must be used (I prefer the plantaris).

After hemostasis is achieved, the tourniquet is reinflated and the graft is pulled into the flexor system by suturing it to the proximal end of the implant and pulling it through the sheath (Figs. 7-39A and 7-40). The implant is then discarded. The distal juncture is created with a technique based on the presence or absence of the FDP stump (see page 248). The finger wound is closed.

Attention is now directed to the proximal juncture. The graft is woven into the motor tendon or tendons (see Fig. 7-39B). When only one motor is used, an end-weave technique is advised (see Fig. 7-25). In instances in which the profundus mass of long, ring, and little fingers is chosen as a common motor, an interweave juncture (see Fig. 7-39B) is created to the common origin of these tendons. Excess sheath is resected so as to allow the juncture to pass distally when the fingers are extended. The need for this will be recognized when the fingers are passively extended and the distal juncture abuts against the proximal sheath.

In the majority of cases, the proximal juncture is placed in the forearm, which is a favorable environment for tendon gliding. In the less common instance in which the palm is not involved in the trauma or in prior surgery, a shorter graft can be used, motored by the FDP tendon at the lumbrical origin.[374] The option of using an adjacent FDS as a motor is also available within the palm if the FDP is not deemed adequate. Proper tension on the graft is essential for success,

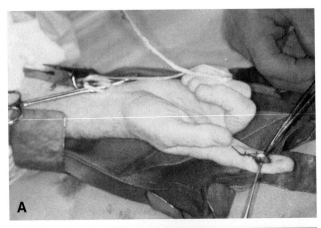

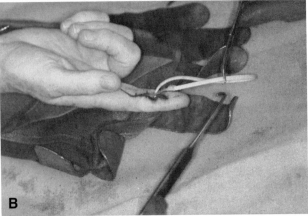

FIGURE 7-40. **A,** Stage II. The tendon graft is secured to the proximal end of the implant. **B,** The implant is removed from the distal incision, pulling the graft into place. The graft is then sutured distally and proximally.

and therefore stage II is ideally done under neuroleptanesthesia (see Chapter 2). With completion of the proximal juncture, wound closure is accomplished. A short-arm dorsal blocking splint is applied, with the wrist kept neutral, the MCP joints in 45 degrees of flexion, and the IP joints neutral.

Postoperative Care: Stage II

Postoperatively, these patients are managed with protected passive range of motion and an early controlled-motion program.[169,266,429] At 2 weeks after surgery, short-arc active extension/flexion and place/hold flexion exercises can be added to the therapy program. Resistance is added to the exercise regimen at 4 to 6 weeks after surgery based on the strength of the repair and the degree of adhesion formation. Dynamic splinting may also be employed at 6 to 8 weeks to combat joint contracture. Therapy must be more aggressive, with active and resisted exercises being instituted earlier in cases where tendon adhesion is observed. Therapy should be carried out in a formal setting where patient education can be reinforced on a regular basis.

If the patient demonstrates less than full cooperation, the hand may be immobilized for 2 to 4 weeks and the mobilization program started after that time. This would include active and passive range-of-motion exercises at 3 weeks with blocking added at 4 weeks. The program is then continued as in the early-mobilization program described previously.

Tissue Response to Silicone Implant

The nature of the sheath formed by silicone and other materials has received much investigation.* Hunter's group, working in the late 1960s, observed an orderly pattern of cellular organization on the surface of the implant when silicone implants were placed in the paravertebral soft tissues of dogs.[189] This was not believed to be a foreign body reaction. A parallel study was designed to evaluate the response to an actively gliding implant in the extensor system of the dog.[190] Evidence was obtained that the system could function as a physiologic sheath capable of supporting a long tendon graft by fluid nutrition and with time through the formation of vascular, yet mobile adhesions. Conway and colleagues[87] and Urbaniak and associates[462] confirmed these findings. Urbaniak's experiments were carried out in the flexor system and actually demonstrated revascularization of the dog tendon by infratendinous vessels within the sheath. At 1 year he believed that these vessels appeared to be normal. In chicken experiments, Farkas and colleagues[116] reported a tissue response that on ultrastructural examination resembled a normal tendon sheath. Farkas agreed with Hunter that motion was most important for adhesion remodeling between the sheath and tendon grafts.

Electron microscopic studies of the silicone rubber–induced sheath in chickens by Salisbury and associates[378] and Takasugi and coworkers[448] showed that the pseudosheath closely resembled normal synovium with respect to

*See references 73, 113, 133, 135, 144, 150, 151, 176, 178, 230, 270, 293, 303, 308, 314, 368, 435, 438, 450, and 512.

CRITICAL POINTS: TWO-STAGE FLEXOR TENDON RECONSTRUCTION: STAGE II

INDICATION

- A patient who underwent stage I of the flexor reconstruction process

PREOPERATIVE EVALUATION

- Interval between stages I and II is approximately 3 months.
- Hand must be soft and joints well mobilized.

PEARLS

- The newly formed sheath is disturbed as little as possible.
- Proximal juncture is placed in the forearm (majority of cases): longer graft is needed (plantaris or toe extensor), motored by the FDP.
- Proximal juncture is placed in the palm (palm not involved in trauma): shorter graft can be used (palmaris), motored by the FDP at lumbrical origin.

TECHNICAL POINTS

- Open distal portion of finger incision to middle of middle phalanx.
- Locate implant at its attachment to profundus stump.
- Reopen proximal incision in the distal forearm.
- Excise forearm fascia and incise sheath.
- Select motor.
- Obtain tendon graft.
- Suture graft to proximal end of implant and pull it distally through sheath.
- Fix distal juncture.
- Create proximal juncture.

PITFALLS

- Proper tension on the graft is essential for success.

POSTOPERATIVE CARE

- Apply short-arm dorsal blocking splint (wrist neutral, MCP joints at 45 degrees, and IP joints neutral).
- Begin therapy in a formal setting.
- Start protected passive range-of-motion and early controlled-motion program.
- Use dynamic splinting for contractures.

---

architecture and biologic properties. In 1976 Rayner[365] pointed out that histologic appearances are deceiving and that the lining of the induced sheath did not fulfill the criteria of normal synovium. He believed that the cell lining is not mesothelial but fibroblastic, although it could secrete a synovial-like fluid. He conceded that this fluid might be helpful in providing nutrition to second-stage tendon grafts, particularly in the first 4 to 5 weeks before blood vessel invasion and adhesion formation. Rayner's studies suggested that grafts should not be done too early, when the fibroblastic potential and vascularity of the sheath are at their highest level of activity. He recommended a delay of 3 to 4 months to wait for the most favorable conditions for grafting.

Eiken and his group concurred with Rayner that the pseudosheath produced in response to silicone rod implantation consisted mainly of connective tissue, which they expected would contract like scar tissue.[106,107] They believed that the rubber induced a foreign body–type reaction in the healing flexor system.[104,108] Although this questioned earlier findings,[87,180,314,462] they agreed that implantation of the material in the muscle[151,365] rather than in synovial systems was not a fair test of the implant's sheath-inducing potential. Placing grafts of synovium about the tendon implant in chickens may improve sheath quality,[104] they reasoned, and success here has prompted them to study this technique in 40 patients.[105] I concur with their conclusion that although silicone rubber is not perfect, it is the best material available for creating a tendon sheath at this time. Farkas and Lindsay[115] showed in experimental conditions in chickens that placing the newly formed sheath over the graft junctures at stage II led to significantly greater flexion recovery.

In summary, the final work on the exact nature of the sheath created in response to a low-reactive, flexible implant used in a passive-gliding program in humans is still debated. Some of the varying observations may be a result of different species and experiment conditions. The presence of a soft, pliable, translucent sheath, seen with frequency in clinical cases and associated with an uncomplicated stage I, encourages us in using this technique in the salvage of severely damaged flexor systems.

THUMB FLEXOR TENDON RECONSTRUCTION

The flexor system of the thumb is considerably less complicated than that of the fingers. The thumb contains one fewer joint than the fingers and only one long flexor tendon is involved. When the long flexor of the thumb is reconstructed, a modest recovery of 30 to 40 degrees of active IP joint flexion may provide a thumb with excellent function. Despite some reluctance to reconstruct lesions in this area,[221] I have felt justified attempting to restore active range of motion at the IP joint.

Indication

Direct repair at all levels of injury may be possible as late as 3 to 6 weeks after injury and even later in cases in which the tendon ends have not widely separated.[11,249,299,312,461,464,468] Reconstructive procedures in flexor pollicis longus injuries are indicated when a satisfactory range of passive IP joint motion exists but the time interval for successful repair has been missed. This may occur for a number of reasons, such as the wound was deemed unfavorable at the time of injury or the significance of the injury was underestimated. In this situation, the surgeon has the following options to restore active thumb range of motion.

Thumb Free Tendon Graft

Free tendon grafting in the thumb has the same indications as was outlined for the fingers. In the case of flexor reconstruction of the thumb, the flexor pollicis longus or one of the superficialis muscles is used as a motor. It must be recognized again that proper tensioning of the graft is critical. Experience with distal laceration advancement has shown that advancement greater than 1 cm[271] will likely have the detrimental effect of creating an IP flexion deformity.

Technique

The same basic technique is used as has been described for free tendon grafting in the fingers.[136] The flexor system is approached through a volar zigzag incision[56] from the distal phalanx proximal to the MCP joint. Pulleys are preserved with care, and the injured tendon is excised. A second incision is made in curvilinear fashion at the volar-radial aspect of the distal end of the forearm starting distally at the wrist crease and proceeding about 6 cm proximally. The musculotendinous junction of the flexor pollicis longus is identified and the tendon is pulled into this incision. The palmaris longus or plantaris is obtained and threaded through the system with a tendon passer. The distal juncture is fashioned by means of a distal pullout suture technique discussed on page 248, and the thumb wound is closed. Interweaving the graft into the tendon of the flexor pollicis longus creates the proximal juncture. Tension in this system is critical. This is estimated by placing the wrist in neutral position, the thumb palmar abducted in front of the index finger metacarpal, and the IP joint of the thumb in 30 degrees of flexion. With tension set at the proximal juncture, the thumb should adopt this position.

After wound closure and dressing, a dorsal splint is applied with the wrist in neutral to 5 degrees of flexion and the thumb protected in about 30 degrees of abduction at the carpometacarpal (CMC) joint. The MCP and IP joints are positioned in 20 to 30 degrees of flexion in the dorsal splint. In my protocol, the patient is instructed to fully flex the thumb passively then fully extend to the limits of the splint for the first 2 weeks postoperatively. Active flexion and extension exercise is added at 2 weeks, with the protective splint reapplied between exercise sessions. At 6 weeks the pullout suture is removed, and more strenuous activities, including blocking techniques, are allowed.

FDS Transfer

An alternative method to tendon grafting, particularly indicated when the flexor pollicis longus muscle is not useful, is utilization of the FDS of the ring finger as both motor and tendon.[342,410]

Technique

The zigzag volar approach to the flexor system of the thumb is used along with a second, curved vertical incision in the distal region of the forearm (Fig. 7-41). The injured tendon is removed with preservation of as much uninjured pulley system as possible. A transverse incision is made at the base of the ring finger, and the FDS is identified and transected about 2 cm proximal to the PIP joint after a suture has been placed in one of the tails. The tendon is then located in the forearm wound and withdrawn into the wound. At times this may be difficult because of synovial interconnections, in which case a second incision in the palm is needed to free these connections. Tagging of the distal end of the FDS tendon with a suture facilitates necessary manipulation to mobilize the donor tendon. With the tendon now in the forearm wound, it can be redirected into the thumb flexor system and a distal juncture carried out as in a free tendon graft. Critical tension is more difficult to establish at the distal juncture, especially if the Bunnell tendon-to-bone technique is planned. For this reason, one of the other techniques that more easily allows readjustment is preferable. In this situation, I prefer the interweave tendon weaving technique described previously. The repair is fixed with one suture, and tension is evaluated before completion of the juncture. The follow-up splint period for 3 to 4 weeks postoperatively is similar to that used in free tendon grafting. Mobilization of the transfer by combining active ring finger flexion with thumb flexion is helpful for patients learning to use the transfer.

Staged Tendon Reconstruction in the Thumb

In patients in whom it is imperative to restore active thumb flexion and in whom prior surgery has failed or there is a severely scarred tendon bed, staged flexor tendon reconstruction offers an opportunity to salvage thumb function. This approach becomes even more of a necessity when the retinacular pulley system has been destroyed. Pulley reconstruction over the implant at the level of the proximal half of the proximal phalanx will usually suffice if the oblique pulley has been destroyed.

Technique

Details of the technique are similar to that in the fingers (see page 255). In the thumb the surgeon can use either a free graft or an FDS transfer at stage II.[410]

Other Options in Flexor Pollicis Longus Disruption

In patients who have lost flexor pollicis longus function but have a stable distal joint, it may be acceptable to do nothing if the time period for direct repair has passed, especially if the CMC and MCP joints are functioning normally. This is certainly reasonable in the aged. When strong pinch is required, especially in the presence of intra-articular damage at the IP joint or in patients with a hyperextensile IP joint, arthrodesis is an acceptable alternative.

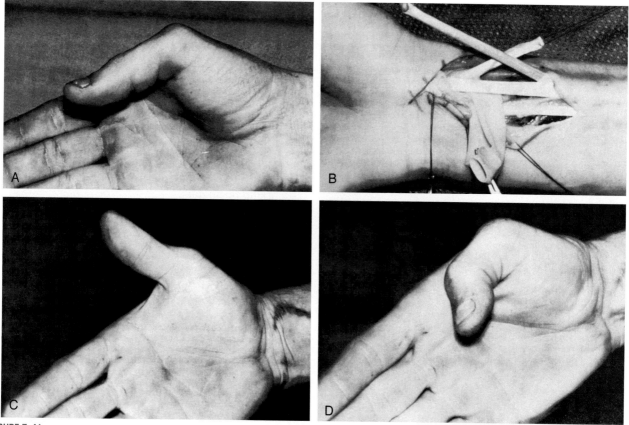

FIGURE 7-41. Flexor pollicis longus reconstruction using the FDS from the ring finger. **A,** Loss of active flexion at the IP joint of the right thumb in a 28-year-old machinist with an old zone V laceration. **B,** The distal flexor pollicis longus stump is obtained and the flexor superficialis brought over into the same wound. An interlace juncture is used. **C** and **D,** Range of extension and flexion after 6 months. The FDS is long enough to use for any level of laceration of the flexor pollicis longus, even out at the insertion.

CRITICAL POINTS: THUMB FLEXOR TENDON RECONSTRUCTION

INDICATIONS

- Repair of flexor pollicis longus is delayed or significant trauma does not allow repair.
- There is satisfactory preoperative range of passive IP joint motion.

PREOPERATIVE EVALUATION

- Free tendon graft: similar indications as for fingers.
- Superficialis transfer: alternative to free tendon graft.
- Two-stage tendon reconstruction: severely scarred tendon bed and/or destroyed pulley system.
- IP arthrodesis: when strong pinch is required, especially in the presence of intra-articular damage at the IP joint or in patients with a hyperextensile IP joint.

PEARLS

- Recovery of 30 to 40 degrees active IP joint flexion may provide well-functioning thumb.

- Tension is critical.
- Tension is estimated by placing the wrist in neutral, thumb in palmar abduction in front of index metacarpal, and IP joint in 30 degrees of flexion.
- Pulley reconstruction over the implant at the level of the proximal half of the proximal phalanx will usually suffice if the oblique pulley has been destroyed.

TECHNICAL POINTS

Free Tendon Graft

- Preserve the pulleys.
- Make a second incision in the distal forearm.
- Identify the musculotendinous junction of the flexor pollicis longus.
- Obtain the graft obtained and thread it through the pulley system.
- Fashion the distal juncture by means of a distal pullout suture technique.
- Interweave the graft into the tendon of the flexor pollicis longus to create the proximal juncture.

Continued

CRITICAL POINTS: THUMB FLEXOR TENDON RECONSTRUCTION—cont'd

Superficialis Transfer

- Use zigzag volar approach to thumb.
- Make longitudinal incision in the distal forearm.
- Remove injured tendon with preservation of uninjured pulley system.
- Make transverse incision at base of ring finger.
- Transect FDS 2 cm proximal to the PIP joint.
- Withdraw tendon into the proximal wound.
- Create distal juncture as in free tendon graft.

PITFALLS

- Proper tension is difficult to create with FDS transfer.

POSTOPERATIVE CARE

- Apply dorsal splint with wrist neutral, thumb in 30 degrees of abduction at CMC, and MCP and IP joints in 20 to 30 degrees of flexion.
- Limit passive flexion and active extension by splint for first 2 weeks.
- Begin active flexion and extension at 2 weeks.
- At 6 weeks, remove pullout suture and begin blocking techniques.

SECONDARY RECONSTRUCTION OF TENDON INJURIES IN ZONES III, IV, AND V

Indications

When flexor tendons are injured in the palm, wrist, carpal tunnel, or distal end of the forearm, direct repair at an early date is desirable. When primary repair fails, secondary reconstruction carries a more favorable prognosis for these more proximal levels than zone II injuries.[478] Impairment from injuries is usually more a function of concomitant nerve injury than flexor tendon dysfunction. Before secondary tendon surgery, the wounds should be well healed and the hand soft and fully mobile. Generous longitudinal, curvilinear incisions are needed to correctly identify and repair the injured structures. The operation is technically easier to do through ample exposure, and the likelihood of additional damage is lessened if all structures are first identified proximally and distally in unscarred areas of normal anatomy and then followed into the area of injury. If synovial connections and adhesions have prevented proximal migration of the tendons, direct end-to-end repairs can be performed. When the tendons cannot be brought together without undue tension, three techniques have proved useful for zones III, IV, and V.

Interposition Graft

When trying to reunite the FDP tendon ends in the palm or wrist after delay, the surgeon often finds that a gap of 2 to 5 cm needs to be bridged to bring the tendons to normal functional length. A short tendon graft is carried out by estimating the length needed and obtaining the graft from a segment of the injured FDS or palmaris longus (Fig. 7-42).[430] A Bunnell crisscross suture is placed in the proximal motor end of the tendon with 3-0 polyester. The graft is threaded on straight needles, and the distal juncture is completed by another crisscross suture in the distal portion to snug up the suture until the appropriate resting posture of the finger is obtained. Proper tension is critical here,

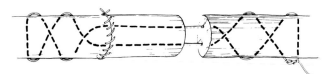

FIGURE 7-42. Interposition graft. By using short segments of available graft material, a gap can be closed in the late repair of zone III, IV, or V injuries.

and in the palm this procedure is often carried out under local anesthesia with active cooperation of the patient (neuroleptanesthesia) to determine the appropriate tension in the system.

FDS Transfer

The gap in the palm or wrist level can be overcome by an end-to-end transfer of an adjacent intact FDS tendon passed deep to the neurovascular bundle or median nerve into the distal segment of the injured tendon (Fig. 7-43).[292,408,409] Any of the techniques described for end-to-end tendon repair can be used. Again, tension is critical and the use of neuroleptanesthesia, if possible, is advocated.[183] In both of the aforementioned techniques, if a juncture is found to be under the proximal pulley when the finger is extended, thereby placing the repair in zone II, the proximal pulley (A1) can be sacrificed. This converts a zone II injury into a more favorable zone III problem. If this is possible, it is recommended over a palm-to-fingertip tendon graft.

End-to-Side FDP Juncture

Occasionally it is possible to attach the distal end of a severed FDP tendon to the side of an intact adjacent FDP,[369] which is best done with an interweave technique (Fig. 7-44). More useful in the zone V area (forearm), this technique should be used with care in the distal portion of zone III (palm) because the juncture could hang up on the A1 pulley in extension.

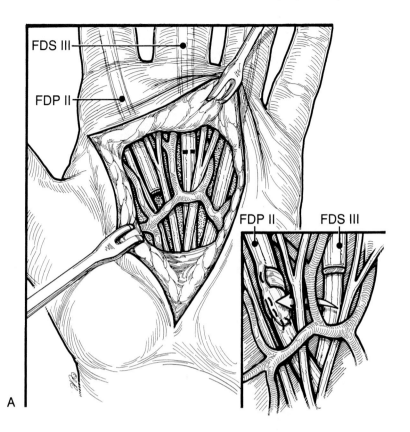

FIGURE 7-43. FDS transfer for FDP injures in another finger. **A,** Illustration of the technique.

Continued

Postoperative Care

A short-arm posterior molded plaster splint is applied from the fingertips to below the elbow. The wrist is maintained in neutral, the MCP joints in 40 to 50 degrees of flexion, and the IP joints in neutral. A program of controlled active range of motion (passive flexion followed by active extension to the limits of the dorsal splint) and protected passive range of motion is begun in a formal therapy setting at the first postoperative visit. Flexion contractures can develop rapidly if full extension at the PIP joint is not achieved early. The patient should be followed closely for development of contractures so that adjustments can be made to the splint and therapy regimen. Active range of motion is introduced at 2 weeks after surgery. Splint protection is discontinued at 4 weeks. Resisted exercise and blocking techniques at each of the IP joints are allowed 4 to 5 weeks after the repair.[66,82]

OBTAINING TENDON GRAFTS

Selection of Graft

The most popular tendon grafts are the palmaris for palm-to-fingertip reconstruction and the plantaris for forearm-to-fingertip reconstruction.[86,207,296,418,419] Other sources of graft material are the long extensors of the three middle toes,[400,505,506] the toe flexors, the extensor indicis proprius, and the extensor digiti minimi.[425] The selection of a graft in any particular instance is determined by its presence and then by the particular demands of the surgical procedure. The use of intrasynovial toe flexor grafts has been investigated by Noguchi and colleagues[319d] and Ark and

associates.[11a] These grafts have demonstrated healing with fewer adhesions in animal models when compared with extrasynovial grafts, but their clinical superiority has not been demonstrated to date. As experience is gained with toe flexor grafts, they may supplant others as the donor graft of choice.

Palmaris Tendon

As a general rule, I prefer the palmaris longus for use in the palm-to-fingertip graft because it is in the same field of surgery and is easily accessible.[311,453] The presence of the palmaris longus is easily determined during preoperative examination. The patient is asked to oppose the thumb to the little finger while flexing the wrist against resistance. The palmaris longus tendon should be readily visible, superficial, and palpable in the midline of the wrist. This tendon is present in 75% to 85% of people.[367,493]

Technique of Palmaris Longus Harvest

A 1- to 2-cm transverse incision is made at the wrist, and the palmaris longus is identified. Care is taken to identify and protect the nearby median nerve during palmaris harvest. After transection at the wrist crease, the distal end of the graft is held with a 4-0 suture or Kocher clamp. The tendon is then mobilized, under direct vision, for 6 to 8 cm and threaded through a circular tendon stripper (Fig. 7-45). With firm, gentle tension held on the graft at its distal end with a clamp, the stripper is slowly advanced with a slight twisting motion. As the stripper advances into the proximal region of the forearm, the muscle belly will fill the circular cutting blade and be divided; this allows the tendon to be withdrawn

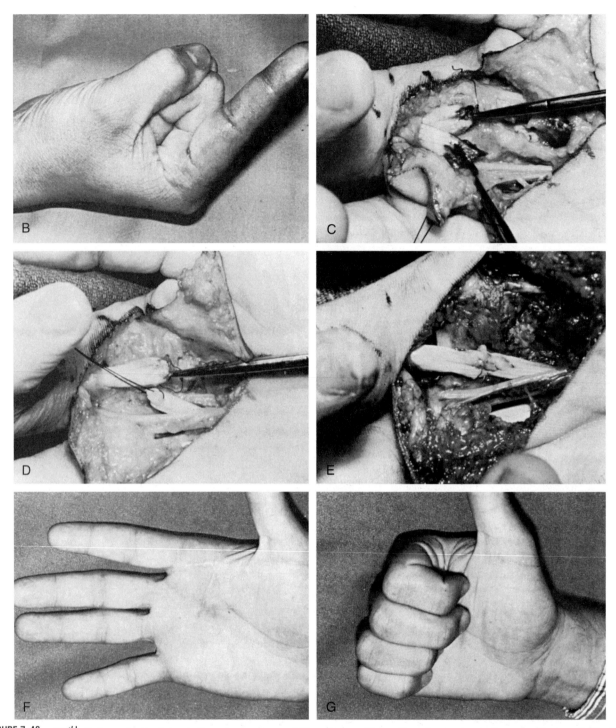

FIGURE 7-43—cont'd. B, Long-standing injury to flexor tendons in zone III in a 20-year-old man. There is no active motion at the IP joints. **C,** The distal tendon stumps have been recovered at the A1 pulley level. There is good distal pull-through of the tendons within the retinacular system. **D,** The superficialis tendon of the long finger is transected and brought over to the profundus of the index finger. **E,** An end-to-end juncture has been created. **F** and **G,** Extension and flexion at 6 months postoperatively.

through one incision. At times a second proximal incision is made over the stripper in the proximal forearm if undue resistance to the stripper is experienced. I prefer this method, but if the appropriate stripper is not available, the tendon can be removed by using a No. 11 knife blade to sever the tendon proximally through a small stab wound at the musculotendinous level as advocated by Saeed and Kay.[375]

Plantaris Tendon

When multiple grafts are needed or one long distal forearm-to-fingertip graft is required, it is necessary to harvest the lower extremity for tendons longer than the palmaris. The presence of the plantaris tendon cannot be predicted preoperatively, and although it is said to be absent in only 7%

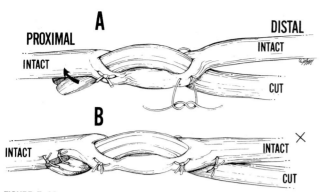

FIGURE 7-44. End-to-side interweave suture technique useful in zone V injuries.

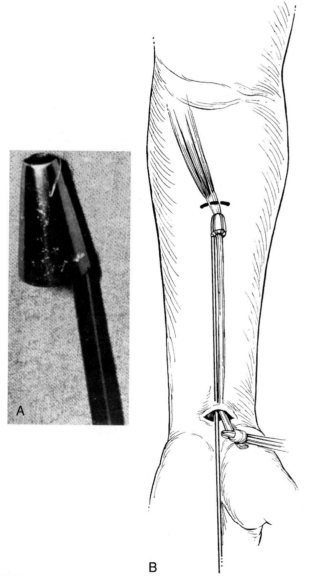

FIGURE 7-45. Palmaris longus graft. My preferred technique for obtaining the graft uses a tendon stripper, which is a circular knife passed along the surface of the tendon. **A,** The stripper. **B,** The stripper is advanced until it cuts off the graft at the muscle belly, or a second proximal incision can be used to obtain the proximal end of the tendon graft.

of cadavers,[92] my experience suggests that it is absent far more frequently. This has been verified by Harvey and associates,[148] who found that the tendon was present in about 80% of limbs. This 80% figure was confirmed by Wehbe.[493] It is also unusable at times because of variations in its girth or by virtue of attachments to the triceps surae, which make its removal in one length impossible. However, at its best, the plantaris is an excellent graft and can supply two and occasionally three palm-to-fingertip grafts or one long distal forearm-to-fingertip graft.

Technique of Plantaris Tendon Harvest

A 5-cm vertical incision is made just anterior to the medial aspect of the Achilles tendon, starting at the insertion and proceeding proximally.[49,505] The tendon is bluntly dissected anterior to the Achilles tendon and divided near its insertion (Fig. 7-46). With a holding suture securely fixed in its cut end, the tendon is mobilized as far as possible under direct vision. This gives the tubular stripper through which the tendon is threaded a straight course up the leg. The stripper should be held parallel to the leg and advanced with a wiggling motion while the tendon graft is held under tension. The knee should be extended. When the belly of the plantaris muscle fills the stripper, the muscle is divided to allow the entire plantaris tendon to be withdrawn from the wound. Care must be taken to keep the stripper parallel to the long axis of the tendon or the tendon may be severed prematurely. As a compartment syndrome after plantaris harvest has been reported, it is recommended that the calf be palpated at the conclusion of the procedure to assess for excessive tension.[449a]

Long-Toe Extensor

The long-toe extensors can provide excellent grafts. Their presence is never in doubt and their diameter is adequate for most needs. As many as three long tendon grafts are available when the tendons to the second, third, and fourth toes are harvested. A frequent problem is that the individual tendons may fuse distal to the ankle and three long grafts may be unobtainable. Although some advise its removal through a large longitudinal incision,[506] I believe that wound morbidity is reduced by using a tendon stripper and multiple transverse incisions.

Technique of Long-Toe Extensor Harvest

A generous transverse incision is made on the dorsum of the foot at the level of the metatarsophalangeal joint (Fig. 7-47). The long-toe extensor is isolated proximal to the hood and prepared for the stripper by placing a holding suture in the tendon and transecting it. After mobilization, a small stripper is advanced proximally but stopped when resistance is encountered. A second transverse incision is made at this level, and the cause of obstruction is checked under direct vision. Further direct dissection can be carried out, the tendon withdrawn into this second wound, and the stripper again used. Distal to the ankle level the cruciate crural ligament encloses the tendons, and this must be opened. It is imperative to make as many transverse incisions as necessary to minimize premature transaction of the graft by forcing the stripper. From this point proximally, the tendon can be stripped up into the leg. In some cases all the long

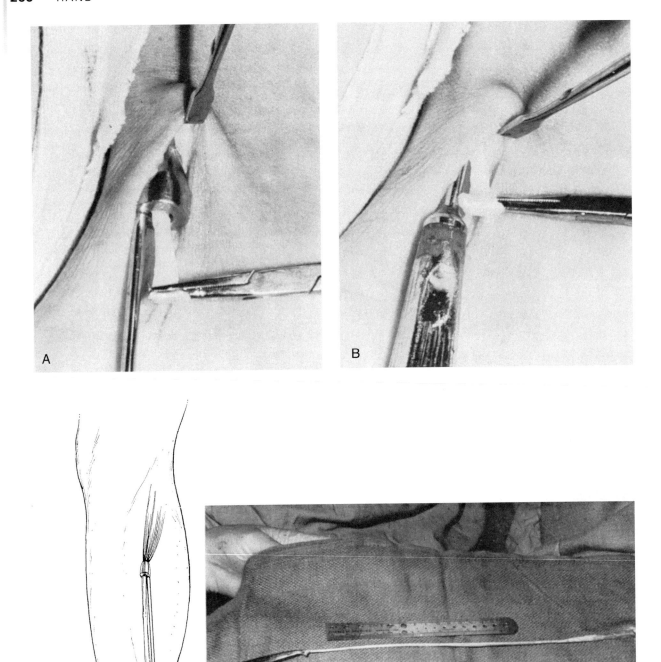

FIGURE 7-46. Plantaris graft. **A,** The tendon is located anterior and medial to the Achilles tendon. After division distally, it is passed through the circular stripper. **B,** The stripper is advanced up the leg. **C,** When the stripper engages the muscle belly, it divides it and the surgeon can withdraw the tendon. **D,** The plantaris graft can supply two fingertip-to-palm grafts.

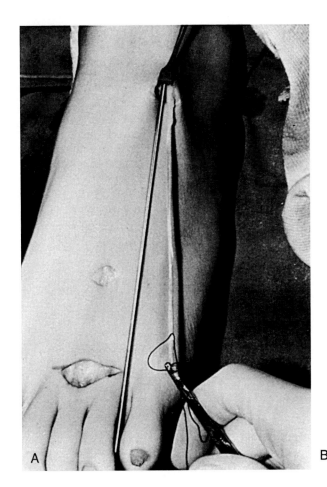

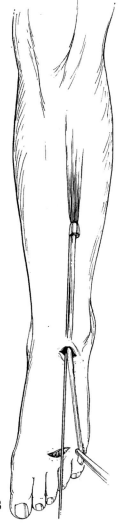

FIGURE 7-47. Long-toe extensors. These tendons are best obtained through multiple transverse incisions on the foot. **A,** Graft obtainable when the long-toe extensor is used. **B,** Once proximal to the ankle, the stripper can be advanced up the leg until the muscle is severed. More than the two incisions shown may be required.

extensors will have merged and thus make it impossible to obtain a high-quality long graft. When this problem is encountered, more and larger incisions are used and the tendons are actually dissected out individually. This, of course, compromises the graft because it will have some raw surfaces created by the dissection.

Extensor Proprius Tendons

The two proprius tendons (extensor indicis proprius and extensor digiti minimi) are available for grafting material. Although each can provide sufficient length for one palm-to-fingertip graft, I rarely use these sources.

Technique of Extensor Indicis Proprius Tendon Harvest

The tendon is exposed through a transverse incision over the MCP joint of either the index or little finger. The extensor indicis proprius tendon lies ulnar to the corresponding extensor digitorum communis tendon and is transected about 1 cm proximal to the hood after a holding suture is placed in the tendon end. The tendon is then mobilized subcutaneously, and a second incision is made over the musculotendinous junction proximal to the wrist. The tendon can usually be pulled into the second wound and transected. If the tendon does not withdraw easily, a third incision halfway between the first and second may be necessary. Synovial connections can be freed under direct vision through this incision. In the case of the proprius extensor to the little finger, usually represented by two tendon slips, Snow recommended taking only the ulnar half as a graft.[425]

Toe Flexors

Recent experiments on intrasynovial toe flexors have shown that these grafts heal with fewer restrictive adhesions than extrasynovial grafts.[1,130,319b,319c,412,412a] The long flexors of the second to fifth toes can be sacrificed with minimal morbidity, and their clinical application has been demonstrated in a small series.[238a]

Technique of Toe Flexor Harvest

The toe flexor is first identified at the base of the toe through a small transverse incision. If only one tendon is required I use the second toe flexor. Next a 6-cm longitudinal incision is curved over the non–weight-bearing portion of the mid foot. The selected tendon is identified and carefully dissected from the coalescence of the toe flexors. Care must be

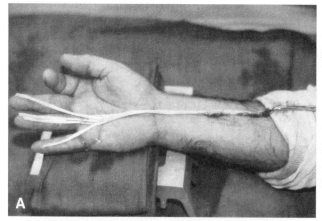

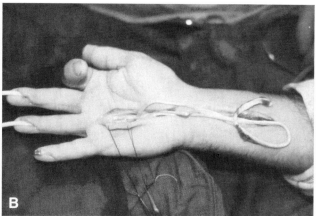

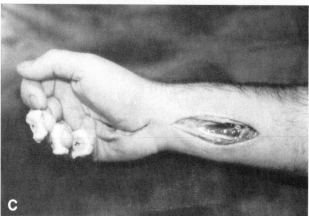

FIGURE 7-48. **A** to **C,** Toe flexor grafts. Multiple digits can be grafted using toe flexors, as illustrated by this case. The ulnar three digits were grafted using the entire long-toe flexor tendons after silicone implants. (Courtesy of David Zelouf, MD.)

taken not to injure the neurovascular structures traversing this region. Resection of the toe flexor from mid foot to toe is suitable for palm-to-fingertip grafts. The entire system of toe flexors can be harvested for grafting multiple digits, leaving the coalescence of the toe flexors intact. This requires more extensive dissection above the ankle (Fig. 7-48). The

tendon graft, once obtained, is handled with the utmost care.[387] It should be placed in a sponge moistened with saline or lactated Ringer's solution to protect it from drying. The graft must be protected from surface injury because careless handling is detrimental. Clamps or suture on each end can be used to facilitate handling of the graft.

CRITICAL POINTS: OBTAINING TENDON GRAFTS

INDICATIONS

- Need for tendon graft is noted during flexor tendon reconstruction.
- Selection of graft is determined by its presence and demands of procedure (primarily, the amount of length required).

PREOPERATIVE EVALUATION

- The presence of the palmaris longus is easily determined through opposition of thumb to little finger while flexing the wrist against resistance.
- Most popular sources: palmaris for palm-to-fingertip reconstruction, plantaris for forearm-to-fingertip reconstruction.
- Other graft options: long extensors of the three middle toes, toe flexors, extensor indicis proprius, and extensor digiti minimi.

PEARLS

- Intrasynovial grafts demonstrate fewer adhesions in animal models.

TECHNICAL POINTS

- Make transverse incision at wrist for palmaris harvest.
- Mobilize tendon under direct vision for 6 to 8 cm.
- Thread tendon through circular tendon stripper.
- If stripper is not available, use multiple incision method.

PITFALL

- Palmaris longus is present in only 75% to 85% of people.
- Plantaris is present in probably about 80%.

RECONSTRUCTION OF THE PULLEY SYSTEM

Successful reconstruction of the flexor tendon system is not only dependent on treatment of the tendon itself but must also involve the important structural aspects of the pulley system and the vincular blood supply.* The long flexor muscles have a maximum shortening capability and through their tendon connection to the fingers pull these into flexion. Because their excursion is constant, the pulley system is charged with maximizing the flexor tendon ability to generate joint flexion.[81,97,158,226,257] The uninjured pulleys prevent tendon translation across the volar aspect of the joint, thereby providing for the most efficient use of flexor tendon excursion. As pulleys are resected, the tendons are displaced volarly and the maximum range of active joint flexion is decreased. Bunnell[57] suggested that pulley loss results in the tendon traversing the shortest distance between two adjacent pulleys and termed this *bowstringing.* When significant, a decreased range of joint motion as well as a flexion deformity at the involved joint will follow.

The relative importance of the individual pulleys has been studied by Doyle and Blythe,[96-98] Hunter and colleagues,[170,171] and others.[51,100,241,243,383,427] They confirmed the work of Barton,[24] who stated that at least two pulleys (A2 and A4) need to be retained or reconstructed. Although this is agreed on, a paper by Savage[383] suggested that mechanically the A2 and A4 pulleys were not more important than the other pulleys, provided that the majority of the sheath was intact. Additionally, the importance of the synovial sheath proximal and distal to the A3 pulley has been shown.[448a] I agree that two pulleys may not be sufficient and realize that a three- or even four-pulley system should be reconstructed for optimal efficiency. Practically, however, because the reconstructive process may interfere with volar plate or collateral ligament function, pulleys should be created just distal to the MCP and PIP joints at the bases of the proximal and middle phalanges as a minimum requirement.[160]

Indications

Proper intraoperative assessment of pulley function during flexor tendon reconstruction is critical. If a one-stage tendon graft is planned, all uninjured pulley material is retained[104,107,180,383] to encourage flexor tendon healing within the uninjured sheath.[107,124,261,263,276,284,285,301] This is in contradistinction to the earlier teachings of Boyes,[39] Brand,[49] Littler,[254] Pulvertaft,[354] Rank and Wakefield,[362] and Tubiana,[459] who believed that only narrow critical bands should be left. If pulley material is absent because of injury or prior surgery, reconstruction must be carried out, at which time, a two-staged tendon reconstruction is recommended.[61,401] During a two-stage reconstruction, it may be acceptable to repair an injured pulley by suturing the ends over the implant. Damaged pulleys that are structurally intact are also useful in two-stage reconstruction because they will not adhere to the implant as they would to a tendon

graft. For this reason, all pulley material is saved at the first stage of the two-stage reconstruction. If a pulley is constricted, the tissue is dilated so that it can accept the implant.

Pulley Reconstruction Using Free Tendon Graft

When doing two-stage tendon reconstruction there is generally sufficient tendon material available to construct free tendon graft pulleys. Various techniques have been described for fixation of this material. Bunnell advocated encircling the phalanx with a free tendon graft.[15,61,267] In his original description,[61] the pulley graft was placed superficial to the extensor apparatus in the middle phalanx and deep to the extensor mechanism in the area of the proximal phalanx. I have found it preferable, however, to place the graft deep to the extensor at all levels (Fig. 7-49A). Although this type of pulley may be bulky, it does not seem to have an adverse effect on the extensor system. In a study by Lin and coworkers[241] it was reported that this type of reconstruction used in a triple loop around the proximal phalanx was very strong and in vitro approached the strength of a normal annulus.[241,323]

Another technique, as described by Kleinert and Bennett,[223] utilizes destroyed pulley remnants for graft fixation. The free graft is woven into the rim itself if this is deemed of adequate size. This method mandates that the graft material is thin and the remnant strong enough to hold the tendon material (see Fig. 7-49B). Doyle and Blythe[98] quoted Riordan as using a technique in which a hole is drilled completely through the bone, upon which the graft is passed and sutured to itself as a pulley. This weakens the phalanx, and the possibility of intraoperative or postoperative phalangeal fracture is of sufficient concern that I do not recommend this method.

Pulley Reconstruction Using FDS Insertion

The FDS tendon tail may be used as a pulley if it is long enough (see Fig. 7-49C). In this technique, its distal attachment is preserved and the free proximal end is sutured over the implant onto the contralateral side. It may be sutured to either periosteum or the original pulley rim or fastened via small holes drilled into bone. This makes an excellent pulley in the A3 area.

Pulley Reconstruction Using Extensor Retinaculum

Lister[250,251] described good results with a technique in which a segment of the extensor retinaculum from the dorsum of the wrist is passed around the phalanx for pulley reconstruction. The advantages of this technique are that (1) the undersurface of the retinaculum is an ideal gliding surface (the broad fourth dorsal compartment segment of the retinaculum is rotated into a position overlying the flexor tendon or silicone implant) and (2) the new pulley is strong enough to allow early motion (e.g., after tenolysis). The major disadvantage is that harvesting the 6- to 8-cm length of retinaculum is technically somewhat difficult and time consuming and also requires a separate incision. Tang and associates[449] used the sheath of the first dorsal compartment

---

*See references 6, 8, 18, 20, 50, 52, 57, 61, 67, 75, 80, 83, 86, 103, 121, 140, 228, 237, 240, 262, 275, 295, 307, 319a, 331, 333, 337, 339, 369a, 422, 437, 447, 453a, 487, 492, 522, and 523.

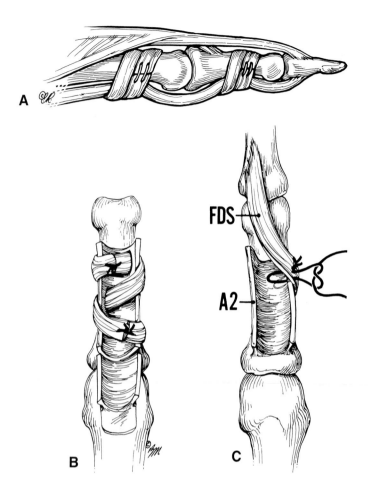

FIGURE 7-49. Methods of reconstruction of the pulley system. **A,** Free tendon graft pulleys encircling the phalanx deep to the extensor mechanism at the proximal and middle phalanges. **B,** A free tendon graft pulley can be constructed by suturing graft material to the rim of the destroyed pulley. This can take the form of an interweave into the rim; or, if the rim is inadequate, the graft can be sutured through drill holes in the bone (not shown). **C,** The tail of the FDS, when left attached to its insertion, can be sutured over the implant to the periosteum or to the rim of the original A2 pulley.

to reconstruct the digital sheath with good results when used in direct delayed tendon repairs.

Pulley Reconstruction Using the Volar Plate

A technique that creates slits in the volar plate for pulley reconstruction has been described by Karev.[209] Recent articles have suggested that this "belt-loop" technique is nearly as strong as a normal annular band[210,243] but does not attain normal joint motion.[241] An excellent comparison of different pulley reconstruction techniques was published by Widstrom and coworkers.[508,509] They showed that among six methods studied in cadaver limbs, mechanically the technique of Karev[210] was the most effective but an encircling technique was the strongest.

Pulley Reconstruction Using Artificial Materials

Artificial materials have been used in the reconstruction of pulleys.[338] These materials include knitted Dacron arterial graft,[518] silicone rubber sheeting,[22] xenograft materials,[76] polytetrafluoroethylene (PTFE),[99,206,413] woven nylon and fascia lata,[100,388] and porcine collagen and peritoneum.[322] Among these, the report by Manske and associates[99] seems most attractive in their application of PTFE. The use of artificial materials may become more pertinent in view of recent work suggesting that tendon grafts used in pulley reconstruction may degenerate and may weaken with time.[94]

However, the availability of tendon remnants that can be used as graft material for pulley reconstruction has allowed us to avoid artificial materials.

Technique of Pulley Reconstruction

I prefer creating a circumferential pulley using the method of Bunnell. Either flexor tendons or tendon grafts are used as material for reconstruction. When exploring a relatively intact system, it appears preferable to enter the tendon sheath at the cruciate pulley areas[171] while bearing in mind that the blood supply to the vincula enters the sheath in these areas as well.[13,321] Removal of the cruciates and A5 pulley, when other annular ligaments are intact, results in no loss of range of motion.

At the proximal phalanx level, the tendon is placed deep to the neurovascular bundles and beneath the dorsal extensor mechanism to prevent compression of the intrinsic system. To best simulate the biomechanics of the A2 and A4 pulleys, I recommend at a minimum two circumferential wraps. If possible, the A2 pulley, which is normally 18 to 20 mm in length, may be re-created by encircling the proximal phalanx four times. When this is performed with a palmaris longus graft with its usual width of 3 to 4 mm, the original dimension of the A2 pulley can be restored. In the A4 region, two wraps will create a pulley approximately 10 mm in length and should adequately simulate the biomechanics of the native pulley (Fig. 7-50). Approximately 6 to 8 cm of

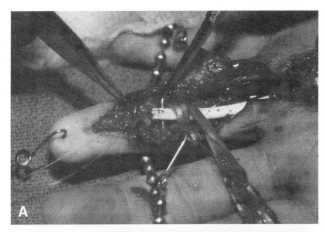

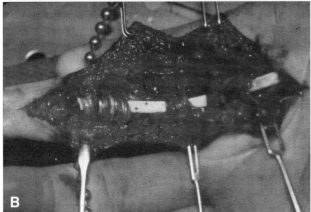

FIGURE 7-50. **A** and **B,** Pulley reconstruction. The resected FDS tendon is used to create a circumferential type pulley around the silicone tendon implant by the phalanx technique.

graft is required to encircle the phalanx one time, so adequate material must be available for reconstruction. Several methods can facilitate placement of tendon material. A curved suture passer may be used to pull sutures placed into the tendon graft around the phalanx. A Penrose drain that is passed with a right-angled hemostat can also be utilized. In this technique, the graft material is slipped into the drain and carried atraumatically around the phalanx as the drain is pulled through. A second dorsal incision that splits the extensor mechanism at the proximal phalanx may be used to allow easier graft placement around the phalanx. A reconstructed pulley should be strong enough to resist breakdown or attenuation.[37,273] Vigorous testing under direct visualization on the operating table is necessary.

Postoperative Care

Postoperatively, the splinting should include an external protective pulley ring, worn for 4 to 6 weeks, to protect the reconstruction. This ring can be rigid and fabricated from moldable plastic or flexible and formed from a simple elastic wrap. The therapist should be apprised of the pulley reconstruction so that this area can be supported during active and resisted exercise performed during the course of rehabilitation.

CRITICAL POINTS: PULLEY RECONSTRUCTION

INDICATION

- Inadequate pulley function during flexor tendon reconstruction

PREOPERATIVE EVALUATION

- During a two-stage reconstruction, it may be acceptable to repair an injured pulley by suturing the ends over the implant.
- Most popular method of pulley reconstruction: Bunnell encircling method.
- Other options: Kleinert technique of weaving graft into remnant of pulley rim, Karev volar plate "belt loop" technique, Lister extensor retinaculum pulley reconstruction.

PEARLS

- Reconstructed pulley must be vigorously tested under direct visualization on the operating table.
- Tendon must be held as close to underlying bone as possible without restricting gliding.

TECHNICAL POINTS

- Enter tendon sheath at cruciate pulley areas.
- Can remove cruciates and A5 with no loss in range of motion.
- Know that encircling method requires 16-cm graft for A2 reconstruction (phalanx encircled twice).
- Place graft deep to extensor mechanism at all levels.

PITFALL

- When encircling phalanx with graft, do not include the neurovascular bundle.

POSTOPERATIVE CARE

- Wear protective external ring for 4 to 6 weeks to protect reconstruction.

FLEXOR TENDON RECONSTRUCTION IN CHILDREN

Indications

Children present a somewhat different problem after flexor tendon injury. The very young, in particular, present difficulties with diagnosis. Careful observation and the use of various tricks geared to stimulate withdrawal of the fingers into flexion will lead to the diagnosis of flexor tendon

CRITICAL POINTS: TENDON RECONSTRUCTION IN CHILDREN

INDICATION

- Same as in adults

PREOPERATIVE EVALUATION

- Direct repair is better procedure than late reconstruction.
- Wait until patient is 7 years of age or older.

PEARLS

- Skin suture is done with absorbable material.
- Children heal rapidly and contractures rarely develop unless the joint is directly injured.
- Plantaris is too thin.

TECHNICAL POINTS

- Use same technique in children as in adults except for distal juncture.

- Do not violate the distal phalanx epiphysis.
- Suture into bone or weave into distal FDP stump.
- Preferred graft material: use palmaris longus or FDS of the injured finger.

PITFALLS

- Children present difficulties with diagnosis.
- Small size of tendon or silicone graft does not hold sutures well.
- Young children cooperate poorly in postoperative care and rehabilitation.

POSTOPERATIVE CARE

- Flexor tendon graft should grow with child's hand.
- Involved finger may remain slightly smaller than uninjured fingers.

---

disruption. Fortunate for children is that they heal rapidly and that contractures rarely develop unless the joint has been directly injured. They also are not constrained by economic considerations that may hinder progress in adults.[91,102,464a]

As a general rule, if wound conditions permit, direct early repair at all levels of injury is encouraged.[110,111,152,246,364,394,485] This is even more pertinent in the youngest age group (younger than 4 to 6 years of age) in whom flexor tendon grafting is particularly difficult.[28] The appropriate time to perform a flexor tendon graft in children has been debated. Although loupe magnification helps eliminate technical difficulties, the physically small size of the tendon or silicone graft does not always hold sutures well, and gap separation may easily occur. Technical difficulties encountered with the small tendon size and the inability of children to cooperate in postoperative care and rehabilitation have been cited as reasons for poorer results.[354] Although one study concluded that age was not a contraindication to grafting[142] and grafts have been successfully placed in young children,[14,179] I agree with a more conservative approach[137] and encourage waiting until the patient is 7 years of age or older.

Technique

The technique in children is essentially the same as that in adults except that the distal juncture is not placed in the distal phalangeal bone. My preferred method in children is a juncture to the distal profundus stump. If no distal stump is present, I have sutured the graft directly into bone with nonabsorbable sutures through drill holes placed distal to the epiphysis. Another technique I have used involves graft placement through a split in the FDP stump that is then passed through the fingertip. This is described in the single-stage tendon grafting section on page 249.

The graft material preferred is the palmaris longus or FDS of the injured finger. I believe that a child's plantaris is

too thin to adequately hold sutures, but this belief is not shared by all. Another important modification in the young is suturing skin with absorbable material, thereby avoiding an unpleasant postoperative confrontation. This also obviates the use of general anesthesia for suture removal, which has been advocated by some surgeons.

As the child grows, the successfully placed flexor tendon graft will probably grow with the child's hand. This clinical observation, however, was questioned by Hage and Dupius,[142] who reported that, despite good function, the involved finger remained slightly smaller than the uninjured fingers.

In general, flexor tendon injuries are difficult problems for both the child and the surgeon. The difficulties encountered with grafting make direct repair a better procedure than late reconstruction.[394]

COMPLICATIONS

Adhesion Formation

The most common problem after flexor tendon grafting, as in all flexor tendon surgery, is adhesion formation. This may occur at the surface of the graft or at the level of the proximal juncture. Adhesions will prevent or tether the free passage of the graft through the tissues and prevent the gliding necessary for finger motion.[53,252,393] To help reduce this problem, the surgeon must practice gentle handling of the tissues, use fine instruments, and adhere to proven surgical indications. Each injury to the surface of the tendon will result in an adhesion at that level. The assistance of a good hand therapy program will often help mobilize adhesions and guide the patient through the critical 8-week period after surgery. Tenolysis, as previously reviewed, is effective in salvaging some tendon grafts with adhesion problems, provided that the patient has reached a plateau and at least 3 to 6 months have elapsed since the grafting procedure.[118]

Mechanical Failure of the Implant

Breakdown of the distal juncture during stage I is rare. The migration of the implant has been reported[515] and could probably have been avoided if the Dacron braid–reinforced implant had been available. The cylindrical silicone unreinforced "rod," which will hold sutures well, is not recommended.[513] One other source of problems after stage I has been seen in patients in whom the surgeon had ill-advisedly sutured the proximal end of the implant, designed for the passive-motion program, to a flexor motor.[167] This juncture will usually disrupt and create additional irritation and scarring in the region of the future proximal tendon graft juncture. If this unnecessary proximal juncture is stronger than the distal juncture, the distal end will most likely break free.

Graft Rupture

Breakdown at the proximal or distal juncture of the graft has been seen in both primary tendon grafting and staged tendon reconstruction.[393] Adhering to excellent surgical technique followed by a closely supervised hand therapy program has, fortunately, made this a rare complication. When rupture at the graft juncture does occur, the patient can usually localize the juncture that has pulled free. If recognized early, the situation can often be salvaged through early reoperation. This complication occurs more frequently at the distal juncture, and if the tendon cannot be advanced to the original insertion, the end of the graft can be attached to the middle phalanx and an FDS finger is created (see page 274).[184] A proximal-level juncture disruption manifests itself usually through distal slippage of the graft interweave. Here, too, early exploration of the distal forearm will often lead to successful reattachment.

Pulley Disruption

Pulley failure is confirmed by a reduction of previously regained range of motion combined with bowstringing of the tendon graft. Early blocking support of the flexor tendon utilizing either the patient's contralateral hand, a wooden block, or an external ring will help maintain necessary tendon gliding while consideration for secondary pulley reconstruction is undertaken. The complication of reconstructed pulley disruption has been virtually eliminated with the common use of an encircling method.

Quadrigia

Quadrigia syndrome manifests as a decrease in flexion of an adjacent normal finger after the proximal excursion of the FDP tendon of the involved digit has been limited.[392] It was first described by Bunnell[60] and later by Verdan[471,473] after the Roman four-horse chariots driven by one charioteer who controlled four horses through individual reins. If injury or a surgical procedure prevents normal proximal excursion of a single FDP, a tethering effect will be experienced by the other FDP tendons that share a common musculotendinous origin. The adjacent FDP tendons then cannot fully flex

their respective digits. The adjacent fingers will lose some distal flexion besides creating a flexion deformity in the operated finger.

The quadrigia syndrome may occur in a number of settings such as when one FDP is advanced too far distally in a reattachment procedure in zone I.[271] Other causes include a tendon graft that is too short, a distal finger amputation in which the flexor is sutured over the tip to the extensor tendon, or an amputation in which the FDP adheres to the proximal phalanx. The patient will complain not only of the flexion deformity in the injured finger but also of weakness of grasp in the adjacent fingers. The adjacent fingers would, on clinical examination, show weakness and deficiency in their FDP function. The treatment is to lengthen, tenolyse, or even sever the offending tendon to allow the other normal adjacent fingers to flex fully.

Hyperextension of the PIP Joint

Absence of the FDS tendon in a grafted finger may, by interfering with the delicate finger balance,[329,423,424,507] result in a hyperextension deformity at the PIP joint and create a problem in initiating flexion at that joint. Surgeons who anticipate this problem in hyperextensile, loose-jointed patients should perform a tenodesis with one slip of the FDS across the PIP joint as part of the grafting procedure.

Lumbrical-Plus Finger

Also notable if the graft is too long is the "lumbrical-plus" finger described by Parkes.[328,329] This occurs because normally the lumbrical origin is pulled proximally with proximal movement of the graft. If the graft is too long, excessive traction is exerted on the lumbrical muscle, which will paradoxically cause extension at the IP joints. This problem can be avoided by ensuring proper length at the time of placement of the graft.[459] Those who advocate wrapping the lumbrical muscle around the proximal juncture in the palm incur an increased risk of creating this problem, and therefore this technique is not advocated.

Synovitis

Synovitis in the sheath forming in response to the implant was formerly recognized in 15% to 20% of post–stage I patients,[360,364] but in a more recent evaluation this complication was reduced to 8%.[496] This problem is characterized by increased heat, crepitus, and obvious swelling with fluid in the sheath and is associated with a thickened, less pliable sheath at stage II (Fig. 7-51). This serious complication is often, but not necessarily always, followed by a less successful end result after stage II. Cultures for bacteria in the fluid found within these sheaths have consistently shown no growth.[393]

Although the inciting cause for this inflammatory reaction is not always apparent, certain circumstances seem to be associated with the development of synovitis. Breakdown of the distal juncture after stage I is usually followed by the clinical picture of synovitis. Careful attention to the details of stage I and use of the Dacron-reinforced implant have all but eliminated this cause of mechanical irritation within the sheath. Buckling or binding of the implant because of tight

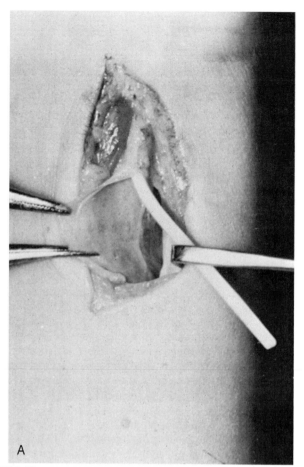 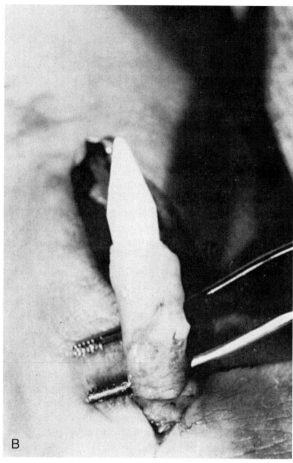

FIGURE 7-51. The sheath formed in response to the implant as seen at stage II. **A,** A soft, translucent sheath seen at 3 months in a patient with a benign postoperative course. **B,** A thickened sheath seen in a patient with synovitis after stage I.

or inadequate pulleys is another situation that may incite synovial reaction in the sheath. Appropriate pulley reconstruction should eliminate this problem. Passive movement of the finger at stage I will usually demonstrate potential problem areas where further dilation or reconstruction of a pulley will be of value. Postoperative lateral radiographs in flexion and extension will identify the amount of excursion present and will often demonstrate buckling, particularly in patients with synovitis.

Minimizing handling of the implant and careful cleansing of the surgeon's gloves reduces the problem of foreign materials such as talc on the implant surface. When synovitis is recognized, the patient's exercise program should be decreased, with return to resting splints except for limited periods of passive range-of-motion exercises. An earlier stage II procedure may be advisable if the problem is not controllable.

Infection

Postoperative infection after stage I is a disastrous complication, as in any implant procedure. When confronted with infection in the sheath, antibiotic irrigation with small-bore catheters has been attempted. In general, however, established infection will necessitate removal of the implant, with a healing period of 3 to 6 months and, if feasible, later replacement with a new implant.

Late Flexion Deformity

A late flexion deformity may develop in the postoperative phase and is related to poor nutritional status, splinting difficulties, or wound contracture. These problems require early intervention and are rarely seen in patients with good initial motion after stage II.[389,393] When noticed early, splinting the digits in extension between therapy sessions and at night can correct this. This program, in combination with gentle stretching exercises, may continue for up to 1 year. Ultimately, capsular release and flexor tenolysis may become indicated. Late flexion deformity is aggravated by inadequate pulley structure and bowstringing. Complete joint release at stage I and the construction of strong pulleys are therefore of great import.

THE FDS FINGER: A SALVAGE PROCEDURE

In flexor tendon reconstruction, an effort is usually made to restore active motion in both the PIP and DIP joints. Occasionally, under specific conditions, efforts are directed at regaining motion only in the PIP joint in a more modest attempt to salvage function. This procedure has been called the FDS finger,[34,79,177,184,325,326,402,403] although most of these reconstructions, in my experience, have been motored by the FDP tendon inserted into the middle phalanx. Perhaps the term *PIP joint finger* would be more appropriate.

In the following three clinical types, where there is flexor system disruption and distal joint motion is likely to be unattainable, consideration for salvage via restoration of motion at the PIP joint might be undertaken:

Type I: digits in which the DIP joint is inadequate because of intra-articular damage or through destruction of the extensor mechanism.

Type II: digits with a gliding flexor system that functions poorly because of bowstringing of the tendon caused by pulley failure or inadequate pulleys.

Type III: digits in which the distal insertion ruptured after tendon grafting.

Technique

In type I, a standard tendon graft is carried out as described earlier, but the graft is inserted into the middle phalanx by the pullout technique as used in the standard tendon graft. Particular attention is directed to padding placed between the button and the skin to distribute skin pressure over as wide an area as possible. Alternately, the graft can be sutured by various techniques: the middle phalanx via use of the pulley remnants, the FDS tail, or local periosteum (Fig. 7-52).

With the patient anesthetized, tension must be adjusted so that with the wrist in neutral, the finger adopts a flexion posture at the PIP joint similar to that of the adjacent fingers. I prefer, whenever possible, to do this procedure with local sedative anesthesia so that the patient can directly cooperate in the setting of distal juncture tension at the middle phalangeal level.

In situations in which the distal joint is not stable, arthrodesis or tenodesis in 20 to 30 degrees of flexion is also carried out.

In types II and III, the motor tendon end is identified through a volar approach to the finger and reattached, preferably to bone. The technique is the same as in type I cases, except that pulley reconstruction is needed in type II. Again, the use of local anesthesia technique to allow active participation of the patient is extremely useful.

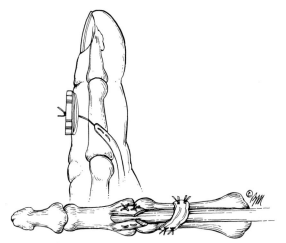

FIGURE 7-52. The FDS finger. The graft is inserted into the middle phalanx by one of several techniques. If the distal joint is not stable, tenodesis or arthrodesis of the DIP joint can be carried out at the same operation.

Postoperative Care

The tendon grafts (type I) are treated exactly as I treat a standard graft. In types II and III, early nonresistive motion is allowed in a splint, combined with gentle rubber band traction on the fingernail. The MCP joints are placed in 70 degrees, with the posterior splint allowing the PIP joints to be fully extended. The wrist is flexed approximately 30 degrees. When a pulley is reconstructed, an Orthoplast ring measuring about 2 cm in width is fabricated and worn to protect the pulley. At 3 to 4 weeks, the splint is removed but the rubber band, attached to a wrist cuff, is continued for a total of 6 weeks. The ring is worn for at least 8 weeks postoperatively.

ANNOTATED REFERENCES

9. Amadio PC, Wood MB, Cooney WP III, Bogard SD: Staged flexor tendon reconstruction in the fingers and hand. J Hand Surg [Am] 13:559-562, 1988.

   In this study of two-stage tendon grafting technique in 30 fingers, 54% achieved good or excellent results and 16% required tenolysis after stage II grafting. Better results were correlated with postoperative therapy supervision by the treating surgeon.

46. Boyes JH, Stark HH: Flexor tendon grafts in fingers and thumbs: A study of factors influencing results in 1,000 cases. J Bone Joint Surg Am 53:1332-1342, 1971.

    The classic paper on flexor tendon grafts, which analyzes the most important factors influencing outcomes after flexor tendon grafts. Pregrafting scar tissue from previous surgery or injury and joint damage were the poorest prognostic factors.

88a. Coyle MP Jr, Leddy TP, Leddy JP: Staged flexor tendon reconstruction fingertip to palm. J Hand Surg [Am] 27:581-585, 2002.

    Staged tendon grafting from palm to fingertip produced 69% good to excellent results. Less favorable outcomes were observed in patients with over 1 year between injury and reconstruction and those with higher injury severity classification.

204a. Jupiter JB, Pess GM, Bour CJ: Results of flexor tenolysis after replantation in the hand. J Hand Surg [Am] 14:35-44, 1989.

    The authors report their results in 41 replanted digits requiring tenolysis after replantation. Total active motion and potential active motion significantly increased after tenolysis using the Strickland formula of assessment.

235. LaSalle WB, Strickland JW: An evaluation of the two-stage flexor tendon reconstruction technique. J Hand Surg [Am] 8:263-267, 1983.

    Preoperative passive motion was compared with postoperative active motion at the PIP and DIP joints to measure outcome after reconstruction. Tenolysis was performed in 47% of the reconstructed digits, whereas overall results showed 40% of the digits achieved at least 60% of their preoperative passive range of motion at the PIP and DIP joints.

298. McClinton MA, Curtis RM, Wilgis EFS: One hundred tendon grafts for isolated flexor digitorum profundus injuries. J Hand Surg [Am] 7:224-229, 1982.

    Single-stage flexor tendon grafts for isolated profundus lacerations had an 87% success rate with average DIP joint motions of 48% postoperatively. This study was the first study to include patients older than 40 years of age as candidates for grafting.

398a. Schneider LH: Tenolysis and capsulectomy after hand fractures. Clin Orthop Rel Res 327:72-78, 1996.

The article reviews basic principles regarding patient selection, operative technique, and postoperative management for extensor and flexor tenolysis.

412. Seiler JG, Gelberman RH, Williams CS, et al: Autogenous flexor tendon grafts: A biomechanical and morphological study in dogs. J Bone Joint Surg Am 75:104-114, 1993.

Intrasynovial and extrasynovial autogenous grafts were compared in dogs. Intrasynovial grafts healed with fewer peripheral adhesions and exhibited greater angular rotation at the PIP joint when compared with extrasynovial tendons at various time intervals after repair.

432. Stark HH, Zemel NP, Boyes JH, Ashworth CR: Flexor tendon grafts through intact superficialis tendon. J Hand Surg [Am] 2:456-461, 1977.

Free tendon grafting with an intact superficialis tendon

resulted in 80% satisfactory results in this series. Ideal candidates include a normal superficialis tendon with normal excursion, good passive range of motion, minimal scar tissue, and younger patients.

496. Wehbe MA, Hunter JM, Schneider LH, Goodwyn BL: Two-stage flexor tendon reconstruction: Ten-year experience. J Bone Joint Surg Am 68:752-763, 1986.

This is a long-term study of 150 fingers over a decade by the surgeons who developed the technique. Range of motion improved an average of 74 degrees when considering the MCP, PIP, and DIP joints. Joint range of motion plateaued by 3 months after stage II.

503. Whitaker JH, Strickland JW, Ellis RK: The role of flexor tenolysis in the palm and digit. J Hand Surg [Am] 2:462-470, 1977.

Improved range of motion after flexor tenolysis was significant regardless of the initial mechanism of injury. PIP joint motion improved in 84% of digits and DIP joint motion improved in 86%.

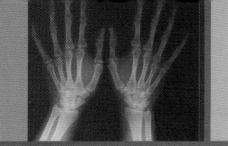

CHAPTER 8

Fractures of the Metacarpals and Phalanges

Peter J. Stern

Fractures of the metacarpals and phalanges are the most common fractures of the upper extremity.[173,239] In a series of 11,000 fractures, Emmett and Breck noted that these fractures accounted for 10% of the total.[120] Hove,[202] in a consecutive series of 1000 carpal, metacarpal, and phalangeal fractures, found that 82% involved the metacarpals or phalanges. The outer rays of the hand (thumb and small finger) were the most frequently injured. Unfortunately, metacarpal and phalangeal fractures are often neglected or regarded as trivial injuries.[463] Swanson aptly stated: "Hand fractures can be complicated by deformity from no treatment, stiffness from overtreatment, and both deformity and stiffness from poor treatment."[434]

The incidence of metacarpal and phalangeal fractures is most common in males and peaks between age 10 and 40 years,[102,335] a time when athletic and industrial exposure is the greatest. In 1980 in the United States there were 16 million upper extremity injuries that resulted in 90 million days of restricted activity and 16 million days off work.[239] The total cost in that year was estimated at $10 billion. Chung and Spilson,[81] using data from the National Hospital Ambulatory Care Survey, estimated that in 1998 there were approximately 1.5 million hand and forearm fractures in the United States. More than 600,000 of these were metacarpal and phalangeal fractures.

Until the early part of the 20th century, these fractures were all managed nonoperatively. In fact, the entire history of operative fixation for hand fractures is limited to the past 80 years[310] and was pioneered by Albine Lambotte.[257] Even today, the majority of these fractures can be successfully managed by nonoperative techniques.[10]

Most fractures are functionally stable either before or after closed reduction and will fare well with protective splintage and early mobilization.[358] Certain fractures require operative fixation (Table 8-1). Selection of the optimum treatment depends on a number of factors, including fracture location (intra-articular vs. extra-articular), fracture geometry (transverse, spiral or oblique, comminuted), deformity (angular, rotational, shortening), whether they are open or closed, whether they have associated osseous and soft tissue injuries, and fracture stability. Additional considerations include the patient's age, occupation, and socioeconomic

Table 8-1
INDICATIONS FOR FIXATION OF METACARPAL AND PHALANGEAL FRACTURES

Irreducible fractures

Malrotation (spiral and short oblique)

Intra-articular fractures

Subcapital fractures (phalangeal)

Open fractures

Segmental bone loss

Polytrauma with hand fractures

Multiple hand or wrist fractures

Fractures with soft tissue injury (vessel, tendon, nerve, skin)

Reconstruction (i.e., osteotomy)

status; the presence of systemic illnesses; the surgeon's skill; and the patient's compliance.

Regardless of the treatment selected, the goal is full and rapid restoration of hand function. Over the past three decades, operative fixation of hand fractures has gained increasing popularity[19,244,423] for the following reasons:

1. Improved materials, implant designs, and instrumentation.[266] Traditionally, implants have been made of 316L stainless steel. Whereas this metal is fully acceptable for fracture fixation, some surgeons prefer titanium, which has a modulus of elasticity that approximates bone. Self-tapping[26] and miniature cannulated screws, with an outer diameter as small as 1 mm, are now available and in selected cases can be inserted in a percutaneous fashion. Plates for the metacarpals and phalanges are low profile, easy to contour and cut, and come in a variety of configurations.
2. Better understanding of the biomechanical principles of internal fixation
3. Greater public expectations
4. Radiographic imaging. Cross-sectional imaging, and particularly computed tomography (CT), permits

multiplanar analysis of any fracture and may be useful in the assessment of intra-articular fractures. In the operating room, the use of portable mini-fluoroscopy units have been shown to reduce operating time substantially. Such units have eliminated much of the guesswork in fracture reduction, are helpful when inserting pins and screws (especially percutaneously), and allow assessment of fracture reduction and fixation in multiple planes (Fig. 8-1).

5. Availability of subspecialists in hand surgery
6. Anesthesia. Many fractures, particularly of the phalanges, can be managed by local nerve blocks and sedation with monitored anesthesia care. In addition, a sterile forearm tourniquet with appropriate sedation can be comfortably inflated for 60 to 75 minutes.
7. Therapy.[54] The hand therapist plays an integral role in both the operative and nonoperative management of hand fractures. Wound management, edema and scar control, fabrication of thermoplastic splints, supervision of therapeutic modalities,[29] and structuring an exercise program all contribute to improved outcomes.

Although prolonged immobilization is to be avoided because of the risk of permanent deformity and stiffness, one should remember that overly aggressive attempts at internal fixation may lead to damage to the soft tissue, tendon adhesion, infection, and the necessity for a secondary procedure for implant removal. Operative fixation must be used judiciously and with the expectation that the ultimate outcome will be as good as, and optimally better than, the outcome after nonoperative management.

METACARPAL FRACTURES (EXCLUDING THE THUMB)

Metacarpal Head Fractures

Fractures of the metacarpal head are rare and are usually intra-articular. In a series of 134 closed articular fractures

Table 8-2
TYPES OF FRACTURES OF THE METACARPAL HEAD

Epiphyseal (all nondisplaced Salter-Harris type III)

Ligamentous avulsions

Osteochondral slices

Two-part fractures occurring in different planes (sagittal, coronal, transverse)

Comminuted fractures

Boxer's fractures with extension into the joint

Fractures with substance loss

Occult compression fractures with subsequent avascular necrosis

of the metacarpophalangeal (MCP) and proximal interphalangeal (PIP) joints, Hastings and Carroll noted five metacarpal head fractures.[192] These fractures are usually the result of axial loading or direct trauma (crush or clenched-fist injury).

McElfresh and Dobyns reported on 103 intra-articular metacarpal head fractures.[304] The injury involved the index metacarpal most frequently, presumably because it is a border digit and its metacarpal base is fixed to the carpus. The fractures were classified into several categories (Table 8-2). Comminuted fractures occurred most commonly. Half the patients with comminuted fractures had loss of more than 45 degrees of flexion at the MCP joint. Articular defects may remodel with time; and unlike weight-bearing joints, an incongruous MCP joint may function satisfactorily with painless motion.

Intra-articular fractures of the metacarpal head can also occur after complex dorsal MCP dislocations. Becton and colleagues[16] noted such a fracture in 7 of 13 patients and recommended open reduction and internal fixation (ORIF) through a dorsal approach.

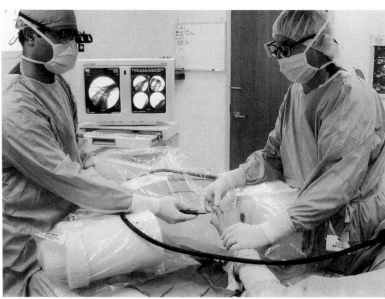

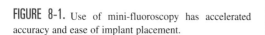

FIGURE 8-1. Use of mini-fluoroscopy has accelerated accuracy and ease of implant placement.

Radiographic evaluation requires three views: postero-anterior, lateral, and oblique. The lateral view is difficult to interpret because of the adjacent overlying metacarpal heads. The Brewerton view (MCP joint flexed 65 degrees with the dorsum of the fingers lying flat on the x-ray plate and the tube angled 15 degrees in an ulnar-to-radial direction) was used by Lane[259] to delineate collateral ligament avulsion fractures of the metacarpal head not seen on routine views. A skyline metacarpal view[122] may be helpful in visualizing the articular profile of the metacarpal head after a clenched-fist injury. The MCP and interphalangeal (IP) joints are fully flexed, and the beam is directed parallel to the dorsal shaft of the proximal phalanx. If operative intervention is contemplated, tomography[299] or CT[199] may be helpful.[299]

Treatment of these fractures must be individualized. Displaced ligament avulsion fractures and osteochondral fractures can be satisfactorily managed by ORIF.[304] Kumar and Satku[253] emphasized that small osteochondral fragments should not be discarded but instead "trapped in place" by larger fragments and not separately internally fixed. Two-part coronal, sagittal, and oblique intra-articular fractures are best managed by ORIF with Kirschner pins or interfragmentary screws (Fig. 8-2).[192,299,304]

Occasionally, an injury occurs with partial loss of a metacarpal head. Boulas[46,47] has reported successful short-term results with osteochondral autografts taken from a corresponding toe.

A comminuted intra-articular fracture is the most difficult to treat. It is often associated with soft tissue injuries and metaphyseal compaction or bone loss. ORIF may be frustrating, if not impossible. Alternative forms of treatment include skeletal traction[15] or silicone arthroplasty (Fig. 8-3).[279,320,424] In a series of 14 patients, Nagle and coworkers[320] recommended immediate silicone arthroplasty for open nonsalvageable intra-articular fractures of the PIP and MCP joints. With slightly over 2 years of follow-up, active range of motion at the MCP joint averaged 60 degrees. There were no deep infections or implant failures, but malrotation was occasionally a problem.

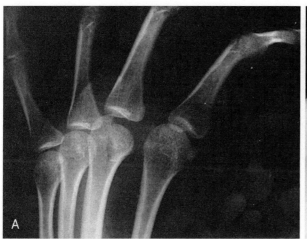
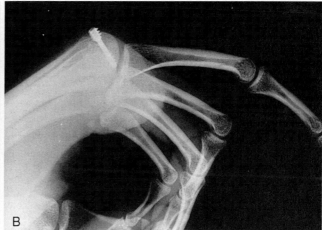
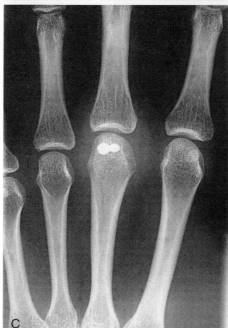

FIGURE 8-2. **A,** Displaced, intra-articular sagittal slice fracture of the middle finger metacarpal head. Postoperative posteroanterior (**B**) and lateral (**C**) views show anatomic reduction and fixation with a Herbert screw. Full MCP mobility was restored.

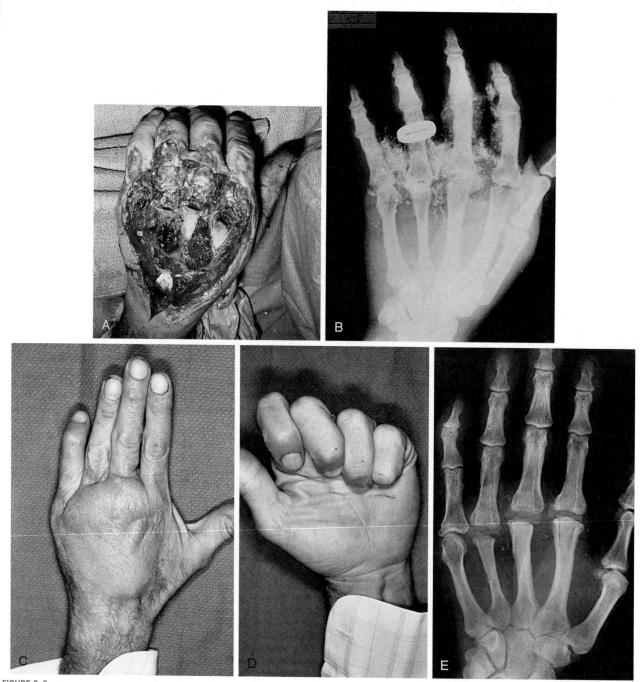

FIGURE 8-3. **A,** Crush/degloving injury to the dorsum of the hand. Note the extensive skin and extensor tendon loss. **B,** Initial radiographs show loss of the index, middle, and ring metacarpal heads. Excellent digital extension (**C**) and flexion (**D**) 9 years after silicone MCP replacements, extensor tendon grafts, and a groin flap. **E,** Radiograph showing the silicone MCP arthroplasties. (From Stern PJ, Amin AK, Neale HW: Early joint and tendon reconstruction for a degloving injury to the dorsum of the hand. Plast Reconstr Surg 72:391-394, 1983.)

The most common complication of intra-articular metacarpal head fractures is stiffness. This may result from extensor tendon adhesions, collateral ligament or dorsal capsular contracture, or articular incongruity. Dibbell and Field[105] reported recurrent locking of the MCP joint secondary to a malunited, impacted metacarpal head fracture.

Epiphyseal arrest can follow children's metacarpal head fractures.[51] To minimize longitudinal growth arrest, Light

and Ogden[275] recommended ORIF of displaced intra-articular metacarpal head fractures. Avascular necrosis[304,484] can also occur, is found predominantly in young adults, and usually involves the index and middle fingers. Buchler and Fischer[57] reported avascular necrosis in 3 of 17 cases when the minicondylar plate was used for metacarpal neck fixation. Whether this was the result of the injury or the fixation was not clear.

Author's Preferred Method of Treatment

Noncomminuted fractures with more than 25% of the articular surface involved or greater than 1 mm of articular stepoff should be treated operatively. I approach these fractures through a dorsal longitudinal incision that splits the extensor tendon to expose the joint. Two-part intra-articular fractures are usually amenable to fixation with headless screws. In performing the reduction, care must be taken to preserve attachments of soft tissue to the articular fragment(s) to avoid devascularization.[253] Fixation with Kirschner pins, although easier, is not as desirable because fixation is less rigid and may delay mobilization of the joint.

Open fractures of a metacarpal head secondary to a clenched fist injury should be treated by formal irrigation and débridement. The wound should be left open and internal fixation, if necessary, delayed until the wound is clean and shows no sign of infection.

Comminuted fractures are problematic. Direct fracture fixation with multiple Kirschner pins or cerclage wire often fails to stabilize the fracture and maintain the reduction. For closed injuries, I prefer immobilization for 2 weeks with the MCP joint flexed 70 degrees, followed by aggressive range-of-motion exercises. Skeletal traction or external fixation may be needed if there are associated comminuted fractures of the adjacent base of the proximal phalanx. For open comminuted head fractures, especially those with bone loss, silicone arthroplasty is a reasonable alternative but should *not* be done under the following circumstances:

1. *Fracture of the head of the index finger*—lateral and shear stresses from pinch will result in implant failure.
2. *Inadequate soft tissue coverage*—the implant cannot be left exposed.
3. *Excessive metacarpal bone loss*—excessive shortening and instability will occur. Under these conditions, external fixation is an alternative that I have used.[475]

MCP arthrodesis is a salvage procedure that results in loss of mobility and length; it should not be done acutely because of the risk of excessive shortening and nonunion.

Metacarpal Neck Fractures

Metacarpal neck fractures (boxer's fracture) are common and usually involve the ring and small metacarpals. "Boxer's fracture" is really a misnomer. Fractures of the fifth metacarpal neck are rarely seen in professional boxers; they are far more common in brawlers and in people who hit solid objects such as walls. Unfortunately, the term *boxer's fracture* seems to be deeply ingrained in the orthopedic literature.

These fractures invariably occur when a clenched MCP joint strikes a solid object and angulates with its apex dorsal. Apex dorsal angulation occurs because (1) the impact occurs on the dorsum of the metacarpal head and causes comminution of the volar metacarpal neck; and (2) the intrinsic muscles that cross the MCP joint lie volar to its axis of rotation and maintain a flexed metacarpal head posture.[309]

Controversy exists regarding the optimum treatment of this fracture, which varies from nonoperative treatment[6,135,349] to a variety of techniques for internal fixation. Nonunion virtually never occurs; however, malunion may be a problem. Patient complaints include a loss of prominence of the metacarpal head, diminished range of motion, a palpable metacarpal head in the palm,[440] and, occasionally, rotatory malalignment.

When deciding on treatment, several factors must be considered: (1) which metacarpal neck is fractured; (2) the degree of angulation; and (3) presence of a rotational deformity.

The ring and small finger carpometacarpal (CMC) joints have 20 to 30 degrees of mobility in the sagittal plane, whereas the index and middle CMC joints have less mobility. Therefore, angulation can be better compensated for in the ring and small fingers.

Leung and colleagues noted that it is difficult to consistently measure the degree of angulation in boxer's fractures. Using lateral radiographs, angulation can either be measured by lines that pass through the shaft (medullary canal) of the metacarpal and center of the metacarpal head or by lines that run tangential to the dorsal cortices of the proximal and distal fragments. When a series of fifth metacarpal neck fracture radiographs were assessed by three observers on two occasions, interobserver reliability was slight and intraobserver reliability was fair.[270]

Several surgeons believe that significant angulation of a small finger metacarpal neck fracture is acceptable without compromising hand function. Hunter and Cowen,[208] Holst-Nielsen,[200] and Kuokkanen and colleagues[255] noted no significant disability with up to 70 degrees of angulation. Both Hunter and Cowen[208] and Eichenholtz and Rizzo[117] did not attempt manipulation of fractures with less than 40 degrees of angulation and noted no increase in angulation during healing. Konradsen and coworkers[249] compared treatment of one group of patients with metacarpal neck fractures using a functional brace that allowed full range of motion of the wrist and digits with another cohort of patients treated with plaster immobilization of the digits and wrist. Those in the functional brace group had a more rapid return to work; however, the overall results were comparable at 3 months. Hansen and Hansen[187] prospectively compared casting, a functional brace, and an elastic bandage in patients with less than 60 degrees of angulation. They found no difference in patient satisfaction but recommended a functional brace because patients became mobile faster and experienced less pain. Similar recommendations were made by Harding and coworkers[188] for fractures angulated less than 40 degrees. Braakman and colleagues[48] prospectively treated 100 fifth metacarpal neck fractures with either cast immobilization or functional taping of the ring to the small finger. The majority of fractures were not reduced, and at the end of treatment functional taping was recommended. In a prospective series of 73 small finger metacarpal neck fractures, Lowdon[288] noted no relationship between the presence of symptoms and residual angulation. Barton[14] used a soft bandage for treating fractures with angulation of less than 50 degrees. McKerrell and associates[306] compared two statistically comparable groups of patients with fifth metacarpal neck fractures treated conservatively and operatively. Failure to correct dorsal angulation was not associated with functional disability despite residual dorsal angulation in the nonoperative group.

Excessive angulation of ring and small finger metacarpal neck fractures is not accepted by everyone. Smith and Peimer[406] believed that persistent angulation of over 30 degrees was unacceptable. The Mayo Clinic group[5] recommended open reduction or percutaneous pinning of ring metacarpal fractures with angulation greater than 20 degrees and small finger metacarpal fractures with angulation greater than 30 degrees. Others have advised accepting only 20 degrees of angulation before recommending internal fixation.[35,243] Flatt[133] and Workman[479] believed that the angulation was unacceptable if pseudoclawing of the small finger was noted on extension.

Because of the lack of compensatory CMC motion, there is almost universal agreement that residual angulation over 10 to 15 degrees in fractures of the index and middle metacarpal necks should not be accepted.[5,35,173,231,234,350,406]

Closed manipulation may not be possible as the fracture heals and stiffens. Brown[52] believed that it was better to accept the deformity if the fracture was more than a few days old. Roberts[369] did not attempt manipulation after 1 to 2 weeks, and Eichenholz and Rizzo[117] used 8 days as the cutoff point. Opgrande and Westphal[333] accepted only 10 degrees of angulation in patients with an acute fracture, but up to 40 degrees was acceptable if the fracture was 7 to 10 days old.

Closed Reduction of Metacarpal Neck Fractures

Jahss[220] recognized that flexing the MCP joint to 90 degrees relaxed the deforming intrinsic muscles and tightened the collateral ligaments, thereby allowing the proximal phalanx to exert upward pressure on the metacarpal head. He applied a cast in two parts, first immobilizing the proximal metacarpal fragment and then flexing the MCP and PIP joints and pushing upward on the flexed PIP joint while applying the second part. He reported 10 cases with uniformly satisfactory results. This method gained wide popularity but has largely been abandoned because persistent PIP stiffness or skin necrosis developed over the dorsum of the PIP joint in some patients. The "Jahss maneuver" today remains the best technique of closed reduction; however, the small finger should never be immobilized in the "Jahss position" (MCP and PIP joints both flexed 90 degrees).

Closed reduction with percutaneous pinning was reported first by Bosworth[42] in 1937. Maintenance of closed reduction by percutaneous transverse Kirschner pin fixation of the fractured metacarpal to the adjacent metacarpal has been a popular method of treatment for metacarpal neck and shaft fractures.[5,74,256,318,433,464,480,483] Percutaneous fixation has the advantage of being minimally invasive and should reduce the likelihood of postoperative swelling and stiffness that frequently follows ORIF.[248] The disadvantage is that it does not provide rigid fixation and some form of external immobilization is necessary. If clawing was present when the patient extended the finger, Green and Rowland[173] advised closed reduction and percutaneous Kirschner pin fixation (obliquely across the fracture or two transverse pins into the adjacent metacarpal). Lord[284] and Heim and associates[198] introduced a Kirschner pin through the flexed MCP joint into the medullary canal to maintain the closed reduction.

Pritsch and colleagues[353,354] inserted bicortical percutaneous pins in the sagittal plane into the proximal and distal fragments. The fracture was then reduced and the pins bonded together with an acrylic resin. Satisfactory results were reported.

Foucher[139] has reported excellent results with the use of "bouquet" osteosynthesis in the management of displaced small finger metacarpal neck fractures (Fig. 8-4). The fracture is reduced in closed fashion, holes are made in the proximal ulnar metaphysis of the metacarpal, and three blunt pre-bent Kirschner pins are passed antegrade down the medullary canal, across the fracture, and into the subchondral bone of the metacarpal head. This has the advantage of avoiding the fracture site; but it can be technically difficult, and pins can migrate either proximally or distally.

Open Reduction of Metacarpal Neck Fractures

Open reduction is indicated when manipulation fails to restore acceptable angulatory or rotational alignment. Smith and Peimer[406] recommended open reduction with crossed Kirschner pins through a transverse dorsal incision for uncorrected angulation over 30 degrees. The hand was splinted for 3 weeks, followed by active motion and pin removal. Heim and Pfeiffer,[197] in the second edition of the AO *Small Fragment Set Manual*, preferred a tension band wire loop when open reduction was required instead of a plate, which had been advocated in the first edition. King[245] advised open reduction maintained with a plate and screws for unstable metacarpal neck fractures. Others have used either an "L" or "T" plate.[393,394] A minicondylar blade plate[57,334] has been used for rigid stabilization of such fractures, especially when there was associated injury to the soft tissues.

Unless there is significant disability, a malunion of the fifth metacarpal neck is usually accepted. Thurston[440] reported good correction in 9 of 10 metacarpal neck osteotomies with a two-cut "pivot" osteotomy. This combined the benefits of an opening wedge osteotomy (no shortening) and a closing wedge osteotomy (no bone graft or tension on soft tissues).

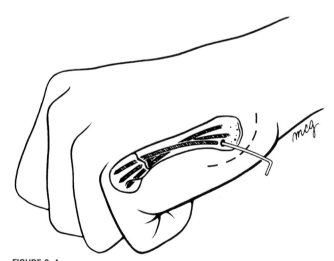

FIGURE 8-4. Technique described by Foucher[139] for antegrade fixation of a metacarpal neck fracture with multiple pre-bent Kirschner pins. Exposure of the fracture site is avoided.

Author's Preferred Method of Treatment

In most cases, closed metacarpal neck fractures (especially of the ring and small finger) should be treated by nonoperative techniques. In the absence of "pseudoclawing" (compensatory MCP hyperextension and PIP flexion) or rotational malalignment, metacarpal neck fractures produce minimal, if any, functional problems despite angulation on the lateral radiograph and shortening in the frontal projection. If no pseudoclawing is present on attempted digital extension, I prefer to use a functional brace. A forearm-based dorsal-ulnar gutter splint using thermoplastic material is fabricated such that the wrist is extended 30 degrees and the proximal phalanges of the ring and small fingers are splinted in approximately 70 degrees of flexion and are buddy-taped to one another. Active range of motion is encouraged. The splint is worn for 2 weeks and is discontinued when pain has resolved.

Reduction of metacarpal neck fractures is clinically indicated when there is "pseudoclawing" or when there is a rotational deformity. A hematoma block or wrist block may be used to achieve anesthesia. Next, closed manipulation of the metacarpal neck fracture is performed by the Jahss maneuver (Fig. 8-5A). This is accomplished by flexing the MCP and PIP joints to 90 degrees and exerting upward pressure through the flexed proximal phalanx and simultaneous downward pressure on the metacarpal shaft. Particular attention is paid to correcting any rotational deformity by using the flexed proximal phalanx as a crank. A forearm-based ulnar gutter plaster cast is applied and includes the adjacent, stable finger. The wrist is placed in 30 degrees of extension, the MCP joints are maximally flexed, and the PIP joints are held extended (see Fig. 8-5B). Radiographs are then obtained to check the accuracy of reduction. Angulation greater than 15 degrees is unacceptable for fractures of the index and middle metacarpal necks. Angulation of 30 to 40 degrees is acceptable in the ring finger, and up to 50 or 60 degrees is acceptable in the small finger. Immobilization can usually be discontinued at 12 to 14 days, and a program of active range of motion with protective splinting is initiated. The patient may return to sports and unrestricted activity at

4 to 6 weeks. Manipulation is not usually worth attempting if the fracture is older than 7 to 10 days.

In fresh metacarpal neck fractures, closed reduction with satisfactory anatomic restoration is usually possible; however, it may be difficult to maintain because of significant volar comminution and intrinsic muscle pull. If the reduction is unacceptable or cannot be maintained, I prefer to percutaneously insert crossed Kirschner pins under fluoroscopic guidance (Fig. 8-6). After closed reduction, the pins are inserted into the lateral nonarticular portion of the metacarpal head and drilled into the metacarpal shaft. Alternatively, two pins can be percutaneously inserted in a transverse fashion from the fractured metacarpal head and fixed to the adjacent intact metacarpal (Fig. 8-7). This technique, however, may cause lateral translation of the fractured metacarpal head.

Should open reduction be necessary, I prefer crossed Kirschner pins, as described earlier by Smith and Peimer.[406] Alternatively, a dorsal tension band wire with a supplemental Kirschner pin or a laterally applied minicondylar plate (Fig. 8-8) can be applied. However, both these techniques require more dissection, which may result in MCP stiffness. Plate application is a last resort. Plates require intracapsular positioning and may interfere with tendon gliding and collateral ligament function, all of which can adversely affect MCP joint mobility. Finally, plates often require secondary removal.

Postoperative management begins with immobilization in an intrinsic-plus position for 5 to 7 days. Radiographs are taken to verify hardware position and fracture alignment, and, if satisfactory, protected active range-of-motion exercises are initiated after internal fixation. Immobilization in an ulnar gutter splint is usually maintained for 2 to 3 weeks after percutaneous pin fixation. If MCP joint transarticular pins have been placed, immobilization is maintained until the pins are removed at 3 weeks postoperatively. Edema control with an elastic garment is also recommended.

Metacarpal Shaft Fractures

Metacarpal shaft fractures are broadly classified into three types: transverse, oblique (spiral), and comminuted.[5,149,173] Each fracture type presents characteristic deformities that

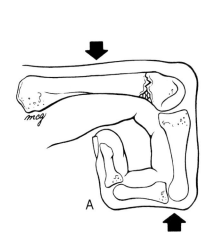

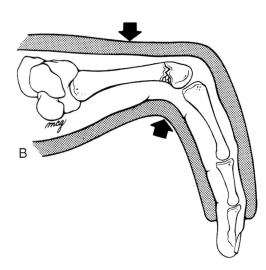

FIGURE 8-5. A, The Jahss maneuver for reduction of a metacarpal neck fracture. Arrows indicate the direction of pressure application for fracture reduction. **B,** After reduction, the fingers are held in an intrinsic-plus (safe) position in an ulnar gutter splint with molding as indicated by arrows.

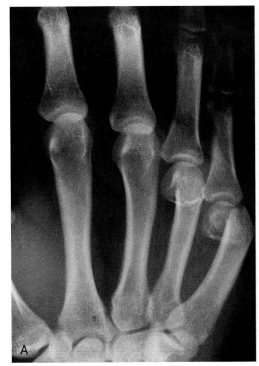

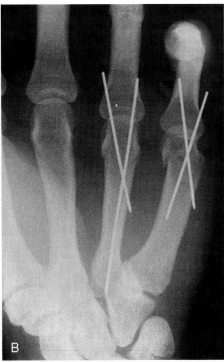

FIGURE 8-6. **A,** Severely displaced neck fractures of the ring and small metacarpals. **B,** Closed reduction using the Jahss maneuver and percutaneous crossed pins.

CRITICAL POINTS: OPERATIVE MANAGEMENT OF BOXER'S FRACTURES

INDICATIONS

- Angulation greater than 70 degrees in lateral view
- Rotatory malalignment
- Associated fractures in fifth ray of hand
- Open fractures with associated soft tissue injury (excluding human bites)
- Presence of pseudoclawing

PREOPERATIVE EVALUATION

- Inquire as to mechanism (human bite).
- Obtain anteroposterior and true lateral radiographs.
- Assess active range of motion and check for presence of pseudoclawing (compensatory MCP hyperextension and PIP flexion).

PEARLS

- Less invasive techniques are preferred.
- Use closed reduction and percutaneous pinning.
- Many patients with this fracture are unreliable, and this may compromise outcome.

TECHNICAL POINTS

- Reduction is accomplished with Jahss maneuver (see Fig. 8-5).
- Under fluoroscopic guidance, insert two 0.9-mm retrograde crossed Kirschner pins from the lateral

(nonarticular portion of the metacarpal head) into the shaft (see Fig. 8-6).
  - Pins should exit through the dorsal metacarpal shaft.
- Other options:
  - Two transverse pins from small to intact ring metacarpal head (see Fig. 8-7)
  - "Bouquet" osteosynthesis: percutaneous antegrade insertion of pre-bent Kirschner pins from small finger metacarpal base into head (see Fig. 8-4)
  - ORIF with a minicondylar plate or "T" plate (see Fig. 8-8)
    - This is the least desirable treatment option (stiffness may occur).
    - Place plate laterally.

POSTOPERATIVE CARE

- Immobilize in ulnar gutter cast no more than 5 to 7 days.
- Then begin protected active range-of-motion exercises stressing MCP flexion.
- Control edema with use of an elastic garment.
- Remove pins at 4 weeks.

ATHLETIC PARTICIPATION

- Surgeon's discretion

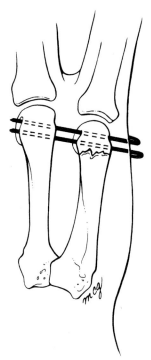

FIGURE 8-7. Percutaneous transverse pinning of a displaced metacarpal neck fracture. After closed reduction, a significantly angulated metacarpal neck fracture can be held with two percutaneous pins extending into an adjacent intact metacarpal.

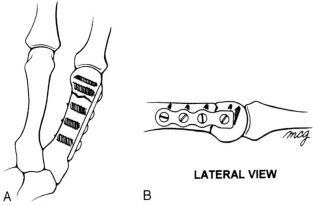

LATERAL VIEW

A   B

FIGURE 8-8. Laterally applied 2.0-mm minicondylar plate for stabilization of a metacarpal neck fracture. **A,** Anteroposterior view. **B,** Lateral view.

may lead to complications if unrecognized or improperly treated.

Although most metacarpal fractures are readily diagnosed with standard biplanar views, oblique views (both in pronation and supination) may be helpful when there is clinical suspicion of a fracture.[260]

Transverse fractures are usually produced by axial loading through the metacarpal head or by a direct blow. The fracture angulates with its apex dorsal; the interosseous muscles are the deforming force. Although significant angulation is functionally well tolerated, some patients consider a residual dorsal bump aesthetically unacceptable.[173] Angulation in excess of 30 degrees for the small finger, 20 degrees in the ring finger, and any angulation in the middle and index fingers is worthy of reduction.

Oblique and spiral fractures are usually the result of torsional forces and can cause rotational malalignment. Five degrees of malrotation in a metacarpal fracture can cause 1.5 cm of digital overlap.[149] Opgrande and Westphal[333] stated that 1 degree of metacarpal shaft rotation could produce 5 degrees of fingertip rotation and result in digital overlap when a fist is made.

Malrotation, which is poorly tolerated and difficult to assess on plain radiographs, is best judged clinically by asking the patient to *simultaneously* flex all the fingers.[62] Royle[376] assessed rotation by placing the palm flat and measuring the fingernail with respect to the horizontal plane. If it was greater than 10 degrees, operative intervention was usually necessary. If significant scissoring is present with composite digital flexion, open reduction must be considered.

Comminuted fractures are usually produced by direct impact, are often associated with soft tissue injury, and may produce shortening. There is considerable controversy as to the degree of shortening that may be accepted. Regardless of fracture geometry, certain fractures may influence the surgeon to perform operative fixation (see Table 8-3). These include the presence of multiple fractures (especially spiral or oblique), fractures of the index or small finger,[480,482] open fractures, especially those with bone loss or concomitant soft tissue injury, and fractures in polytrauma victims who cannot cooperate or tolerate cast immobilization.

Closed Reduction and Plaster Immobilization

Closed reduction with plaster immobilization works well for the majority of metacarpal shaft fractures, and overtreatment is to be avoided.[40,222] Many metacarpal fractures are inherently stable and may be treated with minimal or no immobilization. For example, in athletes, Rettig and associates[365] reported that 82% of the fractures were minimally displaced or nondisplaced and the average time lost from practice or competition was 13.7 days. McMahon and coworkers[308] treated stable metacarpal fractures with either a compression glove or 3 weeks of immobilization. Although the final ranges of motion were comparable, those in the elastic garment had better mobility and less swelling much earlier. Borgeskov[40] noted that immobilization was the chief cause of stiffness. Wright[483] observed that over 60% of patients with fractures of metacarpals that were immobilized for more than 3 weeks had significant loss of hand function. Flatt[134] and Brown[52] advised cast immobilization for approximately 3 weeks. Burkhalter[60] advocated closed treatment for fractures that showed no rotational malalignment on clinical examination. He used a short-arm cast with the wrist in 30 to 40 degrees of extension and added a dorsal extension block to hold the MCP joints flexed 80 to 90 degrees and the IP joints extended.[62] Composite active MCP and IP flexion was initiated and the cast maintained for 4 weeks. When the PIP joints are extended in this splint, the hand assumes the intrinsic-plus or "clam-digger"[474] position (Fig. 8-9). This position limits joint contractures and maintains the intrinsics in a relaxed position. Functional braces[226,454,478] have been designed to provide three-point fixation of the fracture and allow mobility of the wrist and fingers. Some have found the brace ineffective,[409] and others found that if the brace was applied too tightly, skin necrosis could occur.[157]

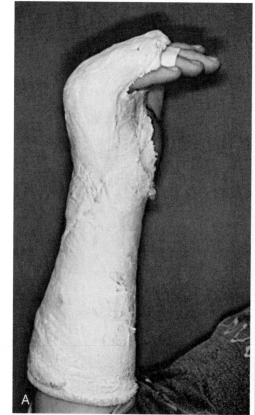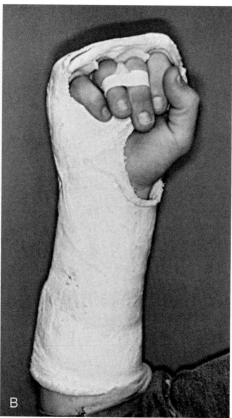

FIGURE 8-9. Clam-digger cast for a metacarpal shaft fracture. The wrist is extended 30 degrees, the MCP joints are flexed 80 to 90 degrees, and the IP joints are extended. Active range of motion is encouraged, and supplemental buddy-taping can help control rotation.

Closed Reduction and Percutaneous Pinning

Closed pinning was first used by Bosworth,[42] and a similar technique has been advocated by others.[25,464,482] Vom Saal[455] introduced intramedullary Kirschner pin fixation for metacarpal and phalangeal fractures in 1953. He left the pin protruding through the skin over the MCP joint and removed it after 4 to 7 weeks. Lord[284] used a 0.062-inch Kirschner pin inserted through the metacarpal head (with the MCP joint flexed 90 degrees), cut the pin off below the skin, and removed it after 3 to 4 weeks. To avoid leaving a pin in the MCP joint, Flatt[134] and Pulvertaft[357] preferred to drill the pin through the metacarpal head and across the fracture and have it emerge in the region of the metacarpal base with the wrist flexed. The pin was advanced until its distal end lay within the metacarpal head and the proximal end was cut off below the skin. The procedure can be difficult, and interference with extensor tendon function from the proximal end of the pin may occur unless it is buried within the medullary canal. Closed intramedullary Kirschner pin fixation for unstable metacarpal fractures has also been advocated.[11,84,107,127,209] The procedure is greatly facilitated by the use of image intensification. Using an awl, a cortical window is made at the ulnar base of the fifth metacarpal or 1 cm distal to the CMC joints of the other metacarpals. Three or four pre-bent (approximately 30 degrees) 0.9-mm pins are inserted and preferably buried proximally within the medullary canal. Posner[350] advised against intramedullary fixation in the belief that it does not control rotation and may produce secondary scarring in the extensor hood. Massengill and colleagues[300] showed that the use of transverse Kirschner pins to fix an experimental pig metacarpal shaft fracture through the adjacent metacarpal

offered a bending stiffness approaching that of plate and screw fixation.

Traction

Traction to maintain a reduction secured by manipulation is generally of historical interest and, today, is rarely used.[36,316,317,435,479]

Open Reduction

Indications for open reduction of metacarpal shaft fractures vary widely. Melone[311] noted that approximately 10% of phalangeal and metacarpal fractures were irreducible by closed manipulation or percutaneous pinning and thus required open reduction. Definite indications for open reduction include:

1. *Open fractures*—particularly those with associated bone loss, soft tissue injury, or additional regional fractures.
2. *Multiple fractures*—in such cases the stabilizing effect of the adjacent metacarpals is lost.
3. *Unstable fractures*—especially those that cannot be satisfactorily held by closed or percutaneous techniques. Fractures of the border metacarpals tend to be more unstable and more difficult to control than fractures of the central metacarpals because of the lack of support for soft tissue on both sides. Freeland and colleagues[145] pointed out that there is a difference between *rigid* and *stable* fixation. *Rigid* fixation is usually unnecessary; however, fixation must be sufficiently *stable* to promote fracture union and early rehabilitation.
4. *Malalignment*—rotational malalignment is unacceptable and is characteristically seen in spiral and oblique frac-

tures. When correction of a rotational deformity by closed techniques or percutaneous pinning is unsatisfactory, open reduction is often indicated.

Dorsal angulation, characteristic of transverse fractures, is better tolerated, particularly when the fracture involves the ring and small metacarpals or when the fracture is in the distal end of the shaft. Dorsal angulation has several undesirable effects:

1. The metacarpal head becomes prominent in the palm and may cause pain on grasping.
2. There may be compensatory hyperextension at the MCP joint that results in a secondary pseudoclaw deformity when the digit is fully extended.
3. Patients find the dorsal prominence aesthetically displeasing.
4. There is metacarpal shortening; and if great enough, the intrinsic muscles may be unable to accommodate and hence are weakened.

Wolfe and Elliott mathematically demonstrated that with the same degree of angulation there is more shortening in shaft fractures than metacarpal neck fractures.[475] However, in contrast to the phalanges, dorsal angulation does not seem to interfere with extensor tendon excursion.

Flatt[134] accepted up to 35 degrees of angulation in the ring and little metacarpals, but not over 10 degrees in the second and third metacarpals. Smith and Peimer[406] and Freeland and associates[149] recommended open reduction if the angulation could not be corrected to under 10 degrees in the second and third metacarpals and under 20 degrees in the fourth and fifth metacarpals. Opgrande and Westphal[333] believed that no angulation should be accepted in fractures of the second and third metacarpals.

Likewise, opinions vary as to the degree of acceptable shortening. Butt[67] and Bloem[35] believed that shortening, even up to 1 cm, was well tolerated without functional impairment. Workman,[479] however, attributed weakness of grip to metacarpal shortening in the belief that the relative decreased length of the musculotendinous unit decreased its efficiency. Burkhalter[61] accepted up to 5 mm of shortening, but both Brown[52] and Freeland and associates[149] advised open reduction if shortening exceeded 3 to 4 mm. Gropper and Bowen[179] performed cerclage wiring if shortening exceeded 2 mm. Eglseder and coworkers[116] demonstrated an average of 3.1 mm of shortening in patients treated for isolated ring metacarpal fractures whether they underwent operative or nonoperative treatment and demonstrated no clinical differences between groups.

Techniques of Open Reduction (Table 8-3)

Kirschner Pins

Kirschner pins may be used in nearly any fracture pattern (Fig. 8-10). Pin fixation is technically easy, requires minimal dissection, and is universally available. Pin configurations can be either single or multiple and may be crossed,[52,115,350,406] transverse, longitudinal (intramedullary), or in combination. They can be used to supplement other forms of fracture fixation and can also be used as a "bailout" if more complicated fixation has failed. On the other hand, Kirschner pins are not rigid, may loosen or even migrate,[182]

and have the potential to distract fracture fragments. Furthermore, pin tract infections may develop secondary to skin irritation or loosening, and pin protrusion may make therapy and splintage awkward. Botte and associates[44] reviewed a series of 422 Kirschner pins placed in the hand and wrist and reported an 18% complication rate. In a series of 590 Kirschner pin fixations, Stahl and Schwartz[415] noted a 15.2% complication rate. The majority were classified as minor (pin loosening, infection, or bending); however, 1.7% were major (osteomyelitis, tendon laceration, or nerve injury). There was no difference between protruding or buried pins. Most of the complications were not serious, and permanent sequelae were infrequent.

For longitudinal fixation, the pin can be drilled in retrograde fashion from the fractured end out the dorsal radial aspect of the metacarpal head and then back down the shaft through the reduced fracture.[455] Retrograde drilling of the proximal fragment is also possible with the wrist acutely flexed.[315,383] After fracture reduction, a pin can also be introduced directly into the metacarpal head on either side of the extensor tendon and driven down the metacarpal shaft to engage subchondral bone at the CMC joint. Transarticular pins are generally bent outside the skin and left in place for 3 weeks. An alternative, but technically more difficult, method is to percutaneously introduce the Kirschner pin through the lateral aspect of the metacarpal head in the area of the collateral ligament origin and then down the shaft.[17,84,236] This technique is indicated primarily for transverse and short oblique shaft fractures.

Composite (Tension Band) Wiring

A combination of Kirschner pins (0.035- or 0.045-inch diameter) and monofilament stainless steel wire (24 or 26 gauge) can also be used. The monofilament stainless steel wire is inserted as a tension band through a small transverse drill hole in the distal fragment and crossed around the Kirschner wires at the bone interface proximally. Composite wiring provides additional stability and fracture compression and superior strength, stiffness, and approximation when compared with crossed Kirschner pins alone.[21,169,176,177] Little, if any, additional dissection is necessary. The technique is rigid enough to allow early motion. Greene and associates[177] reported excellent mobility after fixation of 33 metacarpal fractures and no cases of reduction loss, nonunion, or tendon rupture. The technique is contraindicated when there is bone loss, comminution, or osteopenia. Intraoperatively, care must be taken not to excessively tighten the wire, because this leads to wire breakage.

Cerclage and Interosseous Wiring[278]

Gropper and Bowen[179] reported cerclage (circumferential) wiring with 24-gauge stainless steel wire for oblique and spiral metacarpal shaft fractures. Excellent results were reported in 21 fractures, but this technique has not gained popularity. Gingrass and colleagues[159] achieved six excellent or good results in seven metacarpal fractures treated by double 26-gauge interosseous wires placed in a dorsal-volar direction. A single Kirschner pin was added if the fixation was unstable or bone loss was present (five of seven cases). Haas and Savage[183] reported successful treatment of two oblique metacarpal shaft fractures with 0 nylon cerclage sutures in a patient with severe asthma and metal allergies.

Table 8-3
FRACTURE STABILIZATION TECHNIQUES

Technique	Indications	Advantages	Disadvantages
Kirschner pins	Transverse Oblique Spiral Longitudinal	Available and versatile Easy to insert Minimal dissection Percutaneous insertion	Lacks rigidity May loosen May distract fracture Pin tract infection Requires external support Splint/therapy awkward

Intraosseous wires	Transverse fractures (phalanges)
	Avulsion fractures
	Supplemental fixation (butterfly
	  fragment)
	Arthrodesis
		Available
		Low profile
		Relatively simple
			May cut out (especially
			  osteopenic bone)

Composite wiring	Transverse Oblique Spiral	More rigid than Kirschner pins Low profile Simple and available	Pin/wire migration Secondary removal (sometimes) Exposure may be significant
Intramedullary device	Transverse Short oblique	No special equipment Easy to insert No pin protrusion Minimal dissection	Rotational instability Rod migration
Interfragmentary fixation	Long oblique Spiral	Low profile Rigid	Special equipment Little margin for error

Plates and screws	Multiple fractures with soft tissue
	  injury or bone loss
	Markedly displaced shaft fracture
	  (esp. border metacarpals)
	Intra- and periarticular fractures
	Reconstruction for nonunion, malunion
		Rigid (stable) fixation
		Restore/maintain length
			Exacting technique
			Special equipment
			Extensive exposure
			May require removal
			Refracture after plate
			  removal
			Bulky

External fixation	Restore length for comminution or
	  bone loss
	Soft tissue injury/loss
	Infection; nonunion
		Preserves length
		Allows access to bone and soft
		  tissue
		Percutaneous insertion
		Direct manipulation of fracture
		  avoided
			Pin tract infections
			Osteomyelitis
			Overdistraction: nonunion
			Neurovascular injury
			Fractures through pin holes
			Loosening

Interosseous wiring done without supplemental Kirschner pin fixation is generally not suitable for metacarpal shaft fractures inasmuch as wire loosening and subsequent loss of reduction are real possibilities.

Intramedullary Fixation

Intramedullary fixation is applicable for transverse fractures, is easy to perform, and allows for early active motion (Fig. 8-11). There are no exposed pins and secondary removal is unnecessary. In 1981, Grundberg[181] reported one nonunion in 27 metacarpals treated by open reduction and permanent intramedullary fixation with a large Steinmann pin. Potential disadvantages include rotational instability, pin migration, and occasional fracture distraction. The technique is particularly ill suited for spiral or long oblique fractures.

First, the diameter of the medullary canal is determined with a Steinmann pin and drilled one size larger. Next, the pin is introduced into the proximal fragment (blunt end first to avoid penetration of the subchondral bone) and cut so that it protrudes 1.5 cm. The fracture is distracted, and the pin is introduced into the distal fragment. Finally, the fracture is impacted to achieve rotational stability.

More recently, a technique of closed intramedullary pinning using multiple 0.8-mm flexible pins[163,164,297,452] or pre-bent Kirschner pins has been developed (Fig. 8-12). Advantages include the ability to perform the procedure in a closed fashion and the ability to secure rotational control through three-point fixation. When diaphyseal bone loss is present, insertion of either locked intramedullary rods[163] or plates[98] has been performed. The rod or plate acts as an internal spacer while the defect is bridged with cortico-cancellous autogenous bone graft. Finally, an expandable intermedullary titanium cylinder has been used to treat similar shaft fractures.[272,328] A supplementary Kirschner pin may be necessary.

Interfragmentary Compression Screws

Interfragmentary compression screws provide rigid fixation and are primarily indicated for long oblique and spiral shaft fractures (Fig. 8-13). To ensure success, the fracture length must be a minimum of twice the bone diameter. Technically, there is little margin for error and the appropriate equipment must be available. Interfragmentary compression is accomplished when a screw is passed through a gliding hole

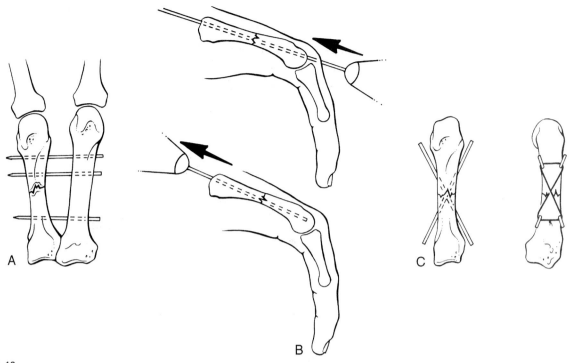

FIGURE 8-10. Techniques for Kirschner pin fixation of metacarpal shaft fractures. **A,** Transverse pins may be inserted percutaneously or open. **B,** Retrograde intramedullary fixation. Note that the pin is backed out so that it does not remain in the MCP joint. **C,** Crossed pins *(left)* and supplemental 25-gauge stainless steel wire (composite wiring) *(right).*

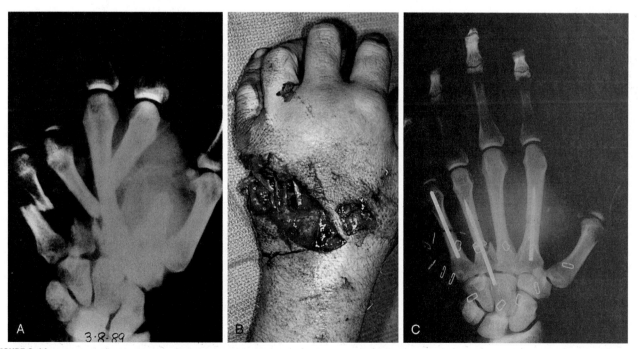

FIGURE 8-11. Intramedullary fixation. **A,** Displaced open metacarpal shaft fractures. **B,** Clinical appearance of the dorsum of the hand. **C,** Intramedullary Steinmann pin fixation. The pin in the ring metacarpal extends into the carpus for more secure fixation.

(nonthreaded and of wider diameter than the threads of the screw) into the far fragment (tapped to the same diameter as the screw threads) such that as the screw is tightened (lagged) the threads grip and draw the far fragment toward the near fragment until compression is achieved.[218] Reduction of the fracture by manipulating it into alignment

and holding the reduction with a specialized clamp must be achieved before attempting interfragmentary compression (see Fig. 8-13).

Ideally, longitudinal compressive (axial) forces are best counteracted by placing the screw 90 degrees to the bone's long axis, and torsional stresses are best resisted by placing

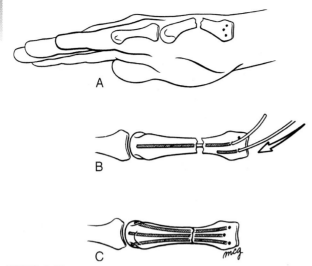

FIGURE 8-12. Intramedullary pins are inserted antegradely through multiple drill holes. The technique is facilitated by fluoroscopy. **A,** Fifth metacarpal shaft fracture. **B,** Antegrade pin insertion. **C,** Pins cut so that they are buried within the medullary canal.

the screw 90 degrees relative to the plane of the fracture. To resist both axial and torsion loading, the screw should be placed in a plane bisecting the fracture plane and longitudinal axis. In large patients, at least two 2.7-mm screws are necessary and in smaller individuals three 2.4- or 2.0-mm screws are necessary.[265] To avoid fragmentation, the screw hole should be a minimum of two screw diameters from the fracture margin.[193] Successful outcomes have been reported by numerous surgeons.[90,107,190,197,198,243,378]

Interfragmentary screw fixation (2.7 mm) of a metacarpal fracture involves six sequential steps (see Fig. 8-13):

1. Bicortical drilling with a 2-mm drill bit (internal diameter of the screw)
2. Countersinking to make the screw as low profile as possible
3. Depth measurement
4. Tapping with a 2.7-mm tap (outside diameter of the screw) (unnecessary if using a self-tapping screw)
5. Creation of a gliding hole; this is done by overdrilling the near cortex with a 2.7-mm drill bit.
6. Screw insertion. It is critical that the screw grab the far cortex to lag and hence compress the fracture. If the screw is inserted through the near cortex and is misdirected such that it hits the endosteal surface of the far cortex, the fracture will splay apart and reduction will be lost. Hence any resistance to screw insertion should alert the surgeon to stop and redirect the screw so that reduction is not lost.

Plate Fixation

In 1970, Simonetta[403] listed indications for plate fixation of the metacarpal shaft: multiple fractures, especially those with soft tissue injury; isolated, unstable transverse fractures; malunions; and pseudarthrosis. Others[144,314] used plates to span defects when there was bone loss requiring grafting. In so doing, the plates provided enough stability so that early mobilization could be initiated, thus minimizing articular stiffness and trophic changes, especially in older

patients. Ruedi and colleagues[378] used AO screws and plates to fix unstable or intra-articular fractures of the mobile first and fifth metacarpals and displaced multiple metacarpal fractures. The AO group[197] recommends plate fixation or rigid interfragmentary compression of the second and fifth (border) metacarpals because each is lacking an adjacent stabilizing metacarpal and thus has a propensity for rotational deformity. Further stability is achieved with supplemental lag screw fixation whenever the obliquity of the fracture permits. In several reports, plate and screw fixation of metacarpal shaft fractures have shown good to excellent results.[82,216,221,315] Stern and colleagues[336,426] reported complications in fractures treated with metacarpal plating. Complications included malunion, nonunion, and stiffness (articular and tendon adhesions). Complications were more frequent when there was associated bone loss, soft tissue injury, and open fractures.

Special plate designs have also been reported. Paneva-Holevich[337] used a nail plate to provide compression primarily for nonunions and malunions. Mennen[312] designed a clamp-on plate that was used to treat 15 fractures. No screws were necessary, and all fractures healed within 6 weeks.

Recently, successful use of microplates taken from maxillofacial sets has been reported.[78,356] Screws are self-tapping and diameters range from 0.8 to 1.7 mm. Because the plates are low profile (approximately 1.0 mm), the periosteum can often be closed with less tendency for adhesion formation. Fracture stabilization, although not rigid, is adequate to allow early mobilization with a low incidence of hardware failure. Prevel and coworkers,[352] using a three-point bending model, experimentally showed that a dorsally applied miniplate provided the greatest rigidity to a dorsal apex load. However, rigidity to three-point bending may not reflect fatigue performance, the usual mode of failure.

Vanik and colleagues[451] and Firoozbakhsh and associates[129] biomechanically compared the strengths of different techniques of internal fixation. When bending forces were applied to human cadaver metacarpal, they found that dorsal plates provided strength comparable to the strongest interosseous loop techniques and were superior to any configuration of Kirschner pins. Others[30,296] have reported that a dorsal metacarpal plate with or without an interfragmentary screw provides more stable fixation than crossed Kirschner pins, an interosseous wire loop alone, or an interosseous wire with a Kirschner pin. One should keep in mind that the minimal amount of strength for stable fixation in the clinical setting has never been determined; hence, biomechanically inferior constructs may be perfectly suitable in some circumstances.

Most implants are made of either stainless steel or titanium. Although titanium is more expensive, Lowka[289] cited some advantages of titanium including no corrosion, no allergic reactions, few infections (not statistically significant), ease of contour, and a modulus of elasticity that approaches that of bone. Great care must be taken when using titanium implants; screws may break, especially when being removed, and plates can break if excessively contoured before application.

External Fixation

External fixation is indicated for severe fractures when anatomic reconstitution of the skeleton is not feasible.

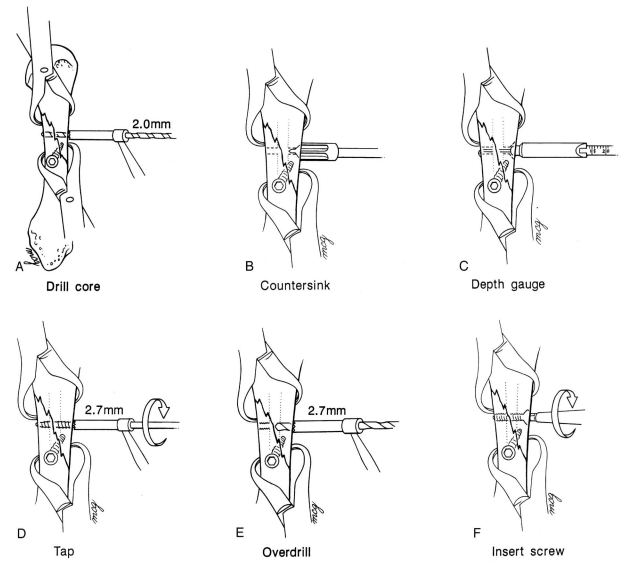

FIGURE 8-13. Fixation of a spiral metacarpal fracture with 2.7-mm lag screws. **A,** A 2.0-mm bicortical hole is drilled. **B,** The near hole is countersunk to accept the truncated screw head and distribute compression. **C,** Screw length is determined with a depth gauge. **D,** Use of a 2.7-mm tap. Care is taken to not angulate the tap so as to avoid missing the far hole, which can cause the fracture to splay apart. **E,** Only the near (gliding) hole is overdrilled. **F,** Insertion of the screw.

Examples include highly comminuted open shaft fractures with or without bone loss; displaced, comminuted intra-articular fractures; and fractures with injury or loss of soft tissue structures.[88,110,191,287,368,396] In addition, external fixation can be used to stabilize septic nonunions when it is necessary to remove infected bone.[7]

The advantages of external fixation were enumerated by Schuind and coworkers.[390] "There is respect of bone biology." Fracture fragments are not stripped of periosteal blood supply and further devascularized. External fixation does not cause the amount of osteopenia seen with more rigid systems such as plating; however, there is adequate stability to permit early mobilization. External fixators are adjustable, and a second reduction can be carried out if the initial reduction is unstable or has secondarily shifted.

Finally, when there has been concomitant soft tissue injury, external fixation permits ready access to the wound for débridement as well as for reconstruction of tendons,

nerves, and blood vessels.[7,88] Moreover, if there has been a delay in fixation such that metacarpal length is compromised, distraction lengthening of the metacarpal with external fixation followed by bone grafting can be performed.[241]

Hastings[191] has listed the complications and disadvantages of external fixation. These include pin tract infection, osteomyelitis, fracture through pinholes after removal, neurovascular injury during insertion, overdistraction with subsequent nonunion, loss of reduction, and interference with adjacent digits by the fixator. Also, pins may transfix extensor tendons or the dorsal apparatus and impair tendon excursion.[390]

The external fixation frame can be homemade by using Kirschner pins and either acrylic resin[94,106,462] or a Charnley toe-fusion clamp[123] to connect the pins. The frame can also be constructed from one of several commercially available mini external fixator sets.[55,88,97,230,339,396] Stuchin and Kummer[431] experimentally studied transverse fractures and found that the most rigid fixation frame consisted of four pins (two above and two below the fracture) held with a wire-reinforced bone cement fixator. Stiffness increased with increasing pin number and diameter.

Author's Preferred Method of Treatment

Most metacarpal shaft fractures can be managed nonoperatively. Fractures that are stable and do not require reduction can be treated in a clam-digger cast or thermoplastic splint until the fracture is clinically nontender. The fractured finger is buddy-taped to an adjacent finger, and immediate finger flexion is initiated.

Transverse shaft fractures are usually easy to reduce but maintenance of acceptable alignment may be difficult. To achieve reduction, a palmarly directed load is applied to the dorsal apex at the fracture site with a counteractive upward (dorsally directed) force on the flexed MCP joint (see Fig. 8-5). A well-padded and well-molded forearm-based cast extending to the IP joints and holding the MCP joints in 60 degrees of flexion is then applied. Special attention must be paid to be sure that the nails are in the same plane and that the flexed fingers converge toward the scaphoid tuberosity. The fracture is monitored radiographically at weekly intervals, and guarded active range-of-motion exercises can be initiated at 3 to 4 weeks. Marked swelling, which is often present in acute metacarpal shaft fractures, does not preclude manipulation and casting. Abundant cotton padding must be used and the cast must be changed at 5 to 7 days when the swelling subsides.

Closed manipulation and percutaneous pinning are indicated when the fracture can be reduced but cannot be maintained in plaster or when there is special reason to avoid casting (concomitant soft tissue injury requiring dressing changes and inspection). Fluoroscopy is invaluable to confirm fracture reduction and assist in pin placement. Reduction can sometimes be further aided by placing a small incision over the fracture and inserting an elevator to help obtain and maintain fracture reduction. I use this technique for transverse fractures of the fifth and/or fourth metacarpal and insert two parallel transverse pins into the distal fragment and one through the proximal fragment (see Fig. 8-10A). The pins should extend into an adjacent unfractured metacarpal.

Open reduction is indicated for transverse fractures that are either significantly displaced or have residual angulation of more than 10 degrees in the second and third metacarpals, 20 degrees in the fourth metacarpal, and 30 degrees in the fifth metacarpal. ORIF (Kirschner wires or screws) is indicated for most spiral and oblique fractures, particularly if there is evidence of a rotational deformity on physical examination, because fracture reduction is difficult to maintain by closed techniques. ORIF is nearly always indicated when there are multiple metacarpal fractures or when the fracture is open and associated with soft tissue injury or bone loss.

Fracture exposure is accomplished through a longitudinal incision just to one side of the extensor tendon overlying the involved metacarpal. If all four metacarpals require reduction, two longitudinal incisions are best, one between the fourth and fifth metacarpals and the other between the second and third metacarpals. Care is taken to preserve the small dorsal sensory branches of the radial and ulnar nerves and the peritenon surrounding the extensor tendons. Occasionally, one of the juncturae tendinum requires division for better fracture visualization; should this be necessary, the junctura should be repaired after fixation. The fracture ends are exposed subperiosteally and cleaned of blood clots with a small curet. Reduction is then accomplished by applying longitudinal traction and is maintained with reduction clamps.

Fixation options include Kirschner pins, composite wiring (a combination of interosseous wire and Kirschner pins), an intramedullary rod, multiple interfragmentary screws, or a plate and screws. The choice of implant is dictated by the fracture configuration and experience of the surgeon (see Table 8-3).

Kirschner pin fixation can be used for nearly all fracture configurations, and the pins are available in nearly all operating facilities in a variety of sizes. I prefer to use the trocar-shaped points. If pin placement or fracture alignment is initially unacceptable, reinsertion is a simple matter. However, multiple passes with the pins should be avoided because this may lead to thermal necrosis of bone and increase the incidence of pin tract infection. In addition, pins may loosen or distract a fracture, and pin tract infection may necessitate premature removal.

I prefer pin fixation for isolated short oblique and transverse fractures and often supplement the pins with composite wiring.[176,177] The pins are placed in a percutaneous fashion and left in place for 3½ to 4 weeks. Patients should be instructed that if there is drainage, early pin removal may be necessary.

I do not use interosseous wires alone for fixation of metacarpal shaft fractures. Despite clinical evidence showing that a dorsal tension band (figure-of-eight wire loop) is satisfactory fixation when there is interlocking of the fracture surfaces[393] and biomechanical evidence that two intraosseous wire loops at 90 degrees to each other are as strong as a dorsal plate and screws,[451] I have found wire fixation alone unsuitable, especially for diaphyseal fractures. Perhaps the *fatigue performance* of the thin wire, not tested in the mechanical studies, is inferior to the larger surface area in contact with the dorsal plate.

Intramedullary fixation using a pre-cut Steinmann pin is particularly useful for multiple open transverse shaft fractures (see Fig. 8-11). In this situation, there is frequently injury to the intrinsic muscles that allows the fracture to be easily distracted, thereby facilitating pin insertion. Pin insertion is easy and takes little time, but rotational stability may be a problem, particularly if the fracture ends fail to interdigitate. If the adjacent metacarpal is not fractured, a transverse wire can be added to control rotation.

Spiral and long oblique fractures are well suited for interfragmentary fixation. The fracture length should be at least twice, and preferably three times, the diameter of the bone at the level of the fracture. Interfragmentary screw fixation is stable enough to allow early active range of motion, but it has the disadvantage of requiring special equipment and being somewhat technically demanding.

Reduction is achieved by anatomically interdigitating the proximal and distal apex of the fracture into its corresponding fragment under direct visualization. After this is done, the reduction is held with two bone clamps and the screws are inserted. Fixation may be achieved by using two 2.7-mm screws or three 2.0- or 2.4-mm screws. The diameter of the bone and configuration of the fracture may dictate mixing screws of different diameters in the same fracture.

In general, I reserve plate and screw fixation for complex situations such as open fractures when there is a combination of diaphyseal bony loss or comminution associated with significant soft tissue injury (Fig. 8-14). Successful plate application is technically gratifying, provides stable fixa-tion, and maintains length when there has been comminu-tion or bone loss. However, plate application is demanding and there is no margin for error. Application requires consid-erable soft tissue mobilization, and the plates are somewhat bulky. Sometimes removal is necessary and a fracture can occur through a screw hole or at the "original" fracture site. Furthermore, application requires a variety of plates and screws, special instrumentation, and power equipment. I prefer a 2.4-mm plate that allows screw fixation of at least four cortices, both proximal and distal to the fracture, to ensure stable fixation. Supplemental fixation with an inter-fragmentary screw (for transverse and short oblique fractures) placed either through a hole in the plate or obliquely across the fracture significantly enhances fracture

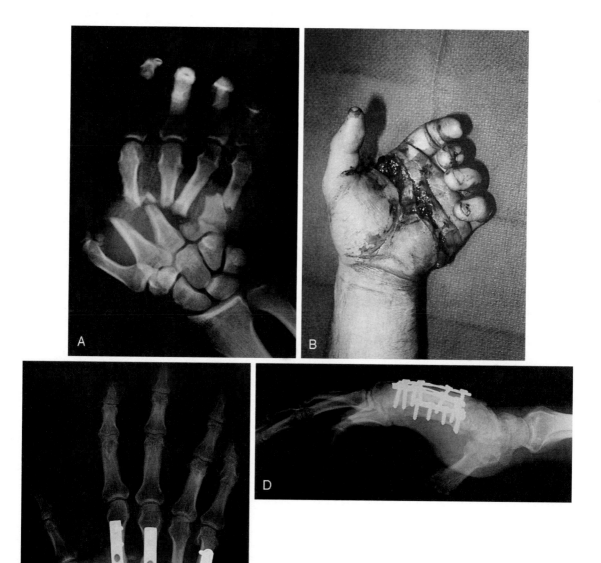

FIGURE 8-14. Plate fixation for metacarpal shaft fractures. **A,** Shaft fractures of all four metacarpals. **B,** The fractures were open and revascularization was required. **C,** Anteroposterior radiograph showing healed fractures. Plate fixation provided a stable framework for microvascular repairs. **D,** Lateral view.

stability.[144] Plate fixation is undesirable if the fracture cannot be covered by local soft tissue or flaps. In such situations, I prefer external fixation.

Whenever possible, after ORIF the periosteum is approximated if possible with an absorbable suture. A forearm-based plaster splint with bulky dressing is applied for 4 to 7 days. Assuming stable reduction, active range of motion is initiated. The wrist is splinted in a slightly dorsiflexed position. Restoration of full MCP flexion may be difficult because of edema, intrinsic muscle injury, and subsequent MCP collateral ligament contracture. To maximize MCP flexion, elastic garments are worn for edema control and the IP joints are splinted in extension when MCP flexion exercises are being carried out.

Hardware removal depends on the type of implant. Generally, Kirschner wires can be removed between 3½ and 6 weeks after fixation. The AO-ASIF group[197] recommends screw and plate removal approximately 6 months after fixation. They note three potential problems if implants are left in place:

1. *The volume factor.* Implants may contribute to tendon adhesions and also to the development of an irritating bursa.
2. *Implant compatibility.* Implants occasionally cause corrosion or allergy.
3. *Alterations in bony structure.* Implants are load bearing and may produce osteopenia beneath the plate, both by stress shielding and by interference with circulation to the bone. Others[373] believe that the screw holes are a more important cause of weakness after plate removal than is bone atrophy.

Despite the aforementioned admonitions, I do not routinely remove plates. If the plate is perceived as bulky or is irritating, I will remove it. Also, if there are restrictive adhesions and a tenolysis/capsulotomy is indicated, I remove the plate. One should tell the patient that refracture may occur after plate removal.

Bioabsorbable Fixation

Although infrequently used in the United States, bioabsorbable implants are commonly used in some European locations. During fracture healing, the implants maintain fracture stabilization; however, over time they hydrolyze, resulting in stresses being transferred to the healing bone and thereby avoiding stress shielding.[131] Furthermore, a second procedure, implant removal, is avoided. The implants are composed of either polyglycolic acid, polylactic acid, or polyparadioxanone[41] and can be fabricated into pins, screws, rods, or plates. The most common complication is a noninfectious inflammatory response that occurs 7 to 30 weeks after fracture fixation in 5% to 25% of cases.

Biomechanical testing in cadaveric metacarpal and phalangeal bone shows that the implants provide fixation stability that is generally comparable to that of metal implants.[131,375,459]

Clinically, bioabsorbable intramedullary rods were compared with metal implants[254] for the fixation of metacarpal and phalangeal shaft fractures. There were no differences in outcome with respect to time to union, range of motion, and return to work. In another series, biodegradable pins (12 patients) were compared with Kirschner wires (11 patients) in the fixation of fractures, arthrodeses, and osteotomies in a prospective randomized study.[224] No difference in time to union or complications was observed. Moreover, there were no inflammatory reactions in the biodegradable cohort.

Segmental Metacarpal Loss

Restoration of metacarpal stability and function after segmental bone loss is a challenge. This situation occurs after an open injury and is nearly always associated with varying degrees of soft tissue injury or loss. Restoration of hand function is usually staged and begins with thorough débridement of devitalized tissue. A discussion of the timing of the soft tissue reconstruction is beyond the scope of this chapter, but it should not begin until a stable osseous framework has been achieved.

There are two philosophies regarding the primary management of acute metacarpal segmental bone loss. The traditional viewpoint espoused by Peimer and associates[340] advocates maintaining metacarpal length with transverse intermetacarpal Kirschner pins and/or external fixation devices, with soft tissue coverage performed as a primary or delayed primary procedure. Bone grafting is performed only after joint motion is regained and healed wounds have matured. They reported nine patients with an average of 2 years elapsed by the time secondary reconstructions by bone, nerve, and tendon grafts or transfers were completed.

Freeland and associates[140,146,148] believe that the best time to restore osseous stability with a bone graft and internal fixation is within the first 10 days of injury ("the golden period of wound repair"). They achieved union without infection in 20 of 21 delayed primary bone grafts after traumatic bone loss in the hand and wrist (11 involved the metacarpals).[148] Initial wound care consisted of débridement and temporary skeletal stabilization. Three to 7 days later the wound was reinspected and if it was judged to be ready for closure or coverage then definitive fracture stabilization, bone grafting, and skin flap coverage (if required) were performed. Calkins and colleagues[70] reported satisfactory functional results in 9 of 10 patients who had traumatic segmental bone defects of the hand. Corticocancellous grafts were inserted within 2½ weeks of injury. The soft tissue wounds were left open, there were no cases of infection, and all grafts went on to incorporate. The authors believed that stable fixation combined with bone grafting promoted optimum return of function by allowing for early mobilization to minimize chronic swelling, pain, tendon adhesions, and articular stiffness. Stahl and associates[414] recommended immediate bone grafting combined with internal fixation and soft tissue coverage when there was segmental bone loss.

Along similar lines, Gonzalez and colleagues[166] reported excellent results in the treatment of 64 metacarpal fractures secondary to low-velocity gunshot wounds treated with early (between 1 and 7 days) stabilization, usually with an intramedullary rod and supplemental iliac crest bone graft. There were no deep infections. The average range of motion at the MCP joint was 65 degrees, and the average shortening was 1.4 mm for high-velocity injuries (72,000 ft/sec). In addition to fracture stabilization, soft tissue débridement and replacement also may be necessary.[344]

Reconstitution of osseous stability involves two steps:

1. *Provisional stabilization* (Figs. 8-15 and 8-16). Maintenance of metacarpal length can be accomplished by a number of techniques, including traction,[161] transfixation pins,[119,256] spacer wires,[340] external fixation,[7,76,106,140,353] methylmethacrylate spacers,[271] and combinations of these techniques.

2. *Bone grafting* with or without internal fixation (Fig. 8-17). Most defects can be bridged with corticocancellous grafts harvested from the iliac crest. Littler[280] advocated cortical bone harvested from the proximal end of the tibia with dowel fixation into the proximal and distal medullary canals. Supplemental fixation could be secured with Kirschner pins. If the MCP joint was destroyed, he fused the proximal phalanx to the remaining metacarpal in 30 degrees of flexion. If more than one metacarpal has segmental loss, a single curved iliac crest graft designed to fit the defects in all metacarpals is useful. In recent years, a bridging plate in conjunction with pure cancellous or corticocancellous graft has gained popularity.[146,148,394]

Rose[372] used a delayed primary vascularized free groin flap to cover a large central hand defect in a 12-year-old boy. Subsequently, he reconstructed the bone loss with a free vascularized second MCP joint and common extensor tendons of the second and third toes.

Author's Preferred Method of Treatment

Generally, when there is metacarpal bone loss, there has been some injury or loss of the dorsal skin and extensor tendons. Following thorough débridement, osseous stability is achieved with an external fixator. The patient is then

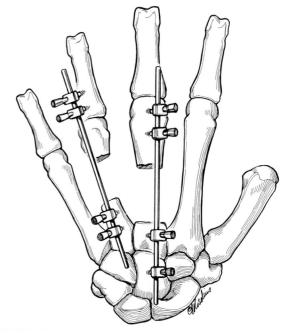

FIGURE 8-15. An external fixator is ideal treatment for metacarpal bone loss. Pins may be placed in carpus or phalanges when necessary.

returned to the operating room for additional débridement over the next 3 to 5 days, until the wound is surgically clean. At that time, a corticocancellous or cancellous bone graft is harvested from the iliac crest and fashioned to fit into the defect, with stabilization accomplished with an appropriately contoured dorsal plate. When there is bone loss from multiple metacarpals, I prefer to use a single block of corticocancellous or pure cancellous graft, rather than individual metacarpal bone reconstruction. Soft tissue coverage is obtained with either a regional, distant, or free flap. I prefer staged tendon reconstruction in which silicone rods are inserted at the time of flap coverage and replaced later with free tendon grafts.

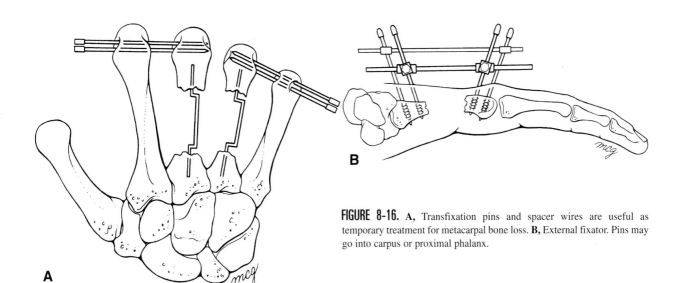

FIGURE 8-16. A, Transfixation pins and spacer wires are useful as temporary treatment for metacarpal bone loss. **B,** External fixator. Pins may go into carpus or proximal phalanx.

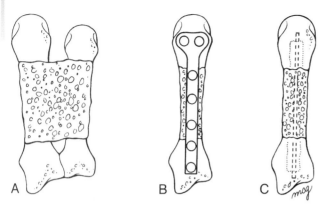

FIGURE 8-17. Techniques of corticocancellous or cancellous bone graft after metacarpal loss. **A,** A block of iliac crest graft is especially useful when there is bone loss in more than one metacarpal. **B,** Corticocancellous graft and plate fixation. **C,** Littler's technique using a corticocancellous dowel and intramedullary Kirschner pin.

Metacarpal Base Fractures and Carpometacarpal Fracture-Dislocations

Avulsion Fractures of the Second and Third Metacarpal Bases

Isolated intra-articular fractures of the base of the second and third metacarpals are rare because of the lack of motion in these joints: hence, there is no consensus regarding optimal treatment. These are usually the result of a fall on a palmar flexed wrist. Avulsion fractures from the dorsal base of the index and/or middle metacarpals have been successfully managed both operatively[104,374,444] and non-operatively.[92,475] Justification for surgical reattachment includes restoration of the integrity of the extensor carpi radialis longus or brevis as a functional wrist extensor, reconstitution of the articular surface of the CMC joint, and elimination of a potentially irritating fragment of dorsal bone.[446]

Fracture-Dislocations of the Small Finger CMC Joint

Intra-articular fractures of the hamate-metacarpal joint are common and are usually associated with proximal and dorsal subluxation of the metacarpal. Kerr[240] was the first to point out the similarities between this injury and Bennett's fracture. The hamate articulates with the ring and small metacarpals by two concave facets separated by a ridge. The base of the fifth metacarpal consists of a concave-convex facet that articulates with the hamate and a flat radial facet that articulates with the fourth metacarpal base. Dorsal and palmar intermetacarpal ligaments and an interosseous ligament stabilize the intermetacarpal joint. The injury results from a longitudinally directed force along the long axis of the fifth metacarpal. Usually the radial fourth to third of the base remains articulated with the hamate, whereas the rest of the metacarpal is subluxated proximally and dorsally. Dommisse and Lloyd[109] coined the terms *bipartite and tripartite fractures* of the metacarpal bone, depending on the number of fragments. The displacement is accentuated by the pull of the extensor carpi ulnaris and the flexor carpi ulnaris through the pisometacarpal ligament. Lilling and Weinberg[276] noted that the pull of the abductor digiti minimi

as well as the oblique slope of the hamate also contributed to the instability of CMC fracture-dislocations of the small finger.

Because the extent of the injury is frequently missed on routine radiographs, Bora and Didizian[39] have recommended an anteroposterior view with the forearm pronated 30 degrees from the fully supinated position. Niechajev[325] recommended a 60-degree supinated view because bony overlap was eliminated and the ring and small CMC joint surfaces could be clearly seen. The diagnosis can also be made by sagittal tomography or CT[298] or by using the Brewerton view.[237]

There is no consensus regarding optimal treatment of these fractures. Options run the gamut from closed reduction and cast immobilization to ORIF. Successful closed reduction and cast immobilization has been reported by Lundeen and Shin[293] and Hsu and Curtis.[204] However, Bora and Didizian[39] found that weakness of grip was the major functional disability resulting from inadequate reduction. Reduction of these fractures may be unstable, and I agree with several authors that have advocated closed reduction and percutaneous pin fixation of the fifth metacarpal to the fourth metacarpal or carpus to maintain reduction.[39,82,109,195,293,360,382,383]

Foster[137] advocated ORIF with intramedullary metacarpal pins for ulnar CMC dislocations. He believed that percutaneous fixation, particularly when the pins were placed transversely across the metacarpals, could lead to fixation failure. Pin insertion was performed by exposing the bases of the fourth and fifth metacarpals and passing a 0.062-inch pin distally through the metacarpal articular surface, down the medullary canal, and exiting dorsally in the distal shaft. The pin was next driven retrograde into the carpus such that it engaged the hamate and either the triquetrum or lunate. Either the proximal or distal end of the pin was left exposed for removal in 5 to 6 weeks. Eight of nine patients regained full digital and wrist motion.

Petrie and Lamb[343] treated 14 fracture-dislocations of the fifth metacarpal-hamate joint by immediate, unrestricted motion and reviewed them at 4½ years. Despite persistent metacarpal shortening, incongruity in the articular surface, and widening of the joint, only one patient had pain significant enough to affect work. They believed that the case for surgical treatment was not strong, inasmuch as arthrodesis of the joint could always be performed for persistent pain. On the other hand, Kjaer-Petersen and colleagues[246] reported that regardless of the method of treatment (closed, percutaneous, or open), 19 of 50 (38%) patients had some symptoms at a median follow-up of 4.3 years. They believed that restoration of the articular surface should be the goal of treatment. Papaloizos and coworkers[338] also advocated open reduction and noted that pain directly correlated with degenerative arthritis, which was attributed to nonanatomic reduction in several of their cases.

Cain and colleagues[69] noted that fracture-dislocations of the fourth and fifth metacarpal joints, in association with comminuted dorsal hamate fractures or coronal fractures through the hamate, were particularly unstable and thus ORIF was uniformly necessary. When the hamate shear fracture is a single fragment, screw fixation of the hamate fragment to the body serves to treat both the fracture and the dislocation.[143,285]

Multiple CMC Dislocations

Multiple CMC dislocations are high-energy injuries that nearly always require ORIF.[24,262,332,428] Lawlis and Gunther[262] reported on 20 patients, 14 of whom had multiple CMC dislocations. Closed reduction was uniformly unsuccessful because of redislocation or subluxation, and open reduction with Kirschner pin fixation was recommended. At 6½ years' follow-up, the only patients who had poor results were those who had isolated second and third CMC dislocations or concomitant ulnar nerve injury.

Schortinghuis and Klasen[389] reported on open reduction of combined fourth and fifth CMC dislocations in 11 patients. They noted that placing a screw or plate across the fourth CMC led to spontaneous reduction of the fifth metacarpal. This permitted early range of motion and satisfactory results in all cases.

Clendenin and Smith[83] reported relief of symptomatic arthritis of the hamate/fifth metacarpal joint when treated by arthrodesis using an iliac crest bone graft. Resection arthroplasty[32,154] and silicone interposition arthroplasty[174] have also been used for post-traumatic hamate-metacarpal arthritis.

Author's Preferred Method of Treatment

Fracture-dislocations of the fifth CMC joint are inherently unstable, and closed reduction and cast immobilization can be risky. Redislocation may not be appreciated because radiographic imaging is difficult, as a result of bony overlap and plaster artifact. Also, many of these injuries occur in unreliable patients. Therefore, for simple fracture-dislocations of the fifth CMC joint, I prefer closed reduction and percutaneous pinning. After adequate regional or general anesthesia, longitudinal traction is applied and downward pressure is exerted on the base of the fifth metacarpal. Under image intensification, the fifth metacarpal shaft is pinned in extra-articular fashion to the fourth metacarpal. A second pin can be obliquely directed across the fifth metacarpal-hamate joint (Fig. 8-18). When multiple fragments or comminution exists, preoperative CT may be useful. If ORIF is elected, a dorsal ulnar incision is used to visualize the joint. Care must be taken to protect the dorsal sensory branch of the ulnar nerve. The joint is débrided of fracture fragments, the articular surface is reduced as best as possible, and reduction is maintained with multiple Kirschner pins or small screws. Occasionally the comminution is so great that restoration of articular integrity of the base of the fifth metacarpal is impossible. In this case, arthrodesis using a corticocancellous bone graft from the distal end of the radius can be accomplished. Postoperatively, a forearm-based ulnar gutter splint is applied. Digital motion is started at 10 to 14 days, and the internal fixation pins are removed at 6 weeks.

For multiple CMC joint dislocations, ORIF is nearly always indicated. The dislocated joints are well visualized through a dorsal longitudinal incision. The reduction is usually simple to accomplish and can be maintained with Kirschner pins extending from the metacarpals into the carpal bones.

If a fracture-dislocation of the fifth CMC joint is seen more than 3 weeks after the injury, I prefer to accept the alignment. If symptomatic arthritis exists a year after the injury, a fusion can be carried out.

For patients with symptomatic CMC joint arthritis, I prefer arthrodesis using a corticocancellous slot graft from the iliac crest (Fig. 8-19). Fixation is accomplished with either Kirschner pins or a plate ("T", "L", or minicondylar design) extending from the hamate to the fifth metacarpal shaft. Fusion of this joint does not significantly compromise hand function.[83]

Complications of Metacarpal Fractures

Malunion

Metacarpal malunions may be classified as either extra-articular or intra-articular. Extra-articular malunions may be *angulatory*, usually as a result of a malunited transverse shaft fracture; *rotational*, as a result of a spiral or oblique fracture; or *shortened,* as a result of a crush injury with bone loss. After crushing injuries or open fractures, there may be shortening and associated soft tissue problems such as tendon adhesions, poor skin coverage, and neurologic deficit.[45] In such cases, one may elect to simultaneously perform an osteotomy and correct the soft tissue problem(s).

In the past there has been pessimism regarding corrective osteotomy. More recently, especially with the use of plates and screws, union rates have approached 100% and there has been a high degree of clinical satisfaction.[292,381,448] Lucas and Pfeiffer[292] reviewed the AO experiences with osteotomies for 26 metacarpal and 10 phalangeal malunions. The osteotomy was done at the site of the deformity and fixation was accomplished with plate and screws. There were no nonunions, and 86% of the patients were satisfied. The failures were due to loss of motion or failure to fully correct the deformity.

Dorsal Angulation

Metacarpal malunion after a transverse fracture results in dorsal angulation in the sagittal plane. This may cause weakness of grip or pain.[292] Healing of second and third metacarpals with angulation is particularly bothersome, both cosmetically (pseudoclawing) and functionally (i.e., prominent metacarpal head in the palm that is painful when gripping). Correction can be accomplished through either an opening or closing wedge osteotomy. A closing wedge osteotomy (Fig. 8-20) is simpler[170] but has the potential disadvantage of metacarpal shortening. Preoperatively, the size of the wedge is calculated by using a template, and intraoperatively the volar periosteum is left intact to act as a hinge. I prefer fixation with a 2.4-mm dorsal plate. Supplemental cancellous bone graft harvested from the distal end of the radius[305] is packed around the osteotomy. Union usually takes longer than after uncomplicated fracture fixation.

If the metacarpal is appreciably shortened because of bone loss, an opening wedge osteotomy (Fig. 8-21) with a trapezoid interpositional iliac crest bone graft is preferable.[397] Stable fixation to allow early motion is accomplished with a dorsal plate.

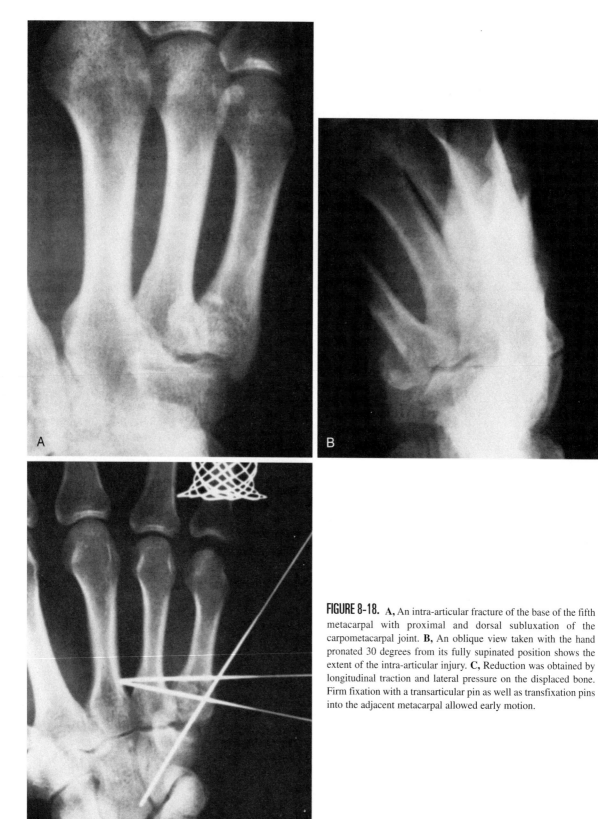

FIGURE 8-18. **A,** An intra-articular fracture of the base of the fifth metacarpal with proximal and dorsal subluxation of the carpometacarpal joint. **B,** An oblique view taken with the hand pronated 30 degrees from its fully supinated position shows the extent of the intra-articular injury. **C,** Reduction was obtained by longitudinal traction and lateral pressure on the displaced bone. Firm fixation with a transarticular pin as well as transfixation pins into the adjacent metacarpal allowed early motion.

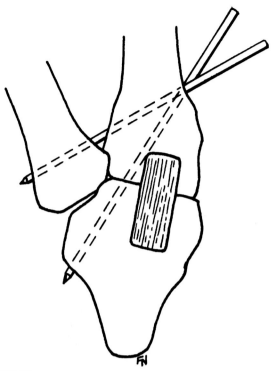

FIGURE 8-19. Method of arthrodesis of the fifth carpometacarpal joint with an inlay graft and pins.

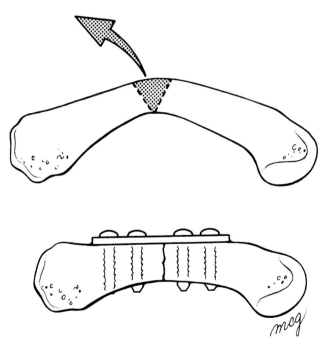

FIGURE 8-20. Metacarpal closing wedge osteotomy for malunion. The volar periosteum is left intact, a precisely calculated triangular wedge is removed, and fixation is provided with an AO plate.

Malrotation

Rotational malunion of a metacarpal results in overlapping of the affected finger over an adjacent finger (scissoring). It usually results from a malunited spiral or oblique fracture. The cosmetic deformity is often marked and grip is impaired. Weckesser[465] advocated a corrective osteotomy through

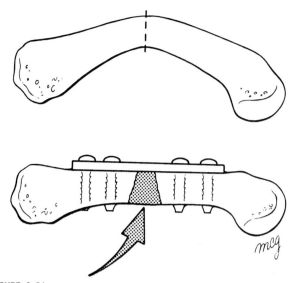

FIGURE 8-21. If there is significant metacarpal shortening, an opening wedge osteotomy and plate fixation will reconstitute metacarpal length, although a bone graft is required.

the base and was able to correct up to 25 degrees in each direction for either metacarpal or phalangeal malunions. Fixation was accomplished with two transverse Kirschner pins through the distal fragment and into the adjacent metacarpal and was supplemented with a longitudinal pin extending across the osteotomy site. Menon[313] reported full correction in 11 of 12 osteotomies through the metacarpal base. Before the osteotomy, he inserted a Kirschner pin into the metacarpal perpendicular and distal to the osteotomy site, carried out the osteotomy, and then used the Kirschner pin as a handle to rotate the distal fragment into the desired position. Fixation was accomplished with crossed Kirschner pins. Gross and Gelberman[180] noted that the maximal phalangeal correction obtained in fresh cadaver metacarpal osteotomies was 18 to 19 degrees for the index, long, and ring fingers and 20 to 30 degrees for the small finger. The transverse metacarpal ligament limited the maximum rotation obtained, but the orientation of the MCP joint did not limit its motion. Butler[66] used a small staple to fix a correctional metaphyseal osteotomy. Reid[363a] performed a corrective osteotomy for metacarpal malrotation in the metacarpal and for phalangeal malrotation in the phalanx. Others[295,345] have used a rotational step-cut osteotomy. Manktelow and Mahoney[295] used this method to successfully correct metacarpal malrotation in ten patients. Two hemitransverse osteotomies on opposite sides of the metacarpal diaphysis are accomplished and connected by a longitudinal dorsal osteotomy. A predetermined longitudinal strip of dorsal cortex (1.3 mm of dorsal bone results in 1 cm of fingertip correction) is removed, and then a longitudinal fracture is created in the volar diaphyseal surface. Tightening with interosseous wires approximates the gap.

I have been pleased with the results achieved when the osteotomy is performed through the metaphyseal base with the technique (Fig. 8-22) described by Weckesser.[465] After rotational correction, the osteotomy is transfixed with a longitudinal Kirschner pin. Correction is then assessed by observing the tenodesis effect of wrist flexion and extension,

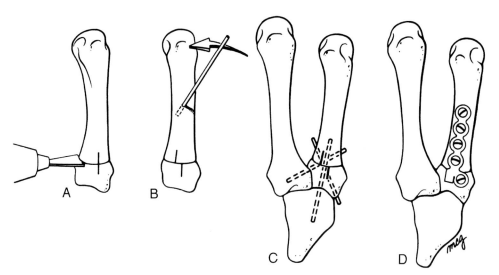

FIGURE 8-22. Metacarpal osteotomy for rotational malunion. **A,** Before osteotomy, a longitudinal mark is placed on the metaphysis with an osteotome. The osteotomy is made with an oscillating saw perpendicular to the mark. **B,** A Kirschner pin in the shaft acts as a "joystick" for correction. Fixation is accomplished with multiple (**C**) Kirschner pins or a (**D**) plate.

assessment of the plane of the fingernails, and checking that the fingertips point to the scaphoid tuberosity. If satisfied with the correction, the osteotomy is held with additional Kirschner pins and supplemented with cancellous bone graft from the distal end of the radius.[305] This fixation technique is appealing because it is simple and forgiving and union usually occurs rapidly. As an alternative, fixation can be secured with a "T"-plate, "L"-plate, or minicondylar plate. This is technically more demanding, and care must be taken to not lose correction when the plate is being applied and to make sure that there is good contact between the bony surfaces.

Intra-articular Malunions

Intra-articular malunions are rarely amenable to corrective osteotomy. If the fracture line can be visualized and bone stock is satisfactory, osteotomy with reconstitution of the articular surface is the optimum treatment.[273,274] Duncan and Jupiter[111] reported successful correction of three malunited metacarpal head fractures by performing an osteotomy through the malunion and maintaining the reduction with either screws and a plate, or screws alone supplemented with cancellous bone graft.

Osteomyelitis

Osteomyelitis occurring after metacarpal fracture fixation is uncommon and treatment must be individualized. In a review of osteomyelitis of the tubular bones of the hand, delay in treatment of more than 6 months or more than three procedures was associated with a very high amputation rate.[364] For metacarpal shaft osteomyelitis, I prefer staged treatment:

1. Remove loose implants and generously débride bone and soft tissue. Then stabilize the proximal and distal segments with an external fixator[114] to preserve length. Stabilization and length preservation can be supplemented with a block of antibiotic-impregnated polymethylmethacrylate. This also provides an open bed for insertion of a future bone graft. Obtain aerobic and anaerobic cultures, and administer appropriate systemic antibiotics for at least 4 to 6 weeks.

2. Re-débride wound until it is surgically clean and allow wound closure by secondary intention.
3. When sepsis has cleared, insert cancellous or corticocancellous bone graft, preferably with plate and screw fixation.

Nonunion

Nonunion after closed metacarpal fractures is uncommon. Nonunions may be classified as either hypertrophic or atrophic.[149] Hypertrophic nonunions are rare in the hand[170]; most are atrophic and hypovascular. Recommended treatment in these cases requires resection of the pseudarthrosis, bone grafting, and stable internal fixation.[149,196]

Nonunions usually occur after bone loss, osteomyelitis, inadequate immobilization, or poor fixation[168,232] (i.e., a metacarpal fracture pinned in distraction) and are extremely rare in children.[214] Prolonged plaster immobilization in the presence of delayed union of a metacarpal fracture is contraindicated because of the attendant MP stiffness.[65] Jupiter and associates[232] advised surgical intervention as early as 4 months. They reported 25 nonunions in 23 patients. Nine occurred in metacarpals, most of which had previously been internally fixed with Kirschner pins. Six of nine nonunions were treated to obtain union, and all healed after bone grafting. Three were fixed with an AO plate and two by Kirschner pins, and one had no fixation. Rigid internal fixation not only allowed early active motion but also permitted concomitant procedures such as capsulotomy and tenolysis.

Management of infected nonunions must be individualized. First, all infected bone and fibrous tissue are débrided. This is followed by skeletal stabilization (external fixation) and appropriate skin coverage. When there is no clinical or hematologic evidence of sepsis (usually 4 to 8 weeks), delayed bone grafting and internal fixation can be accomplished. For persistent nonunions of the border rays, especially those with associated stiffness or contracture, ray amputation should be considered.[210]

Other Complications

Complications are the result of the fracture itself, treatment of the fracture, or a combination of both. Table 8-3 outlines complications inherent to the various techniques of stabilization.

Tendon adhesions occurring after closed metacarpal fractures are uncommon. Usually, adhesions follow tendon lacerations or crush injuries and are most frequently seen between the extensor tendons and the underlying bone. Initial treatment should consist of therapy and include dynamic MCP flexion splinting. Should this fail, tenolysis with or without capsulotomy is indicated.

Intrinsic muscle dysfunction can occur under the following circumstances: loss of innervation, loss of substance, or secondary to contracture. Significant loss of intrinsic muscle substance or denervation can result in clawing, and treatment may require tendon transfers. Intrinsic contractures may also occur, especially after a closed, crushing-type injury associated with an unrecognized hand compartment syndrome, and may require intrinsic releases to improve function.

PHALANGEAL FRACTURES

Fractures of the Distal Phalanx

Distal phalangeal fractures are the most commonly encountered fracture in the hand.[386] The thumb and middle finger are most frequently injured because they extend most distally during work activities.[67] DaCruz and coworkers[100] prospectively reviewed 110 patients with distal phalangeal fractures and noted that fewer than one in three patients had completely recovered at 6 weeks. Numbness, cold sensitivity, hyperesthesia, restricted distal interphalangeal (DIP) joint movement, and nail growth abnormalities frequently occurred. Distal phalangeal fractures can be classified (Table 8-4) into tuft fractures, shaft fractures, and intraarticular injuries.

Tuft Fractures

Tuft fractures usually occur secondary to a crushing injury and are often associated with laceration of the nail matrix

---

Table 8-4
CLASSIFICATION OF DISTAL PHALANGEAL FRACTURES

Tuft Fractures
Simple
Comminuted

Shaft Fractures
Transverse
  Stable
  Unstable

Longitudinal

Articular Fractures
Volar (profundus avulsion)

Epiphyseal
  Child (Salter-Harris type I or II)
  Adolescent (Salter-Harris type III)

Dorsal (mallet fractures)

Modified from Schneider LH: Fractures of the distal phalanx. Hand Clin 4:537-547, 1988.

---

and/or the pulp. Closed tuft fractures are frequently associated with a painful subungual hematoma. Decompression provides dramatic pain relief and can be accomplished with a small drill bit, heated paper clip, or a battery-powered electrocautery. A short period of immobilization (10 to 14 days) is indicated for symptomatic relief. Comminuted tuft fractures rarely require internal fixation. Instead, attention should be focused on carefully approximating associated lacerations of the pulp and nail matrix. In so doing, the underlying bony fragments better reduce and the likelihood of nail abnormalities is lessened. These fractures often fail to unite but are invariably stabilized by a fibrous union.[386,466] Immobilization is rarely indicated for more than 3 weeks and should not include the PIP joint.[173] If the nail plate is intentionally perforated to decompress a hematoma or removed to perform a nailbed repair, a closed fracture is theoretically converted to an open fracture, and a short course of oral antibiotic therapy is generally advised.

Shaft Fractures

There are two types of shaft fractures: transverse and longitudinal. Nondisplaced transverse fractures are sufficiently stabilized by the surrounding soft tissue and do not require internal fixation. Displaced transverse fractures, on the other hand, may be open and are often associated with a transverse laceration of the overlying nail matrix. After débridement, stabilization is accomplished with a longitudinal Kirschner pin or with a small screw.[367]

Epiphyseal Fractures of the Distal Phalanx

Epiphyseal injuries of the distal phalanx result from hyperflexion. Failure to recognize and treat this injury, especially in a toddler, can result in a foreshortened digit that has decreased range of motion at the DIP joint.[460] In preadolescents, a Salter-Harris type I or II injury occurs; and in adolescents, a Salter-Harris type III injury results.[468] The injury may be manifested as an open mallet deformity and mistaken for DIP joint dislocation. The terminal tendon is attached to the proximal epiphyseal fragment, and the profundus tendon, attached to the distal fragment, causes it to flex. In children there is nearly always a transverse laceration of the nail matrix, and the nail plate lies superficial to the proximal nail fold (Fig. 8-23). Seymour[398] and Wood[477] cautioned against discarding the nail plate because it is useful in maintaining fracture reduction. Engber and Clancy[121] recognized that simple reduction without treatment of the soft tissue injury results in loss of reduction and infection. Banerjee reported two cases of irreducible epiphyseal fracture secondary to interposition of a proximally based flap of nail fold.[9] Appropriate treatment consists of irrigation and débridement, fracture reduction, repair of the lacerated nail matrix, and replacement of the nail plate beneath the proximal nail fold to act as a stent in maintaining the reduction. Postoperatively, a splint is applied to hold the distal fragment in extension. Alternatively, a longitudinal Kirschner pin can be placed across the DIP joint to hold the epiphysis in an anatomically reduced position.[1]

Complete dorsal displacement of the distal phalangeal physis (Salter I fracture) is rare and can be missed because its epiphysis does not ossify until 1½ to 3 years of age.[1] Treatment with ORIF within a month can lead to a satisfactory outcome.[32,464] However, when a child presents late,

SEYMOUR FRACTURE

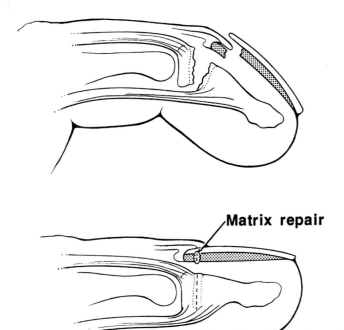

Matrix repair

FIGURE 8-23. An open epiphyseal fracture of the distal phalanx in a child. Note (**top**) the matrix disruption *(stippled)*; the nail plate has been avulsed and is dorsal to the proximal nail fold. Reduction (**bottom**) requires matrix repair and replacement of the nail plate beneath the proximal nail fold.

Table 8-5

FACTORS INFLUENCING OUTCOME AFTER PHALANGEAL FRACTURES

Patient Factors
Age

Associated diseases and arthritis

Socioeconomic status

Motivation and compliance

Fracture Factors
Location
   Intra-articular versus extraarticular

Geometry
   Simple, comminuted, impacted, bone loss
   Transverse, oblique, spiral, avulsion
   Deformity: angulation, shortening, rotation

Stability

Injury to soft tissue sleeve

Associated injuries
   Tendon, ligament, joint, vessel, nerve, other digits

Management Factors
Diagnosis and recognition

Reduction and maintenance

Length of immobilization

Recognition and management of complications

Modified from Strickland JW, Steichen JB, Kleinman WB, Flynn N: Factors influencing digital performance after phalangeal fracture. *In* Strickland JW, Steichen JB (eds): Difficult Problems in Hand Surgery. St. Louis, CV Mosby, 1982, pp 126-139; and Strickland JW, Steichen JB, Kleinman WB, et al: Phalangeal fractures: Factors influencing digital performance. Orthop Rev 11:39-50, 1982.

---

there is a dorsal bump secondary to continued growth of the dorsally displaced epiphysis. Reduction may not restore full DIP joint motion.[460]

Complications
Symptomatic nonunion of distal phalangeal fractures occurs occasionally.[363] Itoh and coworkers[217] reported six patients with nonunions of the waist of the distal phalanx successfully treated with crossed Kirschner pins and bone graft with exposure through a palmar midline approach. Malunion necessitating surgery is also unusual, although Kelikian[238] performed a distal phalangeal osteotomy for a radial deviation deformity in a violinist.

Fractures of the Middle and Proximal Phalanges

Phalangeal fractures that are stable and nondisplaced can be effectively managed by buddy-taping or splint immobilization. However, for successful outcome of many fractures, a sophisticated approach is necessary. Each fracture type has its own characteristics and can be influenced by multiple factors (Table 8-5).[427,428] Improper treatment often leads to stiffness and deformity.

In studies by Strickland and colleagues,[427,428] several factors had a deleterious effect on ultimate digital mobility.

They pointed out that if an extra-articular fracture occurred in the first 2 decades of life, 88% of the mobility was restored; however, in the sixth and seventh decades less than 60% of total active motion was restored. In addition, older patients are more likely to have chronic diseases or underlying osteoarthritis that could contribute to residual stiffness. Uncooperative and noncompliant patients must be identified.[185] They require heavy-duty splints and casts that are not removable, and if surgery is performed, rigid fracture fixation is recommended.

Fracture factors (intra-articular versus extra-articular) have a major influence on the ultimate result. Stark[416] noted that intra-articular fractures have a generally poorer prognosis than extra-articular fractures. More recently, Shibata and associates[400] suggested that stability and alignment are more important than articular congruency in determining outcome. Along similar lines, O'Rourke and colleagues[331] reported a low incidence of late symptomatic osteoarthritis in conservatively treated articular fractures, and they also observed articular reconstitution over time in the small joints of the hand. Likewise, comminuted fractures, those associated with bone loss, and unstable fractures with significant deformity are also prone to residual disability regardless of the method of treatment. Injury to the soft tissue sleeve, usually the result of a crushing injury, may severely compromise digital mobility.[13,134,205,213,221,358,427,428] Duncan and coworkers[112] reviewed 140 *open* fractures at an average time past surgery of 17 months. They found that there was a direct correlation between the severity of the soft tissue injury and the final range of motion at follow-up. In addition, they found that fractures located in flexor tendon zone II had the worst prognosis. Woods[478] points out that the final range of motion after proximal phalangeal fractures depends not only on bony union but also on restoration of flexor and extensor excursion, which may be limited, especially when there is an open fracture with soft tissue compromise. Huffaker and coworkers[205] concluded that flexor tendon injuries have a more serious effect on recovery of digital mobility than do extensor tendon injuries. Prolonged immobilization clearly has a detrimental influence. Most authors[35,221,229,321,483] believe that it is safe to immobilize the digit for three or fewer weeks. Strickland and associates[427,428] pointed out that if immobilization after a phalangeal fracture was less than 4 weeks, final active motion was 80% of normal. However, if immobilization exceeded 4 weeks, total active motion declined to 66% of normal.

Finally, a successful outcome depends on selection of the appropriate treatment. The therapeutic armamentarium is vast and ranges from buddy-taping and short-term splinting to complex methods of internal fixation. Appropriate selection must be tailored to the individual patient and fracture.

It is convenient to divide phalangeal fractures into articular and nonarticular injuries. Articular fractures include condylar fractures; comminuted intra-articular fractures; dorsal, volar, or lateral base fractures; fracture-dislocations; and shaft fractures extending into the joint. Extra-articular fractures include fractures of the neck, shaft, or base.

Articular Fractures of the Phalanges

Condylar Fractures

Condylar fractures were classified by London[283] in 1971. Type I consists of stable fractures without displacement, Type II includes unicondylar, unstable fractures, and type III fractures are bicondylar or comminuted. They are common

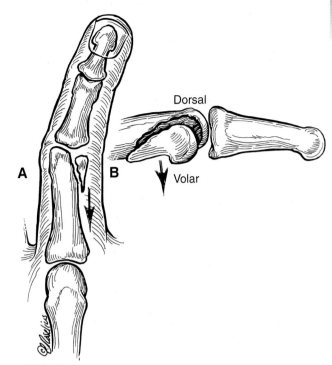

FIGURE 8-24. **A,** Anteroposterior view of condylar fracture. Note articular stepoff. **B,** Lateral view. Note volar displacement of condylar fragment.

athletic injuries, and as Stark[416] pointed out, unicondylar fractures of the proximal phalanx tend to be missed because the athlete can often bend the finger quite well. In addition to standard anteroposterior and lateral radiographs (Fig. 8-24), oblique radiographs[151] are mandatory to properly visualize the fracture geometry and better assess displacement. If the initially undisplaced fracture is misdiagnosed as a sprain and the patient continues to use the hand, subsequent displacement with angulation of the finger and joint incongruity is likely.[35]

Weiss and Hastings developed a useful classification for unicondylar fractures of the proximal phalanx (Fig. 8-25).[470]

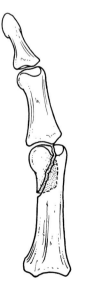
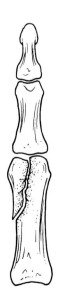
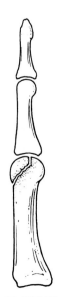
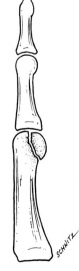

CLASS I
(Oblique Volar)

CLASS II
(Long Sagittal)

CLASS III
(Dorsal Coronal)

CLASS IV
(Volar Coronal)

FIGURE 8-25. Weiss-Hastings classification of unicondylar fractures of the proximal phalanx. These fractures are nearly all unstable and nearly always require operative fixation. (From Weiss APC, Hastings HH: Distal unicondylar fractures of the proximal phalanx. J Hand Surg [Am] 18:594-599,1993.)

They made several significant observations. First, even initially nondisplaced fractures are inherently unstable; five of seven fractures initially treated with a splint became displaced. Therefore, nonoperative management warrants extremely close follow-up. Second, fixation with a single Kirschner pin is inadequate. The preferred fixation techniques include multiple Kirschner pins, mini-screw(s), or a combination of the two. Of these, multiple Kirschner pins provided the best final range of motion at the PIP joint. Finally, regardless of the fracture pattern, full range of motion at the PIP joint was unlikely and was secondary to a flexion contracture and/or extensor lag.

There is a general consensus that displaced unicondylar fractures require ORIF.* The two most popular techniques of fixation are (1) Kirschner pins and (2) a lag screw.

---

*See references 35, 52, 136, 141, 151, 192, 221, 242, 263, 291, 299, 341, 377, 387, 393, 416, 420, 469, and 485.

Rayhack and Bottke[362] reported a combination of interosseous compression wiring and a single Kirschner pin. Fahmy and Harvey[125] expressed concern that ORIF could lead to osteonecrosis and/or comminution of the condylar fragment, as well as stiffness secondary to the surgical manipulation. They reported successful use of a dynamic flexible external fixator. Postoperatively, a 20- to 30-degree PIP flexion contracture[136] or an extensor lag is not infrequent.[471] Some correction of this problem can be obtained by dynamic extension splinting.

Barton and coworkers[10,331] generally recommend nonoperative management for intra-articular phalangeal fractures. They performed ORIF 10% of the time, anticipated articular remodeling, and noted that symptoms and range of motion continue to improve more than 1 year after fracture. Nevertheless, for a displaced condylar fracture, Barton recommends open reduction and pin fixation.

Bicondylar fractures and comminuted intra-articular fractures can be very difficult to fix. Buchler and Fischer

---

CRITICAL POINTS: OPERATIVE MANAGEMENT OF UNICONDYLAR FRACTURES OF THE PROXIMAL PHALANX

INDICATION

- Any displaced condylar fracture

PREOPERATIVE EVALUATION

- Evaluate for angulation or malrotation with flexion.
- Obtain anteroposterior radiograph to assess articular stepoff.
- Check on lateral radiograph to see if fractured condyle is displaced palmarly.
- Check on oblique radiograph for orientation of fracture line.

PEARLS

- This is a highly unstable fracture; err on side of operative intervention.
- Internal fixation *always* requires two screws or two Kirschner pins or one of each.

TECHNICAL POINTS

- Closed reduction by application of longitudinal traction is worth a try.
  - If reduction is achieved, provisionally hold it with one or two towel clips.
  - Confirm reduction with fluoroscopy.
  - Percutaneously fix the fracture with two Kirschner pins (0.7 or 0.9 mm).
- If closed reduction fails, proceed to open reduction.
- Make dorsal longitudinal incision on side of fracture.

- Enter PIP joint by incising between lateral band and central tendon.
- Take care not to detach central tendon.
  - Expose condylar fragment from its apex proximally to articular surface distally.
  - When mobilizing condylar fragment, take care not to detach collateral ligament.
  - Reduction must be anatomic both at the articular surface and proximally so that the condylar apex keys into the phalanx.
  - Provisionally maintain reduction with Kirschner pin or drill bit to later be replaced by a screw.
  - Fix with two Kirschner pins (0.7 or 0.9 mm) or two (lag) screws (2.0 mm or 1.5 mm [1.3 mm]).
  - Confirm reduction with permanent radiographs (three views).

PITFALLS

- One screw or pin may result in loss of reduction from either rotation or loosening.
- Detachment of collateral ligament may produce instability or osteonecrosis of the condylar fragment.

POSTOPERATIVE CARE

- At 5 to 7 days, initiate active range of motion.
- Splint PIP joint in full extension when not exercising.
- Remove Kirschner pins at 3 to 4 weeks.

used a minicondylar plate.[57] Schenck[385] and Stassen and associates[418] used dynamic traction. Steel[420] recommended primary joint arthrodesis, and Fahmy[124] reported success with a spring-loaded external fixation device.

Chin and Jupiter[79] described a *triplane* fracture (coronal, sagittal, and transverse planes) of the head of the proximal phalanx. A satisfactory outcome was achieved with two 1.5-mm interfragmentary screws.

Other Fractures of the Head of the Phalanx

Displaced *collateral ligament avulsion* fractures of the head of the proximal phalanx may be symptomatic if nonunion or fibrous union results. Open reduction or repair of these injuries should be done more often than currently practiced, especially if the injuries are associated with lateral instability. A pseudoboutonnière deformity[303] develops when the ligamentous and the resultant fracture healing causes adhesions between the adjacent lateral band, oblique retinacular ligament, and volar plate.

Extensively comminuted phalangeal head fractures may preclude satisfactory open reduction. These fractures are frequently associated with significant damage to the soft tissue sleeve and are best treated nonoperatively. Treatment can consist of manual molding to restore general alignment, immobilization for 10 to 14 days, and early protected motion or traction.[385]

Dorsal, Volar, or Lateral Base Fractures

Avulsion fractures of the dorsal base of the middle phalanx represent detachment of the insertion of the central tendon and are usually the result of an anterior PIP joint dislocation.[412] If the avulsed fragment is displaced more than 2 mm, accurate reduction is necessary to prevent extensor lag and subsequent boutonnière deformity (Fig. 8-26).

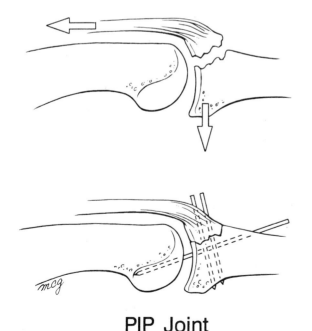

PIP Joint

FIGURE 8-26. Anterior PIP fracture-dislocation. Avulsion fracture from the dorsal base of the middle phalanx results in anterior displacement of the middle phalanx (**top**). Open reduction with Kirschner pins and transarticular pinning (for 3 weeks) is necessary for fracture and joint reduction (**bottom**).

Fractures of the lateral volar base of the proximal or middle phalanx usually represent collateral ligament avulsion injuries. Minimally displaced lateral corner fractures that do not compromise joint stability or result in an incongruous articular surface can be treated by splinting for 10 to 14 days, followed by protected motion. Lee[264] collected 27 corner avulsion fractures of the proximal phalanx. All but two patients were managed nonoperatively by splintage for 2½ weeks, and all but two fractures united in the original displaced position. Significantly displaced lateral corner fractures may compromise joint stability. The recommended treatment is ORIF with either Kirschner pins or tension wire.[233,413] Kuhn and colleagues[252] recommended a volar approach for internal fixation of the fracture. They reported 11 avulsion fractures; and at final follow-up, all patients had full range of motion, a stable MCP joint, and grip strength that was 90% of the opposite side. To expose the fracture, the A1 and proximal portion of the A2 pulley are completely divided and the flexor tendons are retracted to expose the volar plate (Fig. 8-27). The volar plate is longitudinally split in its midline and detached distally from the proximal phalanx on the side of the fracture. The avulsed fragment is now well visualized and reduced. Fixation is accomplished with either small (1.5 mm or less) screws or Kirschner pins. The volar plate is repaired, and the digit is immobilized in partial flexion. With secure screw fixation, protected active range of motion is initiated at the first postoperative visit.

Hastings and Carroll[192] brought attention to lateral plateau fractures of the base of the middle phalanx. They postulated that these are compression injuries that result in articular depression and metaphyseal bony compaction. Open reduction with cancellous bone grafting as a buttress is recommended. More recently, Wolfe and Katz[476] noted that these injuries may be misdiagnosed and treated as a sprain. Using CT scans, they demonstrated impaction of 30% of the articular surface and articular depression between 1 and 4 mm. They reported excellent results in six patients treated by open reduction, bone graft, and pin and tension band fixation.

"T" fractures of the base of the proximal phalanx often require ORIF (Fig. 8-28). These are generally approached through a dorsal extensor tendon-splitting incision to accurately visualize the articular surface. Fixation can be accomplished with a minicondylar plate[57] or Kirschner pins. If the fracture is significantly comminuted and ORIF is precluded, skeletal traction or a spanning external fixator should be considered.

Comminuted intra-articular fractures, particularly those at the base of the middle phalanx, have been termed *pilon fractures*. The fracture is the result of an axial load that causes central articular depression and variable splay of the articular margins. Stern and associates[425] reported 20 injuries treated in three fashions: splintage, traction through the middle phalanx, and open reduction. Splintage resulted in significant stiffness. Skeletal traction through the middle phalanx (Fig. 8-29) and ORIF had similar results. In no case was there anatomic articular restoration, and no patient regained full mobility. Regardless of the treatment, there was significant articular remoding over time. Because of the unpredictable outcome associated with treatment of this injury, a variety of dynamic external fixation devices have been developed.[192,251] These devices are hinged and span the

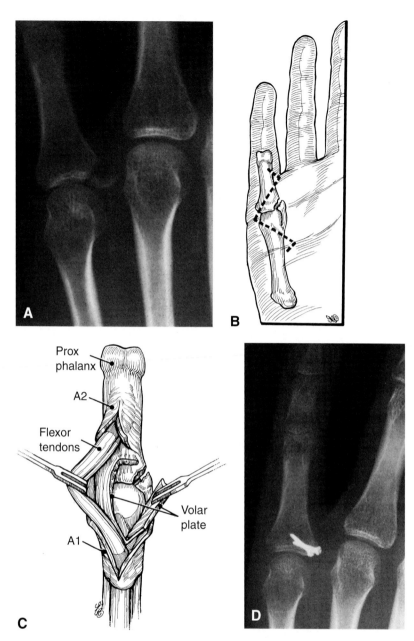

FIGURE 8-27. **A,** Radiograph demonstrating displaced avulsion fracture from radial base of proximal phalanx. **B,** Zigzag incision used to expose fracture. **C,** The A1 pulley (not shown) and proximal part of the A2 pulley are divided. The volar plate is split longitudinally and detached distally from its insertion on the base of the proximal phalanx to expose the fracture. **D,** Radiograph demonstrating fracture reduction and fixation with two mini-screws.

PIP joint to allow early protected range of motion while maintaining reduction of the joint. In addition, when necessary, one can perform limited open reduction and cancellous bone grafting.

Physeal Fractures

Eighty-five to 90 percent of the epiphyseal fractures of the proximal and middle phalanx are Salter-Harris type II. The fracture usually involves the small finger,[2] and angulation is usually in an ulnar[401] direction; as such, it is often referred to as the *extra-octave* fracture. The majority can be treated by closed reduction and splinting. Bogumill[38] pointed out that the collateral ligament inserts exclusively into the epiphysis in the proximal phalanx, whereas the ligamentous insertion into the middle phalanx extends beyond the epiphysis. Reduction is usually easily accomplished by flexing the MCP joint maximally to stabilize the proximal fragment while the deformity is corrected. After reduction (MCP joint

flexed 70 degrees and the IP joints extended), an ulnar gutter splint incorporating the adjacent digit is applied for 2½ to 3 weeks. James[221] used only buddy-taping to maintain stability after reduction. Occasionally, open reduction is necessary. Leonard and Dubravcik[268] cited one patient in whom open reduction of a juxtaepiphyseal fracture was required because of fibrous tissue interposition in the fracture. Von Raffler[456] and Harryman and Jordan[189] each reported a child in whom closed reduction was impossible because the flexor tendons were displaced dorsal to the fracture.

Salter-Harris type III fractures occur at an average age of 14.9 years and are produced by an avulsion force.[93] In a review of pediatric hand fractures by Hastings and Simmons,[194] these fractures, when left unreduced, were prone to deformity and produced the majority of poor functional results. Displaced Salter-Harris type III or IV epiphyseal fractures require accurate open reduction[130,413,421] and fixation with tension band, small pins, or suture.

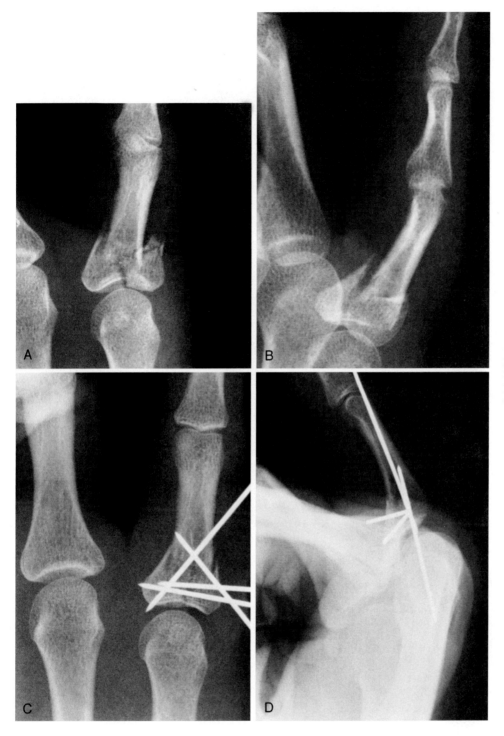

FIGURE 8-28. **A** and **B,** A comminuted T-fracture of the base of the proximal phalanx. **C** and **D,** Open reduction with multiple Kirschner pins. Healing was followed by a 20-degree flexion loss at the MCP joint.

Epiphyseal fractures involving the proximal phalanx are opened through a dorsal tendon-splitting incision. Similar fractures involving the base of the middle phalanx can be approached laterally by incising the interval between the transverse retinacular ligament and the dorsal apparatus.

Leclercq and Korn,[263] in a review of articular fractures in children, noted a high rate of "sequelae" (malunion, osteonecrosis, stiffness, and infection) in displaced articular fractures. They attributed the poor results to the fractures being initially missed, improper treatment (a belief that these fractures will remodel with future growth), and redis-

placement after closed reduction. They recommended surgical treatment for displaced articular fractures. Posttraumatic arthritis in unreduced articular fractures can occur particularly after crush injuries, displaced Salter-Harris type III and IV injuries,[341] and intracondylar and subcondylar fractures of the head of the proximal and middle phalanx.

Shaft Fractures Involving the Joint
A long spiral fracture of the proximal (and sometimes middle) phalanx may project into the retrocondylar space of the IP joint and block flexion. ORIF is usually necessary. If

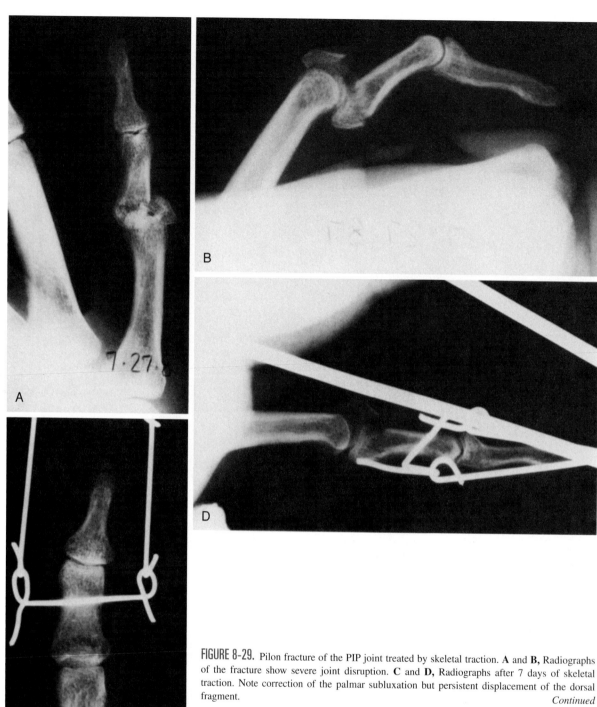

FIGURE 8-29. Pilon fracture of the PIP joint treated by skeletal traction. **A** and **B,** Radiographs of the fracture show severe joint disruption. **C** and **D,** Radiographs after 7 days of skeletal traction. Note correction of the palmar subluxation but persistent displacement of the dorsal fragment.

Continued

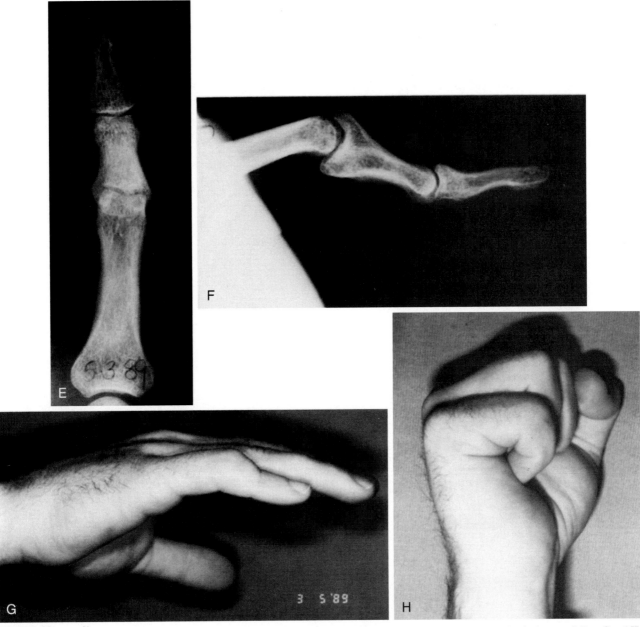

FIGURE 8-29—cont'd. E and **F,** Twenty-one months after injury there has been consolidation of the fracture fragments and articular remodeling. **G** and **H,** At 21 months' follow-up there is excellent flexion. However, there is persistent PIP joint swelling and loss of extension. (From Stern PJ, Roman RJ, Kiefhaber TR, McDonough JJ: Pilon fractures of the proximal interphalangeal joint. J Hand Surg [Am] 16:844-850, 1991.)

the fracture is unreduced and heals with a residual spike that blocks PIP flexion, the bony projection can be removed to improve motion.[170,267]

Author's Preferred Method of Treatment: Articular Fractures

Nondisplaced unicondylar fractures are potentially unstable. Immobilization in a splint is risky and displacement should

be anticipated. If nonsurgical treatment is selected, careful and frequent radiographic follow-up is mandatory to avoid a malunion with articular incongruity. Displaced unicondylar fractures are best managed operatively (Fig. 8-30). Even if closed reduction can be obtained, the fracture is intrinsically unstable and redisplacement is likely. The fracture is exposed through either a dorsal radial or dorsal ulnar curved longitudinal incision. The joint is entered between the central tendon and lateral band. The central tendon should not be detached from its insertion into the dorsal base of the middle phalanx. Fracture hematoma is removed, with care taken to not detach the condyle from its attachment to the collateral ligament. Under direct visualization, the fracture is anatomically reduced with a bone tenaculum and the

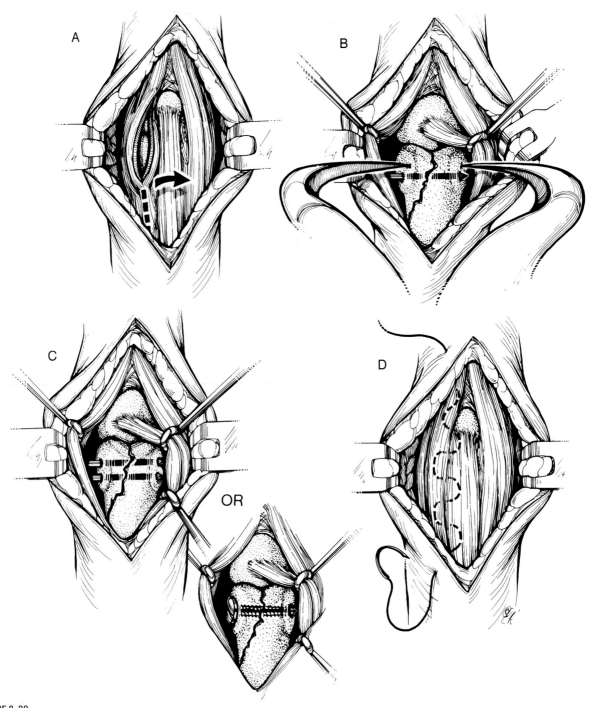

FIGURE 8-30. Method of open reduction of a condylar fracture of the proximal phalanx. **A,** The fracture is exposed between the central tendon and the lateral band. Care must be taken to not disrupt the insertion of the central slip from the middle phalanx and the origin of the collateral ligament from the condylar fragment. **B,** The fracture is reduced and held with towel clips (a specially designed cannulated clamp may also be used). **C,** Internal fixation is accomplished with two transverse Kirschner pins or small screws. **D,** The central slip and lateral band are reapproximated with a running 4-0 suture.

reduction confirmed fluoroscopically. The condylar fragment is fixed with two parallel Kirschner pins (0.028 or 0.035 inch) drilled through the fragment into the intact bone. Interfragmentary screw fixation with two 1.5- or 1.3-mm screws can be used if the fracture fragment is two and one-half to three times the external diameter of the screw. The dorsal apparatus is approximated with either running or inverted nonabsorbable suture. Postoperatively, early active motion is initiated and the PIP joint is splinted in *extension*

to avoid extensor lag. Kirschner wires are removed at 3 to 4 weeks. Screws do not require removal unless they are symptomatic.

Although ORIF is the standard of care for the management of condylar fractures, I have been pleased with the results of closed reduction and percutaneous pin fixation (Fig. 8-31). Using a mini "C"-arm, a pin is placed into the condylar fragment and used as a joystick to manipulate the fragment into its anatomic position. Fingertrap traction is

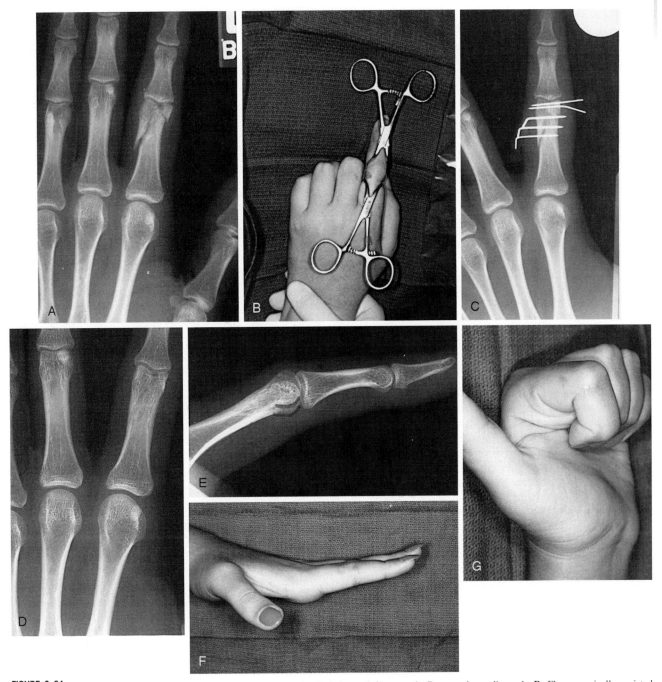

FIGURE 8-31. Percutaneous fixation of an unstable bicondylar proximal phalangeal fracture. **A,** Preoperative radiograph. **B,** Fluoroscopically assisted reduction held with towel clips. **C,** Percutaneous pin fixation. **D,** Anteroposterior view of the healed fracture. Note the small central-radial depression. **E,** Lateral view. Volar condylar surfaces (outlined) should be collinear. They were not in this case. **F and G,** Final extension and flexion.

sometimes helpful to assist in reduction and to free the surgeon's hands for fragment manipulation and fixation. The reduction is provisionally maintained with a bone tenaculum, and the reduction is verified with the image intensifier. Fixation is then secured with two to three appropriately sized Kirschner pins. Miniature cannulated screws of 1.1 and 1.5 mm in diameter are also available for percutaneous management of these fractures. These techniques have the advantage of minimizing soft tissue dissection but can be tedious and do not allow direct visualization of the fracture to verify anatomic reduction.

Bicondylar fractures of the proximal phalangeal head are nearly always displaced and often comminuted. Anatomic restoration of articular congruency usually cannot be accomplished by closed manipulation. Open reduction using the same approach as for unicondylar fractures is advised (Fig. 8-32). First, the two condyles are reduced and fixed to each other with either a screw or Kirschner pins. Next, the head fragment is secured to the shaft in a similar fashion. Supplemental cancellous bone graft may be added if there is significant comminution. Early range of motion is encouraged; however, residual stiffness and/or extensor lag is not

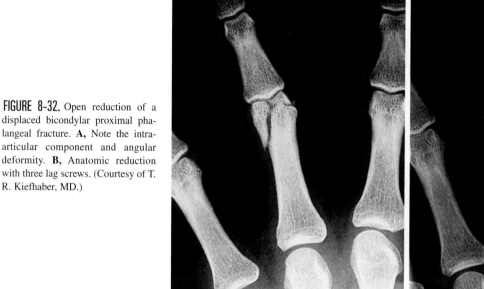
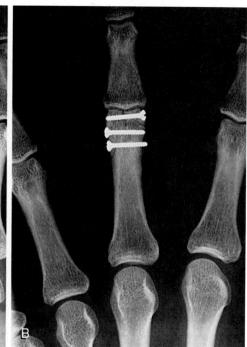

FIGURE 8-32. Open reduction of a displaced bicondylar proximal phalangeal fracture. **A,** Note the intra-articular component and angular deformity. **B,** Anatomic reduction with three lag screws. (Courtesy of T. R. Kiefhaber, MD.)

uncommon. When there is significant comminution, open reduction may be frustrating and restoration of the articular surface may be impossible. In such circumstances, I prefer skeletal traction through the middle phalanx for 3½ to 4 weeks. The traction is secured to a forearm-based splint to immobilize the proximal phalanx but allow active flexion of the PIP joint. Fracture consolidation can be anticipated, and some articular remodeling will occur. Restoration of full motion is unlikely. Primary arthrodesis is unpredictable and may result in excessive shortening.

Because loss of DIP joint mobility is less disabling, bicondylar fractures of the head of the middle phalanx can sometimes be treated by closed reduction, molding, and early protected motion at around 2 weeks, especially if minimally displaced. If open reduction is necessary, a dorsal lateral approach with mobilization of the conjoined lateral bands allows sufficient exposure to perform ORIF with either Kirschner pins or screws. Diminished motion of the DIP joint can be anticipated.

Untreated displaced (> 2 mm) fractures of the dorsal base of the middle phalanx can lead to a boutonnière deformity. I prefer open reduction through a dorsal approach between the central tendon and the lateral band. Fixation can be accomplished with two small Kirschner pins or mini-screws. The fixation must be protected with a transarticular Kirschner pin for 3 weeks.

Displaced fractures of the base of the proximal phalanx require open reduction. I prefer a volar approach in which the A1 and proximal portion of the A2 pulley are divided followed by splitting the volar plate longitudinally. The fracture is easily visualized and anatomic reduction can usually be achieved and preferably held with small screws. Gentle range of motion can be initiated within 1 week of fixation. Isolated fractures of the base of the middle phalanx are unusual; fracture-dislocations and pilon fractures of the PIP joint are covered elsewhere in this volume. If reduction

and fixation of an isolated middle phalangeal base fracture is required, I prefer a midaxial approach with care being taken to maintain the integrity of the collateral ligament. Fixation is accomplished with either small screws or Kirschner pins.

Nonarticular Fractures of the Phalanges

Neck Fractures

Neck fractures (subcapital or subcondylar) of the phalanges are uncommon in adults and can usually be managed either in closed fashion by reduction and splinting or by percutaneous crossed Kirschner pins.

Neck fractures of the proximal or middle phalanx are common in toddlers and result when the child violently attempts to withdraw a finger trapped in a closing door (Fig. 8-33). The serious nature of the neck fracture may be missed unless a true lateral radiograph is obtained. In this view, displacement of the head fragment is best visualized. With lack of tendon attachment, the head fragment displaces dorsally and will rotate 90 degrees such that the fracture surface faces palmarly and the cartilaginous surface faces dorsally. On cursory examination of the anteroposterior view, the rotated head has an ovoid appearance, much like a normal metacarpal head epiphysis, and this may lead to misinterpretation.[243] These fractures are deceptive and have little capacity to remodel in either the coronal or sagittal plane.

Displaced fractures usually require open reduction (Table 8-6). Repeated attempts at reduction may cause further displacement.[210] Fractures involving the head of the middle phalanx can be approached radial or ulnar to the conjoined lateral band, reduced, and pinned with a single Kirschner pin extending longitudinally from the distal phalanx, across the DIP joint and head fragment, and into the middle phalanx. Fractures of the middle phalanx are approached

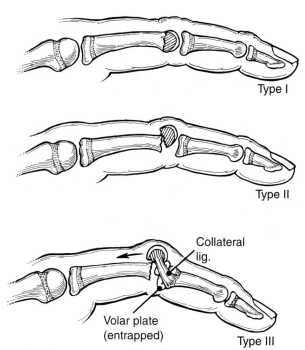

FIGURE 8-33. Classification of fractures of the neck of the proximal phalanx in a child. Type I: Nondisplaced fracture. Type II: Displaced with some bone to bone contact. Type III: Completely displaced, no bone to bone contact. May rotate 180°. (Modified from Al-Quattan MM: Phalangeal neck fractures in children: Classification and outcome in 66 cases. J Hand Surg [Br] 26:112-121, 2001.)

Table 8-6
MANAGEMENT OF PHALANGEAL NECK FRACTURES IN CHILDREN

Author	Comments
Leonard and Dubravick[268]	One redisplacement secondary to premature pin removal; extensor lag frequent
Dixon and Moon[108]	Two acute: one success and one redisplacement, Three late: one no treatment, one satisfactory, one unsatisfactory
Newington, et al.[324]	Five children, all with severely displaced neck fractures, successfully treated with open reduction and internal fixation
Barton[12]	If a "good" closed reduction cannot be achieved under general anesthesia, open reduction and pin fixation is recommended
Segmuller and Schonenberger[395]	Recommend open reduction with one or two pins across DIP joint
Campbell[72]	Recommends open reduction, dorsal approach, two crossed pins (4 weeks)
Hastings and Simmons[194]	Frequently overlooked on radiography
Al-Quattan[3,4]	Poor results from nonsurgical treatment of displacement (type II fractures) Recommends open reduction and pin fixation for all displaced fractures Maintain pin for 4 to 5 weeks

between the lateral band and central tendon, reduced, and immobilized with one or two Kirschner pins, preferably avoiding the base of the middle phalanx. In either case, the pins are left in place for 4 to 5 weeks.

Complications[4] include persistent angulation in either the frontal or sagittal plane, limited extension secondary to injury to the extensor tendon, limited flexion secondary to a bony block, and nonunion.

Delayed open reduction can be successfully carried out as late as 4 weeks; a Freer elevator is used to pry the fracture apart, followed by reduction and pin fixation. If the fracture is healed but PIP flexion is lacking, an ostectomy (Fig. 8-34) of the protruding spike of the proximal fragment can be carried out through a lateral approach.[330,402]

Shaft Fractures

Phalangeal fractures can be transverse, oblique or spiral, and comminuted. Spiral and oblique fractures are more common in the proximal phalanx, whereas transverse fractures tend to be more common in the middle phalanx. McNealy and Lichtenstein[309] accurately described the different fracture deformities in 1935. Proximal phalangeal fractures angulate volarly, the proximal fragment being flexed by the strong interosseous muscles. These same authors were the first to theorize that the deformity in middle phalangeal fractures depended on the relationship of the fracture to the superficialis insertion. They noted that flexion of the proximal fragment by the intact tendon in fractures distal to the superficialis insertion produced volar angulation. Fractures proximal to its insertion resulted in flexion of the distal fragment and dorsal angulation of the fracture. Flatt,[134] disputing the superficialis theory, noted that its insertion covered almost the entire palmar surface of the middle phalanx. He believed that the proximal one-fourth fractures were angulated dorsally because of pull from the unbalanced extensor insertion into the base of the middle phalanx. Middle two-fourth fractures could angulate in either direction, and distal one-fourth fractures were always angulated volarly because of the superficialis pull on the proximal fragment. Butt[67] believed that the type of deformity in displaced middle phalangeal fractures was related to the force and direction of trauma rather than the superficialis pull.

Healing Time

Many authors have commented on the lack of correlation between radiograph and clinical signs of union of phalangeal fractures. Smith and Rider[405] studied phalangeal (toes and hands) fracture healing and found that the average time for complete bony healing was approximately 5 months and that the clinical healing time when the patient could return to work was about one fourth of this. Moberg[317] found that the average time for clinical union was 5 to 7 weeks for the middle portion of the proximal phalanx and up to 10 to 14 weeks for transverse fractures of the exceedingly hard cortical portion of the middle phalanx. Borgeskov's

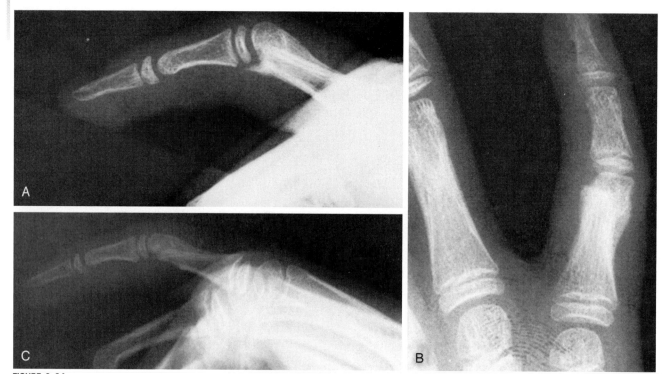

FIGURE 8-34. **A** and **B,** Malunion of a neck fracture of the proximal phalanx in an adolescent. Flexion was blocked by a volar spike at 30 degrees. **C,** Ostectomy of the volar spike restored 95 degrees of flexion.

healing times[40] were very similar to those reported by Moberg. Flatt[134] believed that transverse fractures of the phalanges were clinically healed in 5 to 6 weeks.

Closed Reduction with a Cast or Splint

Prior to 1960, phalangeal fractures were immobilized in a variety of positions, often with the MCP joints in extension and the IP joints flexed.[219,294,318,370,433] Digital stiffness was an almost inevitable sequela. It was James[221,222] who realized the importance of maintaining 70 degrees of MCP flexion to avoid the contracture of the collateral ligaments that occurs with MCP extension. The PIP joints are held in nearly full extension to prevent the collateral ligament and volar plate contracture that occurs in flexion (Fig. 8-35). Even so, almost all of the 58 patients having proximal phalangeal fractures treated by this method had some flexion contracture of the PIP joint with normal MCP motion. Wright[483] reported a large series of patients successfully treated by using James' principles of closed reduction and splint immobilization for 3 weeks for unstable fractures and buddy-taping with immediate motion for stable fractures.

Burkhalter[60,62] advocated treatment of proximal phalangeal shaft fractures by closed reduction and positioning in a short-arm cast with the wrist held in 30 to 40 degrees of extension. A dorsal plaster extension block is added to hold the MCP joints in maximal flexion and to allow full IP extension (intrinsic-plus position). He believed that the dorsal apparatus overlying the proximal phalanx acted as a tension band, and similar positioning of the adjacent digits controlled rotation and angulation. A program of immediate active flexion was then initiated. Reyes and Latta reported 92% satisfactory results using this technique,[366] and Ebinger and colleagues,[113] using a custom-molded two-component thermoplastic splint, also reported satisfactory results.

Barton[14] noted that 75% of phalangeal fractures did not require reduction and could be treated with strapping to the adjacent finger from the start. He found that if the immobilization was prolonged over 3 weeks, 60% of the patients had significant loss of hand function. Strickland and coworkers[427,428] found a return of function to between 75% and 80% of normal in fractured digits mobilized within the first 4 weeks after fracture. However, when mobilization was initiated after 4 weeks, only 66% return of function resulted. Borgeskov[40] stressed the value of early motion and recorded a good functional result in 68% of 485 metacarpal and phalangeal fractures treated without internal fixation.

Traction

Traction can be exerted through the skin, pulp, nail plate, or the skeleton (Table 8-7). It has the advantage of being minimally invasive and simple; however, traction may be difficult to maintain and is cumbersome.

Traction for extra-articular phalangeal fractures has had few advocates and has largely given way to external or internal fixation. Complications relating to the method of application, joint stiffness, difficulty controlling fracture alignment, and counterpressure problems no doubt explain its lack of popularity. Traction may have an occasional role in the management of comminuted fractures, those associated with extensive soft tissue injury, and highly comminuted intra-articular fractures.

External Fixation

External fixation is indicated for open fractures, especially those with concomitant soft tissue injury such as gunshot wounds, highly comminuted diaphyseal fractures, severely

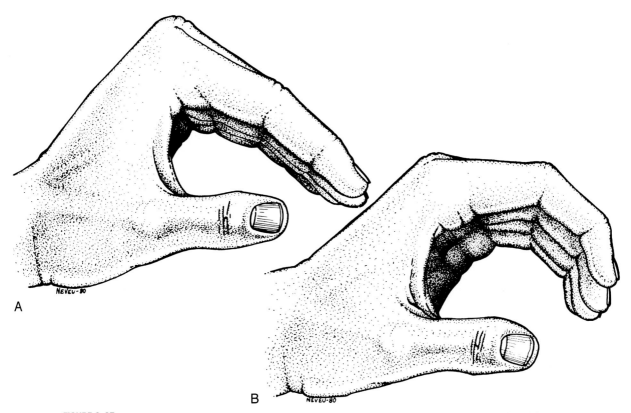

FIGURE 8-35. Positions of hand immobilization. **A,** The "safe" or intrinsic-plus position of James. **B,** Position of function.

Table 8-7
TRACTION FOR PHALANGEAL FRACTURES

Type of Traction	Author/Comment
Skin traction	Rooks[371]: 14 proximal phalangeal fractures; no complications Fitzgerald and Khan[132]: full range of motion in 16/18 fractures; no complications
Nail plate	Moberg[317]: 46 fractures; no complications Weeks and Wray[467]: hook in nail plate with finger in intrinsic-plus position
Pulp	Borgeskov[40]
Skeletal	Lipscomb[277]: wire loop through distal phalangeal tuft

comminuted articular fractures, and fractures with significant loss of bone stock.[7,97,110,230,319,361,396] Advantages include ease of insertion, minimal dissection and devascularization of soft tissue and bone, and preservation of bony length, and it provides access for additional soft tissue care.

Halliwell[186] performed a cadaver study to assess the optimum position for pin placement to maximize extensor tendon gliding. He recommended pin placement just off the dorsal midline of the proximal phalanx and direct dorsal placement over the middle phalanx. On the other hand, Drenth and Klasen[110] recommended pin placement in the transverse plane.

Ashmead and coworkers[7] reported a 90% union rate when using external fixation for acute hand fractures. There were no cases of hardware failure, one pin tract infection, and no iatrogenic tendon or neurovascular injuries, and the device was well tolerated psychologically. Bilos and Eskestrand[28] treated 15 gunshot wounds of the proximal phalanx with a Roger Anderson device. MCP joint motion was well preserved, there were no infections, and wound care was facilitated. Along similar lines, Smith and associates[407] treated nine gunshot fractures of the proximal phalanx (often with intra-articular extension) with external fixation and noted preservation of MCP motion but loss of IP motion. They ascribed the resultant IP joint stiffness to a variety of factors, including the magnitude of the soft tissue injury, pins impaling the dorsal apparatus, and the intra-articular nature of several of the injuries.

Inexpensive external fixators can be made. Godwin and Arnstein[160a] used a 2-mL syringe and four 1.1-mm Kirschner pins. Scott and Mulligan[392] used transverse Kirschner pins proximal and distal to the fracture that were bonded to external longitudinal Kirschner pins on each side with acrylic cement to accomplish the same end. Shehadi[399] treated 11 proximal and middle comminuted phalangeal shaft fractures by closed reduction and external fixation with initiation of active motion at 1 week. Final total range of motion was 84% of normal. Recently, Drenth and Klasen[110] reported the results of treatment of 20 proximal and nine middle phalangeal fractures. Eight of the nine middle phalangeal fractures had a good or excellent result, whereas only 12 of 20 of the proximal phalangeal fractures were in this category.

Another technique for preservation of digital length after bone loss was reported by Stern.[422] He inserted a temporary block of silicone, and after soft tissue healing, the silicone was successfully replaced by a bone graft in three patients.

Freeland[140] emphasized that external fixation is particularly useful in comminuted fractures that require concomitant management of soft tissue injury. He also noted that the device could be replaced with pins, plates, or screws at the time of delayed primary bone grafting and definitive wound coverage.[151]

Percutaneous Pinning

Percutaneous Kirschner pin fixation[19] has the advantage of stabilizing the fracture and allowing early motion while minimizing injury to the soft tissue sleeve. This technique is particularly useful in shaft fractures that are transverse, spiral, or oblique in orientation. Pin insertion should be done in the operating room, preferably with the aid of an image intensifier.[326] Barton[14] noted, however, that it was often difficult to obtain complete reduction, and the Kirschner pin passing through the soft tissue envelope may limit or prevent early mobilization.

A variety of pin configurations have been described for percutaneous placement to stabilize transverse fractures (Fig. 8-36). Vom Saal[455] advised intramedullary Kirschner pin fixation to maintain closed reduction of middle and proximal phalangeal fractures. He introduced the pin through the flexed IP joint distal to the fracture; and despite the fact that the pin protruded through the joint for 4 to 7 weeks, no definite infections were seen. Clifford[84] used Vom Saal's method successfully in 36 patients with phalangeal or metacarpal fractures. Flatt[134] used a single oblique Kirschner pin introduced through the head of the proximal phalanx with the PIP joint flexed 90 degrees. The pin was directed toward the more palmar portion of the head to one side of the midline and aimed to come out the opposite corner of the base of the phalanx dorsally. The wire was then withdrawn proximally until the PIP joint was freely mobile.

Kilgore and Graham[244] introduced transmetacarpal intramedullary Kirschner pin fixation by inserting the pin across

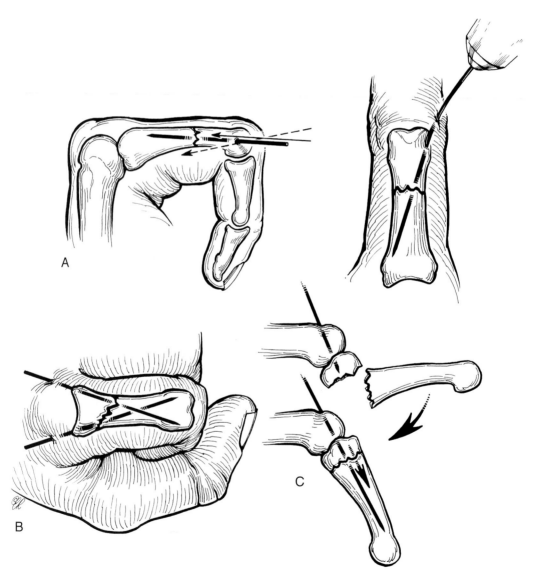

FIGURE 8-36. Three methods of closed reduction and percutaneous pinning of a transverse phalangeal fracture. **A,** The fracture is reduced in a 90-90 fixed position and a Kirschner wire is introduced in the retrocondylar fossa of the proximal phalanx. Slight reverse bowing of the pin while it is being drilled is often necessary. The normal dorsal bow of the proximal phalanx necessitates a slight dorsal direction of the pin. **B,** Alternative method of percutaneous pinning for fractures of the proximal half of the shaft. **C,** Technique for closed reduction and percutaneous pin fixation useful for extra-articular fractures near the base of the proximal phalanx. This method requires plaster immobilization for 3 weeks because the Kirschner pin crosses the MCP joint.

the flexed MCP joint and letting it protrude through the skin. Belsky and colleagues[17-19] used a similar technique in extra-articular transverse shaft fractures at various levels of the proximal phalanx with wrist block anesthesia. After reduction and percutaneous pinning through a flexed MCP joint, the fractures were immobilized for approximately 3 weeks. Good and excellent results were reported in 90% of fractures treated within 5 days of injury. Elmaraghy and associates,[118] using a similar technique, reported good or excellent results in 19 of 25 fractures; however, 8 of 25 patients developed a PIP joint contracture averaging 18 degrees. Hornbach and Cohen[201] reported excellent results in 10 of 12 fractures using two pins for rotational control inserted medial and lateral to the extensor tendon. This method was also advised by Heim and Pfeiffer[197] for a transverse fracture of the proximal phalangeal base. The flexed proximal fragment is immobilized by the pin while the distal fragment is reduced, and the pin is then drilled across the fracture. Joshi[229] avoided the MCP joint by introducing the wire through the base of the proximal phalanx. Using a strict postoperative exercise program, he obtained satisfactory results in 90% of 61 fractures.

Green and Anderson[171] achieved full range of motion in 18 of 22 patients with 26 long oblique fractures of the proximal phalanx treated by closed reduction and two or three percutaneous pins (midlateral) perpendicular to the fracture (Fig. 8-37). They left the pins in for 3 weeks and protected the finger by buddy-taping for an additional 3 weeks. Modified clamps are available[34,160] that not only maintain fracture reduction but also have a cannulated barrel that will accept a Kirschner pin for more accurate placement.

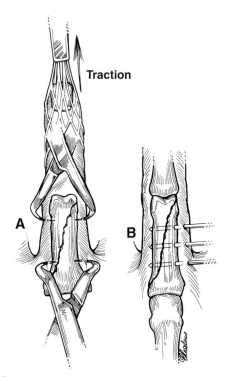

FIGURE 8-37. **A,** Closed reduction and percutaneous pinning of an oblique phalangeal fracture. The fracture is reduced by longitudinal traction and compressed with a towel clips or reduction clamp. **B,** Next, Kirschner pins are drilled transversely across the fracture.

Freeland and associates[142,150] introduced the technique of percutaneous screw fixation for spiral phalangeal fractures. After closed reduction (maintained with bone tenacula), a titanium self-tapping screw is inserted with fluoroscopic guidance through a very small incision. The value of this technique is that it minimizes soft tissue dissection and provides more stable fixation than Kirschner pins; however, more experience will be necessary before it can be recommended.

Open Reduction and Internal Fixation

If an unstable proximal and middle phalangeal fracture cannot be reduced or if percutaneous pinning is not possible, ORIF becomes an option. Ip and colleagues[213] showed that if operative fixation is undertaken, a rigid construct has a significantly better outcome than nonrigid constructs because immediate mobilization was possible.

Surgical Approaches

The desirability of exact anatomic reduction and solid internal fixation to permit early motion has been stressed by many authors.[197,213,242,258,323] Pratt[351] exposed the shaft of the proximal phalanx by splitting the extensor mechanism longitudinally and closing it with a running pullout wire suture (Fig. 8-38). It has the potential disadvantage of causing scarring of the dorsal apparatus to the skin and bone. Posner[350] used a midlateral incision and excised one of the lateral bands to expose the fracture. He opened the finger on the side to which the distal fragment had shifted (Fig. 8-39). Burton and Eaton[64] also found it occasionally necessary to excise a portion of the extensor mechanism to expose the fracture. Heim and Pfeiffer[197] preferred a long dorsal lateral incision with curved ends to expose the proximal phalanx. The proximal portion of the phalanx was then exposed through a longitudinal split in the extensor tendon, and the distal part of the phalanx was exposed by elevation of the lateral extensor tendon. Field and associates[128] recommended a midaxial approach to the proximal phalanx. They argued that scarring of the dorsal apparatus is less likely and PIP extensor lag is minimized. Barton[14] used lateral incisions on both sides of the finger to expose and fix a proximal phalangeal fracture. Jupiter and Silver[234] emphasized preservation of the dorsal veins and paratenon to avoid postoperative adhesions.

Pin Fixation

Smooth Kirschner pins have been by far the most popular technique of maintaining fracture reduction. A pin can usually be inserted with minimal soft tissue stripping, thereby preserving the blood supply to bone and enhancing the potential for healing. In addition, Kirschner pins, when compared with a plate or screws, are less bulky, may be inserted so that the dorsal apparatus is not impaled, and allow for easy closure of soft tissue.

Furthermore, pins are acceptable for nearly all fracture configurations. They have been used longitudinally or obliquely in the medullary canal for transverse or short oblique fractures. London[282] even bundled Kirschner pins together to fill the entire medullary canal. Placement perpendicular to the fracture or bone is recommended for long oblique fractures, and crossed Kirschner pins are best for transverse fractures; however, distraction may be a problem

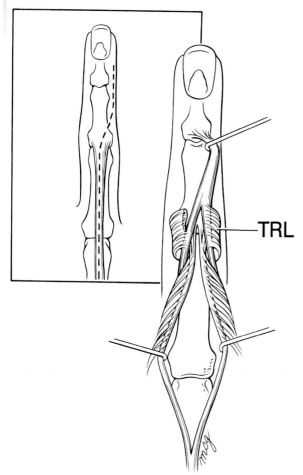

FIGURE 8-38. The author's preferred incision for exposure of proximal and middle phalangeal fractures. For proximal phalangeal exposure, the central tendon is longitudinally split. Care must be taken to not detach its insertion into the dorsal base of the middle phalanx. For middle phalangeal exposure, the transverse retinacular ligament (TRL) is divided at its insertion into the dorsal apparatus, and the fracture is exposed by retracting the conjoined tendon radially or ulnarly.

if the bone ends are not firmly impacted during pin insertion. Pin placement is easier in spiral fractures than transverse fractures because of the small diameter of the diaphysis.[175]

Considerable disagreement exists on whether the ends of the pins should be allowed to protrude through the skin or should be cut off beneath the skin. Kilbourne[242] believed that if the pins were left in for 3 weeks they could protrude but if left longer they should be cut off beneath the skin. Brown[52] preferred to bury the pin if it could be removed; otherwise, he left it protruding through the skin. Stahl and Schwartz,[415] in a series of 590 Kirschner pin fixations, noted no difference in the infection rate between buried and protruding pins.

Kirschner pins are not a panacea. Pun and coworkers[358] prospectively reported on 109 unstable digital fractures treated with Kirschner pin fixation. Nearly 70% had fair or poor results. Open fractures, comminuted fractures, and associated significant soft tissue injuries were unfavorable prognostic signs. These authors did not condemn Kirschner pin fixation but emphasized that there are many determinants of outcome, including stable fracture fixation.

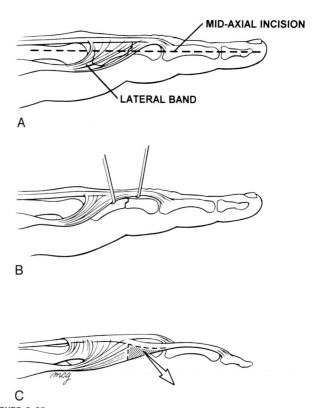

FIGURE 8-39. **A,** The midaxial incision is an approach to the proximal phalanx. **B,** The lateral band is retracted dorsally to expose the fracture. **C,** Alternatively, a triangular portion of the distal lateral band can be excised to facilitate exposure.

Greene and colleagues[175-177] and Safoury[379] have demonstrated that fracture stability is enhanced when the Kirschner pins are supplemented with stainless steel (26-gauge) wire, a technique termed *composite* (or tension band) *wiring* (Fig. 8-40). This technique is particularly useful in spiral and oblique fractures and should be avoided in comminuted fractures. As the stainless steel wire, which is looped under the pins, is cinched down, compression at the fracture site can be achieved. The Kirschner pins are cut so there is a 2- to 3-mm tail.

Screw Fixation

Because a single, longitudinal Kirschner pin does not provide rotational stability and crossed pins may distract the fracture, more rigid methods of fixation have been sought. Screw fixation enhances stability by using the lag technique to achieve interfragmentary compression. Biomechanical testing of an experimentally created spiral fracture of the proximal phalanx demonstrated that a single compression screw was superior to crossed Kirschner wires, interosseous loops, or a dorsal mini-plate when subjected to torsional and cantilever bending.[302] They are particularly useful in oblique and spiral fractures when the fracture length is at least twice the bone diameter.[147] A minimum of two screws is necessary, and they should be inserted at least two screw diameters from the fracture edge. In general, 2.0- and 1.5-mm screws are used in the proximal phalanx and 2.0-mm, 1.5-mm, and 1.3-mm screws are used in the middle phalanx. Even smaller-diameter self-tapping screws of 1.0 to 0.75 mm may be useful on a limited basis.

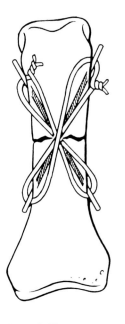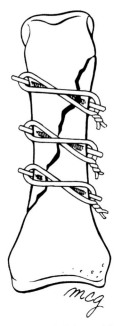

FIGURE 8-40. Technique of composite wiring in the proximal phalanx with 0.035-inch Kirschner pins and 26- to 28-gauge stainless steel wire. The pins are left protruding 2 to 3 mm. **Left,** Transverse fracture. **Right,** Spiral fracture.

Early clinical results of screw fixation were not favorable.[243] With the contributions of the AO/ASIF, results have been good to excellent.[20,90,136,198,211,393] Steel[419] advised AO screw fixation for proximal phalangeal fractures only if the length of the fracture exceeded two times the diameter of the bone. He recommended that the screw bisect the angle between a line perpendicular to the bone and one perpendicular to the fracture to obtain maximum compression and shear protection. In an uncontrolled, retrospective study, Diwaker and Stothard[107] compared Kirschner pin and AO screw fixation of phalangeal and metacarpal fractures. They concluded that screw fixation was superior because it allowed earlier mobilization.

Intramedullary Fixation

Grundberg[181] achieved union in 17 of 18 unstable phalangeal fractures stabilized with a buried intramedullary Steinmann pin introduced through the ends of the fractured fragments. In comminuted fractures, a 30-gauge circumferential wire supplemented fixation. Iselin and Thevenin[215] used a flexible intramedullary screw to provide axial compression in 37 phalangeal fractures. Immediate motion was permitted, and they believed that the results were superior to those of other methods of internal fixation. Gonzalez and coworkers[165] reported excellent results in 28 transverse and short oblique proximal phalangeal fractures treated with multiple pre-bent flexible intramedullary pins. After indirect fracture reduction, the pins were inserted under image intensification in an antegrade fashion through a hole in the dorsal cortex of the proximal phalanx.

Interosseous Wiring

Interosseous wiring can be used alone or as a supplement to Kirschner pin fixation (Table 8-8). It requires minimal exposure, is less prominent than screws and plates, and

Table 8-8
INTEROSSEOUS WIRING

Author	Comments
Lister[278]	Supplement to Kirschner pin fixation of phalangeal fractures; a few technical failures
Gingrass, et al.[159]	Used for articular, comminuted, and transverse fractures; few complications; can supplement with Kirschner pin
Scheker[384]	Used 19-gauge wire as drill to facilitate wire insertion
Gordon and Monsanto[167]	Digital replantation
Zimmerman and Weiland[486]	90-90 wiring for transverse fractures, replantation, and arthrodesis

theoretically minimizes the risk of adhesions to overlying tendons. The technique is most frequently used for transverse phalangeal fractures and in digital replantation.

Plate Fixation

Plate and screw stabilization of phalangeal fractures has the advantage of providing stable fixation, thereby permitting early range of motion.[218] Blair[33] believed that plate application should be used sparingly and that simpler techniques should be used whenever feasible. His primary indication for application was in unstable comminuted diaphyseal fractures (Fig. 8-41). This approach seems justified, inasmuch as plates are relatively high profile and may be difficult to apply and there is no margin for error. Extensive

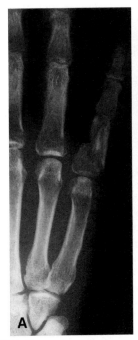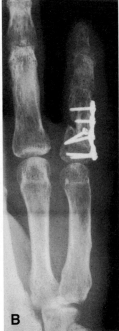

FIGURE 8-41. **A,** Comminuted, open, shaft fracture of the proximal phalanx. **B,** Fixation with 1.5-mm minicondylar plate and interfragmentary lag screw.

dissection of soft tissue may be necessary for exposure, and secondary removal or tenolysis may be necessary.[426] Page and Stern[336] reported complications after plate fixation of 39 phalangeal fractures. Total active digital motion was less than 180 degrees in 62% of fractures. Open fractures carried a particularly poor prognosis.

Dabezies and Schutte[99] reported excellent results in 32 phalangeal fractures stabilized with a lateral plate and screws. Total active motion of more than 220 degrees was seen in nearly all patients. Thaller and coworkers[438] reported encouraging results with a low-profile Vitallium mini-plate. Pun and colleagues[359] prospectively analyzed 42 unstable fractures treated by plate fixation. Results were good in 26%, fair in 33%, and poor in 41% of the fractures. When there was significant soft tissue injury, good results were seen in only 5% of the fractures. When they compared these results with those of a similar series from their institution treated by Kirschner pin fixation,[358] there was no statistically significant difference in the outcome of these two fixation techniques. Gonzalez and colleagues[166] acutely treated 28 proximal phalangeal fractures secondary to low velocity gunshot wounds with either a plate, intramedullary spacer, or both. Supplemental iliac crest bone graft was used in 20 fractures. All of the fractures united, there were no infections, and the average range of motion was 83 degrees and 66 degrees at the MCP and PIP joints, respectively.

Puckett and colleagues[356] applied maxillofacial mini-plates and micro-plates (0.8-mm screws) with excellent results. The screws are self-tapping, there is less periosteal stripping required for application, and the plates are low profile, which may result in less interference with extensor tendon excursion. Supplemental Kirschner pin fixation can be used if the construct is believed to be too fragile.

In 1987, Buchler and Fischer[57] introduced a laterally placed minicondylar plate for the stabilization of periarticular phalangeal (1.5 mm) and metacarpal (2.0 mm) fractures. Technical errors occurred in 18% of the cases, and secondary surgery was frequently necessary. Subsequent biomechanical studies demonstrated that lateral application of this plate resulted in less PIP flexion loss than did dorsally applied plates.[329] Ouellette and Freeland[334] reported 68 metacarpal and phalangeal fractures treated by using the minicondylar design. They noted a high complication rate secondary to technical errors and the severity of the fractures they treated.

Biomechanical Testing

Jones[228] points out that the results of biomechanical testing on various implants may be difficult to compare because investigators use different testing conditions (four-point bending versus three-point or cantilever bending), different bones, dissimilar implant constructs, different fracture patterns, and a variety of loads in different modes. We currently do not have enough information to determine how much stability is *needed* for a given fracture configuration to permit gentle active motion.

Fyfe and Mason[153] produced experimental fractures of the proximal phalangeal shaft and tested five methods of fixation. Straight Kirschner pin fixation proved to be the least rigid. Dorsal plating with ASIF mini-plates and screws allowed bending of the implant under load. Crossed Kirschner pin fixation was more rigid, and intraosseous

wiring supplemented with an oblique Kirschner pin yielded the most rigidity and consistency. Massengill and colleagues,[301] in experimentally produced transverse fractures in the pig metacarpal, found that two pairs of crossed Kirschner pins placed eccentric to the central axis dramatically improved the bending rigidity over one pair of crossed pins placed centrally. In a later article, these authors[300] analyzed various Kirschner pin fixation configurations, again using pig metacarpals. They concluded that Kirschner pins fail as the result of loosening and sliding within the bone. The pins were rated low in overall fixation strength. Plate and screw fixation had maximum bending moments that approached those of intact bone. They noted that volar or lateral plate and screw fixation was considerably stiffer and stronger than any configuration of the wire loop or the Kirschner pins. Gould and coworkers[169] concluded that tension band stabilization provides superior strength, stiffness, and approximation when compared with Kirschner pin fixation. Rayhack and associates[361] from the same laboratory experimentally studied transverse osteotomies and concluded that single-looped tension band wires were superior in strength to figure-of-eight constructs. Black and colleagues[31] studied rigidity and strength in an apex volar bending mode after fixing oblique osteotomies of cadaver proximal phalanges with five commonly used types of internal fixation. They noted that both of the techniques that used interfragmentary lag screws provided more rigidity than did dorsal plating alone or crossed Kirschner pins. Viegas and colleagues[453] biomechanically tested a variety of Kirschner pin fixations in oblique and transverse phalangeal fractures. They concluded that four crossed 0.028-inch Kirschner pins provided the highest rigidity for transverse fractures and three oblique 0.035-inch Kirschner pins provided the highest rigidity in oblique phalangeal fractures. Hung and associates[207] biomechanically tested five different fracture fixation techniques in fifth metatarsal porcine forelimbs. They concluded that an intramedullary Kirschner pin and a cerclage intraosseous wire, which theoretically provides compression as well as bending rigidity, were more stable than crossed Kirschner pins, as stable as a cerclage wire and oblique pin, but not as rigid as a dorsal plate.

Lu and associates[290] evaluated five different fixation techniques for stabilization of comminuted proximal phalangeal shaft fractures and concluded that a lateral (1.5-mm) plate provided the most rigid fixation. If plating was not possible, use of four crossed Kirschner wires was considered a satisfactory alternative.

Author's Preferred Method of Treatment: Phalangeal Shaft Fractures

As with any fracture, many factors enter into the decision for fracture management. Four categories must be considered.

1. *Stability.* Phalangeal fracture stability is determined clinically and radiographically. Fractures that have the potential to rotate, angulate, or shorten are considered to be

unstable. Rotation is difficult to judge radiographically and is best assessed clinically by having patients actively simultaneously flex their fingers while the examiner looks for digital overlap (scissoring). Angulatory malalignment is radiographically apparent in either the coronal or sagittal plane. Clinical angulation in the coronal plane results in digital overlap on flexion. Angulation (apex volar) in the sagittal plane of the proximal phalanx produces compensatory hyperextension at the MCP joint and an extensor lag at the PIP joint (pseudoclawing). Shortening, typically seen in comminuted fractures, is easily assessed both radiographically and clinically.

2. *Open versus closed.* Open phalangeal shaft fractures usually result from direct high-energy trauma and tend to be unstable.

3. *Associated injuries.* Fractures with injuries to adjacent structures such as nerves, vessels, the soft tissue sleeve, or tendons are usually open and generally require internal stabilization. Concomitant fractures either in the same ray or in the hand also necessitate operative fixation because it is difficult to maintain satisfactory alignment of multiple fractures by closed means.

4. *Fracture geometry.* Three basic fracture patterns occur: transverse, oblique and spiral, and comminuted. Transverse fractures tend to produce angulatory deformities in both the lateral and frontal views. Oblique fractures produce rotatory deformities, but they may also angulate or shorten. Comminuted fractures nearly always shorten and may also malrotate or angulate.

Nondisplaced and Stable

Management is nonoperative. If there is discomfort or soft tissue swelling, the digit is immobilized for a week with a dorsal splint (padded aluminum) extending one joint proximal and distal to the fracture. James' position, 70 degrees of MCP flexion and nearly full IP extension (often referred to as the "safe" position), is useful and should be used whenever possible in treating phalangeal fractures. A forearm-based splint with the wrist extended facilitates maintenance of this position. If there is minimal pain, immediate motion with buddy-splinting can be initiated. A nonelastic strap with Velcro on the end is less irritating than tape. Follow-up radiographs should be obtained at weekly intervals to make sure that alignment remains satisfactory.

Displaced: Stable After Closed Reduction

Displaced fractures that are malaligned can often be manipulated into alignment and stabilized. Transverse fractures of the proximal and middle phalanx are especially amenable to closed reduction. First, flex the MCP joint maximally to stabilize the proximal fragment and then flex the distal fragment to correct the volar angulation. Particular attention should be paid to rotation by comparing the planes of the nails. The reduction can be maintained with a clam-digger or short-arm cast (wrist in neutral or slightly extended), with a dorsal plaster extension block holding the MCP joints flexed 70 to 90 degrees and the IP joints extended (see Fig. 8-9). The extension block splint should include the adjacent digits with buddy-taping to help control fracture alignment. Active flexion of the digit should begin within a few days to minimize stiffness and tendon adhesions. Supervised hand therapy with customized splinting and a carefully monitored

rehabilitation program are often required to optimize the final outcome. The splint is maintained for approximately 3 weeks and, following removal, buddy-taping is continued an additional 2 weeks.

Spiral and oblique fractures tend to displace and shorten after reduction and casting and often require internal fixation. These fractures require careful scrutiny if treated with splinting alone. Radiographs can be especially deceptive and difficult to interpret. In addition, once the digit has been immobilized, rotatory malalignment is almost impossible to assess.

The position for immobilization of spiral fractures is similar to that for transverse fractures. However, initiation of early motion will often result in loss of reduction. Therefore, I prefer immobilization for 3 to 3½ weeks, followed by mobilization in an extension block cast or buddy-taping for approximately 2 weeks. Repeated attempts at closed treatment are not warranted. If loss of reduction occurs, or if anatomic alignment cannot be ascertained, I do not hesitate to recommend operative fixation (described later).

Displaced: Unstable After Closed Reduction

Spiral and Oblique Fractures. I have found that closed pinning works particularly well for spiral and oblique fractures treated within 3 to 4 days of injury. I prefer wrist block anesthesia with conscious sedation so that the patient can actively flex the digits to assess rotational alignment after pinning. Provisional reduction is accomplished by applying longitudinal traction and squeezing the fracture fragments together with reduction clamps (see Fig. 8-37). Fluoroscopy greatly facilitates fracture reduction and pin placement. Two or three 0.035- or 0.045-inch Kirschner pins are inserted at right angles to the fracture and should be placed as far apart as possible and engage both sides of the fracture. For additional stability, the pins should not be placed precisely parallel to one another.

After pin insertion, rotational alignment should be checked by asking the patient to actively flex and extend the digits. If malalignment persists (either clinically or radiographically), either remove the pins and make another effort at closed reduction or proceed to open reduction. It is unwise to make more than two or three attempts at closed pinning; otherwise you may create a swollen, "pincushion" finger. Try to use a simple correction to enhance your opportunity for success with the closed technique, but if this is not possible, proceed to open reduction.

A straight dorsal skin incision is my preferred method for exposure of proximal and middle phalangeal shaft fractures (see Fig. 8-38). I believe a midaxial incision makes visualization of the other side difficult and may necessitate either a second midaxial incision or more soft tissue mobilization, including a longer incision (see Fig. 8-39). Generous skin flaps can be elevated, with care taken to preserve the dorsal longitudinal venous system. I approach fractures of the proximal phalanx with a Pratt[351] longitudinal tendon-splitting incision. Fractures of the middle phalanx are satisfactorily approached by dividing the transverse retinacular ligament at its insertion into the dorsal apparatus and mobilizing the dorsal apparatus without splitting it. Next, the periosteum is longitudinally incised and elevated to expose the fracture. To anatomically reduce spiral and oblique fractures one must expose the sharp proximal and distal fracture spikes, key them into the corresponding fragment, and provisionally maintain the reduction with reduction clamps or towel clips. Fixation is accomplished with either Kirschner pins or interfragmentary screws. If interfragmentary screws are used, I prefer two or three 2-mm screws in proximal phalanx fractures and two 1.5-mm or 1.3-mm screws for middle phalangeal fractures. Ideally, the screws should be inserted in the plane that bisects the long axis of the bone and fracture and at least two screw diameters from any fracture line. The screws should be lagged for interfragmentary compression and countersunk to prevent interference with tendon gliding. After screw or pin insertion, an attempt is made to close the periosteum with absorbable suture. If the dorsal apparatus over the proximal phalanx has been divided, it is reapproximated with either a running 4-0 nonabsorbable suture or interrupted inverted sutures.

Postoperatively, a bulky dressing is applied for 3 to 5 days and is followed by an aggressive program of active mobilization. When not exercising, a splint maintaining the MCP joint in flexion and the IP joints extended is preferred to counteract extrinsic deforming forces and minimize extensor lag at the PIP joint. Soft tissue swelling is minimized with an elastic sleeve or Coban. If pins have been inserted, they are removed between 3 to 9 weeks after insertion.

Transverse Fractures. Percutaneous cross-pinning of unstable transverse fractures is difficult even with an image intensifier. The goal is to insert two pins in crossed fashion and avoid the MP and PIP joints. Closed percutaneous cross-pinning of these fractures is frustrating, and I do not recommend it. An easier percutaneous technique is to insert the pin through the flexed MCP joint into the medullary canal of the proximal phalanx (see Fig. 8-36C). The pin penetrates the metacarpal head to either the radial or ulnar side of the exterior tendon and should be driven into the subchondral region of the proximal phalangeal head. Although this technique does not provide rotational stability, I have found it is simple and effective. At the first postoperative visit, an extension block splint or cast is fabricated, maintaining an intrinsic plus position. Active range of motion of the IP joints is encouraged. At 3½ to 4 weeks, the pin is removed and range of motion of the MCP joint is initiated.

Some unstable phalangeal shaft fractures require open reduction to facilitate management of concomitant injuries or because closed reduction and percutaneous pinning are unsatisfactory. In such cases, the fracture can be fixed with two bicortical Kirschner pins inserted in the coronal plane by one of two methods: retrograde cross-pinning or cross-pinning of the reduced fracture. Regardless of the technique, image intensification greatly facilitates the procedure. In the *retrograde cross-pinning method*,[115] after the fracture surfaces are exposed a trial reduction is accomplished (Fig. 8-42). A preview pin held over the dorsal surface of the reduced fracture before pinning helps plan the entrance site of the first fragment drilled and the exit site of the pin in the second fragment. Either the proximal or distal fragment may be drilled first; however, the distal fragment is usually easier to pin because the adjacent digits can be flexed out of the way of the distally protruding pin. An elevator placed beneath the volar cortex is used to lift the fragment up

and make the medullary canal accessible. The pin is drilled in the coronal plane through the middle of the medullary canal. Care must be taken to not angle the pin more than 30 degrees from the long axis of the phalanx because it will not engage adequate cortex of the proximal fragment. Sometimes the pin will bounce off the endosteal cortex when drilling the first fragment. To prevent this, a large-bore 14-gauge hypodermic needle can be used as a drill guide for the 0.035- or 0.045-inch Kirschner pin.[68] The pin is drilled through the cortex and out through the skin where the other end of the pin can be attached to the drill. Ideally, the extensor mechanism should be retracted dorsally so that it is not impaled. A second pin is inserted on the other side of the first fragment in a similar fashion, both pins are backed up flush to the fracture surface, and the fracture is reduced. To prevent distraction, the fracture ends are held firmly together while the two pins are drilled retrogradely into the fragment. It helps to stabilize the proximal fragment by holding it with a towel clip while the pins are drilled.

In the other method, the fracture is held *reduced* while two crossed Kirschner pins are drilled obliquely from the outside across the fracture (Fig. 8-43). This method is more difficult because it is challenging to simultaneously maintain fracture reduction and drive pins. When drilling through the outer cortex, a sharp bone awl can be used to make a starter hole or a 14-gauge hypodermic drill guard can be used to prevent the pin from sliding while being driven in an oblique fashion. Regardless of the technique, pin placement and fracture reduction are confirmed with biplanar radiographs and closure is accomplished as noted earlier.

Intraosseous wires (25 or 26 gauge) work well for the fixation of unstable transverse shaft fractures (Fig. 8-44). The holes for the wire should be drilled at least 3 to 4 mm from the fracture edge so that the wire does not cut out when it is being tightened. In addition, caution should be exercised to avoid kinking because tightening becomes impossible. Intraosseous wire fixation is particularly useful in open or severely displaced fractures in which the fracture has already been circumferentially exposed (secondary to the trauma) because wire passage is facilitated. Supplemental fixation with an oblique Kirschner pin[278] may provide additional stability, particularly in the phalangeal diaphysis, where the bending moment is greatest.

Periarticular phalangeal fractures may be stabilized with a 1.5-mm *minicondylar plate*[57,334] (Fig. 8-45) or a "T"-plate. The technique is exacting and should not be attempted without full knowledge of the implant system.

Plate fixation of noncomminuted transverse phalangeal shaft fractures is technically demanding and there is no margin for error. Considerable exposure is necessary, the plate may interfere with tendon excursion, and secondary removal may be necessary. Despite the secure fixation that plates provide, Kirschner pins, intraosseous wires, and combinations of the two are my preference for the management of unstable, noncomminuted phalangeal shaft fractures.

Displaced: Unstable and Comminuted

These fractures are difficult to manage and usually open and are often associated with soft tissue injury. Instability patterns include angulation, malrotation, and shortening. Fracture stabilization is necessary to restore length and

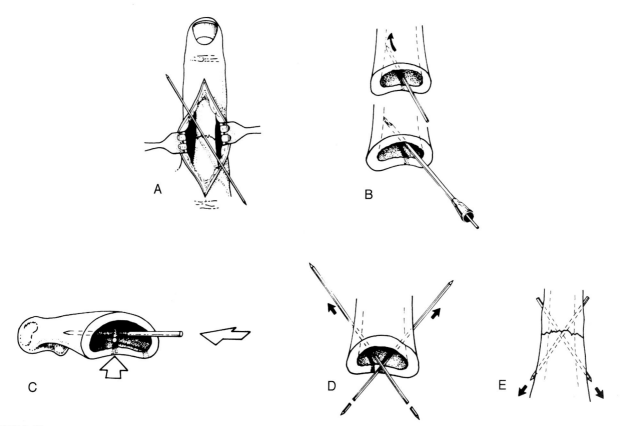

FIGURE 8-42. Open reduction with retrograde cross-pinning of a transverse phalangeal fracture. **A,** A "preview pin" held over the reduced fracture helps plan pin direction and the angle of entry. **B,** Use of a 14-gauge needle as a drill guide to prevent the pin from sliding off the endosteal surface of the cortex. **C,** The pins are drilled so that they are through the middle of the medullary canal in the coronal plane. **D,** The pins are drilled through the cortex and then backed up flush to the fracture surface. **E,** The fracture is then reduced and the fracture ends are compressed while the two pins are drilled retrogradely into the other fragment. (From Edwards GS Jr, O'Brien ET, Heckman MM: Retrograde cross pinning of transverse metacarpal and phalangeal fractures. Hand 14:141-148, 1982.)

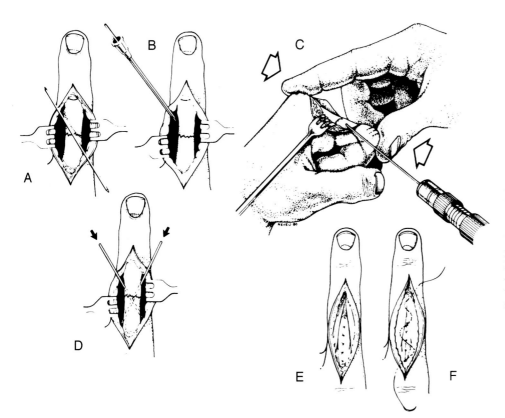

FIGURE 8-43. Open reduction with cross-pinning of a reduced transverse phalangeal fracture. **A,** A "preview pin" held over the reduced fracture to plan pin direction and angle of entry. **B,** Use of a 14-gauge needle as a drill guide for the Kirschner wire. **C,** The fracture must be compressed while the pins are drilled. **D,** Crossed pins drilled across the fracture. **E,** Periosteum closed with interrupted 4-0 absorbable sutures. **F,** Extensor tendon reapproximated with running nonabsorbable suture.

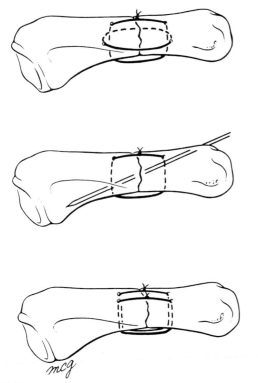

FIGURE 8-44. Intraosseous wire configurations. **Top,** 90-90 wires. **Middle,** Single loop with supplemental Kirschner pin. **Bottom,** Parallel loops.

alignment and to facilitate management of concomitant soft tissue injuries. In nearly all cases operative intervention is necessary.

Application of a mini external fixation device is my preferred treatment. It provides stabilization, allows access to open wounds, and does not risk devitalization of small fracture fragments, which may have a tenuous blood supply. Two transverse pins are placed proximal and distal to the fracture and inserted through midaxial or dorsolateral incisions. If 2-mm half-pins are used, pre-drilling is done bicortically with a 1.5-mm power drill bit and the 2.0-mm pin is inserted. Image intensification facilitates pin insertion, minimizes the risk of articular penetration, and diminishes the chance of further fracture comminution during multiple drill passes. After insertion of the transverse pins, the connecting rods and swivel clamps are applied. Again, with the image intensifier the fracture is reduced and the swivel clamps are tightened to maintain reduction. Usually, stability can be maintained with a single half-frame; if necessary, a second half-frame can be applied. Supplemental Kirschner pins and intraosseous or cerclage wires may increase stability. If there is an osseous void, bone grafting can be considered, assuming that there is adequate soft tissue coverage. The fixator is left in place for 4 weeks, during which time active mobilization of uninvolved joints is encouraged. After the fixator is removed, an aggressive therapy program is initiated. Secondary surgery, including tenolysis and capsulotomy, is frequently necessary but should be delayed until there is solid bony union and the soft tissue sleeve is mature and pliable.

Plates and screws are a popular alternative to external fixation. However, several caveats must be kept in mind:

additional soft tissue mobilization is usually necessary, there is no margin for error (plate malposition may lead to malreduction), the plate may interfere with tendon gliding, and soft tissue coverage (without a flap) may not be possible. For these reasons, plate fixation is my second choice for stabilization of comminuted phalangeal shaft fractures.

Base Fractures of the Proximal Phalanx

Extra-articular fractures at the base of the proximal phalanx occur at the metaphyseal-diaphyseal junction. The fracture is usually comminuted dorsally, impacted, and angulated apex palmward. There also may be mild angulation in the frontal plane; rotational deformity is rare.

In 1969, Coonrad and Pohlman[89] presented a 10-year follow-up of 68 of these fractures. They pointed out that the lateral view provides the most accurate assessment of fracture angulation, even though the degree of angulation is difficult to assess because of the overlap of adjacent digits. Oblique views may be deceptive and may lead the surgeon into underestimating the severity of the fracture.[145] Coonrad and Pohlman,[89] as well as others,[258] pointed out that malunion was associated with immobilization of the digit in insufficient flexion at the MCP joint and resulted in loss of reduction or acceptance of oblique radiographs for the evaluation of angulation. Up to 30 degrees of volar angulation is acceptable in younger children, but uncorrected angulation of 25 degrees or more in adults or older children caused loss of motion and necessitated corrective osteotomy.

Occasionally, reduction may be impossible because of interosseous tendon interposition.[408] A malunion produces "pseudoclawing," which is clinically manifested by hyperextension at the fracture and MCP joint and an extensor lag at the PIP joint. This fracture is reduced by flexing the MCP joint maximally to stabilize the proximal fragment and relax the intrinsic muscles and then correcting the volar angulation by flexing the distal fragment. Immobilization with the MCP joint flexed 70 degrees and the PIP joint extended for 3 to 4 weeks is recommended. In this position, it is believed that the soft tissue attachments to the base of the proximal phalanx confer stability.[472] Closed reduction with pinning, as described by Heim and Pfeiffer[197] and by Belsky and colleagues,[17-19] is an excellent technique to maintain reduction. A Kirschner pin is drilled through the flexed MCP joint into the proximal fragment to stabilize it. After the distal fragment is reduced onto the proximal fragment, the Kirschner pin is drilled across the fracture into the distal fragment.

Strickler and associates[429] have described a novel approach to the management of this fracture. They reported 10 patients in whom the fracture was approached through an extensor tendon-splitting incision; the fracture was disimpacted, and the void was filled with cancellous autograft. Early range of motion was initiated. None of the fractures redisplaced, and 9 of 10 patients were satisfied with the ultimate result.

Complications of Phalangeal Fractures

Malunion

Malunion (Table 8-9) is a common bony complication of phalangeal fractures and has been subclassified into four types: malrotation, volar angulation, lateral angulation, and shortening.[170] Most authors have addressed "established"

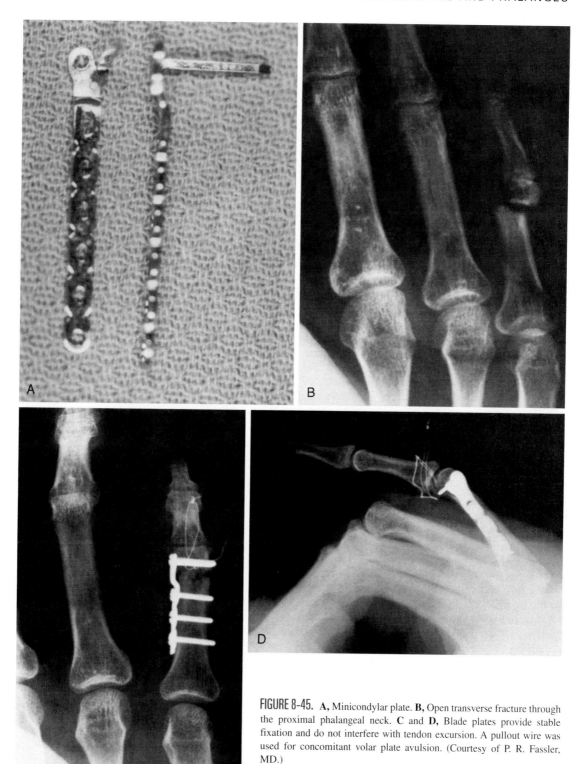

FIGURE 8-45. A, Minicondylar plate. **B,** Open transverse fracture through the proximal phalangeal neck. **C** and **D,** Blade plates provide stable fixation and do not interfere with tendon excursion. A pullout wire was used for concomitant volar plate avulsion. (Courtesy of P. R. Fassler, MD.)

malunions; however, studies by Lester and Mallik[269] have suggested intervention at 4 to 8 weeks.

Buchler and colleagues[58] reviewed 59 extra-articular phalangeal malunions treated by phalangeal osteotomy. There were no nonunions or infections. Full bony correction was achieved in 76% of the digits, and 89% demonstrated increased range of motion. For those digits with an isolated malunion, 83% had excellent and 13% had good results. For digits with "pleuristructural" involvement, there were 45% excellent, 19% good, 13% fair, and 23% poor results. Along similar lines, Trumble and Gilbert[445] reported excellent results in 11 patients using an in situ closing wedge

Table 8-9
PHALANGEAL MALUNION: TREATMENT VARIABLES

Location: proximal vs. middle phalanx; digit involved, level with affected phalanx; intra- vs. extra-articular

Complexity: isolated malunion vs. prior combined injury (compromised integrity of soft tissue sleeve, tendons)

Nature of deformity: angulation, rotation, shortening, translation, gap, step

Bone loss

Functional significance

Modified from Buchler U: Osteotomy for phalangeal malunion. Tech Hand Upper Ext Surg 2:158-165, 1998.

osteotomy to correct either uniplanar or multiplanar deformities. They used a 1.3- or 1.5-mm dorsally applied plate for fixation and saw no major complications.

Malrotation

Malrotation is usually seen after oblique or spiral fractures of the proximal and middle phalanges. It may be difficult to assess radiographically and also may not be appreciated with the digits held in extension. Therefore, malrotation is best assessed by having the patient make a fist and looking for digital overlap. Small amounts of malrotation may be acceptable to many patients. However, significant malrotation results in functional impairment, pain from joint malalignment, and diminished grip strength.[58] Osteotomy is usually required, preferably through the phalanx. Phalangeal osteotomy offers the advantage of correcting the malunion at its site of origin, allows for multiplanar correction, and permits concomitant soft tissue procedures such as tenolysis or capsulotomy. On the other hand, the risk of postoperative adhesions between the dorsal apparatus and phalanx is significant and may result in digital stiffness. Phalangeal osteotomies can be either step-cut[295,345] or transverse[149,152,292,397] and are created with a power saw with a thin blade. Transverse osteotomies can be held with a plate or with Kirschner pins. Step-cut osteotomies are fixed with either small ASIF screws or Kirschner pins.

Before the development of secure internal fixation, malrotation was corrected by an osteotomy through the metacarpal base. Gross and Gelberman[180] experimentally determined that correction of 18 to 19 degrees can be obtained by osteotomy of the index, long, and ring fingers and that 20 to 30 degrees of correction can be achieved in the small finger. The technique was originally described by Weckesser[465] and has subsequently been described by Pieron[346] and Botelheiro.[43] Although metacarpal osteotomy is technically easier, the amount of rotational correction is limited to 25 to 30 degrees and multiplanar correction is not possible. If concomitant tenolysis and capsulotomy are planned, exposing the malunion is necessary anyway, perhaps obviating the potential simplicity of a metacarpal correction.

I prefer phalangeal osteotomy using plate fixation. The use of a supplemental bone graft must be individualized. Postoperatively, an aggressive range-of-motion program is necessary to minimize stiffness.

Volar Angulation

Malunion of adult basilar proximal phalangeal fractures greater than 25 to 30 degrees results in pseudoclawing. This deformity may compromise dexterity, is often aesthetically unacceptable, and can result in a fixed PIP flexion contracture.[170] The osteotomy is performed with an oscillating saw by making an opening or closing wedge at the level of the malunion. I prefer a closing wedge osteotomy (apex dorsal, base volar). Fixation is with Kirschner pins, plates and screws, or intraosseous wires (Fig. 8-46). Preoperatively, a template of the malunited phalanx is made to accurately assess the dimensions of the wedge to be removed. A closing osteotomy is simpler than an opening osteotomy and does not require an intercalated bone graft. If shortening is a concern, an opening osteotomy with insertion of a corticocancellous wedge-shaped graft is recommended.

Lateral Angulation

Lateral angulation can be corrected by either opening or closing wedge osteotomy. A closing osteotomy can be done with an oscillating saw or power burs, as described by Froimson.[152] Alternatively, corrective opening wedge osteotomy can be accomplished (Fig. 8-47). I prefer to leave the opposite cortex intact, use either a pure cancellous or corticocancellous graft, and obtain fixation with a laterally applied plate.

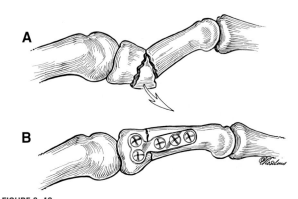

FIGURE 8-46. Closing wedge osteotomy for correction of a malunion of the proximal phalanx with volar angulation.

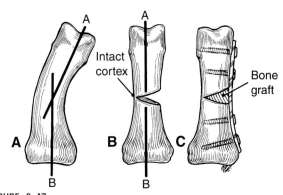

FIGURE 8-47. Technique for lateral opening phalangeal osteotomy. **A,** Angulatory deformity in frontal plane. Lines A and B show alignment of proximal and distal portions of phalanx. **B,** Corrective osteotomy leaving the opposite cortex intact. **C,** Corticocancellous graft inserted with lateral plate fixation.

Shortening

Shortening may occur after a comminuted fracture that is allowed to heal in a collapsed fashion or following a long spiral fracture. Restoration of phalangeal length alone is rarely indicated because of the inherent risks of osteotomy and interposition bone grafting. However, when there is a concomitant rotatory or angular deformity, diaphyseal osteotomy with an appropriately fashioned intercalary graft may be indicated.

Occasionally, a spiral fracture of the proximal phalanx will heal in a shortened position such that the distal spike on the proximal fragment protrudes into the retrocondylar space of the PIP joint and acts as a flexion block.[170,267] In such instances, digital flexion can be restored by removing the spike through a volar approach. This procedure is best performed by using local anesthesia with sedation so that the patient can actively flex the affected digit intraoperatively to ensure that full digital flexion has been restored. Care must be taken to not be overzealous in bony removal because an iatrogenic fracture can occur. Simmons and Peters[402] reported three children who sustained malunited subcondylar fractures through the neck of the proximal phalanx. This resulted in a block to active and passive PIP flexion. They recommended correction through a volar approach by removing a bony block and cautioned against osteotomy because of its difficulty and risk of avascular necrosis of the head fragment.

Intra-articular Malunion

Unreduced condylar fractures that extend into the PIP joint may produce pain, angulatory deformity, stiffness, and, ultimately, degenerative arthritis. Treatment options include corrective intra-articular or juxta-articular osteotomy, arthrodesis, or arthroplasty. Juxta-articular osteotomy corrects alignment but does not address the intra-articular stepoff. Light[273] reported a series of intra-articular malunions treated by osteotomy through the old fracture site and fixation with Kirschner pins and/or intraosseous wires. Six of his cases occurred in patients with intra-articular malunions of the proximal phalanx, five of whom had improved, although not normal, motion after osteotomy and all of whom had relief of pain.

Teoh[437] and colleagues reported excellent results in six patients using a complex type of intra-articular osteotomy that they called a "condylar advancement osteotomy." On the other hand, Gollamudi and Jones[162] reported persistent stiffness after intra-articular osteotomy. In young patients with absence of post-traumatic arthritis, I prefer an intra-articular osteotomy and inform patients that proper alignment can be corrected but restoration of full mobility is unlikely. Furthermore, degenerative arthritis can develop in the future.

Nonunion

Nonunion of phalangeal fractures is uncommon, although delayed union is seen quite often. Infection, bone loss, and

---

CRITICAL POINTS: OSTEOTOMY FOR PHALANGEAL MALUNION

INDICATIONS

- Angulatory or rotatory deformity with or without stiffness
- Pain, weakness

PREOPERATIVE EVALUATION

- Assess plane(s) of deformity.
- Assess integrity of soft tissue sleeve and flexor and extensor tendons.
- Obtain anteroposterior, lateral, and oblique radiographs.
- Assess bone loss (is bone graft necessary?).

PEARLS

- Use plate and screw fixation whenever possible.
- Maintain phalangeal length rather than shorten.
- Consider other options (arthrodesis or amputation) when associated with joint stiffness, unstable soft tissue coverage, or history of osteomyelitis.

PITFALLS

- Inadequate correction
- Poor fixation precluding early range-of-motion exercises
- Shortening more than 3 mm unacceptable

TECHNICAL POINTS

- Use template to assess length, opening vs. closing wedge, or rotational osteotomy.
- Make dorsal incision; preserve veins in skin flaps.
- Place longitudinal line on phalanx to assess rotational correction or temporary Kirschner pins perpendicular to coronal and sagittal planes.
- Create osteotomy with thin saw blade or osteotome.
- If lateral or volar angulation, consider incomplete opening wedge (leave opposite cortex intact) and bone graft.
- Adjust alignment and temporarily hold with Kirschner pin.
- Apply low profile plate (minimum four cortices above and below osteotomy) on lateral surface if possible.
- Perform tenolysis and or capsulotomy if necessary.

POSTOPERATIVE CARE

- Apply bulky dressing for 4 to 7 days.
- Then, begin aggressive active and gentle passive range-of-motion exercises.
- Edema control is done with elastic garment.
- Splint IP joints in extension when not exercising.

(neuro)vascular injury predispose to nonunion.[450] Smith and Rider[405] believed that nonunion could not be diagnosed until at least 1 year had elapsed since the fracture. Jupiter and colleagues,[232] however, advised operative intervention 4 months after the injury because additional immobilization was likely to cause significant stiffness. They reported eight nonunions of the proximal phalanx, four of which were treated with plate fixation. Union was obtained in all patients; however, the earlier motion allowed in the rigid fixation (plate) group resulted in significantly greater total range of motion than in the group fixed with Kirschner pins. Two phalangeal nonunions were treated by arthrodeses, and one required a ray deletion. These procedures were performed in patients with significant soft tissue problems or joint contractures.

In contrast to the work of Jupiter and colleagues,[232] Wray and Glunk[481] reported satisfactory results in 13 patients with delayed union, malunion, or nonunion of the proximal phalanx treated with Kirschner pin fixation and occasional supplemental bone grafting at 3 months post injury. They believed that the key to increased mobility after Kirschner pin fixation was initiation of active motion 2 to 3 weeks after surgical fixation (as opposed to the work of Jupiter and colleagues,[232] who began active motion at 6 weeks). Equally important as the method of fixation for phalangeal nonunions is the surgical resection of the nonunion itself (Fig. 8-48). Fibrous tissue must be removed until there are freshened fracture ends. If a resultant gap produces unacceptable shortening, intercalated corticocancellous bone grafting is indicated. Plate fixation has the advantage of being stable and also affords the opportunity for concomitant tenolysis and capsulotomy when indicated (Fig. 8-49). It is nevertheless a difficult procedure and requires exacting technique.

Loss of Motion

Diminished motion may be the result of tendon adhesions (either flexor or extensor) or capsular contracture. Immobilization greater than 4 weeks,[428] an associated joint injury, more than one fracture per finger, a crush injury, and a soft

tissue injury are all contributing factors to decreased mobility of a fractured digit.[205] In a prospective study of 245 open phalangeal fractures, Chow and colleagues[80] noted that the results directly correlated with the extent of injury to soft tissue, tendon, and nerve. If the fracture was associated with a laceration or isolated digital nerve injury, 40% of the results were good and 25% were poor. If there was an associated extensor tendon injury or extensive skin loss, 18% of the results were good and 50% were poor. If there was an injury to the flexor tendon or more than one component of soft tissue damage, 80% of the results were poor and good results were rare.

The treatment of stiffness should begin with a comprehensive program of hand therapy,[210] including active and passive motion exercises as well as dynamic splinting. In addition, swelling should be controlled with compressive garments. When there has been a plateau in motion and soft tissue induration and edema has been minimized, surgical intervention can be considered. Extensor tendon adhesions restrict passive PIP joint flexion and limit active extension. Passive extension is not usually limited. Extensor tendon adherence is best treated by tenolysis of the dorsal apparatus with or without insertion of an inert material between the tendon and bone. Stark and colleagues[417] recorded improved motion in 10 of 15 patients who had extensor tenolysis and silicone interposition.

Schneider[388] pointed out that the use of tenolysis and capsulotomy after phalangeal fractures must be individualized. I prefer using local anesthesia with sedation. Initially, extensor tenolysis over the proximal phalanx is carried out; and if PIP passive flexion is limited (less than 90 degrees), a dorsal PIP capsulotomy is usually needed. Once full passive PIP flexion has been achieved, the patient is asked to actively flex and extend the digit. If there is a discrepancy between active and passive flexion, that is, if passive flexion exceeds active flexion, flexor tenolysis is performed. Creighton and Steichen[91] found that if a dorsal PIP capsulotomy is performed in addition to an extensor tenolysis, the active PIP extensor lag failed to improve.

Stiffness of the PIP joint may also result from intraarticular incongruity, arthrofibrosis, or soft tissue capsular contracture. A discussion of management of articular stiffness is beyond the scope of this chapter and should be treated according to the principles described by Curtis[96] and Watson and associates.[461] Combined joint stiffness and tendon adhesions can be surgically treated, but the results are not dramatic and surgery is difficult and extensive. Fusion of the PIP joint in a functional position or ray deletion is an option when severe contractures or stiffness exists.

PIP Joint Extensor Lag

Extensor lag at the PIP joint is commonly encountered after proximal phalangeal fractures. Causes include adhesions of the dorsal apparatus to the proximal phalanx, shortening of the proximal phalanx, and an angulatory (apex volar) deformity of the proximal phalanx.

Ideally, prevention of extensor lag is the management of choice. Isolated fractures of the proximal phalanx treated both operatively and nonoperatively should have the PIP joint statically splinted in extension. If an extensor lag is noted, a dynamic PIP extension splint, including a lumbrical

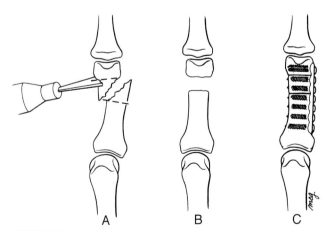

FIGURE 8-48. Technique for the treatment of atrophic nonunion. **A,** The nonunion is resected with an oscillating saw. **B,** The osseous gap after resection. **C,** The gap is filled with a corticocancellous graft, and stabilization is accomplished with a laterally applied plate.

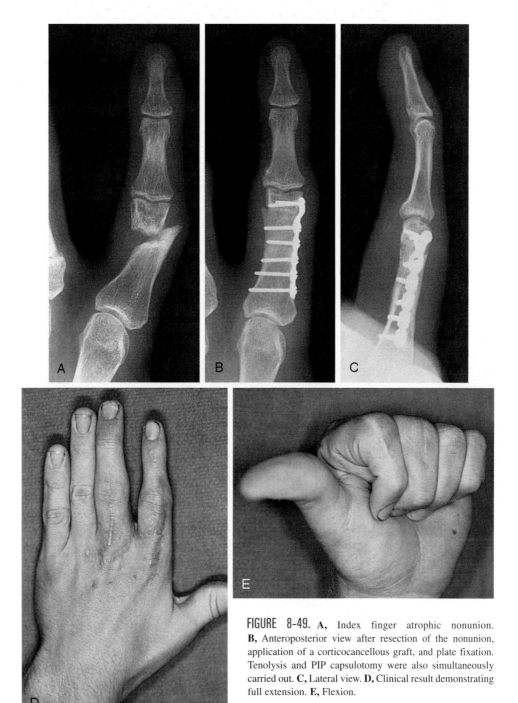

FIGURE 8-49. A, Index finger atrophic nonunion. **B,** Anteroposterior view after resection of the nonunion, application of a corticocancellous graft, and plate fixation. Tenolysis and PIP capsulotomy were also simultaneously carried out. **C,** Lateral view. **D,** Clinical result demonstrating full extension. **E,** Flexion.

bar to prevent proximal phalangeal extension and a sling pulling the middle phalanx into extension, should be applied.

Late management of an extensor lag depends on the cause and the degree of the lag. Most individuals tolerate a lag of less than 15 to 20 degrees. If the lag is symptomatic and adhesions are suspected, extensor tenolysis should be considered.

As noted earlier, an extensor lag can also be the result of apex volar or shortening of the proximal phalanx. Vahey and colleagues[447] in a cadaver study noted that for an average

apex volar angulation of 16, 37, and 46 degrees, a PIP lag of 10, 24, and 66 degrees, respectively, resulted. With respect to proximal phalangeal shortening, for each millimeter of shortening, there was a 12-degree lag. Clinically, however, the intrinsic and extrinsic muscles are capable of compensating for some degree of bone shortening.

Infection

Infection after fracture treatment is rare. The incidence of infection in open fractures varies between 2.04%[80] and 11%,[307] and infection usually occurs after an open injury in which there has been soft tissue injury, a comminuted fracture, or contamination.

Swanson and associates[435] reviewed 200 open hand fractures distal to the carpus in 121 patients. They classified fractures into two types:

Type I
A. Clean wounds without significant contamination or delay in treatment
B. No significant systemic illness

Type II
A. Gross contamination (animal bite, grossly dirty, or barnyard injury)
B. Delay in treatment greater than 24 hours
C. Significant systemic illness

The infection rate in type I injuries was 1.4%, and in type II injuries it was 14%. The incidence of infection was not related to the presence of internal fixation, high-energy injury, or concomitant soft tissue injuries. Swanson and associates recommended primary closure for type I injuries and delayed closure in type II injuries.

Role of Antibiotics

The role of antibiotics in the management of open phalangeal fractures is controversial. Sloan and associates[404] prospectively studied 85 adults with open fractures of the distal phalanx. The infection rate was 30% in the group without antibiotics and less than 3% in those treated with perioperative cephradine. On the other hand, Suprock and colleagues[432] studied 91 open phalangeal fractures without vascular compromise. Antibiotics were administered to alternate patients with open fractures, and the infection rate was the same in both treatment groups. They concluded that irrigation and débridement are adequate treatment for open phalangeal fractures.

I prefer to use "prophylactic" antibiotics for open phalangeal fractures and recommend the intravenous administration of a first-generation cephalosporin in the emergency department and continuation of antibiotic coverage for the first 24 postoperative hours. For grossly contaminated fractures or when there has been a treatment delay, the addition of an aminoglycoside and penicillin is recommended.

Treatment of Infected Fractures

Management of infected fractures includes three goals: (1) eradicating sepsis, (2) obtaining fracture union, and (3) regaining a functional extremity.[436] Sepsis is eliminated by thorough débridement of the infected bone and soft tissue, initiation of appropriate antibiotic therapy, and stabilization of the fracture. I have found a mini external fixation device helpful in stabilization of infected diaphyseal fractures after débridement. Once the infection has been eliminated, bone grafting may be accomplished.

Significant phalangeal osteomyelitis may be difficult, if not impossible, to eradicate. Several operative procedures may be necessary, and the final result is often a painful, stiff, useless digit. In such circumstances, amputation must be considered.

Flexor Tendon Rupture or Entrapment

Flexor tendon rupture is an uncommon complication of phalangeal fractures and is usually iatrogenic. It has been reported after percutaneous pinning[229] and plate fixation.[126] Jones and Schenck[227] reported a patient with a closed, volarly angulated fracture of the proximal phalanx and laceration of the ulnar half of the flexor digitorum profundus tendon that appeared to become entrapped between the ends of the bone when the fracture was reduced. Fracture healing around the tendons resulted in a cyst in the bone and poor flexion of the digit. The entrapped portion of the tendon was excised 5 months after injury and the patient regained good function. More recently, Nogueira[327] and associates reported a child with an irreducible fracture of the proximal phalanx in which the flexor tendons were trapped longitudinally between fracture fragments. Operative relocation of the tendons and internal fixation with pins gave an excellent result.

FRACTURES OF THE THUMB

Because of the compensatory movement of the adjacent joints, the thumb is more forgiving of residual deformity than the fingers. Malrotation is rarely a problem. Angulatory deformities in the frontal plane less than 15 to 20 degrees are functionally acceptable, although cosmetically they may be bothersome. Likewise, angulation less than 20 to 30 degrees in the lateral plane usually causes no functional deficit. Intra-articular fractures must be aggressively treated to avoid loss of motion and post-traumatic arthritis.

Thumb Phalangeal Fractures

Extra-articular Fractures

Fractures of the proximal and distal phalanx of the thumb are often the result of direct trauma and are less common than fractures of the thumb metacarpal.

Distal phalangeal fractures have been classified into three types[5]:

1. Longitudinal shaft fractures
2. Transverse shaft fractures
3. Distal tuft fractures

Tuft fractures are usually comminuted and are nearly always associated with an injury to the nail matrix and/or pulp. The fracture rarely requires reduction or fixation. Treatment should consist of evacuation of painful subungual hematomas and repair of dermal and nail matrix lacerations when indicated. This is followed by splint immobilization for 3 to 4 weeks.

Distal phalangeal transverse shaft fractures are potentially unstable. The fracture angulates with its apex anterior secondary to the pull of the flexor pollicis longus on the proximal fragment. If reduction cannot be held in a splint, it is reasonable to percutaneously insert a longitudinal Kirschner pin across the fracture and into the head of the proximal phalanx.

Vertical extra-articular fractures of the distal phalanx are uncommon. When displaced, the fracture can usually be reduced and percutaneously pinned.

Head and neck fractures of the proximal phalanx are treated according to the same principles used in treating similar injuries in the fingers. Displaced spiral or oblique fractures may be treated by percutaneous pinning or by open reduction with either Kirschner pins or interfragmentary screws. Transverse fractures angulate the apex volarly secondary to the pull of the thenar intrinsics on the proximal fragment and the extensor pollicis longus on the distal fragment. Closed reduction is usually stable. More than 20 to 30 degrees of angulation in the lateral plane is unacceptable because an extensor lag of the IP joint will result. If open reduction of a fracture of the proximal phalanx is required, the fracture is exposed through a dorsal "Y"-shaped incision with the extensor pollicis longus insertion left intact (Fig. 8-50).

Intra-articular Fractures and Avulsions

Intra-articular fractures of the IP or MCP joint may be a single fragment (a sign of a ligament or avulsion injury) or may be significantly comminuted. Comminuted fractures usually occur after blunt trauma. Ideally, articular congruity should be restored. If symptomatic arthritis ensues, IP or MP arthrodesis can be accomplished with little functional impairment.

Avulsion fractures of the dorsal base of the distal phalanx represent a mallet thumb. Unless there is volar subluxation of the distal phalanx, treatment should consist of continuous extension splinting of the IP joint for 6 to 8 weeks. Avulsion fractures of the volar lip of the base of the distal phalanx usually represent impaction fractures after a dorsal IP dislocation or, rarely, avulsion of the flexor pollicis longus. Avulsion fractures from the ulnar base of the proximal phalanx usually represent disruption of the ulnar collateral ligament (gamekeeper's or skier's thumb). If the fragment is displaced more than 2 mm and the MCP joint is unstable to stress, stability needs to be surgically restored. If the fracture fragment is small or breaks during internal fixation, it can be removed and the ligament reinserted with a pullout wire or suture anchor. Larger fragments can be fixed with either Kirschner pins,[286] a tension wire,[233] or a small lag screw. The repair is protected with a transarticular smooth Kirschner pin as well as thumb spica cast immobilization for 4 to 6 weeks.

Fractures of the Thumb Metacarpal

Metacarpal Head Fractures

Metacarpal head fractures are unusual because the longitudinally directed force that produces them is usually dissipated at the proximal metaphysis or trapeziometacarpal joint. Displaced intra-articular fractures require anatomic reduction. Fixation can be obtained by fluoroscopically assisted percutaneous Kirschner pin placement or by open reduction. The fracture is approached by splitting the dorsal apparatus between the extensor pollicis longus and brevis. Avulsion osteochondral fractures of the metacarpal head are usually from the radial side and represent a radial collateral ligament injury. When displaced, open reduction is necessary to ensure joint stability.

Shaft Fractures

Fractures of the thumb metacarpal occur in three locations: shaft and base fractures and intra-articular fractures of the trapeziometacarpal joint.[172] Shaft fractures are uncommon because of the lack of firm fixation of the proximal portion of the bone and because stress applied to the thumb is usually well tolerated by the strong cortical shaft and is dissipated by the soft cancellous bone at its base.[5]

Extra-articular fractures through the base are common and are usually transverse or mildly oblique. They generally occur at the proximal metaphyseal-diaphyseal junction and are referred to as *epibasal*.[231,475] The fracture is angulated with its apex dorsal such that the distal fragment is adducted and flexed (Fig. 8-51). Burton and Eaton[64] believed that the distal fragment may be supinated as well, so when closed reduction is accomplished, they recommend pronating the distal fragment. Radiographs must be carefully evaluated to make sure that the fracture does not extend into the trapeziometacarpal joint. Closed reduction of an extra-articular metacarpal base fracture is usually easy to accomplish by longitudinal traction, downward pressure on the apex of the fracture, mild pronation of the distal fragment, and thumb extension. The reduction is usually stable and can be maintained in a thumb spica cast that excludes the distal phalanx. Angulation less than 20 to 30 degrees is usually well compensated because of the abundant motion at the trapeziometacarpal joint. Angulation greater than 30 degrees, however, results in compensatory hyperextension of the MCP joint and may be unacceptable (Fig. 8-52). Radiographs may not adequately demonstrate the degree of fracture angulation unless a true lateral radiograph of the metacarpal is obtained. Adequacy of the lateral radiograph should be verified by superimposition of the thumb MCP joint sesamoids. In fractures angulated greater than 30 degrees, I prefer closed reduction and percutaneous pinning. Open

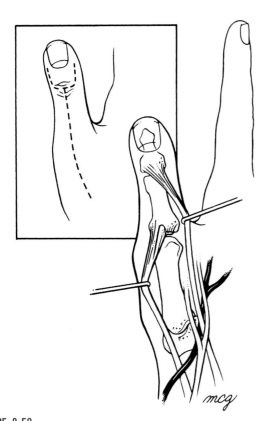

FIGURE 8-50. Exposure of the thumb metacarpal and phalanges. The interval between the extensor pollicis longus and brevis is divided, with both tendons left intact. When exposing the thumb, care must be taken to not injure terminal branches of the superficial radial nerve or radial artery in the anatomical snuff-box.

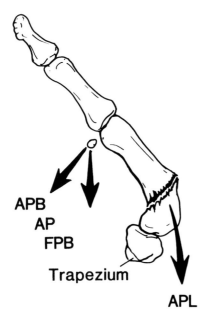

FIGURE 8-51. Deforming forces of a thumb metacarpal shaft fracture. The abductor pollicis brevis (APB), adductor pollicis (AP), and flexor pollicis brevis (FPB) flex the distal fragment, and the abductor pollicis longus (APL) extends the proximal fragment.

reduction for transverse and oblique basilar thumb metacarpal fractures is rarely necessary.

Comminuted thumb metacarpal shaft fractures are usually the result of direct trauma and are often associated with soft tissue injury. Fracture stabilization must be individualized and often requires an external fixator to prevent metacarpal shortening and thumb adduction and to also allow soft tissue healing. Extension of the frame to the index metacarpal will help prevent a thumb/index finger web contracture.

Fractures of the Base of the Thumb Metacarpal: Bennett's Fracture

In 1882, E. H. Bennett[22] presented five pathologic specimens of a healed fracture of the palmar articular surface of the base of the first metacarpal, and in 1886 he published two clinical cases and recommended thumb spica splint immobilization for at least 4 weeks.[23] Since then, many methods of treatment have been advocated, with no consensus on the best technique (Table 8-10).

Accurate radiographs are important in establishing congruity of the CMC joint. Billing and Gedda[27] have described the technique necessary to get a true lateral view of the joint. The palmar surface of the hand is placed flat on the film, and the hand and wrist are pronated 15 to 35 degrees. The x-ray tube is directed obliquely 15 degrees in a distal-to-proximal direction and centered over the trapeziometacarpal joint (Fig. 8-53).

To understand the treatment of intra-articular fractures of the basilar joint of the thumb, one must appreciate its anatomy. The surfaces of the trapezium and thumb metacarpal resemble two reciprocally interlocking saddles[87,322] that allow motion in two planes (perpendicular and parallel to the plane of the palm).

Axial rotation is limited by the joint capsule, ligaments, extrinsic tendons, and geometry of the joint surfaces. Joint stability is maintained by five ligaments: the anterior (volar) and posterior oblique ligaments, the anterior and posterior intermetacarpal ligaments, and the dorsal radial ligament.[184, 212,322,347] During simple pinch and grasp, joint compressive forces are high.[86,87] Thus if significant joint congruency is lost, either secondary to an unreduced intra-articular fracture or from disruption of the soft tissue stabilizers, post-traumatic arthritis may ensue.[49]

Bennett's fracture is really a fracture subluxation. The injury occurs when the thumb metacarpal is axially loaded and partially flexed.[342] The Bennett fragment is of variable size and is pyramidal and consists of the volar-ulnar aspect of the metacarpal base. The anterior oblique ligament,[212] which runs from the Bennett fragment to the trapezium, holds the fragment in anatomic position. The remaining metacarpal base subluxates radially, proximally, and dorsally. The goals of treatment are to (1) restore stability of the CMC joint by rejoining the Bennett fragment (attachment of the anterior oblique ligament) to the thumb metacarpal and (2) restore articular congruity of the thumb metacarpal base.[155]

Prior to the 1970s, nonoperative management was suggested by several surgeons.[37,77,178,348] In recent years the controversy regarding the necessity for anatomic reduction persists. Cannon and coworkers[73] evaluated patients nearly 10 years after nonoperative management of Bennett's fractures and noted little evidence of symptomatic arthritis despite imperfect reduction. Kjaer-Petersen and colleagues[246,247] noted a higher incidence of symptomatic arthritis when articular incongruity persisted after reduction. Livesley[281] observed 17 patients for 26 years after closed

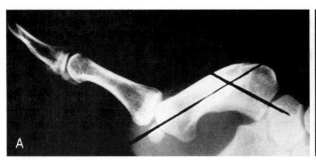
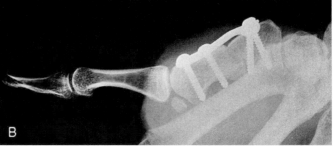

FIGURE 8-52. **A,** Hyperextension deformity after malunion of a thumb metacarpal shaft fracture. **B,** Correction by closing wedge osteotomy and plate fixation.

Table 8-10
TREATMENT ADVOCATED FOR BENNETT'S FRACTURE

Author	Treatment
Robinson (1908)	Cast and continuous skin traction
Cotton (1910)	Goldthwait splint
Roberts and Kelly (1916)	Padded aluminum gutter splint
Key and Conwell (1934)	Roller bandage between thumb and index finger
Roberts (1938)	Cast with traction on a Thomas splint outrigger
James and Gibson (1940)	Plaster immobilization; felt pad over base of thumb
Blum (1941)	No immobilization; early active motion
Johnson (1944)	Closed reduction and Kirschner wire fixation between first and second metacarpals
Ellis (1946)	Buttress pins inserted into trapezium
Wagner (1950)	Closed reduction and Kirschner wire fixation from base of first metacarpal into trapezium
Goldberg (1951)	Pressure pad over base of first metacarpal by outrigger
Gedda and Moberg (1953)	Open reduction: Kirschner wire from thumb metacarpal shaft to Bennett fragment
Wiggins, Bunden, and Park (1954)	Transfixation of carpometacarpal joint with pin
Ross and Sinclair (1954)	Stader splint
Thoren (1955)	Oblique skeletal traction through thumb metacarpal
Iselin (1956)	Intermetacarpal pinning
Badger (1956)	Screw fixation without plaster immobilization
Bunnell (1956)	Skeletal traction or open reduction
Crawford (1976)	ASIF screw fixation
Hughes (1985)	Herbert screw
Foster and Hastings (1987)	Lag screw
van Niekerk and Ouwens (1989)	Intermetacarpal pinning
Dartee, Brink, and van Houtte (1992)	Intermetacarpal pinning
Chabon and Siegel (1993)	Herbert screw
Bruske (2001)	Percutaneous pinning

ASIF, Association for Study of Internal Fixation.

reduction and casting. All patients had diminished mobility and strength, and the majority had radiographic evidence of degenerative arthritis and joint subluxation. He concluded that this fracture should not be managed conservatively.

A number of techniques for closed reduction and percutaneous fixation have been recommended. Cullen and colleagues,[95] in a biomechanical study, simulated a Bennett fracture with 2-mm displacement of the Bennett fragment and then measured contact pressures between the trapezium and metametacarpal. They found that as long as the shaft and Bennett fragments healed in close apposition, despite lack of anatomic restoration of the articular surface, there was no biomechanical basis for the development of posttraumatic arthritis. This study supported closed reduction and percutaneous pinning without anatomic restoration of the articular surface of the metacarpal in the management of a Bennett fracture. With the use of fluoroscopy, this technique has become increasingly popular.[53,203,235,410] Kirschner pin fixation between the first and second metacarpals (intermetacarpal pinning) was advocated by Johnson,[225] van Niekerk and Ouwens,[449] and Dartee and associates (Fig. 8-54).[101] Wiggins and colleagues[473] inserted a pin through the metacarpal head and then directed it across the first CMC joint. Segmuller[393] performed closed reduction and introduced one pin in a lateral-to-medial direction through the base of the metacarpal into the fracture fragment. A second pin was drilled through the second metacarpal into the first metacarpal to maintain abduction. Salgeback and associates[380] and Wagner[457,458] placed two pins from the thumb metacarpal into the trapezium.

Skeletal traction using an oblique pin through the thumb metacarpal has been advocated by several authors.[158,411,439] This technique effectively counteracts both the shortening and varus angulation of the metacarpal.

The generally accepted orthopedic principle of accurate reduction of intra-articular fractures is supported by Gedda and Moberg.[155,156] They monitored 60 patients who had closed treatment of Bennett's fracture for an average of 7½ years. Only those with significant residual displacement were disabled. The 29 patients who had exact open reduction and pin fixation had much less pain and less arthritic change on radiographs. Likewise, Timmenga and associates[442] observed patients nearly 11 years after percutaneous or open reduction of a Bennett fracture. They concluded that exact

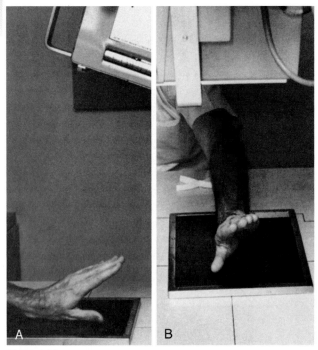

FIGURE 8-53. Hand and x-ray tube position for a true lateral radiograph of the first metacarpal-trapezial joint.

reduction should be the aim of treatment. Interestingly, most of their patients had some degenerative changes radiographically, but there was no correlation with symptoms. Thurston and Dempsey[441] reviewed 21 Bennett's fractures at nearly 8 years' follow-up and noted that results were superior clinically and radiographically when there was less than 1-mm stepoff. The technique by which reduction was achieved was immaterial. Other authors[8,172,416] have substantiated the efficacy of open reduction and secure internal fixation.

If the Bennett fragment is of adequate size, open reduction with either a Herbert[75,206] or conventional screw[90,138,149,]

[197,378,430] has been advocated. Provisional fixation is obtained with a bone tenaculum and/or Kirschner pin, followed by screw placement.[103]

Author's Preferred Method of Treatment

Although some patients with malunited Bennett's fractures remain relatively asymptomatic despite radiographic incongruity and degenerative changes, anatomic reduction is the most reliable method of achieving a satisfactory result. When the Bennett fragment is less than 15% to 20% of the articular surface, I prefer closed reduction and percutaneous pinning of the CMC joint. Under regional or general anesthesia, the thumb metacarpal is extended and pronated while longitudinal traction and downward pressure are applied to the metacarpal base (Fig. 8-55). While the reduction is held, a Kirschner pin is drilled obliquely across the trapeziometacarpal joint under fluoroscopic guidance. The reduction, articular congruity, and pin position are then checked with the image intensifier and confirmed by plain radiographs. If the metacarpal is reduced to the Bennett fragment and there is less than 2-mm of articular stepoff, I will accept the reduction and immobilize the area in a thumb spica cast.

If the Bennett fragment is large (greater than 25% to 30% of the articular surface), I prefer ORIF. The joint is approached through the Wagner[457] incision (Fig. 8-56A). The longitudinal limb of this incision is over the subcutaneous border of the thumb metacarpal (between the abductor pollicis longus and the thenar muscles) and is extended proximally and radially to the radial border of the flexor carpi radialis. The thenar muscles are reflected subperiosteally, the joint capsule is incised, and the fracture is visualized. When articular congruity has been restored, the Bennett fragment is held reduced with either reduction

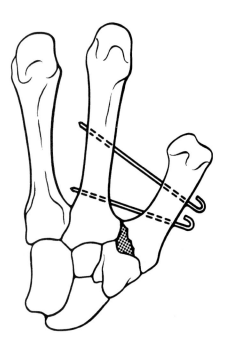

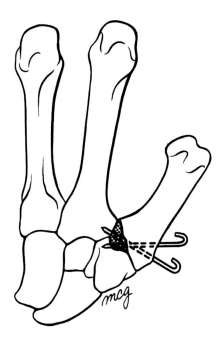

FIGURE 8-54. Percutaneous fixation of Bennett's fracture. **Left,** Intermetacarpal pinning. Pins are inserted between the thumb and index metacarpal. **Right,** Pins from the metacarpal shaft into Bennett's fragment.

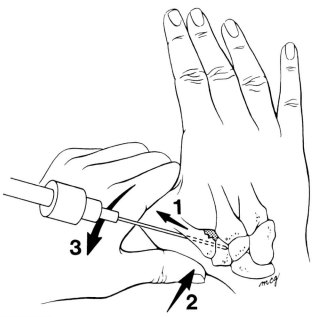

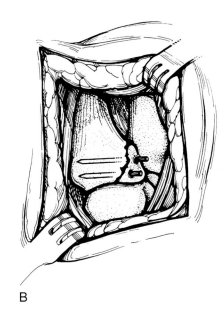

Postoperatively, if pins are used, the thumb is immobilized in a thumb spica cast for 4 weeks and the transarticular pin is removed. The pins holding the fracture fragment are removed at 6 weeks. Screw fixation, although technically more demanding, is more secure, and active range of motion may be initiated 5 to 10 days postoperatively.

Rarely, a Salter-Harris type III epiphyseal fracture involving the thumb metacarpals may occur if there is lateral subluxation of the metacarpal or fracture displacement, and accurate reduction by open means is indicated.[443]

Complications

Malunion may result in recurrent or persistent subluxation of the trapeziometacarpal joint. Clinkscales[85] recommended a closing wedge osteotomy at the base of the first metacarpal to correct the instability from a malunited Bennett fracture if more than 6 weeks has passed since the injury. Wagner[458] noted uniformly poor results when late reduction was attempted and recommended arthrodesis of the CMC joint. If arthritis has not developed, late osteotomy through the old fracture with reduction of the malunited fracture can improve range of motion and strength and provide pain relief.[223] Long-standing instability with painful arthritis is best treated by an arthrodesis. Nonunion is practically unknown. A contracture of the first web can result if the thumb metacarpal has been immobilized in an adducted position.

Rolando's Fracture

In 1910 Rolando[370] presented 12 cases of fracture of the base of the thumb metacarpal and described a fracture pattern with a "Y"- or "T"-shaped intra-articular component. He noted that the prognosis was not good after this injury

FIGURE 8-55. Percutaneous pin fixation of Bennett's fracture. Reduction is performed by (1) longitudinal traction, (2) pressure at the thumb metacarpal base, and (3) pronation. The pin is passed from the metacarpal to the trapezium. It is unnecessary to pin the Bennett fragment.

forceps or a small bone hook. Fixation is secured with either a 2.0- or 2.7-mm lag screw (Fig. 8-57) as advocated by Foster and Hastings.[138] Alternative fixation can be accomplished by passing two 0.035-inch Kirschner pins across the fracture (see Fig. 8-56B). With pin fixation, it is advisable to protect the reduction with a transarticular pin.

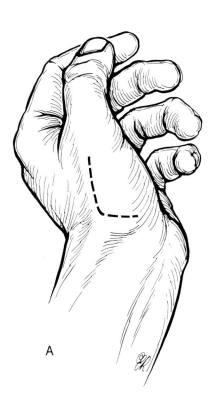

FIGURE 8-56. Incision (**A**) and technique (**B**) of open reduction and internal fixation of Bennett's fracture.

A

B

CRITICAL POINTS: OPERATIVE MANAGEMENT OF BENNETT'S FRACTURE

INDICATIONS

- Failed closed reduction (displacement or stepoff greater than 1 to 2 mm)
- Displaced Bennett fragment greater than 20% of joint surface

PREOPERATIVE EVALUATION

- Obtain *true* anteroposterior (Betts and Roberts views) and lateral radiographs.
- CT is unnecessary unless comminution is suspected.

PEARLS

- Anatomic articular restoration is probably unnecessary but reduction of dislocation is mandatory.

TECHNICAL POINTS

- For Bennett fragment less than 20% of articular surface use closed reduction and percutaneous pinning.
  - Use general or regional anesthesia.
  - Apply longitudinal traction, with downward pressure at base of thumb metacarpal and positioning in pronation.
  - Fluoroscopy greatly facilitates pin placement.
  - Insert two to three 0.9- or 1.1-mm Kirschner pins from thumb metacarpal into carpus or index metacarpal.

- For displaced fragment more than 20% of articular surface, consider open reduction.
  - Use Wagner (volar) approach along subcutaneous border of metacarpal.
  - Elevate thenar musculature off thumb metacarpal.
  - Anatomically reduce fracture with skin hooks or dental probe.
  - Provisionally pin in reduced position with 0.7-mm pin.
  - Fix Bennett fragment to metacarpal with two 2.0- or 1.5-mm screws using lag technique if feasible.
  - Verify anatomic reduction clinically and radiographically.
  - Make sure screws have not penetrated articular surface.

PITFALLS

- Avoid failure to adequately assess reduction intraoperatively such that pins are inappropriately placed or fracture is not reduced.
- Use radiography to confirm misdiagnosis preoperatively. Fracture is either extra-articular or is intra-articular with comminution.

POSTOPERATIVE CARE

- If percutaneous pin fixation is used, immobilize for 4 to 5 weeks in thumb spica cast before removing pins.
- If ORIF is used, begin range-of-motion exercises at first postoperative visit.

despite treatment in a cast or with skin traction. Langhoff and associates[261] noted that there are two controversies associated with the management of Rolando's fracture: (1) open reduction, which is difficult and prone to failure, may be less desirable than closed management; and (2) surgical intervention may not ensure that late symptoms are prevented. Today, the term *Rolando's fracture* has come to include any comminuted intra-articular fracture of the base of the thumb metacarpal.

Techniques of open reduction include multiple Kirschner pins,[155,261] tension band wiring,[21] and plate fixation.[138,197,378] Articular reduction is most likely to be successful when there are two fragments with minimal comminution. The surgical exposure for plate fixation is the same as for a Bennett fracture. Longitudinal traction is applied, and a provisional reduction of the two articular fragments is held with Kirschner pins and/or a reduction clamp. Articular congruity of the metacarpal base is verified by radiographs and by direct visualization. A 2.4- to 2.7-mm "L"- or "T"-plate is applied (Fig. 8-58).

For comminuted intra-articular fractures, Gelberman and coworkers[149,158] recommended oblique traction (Fig. 8-59) through the thumb metacarpal as described by Spanberg and Thoren[411,439] for Bennett's fracture. This technique is appealing for its simplicity and low complication rate. A 1-cm incision is made just distal to the abductor pollicis longus insertion and radial and volar to the extensor pollicis brevis tendon. A 0.062-inch Kirschner pin is drilled obliquely through the thumb metacarpal in a distal and ulnar direction with a slight volar tilt so that it exits in the thumb/index finger web space. The proximal end of the pin is bent 90 degrees, and the incision is closed. A forearm cast with a banjo outrigger is applied with exclusion of the thumb web, and rubber band traction is maintained for 4 to 6 weeks. A satisfactory outcome can usually be anticipated.

For comminuted fractures, Buchler and colleagues[59] recommended the application of a quadrilateral mini external fixation device placed between the thumb and index metacarpal, followed by limited open reduction with Kirschner pins or screws and a cancellous bone graft if there is a metaphyseal void or comminution (Fig. 8-60). At nearly 3 years later, nine patients had a good result and one had a fair result. Focal articular irregularity was common. Alternative techniques for external fixation include a triangular frame with pins in the distal end of the radius, thumb, and index metacarpal[391] or a uniplanar frame

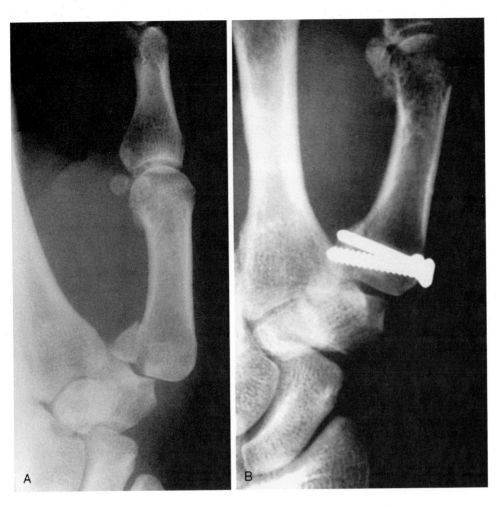

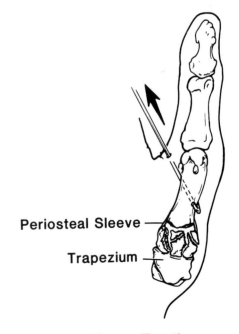

FIGURE 8-57. A, Displaced Bennett's fracture. **B,** Fixation with lag screws.

Periosteal Sleeve

Trapezium

Thoren Traction

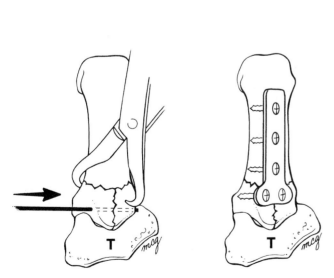

FIGURE 8-58. Rolando's fracture. **Left,** Provisional reduction is held with a clamp and Kirschner pin. **Right,** Final reduction maintained with a "T" (trapezium) plate.

FIGURE 8-59. Oblique skeletal traction for a comminuted fracture of the thumb metacarpal base. Through a small incision, a 0.062-inch Kirschner pin is drilled obliquely through the proximal metacarpal shaft and exits distally through the thumb web. The pin is crimped proximally and distal traction is applied through a banjo outrigger.

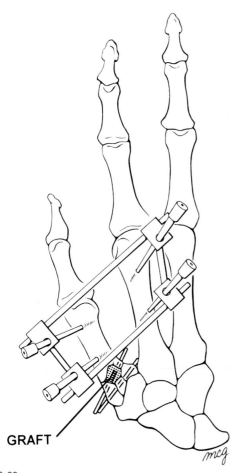

GRAPH

FIGURE 8-60. Quadrilateral frame for a comminuted fracture of the base of the thumb. Two pins each are inserted into the thumb and index finger metacarpals and interconnected with rods and swivel clamps. The thumb metacarpal articular surface is reduced and held with Kirschner pins, and the metaphysis is grafted with cancellous bone.

consisting of one pin in the trapezium and two pins in the thumb metacarpal.[250,355]

Author's Preferred Method of Treatment

The choice of treatment depends primarily on the degree of comminution. This fracture can be deceptively benign on plain radiographs. CT may be helpful in assessing the comminution and extent of articular disruption. If a classic three-part Rolando fracture exists, ORIF with either multiple Kirschner pins or a plate is reasonable. One should also be prepared to perform a bone graft if there is a metaphyseal void secondary to compaction of the cancellous subchondral bone. If there is significant comminution, open reduction may be frustrating and unproductive. Buchler's technique of using quadrilateral external fixation, articular reduction with Kirschner pins, and cancellous bone grafting is a reasonable alternative. The surgeon must keep in mind that anatomic reduction is not usually possible and that prolonged attempts to attain perfect reduction may result in devascularization of the osteochondral fragments and further articular injury.

If, after operative management, there is persistent pain, I prefer no further intervention for a minimum of 6 months. If pain persists, and there is radiographic evidence of articular incongruity, I recommend an arthrodesis of the trapeziometacarpal joint.

ANNOTATED REFERENCES

3. Al-Qattan MM: Phalangeal neck fractures in children: Classification and outcome in 66 cases. J Hand Surg [Br] 26:112-121, 2001.

   This article reviews treatment outcome of 66 phalangeal neck fractures in children. A simple classification that allows a guideline to treatment is also provided. The author makes a convincing argument that all displaced fractures should be treated with open reduction and Kirschner wire fixation and that nonsurgical management should be reserved for nondisplaced fractures.

7. Ashmead D IV, Rothkopf DM, Walton RL, Jupiter JB: Treatment of hand injuries by external fixation. J Hand Surg [Am] 17:956-964, 1992.

   This article makes a strong case for external fixation of metacarpal and phalangeal fractures, particularly if the fracture is open. Application is simple and soft tissue damage is minimal. External fixators stabilize both the fracture and the soft tissues. Union occurred in 20 of 22 acute fractures.

16. Becton JL, Christian JD Jr, Goodwin NH, Jackson JG: A simplified technique for treating the complex dislocation of the index metacarpophalangeal joint. J Bone Joint Surg Am 57:698-700, 1975.

    This article justifies a dorsal approach when managing a complex MCP dislocation and is contrary to E. B. Kaplan's 1957 recommendation for a volar approach. The dorsal approach is simple, permits fixation of associated metacarpal head fracture, and avoids injury to the digital nerves.

19. Belsky MR, Eaton RG, Lane LB: Closed reduction and internal fixation of proximal phalangeal fractures. J Hand Surg [Am] 9:725-729, 1984.

    This technique of percutaneous pin fixation is particularly useful for transverse proximal phalangeal fractures. Reduction is performed with wrist block anesthesia and application of longitudinal traction while the MCP joint is flexed to 60 degrees and the PIP joint is flexed to at least 45 degrees. A Kirschner pin is then passed percutaneously through the metacarpal head and into the medullary canal of the proximal phalanx and into the subchondral bone of the head of the proximal phalanx. This technique led to excellent results in 90% of fractures.

39. Bora FW Jr, Didizian NH: The treatment of injuries to the carpometacarpal joint of the little finger. J Bone Joint Surg Am 56:1459-1463, 1974.

    This is a frequently cited article that accurately describes the deforming forces leading to instability in fractures of the base of the small finger metacarpal. The authors recommend a 30-degree pronated view for optimal visualization of the CMC joint. Reduction and either closed or open Kirschner pinning was recommended for all fracture-subluxations.

44. Botte MJ, Davis JLW, Rose BA, et al: Complications of smooth pin fixation of fractures and dislocations in the hand and wrist. Clin Orthop 276:194-201, 1992.

Despite a reported high complication rate with pin fixation (18%) permanent sequelae were unusual. Infection was the most common complication (7%) followed by loosening without infection (4%) and loss of reduction (4%). Specific management of each complication is outlined.

57. Buchler U, Fischer T: Use of a minicondylar plate for metacarpal and phalangeal periarticular injuries. Clin Orthop 214:53-88, 1987.

    Periarticular fractures around the MCP and PIP joints can be difficult to stabilize. Traditional pin fixation may interfere with ligament stabilization and tendon gliding. The mini-condylar plate, although technically demanding, provides stable fixation in both the acute and reconstructive setting. Such fixation permits early range of motion.

58. Buchler U, Gupta A, Ruf S: Corrective osteotomy for post-traumatic malunion of the phalanges in the hand. J Hand Surg [Br] 21:33-42, 1996.

    Based on a review of 59 phalangeal malunions, the authors conclude that optimal correction can be achieved through the phalanx, rather than through the metacarpal. They point out that many deformities are multiplanar and better correction can be achieved by osteotomy *at the site of the deformity*. Also with stable fixation techniques a concomitant tenolysis or capsulotomy can be performed, thereby permitting early range of motion. Satisfactory correction was achieved in 76% of patients and there were no nonunions.

62. Burkhalter WE, Reyes FA: Closed treatment of fractures of the hand. Bull Hosp Joint Dis 44:145-162, 1984.

    Published in a rather obscure journal, this article emphasizes that most hand fractures can be treated by closed reduction and cast immobilization. Neutralizing the deforming forces of the intrinsics by positioning the fingers in an intrinsic-plus position (MCP flexion and interphalangeal extension) and allowing early range of motion in a cast with an MCP extension block is a reasonable alternative to invasive forms of treatment. "Stability, not rigidity, is the key."

80. Chow SP, Pun WK, So YC, et al: A prospective study of 245 open digital fractures of the hand. J Hand Surg [Br] 16:127-140, 1991.

    This prospective study identifies factors associated with a poor outcome following open hand fractures. One can anticipate a poor result when there is a fracture of the proximal phalanx, comminution, severe soft tissue damage, or flexor tendon injury.

112. Duncan RW, Freeland AE, Jabaley ME, et al: Open hand fractures: An analysis of the recovery of active motion and of complications. J Hand Surg [Am] 18:387-394, 1993.

    Range of motion following an open fracture correlates directly with the degree of associated soft tissue injury. Fracture location, that is, open fractures occurring between the MCP joint and the sublimis insertion (flexor tendon zone II) is also an important determinant of final range of motion. Caution must be exercised when surgically extending the traumatic incision because range of motion may be further compromised. Their findings suggest that application of plates and screws must be done with care because further soft tissue dissection may further jeopardize the outcome.

115. Edwards GS Jr, O'Brien ET, Heckman MM: Retrograde cross pinning of transverse metacarpal and phalangeal fractures. Hand 14:141-148, 1982.

    Although the majority of transverse shaft fractures can be managed closed or by percutaneous pin fixation, operative management using retrograde crossed pins is biomechan-

ically sound. This article describes the technique in detail and illustrates the use of a preview pin, as well as a 14-gauge needle as a pin guide.

127. Faraj AA, Dawson WJ: Percutaneous intramedullary fixation of metacarpal shaft fractures. J Hand Surg [Br] 24:76-79, 1999.

    Percutaneous intramedullary pin fixation of displaced transverse metacarpal shaft fractures has the advantage of providing stability with minimal disruption of the soft tissue sleeve. Disadvantages include the potential for pin migration or bending at the fracture. The authors report generally satisfactory results with few complications.

138. Foster RJ, Hastings H II: Treatment of Bennett, Rolando, and vertical intra-articular trapezial fractures. Clin Orthop 214:121-129, 1987.

    This is an excellent review article of the operative treatment of intra-articular fractures of the base of the thumb.

139. Foucher G: "Bouquet" osteosynthesis in metacarpal neck fractures: A series of 66 patients. J Hand Surg [Am] 20:S86-S90, 1995.

    Stabilization of a significantly displaced 5th metacarpal neck fracture with three pre-bent intramedullary Kirschner pins has the advantage of avoiding the fracture site and risking stiffness (extension contracture) of the MCP joint. The technique is simple, permits early range of motion, and is greatly facilitated with the use of fluoroscopy.

155. Gedda KO: Studies on Bennett's fracture: Anatomy, roentgenology, and therapy. Acta Chir Scand Suppl 193:1-114, 1954.

    This is an early article that points out that *closed management* of Bennett's fractures may lead to long-term disability because anatomic reduction and maintenance of reduction may be difficult to achieve. Open reduction and stabilization of the Bennett fragment to the shaft fragment with a single Kirschner yielded good results.

166. Gonzalez MH, McKay W, Hall RF Jr: Low velocity gunshot wounds of the metacarpal: Treatment by early stable fixation and bone grafting. J Hand Surg [Am] 18:267-270, 1993.

    Low-velocity gunshot fractures of the proximal phalanx are often treated by "benign neglect." Unfortunately, this treatment may lead to nonunion, malunion, or stiffness. The authors demonstrate that in the presence of adequate soft tissue coverage, early *internal fixation* with a plate, intermedullary pin, or both predictably leads to in union with satisfactory range of motion. Supplemental bone graft did not adversely affect outcome.

171. Green DP, Anderson JR: Closed reduction and percutaneous pin fixation of fractured phalanges. J Bone Joint Surg Am 55:1651-1653, 1973.

    A classic article demonstrating the efficacy of closed reduction and percutaneous Kirschner pin fixation of unstable, oblique phalangeal fractures. Pins were left in place for approximately 3 weeks, and the majority of patients gained full range of motion within 8 weeks.

172. Green DP, O'Brien ET: Fractures of the thumb metacarpal. South Med J 65:807-814, 1972.

    This is the classic article on fractures of the base of the thumb. The authors provide a classification and distinguish between intra-articular (Bennett's and Rolando's) and extra-articular (transverse, oblique, and epiphyseal) fractures. They note that extra-articular fractures can usually be managed by closed reduction and casting whereas intra-articular fractures usually require operative stabilization.

181. Grundberg AB: Intramedullary fixation for fractures of the hand. J Hand Surg 6:568-573, 1981.

This is the first article of any size that illustrates the technique of intramedullary fixation of metacarpal and phalangeal fractures. This fixation is particularly applicable to transverse and oblique midshaft fractures. Steinmann pins are used for fixation and are inserted through the fracture site. No hardware is left protruding, and early range of motion can be initiated. Generally satisfactory results were reported.

208. Hunter JM, Cowen NJ: Fifth metacarpal fractures in a compensation clinic population. J Bone Joint Surg Am 52:1159-1165, 1970.

This is a classic article that supports a conservative approach to the fifth metacarpal neck fracture. Fractures angulated up to 70 degrees were treated nonsurgically in an ulnar gutter splint for 10 days, followed by mobilization and early (approximately 4 weeks) return to work in a compensation clinic population. The authors "speak out" against overtreatment (surgical stabilization or prolonged immobilization), a common recommendation before the publication of this article.

220. Jahss SA: Fractures of the metacarpals: A new method of reduction and immobilization. J Bone Joint Surg 20:178-186, 1938.

This is the original description of the reduction maneuver and position of immobilization for a metacarpal neck fracture that today bears the author's name. Ten patients were treated by reduction (upward pressure on flexed PIP joint with downward pressure on MCP joint positioned in maximum flexion) and immobilized in 90 degrees of MCP and PIP flexion for 2½ weeks. On cast removal, the joints were forcefully manipulated (causing considerable pain) and range-of-motion exercises were initiated. The results in all 10 patients were "uniformly good."

221. James JIP: Fractures of the proximal and middle phalanges of the fingers. Acta Orthop Scand 32:401-412, 1962.

This is an article of historic interest. To avoid residual stiffness secondary to collateral ligament contracture during the treatment of a phalangeal fracture, the phalanges must be immobilized in 70 degrees of flexion at the MCP joint and 5 to 10 degrees at the IP joints.

232. Jupiter JB, Koniuch MP, Smith RJ: The management of delayed union and nonunion of the metacarpals and phalanges. J Hand Surg [Am] 10:457-466, 1985.

The authors not only point out that phalangeal nonunions are rare but recognize that they are often secondary to improper or inadequate Kirschner pin fixation. One can anticipate union with stable plate and screw fixation, a technique that also permits concomitant tenolysis or capsulotomy.

252. Kuhn KM, Dao KD, Shin AY: Volar A1 pulley approach for fixation of avulsion fractures of the base of the proximal phalanx. J Hand Surg [Am] 26:762-771, 2001.

Significantly displaced avulsion fractures from the base of the proximal phalanx represent MCP collateral ligament injuries and usually require operative treatment. Traditionally, these avulsions have been treated with open reduction through a *dorsal* approach. This article provides a detailed description of a *volar* approach that is appealing because it is direct and makes anatomic reduction easier.

270. Leung YL, Beredjiklian PK, Monaghan BA, Bozentka DJ: Radiographic assessment of small finger metacarpal neck fractures. J Hand Surg [Am] 27:443-448, 2002.

There is a large volume of literature regarding the management of boxer's fractures based on the *radiographic degree of angulation* (head-shaft angle). Ninety-six sets of radiographs were reviewed by three hand surgeons. They found that the reliability coefficient in measuring this angle between three different observers is *slight* and that consistent measurement within each observer was *fair*. This suggests that clinical assessment, that is, the presence of pseudo-clawing or malrotation, is at least as important as radiographic assessment.

278. Lister G: Intraosseous wiring of the digital skeleton. J Hand Surg 3:427-435, 1978.

The technique of intraosseous wiring for fusion of the IP joints and to stabilize fractures is demonstrated. Forty-seven fractures were treated with this technique; all united. A supplemental Kirschner pin was often necessary.

285. Loth TS, McMillan MD: Coronal dorsal hamate fractures. J Hand Surg [Am] 13:616-618, 1988.

This article brings attention to a rare and often missed entity—a coronal shear fracture of the dorsal hamate associated with a dorsal dislocation of the fourth and fifth metacarpal bases. Treatment consists of open reduction of the metacarpal bases and internal fixation of the hamate fracture with either Kirschner pins or screw(s). Care must be taken not to sever the hamate-metacarpal ligaments.

304. McElfresh EC, Dobyns JH: Intra-articular metacarpal head fractures. J Hand Surg 8:383-393, 1983.

Intra-articular fractures of the metacarpal heads are classified by anatomic involvement based on radiographic evaluation. When technically feasible, the authors favor operative management, especially for large intra-articular fragments.

336. Page SM, Stern PJ: Complications and range of motion following plate fixation of metacarpal and phalangeal fractures. J Hand Surg [Am] 23:827-832, 1998.

Plate and screw fixation of metacarpal and phalangeal fractures is attractive because it provides stable fixation with the potential for an early rehabilitation program. The authors show a high incidence of complications, particularly when plates are used in the treatment of *open* fractures of the phalanges. Plate fixation is not to be condemned, but the surgeon should be aware that this technique is not a panacea, especially for the management of phalangeal fractures with associated soft tissue injury.

343. Petrie PWR, Lamb DW: Fracture-subluxation of the base of the fifth metacarpal. Hand 6:82-86, 1974.

This is a frequently cited article describing the results of nonsurgical management of 14 fracture-subluxations of the base of the fifth metacarpal. They found that their conservatively treated patients had few symptoms at follow-up and concluded that "the case for surgical treatment is not strong," a recommendation that is contrary to most other series in the literature.

359. Pun WK, Chow SP, So YC, et al: Unstable phalangeal fractures: Treatment by A.O. screw and plate fixation. J Hand Surg [Am] 16:113-117, 1991.

Two hundred and 84 digital fractures were studied prospectively. The authors found that *stable* fractures could be managed by free mobilizations but *unstable* fractures did not fare well with splints or Kirschner pin fixation. Poor prognostic factors include open fractures, comminuted fractures, and associated soft tissue injury.

378. Ruedi TP, Burri C, Pfeiffer KM: Stable internal fixation of fractures of the hand. J Trauma 11:381-389, 1971.

This is one of the earliest articles that apply the Swiss ASIF principles of rigid fixation and early mobilization to the small bones of the hand. These surgeons believed that cast immobilization invariably led to joint stiffness and soft tissue atrophy. To permit internal fixation of small bones, special instruments, plates, and screws were designed.

398. Seymour N: Juxta-epiphyseal fracture of the terminal phalanx of the finger. J Bone Joint Surg [Br] 48:347-349, 1966.

The "Seymour" fracture is a Salter I injury that occurs through the physeal plate of the distal phalanx. The patient presents with a mallet deformity. The nail plate and matrix are displaced superficial to the proximal nail fold; if they are not relocated, sepsis frequently occurs. Seymour had uniformly good results with nail plate removal, fracture reduction, and replacement of the nail plate beneath the proximal nail fold.

428. Strickland JW, Steichen JB, Kleinman WB, et al: Phalangeal fractures: Factors influencing digital performance. Orthop Rev 11:39-50, 1982.

Following an analysis of 1418 fractures of the tubular bones of the hands, the authors accurately categorize different factors that influence outcome. Categories include *patient factors* such as age and associated diseases; *fracture factors* such as bone involved and location, as well as associated soft tissue injures; and *management factors*. They found that the important factors influencing outcome include immobilization greater than 4 weeks, open injuries, and increasing age.

439. Thoren L: A new method of extension treatment in Bennett's fracture. Acta Chir Scand 110:485-492, 1955.

Comminuted intra-articular fractures of the thumb metacarpal, as well as Bennett fractures, may be reduced by a traction pin placed obliquely through the thumb metacarpal and into the thumb web. Favorable results were noted in 9 of 10 fractures.

445. Trumble T, Gilbert M: In situ osteotomy for extra-articular malunion of the proximal phalanx. J Hand Surg [Am] 23:821-826, 1998.

Extra-articular malunions of the proximal phalanx have traditionally been corrected by an osteotomy through the base of the metacarpal. More recently, with better internal fixation techniques (small plates and screws), correction can be done at the site of the deformity. Advantages include the ability to correct an angular and rotational deformity simultaneously and, if necessary, perform a tenolysis. Excellent results were reported in 11 patients.

465. Weckesser EC: Rotational osteotomy of the metacarpal for overlapping fingers. J Bone Joint Surg Am 47:751-756, 1965.

This is a classic article that recommends a transverse osteotomy through the *metacarpal base* to correct rotational deformities resulting from malunions of either a metacarpal (six cases) or a phalanx (two cases). Fixation of the osteotomy with three Kirschner pins and early range of motion is recommended. Results were satisfactory, and there were no complications.

470. Weiss APC, Hastings H II: Distal unicondylar fractures of the proximal phalanx. J Hand Surg [Am] 18:594-599, 1993.

In addition to providing a useful classification of unicondylar phalangeal fractures, the authors emphasize that these are unstable injuries and that *displaced* fractures require operative stabilization. Fixation must consist of a *minimum* of two screws or two Kirschner pins or a combination. Even with anatomic reduction, full range of motion may not occur.

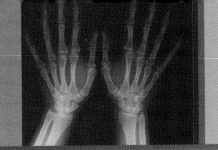

CHAPTER 9

Dislocations and Ligament Injuries in the Digits

Steven Z. Glickel, O. Alton Barron, and Louis W. Catalano III

he hand is our primary tool. It is remarkably well designed to provide sensibility, mobility, and strength sufficient for an almost infinite number of tasks. The adaptability of the hand is a function of its articulations, each well suited to its position in the linear linkage by which power is transmitted from the forearm to the fingertips. Because of our dependency on the hand for creativity, recreation, and livelihood, the hand is subjected to constant use and frequent abuse. The joints, although ingeniously designed for stability and mobility, remain vulnerable to extremes of external force, which may injure the supporting capsule and ligament systems, producing varying degrees of dislocation, subluxation, instability, or contracture.

THE PROXIMAL INTERPHALANGEAL JOINT

The proximal interphalangeal (PIP) joint has been accurately described as the "anatomical and functional locus of finger function."[69] It is not surprising, then, that dislocation of the PIP joint is the most common ligament injury in the hand. The spectrum of PIP joint injuries ranges from the ubiquitous and mundane "jammed" finger to the more complicated and potentially disabling irreducible fracture-dislocation. Many of these ligament injuries are incomplete, and the ligament is only plastically deformed or partially torn, resulting in significant pain, swelling, and stiffness but with maintenance of joint congruity and stability. In certain injuries, such as lateral dislocations and hyperextension injuries, there is complete rupture of one or more supporting structures. However, when the normal alignment of the joint is restored, the extent and precise location of the anatomic lesion are not apparent without specific testing. Treatment is based on an accurate diagnosis of the pathologic lesion and degree of clinical dysfunction.

Anatomy

The PIP joint is a hinge, or ginglymus, joint, having great stability throughout its normal 100- to 110-degree arc of motion.[24] Stability derives from the joint's articular contours and periarticular ligaments, with secondary stabilization provided by adjacent tendon and retinacular systems.[71,162] The head of the proximal phalanx consists of two concentric condyles separated by an intercondylar notch. Slight asymmetry of the condyles imparts up to 9 degrees of conjunct supination through the complete arc of PIP motion.[65,67] The condyles articulate with two concave fossae in the broad, flattened base of the middle phalanx separated by a median ridge. This tongue-and-groove contour and breadth of congruence add stability by resisting lateral and rotatory stress (Fig. 9-1). Minamikawa and coworkers have demonstrated that articular congruence and increased axial load provide additional resistance to lateral angulation when the PIP joint is fully extended.[77]

The lateral joint capsule is largely composed of thick, durable collateral ligaments. These 2- to 3-mm thick ligaments arise from a concave fossa on the lateral aspect of each condyle and pass obliquely and volarly to their insertions. The collateral ligaments have proper and volar accessory components. They are anatomically confluent but distinguished by their points of insertion. The proper collateral ligament inserts on the volar one third of the base of the middle phalanx, and the

The authors would like to acknowledge the enormous contributions made by the original author of this chapter, **Richard G. Eaton, MD.** He developed or perfected several of the techniques described in this chapter and, through his writing and teaching, gave hand surgeons a systematic approach to the treatment of joint injuries. He has been a mentor and friend to a generation of hand surgeons, including the authors.

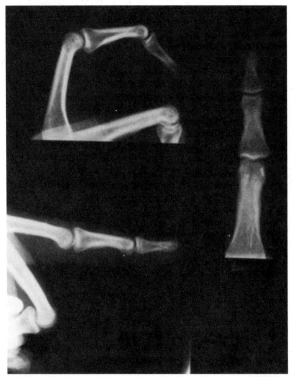

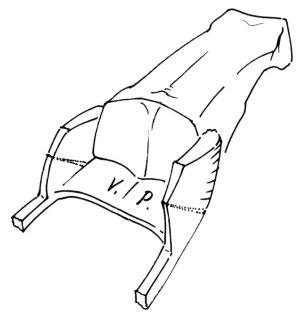

FIGURE 9-2. The three-dimensional ligament-box complex provides strength with minimum bulk. At least two sides of this box must be disrupted for displacement of the joint to occur.

FIGURE 9-1. Radiographs of the IP joints. In the lateral views *(left)*, note the concentric arc of each proximal condyle and the concave base of the middle phalanx that maintains total contact with this condyle through the full 110-degree arc of motion. Full flexion will be blocked by any process, bone spicule, or scar that encroaches on the retrocondylar fossa into which the base of the middle phalanx must fit. In the posteroanterior view *(right)*, the tongue-and-groove articular contours provide additional stability to rotatory and lateral stress.

accessory collateral is directed more volarly, inserting on the volar plate.[65] The collateral ligaments are the primary restraints to radial and ulnar joint deviation, with the actual amount of deviation varying among individuals.[54]

The volar plate forms the floor of the joint and is suspended laterally by the collateral ligaments. The thick fibrocartilaginous distal portion inserts across the volar base of the middle phalanx. This insertion is only densely attached at its lateral margins, where it is confluent with the insertion of the collateral ligament. It is thinner centrally and blends with the volar periosteum of the middle phalanx.[10] The central portion tapers proximally into an areolar sheet and laterally thickens to form a pair of volar check ligaments.[10,23,31,61,68,116] These tough restraining ligaments originate from the periosteum of the proximal phalanx, just inside the walls of the second annular (A2) pulley at its distal margin, and are confluent with the proximal origins of the first cruciate (C1) pulley.[10] The resulting paired, cordlike structures prevent hyperextension of the joint while permitting full flexion, thereby providing remarkable stability with minimum bulk. The volar plate is a secondary stabilizer against lateral deviation, especially with the PIP joint extended, but only when the collateral ligaments are incompetent or torn.[54]

The key to PIP joint stability is the strong conjoined attachment of the paired collateral ligaments and the volar plate into the volar third of the middle phalanx (Fig. 9-2).

This ligament-box configuration produces a three-dimensional strength that strongly resists PIP displacement. For displacement of the middle phalanx to occur, the ligament-box complex must be disrupted in at least two planes.[23]

Load to failure cadaveric studies of the PIP stabilizers have confirmed the clinical observation that the collateral ligaments fail proximally about 85% of the time while the volar plate avulses distally up to 80% of the time.[10,54] However, at lower angular velocities of side-to-side deformation, a less common mechanism of injury, the collateral ligaments tend to fail in their midsubstance.[92]

Evaluation of the Injured PIP Joint

Radiographic Evaluation

Ligament disruptions produce varying degrees of joint instability. Because the goal of treatment is to restore functional stability, it is essential that a systematic evaluation of joint stability be performed. Initial posteroanterior and *true* lateral radiographs of the *digit* must be obtained to determine if recent or preexisting articular involvement is present. Radiographs of the hand alone are not adequate; the "fanned four-finger lateral" is not acceptable. A subtle fracture or dislocation may be missed owing to superimposition of the digits on the lateral view or lack of an optimal oblique view of the digit (Fig. 9-3).[112] Computed tomography or trispiral tomograms are occasionally indicated, especially to assess suspected articular depression.

Clinical Evaluation

The clinician must assess the extent to which the joint widens and the middle phalanx deviates with lateral stress.[54,77] However, the ultimate determinant of treatment is whether the joint remains concentrically reduced with active motion. A simple test to determine the condition of the joint is to load and passively move the PIP joint while feeling for joint

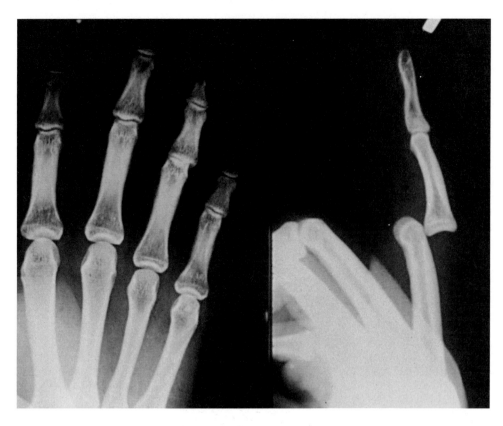

FIGURE 9-3. Posteroanterior and lateral radiographs of a dorsal dislocation of the ring finger PIP joint. The dislocation is barely recognizable on the posteroanterior view but clearly seen on the lateral view, where the middle phalanx is in bayonet apposition to the proximal phalanx.

crepitus. Functional stability may be determined by the following simple two-phase test, performed under the digital or wrist block anesthesia.[25]

1. *Active stability.* The patient voluntarily moves the digit through its normal range of motion. Completion of a full or near-full range indicates that, despite ligament disruption, adequate joint stability remains. Treatment requires only brief immobilization (mean, 5 to 7 days) to allow sufficient soft tissue recovery to begin protected range of motion exercises. Re-displacement with motion, however, indicates significant ligament disruption (i.e., at least two sides of the "box"). The position at which displacement occurs is a clue to the specific site of ligament injury, as well as the optimum position for joint immobilization.
2. *Passive stability.* Final assessment of stability is determined by passive manipulation. Gentle lateral stress is applied to each collateral ligament in full extension and 30 degrees of flexion, and the angle of deviation of the middle phalanx from the longitudinal axis is assessed.[54,77] Dorsovolar stability is tested by shearing the joint surfaces dorsally and volarly. Increased mobility in any plane should always be compared with an uninjured digit.

Determination of the degree of joint stability allows the examiner to codify the injury into one of three grades of ligament sprains. The mild grade I sprain implies macroscopic continuity but microscopic tearing of the ligament(s), without instability. At the other end of the spectrum is the grade III sprain, which is a complete tear of the collateral ligament and gross instability. Grade II includes all injuries in which the ligaments, although grossly intact, have a moderate degree of fiber disruption and may have some abnormal laxity

when stressed. The diagnosis of grade I and mild grade II sprains is inferred when the joint is stable to active and passive stress but is significantly swollen and pain is elicited on stress and palpation of the involved ligament(s).

DISLOCATIONS OF THE PIP JOINT

The PIP joint may dislocate in one of three directions: dorsal, lateral, and volar. These refer to the position of the middle phalanx when joint deformation occurs.

Acute Dorsal PIP Dislocations

The mechanism of injury in dorsal dislocations is usually PIP joint hyperextension combined with some degree of longitudinal compression, which frequently occurs in ball-handling sports if the tip of the digit is hit with the ball. In the majority of cases, dorsal dislocation produces a soft tissue or bone injury to the distal insertions of the three-dimensional ligament-box complex. The greater the longitudinal force, the more likely the volar lip of the middle phalanx will be sheared off or impacted, producing a fracture-dislocation. On rare occasions, the volar plate ruptures proximally and can become interposed, perhaps with an osteochondral fragment, between the head of the proximal phalanx and the base of the middle phalanx. This results in an irreducible dislocation and necessitates an open reduction.[13,36,55,57,82,84] The volar fracture fragment may even become trapped within the flexor sheath and inhibit motion.[29] Dorsal displacement of the middle phalanx produces specific lesions of the ligament system that can be classified into three major types (Fig. 9-4). Each lesion represents a specific disruption of this ligament-box complex. Types I (hyperextension) and II (dorsal dislocation) rarely require surgical treatment, whereas type III (fracture-dislocation) injuries may require a more intensive, often surgical, treatment regimen.

Type I (Hyperextension)

Hyperextension injuries are characterized by partial or complete avulsion of the volar plate from the base of the middle phalanx, with or without a bone fragment, and minor longitudinal rents in the collateral ligaments. In cases where the initial deformity has been severe, the middle phalanx may actually become locked in 70 to 80 degrees of hyperextension. The articular surfaces remain congruent, but with the middle phalanx articulating with the dorsal third of the condyle of the proximal phalanx (Fig. 9-4A). True lateral radiographs will often reveal a small, minimally displaced avulsion fragment from the base of the middle phalanx that should have no impact on treatment.

Type II (Dorsal Dislocation)

With complete dorsal dislocation of the PIP joint, avulsion of the volar plate is accompanied by a major bilateral split in the collateral ligament system. The base of the middle phalanx rests dorsally on the condyles of the proximal phalanx, usually in bayonet apposition with the shafts of the phalanges essentially parallel. There is no contact between the articular surfaces (see Fig. 9-4B).

Type III (Fracture-Dislocation)

Occasionally, the compressive force is of sufficient magnitude to shear off or impact the volar base of the middle phalanx, producing a fracture-dislocation (see Fig. 9-4C).[40] Fracture-dislocations can be subdivided into two types, stable and unstable, which have very specific implications for reduction and treatment (Fig. 9-5).

Stable Fracture-Dislocation. Fracture-dislocation with a small triangular fragment representing less than 40% of the volar articular arc results in a dorsal displacement much like simple dorsal dislocations. The transverse disruption, however, occurs through the base of the phalanx rather than at the insertion of the volar plate. The dorsal portion of the collateral ligaments remains attached to the middle phalanx, which is what renders these injuries inherently stable on reduction (see Fig. 9-5A).

Unstable Fracture-Dislocation. Fracture or impaction of a larger segment of the volar articular surface of the middle phalanx may also result in dorsal dislocation. However, this represents a major loss of articular and ligamentous support for the PIP joint. With disruption of greater than 40% of the volar articular segment, the majority of the collateral ligament-volar plate complex is attached to the fragment, not the remaining intact base of the middle phalanx. Accurate closed reduction is difficult to achieve and even more difficult to maintain. Adding to the instability is the loss of the buttressing effect of the volar margin of the middle phalanx that partially cups the proximal phalangeal condyles (see Fig. 9-5C). Treatment is described in the section on open reduction.

Schenck introduced a 16-component classification system in an effort to more specifically characterize the type III

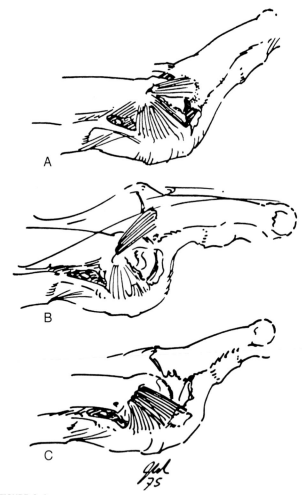

FIGURE 9-4. Pathology of dorsal dislocations of the PIP joint. **A,** Type I (hyperextension). The volar plate is avulsed and an incomplete longitudinal split occurs in the collateral ligaments. The articular surfaces maintain congruous contact. **B,** Type II (dorsal dislocation). There is complete rupture of the volar plate and a complete split in the collateral ligaments, with the middle phalanx resting on the dorsum of the proximal phalanx. The proximal and middle phalanges lie in almost parallel alignment. **C,** Type III (fracture-dislocation). The insertion of the volar plate, including a portion of the volar base of the middle phalanx, is disrupted. The major portion of the collateral ligaments remains with the volar plate and flexor sheath. A major articular defect may be present. (From Eaton RG, Littler JW: Joint injuries and their sequelae. Clin Plast Surg 3:85-98, 1976.)

(fracture-dislocation) injuries just discussed.[98] The PIP joint is examined on the lateral radiograph and assigned one of four fracture grades (I to IV) and one of four subluxation grades (A to D). The injury is thereby classified into one of the 16 possible permutations. This was devised as an attempt to standardize published reports and facilitate comparative analyses of different treatment methods for the specific PIP injury patterns.

Pilon Fracture. Fracture-dislocations of the PIP joint usually occur when the vector force of compression is not directly axial and the PIP joint is flexed to some degree. When an axial compressive force occurs with the proximal and middle phalanges being collinear, a pilon fracture may occur. (See Chapter 8 on fractures of the metacarpals and

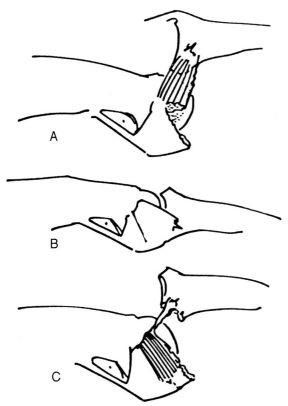

FIGURE 9-5. Comparison of type III stable and unstable fracture-dislocations. **A,** Stable. Fracture of less than 40% of the volar base of the middle phalanx leaves a significant portion of the collateral ligaments still attached. This portion will guide the displaced middle phalanx to a congruous reduction. **B,** Normal. Collateral ligament insertion into the volar third of the middle phalanx and volar plate. **C,** Unstable. Fracture of greater than 40% of the volar base of the middle phalanx leaves little or no collateral ligament attached. Congruous reduction is unlikely without these ligaments. Frequently the articular surface is impacted into the subcondylar bone and produces an irregular, depressed volar articular defect.

phalanges.) This fracture is primarily intra-articular without dislocation or subluxation of the joint, but there is often widening of the base as dorsal and volar fragments are driven apart and more central cartilage surfaces are impacted into the cancellous bone of the base.[106a,123] Treatment modalities such as those used for fracture-dislocations may be necessary.

Depression of the concave articular surface of one or both condylar fossae of the middle phalangeal base mimics certain tibial plateau fractures. Angular deformities are common especially if only one condyle is involved. These fractures are subtle on plain radiographs of the involved digit, and the clinician should maintain a low threshold for obtaining a CT scan of the PIP joint to better visualize the articular depression. Aggressive treatment should lessen the risk of persistent or worsening angular deformity, stiffness, and arthritis. Nevertheless, excellent results are difficult to achieve, with residual stiffness likely.[106a]

Treatment of Stable PIP Joint Injuries

The PIP joint is contaminated in an open dorsal dislocation. Therefore, adequate débridement and irrigation should be performed under ideal conditions, usually in the operating room, and antibiotics given based on the condition of the wound and the nature and location of the injury.[106]

Type I (hyperextension) injuries may be quite painful but are relatively benign injuries in the majority of cases.[44] The two most important aspects of treatment are patient education and the avoidance of prolonged immobilization. Patients must be reassured that most of these injuries will return to normal function but that the swelling and stiffness may persist for several months, and occasionally for more than 6 months. These injuries are stable and should be immobilized for comfort and soft tissue recovery for no more than 1 week. It is rare to see problems arising from premature mobilization and common to see stiffness and contracture as a result of prolonged immobilization.

Few clinical studies have been performed on these ubiquitous injuries. Jesperson and associates prospectively evaluated 57 PIP joint hyperextension injuries, 57% of which occurred during ball-handling sports.[48] The ring finger PIP joint was most commonly affected, and 44% had associated avulsion fractures. The four patients with persistent pain and instability all had hyperextension instability on the initial examination.

Type II (dorsal dislocation) injuries are usually stable to active and passive testing and require more protection than simple hyperextension injuries but still no more than 2 to 3 weeks of immobilization or controlled mobilization[101] (see Authors' Preferred Methods of Treatment).

Type III (fracture-dislocation) injuries must be carefully assessed to determine whether the dislocation is stable or unstable. Stable fracture-dislocations can generally be treated conservatively with 3 weeks of dorsal block splinting followed by range of motion exercises. Intermittent static or dynamic splinting may be necessary to overcome the natural tendency to develop stiffness and flexion contracture.[49,122] Most patients will require formal hand therapy to regain full motion and function. In our experience, the patient's personality and initial response to the injury may play more of a role than the specific injury in determining the extent to which therapy is needed.

Treatment of Unstable PIP Joint Injuries

Unstable type III PIP fracture-dislocations must be evaluated and treated with great attention to detail, because in the best of circumstances these injuries may still lead to complications, permanent dysfunction, and dissatisfaction. The continuing development of new treatment techniques for these injuries may imply that none of the current techniques produces consistently good to excellent results in a majority of patients for a majority of hand surgeons.

Specific Techniques

Dynamic Skeletal Traction. Variations on this theme have been recommended for several decades.[3,4,16,81,93] Both early and current devices are founded on the principle of *ligamentotaxis* through which the fracture fragments and the articular surface are reduced as longitudinal traction tightens the intact components of the attached soft tissue envelope. Early range of motion may be instituted with the traction maintained.[4,43,79,97,107] However, care must be taken to ensure that joint subluxation does not occur during any part of the motion arc. A review of several recent reports showed an average range of motion of approximately 85 degrees at 1- to 2-year follow-up.[4,43,79,107] Pin tract complications ranged from 0% to 74% but rarely affected final outcome. The best results were achieved in fractures with less articular involvement and those treated acutely. Although design specifics vary, the effective application of certain of these devices can be difficult even for experienced hand surgeons.[4,43,79,97,107] Dynamic traction devices can be cumbersome to wear and do not necessarily ensure optimal restoration of the articular surface, particularly when impaction of articular fracture fragments is present. Nevertheless, in certain fracture-dislocations and articular impaction and pilon fractures a dynamic traction device may be the only option. For pilon fractures, the dynamic traction device can help to neutralize the joint reactive forces after open elevation of the depressed articular surface and bone grafting of the resultant defect. Dynamic traction devices vary in design, one type deriving the distraction force from rubber bands and the other from coiled Kirschner wires.[4,43,79,100a,100b,107] Regardless of which particular device is used, care must be taken to prevent creating a moment arm about the middle phalanx leading to re-subluxation.

Krakauer and Stern used a hinged device to allow early active range of motion after surgical procedures on the PIP joint that combined distraction arthroplasty with other techniques, including closed reduction, open reduction and internal fixation (ORIF), and volar plate arthroplasty.[59] Satisfactory results in 20 patients led the authors to recommend the selective use of this device in the treatment of fractures about the PIP joint.

Extension Block Splinting. McElfresh and colleagues reported good results with active flexion using a dorsal splint to block extension beyond the point of potential redisplacement.[75] The PIP joint is brought into extension incrementally by reducing flexion in the splint by 10 to 15 degrees per week. However, in their series of 17 fingers, only four patients had a fragment size greater than 30% of the articular surface. This suggests that the technique is most useful in fractures with small volar fragments in which the majority of the collateral ligament remains attached to the middle phalangeal base.[20,75] Hamer and Quinton prospectively followed 27 patients for less than 2 years, with fracture-dislocations involving an average of 50% of the articular surface treated by extension block splinting.[38] They reported a mean of 87 degrees of active PIP motion and good results in 70% of patients. Green also advocated this technique.[35] Unstable fracture-dislocations tend to become stable only in marked flexion, and several authors have recommended immobilization or fixation in up to 75 degrees of PIP flexion.[14,21,100,104,122] This, however, dramatically increases the risk for late flexion contracture. Short, small, fingers make the fixation of the extension block splint more difficult, and thick swollen fingers decrease the efficacy of this technique, given that re-subluxation and even re-dislocation may occur. Serial radiographs must be obtained to document the ongoing effectiveness of this technique in maintaining joint congruity.

Extension Block Pinning. With this technique, a Kirschner wire is placed into the head of the proximal phalanx at an angle to mechanically block extension of the PIP joint and prevent dorsal subluxation of the middle phalanx.[111,114] However, reports of this technique include only a small number of cases, and its clinical efficacy must be substantiated through further study.

Trans-articular Pinning. Simple reduction and pinning of the PIP joint with no attempt at articular reconstruction has been advocated in a retrospective report by Newington and associates.[83] Although preoperative data were limited, the authors used this technique for articular involvement greater than 25% and less than 60%. In 11 fingers with long-term follow-up, all of the PIP joints were congruent, average PIP motion was 85 degrees, and 3 of 10 patients had some residual pain.

Open Reduction with Internal Fixation. This method has many advocates* and is most likely to be successful in acute cases with a single, large fragment. Anatomic restoration of the articular surface is technically difficult even with a large, single fragment, especially because the remaining articular contour may be disrupted secondary to impaction of subchondral cancellous bone. As with dynamic digital traction, the relatively small series and short follow-up leave unanswered the question of whether the articular reductions are adequate to prevent late post-traumatic arthrosis. If early active motion is not instituted, the risk for joint contracture is greatly increased after open treatment, especially if pins are placed in positions that impale or tether the extensor mechanism.[37]

Using a novel technique introduced by Hasting in 1999 (Scientific presentation, American Society for Surgery of the Hand, Annual Meeting, 1999) William and associates reported on 13 consecutive patients treated with a hemihamate autograft. The autograft is harvested from the dorsal distal aspect of the hamate centered at the fourth and fifth carpometacarpal articulations, spanning approximately one-half of each in both the radioulnar and dorsovolar planes. The graft is then rotated 180 degrees in two planes, keyed into the prepared bed at the volar base of the middle phalanx, and stabilized with two or three mini-fragment lag screws.

All 13 patients in this study had unstable dorsal PIP fracture-dislocations with 40% to 80% loss of the middle phalangeal articular base. These retrospectively studied patients achieved a mean of 85 degrees (range, 65 to 100 degrees) of PIP motion at an average of 17 months. Eleven of 12 patients were "very satisfied," with two of 12 cases complicated by re-subluxation and four of 12 patients noting some pain at the donor site. The authors expressed cautious optimism as to the longevity of the procedure. The authors maintained that while indications for this procedure largely parallel those of volar plate arthroplasty, the increased risk of re-subluxation with volar plate arthroplasty in the face of more extensive articular comminution may make the hemihamate graft a better option.

Volar Plate Arthroplasty. Multiple authors have reported on the technique and efficacy of using the distal aspect of the fibrocartilaginous volar plate to resurface the comminuted volar articular surface of the middle phalanx, especially when other techniques are not feasible.[8,22,26,46,47,72] The technique is described in detail in Authors' Preferred Methods of Treatment.

As a variation on the theme of volar plate arthroplasty, Wiley proposed débridement of the fragments and insertion of a slip of flexor superficialis tendon into the defect to

---

*See references 34, 46, 47, 64, 66, 70, 74, 78, 103, 117, 121, 123, 125, and 126.

reduce the displacement by active tendon tone.[119,120] The irregularity of the articular surface was not specifically corrected in his series.

Authors' Preferred Methods of Treatment

Stable Injuries. Most dorsal dislocations and fracture-dislocations of the PIP joint are amenable to nonoperative treatment. PIP joint injuries that are stable with active motion can be treated by immobilization with a dorsal splint usually in 20 to 30 degrees of flexion for comfort and to rest the soft tissues. The period of immobilization ranges from as little as 3 to 5 days for mild to moderate type I hyperextension injuries to 7 to 14 days for dislocations and stable fracture-dislocations. Duration of immobilization is individualized depending on the extent of the injury and resultant amount of soft tissue swelling; higher energy injuries with more swelling are rested longer. The PIP joint should not be immobilized in more than 30 degrees of flexion or a flexion contracture is likely to develop. After full-time splinting, the finger can be buddy-taped to an adjacent digit for further protection while active use and range-of-motion exercises are begun. Stiffness and swelling may persist for many months, and if patients are advised of this at the outset, they will better accept this slow but normal improvement.

Unstable Injuries. Several satisfactory and no perfect treatment options exist for the treatment of unstable PIP joint fracture-dislocations. We are not wedded to a particular modality of treatment and allow the injury characteristics to guide our approach. The rare unstable pure dislocation without fracture is usually treated with extension block splinting and only with extension block pinning if subluxation occurs in the splint. Timely follow-up care with radiographs to document reduction and pin position are necessary for good outcomes. On the rare occasions that we use an extension block pin, the digit is splinted to decrease the risk for pin migration or pin tract infection. Gentle active motion exercises are possible with an extension block pin in place, but the pin must be placed obliquely between the central tendon and lateral bands, and patient compliance must be substantiated.[111,114]

Operative treatment is indicated only for those unstable fracture-dislocations in which a congruous closed reduction is not possible. These are usually type III unstable fracture-dislocations that have more than 40% of the volar articular surface fractured, leaving little if any collateral ligament attached to the middle phalanx. The goals of treatment are congruous reduction of the PIP joint, restoration of the articular surface, and active motion as soon as possible.

For fracture-dislocations, the only treatment option we do not use is transarticular pinning without articular reduction.[83] We have found extension block splinting to be quite effective for cases where subluxation is relatively mild and articular involvement is less than 40%[20] (Fig. 9-6). There are two important caveats in using this technique: (1) the joint must be reduced before applying the splint, and (2) care must be taken to ensure that dorsal subluxation (loss of reduction) does not occur during the course of treatment with the splint in place. If the PIP joint injury is amenable to extension block splinting, but the digit is too short, stocky, or swollen for such treatment, then we will occasionally use an extension block pin.

We find dynamic skeletal traction methods useful in select cases, especially with increased comminution and nondisplaced fracture lines extending dorsally through the base of the middle phalanx. We have tried most of the methods noted earlier and have found the device reported by Suzuki and colleagues to be the most reproducible in our hands[43,107] (Fig. 9-7).

ORIF is an excellent form of treatment when there is a single large volar fragment.[34] The procedure is performed through a volar zigzag incision, based radially in the index and long fingers and ulnarly in the ring and small fingers to reduce the potential for contact hypersensitivity. The PIP joint is entered in the interval between the flexor sheath and accessory collateral ligaments on one or both sides of the

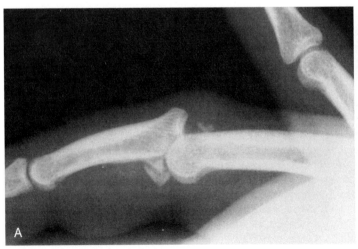

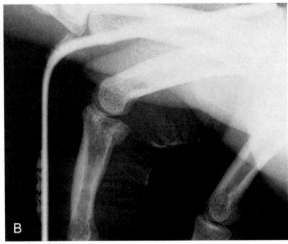

FIGURE 9-6. **A,** Type III fracture-dislocation of the PIP joint in which approximately 40% of the volar articular surface is displaced with the fracture fragment. **B,** Fracture-dislocations with 40% or less of the articular surface involved may be successfully treated with dorsal extension block splinting. The patient is allowed to actively flex the PIP joint, which is progressively extended over the course of approximately 4 weeks. The key to this mode of treatment is concentric reduction of the PIP joint.

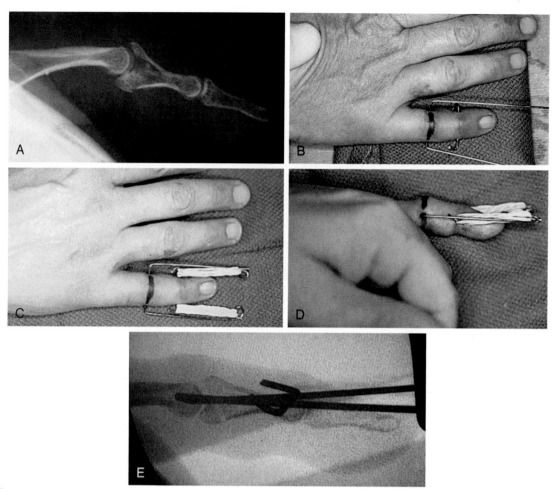

FIGURE 9-7. **A,** Lateral radiograph shows a pilon-type fracture of the middle phalangeal base. **B,** The wires of a dynamic traction device are placed in the proximal and middle phalanges in a manner similar to that described by Suzuki and associates.[107] **C,** The two wires are connected by rubber bands. **D,** Lateral view of the traction device. **E,** Postreduction lateral radiograph shows significantly improved position of the articular fragments. (Courtesy of Benjamin Rosenstadt, MD, New York, NY.)

joint. Careful preoperative evaluation of the lateral radiograph will have revealed any impaction of the remaining dorsal articular surface. This is elevated with a dental pick or Freer elevator, and the remaining void is filled with a small autologous or allograft cancellous crouton.

A single, large fragment may then be reduced and held with one or two small Kirschner wires, the goal being an anatomic, stable reduction. Mini-fragment lag screw fixation may be performed, if preferred over Kirschner wire fixation. In hard bone, the small screw head(s) are counter-sunk to decrease flexor sheath irritation and care is taken to avoid screw tips extending beyond the dorsal cortex and irritating the extensor mechanism. Excision of the collateral ligaments attached to the fragment greatly improves visualization and ease of manipulation, but preserving the volar plate insertion on the fragment seems to maintain sufficient blood supply for fracture healing to occur. Protected early motion is the goal. (See Chapter 8 for more detailed description of ORIF techniques.)

The majority of unstable PIP dorsal fracture-dislocations are not amenable to ORIF, and we prefer to treat these with volar plate arthroplasty.[8,22,26,46,47,72] Although not necessarily apparent radiographically, the volar fragment is frequently comminuted, making ORIF difficult or impossible. Through the same exposure, the feasibility of ORIF is assessed. If ORIF

is impossible, then resurfacing of this depressed, irregular area can be achieved by advancement of the fibrocartilaginous volar plate.

Technique of PIP Volar Plate Arthroplasty. The PIP joint is exposed using a radially based flap through a chevron-shaped incision with its apex at the ulnar midaxial point. The flexor sheath is excised between the A2 and A4 pulleys, and the flexor tendons are atraumatically retracted with a Penrose drain. The articular surfaces are very difficult to assess with the joint reduced. Hyperextension of the joint will usually expose the distal edge of the fracture fragment, facilitating entrance into the joint. To gain optimal exposure, the collateral ligaments that remain attached to the middle phalanx are excised except for the most volar remnants. These are preserved for later use in the procedure to suture each corner of the volar plate margin after advancement. Excising the collateral ligaments allows the joint to be maximally hyperextended, as one would open a shotgun. With both articular surfaces completely exposed, the feasibility of reduction and fixation of the fragments can be determined.

Congruous reduction may not be possible if the fracture fragments are markedly comminuted or impacted. Loose bone fragments and the segment attached to the volar plate are

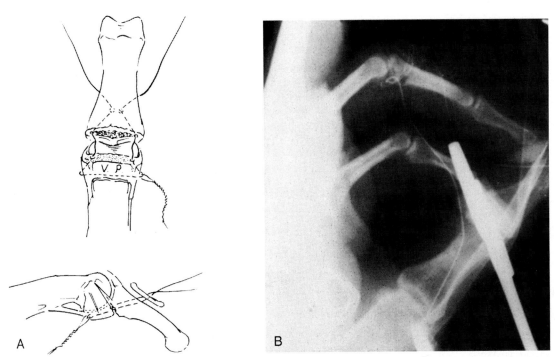

FIGURE 9-8. **A,** Technique of volar plate arthroplasty (see the text). **B,** Intraoperative lateral radiograph confirming congruous reduction of a volar plate arthroplasty. The pull-out suture marks the position of the volar plate within the articular defect.

débrided. The defect in the volar rim of the middle phalanx is shaped into a transverse groove perpendicular to the long axis of the phalanx. Deeply impacted fragments may be left undisturbed to serve as a buttress for the volar plate. The interval between the volar plate and both collateral ligaments is incised, and the fibrocartilaginous plate is mobilized if necessary to allow its advancement 4 to 6 mm distally into the defect in the middle phalanx. The more recent the injury, the more easily the plate will advance. In late cases, it is usually necessary to partially release the proximal checkrein ligaments to gain sufficient length for advancement.

The volar plate is advanced into the middle phalangeal defect by means of a pull-out wire or suture, which spirals along the lateral margins of the volar plate and is then passed through drill holes in the lateral margins of the middle phalangeal defect (Fig. 9-8A). The holes are made by drilling a Keith needle from volar to dorsal, and the needles are threaded with the suture and pulled out dorsally. These holes should be as proximal as possible to draw the plate against the edge of the remaining articular cartilage. They should exit the dorsum of the middle phalanx more centrally through the triangular ligament of the extensor mechanism to avoid binding down the lateral bands. The DIP joint should be flexed 30 degrees as the suture is passed through the extensor mechanism to avoid tethering the tendon. Traction on the sutures emerging from the dorsum of the middle phalanx facilitates reduction of the joint as the plate is advanced into the defect.

Lateral radiographs are obtained to confirm that a congruous reduction has been achieved (see Fig. 9-8B). Maintenance of the reduction with articular gliding through the flexion arc (as opposed to hinging on the dorsal articular surface) must be documented. This is particularly true in chronic fracture-dislocations with dorsal adhesions. If hinging is present, then additional release is necessary, usually of the dorsal capsule, which may have become scarred and

inelastic over time. Once a congruous reduction and arc of motion is ensured, the pull-out sutures are tied over felt and a button. A secondary suture is placed between each lateral margin of the volar plate and its adjacent remaining collateral ligament remnant. This reestablishes three-dimensional stability and ensures broad coverage of the condyles and phalangeal base. If there is too much laxity in the volar plate with the joint reduced, additional tightening sutures may be placed to further tie the sides of the volar plate to the accessory collateral ligaments, although this is rarely necessary. An oblique Kirschner wire is used to maintain the reduced joint in 20 to 30 degrees of flexion. On rare occasions, a perceived lack of osseous support distal to the volar plate insertion may be corrected with cancellous bone graft or even the fracture fragments that are not otherwise reconstructable.

Postoperative Management

DIP joint motion is started immediately. Three weeks after surgery, the Kirschner wire is removed and active, unlimited flexion of the PIP joint is begun using a dorsal extension block splint. Unrestricted active extension is permitted at 4 weeks after surgery, and dynamic extension splinting is begun if full active extension is not regained by 5 weeks after surgery. Unlimited sports activities are allowed at 8 weeks with buddy taping, and buddy taping is continued for 4 to 6 months. Swelling may persist for several months, and it may take up to 6 to 8 months to achieve final range of motion.[26,46,47]

Expected Outcome

The hand surgeon will often see PIP fracture-dislocations after patients have been initially treated elsewhere, and the true nature of this complicated injury may not have been appreciated or conveyed to the patient. The patient must understand from the outset that while normal PIP joint func-

CRITICAL POINTS: VOLAR PLATE ARTHROPLASTY FOR DORSAL FRACTURE-DISLOCATIONS OF THE PIP JOINT

INDICATION

- Unstable dorsal PIP fracture-dislocations with more than 40% articular surface involvement and not amenable to ORIF

PREOPERATIVE EVALUATION

- Standard radiographs (anteroposterior, lateral, oblique) of digit
- Determination if remaining dorsal articular surface is anatomic or impacted
- Age of the injury

PEARLS

- It may be used as a bailout through same approach if ORIF is not possible.

TECHNICAL POINTS

- Use volar approach with chevron incision.
- "Shotgun" joint after proper collateral ligament excision.
- Excise comminuted fragments and elevate dorsal, impacted articular surface.
- Place holes for pull-out sutures as proximal as possible and avoid lateral bands dorsally.
- Establish ideal length of volar plate with joint reduced.

- Reduce joint, tie sutures with DIP flexed, and document congruency radiographically in flexion and extension.
- Pin in 20 to 30 degrees of flexion for 3 weeks only.

PITFALLS

- Leaving stable but impacted dorsal articular surface unaddressed
- Impaling lateral bands with pull-out sutures
- Failing to spread volar plate broadly across condyles
- Failing to identify hinged versus gliding flexion via dorsal adhesions

POSTOPERATIVE CARE

- Immobilize joint with Kirschner wire and splint for 3 weeks.
- Remove pin at 3 weeks with radiographs after pin removal.
- Use extension block flexion for 1 to 3 weeks and then unlimited extension.
- Use a dynamic extension splint at 5 to 6 weeks as needed.

ATHLETIC PARTICIPATION

- Contact sports including basketball can be resumed at 8 weeks with buddy-taping.

---

tion (as compared with the contralateral or adjacent digits) is possible, it is highly unlikely. They can be reassured that carefully planned treatment and compliance with postoperative regimens will likely lead to long-term satisfactory to good results. Of course, overall results diminish with increased time from injury to treatment, especially beyond 6 weeks.[17a,26]

Eaton and Malerich reported on 24 patients who underwent volar plate arthroplasty for both acute and chronic PIP fracture-dislocations, with a 10-year average follow-up.[26] The seven cases performed within 6 weeks of injury attained an average of 95 degrees of motion and a 6-degree flexion contracture. In contrast, the 17 patients with chronic (>6 weeks after injury) disease achieved 78 degrees of motion and 12 degrees of contracture. Only 3 patients reported any pain, and only with strenuous use. More recent reports have confirmed the reliability of this procedure in producing good results in a majority of patients.[8,22]

Dionysian and Eaton have reviewed the results of 17 volar plate arthroplasties at a mean follow-up of 11.5 years and found that the long-term benefit of the procedure endured with an average arc of PIP motion of 85 degrees and no residual pain.[19]

Complications

Careful preoperative planning, intraoperative attention to detail with awareness of potential pitfalls, and good patient compliance will minimize the risk of complications associated with treatment of these injuries.

Redisplacement. Failure to achieve a stable reduction, pull-out suture failure, or inadequate protection to prevent extension during mobilization may result in recurrent dorsal subluxation. One cause of pull-out suture failure is damage from the transarticular Kirschner wire fixation. This complication may be obviated by pre-positioning of the wire in the middle phalanx after Keith needle passage but before the sutures are pulled through. With close clinical and radiographic follow-up, such problems can be more expeditiously addressed and their effects minimized.

Angulation. Asymmetrical impaction of the base of the middle phalanx or failure to create a trough for the volar plate that is perpendicular to the long axis of the middle phalanx will occasionally result in angulation of the middle phalanx. Although postoperative angular deformity is usually mild and not functionally significant, patient satisfaction may be compromised and secondary corrective osteotomy at the base of the middle phalanx may become necessary.[26]

Flexion Contractures. Immobilization of the PIP joint in more than 30 degrees of flexion and failure to begin dynamic extension splinting by 5 weeks may result in lack of full extension. Recognition of this potential and common problem should help minimize it. Even with early motion and formal hand therapy, a certain percentage of patients will develop a PIP flexion contracture.

DIP Stiffness. Failure to flex the DIP joint approximately 30 degrees or impaling the lateral bands while passing the pull-out suture through the extensor mechanism on the dorsum of the middle phalanx may cause limitation of DIP flexion. Modifications in the technique help to decrease the risk of DIP stiffness. These include using two separate sutures for each side of the volar plate, tying the suture knots beneath the skin dorsally, or using small suture anchors in lieu of the pull-out suture. It is imperative to start DIP motion immediately postoperatively to regain the maximal motion possible.

CHRONIC PIP SUBLUXATIONS (HYPEREXTENSION)

Untreated or underdiagnosed type I (hyperextension) injuries will occasionally result in PIP hyperextension or a swan neck deformity. There may be pain as the lateral bands snap dorsally and volarly around the condyles of the proximal phalanx in moving to and from the hyperextended position. In swan neck deformities, the examiner must distinguish primary volar plate laxity from extensor mechanism imbalance, such as that after a severe mallet finger injury. The distinction can usually be made by stabilizing the PIP joint in full extension as the patient attempts to actively extend the distal joint. If there is a significant lag in active distal extension with the PIP joint stabilized in neutral, the problem is primarily with the extensor mechanism. If the distal joint extends normally, the problem is primarily with the volar support of the PIP joint, and surgical stabilization is indicated if the patient is sufficiently symptomatic.

Treatment

There is no effective nonoperative treatment for symptomatic chronic hyperextension deformities other than figure-of-eight ring splints that are custom made or dorsal extension-block splinting. Surgical correction of these deformities involves either late reattachment or reconstruction of the volar plate.

Reattachment procedures include direct suture of the volar plate or advancement of the avulsed distal margin of the plate using a pull-out wire technique or suture anchors, similar to that described earlier for volar plate arthroplasty, following scarification of the base of the middle phalanx.[9,86,88] Reconstruction by tenodesis of one or both slips of the flexor digitorum superficialis (FDS) tendon is a more predictable means of preventing hyperextension.[16,63,67,74,86,108] Use of both slips is reserved for hyperextension deformities created by a severe chronic imbalance of forces, as in cerebral palsy or in some cases involving the small finger where the FDS slips may be quite thin. Hyperextension with less dynamic deforming force, such as that resulting from loss or transfer of the FDS or an old partial volar plate tear, may be stabilized by reattachment of the accessory collateral ligaments into the volar plate[6,58] or restoration of a passive restraint to extension beyond neutral using a free tendon graft.[2]

Authors' Preferred Method of Treatment

The techniques of tenodesis or capsulodesis to prevent PIP hyperextension have the potential to attenuate and elongate over time with repetitive stress. The simplest, most predictable procedure is a superficialis hemitenodesis in which one slip of the FDS tendon is divided proximally and then fixed by passing it through a transverse hole in the base of the proximal phalanx. This passage provides strong bony fixation of the tendon and allows precise adjustment of the tension on the tenodesis to a few degrees of flexion.

Technique of FDS Tenodesis ("Sublimis Sling")

The A1 pulley of the flexor tendon sheath is exposed through a short oblique incision in the palm. Proximal traction is applied to the superficialis tendon, and the radial slip is transected obliquely as far proximally as possible. This provides an ample amount of free tendon proximal to the PIP joint. The volar aspect of the PIP joint is then exposed through a chevron-shaped incision creating a radially based flap, as described for volar plate arthroplasty. When the tendon is split distally, the vincula to the ulnar slip of the superficialis should be left undisturbed. A transverse bicortical gouge channel is made from the more easily accessible ulnar aspect to the radial aspect of the broader proximal third of the proximal phalanx. The tendon should be placed between the remaining superficialis slip and the proximal phalanx, avoiding the vincula, to reach the ulnar end of this channel. The tapered end of the radial slip of the superficialis tendon is passed through the gouge hole from the ulnar to the radial side using a 28-gauge stainless steel wire as a guide to its passage. Tension is adjusted so that the PIP joint cannot extend beyond 5 degrees short of neutral (5 degrees of flexion). The tendon is sutured to the periosteum at the entrance and exit of the tunnel. Alternatively, this anchor point can be reinforced using a small suture anchor adjacent to the gouge hole. If enough length is available, the free proximal end is then passed distally, where it is sutured to reinforce the volar plate middle phalangeal juncture. This is an extremely secure tenodesis.

Postoperative Management

On the first postoperative day a dorsal extension block splint is applied in 5 degrees of flexion at the PIP joint to allow immediate active flexion while preventing extension of the joint to neutral. Unrestricted motion is permitted at 6 weeks. Unlimited sports activities are possible at 8 to 10 weeks with buddy-taping until 3 months after the surgery.

Expected Outcomes

Patients seek treatment for PIP hyperextension deformities because of significant dysfunction in daily activities. We

CRITICAL POINTS: FDS TENODESIS FOR CHRONIC HYPEREXTENSION DEFORMITY OF THE PIP JOINT

INDICATION

- Symptomatic hyperextension deformity of PIP joint with intact extensor mechanism

PREOPERATIVE EVALUATION

- Obtain standard radiographs (anteroposterior, lateral, oblique) of digit.
- Confirm competence of extensor mechanism by stabilizing PIP joint in neutral and then confirming full DIP joint extension.

PEARLS

- Both slips of the FDS may be necessary at times, owing to very little tendon substance, especially in the small finger.

TECHNICAL POINTS

- Volar approach with chevron incision at PIP joint
- Small palmar incision to release radial slip of superficialis tendon
- Gouge hole within proximal flare of proximal phalanx
- Tension to no more than 5 degrees of flexion
- Immediate flexion with extension block splint

PITFALL

- Tensioning too tightly leads to flexion contracture.

POSTOPERATIVE CARE

- Immediate flexion with extension block splinting
- Unrestricted motion at 6 weeks

ATHLETIC PARTICIPATION

- Contact sports including basketball are allowed at 12 to 16 weeks with buddy-taping for 1 additional month.

Complications

In spite of the intraosseous passage of the tendon slip and postoperative splinting, the final tenodesis position may not correspond to that which was set at surgery. There is more of a tendency toward a flexion contracture than residual hyperextension. Therefore, it is important to set the tension on the tenodesis in no more than 5 or 10 degrees short of full extension. In an effort to avoid this complication, particular attention should be paid to early extension block splinting and active flexion as well as progressive mobilization of the PIP joint, preferably under the supervision of a hand therapist who can monitor the position of the joint and focus on correcting impending problems. In our series of 12 patients, 5 had a mild residual flexion contracture of less than 15 degrees.[13a] Two patients, both of whom were noncompliant with postoperative therapy, had flexion contractures of 30 and 60 degrees. There were no other complications that occurred with this procedure.

CHRONIC PIP FRACTURE-DISLOCATIONS

Occasionally, fracture-dislocations of the PIP joint remain untreated or the initial closed reduction is lost, resulting in a fixed dorsal subluxation with a mal- or non-united volar buttress of the middle phalanx. Stiffness and progressive pain are inevitable.

Donaldson and Millender proposed a method of treatment that incorporates open reduction, temporary Kirschner wire fixation (for 10 or 11 days) at 90 degrees of flexion, and subsequent "early" active range of motion protected by an extension block splint.[21] Success of this technique is predicated on the accurate reduction of the joint in chronic injuries. Open reduction with a corrective osteotomy with or without bone graft of malunited fractures has also been advocated.[16,74,121,125,126] These procedures attempt to provide stable reduction and restore articular congruity but cannot predictably prevent the development of degenerative disease in the severely injured joint. Resurfacing an interphalangeal (IP) joint with costal cartilage and perichondrium (perichondrial arthroplasty) has been used in a small number of chronic intra-articular PIP joint fractures.[40,53] The efficacy of this technique for chronic fracture-dislocations has yet to be shown. Other treatment options include implant arthroplasty and arthrodesis, both of which are less than ideal in the relatively young patient population in whom this problem most often occurs.

have found this procedure to be extremely reliable with generally good results and feel confident in relaying this information to the patients. Immediate postoperative pain is mild, and recovery is brief with a rapid return to function. There are no published data of which we are aware reporting on the use of this procedure for post-traumatic PIP hyperextension deformities.

A recent review of 12 of our patients treated with an FDS tenodesis for an unstable PIP joint revealed five excellent, five good, and two fair results, with all 12 patients returning to their original occupations and recreational activities.[13a]

Authors' Preferred Method of Treatment

Volar plate arthroplasty restores a smooth fibrocartilaginous surface to the base of the middle phalanx and maintains a stable reduction. This technique can be used for major PIP reconstruction provided the concentric arc of the proximal phalangeal condyles remains intact and there is enough intact articular surface on the dorsum of the base of the middle phalanx with which to form a congruous articulating facet. Adequate advancement of the volar plate may require fractional lengthening of the proximal checkrein ligaments by making several 2- to 3-mm incisions in both lateral margins at intervals along their length. Complete *excision* of both PIP collateral ligaments is essential to achieve adequate exposure, a congruous joint reduction, and maximal postoperative motion. In long-standing dislocations, a release of the dorsal capsule may be needed to regain flexion. Surgical technique, aftercare, and complications are the same as those for the acute fracture-dislocation. Surgical outcomes are less predictable than for acute injuries.[26]

LATERAL PIP DISLOCATIONS

The critical anatomic lesions in a lateral dislocation of the PIP joint are a rupture of one collateral ligament and at least partial avulsion of the volar plate from the middle phalanx. Failure probably begins with disruption of the origin of the collateral ligament from either the proximal phalangeal head or the middle phalangeal base,[92] proceeds through the junction of the collateral and accessory collateral ligaments, and finally detaches the insertion of the volar plate on the middle phalanx. To assess PIP stability after spontaneous or manual reduction of the joint, the examiner must test the joint in extension to assess not only the collateral ligaments but also the secondary stabilizers (e.g., volar plate, articular contour).[76] More than 20 degrees of deformity on gentle static lateral testing indicates complete collateral ligament disruption and injury to at least one other secondary stabilizer.[54,77] This is a major disruption of the four-sided ligamentous box, but with few exceptions the ligaments heal when the joint is reduced and early controlled motion begun.[105,113] The joint should be protected with buddy-tapes to an adjacent uninjured digit. On occasion, these injuries may benefit from a malleable splint placed along the same side as the ligament tear to prevent inadvertent lateral deviation.

Repair of the ruptured collateral ligaments has been frequently reported after PIP dislocations in general and lateral dislocations in particular.[5,11,35,46,47,74,91,94] Most of these series involve athletes, and surgery can be performed in selected patients to provide more predictable stability with reduced length of disability. Kato and colleagues reported on 11 primary repairs of acute PIP joint collateral ligament tears in athletes and manual laborers.[52] Suture anchors were utilized in the repair, active motion was initiated at 2 to 3 weeks, and unlimited activities were allowed at 6 weeks.

Nevertheless, because the usual sequela of ligament injury of the PIP joint is stiffness and not instability, the surgical trauma of ligament repair may have an adverse effect on the ultimate range of motion after lateral dislocations. A clearer indication for surgical repair or reconstruction is the subacute or chronic collateral ligament rupture with persistent PIP instability and dysfunction.

VOLAR PIP DISLOCATIONS

Volar dislocations of the PIP joint are rare injuries. The base of the middle phalanx may dislocate volarly without rotation (volar dislocation) or may rotate on one intact collateral ligament so that the opposite side subluxates in a volar direction (volar rotatory subluxation). Appreciating the difference between these two related injuries and identifying them clinically can help ensure appropriate management.[34] Volar rotatory subluxation of the PIP joint is a rare injury.

The mechanism of injury is usually a rotatory longitudinal compression force on a semiflexed middle phalanx that results in unilateral disruption of a collateral ligament and partial avulsion of the volar plate. One of the most common causes is catching the involved digit in a spin dryer that has not stopped spinning.[33] As the middle phalanx displaces volarly, the involved condyle ruptures through the extensor mechanism. Usually this rupture occurs between the central slip and the ipsilateral lateral band. The involved condyle may buttonhole between the central slip and the thickened volar fibers of the lateral band. These fibers are caught behind the volar flare of the condyle, routing the distal lateral band through the joint as it remains in continuity with the central tendon over the middle phalanx. Because of this interposition, the usual reduction maneuver of traction and middle phalanx extension tends to further tighten this encirclement of the condyle and block reduction.

Occasionally, when a volar dislocation occurs without a rotatory component, the central slip is ruptured. If the dislocation is irreducible, there is a high likelihood of an interposed structure such as the central slip, a collateral ligament, or a fracture fragment.[15,45] If the joint reduces easily, one must still be wary of a more profound injury that may have occurred to the extensor mechanism. This must be taken into account when deciding on the position of immobilization for the PIP joint.[35]

Volar fracture-dislocations are also rare. Rosenstadt and coworkers reported on 13 cases treated surgically, of which 9 involved acute injuries.[96] Variations in the size of the dorsal fragment and age of the injury dictated specific treatment (closed pinning versus ORIF). At an average of 4½ years of follow-up, the acute injuries fared better than those that presented at 4 or more weeks. Average arc of motion was 91 degrees for the acute injuries and 70 degrees for the chronic injuries. Five patients had an average 25-degree extensor lag at final follow-up.

Volar fracture-dislocations with a large dorsal fragment may be treated with ORIF via mini-fragment lag screw fixation. Tekkis and coworkers reported two such cases with excellent clinical outcomes[109] and attributed their success to rigid screw fixation and immediate active motion. Care must be taken to avoid distal thread extension into the flexor sheath; similarly, dorsal screw head prominence may require later screw removal.

The management of chronic volar dislocations of the PIP joint is complex and requires the simultaneous surgical correction of an incongruous and contracted joint as well as an incompetent extensor mechanism.[87] There may be degeneration of the articular cartilage; if so, the prospect of restoring normal joint function is greatly diminished. Therefore, it is important to recognize a volar PIP joint dislocation at the time of injury and adequately treat the disrupted extensor mechanism.[30,35,87,89] Peimer and colleagues also pointed out the necessity of repair of the ruptured collateral ligament.[87] In this relatively large series of 15 patients with volar PIP dislocations, inspection at the time of surgery revealed disruption of the extensor mechanism, the volar plate, and one collateral ligament in all patients. In each, the extensor mechanism and collateral ligament were repaired, and motion with therapy was started at 4 weeks after removal of the Kirschner wire that transfixed the joint. Although all patients had painless, stable PIP motion, no patient achieved preinjury PIP motion.

Authors' Preferred Method of Treatment

The management of volar rotatory dislocations of the PIP joint is controversial. Volar rotatory dislocation has been described as irreducible or trapped by many authors and one that necessitates open reduction.* Open reduction is advocated not only to reduce the interposed extensor mechanism but also to repair the rent in this mechanism. Others feel compelled to repair the torn ligaments and volar plate as well.[74,102,124] We believe that open reduction is necessary only if closed reduction fails and have a great deal of success using the specific reduction maneuver described next.[45-47,87]

The majority of volar rotatory dislocations can be reduced without surgery by applying gentle traction while holding both the MP and PIP joints flexed.[110] This maneuver relaxes the volar-displaced lateral band so that with a gentle rotatory motion the intra-articular portion can be disengaged from behind the condyle and reduction accomplished. If necessary, further relaxation of the extensor mechanism can be gained by moderate wrist extension. Once the joint is reduced, active motion is tested. Because the ligament lesion is a collateral ligament disruption, when the joint is reduced the ligaments are usually restored to their anatomic alignment. Postreduction radiographs should confirm congruous reduction. After reduction of a volar rotatory dislocation, full active extension is usually possible (under digital block) because the contralateral lateral band and at least a portion of the central slip usually remain intact. If the patient cannot actively extend to neutral, the PIP joint should be immobilized in full extension for 6 weeks, just as one would treat a closed boutonnière deformity. The only indication for open reduction, therefore, would be failure to obtain a completely congruous reduction, confirmed by radiographs, and presumably due to the presence of ligament, capsule, or extensor mechanism trapped within the joint.

In volar dislocations without a rotatory component, the reduction is easily accomplished. However, one must assume an injury to the central slip of the extensor mechanism has occurred and thus treat the finger in the postreduction period as one would treat an acute boutonnière deformity, in full extension for 4 to 6 weeks.

Technique of Open Reduction of Volar Rotatory PIP Dislocation

Open reduction is approached through a midaxial incision on the side of the major ligament disruption. The lateral band is atraumatically extricated from the joint and reduction is easily accomplished. With the patient under local or wrist block anesthesia it is then possible to test active extension. If the lateral band is not severely traumatized, it may be carefully repaired. Should the band be ragged, it is best to excise it because the normal contralateral lateral band is sufficient to provide intrinsic extensor power. If full extension is demonstrable on examination, the finger should be immobilized in extension for 5 to 7 days until the wound has stabilized and then active range of motion begun. Dynamic extension splinting is alternated with a resting extension splint to protect the extensor mechanism.

POST-TRAUMATIC FIBROSIS AND CONTRACTURE

The inevitable consequence of a PIP joint dislocation is collateral ligament fibrosis. The degree of fibrosis is generally proportional to the extent of ligament disruption, the post-traumatic rehabilitation efforts, and, to some degree, the patient's intrinsic healing response. The characteristic fusiform swelling of the PIP joint is initially due to acute hemorrhage and edema, which is gradually replaced by ligament fibrosis and, finally, mature inelastic scar. This process evolves over a period of 10 to 12 months.

To minimize fibrosis of the injured ligament and the associated loss of joint mobility, motion should be instituted as soon as joint stability is ensured. Most patients with PIP dislocations may begin guarded motion immediately, avoiding the arc of motion within which the joint is likely to re-dislocate. Even joints with surgically repaired ligaments should be moved within 3 to 4 weeks if optimal motion is to be expected. Use of systemic low-dose corticosteroids at 4 weeks after dislocation may be considered to reduce excessive soft tissue swelling and to enhance recovery of movement. Prednisone is administered in a convenient, pharmaceutical-prepared schedule or, alternatively, in the dose of 5 mg every 6 hours for 4 days, followed by a 5-mg daily taper over the next 3 days.

The most frequent complication of a PIP joint dislocation is late stiffness. When significant loss of motion (<60 degree arc) persists despite dynamic splinting and a well-attended rehabilitation program, consideration should be given to PIP joint release by one of several techniques. Established contracture of these small joints is usually resistant to non-surgical or closed surgical treatment, such as the hinged external fixator. In one series of 27 cases, there was a 50% complication rate, and modifications to the fixator design were recommended.[42] Total collateral ligament excision and, if necessary, a distal volar plate release have engendered good results.[18,72] Abbiati and associates recommended sparing the proper collateral ligaments while releasing the volar plate and accessory collateral ligaments.[1] Mansat and Delprat recommended a technique in which the volar plate and capsule are released and then the origins of the collateral ligaments are incised but not excised.[73] Diao and coworkers demonstrated no long-term collateral ligament insufficiency

---

*See references 15, 17, 33, 46, 47, 50, 51, 56, 76, 80, 85, 90, 99, 102, 118, and 124.

after complete excision of the collateral ligaments during joint release.[18]

Preoperative Evaluation

Stiffness and contractures of the PIP joints are common in an active, laboring, and athletic culture. Most PIP contractures, even if chronic, do not require any further treatment once maximal motion is achieved through exercises, static or dynamic splints, and active use.[7] Those patients desiring more aggressive treatment of their PIP contractures may feel functionally impaired from doing specific work-related or recreational activities that require forceful grasp or more mundane daily activities such as reaching into one's pants pocket for change.

Specific functional deficits and their impact on patients' quality of life must be determined, and the patients' expectations for the outcome of any surgery must be clear to the treating physician. The cause of the contracture should be determined. A patient who was noncompliant with the treatment regimen for his or her initial PIP dislocation is probably not a good candidate for joint release, because the results are critically dependent on postoperative compliance and rehabilitation.

The timing and mechanism of the initial injury, prior treatment, history of other joint contractures, and underlying medical problems must be determined. Patients with underlying diabetes are at greater risk for post-traumatic joint stiffness.

Examination should include a comparison of active and passive PIP joint motion in the involved and contralateral digits. Radiographs must be obtained to rule out mechanical motion block resulting from osteophytes, heterotopic ossification, or degenerative joint narrowing.

Authors' Preferred Method of Treatment

Lack of response to conservative treatment of a PIP flexion contracture is an indication for collateral ligament excision. This can be done using digital block anesthesia and a brachial or forearm tourniquet. This allows active motion after joint release and may eliminate the need for proximal tendon exposure and tenolysis.

The PIP joint is approached through midaxial incisions, with care taken to spare the obliquely coursing dorsal sensory nerves. The lateral bands of the extensor mechanism are usually congealed in extensive scar formation superficial to the thickened collateral ligaments. An oblique incision parallel to the normal alignment of the lateral band fibers is made midway between the dorsal and volar borders of the lateral band scarring. The thickened segment of the extensor mechanism, including both the oblique and transverse retinacular fibers, is peeled dorsally and volarly using sharp dissection, to expose the thickened collateral ligaments. Excision of these ligaments is begun by sharply dividing the proximal origins from the condylar fossa and continuing distally to the broad insertion of the ligaments across the

lateral and volar margins of the middle phalanx and volar plate. As a general rule, if the degree of PIP stiffness was sufficient to warrant surgical treatment in the first place, both collateral ligaments will need to be excised. These ligaments will eventually re-form, but it is hoped that they do so in a more elastic and relatively lengthened state.[27]

Occasionally, if débridement of the clinically most thickened side yields complete restoration of motion, the opposite ligament is left undisturbed. Usually, the ulnar collateral ligament (UCL) is excised first and then the radial side is addressed. If only flexion is limited, one may choose to excise only the dorsal half of the radial collateral ligament (RCL). If extension is limited, excision of the volar half may be sufficient to restore full motion. However, extension may be unchanged because of restraint by the volar plate. If extension is not complete, the flexor sheath should be opened at the level of the middle phalangeal base and the flexor superficialis tendon protected as the distal insertion of the volar plate is released. Passive range of motion will demonstrate the need for additional release or gentle stretching, usually of the tight dorsal capsule. Full relaxed passive motion *must* be achieved before active motion is tested. Active motion should equal passive motion unless additional fixation of the extensor or flexor tendon is present.

With this direct and carefully planned surgical strategy, it should be possible to reach this stage of the operation before the tourniquet becomes painful or ischemic motor paralysis develops. If not, the tourniquet can be released and later reinflated or the final dissection can be completed without the tourniquet. If necessary, limited extensor and flexor tenolysis at the level of the proximal phalanx can be performed through these midaxial incisions. Occasionally, release of the flexor superficialis tendon at the proximal PIP joint level is necessary if a significant flexion contracture persists after volar plate release. Frayed, ragged edges of the scarred lateral bands are conservatively débrided. Only skin sutures are required.

Postoperative Management

Active PIP motion is begun the day after surgery with appropriate dynamic splinting when wound sensitivity permits but no later than 7 days postoperatively. Some part-time and/or night splinting may be required for 3 to 4 months after surgery to maximize maintenance of the early correction. Immediate, active hand use is encouraged as symptoms allow.

Expected Outcomes

A careful preoperative assessment of the PIP contracture, maximal correction at the time of surgery, postoperative patient compliance, and realistic expectations by both the patient and surgeon will optimize patient satisfaction and outcomes. Extension contractures generally have better outcomes after surgical release as long as the extensor mechanism is competent. Because the flexors are more powerful than the extensors, maintenance of increased intraoperative flexion is more likely.

Ghidella and associates reported on 68 PIP joint contracture releases in 44 patients at minimal 2-year follow-up with some sobering results.[32] For their total population on average, there was no significant improvement. However, the patients younger than 28 years old with simple contractures did the best and did improve to a significant degree. Bruser and coworkers have reported better overall results in 45 fingers, especially when they utilized the midlateral incision instead of a volar incision.[12] The results reported by Bruser have more closely paralleled our own experience.

Complications

Exact knowledge of the anatomy, which is frequently distorted in the post-traumatic PIP joint, will generally prevent injury to the lateral bands or adjacent sensory nerves. No surgical complications were reported in a recent review of 68 PIP contracture releases.[32]

CRITICAL POINTS: COLLATERAL LIGAMENT EXCISION FOR PIP CONTRACTURE RELEASE

INDICATION

- Functional deficit secondary to a mature contracture in a compliant patient

PREOPERATIVE EVALUATION

- Complete problem-specific history of injury and treatment.
- Obtain plain radiographs.

PEARLS

- You will never gain more motion and usually will gain less than that achieved intraoperatively.

TECHNICAL POINTS

- Ideally done under local anesthesia
- Midaxial incisions
- Preserve lateral bands
- In general, completely excise both collateral ligaments
- Must have full passive motion before active motion attempted

PITFALLS

- Failure to identify and remove osteophytes blocking motion
- Failure to test active motion intraoperatively

POSTOPERATIVE CARE

- Immediate active motion as pain allows
- Dynamic splints
- Nonsteroidal anti-inflammatory drugs or prednisone (taper) as needed for swelling

ATHLETIC PARTICIPATION

- Gradually progressive as symptoms allow

Concerns for PIP joint instability after collateral ligament excision are unfounded. After 2 months, the joints are stable to lateral stress in all positions of flexion. By 3 months, characteristic thickening is palpable on the lateral aspect of the condyles of the proximal phalanges, in distinct contrast to the concavity noted immediately postoperatively. A review of 16 patients who had total ligament excision and volar plate release for isolated post-traumatic PIP fibrosis showed an increase in total active motion from 38 degrees preoperatively to 78 degrees postoperatively at 1-year follow-up. In all patients, the joints were stable to lateral stress in all positions of flexion by 3 weeks.[18]

THE FINGER DIP AND THUMB IP JOINTS

The ligamentous anatomy of the distal articulation of the finger and thumb is analogous to that of the PIP joint of the finger. However, owing to the shorter lever arm of the distal phalanx and the enhanced stability provided by the adjacent insertions of the flexor and extensor tendons, dislocations are not as frequent. Dislocations of the DIP joint are usually dorsal or lateral and often associated with an open wound because of the snug skin fixation about the joint.

Treatment of these dislocations consists of closed reduction under digital or wrist block anesthesia. The reduction maneuver consists of longitudinal traction, direct pressure on the dorsum of the distal phalanx, and manipulation of the distal phalanx into flexion. If the dislocation is open, the joint is contaminated by definition and treatment should include thorough irrigation and débridement in a controlled, sterile setting.[132] After reduction, joint stability should be tested actively with range of motion by the patient and passively by the examiner to gently stress the collateral ligaments. Postreduction radiographs are mandatory to confirm congruous reduction. Instability after pure dislocations is rare, and the joint is immobilized in slight flexion using a dorsal splint for 2 to 3 weeks. After the first week, the patient should be encouraged to remove the distal tape or Velcro fixation of the splint and actively flex the DIP joint while avoiding the last 20 degrees of extension.

Digital DIP and thumb IP dislocations are rarely irreducible. When they do occur, it is most commonly the result of proximal disruption of the volar plate, which then becomes interposed between the head of the digital middle or thumb proximal phalanx and the base of the distal phalanx, preventing reduction (Fig. 9-9).[136,145,152,153,159,161,165] Interposition of the flexor tendon,[142,150,154,156,159,165,167] a fracture fragment,[161,163,169] and a sesamoid bone[146] have also been reported, and the condyles of the middle phalanx can become entrapped in a longitudinal rent in the flexor digitorum profundus (FDP) tendon.[135] Irreducible dislocations require surgical removal or manipulation of the offending anatomic structure(s) to facilitate reduction.

Rarely, a dorsal dislocation may be associated with a fracture of the volar lip of the distal phalanx, akin to a PIP joint dorsal fracture-dislocation.[140] If the volar fragment is not avulsed with the FDP tendon, then the goal of treatment remains a stable closed reduction. If the profundus tendon is avulsed, however, it must be reattached surgically. Even if the volar fragment is proximal to the FDP insertion, it can still be large enough to render the joint unstable despite

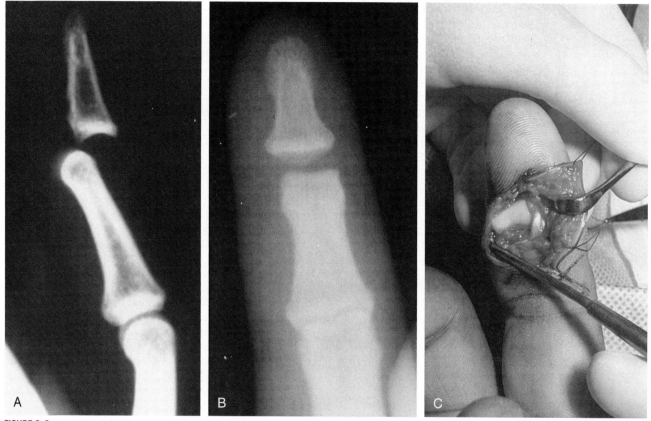

FIGURE 9-9. **A,** Irreducible dorsal dislocation of an index DIP joint. **B,** The posteroanterior view shows a wide gap between the middle and distal phalanges suggestive of soft tissue interposition. This appearance is typical of an irreducible dislocation in which the interposed soft tissue prevents reduction of the joint. These injuries are commonly open, and, at exploration **(C),** the head of the middle phalanx was seen ulnar to the displaced flexor tendon. The volar plate was interposed between the base of the distal phalanx and the head of the middle phalanx.

closed manipulation. If mild to moderate flexion of the DIP joint is insufficient to keep the joint reduced and especially if more than 40% of the articular surface has been fractured, then a volar plate arthroplasty is indicated.

We have found volar plate arthroplasty to be a very effective treatment for this problem, as did Rettig and associates in their report of 10 patients who underwent volar plate arthroplasty for chronic dorsal fracture-subluxation of the DIP joint.[157] At mean 25-month follow-up, the four thumb IP joints and six finger DIP joints had an average of 51 and 42 degrees, respectively, of stable active motion. All patients had a flexion contracture, which averaged 12 degrees. Patient satisfaction was high, and there were no complications.

Dorsal dislocation of both IP joints of a single digit, most often the small finger, is rare enough to have prompted a number of case reports.* The force required to cause this double dislocation implies more extensive soft tissue injury. Aggressive hand therapy is instituted soon after stable reduction to maximize range of motion.

Pure volar dislocations of the DIP joint are rare and probably spontaneously reduce. These are essentially mallet injuries and require splinting in full extension for 6 weeks followed by progressive mobilization. However, an irreducible volar dislocation of a DIP joint has been reported in which the extensor mechanism was longitudinally split with interposition of the terminal lateral bands within the joint surface, preventing reduction.[144]

THE FINGER METACARPOPHALANGEAL JOINT

 Anatomy

The MP joints of the fingers are relatively resistant to ligament injury and dislocation because of their intrinsic ligamentous structure, their surrounding supporting structures including flexor and extensor tendon systems, and their protected position at the base of the fingers. They are most vulnerable to injury from forces directed ulnarly and dorsally. The articular surfaces form a condyloid joint. The metacarpal head is narrow dorsally, with a widened volar flare giving progressively more contact with the base of the proximal phalanx with increasing flexion (Fig. 9-10).

The capsule of the MP joint extends from the metacarpal neck to the base of the proximal phalanx and is reinforced by specialized structures on all sides. The capsule is composed of areolar tissue dorsally and is reinforced by the loose insertion of the common extensor tendon. On the volar

---

*See references 28, 39, 60, 95, 115, 127-131, 133, 134, 137-139, 141, 143, 147-149, 151, 155, 158, 160, 164, 166, and 168.

side, the joint is supported by the volar plate, which is continuous laterally with the deep transverse metacarpal (intervolar plate) ligament (see Fig. 9-10). The volar plate has a thick fibrocartilaginous distal portion and a thin membranous proximal portion. It does not have strong proximal checkrein ligaments comparable to those of the PIP joint. Lateral reinforcement for the volar plate is afforded by the collateral and intervolar plate ligaments, which insert into its lateral margins to produce a linked ligament-box support from one MP joint to adjacent one(s).[235] The sagittal bands and the tendons of the intrinsic muscles provide additional, secondary support.[255] The collateral ligaments are more taut in flexion than in extension because of the cam effect created by the nonspherical shape of the metacarpal head, which is wider volarly than dorsally (Fig. 9-11). There is

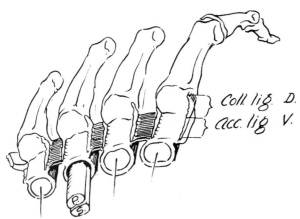

FIGURE 9-10. The intervolar plate ligaments that reinforce the ligament-box complex at each MP joint. Because the volar plate is most securely attached to the proximal phalanx, this transverse ligament primarily supports the proximal phalanges. (From Eaton RG, Littler JW: Joint injuries and their sequelae. Clin Plast Surg 3:85-98, 1976.)

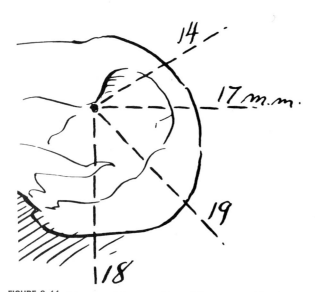

FIGURE 9-11. Diagram of the cam effect of the metacarpal head contour and relative length of the collateral ligaments with increasing flexion. Shortening or loss of elasticity of the collateral ligaments will limit flexion. Therefore, the MP joint must be splinted in at least 50 degrees of flexion to maintain ligament length.

also broader and more stable articular contact between the metacarpal head and base of the proximal phalanx beyond 70 degrees of flexion. Therefore, the joint is stable laterally in full flexion but allows some abduction and adduction in full extension.[254]

DORSAL MP DISLOCATIONS

Dorsal dislocations of the MP joints of the fingers are relatively uncommon injuries. The most frequently involved digit is the index followed by the small finger. With few exceptions,[195,216,228,229,239] dorsal dislocation of the central digits has been seen only with concomitant dislocation of a border digit.* Dorsal dislocation of a DIP and MP joint in the same finger has been reported.[215]

The mechanism of injury is usually forced hyperextension of the digit as might occur from falling on an outstretched hand. The pathology of complete dislocation of the index and small fingers is similar but not identical. In both instances, the volar plate ruptures in its membranous proximal portion and becomes interposed dorsally between the base of the proximal phalanx and the dorsal metacarpal head. If this was the only structure blocking reduction, it could be accomplished by using traction sufficient to draw the proximal edge of the volar plate over the metacarpal head. This is not possible, however, because of the taut medial and lateral structures drawn tightly around the narrow metacarpal neck, which become even more taut with traction.

 Anatomy

Kaplan, in 1957, described the pathomechanics of the volar structures that block reduction of the dislocated MP joint.[222] The anatomic basis for complete, irreducible dislocation of the MP joint involves the following structures: the volar plate, the A1 pulley, the flexor tendons, the lumbricals, and, in the small finger, the abductor and flexor digiti quinti. As the volar plate is drawn distally over the metacarpal head by the dislocating proximal phalanx, the periarticular tendons are drawn dorsally past the metacarpal head. In this manner, a tendon noose has been formed around the metacarpal head that only tightens further with closed reduction maneuvers. In the index finger, these structures include the lumbrical muscle radially and the flexor tendons ulnarly. The latter remain in the proximal flexor pulleys, which are attached to the dorsally displaced volar plate (Fig. 9-12). In the small finger, the entrapping structures include the common tendon of the abductor digiti quinti and the flexor digiti minimi ulnarly and the lumbrical muscle and flexor tendons radially.[176,178] The tendons are also drawn taut by the dorsally displaced volar plate and pulley.

Distinction must be made between subluxation (simple) and complete (complex) dorsal dislocations. Understanding this anatomic distinction is important in planning treatment,

---

*See references 170, 175, 183, 201, 204, 211, 230, 240, 245, 247, 264, and 269.

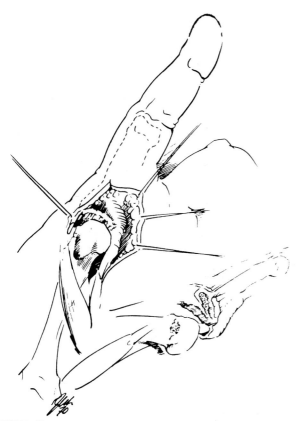

FIGURE 9-12. Pathology of irreducible (complex) dislocations of the index MP joint. The metacarpal head protrudes volarly between the lumbrical (radially) and flexor tendons (ulnarly). The proximal phalanx and volar plate displace dorsal to the metacarpal head, and the plate is folded and impinged within the previously congruous articular surfaces. The flexor tendons remaining in the fibrous sheath attached to the volar plate are kept taut by this displacement and thus maintain the tight tendon-lumbrical encirclement around the narrow metacarpal neck. Traction applied to attempt reduction further tightens this entrap-ment and makes closed reduction impossible.

because the former is reducible by closed means whereas the latter is not. Similarly, an incomplete dislocation can be converted into a complete dislocation by an inappropriate attempt to reduce the finger by exaggerating the hyperextension deformity.[194,200,206,208,209,231]

Simple MP Subluxation

Subluxation differs anatomically from complete dislocation because the volar plate is draped over the metacarpal head instead of entrapped within the joint and the base of the proximal phalanx is locked in 60 to 80 degrees of hyperextension. If either hyperextension or traction is employed as part of the reduction maneuver of this incomplete lesion, it is possible to draw the entire volar plate dorsally, where it becomes folded between the base of the proximal phalanx and the metacarpal head, converting a subluxation into a complete or irreducible dislocation. The reduction maneuver for incomplete dislocations should therefore be performed by flexing the wrist to relax the flexor tendons and applying simple distal- and volar-directed pressure to the dorsal base of the proximal phalanx. This *slides* the proximal phalanx and its attached volar plate over the metacarpal head into a

reduced position.[231] Early range of motion is then encouraged, with a dorsal extension block splint to prevent extension beyond neutral.

Complete (Complex) MP Dislocation

Preoperative Evaluation

Patients with complete (complex) dislocations present with the MP joint of the digit held in slight extension; flexion is impossible. The distal joints are slightly flexed, and the digit itself is mildly deviated toward the adjacent, more central digit. A prominence is felt in the palm corresponding to the metacarpal head, and the adjacent skin may be puckered. Dorsally, a hollow can be palpated proximal to the base of the proximal phalanx. In contrast, the subluxated proximal phalanx is markedly hyperextended and the articular surface of the base of the proximal phalanx lies directly dorsal and still articulates with the metacarpal head.

Posteroanterior radiographs of complete dislocations show widening of the joint space (Fig. 9-13). The identification of a sesamoid within the joint confirms the presence of an entrapped volar plate.[194,208,240,257] In the lateral view, the dorsal dislocation is obvious and a large osteochondral shearing fracture from the metacarpal head may be identified.[184,185,203,208,231,250,260] A Brewerton view may help demonstrate a fracture of the metacarpal head.[224,251,265] This radiographic view is produced by placing the palm up and the dorsum of the MP joints against the x-ray plate. With the MP joints flexed approximately 65 degrees, the x-ray beam is tilted 15 degrees in an ulnar to radial direction.[208]

Historical Review of Surgical Procedures

Farabeuf introduced the dorsal approach for irreducible dorsal MP dislocations in the late 19th century.[185] His assumption and that of others was that the volar plate is the only structure blocking reduction and that, if it were longitudinally split, the joint could be reduced without difficulty.* In 1975, Becton and colleagues described a modification of Farabeuf's technique that they used with no complications in 13 patients with complex index MP dislocations.[185] Two patients in his series had radial digital nerve anesthesia attributed to previous volar approaches performed by other surgeons.

Becton's technique uses a 4-cm straight dorsal incision to expose the extensor tendon and joint capsule, which are split longitudinally to access the interposed volar plate. After dividing the volar plate longitudinally in the midline, the two halves fall away as the proximal phalangeal base is gently reduced onto the metacarpal head. The dorsal approach facilitates reduction and fixation of any osteochondral fragment that may be present. Osteochondral fractures associated with MP dislocations have a reported incidence of up to 50% but occur much less frequently in our experience.[185,188]

Difficulty reaching the volar structures from the dorsal approach has led many to recommend the volar or volar midaxial approach.* The presence of a complex dorsal fracture-dislocation may make reduction significantly more difficult than for a dislocation alone. A combined dorsal and volar approach may be necessary.

---

*See references 173, 181, 184, 188, 222, 229, 238, 240, 249, 250, and 259.

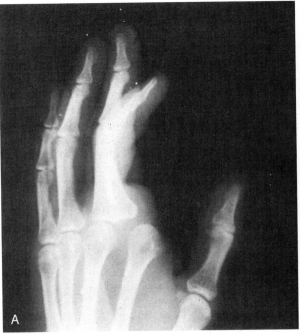
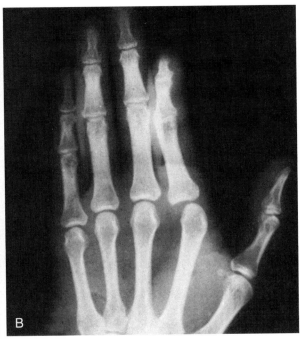

FIGURE 9-13. Radiographs of a dorsal irreducible (complex) dislocation. **A,** An oblique view shows the dorsal dislocation and widened joint space caused by interposition of the volar plate. **B,** The ulnar shift of the proximal phalanx suggests rupture of the radial collateral ligament.

The longer a dorsal dislocation remains unreduced, the more likely is the development of degenerative arthritis and the less satisfactory the result of surgery in terms of pain and ultimate range of motion. That notwithstanding, fair results have been reported after open reduction as long as 5 months after the original dislocation. This generally also requires a combined volar and dorsal approach to release the contracted collateral ligaments.[207,226,237]

Authors' Preferred Method of Treatment

Open reduction is indicated for acute complete (complex) dorsal dislocations. Although the surgery can be performed under local anesthesia, relaxation of extrinsic flexors via regional anesthesia (e.g., Bier or axillary block) is preferable. The index finger is exposed through an oblique palmar incision running between the proximal and distal palmar creases and extending to the radial midaxial line. A mirror image incision is used for the small finger extending to the ulnar midaxial line. The radial neurovascular bundle is invariably tented over the protruding index metacarpal head and lies immediately beneath the skin. It may be easily damaged if the incision is not made with great care. Similarly, the ulnar neurovascular bundle is displaced in dislocations of the small finger MP joint. Once the skin is incised, the metacarpal head is immediately obvious in the subcutaneous tissue, herniated between the entrapping structures.

*See references 174, 176, 179, 180, 182, 190-192, 194, 200, 203, 206, 207, 210, 214, 219, 220, 222, 231, 232, 237, 257, 262, 263, and 267.

CRITICAL POINTS: THE VOLAR APPROACH TO COMPLEX MP DISLOCATIONS

INDICATION

- Irreducible MP dislocations with or without osteochondral fractures

PREOPERATIVE EVALUATION

- Document sensibility, because digital nerves are at risk in approach.
- Obtain standard radiographs as well as Brewerton views (see text).
- Tomography is rarely indicated for osteochondral fractures.

PEARLS

- These injuries are a classic study in anatomy, which should be reviewed before surgery.
- With osteochondral fractures, combined dorsal-volar approach may be necessary.

TECHNICAL POINTS

- Make an oblique palmar incision over the metacarpal head.
- Incise *skin only* to avoid division of nearby digital nerves.
- Use blunt dissection to identify and retract nerves.
- Release A1 pulley.

CRITICAL POINTS: THE VOLAR APPROACH TO COMPLEX MP DISLOCATIONS—CONT'D

- Use blunt elevator or hemostat to leverage tendons away from metacarpal head as joint is reduced.
- No soft tissue repair is necessary. Close skin.

PITFALLS

- Digital nerve laceration
- Failure to identify chondral or osteochondral fracture

POSTOPERATIVE CARE

- Immobilize in 30 degrees of flexion for 2 weeks.
- Begin active motion with extension block splint at 10 degrees of MP flexion for 2 more weeks.
- Buddy-tape to adjacent digit at 8 weeks.
- Unlimited use is allowed at 12 weeks.

ATHLETIC PARTICIPATION

- Unlimited contact sports are allowed at 12 weeks.

The main deterrent to reduction is the tension in the previously described muscle-tendon noose around the narrow metacarpal neck. This tension is maintained by the dorsal displacement of the flexor tendon that remains within the flexor sheath, which has been displaced dorsally with the volar plate. Reduction can be accomplished atraumatically by releasing the A1 pulley. This relaxes the tension of one tendon limb of the noose mechanism and allows the proximal phalanx and the attached volar plate to fall back or be gently manipulated into their normal anatomic position.

Postoperative Management

Immobilization of the joint in 30 degrees of flexion is continued for 2 weeks, after which active range of motion is begun using a removable 10-degree dorsal extension block splint. At 4 weeks the splint is used only for protection and at 6 weeks is discontinued. Unlimited activity is allowed at 12 weeks.

Complications

Complex dorsal MP joint dislocations are not uncommon in children. Closure of the metacarpal head physis has been reported as a rare sequela of this injury.[226] Therefore, the family should be warned of this possibility at the time of treatment.

Repeated attempts at closed reduction, traumatic open reduction (i.e., prying the proximal phalanx volarly), or late reduction may lead to degenerative arthritis and, occasionally, osteonecrosis of the metacarpal head.[205] Failure to recognize the very superficial position of the neurovascular bundle tented over the metacarpal head may lead to its division during surgical exposure of the joint. Prolonged immobilization, late reduction, or severe adjacent tissue injury may pro-

duce excessive fibrosis and reduce the final range of motion. However, motion may continue to improve for as long as 6 to 8 months.

Expected Outcomes

Timely open treatment of irreducible MP dislocations is the single most important factor in determining patient outcomes and will lead to good results in a majority of patients. The potential sequelae of treatment delays should be discussed with patients, including residual stiffness and late degenerative arthrosis.

VOLAR MP DISLOCATIONS

Irreducible volar dislocations of the MP joints of the fingers have been reported but are extremely uncommon.[223,231,234,248,268] Four different anatomic structures have been reported to prevent reduction.[186,241,248] The dorsal capsule may be avulsed from the metacarpal proximally and become interposed between the base of the proximal phalanx and the metacarpal head.[268] The distal insertion of the volar plate and/or collateral ligament can be avulsed and become lodged between the dislocated articular surfaces and prevent reduction.[186,236,248] In a border digit, a junctura tendinum may slip distal and volar to the metacarpal neck, also leading to an irreducible MP joint.[241] Successful closed reduction has been described and should be attempted under adequate anesthesia; failure necessitates an open reduction through a dorsal approach.

ISOLATED RADIAL COLLATERAL LIGAMENT RUPTURES OF THE MP JOINTS

While isolated MP ulnar collateral ligament ruptures are extremely rare, isolated RCL ruptures of the MP joints of the fingers are seen with increasing frequency as aggressive athletics are pursued by a larger percentage of the population.[171] These injuries generally occur in the three ulnar digits. The mechanism of injury is forced ulnar deviation with the MP joint flexed. Patients will often present late for evaluation and treatment owing to persistent swelling and dysfunction. The clinician should first examine the contralateral digit to determine normal tension in the RCL with MP joint flexion. In the injured digit, there will be tenderness along the radial aspect of the joint, most notably at the volar base of the proximal phalanx, near the RCL insertion. Passive MP flexion of the injured digit will usually cause pain, and then ulnar deviation of the proximal phalanx will demonstrate the instability and exacerbate the pain. Radiographic evaluation should include a Brewerton view to look for avulsed bone fragments, which are not uncommon.[224,265] Arthrography or magnetic resonance imaging (MRI) has been suggested to help identify the nature and location of the ligament disruption, although we have not found this necessary.[197,221]

Initial treatment usually consists of immobilization of the joint in 30 degrees of flexion for 3 weeks for comfort or occasionally immediate protected motion with a buddy strap or tape to the adjacent radial digit. Clinical reassessment with gentle RCL stress is performed at 3 weeks, and, if notable tightening or stability of the RCL is appreciated, then primary healing of the ligament is likely. The involved finger is then buddy-taped for an additional 2 to 3 weeks while gentle motion is instituted. For the index finger, which cannot be effectively buddy-taped, a custom hand-based splint is fashioned with an ulnar loop around the proximal phalanx to prevent ulnar deviation. This treatment is usually successful, but even with a stable MP joint, pain with maximal MP flexion and forceful gripping may continue for up to a year. If instability or pain is present at 6 weeks or beyond, surgical repair or reconstruction may be considered and will give satisfactory results.[199,213]

On initial presentation, if the joint is grossly unstable, or if there is a large displaced avulsion fragment off the base of the proximal phalanx, consideration should be given to primary surgical repair, particularly in the less protected index and small fingers.[189,197,219,220,221,253,266] The ligament disruption may occur proximally or distally, and, in the latter, Stener-like lesions have been reported.[221,253,266]

If a patient presents with a subacute or chronic RCL injury, conservative treatment with splint immobilization or partial immobilization with buddy-taping and reduced activity may yield satisfactory results. Surgical reconstruction is indicated for continued symptomatic instability.

LOCKED METACARPOPHALANGEAL JOINTS

Locking of the MP joint of a finger is an unusual entity characterized by a moderate flexion deformity of the joint, with the PIP and DIP joints continuing to function normally. The deformity most often results from hyperflexion of the MP joint caused by muscular contraction or trauma to the dorsum of the proximal phalanx. Patients may awaken with an MP joint locked in such a manner. The locked MP joint must be differentiated from a locked trigger finger. This should not be difficult, because in a locked trigger finger, full active extension of the IP joints is not possible.

Although various causes have been reported such as sesamoid entrapment and periarticular exostoses,[187,193,202,227,244] the usual cause of locking is the restriction of collateral or accessory collateral ligament excursion by a prominent metacarpal head radial condyle or actual impalement on a marginal degenerative osteophyte.* Most commonly, the index and long fingers are involved because of their prominent metacarpal head radial condyles. The condition can be degenerative or idiopathic. In the former group, the patients tend to be older, and oblique or specialized radiographs will usually demonstrate degenerative changes and a marginal osteophyte. Although any finger may be involved, the long finger is the most frequently affected. In the idiopathic group, the patients are younger and have no degenerative disease. The index finger is usually involved, and the pathologic structure is a very prominent radial condylar margin of the metacarpal head that entraps the RCL.[198,212,218,243]

Historically, definitive treatment is usually surgical, regardless of the cause. However, nonoperative treatment should first be attempted by insufflating the joint with local anesthetic to disengage the impaled collateral ligament before

gentle manipulation.[209] Care should be taken to not fracture the osteophyte or prominent (usually radial) condyle.[217] Only if this maneuver is unsuccessful, or if there has been a previous episode of locking, is it necessary to acutely explore the joint and remove the offending osteophyte or condylar margin.[198,218,243] MRI is able to delineate these structures about the MP joint but is usually not necessary to make the diagnosis or plan treatment.[252] Occasionally, a patient will present with a chronically locked MP joint. Because the collateral ligaments are at full length in flexion, good to excellent motion is still usually achieved after surgery.

FINGER CARPOMETACARPAL JOINTS

Anatomy

The carpometacarpal (CMC) joints of the digits form the base of the transverse metacarpal arch of the hand. The fixed central unit of the arch, the index and long metacarpals, has interdigitating articulations with the trapezoid and capitate bones and is quite stable. On the ulnar side of the arch, the fourth and fifth metacarpals demonstrate approximately 10 and 20 degrees of flexion and extension, respectively, and a few degrees of rotation when opposing the thumb. The slightly convex base of the fifth metacarpal articulates with a mildly concave facet of the hamate to permit this type of motion. The strong dorsal, volar, and interosseous ligamentous support of these joints is reinforced by the broad insertions of the wrist flexors and extensors. The volar ulnar aspect of the fifth metacarpal joint is also reinforced by the pisometacarpal ligament, an extension of the flexor carpi ulnaris insertion. In addition to the articulations with the distal carpal row, each metacarpal has a small facet for articulation with its adjacent metacarpal. It is this periarticular soft tissue reinforcement that makes the CMC fracture-dislocation much more common than a pure dislocation.

The most frequently injured CMC joint is the fifth. Although volar dislocations have been reported,* the overwhelming majority of these injuries are dorsal fracture-dislocations.† If the fracture fragment is small, the diagnosis may easily be missed in the posteroanterior radiograph. Careful attention to the parallel lines of the CMC articular surfaces can help avoid this pitfall.[281,286,287,302] In the lateral radiograph, displacement is obscured by superimposition of the central metacarpals. The key diagnostic radiograph is a 30-degree pronated lateral view in which the fifth CMC joint is projected in profile to demonstrate displacement (Fig. 9-14).[286,287] This diagnosis is most easily established when large or comminuted fracture fragments are present. These injuries are analogous to Bennett fracture-dislocation of the thumb metacarpal[331] and have been referred to as reverse-Bennett fracture-dislocations. The injury may require open reduction if closed reduction is inadequate.

---

*See references 172, 177, 196, 198, 212, 225, 233, 242, 243, 246, 256, 258, 261, and 270.

*See references 271, 276, 278, 282, 284–287, 297, 320, 322, 337, and 343.
†See references 223, 225, 279–282, 284–287, 300, 305, 307, 310, 313, 321, 326, 327, 338, and 342.

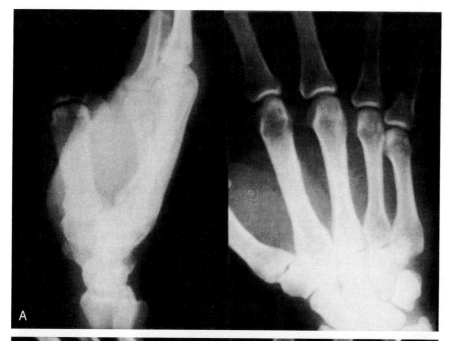

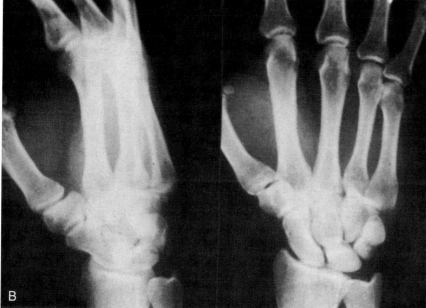

FIGURE 9-14. Radiographs of dorsal displacement of the fifth CMC joint. **A,** Routine posteroanterior and lateral views may not clearly demonstrate dorsal displacement of the fifth metacarpal base, although it should be suspected by the angulation of the fifth metacarpal in the lateral view *(left)*. **B,** A 30-degree pronated view of the hand demonstrates dorsal displacement of the metacarpal base and a shearing fracture of the dorsal lip of the hamate.

Isolated dislocations or fracture-dislocations of the remaining CMC joints are substantially less common.* These may be accompanied by diaphyseal fractures of adjacent metacarpals, which permit shortening and increased displacement of the dislocations. Isolated dorsal dislocation or fracture-dislocation occurs when a longitudinal compressive force strikes the dorsum of the metacarpal head causing simultaneous flexion and longitudinal compression. As the head toggles volarly, the base is driven out dorsally, frequently shearing off a portion of the dorsal lip of the opposing carpal bone. One case of simultaneous isolated dorsal dislocation of both the index MP joint and the second CMC joint via this mechanism has been reported.[283] In the presence of an associated carpal fracture, the CMC joint usually remains unstable after closed reduction (unless the fragment

comprises only a small percentage of the articular surface), precluding closed reduction alone as a treatment option.[288,301]

Multiple dislocations or fracture-dislocations are rare and usually are the result of injuries of greater force than those causing isolated dislocations. Motorcycle accidents are frequent causes of these injuries owing to the great energy imparted directly to the extended mid palm through the handlebars on impact.[311] Multiple dislocations or fracture-dislocations are frequently accompanied by fractures of adjacent carpal or metacarpal bones, additional orthopedic injuries, and extensive soft tissue trauma.[327] Displacement is

---

*See references 276, 282, 295, 300, 304, 308, 312, 314, 316, 319, and 332.

usually dorsal, but volar displacement has been reported.* Associated neurapraxia of the ulnar[276,291,327,325,344] or median[340] nerve may occur.

Treatment

Maintenance of a stable reduction is essential to prevent the muscle imbalance, weakness of grasp, and, eventually, traumatic arthritis, which may complicate chronic dislocations of the CMC joints of the fingers.[292,306,309] The traditional treatment of acute injuries has been either closed reduction with plaster immobilization, closed reduction with percutaneous Kirschner wire fixation, or ORIF.[290,294,311] Primary fusion of *acute*, unstable central (second and third) CMC fracture-dislocations has been reported for 5 patients, with four excellent and one good result.[296,311] Injuries seen late require ORIF or arthrodesis, depending on the integrity of the articular surfaces, the specific joint involved, and the preference of the surgeon. A possible alternative to arthrodesis for late post-traumatic arthrosis of the fifth CMC joint is interposition arthroplasty. In a series of 8 patients, there were three excellent and five good results.[289]

Garcia-Elias and coworkers retrospectively reviewed 13 cases of multiple CMC fracture-dislocations in the same hand.[290] In only 8 of the 13 cases was an accurate diagnosis made initially. Those patients were treated with ORIF and had excellent functional results with no complications. In the remaining five patients, the diagnosis was made 1 week to 8 months post injury, and they were treated with ORIF and bone grafting. One patient had a good result.

Lawlis reported on 20 patients with fracture-dislocations of the CMC joints, 15 of which involved multiple joints.[311] Of the 15 patients treated with ORIF between 1 and 17 days post injury, there were 13 excellent, 1 satisfactory, and 1 unsatisfactory result. One patient was treated with primary arthrodesis, and two others underwent arthrodesis as a late reconstructive procedure. Five patients were treated late, including 3 with primary arthrodesis. The authors recommended that arthrodesis remain a salvage procedure for CMC joint injuries.

Authors' Preferred Method of Treatment

Although irreducible CMC joint dislocation has been reported due to tendon interposition,[303] closed reduction is usually successful when performed within 24 to 48 hours of the injury. Adequate regional anesthesia (brachial or intravenous block) should be used to provide muscle relaxation as well as analgesia. Traction in flexion with simultaneous longitudinal pressure on the dorsally displaced metacarpal base, followed by extension of the metacarpal head when length has been restored, will generally accomplish reduction. Interposition of capsule or loss of the dorsal lip of the

adjacent carpal bone may impede stable reduction, making open reduction necessary. Whether the reduction is achieved open or closed, longitudinal and/or oblique Kirschner wire fixation is advisable to ensure adequate stability. Immobilization in plaster is continued for 4 to 6 weeks, at which time the wire is removed. IP and MP joint motion is permitted during the period of immobilization.

For dorsal fracture-dislocations of the fifth metacarpal, internal fixation is usually necessary, even if treated initially with closed reduction, because re-displacement tends to occur because of the pull of the extensor carpi ulnaris on the metacarpal base. Open reduction is indicated if closed reduction fails to yield a congruent articular surface or if a large fragment remains displaced. Exposure is through a small lazy-S incision, with the transverse limb directed over the dorsal aspect of the fifth CMC joint. Care is taken to avoid damage to the dorsal sensory branches of the ulnar nerve. The dislocated base of the fifth metacarpal is identified, and any invaginating capsule or avulsed fragments from the hamate that are blocking reduction are removed. The fracture-dislocation is then reduced and fixed with a longitudinal Kirschner wire as previously described. A transverse Kirschner wire to transfix the small avulsed fragment to the metacarpal may be used. Radiographs confirm adequate reduction, and postoperative management is the same as when the injury is treated with percutaneous pin fixation only.

Complications

The late sequelae of dislocations or fracture-dislocations are pain and weakness from traumatic arthritis at the CMC or intermetacarpal articular surfaces. Symptoms can be relieved by either CMC fusion or interpositional fascial arthroplasty.

THE THUMB METACARPOPHALANGEAL JOINT

 Anatomy

The MP joint of the thumb combines characteristics of both a condyloid and ginglymus joint.[376] The primary arc of motion is in the flexion/extension plane with secondary, minor arcs of abduction/adduction and pronation/supination. The radial condyle of the metacarpal head has greater dorsopalmar height than the ulnar condyle, which allows an element of conjunct rotation in pronation with increasing flexion. Range of motion of the thumb MP joint is the most variable of any joint in the body, resulting from different radii of curvature of metacarpal heads. More spherical heads are associated with a greater range of motion in flexion and extension than flatter heads.[373,393,412,475] There is some evidence for an inverse relationship between range of motion and the incidence of injury (i.e., limited range of motion is associated with an increased frequency of joint injury).[475] Coonrad and Goldner[368] found that there is even variability in range of motion from one side to the other in the same patient. The range of abduction and adduction also varies depending on the degree of ligamentous laxity.

---

*See references 272, 275, 277, 280, 282, 284, 285, 290-293, 295, 298-300, 302, 304, 305, 309, 311, 315, 317, 318, 324, 329, 330, 333-336, 339, and 341.

Because of the relatively large radius of curvature of the base of the proximal phalanx, the MP joint of the thumb has little intrinsic stability and depends instead on a complex arrangement of capsular, ligamentous, and musculotendinous structures. It is supported laterally by the strong proper collateral ligaments, which arise from the lateral condyles of the metacarpal and pass obliquely to insert on the volar third of the proximal phalanx. The accessory collateral ligaments originate from a more volar site on the metacarpal head and insert on the volar plate and sesamoids on either side of the joint.[478] The proper collateral ligaments are tight in flexion and loose in extension and, conversely, the accessory collateral ligaments are tight in extension and loose in flexion.[481] The floor of the joint is formed by the volar plate, creating a three-sided ligament-box configuration similar to that described previously at the PIP joint. However, it differs from the PIP complex because there is no flexor sheath proximal to the plate and, consequently, no strong checkrein ligaments present. In addition to the fibrocartilaginous plate, volar support is provided by the thenar intrinsic muscles that insert into a pair of sesamoid bones, embedded in the thickened distal volar plate. The adductor pollicis inserts on the ulnar sesamoid, and the flexor pollicis brevis and abductor pollicis brevis insert on the radial sesamoid.[416] Both muscles also have secondary insertions into the extensor mechanism via the adductor and abductor aponeuroses, which provide additional dynamic lateral stability.[481]

Acute Ulnar Collateral Ligament Injuries (Skier's Thumb)

Preoperative Evaluation
Injuries to the UCL of the MP joint of the thumb are common, particularly among skiers[369] and ball-handling athletes. In one series, UCL injuries made up 7% of 9749 ski injuries and 33% of all upper extremity injuries in 12 seasons at a popular ski resort.[490] Ulnar collateral injuries occur with significantly greater frequency than do RCL injuries[368,380,382,448,449,470,472,477,496]; Moberg and Stener[448] noted UCL injuries to be 10 times more common. The mechanism of injury is sudden, forced radial deviation (abduction), often resulting from a fall on an outstretched hand with the thumb abducted. Skiing injuries may occur from this mechanism, or from falling while gripping the ski pole so that its handle abducts the thumb.[367,381,462] Most modifications in ski pole design, including elimination of the strap, have not been shown to substantially reduce the incidence of thumb injuries.[381] Associated injuries include tears of the dorsal capsule and ulnar aspect of the volar plate and occasionally a rent in the adductor aponeurosis.[362,368,415,477,481,485] Volar subluxation of the MP joint may result from concomitant tears of the dorsal capsule and UCL. Distal tears of the UCL at its insertion are five times more common than proximal tears according to Bowers and Hurst.[358] Ruptures within the substance of the ligament or avulsion of the ligament from the metacarpal head occasionally occur.[358,368,428,485]

Smith[477] observed that not only do the collateral ligaments of the thumb MP joint afford lateral stability but they also resist volar subluxation. If one ligament is torn, the proximal phalanx tends to rotate volarly on the side of the tear, with the opposite intact ligament serving as the axis. In the case of an isolated UCL rupture, the proximal phalanx rotates in supination around the intact RCL. Conversely, if the RCL is torn, the proximal phalanx pronates relative to the metacarpal.

Several fracture patterns may be associated with UCL injuries. An avulsion fracture of the ulnar base of the proximal phalanx at the insertion of the ligament is most common.* Typically, the fracture fragment is small and includes little of the articular surface. Fractures involving greater than 10% of the articular surface can occur,[382,477] and larger fragments have implications for treatment. Large fractures necessitate ORIF if they are displaced 2 mm or more and associated with articular incongruity.[405,426] Somewhat surprisingly, there is incomplete agreement about the optimal treatment for small, minimally displaced or nondisplaced avulsion fractures. Cast immobilization is generally believed to be adequate,[427] but one series found that nine of nine patients with small avulsion fractures and displacement of less than 2 mm had persistent pain after immobilization, and all required secondary ORIF.[371] Avulsion fractures from the metacarpal head and intra-articular shearing fractures of the volar surface of the radial condyle of the metacarpal head have also been reported.[482] An interesting fracture pattern that is rare but potentially problematic is one in which there is an avulsion of the UCL with or without an avulsion fracture attached to the ligament and a simultaneous articular shear fracture of the proximal phalangeal base.[417,421] If attention is directed solely to the shear fracture, a complete tear of the UCL might be missed. In the skeletally immature individual, isolated rupture of the UCL without a Salter fracture of the proximal phalanx is rare but does occur.[366,419,444,484,489,493,495]

The Stener Lesion

In 1962, Stener[481] described the lesion that has come to bear his name, which he observed in 25 of 39 cases of complete rupture of the UCL of the thumb (Fig. 9-15). At surgery he found the adductor aponeurosis interposed between the distally avulsed ligament and its insertion into the base of the proximal phalanx. He concluded that without contact at the site of rupture, ligament healing would be imperfect and result in ulnar laxity regardless of the period of immobilization.[481] These findings have been repeatedly confirmed.[358,428,440,454,488]

Adductor aponeurosis interposition does not occur in partial ruptures. Therefore, it is critical to distinguish between acute complete and partial ruptures of the UCL. That differentiation can usually be made clinically, although there is no absolute consensus in the literature concerning the criteria for making the diagnosis. Smith and Peimer[479] used 45 degrees of laxity of the ulnar side of the joint when stressed in flexion and extension, Osterman and colleagues[456] suggested 40 degrees of laxity in extension and 20 degrees in flexion, and Palmer and Louis[458] advocated 35 degrees of laxity when the joint is stressed in full flexion. Heyman and coworkers[398] determined that 35 degrees of laxity in full extension, or 15 degrees of increased laxity when compared with the opposite side, indicated a complete tear of the proper and accessory collateral ligaments.

---

*See references 358, 362, 380, 382, 384, 419, 428, 440, 477, 481, and 485.

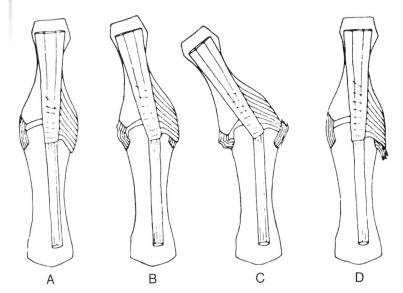

FIGURE 9-15. Diagram of the displacement of the ulnar collateral ligament of the thumb MP joint. **A,** Normal relationship with the ulnar ligament covered by the adductor aponeurosis. **B,** With slight radial angulation the proximal margin of the aponeurosis slides distally and leaves a portion of the ligament uncovered. **C,** With major radial angulation, the ulnar ligament ruptures at its distal insertion. In this degree of angulation the aponeurosis has displaced distal to the rupture and permitted the ligament to escape from beneath it. **D,** As the joint is realigned, the proximal edge of the adductor aponeurosis sweeps the free end of the ligament proximally and farther away from its insertion. This is the Stener lesion. Unless surgically restored, the ulnar ligament will not heal properly and will be unstable to lateral stress. (From Stener B: Skeletal injuries associated with rupture of the ulnar collateral ligament of the metacarpophalangeal joint of the thumb: A clinical and anatomic study. Acta Chir Scand 125:583-586, 1963.)

Patients with injuries to the UCL usually have tenderness, ecchymosis, and swelling along the ulnar border of the joint. We have adhered to the criteria of 30 degrees laxity of the ulnar side of the joint when stressed radially in extension and in 30 degrees flexion, as well as 15 degrees more laxity when compared with the contralateral thumb. It is hard to imagine that clinical testing is sufficiently precise to determine the difference between 30 and 35 degrees of laxity. A more helpful criterion for assessing instability may be the presence of an end point to valgus stress.[444] If the ligament is completely torn, the joint can be opened without resistance and without a clear end point. A partially torn ligament (grade II sprain) usually has a discrete end point even if there is some laxity with stress. Rarely, patients have too much pain and guarding to allow an adequate assessment of stability. In that case, the MP joint can be anesthetized with either median and radial nerve blocks at the wrist[391] or an intra-articular injection of local anesthetic[350,466] before stressing the joint.

Standard posteroanterior, lateral, and oblique radiographs should be obtained in all patients with suspected UCL injury to identify an accompanying avulsion or condylar fracture. Radiographs should be done before stressing the joint. In the absence of a fracture, the posteroanterior view is usually normal. A rare exception is when the joint is so unstable that there is radial deviation of the proximal phalanx at rest. Volar subluxation of the proximal phalanx in the lateral view suggests a significant dorsal capsular tear or extensor insertion injury that may require repair. For some patients with generalized ligament laxity, a small degree of volar subluxation is normal. To be certain that the subluxation is pathologic, comparison should be made with radiographs of the contralateral thumb. Stress radiographs are recommended by many authors.[358,373,408,433,456,482] The presence of a fracture does not necessarily obviate the need for stress views, but it does suggest that they should be done very gingerly to prevent displacement. Diagnosis of a torn UCL remains primarily a clinical diagnosis. Stress radiographs are at best an adjunct to physical examination and are ideally performed by a clinician who knows how much force may

safely be used to deviate the joint. Arthrograms have been recommended for diagnosing UCL tears.[358,379,414,431,465] Dye injected into the MP joint will leak out of the joint and outline the torn end of the collateral ligament if there is a capsular tear. The use of arthrograms is less common than in years past and might best be reserved for patients with uncertain physical findings. The use of diagnostic ultrasound and MRI has received considerable attention in recent years, particularly in the radiology literature. Ultrasound is noninvasive, relatively inexpensive, and reasonably accurate in a few small in vitro[461] and clinical series.[395,396,401,422,453,454] In one series, ultrasound accurately diagnosed the Stener lesion in 32 of 39 patients in whom there was operative confirmation of the findings. There were four false-positive results and three false-negative results.[401] Similar findings were reported in a series of 43 patients: Stener lesions were diagnosed accurately in 37 patients, with six false-negative findings.[422] In another group of 15 patients,[422] the sensitivity was 88% and the specificity 83% for Stener lesions, whereas the sensitivity was 91% for non-Stener lesions. More recent studies have shown comparable specificity and sensitivity rates in the range of 75% to 95% and have noted that accuracy diminishes if the procedure is delayed.[395,411] MRI is slightly more accurate but considerably more expensive. In one in vitro model, MRI was 100% sensitive and 67% specific for all tears but 94% specific for Stener lesions[480]; and in another, the sensitivity was 63% and the specificity was 50%.[392] One series found MRI more effective in distinguishing Stener from non-Stener lesions in 8 of 11 patients,[399] and another showed 100% sensitivity and specificity in a group of 15 patients.[365] MRI may be a helpful adjunct in the evaluation of selected cases[432] but is likely highly dependent on the available equipment and radiologist's experience. Ahn and associates[348] showed MR arthrograms were more accurate than standard MRI and conventional arthrograms for distinguishing between Stener lesions and nondisplaced complete UCL tears. The three diagnostic modalities were comparably accurate in determining the presence of a complete tear. However, the expense of MR arthrography is not insignificant and remains a consideration in clinical practice.

Historical Review

Watson-Jones[491] indicated the importance of the UCL in the stability of the thumb MP joint. He recommended conservative treatment with cast immobilization for UCL tears. Campbell[364] described the injury as a "gamekeeper's thumb," although the pathologic process that he was describing was chronic repetitive attenuation of the ligament by a radially directed force on the ulnar side of the thumb among Scottish gamekeepers who fractured the necks of rabbits between their thumbs and index fingers. The phrase *gamekeeper's thumb* describes chronic instability of the UCL, although it has been repeatedly misapplied in the literature when referring to any instability of the UCL, acute or chronic. Stener,[482–484] in addition to describing the adductor interposition,[481] also wrote extensively about the ligamentous anatomy and pathoanatomy of the MP joint. Moberg and Stener[448] recommended immobilization for incomplete tears and surgical repair for complete tears of the UCL. Alldred[349] outlined the findings on physical examination in patients with acute UCL tears, including tenderness, fullness on the ulnar side of the metacarpal head, and joint laxity. Frykman and Johansson[382] reported excellent results with UCL repair. Smith[477] made several important observations about the pathophysiology of ulnar collateral ligament instability by suggesting that the ligaments not only provided lateral but also dorsovolar and rotational stability. Bowers and Hurst[358] mentioned the use of arthrography for diagnosis of complete UCL tears. Palmer and Louis[458] identified the anatomic structures that have to be torn to allow complete instability of the MP joint and suggested parameters for the physical examination diagnosis of UCL instability.

Treatment

There is general agreement that acute partial ruptures of the UCL can be effectively treated by a 4-week period of continuous immobilization in a thumb spica cast, hand-based glove spica cast,[365] or a custom-molded, hand-based thumb cone thermoplastic splint to immobilize only the MP joint while leaving the IP joint free. This is followed by an additional 2-week period of splint immobilization, during which active range-of-motion exercise is begun. Alternatively, a functional splint allows earlier range of motion while protecting the thumb from lateral stress. Because the injured ligament maintains its normal anatomic relationship, healing with full recovery can be expected. Strenuous activity with the thumb is avoided for 3 months after the injury. It is common for patients to have a degree of aching pain on the ulnar side of the MP joint for 2 to 3 months after the injury despite having no laxity on examination.

There is less consensus concerning the treatment of acute *complete* ruptures of the UCL. Some authors advise immobilization in a well-molded thumb spica cast[366,452] or splint.[430] Others recommend operative treatment only if there is a palpable mass adjacent to the thumb metacarpal head strongly suggesting the presence of a Stener lesion.[345] Most, however, believe that the results of nonoperative treatment are unpredictable and only surgical exploration and repair ensure that anatomic ligament-bone continuity has been restored.*

Types of Operations

The technique used for repair of complete tears of the UCL depends, in part, on the location of the tear within the ligament. Intrasubstance tears are less common and can be fixed by direct suture of the ligament to itself or the periosteum.[368,380,382,424,477,485,488] The more common distal avulsion of the ligament necessitates reattachment of the ligament to its bony insertion using any of a number of techniques, including a pull-out suture,† bone anchor,[354,357,413,418,424] Acier cable (premade pull-out steel suture),[468] or "fishhook" pull-out wire technique.[384] Open repair of the torn UCL is a time-tested technique with good results in most reported series.[356,380,384,410,414,424,436,456,477] Complications are infrequent. After repair, the joint is immobilized for approximately 4 weeks, after which range of motion is begun.

Ryu monitored eight patients in whom complete tears of the UCL were treated successfully by arthroscopic reduction of Stener lesions without suture repair.[467] The results were good but the series was small and the follow-up averaged only 39 months. Slade and Gutow[476] performed arthroscopic-assisted repair of the ligament using a bone anchor for bony reattachment or direct arthroscopic suture for midsubstance tears. The theoretical advantage of arthroscopic repair is the decreased manipulation of the adductor aponeurosis and capsule, which may result in less postoperative scarring and more rapid restoration of motion. A potential disadvantage includes the limited visualization of the dorsal sensory nerve branches, which are susceptible to injury. Introduction of arthroscopic instruments into a small joint by an inexperienced operator has the potential to traumatize the articular cartilage. There are no comparative studies to assess whether the technique is time efficient or clinically advantageous.

Ryu's[467] technique of arthroscopic UCL repair involves visualization of the ligament from the radial side of the joint and replacement of the proximal stump of the UCL in its anatomic position beneath the adductor aponeurosis. Because the ligament is not repaired, arthroscopic visualization and manipulation of instrumentation is from the radiodorsal and radiovolar aspects of the joint, respectively. The extremity is exsanguinated, and the tourniquet is inflated. The thumb is placed in finger trap traction using an arthroscopic tower with the weight of the arm used for countertraction. The joint is insufflated with approximately 2 mL of normal saline. The skin on the radiodorsal aspect of the thumb at the level of the MP joint is incised with a No. 11 scalpel. A blunt trocar is introduced into the joint followed by a 1.7-mm, 15-degree angled arthroscope. A radial volar portal is created just volar to the RCL. A hook is introduced into the joint. Excessive synovium is débrided with a 2-mm full-radius shaver. The inner surface of the adductor aponeurosis is identified. The probe is passed along the proximal edge of the aponeurosis and pulled toward the joint in an effort to deliver the retracted UCL deep to the adductor aponeurosis. The distal end of the torn ligament is manipulated so that it is adjacent to its site of insertion on the base of the proximal phalanx. The MP joint is maintained in 20 to 30 degrees of flexion. A thumb spica cast is placed.

---

*See references 376, 380, 384, 385, 388, 391, 407, 408, 431, 433, 440, 443, 446, 448, 461, 477, 485, 488, and 494.

†See references 358, 362, 372, 373, 380, 448, 449, 477, 485, and 488.

Slade and Gutow[476] place the arthroscope radially and operative instrumentation ulnarly to perform arthroscopic-assisted UCL repair. The thumb is placed in fingertrap traction with 8 to 12 pounds of distraction. The extremity is exsanguinated, and the tourniquet is inflated. Nineteen-gauge needles are used to establish the location at the dorsoradial and dorsoulnar portals. The skin is incised with a No. 11 scalpel blade, and blunt dissection is carried down to the level of the joint capsule to avoid injury to the sensory branches of the dorsal sensory branch of the radial nerve. A blunt trocar is introduced into the joint through the dorsoradial portal. A 2.3-mm, 30-degree angled arthroscope is placed through the cannula. A second, dorsoulnar portal is established in a similar manner for placement of instruments. The joint is examined arthroscopically, and the torn ends of the ligament are identified. Usually, the ligament is torn from its insertion on the ulnar base of the proximal phalanx. The distal end of the ligament and its bony insertion are débrided with a shaver. The site of repair is identified with another 19-gauge needle at the level of the midlateral joint line. A skin incision is made, and blunt dissection is carried down to and through the adductor aponeurosis and the suture for repair is passed either using a 19-gauge "Touhy" spinal needle or a TFCC repair instrument. A braided synthetic suture such as 2-0 Ethibond (Ethicon Inc., Sommerville, NJ) is passed through the distal end of the ligament. The end of the suture is retrieved with a suture grabber or hemostat. The suture is threaded onto a mini Mitek bone anchor (Mitek Products, Westwood, MA). Through the same ulnar incision, a hole is drilled in the ulnar base of the proximal phalanx to accommodate the bone anchor; this is checked fluoroscopically. The bone anchor is inserted in the hole. Traction is removed from the thumb, and the ligament is advanced to its insertion site. The suture is tied. A second anchor may be used if deemed necessary to secure the ligament. The portals are sutured. A thumb spica cast is used for 3 to 4 weeks, after which flexion and extension exercises are begun and a splint used when not exercising.

Authors' Preferred Method of Treatment

Patients having less than 30 degrees laxity of the UCL, less than a 15-degree differential in laxity compared with the contralateral side, and a discrete end point to joint opening are assumed to have incomplete tears. Nonoperative treatment consists of immobilization of the MP joint for 4 weeks in neutral varus/valgus alignment and slight flexion. Adams has shown that excessive flexion and premature range of motion increase the strain on the healing ligament.[346] The IP joint is left free and IP range of motion encouraged to avoid adherence of the extensor tendons to the injured MP joint capsule. The MP joint can be immobilized either with a custom-molded thermoplastic splint or a cast. The splint may be a short opponens that extends to just proximal to the thumb CMC joint or a shorter splint that leaves the CMC joint completely free. We refer to the latter as a thumb "cone" splint.

Cast immobilization is the time-honored way to immobilize the thumb MP joint and is optimal treatment for patients who may be noncompliant with splint wear. The cast may either extend across the wrist to the junction of the middle and distal thirds of the forearm or stop at the wrist as a "glove spica" cast. Great care must be taken when molding the spica cast to avoid the natural tendency to abduct the thumb ray and to be certain that no radial deviation occurs through the unstable MP joint. The functional results of splint and cast immobilization have been shown to be comparable, and most patients prefer splinting.[345] In rare instances with more swollen unstable thumbs, consideration might be given to transfixing the MP joint with a percutaneous Kirschner wire in a neutral or even a slightly overcorrected position before applying the cast.

Technique of Open Repair of the Thumb MP Ulnar Collateral Ligament

If clinical evaluation confirms that an acute complete rupture of the UCL is present, surgical repair is indicated. A "lazy-S"-shaped incision is used that parallels the ulnodorsal border of the thumb metacarpal to the MP joint, curving sharply in a volar direction to parallel the joint and extending distally along the ulnar midaxial line (Fig. 9-16). The distal limb of the incision should be sufficiently volar to give easy access to the volar base of the proximal phalanx and the volar plate. Branches of the superficial radial nerve lying in the deep subcutaneous plane should be identified and protected. The proximal edge of the adductor aponeurosis is identified. When a Stener lesion is present, it appears as an edematous, rounded mass that may obscure this otherwise well-defined proximal border (Fig. 9-17). A longitudinal incision is made in the adductor aponeurosis parallel and approximately 3 mm volar to the ulnar border of the extensor pollicis longus (EPL). The aponeurosis is reflected volarly to expose the ulnar aspect of the MP joint, including the volar base of the proximal phalanx. The joint should be examined to determine the extent of the soft tissue injury and the condition of the articular cartilage. A small cartilaginous shear fragment will occasionally be found and should be removed if loose.

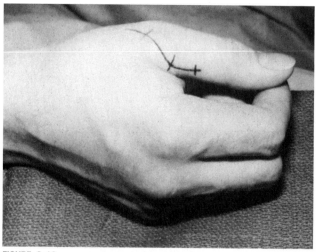

FIGURE 9-16. Incision for repair or reconstruction of a ruptured ulnar collateral ligament of the MP joint of the thumb. Exposure is excellent, and the healing leaves an almost imperceptible scar.

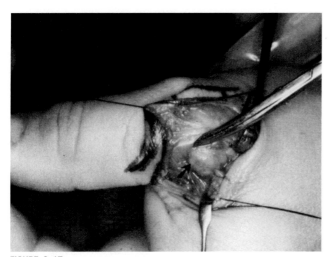

FIGURE 9-17. Displaced edematous end of the ulnar collateral ligament *(arrow)* lying proximal to the edge of the adductor aponeurosis.

Tears in the middle two thirds of the ligament can be reapproximated with interrupted figure-of-eight or horizontal mattress sutures using nonabsorbable braided synthetic suture material such as 4-0 Ethibond. However, the ligament is usually avulsed distally and can be approximated to the distal stump or into the bone defect from which it was avulsed with a pull-out suture technique or a small bone anchor (Fig. 9-18).

Secure fixation of the ligament to bone can be achieved by pull-out suture technique after scarifying the bone at the site of reattachment with a curet or rongeur. A monofilament synthetic suture such as 3-0 nylon, Prolene, or stainless steel wire is placed in the proximal stump of the UCL with a modified Kessler technique. Keith needles are drilled using a Kirschner wire driver across the base of the proximal phalanx in an ulnoradial direction, exiting percutaneously on the radial side. The ends of the suture in the UCL stump are threaded through the eye of the Keith needles, which are then pulled through the proximal phalanx. The ligament is pulled up to the shallow trough previously made in the ulnar base of the phalanx and the ends of suture then tied over a felt-padded button or rubber catheter. The repair can be supplemented by suturing the proximal stump of the ligament to any remnants of the distal stump or periosteum.

An alternative is to secure the avulsed ligament with a bone anchor. The pilot hole for the anchor is hand-drilled in the ulnar base of the proximal phalanx. If a single anchor is used, it is placed volar to the axis of the joint. If two anchors are used, one is placed ulnovolarly and the other more dorsally. Bone anchors generally come prethreaded with 0 or 2-0 braided suture, the latter being more than sufficient to secure the ligament. The anchors are advanced into the drill holes and the sutures threaded into the proximal stump of the ligament, separated as widely as possible to spread out the ligament. A single simple throw may be placed in the suture and tightened down to check range of motion and ensure satisfactory tension on the repair before completing the knots. This repair may also be supplemented with sutures in local tissue.

If a fragment of bone accompanies the avulsed ligament, the repair depends on the size of the fragment. If the fragment is small (less than 10% to 15% of the articular surface), it may be excised and the ligament inserted directly into the defect with a pull-out suture. If the fragment is large, it is reduced anatomically into the defect with a pull-out suture, Kirschner wires, one or more mini-fragment screws, or an interosseous wire.

Regardless of the pathologic process, additional steps should be considered before closure. First, a suture should be placed between the distal volar portion of the repaired ligament and the volar plate to secure this vital three-dimensional complex. Second, meticulous repair of the dorsal ulnar capsule is performed to prevent volar subluxation or rotation of the joint. Third, gentle radial stress is applied to the joint to test the stability of the repair. Finally, the joint may be transfixed

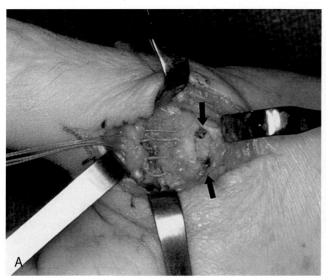
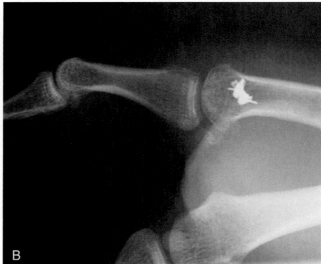

FIGURE 9-18. Collateral ligaments avulsed from their insertions may be reattached with bone anchors. In this unusual example of the ulnar collateral ligament avulsed from its *proximal* origin on the metacarpal head, Mitek bone anchors with 2-0 nonabsorbable braided synthetic suture were used to reattach the ligament. The repair was supplemented with additional sutures in the adjacent periosteum and capsule. **A,** The holes in the metacarpal neck *(arrows)* indicate the points of insertion of the bone anchors. **B,** Bone anchors are seen in the metacarpal neck on the postoperative radiograph.

CRITICAL POINTS: ACUTE UCL REPAIR

INDICATIONS

- Complete UCL tear with Stener lesion; absolute
- Complete UCL tear without Stener lesion; relative

PREOPERATIVE EVALUATION

- Physical examination is usually adequate for diagnosis.
- Obtain posteroanterior, lateral, and oblique radiographs.
- Stress radiographs are rarely helpful.
- Arthrography is primarily of historical interest.
- Ultrasound and MRI used to assess a Stener lesion are rarely necessary.

PEARLS

- Physical examination alone is usually sufficient to make the diagnosis.
- Absence of an end point to joint opening is important for diagnosis.
- Avulsion fracture and complete UCL tears can occur in the same thumb.
- Avulsion fracture is not a contraindication to stress joint gently.
- Suture anchor placement in volar base of proximal phalanx.
- Use of a Kirschner wire is unnecessary.

TECHNICAL POINTS

- Avoid injury to branch of dorsal sensory branch of radial nerve.
- Reattach ligament avulsions to physiologic insertion.
- Suture intrasubstance tears with 3-0 or 4-0 braided synthetic suture.
- Reattach ligament avulsions with bone anchors using 2-0 braided synthetic suture.
- Repair adductor aponeurosis with 4-0 Vicryl or monocryl.
- Avoid stress on repair when molding splint or cast.

PITFALLS

- Do not make repair too tight.
- Avoid too dorsal placement of suture anchor.
- Avoid prolonged immobilization.

POSTOPERATIVE CARE

- Wear short-arm thumb spica cast for 4 weeks.
- Wear thermoplastic splint for 2 additional weeks.
- Begin range-of-motion exercises when cast is removed.
- Avoid radially directed stress on thumb tip for 12 weeks.

ATHLETIC PARTICIPATION

- Protect with splint or tape for 4 months.

---

in a slightly overcorrected ulnar-deviated position in mild flexion with an oblique Kirschner wire to prevent tension on the repair, although we have eliminated this last step several years ago without any untoward consequences.

The adductor aponeurosis is repaired with a slowly absorbable suture. The skin is reapproximated with a running subcuticular suture of 4-0 monofilament suture. The thumb is immobilized in a thumb spica cast with the IP joint left free to prevent adhesions of the extensor mechanism during healing. Cast immobilization is continued for 4 weeks, after which a hand-based custom-fabricated thermoplastic splint is used to protect the MP joint. The splint is removed approximately four times per day for controlled active range-of-motion exercise, preferably under the supervision of a hand therapist. Splint protection is discontinued 6 weeks postoperatively. Activities that stress the UCL are avoided, and unrestricted use is not recommended for 3 to 4 months after surgery. Vague discomfort and some tenderness and thickening on the ulnar side of the joint can be expected to persist for as long as 1 year.

Postoperative Management and Expectations

We advise patients that when the cast is removed at 4 weeks postoperatively, they will be extremely stiff and that it will take several weeks to work out that stiffness with therapy and exercise. Ultimately, they can expect range of motion of the MP joint averaging 80% to 90% of the uninjured thumb and nearly full range of motion of the IP joint. Pinch and grip strength are usually regained to within 5% to 10% of the contralateral, unoperated side. Patients are often concerned about whether they will be able to return to preinjury sporting activities. In the majority of cases, full athletic participation, including contact sports, can be resumed by approximately 4 months postoperatively. Some competitive athletes will return sooner but only if the thumb is protected with a splint.

The postoperative cast remains on for 4 weeks. The use of subcuticular or absorbable sutures obviates the need for a cast change for suture removal. When the cast is removed the patient is referred to the hand therapist for a customized, thermoplastic "thumb cone" splint designed to immobilize only the MP joint. The IP and CMC joints are free to move. Range-of-motion exercises are begun under the supervision of the therapist. MP and IP flexion and extension and full range of motion in the CMC joint and wrist are encouraged. Radially directed force on the tip of the thumb and resisted activities with the thumb are prohibited. The splint is worn full time except for bathing and exercise.

During the ensuing 2 weeks (weeks 4 to 6) the patient gradually weans from the splint. During the first week it is off primarily at mealtimes and during sedentary activity. In the second week, nonstrenuous activities at home and in an office are allowed and patients begin light resisted activities such as manipulating zippers and buttons. Flexion of the IP joint against slight resistance is begun with the therapist. By the seventh postoperative week, full active range of motion of the thumb is encouraged. The patient works on wrist and forearm strengthening exercise using 1- to 2-pound weights. The therapist initiates gentle strengthening of the thumb against light resistance, including the use of the "thumb-cisor," which is essentially a small plunger with rubber bands for resistance.

By 9 to 10 weeks postoperatively, the patient should have regained nearly full active range of motion. Focused exercises compensate for any deficit in that range. The patient is expected to have between 60% and 75% of normal pinch strength. The only activities that are restricted are forceful torque and radially directed pressure on the thumb tip. Full, unrestricted activity is allowed at 3 months, with the exception of contact sports, which can be played, if necessary, with taping or semi-rigid splinting of the MP joint.

The most common complication of UCL repair is neurapraxia of the crossing branches of the dorsal sensory branch of the radial nerve. Traction on the nerve during the procedure causes numbness and tingling on the dorsoulnar aspect of the thumb distal to the incision. These symptoms are usually self-limited but can last from days to weeks and can be disconcerting, particularly if the patient is not forewarned. The likelihood of the problem arising can be diminished by fully mobilizing the nerve during the exposure and retracting gently. If vessel loops are used for retraction, there should not be a heavy instrument like a hemostat securing it. The weight of the instrument creates too much traction on the nerve. Another potential complication is stiffness, which can result from reattaching the ligament too distally on the base of the proximal phalanx or inserting it in a nonanatomic or nonisometric location, particularly too dorsal relative to the axis of the joint. This complication can be avoided by careful attention to the detail of where the sutures or suture anchors are placed in reattaching the ligament and testing with a single knot so that adjustments can be made as needed.

Chronic Ulnar Collateral Ligament Injuries (Gamekeeper's Thumb)

Preoperative Evaluation

Causes of chronic instability of the UCL include lack of or inadequate treatment of an acute tear, failure to recognize a Stener lesion, or progressive attenuation of the ligament. Patients with chronic instability usually present with pain, swelling, and weakness of the involved thumb. The pain tends to be exacerbated by forceful pinch and activities requiring torsional motions of the hand, such as unscrewing jar tops. Holding large objects like a half-gallon container of milk may be painful and, in addition, cause a feeling of instability or lack of power because the thumb's ability to resist counterpressure on the object by the hand is compromised.

Preoperative evaluation of patients with chronic instability of the UCL is similar but less challenging than that of patients with acute instability. Chronic instability almost invariably occurs with untreated complete tears. Partial acute tears usually heal without significant laxity. The presence of a Stener lesion in chronic instability is a moot point, because symptomatic chronic tears require UCL reconstruction by definition. The criteria for assessing instability on physical examination parallels that described previously for acute tears, and the authors prefer the criteria recommended by Heyman and coworkers.[398] The resting posture of the thumb should be observed for volar subluxation or radial deviation of the MP joint. Crepitus with active motion suggests degenerative disease.

Radiographic assessment includes posteroanterior, lateral, and oblique views of the thumb. Specific attention should be paid to volar subluxation of the joint and radial deviation of the proximal phalanx. In addition, osteoarthritis of the joint needs to be ruled out if consideration is to be given to reconstruction. Stress views occasionally help clarify the degree of laxity when clinical examination is not definitive. Additional imaging studies are not indicated to define a Stener lesion, but they may be helpful to determine the adequacy of remaining ligament tissue and the potential need for tendon graft augmentation of the repair.

It is worthwhile to treat patients with splint immobilization, avoidance of strenuous activity, and nonsteroidal anti-inflammatory medication. In some, this will diminish their pain to the point of tolerance and, particularly for sedentary patients, this may be adequate. In others, this is a temporizing measure that postpones the inevitable need for reconstruction.

Historical Review

Among the causes of chronic instability is an unrecognized or untreated acute tear. The longer a complete rupture has existed, the less likely that restoration of stability by anatomic repair will be successful.[394] Some surgeons, however, have been successful in restoring stability by mobilizing and using the remnant of the torn ligament.[407,408,441,442,449,459,485] Techniques of reconstruction have included dynamic and static procedures. Kaplan[415] used the extensor indicis proprius tendon as a dynamic tendon transfer inserted into the extensor mechanism and ignored the UCL. Sakellarides and DeWeese[469,470] and Ahmad and DePalma[347] detached the extensor pollicis brevis (EPB) dorsally and reinserted it ulnarly. Neviaser[452] and other authors[362,388,440,457] have achieved good results with adductor advancement by transferring the adductor pollicis from its insertion on the ulnar sesamoid to the ulnar base of the proximal phalanx 1 cm distal to the joint. This is combined with a proximal reefing of the fibrotic stump of the UCL. Static reconstructions have included descriptions of "static" tendon transfers, such as leaving an adjacent tendon like the EPB,[485] abductor pollicis longus (APL),[382] or palmaris longus[429] attached distally, dividing it proximally, and rerouting it through the metacarpal or proximal phalanx. This method leaves a length of tendon free for reconstruction of the ligament with a theoretical advantage of some intrinsic blood supply. Several authors have reported good results from reconstructing the ligament with a free tendon graft passed in one of a variety of configurations, including a figure of eight,[359,382,387,446,456,459,474,485] rectangle,[456] single tail longitudinally across the joint,[477] and triangle with the apex proximally.[349,435] Some surgeons recommend MP arthrodesis as the preferred procedure for chronic instability,[380,428,464] whereas others reserve fusion for patients with concomitant arthritis of the MP joint or after ligament reconstruction has failed.[447,453,459,477]

Types of Operations

Currently, the techniques commonly used for UCL reconstruction are adductor advancement[452] or reconstruction with a free tendon graft. There are technical modifications of how the graft is passed through or attached to the metacarpal and proximal phalanx. Space does not permit description of each of these techniques in this chapter.

Adductor advancement was described by Neviaser in 1971. It is an effort to replace the static restraint normally provided by the UCL with a dynamic tendon transfer. The ulnar side of the MP joint is exposed through a chevron incision extending from the center of the first web and extending to just proximal to the IP joint. The branches of the dorsal sensory branch of the radial nerve are mobilized and protected. The adductor aponeurosis is incised and reflected volarly. The scarred ligament and capsule are identified, and the joint is exposed. The adductor pollicis tendon is detached from its insertion on the ulnar sesamoid. A "U"-shaped flap of the remnant of the UCL is mobilized and "reefed."[452] A hole is made in the ulnar cortex of the base of the proximal phalanx 1 cm distal to the MP joint. The distal end of the adductor tendon is advanced and inserted into the bone where it is fixed with a pull-out wire. The thumb is immobilized for 1 month after which the patient begins progressive range of motion of the thumb.

Smith[477] treated chronic UCL instability with reconstruction using a free tendon graft. The ulnar aspect of the MP joint is exposed with a midaxial incision. The adductor aponeurosis is incised longitudinally and mobilized from the underlying soft tissue exposing the capsule. A 2.8-mm hole is drilled in the ulnar base of the proximal phalanx in the area of the anatomic insertion of the UCL. A tendon graft is obtained (Smith preferred the palmaris longus), and a figure-of-eight suture is placed in the free end of the graft. The two ends of that suture are placed on needles and passed through the hole in the base of proximal phalanx and through the radial cortex where the sutures are brought out through the skin and tied over a button. The torn UCL is identified and dissected free of surrounding scar. If a proximal stump of ligament remains on the metacarpal head, the graft is woven into the ligament remnant through parallel longitudinal incisions. If there is no usable remnant of ligament, the tendon graft is fixed to the metacarpal through adjacent drill holes in the metacarpal head. The graft is placed through the holes, and the free end of the graft is placed adjacent to the primary limb to which it is sutured. The abductor aponeurosis is repaired and the skin is reapproximated. A thumb spica cast is worn for 4 weeks postoperatively. Thereafter, the thumb is protected for an additional 5 weeks in a splint. Mitsionis and colleagues[445] devised a modification of this technique in which the free tendon graft is fixed to both the metacarpal and proximal phalanx with bone anchors. Bean and associates[352] emphasized in a cadaver model the importance of anatomic positioning of the origin and insertion of the tendon graft. They found that the center of origin of the ligament is 7 mm from the joint, 3 mm from the dorsal border, and 8 mm from the volar border of the metacarpal head. The phalangeal insertion is 3 mm from the joint, 3 mm from the volar border, and 8 mm from the dorsal border of the phalangeal base. Even small variations from these positions had the effect of limiting motion.

There has been preliminary interest in the bone-ligament model for joint reconstruction. Fusetti and coworkers[383] described bone-tendon ligamentoplasty in which a strip of the extensor carpi radialis longus (ECRL) tendon with an attached bone block is used to replace the incompetent UCL. A "lazy S"-shaped incision exposes the adductor aponeurosis, which is incised longitudinally. The remnant of the scarred UCL is resected. A 4-cm-long strip of half of the width of the ECRL tendon just proximal to its insertion is harvested along with a 5-mm square block of bone at its insertion. A 5-mm square trough is cut in the cortex on the ulnar side of the metacarpal head at the point of origin of the UCL. The bone block in continuity with the UCL strip is placed into the trough and secured with a 1.5-mm titanium cortical screw. The strip of ECRL is split longitudinally so that one half can be used to reconstruct the proper collateral ligament and the other half, the accessory collateral ligament. The more dorsal segment is attached using a bone anchor to the ulnar side of the base of the proximal phalanx at the normal point of attachment of the UCL. The more volar strip of the tendon is sutured to the volar plate with 3-0 braided synthetic suture. The adductor aponeurosis is closed with a 5-0 running absorbable suture, and the skin is reapproximated. The thumb is placed in a cast for 6 weeks postoperatively. No long-term or comparative results are available to assess this method of reconstruction.

Adductor advancement replaces a static structure with a dynamic tendon transfer. The procedure as described by Neviaser includes reefing the scarring ulnar collateral ligament and ulnar capsule. This portion of the procedure may add a static restraint to radial instability of the proximal phalanx. We see no advantage to using an isolated dynamic transfer when static replacements for the incompetent UCL are available, especially in light of the potential disadvantage of weakening the adductor pollicis muscle.

The use of free tendon grafts to reconstruct chronic instability addresses a deficient static joint restraint with a static replacement. Smith reported excellent results with his technique using a double thickness of tendon. Mitsionis and associates[445] modified the technique of graft fixation, but conceptually the operation is very similar to Smith's and the results are comparably good. The bone-tendon bone model for ligament reconstruction has been efficacious in other situations, such as anterior cruciate ligament replacement, and has theoretical appeal in upper extremity reconstruction as well. The only absolute contraindication to any of these procedures is advanced osteoarthritis of the MP joint. A relative contraindication is marked volar subluxation and/or supination of the MP joint, which may not be adequately addressed by these reconstructive procedures.[403]

Authors' Preferred Method of Treatment

We use 6 weeks as a general criterion for distinguishing between acute and chronic UCL injuries. It is certainly the case that local tissue can sometimes be used for reconstruction, particularly if the duration from injury to reconstruction is relatively short (i.e., in the range of 6 to 12 weeks). The remnant of the torn ligament must be supple. Characteristically, the proximal stump of the ligament is shortened, retracted, and surrounded with a layer of fibrous tissue. To use the ligament for reconstruction, that layer of fibrous tissue needs to be mobilized and the substance of the ligament brought out to its physiologic length. It is reattached to the base of the proximal phalanx with a bone anchor, which we use now in preference to a pull-out suture. Using local tissue for reconstruction beyond the time frame noted has yielded unpredictable and, sometimes, less than optimal results in our hands.

Our preferred technique[386,387,435] for late reconstruction of an incompetent UCL is to replace the static restraint with a free tendon graft anchored in the medullary canals of both the metacarpal and the proximal phalanx. The technique of passage of the tendon graft very nearly recapitulates the normal anatomy of the UCL and attempts to resist the volar and rotatory translation by the triangular configuration of the graft.[386,387,435] The exposure is the same as that described earlier for repair of acute ligament ruptures. The adductor aponeurosis is exposed, and an attempt is made to preserve the sagittal fibers of the extensor mechanism. A volar-based triangular flap of the adductor aponeurosis distal to the sagittal band is reflected to expose the MP joint and base of the proximal phalanx. The scarred, redundant UCL and capsule are resected from the concavity of the metacarpal head to the base of the proximal phalanx. Holes approximately 3 mm in diameter are made with progressively larger hand-held gouges at approximately the 1- and 5-o'clock positions through the ulnar cortex of the phalangeal base (Fig. 9-19A). These holes are directed obliquely to connect within the medullary canal of the proximal phalanx 3 to 4 mm distal and parallel to the articular surface. Particular attention is directed toward keeping the holes sufficiently far apart to avoid fracturing the cortical bone bridge between them. A 28-gauge stainless steel wire is threaded through

this channel for subsequent passage of the tendon graft. Another gouge tract about 4 mm in diameter is made in the metacarpal starting at the ulnar concavity of the metacarpal head (the UCL origin) and extending slightly obliquely in a dorsoradial direction across the medullary canal, through the radial cortex to emerge subcutaneously on the radial side of the thumb. A small incision is made in the skin at this site, and a second 28-gauge wire is passed through this channel with the concavity of the gouge used as a guide.

A palmaris longus tendon graft is then obtained if available. In the absence of the palmaris longus, a longitudinal strip of the flexor carpi radialis (FCR), the APL, the plantaris, or a toe extensor may be used. The end of the stainless steel wire that emerges from the volar end of the proximal phalangeal channel is tied in a loop around the narrowest end of the tendon graft. The end of the tendon is drawn into the gouge hole using a dental probe to direct its passage. Traction on the wire allows the tendon to be pulled through the channel in the medullary canal and emerge through the dorsal hole. The two free ends of the tendon are equalized in length and secured within a loop of the wire in the ulnar metacarpal hole. The two ends of the graft are drawn simultaneously through the metacarpal into the incision on its dorsoradial aspect. Tension is adjusted in the reconstruction by traction on the ends of the tendon. The traditional method of fixation of the graft was to tie the ends in a knot over a button backed with felt or a section of a rubber catheter and suture the limbs of the knot with nonabsorbable suture (see Fig. 9-19B). A preferable alternative, which we use, is to secure the tendon to local tissue (i.e., periosteum) and supplement that fixation with a bone anchor if necessary. The anchor is placed about 5 mm proximal to the hole to avoid disrupting the bridge of cortex between them. After tension is set on the reconstruction, the ends of the tendon are tied in a single throw knot, which is then sutured to itself and to adjacent periosteum. The sutures from the bone anchor are also placed into the knotted graft to keep it from slipping back into the hole. The configuration of the reconstructed

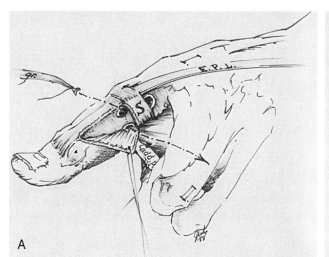
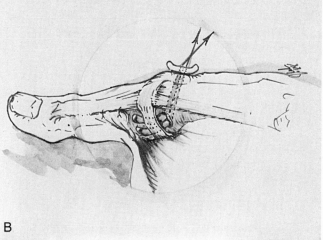

FIGURE 9-19. Authors' preferred method for reconstruction of the ulnar collateral ligament with a free tendon graft. **A,** Gouge holes are made at the 1-o'clock and 5-o'clock positions on the ulnar side of the base of the proximal phalanx. A second gouge hole is made slightly obliquely across the metacarpal neck. **B,** The tendon graft is passed through the hole in the base of the proximal phalanx, beneath the sagittal band, and then both limbs of the graft are passed through the metacarpal neck. They are secured on the radial side of the metacarpal either with percutaneous fixation over a button or catheter or by fixation to adjacent periosteum. Fixation of the graft may also be supplemented with a bone anchor.

ulnar ligament is that of a distally based "V", with the apex converging on the concavity in the ulnar condyle of the metacarpal head. The stability of the reconstruction is tested with stress in radial deviation. If the ulnar side of the joint opens more than 10 degrees, the tension on the reconstructed ligament must be adjusted. The MP joint is transfixed with a 0.045-inch Kirschner wire, and care is taken to reduce any element of volar subluxation before joint fixation.

Postoperative Management and Expectations

Postoperative management of the reconstructed ulnar collateral ligament is nearly identical to that for acute UCL repair but the process is begun 2 weeks later for reconstruction than repair. The cast placed in the operating room is removed at 6 weeks rather than 4 weeks. The Kirschner wire is extracted when the cast is removed. The patient is referred to the hand therapist for a thumb cone splint and to begin the protocol described previously. Full activity including contact sports should be postponed for at least 4½ months postoperatively.

The expected outcomes of UCL reconstruction are similar to those for repair with a few exceptions. The thumb is rendered stable by the reconstruction to within greater than 90% of the unoperated side. Two thirds of patients who have the procedure have no pain postoperatively, and one third have mild, occasional pain. Approximately 80% of the motion of the MP joint and more than 90% of the motion of the IP joint is regained compared with the contralateral side. There is mild loss of key pinch strength and mild weakness with radially directed pressure on the ulnar aspect of the thumb tip. The overall satisfaction rate among patients who have had the procedure is very high.

Radial Collateral Ligament Injuries

Injuries to the RCL are substantially less common but may be as debilitating as tears of the UCL. Moberg and Stener[448] observed, and many authors[363,366,421,428,477] have confirmed, that the UCL is injured about 10 times more often than the RCL, although some have found a higher incidence, ranging from 23%[477] to as high as 35%.[363] The principles of diagnosis and treatment of RCL and UCL injuries are similar and therefore only their differences will be highlighted in this discussion.

 Anatomy

The principal difference between the anatomy on the radial and the ulnar sides of the thumb is that the abductor aponeurosis is broad and covers most of the radial side of the MP

CRITICAL POINTS: CHRONIC UCL REPAIR

INDICATIONS

- Chronic complete UCL tear with or without Stener lesion
- Persistent pain despite conservative treatment

PREOPERATIVE EVALUATION

- Physical examination is usually adequate for diagnosis.
- Obtain posteroanterior, lateral, and oblique radiographs.
- Rule out degenerative disease.
- Stress radiographs may be helpful.

PEARLS

- Physical examination alone is usually sufficient to make the diagnosis.
- Preserve large bone bridge between gouge holes in base of proximal phalanx.

TECHNICAL POINTS

- Avoid injury to branch of dorsal sensory branch of radial nerve.
- Incise adductor aponeurosis.
- Resect remnant of collateral ligament.
- Make gouge holes in base of proximal phalanx at 1 and 5 o'clock positions.
- Make gouge hole in metacarpal neck.
- Use 28-gauge stainless steel wire through gouge holes to pass graft.
- Harvest tendon graft.
- Pass tendon graft using 28-gauge wire.
- Set tension on graft.
- Tie ends of the graft in a knot and suture to adjacent periosteum.
- Repair adductor aponeurosis.
- Transfix the MP joint with 0.045-inch Kirschner wire.

PITFALLS

- Do not make reconstruction too tight or too loose.
- Avoid fracturing bony bridge.

POSTOPERATIVE CARE

- Place in short-arm thumb spica cast for 6 weeks.
- Use thermoplastic splint for 2 additional weeks.
- Begin range-of-motion exercises when cast is removed.
- Avoid radially directed stress on thumb tip for 12 weeks.

ATHLETIC PARTICIPATION

- Begin sports at 8 to 12 weeks protecting MP joint with splint or tape for 16 weeks from surgery.

joint whereas the adductor aponeurosis is a narrower sheet of tissue that is easily interposed between the torn UCL and its insertion (i.e., the Stener lesion).[439] There is no potential interposition lesion on the radial side comparable to the Stener lesion on the ulnar side.[351] The mechanism of RCL injuries is forced adduction or torsion on the flexed MP joint. The ligament is torn with about equal frequency proximally and distally[351,363,477] and, somewhat more commonly than the UCL, is attenuated in its midsubstance.[363,374,477] The abductor aponeurosis may be attenuated as well.[374,477] A tear in the RCL, as noted previously for the UCL, creates a rotatory deformity of the MP joint in which the proximal phalanx shifts volarly on the radial side and rotates around the intact UCL into pronation. This is responsible for dorsoradial prominence of the metacarpal head, a common physical finding seen with RCL rupture.

Preoperative Evaluation

The differentiation between partial and complete tears of the RCL is made in much the same way as for the ulnar collateral ligament. Partial tears are characterized by swelling, tenderness, and sometimes ecchymosis over the radial side of the joint and metacarpal head. There may be little or no laxity with stress of the RCL, but if laxity is present there usually remains a clear end point to opening of the joint. Patients with complete radial ligament ruptures generally have localized tenderness, particularly at the dorsoradial joint line where the tear in the ligament and dorsal capsule is subcutaneous. The same criteria used to assess UCL instability can be applied to the RCL as well. Laxity of 35 degrees in full extension or 15 degrees of increased laxity when compared with the contralateral thumb are indicative of a complete tear. The other useful diagnostic finding is the absence of a firm end point to the joint opening.

Radiographic evaluation should include standard posteroanterior, lateral, and oblique views. Volar subluxation of the proximal phalanx, best detected on the lateral radiograph, usually accompanies the more extensive radial ligament tears and is strongly suggestive of an extension of the tear into the dorsal capsule. The posteroanterior radiograph occasionally shows ulnar angulation of the proximal phalanx at rest and suggests gross instability. Avulsion fractures are best seen on the posteroanterior view. Stress radiographs may help confirm a presumptive diagnosis of a complete tear based on physical examination. A variation of the standard stress view done by the examiner is to use the basal joint stress view recommended by Eaton[501,502] in which the radial side of the thumb tips are pushed against each other while a posteroanterior radiograph of both thumbs is obtained. Laxity of the RCL will cause ulnar deviation of the proximal phalanx. Special studies such as arthrograms, ultrasound, and MRI are rarely indicated because the Stener lesion does not occur on the radial side.

Historical Perspective

Partial tears of the RCL can be treated much the same as partial tears of the UCL, that is, with a cast or splint. There is no consensus about the treatment of acute, complete RCL ruptures. Some authors, including Lamb and associates,[428] Kessler,[419] Coonrad and Goldner,[368] and Camp and colleagues,[363] believe that immobilization alone produces satisfactory stability. Basuk and Melone,[351] Frank and Dobyns,[380] Miller,[443] and Smith[477] recommend early operative repair as a more predictable way

of ensuring superior results. Reports have included the use of bone anchors for fixation of the ligament.[437] For chronic instability, some authors prefer repair of the scarred ligament only. Camp and colleagues[363] and Green[388] recommend local repair in conjunction with tendon advancement. Ligament reconstruction with a tendon graft is recommended by Smith,[477] Brewood and Menon,[360] and Glickel.[385]

Types of Operations

There is a paucity of literature specifically addressing the treatment of acute tears of the radial collateral ligament, and the few studies that do[351,374,380,443,477] simply refer to repairing or reattaching the ligament. The treatment options for reconstruction of chronic radial instability are also somewhat sparsely documented. Camp and colleagues[363] and, then, Durham and associates[374] used the technique of abductor advancement, a mirror image of Neviaser's adductor advancement, either alone or in combination with repair and/or reefing of the remnant of the RCL.

The radial side of the thumb is exposed through a midaxial incision. The abductor aponeurosis and tendon are mobilized from the underlying collateral ligament and capsule, and the muscle belly is freed up proximally. The dorsoradial joint capsule is incised, and the location of the tear in the RCL is identified. The ligament is mobilized as a proximally or distally based flap depending on the site of rupture. Drill holes are made at the location of origin or insertion of the normal RCL to accommodate sutures to be placed into the ligament. A ³⁄₁₆-inch unicortical hole is drilled in the radial side of the base of the proximal phalanx 10 to 12 mm distal to the articular surface into which the abductor tendon will be advanced. Through this hole, two smaller holes are made in the ulnar cortex to accommodate pull-out sutures. The ligament is repaired with a 2-0 or 3-0 braided nonabsorbable suture. A similar suture is placed in the distal end of the abductor pollicis brevis tendon. Straight needles are then used to pass the sutures in the end of the tendon through the radial-sided hole and out through the ulnar holes. A small counterincision is made over the ulnar holes. The abductor pollicis brevis tendon is advanced into the radial drill hole, and the sutures are tightened and tied over the ulnar bony bridge beneath the skin. The aponeurosis is repaired with 4-0 braided nonabsorbable suture. A thumb spica splint is applied in the operating room and replaced in a few days with a thumb spica cast that is worn for 4 weeks. After the cast is removed patients are allowed to resume activity gradually and, at 8 weeks, full activity is allowed.

Smith[477] reconstructed chronic instability of the RCL using a free tendon graft in the same manner in which he recommended reconstruction of UCL laxity. The radial side of the joint is exposed through a midaxial incision. The branches of the dorsal sensory branch of the radial nerve are protected. The abductor aponeurosis is incised longitudinally and mobilized from the underlying soft tissue exposing the capsule. If the ligament is torn proximally, a 2.8-mm hole is drilled in the radial base of the proximal phalanx in the area of the physiologic insertion of the RCL. A figure-of-eight suture is placed in the free end of a tendon graft. The two ends of that suture are placed on Keith needles, which are passed through the hole in the base of the proximal phalanx and through the ulnar cortex, where they are brought out through the skin and tied over a button. The end of the tendon graft is pulled into the medullary canal of the proximal phalanx with this pull-out suture. The remnant of the torn RCL is identified and mobilized. If a proximal stump of ligament remains on the metacarpal head, the graft is woven into the ligament remnant using parallel longitudinal incisions. If there is no usable remnant of ligament, the tendon graft is fixed to the metacarpal through two adjacent drill holes in the metacarpal head. The graft is placed through the drill holes, the free end of the graft placed parallel to the primary limbs, and the two are sutured to each other. If the RCL is torn proximally, the tendon graft is anchored to the metacarpal through the two adjacent drill holes noted previously. The distal end of the tendon graft is either woven into the distal stump of the torn ligament, or it is advanced into the medullary canal of the proximal phalanx with a pull-out suture. The abductor aponeurosis is repaired, and the skin is reapproximated. Smith did not routinely transfix the joint with a Kirschner wire. A thumb spica cast is worn for 4 weeks postoperatively. Thereafter, the thumb is protected for an additional 5 weeks in a splint.

The indication for both of these procedures is chronic symptomatic RCL laxity; patients with moderate to advanced osteoarthritis of the MP joint should be offered an arthrodesis instead. The abductor advancement procedure has the same shortcomings as the adductor advancement for UCL instability; it is a dynamic reconstruction that is used to replace a static restraint. The procedure involves ligamentous or capsular reefing, which may compensate for the dynamic component of the reconstruction. Smith's and others' techniques of RCL reconstruction with a free tendon graft address the lack of a static joint restraint by replacement with a static joint restraint; this seems intuitively more physiologic than an advancement. Neither of these techniques addresses the tendency toward pronation or volar translation, which tends to occur when the dorsal capsule and volar plate are torn in addition to the RCL.

Authors' Preferred Method of Treatment

The principles of treatment are similar to those for the UCL. Partial tears of the RCL are best treated by immobilization of the MP joint full time for 4 to 5 weeks in either a thumb cone splint, thumb spica cast, or glove spica cast. A thumb cone splint is worn the majority of the time for an additional 2 weeks during which active range of motion in flexion and extension is begun. The literature does not resolve the question of whether all complete tears of the RCL need to be repaired. Nonoperative treatment of an isolated complete tear should consist of the same immobilization program described for partial tears. Complete tears with volar subluxation of the MP joint should be repaired, because Lyons and colleagues demonstrated in a cadaver model that this finding connotes additional injury to the dorsal capsule and/or volar plate.[434]

Patients with chronic RCL instability usually present with pain, weakness, and a sensation of instability of the thumb with certain activities, particularly those that require twisting motions like unscrewing jar tops. They may benefit from a period of rest with splint immobilization and nonsteroidal anti-inflammatory medication. In some, this may diminish their symptoms to a tolerable level or temporize during their decision to proceed with surgical reconstruction.

Operative repair is indicated for acute complete lesions with symptomatic instability and/or volar subluxation. The radial side of the MP joint is exposed using a "lazy S" incision in which the proximal limb is along the dorsoradial aspect of the thumb metacarpal and the central limb extends from dorsal to volar and parallel to the joint line. The distal limb parallels the radial volar base of the proximal phalanx in the midaxial line. A longitudinal incision is made in the abductor aponeurosis just radial to the EPB. The aponeurosis is reflected volarly to expose the radial side of the joint. Ligament repair is similar to that for the ulnar ligament. Mid-substance tears are repaired with figure-of-eight or mattress sutures using a 3-0 or 4-0 braided synthetic suture. Avulsions of the ligament from the metacarpal or proximal phalanx can be fixed with a pull-out suture or bone anchor. We prefer the use of one or two anchors placed in the manner described for UCL repair. Subluxation of the proximal phalanx must be reduced and the dorsal capsule accurately repaired. If present, disruption of the insertions of the EPB and the extensor mechanism at the base of the proximal phalanx must also be repaired. In the setting of marked volar subluxation of the joint, the repair can be supplemented with a 0.045-inch Kirschner wire to transfix the joint. The thumb is immobilized for 5 weeks in a short-arm thumb spica cast.

The treatment of chronic complete ruptures is similar to that for the UCL. Unlike the UCL, the torn RCL always lies beneath the abductor aponeurosis. Consequently, it is more likely that the ends of the RCL can be mobilized and repaired in the chronic situation by using the same technique as described for acute tears. The joint should be immobilized for an additional week because healing of chronically torn ligament is not as rapid or as strong as a ligament repaired acutely. If the ruptured RCL is too fibrotic or shortened to be repaired, ligament reconstruction with a free tendon graft is our procedure of choice (Fig. 9-20). The technique of reconstruction is the mirror image of that described earlier for the ulnar side. It is sometimes more difficult to preserve the sagittal band inasmuch as the scarred ligament invariably lies immediately beneath and is often adherent to it. In that case, the sagittal band can be incised longitudinally along with the abductor aponeurosis and repaired at the end of the procedure. The gouge holes in the proximal phalanx and route of passage of the tendon are the same. The MP joint is transfixed with a 0.045-inch Kirschner wire until cast removal at 6 weeks.

Postoperative Management and Expectations
The postoperative management of acute RCL repairs and RCL reconstructions is identical to that described previously for UCL repairs and reconstructions with the single exception that the acute RCL repairs are immobilized for an additional week, beginning rehabilitation at 5 weeks postoperatively. Chronic UCL and RCL reconstructions are immobilized for 6 weeks before beginning their therapy protocol.

Postoperative expectations are also similar to those for UCL repair and reconstruction. Some patients will have a persistent prominence of the radial side of the thumb metacarpal head postoperatively. This results from fibrosis of the soft tissue in the area of the repair or reconstruction.

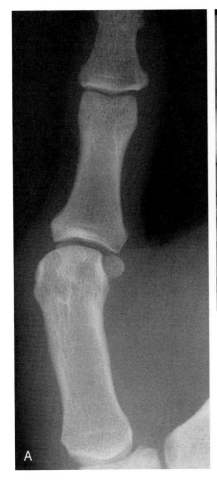

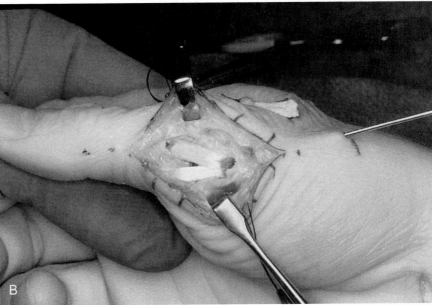

FIGURE 9-20. A, The typical radiographic appearance of chronic radial collateral ligament instability is ulnar deviation of the proximal phalanx even at rest. **B,** Chronic radial collateral instability may be reconstructed with a free tendon graft by using a mirror-image technique similar to that described for ulnar collateral ligament instability (see Fig. 9-19).

It may represent a mild degree of laxity of the ligament that, however, has not, in our experience, been a functional problem. Patients are advised that they will most likely be free of pain or have mild pain with exertion. They will regain approximately 80% of the range of motion of the MP joint on average and 90% of their pinch strength. They will be able to participate in all activities, including athletics.

Dorsal MP Dislocations

Historical Perspective

Most dislocations of the thumb MP joint are dorsal, although palmar dislocation has been reported and may be irreducible.[419,447,450] Coonrad and Goldner's series[368] included 26 dorsal and no palmar dislocations. The mechanism of dorsal dislocation is hyperextension that produces complete rupture of the volar plate and capsule and at least part of the collateral ligaments.[483] Rupture of the volar plate usually occurs proximally but can be through or distal to the sesamoid bones (Fig. 9-21). Most dorsal dislocations are reducible, although some are more complex injuries and are irreducible. McLaughlin[438] described 132 thumb MP dislocations, 22 of which were irreducible by closed measures. There have been several other reports of irreducible dislocations caused by soft tissue interposition, including the flexor pollicis longus (FPL) tendon[404,456] or, more commonly, the volar plate.[375,389] The FPL tendon more often remains within the flexor tendon sheath and displaces to the ulnar side of the metacarpal head, creating a "noose" around the metacarpal

neck together with the radially displaced thenar intrinsic musculature.[353,376,388,443,458]

Preoperative Evaluation

Diagnosis of an MP joint dislocation is generally not difficult. Clinically, the MP joint has an obvious hyperextension deformity and the metacarpal is adducted. There may be dimpling of the skin on the volar aspect of the MP joint that is suggestive of a complex dislocation.[457] Radiographs typically show the MP joint to be hyperextended with the proximal phalanx dorsal and sometimes lying in "bayonet" apposition to the metacarpal. There may be an increased space between the metacarpal head and the proximal phalanx suggestive of interposed soft tissue. Interposition of the sesamoids between the metacarpal head and the proximal phalanx is strong evidence of a complex, irreducible dislocation. Stener pointed out that fracture of the sesamoids implies that the dislocation is likely to be simple.[483]

Treatment Options

The majority of dorsal dislocations can be easily reduced without surgery. Most authors argue against the use of longitudinal traction as a reduction maneuver for concern that a simple dislocation might be converted into a complex one.[375,389,438] The preferred reduction technique is hyperextension of the MP joint with direct pressure on the dorsal base of the proximal phalanx to gently push it over the metacarpal head. This may be combined with a rocking motion of the proximal phalanx to extricate any inter-

CRITICAL POINTS: CHRONIC RCL REPAIR

INDICATIONS

- Chronic complete RCL tear
- Persistent pain despite conservative treatment

PREOPERATIVE EVALUATION

- Physical examination is usually adequate for diagnosis.
- Obtain posteroanterior, lateral, and oblique radiographs.
- Rule out degenerative disease.
- Stress radiographs or "basal joint stress view" may be helpful.

PEARLS

- Physical examination alone is usually sufficient to make the diagnosis.
- Preserve large bone bridge between gouge holes in base of proximal phalanx.

TECHNICAL POINTS

- Avoid injury to dorsal sensory branch of radial nerve.
- Incise abductor aponeurosis.
- Resect remnant of collateral ligament.
- Make gouge holes in base of proximal phalanx.
- Make gouge hole in metacarpal neck.

- Use 28-gauge stainless steel wire through gouge holes to pass graft.
- Harvest tendon graft.
- Pass tendon graft using 28-gauge wire.
- Set tension on graft.
- Tie ends of the graft in a knot and suture to adjacent periosteum.
- Repair abductor aponeurosis.
- Transfix the MP joint with 0.045-inch Kirschner wire.
- Avoid stress on repair when molding splint or cast.

PITFALLS

- Do not make reconstruction too tight or too loose.
- Avoid fracturing bony bridge.

POSTOPERATIVE CARE

- Place in short-arm thumb spica cast for 6 weeks.
- Use thermoplastic splint for 2 additional weeks.
- Begin range-of-motion exercises when cast is removed.
- Avoid forceful pinch, torsional activities and ulnarly directed stress on thumb tip for 12 weeks.

ATHLETIC PARTICIPATION

- Begin 8 to 12 weeks of protecting the joint with splint or tape for 16 weeks from surgery.

posed tissue from the joint.[375] Failure to achieve closed reduction because of interposition of the volar plate, sesamoid bones, or the FPL tendon is an indication for open reduction.[366,419,446,455] Stener emphasized the difference between dorsal dislocations with proximal versus distal rupture of the volar plate.[483] When the rupture of the volar plate is distal or through the sesamoids, both the active restraints (adductor pollicis and flexor pollicis brevis tendons) as well as the passive restraint (volar plate) to hyperextension are lost. When the rupture of the volar plate occurs proximal to the sesamoids, only passive restraint to hyperextension is lost. He favored surgical repair only in the former.

Less severe hyperextension injuries can cause dorsal subluxation of the MP joint rather than frank dislocation. This may present as a locked MP joint in which the joint cannot be flexed actively or passively.[390,487] The pathoanatomy is thought to be entrapment of the radial condyle in a tear of the radial part of the volar plate, proximal to the sesamoid.[409] Closed reduction may be attempted with wrist block anesthesia, supplemented by local joint insufflation. The examiner applies volar-directed pressure on the proximal phalanx while twisting it on the metacarpal head.[423] Closed reduction was successful in fewer than a third of the patients in one large series.[390] If closed reduction fails, open reduction may be necessary[406] and can be done through several approaches.

The surgical approach may be dorsal,[355,375] volar,[404,438,442] or lateral.[455] Dutton and Meals[375] and Bohart and colleagues[355] prefer the dorsal approach. A longitudinal skin incision exposes the extensor tendons. The interval between the EPL and EPB tendons is developed. The dorsal capsule is incised. The tissue interposed in the joint is identified and mobilized using blunt instruments such as hooks, forceps, and periosteal elevators. The tissue is pushed over the metacarpal head and the joint is reduced. McLaughlin,[438] Milford,[442] and Hughes and Freiberg[404] recommend a volar approach. The proximal phalanx is hyperextended, and the interposed soft tissue is extricated from the joint. Once reduced, the joint is usually stable but, if not, direct ligament repair or pull-out suture repair can be performed.[421,449] If the joint is stable, immobilization for 2 weeks before initiating range-of-motion exercise is believed to be adequate for most cases,[375,442,455,457] although Green and Terry[389] and McLaughlin[438] recommend immediate range of motion.

Occasionally, a dorsal MP dislocation will present as a volar laceration that necessitates débridement and extension of the volar wound. The advantage of the volar approach is that it allows the interposed structures to be pulled from between the metacarpal head and base of the proximal phalanx and affords an excellent view of all of the structures likely to be interposed, including the volar plate and sesamoids. If volar structures need to be repaired, they are easily acces-

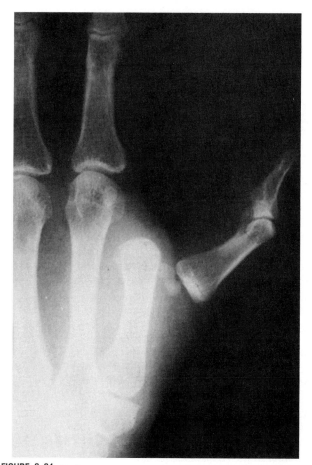

FIGURE 9-21. Radiograph of dorsal dislocation of the thumb MP joint. Sesamoid proximity to the proximal phalanx indicates that the plate remains attached distally. The metacarpal head lies herniated between the muscles that insert into these sesamoids.

sible after reduction. The advantage of the dorsal approach is that it allows the structures preventing reduction to be gently pushed over the metacarpal head, which may, in fact, be somewhat easier than pulling them from the volar side. However, once the joint is reduced the injured volar structures can no longer be visualized. For that reason, the authors prefer a volar approach.

 ## Authors' Preferred Method of Treatment

Closed reduction is usually successful if the following technique is used. Under radial and median nerve wrist block or Bier block anesthesia, distally directed pressure is applied to the base of the proximal phalanx with the metacarpal in a position of flexion and adduction. This maneuver relaxes the "noose" that the thenar muscles and FPL occasionally create around the metacarpal neck. If necessary, flexing the IP joint and the wrist will relax an entrapped FPL tendon that is blocking reduction. After reduction, collateral ligament stability is tested and a congruous reduction con-

firmed by radiographs. In the usual situation, the collateral ligaments are stable and the joint is splinted or placed in a cast in 20 degrees of flexion for 2 weeks. Flexion exercises with a 20-degree extension block splint can safely be initiated at 2 weeks. If there is significant collateral ligament instability, consideration should be given to immobilization of the MP joint for 4 weeks. Open reduction is required when closed reduction fails, particularly in late cases. The joint is exposed through a volar modified Bruner incision with its apex at the radial midaxial line. Interposed or entrapped structures are reduced with blunt instruments, avoiding injury to the metacarpal head. Once a congruous reduction has been achieved, minimal additional tissue manipulation is necessary to ensure stability. Stabilization of the joint in 25 degrees of flexion with a Kirschner wire should be done if the joint does not feel completely stable. In the rare situation in which the volar plate is detached from the base of the proximal phalanx, open surgical repair using bone anchors is recommended after closed reduction.

Postoperative Management and Expectations

Patients are advised that they will most likely have a stable joint after closed or open reduction. However, stiffness is a possible sequela of any dislocation and the chance of stiffness is greater if the joint needs to be opened. Recovery of motion can be slow and require several weeks of therapy. Patients should be counseled at the time of injury that stability is a more important consideration than full range of motion of the MP joint of the thumb. The protocol for rehabilitation is similar to that for acute collateral ligament injury of the MP joint, with a focus on avoidance of forceful extension while the volar plate is healing during the initial 6 to 8 weeks after the injury.

Chronic Volar Instability of the Thumb MP Joint

Preoperative Assessment

Chronic laxity of the thumb MP joint occurs most commonly in the context of generalized ligament laxity and is rarely symptomatic. Symptomatic laxity may be a manifestation of systemic conditions such as collagen vascular disease, congenital or acquired paralytic disorders, collapse deformity secondary to basal joint arthritis, or trauma. Post-traumatic hyperextension of the MP joint is infrequent and may be the consequence of an unrecognized or undertreated tear of the volar plate or dislocation of the MP joint. Patients with instability caused by generalized ligament laxity are able to volitionally maintain the joint in flexion during pinch and grip, whereas those with post-traumatic laxity cannot, and the resultant collapse of the joint may be painful and cause weakness.[460] If the injury is relatively recent, the patient may have tenderness, swelling, and ecchymosis of the volar aspect of the MP joint. If the injury is more than a few weeks old, the only manifestation may be painful active and passive hyperextension of the MP joint. Radiographs are usually normal but may show an avulsion fleck of bone at the site of the volar plate injury.

Types of Operations

Several techniques have been described to treat symptomatic hyperextension of the MP joint. Capsular reefing, supplemented with the volar edge of the first dorsal interosseous muscle, was proposed by Milch[441] in 1929. Kessler[420] transected the EPB proximally and reconstructed the volar plate with the distally attached segment. The graft was directed in a dorsovolar direction along the radial side of the MP joint and then passed along the volar aspect of the joint in a radioulnar direction. The tendon is then passed through a hole in the metacarpal neck from ulnar to radial and again passed across the volar aspect of the MP joint to the ulnar side, where it is sutured to the adductor tendon. This creates a static restraint to hyperextension. Eaton and Floyd[377] used a volar capsulodesis as an adjunct to basal joint arthroplasty for osteoarthritis in patients with MP hyperextension of 30 degrees or more. They incised the interval between the volar plate and the RCL. The cortex of the retrocondylar fossa is decorticated, and the volar plate is advanced proximally into this area. The authors place a bone anchor in the decorticated retrocondylar fossa and use it to fix the proximally advanced volar plate. The RCL is sutured to the volar plate and the joint transfixed with a 0.045-inch Kirschner wire for 4 weeks, after which range of motion is begun. The joint is protected in a splint for 2 more weeks. A similar technique of volar plate proximal recession has been described in which sutures are placed in both corners of the volar plate, which is advanced into a decorticated groove in the metacarpal neck. The sutures are secured by interosseous passage from the volar to the dorsal surface.[473] Tonkin[486] reported good results with sesamoid arthrodesis to the metacarpal head for 42 thumbs in 37 patients with either cerebral palsy or osteoarthritis of the CMC joint. Posner[460] used a technique somewhat analogous to the adductor advancement for UCL instability in which the abductor pollicis and flexor pollicis brevis muscles are advanced 1.5 cm distally along the radiovolar surface of the proximal phalanx where they are fixed with a pull-out suture. A procedure used by Littler has been cited[385] in which a free tendon graft provides a passive restraint to MP extension beyond neutral. Two holes are made in the volar base of the proximal phalanx on either side of the flexor tendon sheath, and a single hole in a volar-to-dorsal direction is made in the metacarpal neck. A free tendon graft is placed through the holes in the base of the proximal phalanx. Both ends of the graft are passed through the hole in the metacarpal and emerge dorsally just radial to the EPB tendon, where they are secured. The thumb is immobilized in a cast for 5 weeks, after which range of motion is begun with the joint protected for 2 more weeks in a splint.

If there has been a relatively recent hyperextension injury of the MP joint, it may be possible to reattach the volar plate to its metacarpal origin. A zigzag incision is used to expose the volar aspect of the MP joint. The volar plate is identified and mobilized. Its proximal end is minimally débrided and reattached to the volar aspect of the metacarpal neck with two bone anchors. The MP joint is immobilized in a cast for 1 month, after which range of motion with a 20-degree extension block splint is encouraged for an additional 2 weeks. The procedure is unlikely to be successful if the injury is chronic and the volar plate attenuated.

THUMB CARPOMETACARPAL JOINT

Carpometacarpal Joint Dislocations

 Anatomy

The articular surfaces of the CMC joint of the thumb resemble two reciprocally opposed saddles whose transverse axes are perpendicular.[503] The CMC joint has motion in three principal planes: flexion-extension, abduction-adduction, and pronation-supination (or opposition-retropulsion). There is an element of conjunct rotation in pronation that results from the asymmetrical height of the radial and ulnar condyles of the trapezial articulating surface.[515] These concavoconvex contours by themselves produce a degree of intrinsic stability, but the ligaments and joint capsule play the principal role in stabilization.[504,518] There are four major ligaments: volar (anterior oblique), intermetacarpal, dorsoradial, and dorsal oblique (posterior oblique). Although there is some disagreement,[497,518,519] several authors believe that the ligament that is most significant in maintaining CMC stability is the volar ligament, which passes from the trapezium to the volar beak of the thumb metacarpal (Fig. 9-22). Dorsal subluxation force is inherent with pinch and is resisted by this volar ligament.[501] The dorsal ligament is thin but is reinforced by the expanded insertion of the APL.

Historical Review

Dislocation of the CMC joint is rarely reported in the English-speaking literature.* It is particularly rare in children and adolescents.[525] All of the reported dislocations have been dorsal. It is generally believed that the mechanism of injury is axial compression on a flexed thumb metacarpal, driving the metacarpal base out dorsally.[517,523] There is some disagreement concerning which ligaments

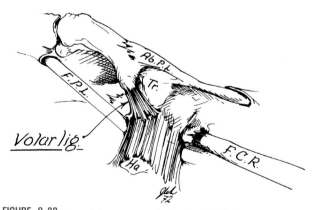

FIGURE 9-22. Essential anatomy of the thumb CMC joint. The key structure is the volar ligament, a short reflection of the transverse carpal ligament that maintains the thumb metacarpal in the biconcave contour of the trapezium. Ab.P.L., abductor pollicis longus; Tr., trapezium; F.P.L., flexor pollicis longus; F.C.R., flexor carpi radialis; Ha, hamate. (From Eaton RG, Littler JW: Joint injuries and their sequelae. Clin Plast Surg 3:85-98, 1976.)

must be injured to allow complete dislocation to occur. It has been suggested that the dorsoradial ligament has to be torn for a dorsal dislocation to occur but that the volar ligament is often sheared off of its insertion on the metacarpal base as well.[498,507,520,523,528] Shah and Patel[520] and Hooper[507] found that the dorsal ligaments were disrupted and the volar ligament was in continuity but had been stripped off the base of the metacarpal subperiosteally. Wee and associates[528] and Burkhalter[498] also found that the volar ligament was intact but stripped subperiosteally. Strauch and colleagues[523] made similar observations using a ligament-cutting cadaver model and concluded that the dorsoradial ligament had to be disrupted for a complete dislocation to occur and that the volar ligament was insufficient to resist dislocation.

Preoperative Evaluation

Injuries to the ligaments of the thumb CMC joint may be complete or partial. Complete rupture permits the thumb metacarpal to dislocate dorsally (Fig. 9-23). Partial rupture of the ligaments permits varying degrees of displacement.

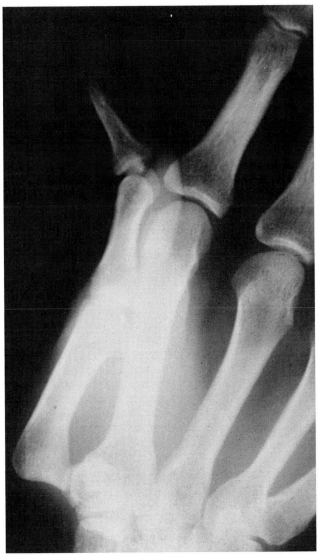

FIGURE 9-23. Dislocations of the thumb CMC joint are uncommon and are invariably dorsal and usually very unstable. The thumb is generally adducted.

The more extensive the tear, the greater the displacement and, hence, the more obvious the diagnosis. Less severe tears are particularly difficult to diagnose because the contours of the joint tend to maintain gross alignment of the metacarpal in the concavity of the trapezium. There may be minimal detectable dorsal translation of the metacarpal on clinical and radiographic examination. The difference between normal mobility and hypermobility is difficult to measure because these structures are at least partially enclosed within the thenar muscles.

Standard posteroanterior and true lateral radiographs must be taken to rule out existing joint pathology and the relatively more frequent Bennett fracture-dislocation. Widening of the joint space or a slight dorsoradial shift of the metacarpal may be apparent on these routine radiographs. A useful diagnostic technique is the stress radiograph, which is a posteroanterior view of both thumbs positioned parallel to the x-ray plate with the distal phalanges pressed firmly together along their radial borders. This tends to lever the base of the metacarpal laterally, and in the presence of a capsular tear or laxity, radial shift of the metacarpal on the trapezium will occur. Because both thumbs are included on the film, a comparison with the uninjured joint is possible.[502,504]

Treatment

Because acute complete dislocations are quite rare and partial tears of the CMC joint are rarely recognized, the relevant literature is composed largely of case reports with few specific recommendations about the management of these injuries.[498,499,509,527] Shah and Patel[520] treated three patients with open reduction and Kirschner wire internal fixation and one with closed reduction and Kirschner wire fixation. Watt and Hooper[527] treated nine patients with closed reduction and cast immobilization and three with closed reduction and percutaneous Kirschner wire fixation. Three in the first group and one in the second had persistent instability. Simonian and Trumble[521] reported persistent instability in four of eight patients after closed reduction and percutaneous Kirschner wire fixation of acute CMC dislocations and significantly better results with early ligament reconstruction. There have been several reports of various techniques of ligament reconstruction for persistent or recurrent instability after an acute injury.[497,500,501,505,512,513] The only ones that are used commonly are those described by Eaton and Littler[501,502,504,506,513] and Brunelli and associates.[497]

Authors' Preferred Method of Treatment

Patients with acute post-traumatic pain in the CMC joint of the thumb but without gross clinical instability or radiographic subluxation should be considered to have a partial volar ligament tear and immobilized in a long opponens or thumb spica splint with the metacarpal in palmar abduction-extension for 4 to 6 weeks. The thumb should be positioned to prevent its tip from opposing the digits, which would create axial compression along the thumb ray.

Patients with a documented dislocation or with clinical instability and radiographic subluxation require special consideration. If postreduction radiographs show the metacarpal to be well reduced initially and at 5 to 7 days thereafter, cast immobilization may be adequate treatment. However, if the metacarpal is not well seated radiographically or is clinically loose or "sloppy," surgical reduction is indicated. In light of the study by Simonian and Trumble,[521] the indications for closed reduction and percutaneous Kirschner wire fixation of the CMC joint should be narrow. A possible exception might be in a patient in whom secondary reduction in the operating room resulted in a stable joint, suggesting that interposed soft tissue was extricated by manipulation. The joint may then be transfixed with a percutaneous 0.045-inch Kirschner wire down the medullary canal or obliquely across the base of the metacarpal. When the pin is driven across the joint, the metacarpal should be held in abduction and extension as the joint is held manually reduced. Pressure at its dorsoradial base seats the metacarpal and approximates the metacarpal beak to the volar ligament, to encourage ligament healing. If the metacarpal will not reduce congruously but remains dorsally or laterally translated, or if the joint continues to feel grossly unstable, it must be assumed that soft tissue is interposed or that a small, undetected bony or chondral fragment is preventing reduction. Open reduction is indicated, and the volar ligament is reconstructed with a tendon graft.

Technique of Volar Ligament Reconstruction of the Thumb CMC Joint

The CMC joint of the thumb is exposed through a modified Wagner volar approach that curves ulnarly into the distal wrist flexion crease.[502,504,514,526] Care is taken to avoid injury to the palmar cutaneous branch of the median nerve, the superficial radial artery, as well as branches of the lateral antebrachial cutaneous and radial nerves. The thenar muscles are elevated extraperiosteally. The intact volar and radial capsule is incised, and any interposed tissue is removed from the joint. The FCR tendon is identified at the wrist flexion crease and unroofed distally as far as the midportion of the trapezium.

Reconstruction of the volar ligament is begun by first creating a channel in the base of the metacarpal in a sagittal plane perpendicular to the thumbnail. A small incision is made in the dorsal periosteum through which a hole is made in the metacarpal base and enlarged with progressively larger hand-held gouges. It emerges just distal to the volar beak, at the site of the volar ligament insertion. A 28-gauge stainless steel wire is placed through this channel for subsequent passage of the tendon graft used for ligament reconstruction (Fig. 9-24).

The radial half of the FCR is then mobilized beginning 6 to 8 cm proximal to the wrist and continuing distally via a series of short transverse incisions over the tendon to emerge at the level of the trapezium (Fig. 9-25). Alternatively, a looped monofilament suture or an arthroscopic suture passer can be passed from the incision at the wrist crease, beneath the skin bridge, to emerge through a proximal forearm incision and thereby avoid the need for multiple incisions on the forearm. The loop of the suture or the suture passer is placed through a split in the FCR tendon and firmly pulled distally into the distal wound to continue the split longitudinally. The distal end remains in continuity with the index metacarpal insertion, and the transected proximal end is passed through the channel in the volar base of the metacarpal to emerge dorsally. The metacarpal is held reduced under direct vision as the tendon is drawn tight to remove any kinks along its passage, and then traction is relaxed slightly to keep the reconstruction from being too tight. The tendon is sutured to the dorsal periosteum to set proper tension in the new ligament, and its free end is passed deep to the insertion of the APL on the metacarpal base. It is sutured at this point to reinforce the dorsal capsule. The free end is further passed volarly around the intact FCR tendon and finally reflected

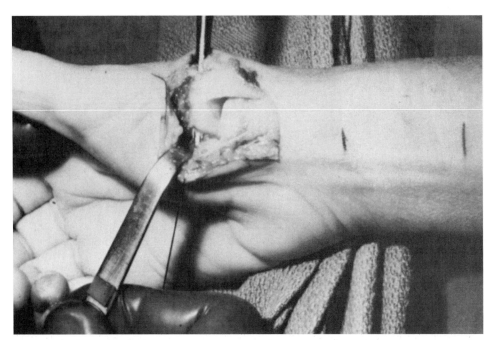

FIGURE 9-24. Reconstruction of the volar ligament of the thumb CMC joint. A midsagittal channel is gouged from the dorsum to the volar beak of the metacarpal. A wire is threaded through this channel for subsequent passage of a tendon strip. (From Eaton RG, Littler JW: Ligament reconstruction for the painful thumb carpometacarpal joint. J Bone Joint Surg Am 55:1655-1666, 1973.)

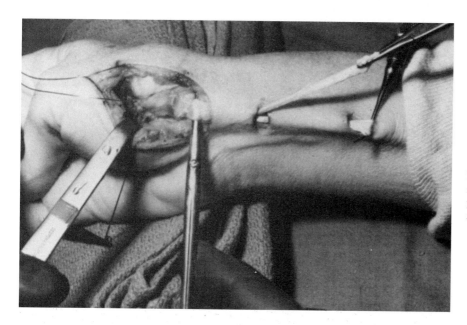

FIGURE 9-25. A distally based strip of flexor carpi radialis tendon is separated to the level of the trapezium, where it is then passed from the volar to the dorsal surface to create a new volar ligament. (From Eaton RG, Littler JW: Ligament reconstruction for the painful thumb carpometacarpal joint. J Bone Joint Surg Am 55:1655-1666, 1973.)

distally across the radial aspect of the joint, where it is sutured to a remnant of the capsule (Fig. 9-26). Kirschner wire fixation of the trapeziometacarpal joint is optional. It is important that the new volar ligament not be sutured with excessive tension, which may restrict joint motion, particularly rotation. The thenar muscles are reattached. Immobilization is continued for 4 weeks, at which time the cast and Kirschner wire are removed and gentle progressive motion is begun.

Postoperative Management and Expectations

Patients are advised that volar ligament reconstruction predictably stabilizes the unstable basal joint, whether due to dislocation, subluxation, or stage 1 symptomatic atraumatic laxity of the basal joint. The vast majority of patients who have undergone CMC ligament reconstruction are either pain free or have mild, intermittent pain postoperatively. It is very unlikely for laxity or pain to recur in the short and intermediate term, and patients should have essentially full function of their thumb and hand and be able to participate in all activities including athletics. However, dislocation of the thumb CMC joint represents a significant injury not only to the ligaments but to the articular cartilage as well and raises the possibility of long-term degenerative arthritis.

Postoperative mild limitation in range of motion of the basal joint is not uncommon, including the possibility the patient will not be able to fully flatten the palm on a countertop. This can usually be avoided by ensuring that the reconstruction is not overly tightened.

During the 4 weeks of immobilization after volar ligament reconstruction, patients are encouraged to move the digits and thumb IP joint within the limits of the cast. The cast and Kirschner wire are removed after 4 weeks, and patients are referred to a hand therapist. A custom-molded thermoplastic long opponens splint is worn for 2 weeks and removed for range-of-motion exercises. Patients are encouraged to oppose the tip of the thumb to the index and long fingers during the first 2 weeks. In the ensuing 2 weeks (beginning at 6 weeks' postoperatively), they oppose the tip of the thumb to the ring and small fingers. Strengthening of the thenar musculature begins 2 months postoperatively and strengthening of pinch and grasp at 10 to 12 weeks postoperatively. It is important that the therapist not be overly aggressive with strengthening during the first 2 months postoperatively, because this may contribute to the reconstruction "stretching out." Patients are allowed essentially full use of the thumb at 3 months.

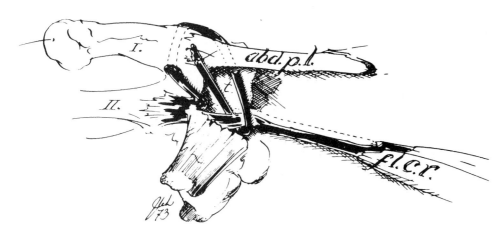

FIGURE 9-26. Schema for routing of the flexor carpi radialis (fl.c.r.) tendon in reconstruction of the volar ligament of the CMC joint of the thumb. The volar, dorsal, and radial capsules are reinforced by this routing. abd.p.l., abductor pollicis longus. (From Eaton RG, Littler JW: Ligament reconstruction for the painful thumb carpometacarpal joint. J Bone Joint Surg Am 55:1655-1666, 1973.)

CRITICAL POINTS: VOLAR LIGAMENT RECONSTRUCTION

INDICATIONS

- Acute, irreducible dislocation of the thumb CMC joint
- Redislocation of the CMC joint after reduction
- Subacute or chronic post-traumatic instability of CMC joint
- Chronic symptomatic atraumatic laxity of CMC joint
- Persistent pain despite conservative treatment

PREOPERATIVE EVALUATION

- Dorsal prominence of thumb metacarpal base is evident on physical examination.
- Obtain posteroanterior, lateral, and oblique radiographs.

PEARLS

- Inspect CMC joint for chondral fractures or interposed soft tissue in post-traumatic instability.
- Do not make gouge hole too distal to metacarpal base.
- FCR spirals through its course, to end radially started division of tendon ulnarly.
- Pull tightly on FCR but then relax 2 to 3 mm to set tension.

TECHNICAL POINTS

- Use modified Wagner incision.
- Avoid injury to branch of dorsal sensory branch of radial nerve.
- Elevate thenar musculature extraperiosteally.
- Inspect CMC joint through transverse arthrotomy.
- Make dorsovolar hole in metacarpal base perpendicular to the plane of the thumbnail.
- Place 28-gauge stainless steel wire through hole for later passage of tendon graft.

- Harvest distally based slip of FCR tendon.
- Tie volar end of 28-gauge wire to proximal end of FCR tendon slip.
- Pull tendon through hole from volar to dorsal.
- Position thumb in abduction and extension.
- Set tension on FCR graft.
- Suture graft to periosteum adjacent to dorsal hole with 3-0 Ethibond.
- Place free end of graft beneath APL to which it is sutured.
- Loop graft around the intact FCR and then back dorsally.
- Reattach thenar musculature.

PITFALLS

- Do not make reconstruction too tight.
- Create gouge hole at isometric point to avoid limitation of motion.

POSTOPERATIVE CARE

- Place in short-arm thumb spica cast for 4 weeks.
- Use a thermoplastic long opponens splint for 2 additional weeks.
- Begin range-of-motion exercises when cast is removed.
- Begin gentle strengthening at 8 weeks.
- Avoid strenuous pinch and torsional motions for 3 months.

ATHLETIC PARTICIPATION

- Begin sports at 12 weeks protecting the CMC with splint or tape for 16 weeks from surgery.

It is not uncommon for patients to have some numbness on the dorsal radial aspect of the thumb after volar ligament reconstruction. Most often it is due to traction on the branch of the dorsal sensory branch of the radial nerve that crosses the operative field. This complication can be avoided by being particularly attentive to identification and gentle retraction of the nerve(s) throughout the procedure. Heavy clamps attached to vessel loops around the nerve should be avoided. Occasionally, the nerve can become entrapped in scar tissue at the site of the fixation of the FCR tendon slip to the periosteum of the thumb metacarpal base. Neurapraxia due to traction almost invariably resolves completely over the course of weeks to months. Rarely, entrapment of the nerve in scar may require neurolysis and transposition of the nerve away from the previous point of fixation.

ANNOTATED REFERENCES

PIP Joints

4. Agee JM: Unstable fracture dislocations of the proximal interphalangeal joint: Treatment with the force couple splint. Clin Orthop 214:101-112, 1987.

    The author describes the use and surgical technique of a force couple splint to treat PIP joint fracture-dislocation in 16 patients. The force couple allows for early active PIP joint motion while maintaining a concentric joint. Nine patients were treated acutely whereas seven were treated late (average, 7 weeks). Follow-up averaged 21 months. The total active PIP joint motion in the acute group was 95 degrees, and it was 68 degrees in the late treated group. Three patients had recurrent subluxations.

8. Bilos ZJ, Vender MI, Bonavolonta M, Knutson K: Fracture subluxation of proximal interphalangeal treated by pal-

mar plate advancement. J Hand Surg [Am] 19:189-196, 1994.

The authors describe use of a modified volar plate arthroplasty technique to treat 11 patients with fracture subluxation of the PIP joint. Their two modifications to the original technique included using two sutures to attach the volar plate (one at each lateral edge) and tying the suture beneath the skin. Reduction was maintained in all patients and no infections developed.

17a. Deitch MA, Kiefhaber TR, Comisar BR, Stern PJ: Dorsal fracture-dislocation of the proximal interphalangeal joint: Surgical complications and long-term results. J Hand Surg [Am] 24:914-923, 1994.

Retrospective study evaluating treatment of 56 acute PIP joint fracture-dislocations with volar plate arthroplasty (23 patients) or open reduction and internal fixation (33 patients). Twenty-four patients returned for follow-up evaluation; 83% of the patients had little or no pain despite radiographic evidence of degenerative changes in 96% of the patients. In six cases, redislocation occurred (3 patients in each group), and in each case, the middle phalanx fracture involved more than 50% of the articular surface.

22. Durham-Smith G, McCarten GM: Volar plate arthroplasty for closed proximal interphalangeal joint injuries. J Hand Surg [Br] 17:422-428, 1992.

The authors present results of 71 cases of volar plate arthroplasty performed over a 5-year period to treat fracture-subluxation of the PIP joint. An important technical difference from the originally described technique is tying the suture beneath the extensor mechanism, directly on the dorsum of the middle phalanx. Eighty-seven percent of patients achieved a stable, pain-free PIP joint with an average arc of motion of 5 to 95 degrees.

26. Eaton RG, Malerich MM: Volar plate arthroplasty of the proximal interphalangeal joint: A review of ten years' experience. J Hand Surg [Am] 5:260-268, 1980.

Ten-year follow-up of seven patients who were treated within 6 weeks of injury (average, 7 days) and 17 patients who were treated at greater than 6 weeks (average, 7 months) after the injury with volar plate arthroplasty. At an average follow-up of approximately 3 years, the final arc of PIP joint motion was 95 degrees for the acutely treated patients and 78 degrees for the late treated group. Radiographs taken at follow-up demonstrated marked remodeling of the volar articular portion of the middle phalanx.

59. Krakauer JD, Stern PJ: Hinged device for fractures involving the proximal interphalangeal joint. Clin Orthop 237:29-37, 1996.

Evaluated the use of a Compass PIP Hinge, a dynamic external fixation device, combined with a variety of more standard treatment modalities in the treatment of PIP joint fractures or fracture-dislocations. Twelve patients were treated within 2 weeks of the injury, and an additional eight patients were treated more than 4 weeks after the injury. The average arc of PIP joint motion for the acutely treated patients was 9 to 82 degrees whereas the arc was 21 to 77 degrees for the late-treated group. One patient from the late-treated group required a PIP joint silicone arthroplasty due to painful degenerative arthritis.

87. Peimer CA, Sullivan DJ, Wild DR: Palmar dislocation of the proximal interphalangeal joint. J Hand Surg [Am] 9:39-48, 1982.

Retrospective review of 15 patients with PIP joint palmar dislocations at an average follow-up of 17 months. In all cases, disruption of the central slip, palmar plate, and one collateral ligament had occurred. Importantly, the delay from injury to referral averaged more than 11 weeks. Although joint stability was restored in all patients, a full range of motion was not recovered in any case.

96. Rosenstadt BE, Glickel SZ, Lane LB, Kaplan SJ: Palmar fracture-dislocation of the proximal interphalangeal joint. J Hand Surg [Am] 23:811-820, 1998.

Nine patients with this unusual injury were treated acutely with either closed (seven patients) or open reduction (two patients) and internal fixation. Four patients whose injury was at least 1 month old were treated with open reduction and internal fixation with additional repair of the central slip in two patients. At a mean follow-up of 55 months, the average arc of PIP joint motion was 91 degrees for the acutely treated group and 70 degrees for the chronically treated group.

97. Schenck RR: Dynamic traction and early passive movement for fractures of the proximal interphalangeal joint. J Hand Surg [Am] 11:850-858, 1986.

Review of 10 patients with comminuted intra-articular fractures of the proximal interphalangeal joint treated with a new technique of dynamic, distal traction and early mobilization. Follow-up at an average of 16 months revealed an average arc of motion of 87 degrees and no radiographic evidence of degenerative changes was present.

106a. Stern PJ, Roman RJ, Kiefhaber TR, McDonough JJ: Pilon fractures of the proximal interphalangeal joint. J Hand Surg [Am] 16:844-850, 1991.

The results of 20 patients with PIP joint pilon fractures treated with either splinting (4 patients), skeletal traction (7 patients), or open reduction (9 patients) are presented. Clinical and radiographic follow-up averaged 25 months. Anatomic restoration of the articular surface was not restored in any joint, regardless of technique, and no patient regained full motion at either IP joint. The authors state that treatment with immobilization is "undesirable."

Thumb MP Joint

363. Camp RA, Weatherwax RJ, Miller EB: Chronic post-traumatic radial instability of the thumb metacarpophalangeal joint. J Hand Surg [Am] 5:221-225, 1980.

Retrospective review of 26 patients with thumb instability over a 3-year period. It was determined that RCL injuries constituted 35% (9 patients) of the total. In all 9 patients who were identified, surgical treatment included RCL repair, distal advancement of the abductor pollicis brevis tendon, and repair of the abductor aponeurosis. Functional and clinical stability was restored in all patients.

364. Campbell CS: Gamekeeper's thumb. J Bone Joint Surg Br 37:148-149, 1955.

Classic original description of the development of chronic thumb MP joint ulnar collateral ligament insufficiency in gamekeepers. The mechanism of injury is described as repetitive ulnar-opening forces at the MP joint produced while fracturing the necks of rabbits with their thumbs.

374. Durham JW, Khuri S, Kim MH: Acute and late radial collateral ligament injuries of the thumb metacarpophalangeal joint. J Hand Surg [Am] 18:232-237, 1993.

Eighteen cases of RCL instability (6 treated acutely, 12 treated late) were treated surgically. The late repairs were treated with abductor advancement, capsular imbrication, free tendon graft reconstruction, or a combination thereof. At mean follow-up of 6 years, the authors found an overall 94% satisfaction rate with no difference in satisfaction between groups. The sole difference was "slightly more" motion loss in the late group.

375. Dutton RO, Meals RA: Complex dorsal dislocation of the thumb metacarpophalangeal joint. Clin Orthop 164:160-164, 1982.

Case report of a complex dorsal thumb MP joint dorsal dislocation with surgical exploration revealing an interposed volar plate (and sesamoids) within the MP joint. The volar plate had ruptured proximally from the metacarpal neck and the joint reduced immediately after the volar plate was withdrawn. A comprehensive review of the literature is also included.

387. Glickel SZ, Malerich M, Pearce SM, Littler JW: Ligament replacement for chronic instability of the ulnar collateral ligament of the metacarpophalangeal joint of the thumb. J Hand Surg [Am] 18:930-941, 1993.

Retrospective review of 26 patients followed for an average of 4.5 years who were treated with ligament reconstruction using a free tendon graft. The graft is placed through two gouge tracks in the proximal phalanx and one in the metacarpal in an attempt to replicate normal anatomy. Results were excellent in 20 patients, good in 4, and fair in 2.

398. Heyman P, Gelberman RH, Duncan K, Hipp JA: Injuries of the ulnar collateral ligament of the thumb metacarpophalangeal joint: Biomechanical and prospective clinical studies on the usefulness of valgus stress testing. Clin Orthop 292:165-171, 1993.

In the anatomic portion of the study, the authors demonstrated that only with division of both the proper collateral ligament and accessory collateral ligament/palmar plate was the MP joint unstable in full extension. In the clinical study, valgus instability of greater than 35 degrees in extension indicated tears of both the proper and accessory collateral ligaments. The authors recommended surgery if this criterion was met and found a Stener lesion was present in 15 of 17 such cases.

438. McLaughlin HL: Complex "locked" dislocation of the metacarpophalangeal joints. J Trauma 5:683-688, 1965.

The author reports on his 35-year experience of 160 MP joint dislocations, 132 of which involved the thumb MP joint. Twenty-two of these were "locked" and required open reduction. The author emphasizes that traction on the dislocated digit can convert a simple lesion into a complex dislocation requiring open treatment.

452. Neviaser RJ, Wilson JN, Lievano A: Rupture of the ulnar collateral ligament of the thumb (gamekeeper's thumb): Correction by a dynamic repair. J Bone Joint Surg Am 53:1357-1364, 1971.

Original description of capsulorrhaphy and adductor advancement for the treatment of chronic UCL instability. The authors treated eight patients in this manner and, at 1-year follow-up, six patients had stable, painless, mobile thumbs. One patient had persistent pain and the other had "partial recurrence of instability."

481. Stener B: Displacement of the ruptured ulnar collateral ligament of the metacarpophalangeal joint of the thumb: A clinical and anatomical study. J Bone Joint Surg Br 44:869-879, 1962.

Classic, original description of the pathoanatomy of the Stener lesion including several illustrative cases. Ligament displacement with adductor aponeurosis interposition was found in 25 of 39 consecutive cases.

Thumb CMC Joint

504. Eaton RG, Littler JW: Ligament reconstruction for the painful thumb carpometacarpal joint. J Bone Joint Surg Am 55:1655-1666, 1973.

Eighteen patients treated with a volar ligament reconstruction were reviewed. The manuscript includes the original description of the surgical technique and a grading system based on plain radiographs for CMC joint arthrosis. The authors demonstrated that the surgical results were directly related to the extent of degenerative changes at the CMC joint, with improved results found in patients with minimal articular degeneration.

527. Watt N, Hooper G: Dislocation of the trapeziometacarpal joint. J Hand Surg [Br] 12:242-245, 1987.

Review of 12 patients over a 10-year period who sustained an acute, traumatic trapeziometacarpal joint dislocation. The authors emphasize that the stability of the CMC joint should be assessed after closed reduction of a dislocation. If instability exists, they recommend supplemental Kirschner wire fixation across the CMC joint. Long-term instability and pain was noted in 5 of the 12 patients, all of whom presented at least the day after the injury.

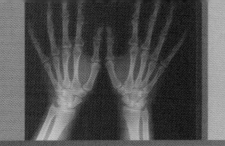

CHAPTER 10

The Perionychium

Nicole Z. Sommer and Richard E. Brown

The fingernail serves many functions that are taken for granted in everyday use of the hand, such as scratching. However, the nail also protects the fingertip, helps in regulation of peripheral circulation, and contributes to tactile sensation that assists us in picking up small objects. An abnormal nail is thus both a functional and a cosmetic problem. Unfortunately, because of the prominence of the nail on the tip of the finger, the perionychium is the most frequently injured part of the hand.

Anatomy

The anatomic landmarks of the nail are shown in Figure 10-1. The perionychium includes the nail bed, nail fold, eponychium, paronychium, and hyponychium. The nail bed, the soft tissue beneath the nail, includes the germinal matrix proximally and the sterile matrix distally. The nail fold, the most proximal extent of the perionychium, consists of a dorsal roof and a ventral floor. The ventral floor is the germinal matrix portion of the nail bed. Paronychium and hyponychium describe the skin on each side of the nail and the skin distal to the nail bed, respectively. The eponychium is the skin proximal to the nail that covers the nail fold. Extending distally from the eponychium onto the nail is the nail vest or cuticle. The white arc of the nail just distal to the eponychium, known as the lunula, is the distal extent of the germinal matrix.

The germinal matrix produces about 90% of the nail,[61] an important point in reconstruction of the nail bed. The sterile matrix adds a thin layer of cells to the undersurface of the nail, thereby keeping the nail adherent to the nail bed.[11,28,50] Injury of the germinal matrix leads to nail absence, whereas injury to the sterile matrix leads to nail deformity. The dorsal roof of the nail fold produces the shine on the nail.

The blood supply of the perionychium comes from the terminal branches of the radial and ulnar volar digital arteries that course longitudinally as well as from capillary loops (Fig. 10-2).[45] The veins drain into the proximal nail bed and nail fold, then course randomly over the dorsum of the finger.[68,102] Sensation to the nail bed is supplied by dorsal branches of the volar radial and ulnar digital nerves as well as the most distal extent of the dorsal radial digital nerve branches.[93]

The numerous lymphatics of the nail bed roughly parallel the veins. The hyponychium contains the greatest density of lymphatics of any dermal area in the body,[87] which aids in deterring infection in this frequently exposed area.[98]

PREOPERATIVE EVALUATION

Evaluation of the perionychium usually begins in the office or emergency department with the patient history. Evaluation of an injured perionychium includes assessment for associated injuries. We recommend a radiograph of the involved finger because of the 50% chance of bone involvement with a nail bed injury.

Doors are the most common source of trauma to the perionychium, followed by smashing the finger between two objects and lacerations from yard or workshop tools. Patients are most often older children or young adults. The long finger is most frequently injured because of its increased exposure distal to the other digits. Similarly, the most distal part of the nail bed is the most frequently injured part of the perionychium, and often the hyponychium is involved as well.

The majority of nail bed trauma falls into the classification of simple lacerations, stellate lacerations, severe crush, or avulsions (Fig. 10-3).[42,101] These injuries occur in this same order of frequency. A fifth category of injury is the subungual hematoma. Because of the inability to see the extent of the nail bed laceration, subungual hematomas can be the most challenging injury to treat.

TYPES OF OPERATIONS

Subungual Hematoma

Compression of the nail onto the underlying distal phalanx can lead to a laceration in the nail bed and bleeding beneath the nail, known as a subungual hematoma. If the nail is intact, the pressure of the blood within this confined space frequently causes severe throbbing pain, and evacuation of the hematoma is indicated.

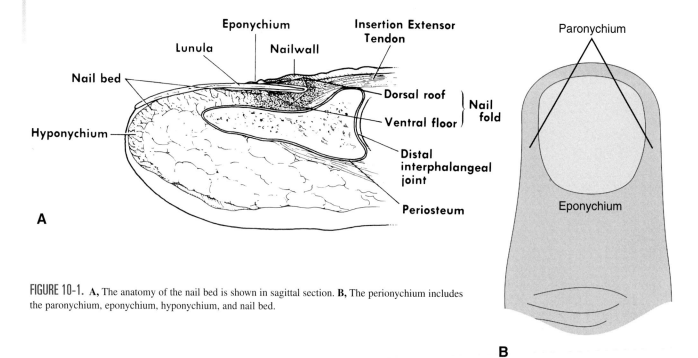

FIGURE 10-1. **A,** The anatomy of the nail bed is shown in sagittal section. **B,** The perionychium includes the paronychium, eponychium, hyponychium, and nail bed.

Before evacuation of the hematoma, the finger should be surgically prepped. This is essential to decrease the chance of bacterial inoculation of the subungual space on trephination of the nail. We prefer a povidone-iodine (Betadine) soap scrub. Trephination of the nail has been performed with drills, needles, and paperclips heated in a Bunsen burner until red hot. We prefer the battery-powered microcautery unit available in most emergency departments (Fig. 10-4). The heated tip is passed through the nail and is cooled by the hematoma, thus avoiding injury to the nail bed. The hole must be large enough to allow continued drainage or the hematoma will recur once a clot seals the hole.

In the past, we recommended removal of the nail and repair of the nail bed if greater than 25% to 50% of the nail was undermined by blood.[91,100] However, a prospective 2-year study of 48 patients with hematomas showed no complications of nail deformity with drainage only, regardless of hematoma size or the presence of a distal phalangeal fracture.[82] Our cutoff for nail removal and repair subsequently became greater than 50%. At the present time, decision for removal of the nail is based primarily on evaluation of the nail edges rather than the percent of hematoma. In general, if the nail edges are intact, we recommend drainage only. If the nail is broken or the edges disrupted,

FIGURE 10-2. The *small arrowhead* shows the common volar digital artery, the *medium-sized arrowhead* indicates the dorsal branch to the nail fold, and the *large arrowhead* points to the artery that progresses along the perionychium and sends branches to the nail bed. The terminal branch to the pad of the finger is not shown. (From Zook EG, Van Beek AL, Russell RC, Beatty ME: Anatomy and physiology of the perionychium: A review of the literature and anatomic study. J Hand Surg [Am] 5:528-536, 1980, with permission.)

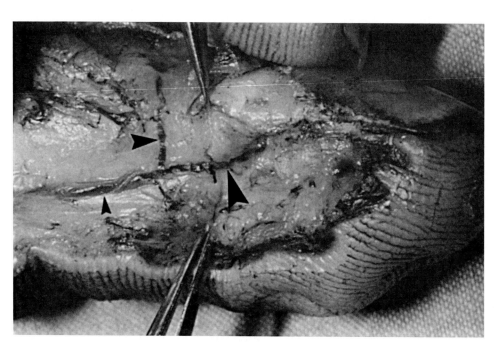

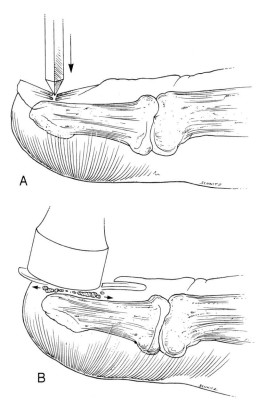

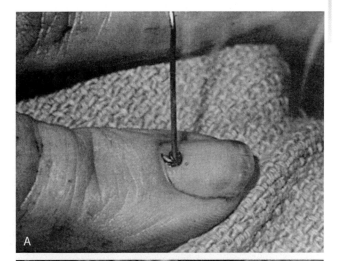

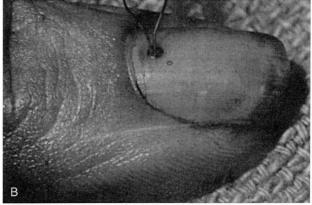

FIGURE 10-3. **A,** A relatively sharp object compressing the nail between the nail and bone causes a splitting laceration (simple). **B,** A wider area of compression of the nail bed between the nail and the bone causes an exploding-type injury that results in multiple fragments (stellate or crush).

we recommend removal of the nail with exploration and repair of the nail bed.

Nail Bed Repair

This discussion on nail bed repair will include the various points pertinent for treatment of simple lacerations, crush injuries, and avulsion injuries.

A finger block is performed with 1% plain lidocaine. The finger and often the entire hand is surgically prepped and draped. After exsanguination, a finger tourniquet is placed around the proximal phalanx to allow for hemostasis and adequate visualization of the nail bed. The nail is removed with a periosteal elevator or iris scissors. The scissors are inserted beneath the free edge of the nail and gently opened and closed working them proximally. If curved scissors are used, the tips are pointed superficially toward the nail to avoid injury to the nail bed. Caution must be used with an elevator because blunt force can tear the nail bed. We recommend a Kutz elevator because it is smaller than the Freer elevator and does less damage to the nail bed. The nail is cleaned by scraping the undersurface to remove the residual fibrinous tissue and soaked in povidone-iodine during the repair of the nail bed laceration.

The nail bed is examined under loupe magnification. Irregularities of the edges are trimmed if it is possible to do so without compromising the repair. However, débridement must remain conservative. The nail bed is adherent to the distal phalanx and difficult to mobilize. Undermining the edges approximately 1 mm allows for slight eversion but

FIGURE 10-4. **A,** A time-honored method of burning a hole through the nail is with a heated paperclip. **B,** The authors' preferred method of burning a hole through the nail is with an ophthalmic battery-powered cautery.

minimal to no mobilization. It is better to leave contused edges in place if there is doubt of closure rather than to leave a defect because of aggressive débridement. The wound is copiously irrigated with normal saline. The nail bed is repaired with a 7-0 chromic suture on a micro-point spatula, double-arm, GS-9 ophthalmic needle (Ethicon). The curve of this needle allows easier passage through the nail bed, which is adherent to the periosteum. The double needle provides a spare in case one is bent or broken. Simple nonburied sutures are placed.

With stellate lacerations and especially with crush injuries, the nail is often fragmented. Therefore, the nail is removed very cautiously to avoid injury to the small segments of adherent nail bed. With meticulous approximation of the multiple segments, stellate lacerations have a surprisingly good outcome (Fig. 10-5). Crush injuries have a poorer prognosis likely because of the presence of greater contusion along with the complicated laceration.

After repair of simple or complex lacerations or placement of a graft, the nail bed must be protected. The best option is the native nail if this is available. The nail also acts as a perfect mold for the repaired nail bed.[80] The nail is removed from the povidone-iodine soak and irrigated with normal saline. A hole is then cut in the nail with a pair of fine scissors or burned with a battery-operated cautery to allow drainage of serum or hematoma from the subungual

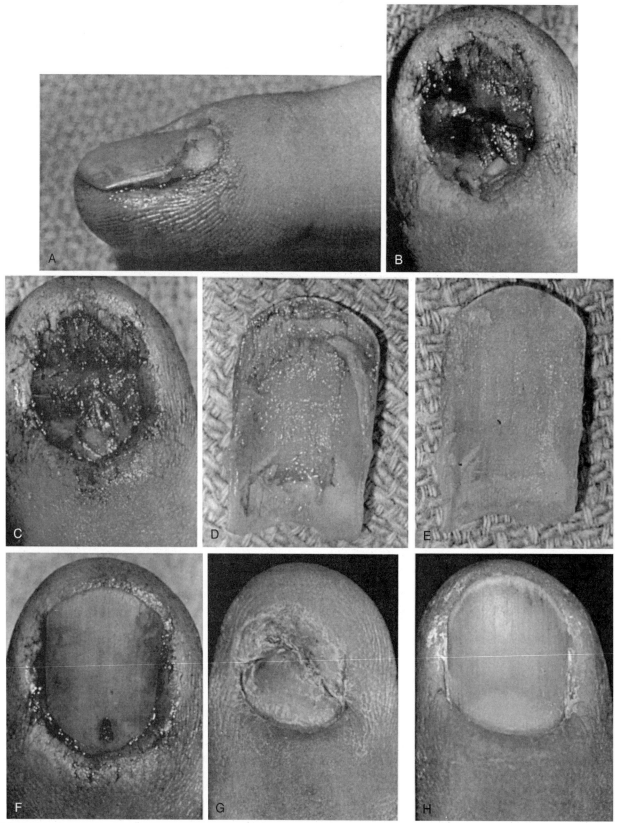

FIGURE 10-5. A, Avulsion of the proximal end of the nail from the nail fold. **B,** A stellate laceration of the nail bed is visible only after the nail has been removed. **C,** The lacerations are approximated as accurately as possible with fine 7-0 chromic sutures under magnification. **D,** The undersurface of the nail after it has been removed from the nail bed shows the residual soft tissue that is usually present. **E,** The undersurface of the nail after it has been cleaned and soaked. **F,** A hole large enough to allow drainage has been burned through the nail, and the nail has been inserted back into the nail fold. **G,** The nail 2 months after the injury. **H,** The nail 1 year after injury. (From Zook EG: The perionychium: Anatomy, physiology and care of injuries. Clin Plast Surg 8:21-31, 1981, with permission.)

space. We prefer to place the hole away from the repair when possible. The nail is secured in place with a 5-0 nylon mattress suture through the nail and nail fold or a simple suture through the edge of the nail and hyponychium. The nail prevents scar formation between the ventral and dorsal surface of the nail fold. The nail stiffness prevents it from flipping out of the nail fold when the hyponychium suture is used. Dermal adhesives[43,88] have been advocated for nail adhesion, but we have no experience with this technique. If the nail is not available or is too badly damaged, a nail-shaped piece of 0.020-inch reinforced silicone sheeting may be substituted. Silicone is less stiff and therefore requires a nail fold suture to hold it in place beneath the nail fold (Fig. 10-6). We believe that the silicone is able to mold the edges of the repair more accurately than firmer prosthetic materials recommended by Ogunro.[72] If neither nail nor silicone is available, a single thickness of nail-shaped nonadherent gauze may be placed in the nail fold.

The finger is wrapped in nonadhesive gauze and small gauze bandages and wrapped with a small gauze roll. We recommend a four-prong or volar aluminum splint for protection of the repair and reduction of pain. The splint is worn for 2 to 3 weeks, or longer if a fracture is present. Immobilization of the distal interphalangeal (DIP) joint is only necessary if a significant distal phalanx fracture is present. Patients are instructed to keep the finger and dressing dry until follow up and to keep the hand elevated. If a graft is taken, the donor site is treated in a similar fashion with replacement and stabilization of the nail and a protective dressing.

Avulsion

Nail bed avulsion often leaves a fragment of nail bed attached to the undersurface of the avulsed nail and often involves most of the nail bed. An avulsion commonly presents as laceration of the nail bed within the nail fold with the nail bed attached distally. In a child, avulsion of the nail bed out of the nail fold suggests a Salter I fracture. Radiographic evaluation, especially in the lateral view, is recommended.

Adequate visualization and repair requires an incision in the eponychium. The incision is made perpendicular to the lateral curved portion of the eponychial fold and may be necessary on both sides (Fig. 10-7). The nail bed is repaired under direct visualization, and the eponychial incisions are closed with 6-0 nylon.

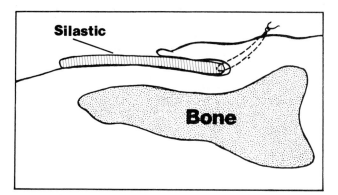

FIGURE 10-6. A horizontal mattress suture through the nail wall is used to hold a silicone sheet in the nail fold.

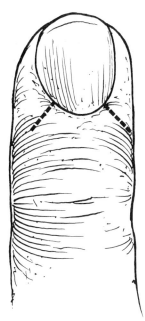

FIGURE 10-7. When incisions are made in the eponychium, they should be made at 90-degree angles from the eponychium to prevent deformity.

An attempt should be made to find the nail if it does not accompany the patient. The avulsed nail bed is replaced as a nail bed graft with the nail acting as an optimal graft bolster. If the fragment is large, the nail is trimmed back 1 to 2 mm from the outer edge of the nail bed to allow suturing of the nail bed (Fig. 10-8). Small fragments of nail bed are removed from the nail and replaced as nail bed grafts. A graft of 1 cm in diameter will usually take by inosculation and vascular ingrowth from the periphery. The distal phalanx is one of the few sites where a graft will survive on bare cortex. Nail bed fragments less than 1 cm may be more difficult to remove. Although rarely the case, if there is concern about further injury to the nail bed fragment on attempted removal, the entire nail is replaced without separation of the nail bed fragment from the nail or suturing of the nail bed.

Nail Bed Defect

A split-thickness injury resulting in loss of the nail bed will regenerate and does not need closure. Small areas of full-thickness nail bed loss have been left to heal by secondary intention; however, this generally results in scarring and nail deformity. Johnson[50a] advocated releasing incisions in the lateral paronychial folds with advancement of the germinal matrix toward the center of the nail. Favorable features that increase success of this lateral mobilization include a defect less than one third of the nail width, good condition of the matrix to be mobilized, and careful elevation and advancement of the matrix.[3] We have found this technique useful in the acute setting with a defect of 3 to 5 mm.

There are several other options for closure of these defects, including split-thickness or full-thickness nail bed grafts.[79] Use of a split-thickness nail bed graft[85] allows for harvest of nail bed from adjacent uninjured nail bed without altering nail growth at the donor site. It has been our experience that if there is inadequate undamaged area on the injured nail bed from which to harvest such as a defect greater than

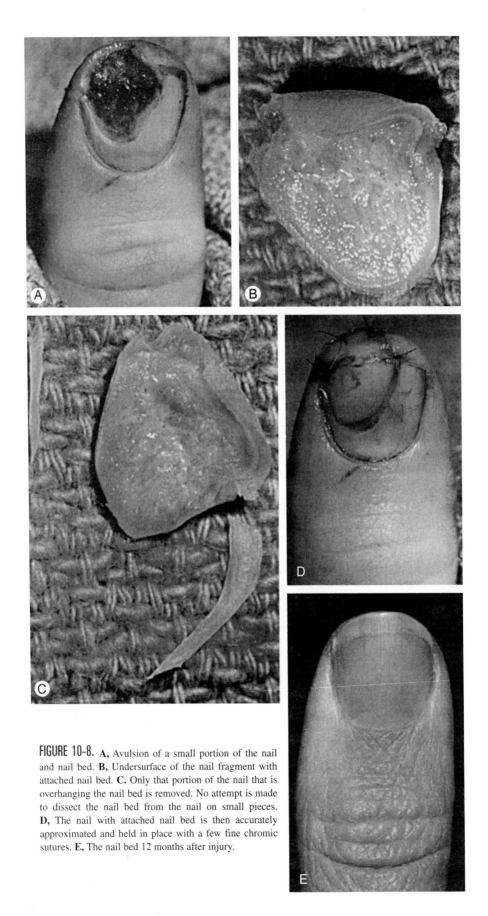

FIGURE 10-8. **A,** Avulsion of a small portion of the nail and nail bed. **B,** Undersurface of the nail fragment with attached nail bed. **C.** Only that portion of the nail that is overhanging the nail bed is removed. No attempt is made to dissect the nail bed from the nail on small pieces. **D,** The nail with attached nail bed is then accurately approximated and held in place with a few fine chromic sutures. **E,** The nail bed 12 months after injury.

50% of the nail bed, then the nail bed graft should be harvested from an adjacent finger or toe. Patients often choose to have a graft harvested from the toe rather than another finger. From a clinical standpoint, the toe is likely a better option, owing to the small risk of donor site nail deformity if the graft is harvested too deeply (Fig. 10-9).

Full-thickness nail bed grafts are rarely used except when there are salvageable spare parts that would otherwise be discarded. Otherwise, a full-thickness graft would leave a deformity of the nail at the donor site. A second situation in which full-thickness grafts are chosen involves injury to the perionychium surrounding the nail bed. Zaias has shown that there are no living cells in split-thickness nail bed grafts, and the recipient site is actually resurfaced with cells from the surrounding hyponychium, eponychium, and paronychium.[95] Therefore, if the surrounding perionychium is also missing, a full-thickness nail bed graft, which possesses living cells, will yield superior results compared with a split-thickness graft.

Harvest of Nail Bed Graft

The finger or toe to be used as the donor is anesthetized with a digital block. After exsanguination, a digital tourniquet is placed for hemostasis and the nail removed. If possible, only a portion of the nail is removed, leaving the proximal nail intact within the nail fold. If a sterile marker is available, it is helpful to mark the area of graft needed on the donor site.

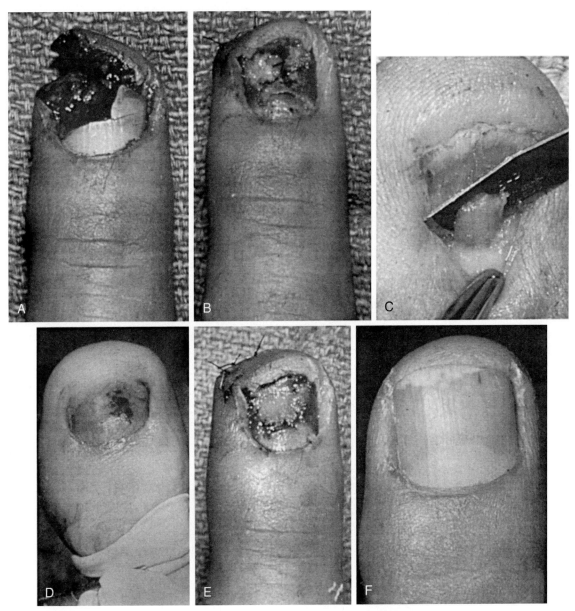

FIGURE 10-9. A, A nail bed and fingertip injury with avulsion of approximately 25% of the nail bed. **B,** The tip skin and nail bed surrounding the avulsion have been repaired. The white area at the distal left portion of the nail bed is bare cortical bone of the distal tuft. **C,** The technique of harvesting a small, split-thickness nail bed graft. **D,** The large toe after the nail has been removed and a split-thickness graft has been removed from the sterile matrix. The germinal matrix should not be included in a split-thickness graft. **E,** The split-thickness graft of sterile matrix is sutured in place on the nail bed. **F,** The fingernail 1 year later.

A split-thickness nail bed graft (approximately 0.010 inch thick) is harvested with a No. 15 scalpel (see Fig. 10-9C). Harvesting must be done carefully and slowly. The scalpel is placed parallel to the nail bed and a back-and-forth sawing motion is used. To ensure thinness of the graft, we recommend visualization of the blade through the graft. It is better for the graft to be too thin than too thick. If a thick graft results in full-thickness donor loss, donor site deformity is likely. A large graft is more difficult to harvest owing to the curve of the nail and increases the chance of an accidental full-thickness harvest. To avoid this, we use the tip of the blade while picking up the edge of the graft with fine forceps. The graft is sutured into the defect with 7-0 chromic sutures.

Fracture

Fifty percent of nail bed injuries will have an associated distal phalanx fracture.[101] Nondisplaced fractures and distal tuft fractures are treated with repair of the nail bed and replacement of the nail as a splint. The curve of the nail and its close approximation to the underlying bone makes an excellent splint to maintain fracture reduction. A tension band suture over the replaced nail can provide further stability to the fracture (Fig. 10-10).[15] If the nail is missing, the fracture may need to be pinned for better stabilization.

Displaced fractures, especially those proximal to the nail fold, are accurately reduced and fixed with 0.028 longitudinal or crossed Kirschner wires (Fig. 10-11). The use of a single wire is not recommended, because although it can reduce the fracture, it cannot eliminate axial rotation. If only a small nail bed laceration is present, wires are passed in a retrograde fashion. However, with large nail bed lacerations, the wires are passed antegrade through the distal fragment then retrograde into the proximal fragment. Crossing the DIP joint should be avoided if possible. With crush injuries, the distal phalanx fracture is often comminuted with small fractured pieces adherent to the nail bed. In this case, the bony fragments are reduced with reapproximation of the nail bed using the nail as a splint. If the nail is not available

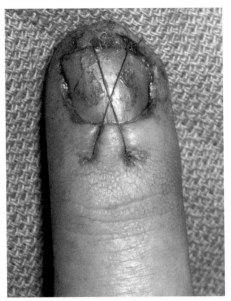

FIGURE 10-10. A figure-of-8 stitch holds the nail in place and adds stability to the fracture. (From Brown RE: Acute nail bed injuries. Hand Clin 18:561-575, 2002.)

for use as a splint, a piece of reinforced silicone is recommended. The goals of distal phalanx reduction are bony union and an even dorsal cortex. An uneven cortex will impair nail bed healing and lead to a nail deformity.

Salter I fractures are often reduced with repair of the nail bed alone. Pinning of the fracture should be avoided unless it is unstable. The patient and parents should be informed that growth of the distal phalanx may be affected, even with adequate reduction.

Amputation

Amputation can be treated in multiple ways, usually based on the remaining proximal tissue and the presence and quality of the amputated piece. Options include revision

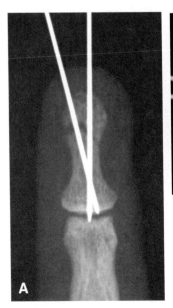

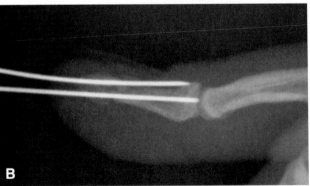

FIGURE 10-11. **A** and **B,** Distal phalanx fractures with Kirschner wire fixation. (From Brown RE: Acute nail bed injuries. Hand Clin 18:561-575, 2002.)

amputation, closure with flaps and grafts, or replantation. Our preference for treatment is discussed for a distal to proximal direction of injury.

On the rare occasion that the distal phalanx is covered by a layer of soft tissue, the amputated piece can be defatted and replaced as a skin/nail bed graft. If the distal phalanx is exposed, the options consist of trimming back the bone to allow for primary closure or rotation of local or regional skin flaps to preserve length. In both cases, when suturing the fingertip skin to the distal nail bed, tension should be avoided. Tension at the closure causes volar curvature of the distal nail bed and plate, leading to a hook nail. If a portion of the distal phalanx is absent, the nail bed should be shortened to the end of the remaining distal phalanx before repair. This will avoid hooking of the nail from loss of bony support.

More proximal amputations involving the midportion of the nail bed can be managed with local and regional flaps.[19] We use local volar and lateral "V-Y" advancement flaps as well as regional cross-finger and thenar flaps to provide tip coverage (Figs. 10-12 and 10-13).[18] It is important to remember that "V-Y" advancement flaps cannot be advanced more than 5 to 10 mm.[18] These flaps can be used to close defects primarily involving the volar and distal fingertip or can be used with nail bed grafts to reconstruct the entire fingertip. Such flaps provide excellent tip coverage and can be de-epithelialized to provide a vascularized bed for placement of the nail bed graft. Full-thickness nail bed grafts from the amputated part or a split-thickness nail bed graft from an adjacent finger or toe may be used.

Amputations through the eponychium may be replanted, but success is variable. We tend to perform revision amputation at the level of the eponychium. If 25% or greater of the nail bed distal to the eponychium is present, the patient will benefit from maintaining that nail. However, if less than 25% remains, we recommend resection of the remaining nail bed. This requires removal of the dorsal roof and ventral floor of the nail fold as well. The eponychial skin is left intact to use for coverage. Netscher describes success with

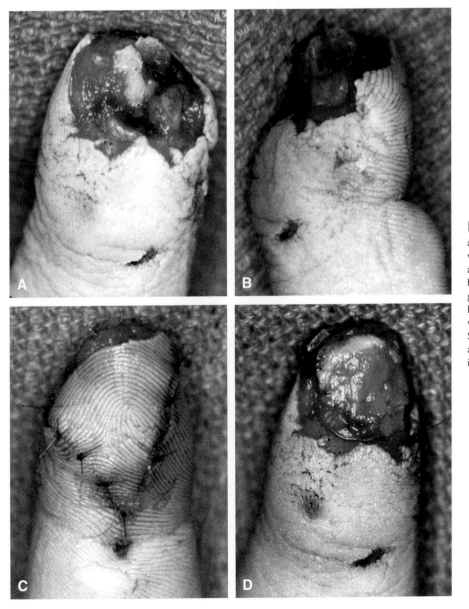

FIGURE 10-12. **A,** Fingertip injury with avulsion of nail bed. **B,** Dorsal tip defect with intact volar skin. **C,** "V-Y" volar advancement flap for coverage and nail bed support. **D,** Nail bed replaced as graft. (**A** and **D** from Brown RE, Zook EG, Russell RC: Fingertip reconstruction with flaps and nail bed grafts. J Hand Surg [Am] 24:345-351, 1999; **B, C, E, F** and **G** from Brown RE: Acute nail bed injuries. Hand Clin 18:561-575, 2002.)

Continued

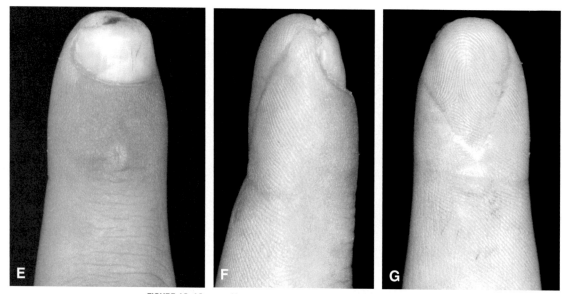

FIGURE 10-12—con'd. **E** to **G,** Results after partial nail regrowth.

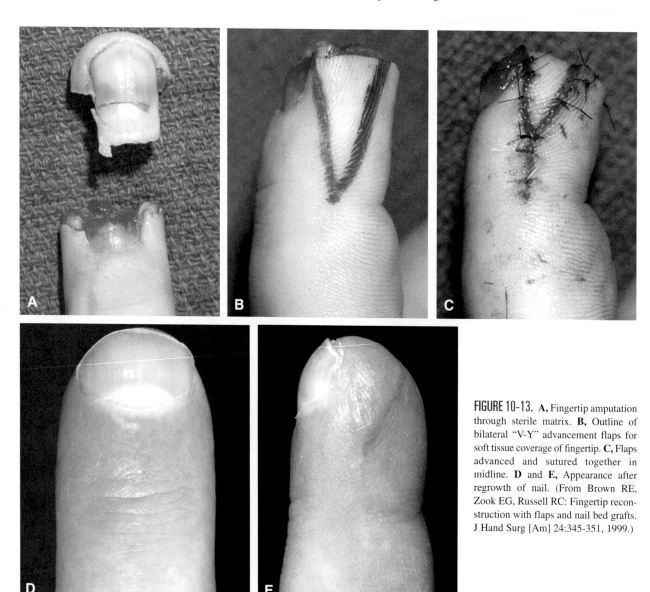

FIGURE 10-13. **A,** Fingertip amputation through sterile matrix. **B,** Outline of bilateral "V-Y" advancement flaps for soft tissue coverage of fingertip. **C,** Flaps advanced and sutured together in midline. **D** and **E,** Appearance after regrowth of nail. (From Brown RE, Zook EG, Russell RC: Fingertip reconstruction with flaps and nail bed grafts. J Hand Surg [Am] 24:345-351, 1999.)

the use of full-thickness graft of hyponychium, nail bed, and perionychium for amputations between the midportion of the nail and just proximal to the eponychium.[71] In several cases, the distal phalanx was replaced as a graft and covered with regional flaps. The graft was then placed onto the de-epithelialized flaps. This would allow for preservation of length when successful.

Replantation is most successful when the amputation is proximal to the area of the paronychium through the proximal aspect of the distal phalanx. Amputations through the nail bed are less successful because of the size of the vessels.

In children, the tip of the finger is often avulsed with the nail bed. In these cases, we approximate the edges of the nail bed and tip skin as a composite graft. Débridement of this composite graft is minimal to allow for maximum inosculation effect. Longitudinal or crossed pins are used to hold the bone in place. With young children, we occasionally use hypodermic needles in place of Kirschner wires for the bony reduction. The younger the child, the better chances for "take" of a composite graft of skin and nail bed. Our greatest success rate is for children ages 3 and younger. Alternatively, in an older child, a "cap" graft[78] will likely have greater success. This includes removal of the bone fragment and defatting of the skin for use of the piece as a full-thickness skin/nail bed graft.

Delayed Treatment of Acute Injuries

Occasionally a nail bed injury will be seen hours or days after the injury, with or without previous treatment. The first decision must be whether the initial care was adequate and, if it was not, whether more should be done.

If there is any question, the nail bed is explored and accurately approximated. This can usually be done up to 7 days after injury. Any untreated or maltreated distal phalangeal fractures should also be treated appropriately and the patient placed on perioperative antibiotics. Although the chance of infection may be greater with delayed treatment, a nail deformity will occur if nothing is done. Therefore, we believe the risk is worth taking.

POSTOPERATIVE MANAGEMENT

Patients are seen at 5 to 7 days after surgery. It is usually necessary to soak the finger with normal saline and peroxide to remove the dressing. The bandage is removed gently and slowly to protect the repair. This is especially difficult when nonadherent gauze alone is used for the nail fold because it adheres to the nail bed. If it does not loosen, we instruct the patient to perform warm soapy soaks at home several times a day. It will generally separate as the nail grows.

The nail is checked for subungual seroma or hematoma. If either is present, the hole is reopened or the nail very gently raised at the paronychium to permit drainage. The suture used to hold the nail or silicone sheet in place within the nail fold should be removed 5 to 7 days after injury to avoid a sinus tract formation through the nail fold. Sutures placed through the hyponychium or the paronychium (lateral skin) may be left in longer and removed in 10 to 14 days as would be customary for sutures in the hand. The old nail will likely adhere to the nail bed for 1 to 3 months until pushed off by the new nail. Silicone sheeting will fall off sooner.

The nail bed repair is protected and distal phalangeal fractures are immobilized with a splint dressing for the first 3 to 4 weeks. After this time, a bandage is adequate for protection of the repair and for assisting in retention of the old nail. Retention of the nail protects the nail bed as well as creates a much less tender fingertip while the new nail grows.

Scarring of the nail bed is reduced with surgical repair, and growth of a normal new nail is expected. However, nail bed scarring and nail deformities do occur, and the patient should be reminded of this at the postoperative visit.

The nail grows at approximately 0.1 mm per day[6] or 2 to 3 mm per month. After removal of the nail for nail bed repair there is a delay of new growth for 3 to 4 weeks.[6] If the proximal nail was uninjured and left in place during repair of a distal nail bed injury, growth of that nail will occur at a normal rate without delay. As the nail grows, there is a bulge on the leading edge. This distal end is expected to reach the distal finger at 6 to 9 months after injury. Toenail growth occurs four times more slowly than fingernail growth.[73]

COMPLICATIONS

Postoperative complications can be divided into problems at the site of nail growth (i.e., the germinal and sterile matrix and nail fold) and the site of nail support, the distal phalanx. Scar within the sterile matrix results in various deformities, including notching, splitting, elevation, and nonadherence because the nail will not grow over or adhere to a nail bed scar.[46] Scar within the germinal matrix may lead to absence of nail growth. Splitting or absence of the nail may also be caused from scarring of the nail fold dorsal roof to the ventral floor, which again emphasizes the importance of placing the nail or a silicone sheet under the nail fold after acute repair. All of these deformities can be functional as well as cosmetic. Bony complications include an uneven dorsal cortex and loss of bony support secondary to overdébridement of the distal phalanx, nonunion of the distal phalanx, or osteomyelitis.

Late reconstruction of the nail bed is commonly not as successful as the surgeon or the patient would desire. These less than satisfactory results have discouraged and hindered progress in reconstruction of the perionychium. Every reconstructive problem of the nail bed is different and must be approached individually. A thorough understanding of the anatomy and physiology of the nail bed of the fingers and toes is essential to devise and carry out a treatment plan.

Nail Ridges

Nail ridges are caused by an uneven dorsal cortex or scar beneath the nail bed. Because nail growth follows the shape of the nail bed, an uneven surface beneath the nail bed leads to an irregular nail bed and a subsequent nail ridge. A transverse nail ridge can raise the nail off of the nail bed preventing distal adherence. Ridging is typically a cosmetic problem except in the instance of nonadherence, where the free nail edge can catch on objects such as clothing, making this a functional problem as well. Correction requires elevation of the nail bed off of the distal phalanx and surgical excision of the scar and/or leveling of the uneven dorsal cortex to create a flat nail bed.[4,89]

We have noted minor transverse ridges of the nail after general hypoxic illness and local hypoxia from use of an arm tourniquet for upper extremity procedures. Hypoxia leads to temporary abnormality of germinal matrix cells and the ridges resolve as the nail grows.

Split Nail

A split nail may be caused by a ridge or longitudinal scar in the germinal or sterile matrix. Because scar does not produce nail cells there is a blank area between the regions of normal nail production, thus producing a split.

If the split is due to scar in the germinal matrix with lack of nail production, the scar must be removed and the nail bed repaired or replaced. The eponychium is elevated with incisions at right angles to the corners to expose the germinal matrix. The nail is removed; and under loop magnification, the scar is identified and resected. Rarely, the defect

is small enough (less than 2 mm) to be closed primarily. Therefore, if there is any tension, a nail bed graft should be used instead. We have found lateral mobilization of the matrix,[50] as mentioned earlier, to be mostly unsuccessful in the case of late reconstruction owing to the interference of the scarring with flap rotation.

A larger defect must be closed with a nail bed graft. Our preference is to use a germinal matrix graft from a toe that is similar in size and shape to the resected scar (Fig. 10-14). The germinal matrix must be taken as a full-thickness graft for it to produce nail at the recipient site. Because this frequently requires the elimination of nearly an entire toenail bed, the second toenail is more acceptable to most individuals rather than having a significant deformity of the large toenail.[25] The third through fifth toes usually do not have enough germinal matrix available for a graft.

If the scar involves the sterile matrix, rarely can it be treated with resection and primary closure. In our experience, the scar is frequently too wide to approximate the edges without significant tension and recurrence of the scar

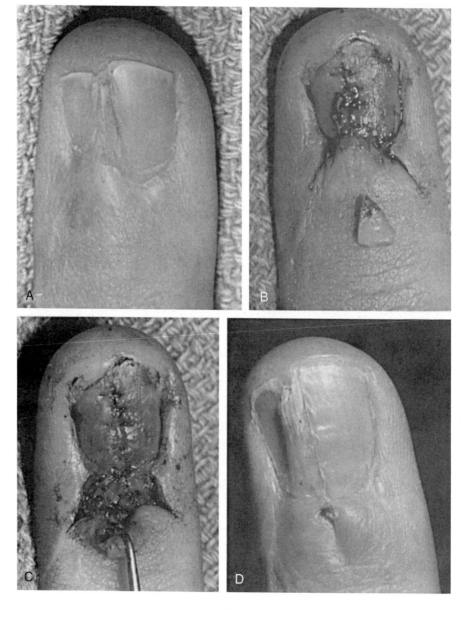

FIGURE 10-14. **A,** A split nail with a pterygium caused by scarring of the germinal matrix. **B,** The scar of the germinal matrix has been removed and a fragment of germinal matrix from the second toe cut to shape to fit the defect. **C,** The germinal matrix graft sutured in place. **D,** Six months later, nail can be seen growing from the germinal matrix graft.

and subsequent split. We recommend resection of the scar and replacement with a split-thickness nail bed graft. A defect in the sterile matrix does not require a full-thickness graft as does the germinal matrix. Therefore, harvest of the graft should cause no donor site deformity.[75,84] Donor site options include adjacent nail on the injured finger, an adjacent finger, or the first or second toe (Fig. 10-15).

Nonadherence

The sterile matrix adds nail cells to the undersurface of the nail, resulting in adherence of the nail to the nail bed. Scars within the sterile matrix do not produce nail cells, thus allowing for loosening of the nail attachments. The nail is lifted off of the nail bed by transverse and diagonal scars and is unable to adhere distally. Resection of the scar is essential for correction. Our preference for replacement is a split-thickness sterile matrix graft from either an adjacent area of the nail bed or a toenail bed (Fig. 10-16).[75,96,99]

Chronic nonadherence of the nail to the distal nail bed can also occur with repetitive trauma, such as using the fingernails to pry open objects. Cutting back or avoiding the activity is advised. If no improvement is seen, replacement of this distal nail bed segment with a split-thickness sterile matrix graft is recommended.

Absence

Absence of a nail may be congenital or may result from avulsion, severe crush, infection, or burn and is a

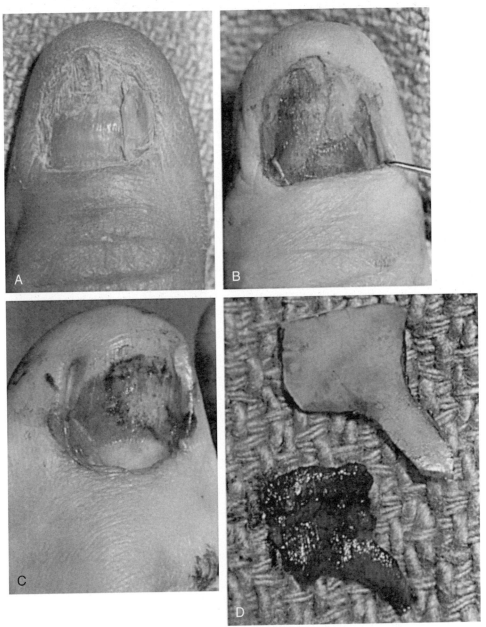

FIGURE 10-15. **A,** Preoperative view of a thumbnail following injury by a car door. The nail grows out and becomes nonadherent every 2 to 3 months. **B,** The nail remnant has been removed and scar can be seen in the nail bed on the right side. **C,** The scar of the nail bed is marked for excision. **D,** An exact template in the configuration of the scar is used to shape a split-thickness nail bed graft from sterile matrix of the toe.   *Continued*

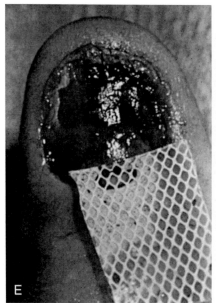

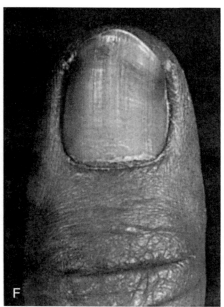

FIGURE 10-15—cont'd. **E,** The split-thickness nail bed graft has been sutured in place and a silicone sheet placed over it and into the nail fold. **F,** The nail 11 months postoperatively with complete adherence of the nail.

disconcerting deformity to the patient. Absence may be partial or complete. Absence of nail distal to the germinal matrix is treated with removal of the scar and replacement with a split-thickness sterile matrix nail bed graft. Lemperle and associates[60] reported success with serial excisions of 4-mm wide, crescent-shaped full-thickness scars at 2-month intervals that resulted in distal migration of the nail bed by wound contraction. This technique appears to eliminate morbidity of a donor graft site while increasing the number of procedures required in serial excision.

Complete absence is more difficult to reconstruct especially when the proximal nail fold is absent along with the germinal matrix. A simple but suboptimal treatment is resection of an area of skin in the shape of a slightly larger than normal nail.[44] A full- or split-thickness skin graft is used to mimic the appearance of a nail. Artificial nails

applied with glue have not been successful.[13] Buncke and Gonzalez advocated reconstruction of a nail fold pouch to aid in artificial nail adherence.[22] However, as time passes, the pouch becomes obliterated and no longer holds the edge of the prosthetic nail.[13] The use of titanium implants inserted into the distal phalanx has been described by Baruchin and colleagues[12] as a method of artificial nail fixation. A small patient series demonstrated favorable results.

Composite toenail grafts that include germinal and sterile matrix and the dorsal roof have been used for nail reconstruction (Fig. 10-17). The few reported cases have produced unpredictable results. In our experience, the results do not appear to be directly related to patient age or size of the graft.[62] Therefore, we inform the patients of the expected toenail deformity and the potentially suboptimal fingernail outcome. In selecting a donor site for composite grafts, we

FIGURE 10-16. **A,** A finger with normal germinal matrix but absent sterile matrix and nonadherence of the nail. The patient had had repeated infections beneath the nail. **B,** The scarred nail bed has been removed and a full-thickness sterile matrix graft from the second toe has been used to replace it. **C,** One year later, the nail adheres to the full-thickness toenail graft but does not adhere to the distal scar. (From Zook EG: The perionychium: Anatomy, physiology and care of injuries. Clin Plast Surg 8:21-31, 1981, with permission.)

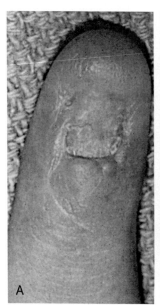

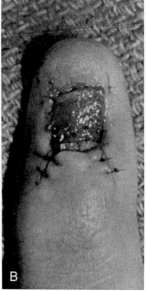

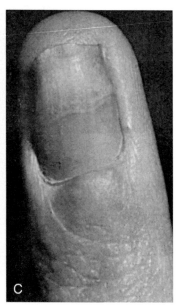

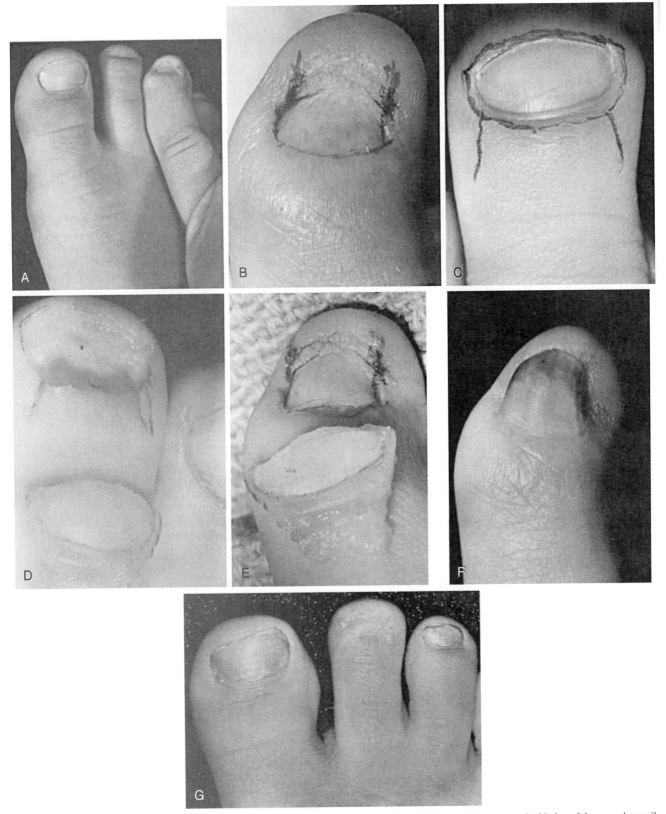

FIGURE 10-17. **A,** A 7-year-old child with post-traumatic absence of the index nail; the width of the fingernail is compared with that of the second toenail. **B,** The nail bed is seen close-up at the time of surgery. **C,** The second toe is marked for removal of the composite nail and nail bed graft. **D,** The composite graft is excised. **E,** The composite graft is placed on the dorsum of the finger after the nail fold has been created. Note that the toenail does not have as much length as a normal fingernail. The sterile matrix was advanced distally to create a recipient site for the graft. **F,** The nail 1 year postoperatively. **G,** Postoperative view of the second toe. A split-thickness skin graft was applied to the periosteum.

prefer to use the second toe because it is usually approximately the width of the fingernail. A toenail is, however, not as long as the fingernail, and a split-thickness sterile matrix graft from another toe needs to be placed distal to the composite graft to lengthen the attachment area. The large toenail or a portion of it is necessary for thumbnail reconstruction with composite grafts.

The most reliable treatment to produce a growing nail is a free microvascular transfer of the dorsal tip of the toe, including the nail bed (Fig. 10-18).[31,66,67,86,92] This requires very skilled microvascular technique, has some risk of failure, and leaves significant scars on the foot, toe, and finger. Nakayama[70] and Iwasawa and coworkers[48] have described microsurgical transfer of small toe nail flaps that result in less donor and defect site morbidity than the larger wraparound flaps. Nakayama successfully transferred a venous flap based on the venous system only,[70] and Iwasawa and coworkers reported a case of a venous flap anastomosed to a digital artery and vein.[48] Nail flaps with short vascular pedicles have been reported for decreased scarring owing to less dissection at both sites but require expert microsurgical skill because of the small size of the vessels.[26,32,33,57]

Nail Spikes, Cysts, and Cornified Nail Bed

Nail cysts most commonly occur from failure to remove the entire germinal matrix from the nail fold during revision amputation. The skin is closed over the germinal matrix, producing a cyst wall, which continuously produces nail. They present as painful, enlarging masses at the site of the previous nail fold. Treatment consists of complete resection of the nail cyst and wall (Fig. 10-19).

Nail spikes also result from incomplete removal of the germinal matrix. However, they are unenclosed and produce nail, which grows distally. They are a frequent occurrence after removal of the side of the nail and nail bed for an ingrown toenail. Treatment is complete removal of the spike and the residual germinal matrix.

A cornified nail bed occurs in patients whose germinal matrix has been removed to eliminate nail growth but the sterile matrix has been left intact. The nail bed does not produce nail, but the sterile matrix continues to produce the keratinizing material, which in a normal nail bed maintains nail adherence. To relieve this, the sterile matrix is excised and a split-thickness skin graft is applied.

Eponychial Deformities

Traumatic loss of the eponychium exposes more of the proximal nail and leads to loss of the nail shine, which is produced by the dorsal roof of the nail fold. This is commonly an aesthetic defect only because there is no alteration to actual nail growth. Notching of the eponychium is often a primarily aesthetic concern but can be functional if the free edge is frequently caught on objects. Notching is usually secondary to loss of part of the eponychium or failure to repair an eponychial laceration.

Scarring of the eponychium and nail fold to the nail bed, also known as pterygium, leads to functional as well as aesthetic deformities, such as absence of nail growth and splitting of the nail. This webbing between the eponychium and the nail bed most commonly occurs secondary to trauma but has also been associated with ischemia and collagen vascular diseases. In trauma, scarring is minimized with precise repair of the nail bed within the fold and separation of the dorsal and ventral layers of the nail fold during healing, as previously mentioned. However, scarring remains a possible complication. Absence or splitting of the nail occurs with scarring of the eponychium to the germinal matrix. The nail is either unable to grow in the area of scar, leading to absence, or the nail grows around the scar, leading to splitting.

For a persistent pterygium of the eponychium, we recommend freeing the dorsal roof of the nail fold from the nail and inserting a small piece of silicone sheet into the nail fold with a horizontal mattress suture. The undersurface of the nail fold epithelializes and releases the adherence. If this is unsuccessful, it may be necessary to separate the dorsal roof from the nail and to place a thin split-thickness sterile matrix graft on the undersurface of the eponychium to prevent the adherence.[83] The nail bed must also be examined for scarring, especially in patients with absence of nail growth.

The eponychium may be reconstructed by a composite toe eponychial graft,[62] the helical rim of the ear,[77] or rotation flaps.[1] We recommend use of a composite eponychial graft from an appropriate toe to replace missing eponychium. A template of the eponychial defect is used to plan the composite graft of eponychium and underlying dorsal roof. With this graft, there is only a small area of raw surface on the proximal end for revascularization. Therefore, to improve the chance of graft take, we harvest a larger area of dorsal skin with the graft that corresponds to a de-epithelialized area on the finger, which lies just proximal to the defect. This leaves a slightly larger area on the toe that is left to heal secondarily. The resultant toe deformity has been minimal.

Hyponychial Deformities

Pterygia can also occur within the hyponychium secondary to trauma. Other sources of scarring within the hyponychium include denervation and ischemia. The tip of the finger may become painful and tender. We recommend removal of the distal 5 mm of nail from the nail bed and hyponychial area. A narrow strip of nail bed and hyponychium, 3 to 4 mm wide, is resected and replaced by a split-thickness skin graft. This causes nonadherence in the hyponychial area and usually provides relief of pain.

Hooking of the nail occurs with tight closure of a fingertip amputation and/or loss of bony support under the nail bed, which leads to curving of the matrix in a volar direction (Fig. 10-20). Because the growing nail follows the nail matrix, any alteration in the support of the distal finger will alter the direction of nail growth. To avoid this, the nail should not be pulled over the distal phalanx. Acutely, when the distal bone is absent, it must be replaced or the nail bed trimmed back to the end of the bone so the nail bed does not curve over the end.

After a hooked nail has developed, a decision must be made whether to shorten the bone or attempt to add support to the nail bed. If the distal nail bed had been pulled over the end of the finger, a "V-Y" advancement flap, cross-finger flap, or full-thickness skin graft can be used to replace the

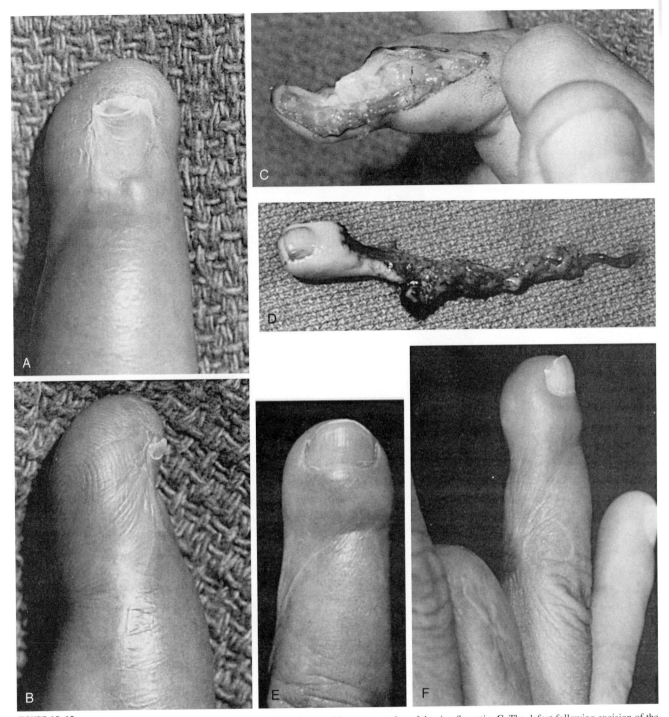

FIGURE 10-18. **A** and **B,** Minimal nail growth and soft tissue loss after an oblique amputation of the ring fingertip. **C,** The defect following excision of the scarred nail bed and tip. **D,** Partial second-toe free flap. **E** and **F,** Postoperative appearance of the ring finger.

soft tissue for the tip and allow replacement of the nail bed onto the dorsum of the bone.[59] This usually improves the hook, although complete correction is uncommon. Correction of a hooked nail with maintenance of nail length requires replacement of the distal phalanx or tuft with a bone graft. This may require additional tip soft tissue before or at the time of bone grafting. Initially, bone grafts support the nail bed satisfactorily, but as with most bone grafts that do not have bone apposition on both ends, in time they tend

to resorb and the correction is lost. A free vascularized transfer of second-toe tip, including the distal phalanx and nail, is the best, although most complex, solution.[56] A prosthesis, rather than reconstruction, is a simple solution that may give very satisfactory results.[13]

Hyponychial nonadherence occurs with loss of the hyponychial barrier from exposure of the fingertips to acids or alkali or chronic exposure to fluid. Without the barrier, fungus, bacteria, and dirt have direct access to the subungual

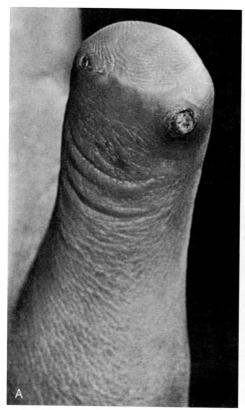
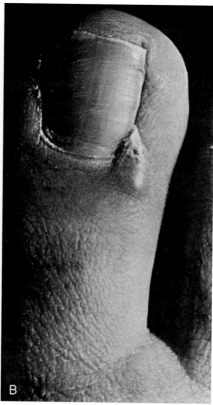

FIGURE 10-19. **A,** Nail cysts after amputation of the fingertip without complete removal of the nail bed. **B,** A nail spike resulting from incomplete removal of nail bed after resection of an ingrown toenail.

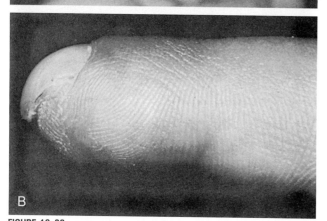

FIGURE 10-20. **A,** A hooked-nail deformity caused partially by some loss of bony support but primarily by the nail bed being pulled over the tip to close the amputation. **B,** Loss of bony support to hold the nail bed flat.

space, causing nonadherence of the nail. If removing the cause does not result in readherence, it is usually secondary to the presence of keratinous material. The nail is then removed to a point just proximal to the nonadherence and the keratin scrapped from the nail bed to allow for adherence as the nail grows distally. The nail may need to be scrapped multiple times as the nail grows to the desired length.

Dull Nail

A dull nail is another minor complication that is cosmetic in nature. The dorsal roof of the nail fold is responsible for the shiny surface to the nail. Scar within the dorsal roof may lead to a dull streak within the nail.[102] No treatment is necessary as long as there are no associated functional problems.

PINCER NAIL

Although the pincer or trumpet nail deformity has been attributed to several causes, the exact etiology of this deformity remains uncertain. It consists of excess transverse curvature of the nail and progressive pinching off of the soft tissue of the distal fingertip with resultant pain and an unaesthetic deformity. Although partial or complete nail ablation may provide symptomatic relief, various nail-preserving methods have been reported. Our preferred treatment consists of nail plate removal, elevation of the sides of the nail bed from the distal phalanx, and placement of autogenous dermal grafts[21] or Alloderm under the lateral portions of the nail bed, between the nail bed and periosteum (Fig. 10-21). Kosaka[55] demonstrated satisfactory

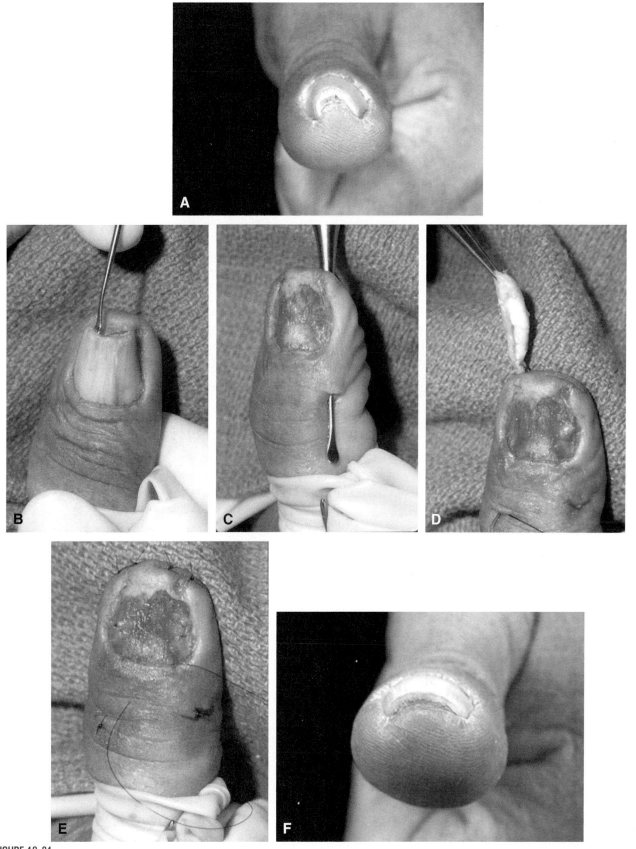

FIGURE 10-21. **A,** Pincer nail deformity with tubing of the nail. **B,** Removal of the nail. **C,** Elevation of the sides of the nail bed from the underlying distal phalanx. **D,** Placement of dermal graft into the created tunnel. **E,** Closure of distal and proximal tunnel wounds after placement of graft. **F,** Improvement of pincer nail 1 year after surgery. (Courtesy of Nicole Z. Sommer, MD, and Richard E. Brown, MD.)

CRITICAL POINTS: PINCER NAIL TREATMENT

INDICATIONS

■ Painful nail
■ Disfigured nail

TECHNICAL POINTS

■ Use digital block and apply tourniquet to finger.
■ Remove nail with elevator or curved iris scissors.
■ Perform stab incisions to radial and ulnar hyponychium.
■ Place Kleinert-Kutz elevator into stab incisions.
■ Carefully elevate nail bed from underlying periosteum.
■ Harvest dermal graft or prepare alloderm.
■ Cut graft or alloderm to length and tube.
■ Perform stab incision to ulnar and radial proximal eponychium.
■ Pass dull end of Keith needle proximal to distal beneath the nail bed, leaving needle within wound.
■ Thread 5-0 nylon suture through end of graft/Alloderm.
■ Thread suture into Keith needle.
■ Pull needle proximally to pull graft/Alloderm into space beneath nail bed.
■ Close stab incisions with superficial stitches.

PITFALL

■ Tearing radial or ulnar paronychium on nail bed elevation

success in treatment of severe pincer deformity with a contracted hyponychium. This method involves a fish-mouth incision near the nail margin, elevation of the nail bed, flattening of the distal phalanx dorsal surface, widening of the contracted hyponychium, and a "W"-plasty type closure between the distal nail bed flap and hyponychium.

INFECTIONS

Fungal

Perionychial infections of the subungual area are the most common infections in the hand. These are most frequently onychomycosis or chronic fungal infections (although superimposed bacterial infections may occur) and are usually treated medically by primary care physicians or dermatologists.[8] Treatment usually starts with topical therapy with nail lacquer placed over the nail. Systemic treatments are started if this is not successful after 6 months. Options include terbinafine (250 mg/daily for 6 weeks for fingernails and 12 weeks for toenails), itraconazole (200 mg twice a day for 1 week every month for 2 months for fingernails and 4 months for toenails), or fluconazole (150 to 300 mg once a week for 6 to 9 months). Twenty-five percent of patients do not respond to systemic treatment and require surgical intervention.[8]

We most commonly see patients after these first lines of treatment have not been successful. At this point, we recommend removal of the nail and application of 4% Mycolog cream twice a day to the nail bed until the nail has completely regrown. This allows for exposure of the subungual fungal infection and, if needed, debulking of the onychomycosis for improved penetration. Occasionally, we have performed total ablation of the nail for recurrent or persistent fungal infections.[104]

Bacterial

Bacterial infections of the nail most commonly involve the paronychium. The dermal and epidermal layers of the paronychium are arranged in an overlapping fashion, much like the shingles of a house. When one of these layers is pulled up, an open wound (hangnail) is created. Subsequent infection produces a paronychia. *Staphylococcus aureus* is the most frequent organism isolated.[64] If the infection involves the paronychium but is above the nail, it can be drained by lifting the paronychium away from the nail, followed by soaks to encourage adequate drainage. If the infection and purulence have progressed beneath the edge of the nail, a portion of the nail must be removed to permit drainage (Fig. 10-22). The nail is dissected from the underlying nail bed and the overlying proximal eponychium with fine scissors or a periosteal elevator. The nail is then split longitudinally and the undermined portion removed to allow drainage. Adequate open drainage is maintained by soaking the digit in warm soapy water three to four times per day. Antibiotics are indicated if tissue cellulitis is present. If the abscess dissects beneath the dorsal roof of the nail fold or beneath the nail in the nail fold, the proximal portion of the nail must be removed. The distal portion of the nail may be left in place to decrease discomfort. In neither of these instances should incisions be made in the eponychium to drain the infection. Such incisions will frequently not heal primarily in the presence of infection, and a notch or square corner in the eponychium may result. We have never seen a paronychia or abscess that required incision in the eponychium for adequate drainage.

Chronic paronychia usually occurs between the nail and the dorsal roof of the nail fold and results in a tender, erythematous, and swollen fingertip. The infection is most commonly caused by gram-negative organisms and fungus, primarily *Candida*.[7] Treatment involves topical and/or oral antifungal agents as well as preventive measures such as avoidance of moisture, of trauma from cuticle treatments, and of irritants such as citrus fruits and cosmetic nail products.[95] For resistant cases, treatment is a Keyser-Eaton marsupialization of the nail fold.[1,14,51,52] A 3- to 4-mm wide crescent is excised from the proximal nail fold, preserving the cuticle. The skin and dorsal roof of the nail fold are excised down to the nail, taking care not to injure the germinal matrix (Fig. 10-23). The wound is allowed to heal

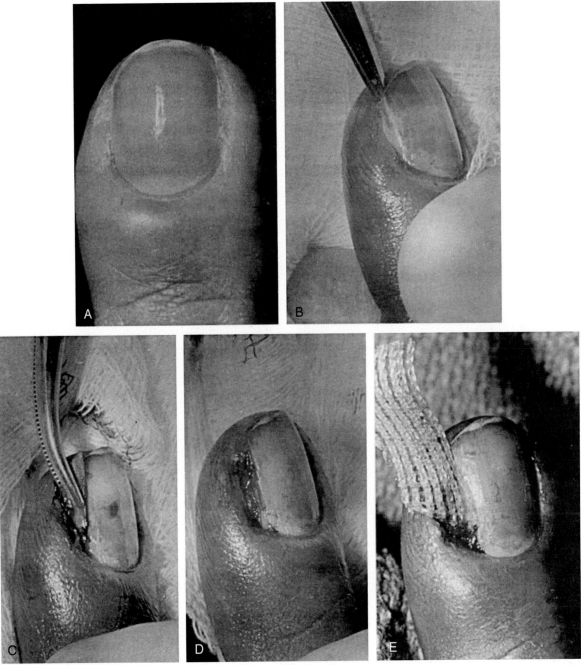

FIGURE 10-22. **A,** Paronychia is seen on the left side of this nail, with pus extending beneath the nail. **B,** A fine pair of iris scissors is used to elevate the side of the nail from the nail bed and the eponychium from the dorsum of the nail. **C,** The loosened fragment of nail is then split longitudinally and removed from the nail fold. **D,** Adequate drainage is performed after partial removal of the nail. **E,** A small wick of gauze is used to promote drainage.

secondarily. We have found this treatment generally successful.

TUMORS OF THE PERIONYCHIUM

Benign

Pyogenic Granuloma

Pyogenic granulomas manifest as rapidly growing lesions with a round, red, elevated area similar to granulation tissue growing through the nail. They are usually the result of perforations of the nail by trauma or iatrogenic causes

(Fig. 10-24). The most common treatment is repeated silver nitrate cauterization, which may result in some nail deformity. Excision is also an option but will likely require a nail bed graft for closure. Differential diagnosis for these lesions include squamous cell carcinoma or amelanotic melanoma. Therefore, if the lesion is persistent or recurrent after cauterization, biopsy is needed.

Subungual Nevi

Nevi of the nail bed are not uncommon. The nail produced by a nail bed with a pigmented nevus will also be pigmented because the nevus cells are added to the nail as it grows

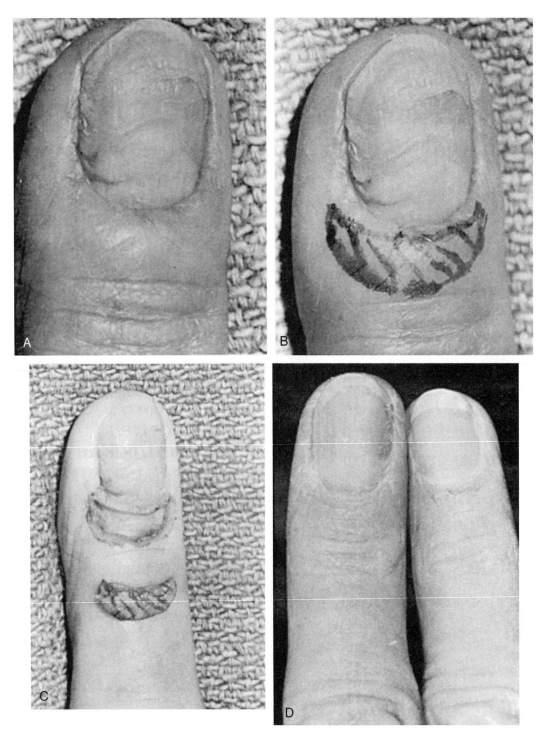

FIGURE 10-23. **A,** Chronic paronychia that has been present for 2 years. **B,** The area on the dorsal roof is marked for excision. **C,** The dorsal roof of the nail fold has been removed down to the nail. **D,** Appearance 1 year after injury with no further infection.

distally (Fig. 10-25). Roughening of the nail surface usually does not occur, but elevation and ridging of the nail may. A nevus is frequently present at birth and first noticed in childhood. As years pass, it may become lighter or darker.

In the past, nevi of the nail bed were commonly observed owing to the potential deformity of the nail on nail bed biopsy. Because of a greater potential for malignant degeneration within the nail bed, we generally recommend incisional biopsy of the nevi. However, watching the nevi for

changes and delaying the biopsy until the child is older is also a reasonable option. We discuss the options with the patient and parents. On biopsy, if atypical cells are present, the involved portion of the nail bed is removed and the nail bed reconstructed as needed.[35]

It is important to remember the other causes of subungual pigmentation, including melanonychia striata and hematoma. Melanonychiae are benign longitudinal bands of pigmentation most often seen in African Americans and are usually

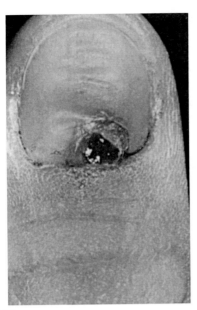

FIGURE 10-24. Pyogenic granuloma growing through the nail after perforation of the nail with cuticle scissors.

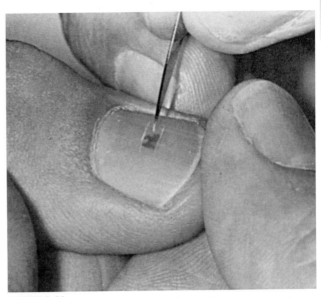

FIGURE 10-26. Marking the nail over a pigmented area to measure changes in relation to growth (see text).

present on multiple nails. They can be difficult to diagnose, and Glat and colleagues recommend biopsy in whites of any longitudinal pigmented band and in African Americans if only one digit is involved.[37] A subungual hematoma is the most common cause of subungual pigmentation in an adult, even when there is no history of trauma. These areas of pigmentation should be monitored closely for resolution. We make a scratch into the surface of the nail at the proximal and distal borders of the pigmented area (Fig. 10-26) and monitor the pigment in relation to the scratches for approximately 3 weeks. If the pigment is from a hematoma, it will progress toward the free edge of the nail with the scratches. If the pigment is a foreign body, nevus, or

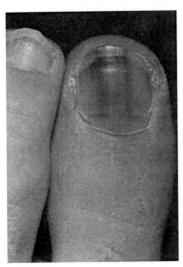

FIGURE 10-25. A pigmented nevus of the large toenail present since birth on which biopsy was performed at puberty and showed atypical melanocytes. The entire nail bed was excised.

melanoma in the nail bed, the scratches will progress distally away from the area of pigmentation, necessitating a biopsy.

Verruca Vulgaris

Hand surgeons usually see patients with verruca vulgaris (viral warts) of the perionychium after they have been treated by their primary physician or dermatologist. We recommend laser therapy for patients with persistent warts. The keratin outer layer is shaved off to allow better penetration, and a vascular laser is used to target the vessels within the wart. To avoid injury to the nail bed, laser treatment should remain superficial. Therefore, multiple treatments may be necessary. Our estimated success with this has been 50% to 75% resolution.

We also see patients with nail deformity that occurred from treatment of the wart. The resulting scar tissue in the nail bed prevents return of normal nail growth. Reconstruction consists of surgical excision of the nail bed scar and nail bed grafting, usually from the toes, as previously discussed.

Ganglion

Ganglions of the DIP joint, incorrectly known as mucous cysts, are the most common tumors that deform the nail bed. Kleinert and coworkers[54a] reported a communication between these cysts and the DIP joint in the area of an arthritic spur (osteophyte). When the cystic expansion of the ganglion is between the floor of the nail and the periosteum, upward pressure on the nail bed causes a ridged, curved, or ragged nail (Fig. 10-27). If the cyst lies dorsal to the nail bed within the nail fold, the pressure is downward on the nail, causing grooving, thinning, or roughening of the nail (Fig. 10-28). If there is severe nail deformity, we believe that the best treatment is removal of the nail followed by débridement of the DIP osteophytes and drainage of the cyst through a "T"-shaped incision over the joint (Fig. 10-29). A

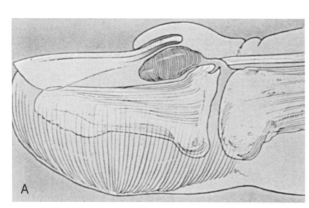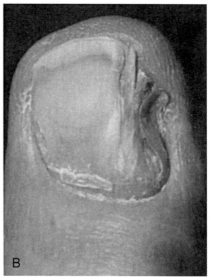

FIGURE 10-27. A, Dissection of a ganglion between the periosteum of the distal phalanx and the nail bed. **B,** The typical (but somewhat extreme) longitudinal groove deformity that results when the ganglion is located as shown in **A.**

piece of 0.020-inch silicone sheet is placed into the nail fold to help mold the nail bed back into its normal position. For minor grooves or flattening, removal of the deformed nail is not necessary. In our early experience, débridement of the osteophytes and removal of the cyst wall resulted in a residual minor nail deformity in 36% of cases.[20] Our more recent experience with only débridement of the osteophytes and evacuation of the cyst through the incision resulted in minor nail deformity in 10% with no recurrence of the cyst.[36] We thus believe that osteophyte débridement is the key to preventing recurrence. Therefore, removal of the cyst

wall is not necessary and increases the risk of nail deformity owing to possible nail bed damage.

Ganglions occasionally rupture and drain through the nail fold of the overlying skin. If infection occurs, permanent nail deformity and limitation of joint motion may result. If the ganglion ruptures, the appropriate treatment is antibiotics until the skin is closed, followed by surgical removal of the osteophyte before the ganglion re-ruptures. A ganglion should not be surgically treated while it is actively draining because of an increased risk of subsequent infection and deformity.

CRITICAL POINTS: TREATMENT OF DIP GANGLION

INDICATIONS

- Pain
- Recurrent ganglion rupture/infection
- Significant nail deformity

PEARLS

- Nail deformity resolves with removal of osteophyte and ganglion drainage.
- Chance of nail deformity is decreased with drainage rather than excision of ganglion.
- Infection of draining cyst must be resolved before definitive treatment.

TECHNICAL POINTS

- Use "T"- or "H"-shaped incision over dorsal DIP joint.
- Elevate and retract extensor tendon without disrupting the insertion.
- Identify and drain the ganglion.
- Excise osteophyte with small rongeur.
- Irrigate joint and wound with normal saline.
- Use superficial interrupted closure of skin.
- Apply volar DIP joint digital splint for comfort.

PITFALLS

- Extensor lag may develop with too aggressive extensor tendon elevation.
- Patients must be willing to accept lengthy recovery with a painful joint and swollen finger.
- Healing difficulties may occur at "T" junction.

POSTOPERATIVE CARE

- Use a splint for 1 week if there is minimal retraction of extensor.
- Use a splint for 3 to 4 weeks if extensor tendon is attenuated during retraction.
- Begin active range-of-motion exercises after splint is removed.

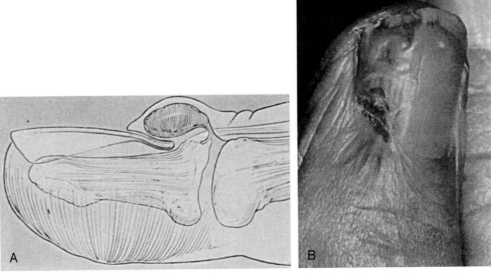

FIGURE 10-28. **A,** Dissection of a ganglion into the dorsal roof of the nail fold compresses the nail bed volarly. **B,** Irregular breakup of the nail (or a longitudinal groove) is the deformity frequently caused by a ganglion.

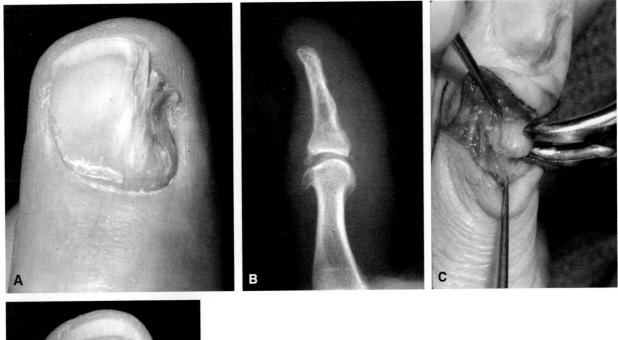

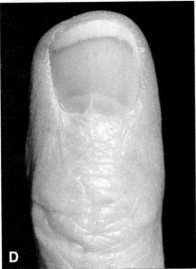

FIGURE 10-29. **A,** DIP joint ganglion causing nail deformity. **B,** Radiographic evidence of osteophytes of DIP joint. **C,** The offending osteophyte is excised and the ganglion decompressed. **D,** One year follow-up with normal nail growth. (From Sommer N, Neumeister MW: Tumors of the perionychium. Hand Clin 18:673-689, 2002.)

Glomus Tumor

A glomus tumor arises from the glomus body that regulates blood flow and temperature in the finger.[10] Although not limited to the nail bed, 50% do occur subungually. Proliferation of this angiomatous tissue within the confined space of the nail bed results in exquisite pain. On presentation, the patient may have a bluish discoloration beneath the nail. The nail may be exquisitely tender to pressure and sensitive to temperature changes, especially cold. Thus, an ice cube held over the nail bed may reproduce the pain. Both ultrasound[24] and magnetic resonance imaging[29] have been reported as highly successful in identifying subungual glomus tumors.

Treatment consists of removal of the nail, identification of the glomus tumor or tumors, and surgical excision. The entire nail bed should be carefully examined for multiple tumors after the nail is removed. A longitudinal incision is made over the glomus tumor and the tumor is dissected out from the surrounding tissue. The tumor frequently "shells out," much like a lipoma (Fig. 10-30). This allows primary closure of the nail bed incision. Alternatively, the nail bed

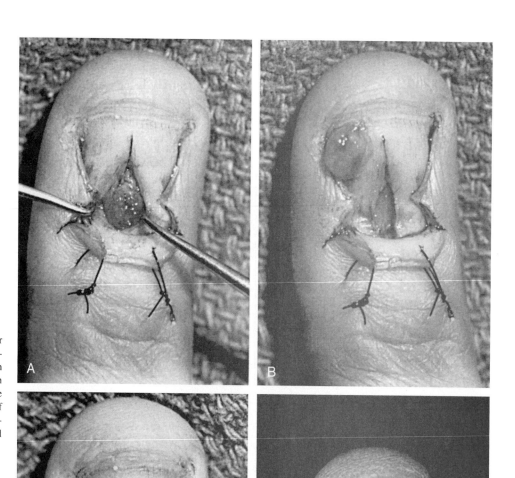

FIGURE 10-30. A, A glomus tumor exposed at the junction of the germinal and sterile matrices. The approach is through a longitudinal incision in the nail bed after removal of the nail. **B,** Appearance after excision of the tumor. **C,** The nail bed is meticulously repaired. **D,** Normal nail growth 6 months later.

may be raised up as a flap from distal to proximal to provide exposure for tumor excision.

Malignant Tumors

Basal cell carcinoma (BCC) is rare in the hand and even more so in the finger. Only 11 cases have been reported.[53] They most frequently occur after radiation exposure or other chronic trauma or exposure. Arsenic exposure is also thought to be a risk factor.[53] Complete resection of the tumor with frozen section examination of the margins is recommended to ensure complete removal. If the distal phalanx is involved, amputation at the DIP joint level is recommended. Repair consists of nail reconstruction with a split-thickness nail bed graft or skin graft closure.

Squamous cell carcinomas (SCC), although uncommon, are the most common malignant tumor of the perionychium[49] and can also be secondary to radiation exposure (Fig. 10-31).[2,23,63] In the past, dentists' hands were commonly involved, owing to chronic radiation exposure. This became much less common with the knowledge of radiation-induced tumor formation. Other predisposing factors include repeated trauma, infection, arsenic exposure, or presence of human papillomavirus.[23,69,81] In a retrospective review at the Cleveland Clinic of 12 patients in 10 years with SCC of the nail, only two causes were clearly defined: human papillomavirus and radiation.[40] SCC tumors may present as a raised, red, sometimes ulcerated, bleeding lesion or as a simple nail deformity. They are slow growing and are frequently misdiagnosed as paronychia. Carroll showed that the average length of time between appearance and treatment was 4 years.[23] This tumor is seen more commonly in males and usually involves the thumb. A lesion without bony involvement requires resection of the entire lesion with adequate margins, frequently requiring a nail bed or skin graft. If the carcinoma has been present for a long time, is large, or involves the bone, amputation at the DIP joint or even more proximally is indicated. Node dissection is indicated only if the nodes do not disappear after amputation because most nodal enlargements appear to be inflammatory.

Melanomas of the hands and feet have a poorer prognosis than those elsewhere on the body.[27] They are almost always pigmented and may or may not have nail deformity (Fig. 10-32). Fungal infection, paronychia, warts, pyogenic granuloma, foreign bodies, subungual hematoma, and melonychiae striata may mimic a melanoma of the perionychium. Consequently, the diagnosis is often missed initially and delayed up to 2 to 3 years.[58,65]

Any pigmented lesion that does not advance with nail growth, such as the case with foreign bodies or subungual hematoma, should raise suspicion. If the lesion has not changed in 4 to 6 weeks, biopsy with permanent pathologic examination is recommended.[17] Margins of excision are based on thickness of the skin melanoma, but thickness is difficult to determine in cases of subungual melanoma.[34] We recommend complete excision with clear margins for lesions with dysplasia or atypia. Melanoma in situ requires excision with 5-mm margins. For invasive melanoma, early studies recommended metacarpal or metatarsal ray amputation for stage I (local) disease.[16,39] However, more recent recommendations include more conservative amputation[34] at the proximal interphalangeal joint[47] or at the joint just proximal to the nail bed melanoma[38] with preservation of as much function as possible.

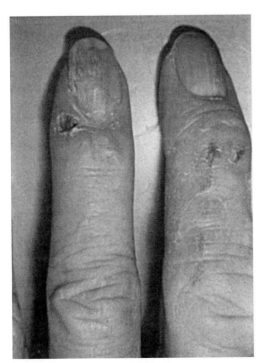

FIGURE 10-31. A veterinarian with many years of radiation exposure to his fingers contracted squamous cell carcinoma of the perionychium.

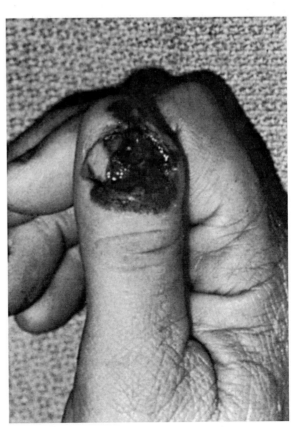

FIGURE 10-32. Malignant melanoma of the nail bed.

Evaluation for metastatic disease should include physical examination of the regional lymph nodes along with a chest radiograph and liver function tests. Opinions have varied regarding the advisability and timing of lymph node dissections in subungual melanoma. As in other areas of the body, elective lymph node dissection in the absence of palpable nodes is controversial and is still being evaluated whereas therapeutic lymph node dissection is indicated for palpable nodes. Glat and colleagues have recommended lymph node dissection for lesions greater than 1.0 mm in thickness, which is in line with the recommendation for intermediate cutaneous melanomas (1.0 to 4.0 mm). The use of sentinel node biopsies has shown promising results for the detection of lymph node metastases while potentially preventing unnecessary nodal dissections. With a negative sentinel node, the chance of regional lymph node metastasis was found to be less than 1%.[5]

Survival rates for subungual melanomas are varied. Park found a poorer 5-year survival for subungual melanomas (41%) versus cutaneous melanomas (72%).[74] Klausner reported 5-year survival of 28% to 30% and 10-year survival of 0% to 13%.[54]

ANNOTATED REFERENCES

8. Baran R: Nail fungal infections and treatment. Hand Clin 18:625-628, 2002.

   Dr. Baran is head of the Nail Disease Center in Cannes, France, which gives him an extensive opportunity to treat diseases of the nail. In this brief chapter, he concisely reviews recommended treatment for the common problem of onychomycosis.

15. Bindra RR: Management of nail bed fracture-lacerations using a tension-band suture. J Hand Surg [Br] 21:1111-1113, 1996.

   This rather obscure article published in the British literature describes a simple technique to help stabilize distal phalangeal fractures associated with nail bed injuries. Although it does not replace Kirschner wire fixation for the more proximal distal phalangeal fracture, it uses the intact nail plate to provide fixation when pins are not needed. It is a technique the authors are definitely passing on to their residents.

18. Brown RE: Acute nail bed injuries. Hand Clin 18:561-575, 2002.

   The author draws on his extensive experience at an institution known for its state of the art management of nail bed injuries. Detailed guidelines and illustrative cases are provided that should enable the reader to accurately and easily manage this common fingertip injury.

21. Brown RE, Zook EG, Williams J: Correction of pincer-nail deformities using dermal grafting. Plast Reconstr Surg 105:658-1661, 2000.

   The authors present a relatively simple but successful method of preserving the nail in the treatment of this not uncommon but yet frequently overlooked nail deformity. Their treatment and success have been unparalleled in previous studies.

33. Endo T, Nakayama Y: Microtransfers for nail and finger tip replacement. Hand Clin 18:615-622, 2002.

   Perhaps nowhere else in the world than Japan is importance placed on having five complete digits on a hand. The authors therefore have the unique opportunity to perform many microsurgical fingertip reconstructions. Great attention should therefore be given to their recommendations.

34. Finley RK, Driscoll DL, Blumenson LE, Karakousis CP: Subungual melanoma: An eighteen year review. Surgery 116:96-100, 1994.

   Data from a known cancer institute is generally very useful to the practicing hand surgeon when it comes to managing uncommon tumors of the hand. This paper from the Roswell Park Institute provides just such data on the management of subungual melanomas. Although more than 10 years old, it still provides useful guidelines.

36. Gingrass MK, Brown RE, Zook EG: Treatment of fingernail deformities secondary to ganglions of the distal interphalangeal joint. J Hand Surg [Am] 20: 502-505, 1995.

   Ganglions of the DIP joint are very common and frequently associated with nail deformities. Unfortunately such ganglions are often treated inappropriately. In this paper the appropriate management of nail deformities associated with DIP ganglions is clearly defined.

47. Heaton KM, el-Naggar A, Ensign LG, et al: Surgical management and prognostic factors in patients with subungual melanoma. Ann Surg 219:197-204, 1994.

   The authors review an extensive experience with subungual melanoma over a 32-year period. Prognostic factors and treatment recommendations from such an extensive experience cannot be ignored.

55. Kosaka M, Kamiishi H: New strategy for the treatment and assessment of pincer nail. Plast Reconstr Surg 111:2014-2019, 2003.

   This paper from Japan describes a technique for surgical treatment of this often overlooked nail deformity. It reshapes the nail without grafting and appears to provide a long-term correction.

62. Lille S, Brown RE, Zook EG, Russell RC: Free nonvascularized composite nail grafts: An institutional experience. Plast Reconstr Surg 105:2412-2415, 2000.

   Although composite nail bed grafts are technically much easier to perform than free vascularized grafts, there have been little published data to rely on. The authors' extensive experience with management of nail bed reconstruction makes this article a must-read before embarking on this challenging reconstruction.

83. Shepard GH: Treatment of nail bed avulsions with split thickness nail bed grafts. J Hand Surg 8:49-54, 1983.

   A study of nail bed reconstruction without a review of Shepard's pioneering work is incomplete. His early work led to the appropriate treatment of nail bed loss.

93. Yates YJ, Concannon MJ: Fungal infections of the perionychium. Hand Clin 18:631-642, 2002.

   The authors extensively discuss the management of the common problem of onychomycosis. Readers should not have to look further for help with management of this often frustrating problem.

99. Zook EG, Guy RJ, Russell RC: A study of nail bed injuries: Causes, treatment and prognosis. J Hand Surg [Am] 9:247-252, 1984.

   This classic paper from two decades ago began the modern treatment of nail bed injuries. It still bears reading today by all who treat nail bed and fingertip injuries.

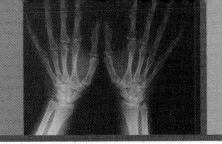

CHAPTER 11

Stiff Finger Joints

Alexander Y. Shin and Peter C. Amadio

An ever-present menace in hand surgery is the decided tendency for the hand to stiffen and to stiffen in the position of nonfunction.[26]

STERLING BUNNELL

The restoration of motion to the joints of the hand is one of the most common problems in reconstruction of the hand. Stiff finger joints may result after injury even though the initial injury was distant to the digits. Whether the etiology is direct or indirect injury, infection, excessive immobilization, or arthrosis, the ensuing adverse sequelae of joint stiffness can result in significant disability.

Overcoming stiff and painful joints is essential if the hand is to function properly, and this salient fact creates a formidable challenge for the hand surgeon.

Essential in the evaluation of the stiff finger is the understanding of the concept that the hand is an organ whose parts affect its entire function.[101] One stiff finger can impair the function of the entire hand and jeopardize a patient's career. In this chapter we review the causes and treatment for stiff finger joints, emphasizing those factors associated with the finger joints themselves as well as certain afflictions of the intrinsic muscles of the hand. Other problems that may result in stiff finger joints, such as those associated with rheumatoid arthritis and tendon injury, are discussed elsewhere in this text.

PATHOPHYSIOLOGY OF JOINT STIFFNESS

The initial response to nearly any injury to the hand or finger is edema.[17,26,101] The injured hand and digit are bathed in a macrophage- and protein-rich fluid that not only encompasses the injured structure but surrounds and bathes adjacent uninjured structures as well. The accumulation of edema fluid or hematoma within the layers of tendons, sheaths, or capsular structures of the joint or within synovial spaces acutely impairs the function of the joint.[2,16,17,26] With continued edema, the synovial spaces are distended with excess fluid and the capsular structures and collateral ligaments effectively become shortened. Eventually the changes become fixed, and joint contractures are the result.

The swollen hand assumes a characteristic posture. The key to the development of this posture is the metacarpopha-langeal (MP) joint.[165] After an insult, the edema fluid acts as a hydraulic pump, filling the joint spaces. The intracapsular fluid capacity of the MP joint is maximized when the joint is fully extended. In this position, the MP joint is also at its most unstable, with the contact of articular surfaces minimized and the capsular structures most lax (Fig. 11-1).

In contrast to the MP joint, the capacity of the interphalangeal (IP) joints is affected little by joint position and is

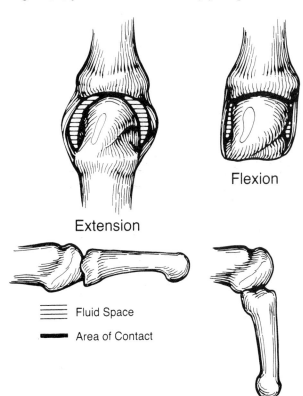

FIGURE 11-1. Anatomy of the extended MP joint differs significantly from that of the fully flexed MP joint. In extension, the bone contact surface area is minimal. The collateral ligaments are loose, the intra-capsular fluid space is at a maximum, and the joint is relatively unstable. The proximal phalanx rotates, abducts, and adducts on the metacarpal. In full flexion, the metacarpal condylar surface is broad and the contact area is maximal between the metacarpal and proximal phalanx. The collateral ligaments are tight secondary to a cam effect and the necessity of the collaterals to pass around the metacarpal head prominences. The intracapsular fluid space is minimal, and the joint is highly stable secondary to bone and ligament configurations in the flexed position.

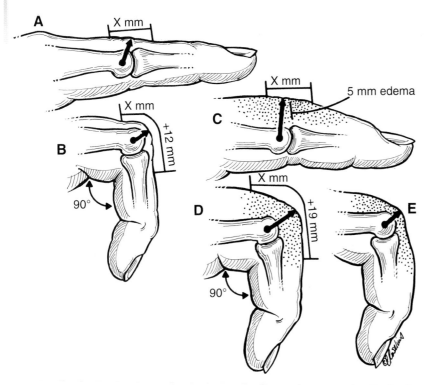

FIGURE 11-2. **A** and **B,** The dorsal skin requires 12 mm of lengthening for 90 degrees of flexion. **C** and **D,** With 5 mm of thickness secondary to edema, skin requires 19 mm of lengthening for 90 degrees of flexion. **E,** With application of slowly applied torque, the edema fluid shifts allowing the skin to cross closer to the joint axis, requiring less stretch. (Adapted from Brand PW: Clinical Mechanics of the Hand. St. Louis, Mosby, 1985, pp 61-87.)

minimally affected by the hydrostatic effect of edema, although skin tension does have some limiting effect (Fig. 11-2). In a normal IP digit, the dorsal skin requires 12 mm of lengthening for 90 degrees of flexion.[16,17] With as little as a 5-mm increase in thickness of the dorsal tissues secondary to edema, a digital joint needs 19 mm of lengthening to obtain 90 degrees of flexion. This is often impossible, owing not only to the limits of elasticity of normal skin but also to the secondary inelasticity of edematous skin and soft tissues.

Edema limits IP joint motion, but it has no effect on the position in which this stiffness occurs. Rather than edema, it is the MP joint that drives the characteristic position of the proximal interphalangeal (PIP) joint. The increase in flexor tension and decrease of extensor tension from MP joint extension causes the IP joints to flex, limited somewhat by the effect of edema discussed earlier. If left untreated, the posture of MP joint extension and IP flexion will result in fixed changes to both articular and extra-articular structures.[165]

Anatomy

Metacarpophalangeal Joint

The MP joint is a multiaxial condyloid joint that permits flexion, extension, abduction, adduction, and a slight degree of circumduction.[76] The joint consists of a capsule, two collateral ligaments, two accessory ligaments, and a volar plate (Fig. 11-3). The capsule about the joint is loose and is attached to the crest surrounding the articular surface of the head of the metacarpal and at the base of the proximal phalanx. The redundant capsule allows for the extensive motion of the

proximal phalanx on the metacarpal head and also allows for distraction as well as a minimal amount of rotation.

The collateral ligaments are situated on the radial and ulnar aspect of the joint and are quite substantial, measuring 1.5 to 3.0 mm thick and 4.0 mm to 8.0 mm wide. The collateral ligament arises from the depression in the subcapital area of

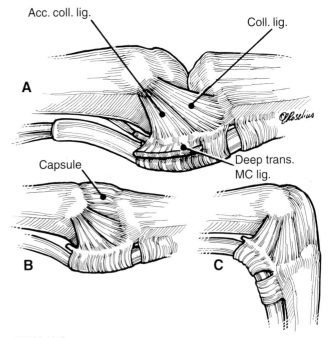

FIGURE 11-3. Ligament anatomy of the MP joint. **A,** The MP joint has an accessory and a proper collateral ligament on the radial and ulnar aspects of the joint. A capsule covers the dorsal aspect. **B,** In extension, the proper collateral ligament is lax, as is the dorsal capsule. **C,** In flexion, the proper collateral ligament and dorsal capsule are taut.

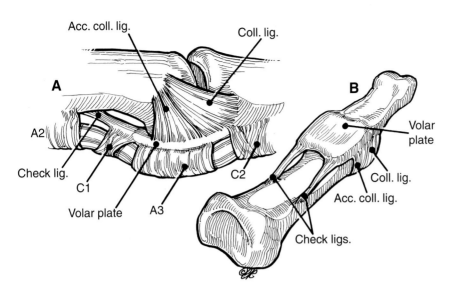

FIGURE 11-4 Anatomy of the PIP joint. **A,** Similar to the MP joint, the PIP joint has an accessory and proper collateral ligaments. **B,** The volar plate of the PIP joint is more defined and has two proximal extensions called checkrein ligaments.

the dorsal metacarpal head, courses distally toward the volar proximal phalanx, and has a length of 12 to 14 mm. The accessory ligament courses volar to the collateral ligament origin on the metacarpal head and fans out to blend in with the collateral ligament, attaching to the proximal phalanx and the volar plate.

The volar plate of the MP joint is composed of crisscrossing fibers that have the ability to collapse from the fully extended to the fully flexed position, diminishing its longitudinal length by one third to one half in full flexion.[165] The volar plate is the structure that ultimately restrains hyperextension. Normally, some degree of hyperextension is possible, but this varies considerably from one person to the next.

The shape of the metacarpal head is that of a cam with a volar flare. As the proximal phalanx is flexed, the cam and volar flare displace and lengthen the collateral ligaments and thus place them in the position of the greatest tension and the joint in its position of greatest stability.[165] Although the contours of the cam vary slightly from digit to digit, recognition of this cam effect is essential to understanding MP joint pathology.

Proximal Interphalangeal Joint

The PIP joint is a hinge, or ginglymus, joint whose configuration facilitates a wide arc of flexion and extension while resisting motion in the coronal plane. The stability of the joint is afforded not only by the geometry of the articular surfaces but also by the collateral ligaments and the volar plate (Fig. 11-4). The PIP joint is supported laterally by two layers of soft tissues. The superficial layer is thin and is made of the transverse and oblique fibers of the retinacular ligament of Landsmeer. The deeper and stouter layer is made of the collateral ligaments, which arise from the small recess in the proximal phalanx head and insert into the volar third of the middle phalanx and the volar plate. The accessory ligaments follow a similar path but run more obliquely and insert onto the sides of the volar plate. Unlike the MP joint, there is no cam or volar flare of the proximal phalanx head and the tension of the collateral ligaments is uniform throughout the arc of motion.

The volar plate of the PIP joint is also different from that of the MP joint (Fig. 11-5). There are two distinct regions of

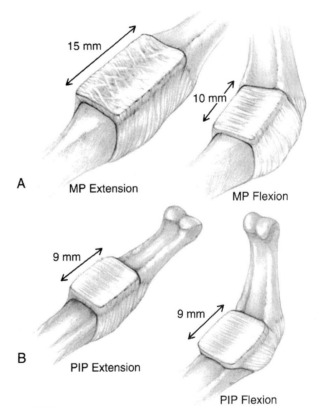

FIGURE 11-5. The volar plate. **A,** The volar plate of the MP joint is composed of crisscrossing fibers that have the ability to collapse from the fully extended to the fully flexed position. In flexion, the volar plate collapses to one third to one half of its length in full extension. The volar plate pocket behind the MP volar plate is smaller than at the IP joint; thus, there is no tendency for the development of checkreins. (Sagittal microscopic views demonstrate these bundles of fibers as compared with the more homogeneous collagenous arrangement in the IP volar plate.) **B,** The IP joint volar plate is similar to a unit in a suit of armor. It slides proximally and distally, protecting the joint. The volar plate is thick, allowing for extreme external loading over the joint. The pocket behind the proximal volar plate is large. The excursion of the volar plate between flexion and extension is significant, and collapse of the volar plate itself between extension and flexion is minimal. Any limitation or fixation of the proximal volar plate, as with the development of checkreins, produces a significant restriction in extension of the IP joint.

the volar plate of the PIP joint.[98,99] The distal portion is the articular portion, which is fibrocartilaginous and quadrangular; the proximal portion is thin and membranous. The distal lateral portions of the quadrangular volar plate form a confluence that anchors the collateral ligament and volar plate to the middle phalanx.

On either side of the volar plate there is an expansion that extends proximally and onto the volar margins of the proximal phalanx. These proximal extensions cross the transverse digital artery just proximal to the PIP joint and are variously referred to as checkreins, check ligaments, or swallowtail extensions (see Fig. 11-4).[43,163] This volar plate, unlike that of the MP joint, does not contract with flexion but rather slides proximally and distally with flexion and extension of the joint.[165] Thus, any limitation or adhesions of the proximal volar plate or contraction of the checkrein ligaments can result in significant limitation to extension of the PIP joint. Moreover, the checkrein structure limits hyperextension much more effectively than the looser arrangement of fibers at the MP joint, so that the IP joints typically hyperextend much less than the MP joints do.

Finally, dorsally, the joint capsule is closely connected to the central tendon, which provides a dorsal stabilizing force. The relationship is so intimate that the undersurface of the central tendon undergoes a fibrocartilaginous metaplasia and serves as an additional articulating structure for the proximal phalangeal head in flexion.[87,105]

Distal Interphalangeal Joint

The distal interphalangeal (DIP) joint is also a hinge, or ginglymus, joint (Fig. 11-6). A capsule surrounding the DIP joint is reinforced laterally by collateral ligaments that insert into the sides of the head of the middle phalanx and run in a distal and volar direction to insert into the volar lateral tubercle of the distal phalanx. Accessory ligaments are more volar and extend from the sides of the middle phalanx head to the sides of the volar plate. The volar plate serves as an accessory insertion point for the flexor digitorum profundus. Proximally the plate extends and is attached to the neck of

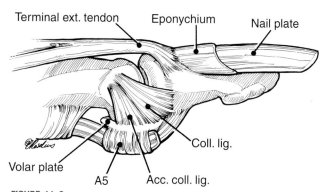

FIGURE 11-6. Anatomy of the DIP joint. The DIP joint is bound on the radial and ulnar sides by the accessory and proper collateral ligaments. The dorsal aspect of the joint is covered by the terminal extensor tendon, which inserts onto the distal phalanx.

the middle phalanx but, unlike the PIP joint, does not have lateral volar extensions. Not having checkrein ligaments, the DIP joint volar plate can hyperextend.[76] The dorsal aspect of the joint has no reinforcing ligament, but the terminal portion of the extensor mechanism attaches from the dorsal edge of one collateral ligament to the other and blends into the capsular fibers and the periosteum of the distal phalanx.

Intrinsic System

Anatomy of the hand does not change. Although our understanding of the meaning and fine details of that anatomy does change, the classic description of the intrinsic system of the hand by the late Richard J. Smith, MD, in previous editions of this textbook remains, in our opinion, the gold standard. In tribute to Dr. Smith's enduring contribution to hand surgery, we have preserved his description of the anatomy of the intrinsic system here, in his words.

The Interossei and Hypothenars

There are seven interosseous muscles: four dorsal and three volar (Fig. 11-7). The dorsal interossei are abductors. As the

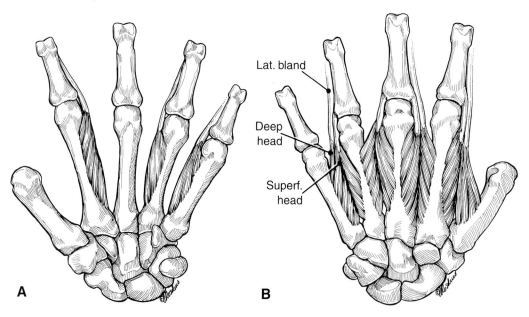

FIGURE 11-7. Anatomy of the interosseous muscles. **A,** The palmar interossei muscles are located on the ulnar side of the index metacarpal and on the radial aspect of the ring and small metacarpals and extend to the lateral bands of their respective digits. The middle finger has no palmar interosseous muscles. **B,** The dorsal interosseous muscles are bipennate muscles originating from the adjacent metacarpals of each web space.

anatomic axis of the hand coincides with the axis of the third metacarpal, the dorsal interossei lie to the radial side of the index and middle fingers and the ulnar side of the middle and ring fingers. The little finger is abducted by the abductor digiti quinti, which functions like an interosseous muscle. The volar interossei are adductors and lie to the ulnar side of the index finger and the radial side of the ring and little fingers. The middle finger therefore has two dorsal interossei (abductors) and no volar interossei (adductors) since the central axis of the hand lies within it.[76,133]

Each *dorsal interosseous muscle*, with the exception of the third, has two muscle heads. The *superficial head* arises most dorsally from the shaft of contiguous metacarpals and is inserted deeply by a *medial tendon* onto the lateral tubercle of the base of the proximal phalanx. The superficial head abducts and weakly flexes the proximal phalanx. It has no direct effect on the middle or distal phalanges. The *deep head* of each dorsal interosseous muscle forms a *lateral tendon*, or *lateral band*, at the level of the MP joint. The deep head flexes and weakly abducts the proximal phalanx and extends the middle and distal phalanges. At the level of the middle of the proximal phalanx, *transverse fibers* arch dorsally from each lateral band to join each other over the dorsum of the finger. These fibers flex the proximal phalanx. More distally, *oblique fibers* (spiral fibers) from the lateral bands sweep over the distal third of the proximal phalanx to insert onto the lateral tubercles at the base of the middle phalanx. The oblique fibers extend the middle phalanx. More distally the lateral bands are joined by the *lateral slips* of the extensor tendon to form the *conjoined lateral band*. The two conjoined lateral bands to each finger unite at the distal third of the middle phalanx to form the *terminal tendon*. The terminal tendon inserts at the base of the distal phalanx to extend it[83] (Figs. 11-8 and 11-9).

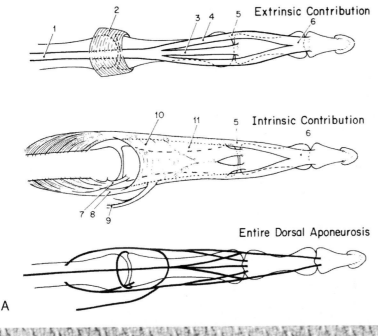

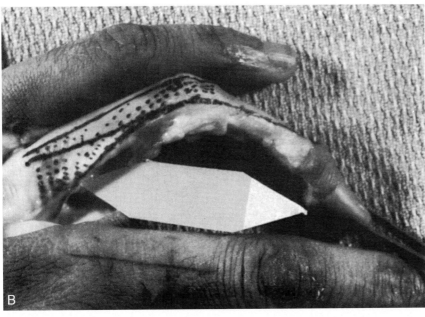

FIGURE 11-8. Lateral view of the dorsal aponeurosis of the finger. **A,** Diagram of the extrinsic contribution, the intrinsic contribution, and the entire dorsal aponeurosis of the finger. 1, Extensor tendon; 2, sagittal band; 3, central slip; 4, lateral slip; 5, conjoined lateral band; 6, terminal tendon; 7, superficial head and medial tendon of dorsal interosseous; 8, deep head and lateral tendon of dorsal interosseous; 9, lumbrical muscle and tendon; 10, transverse fibers of dorsal aponeurosis; 11, oblique fibers of dorsal aponeurosis. **B,** Dissected specimen showing the dorsal aponeurosis of the finger. The cardboard arrow points to the lateral band lying between the lateral tendon and the conjoined lateral band. Transverse and oblique fibers are dotted. Central slip, lateral slip, lateral band, and conjoined lateral band are identified by the continuous dark lines. The sagittal bands lie proximal to the dotted transverse fibers of the dorsal aponeurosis.

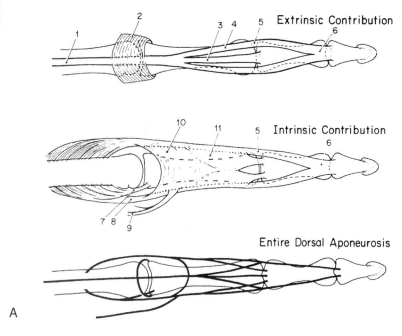

Extrinsic Contribution

Intrinsic Contribution

Entire Dorsal Aponeurosis

A

FIGURE 11-9. Dorsal view of the dorsal aponeurosis of the finger. **A,** Diagram of the extrinsic and intrinsic contributions of the dorsal aponeurosis. 1, Extensor tendon; 2, sagittal band; 3, central slip; 4, lateral slip; 5, conjoined lateral band; 6, terminal tendon; 7, superficial head and medial tendon of dorsal interosseous; 8, deep head and lateral tendon of dorsal interosseous; 9, lumbrical muscle and tendon; 10, transverse fibers of dorsal aponeurosis; 11, oblique fibers of dorsal aponeurosis. **B,** Dissected specimen showing the dorsal aponeurosis of the finger. The central slip, lateral slips, lateral band, and conjoined lateral band are identified by solid lines over the proximal phalanx. The conjoined lateral bands and terminal tendons are identified with continuous lines over the middle phalanx. The *dotted lines* represent the transverse fibers (proximally) and oblique fibers (distally) of the dorsal aponeurosis overlying the proximal phalanx.

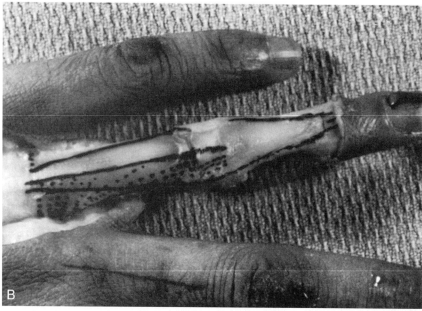

B

The *flexor digiti quinti brevis* is structurally and functionally similar to the deep head of the dorsal interossei. It forms the ulnar lateral band of the little finger.

The three *volar interossei* arise from adjacent surfaces of contiguous metacarpal shafts. Unlike the dorsal interossei, they each have only one muscle head; none of them inserts onto the proximal phalanx. The volar interossei form the ulnar lateral band of the index finger and the radial lateral band of the ring and little fingers. As with the lateral bands of the dorsal interossei, transverse fibers arch over the dorsum of the proximal phalanx and join those of the opposite lateral band to flex the proximal phalanx. All send oblique or spiral fibers to insert onto the base of the middle phalanx at its lateral tubercle. All lateral bands are joined by the lateral slips of the extensor tendon to form a conjoined lateral band and finally a terminal tendon that extends to the distal phalanx.

Of the *hypothenar muscles*, the *abductor digiti quinti* and *flexor digiti quinti brevis* have been described. These muscles are similar in both structure and function to the superficial and deep heads of the dorsal interossei, respectively, and arise from the fifth metacarpal. The abductor inserts onto the ulnar lateral tubercle at the base of the proximal phalanx of the little finger. The flexor digiti quinti forms the ulnar lateral band. A third muscle, the *opponens digiti quinti*, lies deepest. It arises from the pisohamate ligament and the hook of the hamate and inserts onto the ulnar side of the diaphysis of the fifth metacarpal, which it flexes and supinates.

The Lumbricals

The lumbrical muscles arise from the flexor digitorum profundus tendons in the palm. The lumbricals to the index and middle fingers arise from the radial side of the profundus tendons to these fingers (Fig. 11-10). The lumbricals of the

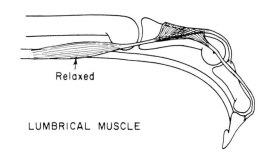

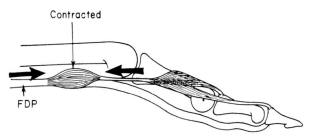

FIGURE 11-10. The lumbrical muscle arises from the FDP tendon. When the lumbrical is relaxed and the flexor profundus contracts, the IP joints flex. When the lumbrical contracts, it extends the IP joints through both relaxation of the profundus tendon distal to the lumbrical origin and the proximal pull on the lateral band and dorsal aponeurosis. (From Smith RJ: Intrinsic muscles of the fingers: Function, dysfunction and surgical reconstruction. *In* AAOS Instructional Course Lectures, vol 24. St. Louis, CV Mosby, 1975, pp 200-220.)

ring and little fingers arise from the profundus tendons of adjacent fingers. The tendon of each lumbrical passes volar to the deep transverse metacarpal ligament and joins the radial lateral band at the middle of the proximal phalanx. The lumbricals extend the PIP and DIP joints. They also assist in flexing the MP joint. When a lumbrical muscle contracts, it pulls the profundus tendon distally and the lateral band proximally. Thus, lumbrical contraction decreases the flexion force of the flexor digitorum profundus on the distal phalanx, and it can more effectively extend the IP joints.[6,76] By contrast, when the flexor profundus contracts and the lumbrical contracts as well, IP joint flexion may be limited (see Fig. 11-10).

Extrinsic Extensors

The *extrinsic extensors* join the dorsal aponeurosis at the level of the MP joint (Fig. 11-11).[59] The four extensor digitorum communis tendons and the extensor indicis proprius and extensor digiti quinti proprius tendons are the only extensors of the proximal phalanges. These tendons are loosely tethered to the dorsal joint capsule and the base of the proximal phalanx by a short leash of articular fibers, which helps hold the extensors at the midline of the MP joint. Normally, the articular fibers have little effect on MP joint extension.[76] In the region of the MP joint, a sling of sagittal (transverse) fibers, the *sagittal bands*, pass toward the palm from the extensors to insert onto the volar plate and the volar base of the proximal phalanx. The sagittal bands lie

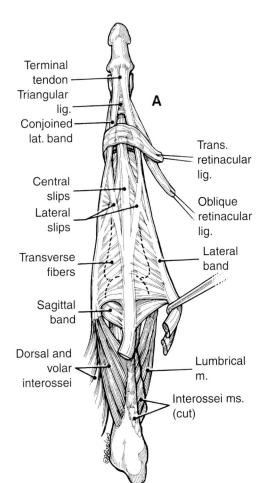

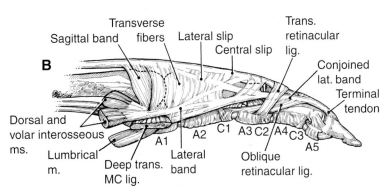

FIGURE 11-11. Dorsal (**A**) and lateral (**B**) extensor tendon anatomy.

deep to the lateral tendons of all the interossei and are superficial to the medial tendon of the dorsal interossei and to the joint capsule. When the extensor communis muscle contracts, the extensor tendons lift the proximal phalanx into extension through the sling of sagittal bands. Hyperextension of the proximal phalanx is restricted by the volar plate and the normal tone of the intrinsic muscles of the fingers.

On dissecting the dorsum of the finger, one might confuse the sagittal bands for the transverse fibers. Both structures are directed transversely and both lie in approximately the same plane at the dorsum of the finger. However, the sagittal bands arise from the extensor tendon at the MP joint and pass volarly into the volar plate and the base of the proximal phalanx; they extend the finger. The transverse fibers, more distally, arch dorsally from the lateral bands. They are not inserted onto bone; they flex the proximal phalanx.[129]

Distal to the MP joint the extensor tendon divides into three slips (see Fig. 11-11). The *central slip* inserts onto the base of the middle phalanx to extend it. The two *lateral slips* diverge beneath the oblique fibers of the dorsal aponeurosis and join the lateral bands at the distal end of the proximal phalanx. The combined tendon distal to the juncture of the lateral slip and lateral band is called the *conjoined lateral band*. The two conjoined lateral bands of each finger join each other proximal to the DIP joint and form the terminal tendon. The conjoined lateral bands are held dorsally by the *triangular ligament* that passes between them. Thus, the borders of the triangular ligament include the medial and lateral tubercles at the base of the middle phalanx and the conjoined lateral bands at its sides. The apex of the triangle is the juncture of the conjoined lateral bands where they form the terminal tendon. Laterally, the *transverse retinacular ligament* prevents the bands from bowstringing dorsally. These ligaments extend from the lateral sides of the conjoined bands to the fibro-osseous tunnel.[83,127,155]

EXAMINATION AND ETIOLOGY OF THE STIFF JOINT

The most important aspect in determining a treatment protocol, whether it be conservative or surgical, is the determination of the factors contributing to joint stiffness or contracture.* Those factors that limit flexion include scar contracture of the skin over the dorsum of the joint, contracted or adherent extensor tendons, contracted or adherent interosseous muscles, retinacular ligament adherent to the lateral capsular ligament, contracted collateral ligaments, volar plate adherence or contracture, bony block or exostosis, and joint incongruity.[40,41] The factors that limit extension include volar skin scarring, contraction or adhesion of flexor tendons, contraction of superficial fascia (Dupuytren's contractures), adherence of the retinacular ligament to the collateral ligaments, adhesions of lateral bands after their subluxation, and bony blocks or exostosis.[40,41] *The stiff finger secondary to flexor or extensor tendon adhesions, rheumatoid arthritis, Dupuytren's disease, neurologic causes, thermal injuries, congenital abnormalities, or chronic regional pain syndrome are addressed in their respective*

chapters. Finger stiffness secondary to intrinsic muscle contracture and articular and periarticular pathology is the focus of this chapter.

The first priority in examining the stiff finger joint is to note whether the limitation of joint movement is fixed or varies in response to the position of adjacent joints or muscle activation. In the presence of a joint that cannot move at all, it is difficult and often impossible to tell if the problem is due to joint incongruity, capsular contracture, tendon adhesions, or some combination of factors. If movement is possible but limited in flexion, extension, or both, it may be possible to begin localization of the etiology of stiffness but still may be difficult. As is shown later, often different elements of contracture are revealed only as others are released or otherwise resolved.

Active Versus Passive Motion

It is imperative to examine both active and passive motion. If passive motion exceeds active motion, one can be confident that the problem is at least in part musculotendinous: either the motor unit is incompetent or adherent or both. The presence of a contracture in this setting lends support to the presence of adhesions, but one cannot rule out incompetence (paralysis or tendon rupture). The adequacy of a motor unit can only be fully assessed once all contractures are resolved. Muscle testing can help identify any motor weakness. Magnetic resonance imaging (MRI) or ultrasound may be useful in identifying tendon or capsular injury.[44]

Of course, a contracture may also be present in circumstances in which active and passive motion are equal. In this case, the problem is more likely to be capsular or the result of a bony block to motion.[51,52] Radiographs may help identify articular incongruity or heterotopic ossification within the capsule. With the advent of 3-Tesla MRI, and the increased detail and definition it affords to cartilage and ligament structures, MRI will no doubt play an increasingly important role in the preoperative evaluation of the stiff finger joint (Fig. 11-12).

Intrinsic Contracture

In addition to a detailed examination of joint motion and motor function, a careful assessment of the effect of the position of adjacent joints is also important.[73,84] When a nonarticular contracting structure spans two joints, the *seesaw effect*, described by Watson and Weinzweig, can be seen.[165]

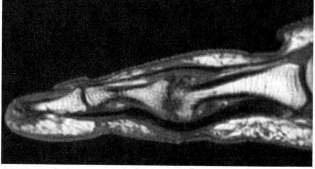

FIGURE 11-12. Three-Tesla MRI of a PIP joint shows the high-resolution imaging of the volar plate avulsion and articular cartilage changes.

---

*See references 40, 41, 63, 98, 99, 131, 132, 163, and 165.

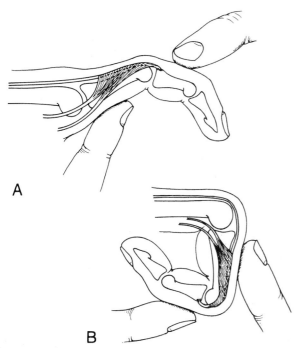

FIGURE 11-13. Intrinsic tightness (IT) test. In most cases of intrinsic tightness there is less flexion of the PIP joint when the MP joint is held extended (**A**) than when the MP joint is flexed (**B**). (From Smith RJ: Intrinsic muscles of the fingers: Function, dysfunction and surgical reconstruction. *In* AAOS Instructional Course Lectures, vol 24. St. Louis, CV Mosby, 1975, pp 200-220.)

When one joint is flexed, the other can be extended, and vice versa. By understanding this phenomenon, Bunnell described the intrinsic tightness tests.[25,27] The *Bunnell intrinsic tightness test* examines the effect of MP joint position on PIP joint flexion (Fig. 11-13). The test is considered positive when there is less flexion of the PIP when the MP joint is held extended than when the MP joint is flexed. A positive intrinsic test indicates that there is some element of intrinsic muscle tightness contributing to finger stiffness.

Lumbrical Contracture

It is not possible by this test to determine if the tightness is due to interosseous muscle pathology alone or to a combination of lumbrical and interosseous muscle pathology.[36] One can get an idea, however, by performing the test with the MP joint alternately radially and ulnarly deviated. If the tightness is symmetrical, then clearly more than the lumbrical is involved. If there is more tightness with ulnar deviation, however, a component of lumbrical tightness can be suspected. Additional information on lumbrical tightness can also be obtained if the Bunnell test result is normal. In such cases, limited active finger flexion may be present in the absence of a passive joint contracture due to lumbrical tightness alone. According to Colditz and colleagues, because the lumbrical fibers are most palmar, they participate more in distal joint extension.[36] Thus, lumbrical tightness can be evaluated by passively flexing not just the PIP joint, as in the Bunnell test, but in addition the DIP joint, making a passive hook grip. If this lumbrical tightness test is positive, and the Bunnell test is normal, then a specific contracture of the lumbrical muscle may be present.

Extrinsic Contracture

Extrinsic tightness of the extensor tendons or flexor tendons can be examined in a similar fashion.[40,41] To test for extensor tendon tightness, the wrist and the MP joints are flexed and passive flexion of the IP joints is assessed. In the normal state there is easy passive flexion of the IP joints. If extensor adhesions or tightness exists, the IP joints will have limited (or tight) flexion. Similarly, if IP extension is less with the wrist and MP joints extended, then an extrinsic flexor tightness may be the problem.

Oblique Ligament Tightness

Similar to the Bunnell intrinsic tightness test is the Landsmeer test, which elicits the findings of a tight oblique ligament of Landsmeer.[83] The ligament of Landsmeer extends from the dorsal insertion of the extensor tendon to the volar bony ridge of the proximal phalanx.[51,52,83] The ligament inserts dorsal to the axis of rotation of the DIP joint and is an extensor and originates volar to the axis of rotation of the PIP joint, where it is a flexor. Thus, DIP joint flexion can occur only if the PIP joint is flexed. Passive extension of the PIP joint brings the DIP joint into full fixed extension. As this ligament shortens, from injury or disease, it results in a combination of DIP joint extension and PIP joint flexion, similar to what one would see with a boutonnière deformity.

Application of these simple tests can assist in determining whether the etiology is within the intrinsic or extrinsic system or within the capsule and collateral ligament system.

Nonoperative Intervention

Nonoperative treatment of the stiff finger and hand should always precede any consideration of operative intervention. This involves a combination of modalities to decrease the edema within the digit, to rest the injured part to reduce inflammation, and then to obtain motion of the finger by application of low-load, prolonged stress to soft tissue through continuous or consecutive advancing adjustments.[54,81] Principal among these modalities are active and passive exercise, heat, cold, and splinting.

There are four types of splints available to the surgeon or therapist treating joint contractures in the hand. *Static* splints are used to maintain the hand and digits in one position and are worn either continuously to support healing tissue or removed periodically to exercise the injured hand. They are effective in minimizing external stresses and, when used as blocking splints, in confining movement within a specified range. *Serial static* splints are applied with the tissue at its maximum excursion and worn for a period of time. The splint is then removed after the tissues have accommodated to it, and additional stretching force is applied. A new splint is then applied again with the tissues at their new maximum excursion. *Dynamic splints* apply some sort of elastic traction, either through springs or rubber bands typically, and thus apply load while permitting motion (Fig. 11-14). Dynamic splinting is the treatment of choice when passive motion is responsive to manual stretch and when inflammation has subsided.[26] *Static progressive splints* are similar to dynamic splints except that motion is not possible within the splint. These splints often use the principle of three-point

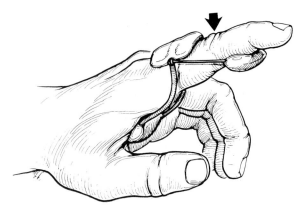

FIGURE 11-14. The LMB spring finger extension splint exerts its action solely on the PIP joint. Being less bulky than some other splints, it may be more acceptable for daytime use in the active or employed individual. Single or multiple splints of this type can be worn either as the sole splint or in conjunction with the Joint-Jack, with the latter being used at night.

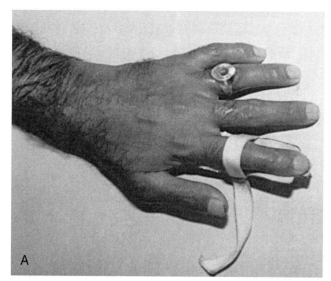

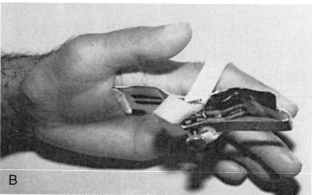

FIGURE 11-15. The Joint-Jack splint is an effective passive extension splint for PIP and DIP joint contractures. The splint produces a steady three-point extension moment on either the PIP or DIP joint. The pressure is vernier-controlled by the screw mechanism and will not produce skin necrosis, except in a digit that is lacking sensation.

force application. Examples of commercially available static progressive splints include the Joint Jack splint and Knuckle-Jack splint (Joint Jack Company, East Hartford, CT) (Fig. 11-15).

The different types of splints described are effective in the various stages of healing of the injured finger. Static splints are best applied during the acute phase, to allow soft tissues to heal and protect injured structures. Dynamic splinting is best applied at the end of the acute phase and during the proliferative stages of healing. Although dynamic splinting can be used in the early chronic phase, they are not as successful as the serial static splinting or static progressive splinting. Static progressive splinting is most useful in the chronic proliferative stages, whereas serial static splinting can be used in any phase of injury/healing. Our recommendation is to use static splints in the acute phase, and we prefer the static progressive splinting combined with dynamic splinting with night-time static splinting.

Alternating modalities to diminish edema and promote mobilization, with application of low-load, prolonged stress, coupled with active exercise with encouragement of functional use of the hand in light and moderate activities can often result in satisfactory results. It has been estimated that 87% of MP joint and PIP joint contractures can be successfully managed nonoperatively.[166] As long as there is continued positive progress, nonoperative treatment should continue. Only if a plateau has been reached and several weeks pass with no further improvement in range of motion, either active or passive, and the result is functionally unacceptable should surgical options be considered.

Nonoperative Treatment of MP Joint Contractures

As previously described, the anatomy of the MP joint is unique in that, in the extended position, the collateral ligaments are loose, the capsule is lax, and the joint contact area is minimal. This results in a large intrasynovial space and allows the joint to have motion in the coronal plane as well as rotational movement. When there is injury to this joint, the effect of soft tissue edema and intrasynovial joint fluid accumulation is to maneuver the joint into extension. If the injury is left untreated, an extension contracture of the MP joint will occur as fibrosis of the collateral ligaments and

capsule develops. Splinting the MP joint in the flexed position results in a diminished intrasynovial space and increased collateral ligament and capsular tension, which effectively maintains length of the collateral ligaments. Thus the best preventive treatment to reduce the risk of extension contracture of the MP joint is aggressive edema control, splinting (or occasionally even pinning) of the joint in flexion, and controlled mobilization once soft tissues and skeletal structures are stabilized. The converse problem of flexion contracture is much less common in the MP joints. When flexion contractures do occur, they are typically secondary to external abnormalities such as intrinsic muscle tightness or other extra-articular causes.

When confronted with a contracture of the MP joint that clinical examination and radiographs suggest is from collateral ligament or capsular fibrosis, splinting and aggressive hand therapy is the first line of treatment. Weeks and colleagues evaluated the conservative management of 212 patients with 789 stiff joints of the hand, of which 336 were MP joint contractures, using exercise and dynamic splinting.[166] There were 173 patients, or 87%, who responded favorably within 2 weeks of therapy with no further treatment necessary. The index finger gained an average of 35 degrees, the long finger an average of 40 degrees, the ring finger an average of 11 degrees, and the small finger an average of 42 degrees.

Our preference for conservative treatment of MP joint extension contractures is the use of a combination of dynamic daytime and static progressive night-time splinting. Whether the splints are custom made or are commercially available, when used by a diligent patient and knowledgeable therapist, improvement of motion is generally the norm. As long as improvement continues, nonoperative treatment should be continued.

Although in most normal hands the MP joint can be passively flexed to 90 degrees, it is important to recognize that this degree of flexion is rarely needed functionally. In grasp, the index and long MP joints flex usually to 75 degrees, while the ring and small MP joints flex to 80 or 85 degrees. Provided that the IP joints are supple, it is unusual for a patient whose MP joints can flex as much as 60 degrees to request or benefit from surgical release. Again, somewhat less flexion can be tolerated in the radial digits than in the ulnar ones.

Nonoperative Treatment of PIP Joint Contractures

Flexion Contractures. Limited extension, or flexion contractures, of the PIP joint can result from a variety of causes. The structures involved may include scar of the volar surface of the finger, contractures of the superficial fascia of the finger (as in Dupuytren's disease), contraction of the flexor tendon sheath within the finger, adherent flexor tendons or contracted flexor muscles, adherence of the retinacular ligaments of Landsmeer to the collateral ligaments, contraction of the volar plate, adherence of the collateral ligaments with the finger in the flexed position, a bony block or exostosis, or joint incongruity.[40] The treatment of Dupuytren's contractures and flexor tendon injuries and their complications are detailed in Chapters 5 and 7, respectively. Regardless of cause, however, the most common final pathway to flexion contracture is pathology of the volar plate complex. The anatomy of the volar plate of the PIP joint is unique in that its fibers are transverse and that there is little to no excursion of the volar plate in flexion or extension. On the most lateral margins of the volar plate are proximal-distal expansions known variously as the swallowtail ligaments or checkrein ligaments. After injury, these ligaments form thick collagenous bands linking the volar plate and the proximal phalanx and restrict extension of the joint.[163] Any injury that results in even slight shortening of these capsular structures can result in fibrosis and contracture,[26] despite the most rigid attention to proper splinting and hand therapy protocol.[40,41]

Splinting with dynamic techniques or serial casting is the mainstay of conservative treatment of PIP joint contractures. Although there are many splint designs, all rely on the principle that applied tension alters cell proliferation and elasticity of contracted tissues.[17,81,172] These splints vary in design, but the principle of proper use is invariable—the slow, steady application of an extension force perpendicular to the position of the flexed middle phalanx (which means constant adjustment of the line of pull as the contracture improves). Dynamic splinting should be applied for at least 1 hour several times per day. Pain that limits dynamic splinting to shorter times, or that requires narcotic medication for control, is a good sign that the applied load is too large and that the scar is being torn rather than stretched.

Static splinting is useful at night to maintain the gains obtained in the daytime. It is not advisable to wear dynamic splints at night because the position may slip during sleep and pressure sores may develop. So long as there is measurable progress, splinting should continue. As time passes, the force needed to obtain extension diminishes and flexion deformity of the digit occurs more slowly and less severely. Often several months are needed to achieve maximal correction. The surgeon should re-examine the patient at least monthly, continuing nonoperative treatment until improvement has reached a plateau.

An alternative nonoperative approach to the difficult flexion contracture is serial "casting" (with plaster, fiberglass, or thermoplastic material). Casts should be applied with sufficient force to obtain some correction but not so much that the digit is painful. The casts should be changed every few days so long as progress is being made.

The results of nonoperative management of PIP joint contractures have been reported by several authors. Weeks and colleagues reported on 453 PIP joint flexion contractures treated with active, passive, and resistive exercises in addition to dynamic and static splinting.[166] Eighty-seven percent of the joints responded to treatment such that no further treatment was necessary. Their pretreatment arc of range of motion improved from 42 to 76 degrees in the long finger, 40 to 75 degrees in the ring, and 39 to 71 degrees in the small finger.

Prosser published an outcome study of 20 patients with PIP joint flexion contractures, comparing a program of dynamic splinting with a Capener splint versus a low-profile outrigger splint.[115] Although there was no statistical difference between splint types, there was a statistically significant relationship between splinting time and final range of motion.

Hunter and colleagues[68] also demonstrated the efficacy of nonoperative treatment.

Extensor Contractures. Extensor tendon adhesions are the most common cause of extension contractures and are detailed in Chapter 6. The other structures that may limit flexion include scar contractures of the skin over the dorsum of the finger, dorsal capsular fibrosis, contracted or adherent intrinsic muscles and tendons, and bony deformity.[40] Clinical examination will elucidate if there are skin problems, extensor tendon adherence, or intrinsic tightness, whereas radiographs will determine if there is a joint incongruity.

Although PIP extension contractures are not uncommon, there are few published reports of results of conservative management.[68,166] As with flexion contractures, a combination of static and dynamic splints and stretching exercises is often helpful. Interosseous muscles can be stretched by putting the hand in the intrinsic minus position of MP extension and IP joint flexion. Both isolated PIP and combined PIP and DIP joint flexion stretches can be used.

Operative Treatment

Release of Contractures

The release of soft tissue contractures is indicated when residual joint motion is functionally disabling, there is a normal or relatively normal articular surface of the joint, the joint motors are intact, and all nonoperative modalities have been correctly applied and exhausted. Finally, surgical release of contracture requires a diligent, educated, and compliant patient who will follow the postoperative therapy regimen. Even with proper therapy, contractures often recur. Without dedicated compliance with the postoperative rehabilitation program, contracture recurrence is practically a certainty.

Release of MP Joint Extension Contractures

When nonoperative measures fail to gain flexion in the stiff MP joint, surgical intervention is often required.[21] Although it is true that the results of the surgical intervention often depend on the status of the articular cartilage, this is less true, at least in our experience, for the MP joint. Although there may be radiographic changes consistent with cartilage loss, if the MP joint remains congruent, it is frequently possible to salvage good range of motion.[40,41]

Capsulotomy and Collateral Ligament Release. In 1974, Buch[21] published the anatomic characteristics of the joint and ligaments and detailed the technique of capsulotomy and collateral ligament release using a technique first described by Curtis in Flynn's *Hand Surgery* in 1966.[40a] This technique uses a dorsal exposure, dividing the sagittal band off the extensor tendon to expose the capsule. A capsulotomy is made and the volar pouch is recreated using an elevator. The collateral ligaments are detached from their attachment from the metacarpal head and the joint is then flexed to 90 degrees. A meticulous closure is performed, being careful to maintain centralization of the extensor tendon. Postoperatively the MP joints are splinted in flexion. Mobilization is started 5 to 7 days after surgery.

Young and colleagues described a technique that involved use of Kirschner wire fixation of the joint in flexion for 2 weeks after the operation.[175] They described both volar and dorsal approaches. Their dorsal technique was similar to Buch's, with the exception that the extensor tendon is split longitudinally and the volar half of the collateral ligaments and accessory collateral ligaments preserved to maintain joint stability. The joint is pinned with a transarticular Kirschner wire in 90 degrees of flexion for 2 weeks, after which it is removed and therapy initiated. Their volar technique is used if the dorsal skin is moderately deficient but adequate to preclude skin grafting, flexor tenolysis is required, or later extensor tendon reconstructive surgery is planned. The volar technique uses a 2-cm longitudinal incision between the metacarpal heads. The lateral bands are traced proximally to the MP joint. The insertions of the collateral ligaments are detached and a segment excised. In comparing the dorsal and volar approaches, Weeks and colleagues reported that 44% of the joints in the volar approach gained more than 50 degrees of active motion, compared with just 16% in the dorsal group.[167]

Gould and Nicholson evaluated 105 MP joint capsulotomies performed in 37 patients using a dorsal approach similar to Buch's technique.[57] The average gain of flexion was 21 degrees. When only fracture and crush injuries were considered, the average gain of flexion was 18 degrees, despite obtaining 90 degrees of flexion at the time of surgery. They concluded that (1) the end result is a lot less than the gain obtained at surgery but (2) the small gain makes the operation worthwhile.

Authors' Preferred Method of Treatment For MP Extension Contractures

Despite Weeks and colleagues' results, showing that a volar approach was superior to a dorsal approach, we prefer a dorsal approach to the MP joint to release the collateral ligaments and perform a capsulotomy (Fig. 11-16). The approach is direct and allows direct visualization of the collaterals, the dorsal capsule, and the joint. Longitudinal incisions over the MP joint will allow exposure of the extensor mechanism, the joint, and collateral ligaments. If multiple MP joints are to be approached, we prefer to approach each joint through its own longitudinal incision rather than a transverse incision across the MP joints. Transverse incisions may gap or restrict flexion under the stress of postoperative therapy. Unless very extensive surgery on multiple fingers is advised, we prefer local anesthesia with sedation, because this allows an assessment of active motion intraoperatively.

Through the dorsal incision, the extensor tendon is split sharply in the midline and elevated off the capsule, reflecting the extensor tendon and sagittal band radially and ulnarly. A "T"-shaped incision is made into the dorsal capsule, taking care not to injure the articular surfaces. The

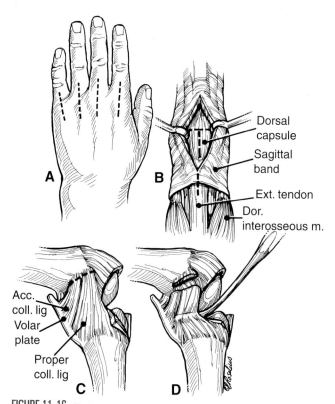

FIGURE 11-16. Technique for MCP capsulotomy, collateral ligament release. **A,** Through longitudinal dorsal incisions centered over the MP joints, the skin is incised and mobilized. **B,** The extensor tendon is split and carefully elevated with the sagittal band exposing the dorsal joint capsule. A transverse incision is made in the distal aspect of the capsule, and a longitudinal incision is made to create a "T" capsulotomy. **C,** The collateral ligament insertions are released off the metacarpal. **D,** An elevator is used to re-create the pouch between the volar plate and the metacarpal.

dorsal capsule and dorsal half of the collateral ligaments are excised. The joint is then passively flexed. If the remaining collateral ligament is unable to pass over the condyles of the metacarpal head, they are detached from their origin on the metacarpal head. Although satisfactory flexion can be obtained by detaching the ulnar collateral ligament alone, it is often necessary to detach both collateral ligaments to prevent abnormal rotation as flexion occurs.

Once the collateral ligaments have been released, an elevator is used to free any adhesions between the volar plate and the volar capsule. Passive motion is tested again. Occasionally the MP joint will jump or trigger as the joint reaches full extension. In such cases, any remaining accessory collateral ligament should be divided.

The extensor tendons are then examined for their excursion and possible adhesions. The operation should be done under neurolept anesthesia (see Chapter 2), for ideally the completeness of the release is ascertained by releasing the tourniquet and asking the patient to actively move the affected finger. If a block or general anesthesia has been used, a proximal traction check will be needed. In either case, if the extensor tendons do not glide freely, a tenolysis should be performed.

The extensor tendon incision is then closed with buried and interrupted 4-0 nonabsorbable suture, and the hand is placed in a bulky dressing with dorsal and volar plaster splints holding the MP joints in 70 degrees of flexion. Although other authors have recommended pin fixation of the MP joints to maintain flexion,[175] we do not routinely use pin fixation after contracture release (although we do occasionally find it useful in the acute management of the massively swollen hand, such as after a severe crush injury).

Postoperative Management. Elevation of the hand is encouraged for the next 72 to 96 hours, at which time the dressing is removed and two custom-made orthoplast splints are fabricated. A resting volar static splint holds the MP joints in the maximum flexion obtained in surgery. This splint is used at night. A dynamic flexion assist splint is used during the day. The splints are used in conjunction with a closely monitored therapy program until the patient is able to actively obtain the range of motion, it is hoped, to the degree that was obtained intraoperatively. Generally, this takes several months. Although many authors state that passive range of motion obtained at the time of surgery is approximately the active range of motion that can be expected at the conclusion of postoperative therapy, our personal experiences have not been as gratifying. Despite obtaining full passive motion at the time of surgery, our experience has been that the final active range of motion has been approximately half of what was obtained intraoperatively.

Complications. Complications can occur secondary to surgical technique, postoperative therapy, patient compliance and selection, or surgical timing. With respect to surgical technique, ulnar deviation of the digits may occur if there is imbalance in release of the collateral ligaments, especially if the radial collateral ligament is released to a greater degree than the ulnar ligament. Disruption of the extensor tendon mechanism can occur if therapy is too aggressive, if sufficient extensor tenolysis is not performed, or if the suture technique to close the extensor tendon is inadequate. The

joint may become stiff or ankylose if the contractures were not properly or adequately released during surgery or if there were difficulties with compliance with therapy after surgery. In the current medical environment, this latter problem may be a result not only of patient attendance or therapist competence but also of insurance denials. Thus we consider it essential to confirm preoperatively that a compliant patient and competent therapist will be permitted to work together and that the postoperative therapy visits are indeed recognized by all concerned parties as being an essential part of the treatment plan. If all three conditions (i.e., willing patient, capable therapist, third party approval where that is required) are not met, the decision to proceed with surgery should be reconsidered.

PIP Joint Flexion Contractures

When conservative measures fail to improve a flexion contracture of the PIP, and the joint remains functionally inadequate, surgical intervention may be indicated. If there are volar skin contractures, "Z"-plasties or excision of scar and coverage with vascularized skin flaps such as a cross-finger flap should be considered.[72] Flexor tendon pathology should also be addressed. However, whereas there are many causes for flexion contractures, the main problem is typically the volar plate and its proximal checkrein expansions.*

Surgical approaches to the PIP joint have been well described in the literature. All use either the volar zigzag Bruner incision or the midaxial approach.

The use of local anesthesia with intravenous sedation (neurolept anesthesia, see Chapter 2) is preferred to allow the patient to actively flex and extend the joint after release of contractures. This enables immediate evaluation of the effectiveness of the procedure and any fine tuning or additional releases can be performed if full extension is not obtained. If neurolept anesthesia with sedation is not possible, an arm block or general anesthesia can be used but then the effectiveness of the releases cannot be thoroughly evaluated intraoperatively.

Volar Surgical Approach. A standard Bruner incision is made from the distal phalangeal crease to the digital-palmar skin crease, and the skin flaps are elevated, taking care not to devitalize the corner. The radial and ulnar neurovascular bundles are identified and protected. The flexor tendon sheath is opened on a lateral hinge from the distal aspect of the A2 pulley to the proximal aspect of the A4 pulley, and the flexor tendons are carefully retracted, preserving the vincula. The checkrein ligaments are identified (Fig. 11-17).[163] An anatomic landmark to the checkrein ligaments is the transverse digital artery, which passes underneath the checkrein ligament 3 mm proximal to the joint. The checkrein ligaments are released, sparing the transverse digital arteries. An attempt at passive extension of the joint is then made. If full passive extension is not achieved, a capsular release is then performed, releasing the volar plate complex and accessory collateral ligaments. If the contracture still persists, the rest of the collateral ligament is detached from the proximal phalanx. It is very valuable at this point to check

---

*See references 40, 41, 98, 99, 116, 131, 132, 163, 165, and 167.

CRITICAL POINTS: MP JOINT EXTENSION CONTRACTURE RELEASE

INDICATIONS

- Failure to obtain MP joint flexion after dedicated hand therapy protocol
- Absence of arthritic changes within the MP joint
- Absence of external abnormalities—intrinsic contractures, extensor tendon adhesions

PREOPERATIVE EVALUATION

- Perform a thorough clinical examination.
- Rule out causes external to the joint.
- Obtain radiographs to evaluate for degenerative changes.

PEARLS

- It is imperative to confirm preoperatively that a compliant patient, a competent therapist, and third party approval (when required) are present before proceeding with surgery.
- The patient must understand that postoperative care is an essential part of the treatment plan.
- Range of motion at surgery overestimates the final outcome.

TECHNICAL POINTS

- Local anesthesia with sedation allows assessment of active motion intraoperatively.
- Authors prefer a dorsal extensor tendon splitting approach.
- Excise the dorsal capsule and dorsal half of collaterals.

- If unable to obtain full flexion, detach remaining collaterals off metacarpal heads.
- Release adhesions between the volar plate and volar capsule with a Freer elevator.
- Test motion. If jumping exists, release accessory collaterals as needed.
- Examine extensor tendons for excursion, because they may also prevent full flexion.
- Assess active motion by patient.
- Closure of the extensor tendon is with nonabsorbable sutures.
- Plaster splints (dorsal and volar) are used to maintain 70 degrees of flexion at MP joints.

PITFALL

- Motion obtained intraoperatively will be the "best case" scenario.

POSTOPERATIVE CARE

- Elevation of the finger for 3 to 4 days
- Early removal of dressings (4 to 5 days) with fabrication of two custom-made splints, volar static with MP joints at maximum flexion, and dynamic flexion splint
- Aggressive supervised therapy

ATHLETIC PARTICIPATION

- Protect in splints until stable range of motion is obtained (typically 2 to 3 months).

---

active motion, provided the patient has agreed to surgery under local anesthesia with sedation. It is impossible to know if an extensor tenolysis will be needed in the presence of a flexion contracture. Thus, active extension always needs to be checked after flexion contracture release, and the patient must be advised preoperatively of the possible need of extensor tenolysis.

The tourniquet is then deflated and hemostasis is achieved. Any hematoma will encourage the formation of a new contracture, and the swelling will impair postoperative rehabilitation. The vascularity of the digit must be carefully monitored during closure and postoperative positioning, because overstretching of the neurovascular tissues may result in spasm and an ischemic digit.[165] Postoperatively, the finger should be splinted in the maximum safe extension for 3 to 5 days. Kirschner wire fixation of the joint in extension is used only occasionally to maintain the release for a short period of time while soft tissues accommodate to the new position. If there is excessive pressure to maintain extension on the joint, placement of the Kirschner wire can result in cartilage necrosis.[48,51,52]

After the dressings are removed, a light dressing is applied and active range-of-motion exercises are begun. Dynamic and static resting splints are fabricated and used for 3 to 4 months, or until gains in motion plateau.

Surgical Midlateral Approach (Fig. 11-18). A midlateral skin incision is made extending from the midshaft of the proximal phalanx to the midshaft of the middle phalanx. The neurovascular bundle is identified and retracted palmarly. The transverse retinacular ligament is divided, and the accessory collateral ligament and volar plate are visualized. Although a unilateral incision is preferred, a bilateral incision can be utilized if exposure of the contralateral collateral ligament is difficult. Once exposure is achieved, the operation proceeds as described for the volar approach.

A variation of the midaxial approach is the total anterior tenoarthrolysis (TATA) procedure described by Saffar and associates.[55,114,120] In the TATA procedure, a midaxial approach that extends from the web space to the fingertip is utilized. Dissection is carried down to the middle and proximal phalanges, dorsal to the neurovascular bundle and deep to

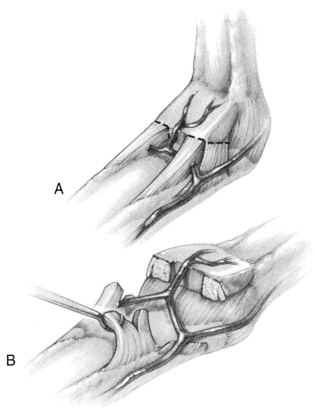

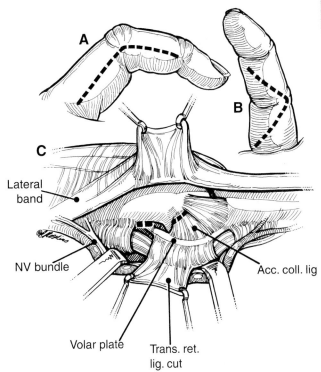

FIGURE 11-17. Checkrein pathologic bands. **A,** The checkreins attach proximally to the assembly line and distally to the volar plate on both the radial and ulnar sides. The transverse communicating vessels traverse the collagen band approximately 2 mm proximal to the volar plate. **B,** Complete excision of the checkreins often requires resection dorsal as well as volar to the transverse communicating vessels. These vessels should be preserved.

FIGURE 11-18. Flexion contracture release at the PIP joint can be performed through a midlateral approach (**A**) or a volar Bruner approach (**B**). Although technically easier, the results of a volar Bruner approach have been shown to result in less favorable results. Therefore, a midlateral or a bilateral midlateral approach is favored by the authors. **C,** The transverse retinacular ligament is divided and the lateral aspect of the joint is visualized. The volar plate checkrein ligaments are released first and then the accessory collateral ligaments are cut at their origins on both the radial and ulnar aspects of the joint. If motion is not improved, the proper collateral ligament is also released.

the extensor mechanism. The periosteum is incised and is elevated from the anterior surface of the middle and proximal phalanges. The insertion of the flexor digitorum superficialis is released, but the pulleys are left intact. The PIP joint is released via a lateral approach to the joint. The volar plate is released along with its periosteal attachments, and the accessory collateral ligaments are released on the radial and ulnar aspects of the joint. The DIP joint volar plate and the insertion of the profundus tendon may also need to be released to obtain full extension. Occasionally, it may be necessary to gain extension by completely releasing the true collateral ligaments.

Postoperatively, the dressing is removed at 3 days and active motion is encouraged. Two splints are made at that time, one for extension and one for flexion, and are alternated every 8 hours. At the end of the first postoperative week, formal hand therapy is instituted. The splints are used for 2 months, and night-time splinting is continued for 6 months.

Results of Surgical Treatment of Flexion Contracture of the PIP Joint. In 1954, Curtis reported on 25 patients with PIP flexion contractures who had a midlateral exposure, capsulectomy, collateral ligament excision, and volar plate

elevation followed by Kirschner wire fixation for 5 to 7 days.[40] He reported that the more anatomic structures that were involved in the limitation of motion, the poorer the end result. If the only limiting factor was the capsular ligaments, then release of the collateral ligaments gave a good result. Curtis summarized his findings by stating that restoration of complete motion by his technique is not expected but that improvement of function can be anticipated. Typically about half of the intraoperative gain is maintained. Using Curtis's technique, Rhode and Jennings [116] were able to obtain similar results. Sprague was not as enthusiastic in his reports of the Curtis technique[131,132] but echoed Curtis's finding that the more structures involved, the worse the outcome.[4,40,41,131,132] In joints that had had capsulotomy, excision of collaterals, volar plate excision, and release of extensor mechanism adhesions, the results were disheartening. The initial gain intraoperatively was just 30 degrees, of which 90% was lost in the postoperative period. Sprague concluded, and others have agreed, that surgical release of the severely contracted PIP joint yields unpredictable results and should be considered only when both surgeon and patient understand its limitations clearly.[60,121,131,132]

Saffar reported on 72 cases of the TATA procedure. Of the 72 cases, only 56 patients had enough follow-up to be reported. He reported that the PIP gained an average extension of 40 degrees.[119] However, the preoperative contractures were not reported, and the report also included patients with Dupuytren's contractures. Complications included skin necrosis and early recurrence when therapy was neglected.

Bruser and associates compared the use of a midlateral versus a palmar incision in contracture releases for the PIP joint in 1999.[20] Their study of 45 joints demonstrated an average of 30 to 50 degrees of increased motion at 1.5 years of follow-up. The midlateral group had an average improvement of 50 degrees, whereas the volar group had an increase of 30 degrees. The differences were found to be statistically significant.

In an effort to identify which demographic, preoperative, and intraoperative factors affected outcome of contracture release, Ghidella and colleagues performed a review of 68 PIP joints that had been released.[56] The average improvement with a minimum of 24-month follow-up was 7.5 degrees. Based on their analysis, the best candidates for surgical release were younger than 28 years of age with an uncomplicated contracture who had a preoperative maximal flexion of less than 43 degrees.

External Fixation Devices. The benefit of external fixation is the ability to apply a constant force to the contracted tissues through bone, rather than through application of pressure through the skin. The use of external fixation devices for flexion contractures secondary to Dupuytren's disease has been reported with good success.[7-9,35,64,77,102,103] The continuous extension technique (TEC) device, introduced in 1986 and reported on in 1991 by Messina, has been applied to significant Dupuytren's contractures of the PIP joint (Fig. 11-19). The results in resolving contractures of this joint were impressive.[102,103] The application of external fixation to flexion contractures not associated with Dupuytren's disease has not been as well described.[8,121]

The use of the Compass Hinge (Smith & Nephew Richards, Memphis, TN) in 20 patients with joint contractures of the PIP joint secondary to fractures, dislocations, and contractures was published in 1998.[8] Although the initial range of motion was not reported, the final range of motion after a mean wearing of the device for 42 days averaged 12 to 86 degrees. Complications included septic arthritis, pin tract infections, and breakage of the hinge. In 2002, 27 patients with contractures treated with the Compass Hinge alone were reported by Houshian and associates.[66] After an average application of 33 days, the mean extension gain was 38 degrees and the mean flexion-extension arc improved by 42 degrees. Complications included superficial pin tract infection in 11 cases and pin loosening in four cases.

A device that utilizes extension torque rather than a distractive force like the previously described devices was introduced in 2001 (Agee J, personal communication). This device, called the Digit Widget (Hand Biomechanics Laboratory, Sacramento, CA), allows range of motion of the PIP joint during the application of extension torque via a series of rubber bands that are applied to the device (Fig. 11-20). The results of the Digit Widget have yet to be reported, but in the authors' personal experience in a small number of cases the device has been simple to apply and maintain and good results have been obtained.

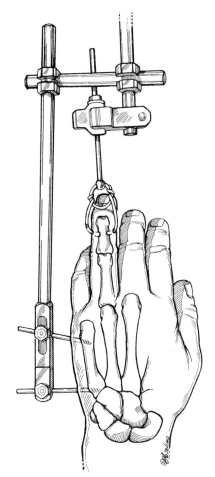

FIGURE 11-19. The Messina device is an external-type fixator that is anchored to the metacarpal and the middle phalanx. Sequential extension results in stretching of the PIP joint contracture.

Authors' Preferred Method of Treatment for DIP Flexion Contractures

Before an open release, application of the Digit Widget is preferred by one of us (AYS). In our experience with this device, we have successfully avoided open release in a majority of flexion contractures of the PIP joint. Once the Digit Widget is applied, sequential rubber bands are applied over a 3- to 4-week period and range-of-motion therapy is performed daily. The device is then removed, and dynamic splinting is applied during the daytime and static extension splinting is used at night for an additional 4 to 8 weeks. Although the results and the maintenance of motion of the Digit Widget have yet to be reported, our experience has been favorable.

If an open release is to be performed, we prefer a midlateral approach to the PIP joint as described by Bruser and colleagues.[20] The checkrein ligaments are released, sparing the transverse digital arteries. An attempt at passive extension of the joint is then made. If full passive extension is not achieved, a capsular release is then performed, releasing the volar plate complex and accessory collateral ligaments. If

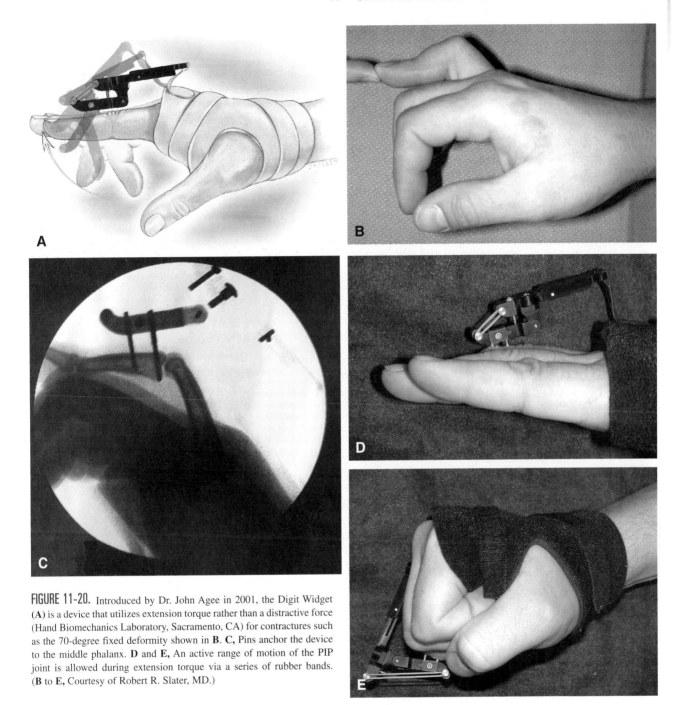

FIGURE 11-20. Introduced by Dr. John Agee in 2001, the Digit Widget (**A**) is a device that utilizes extension torque rather than a distractive force (Hand Biomechanics Laboratory, Sacramento, CA) for contractures such as the 70-degree fixed deformity shown in **B**. **C,** Pins anchor the device to the middle phalanx. **D** and **E,** An active range of motion of the PIP joint is allowed during extension torque via a series of rubber bands. (**B** to **E,** Courtesy of Robert R. Slater, MD.)

the contracture still persists, the rest of the collateral ligament is detached from the proximal phalanx.

Authors' Preferred Method of Treatment for PIP Extension Contractures

Surgery for extension contractures of the PIP joint is best performed under local anesthesia with sedation (neurolept anesthesia). This enables testing of the contracture release using the patients own volitional control of his or her muscles and allows fine tuning of contracture releases. Active motion by the patient is also the best way to determine if a flexor tenolysis is required. The operative approach for extension contractures can be from a dorsal or midlateral approach (Fig. 11-21). The extensor mechanism is exposed, and the transverse fibers of the retinacular ligament are identified and longitudinally divided on either side of the central tendon. The extensor tendon is then elevated, with care being taken to avoid injury to the central slip insertion. This provides exposure of the dorsal capsule and the collateral ligaments. An extensor tenolysis can also be done at this time, continuing as far proximal and distal as needed to free the tendon from underlying bone and overlying skin. The dorsal

CRITICAL POINTS: PIP JOINT FLEXION CONTRACTURE RELEASE

INDICATIONS

- Failure to obtain PIP joint flexion after dedicated hand therapy protocol
- Absence of arthritic changes within the PIP joint
- Absence of external abnormalities—flexor tendon adhesions, volar skin contractures

PREOPERATIVE EVALUATION

- Perform a thorough clinical examination.
- Rule out causes external to the joint.
- Obtain radiographs to evaluate for degenerative changes.

PEARLS

- It is imperative to confirm preoperatively that a compliant patient, a competent therapist, and third party approval (when required) are present before proceeding with surgery.
- The patient must understand that postoperative care is an essential part of the treatment plan.
- Range of motion at surgery overestimates final outcome.

TECHNICAL POINTS

- Surgical exposure: volar is easier to visualize and release structures; midlateral has better reported range of motion but is more difficult to release opposite side.
- Local anesthesia with sedation allows assessment of active motion intraoperatively.

- Visualization of the checkrein ligaments is essential. Landmark is the transverse digital artery that passes underneath the ligament 3 mm proximal to the joint.
- Divide checkrein ligament—check motion.
- If full passive extension is not obtained, release the volar plate and then the accessory collateral ligaments from the proximal phalanx.
- Complete collateral ligament release may be necessary if full extension is not obtained after releasing the volar plate and accessory collateral ligaments.
- Protective soft dressing with volar plaster splint is applied, avoiding overstretching of the neurovascular bundles.

PITFALLS

- Evaluate flexor tendon excursion and perform tenolysis as needed.
- Perform meticulous hemostasis before closure.

POSTOPERATIVE CARE

- Elevation of the joint for 3 to 4 days
- Early removal of dressings (4 to 5 days) with fabrication of two custom-made splints, volar static with PIP joints at maximum safe extension, and dynamic extension splint
- Aggressive supervised therapy

ATHLETIC PARTICIPATION

- Protect in splints until stable range of motion is obtained (typically 2 to 3 months).

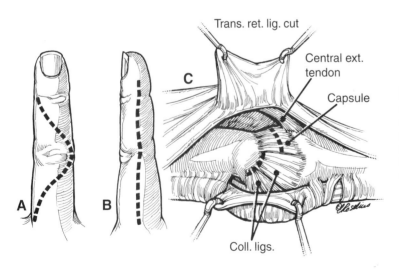

FIGURE 11-21. Extension contracture release of the PIP joint can be performed through a dorsal curvilinear (**A**) or midlateral (**B**) approach. Once the skin is elevated and mobilized, the transverse retinacular ligament is divided, exposing the joint (**C**). An extensor tenolysis is performed, and a dorsal capsulotomy is made. The collateral ligaments are then released at their insertion on the proximal phalanx.

capsule is excised, and range of motion of the joint is assessed. If full easy flexion is not possible, the most dorsal fibers of the collateral ligaments should be released. If full flexion is still not obtained, the rest of the collateral ligaments are released off the proximal phalanx origin. Diao and Eaton[42a] have shown that complete excision of both collateral ligaments can be done to correct extension contractures without creating joint instability.

Once passive flexion is satisfactorily obtained, the patient is asked to voluntarily flex the digit to determine if there are any extrinsic causes of blocked flexion. It is impossible to know if a flexor tenolysis will be needed in the presence of an extension contracture. Thus, active flexion always needs to be checked after contracture release and the patient must be advised preoperatively of the possible need of flexor tenolysis. If the patient does not tolerate local anesthesia with sedation, the procedure can be done under regional or general anesthesia and a small incision in the distal forearm can be made and the flexor tendons manually pulled to verify the joint's ability to fully flex.

No discussion of PIP extension contractures is complete without mentioning the possibility of intrinsic contractures. After surgical release is performed, Bunnell's intrinsic tightness test is performed to determine if there is contracture of the intrinsic elements. If positive, release of the intrinsics should be performed as described in the intrinsic tightness section (see p. 425).[98] Again, if possible, active hook grip should also be tested, to detect more subtle degrees of intrinsic tightness that might respond to stretching postoperatively.

An alternative to capsulotomy is the release of lateral bands on either side of the central slip, followed by a gentle passive flexion maneuver described by Inoue.[70] In this technique, the passive flexion breaks up adhesions of the extensor tendon and intra-articular adhesions. A dorsal extension block Kirschner wire prevents active extension beyond the desired flexed position, and active flexion exercises are initiated immediately postoperatively. The wire is removed at 2 weeks, and vigorous flexion exercises are initiated with a dynamic flexion splinting device. The results of 10 patients treated in this manner demonstrated an average gain of 47.5 degrees of flexion without complications.

Results of release of extension contractures have been reported by Mansat and Delprat.[98] In a multicenter study in 10 institutions in France, 246 contracture releases were performed of the PIP joint, of which extension contractures comprised 45% of cases. The average improvement of flexion was 28 degrees, with a preoperative range of motion of 19 to 34 degrees as compared with a postoperative range of motion of 8 to 62 degrees.

Contractures of the DIP Joint

Stiffness or contractures of the DIP joint are seldom problematic unless a fixed flexion or hyperextension deformity exists.[165] Treatment of the underlying etiology of the deformity, such as a swan neck or boutonnière deformity, will often resolve the stiffness of the DIP joint. Fixed extension contractures can be treated by dividing the most dorsal and lateral fibers of the extensor tendon. Fixed flexion contractures, such as chronic mallet deformities, are best managed by arthrodesis rather than tendon reconstruction. The role of contracture release about the DIP joint is very limited.

Release of Intrinsic Contractures

The classic description of the surgical treatment of intrinsic contractures of the hand by the late Richard J. Smith, MD, in previous editions of this textbook remains, in our opinion, the gold standard on this subject. Again, in tribute to Dr. Smith's enduring contributions to hand surgery, we have included his description of the surgical techniques for release of intrinsic contractures of the hand, in his own words.

Intrinsic Contracture After Trauma. Post-traumatic interosseous contracture is usually caused by edema, prolonged immobilization, or muscle ischemia. *Hematoma* and *edema* fluid envelop the interosseous muscles after severe hand injuries. This fluid fills the interosseous muscle compartment and is trapped by the firm dorsal and volar interosseous fascia. Capillary compression and venous stasis add to the congestion. The fingers move little because of pain. If a compressive bandage or circular cast further impedes venous drainage, the interossei develop a myostatic contracture in their viscid environment. When edema finally subsides, fibrosis supervenes.

Late Post-traumatic Intrinsic Contracture of the PIP Joint. Several months after injury to the wrist or hand, many patients will have persistent limited flexion of the PIP joints. The surgeon may suspect that the limited motion is due to intra- or periarticular adhesions or post-traumatic synovitis. Often the cause is residual intrinsic contracture. In order to flex the MP joints, intrinsics must stretch the collateral ligaments. With diffuse edema these ligaments are tight and resist stretching. However, there is no resistance to PIP extension, because the collateral ligaments relax with extension. The swollen collateral ligaments of the injured finger therefore resist MP flexion but not PIP extension. The MP joint is unaffected. There is an extension contracture at the PIP joint, and the intrinsic tightness test is positive.

It is not necessary to release the entire intrinsic aponeurosis in these patients. Because only PIP joint flexion is limited, only the oblique fibers of the lateral bands are resected. This is known as a *distal intrinsic release*[58] (Fig. 11-22).

Technique of Distal Intrinsic Release. Local anesthesia is infiltrated dorsal to the proximal phalanx. A longitudinal incision is made along the dorsal midline of the distal half of the proximal phalanx. The lateral bands, oblique fibers, and central and lateral slips of the dorsal aponeurosis are identified. The lateral band and oblique fibers are resected at the distal third of the proximal phalanx. The central slip, the lateral slips of the extensor tendon, and the transverse fibers of the intrinsic aponeurosis should not be resected.[58] Postoperatively, the MP joints are splinted in extension for 3 weeks. Active and passive assisted interphalangeal flexion exercises are begun within 1 day of surgery.

Late Post-traumatic Interosseous Contracture of the MP and PIP Joints. Severe prolonged deep-space edema of the hand will cause interosseous muscle necrosis and fibrosis.[25,27] With unrelenting contracture of the scarred muscle remnant, deformities develop at both the MP and IP joints. When there has been extensive edema of the hand, the collateral ligaments of the MP joints are swollen and resist stretching. Thus, it is only with the most severe interosseous

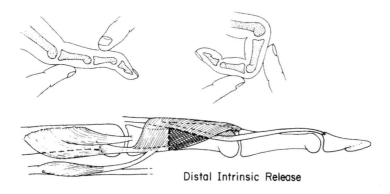

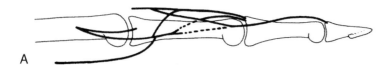

Distal Intrinsic Release

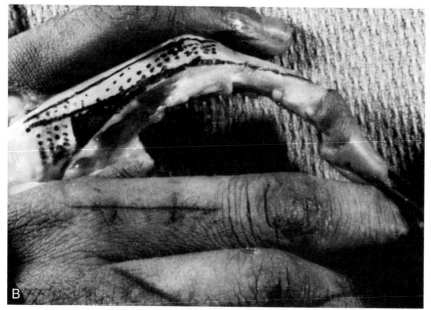

A

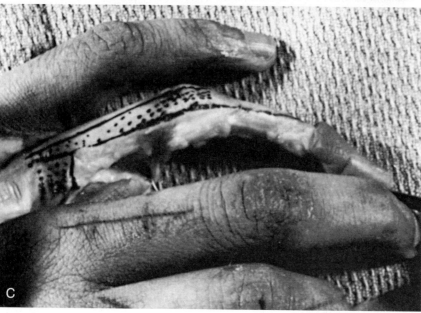

FIGURE 11-22. Distal intrinsic release is indicated for late post-traumatic interosseous contracture with PIP joint stiffness when the IT test is positive but there is no MP joint contracture. **A,** The lateral band and oblique fibers of the dorsal aponeurosis are removed proximal to the juncture of the lateral band with the lateral slip of the extensor tendon. Strong MP flexion and DIP extension are preserved by the distal intrinsic release. **B,** In this dissected specimen the portion of the dorsal aponeurosis that was removed with the distal intrinsic release is blackened. **C,** The oblique fibers and lateral band have been resected lateral to the lateral slip and proximal to the conjoined tendon. Transverse fibers to the dorsal aponeurosis remain intact.

CRITICAL POINTS: PIP JOINT EXTENSION CONTRACTURE RELEASE

INDICATIONS

- Failure to obtain PIP joint extension after dedicated hand therapy protocol
- Absence of arthritic changes within the PIP
- Absence of external abnormalities—extensor tendon adhesions, extensor skin contractures

PREOPERATIVE EVALUATION

- Perform a thorough clinical examination.
- Rule out causes external to the joint.
- Obtain radiographs to evaluate for degenerative changes.

PEARLS

- It is imperative to confirm preoperatively that a compliant patient, a competent therapist, and third party approval (when required) are present before proceeding with surgery.
- The patient must understand that postoperative care is an essential part of the treatment plan.
- Range of motion at surgery overestimates final outcome.

TECHNICAL POINTS

- Surgical exposure: dorsal or dorsolateral approach
- Local anesthesia with sedation allows assessment of active motion intraoperatively.
- Transverse fibers of the retinacular ligament are identified and divided longitudinally on either side of the central tendon.

- Extensor tendon is elevated, preserving central slip.
- Extensor tenolysis is performed as needed.
- Excise dorsal capsule; assess motion.
- Collateral ligaments are released off the proximal phalanx if full flexion is not obtained.
- Protective soft dressing with volar plaster splint is applied, avoiding overstretching of the neurovascular bundles.

PITFALLS

- Flexor tendon adhesions may be required to obtain full motion; be prepared to do this if full active motion is not obtained.
- Potential for concomitant intrinsic contractures; test for tightness, and release as needed.

POSTOPERATIVE CARE

- Elevation of the joint for 3 to 4 days
- Early removal of dressings (4 to 5 days) with fabrication of two custom-made splints, volar static with PIP joints at maximal safe extension and one in maximal safe flexion. Splints are alternated every 8 hours for 1 week.
- Aggressive supervised therapy

ATHLETIC PARTICIPATION

- Protect in splints until stable range of motion is obtained (typically 2 to 3 months).

muscle contracture that the shortened collateral ligaments yield, permitting the proximal phalanx to be pulled into flexion. The PIP joint is held in extension by the oblique fibers of the contracted interossei. Secondary para-articular changes may include contracture of the volar plate and accessory collateral ligaments of the MP joints and of the collateral ligaments of the PIP joints. This deformity causes serious disability. Large objects cannot fit in the palm, the grip is weak, and pulp-to-pulp pinch is impossible (Fig. 11-23).

To correct severe intrinsic contractures that involve both the MP and IP joints, extensive release of the dorsal aponeurosis is necessary. If the interossei retain their contractility but are fibrotic and tight, they may be released by muscle slide. With more severe ischemia, the interossei are necrotic and nonfunctional. Lumbrical function may be preserved and the interosseous muscle contracture released by transecting the interosseous tendons proximal to the MP joints (Fig. 11-24).

Para-articular structures that have become secondarily contracted are also transected to improve passive motion of the MP and IP joints. The surgeon need not fear overcorrec-

tion or a claw deformity. MP joint hyperextension rarely develops even with the most thorough soft tissue release.

Technique of Release of Severe Post-traumatic Intrinsic Contractures With Muscle Fibrosis. A dorsal transverse incision is made just proximal to the MP joints. The lateral tendons of all interossei and the abductor digiti quinti tendon are resected at the level of the MP joints. If the MP joints remain flexed, the sagittal bands are retracted distally and each accessory collateral ligament is divided at its insertion into the volar plate. The volar plate is freed from its attachments to the base of the proximal phalanx. With a blunt probe, any adhesions between the volar plate and the head of the metacarpal are separated. If it is difficult to maintain extension of the proximal phalanx after soft tissue release, a Kirschner wire is inserted obliquely through the MP in maximum extension. When the phalanx is extended, it is important to be certain that the base of the proximal phalanx articulates properly with the metacarpal head before inserting the Kirschner wire. If passive PIP flexion is incomplete with the MP joint extended, the lateral bands are resected at the distal half of the proximal phalanx through a separate

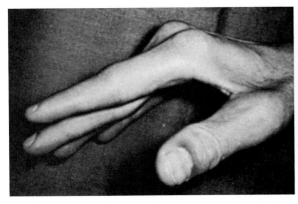

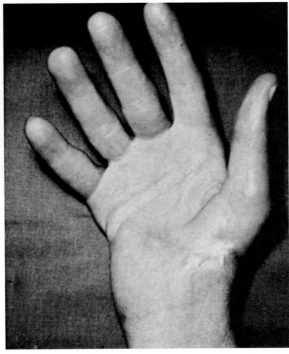

FIGURE 11-23. Late post-traumatic interosseous contracture involving both the MP and PIP joints is often associated with interosseous ischemia and necrosis. The fingers are flexed at the MP joints and extended at the IP joints. The contracture in this patient was due to severe edema after the application of a tight cast for a fracture of the wrist.

dorsal incision. Postoperatively, passive and active PIP flexion exercises should begin within 1 day of surgery. The Kirschner wire is usually removed at about 3 weeks.

ARTHROPLASTY

The indications for joint arthroplasty of the fingers include an incongruent joint with pain, deformity, or stiffness. There are several types of arthroplasty, ranging from simple resection of the injured joint to cemented total joint surface replacement. The general principles of each type are described, and

the details of technique and results of treatment are reviewed by joint. It is important to understand that arthrodesis is almost always the major alternative to arthroplasty and should be considered in lieu of arthroplasty in all cases where the bone stock is poor or the supporting soft tissue is severely damaged or significantly unbalanced.

Resection arthroplasty of the finger joints was first reported in 1954 when Taber described Carroll's method of resection arthroplasty for the PIP joint (Fig. 11-25).[31] Although soft tissue interposition arthroplasty using portions of the extensor tendon or volar plate has been described,[15,159,160,170] currently silicone elastomer spacers are most commonly used

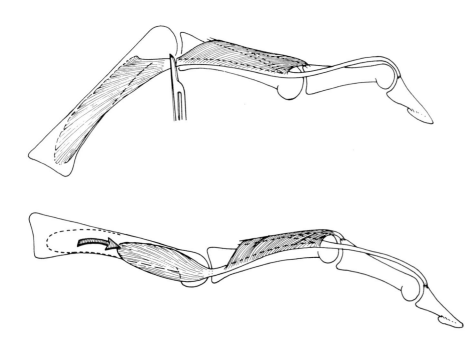

FIGURE 11-24. MP and PIP deformity after late post-traumatic interosseous contracture may be relieved by transecting the lateral tendon proximal to the MP joint (**top**) if the muscles are necrotic. If some function remains, the muscles may be relaxed by an interosseous muscle slide (**bottom**).

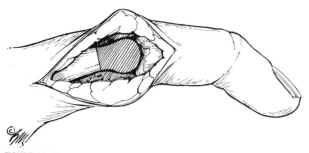

FIGURE 11-25. Resection arthroplasty of the PIP joint (Carroll and Taber). The proximal phalanx is exposed laterally and the head is resected at its neck. (Adapted from Carroll RE, Taber TH: Digital arthroplasty of the proximal interphalangeal joint. J Bone Joint Surg Am 36:912-920, 1954.)

for resection arthroplasty of the digits.[139-143,145,146,148,150,151] The stemmed silicone elastomer spacer can be applied to all joints of the finger and has enjoyed good success when implanted for the appropriate indication and in the proper individual. Because the vast majority of these devices are used for joints affected by rheumatoid or other inflammatory arthropathy, the results of silicone elastomer implant arthroplasty are discussed in that chapter and are reviewed only superficially here (see Chapter 59).

In the presence of adequate bone stock, damaged articular surfaces of the joints can be resurfaced with transplanted perichondrium.[117] Perichondrial resurfacing arthroplasty was described by Engkvist, Jackson, Sully, Ohlsen, and Skoog in Western Europe during the 1970s[45-47,111,112,128,138] as an alternative to implant arthroplasty in young adults with traumatic arthrosis, but the reported results have been disappointing.[61,125] Some authors have also reported on the use of extensor retinaculum as a resurfacing arthroplasty.[110] Thus, while theoretically an option, the long-term results of perichondrial resurfacing arthroplasty do not suggest that it is, in most cases, a viable alternative to other types of arthroplasty or to arthrodesis.

Total joint replacement arthroplasty of the digits became popular after the success of total hip arthroplasties that used metal and high-density polyethylene as articular components.[37,38,88,90,92-94,122,134,158] The advantages of the surface replacement arthroplasties include reconstruction of an anatomic joint with a virtual rather than a fixed axis at its instant center of rotation.[38,88,122,158] The virtual center of rotation allows a combination or rolling and sliding motions at the extremes of motion that gives the agonist muscles an improved mechanical advantage. Minimal bone resection leaves wider cortical contact surface area for distribution of compressive loads and preserves the capsular ligaments that assist in stabilizing the prosthesis by partially diverting the out of plane forces away from the prosthesis. The disadvantages include a higher risk of subluxation or dislocation, increased technical difficulties of tendon balancing, and the great difficulty in revision of a failed arthroplasty. The total joint replacement arthroplasties are technically much less forgiving than silicone elastomer joint replacement.

Metacarpophalangeal Joint Arthroplasty

When injury to the MP joint results in destruction of the articular surfaces or in cases where appropriate surgical release and application of hand therapy does not restore functional motion and significant pain with motion exists, arthroplasty can be considered in the appropriate patient. Currently there are three types of implants that are commercially available in the United States: (1) a variety of silicone elastomer implants, all essentially used as hinged spacers after resection arthroplasty; (2) a more classic metal and plastic surface replacement arthroplasty designed for cement fixation (SR MCP Implant, Avanta, San Diego, CA), which, however, is currently (in 2003) approved in the United States only under a Humanitarian Device Exemption and which requires Institutional Review Board approval from any hospital where the surgery will be performed; and (3) a unique uncemented surface replacement design made of graphite coated with pyrolytic carbon.

Silicone Elastomer Arthroplasty

Silicone elastomer implant arthroplasty of the MP joint has been used since the 1960s and, with a known material and long track record, is predictable and dependable in patients with low demands.[104,141,143,145,147] The results fall far short of the normal but are often serviceable and remain the benchmark with which other implants must be compared. Silicone elastomer implants have traditionally been used for rheumatoid arthropathy and less commonly in the setting of trauma or isolated degenerative arthritis. There is a paucity of literature regarding the long-term results of Silastic metacarpal joint replacement for degenerative arthritis with significant numbers. There are also a few reports of Silastic MP joint replacement in traumatic injuries. Nagle and colleagues reported that the average range of motion in 6 patients with nonsalvageable MP fractures treated with Silastic arthroplasty was 60 degrees at an average of 24 months follow-up.[109]

Although silicone elastomer joint spacers have provided a means of treatment for painful and stiff arthritic degenerative MP joints, they have been criticized because of limits of range of motion and stability. The highly deformable silicone implants are subject to rotation and lateral deformation and depend solely on the integrity of surrounding soft tissue for stability. Implant fracture is common, although fracture does not necessarily require a revision. Reactive synovitis secondary to silicone particulate debris (the so-called silicone synovitis) has also been described around the stems of finger joint implants, but with far less frequency and severity than it has been with carpal implants.[11,32,113,144,149,150]

Surface Replacement Arthroplasty (SRA)

Surface replacement arthroplasty (SRA) attempts to re-create the normal geometric articulation found in the premorbid joint and has been used in other joint systems such as the knee, where precise kinematics, in addition to stability and load bearing, are highly desirable. Although the concept of SRA is logical, the development of a reliable device for the MP joint has proved difficult, largely because of problems associated with stability. Linscheid and Cooney developed a system of SRA components for the MP joint that is based on a large series of anatomic and histologic evaluations of the normal geometry of the articular surfaces of the joint (Fig. 11-26).[88,90,91,94] The design provides a substantial amount of mediolateral stability in flexion, and the radius of curvature of the articular surfaces of both the proximal and distal components allows a potential for a nearly normal arc of motion.

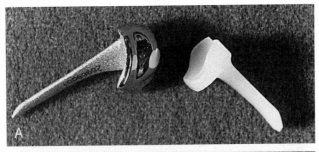

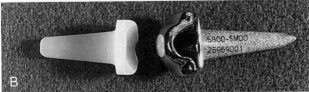

FIGURE 11-26. A and B, Surface replacement (SR) arthroplasty components for the MP joints. (Courtesy of Avanta Orthopedics, San Diego, CA, 1998.)

The components are currently designed to be cemented in place, but future designs are being considered for non-cemented implantation. The proximal component is composed of a chromium-cobalt alloy, and the distal component is made of ultrahigh-molecular-weight polyethylene. The stems are rectangular to maximize rotational stability and are slightly curved to match the curvature of the medullary canal. The components are paired in extra small, small, medium, and large sizes. The indications for implantation of an SRA metacarpophalangeal device are proposed to be the same as for a silicone arthroplasty, including the importance of intact soft tissue to cover the implant and the need for functioning flexor and extensor tendons, but the need for

functioning collateral ligaments is far more absolute with the SRA design.

Carbon Implants

Pyrolytic carbon is a synthetic material formed by the pyrolysis of a hydrocarbon gas at about 1300° C.[38] In 1969 this material was successfully used to make components of artificial heart valves and since then has demonstrated exceptional reliability in more than 15 million patient-years of experience.[62] The mechanical properties of pyrolytic carbon have demonstrated a modulus of elasticity similar to cortical bone,[39] and wear models have revealed no evidence of wear or wear debris, no evidence of inflammatory reaction, and excellent bone implant incorporation.[37,38]

Pyrolytic carbon finger joint arthroplasty was introduced in 1979. Short-term results demonstrated an improvement in the range of motion, relief of pain, adequate biological fixation, and few complications.[10] In a population of 53 patients, most with inflammatory arthritis, overall survivorship at 16 years was 70.3%.[38] The material properties of pyrolytic carbon make it an attractive alternative for surface replacement arthroplasty in the patient with degenerative or traumatic arthritis of the MP joint (Fig. 11-27).

Surgical Technique

The surgical technique for Silastic MP arthroplasty is discussed in Chapter 59. Details that pertain to the use of surface replacement and pyrolytic carbon implants are discussed here. Participation in a laboratory course on cadavers is strongly recommended before attempting these operations in a clinical setting.

If metal and plastic or pyrolytic carbon implants are being used, it is important to use the templates supplied by the manufacturer to estimate component size preoperatively. The templates are applied to the standard true posteroanterior and

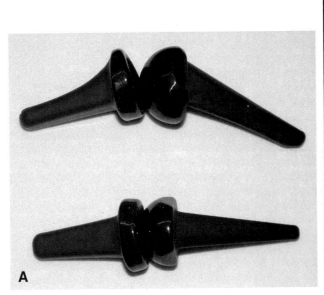

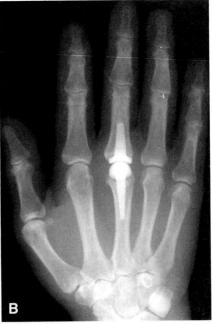

FIGURE 11-27. A, The Ascension carbon pyrolytic MP joint. B, An illustrative radiograph of replacement of post-traumatic degenerative arthritis of the MP joint. (A, Courtesy of Ascension Orthopaedics, Austin, TX.)

lateral radiographs of the MP joint under consideration for arthroplasty. Even so, it is wise to have the entire spectrum of component sizes available at the time of surgery in the event that upsizing or downsizing is necessary secondary to soft tissue constraints.

For SR MP or pyrolytic carbon MP arthroplasty, the osteotomy at the end of the metacarpal is carried out through subchondral bone, just distal to the insertion of the collateral ligaments, perpendicular to the long axis of the metacarpal (Figs. 11-28 and 11-29). The angle will depend on the type of implant used: perpendicular to the long axis of the metacarpal for silicone implants, 45 degrees for the Avanta SR MCP, and 27.5 degrees for the Ascension pyrolytic carbon MP implant. Cutting guides are available with the implants to make precise angled cuts. A 1- to 2-mm resection of the base of the proximal phalanx is then also performed. Care must be taken to preserve the collateral ligament attachments, because ligamentous stability is essential to the success of replacement arthroplasty.

The bony canals must be rasped and sized carefully. The importance of the trial reduction cannot be overemphasized. Intraoperative radiographs or fluoroscopy will verify trial placement and orientation of the stems to confirm alignment and fit. The pyrolytic carbon implant is used without cement. Pyrolytic carbon implants are brittle and should be impacted only with the special plastic impactors provided by the manufacturer.

For SR MCP arthroplasty, polymethylmethacrylate cement is mixed and while relatively watery is packed

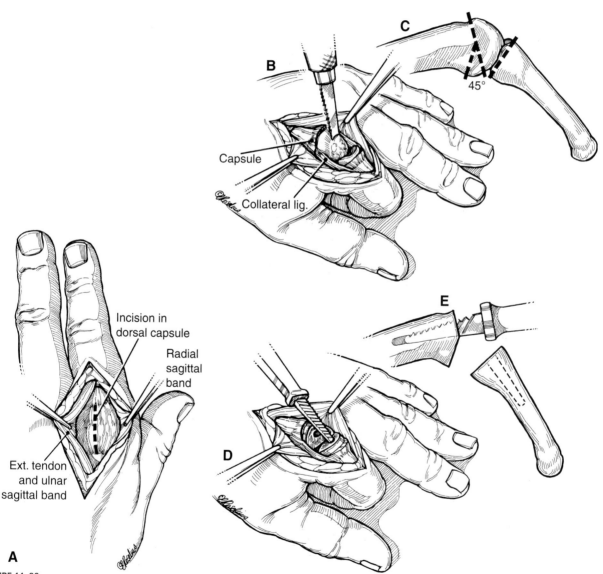

FIGURE 11-28. Technique of SR MP arthroplasty. **A,** A longitudinal incision centered about the MP joint is made under tourniquet control. The sagittal band is divided and elevated, exposing the dorsal capsule, which is longitudinally incised to expose the joint. **B,** The metacarpal head is removed with a vertical saw cut just distal to the collateral ligaments. **C,** A second cut at 45 degrees is made in a proximal-volar direction removing the remainder of the metacarpal head. The base of the proximal phalanx is osteotomized to remove only the articular cartilage. **D,** An awl is inserted into the dorsal aspect of the metacarpal intramedullary canal. **E,** Sequential broaching is performed until proper fit is established. A similar procedure is performed for the proximal phalanx.

Continued

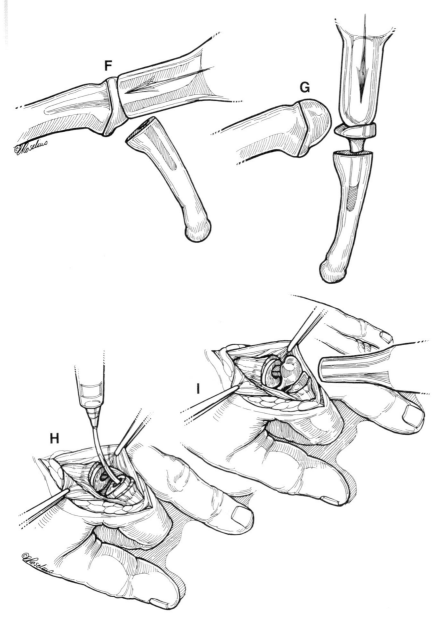

FIGURE 11-28—cont'd. **F** and **G,** Trial components are placed, and the range of motion and the stability of the joint are assessed.

After the canals are cleaned of debris and blood, polymethylmethacrylate cement is injected into the intramedullary canals in a liquid state using a syringe and Intracath guide (**H**), and the distal component inserted, followed by the proximal component (**I**). The joint is compressed and excess cement is removed. Once the cement is hardened, range of motion is assessed. The joint capsule is closed, the extensor mechanism repaired or reconstructed, and a bulky dressing is applied with the digit in extension.

into a syringe with a large-bore plastic needle (14-gauge Intracath). The tip of the plastic needle is introduced into the proximal phalanx and metacarpal canals, and the cement is injected slowly until the canal is filled. Using a no-touch technique, the distal component is inserted. Care must be taken to ensure that proper alignment and rotation of the component is maintained during insertion. The metacarpal component is inserted with similar care. The joint is reduced and held in extension until the cement hardens. Residual cement is then removed, and the range of motion and stability of the joint are again assessed. Final radiographs are obtained to verify component placement and to evaluate for extruded cement.

Postoperative Rehabilitation

For the SR MCP implant, the postoperative dressing is removed at 2 to 4 days and a dynamic splint is applied for daytime exercise and a static splint to hold the digits in the corrected position at the other periods of time for 4 to 6 weeks. A supervised rehabilitation program with daily sessions for the first 2 weeks, followed by interval visits, is essential in obtaining optimal outcome.

For the pyrolytic carbon implant, at the first postoperative visit the dressings are removed and a plaster splint is applied to maintain the joint in full extension, while allowing PIP joint flexion. Between the first and third week, the patient is evaluated twice a day and undergoes an exercise program that emphasizes edema control and guided range of motion preventing MP joint motion past 45 degrees for 3 weeks. Dynamic splints are designed to hold the MP joint at 0 degrees and proper rotation while allowing PIP joint motion. A static resting splint is also fabricated to hold the MP joints in full extension and the PIP joints in moderate flexion. Between the third and fourth week, active flexion to 45 degrees in the splints is emphasized, and by 4 to 6 weeks, guarded active range of motion outside the splint is performed. Deviation stresses to the joint are avoided. Between 6 and 12 weeks, gradual weaning from the dynamic splints

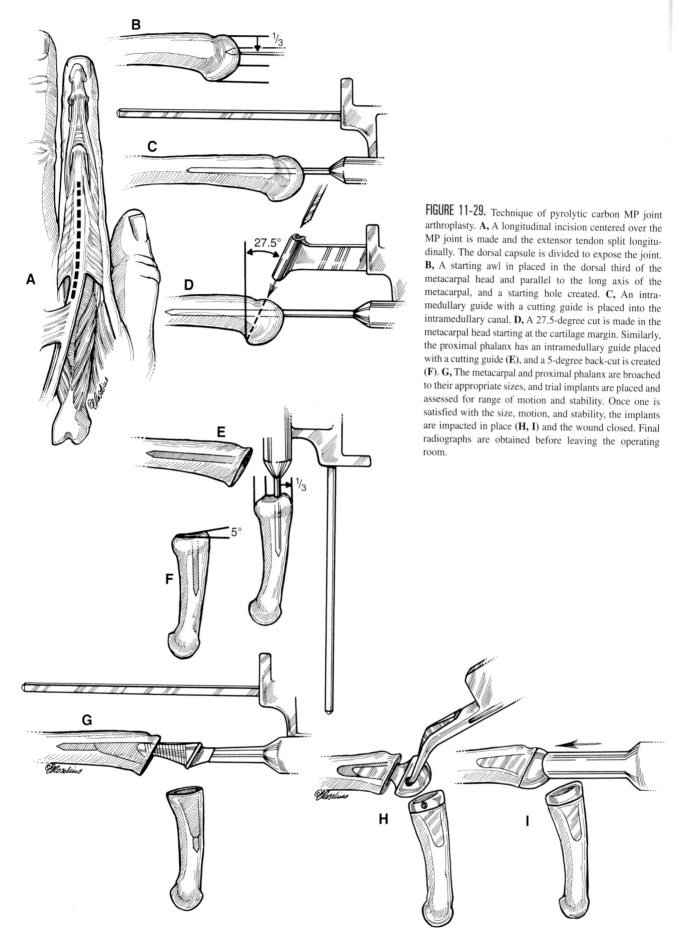

FIGURE 11-29. Technique of pyrolytic carbon MP joint arthroplasty. **A,** A longitudinal incision centered over the MP joint is made and the extensor tendon split longitudinally. The dorsal capsule is divided to expose the joint. **B,** A starting awl in placed in the dorsal third of the metacarpal head and parallel to the long axis of the metacarpal, and a starting hole created. **C,** An intramedullary guide with a cutting guide is placed into the intramedullary canal. **D,** A 27.5-degree cut is made in the metacarpal head starting at the cartilage margin. Similarly, the proximal phalanx has an intramedullary guide placed with a cutting guide (**E**), and a 5-degree back-cut is created (**F**). **G,** The metacarpal and proximal phalanx are broached to their appropriate sizes, and trial implants are placed and assessed for range of motion and stability. Once one is satisfied with the size, motion, and stability, the implants are impacted in place (**H, I**) and the wound closed. Final radiographs are obtained before leaving the operating room.

continues and motion is increased to 60 degrees or greater of flexion.

Authors' Preferred Method of Treatment for MP Arthroplasty

There are few reports on the results of arthroplasty for the nonrheumatoid degenerative MP joints. Swanson silicone elastomer implants certainly do not yield normal results but are a known quantity. The published results of other silicone elastomer devices and surface replacement arthroplasty appear to offer little improvement in final range of motion, and the follow-up of these newer devices, with the exception of a single series of pyrolytic carbon implants, is too short to comment meaningfully on reoperation rates. In the past, many implants have been tried, each being touted as an improvement over silicone elastomer implants but then falling from favor as the hoped-for outcomes did not materialize. Meanwhile, the Swanson design silicone elastomer implants soldier on and remain by far the most commonly used devices as of this writing (2004). Conscious of the available evidence and this historical perspective, one of us (PCA) still prefers the use of silicone elastomer implants, while the other (AYS), ever hopeful for the future, prefers the use of the pyrolytic carbon surface replacement arthroplasty.

Proximal Interphalangeal Joint Arthroplasty

When consideration is made for arthroplasty of the PIP joint, affected digit, handedness, occupation, and avocations of the patient are important to consider in the decision-making process. For example, the needs of a laborer, who requires power grip, stability, and longevity are much different than that of a sedentary individual who requires light general hand function for activities of daily living. Loads on the ulnar digits, primarily used for grip, are different from those on the index finger, where pinch adds considerable lateral-bending loads. Realistic patient and surgeon expectations are an absolute prerequisite in obtaining good outcomes.

The average arc of motion after PIP joint arthroplasty is between 40 and 60 degrees in most series. If the arc of motion is already in this range, restoration of additional motion is an unrealistic goal. A patient with a painless arc of 60 degrees of PIP motion in good position should therefore be advised to avoid surgery. Arthroplasty may of course be appropriate to relieve pain or to redirect an arc of motion that is otherwise acceptable to a more functional zone, such as to improve grip. In patients with fixed deformities, poor bone stock, or joint destruction, however, arthrodesis may be a better alternative than arthroplasty.

Absolute prerequisites to PIP joint arthroplasty include good bone stock to receive the stems of the implant, supple, full-thickness skin coverage, adequate sensibility and circulation, and normal or functional tendons. Stability of the collateral ligaments needs to be determined preoperatively.[80]

If they are deficient, reconstruction should be considered at the time of surgery, or another option chosen, especially with any surface replacement implant.

The selection of PIP joint implants available for use today include the silicone elastomer one-piece flexible implant and surface replacement arthroplasty. The results of silicone elastomer implant arthroplasty for the PIP joint have been reported by many investigators. In 1985, Swanson published his personal series of 424 implants with a minimum of 1-year follow-up.[151] Over two thirds of these fingers had more than 40 degrees of motion, averaging between 38 and 60 degrees, depending on the etiology. Best results were in fingers with minimal deformity, and worst results were in those with rheumatoid swan neck deformities. When performed for degenerative and post-traumatic arthritis, Moore and associates reported that at a 2-year follow-up there was an approximately 40% revision rate as well as a nearly 15% implant fracture rate.[107] Ferencz and Millender reported 11 patients with post-traumatic arthritis observed for a minimum of 18 months.[50] In this series, there were no fractures or revisions and motion averaged 64 degrees. Iselin and Pradet, in a series of 120 arthroplasties in fingers with post-traumatic contractures observed for at least 2 years, had satisfactory results in two thirds.[71]

Stern and Ho cautioned against the use of Swanson silicone implants in the index and middle finger PIP joints, especially in the young, active patient.[137] They highlighted the usual necessity of detaching the radial and ulnar collateral ligament origins from the proximal phalanx to resect the proximal phalangeal head through its neck. They contended that resultant stresses on the radial collateral ligament are significant in key pinch and may lead to implant failure. They recommended arthrodesis of the index and long PIP joints when these joints are destroyed, reserving arthroplasty for the ring and small PIP joints. Others, however, continue to advocate the use of Swanson hinged interposition implant arthroplasty for the painful, arthritic index and middle finger PIP joints as long as these digits are well aligned and the collateral ligaments are in good condition[92-94,107] or in low demand patients.

The use of flexible silicone elastomer implants such as the Swanson (Wright Medical, Arlington, TN), Neuflex (DuPey, Warsaw, IN), or Avanta (Avanta Orthopedics, San Diego, CA) devices for nonrheumatoid arthritis of the PIP joint remains a viable alternative to arthrodesis or other surface replacement arthroplasties. The surgeon must take into account the patient's expectations as well as occupational and avocational needs and realistically determine if flexible Silastic implants are suitable. The surgical technique for silicone elastomer PIP implants is described in Chapter 59.

Similar to the SR MCP system, an SR PIP system has been developed. Like its MP analogue, this device is only available for humanitarian use under IRB supervision. The proximal component is composed of a chromium-cobalt alloy, and the distal component is made of ultrahigh-molecular-weight polyethylene (Fig. 11-30). The stems are rectangular to maximize rotational stability and are slightly curved to match the curvature of the medullary canal. The components are paired in extra small, small, medium, and large sizes.

A pyrolytic carbon surface replacement arthroplasty is also available. The PIP joint pyrolytic carbon implant has a

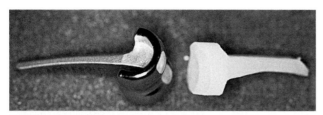

FIGURE 11-30. Surface replacement arthroplasty components for the PIP joint. (Courtesy of Avanta Orthopedics, San Diego, CA, 1998.)

bicondylar anatomic design with a dorsal groove that allows the central slip to track in (Fig. 11-31). There are four sizes that are interchangeable such that upsizing or downsizing of the proximal and distal components can occur. The indications for implantation of either of these surface replacement devices are the same as for a silicone arthroplasty, including the importance of intact soft tissue to cover the implant, the need for functioning flexor and extensor tendons, and the desirability of functioning collateral ligaments. As with the MP joint, however, while there are hypothetical advantages to the SRA and pyrolytic carbon implants, including the enhanced lateral stability that makes implantation into an index finger more attractive, there are few published results that allow the surgeon to compare these devices with their silicone elastomer alternatives.

Surface Replacement PIP Implant Technique
(Figs. 11-32 and 11-33)
Preoperative Planning
Templates supplied by the manufacturer can be used to estimate implant component size preoperatively. The templates are applied to standard true posteroanterior and lateral radiographs of the digit under consideration for arthroplasty.

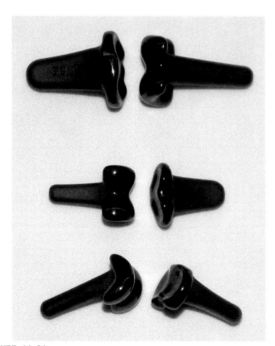

FIGURE 11-31. Examples of carbon pyrolytic PIP joints. (Courtesy of Ascension Orthopaedics, Austin, TX.)

Having all component sizes available during the time of surgery is recommended in the event that upsizing or downsizing is necessary because of soft tissue constraints and the other factors.

Dorsal Approach
A generous dorsal linear or curvilinear incision is made, followed by creation of full-thickness flaps of skin. The extensor mechanism can be split longitudinally down the midline if no need for length adjustment of the extensor mechanism is anticipated. The edges of the tendon are gently retracted away from the midline, with care taken to ensure that the insertion of the central slip into the base of the middle phalanx is preserved. If length adjustments for a mild boutonnière or swan neck deformity are anticipated, the Chamay incision is used.[33] This is created by longitudinally incising the extensor mechanism along the medial and lateral edges of the central slip and then connecting the incisions just proximal to the merger of the medially directed fibers of the lateral bands and the central slip. The slip of tendon is then gently elevated distally as far as the insertion of the central slip into the base of the middle phalanx. The dorsal capsule of the PIP joint is very thin and often compromised in severe inflammatory or degenerative arthritis. If present, it is incised longitudinally to expose the joint surfaces. The marginal attachments of the collateral ligaments may be carefully undermined to allow adequate exposure of the joint surfaces.

Osteotomy
An osteotomy at the base of the middle phalanx through the subchondral bone perpendicular to the long axis of the bone is made, preserving the collateral ligament attachment. It may be necessary to slightly undermine the ligament insertion to fully resect the subchondral bone, but an effort should be made to preserve the bulk of the ligament insertion. Attention is then directed to the proximal phalangeal osteotomy, which is carried out through the base of the head, just distal to the proximal attachment of the collateral ligaments. Occasionally it may be necessary to make the osteotomy slightly oblique, angled in a dorsal distal-to-proximal palmar direction, to ensure the best fit of the proximal component. A side-cutting bur is used to resect the bulk of the cancellous bone at the level of the osteotomy and allow introduction of the broach system to prepare the medullary canal for introduction of the components. Broaching starts with the smallest broach and is incrementally increased until a size smaller than the templated prosthetic component is introduced in a reciprocating fashion into the medullary canal while making certain that it is advanced into the canal parallel to the long axis of the bone. Trial components are advanced into the proximal and distal phalanges, and the joint is reduced. Joint stability, range of motion, and stiffness are assessed with the trial components in place. If the joint is unacceptably lax, a decision is made to increase the trial size. If it is too tight, even to the point where the joint is irreducible, consideration should first be directed at decreasing the trial component size. If still unsuccessful, an additional resection osteotomy should be carried out. The proximal phalanx can tolerate more resection than the middle phalanx, simply because of the anatomy of the collateral ligament insertions. Intraoperative

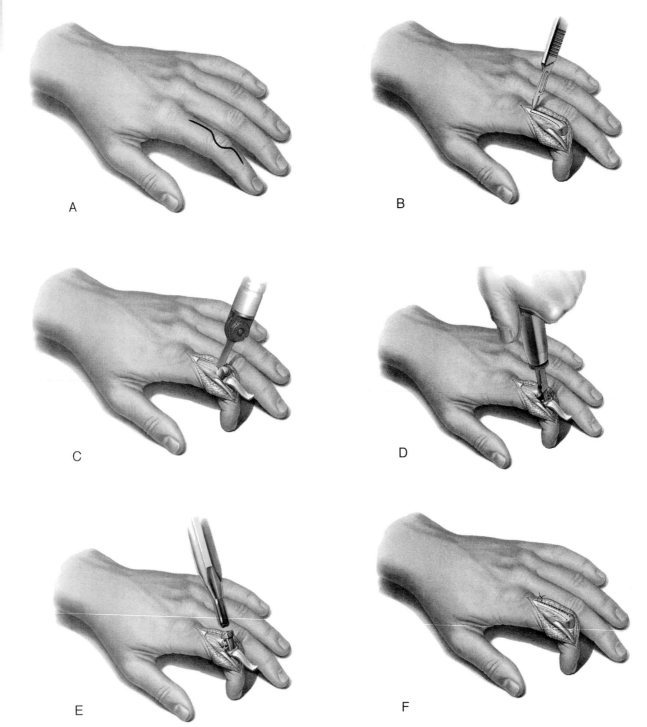

A

B

C

D

E

F

FIGURE 11-32. Technique for implantation of surface replacement arthroplasty for the PIP joint. **A,** A dorsal curvilinear incision centered over the PIP joint is made. **B,** The extensor mechanism is incised in a manner to create a distally based flap while preserving the distal attachment of the central slip. **C,** A transverse osteotomy is carried out through the head of the proximal phalanx, just distal to the collateral ligament attachments. The base of the middle phalanx is osteotomized just proximal to the collateral ligament insertion. **D,** Special broaches are used to prepare and size the medullary canals of the proximal and middle phalanges. **E,** The components are implanted, after injection of cement into the medullary canals, and seated with special push rods. **F,** The extensor mechanism is repaired with nonabsorbable suture. (From the Mayo Foundation, with permission, courtesy of Avanta Orthopedics, San Diego, CA.)

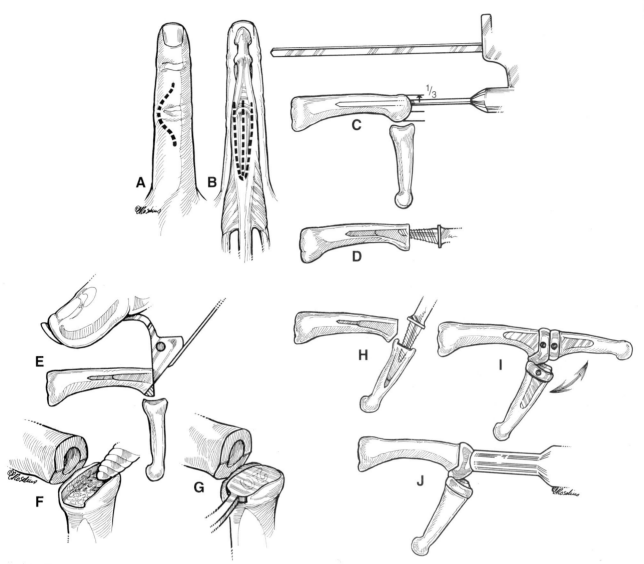

FIGURE 11-33. **A** and **B,** Carbon pyrolytic PIP joint replacement is performed through a dorsal approach or a Chamay approach. **C,** Once the joint is exposed, the proximal phalanx has a starting hole placed in the dorsal third of the joint in line with the longitudinal axis of the dorsal cortex. A perpendicular osteotomy is made using the cutting guide. **D,** The canal is broached to the appropriate size and a second cutting guide is placed into the proximal phalanx. **E,** The volar lip is then osteotomized using the second cutting guide. **F,** A side-cutting bur or saw is used to remove the cartilage from the middle phalanx. **G** and **H,** A starting hole is created and the middle phalanx is broached. **I,** Trial components are placed, stability, range of motion and component size are assessed. **J,** The implants are then gently impacted into place. The wound is closed with nonabsorbable sutures.

radiographs should be taken at the point where the joint seems stable with the trial implants in place to verify the orientation of the stems and to confirm that alignment and component placement are optimal. If excessive undermining of the collateral ligament attachments was required during preparation of the joint, it may be necessary to reattach the ligaments with a multifilament nonabsorbable suture passed through the ligament into a drill hole in the bone created with a 0.045-inch Kirschner wire.

Trial reduction is an important component of surface replacement arthroplasty. The distal trial is inserted with the joint hyperflexed and impacted into place to ensure a press fit. The collar of the trial should abut the cut surface. The proximal trial is inserted in a similar fashion. The joint is reduced and checked for proper sizing, stability, and range of motion. The finger should extend and flex passively with

ease; there should be minimal lateral laxity. Fluoroscopic imaging is used to confirm accurate alignment of the trials. If the joint does not fully extend or is too tight, the proximal phalanx osteotomies should be adjusted first in small increments.

Implantation

Once the appropriate component sizes are determined, the medullary canals are irrigated to remove any residual debris. For metal and plastic devices, polymethylmethacrylate is mixed in the usual manner and, while relatively fluid, is packed into a syringe with a large-bore plastic needle. The tip of the needle is sequentially advanced into the medullary canal of both the proximal and middle phalanges, and cement is injected slowly until the canal is filled. The components are then advanced by using a "no-touch" technique for the articular surfaces, with the proximal component typically placed first. Excess cement is removed, and the joint surfaces are reduced and held in full extension until it is verified that the cement has cured. Final radiographs are obtained at this point to verify component placement and to attempt to look for extruded cement (Fig. 11-34). An assessment of joint stability and range of motion is now possible. For pyrolytic carbon implants, after successful sizing of the trials, the distal implant is inserted with the intercondylar notch dorsally placed and impacted with the impactor. The proximal implant is then inserted and impacted. The implant

collars should abut the cut surfaces. The joint is reduced, and stability and range of motion are assessed clinically and with radiographs (Fig. 11-35).

Closure

If sufficient joint capsule is present dorsally, it may be closed as a separate layer with 3-0 multifilament absorbable suture. Appropriate tension of the extensor mechanism is estimated, and side-to-side primary closure of the tenotomy is performed. Hemostasis is obtained by electrocautery, and the skin is closed, typically with monofilament suture.

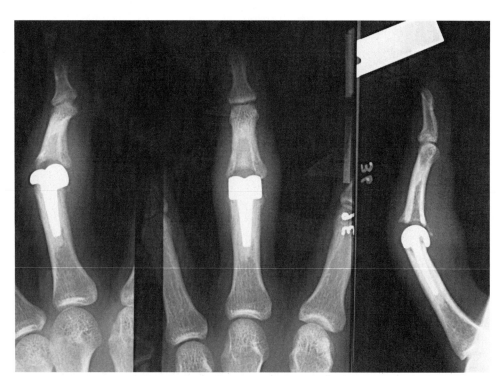

FIGURE 11-34. Radiographs demonstrating proper implantation of the PIP surface replacement prosthesis.

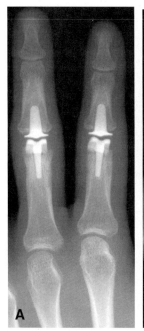 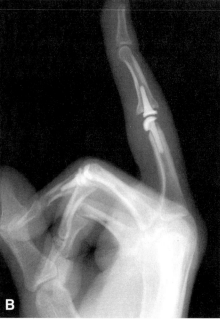

FIGURE 11-35. A and **B,** Radiographs of PIP carbon pyrolytic implant in place.

Postoperative Rehabilitation

A supportive dressing is applied, and in 3 to 5 days a monitored daily therapy protocol is initiated. Active flexion and dynamic passive extension are begun with splint protection. Splint protection is maintained for at least 4 weeks postoperatively. Motion in a limited arc of 0 to 30 degrees is initiated in the dynamic splint. If hyperextension of the joint is noted, an extension block is added. By 7 to 8 days, if full active extension of the joint is achieved and no extension lag is present, the arc of motion is increased to 45 degrees in the dynamic splint. If active flexion is less than 30 degrees and full active extension is maintained, the dynamic extension can be removed and motion can be increased to 45 degrees. The goal is to achieve 0 to 45 degrees by the fourth week postoperatively. By 6 weeks, motion should achieve 0 to 75 degrees of motion and gentle stretching is initiated. By 3 months, the goal should be 0 to 75 degrees and activity as tolerated.

Results

The preliminary results of the SR PIP joint arthroplasty were reported in 1997.[94] The average range of motion increased from 35.5 degrees preoperatively (extension, −13.0 degrees; flexion, +48.9 degrees) to 47.5 degrees (extension, −16.3 degrees; flexion, +63.8 degrees) postoperatively. Component failure has not been a problem. Frank loosening has occurred in two fingers in this series. The stability of the index PIP joint has been maintained with the use of this prosthesis. Complications have included boutonnière and swan neck deformities and joint subluxation. The major complication rate is currently 20%, compared with a 10% reoperation rate in a concurrent series of Swanson implants at the Mayo Clinic.[89] At the time of writing of this chapter, there are no published reports of the results of pyrolytic carbon PIP arthroplasty, although several clinical trials are in progress.

Authors' Preferred Method of Treatment for PIP Arthroplasty

The use of silicone implants for PIP joint replacement in degenerative and post-traumatic injuries has demonstrated good range of motion but a higher incidence of implant failure and revision surgery compared with rheumatoid joint replacement. The advances in surface replacement arthroplasty may eventually relegate silicone elastomer implants to rheumatoid disease, but further investigation with prospective clinical trials comparing the SRAs to silicone implants in degenerative and post-traumatic arthritis is necessary. Based on the current state of knowledge and anticipation for the future, and mindful again of the history of new implants failing the test of time in the past, one of us (PCA) prefers silicone elastomer PIP joint replacement, while the other (AYS) prefers the SRA.

Distal Interphalangeal Joint Arthroplasty

The DIP joint is the joint most commonly involved by degenerative arthritis. Fortunately, pain in these joints usu-

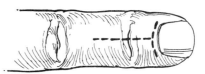

FIGURE 11-36. Incision for exposure of the distal interphalangeal joint. (Courtesy of A. B. Swanson.)

ally abates with time, deformities remain generally mild to moderate, and hand function is usually minimally compromised by decreased motion at this level.[1,146] When surgery is indicated at the DIP joint, pain is the most likely indication. In such cases, arthrodesis is generally the preferred method.

If pain is associated with a need for motion, Swanson has used a double-stemmed implant for arthroplasty of the distal joint of the index finger and thumb. A single-stemmed silicone elastomer implant is also available for hemiarthroplasty but is less effective in maintaining alignment. The goal of both procedures is limited pain-free motion. Excessive motion favors instability.[147,148]

This type of distal joint arthroplasty can offer 25 to 30 degrees of motion, pain relief, and acceptable stability.[19,176] Extension lag of 10 to 30 degrees is common.

Swanson Double-Stemmed Implant for the DIP Joint

A distally based "T"-shaped incision is made on the dorsum from the middle of the middle phalanx to the base of the nail (Fig. 11-36). The extensor tendon is divided 0.5 cm proximal to the joint and retracted distally (Fig. 11-37). The joint is flexed sharply and the dorsal half of the collateral ligament is incised as necessary for exposure. The head of the middle phalanx and base of the distal phalanx are removed and the osteophytes trimmed. The medullary cavities are reamed to accept the implant stems. The joint should easily extend fully. The extensor tendon is repaired anatomically and snugged up to maintain extension. One of the problems with this operation is that the extensor tendon inserts directly on the large dorsal osteophyte, and concomitant removal of the osteophyte and preservation of the extensor tendon integrity are often difficult.

Postoperatively, the PIP and DIP joints are maintained in extension for 2 weeks and then only the DIP joint for an additional 4 to 6 weeks. Gentle active flexion is progressively begun during the day, but night-time splinting in extension is continued for an additional 6 weeks.[148] Zimmerman and associates prefer to immobilize the DIP joint in extension full time for 8 weeks with gradual weaning from extension splints.[176]

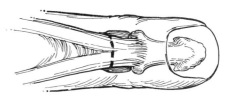

FIGURE 11-37. The central tendon is divided proximal to the DIP joint and then retracted distally to expose the joint. After repair, the finger is immobilized as for a mallet deformity. (Courtesy of A. B. Swanson.)

ARTHRODESIS

The general indications for arthrodesis of joints of the hand include pain, instability, or deformity combined with a loss of motor control[13] or bony stock sufficient to support an arthroplasty. When all previous attempts at restoring painless effective motion fail, arthrodesis of the joint should be considered. Improvement of hand function occurs with elimination of pain and restoration of stability when the injured joint is arthrodesed.[168] The most commonly arthrodesed finger joints are the DIP and PIP joints. With newer and more sophisticated arthroplasty designs and implants, arthrodesis of the MP joint is usually reserved for failed arthroplasty or in cases where there is not enough bone stock to support an arthroplasty.

The position of arthrodesis of joints should be individualized depending on the patient's needs. A detailed preoperative discussion regarding the position of arthrodesis is imperative. It is frequently helpful to splint the affected joint in the proposed position of arthrodesis or to fix it temporarily with a Kirschner wire, to allow the patient an opportunity to test hand function with the joint in that position. As a general guideline, the finger MP joints should be positioned in increasing flexion as one goes from a radial to ulnar direction, beginning with 25 degrees of flexion for the index finger and adding 5 degrees for each finger as one goes ulnarly (Fig. 11-38).[168] Thus, the middle finger MP joint should generally be arthrodesed in approximately 30 degrees of flexion, the ring finger at 35 degrees, and the small finger at 40 degrees. Rotation or radial/ulnar deviation is poorly tolerated and should be avoided.

Techniques of Finger Joint Arthrodesis

The critical elements of a successful joint arthrodesis are surface preparation and fixation. Optimally, the surface preparation should result in good cancellous to cancellous bone contact and should not shorten the digit excessively. The types of surface preparation include the "cup and cone"[164] (Fig. 11-39) and osteotomy flat surface techniques. Advocates of the cup and cone technique believe that this type of preparation is more forgiving and allows for fine adjustment of the position of the arthrodesis in all planes; it is also compatible with a wide variety of fixation techniques.[30,154,168,169] Essentially, after the bone ends of the joint are exposed and all the articular cartilage is meticulously removed, the proximal end is shaped, either by hand or with a power tool, into a rounded hemisphere, to form the cone. The distal surface is shaped into a concave surface with curets, bur, or a matching power reamer, to form the cup. The surfaces are then trimmed by hand as needed to fit within each other in the proper alignment and flexion. Fixation technique of the surgeon's choosing is used to secure the cup and cone arthrodesis.

Surface preparation with flat angled resections of the articular surface or the creation of chevrons require thoughtful preoperative planning and precision cuts, because slight deviations can result in an undesirable position of the arthrodesed digit.[168,169] Correction of these deviations can result in excessive bone loss or shortening. Despite this, flat angled resection of articular surface for arthrodesis remains a popular technique.

Methods of fixation of finger joints are numerous and range from simple Kirschner wire fixation to plate fixation, each with its advocates and indications. Kirschner wire technique usually involves retrograde advancement of the wires across the proximal bone end, followed by adjustment of the desired joint position, and then antegrade advancement of the wires across the arthrodesis site. The simplest and most commonly used methods are the crossed wire technique and the axial wire combined with an oblique wire configuration (Fig. 11-40).[100,164] Any bone chips obtained from the surface preparation can be placed into the arthrodesis site as bone graft if needed. The Kirschner wires can be bent, advanced with a tamp, and buried or alternatively left through the skin and removed after union.

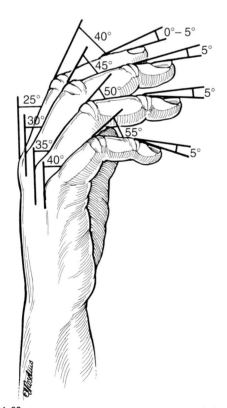

FIGURE 11-38. The authors' preferred positions for arthrodesis of the finger joints.

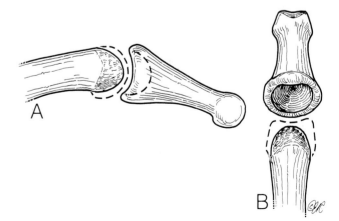

FIGURE 11-39. **A** and **B,** Contouring the bone ends as a proximal cup and distal cone allows good bony apposition in any position.

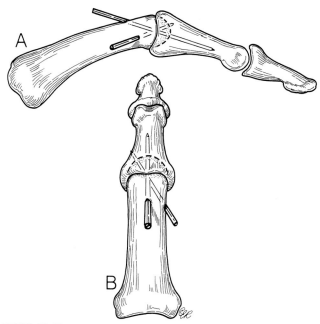

FIGURE 11-40. Kirschner wire fixation using one longitudinal and one obliquely oriented wire. **A,** Lateral view. **B,** Anteroposterior view.

Interosseous wiring with two orthogonal loops of 26-gauge surgical steel is stronger than Kirschner wire fixation (Fig. 11-41).[97,161] After the bone ends are prepared, a 0.035-inch wire is used to drill parallel holes in the ulnoradial and dorsovolar planes 3 to 4 mm from the end of the prepared bone ends. A 20-gauge hypodermic needle is passed through the sets of the drill holes and facilitates the passage of 26-gauge surgical steel through the drill hole to form a loop around the arthrodesis site. Once both wires are passed, they are tightened, cut short, and bent. Although simplistic and biomechanically strong, interosseous wiring with the 90-90 technique requires greater surgical exposure and soft tissue stripping than do other techniques of fixation.

Tension band wiring of finger joint arthrodesis adds to the strength of parallel placed Kirschner wires across an arthrodesis site (Fig. 11-42).[3,69,79,136,173] The principle of tension band wiring is to create a compressive force from a distracting force. As the finger flexors exert a distracting force across an arthrodesis site, placement of a tension band wire can redirect the force to a compressive one. Joint surfaces are typically prepared by flat angled resection with a microsagittal saw. A transverse drill hole using a 0.035-inch Kirschner wire is placed in the distal bone, 8 to 9 mm distal to the joint surface. A 26-gauge surgical steel wire is passed through the drill hole. The passage of the wire can be facilitated with the use of a 20-gauge hypodermic needle. Two parallel 0.035-inch Kirschner wires are placed retrograde into the center of the proximal bone end, exiting the dorsal cortex. The bone ends are coapted and the wires are advanced across the fusion site. The 26-gauge surgical steel is passed around the two Kirschner wires in a figure-of-eight configuration and tightened to rigidly fix the bone ends. The wires are adjusted under fluoroscopic guidance and are bent, cut, and tamped down to bone. The tension band wire is cut and bent. A small drill hole can be placed next to the end of the

tension band wire, and the cut end can be placed into this hole to prevent irritation to the dorsal soft tissues.

Screw fixation for small joint arthrodesis of the hand can include the use of cortical, lag, or headless screws. After the bone ends are prepared a single 2.0- to 2.7-mm screw can be lagged across the joint from the dorsal proximal segment into the intramedullary canal distally (Fig. 11-43) [123] or from an oblique direction across the joint.[152] One of the problems with axial screw fixation for finger joint arthrodesis is the prominence of the screw head subcutaneously. Headless compression screws, such as the Herbert screw (Zimmer, Warsaw, IN) or Acutrak screw (Acumed, Beaverton, OR), provide a lower profile fixation and have been used for finger joint arthrodesis with excellent reported success.[5,49,78,86,173]

Plate fixation using dorsal mini-plates, ranging from 1.5 to 2.7 mm, have been used for arthrodesis of the MP and PIP joints (Fig. 11-44).[22,85,171] Plate fixation requires extensive soft tissue dissection compared with other techniques and is best applied when there is segmental bone loss.[22] The technique is demanding and often requires a second operation for removal of prominent hardware and/or extensor tenolysis.[85,168,169] A compression plate is bent to the desired angle with a minimal of three holes distal and three proximal to the fusion site. The plate is first secured distally and is then secured proximally using a compression technique.

Fixation of carpal bone arthrodesis by power staple was described in 1987.[126] The technique has also been applied to the finger joints as well, with proponents of the technique stating that it reduces operative time.[28,65,96,118,126] Ritt and associates demonstrated that two or three 7 × 7-mm staples placed across the fusion site had inferior biomechanical properties to tension band wiring and recommended tension band wire techniques, despite the increase in operative times.[118]

External fixation devices can also be used for arthrodesis (Fig. 11-45). Before the introduction of the commercially available mini-external fixator, Braun used parallel proximal and distal 0.0625-inch Kirschner wire about the arthrodesis site and compressed the ends of the wires in methylmethacrylate cement.[18] Others have used external fixators made from dental screws and Kirschner wires to achieve union.[157] Although the mini-external fixator has union rates comparable to other techniques,[124] its use should be limited to special circumstances because of the complications that occur with external fixation (e.g., pin tract infection, interference of motion of adjacent digits).[13] These circumstances include severe bone loss or soft tissue loss, septic arthritis or osteomyelitis, failed prior arthrodesis, and fixed deformity.[13,168]

Bioabsorbable fixation devices have the major advantage of the elimination of the need for a second operation for hardware removal. The use of absorbable lactide-glycolide copolymer, polyglycolide acid, and polylactic acid implants for biofixation of fractures has been well described.* Despite this, their use for fixation of arthrodesis in the hand is limited to one report.[162] Although biomechanical studies show comparable strengths and rigidity of absorbable implants compared with metallic ones, the ultimate role of this method of fixation appears to us unclear, given the limited clinical data available.[34,42,108]

---

*See references 12, 14, 23, 34, 42, 67, 153, 156, and 174.

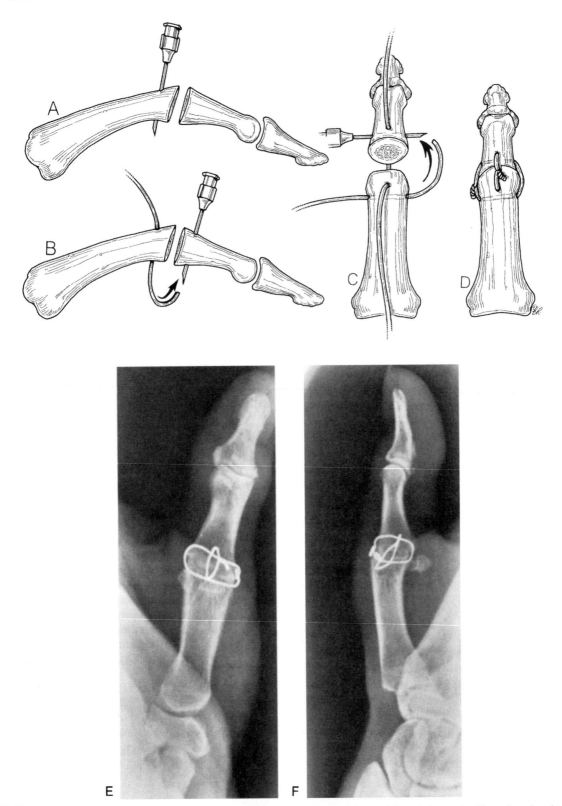

FIGURE 11-41. Interosseous wiring. **A,** With the use of a 20-gauge needle, a 26-gauge wire is inserted through the proximal bone from dorsal to palmar. **B,** The wire is then passed through the needle now in the distal fragment from palmar to dorsal. **C,** The procedure is repeated for a transversely placed wire. **D,** The bone surfaces are brought together, and the wires are twisted until tight. **E** and **F,** Example of 90-90 interosseous wiring for osteoarthritis of MP joint of the thumb. (A to D Adapted from Zimmerman NB, Weiland AJ: Ninety-ninety intraosseous wiring for internal fixation of the digital skeleton. Orthopedics 12:99-104, 1989.)

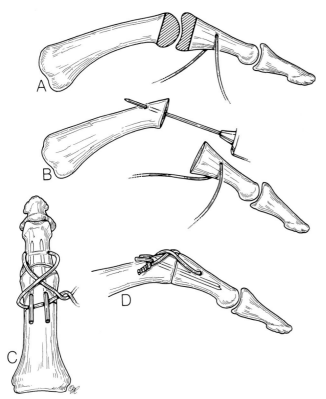

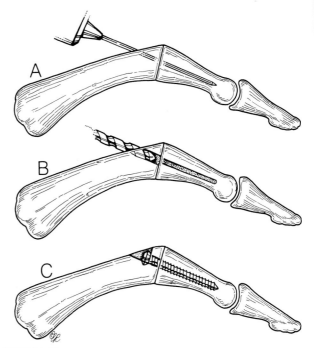

FIGURE 11-42. **A** to **D,** Tension band technique. (Adapted from Allende BT, Engelem JC: Tension-band arthrodesis in the finger joints. J Hand Surg [Am] 5:269-271, 1980.)

FIGURE 11-43. **A** to **C,** AO lag screw technique. (Adapted from Segmuller G: Surgical Stabilization of the Skeleton of the Hand. Baltimore, Williams & Wilkins, 1977, pp 42-59.)

Biomechanical Considerations

Biomechanical studies of the methods of fixation described previously have been cited by both proponents and opponents of the various techniques. In a bending study in cadavers, Vanik and colleagues[161] evaluated the biomechanical properties of a variety of Kirschner wire fixation techniques, looped wire techniques, and plating techniques for simulated diaphyseal transverse metacarpal fractures. Of the Kirschner wire fixation techniques, the crossed 0.045-inch Kirschner wire technique was the strongest, but the 26-gauge interosseous wire techniques were all stronger than Kirschner wires. The 90-90 interosseous wire technique was stronger than two dorsal-palmar wires, and both were stronger than a single transverse interosseous wire. The dorsal plating technique with a five-hole plate was comparable to the 90-90 interosseous wiring with 26-gauge wire. The addition of an oblique Kirschner wire across the fracture site did not significantly improve the strength of fixation of the interosseous wire techniques. In a study comparing crossed Kirschner wires, tension band wire technique, and a single interosseous wire supplement with an oblique Kirschner wire, Kovach and colleagues[82] found that tension band wiring was the strongest in a biomechanical PIP joint arthrodesis model. With respect to the bioabsorbable implants, biomechanical models have demonstrated that bioabsorbable rods are comparable to similar size Kirschner wires in all modes except torsion.[53] Although comparable in a nonbiologic system (cadaver bone), there are no studies that evaluate the in vivo characteristics of these bioabsorbable implants with respect to strength over time.

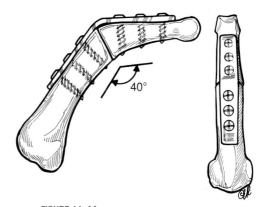

FIGURE 11-44. Plate fixation of the PIP joint.

Complications of Arthrodesis of Small Joints of the Hand

Because arthrodesis of finger joints is such a commonly performed procedure, it is often viewed as a predictable operation. This is far from true. A significant number of complications can occur, including infection (pin tract and deep infection), nonunion, malunion, vascular insufficiency, skin necrosis, prominent hardware, and cold intolerance.[74,135,168] In a review of complications of DIP joint arthrodesis, Stern and Fulton reported that, of 181 arthrodeses, 20% had a major complication of nonunion, malunion, and deep infection or osteomyelitis. An additional 16% had minor complications such as skin necrosis, cold intolerance, PIP joint stiffness, paresthesias, superficial wound infection, or prominent hardware.[135] The nonunion rate of the DIP joint

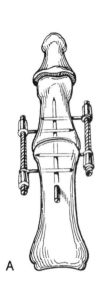

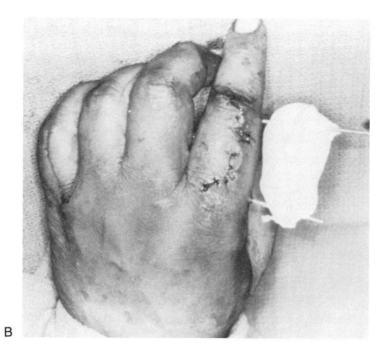

A   B

FIGURE 11-45. External fixators. **A,** Commercial type. **B,** A "homemade" external fixator created from Kirschner wires and methylmethacrylate. (**A** Adapted from Tupper JW: A compression arthrodesis device for small joints of the hands. Hand 4:62-64, 1972.)

arthrodeses in this series was similar for the techniques of crossed Kirschner wires, interfragmentary wire and Kirschner wires, and Herbert screw fixation. Successful arthrodesis was dependent on the quality and quantity of bone stock before the arthrodesis. Moberg and Hendrickson reported similar complications.[106] Hogh and Jenson reported that in primary arthrodesis for traumatic conditions, in which comminution and bone loss played a more prominent role, the nonunion rate was 38%.[65a] A comparison of fixation techniques, time to union, and failure rates for IP arthrodesis is detailed in Table 11-1.

Author's Preferred Method of Treatment of MP Joint Arthrodesis

The position and techniques of MP arthrodesis have been discussed earlier. We prefer to avoid MP arthrodesis in most cases, preferring arthroplasty. When arthrodesis is unavoidable, owing to tendon loss, then fixation in 25 degrees of flexion for the index finger, 30 degrees for the long finger, 35 degrees for the ring ringer, and 40 degrees for the small finger[168,169] is preferred. When applicable, a cup and cone technique or flat coapting surfaces is preferred, typically with tension band wire fixation. In cases in which wires cannot be applied (poor periarticular bone quality), plate fixation is preferred (Fig. 11-46).

Proximal Interphalangeal Joint Arthrodesis

Although many techniques for arthrodesis of the PIP joint exist, the basic tenets of surface preparation followed by

rigid fixation must be adhered to for successful outcome. Arthrodesis of the PIP joint reliably decreases pain and often improves function, especially for the index and middle fingers, where strong lateral pinch is an important element and flexion for grasping less critical than in the ulnar digits. However, with the introduction of the newer surface replacement arthroplasties, this distinction between the radial and ulnar sides of the hand may not necessarily be as valid. Nonetheless, in cases that do not meet the indications for arthroplasty, or in patients who require a durable solution to the stiff or arthritic PIP joint, arthrodesis is still recommended. This is particularly true for the index finger, which does not participate in power grip. For the ulnar three fingers, arthrodesis of the PIP joint may have a deleterious effect on grip strength, especially in patients with degenerative or traumatic arthritis, where adjacent fingers may be normal. In such cases, arthrodesis should truly be considered the last option in our opinion.

The optimal position of arthrodesis of the PIP joint is debatable, with some authors advocating a cascade from 40 degrees for the index finger to 55 degrees for the small finger[24,154] whereas other authors recommend a constant 40-degree angle for all fingers.[29] As with the MP joint, rotational malalignment and deviation in the coronal plane are poorly tolerated and should be avoided.

Our preference is the use of longitudinal Kirschner wires with an additional tension band wire. Exposure of the PIP joint is through a dorsal longitudinal incision over the joint. The extensor tendon is split longitudinally in the midline and elevated radially and ulnarly. The central tendon is released as well as the proximal origins of the collateral ligaments. The bone ends are prepared by flat resection with a microsagittal saw such that when the ends are coapted the angulation is appropriate for the digit and the varus/valgus alignment is in neutral position. A transverse hole is drilled in the middle phalanx with a 0.035-inch Kirschner wire

Table 11-1
RESULTS IN THE LITERATURE ON INTERPHALANGEAL ARTHRODESIS

Study	Fixation Technique	Time to Union (wk)	Failure Rate (%)
McGlynn, et al.[100]	Cup and cone, Kirschner wire	~8	0
Lewis, et al.[87]	Tension & mortise, Kirschner wire	~8	2
Khuri[79]	Tension band wire	7	0
Hogh and Jensen[65a]	Kirschner wire/cerclage	8	7-16
Granowitz and Vaino[57a]	Crossed Kirschner wire		7
Carroll and Hill[30]	Cup and cone, Kirschner wire	6-8	10 (all cases)
Lister[97]	Intraosseous wire	10	13
Burton, et al.[27a]	Kirschner wire	8	0
Buchler and Aikin[22]	Plate		8
Ayres, et al.[5]	Herbert screw		2
Moberg and Hendrickson[106]	Bone peg	~6	6
Allende and Engelem[3]	Tension band wire		0
Wright and McMurty[171]	Plate		0
Potenza[114a]	Bone peg and Kirschner wire	7	
Ijsselstein, et al.[69]	Kirschner wire	~6	8
Ijsselstein, et al.[69]	Tension band wire		3
Stern and Fulton[135]	Kirschner wire		12
Stern and Fulton[135]	Interosseous wire		12
Stern and Fulton[135]	Herbert screw		11
Katzman, et al.[78]	Herbert screw	8	0
Stern and Gates[136]	Tension band wire		3
Braun and Rhoades[18]	External fixator	~8	0
Seitz, et al.[124]	External fixator	6	9
Teoh, et al.[152]	Compression screw	8.2	4
Watson and Shaffer[164]	Kirschner wire	6	0
Leibovic and Strickland[86]	Kirschner wire	10	21
Leibovic and Strickland[86]	Tension band wire	11	5
Leibovic and Strickland[86]	Herbert screw	9	0
Leibovic and Strickland[86]	Plate	12	50+

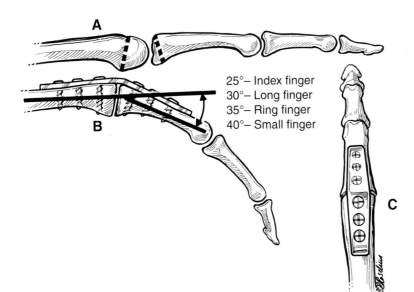

25°– Index finger
30°– Long finger
35°– Ring finger
40°– Small finger

FIGURE 11-46. **A** to **C,** Plate fixation for MP arthrodesis.

8 to 9 mm from the joint surface and a 20-gauge needle is passed through the drill hole. Through the tip of the needle a 26-gauge stainless steel wire is passed and the needle is removed. Two parallel 0.0035-inch Kirschner wires are passed retrograde from the center of the proximal anterior surface through the dorsal cortex. The prepared surfaces are coapted in the appropriate position, and the two parallel Kirschner wires are advanced across the fusion site engaging into the middle phalanx. The tension band wire is crossed in a figure-of-eight fashion around the protruding Kirschner wires and tightened, cut, and bent flush with the dorsal cortex. The protruding Kirschner wire lengths

CRITICAL POINTS: MP JOINT ARTHRODESIS

INDICATIONS

- Painful joint
- Arthritic changes
- Arthroplasty contraindicated

PREOPERATIVE EVALUATION

- Obtain radiographs.
- Relieve pain with intra-articular injection of anesthetic.

PEARLS

- Precise preparation of bone surfaces is essential to successful arthrodesis.
- There are multiple methods of bone fixation. Choose the technique that is appropriate for bone size, patient, and surgeon.

TECHNICAL POINTS

- A longitudinal, extensor tendon–splitting incision is used.
- Preserve joint capsule to close over hardware and arthrodesis site to prevent adhesion of extensor tendon.

- Preparation of bone surfaces: denude all cartilage, whether cup and cone or flap coapted surfaces.
- Obtain 25 degrees of flexion for index finger, 30 degrees for long finger, 35 degrees for ring finger, and 40 degrees for small finger.
- Occasionally, degree of flexion may be changed for occupational/recreational endeavors.

PITFALL

- Avoid radioulnar deviation and rotational deformity.

POSTOPERATIVE CARE

- Immobilize in bulky dressing with protective plaster splint.
- Replace with cast, which is worn until bony union is visible on radiographs.

ATHLETIC PARTICIPATION

- When solid union is visible on radiographs

---

are adjusted, bent, and cut such that they do not irritate the overlying skin. The extensor tendons are reapproximated with a 4-0 multi-filament nonabsorbable suture, and the skin is closed with a 4-0 monofilament nonabsorbable suture.

The hand is immobilized for 10 days, skin sutures are removed, and active range of motion of the hand and digits is encouraged with custom-made splint immobilization of the fused joint. Arthrodesis typically occurs between 4 and 6 weeks.

Distal Interphalangeal Joint Arthrodesis

Stiffness of the DIP joint is most often secondary to degenerative arthritis and is most easily addressed by arthrodesis. Similar to arthrodesis of the PIP, there are many techniques and recommendations regarding optimal position of DIP arthrodesis. The recommended position for DIP joint arthrodesis varies from 0 to 25 degrees of flexion for all fingers.[30,74,154,168] We prefer 0 to 5 degrees. Either tension band wiring, as previously described, or the use of a headless screw is our preferred technique of fixation for DIP arthrodesis.

The surgical approach we prefer is a "T"-shaped incision where the transverse limb is midway between the nail fold and the DIP joint line (see Fig. 11-36). Full-thickness flaps are created down to the epitenon and reflected. The extensor tendon insertion is divided at the base of the distal phalanx,

the joint capsule is incised transversely, and the collateral ligaments are divided (see Fig. 11-37). The joint surfaces are exposed by flexing the joint. If tension band wiring is to be performed, flat resection of the surfaces is prepared such that 5 degrees of flexion will result when the surfaces are coapted. If a cannulated scaphoid screw is to be used, the surfaces are prepared and the guide wire for the screw is inserted through the intramedullary canal of the distal phalanx and through the skin at the tip of the finger (Fig. 11-47). The joint is reduced in 0 degrees of flexion and the guide wire advanced across the fusion site and into the middle phalanx. Fluoroscopy is used to confirm the position of the wire and its length. Once proper length is determined, an incision is made at the tip of the finger around the guide wire and a fine hemostat is used to spread a tract for the screw and drill. The cannulated drill is advanced over the guide wire and drilled to the proper depth, and the cannulated screw is then advanced across the fusion site. Alternatively, a noncannulated headless screw can be inserted freehand. In either case, proper position is confirmed radiographically and the joint capsule is closed with nonabsorbable multifilament suture, as is the extensor tendon. The skin is reapproximated with 4-0 monofilament nonabsorbable suture, and the digit is immobilized in a bulky dressing with a plaster splint. The dressing is removed at 10 days, the sutures are removed, and mobilization of the nonfused joints of the hand is initiated. A custom-made splint immobilizing the fused joint is fabricated and used to immobilize the fusion site until union.

CRITICAL POINTS: PIP JOINT ARTHRODESIS

INDICATIONS

- Painful joint
- Arthritic changes
- Arthroplasty contraindicated (majority of cases)

PREOPERATIVE EVALUATION

- Obtain radiographs.
- Relieve pain with intra-articular injection of anesthetic.

PEARLS

- Precise preparation of bone surfaces is essential to successful arthrodesis.
- There are multiple methods of bone fixation. Choose the technique that is appropriate for bone size, patient, and surgeon.

TECHNICAL POINTS

- Use a longitudinal, extensor tendon–splitting incision.
- Preserve the joint capsule to close over hardware and arthrodesis site to prevent adhesion of extensor tendon.

- Preparation of bone surfaces: denude all cartilage, whether cup and cone or flap coapted surfaces.
- Obtain 40 degrees of flexion for index finger, 45 degrees for long finger, 50 degrees for ring finger, and 55 degrees for small finger.
- Occasionally, degree of flexion may be changed for occupational/recreational endeavors.

PITFALLS

- Avoid radioulnar deviation and rotational deformity.
- Avoid excessive shortening of bone.

POSTOPERATIVE CARE

- Immobilize in bulky dressing with protective plaster splint.
- Replace with orthoplast splint, which is worn until bony union is visible on radiographs.

ATHLETIC PARTICIPATION

- When solid union is visible on radiographs

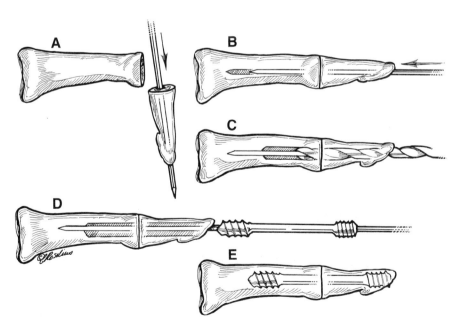

FIGURE 11-47. A to **E,** Herbert Whipple screw fixation for DIP joint arthrodesis.

ANNOTATED REFERENCES

20. Bruser P, Poss T, Larkin G: Results of proximal interphalangeal joint release for flexion contractures: Midlateral versus palmar incision. J Hand Surg [Am] 24:288-294, 1999.

A comparison of a midlateral versus palmar incision was retrospectively performed in comparably matched groups with respect to degree of contracture and demographic characteristics. In the palmar incision group, preoperative median PIP joint range of motion was 60 to 90 degrees (extension/flexion) and 30 to 90 degrees at the 3-year follow-up examination. In the midlateral incision group, preoperative median PIP joint range of motion was 50 to 90 degrees (extension/flexion) and 0 to 90 degrees at the 1.5-year follow-up examination. The improvement in range of motion was significantly better in the midlateral incision group than in the palmar incision group.

21. Buch VI: Clinical and functional assessment of the hand after metacarpophalangeal capsulotomy. Plast Reconstr Surg 53: 452-457, 1974.

An elegant anatomic, radiographic, and clinical study of MP joint stiffness. The author concisely details his anatomic and radiographic findings of the properties of the proper and accessory collateral ligaments and the tension on each during flexion and extension. A description of his method of capsulotomy and collateral ligament release to regain flexion is provided.

25. Bunnell S, Doherty DW, Curtis RM: Ischemic contracture, local, in the hand. Plast Reconstr Surg 3:424-433, 1948.

The classic article of ischemic contractures of the hand. A "must read" for every student of hand surgery.

27a. Burton RI, Margles SW, et al. Small-joint arthrodesis in the hand. J Hand Surg [Am] 11:678-882, 1986.

A review of 171 consecutive arthrodeses of small joints in 134 patients. Emphasis was placed on the accurate coaptation of bone surfaces, the use of cancellous bone graft when needed, maintenance of the coaptation with Kirschner wires, and the need for postoperative immobilization. This technique resulted in union of 170 of 171 arthrodeses (a nonunion rate of 0.6%). There were no infections. There were four delayed unions.

30. Carroll RE, Hill NA: Small joint arthrodesis in hand reconstruction. J Bone Joint Surg Am 51:1219-1221, 1969.

A classic article describing the cup and cone technique for small joint arthrodesis as well as the recommended positions of joint fusions.

38. Cook SD, Beckenbaugh RD, Redondo J, et al: Long-term follow-up of pyrolytic carbon metacarpophalangeal implants. J Bone Joint Surg Am 81:635-648, 1999.

A review of 151 pyrolytic carbon MP joint arthroplasties performed in 53 patients, mostly with rheumatoid arthritis. The background of pyrolytic carbon and the rationale for its use is eloquently described. Follow-up of an average of 11.7 years was obtained. The implants improved the arc of motion of the fingers by an average of 13 degrees and elevated the arc by an average of 16 degrees. As a result, fingers were in a more functional, extended position. There was a high prevalence of joint stability. No adverse remodeling or resorption of bone was seen. Survivorship analysis demonstrated an average annual failure rate of 2.1% and a 16-year survival rate of 70.3%. The 5- and 10-year survival rates were 82.3% (95% confidence interval, 74.6% to 88.2%) and 81.4% (95% confidence interval, 73.0% to 87.8%), respectively. None of the revised implants had any visible changes of wear or deformity of the surfaces or stems. The results of this study demonstrate that pyrolytic carbon is a biologically and biomechanically compatible, wear-resistant, and durable material for arthroplasty of the MP joint.

40. Curtis M: Capsulectomy of the interphalangeal joints of the fingers. J Bone Joint Surg Am 36:1219-1232, 1954.

The classic description of the etiology and treatment of contractures of the IP joints of the hand. The surgical treatment described remains one of the most common methods of treatment nearly 50 years since it was described in this article.

56. Ghidella SD, Segalman KA, et al: Long-term results of surgical management of proximal interphalangeal joint contracture. J Hand Surg [Am] 27:799-805, 2002.

To evaluate the long-term results of surgical treatment of PIP joint contractures, 68 PIP joints were retrospectively reviewed with a minimum follow-up period of 24 months. Preoperative and intraoperative factors were studied for outcomes and subjected to statistical analysis. Among the total group the average improvement was 7.5 degrees. When grouped by diagnosis into simple (less severe diagnoses) and complex (more severe diagnoses) the average degrees gained were 17.2 degrees and 0.5 degree, respectively. The statistically significant factors that were identified that affected results were age, number of prior procedures, preoperative flexion, removal of an exostosis, number of structures addressed, and preoperative arc of motion. The second surgery (joints requiring repeat release or salvage procedure) rates were 35% overall, 29% simple, and 39% complex; the difference was not significant. The best surgical candidate is a patient younger than 28 years with a less severe diagnosis and who has preoperative maximum flexion measurement less than 43 degrees.

66. Houshian S, Gynning B, Schroder HA: Chronic flexion contracture of proximal interphalangeal joint treated with the Compass Hinge External Fixator: A consecutive series of 27 cases. J Hand Surg [Br] 27:356-358, 2002.

Twenty-seven chronic flexion contractures of the PIP joint were treated with the Compass Hinge external fixator without open surgery. The fixator was removed after a mean of 33 (range, 14 to 68) days. The mean time from injury to operation was 4 (range, 1 to 19) years, and all patients were reviewed at a mean follow-up of 21 (range, 12 to 50) months. The mean extension gain was 38 degrees (range, 0 to 70 degrees), and the mean flexion-extension arc improved by 42 degrees (range, 0 to 80 degrees). Complications included superficial pin tract infection in 11 cases and pin loosening in four cases.

68. Hunter E, Laverty J, Pollock R, Birch R: Nonoperative treatment of fixed flexion deformity of the proximal interphalangeal joint. J Hand Surg [Br] 24:281-283, 1999.

Sixty-one stiff, stable PIP joints were treated by exercise and splinting. The average range of movement was 24 to 67 degrees before treatment; this increased to 8 to 98 degrees after treatment. The indications and technique are described.

70a. Iselin F: Arthroplasty of the proximal interphalangeal joint after trauma. Hand 7:41-42, 1975.

The results of 238 PIP joint arthroplasties performed for post-traumatic joint stiffness. The long-term results of 25 patients were reviewed and found to have 67% good results versus 36% fair and poor results. The author states that Silastic arthroplasty for post-traumatic joint stiffness is useful.

83. Landsmeer JMF: The anatomy of the dorsal aponeurosis of the human finger and its functional significance. Anat Rec 104:31, 1949.

The classic description of the extensor tendon anatomy of the finger.

102. Messina A, Messina J: The continuous elongation treatment by the TEC device for severe Dupuytren's contracture of the fingers. Plast Reconstr Surg 92:84-90, 1993.

Although not applied to the "stiff finger" secondary to traumatic conditions, the continuous elongation technique that was described for Dupuytren's contracture has been applied to non-Dupuytren's etiologies for joint stiffness. In this article the results of the TEC device are described. As a preparatory step for excision of the pathologic palmar fascia for severe Dupuytren's contracture of the hands, the application of the TEC device results in physiologic, painless, and atraumatic elongation of contracted tissues that is obtained by means of a device fixed on the fourth and fifth metacarpal bones by two self-tapping pins. This paper described the rationale and the results of treatment in patients with Dupuytren's contractures.

128a. Smith RJ: Non-ischemic contractures of the intrinsic muscles of the hand. J Bone Joint Surg [Am] 53:1313-1331, 1971

The classic description of intrinsic contractures, anatomy, and treatment.

163. Watson HK, Light TR, Johnson TR, et al: Checkrein resection for flexion contracture of the middle joint. J Hand Surg 4:67-71, 1979.

The classic description of the checkrein ligament release for flexion contractures of the proximal interphalangeal joint.

166. Weeks PM, Wray RC Jr, Kuxhaus M: The results of nonoperative management of stiff joints in the hand. Plast Reconstr Surg 61:58-63, 1978.

A large series of conservatively managed contractures of the hand, in which 173 of the 212 patients treated and 686 of 789 stiff joints responded sufficiently to this treatment alone. The results of this regimen of nonoperative treatment of stiff joints provide excellent functional improvement in most patients, with a large saving of money through the reduction in disability payments required.

167. Weeks PM, Young VL, Wray RC Jr: Operative mobilization of stiff metacarpophalangeal joints: Dorsal versus volar approach. Ann Plast Surg 5:178-185, 1980.

The effectiveness and merits of the dorsal and volar approaches for release of structures contributing to MP joint stiffness were studied. Seventy-six percent of the joints in the volar group gained greater than 50 degrees passive motion compared with 29% in the dorsal group. Forty-four percent of the joints in the volar group gained greater than 50 degrees of active motion compared with 16% in the dorsal group. Discussion of surgical technique and postoperative management reveals that the advantages of the volar approach are most evident during postoperative management, whereas the main advantage of the dorsal approach is better operative exposure.

175. Young VL, Wray RC Jr, Weeks PM: The surgical management of stiff joints in the hand. Plast Reconstr Surg 62:835-841, 1978.

Significant and lasting improvement in stiff MP and PIP joints can be achieved by operative management. Operative intervention should be considered only after persistence of stiffness following a vigorous program of nonoperative therapy. In this series of 135 such stiff finger joints, capsulotomy increased the range of motion in MP joints by more than 30 degrees in 68% of the patients, more than 50 degrees in 57%, and more than 70 degrees in 32%. The increased range of motion for the PIP joints was more than 30 degrees in 63% of the patients, more than 50 degrees in 41%, and more than 70 degrees in 25%.

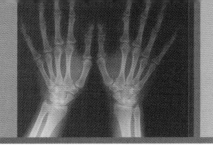

CHAPTER 12

Thumb Basal Joint Arthritis

Matthew M. Tomaino, John King, and Michel Leit

The term *osteoarthritis* has been rather loosely used to refer to all degenerative conditions of articular cartilage other than the classically described inflammatory arthropathies, such as rheumatoid disease and the seronegative spondyloarthropathies. *Osteoarthritis* is best reserved to describe the degeneration of articular cartilage that occurs without clear etiology, and, indeed, *primary idiopathic osteoarthritis* has been suggested as a more descriptive name for this condition.

Both clinical and radiographic examinations of the hand are fundamental to making the diagnosis of primary idiopathic osteoarthritis. Although the trapeziometacarpal (TM) joint is the second most commonly involved site of disease, after the distal interphalangeal (DIP) joint, its involvement causes, potentially, far more significant functional disability secondary to painful, weakened pinch and grip.

Accordingly, we exclusively address the subject of thumb "basal joint" arthritis in this chapter—terminology aptly chosen in light of the fact that degeneration is not restricted to the TM joint alone but may involve all five articulations of the pantrapezial "basal joint" (Fig. 12-1).[84]

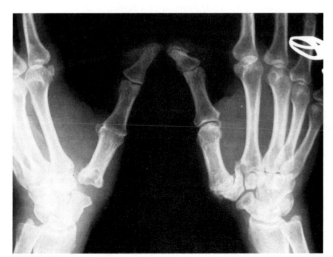

FIGURE 12-1. A 30-degree oblique radiograph shows the five trapezial articulations that may be involved in "basal joint arthritis": trapeziometacarpal, scaphotrapezial, scaphotrapezoidal, trapezium-index metacarpal, and trapezium-trapezoid.

The management of symptomatic thumb basal joint arthritis requires an understanding of normal functional imperatives for the thumb, its ligamentous anatomy and kinematics, pathomechanics, and pathoanatomy, the effect of hyperextensibility at the thumb metacarpophalangeal (MP) joint, radiographic staging, and, lastly, treatment options and expected surgical outcomes. Indeed, there are many surgical options and a plethora of articles that address treatment options. We provide needed historical, anatomic, and biomechanical background and then proceed to diagnosis, treatment options and outcomes, revision surgery, and finally new developments.

THE FOUNDATION

Historical Perspective

Evolution of the human hand has revolved around the refinement of a prehensile thumb such that more consummate stability has been compromised in the interest of mobility. Indeed, the basal joint of our simian ancestors functioned as a single-axis hinge, providing only thumb flexion-extension in the plane of the palm.[90] The evolution of a biconcave saddle joint along with the muscles to provide active opposition has increased the importance of stabilizing ligaments during lateral pinch, which, when incompetent or injured, may lead to arthritic degeneration.[91]

Gervis has frequently been referenced for his review of trapeziectomy in 1949 as treatment for basal joint arthritis,[45] partly because he himself underwent the procedure. Interestingly, despite less than ideal long-term durability and pain relief, and now well-documented favorable results when ligament reconstruction is combined with trapezium excision,[109,113] the operation performed on and by Gervis more than 50 years ago is not only still performed today but with renewed popularity.[59,65]

Ligamentous Anatomy and Thumb Kinematics

The complex anatomy of the TM joint permits prehension, opposition, and circumduction. An appreciation of the specific architecture of the thumb axis is fundamental to understanding the role of ligament incompetence in the development of pathologic translation and arthritic degeneration.

The TM joint is a biconcave-convex saddle joint with minimal bony constraints.[52] Although the incongruity in the radii of curvature between the thumb metacarpal articulation and trapezium provides increased mobility, limited bony constraint exists except at the extremes of motion.[81] The function and kinematics of the three joints of the thumb as a unit is a function, in large part, of eight musculotendinous units acting on it.[22] Biomechanical studies by Cooney and Chao underscored the importance of strong supporting ligaments, particularly during pinch and grasp, when large axial and cantilever loads are transmitted to the TM joint.[22] These authors have reported the motion of a normal TM joint.[22] The arc of active flexion-extension is 53 ± 11 degrees, and the arc of active abduction-adduction is 42 ± 4 degrees. The most common position of the first metacarpal during normal thumb function is flexion, adduction, and pronation.

There is only minimal constraint of the joint from a bony standpoint, and thus ligamentous support is extremely important, especially considering the compressive forces transmitted across the joint during functional pinch.[22] Cooney and Chao showed that the extrinsic tendon forces during pinch and grasp are four to five times the applied external forces. Most of these forces in pinch are transmitted dorsoradially and proximally. The intrinsic tendon forces are one and one-half to three times the applied external force. A pinch force of 1 kg at the thumb tip is magnified up to 3.68 kg at the interphalangeal (IP) joint, up to 6.61 kg at the MP joint, and up to 13.42 kg at the TM joint.[22] Cantilever bending significantly contributes to the forces across the TM joint, which may contribute to tangential dorsoradial subluxating forces and cartilage erosion.[7]

Prior to more contemporary anatomic studies,[7,57] Eaton and Littler[36] identified the anterior oblique "beak" ligament, so called for its attachment on the palmar beak of the thumb metacarpal, as the primary stabilizer of the TM joint (Fig. 12-2). Furthermore, they identified that the weakest portion of the capsule was between the beak ligament and the dorsal ligaments. The beak ligament is intracapsular and attaches to the beak on the ulnar side of the first metacarpal. It originates from the palmar aspect of the trapezium, and in this position it is an effective restraint against dorsal translation of the metacarpal on the trapezium, which is of particular importance during pinch and grip.

With the assistance of arthroscopy of the TM joint, Bettinger and colleagues[7] have further defined the anterior oblique ligament (AOL) into a superficial (sAOL) and deep ligament (dAOL) (see Fig. 12-2). The dAOL, which is intracapsular, is in fact the beak ligament. The dAOL plays an important role in the kinematics of thumb opposition. It acts as a pivot point and becomes tight during pronation, opposition, and palmar abduction. The dAOL limits pronation in flexion and both pronation and supination in extension.[7] The sAOL, which also originates from the volar aspect of the trapezium, inserts broadly about 2 mm distal to the articular surface on the volar aspect of the first metacarpal. The sAOL, which appears to be lax in both the normal and pathologic state, along with the dAOL, functions to limit volar subluxation of the TM joint. Laxity of the sAOL permits pronation to occur during opposition.

In their comprehensive assessment of the ligamentous anatomy of the TM joint, Bettinger and colleagues[7] described a total of 16 ligaments that stabilize the trapezium and TM. Seven of these ligaments, including the sAOL, dAOL "beak" ligament, dorsoradial (DRL), posterior oblique (POL), ulnar collateral (UCL), intermetacarpal (IML), and dorsal intermetacarpal ligament (DIML), are responsible for directly

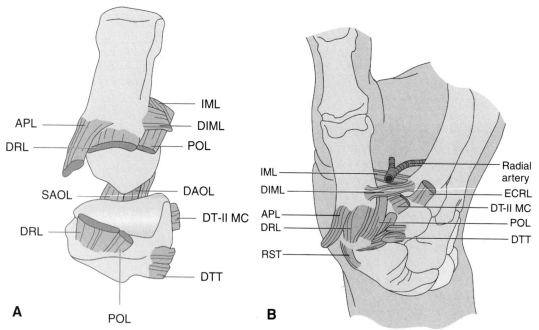

FIGURE 12-2. Trapeziometacarpal (TM) ligaments. **A,** Volar ligaments. The TM joint has been hinged open from the dorsum to reveal the deep anterior oblique ligament (DAOL; beak ligament) lying within the joint ulnar to the volar tubercle of the metacarpal. **B,** Dorsal ligaments (the ECRL has been reflected distally). APL, abductor pollicis longus tendon; DIML, dorsal intermetacarpal ligament; DRL, dorsoradial ligament; DT-II MC, dorsal trapezio-II metacarpal ligament; DTT, dorsal trapeziotrapezoid; IML, intermetacarpal ligament; POL, posterior oblique ligament; RST, radial scaphotrapezial ligament. SAOL, superficial anterior oblique ligament. (Redrawn from Bettinger P, Linschied RL, Berger R, et al: An anatomic study of the stabilizing ligaments of the trapezium and trapeziometacarpal joint. J Hand Surg [Am] 24:786-798, 1999.)

stabilizing the TM joint. The remaining nine ligaments stabilize the trapezium, providing a stable base for the TM joint. These ligaments are tight without any load. Some of these ligaments may function as tension bands to resist cantilever-bending forces of the metacarpal on the trapezium, thus providing a stable base for the TM joint. We recommend further study of Bettinger and colleagues' article for more detail.[7]

Although earlier work by Imaeda and Cooney[57] did not establish an important role for the DRL in joint stability, Bettinger and colleagues[7] showed that the DRL is an important joint stabilizer. The DRL, which covers a large percentage of the posterior aspect of the joint, is a wide thick ligament that attaches to the trapezium and inserts on the dorsum of the metacarpal base (see Fig. 12-2). This ligament tightens with dorsoradial and dorsal translational forces in all positions except full extension. It also tightens in supination and in pronation with joint flexion. The Eaton and Littler ligament reconstruction using a dorsal metacarpal drill hole in effect reconstructs the DRL.[36]

The POL, UCL, IML, and DIML provide additional support. The POL originates on the dorsoulnar aspect of the trapezium and inserts onto the dorsoulnar aspect of the thumb metacarpal and the palmar-ulnar tubercle with the IML. The POL resists ulnar translation of the metacarpal base during abduction and opposition. The UCL originates from the transverse carpal ligament and inserts superficial and ulnar to the sAOL on the palmar-ulnar tubercle of the metacarpal. The UCL limits volar metacarpal subluxation. The IML originates on the dorsoradial aspect of the index metacarpal radial to the ECRL and inserts on the palmar-ulnar tubercle of the base of the thumb metacarpal. According to Bettinger and colleagues,[7] the IML resists radial subluxation and volar subluxation. The DIML also originates on the dorsoradial aspect of the index metacarpal but superficial to the ECRL insertion. It inserts on the dorsoulnar aspect of the thumb metacarpal. It appears to constrain metacarpal pronation.

The versatile ligamentous anatomy of the TM joint of the human thumb permits prehensile activities. The evolutionarily unique articular configuration and complex ligament system of this joint initially appreciated by Eaton and Littler,[36] and explored more recently by Bettinger and colleagues,[7] allows motion in multiple planes. An in-depth understanding of these ligaments clearly assists in understanding the rationale behind clinically successful ligament reconstruction procedures to date[113] and may stimulate new approaches in the future.

Pathomechanics and Pathoanatomy

The etiology of osteoarthritis involves many factors. A complex interplay between biomechanical and biochemical factors certainly contributes to the production of clinical disease at the basal joint.[91] Synovially derived cytokines such as interleukin-1 have been shown to activate degradative enzyme synthesis in the chondrocyte, which result in breakdown of the proteoglycan matrix components. Neutral proteases and metalloproteoglycanases play a central role in catabolism of the matrix, resulting in decreased hydrophilic properties and a smaller volume of hydration of cartilage. These biochemical events significantly alter the mechanical properties of hyaline cartilage, making it more susceptible to failure under

load and less effective in buffering the subchondral trabeculae from impact loading and fracture.[95] Furthermore, hyaline cartilage and the surrounding collagenous tissues may be sensitive to estrogen-related compounds, potentially clarifying our understanding of the gender predisposition of this disease.

Pellegrini's analysis of both surgical and postmortem specimens of the TM joint revealed the chondromalacic nature of the articular cartilage in the dorsal compartment, but, more importantly, that the palmar joint surfaces were often found to be polished to eburnated bone.[88,89] Eburnation always began at the most palmar perimeter of the joint and spread dorsally with progressive disease, sparing only a small peripheral rim of pitted and softened cartilage in the dorsal compartment of end-stage joints. Palmar cartilage surface degeneration was closely associated with degeneration of the beak ligament from the articular margin of the metacarpal.[30] In all cases of eburnation there was frank detachment of the ligament from its normal position confluent with the joint surface, effectively reducing its mechanical efficiency in checking dorsal migration of the metacarpal on trapezium during dynamic flexion-adduction of the thumb.

Pellegrini also showed that the primary loading areas during lateral pinch are in the same palmar regions of the joint as the eburnated surfaces in diseased joints.[93] Division of the beak ligament in specimens with healthy cartilage surfaces altered the contact patterns and reproduced the topography of the eburnated lesions observed in the arthritic joints. Furthermore, contact patterns in specimens with end-stage arthritic disease were notable for pathologic congruity with total contact of joint surfaces, hypertrophic marginal osteophytes, and diffuse eburnation. Biochemical analysis of hyaline cartilage from arthritic TM joints revealed preferential loss of glycosaminoglycan from the extracellular matrix with relative sparing of the collagen framework in the palmar regions of the joint where osteoarthritic lesions first appear.[88]

This is consistent with the aforementioned suggestion that a selective biochemical degradation of the extracellular matrix contributes to the development of osteoarthritis of the TM joint. The unique feature of this observation in this joint is the localization of this process to the palmar contact areas of the joint where mechanical abrasion and shear are most severe. Scanning electron microscopy of TM surfaces has demonstrated disruption of the protective superficial cartilage lamina in these same palmar contact regions where glycosaminoglycan loss and eventual osteoarthritic disease are known to occur.[91] Furthermore, histologic study has shown that attritional changes in the POL where it attaches to the palmar lip of the metacarpal precede degeneration of cartilage.[30]

Thus, in summary, degeneration of the TM joint POL has been linked to the development of osteoarthritis. Functional incompetence of the POL results in pathologic laxity, abnormal translation of the metacarpal on the trapezium, and generation of excessive shear forces between the joint surfaces, particularly within the palmar portion of the joint during grip and pinch activity.[93] Because the POL appears to be the primary stabilizer of the TM joint, and because its detachment results in dorsal translation of the metacarpal, its reconstruction has been recommended to restore thumb stability not only in cases of end-stage osteoarthritis but also for early-stage disease.[34,36,41]

Such a mechanism of osteoarthritis, predicated on instability of the TM joint, is consistent with the empirical clinical observations of amelioration of synovitis and retardation of the progression of arthritic disease in young women with symptomatic hypermobile joints after palmar beak ligament reconstruction procedures.[41]

THE CLINICAL SCENARIO

Epidemiology

Basal joint arthritis may present as mild symptoms beneath the thenar cone at the level of the TM joint, particularly during pinch and grip. Ultimately the greatest functional impairment occurs with advanced disease-limiting breadth of grasp and forceful lateral pinch activities such as brushing teeth, turning a key, opening a jar, or picking up a book. Complaints are directed toward the base of the thumb, and pain is frequently associated with a sensation of movement or "slipping" within the joint. An enlarging prominence, or "shoulder sign," inevitably develops at the base as the clinical manifestation of dorsal metacarpal subluxation on the trapezium and metacarpal adduction (Fig. 12-3).

Women with the disorder outnumber men by a ratio of 10 to 15:1, but work-related mechanical loading has long been thought to influence the frequency and pattern of osteoarthritic disease.[61] Geographic and racial differences also appear to have a strong influence on the prevalence of osteoarthritis in the hand, particularly relative to the observed differences in TM disease among Asian and white populations.[90] Post-mortem material from whites has consistently demonstrated a prevalence of severe disease, with eburnation of joint surfaces in 50%, chondromalacia in 25%, and grossly normal hyaline cartilage in 25% of specimens.[22] In contrast, a review of published studies in the Japanese literature, accounting for more than 500 specimens, shows evidence for eburnation in only 8%, chondromalacia in 48%, and normal joint surfaces in 44% of specimens.[43]

Physical Diagnosis

Physical examination characteristically reveals tenderness along the thumb TM joint, and the traditional grind test, performed with axial compression, flexion, extension, and circumduction, causes crepitance and pain (Fig. 12-4). Patients with early involvement may present with pain on TM stress and palpation beneath the thenar cone, without deformity, instability, subluxation, or crepitance.[36] The decision for operative treatment is not based solely on radiographs, because patients may be quite asymptomatic despite significant radiographic evidence of joint degeneration. Conversely, patients with relatively mild radiographic changes may be very symptomatic.

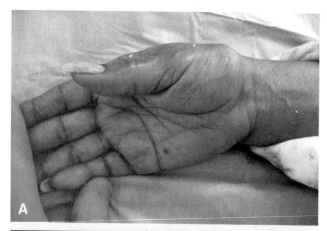

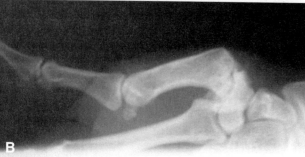

FIGURE 12-3. A, Clinical photograph of the typical basal joint "shoulder sign." Note the dorsal prominence of the base of the thumb metacarpal. **B,** Corresponding lateral radiograph showing TM dorsal subluxation.

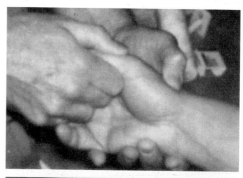

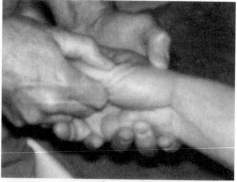

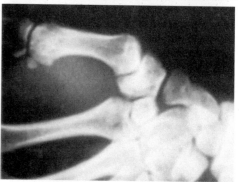

FIGURE 12-4. The grind test.

It is critical to evaluate the entire hand for signs and symptoms of carpal tunnel syndrome; stenosing flexor tenosynovitis; DeQuervain's disease; and scaphotrapezial, scaphotrapezoidal,[58,84,114] and subsesamoid arthritis.[76] Allen's test should be performed because exposure of the basal joint during surgery may involve mobilization of, and potential injury to, the radial artery. Swelling after basal joint arthroplasty may exacerbate even mild cases of carpal tunnel syndrome, which may coexist with basal joint arthritis in up to 43% of cases.[39] Concomitant carpal tunnel release is recommended in such patients because basal joint surgery alone does not appear to significantly increase carpal tunnel volume based on magnetic resonance imaging (MRI) estimates.[49]

Pain secondary to the other conditions mentioned earlier may compromise compliance with postoperative hand therapy in the short term and pain relief and functional improvement in the long term. It is important, therefore, to treat these entities should they coexist with basal joint arthritis. Scaphotrapezoidal arthritis, in particular, may be underappreciated on preoperative radiographs, which have a sensitivity of only 44% and a specificity of 86%[114] (Fig. 12-5). A prevalence of over 60% in patients requiring basal joint arthroplasty[114] and the potential that unaddressed scaphotrapezoidal arthritis may be cause residual pain postoperatively[58] support routine intraoperative assessment of this articulation and excision of the proximal trapezoid if degeneration is present.[25]

The thumb MP joint should also be carefully assessed preoperatively for the presence of hyperextensibility, particularly during lateral pinch (Fig. 12-6). Thumb MP joint hyperextensibility may cause or exacerbate metacarpal adduction. Thus, after trapezium excision, if MP joint hyperextension occurs during pinch and grip, dorsally directed vectors at the base of the metacarpal might inordinately stress a ligament reconstruction, if performed, or lead to frank dorsal subluxation after trapeziectomy alone. When hyperextension deformity exceeds 20 degrees, either fusion or volar capsulodesis is recommended.[72]

Radiographic Staging

Radiographic evaluation includes posteroanterior 30-degree oblique stress view, lateral view, and Robert (pronated anteroposterior) view (Fig. 12-7). Osteoarthritis may be confined to the TM joint, or it may involve the pantrapezial joint complex. Indeed, the staging system originated by Eaton and Littler[36] described four stages:

- Stage 1: a normal joint with the exception of possible widening from synovitis
- Stage 2: joint space narrowing with debris and osteophytes less than 2 mm
- Stage 3: joint space narrowing with debris and osteophytes greater than 2 mm in size
- Stage 4: scaphotrapezial joint space involvement in addition to narrowing of the TM joint

They underscored the importance of diagnosing scaphotrapezial arthritis (stage 4) because hemitrapeziectomy alone, in such cases, will be complicated by residual pain. The staging system neglects any mention of the scaphotrapezoidal joint, but North and Eaton identified degenerative changes at this articulation in 16 of 68 cadaver hands (24%).[84] Irwin and coworkers, in 1995, heightened our appreciation of

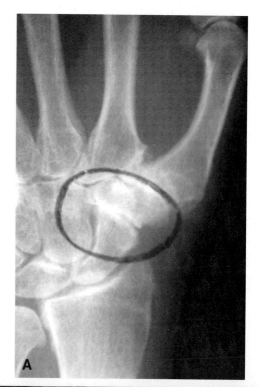

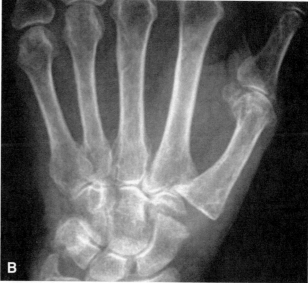

FIGURE 12-5. Stage 5 disease (pantrapezial arthritis). **A,** Preoperative radiograph. **B,** LRTI arthroplasty and proximal resection of the trapezoid have been performed.

unaddressed scaphotrapezoidal arthritis as a potential cause of residual pain after the ligament reconstruction tendon interposition (LRTI) arthroplasty.[58] Because the x-ray sensitivity and specificity for disease at the scaphotrapezoidal joint are only 44% and 86%, respectively,[114] routine intraoperative assessment of the scaphotrapezoidal joint is mandatory at the time of arthroplasty by pulling on the index and long fingers. Inspection of the scaphotrapezoidal joint is further facilitated by inserting a Freer elevator into the joint to gently wedge the joint open. When arthritis is present, what may be considered "stage 5 disease" (see Fig. 12-5), 2- to 3-mm excision of the proximal trapezoid can be per-

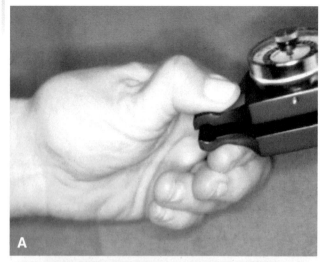

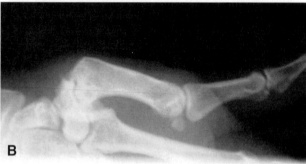

FIGURE 12-6. MP joint hyperextensibility. **A,** Pinch increases thumb MP joint hyperextensibility, which in turn accentuates metacarpal adduction. **B,** Radiograph shows hyperextension of the MP joint and adduction of the thumb metacarpal.

formed without morbidity to avoid the potential for residual pain in the postoperative period after arthroplasty.[58,114]

Operative Indications

Indications for surgical intervention of basal joint disease of the thumb include pain, deformity, and/or weakness that interfere with daily function and are unresponsive to nonoperative measures. Historically, radiographic staging has facilitated a "stage-dependent" treatment approach in which ligament reconstruction was recommended for stage 1 disease; hemitrapeziectomy, TM fusion, or implant arthroplasty for stages 2 and 3 (TM arthritis only); and complete trapezium excision with or without ligament reconstruction for stage 4 disease (pantrapezial arthritis).

Stage 1 disease continues to deserve special mention (see next section on surgical options), but the treatment of all remaining stages can be grouped together, because few surgeons today preferentially perform a hemitrapeziectomy for stages 2 and 3 because of the technical ease and the benefit of improved restoration of the breadth of the thumb-index web when complete trapeziectomy is performed. Obviously, pantrapezial involvement contraindicates procedures such as TM arthrodesis or hemitrapeziectomy alone. Surgical treatment options and their rationale, indications, contraindications, and expected outcomes are discussed in detail later in this chapter.

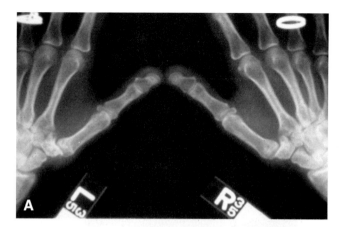

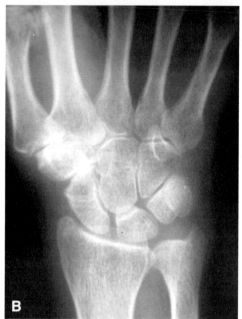

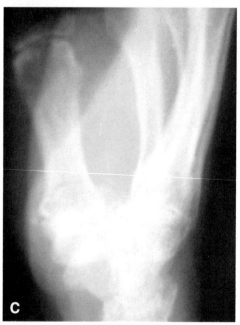

FIGURE 12-7. Standard basal joint radiographic series. **A,** A 30-degree oblique stress view (note thumb tips pressing against each other). **B,** Lateral view. **C,** Robert view (true anteroposterior view of the TM joint).

Nonoperative Treatment

Nonoperative treatment includes anti-inflammatory medication, intra-articular corticosteroid injection, hand- or forearm-based thumb spica splint immobilization, and thenar muscle isometric conditioning.[6,107,120] Although none of these measures may provide permanent or even long-lasting relief from symptoms, they may indeed provide temporary relief and, in so doing, allow the patient a more active role in participating in the acceptance and timing of surgical intervention. Swigart and colleagues reported that 76% of patients with stage 1 and 2 disease and 54% with stage 3 and 4 disease had improvement in their symptoms with splinting.[107] Six months after the initiation of a splinting program the symptom severity scores improved an average of between 54 and 61%.[107] A short opponens splint may be preferable to a long opponens splint,[120] and Berggren and associates reported that longitudinal analysis of 33 patients over 7 years showed that occupational therapy and splinting were successful in helping 70% to avoid surgery altogether.[6]

OPERATIVE TREATMENT

Stage 1 Disease

Until recently, surgical treatment has centered around reconstruction of the palmar beak ligament with a slip of flexor carpi radialis (FCR) tendon as described by Eaton and Littler[36] (Fig. 12-8). However, for this stabilizing procedure to provide pain relief, the joint surfaces must be free of eburnation and demonstrate only the earliest changes of chondromalacia in the contact areas of the palmar compartment. Such a complete assessment of the articular surfaces is best afforded intraoperatively by the exposure gained through a Wagner approach, detaching the origin of the thenar musculature to reveal the membranous capsule between the abductor pollicis longus (APL) and the palmar beak ligament.

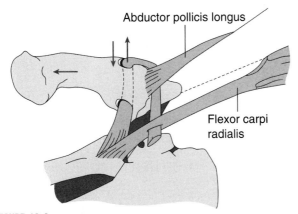

Abductor pollicis longus

Flexor carpi radialis

FIGURE 12-8. Littler-Eaton ligament reconstruction. This utilizes half of the flexor carpi radialis (FCR) tendon, passed through a bony channel in the metacarpal base to its dorsum. The tendon is then routed proximally to pass beneath the abductor pollicis longus tendon, around or through the FCR, and back across the radial margin of the TM joint. It reinforces the volar, dorsal, and radial aspects of the TM joint. (Redrawn from Tomaino MM: Treatment of Eaton stage 1 trapeziometacarpal disease: Ligament reconstruction or thumb metacarpal extension osteotomy? Hand Clin 17:197-205, 2001.)

Therefore, the plan to perform ligament reconstruction without an arthroplasty procedure must always be contingent on intraoperative confirmation of satisfactory articular surfaces, and both surgeon and patient must be prepared to exercise an alternative treatment option should this not be the case.

The objective of ligament reconstruction in the treatment of the hypermobile TM joint is the restoration of a static restraint to dorsal translation. Even before the availability of contemporary anatomic reports,[7,57] Eaton and Littler recognized that the anterior oblique (beak) ligament, which inserts on the palmar beak of the metacarpal, is the key structure responsible for maintaining thumb stability.[36] They also noted that the weakest portion of the TM capsule spanned between the palmar beak ligament and the dorsal ligaments in a plane perpendicular to the former. Indeed, the ligament reconstruction described by these authors reconstructs the beak ligament and reinforces the membranous radial capsule.[36] As evidence becomes available that supports the importance of the dorsal ligaments as well,[7] this ligament reconstruction, through exit of the FCR tendon at the dorsum of the metacarpal base and its passage around the APL tendon, provides reinforcement dorsally as well (see Fig. 12-8).

Many alternative techniques for ligament reconstruction have been reported.[9,11,19,97] Brunelli and coworkers preferred to use the APL tendon, noting that its use removed a "dislocating force" on the base of the first metacarpal.[11] At an average follow-up of 21 months, Roberts and colleagues reported a favorable outcome in 13 of 14 patients using Brunelli and coworkers' technique.[97]

In 1984, Eaton and associates reported long-term follow-up on 50 thumbs after the procedure.[34] For eight thumbs with stage 1 disease, that is, with a normal TM joint space, excellent pain relief and complete restoration of pinch strength resulted. In 1987, Lane and Eaton reported the results of ligament reconstruction in 25 prearthritic (stage 1) thumbs, with an average follow-up of 5.2 years.[67] All patients had a good or excellent result. Eighteen patients (72%) had no pain postoperatively; 7 (28%) experienced rare discomfort with repeated or heavy use. Pinch strength was equal to or greater than the contralateral side in 19 patients (76%), 90% or more than the opposite side in 4 (16%), and between 70% and 90% of the opposite side in only 2 patients (8%).[67] Follow-up radiographs at least 1 year after surgery in 21 revealed no evidence of degenerative change.

Most recently, Freedman and coworkers showed that ligament reconstruction restored pain-free TM stability and prevented the development of TM osteoarthritis in 15 of 23 thumbs (65%) at an average follow-up of 15 years.[41] Only 8% of thumbs advanced to show radiographic evidence of arthritic disease and 15 patients were at least 90% satisfied with their long-term results. Among the 15 thumbs classified as stage 1 at final follow-up, pain was noted in 10, although all were able to return to their preoperative occupation. Eight of the 15 thumbs had no tenderness at the TM joint on physical examination. Overall, pinch and grip strength averaged 108% and 105% of the contralateral side, respectively.[41]

Pellegrini and colleagues' biomechanical analysis of the effects of thumb metacarpal osteotomy[94] inspired Tomaino's prospective investigation of the efficacy of this procedure for treatment of stage 1 disease[111] (Fig. 12-9). The rationale for thumb metacarpal extension osteotomy involves dorsal load transfer and a shift in force vectors during pinch.

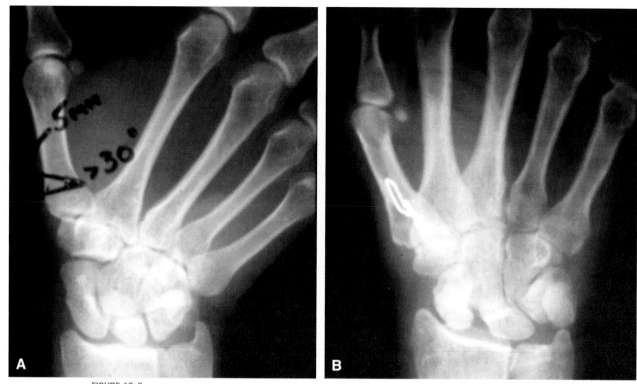

FIGURE 12-9. Extension osteotomy. **A,** A 30-degree closing wedge is planned. **B,** Postoperative radiograph.

Pellegrini and colleagues showed that a 30-degree closing wedge extension osteotomy effectively unloaded the palmar compartment when eburnation involved less than one half, and optimally only one third, of the palmar joint surfaces.[94] Osteotomy in this setting shifted the contact areas to the intact dorsal articular cartilage. The most recent biomechanical assessment of metacarpal osteotomy suggested that joint laxity is reduced in lateral pinch because of obligatory metacarpal flexion and resulting increased tightening of the dorsal radial ligament.[100]

Tomaino's report of metacarpal osteotomy in 12 patients with an average follow-up of 2.1 years showed that all osteotomies healed at an average of 7 weeks and 11 patients were satisfied with outcome.[111] Grip and pinch strength increased an average of 8.5 and 3 kg, respectively. No long-term follow-up studies are yet available on metacarpal osteotomy, but early reports suggest that thumb metacarpal extension osteotomy may be an effective "biomechanical alternative" to ligament reconstruction as treatment for Eaton stage 1 disease of the TM joint.[110]

Methods of Treatment: Stage 1
Ligament Reconstruction[36]
The TM joint is exposed through the so-called Wagner approach. An incision is made along the radial border of the metacarpal, at the junction of the more dorsal, hair-bearing skin and the glabrous skin. At the base of the thumb it curves ulnarly at the wrist crease as far as the FCR tendon. Care should be taken to identify and protect branches of the radial sensory nerve. The volar branch of the radial artery can be coagulated and divided if necessary.

The thenar muscles are reflected extraperiosteally from the metacarpal and volar aspect of the trapezium. At the proximal border of the trapezium transverse fascia fibers overlying the FCR are incised longitudinally and released, thus exposing the course of the tendon, which disappears distally beneath a horizontal projection of the trapezium. The FCR is freed by sharp dissection approximately 0.5 cm distal to this point.

An arthrotomy of the TM joint between the APL dorsally and the volar beak ligament allows synovectomy, débridement of small osteophytes if present, and inspection of the articular cartilage. A bony channel is then created from the dorsum of the metacarpal, beginning in a plane perpendicular to the nail, to the apex of the volar beak of the metacarpal (see Fig. 12-8). Initial placement of a Kirschner wire to get a sense of the appropriate position of the channel is an option; handheld gouges or a small motorized bur is preferred over drilling a hole to create the channel. Supination of the metacarpal facilitates exposure. Obviously the joint should not be entered.

To obtain a "new ligament" from the FCR, two transverse incisions are used 3 cm and 6 cm proximal to the wrist crease over the course of the tendon. A strip composed of half its width is split away radially and tunneled beneath skin bridges to emerge beyond the wrist crease, remaining in continuity distally. The split continues distal to the crest of the trapezium, at which point the free end is redirected across the crest to enter the volar entry point of the bony channel. The tendon is drawn dorsally using either a wire suture or a small tendon passer. At this point the TM joint is accurately reduced under direct vision and stabilized by the insertion of a Kirschner wire inserted from the dorsum of the metacarpal into the trapezium or ulnar carpus.

The tendon strip is pulled tight, sutured to the dorsal periosteum, and routed proximally with its residual length. It is passed over the dorsal capsule of the TM joint, then beneath the APL and extensor pollicis brevis (EPB), around the FCR* just proximal to the trapezium, and back across the radial margin of the joint to insert into the metacarpal periosteum.

After 4 weeks of immobilization the Kirschner wire is removed and the basal joint is splinted for an additional week. Over the next 6 to 8 weeks a motion and strengthening program is carried out.

Metacarpal Extension Osteotomy[111]

Regional, axillary block anesthesia is performed, and a non-sterile tourniquet is placed. After exsanguination with an Esmarch bandage and inflation of the tourniquet to 250 mm Hg, a Wagner incision is aligned over the radial aspect of the thumb at the junction of the glabrous and more dorsal hair-bearing skin, extending proximally into the wrist flexion crease. In the subcutaneous tissue the sensory branches of the radial and lateral antebrachial cutaneous nerves are identified and protected. The origin of the thenar musculature is incised along the radial aspect of the metacarpal shaft distally and in a curvilinear fashion across the base of the thumb proximally onto the trapezium. The muscle fibers are sharply dissected extraperiosteally from the thumb metacarpal and TM joint capsule. If assessment of the articular surfaces is desired and if synovectomy is planned, an arthrotomy of the TM joint is performed with the metacarpal held in supination between the dorsally located APL and the palmar beak of the metacarpal at the location of the POL. A hand probe is used with gentle distraction on the thumb to assess pathoanatomy. A formal closure of the capsule is not performed.

Dorsally, approximately 1 cm distal to the TM joint, the extensor tendons are elevated subperiosteally from the metacarpal, and near-circumferential access around the metacarpal is obtained in anticipation of the osteotomy. The volar extent of the metacarpal is visualized at this location to facilitate

accurate resection of a dorsally based 30-degree wedge of bone (see Fig. 12-9A). A microsagittal saw is used to score the metacarpal 1 cm distal to its base transversely, but a complete cut through the volar cortex is not done. The saw blade is left in that partial osteotomy site, and a second blade is used approximately 5 mm distal to the first cut at an angle of 30 degrees so that the two blades intersect at the volar cortex. The wedge of bone is removed, and a 0.045 Kirschner wire is used to create a transverse hole on either side of the osteotomy. A 22-gauge wire is passed radial to ulnar and ulnar to radial. The 0.045 Kirschner wire is placed retrograde through the distal osteotomy site, exiting out the ulnar aspect of the thumb, and the osteotomy is compressed by extending the distal metacarpal. With an assistant maintaining compression, the 22-gauge wire is tightened, cut, and bent beneath the thenar musculature (see Fig. 12-9B). The Kirschner wire is then advanced anterograde. The Kirschner wire is cut external to skin to facilitate removal, and the periosteal origin of the thenar musculature is repaired with absorbable suture.

The wound is closed after inspection of the sensory nerves, and a postoperative dressing and overlying thumb spica splint are worn for 10 days. At that time sutures are removed and a thumb spica cast, or orthoplast splint, with the IP joint of the thumb left free, is worn for an additional 4 weeks. Approximately 6 weeks after surgery the Kirschner wire is removed. The patient is instructed to begin gentle TM motion, because in most cases union is either complete or nearly complete at that time. Grip and pinch exercises are started approximately 8 weeks after surgery unless union is delayed.

Advanced Stage Disease

Alternative Methods of Treatment

Advanced disease implies end-stage degeneration of the TM joint (stages 2 to 4) salvageable only by a procedure that removes or replaces the entire articular surface. Although TM fusion (Fig. 12-10) provides superlative pain relief[44] and

---

*The tendon strip may be passed either around the FCR or through a slit, as shown in Figure 12-8.

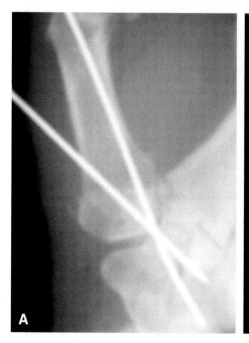
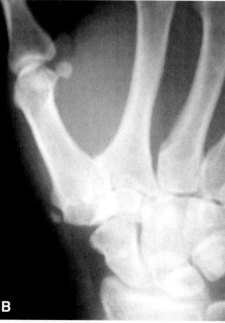

FIGURE 12-10. TM fusion. **A,** Intraoperative radiograph showing Kirschner wire fixation. **B,** Radiograph after union.

outcomes potentially comparable to ligament reconstruction,[54] mobility is limited, and abnormal wear at adjacent unfused joints can develop.

Simple trapezium excision[27,45,46] avoids the problems associated with fusion, as well as the now well-understood complications of material wear and instability associated with implant arthroplasty,[92] but weakness, instability, and proximal metacarpal migration have historically compromised long-term functional results in the absence of ligament reconstruction (Fig. 12-11). Even the addition of fascial or tendon interposition by Froimson in 1970, in an effort to improve grip strength and reduce metacarpal shortening, failed to improve long-term results.[42] Simple trapezium excision in conjunction with temporary distraction and pinning

has gained recent popularity—the so-called hematoma-distraction arthroplasty—but long-term follow up has not yet been reported, and the potential for a decline in pinch strength with time seems inevitable, at least in higher demand thumbs.[59,65]

Cemented arthroplasty has been associated with an unacceptably high loosening rate and has fallen from favor.[98] Recently the de la Caffiniere prosthesis has undergone design revisions intended to reduce the incidence of early metacarpal loosening by enlarging the stem diameter, adding a circumferential collar, and providing a modular head-neck segment. The polyethylene trapezial component remains unchanged. Meaningful results using this new component design will not be available for several years (see Fig. 12-11).

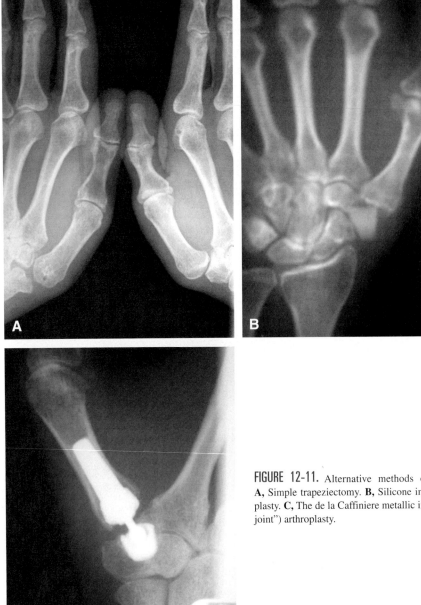

FIGURE 12-11. Alternative methods of treatment. **A,** Simple trapeziectomy. **B,** Silicone implant arthroplasty. **C,** The de la Caffiniere metallic implant ("total joint") arthroplasty.

To the extent that the literature can be used to identify what is the most common treatment used to treat basal joint arthritis today, clearly the LRTI arthroplasty procedure (Fig. 12-12) prevails as most popular.[69,85,96,109,113,118] However, other "suspensionplasty" procedures[64,86,101,115,119] appear to be successful as well, thus emphasizing the importance of common principles:

* Trapezium excision
* Ligament reconstruction/metacarpal suspension

Tissue interposition appears to promote the repopulation of the arthroplasty space with denser, less "fatty" scar tissue, thus providing (theoretically) a more effective "secondary restraint" to proximal metacarpal migration over time.[99] However, Gerwin and Weiland showed us that tissue interposition probably does not matter, at least in the short term.[47] Furthermore, there appears to be no correlation between some degree of proximal migration of the metacarpal and outcome, unless actual scaphometacarpal impingement occurs, which is more likely when no ligament reconstruction has been performed.[60,69]

In that light, in addition to the LRTI procedure, for which the entire width of the FCR tendon is commonly used without morbidity,[112] and a bony channel is made through the metacarpal base,[109] Thompson has been credited with describing use of a slip of the APL tendon using tunnels through both thumb and index metacarpal bases.[108] Diao described using a suture anchor in lieu of the index metacarpal tunnels,[29] and others have avoided the use of any bony tunnel, simply weaving a slip of APL around the FCR and sewing it back dorsally to itself and/or periosteum.[101] Weilby originated this variant by describing a suspension weave of one half of the FCR looped around the APL.[86,119] In general, mostly favorable outcomes have been reported after such suspensionplasties, characterized by excellent pain relief and significant improvement in strength. Patients have been very satisfied with the performance of their thumbs during activities that involve forceful grasp and lateral pinch.

With respect to the LRTI arthroplasty, in particular, results seem to improve for several years after the operation,[113] underscoring the protracted time necessary to achieve maximum strength recovery after the procedure. Documentation of such durable long-term performance after this procedure contrasts markedly to the experiences of prosthetic trapezium replacement and trapezium excision with fascial interposition, after which stability and strength decline with time.

The Thumb MP Joint and Implications of Hyperextensibility

The status of the thumb MP joint is of critical importance to the long-term stability of the more proximal basal joint reconstruction,[72] and any propensity for hyperextension to occur in excess of 30 degrees during lateral (key) pinch requires either fusion or volar capsulodesis of the MP joint. Failure to address a hyperextensile MP joint may result in the longitudinal collapse of the thumb during pinch, which imposes thumb metacarpal flexion and adduction and increases stresses on the ligament reconstruction (see Fig. 12-6). Accordingly, if there is more than 30 degrees of hyperextension instability during pinch, and metacarpal adduction occurs secondarily, arthrodesis in 5 to 10 degrees of flexion is recommended. Although volar capsulodesis is an alternative, arthrodesis is simpler, durable, and predictable. If hyperextension stability is less than 30 degrees, temporary stabilization in flexion with a Kirschner wire is used for a period of 4 weeks.

OUTCOMES AND TECHNIQUES

Treatment options for stage 2 and 3 disease include trapezium excision with or without tendon interposition, ligament reconstruction with or without tendon interposition, implant arthroplasty, and arthrodesis. In stage 4 disease, options change because of the degeneration of the scaphotrapezial articulation. Accordingly neither TM arthrodesis nor procedures that do not resect the entire trapezium are indicated, although Barron and Eaton have advocated saving the trapezium even in these cases by using a double tendon interposition.[4] Their belief that complete resection of the trapezium may result in proximal migration even when suspensionplasty is performed is not shared by the majority.

The results at long-term follow-up must be critically reviewed when making a decision concerning which procedure to perform. Each of these alternatives, and their outcomes, are discussed, but a description of technique is limited to only hematoma and distraction arthroplasty,[59,65] arthrodesis,[44,68] and LRTI arthroplasty[109,113] because these are most commonly selected.

Trapezium Excision

Gervis first described simple excision of the trapezium in 1949.[45] Results were promising, but his reports were largely anecdotal.[45,46] Other, more balanced reviews showed acceptable pain relief but problematic weakness and instability.[27,66,80] Thus, over the past few decades simple excision of the trapezium became less popular, and the focus shifted to more complicated procedures.

By contrast, several subsequent studies have revealed that strength improves approximately 40% from preoperative values despite remaining weaker than the nonoperative thumb.[28,48,116] Two recent reports compared outcomes after

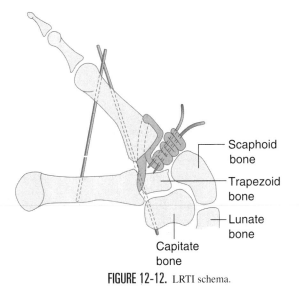

Scaphoid bone

Trapezoid bone

Lunate bone

Capitate bone

FIGURE 12-12. LRTI schema.

simple excision, excision with tendon interposition, and excision with ligament reconstruction and tendon interposition.[25,31] In an attempt to lessen instability and weakness as a problem, a Kirschner wire was used to stabilize the thumb metacarpal for 4 weeks in all patients. No statistical difference in pain relief was noted, and outcomes with respect to stiffness, function, grip and pinch strength were similar as well. The shortcoming of both studies was follow-up of only 1 year. Indeed, we might anticipate that thumbs in which ligament reconstruction was performed would be more durable with time.

Bringing us full circle from Gervis's first report[45]—through a period of relative unpopularity because of weakness—trapezium excision has reappeared, of late, as a "recommended" option, remarketed, if you will, under the name "hematoma and distraction arthroplasty" (HDA).[59,65] In an attempt to address thumb metacarpal subsidence, which may have played a part in poor outcomes after simple excision in the past, HDA proponents recommend pinning the metacarpal in a distracted position for 5 weeks. Kuhns and coworkers reported on 26 patients, prospectively evaluated at 6 and 24 months after surgery.[65] Complete pain relief was reported by 73% at 6 months and by 92% at final follow-up. Two-year follow-up evaluation showed a 47% increase in grip strength, a 33% increase in key pinch strength, and a 23% increase in tip pinch strength. Proximal migration of the metacarpal averaged 51% on radiographs at 2-year follow-up, which increased an additional 10% with pinch. Twenty-four of 25 patients questioned 2 years after HDA reported that they were very satisfied with the outcome.[65]

The short-term results, at 2 years, appear to compare favorably to the early results of the LRTI arthroplasty reported by Burton and Pellegrini.[13] Tomaino's long-term evaluation shows, however, clearly superior strength data at a minimum of 9 years and markedly less subsidence.[113] And so, although pinning of the thumb metacarpal in a distracted position may allow the trapezium space to fill with hematoma fluid, which may later organize and fibrose, durability in the long term may be better when ligament reconstruction is combined with trapezial excision.

Furthermore, despite the observation that use of a Kirschner wire for fixation has diminished problems with instability and weakness, all studies addressing simple trapezium excision have been short term.[25,31,59,65] Although several authors have confirmed that there is no correlation between the height of the trapezium space and function or pain relief,[31,60,69] proximal migration may continue long term and lead to painful scaphometacarpal impingement (see Fig. 12-11A).

When impingement of the thumb metacarpal base on the scaphoid occurs, such profound loss of the trapezial space undoubtedly compromises outcome. Connolly and Rath treated seven patients with scaphometacarpal arthrosis, all requiring surgical intervention at 8 to 18 years after trapezial excision.[21] Neither the prevalence nor incidence of this complication are known. Certainly the incidence—"rate of future occurrence"—should be tracked if more surgeons preferentially select HDA as their treatment method. The average surgical time of 35 minutes that Kuhns and coworkers reported[65] is, in actuality, not much less than what is needed typically to perform a ligament reconstruction,[109] thus we are hard pressed *not* to recommend the latter simply on the basis that long-term outcome is likely better. Time will tell.

Until long-term studies of the HDA arthroplasty are available, enthusiasm for the procedure should be guarded.

One principle appears to be well established: if trapezium excision alone is selected, Kirschner wire fixation should be used. At 5-year follow-up, without use of a Kirschner wire at surgery, Varley and associates noted a trapezial space of only 1 mm, and only 3 of 30 cases maintained a height of greater than or equal to 2 mm.[116] In addition, 11 of 27 developed degenerative changes at the distal pole of the scaphoid that were not present preoperatively.

"Hematoma and Distraction" Arthroplasty[65]

A longitudinal or curvilinear incision is made along the radial aspect of the wrist at the base of the thumb metacarpal. Cutaneous branches of the radial nerve are identified and retracted gently. The first dorsal extensor compartment is released, and the interval between the APL and EPB tendons is developed. The dorsal branch of the radial artery is identified in the anatomic snuffbox, mobilized, and retracted. A longitudinal incision is made over the trapezium into the soft tissue. A capsulotomy is performed creating dorsal and volar flaps. The trapezium, the base of the thumb metacarpal, the TM joint, and the scaphotrapezial and scaphotrapezoidal joints are exposed.

The capsular edges are tagged with suture for later identification and to assist with retraction. A cruciate osteotomy of the trapezium is performed using an oscillating saw and/or osteotome. The trapezium is removed piecemeal. Care is taken to preserve the FCR tendon, which runs through a groove within the trapezium. All bone fragments and loose bodies must be removed. Large osteophytes on the base of the metacarpal should be débrided.

Longitudinal traction is applied to the thumb with slight pronation. The metacarpal is fixed to the index metacarpal with one or two 0.045- or 0.062-inch Kirschner wires placed percutaneously. Thumb position is rechecked so that an adequate trapezial space is created by the distraction. The joint capsule is repaired, and the remaining closure follows routine fashion. A short-arm thumb spica splint is applied, leaving the thumb IP joint free for motion. At 2 weeks after the surgery the wound is inspected and the sutures are removed. A thumb spica cast is worn for 5 to 6 weeks when Kirschner wires are removed. Active range-of-motion exercises are begun at this time. A short opponens splint is used for an additional 2 weeks after cast removal.

Trapezium Excision With Tissue Interposition

After early reports of simple excision of the trapezium identified difficulties with loss of strength, instability, and shortening of the thumb ray, interposition material was added in an attempt to alleviate these problems. Carroll began using tendon interposition to treat basal joint arthritis in 1951.[15] Froimson reported using one half of the FCR or palmaris longus tendon.[42] Uniform pain relief was noted at 6-year follow-up, but weakness and metacarpal subsidence were still a problem. Menon and associates noted the same findings[75]; all patients showed considerable migration of the thumb metacarpal proximally. Several comparative studies have shown, in fact, that the addition of tendon interposition at the time of trapezial excision makes no significant difference.[25,27,31] Thus, interposition seems to provide no additive benefit to the results of trapeziectomy alone. Interestingly, Gerwin and colleagues have shown that interposition may not make a difference when performing ligament reconstruction either, at least in the short term.[47]

Trapeziometacarpal Arthrodesis

Arthrodesis of the TM (or CMC) joint was first described by Muller in 1949,[78] the same year in which Gervis reported simple excision[45] (see Fig. 12-10). Arthrodesis has traditionally been recommended in younger patients with isolated TM arthritis in whom the retention of power and long-term durability were considered more important than the retention of motion. As motion-preserving arthroplasty techniques have evolved, however, and longer-term outcomes have proven satisfactory, fusion has become less popular.

Concerns regarding the TM arthrodesis have included actual and perceived shortcomings, including limitation of motion, the development of compensatory hypermobility at the MCP joint, the risk of degenerative changes at adjacent joints, the need for prolonged immobilization postoperatively, hardware complications,[40] and the risk of nonunion.[3]

Patients may complain of the inability to flatten the palm, trouble with dexterity, and difficulty putting on gloves or placing the hand into small spaces, such as a pocket.[3,28] Chamay and coworkers[18] and Lisanti and associates[70] reported that greater than 40% of their patients had an inability to flatten the hand and a significant amount of difficulty handling small objects. In contrast, many authors have noted that thumb mobility was not dramatically altered and that, when motion was lost, it was not perceived as a problem by patients.[14,16,35,68,104] Indeed, recent comparison between TM arthrodesis and the LRTI arthroplasty showed little difference with regard to thumb mobility.[54] The patient's occupation should be considered when contemplating arthrodesis as a treatment choice. Those with jobs requiring fine manipulation, or which require maneuvering the hand into tight spots, may be better served with another option.

Leach and Bolton described what they considered the ideal position for TM arthrodesis.[68] When making a fist, the thumb should contact the middle phalanx of the index finger. The thumb metacarpal is positioned at 35 to 40 degrees relative to the index metacarpal when viewed from the radial side (palmar abduction) and at 10 to 15 degrees when viewed from the dorsum. Excessive abduction and extension may limit functional opposition and should be avoided.[12] Carroll taught his fellows to fuse the joint in "45-45-45" (45 degrees of palmar abduction, 45 degrees of radial abduction, and 45 degrees of nail rotation) (Carroll RE: Personal communication to the editor [DPG], 1970.)

Others have suggested that position is not absolutely critical because of the potential for compensatory motion at the MP and scaphotrapezial joints.[3,18,70] In light of the fact that Carroll reported that 75% of compensatory motion occurs at the MP joint and 25% at the scaphotrapezial joint, arthrodesis may be relatively contraindicated when MP joint stiffness, hyperextension deformity, or a zigzag collapse deformity exists because the loss of thumb dexterity in such cases may be more limiting.[16]

As mentioned earlier, another concern with TM arthrodesis has centered on the risk of adjacent joint degeneration.[12,16,18]

Chamay and Piaget-Morerod found arthrosis at the scaphotrapezial joint in 25% at 6.5 years follow-up.[18] Nevertheless, others have not regarded acceleration of degenerative changes at the scaphotrapezial joint as a common problem.[35,37,104] Stark and associates found progression in only 1 of 30 patients.[104] Degeneration was noted in this patient preoperatively, and it was thought that progression was secondary to a Kirschner wire placed within the joint. Other patients re-examined at 8 to 12 years after fusion showed no progression.[104] Eaton and Littler found no changes in adjacent joints as long as 11 years postoperatively.[35] Although minimal preoperative degeneration at the ST joint may not contraindicate TM fusion, another procedure should be chosen if there is more advanced arthrosis. Degenerative changes at the MP joint should be regarded seriously, as well, because the significant increase in compensatory mobility after surgery may be a source of discomfort.[70]

Because prolonged immobilization after arthrodesis has caused many to shy away from arthrodesis, more rigid techniques of internal fixation have been used. In addition, more rigid methods of fixation, one would think, might minimize the occurrence of nonunion. Methods of fixation used have included a cortical strut with or without Kirschner wire fixation,[68,78] a single Kirschner wire,[16] crossed Kirschner wires,[3,18,35,104] tension band wiring,[32] cerclage wiring,[73] staple fixation,[3,14,18] Herbert screw fixation,[14,18,20] and plate and screw fixation.[18,53] Obviously the more rigid the fixation, the less time that immobilization is required. But, complications also appear to be more likely.[40] Use of the Herbert screw has been abandoned because of an exceedingly high rate of nonunion.[14,20]

Forseth and Stern have shown that union rates were comparable between groups treated with either plates and screws or Kirschner wires, but patient satisfaction was lower, and a second surgery more common, after use of the former.[40] All forms of fixation can lead to complications attributable to the hardware. These complications may include hardware intolerance caused by prominence, tendon irritation or rupture, and joint penetration. Penetration of the joint can lead to secondary degenerative changes. We recommend Kirschner wire fixation over more rigid plate and screw fixation in light of Forseth and Stern's timely report.[40]

Interestingly, studies comparing soft tissue arthroplasty and arthrodesis reveal similar results with regard to pain relief and patient satisfaction.[54,66,79] Soft tissue arthroplasty appears to decrease immobilization time and increase range of motion.[54] Arthrodesis may give stronger pinch strength but leads to a higher rate of, and more serious, complications.[54,79] In the final analysis, the decision to perform soft tissue arthroplasty or arthrodesis depends largely on the preference of the surgeon and the needs and wants of the patient.

Authors' Preferred Method of TM Arthrodesis

A longitudinal incision is made over the first dorsal extensor compartment extending from the midportion of the thumb metacarpal to just proximal to the radial styloid. Branches of the radial nerve are identified and gently retracted. The first dorsal extensor compartment is identified and released dorsally. The interval between the APL and the EPB is developed, and the tendons are retracted. The dorsal branch of radial artery, which runs obliquely from volar to dorsal beneath the tendons, is mobilized and retracted. An incision is made into the periosteum over the base of the metacarpal dorsally and carried proximally until the TM joint is located. A capsulotomy is performed, releasing soft tissue from the base of the metacarpal and the distal trapezium. Dissection of the soft tissue from the metacarpal base must be circumferential to allow the bone to be elevated from the wound. The metacarpal shaft is flexed and adducted to deliver the base. The proximal metacarpal is decorticated, removing remaining cartilage, subchondral bone, and osteophytes so that a cone type configuration is accomplished. The trapezial surface is fashioned into a cup to match the base of the metacarpal. Three 0.045-inch Kirschner wires are driven antegrade through the base of the metacarpal exiting the dorsal cortex. The first is placed in line with the shaft. The remaining two are drilled in a divergent manner at approximately 15 degrees to the first pin. The bony surfaces are opposed, and axial compression is applied manually. An assistant then drills the pins proximally into the trapezium. An attempt is made not to cross the scaphotrapezial joint unless the bone is osteoporotic and additional support for fixation is needed. Position of the arthrodesis should be planned so that the thumb is placed in approximately 35 degrees of palmar abduction and in slight pronation. With the fist clenched, the thumb should overlie the middle phalanx of the index finger. Position and bony apposition are confirmed with radiographs. If bony apposition is poor, the position is adjusted or bone graft is harvested from the distal radius, and gaps in the fusion site are filled with bone graft. Closure is accomplished in a routine fashion, and a thumb spica splint is applied. The wound is inspected and sutures are removed at approximately 2 weeks postoperatively. If fixation is secure, a removable orthoplast splint may be worn and removed for bathing; otherwise, a short-arm thumb spica cast is worn until fusion is complete. Pins are routinely removed between 6 and 8 weeks after surgery if radiographs confirm union and the site is nontender to palpation. After pin removal, range-of-motion exercises are begun; strengthening is allowed after a few additional weeks.

An alternative to the cone-and-cup arthrodesis of this joint is to create flat cuts at the base of the metacarpal and the distal surface of trapezium. This technique provides a broader fusion surface but can be difficult because the cuts must be made absolutely correct to ensure precise coaptation of the two surfaces in the desired angle of arthrodesis.

Achieving solid bony union of the basal joint of the thumb in the correct position is not an easy operation by either technique.

Implant Arthroplasty

The use of implant arthroplasty as treatment for basal joint arthritis of the thumb first began in the 1960s. Concerns over shortening of the thumb ray and instability after trapeziectomy and problems with stiffness and nonunion after arthrodesis led to the development of joint replacement. Two types of implants were developed. The first involved arthroplasty of only the TM joint, using either a spacer or total joint replacement. The second type, which has more commonly been used, addressed pantrapezial arthritis and involved replacement of the entire trapezium. This type is discussed first.

Silicone Replacement Arthroplasty

Swanson and Niebauer independently introduced silicone implant arthroplasty after complete trapeziectomy as an alternative to treatment of basal joint arthritis.[83,105] The procedure became very popular during the 1970s because thumb length was maintained and early results revealed good pain relief and restoration of strength.[51,105]

When the complication of dorsoradial subluxation of the implant was first recognized, it was thought to be secondary to implant design and technical errors. The implant was modified, and the surgical technique was refined. Swanson recommended a precise surgical technique including adequate resection of the bony structures to allow proper seating of the implant and capsular preservation and reinforcement with tendon grafts. He urged correction of the deforming forces secondary to hyperextension of the MP joint, release of first web space contracture, and adequate immobilization postoperatively.[105,106] Eaton developed a cannulated implant to allow passage of the APL through it in an effort to provide additional stability.[33] Even with this modification, however, instability remained a problem: subluxation approached 20% to 25% at early follow-up.[33,51,106]

In addition, reports began to emerge regarding implant wear and tissue response to silicone particulate matter.[87,92] Studies of silicone *carpal* implants noted late osseous complications including focal zones of osteolysis and erosions in bone adjacent to the implant. As time from the index procedure increased, lytic lesions appeared to be progressive and began to appear in noncontiguous extra-articular bones.[87] This so-called silicone synovitis was noted to occur usually more than 2 years after the initial surgery and was associated with pain, swelling, and radiographic lucencies. Persistent symptoms and radiographic findings necessitated synovectomy, implant removal, and curettage of lytic defects.[87] These findings tempered enthusiasm for silicone implants in other small joints of the hand.

Notwithstanding the prevalence of silicone synovitis with carpal implants, rates of silicone synovitis have not been as significant after silicone trapezium arthroplasty. Pellegrini and Burton reviewed a subset of 32 silicone implant arthroplasties in osteoarthritic thumbs with nearly a 4-year follow-up.[92] The implants lost nearly 50% of their vertical height, with the wear consistently being worse along the ulnar margin. Subluxation was, on average, 35% of the width of the prosthesis. Four different types of implants were reviewed in the study. Swanson trapezium implants did not experience as much wear, but subluxation was worse (see Fig. 12-11B). At the time of revision, required in 16%, proliferative synovitis was associated with silicone particulate matter.[92] In spite of these implant complications, 75% of patients in whom the diagnosis was osteoarthritis and all of those with rheumatoid thumbs were satisfied with outcome.[92]

Although instability, implant wear, and radiographic erosions may complicate silicone trapezium arthroplasty, these findings appear not to correlate with subjective results. Bezwada and coworkers noted 84% good to excellent results at 16.4-year follow-up.[8] These authors reported that subluxation and bony radiolucencies were not clinically important. Implant fractures were noted in only 6% and, when addressed early, led to good long-term outcomes. No evidence for frank silicone synovitis was found.

Notwithstanding the observation that good or excellent results can be obtained after silicone trapezium implant arthroplasty, results may deteriorate with time.[102] Silicone implant arthroplasty is currently recommended only in the low demand rheumatoid thumb[92] and even in that population alternative procedures may be preferable.

Silicone Hemiarthroplasty

The second type of implant utilized for basal joint arthritis involves replacement of only the TM joint. These devices are limited to those cases in which degeneration affects only that joint and scaphotrapezial-trapezoid arthritis is not present. Kessler devised a thin silicone disc to be interposed between the trapezium and metacarpal,[62] but synovitis and instability were problematic in the majority. Ashworth and Blatt utilized a modified neurosurgical bur hole cover as a trapeziometacarpal spacer.[2] These, too, were unsuccessful, and thin silicone implants were abandoned.

Swanson developed a titanium hemiarthroplasty for the TM joint in 1985. The stemmed component is placed into the base of the metacarpal without cement, but long-term outcomes have not been reported.

The Orthosphere (Wright Medical Technology, Inc., Arlington, TN) has been utilized as a spacer at the TM joint. The developers suggest that the best results are achieved in male patients between the ages of 45 and 60 in which strong pinch strength is desired. Good results have been reported, but follow-up has been short; and complications have included dislocation, trapezium fracture or erosion, and severe pain. Based on limited data, mostly from personal communication and presentations, this implant may show long-term problems.

Total Joint Arthroplasty

Total joint arthroplasty has also been utilized in treatment of basal joint arthritis involving only the TM joint. In 1971, de la Caffiniere introduced a cemented ball and socket type implant (see Fig. 12-11C). Surgical indications included rheumatoid disease, osteoarthritis, and trauma. In his 1979 report of 34 operations, the best results were obtained for pain or instability. When the indication was stiffness, results were less satisfying.[26] The design resembles total hip components with a polyethylene cup placed into the trapezium and a stemmed cobalt-chromium ball inserted into the shaft of the thumb metacarpal.[26]

The Caffiniere prosthesis has been the most widely utilized joint replacement, but other designs have been used.[10,38,74] Cooney and colleagues developed a second type of cemented total joint arthroplasty.[23] The ball-and-socket components were reversed with this device. The trapezium component was a metallic implant with a pedestal and with a sphere protruding from the bony surface, and the metacarpal component was a polyethylene-stemmed socket.

Early results of the total joint designs have been similar; most authors have reported rapid functional recovery with good or excellent results at short-term follow-up.[10,23,38,74] Cooney and colleagues noted that formation of heterotopic bone in 36% of implants negatively affected the outcome.[23]

They emphasized that heterotopic bone noted preoperatively may contraindicate total joint arthroplasty.[23] Use of these prostheses, in general, requires good bone stock, especially when assessing the trapezium for implantation. Arthrodesis of either the MP or scaphotrapezial-trapezoid joint has led to early rapid loosening of both components, and the presence of either contraindicates use of the prosthesis. Radiographic evaluation in early follow-up periods has revealed a high incidence of radiolucent lines, particularly around the trapezial component.[38] As with other cemented joint replacements, these radiolucent lines at the bone-cement interface are associated with an increase in aseptic loosening at long-term follow-up.

Long-term outcome after use of the Caffiniere prosthesis has been reported.[17,82,103,117] At a median of 9 years after operation in 20 patients (22 thumbs), Sondergaard and associates reported that 82% of the prostheses were still in place.[103] Three had been revised because of aseptic loosening. Functional results were believed to be durable overall for this time interval.[103] In 1992, Nicholas and Calderwood reported on 20 arthroplasties performed for osteoarthritis and followed for up to 10 years.[82] Failure in 2 patients was believed to be due to over-reaming of the trapezium and traumatic dislocation, respectively. Pain relief and range of motion were satisfactory, and one case with radiolucencies on radiography was asymptomatic.[82]

Use of the Caffiniere prosthesis has been discouraged in men of working age because of a higher prevalence of aseptic loosening of the trapezial component.[17] Chakrabarti and coworkers reported an 89% survival rate at 16 years for 93 replacements performed in 71 patients.[17] In 1999 van Cappelle and associates reported long-term results of 77 Caffiniere arthroplasties for osteoarthritis.[117] The mean follow-up period was 8.5 years (range, 2 to 16 years), and the survival rate at 16 years was 72%. The total loosening rate was 44%, and half of these required revision. These authors also noted a higher revision rate among men, presumably because of increased demands on the prosthesis. They advised its use only in women, preferably those older than 60 years.[117]

In 2003, total joint arthroplasty appears not to offer any compelling functional advantage or durability over trapezium excision and ligament reconstruction and is clearly fraught with a higher complication rate.

Trapezium Excision and Ligament (LRTI) Reconstruction

The combination of ligament reconstruction and tendon interposition with trapezium excision (LRTI arthroplasty) reflects, as mentioned earlier, the consolidation of three fundamental principles: trapezium excision to remove arthritic joint surfaces, anterior oblique ligament reconstruction to restore thumb metacarpal stability and prevent axial shortening, and fascial interposition to reduce the likelihood of impingement between neighboring bony surfaces (see Fig. 12-12). As originally described by Burton and Pellegrini in 1986,[13] the ligament was reconstructed with one half of the width of the FCR tendon. Many surgeons, including Burton, have altered this procedure to include its entire width to facilitate harvest and provide a bulkier tendon for interposition. Indeed, Tomaino and Coleman have reported that no morbidity accompanies use of the entire tendon.[112] Although many surgeons have elected to use alternative methods of suspending the metacarpal and have stopped pinning it for 4 weeks, appreciation of the underlying principles will increase the likelihood of functional improvement, which should be measured against very favorable long-term outcomes.[113]

Based on the favorable results after ligament reconstruction for the hypermobile TM joint without arthritis,[36] Burton combined trapezium excision, as first recommended by Gervis,[45] with fascial interposition as described by Froimson,[42] in an attempt to rectify the long-term problems of instability and particulate synovitis that were associated with silicone implant arthroplasty.[92] Since that time, his technique has evolved to include routine use of the entire width of the FCR tendon and resection of the entire trapezium.[109]

Only five series in the literature report outcome after the LRTI arthroplasty, for which the average follow-up exceeds 3 years.[69,85,96,113,118] Improvements in grip strength typically have exceeded improvements in key pinch strength. In 1995, Tomaino, Pellegrini, and Burton detailed that key pinch strength took at least 6 years to equal preoperative measurements but, by long-term follow-up, improvements averaged 34%.[113] At an average follow-up of 9 years (range, 8 to 11 years), these authors reported on 24 thumbs in 22 patients and identified that average grip strength increased 93%, average key pinch strength, 34%, and tip pinch strength, 65%, compared with preoperative values. In contrast to the other studies, stress radiographs showed an average subluxation of the metacarpal base of 11% and subsidence of only 13%.[113] This compares favorably with the radiographic outcomes following an HDA.[65] It is worthwhile noting, however, that even in series in which proximal migration of the metacarpal base averaged greater than 20%,[60,69,96] there has been no significant correlation between maintenance of arthroplasty space height and objective or subjective clinical outcome.

In 1996, Lins and coworkers reported on 30 thumbs in 27 patients with an average follow-up of 3.5 years and observed an average 50% improvement in grip strength and 43% improvement in key pinch.[69] The results of their investigation paralleled Tomaino and colleagues' observations,[113] and their seminal contribution centered around the use of the "trapezial space ratio" reported earlier by the same group.[60]

In 1997, Rayan and Young reported on 30 thumbs (in 28 patients), with an average follow-up of 3.2 years.[96] They reported a more modest 13% improvement in grip strength and a 27% decline in key pinch strength. These results are mitigated somewhat by the authors' acknowledgment that comparison, in the majority of patients, was to the contralateral hand as opposed to preoperative values. Like Lins and coworkers,[69] they reported patient satisfaction and pain relief in more than 85%.[96] They did report, however, significant difficulty opening jars in 63% of patients.[96]

The largest series in the literature were reported by Nylen and colleagues[85] in 1993 (100 operations) and by Varitimidis and coworkers[118] in 2000 (62 thumbs). Both series compare favorably with the three reports already mentioned with respect to pain relief, functional return, and patient satisfaction.

In the report of Tomaino and colleagues from 1995,[113] the availability of data for each patient from before operation and at an average of 2, 6, and 9 years postoperatively provid-

ed the unique opportunity to track thumb function with time. Long-term evaluation convincingly showed that the function of the thumb continued to improve for as long as 6 years after ligament reconstruction and tendon interposition. This underscores the protracted time that is necessary for maximum recovery of strength after the procedure.

This durable long-term performance contrasts markedly to reported experiences with prosthetic replacement of the trapezium and to excision of the trapezium alone or in combination with fascial interposition. The literature unequivocally supports the LRTI arthroplasty. Indeed, thumb stability, pain relief, and improvements in strength are the expected outcomes. Although some investigators continue to believe that ligament reconstruction is not necessary,[59,65] trapezium excision alone, or in combination with tendon interposition or distraction, appears to be less likely to provide long-term stability or restore satisfactory pinch and grip strength.

Some hand surgeons may be apprehensive about harvesting the entire width of the FCR tendon because of fear that wrist function may be impaired or that a larger bony channel in the metacarpal might result in fracture. However, Tomaino and Coleman reported rather convincingly that there was no morbidity accompanying harvest of the entire FCR tendon from the standpoint of wrist strength or endurance.[112] Furthermore, technical modification by which the end of the FCR is tapered or trimmed obviates the need for an excessively large bony channel through the metacarpal.[109] Pin fixation of the metacarpal in the fisted position, with its base suspended at the level of the index carpometacarpal joint, is still recommended to allow accurate tensioning of the new ligament and protection in the early postoperative period. Proximal migration of only 13% at an average of 9 years after surgery may very well reflect the value of pin fixation.[113]

Authors' Preferred Method of LRTI Arthroscopy

Incision and Superficial Dissection

A triradiate line is drawn on the skin before the tourniquet is inflated to allow palpation of the radial pulse in the vicinity of the anatomic snuffbox; this typically identifies the scaphotrapezial joint (Fig. 12-13A). When a significant shoulder sign exists, it can be difficult to identify the TM joint. In these cases, palpation of the scaphoid tuberosity is helpful to ensure that the incision is neither too distal nor too proximal. I have found that the triradiate incision facilitates dissection of the radial artery off of the dorsal capsule, and I continue to prefer a dorsal approach during this operation because it provides a safer exposure of the FCR tendon. When a first extensor compartment release is planned, however, a longitudinal incision may be preferred.

At the outset, it is imperative that the radial sensory nerve be identified and that small branches not be skeletonized or divided. This may cause postoperative radial sensory neuritis and even transient reflex sympathetic dystrophy. Blunt retractors are placed beneath the extensor pollicis longus (EPL) in a dorsal and ulnar position and APL radially and volarly. The radial artery courses within this interval, and deep perforators to the dorsal capsule must be coagulated and divided so the artery can be retracted dorsally and ulnarly.

Capsular Incision

With gentle traction on the thumb, longitudinal capsulotomy is done, and subperiosteal exposure of the trapezium and the base of the metacarpal is obtained. The capsulotomy must be extended proximally so that the scaphotrapezial joint can be identified. Either retractors or placement of tag sutures of 3.0 Vicryl are used to retract the capsule.

Trapezial Excision

Before the trapezium is excised, a microsagittal saw is used to remove a thin sliver of bone at the base of the metacarpal (see Fig. 12-13B). This facilitates exposure of the distal extent of the trapezium and, with further traction on the thumb, provides a safer window for excision of the trapezium. The trapezium is cut into quadrants, beginning with the limb that parallels the expected course of the FCR tendon. Injury to the tendon during this portion of the procedure is unlikely if the saw is not brought completely through the trapezium. After perpendicular cuts in the trapezium are made, an osteotome is placed and twisted to separate the bone into its four quadrants. Removal of the trapezium in pieces with a rongeur is facilitated by sharp dissection of remaining capsule, particularly volarly and around loose bodies. Inordinate ripping and pulling with the rongeurs is avoided because damage to the underlying capsule can increase postoperative discomfort, particularly where it abuts the carpal tunnel. It is imperative to remove osteophytic bone between the base of the thumb and index metacarpal so that pain does not accompany key pinch after the procedure (see Fig. 12-13C). It is also important to identify the FCR tendon at the base of the arthroplasty space so it is not injured; it must be remembered that the trapezium may encircle the FCR tendon at its volar extent.

At this portion of the procedure, I routinely have an assistant place traction on the index and long fingers to

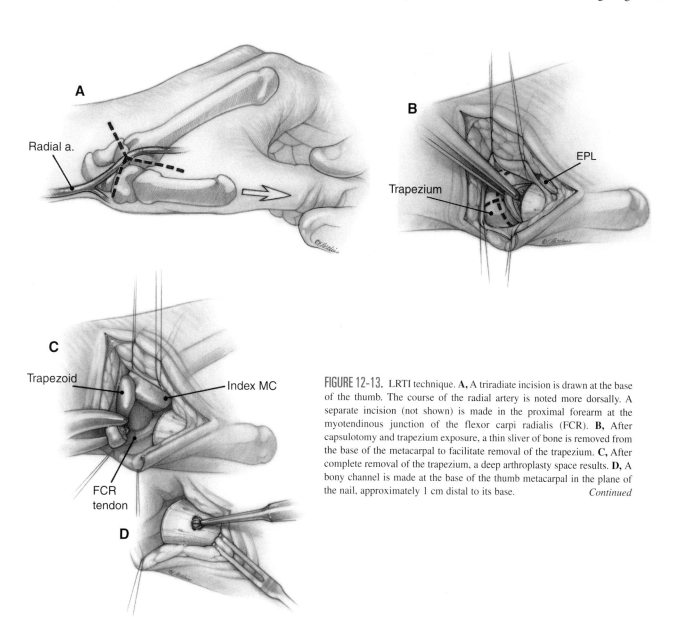

FIGURE 12-13. LRTI technique. **A,** A triradiate incision is drawn at the base of the thumb. The course of the radial artery is noted more dorsally. A separate incision (not shown) is made in the proximal forearm at the myotendinous junction of the flexor carpi radialis (FCR). **B,** After capsulotomy and trapezium exposure, a thin sliver of bone is removed from the base of the metacarpal to facilitate removal of the trapezium. **C,** After complete removal of the trapezium, a deep arthroplasty space results. **D,** A bony channel is made at the base of the thumb metacarpal in the plane of the nail, approximately 1 cm distal to its base. *Continued*

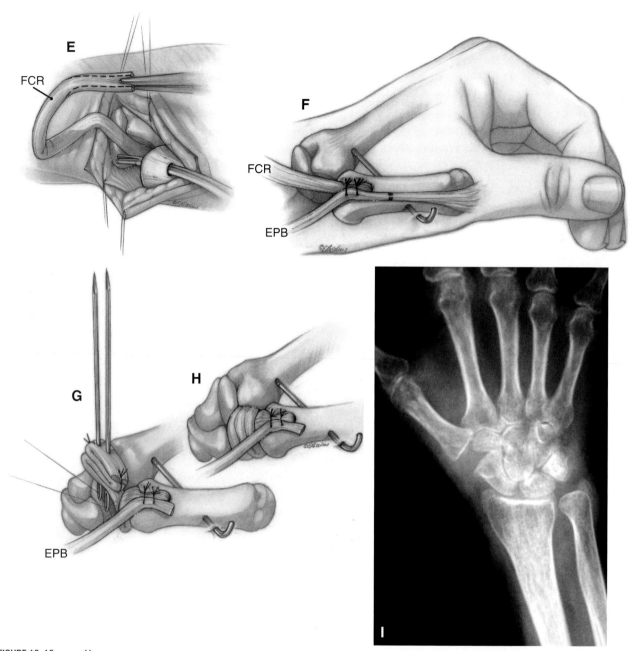

FIGURE 12-13—cont'd. **E,** The FCR tendon has been released in the forearm and delivered more distally into the arthroplasty space. A Carroll tendon passer is placed through the bony channel, grasping the tapered end of the FCR tendon. The tendon is successfully passed through the bony channel. **F,** The thumb is placed in the fisted position as if engaged in key pinch. The base of the metacarpal is suspended at the level of the index carpometacarpal joint, co-linear with the scaphoid articular surface. After placement of a stabilizing Kirschner wire, the exit point of the FCR tendon is secured to adjacent periosteum and soft tissues. The extensor pollicis brevis (EPB) tendon is included in that closure, effectively rendering it an abductor of the metacarpal. **G,** The FCR tendon is folded on itself like ribbon candy, secured at its corners with suture, and then passed over two Keith needles to facilitate delivery of this "anchovy" into the arthroplasty space. **H,** The anchovy is placed into the depth of the arthroplasty space and secured with a previously placed suture. **I,** Postoperative posteroanterior radiograph of the hand shows trapezium resection and suspension of the thumb metacarpal at the level of the index carpometacarpal joint, after pin removal.

allow inspection of the scaphotrapezoidal joint. If there is cartilage fraying or eburnation, a motorized bur or rongeur is used to remove 2 to 3 mm of proximal trapezoid so that, with axial compression applied to the index and long finger metacarpals, there is no contact between the remaining trapezoid and scaphoid. I do not interpose soft tissue or FCR tendon into the space. Care must be taken not to remove bone from the capitate.[114]

Creation of the Bony Channel Through the Metacarpal Base

One centimeter distal to the squared off base of the metacarpal, in the plane of the nail, a bone tunnel is created with a motorized 3-mm bur that exits at the volar base of the metacarpal. This position is selected rather than a central exit point in the metacarpal base because passage of the FCR tendon volarly more closely simulates the original attachment of the beak ligament. The bony channel is enlarged with two curets of increasing size but is not made large enough for the entire width of the leading edge of the FCR tendon (see Fig. 12-13D). Rather, the tip of FCR tendon is trimmed to facilitate passage with a Carroll tendon passer. In that light, the bony channel needs to be large enough only for the Carroll tendon passer to be used (see Fig. 12-13E).

Flexor Carpi Radialis Harvest

The FCR tendon is palpated at the wrist level during passive flexion and extension of the wrist, where it is clearly tendinous. More proximally in the forearm the tendon becomes less discrete. This generally correlates with the proximal one third to one half of the forearm, and, at that location, a 1.5-cm transverse incision is made. The fascia is opened, the wrist is maximally flexed, and the interval between the FCR tendon and muscle is identified, lifted into the wound with a curved clamp, and divided. This wound is now closed with 5.0 nylon sutures. With retraction of the capsular flaps, ensuring protection of the overlying radial artery dorsally and ulnarly, a curved hemostat is placed beneath the FCR tendon and pulled. This typically delivers the entire tendon into the arthroplasty space.

It is imperative at this point that the tendon be grasped at its tip and mobilized to its insertion at the base of the index metacarpal without violating small blood vessels that perfuse the tendon insertion itself. If adhesions between the FCR and the volar capsule are not released, the vector of the ligament reconstruction is based more proximally and will not truly simulate the original vector of the beak ligament. This is a potential cause of early subsidence after ligament reconstruction. The tendon is then tapered for 2 to 3 cm so the diameter of the tip of the tendon can easily be pulled through the bone tunnel with the Carroll tendon passer (see Fig. 12-13E). At this point, a 4.0 Vicryl suture on a small needle is used to grasp the volar capsule for subsequent stabilization of the tendon interposition. If there are rents in the volar capsule, this same suture can be used to repair them, but I am no longer inordinately preoccupied with repairing small tears in the volar capsule because there is little risk, if any, of the tendon interposition extruding into the carpal canal or, for that matter, into the base of the metacarpal.

Stabilization of the Thumb Metacarpal and FCR Tendon Tensioning

A 4-week period of Kirschner wire stabilization of the metacarpal continues to be a mainstay of the surgical technique for two reasons. First, it ensures accurate positioning of the thumb metacarpal before ligament (FCR) tensioning. Second, it protects the ligament reconstruction during placement of the postoperative dressing at the completion of the operation and 2 weeks later at the time of suture removal and new thumb spica cast application. Kirschner wire placement is one of the more tedious parts of the procedure and must be performed skillfully so that the bony channel is not violated. If the Kirschner wire inadvertently impales the FCR tendon within the bony channel in the metacarpal, it will impair the ability to pull it tight and properly tension the new ligament. Usually a 0.045-inch wire is used (a 0.054-inch wire is preferred in larger hands) that begins

obliquely at the dorsoradial aspect of the metacarpal and purchases the ulnar carpus. The thumb is placed in the "fisted" position as if engaged in key pinch (see Fig. 12-13F). The thumb metacarpal is suspended at the level of the index metacarpal. Its base should be co-linear with the scaphoid articular surface, and the thumb tip should rest on the index finger, neither too extended nor too flexed at its base. Ideally, this positions the thumb intrinsic muscles optimally on the Blix curve and ensures optimal restoration of pinch strength. The wire is bent external to skin and cut.

At this point, it is imperative that a hand probe or similar instrument be used to hook the FCR tendon at the base of the metacarpal and pull it proximally. This is done to ensure that the Kirschner wire does not prevent free excursion of the FCR through the bone channel. The tendon is then pulled tightly as it exits the dorsum of the thumb metacarpal tunnel and sutured to adjacent periosteum and soft tissue with 3.0 Vicryl. The EPB tendon is attached more radially and divided distally. This completes the EPB tenodesis, rendering it an abductor of the metacarpal and lessening its effect as a potential hyperextender of the MP joint. A second suture is placed slightly more proximally, the ligament reconstruction is stabilized adequately, and tissue interposition is performed.

Tissue Interposition

Although Burton's original technique "resurfaced" the metacarpal base to minimize the chance that interposition material may extrude through the channel,[113] this is unlikely, and, from a technical standpoint, a nuisance. In that light, I prefer to fold the tendon into the volar aspect of the arthroplasty space to ensure that it will sink into its depth, and from that point distally, it is folded back and forth approximately four times on a single Keith needle, like ribbon candy. A 4.0 Vicryl suture is used to stabilize each corner of the tendon "anchovy," and then a second Keith needle is placed through it, parallel to the first (see Fig. 12-13G). Apertures in each needle should be volar, the tip of each needle should be dorsal, and, with the previously placed volar capsular suture, each limb is threaded and the anchovy is slid down and delivered into the arthroplasty space. The two Vicryl limbs are tied, securing the tissue interposition (see Fig. 12-13H).

Capsular Repair

The capsule is tightly repaired with 3.0 Vicryl. I prefer to place a suture at the level of the metacarpal base and at the scaphoid tuberosity, tagging these with clamps to allow better exposure of the intervening capsule during closure. If redundant capsule is present, a pants-over-vest closure can be performed. When closing the capsule, it is important that the radial artery and neighboring radial sensory nerve branches be protected to avoid damage.

Wound Closure

The incisions are closed with 4.0 nylon; and, again, identification of underlying radial sensory nerve branches is important so that inadvertent injury is avoided during skin closure. This may be a cause of dystrophic pain postoperatively. A wet and dry bulky thumb spica dressing is placed, followed by volar and thumb spica splints. The hand is elevated in a Carter pillow or the like for 3 to 4 days postoperatively.

POSTOPERATIVE THERAPY PROGRAM

First Month

At 2 weeks, the patient returns for suture removal, wound inspection, and application of a fiberglass thumb spica cast that allows full motion of the thumb IP joint, unless MP joint fusion has been performed. At 4 weeks, the Kirschner wire is removed and a forearm-based thumb spica orthoplast splint is fashioned by the hand therapist. Gentle wrist and thumb MP range of motion exercises are initiated, as well as thenar isometric exercises. The latter are performed with the thumb in the splint.

Second Month

At 6 weeks, if the patient is comfortable, gentle pinch and grip strengthening exercises are initiated and, by 8 weeks, flexion-adduction and opposition exercises are begun.

Third Month

By this time, the patient is usually doing well enough that the splint can be discarded. Grip and pinch exercises are typically continued by the patient on a self-administered basis. No rigorous attempt is made for the thumb to reach the ring and small finger bases because there is no functional relevance to these activities, and they risk stretching the ligament. In that light, passive range of motion is not a part of the regimen. The patient typically returns at approximately 3 months postoperatively (the third postoperative visit) and a posteroanterior radiograph of the hand is obtained to assess the arthroplasty space height (see Fig. 12-13I).

Three to Six Months

During these months, the patient is encouraged to use the hand and to push the exercises vigorously. Typically, patients return to work with little restriction. Work-simulating machines may be helpful in therapy if return to work has been difficult.

Long Term

Occasionally, a patient returns with a complaint of some pain or decrease in function. Burton has noted that grip and pinch measurements may reveal loss of strength, but, in every case, resumption of a strengthening program with putty has been successful in eliminating pain and restoring function.[109]

CRITICAL POINTS: LRTI ARTHROPLASTY

INDICATIONS

- Eaton stage 2 to 4 disease
- As revision for failed trapeziectomy

TECHNICAL POINTS

- Make a longitudinal or triradiate incision over the TM joint, dorsally.
- Mobilize and retract the radial artery, and protect radial sensory nerve branches.
- Open the capsule and visualize the TM and scaphotrapezial-trapezoid joints.
- Square off the base of the thumb metacarpal.
- Cut the trapezium into quadrants and remove with rongeur.
- Make a bony channel through the metacarpal, 1 cm from the base, exiting through the base in the plane of the nail.
- Inspect the scaphotrapezoid joint and resect the proximal 2 mm of the trapezoid if arthritis exists.
- Release the FCR in the midproximal forearm through a single transverse incision.
- Deliver the FCR into the arthroplasty space by putting a curved clamp beneath the tendon at the base of the arthroplasty space.
- Mobilize the tendon to its insertion at the base of the index metacarpal.
- Taper the tip of the tendon and pass through the channel with a Carroll tendon passer.
- Suspend the thumb metacarpal at the level of the index CMC joint, in the key pinch position, and place a Kirschner wire into the ulnar carpus.
- Pull the FCR tight and suture to EPB and ulnar periosteum.
- Divide the EPB to complete the EPB tenodesis.
- Secure the residual tendon length into an "anchovy" and place in the arthroplasty space with deep capsular suture (optional).
- Close capsule and skin.
- Apply a short-arm spica splint for 10 days.

POSTOPERATIVE CARE

- Apply new thumb spica cast at 10 days for 3 weeks.
- Remove short-arm thumb spica cast at 1 month; forearm-based orthoplast spica splint is placed for 6 weeks.
- At 4 to 6 weeks begin wrist and thumb range-of-motion exercises (no opposition).
- Begin thenar isometric exercises at 6 weeks and pinch and grip strengthening at 8 weeks.

ATHLETIC PARTICIPATION

- Resume tennis and golf at 10 to 12 weeks.

REVISION SURGERY

Potential Complications and Principles

One cause of unsatisfactory outcome after basal joint arthroplasty is residual pain because of failure to address scaphotrapezial or scaphotrapezoidal disease. Routine complete excision of the trapezium certainly precludes the former and also allows adequate intraoperative observation and treatment of the latter by partial excision of the proximal trapezoid, as has been mentioned[58,114] (see Fig. 12-5).

Unaddressed hyperextension instability of the MP joint can also impair functional outcome after ligament reconstruction. During lateral pinch, MP hyperextension causes reciprocal deformity more proximally, imposing metacarpal adduction and stressing the reconstructed ligament (see Fig. 12-6). Accordingly, early identification of hyperextension in excess of 30 degrees should prompt stabilization to protect the integrity of the basal joint ligament reconstruction. Even with a sound ligament reconstruction and appropriate stabilization of the MP joint, it is theoretically possible to develop recurrent laxity at the basal joint owing to stretching of the FCR tendon, in the case of the LRTI arthroplasty, or attenuation of other alternative suspensionplasty techniques using a slip of APL or FCR.[101,119]

When thumb metacarpal subsidence occurs, whether because of failure of ligament reconstruction or when trapezium excision alone was performed, effective revision is possible (Fig. 12-14). If only one half of the FCR tendon had been harvested, the other half may be a potential source for a second reconstruction of the ligament. As with the initial procedure, correction of any adduction contracture becomes important, as well as close scrutiny of the status of the MP joint.

If the residual FCR tendon is insufficient, or is too scarred in the arthroplasty bed, alternative suspensionplasty techniques can be used.[86,101,108,115,119] A slip of the APL tendon can be used, as described by Thompson as a salvage procedure for the revision of a failed silicone implant arthroplasty[108] or as described as a modification of Weilby's technique.[86,101] Alternatively, when the MP joint has been fused, the distally based EPB tendon can be used.

Lastly, in cases in which only hemitrapeziectomy was performed originally, fusion between the metacarpal and the hemitrapezium can be performed. Fusion is relatively contraindicated if the MP joint has been previously fused. If a trapezial remnant does not exist, fusion to the distal pole of the scaphoid would dramatically alter normal carpal kinematics and is not recommended.

NEW DEVELOPMENTS

Biomechanical

The results of biomechanical research may not necessarily have immediate clinical relevance, but two investigations that improve our understanding of TM mechanics may also impact on future treatment.[77,100] Shrivastava and colleagues simulated extension osteotomy of the thumb metacarpal and showed that carpometacarpal joint laxity during lateral pinch was reduced. They suggested that first metacarpal osteotomy results in obligatory metacarpal flexion, which effectively tightens the dorsal radial ligament.[100]

Moulton and coworkers proposed that a hypermobile MP joint might have a causative role in the development of TM osteoarthritis by concentrating forces on the palmar aspect of the TM joint.[77] Pressure-sensitive film was used to study the contact at the TM joint in cadaver thumbs during lateral pinch with the MP joint unrestrained, pinned in neutral, pinned in 30 degrees of flexion, and pinned in maximal hyperextension. The center of pressure in nonarthritic TM joints moved dorsally when the MP joint was flexed 30 degrees. The authors reported that MP joint flexion effectively unloaded the most palmar surfaces of the TM joint regardless of the presence or severity of arthritic disease and intimated that MP joint arthrodesis in flexion might be an early preventive intervention in thumbs with TM hypermobility or early degenerative disease.[77]

Biologic

Pellegrini and coworkers detailed the pathobiology of articular cartilage in TM osteoarthritis in 1994, showing preferential loss of glycosaminoglycan, retention of collagen, and an increase in chondroitin sulfate/keratan sulfate ratio in the volar surfaces of the joint affected by chondromalacia.[95] Still, the exact mechanisms by which mechanical forces lead to articular degeneration remain elusive.

Nevertheless, the observation of such selective glycosaminoglycan depletion localized to the contact areas of the joint suggests an interdependent relationship between mechanical factors and biochemical matrix degradation[95] and raises hope that pharmacologic intervention may be possible in the future to interrupt, slow down, prevent, or even possibly reverse the cartilage lesion of TM osteoarthritis.

Clinical: TM Arthroscopy

TM arthroscopy is, arguably, the newest tool available for treating basal joint disease, particularly stage 1 synovitis and TM instability. Although the technical pearls of TM arthroscopy have been published,[5,24,50] and many surgeons can attest to the technical feasibility of the procedure, little is available in the literature to guide assessment of this tool's efficacy and advisability.[24]

The use of radiofrequency energy in medicine is not new, but the notion of capsuloligamentous shrinkage to treat instability and other applications in orthopedics have only recently emerged. Monopolar and bipolar radiofrequency probes are available commercially. This process produces molecular friction in tissue fibers, resulting in tissue heating and histologic changes. A characteristic hyalinization of collagen occurs, and transmission electron microscopy shows alterations to the collagen architecture, including contracture in fibril length and expansion in fiber diameter.[55] Longitudinal sections of heated collagen fibrils also demonstrate destruction of the triple-helical structure and loss of cross striation.[56,71] The degree of this reaction or shrinkage depends on the duration of exposure as well as the temperature.[56]

Some surgeons advocate arthroscopic synovectomy, ligament thermal shrinkage, and temporary TM pinning for

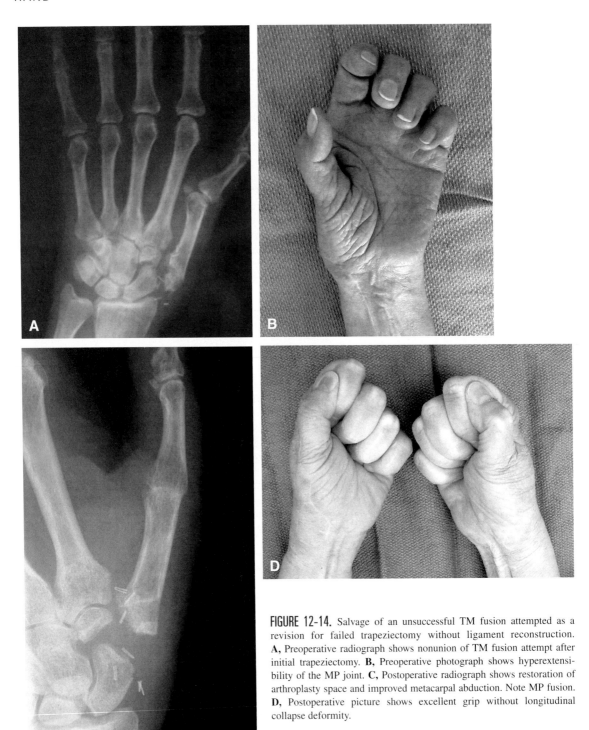

FIGURE 12-14. Salvage of an unsuccessful TM fusion attempted as a revision for failed trapeziectomy without ligament reconstruction. **A,** Preoperative radiograph shows nonunion of TM fusion attempt after initial trapeziectomy. **B,** Preoperative photograph shows hyperextensibility of the MP joint. **C,** Postoperative radiograph shows restoration of arthroplasty space and improved metacarpal abduction. Note MP fusion. **D,** Postoperative picture shows excellent grip without longitudinal collapse deformity.

stage 1 disease. More daring surgeons continue to advance arthroscopic techniques by treating more advanced disease. Culp and Rekant have reported that results after arthroscopic hemi- and complete trapeziectomy and electrothermal shrinkage have been successful, but they have yet to provide much objective follow-up data.[24] Among 24 thumbs in 22 patients, 88% excellent or good outcome scores were obtained with follow-up of 1.2 to 4 years. Subsidence of the thumb metacarpal was 2 to 4 mm, and pinch strength improved 22%.

They reported that 8 patients actually preferred their arthroscopic procedure over their standard open arthroplasty on the contralateral side.[24]

The absence of published reports of outcome justifies a modicum of restraint before adopting these alternatives, but it is hoped that prospective assessment of outcomes of TM arthroscopic techniques for various stages of disease will be forthcoming. One report, which addressed the efficacy of arthroscopic débridement for isolated scaphotrapezial-

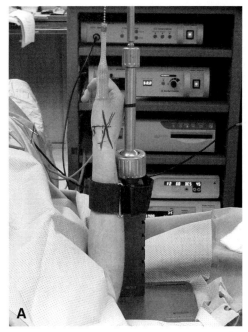

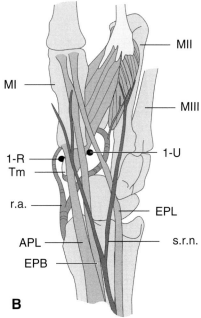

FIGURE 12-15. TM arthroscopy. **A,** Setup. **B,** Portals. At the level of the TM joint, the 1-R portal is radial to the APL and the 1-U portal is ulnar to the EPB. Note the proximity of the radial artery (r.a.) to both portals. APL, abductor pollicis longus; EPB, extensor pollicis brevis; EPL, extensor pollicis longus; s.r.n., radial sensory nerve; Tm, trapeziometacarpal joint. (From Berger RA: A technique for arthroscopic evaluation of the first carpometacarpal joint. J Hand Surg 22:1077-1080, 1997.)

trapezoid arthritis, showed favorable pain relief in 9 of 10 patients.[1]

Operative Technique

TM Arthroscopy[5]

Equipment and setup are similar to what is used for standard wrist arthroscopy with minor exceptions. A single fingertrap is placed on the thumb, and traction is limited to between 5 and 10 pounds (Fig. 12-15A). A short barrel 1.9-mm arthroscope is recommended by Berger, with inflow via manual delivery through a 20-mL syringe.[5] I have been satisfied with gravity inflow exactly as is done in wrist arthroscopy. The 2.0-mm shavers are recommended.

Arthroscopic portals are marked with a pen once the tourniquet has been inflated and the thumb is distracted. The proximal radial edge of the metacarpal and the APL and EPB tendons are palpated and marked. To estimate the angle of entry, a 20-gauge needle is advanced into the joint at the line drawn to indicate the location of the distracted TM joint. Insufflation with 1 to 2 mL of normal saline is then performed. The portals are located on the radial side of the APL (1-R) and the ulnar side of the EPB (1-U)[5,50] (see Fig. 12-15B). A No. 11 blade is used to make a 3-mm long incision at each portal site, oriented proximodistally, and blunt separation of the subdermal tissues is performed with a small straight clamp. We use a tapered blunt trocar and sheath combination and, once through the skin, carefully advance in combination with a gentle sweeping motion to find any natural division between the capsuloligamentous structures. Because the 1-U portal allows excellent visualization of the palmar oblique (beak) ligament, we preferentially insert the scope through this portal and use the 1-R portal as a working portal initially. The 1-R portal affords excellent visualization of the dorsoradial, posterior oblique, and ulnar collateral ligaments.[5]

When the synovial lining of the joint capsule or frank synovitis obscures visualization of the capsular ligaments or articular surfaces, a 2.0-mm shaver is initially used to perform a synovectomy.

ANNOTATED REFERENCES

5. Berger RA: A technique for arthroscopic evaluation of the first carpometacarpal joint. J Hand Surg [Am] 22:1077-1080, 1997.

    Berger describes the technique, indications, and potential complications of first CMC arthroplasty.

7. Bettinger P, Linschied RL, Berger R, et al: An anatomic study of the stabilizing ligaments of the trapezium and trapeziometacarpal joint. J Hand Surg [Am] 24:786-798, 1999.

    This paper details the most current understanding of the complex ligamentous anatomy of the basal joint.

40. Forseth MJ, Stern PJ: Complications of trapeziometacarpal arthrodesis using plate and screw fixation. J Hand Surg [Am] 28:342-345, 2003.

    Union rates were comparable between groups treated with plates and screw fixation or Kirschner wires, but patient satisfaction was lower, and a second surgery more common, after use of the former.

41. Freedman DM, Eaton RG, Glickel SZ: Long-term results of volar ligament reconstruction for symptomatic basal joint laxity. J Hand Surg [Am] 25:297-304, 2000.

    Ligament reconstruction restored pain-free TM stability and prevented the development of TM osteoarthritis in 15 of 23 thumbs (65%) at an average follow-up of 15 years. Only 8% of thumbs advanced to show radiographic evidence of arthritic disease, and 15 patients were at least 90% satisfied with their long-term results.

42. Froimson AI: Tendon arthroplasty of the trapeziometacarpal joint. Clin Orthop Rel Res 70:191-199, 1970.

    Froimson was among the first to combine excision of the trapezium with placing a portion of the flexor carpi radialis tendon in the trapezial void. Uniform pain relief was noted in the short term, with little joint space collapse, but longer-term follow-up (4 years) showed decline in grip strength and stability.

47. Gerwin M, Griffith A, Weiland AJ, et al: Ligament reconstruction basal joint arthroplasty without tendon interposition. Clin Orthop 342:42-45, 1997.

   The authors questioned the necessity of tendon interposition for the maintenance of joint space after basal joint resection arthroplasty with ligament reconstruction. In their prospective, randomized study, tendon interposition was found to be not necessary for maintenance of joint space after basal joint resection arthroplasty if ligament reconstruction is performed.

54. Hartigan BJ, Stern PJ, Kiefhaber TR: Thumb carpometacarpal osteoarthritis: Arthrodesis compared with ligament reconstruction and tendon interposition. J Bone Joint Surg Am 83:1470-1478, 2001.

   Similar results were shown comparing fusion and LRTI arthroplasty with regard to pain relief and patient satisfaction. Soft tissue arthroplasty appeared to decreased immobilization time and increase range of motion, whereas arthrodesis appeared to result in a stronger pinch strength but led to a higher rate of, and more serious, complications.

58. Irwin AS, Maffulli N, Chesney RB: Scapho-trapezoid arthritis: A cause of residual pain after arthroplasty of the trapeziometacarpal joint. J Hand Surg [Br] 20:346-352, 1995.

   These authors heightened our appreciation of unaddressed scaphotrapezoidal arthritis as a potential cause of residual pain after the LRTI arthroplasty. Partial resection of the trapezoid restored satisfactory pain relief.

60. Kadiyala RK, Gelberman RH, Kwon B: Radiographic assessment of the trapezial space before and after ligament reconstruction and tendon interposition arthroplasty. J Hand Surg [Br] 21:177-181, 1996.

   A radiographic method of measuring the change in scaphometacarpal space following trapezial excision arthroplasty is described. The authors report that ligament reconstruction tendon interposition arthroplasty is not entirely successful in either restoring or maintaining the length of the thumb ray.

65. Kuhns CA, Emerson ET, Meals RA: Hematoma and distraction arthroplasty for thumb basal joint osteoarthritis: A prospective, single-surgeon study including outcomes measures. J Hand Surg [Am] 28:381-389, 2003.

   In an attempt to address thumb metacarpal subsidence, which may have played a part in poor outcomes after simple excision in the past, proponents of this procedure recommend pinning the metacarpal in a distracted position for 5 weeks. This report assessed outcome in 26 patients prospectively evaluated at 6 and 24 months after surgery. Complete pain relief was reported by 74% at 6 months and 92% at final follow-up. Two-year follow-up evaluation showed a 47% increase in grip strength, a 33% increase in key pinch strength, and a 23% increase in tip pinch strength. Proximal migration of the metacarpal averaged 51% on radiographs at 2-year follow-up, which increased an additional 10% with pinch. Twenty-four of 25 patients queried 2 years after hematoma and distraction arthroplasty reported that they were very satisfied with the outcome.

69. Lins RE, Gelberman RH, McKeown L, et al: Basal joint arthritis: Trapeziectomy with ligament reconstruction and tendon interposition arthroplasty. J Hand Surg [Am] 21:202-209, 1996.

   This qualitative and quantitative outcomes assessment of ligament reconstruction and tendon interposition arthroplasty revealed that 89% of patients were satisfied with the pain relief provided by the arthroplasty, 67% noted improvement in the ability to perform activities, and significant improvements were noted in web space measurements as well as grip and pinch strength. A trapezial height decrease of 33% was noted but did not correlate with objective and subjective clinical outcome.

89. Pellegrini VD: Osteoarthritis of the thumb trapeziometacarpal joint: A study of the pathophysiology of articular cartilage degeneration: II. Articular wear patterns in the osteoarthritic joint. J Hand Surg [Am] 16:975-982, 1991.

   Analysis of both surgical and post-mortem specimens of the trapeziometacarpal joint revealed the chondromalacic nature of the articular cartilage in the dorsal compartment but, more importantly, that the palmar joint surfaces were often found to be polished to eburnated bone.

92. Pellegrini VD Jr, Burton RI: Surgical management of basal joint arthritis of the thumb: I. Long-term results of silicone implant arthroplasty. J Hand Surg [Am] 11:309, 1986.

   Subluxation and wear after use of the Swanson implant at average follow-up of 3.9 years was greater in osteoarthritis patients than in rheumatoid patients. The implant wear was seen primarily at the ulnar margin where a 50% loss of height was found. The authors recommended use of this implant in the low-demand patient.

94. Pellegrini VD, Parentis M, Judkins A, et al: Extension metacarpal osteotomy in the treatment of trapeziometacarpal osteoarthritis: A biomechanical study. J Hand Surg [Am] 21:16-23, 1996.

   The biomechanical effects of extension metacarpal osteotomy on contact pressures in the TM joint during lateral pinch were studied in 20 anatomic specimens using pressure-sensitive film. Extension metacarpal osteotomy effectively unloaded the palmar contact area in nonarthritic and moderately arthritic specimens; primary contact areas and zones of peak pressure were shifted from the disease palmar compartment to the normal dorsal compartment. In contrast, the pathologically congruent contact pattern seen in end-stage osteoarthritic joints was unaffected by osteotomy. The data demonstrated the efficacy of extension metacarpal osteotomy in unloading the palmar contact areas of normal and moderately arthritic joints but provided no biomechanical rationale for metacarpal osteotomy as originally described in treatment of advanced TM osteoarthritis.

101. Sigfusson R, Lundborg G: Abductor pollicis longus tendon arthroplasty for treatment of arthrosis in the first carpometacarpal joint. Scand J Plast Reconstr Hand Surg 25:73-77, 1991.

   The authors describe a technique in which a portion of the abductor pollicis longus (APL) was used in a figure-of-eight fashion around the FCR and remaining portion of the APL. Grip and pinch strengths over 80% of the estimated normal hand were found. Scaphometacarpal height reduced to about 2 mm with pinch. Arthrosis of the scaphotrapezoid joint was a presumed potential cause of suboptimal results.

104a. Stern PJ: Trapeziometacarpal joint arthrodesis in primary osteoarthritis: A minimum two-year follow-up. J Hand Surg [Am] 26:109-114, 2001.

   A retrospective review of 59 TM arthrodeses with follow-up from 2 to 20 years. Only four nonunions (7%) occurred, and only one of these was symptomatic and required reoperation. Peritrapezial arthrosis was seen in seven patients at the last follow-up.

111. Tomaino MM: Treatment of Eaton stage I trapeziometacarpal disease with metacarpal extension osteotomy. J Hand Surg [Am] 25:1100-1106, 2000.

   This study prospectively evaluated the efficacy of a 30-degree extension osteotomy of the thumb metacarpal as treatment for Eaton stage I basal joint arthritis in 12 patients. The osteotomy redistributes trapeziometacarpal contact area and load, obviating the need for ligament reconstruction. All osteotomies healed at an average of 7 weeks. Eleven patients were satisfied with the outcome. Grip and pinch strength increased an average of 8.5 and 3.0 kg, respectively. Thumb metacarpal extension osteotomy was thought to be an effective biomechanical alternative to ligament reconstruction in the treatment of Eaton stage I disease of the TM joint, although the follow-up was somewhat short (average 2.1 years; range, 6 to 46 months).

112. Tomaino MM, Coleman K: Use of the entire width of the flexor carpi radialis tendon for the LRTI arthroplasty does not impair wrist function. Am J Orthop 29:283-284, 2000.

There appeared to be no morbidity associated with harvesting the entire tendon, evaluated 1 year after LRTI arthroplasty. The authors recommend use of the whole tendon, which provides a stouter ligament reconstruction and facilitates execution of the procedure.

113. Tomaino MM, Pellegrini VD Jr, Burton RI: Arthroplasty of the basal joint of the thumb: Long-term follow-up after ligament reconstruction with tendon interposition. J Bone Joint Surg Am 77:346-355, 1995.

Follow-up averaged 9 years (range, 8 to 11 years) in this study of LRTI in 24 thumbs (22 patients) for osteoarthritis. Ninety-five percent had excellent relief of pain. Grip strength increased 93% and tip pinch, 65%. Improvements in key pinch strength were first noted at the 6-year follow-up and then tapered slightly but were not significantly different from the preoperative values. Radiographs demonstrated an average 13% height loss, which was not indicative of a poorer outcome.

114. Tomaino MM, Vogt M, Weiser R: Scaphotrapezoid arthritis: Prevalence in thumbs undergoing trapezium excision arthroplasty and efficacy of proximal trapezoid excision. J Hand Surg [Am] 24:1220-1224, 1999.

These authors showed that x-ray sensitivity and specificity for disease at the scaphotrapezoidal joint were only 44% and 86%, respectively. They recommend routine intraoperative assessment of the scaphotrapezoidal joint at the time of arthroplasty by pulling on the index and long fingers. When arthritis is present—what may be considered "stage 5 disease"—2- to 3-mm excision of the proximal trapezoid can be performed without morbidity to avoid the potential for residual pain in the postoperative period after arthroplasty.

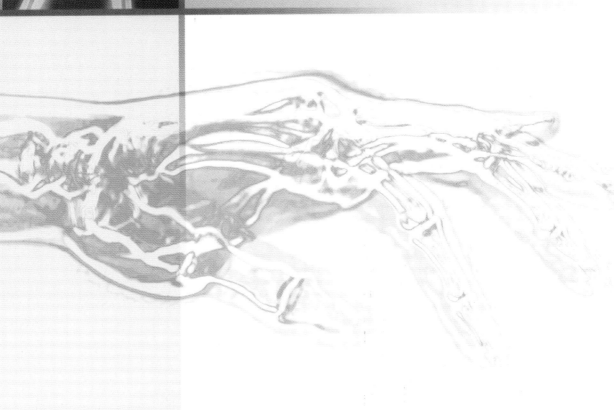

PART III

Wrist

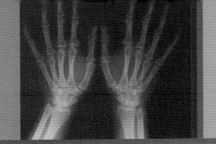

CHAPTER 13

Arthrodesis (Partial and Complete)

Hill Hastings II

The wrist joint may become painful and deformed by trauma, such as fracture, dislocation, or ligament injury, which causes instability, or by insidious disease of an inflammatory nature, infection, or tumor. Partial or total wrist arthrodesis remains one of the important tools for the reconstructive hand surgeon through its ability to render stability, alignment, and pain relief. In general, pain relief and stability have precedence over maintaining wrist range of motion.

Although the "normal" wrist enjoys a large arc of motion through its three degrees of freedom (flexion/extension, radioulnar deviation, and rotation), the majority of activities in daily living can be accomplished with only a small percentage of the total motion. Normal functional range of wrist motion is 5 degrees of flexion, 30 degrees of extension, 10 degrees of radial deviation, and 15 degrees of ulnar deviation.[87] The functional range of motion needed to perform activities of daily living with satisfactory outcome and minimum difficulty in fact is much lower than this and only requires about 5 degrees of flexion, 6 degrees of extension, 7 degrees of radial deviation, and 6 degrees of ulnar deviation.

Several authors have studied the range of motion used in activities of daily living. Brumfield and Champoux[14] found that in accomplishing 15 activities of daily living, 10 degrees of wrist flexion and 35 degrees of wrist extension were used. Similarly, Palmer and colleagues,[87] in 1985, evaluating 52 standardized tasks of activities of daily living and activities of work, found that "normal functional range of motion" was 5 degrees of flexion, 30 degrees of extension, 10 degrees of radial deviation, and 15 degrees of ulnar deviation. Ryu and coworkers,[100] in 1991, in evaluating 24 activities of daily living found that the "ideal range of motion" was 54 degrees of flexion, 60 degrees of extension, 17 degrees of radial deviation, and 40 degrees of ulnar deviation. All these studies evaluated motion used for certain activities. One must recognize that the range of motion used in accomplishing activities is not necessarily equal to that which is needed. Nissen and coworkers,[84] for example, found that patients could perform a complete list of 123 activities of daily living successfully wearing a splint that limited flexion to 5 degrees, extension to 6 degrees, radial deviation to 7 degrees, and ulnar deviation to 6 degrees. This underscores that while range of motion is desirable, very little motion in fact is needed to perform almost all activities of daily living. Those activities that showed minimal difficulty or only slight modification of the activity were fastening a brassiere, dusting low surfaces, washing one's back, using a manual can opener, writing one's name, or handling a sharp knife. Activities of work and activities of recreation may require a greater arc of motion.

PREOPERATIVE EVALUATION

Radiographic Evaluation

The first and most important decision involves determining which joint components of wrist motion are deformed, because this principally will determine whether a total arthrodesis or a partial arthrodesis is required. About 95% of degenerative arthritis involving the wrist occurs around the scaphoid.[127,133] Fifty-five percent occurs secondary to scapholunate advanced collapse (SLAC), 26% by scaphotrapezial-trapezoid (STT) arthritis, and 14% as a combination of both. With a SLAC pattern of arthritis, the radiolunate joint is invariably spared. In metabolic disease, such as calcium pyrophosphate deposition disease (CPDD), the radiolunate joint may be involved.[95] Radiographs should carefully evaluate the alignment of the wrist to rule out significant palmar or ulnar translation and to stage the presence or absence of arthritic involvement of the radioscaphoid (RS) joint, radiolunate (RL) joint, STT joint, and the midcarpal articular surfaces of the capitate and triquetrum.

The author would like to acknowledge the previous contributions of **Harold M. Dick** (total wrist arthrodesis) and **H. Kirk Watson** (intercarpal arthrodesis); some illustrations and text in this chapter are reprinted from their work in earlier editions.

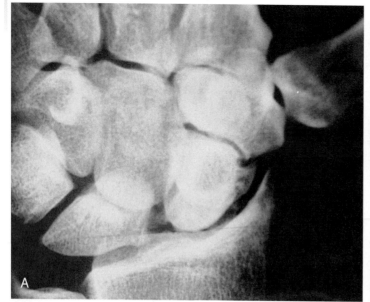

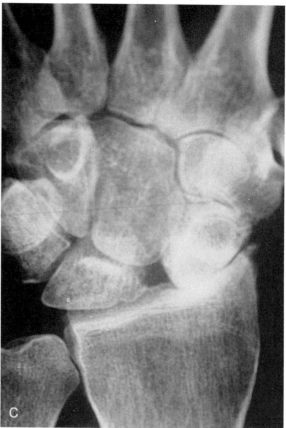

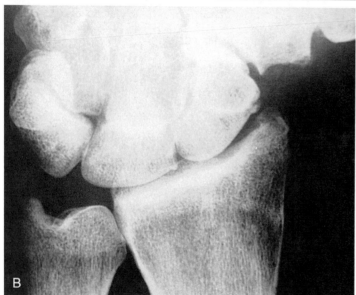

FIGURE 13-1. Stages of scapholunate advanced collapse (SLAC) wrist. **A,** SLAC changes are seen earliest at the radial aspect of the radioscaphoid joint beginning at the radial styloid (stage IA). **B,** Subsequently, the remainder of the radioscaphoid joint is involved (stage IB). **C,** Finally, destruction of the capitolunate joint occurs (at age II). Isolated involvement of the capitolunate joint may also be seen and is referred to as midcarpal SLAC.

Standard radiographs should include a supinated antero-posterior (AP) view, a lateral view, and a zero-rotation view. The AP view is best for assessment of the radiocarpal and midcarpal joint spaces and relationship of the scaphoid to the lunate (Figs. 13-1 and 13-2). The lateral radiograph should be taken in neutral flexion/extension to show the midcarpal and scapholunate (SL) alignment (see Fig. 13-2B). The zero-rotation radiograph better reveals the triquetral-lunate joint relationship and relative length of the ulna. Radial and ulnar deviation views can assist in assessment of the RS and STT joints for potential joint space narrowing.

Arthritis of the radiocarpal and/or midcarpal joints can be associated with instability or arthritis of the distal radioulnar joint (DRUJ). The DRUJ should be carefully assessed to rule out arthritis instability or deformity that would require simultaneous treatment (see Chapter 15).

Physical Examination*

Because the vast majority of carpal pathology originates on the radial aspect of the wrist, a systematic clinical examination consisting of five maneuvers has evolved.[136] None of these maneuvers is necessarily diagnostic of a specific entity by itself, nor intended to be. However, a diagnosis can almost always be derived by coupling the entire picture of the patient's wrist mechanics and pathomechanics with the history, symptomatology, and radiographic examination. Before performing these maneuvers, wrist motion should be thoroughly assessed. In our experience, any loss of passive flexion consistently represents a sign of underlying organic carpal patho-

*This section is from the chapter on intercarpal arthrodesis in the previous edition of this book, authored by H. Kirk Watson and Jeffrey Weinzweig.

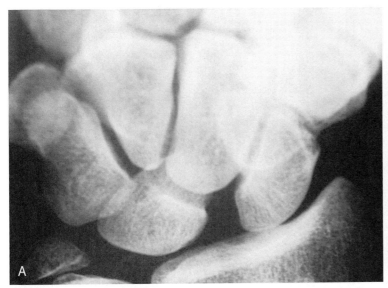

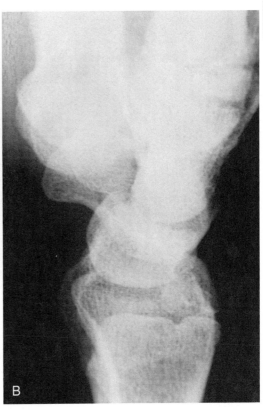

FIGURE 13-2.   Static rotatory subluxation of the scaphoid. **A,** Radiographic findings on the neutral AP view are foreshortening of the scaphoid, a positive ring sign, and an increased scapholunate gap. **B,** Radiographic findings on the neutral lateral view are a scapholunate angle greater than 70 degrees (90 degrees in this case), with or without DISI of the lunate (present in this case).

logy. It is rare, for example, that a patient with Kienböck's disease, even stage I, does not present with some degree of loss of passive flexion.

Watson's radial wrist examination consists of the following five maneuvers.

Dorsal Wrist Syndrome/Scapholunate Joint

Identification of the SL joint is facilitated by following the course of the third metacarpal proximally until the examiner's thumb falls into a recess (Fig. 13-3). That recess lies over the capitate with the wrist in flexion. The SL articulation is readily palpable just proximal between the extensor carpi radialis brevis (ECRB) and the extensors of the fourth compartment. A normal joint produces no pain with palpation. SL dissociation, Kienböck's disease, dorsal wrist syndrome, or other pathologic process involving the SL or RL joints, or the lunate itself, will elicit pain with direct palpation.

Finger Extension Test (FET)

The increased mechanical advantage of carpal loading during the FET produces a reliable indicator of carpal pathology. With the patient's wrist held passively in flexion, the examiner resists active finger extension (Fig. 13-4). In patients with significant periscaphoid inflammatory change, radiocarpal or midcarpal instability, symptomatic rotatory subluxation of the scaphoid (RSS), or Kienböck's disease, the combined radiocarpal loading and pressure of the extensor tendons cause considerable discomfort. In our experience, patients with these carpal disorders always demonstrate a positive FET. The FET has become a very reliable indicator of problems at the SL joint. Full-power finger extension against resistance (i.e., a negative FET) eliminates dorsal wrist syndrome, RSS,

Kienböck's disease, midcarpal instability, and SLAC from the patient's differential diagnosis.

Articular-Nonarticular (ANA) Junction of Scaphoid

The proximal pole of the scaphoid articulates with the radius within the radiocarpal joint. The articular surface of the proximal scaphoid continues distally toward a junctional point along the radial aspect where the cartilage changes from articular to nonarticular. With the wrist in radial deviation, that ANA junction is obscured by the radial styloid. With the wrist in ulnar deviation, the ANA junction is easily palpated just distal to the radial styloid. The ANA maneuver is performed with the examiner's index finger firmly palpating the radial aspect of the patient's wrist just distal to the radial styloid with the wrist initially in radial deviation (Fig. 13-5). Pressure is maintained as the patient's wrist is brought into ulnar deviation with the examiner's other hand. The normal asymptomatic wrist demonstrates mild to moderate tenderness and discomfort at the ANA junction with direct palpation in almost every individual. However, the patient with periscaphoid synovitis, scaphoid instability, or SLAC changes at the styloid will experience severe pain with this maneuver. For purposes of comparison, it is necessary to perform this maneuver as a bilateral examination.

Scaphotrapezial-Trapezoid (STT) or Triscaphe Joint

Identification of the triscaphe joint is facilitated by following the course of the second metacarpal proximally until the examiner's thumb falls into a recess (Fig. 13-6). That recess is the triscaphe joint. A normal joint produces no pain with palpation. Any triscaphe synovitis, degenerative disease, or

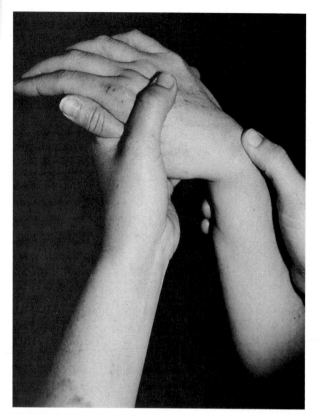

FIGURE 13-3. Dorsal wrist syndrome (DWS)/scapholunate joint. Identification of the scapholunate (SL) joint is facilitated by following the course of the third metacarpal proximally until the examiner's thumb falls into a recess. The SL articulation is readily palpable between the ECRB and the extensors of the fourth compartment. (From Watson HK, Weinzweig J: Physical examination of the wrist. Hand Clin 13:17-34, 1997.)

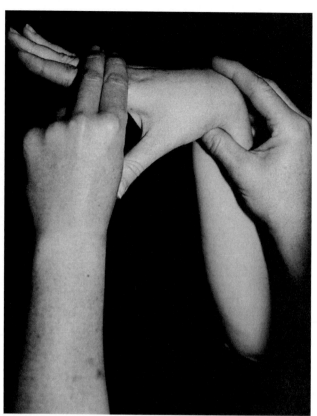

FIGURE 13-4. Finger extension test (FET). With the patient's wrist held passively in flexion, the examiner resists active finger extension. (From Watson HK, Weinzweig J: Physical examination of the wrist. Hand Clin 13:17-34, 1997.)

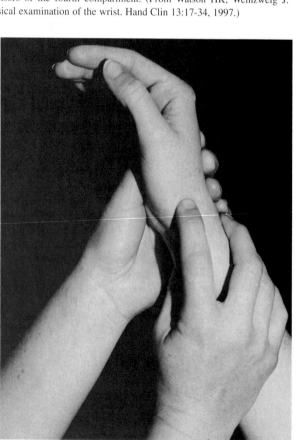

FIGURE 13-5. Articular-nonarticular (ANA) junction of scaphoid. With the wrist in ulnar deviation, the ANA junction is easily palpated just distal to the radial styloid. The ANA maneuver is performed with the examiner's index finger firmly palpating the radial aspect of the patient's wrist just distal to the radial styloid with the wrist initially in radial deviation. Pressure is maintained as the patient's wrist is brought into ulnar deviation with the examiner's other hand. (From Watson HK, Weinzweig J: Physical examination of the wrist. Hand Clin 13:17-34, 1997.)

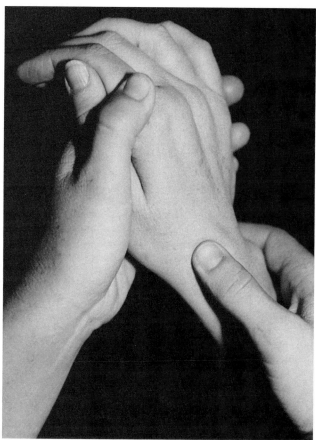

FIGURE 13-6. Scaphotrapezial-trapezoid (STT) or triscaphe joint. Identification of the triscaphe joint is facilitated by following the course of the second metacarpal proximally until the examiner's thumb falls into a recess, just ulnar to the anatomic snuffbox. (From Watson HK, Weinzweig J: Physical examination of the wrist. Hand Clin 13:17-34, 1997.)

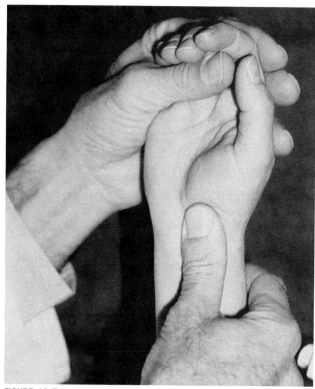

FIGURE 13-7. Scaphoid shift maneuver. The examiner grasps the wrist from the radial side, placing the thumb on the palmar prominence of the scaphoid while wrapping the fingers around the distal radius. This enables the thumb to push on the scaphoid with counterpressure provided by the fingers. The examiner's other hand grasps the patient's hand at the metacarpal level to control wrist position. Starting in ulnar deviation and slight extension, the wrist is moved radially and slightly flexed with constant thumb pressure on the scaphoid. (From Watson HK, Weinzweig J: Physical examination of the wrist. Hand Clin 13:17-34, 1997.)

other pathologic process involving the joint or scaphoid will elicit pain with direct palpation.

Scaphoid Shift Maneuver

The scaphoid shift maneuver provides a qualitative assessment of scaphoid stability and periscaphoid synovitis when compared with the contralateral asymptomatic wrist.[126] This examination, therefore, is meaningful only when performed bilaterally.

With the patient's forearm slightly pronated, the examiner grasps the wrist from the radial side, placing the thumb on the palmar prominence of the scaphoid while wrapping the fingers around the distal radius. This enables the thumb to push on the scaphoid with counterpressure provided by the fingers (Fig. 13-7). The examiner's right thumb is used to examine the patient's right scaphoid; the left thumb is used to examine the left scaphoid. The examiner's other hand grasps the patient's hand at the metacarpal level to control wrist position. Starting in ulnar deviation and slight extension, the wrist is moved radially and slightly flexed with constant thumb pressure on the scaphoid.

When the wrist is in ulnar deviation, the scaphoid axis is extended and lies nearly in line with the long axis of the forearm (Fig. 13-8). As the wrist deviates radially and flexes,

the scaphoid also flexes and rotates to an orientation more nearly perpendicular to the forearm, and its distal pole becomes prominent on the palmar side of the wrist. The examiner's thumb pressure opposes this normal rotation and creates a subluxation stress, causing the scaphoid to shift in relation to the other bones of the carpus. This scaphoid shift may be subtle or dramatic. In a patient with rigid periscaphoid ligamentous support, only minimal shift is tolerated before the scaphoid continues to rotate normally, pushing the examiner's thumb out of the way. In patients with ligamentous laxity, the combined stresses of thumb pressure and normal motion of the adjacent carpus may be sufficient to force the scaphoid out of its elliptical fossa and up onto the dorsal rim of the radius (Fig. 13-9). As thumb pressure is withdrawn, the scaphoid returns abruptly to its normal position, sometimes with a resounding "thunk."

The scaphoid may shift smoothly and painlessly or with a gritty sensation or clicking, accompanied by pain. Grittiness suggests chondromalacia or loss of articular cartilage, and clicking or catching may indicate bony change sufficient to produce impingement. Pain is a significant finding, especially when it reproduces the patient's symptoms. Pain associated with unilateral hypermobility of the scaphoid is virtually diagnostic of rotatory subluxation or scaphoid nonunion. A

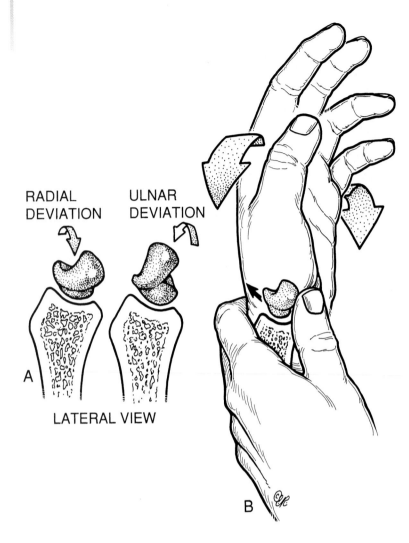

RADIAL
DEVIATION

ULNAR
DEVIATION

A

LATERAL VIEW

B

FIGURE 13-8. Mechanism of scaphoid shift. **A,** When the wrist is in ulnar deviation, the scaphoid dorsiflexes and its long axis approaches alignment with the axis of the radius. In radial deviation, the scaphoid volar flexes. Its long axis lies more perpendicular to the axis of the radius, and its distal pole becomes prominent on the palmar side of the wrist. **B,** During the scaphoid shift maneuver, the examiner's thumb resists the normal volar tilt of the scaphoid.

less-well-localized pain associated with normal or decreased mobility is encountered in patients with periscaphoid arthritis, whether of triscaphe or SLAC pattern.

Experience performing the scaphoid shift maneuver is essential for obtaining useful diagnostic information and distinguishing the normal wrist from the pathologic one. Of 1000 normal asymptomatic subjects examined, 209 demonstrated a unilateral abnormal scaphoid shift maneuver with hypermobility of the scaphoid and/or pain.[118] This represents 21% of examined subjects and 10% of examined wrists and makes the point that some degree of periscaphoid ligamentous injury is extremely common.

Summary Guidelines

The following are summary guidelines I (Watson) have found helpful in diagnosing the most common situations requiring limited or total wrist arthrodesis:

Radioscaphoid Arthritis

Clinical examination will reveal tenderness and/or prominence to the tip of the radial styloid and swelling palpable over the RS joint between the first and second dorsal compartments. Watson's scaphoid shift test[58,126] will increase pain and will frequently demonstrate crepitus. Radiographic examination will show enlargement of the RS joint and most commonly RSS with an increased SL angle caused by SL instability. A radial-deviation view will show narrowing or absence of the cartilage space between the scaphoid and the distal radius.

Scaphotrapezial-Trapezoid Arthritis

Clinical examination will show swelling and fullness in the dorsal radial wrist in the region of the snuffbox and frequently a visible swelling about the volar radial wrist. The volar scaphoid and flexor carpi radialis (FCR) tunnel may demonstrate tenderness that is exacerbated by grip and radial deviation. Volar palpation of the scaphoid, as in performing a scaphoid shift test, will cause pain. A hyperpronated view of the wrist may show narrowing, subchondral cysts, or irregularity of the STT joint.

Scaphocapitate or Capitolunate Arthritis

Scaphoid nonunion will frequently lead to arthrosis at the SC joint. At a late stage, SLAC wrist deformity will also affect the capitolunate joint. Clinical examination may reveal tenderness or swelling over the midcarpal joint. Preservation or loss of cartilage space (height) between the lunate and capitate and between the scaphoid and capitate may be appreciated on AP and lateral radiographs. Standard radiographs may not always be adequate to confirm or rule out arthritic

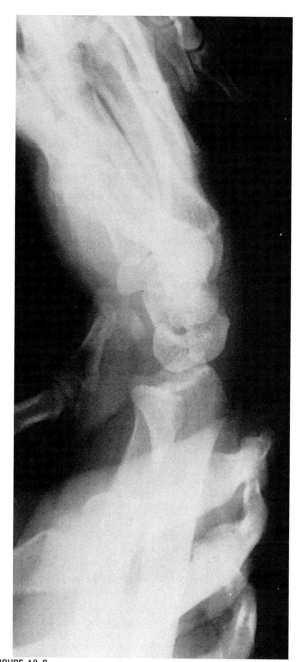

FIGURE 13-9.   Scaphoid shift dynamics. The examiner's thumb pressure has prevented the normal palmar tilt of the scaphoid, and, in this patient with ligamentous laxity, the scaphoid has been forced out of the elliptical fossa and up onto the dorsal rim of the radius. (From Watson HK, Weinzweig J: Physical examination of the wrist. Hand Clin 13:17-34, 1997.)

involvement of the capitolunate joint. Special studies may be helpful (see later). At present, the only way to definitively confirm that the capitate has a normal preserved cartilage surface free of significant wear is to directly inspect it by operative arthroscopy or arthrotomy.

Radiolunate and Ulnocarpal Joints

Ligamentous disruption by trauma or inflammatory disease may lead to ulnar translation of the carpus. On AP radiographic views, the position of the lunate with respect to the lunate fossa is assessed. In a neutral position, two thirds of the lunate should lie contained within the lunate fossa. Zero-rotation radiographs should be obtained to assess ulna variance, the space between the distal ulna and the lunate and triquetrum, alignment of the proximal articular surfaces of the lunate and triquetrum, and presence or absence of inflammatory, induced radiolucenies within the proximal lunate and triquetrum.

Rheumatoid Wrist Deformity

See the discussion in Chapter 59.

Evaluation of Associated Soft Tissue Lesions

The presence or absence of previous incisions should be identified. Recent incisions may require incorporation into the surgical approach for total or limited wrist arthrodesis. Composite wrist and digital range of motion is measured, both actively and passively, to rule out concomitant extensor or flexor adhesions. The presence of associated neuromas of the dorsal sensory branch of the radial nerve (DSBRN) or the ulnar nerve (DSBUN) is ruled out through the presence or absence of Tinel's sign. Lastly, wrist deformity is frequently associated with compression neuropathy of the median and/or ulnar nerves. Hence, carpal tunnel syndrome and ulnar tunnel syndrome, which might require concomitant treatment, should be carefully ruled out (see Chapter 28).

Special Procedures

Special procedures are rarely indicated. To best evaluate the radiocarpal joint by standard radiographs, views taken tangential to the joint surfaces may be useful. A modified lateral radiograph is taken with the x-ray tube aimed 23 degrees cephalad to obtain a tangential view of the RL joint ("fossa lateral view") (Fig. 13-10). A modified AP view is obtained,

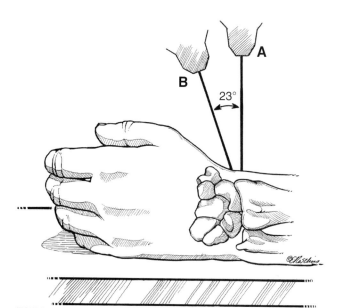

FIGURE 13-10.   Fossa lateral radiography. The normal lateral radiograph of the wrist does not show well the surface of the scapholunate fossa. To better evaluate the scaphoid fossa and lunate fossa, the x-ray incident beam angle is aimed slightly distal to proximal according to the ulnar inclination of the radius. A slightly wider angle is needed for assessment of the scaphoid fossa, and a slightly narrower one is needed for the evaluation of the lunate fossa.

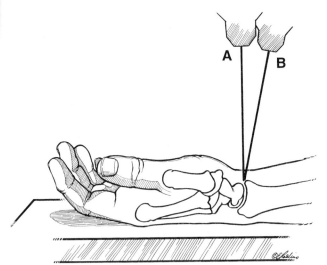

FIGURE 13-11.   Modified anteroposterior radiography. An AP radiograph (*A*) will not show well the surface of the lunate or scaphoid fossa because it will not be parallel to the surface. In a normal wrist, the x-ray beam is angled 11 degrees cephalad (proximal to distal) (*B*). In a distal radius fracture deformity, the beam will have to be adjusted so as to match the tilt of the distal radius surface. If the radius has settled into dorsal tilt, the x-ray unit will be angled distal to proximal by the amount of dorsal tilt.

adjusting the x-ray beam to the amount of volar or dorsal distal radius tilt (Fig. 13-11). Computed tomography (CT) is most often helpful in assessing the presence or absence of articular deformity of the radiocarpal joint and DRUJ by coronal and sagittal views of the radiocarpal joint and by coronal and axial views of the DRUJ. At times, magnetic resonance imaging (MRI) can be helpful in assessing the integrity of the cartilage surface of the head of the capitate. The most accurate method of staging the extent of cartilage damage is through diagnostic wrist arthroscopy or by direct inspection either as a preliminary surgical procedure or at the time of definitive wrist reconstruction.

 ## Anatomy

The wrist extends from the carpometacarpal (CMC) joints to the distal volar border of the pronator quadratus. It is a complex hinge joint, with flexion and extension as the major motions, modified by radial and ulnar deviation. During wrist flexion and extension, the scaphoid and lunate move mainly in the plane of flexion and extension. In radial and ulnar deviation, the scaphoid and lunate move in both radial and ulnar deviations, as well as flexion and extension.[107] The bones of the distal carpal row show little intercarpal motion. The bones of the proximal carpal row are less tightly connected. A normal arc of wrist flexion is 79 degrees, with wrist extension of 59 degrees, radial deviation of 21 degrees, and ulnar deviation of 38 degrees.[100] The RL joint contributes more motion to flexion than does the capitolunate joint. Dorsiflexion is achieved more through the capitolunate joint

than the RL joint.[88] (The biomechanics of wrist motion is further discussed in Chapter 14.)

The distal ulna is an integral part of the anatomy of the wrist joint because of its relationship to the carpus and the distal radius. The anatomy and treatment of radioulnar derangements are discussed in Chapter 15.

HISTORICAL REVIEW

One of the oldest and most successful reconstructive procedures in medical literature in the western world is partial* or total† wrist arthrodesis. Early articles pertained mostly to total wrist arthrodesis as a reconstructive procedure for deformities induced by poliomyelitis or tuberculosis.[30,112] Earliest techniques involved using an inlay graft, which provided both osteogenic and osteoconductive potential for healing, with the technique serving to provide some initial stability.[18,19,40] With the advent of internal fixation devices, staples, then plates, were used, with the latter no longer requiring a stable, interposed graft. The stability of current fixation devices in most instances precludes the necessity for distant autogenous graft. Bone graft substitutes and synthetic composites are increasingly replacing the need for autogenous bone graft. (See Table 13-1 for a historical review.)

With the improved understanding of wrist biomechanics, motion-preserving techniques of reconstruction, such as limited arthrodesis or proximal row carpectomy, have increasingly been employed. A variety of internal fixation devices have been adapted, and special implants (e.g., Acutrak screws, the spider plate, Shapiro staples, and Kirschner wires) were designed to facilitate intercarpal arthrodesis and enhance union rates.

Limited Versus Complete Wrist Arthrodesis

For obvious reasons few patients or surgeons will choose a total wrist fusion over a motion-preserving procedure for first-time reconstruction. Reconstruction will not reliably improve wrist motion but may provide diminished pain and improved strength. The potential advantage of limited wrist fusion in preserving a useful arc of motion may be offset by risks of nonunion or by continued pain despite successful fusion.

In a meta-analysis of nonunion rates of limited carpal arthrodesis analyzed by Larsen and colleagues,[59] nonunion for 385 STT fusions was 14%, with a confidence level of 95%. Nonunion after lunotriquetral fusion was 27%. Joints not included in the fusion, if damaged, can experience increased load, deteriorate, and cause persistent or new pain. For example, in 15 cases of radioscapholunate (RSL) fusion, Nagy and Büchler reported a 27% nonunion rate.[83] Seven cases showed secondary degenerative changes of the midcarpal joint, two of which were progressive. Five cases (33%) later required total wrist fusion. Four patients with nonunion treated by revision fusion continued to experience pain despite successful bony healing in three cases, underscoring that good pain relief cannot always be achieved with successful fusion that follows multiple previous failures.

---

*See references 6, 7, 38, 89, 118, 125, 128, 135, and 140.
†See references 1, 2, 4, 13, 16, 18, 19, 23, 31, 32, 98, 101, and 116.

Table 13-1
HISTORICAL REVIEW: WRIST ARTHRODESIS

Early Descriptions

Steindler[112]	1918	Drew attention to wrist arthrodesis for stabilizing the wrist in poliomyelitis reconstruction and in spastic hemiparesis of young adults
Ely[30]	1920	Reported its use for tuberculosis of the wrist

Use of Bone Graft

Gill[111]	1923	Devised method of corticocancellous graft to provide stability
Liebolt[65]	1938	Further popularized wrist fusion by corticocancellous graft
Smith-Petersen[109]	1939	Described ulnar approach with excision of distal ulna
Abbott, et al.[1]	1940	Advocated wrist arthrodesis and discussed procedures and results in articles written between 1920 and 1942
Butler[16]	1949	Described the autogenous iliac graft as a donor site
Campbell and Keokarn[18]	1964	Outlined the inlay technique of radiocarpal arthrodesis
Haddad and Riordan[40]	1967	Combined the above two procedures in their techniques
Carroll and Dick[19]	1971	Described radial approach and inclusion of second and third carpometacarpal joints in the fusion

Fixation—Plate, Wires, Staples

Wood[144]	1967	Introduced modification of the Gill technique involving compression wire fixation
Larsson[60]	1974	Reported 23 cases of plate fixation by Arbeitsgemeinschaft Osteosynthesefragen (AO) method
Benkeddache, et al.[9]	1984	Reported use of multiple staples as fixation
Hastings, et al.[44,43]	1993, 1996	Described modifications to the AO method with compression plating
Weiss and Hastings[141]	1995	AO fusion results with plate and only local bone graft

Fixation—Intramedullary

Robinson and Kayfetz[96]	1952	Described techniques in rheumatoid patients with intramedullary rods
Clayton[21]	1965	Outlined techniques in rheumatoid patients without fixation
Mannerfelt and Malmsten[70]	1971	Popularized use of Steinmann pin in rheumatoid patients
Millender and Nalebuff[74]	1973	Intramedullary Steinmann pin and sliding radial graft

Limited Wrist Fusion

Chamay, et al.[20]	1983	Radiolunate arthrodesis
Watson and Ballet[127]	1984	SLAC wrist deformity and surgical correction
Pisano, et al.[91]	1991	Scaphocapitate arthrodesis
Minamikawa[77]	1992	Ideal radioscaphoid angle for STT or scaphocapitate fusion
Kirschenbaum, et al.[54]	1993	Scaphoid excision and capitolunate fusion for SLAC wrist
Kirschenbaum, et al.[53]	1993	LT instability diagnosis and treatment
Tomaino, et al.[117]	1994	Proximal row carpectomy versus four-corner arthrodesis for SLAC wrist
Wyrick, et al.[146]	1995	Proximal row carpectomy versus four-corner arthrodesis for SLAC wrist
Larsen, et al.[59]	1997	Nonunion rates of limited carpal arthrodesis: a meta-analysis of the literature
Nagy and Büchler[83]	1997	Radioscapholunate fusion
Calandruccio, et al.[17]	2000	Capitolunate fusion with excision of scaphoid and triquetrum for SLAC wrist
Cohen and Kozin[25]	2001	Proximal row carpectomy versus scaphoid excision and four-corner arthrodesis for SLAC wrist

Function After Wrist Arthrodesis

Kraft and Detels[55]	1972	Ideal angle of wrist to allow greatest hand function
Pryce[92]	1980	Grip strength with respect to position of wrist radial deviation/ulnar deviation
Palmer, et al.[87]	1985	Biomechanical study of functional wrist motion
Weiss, et al.[142]	1995	Analysis of upper-extremity function after wrist arthrodesis

Kinematics

Youm and Flatt[147]	1978	Kinematics of the wrist
Douglas, et al.[28]	1987	Motion after simulated limited wrist fusion
Meyerdierks[72]	1987	Laboratory study of limited wrist fusion
Garcia-Elias, et al.[35]	1989	Wrist kinematics after limited intercarpal arthrodesis

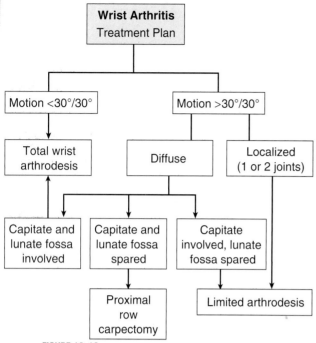

FIGURE 13-12. The author's wrist treatment algorithm.

Because reconstruction by limited fusion cannot be counted on to improve motion and it still carries a significant risk of nonunion or continued pain in a third of patients, it should be reserved for those with a reasonable likelihood for success and who absolutely require wrist motion for occupation or sport. Positive expectant factors include those who have arthritis or instability limited to one or two joints, have a functional preoperative arc of motion, and have not experienced two or more previous failed procedures. Limited fusion may not be the right choice for the patient only willing to undergo one surgical reconstruction or for those patients with a very restricted preoperative arc of wrist motion. I use the algorithm in Figure 13-12 as a basis for planning management of the arthritic wrist.

TYPES OF OPERATIONS

Radioscapholunate Arthrodesis

Indications

Destruction of the radiocarpal joint involving RS and RL portions most commonly occurs from comminuted intraarticular distal radius fractures. In younger individuals, attempts to preserve midcarpal joint motion may be warranted by RSL fusion with preservation of midcarpal joint motion.

Contraindications

Relative contraindications include patients who have undergone more than two previous operative procedures and those with normal or high range of motion.[83] Absolute contraindications include deformity or early degeneration of the midcarpal joint, which must be normally preserved to function after RSL fusion.

Adjunctive Procedures

Although fusion of the RSL joint can successfully be obtained, nonunion rates remain high (27%) and motion limited.[83] After RSL fusion the scaphoid fixed to the radius prevents motion of the distal carpal row, preventing flexion and radial deviation. With radial deviation the STT joint experiences high compressive forces that may lead to progressive joint degeneration. Two patients in the series by Nagy and Büchler developed scaphoid fracture after successful RSL fusion, one of which failed to heal. Enhanced union rates of RSL fusion, improved motion, and diminished STT degeneration can be expected from excision of the distal scaphoid[36] or along with excision of the triquetrum (personal experience).

Author's Preferred Method of Treatment for Radioscapholunate Arthrodesis

The joint is exposed through a longitudinal dorsal incision centered over Lister's tubercle. The extensor pollicis longus (EPL) is released from the third dorsal compartment and transposed radially. The capsule is longitudinally incised distal to Lister's tubercle, and the distal scaphoid and triquetrum are exposed by transverse capsular extensions. The capitolunate joint is inspected.

The second dorsal compartment with its tendons (i.e., extensor carpi radialis longus [ECRL] and ECRB) is subperiosteally elevated from the radius and retracted radially. The fourth dorsal compartment with its extensor tendons is subperiosteally elevated from the dorsal radius and retracted ulnarly.

The scaphoid is transected distal to the waist and the distal 30% to 40% excised distal to the waist. A large curet is used to dissect between the volar scaphoid and volar ligaments, preserving the radial and volar ligaments. The lunotriquetral ligament is sharply divided and the triquetrum removed by scalpel dissection.

Fusion surfaces are prepared by removal of the cartilage and subchondral bone from the RS and RL joints. Because the triquetrum has been excised there is no need to maintain the height of the scaphoid and lunate with interpositional graft to avoid ulnocarpal abutment. The scaphoid and lunate can be inset slightly into the distal radius, optimizing contact and providing relative stability. The lunate is fixed to the radius in neutral flexion/extension with two Kirschner wires inserted from the dorsal radius and advanced through the lunate to the resected surface of the RL joint. The scaphoid similarly is fixed to the radius with two Kirschner wires in a position approximating a lateral 47-degree RS angle. The Kirschner wires similarly are directed to the distal resected surface of the scaphoid. The proximal Kirschner wires are bent, cut, and tamped into the dorsal surface of the radius to prevent migration and interference with the extensor compartment. They should lie in the vicinity of the empty third dorsal compartment radial to the repositioned second dorsal compartment and ulnar to the repositioned fourth compartment (Fig. 13-13).

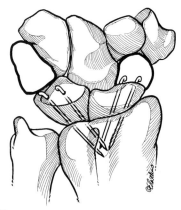

FIGURE 13-13. Radioscapholunate fusion with excision of scaphoid and triquetrum. Excision of the triquetrum and distal scaphoid "unlocks" the midcarpal joint for better motion and less stress on the evolving radioscapholunate fusion. With excision of the triquetrum, the scaphoid and lunate may be inset into the scaphoid and lunate fossae of the distal radius, obviating the significant need for graft and enhancing contact and union rate.

The capsule is closed over a suction drain with 3-0 braided nylon. The third dorsal compartment radial and ulnar retinacular leaves are sutured back together with 3-0 braided nylon, leaving the EPL transposed. The skin is closed with 4-0 or 5-0 monofilament nylon.

Case Study (Fig. 13-14)

A 50-year-old, right-hand–dominant woman fell, fracturing her distal radius. Percutaneous Kirschner wire fixation and external fixation were applied, but an anatomic reduction was never obtained. She developed severe stiffness of her shoulder, wrist, and hand requiring reconstruction of the DRUJ, extensor tenolysis, and dorsal proximal interphalangeal joint (PIP) capsulectomies. Persistent radiocarpal incongruity led to pain, requiring RSL arthrodesis. The distal scaphoid and entire triquetrum were excised. After successful fusion, pronation was 85 degrees, supination 70 degrees, wrist extension 30 degrees, flexion 30 degrees, radial deviation 15 degrees, and ulnar deviation 10 degrees.

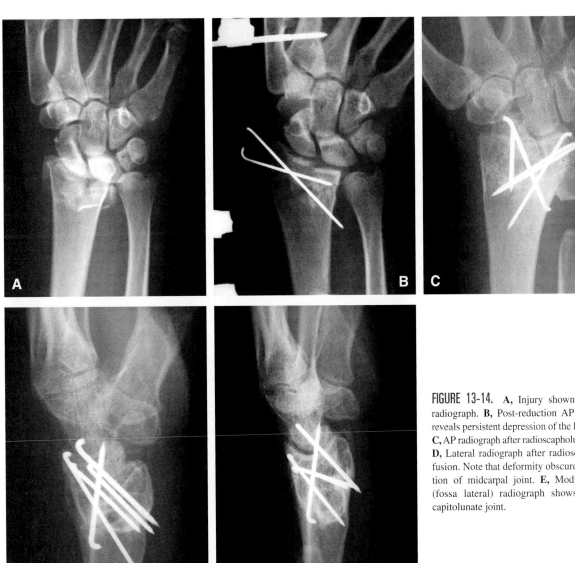

FIGURE 13-14. A, Injury shown on an AP radiograph. **B,** Post-reduction AP radiograph reveals persistent depression of the lunate fossa. **C,** AP radiograph after radioscapholunate fusion. **D,** Lateral radiograph after radioscapholunate fusion. Note that deformity obscures visualization of midcarpal joint. **E,** Modified lateral (fossa lateral) radiograph shows preserved capitolunate joint.

Postoperative Management

The hand and wrist are immobilized in a safe position with a bulky dressing and splint. At 10 days, sutures are removed and a short-arm thumb spica cast is applied. Active and passive motion is encouraged in all digits. At 6 weeks the cast is removed and radiographs are taken to assess fusion status. Active range-of-motion exercises of the wrist are initiated six times a day with interval splint protection between exercises. By 8 weeks postoperatively motion should approximate 30 to 40 degrees of extension and 30 to 40 degrees of flexion. If this motion is deficient, passive and weighted stretching exercises are begun. Light strengthening is initiated with putty. At 10 weeks postoperatively strengthening of the wrist is initiated. If a 70- to 80-degree arc of flexion/extension has been achieved, no additional modalities are needed to improve motion. If not, dynamic splinting is applied.

Special Considerations

Whereas fusion is mature enough in most cases by 8 to 10 weeks to allow full use, most patients still experience intermittent swelling, discomfort with exercise, and insufficient protective strength to handle repetitive forceful use. If the patient needs to return to an occupation requiring heavy lifting, a formalized strengthening therapy program is advised. Full, unrestricted use is allowed by 12 weeks after surgery, including work and sport. Some patients find a supporting splint to be helpful for heavier lifting and protection against sudden extremes of motion for an additional 1 or 2 months.

What the Literature Suggests

Most studies have included insufficient numbers of patients with varying methods of treatment from which to gauge expected outcomes. Motion after RSL fusion alone is markedly limited, based on obligate interference of midcarpal motion. Of successful fusions, Nagy and Büchler reported that flexion averaged 18 degrees; extension, 32 degrees; radial deviation, 3 degrees; and ulnar deviation, 25 degrees.[83] The arc of motion expected is in a "dart-throwing" plane of motion, with the wrist extending into radial deviation and flexing into ulnar deviation. This is the most functionally used plane of motion. I believe that excision of the triquetrum expands the motion out of this restricted dorsoradial to palmar-radial plane.

RSL fusion places a very high load on the scaphoid, which is evident by later difficulty obtaining RS fusion and RL fusion and by the occasional occurrence of a scaphoid fracture after solid fusion. This is best avoided by partial exci-

---

CRITICAL POINTS: RSL ARTHRODESIS

INDICATIONS

- RS or RSL joint arthritic deformity due to fracture
- Radiocarpal ulnar translation instability

PREOPERATIVE EVALUATION

- Special radiographic views are not always needed.
- Obtain "fossa-lateral" and volar tilt AP radiographs for best look at RSL joint.
- Assess CL joint integrity on AP and lateral radiographs.

PEARLS

- The midcarpal joint must be normal.
- More rigid fixation may be used such as blade plate, screws, or staples, but this is not necessary if the distal scaphoid and triquetrum are excised (unloads scaphoid and lunate from flexion and extension forces).

TECHNICAL POINTS

- Transpose EPL radially.
- Elevate second and fourth dorsal compartments without opening them.
- A power osteotome can assist in transecting the scaphoid distal to the waist.
- It is easiest to decorticate scaphoid and lunate with a rongeur.

- If difficulty is encountered penetrating the scaphoid and lunate fossae, make multiple drill holes or Kirschner wire holes into the surface before using a rongeur.
- A curet may assist further decortication of the scaphoid and lunate fossae.
- Leave the transverse capsulotomy unrepaired to facilitate postoperative motion.

PITFALL

- Avoid Kirschner wire penetration of the SC and CL joints.

POSTOPERATIVE CARE

- Apply short-arm thumb spica cast at 10 days. Remove at 6 weeks to begin active range of motion. Allow full use after 10 weeks.

ATHLETIC PARTICIPATION

- Work to restore full potential wrist motion and strength before return to full work or sports.
- Expect the reconstruction to be secure by 10 to 12 weeks, but full symptomatic recovery and plateau of recovery with respect to strength and comfort may ultimately require 12 months.

sion of the distal scaphoid and simultaneous excision of the triquetrum at the time of RS fusion. Excision of the distal scaphoid and triquetrum unlocks the midcarpal joint for improved motion. In doing so, this also improves wrist range of motion.[36] With additional excision of the distal scaphoid, Nagy and Büchler found wrist motion improved to an average 71 degrees with extension of 37 degrees and flexion of 34 degrees.[36]

What I Tell Patients About Expectations

The literature shows RSL fusion to be successful in only about 73% of cases. I expect higher success with respect to union and motion with the addition of distal scaphoid and triquetral excision. The need for secondary surgery is a real possibility. A 60-degree arc of flexion/extension can be expected in most cases. Grip strength will improve over a year's time and should approximate 60% to 70% of normal.

Radiolunate Arthrodesis

Indications

Arthrodesis of the RL joint is most commonly indicated for fracture-related deformity of the lunate fossa. Most commonly, this occurs from an intra-articular die punch distal radius fracture that disrupts the cartilaginous surface of the lunate fossa. Residual incongruity leads to pain and altered kinematics of the RL joint. Similar arthritic disruption can occur in inflammatory arthropathy such as rheumatoid arthritis (see Chapter 59), for which this procedure was first popularized by Chamay.[20] RL fusion may also be required to correct ulnar translation instability of the radiocarpal joint after severe ligamentous disruption.

Contraindications

RL fusion alone is contraindicated in the presence of arthritis or abnormalities of the CL joint. The procedure depends on a normal CL joint for wrist motion after RL arthrodesis.

Techniques

Many different techniques have been reported to achieve RL fixation. Fixation can be accomplished by Kirschner wires, staples, blade plate, or screws. Interpositional bone graft is usually required to maintain proper RL height and to prevent increased joint forces on the RS and ulnocarpal joints.

Author's Preferred Method of Treatment for Radiolunate Arthrodesis

The RL joint is exposed through a longitudinal incision centered over Lister's tubercle. The third dorsal compartment is opened, and the EPL is transposed radially. The capsule is incised in a longitudinal fashion between the third and fourth dorsal compartments. The fourth dorsal compartment is elevated subperiosteally from the radius and reflected ulnarward to expose the RL joint.

The cartilaginous and subchondral surfaces of adjacent lunate fossa and radius are decorticated. Bone graft is insert-

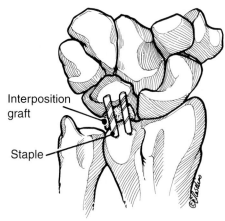

FIGURE 13-15.   Radiolunate fusion with staples. Normal dimensional relationships are maintained between the radius and lunate by interpositional graft. Fixation is accomplished with staples.

ed between the radius and lunate to elevate the lunate to its normal height. A slight overcorrection is better tolerated than undercorrection. Failure to do so will lead to abnormal forces on the adjacent scaphoid and triquetrum, ulnocarpal abutment, and diminished wrist motion. At times, lunate fossa derangement coexists with degenerative changes of the DRUJ, requiring concomitant distal ulnar reconstruction (see Chapter 15). Excision of the distal ulna will serve as a useful source of interpositional bone graft.

A 0.062-inch Kirschner wire is inserted into the dorsal lunate to use as a joystick for reduction of the lunate. The lunate is reduced into collinear alignment with the radius and provisionally fixed with 0.054-inch Kirschner wires. One wire is inserted from the ulnar dorsal lunate into the volar radius. A second is inserted from the region of Lister's tubercle to the volar distal lunate. Both Kirschner wires are bent and cut flush with the surface of the radius. Fixation is supplemented with one or two centrally placed staples (Fig. 13-15). If the bone quality is poor or delayed healing anticipated, more rigid stabilization can be accomplished with an AO 2.7-mm fixed-angle blade plate or 2.4-mm combi plate (Synthes, Paoli, PA), which allows for both a 2.4-mm screw and a 2.0-mm fixed angle pin in the lunate and 2.4-mm screws proximally.

The radial and ulnar leaves of the third dorsal compartment are closed with 3-0 braided nylon. The skin is closed with 4-0 monofilament nylon. The wrist is immobilized in a short-arm bulky dressing and volar short-arm thumb spica splint.

Pitfalls

Internal fixation can violate the CL joint, leading to degeneration and arthritis. The CL joint should be inspected to be sure that fixation has not violated its cartilaginous surfaces.

Overcorrection of the lunate is preferred to undercorrection. Undercorrection of lunate height will lead to excessive forces on the RS joint and ulnocarpal joint, with resultant pain and diminished motion.

The radial Kirschner wire must enter the dorsal distal radius radial to the normal position of the fourth dorsal compartment so as to not interfere with the gliding of its tendons.

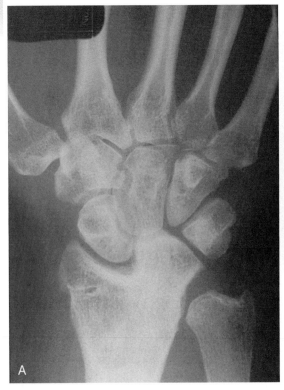

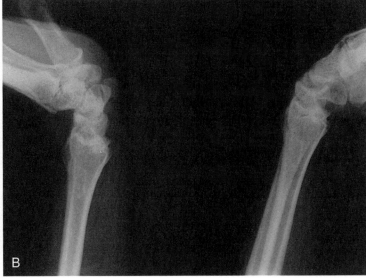

FIGURE 13-16. Radiolunate arthrodesis. **A,** AP radiograph demonstrates the radiolunate arthrodesis maintaining or accentuating the normal distance between radius and lunate. Note distal lunate positioning. **B,** Lateral radiograph of this radiolunate fusion demonstrates the significant flexion-extension arc available with proper lunate positioning.

Postoperative Management

At 10 days sutures are removed and AP, lateral, and zero-rotation radiographs are obtained to check the positions of the fusion and implants. A short-arm thumb spica cast is applied that is well molded in the palm. At 6 weeks from surgery, the cast is removed and additional radiographs are obtained. If good position and apposition of the RL fusion is present, a short-arm removable splint is applied for work and sport protection, and active range-of-motion exercises are initiated. At 10 weeks hand strengthening is initiated with putty. At 12 weeks the fusion is checked with radiographs. If healing has occurred, unprotected activity is allowed out of the splint (Fig. 13-16).

What the Literature Suggests

Combining the results of six studies, an overall nonunion rate of 9% is seen.[59] With a 95% confidence level, a nonunion rate between 4% and 15% can be expected. At least a 50% reduction in flexion/extension can be expected. By simulated fusion in the laboratory, Myerdierks and coworkers found a 47% loss of flexion/extension and a 37% loss of radioulnar deviation.[72]

What I Tell Patients About Expectations

RL fusion will diminish potential wrist motion by over 50%. Most patients presenting for surgery already have substantial loss of motion so in most cases postoperative motion should be similar to or slightly further diminished from the preoperative arc of motion. Surgery should diminish pain but may not remove it entirely. Return of grip strength will relate to adequacy of pain relief and will take 1 year to approximate to 60% to 80% of normal.

CRITICAL POINTS: RL ARTHRODESIS

INDICATIONS

- Isolated RL arthritis most commonly from die punch fracture
- Radiocarpal ulnar translation instability

PREOPERATIVE EVALUATION

- Obtain AP and lateral radiographs to be certain the surrounding joints (particularly the midcarpal joint) are normal.
- Rule out concomitant arthritis or instability of the DRUJ by clinical examination and AP, zero-rotation, and lateral radiographs.

PEARLS

- Protect the extensor digitorum communis tendons by elevating the fourth dorsal compartment without opening it.
- A Kirschner wire is inserted dorsal to volar through the lunate and when checked on lateral radiographs and by direct visualization of the CL joint can help identify the proper location for dorsal staples or blade plate.

TECHNICAL POINT

- Reduce the lunate to normal height to avoid excessive pressure on the RS joint and ulnocarpal joint.

CRITICAL POINTS: RL ARTHRODESIS— cont'd

PITFALL

■ The normal concavity of the distal lunate predisposes to hardware penetration into the CL joint if placed too distal in the lunate.

POSTOPERATIVE CARE

■ Avoid radioulnar deviation postoperatively. The scaphoid will impart flexion to the lunate with wrist radial deviation and flexion to the triquetrum extension with ulnar deviation.

■ Apply a short-arm thumb spica cast with good palmar mold.

ATHLETIC PARTICIPATION

■ At least 12 weeks of healing is usually needed before returning to full sports participation.

■ Use more rigid methods of internal fixation such as a blade plate when early return to activity is required.

Scapholunate (SL) Arthrodesis

Indications

In my opinion, there are no indications for SL arthrodesis at this time. It has represented an obvious approach to the management of SL dissociation, but numerous problems prevent it from becoming a useful procedure.

Successful fusion is very difficult to obtain. There are small adjacent articular surfaces of the scaphoid and lunate that provide inadequate cancellous contact for successful fusion. Second, the small, banana-shaped scapholunate surface has inadequate surface area to carry load after fusion. Lastly, this joint shares a small degree of motion, which is very difficult to prevent given the flexed and longer attitude of the scaphoid. The scaphoid and lunate reside in different fossae with a prominent sagittal ridge separating the two. Fusion would remove the small but necessary motion between the two bones and potentially lead to degenerative change in the radiocarpal joint. Compiling the reports of four papers, a 59% nonunion has been reported.[59] With a 95% confidence, a nonunion rate of 56% to 83% can be expected.

Lunotriquetral Arthrodesis

Indications

Isolated lunotriquetral (LT) arthrodesis is indicated for complete lunotriquetral instability without volar flexed intercalated segment instability (VISI). This most commonly occurs from traumatic injury. It can be due to degenerative arthritis from long-standing ulnocarpal impingement, incomplete congenital synchondrosis (Fig. 13-17), or incomplete separation of the lunate and triquetrum, which over time can become symptomatic.

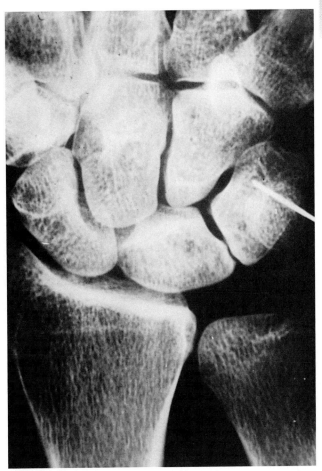

FIGURE 13-17. Carpal coalition of the lunotriquetral joint. The pathognomonic "champagne flute" appearance occurs secondary to degenerative joint disease of the incompletely developed proximal portion of the joint, in contrast to the distal portion of the joint where normal articular cartilage has formed.

Complete ligamentous disruption of the LT joint is rare. Disruption of the dorsal and palmar LT ligaments alters mechanics but does not lead to static VISI without injury also to the dorsal radiotriquetral and dorsal scaphotriquetral ligaments. Instability without VISI can be treated by either fusion or ligament reconstruction with tendon graft. LT instability with static VISI deformity is best treated by LT arthrodesis in conjunction with inclusion of the triquetral-hamate joint or the entire ulnar midcarpal joint (lunate, triquetrum, capitate, and hamate) (see Chapter 14 for a more detailed discussion of LT instability).

Contraindications

LT arthrodesis is contraindicated in the presence of midcarpal arthrosis. Because it will not correct static deformity, it alone should not be used in the presence of VISI pattern. It will not correct the static deformity. Relative contraindications may also include partial LT ligament tears associated with low-grade instability best managed by ulnocarpal decompression along with arthroscopic débridement of the triangular fibrocartilage complex and/or LT joint surfaces (see Chapter 19).

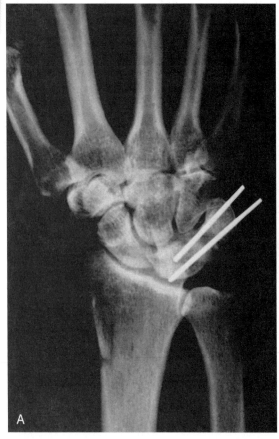

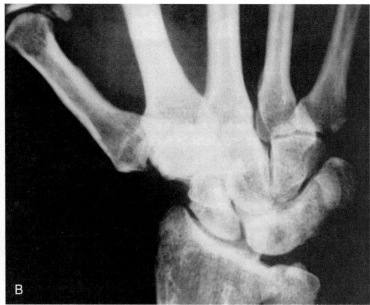

FIGURE 13-18. Lunotriquetral arthrodesis. **A,** Postoperative radiographic examination 6 weeks after LT arthrodesis demonstrates typical pin placement and bony consolidation. **B,** At 3 months after LT fusion, the arthrodesis is radiographically solid.

Techniques

A number of methods have been used to obtain fusion of the LT joint, all with some incidence of pseudarthrosis. Compression screws have been advocated[90] but alone may not control rotational motion between the lunate and triquetrum. Of 11 patients treated by LT fusion with compression screw, fusion was obtained at between 2 and 5 months. Only 4 patients were free of pain, with 4 experiencing painful extremes of motion and 3 with persistent pain. Multiple Kirschner wires have been advocated because of their ease of use and ability to resist rotational motion between the lunate and triquetrum (Fig. 13-18). Of 14 cases reported by Kirschenbaum and colleagues,[53] successful fusion was obtained in 12. Of the two pseudarthroses, one was symptomatic, requiring a second procedure.

Additional methods that have been employed include staples and a combination of Kirschner wires and screw fixation. Bone graft methods employed have included both vascularized and nonvascularized grafts.

Author's Preferred Method of Treatment for Lunotriquetral Arthrodesis

The LT joint is exposed through a transverse dorsoulnar incision centered over the joint. Dorsal veins and the dorsal sensory branches of the ulnar nerve are mobilized and protected. The fifth dorsal compartment is opened to expose the underlying capsule. The capsule is incised between the lunate and triquetrum in the interval between the converging dorsal radiotriquetral and dorsal scaphotriquetral ligaments.

For placement of Kirschner wires, the ulnar aspect of the triquetrum is exposed dorsal and volar to the sixth dorsal compartment. The lunate and triquetrum are reduced using their articular surfaces as a guide to anatomic reduction. A 0.045-inch Kirschner wire is advanced from the distal volar-ulnar triquetrum into the volar lunate under fluoroscopic guidance. Similarly, a pin is placed across the more proximal volar triquetrum into the lunate. Fluoroscopy is used to confirm and guide any needed adjustment in pin position. A third pin is prepositioned more dorsally between the triquetrum and lunate but not advanced as yet across the joint.

A rectangular trough is created between the lunate and triquetrum with a 4-mm sagittal saw. The distal, volar, and most proximal cartilaginous surfaces of the lunate and triquetrum are left intact to preserve the relationship between the two bones and protect the radiocarpal and midcarpal joints. The trough of decorticated bone should extend down to the volar portion of the joint (Fig. 13-19).

A corticocancellous graft is harvested from the volar radius. The depths of the trough are packed with cancellous bone. The graft is trimmed to the dimensions of the prepared trough between the lunate and triquetrum and tamped firmly into position. This achieves stability of the graft and provides additional stability to the fusion construct. The dorsal prepositioned Kirschner wire is then advanced across the LT joint. After confirmation of hardware position, the Kirschner wires

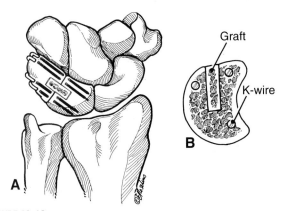

FIGURE 13-19. Lunotriquetral fusion. **A** and **B,** A tenon-and-mortise-type graft is prepared between the lunate and triquetrum. Four Kirschner wires are utilized, two dorsal and two palmar, between the triquetrum and lunate to maintain alignment and resist rotational motion.

are bent, cut, and recessed into a protected position. Two will lie volar to the extensor carpi ulnaris tendon, whereas the third will usually lie dorsally.

The capsule is repaired with 3-0 braided nylon suture and the skin is closed with a subcuticular 3-0 monofilament suture and Steri-Strips. A short-arm bulky dressing and protective splint is applied incorporating the digits.

Postoperative Management

At 10 to 14 days the dressing is removed, radiographs are obtained, and a short-arm thumb spica cast is applied. At 8 weeks postoperatively the cast is removed, radiographs are checked, and active range of motion exercises are begun. A short-arm splint is used for additional protection between exercises until 10 weeks, when it is discontinued and strengthening initiated. Full, unrestricted use is allowed by 12 weeks postoperatively.

Pearls

The lunate and triquetrum are reduced before decorticating the joint surface. The 0.062-inch Kirschner wires are passed dorsal to volar into the lunate and triquetrum to be used as joysticks in obtaining reduction.

The provisional Kirschner wire is inserted palmarly, making sure it does not interfere with the major part of the joint decortication.

I have found percutaneous Kirschner wires poorly tolerated around the wrist, presenting comfort problems with the cast and at times leading to pin tract infection. It is safer for the wires to be cut and buried so that they do not lead to postoperative wound problems. As well, they serve as continued immobilization in the case of delayed union.

Pitfalls

Kirschner wires may protrude through the proximal lunate surface. They should be adjusted carefully under fluoroscopy and under direct vision or palpation, with a Freer elevator inserted between the radius and lunate. Also, the midcarpal joint should be carefully inspected between the lunate and triquetrum.

LT arthrodesis frequently fails in the presence of positive ulnar variance. When associated with positive ulnar variance,

CRITICAL POINTS: LT ARTHRODESIS

INDICATION

- Complete LT instability or arthrosis without VISI deformity

PREOPERATIVE EVALUATION

- Rule out VISI with lateral wrist radiographs.
- Assess ulnar variance with zero-rotation radiographs.

PEARLS

- Untreated positive variance may favor nonunion and residual symptoms from ulnocarpal abutment.
- Several Kirschner wires better resist rotational motion than a single screw and take up less room across the limited fusion surface.
- Cancellous bone graft alone can resorb in a synovial environment. The use of corticocancellous graft is more resistant to resorption.

TECHNICAL POINTS

- Maintain cartilage surfaces at the volar LT, RL, and midcarpal joints to preserve normal space relationships.
- Corticocancellous graft better resists graft resorption than cancellous graft alone.

PITFALLS

- Assess Kirschner wire position by fluoroscopy to be sure Kirschner wires have not penetrated proximal and distal lunate articular surfaces.
- Kirschner wires are more safely tolerated and pin tract infection avoided by a buried position.

POSTOPERATIVE CARE

- Pins are left in place unless symptomatic.

ATHLETIC PARTICIPATION

- Solid fusion usually requires 10 to 12 weeks before return to unrestricted work can be initiated. Most patients will have significant residual comfort and strength deficiencies for several additional months.

the positive variance should be corrected at the same time as LT arthrodesis (see Chapter 15).

What the Literature Suggests

While patients with asymptomatic congenital synostosis of the lunate and triquetrum usually present with uncompromised or normal wrist range of motion, normal motion should not be expected after LT fusion. In 14 cases reported by Kirschenbaum and colleagues,[53] wrist range of motion compared with the contralateral side averaged 85% for palmar flexion, 88% for extension, 83% for ulnar deviation, and 80% for radial deviation. Grip averaged 93% of the opposite side. Eleven patients reported by Pin and associates[90] reported change in mean wrist motion from preoperative to postoperative as follows: flexion changed from 53 to 45 degrees, extension from 60 to 49 degrees, radial deviation from 17 to 21 degrees, and ulnar deviation from 25 to 18 degrees. Grip strength as a percentage of the uninjured side preoperatively was 73%, and postoperatively it was 59%.

Combining the results of eight studies, an overall nonunion rate of 28% is seen.[59] With a 95% confidence level, a nonunion rate between 19% and 36% can be expected. At least an 11% reduction in flexion/extension can be expected. By simulated fusion in the laboratory, Meyerdierks and coworkers[72] found an 11% loss of flexion/extension and a 17% loss of radioulnar deviation.

What I Tell Patients About Expectations
This is a pretty successful procedure if fusion is successfully obtained, but nonunion can occur in up to 30% of cases. Maximal range of motion should be obtained by 12 to 14 weeks and is approximately 80% of normal. Maximal grip strength takes at least 9 to 12 months to obtain and, when pain relief has been obtained, will approximate 60% to 80% of normal.

SLAC Wrist Reconstruction (Scaphoid Excision and Arthrodesis of Capitolunate Joint or Capitate-Lunate-Hamate-Triquetrum)

The most common pattern of arthritis in the wrist evolves from instability or rotatory subluxation of the scaphoid or chronic fracture nonunion of the scaphoid. Both dynamic and static rotatory subluxation of the scaphoid can, over a period of time, lead to degenerative wear of the RS joint and in later stages affect the capitolunate (CL) joint. Cases presenting with periscaphoid arthritis invariably have preservation of the RL joint, which is preserved in all stages of SLAC wrist involvement and represents the key to preserving a reasonable range of motion.

Indications
Indications most commonly include stage III SLAC wrist deformity (see Chapter 14) with degeneration of the RS and CL joints (Fig. 13-20). Some surgeons recommend its application to stage II disease with degeneration of the RS joint but preservation of the CL joint, where proximal row carpectomy is usually the preferred option. In stage II disease proximal row carpectomy is a simpler and easier operative option with equal or better results.[25,48,56,146] Chronic SL dissociation, scaphoid nonunion, and Preiser's disease all can lead to SLAC wrist, requiring reconstruction.

Contraindications
SLAC wrist reconstruction is contraindicated in more generalized wrist arthropathy that may compromise the integrity of the RL joint. The most commonly seen is CPDD. Contraindications also include trauma or generalized inflammation that has led to radiocarpal instability with ulnar translation.

The RL joint must be normal for SLAC wrist reconstruction to succeed.

Types of Operations
All techniques involve excision of the scaphoid, the cornerstone to removing periscaphoid arthritis. All involve stabilization of the midcarpal joint. This can be achieved either through isolated CL fusion or entire midcarpal fusion of the capitate, lunate, triquetrum, and hamate. The latter has been more commonly recommended as a way to expand the fusion mass and increase the likelihood of successful fusion. There is no additional motion loss from including the triquetrum and hamate.

Author's Preferred Method of Treatment[7,127,137] for SLAC Wrist Reconstruction

Two parallel transverse incisions are made (this is Watson's technique; I prefer a single longitudinal incision), one over the radiocarpal joint and one proximally over the distal radius for harvest of cancellous bone graft. The extensor retinaculum is incised over the third compartment. The capsule is incised transversely at the level of the CL joint. The ECRL is retracted radially and the ECRB retracted ulnarly to extend the capsulectomy more radially and expose the scaphoid. The scaphoid is removed in a piecemeal fashion with a rongeur. In doing so, care is taken to preserve the radioscaphocapitate and long RL ligaments.

With traction on the wrist, the RL joint is inspected to confirm that it is well preserved. With confirmation of its preservation, the midcarpal joint is decorticated. Articular cartilage and subchondral bone are removed from the adjacent surfaces of capitate, lunate, hamate, and triquetrum until a broad cancellous surface is obtained.

Through the transverse incision, bone graft is harvested from a window in the dorsal radius just proximal to Lister's tubercle. Because it is not essential to maintain carpal height in the original dimensions of the capitate-lunate-hamate-triquetrum joints, only a modest amount of bone graft is required.

The 0.045-inch Kirschner wires are percutaneously preset through the capitate, hamate, and triquetrum to line up with the more proximal lunate. A fourth wire is passed into the triquetrum directed toward the capitate (Figs. 13-21 and 13-22). Cancellous graft is packed into the deep interval between the capitate and lunate.

The most important step in SLAC wrist reconstruction is to reduce the dorsiflexed position of the lunate. The capitate must be volarly displaced onto the lunate for proper alignment (Figs. 13-23 and 13-24). This will tend to rotate the lunate into neutral or slight palmar flexion. A 0.062-inch Kirschner wire inserted into the dorsal lunate is used as a joystick for reduction. With the lunate reduced into neutral alignment or very slight flexion, the capitate is translated ulnarward to center it with the lunate. The preset pins are advanced into the lunate from the capitate, hamate, and

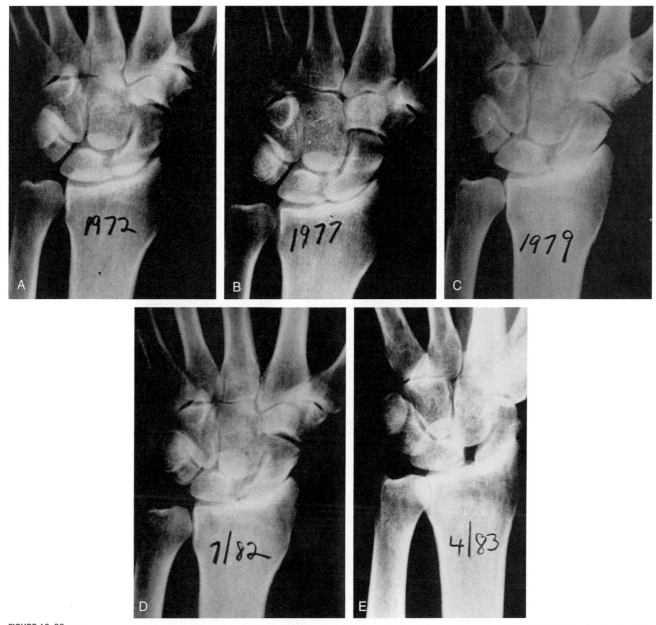

FIGURE 13-20.   The natural progression of SLAC wrist. This 11-year sequence of radiographs demonstrates the progression to SLAC wrist, beginning with symptomatic dorsal wrist syndrome. **A,** In 1972, the patient is symptomatic from scapholunate overload without significant radiographic changes. **B,** The scaphoid is rotating under load, and early narrowing of the radioscaphoid joint is present. **C,** By 1979, complete destruction of the radioscaphoid joint and early narrowing of the capitolunate joint have occurred. **D,** By 1982, there is complete loss of the capitolunate joint space. **E,** By 1983, the scaphoid is now static in its displacement. There is erosion of the scaphoid into the radius, capitolunate joint destruction, hamate-lunate joint narrowing, and proximal migration of the capitate. The radiolunate joint, however, remains normal.

triquetrum, followed by the Kirschner wire from the triquetrum into the capitate. Additional cancellous bone is packed into the intercarpal spaces using a curet or dental tamp. All pins are cut off below skin level. The capsule is closed with 3-0 braided nylon and the skin is closed with a subcuticular monofilament 3-0 nylon followed by Steri-Strips.

Postoperative Management
The extremity is immobilized in a bulky noncompressive dressing incorporated with a long arm plaster or fiberglass splint. The wrist is maintained in neutral to slight extension,

and the elbow is flexed 90 degrees. At 5 to 10 days after surgery, the bulky dressing is removed and a long-arm thumb spica cast is applied. The metacarpophalangeal (MP) joints of the index and middle fingers are included in the cast in 80 to 90 degrees of flexion, with the interphalangeal joints left free for range of motion. At 4 weeks after surgery, the long-arm cast is removed and a short-arm thumb spica cast applied for an additional 2 to 3 weeks. The index and middle digits are left free. In patients older than age 55 years, a long-arm cast is worn for 3 weeks, followed by a short-arm cast for an additional 3 weeks.

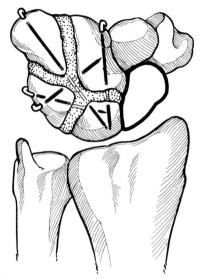

FIGURE 13-21. Depiction of four-corner fusion with Kirschner wires.

Alternative Methods of Fixation

In recent years a number of internal fixation devices have been designed and applied to limited wrist fusion in an attempt to provide more rigid fixation. All intend to simplify fixation, enhance union rates, allow for earlier initiation of range of motion, avoid interference or irritation of soft tissues, and avoid the necessity for subsequent implant removal. It remains to be proven if more rigid fixation will deliver improved results over Kirschner wires and more prolonged immobilization.

Staple Fixation

Power fixation devices have facilitated placement of staples with both improved accuracy of placement and improved biomechanical properties.[105] The capitate, lunate, hamate, and triquetrum are prepared as described earlier and provisionally held with Kirschner wires. The 3M Staplizer (3M, Minneapolis, MN) is used for staple placement. This air-powered stapler/impactor applies staples efficiently and with greater pullout strength as compared with manually driven staples. One staple is placed between the capitate and hamate, a second between the hamate and triquetrum, and a third between the lunate and capitate (Fig. 13-25). Although a fourth staple can be placed between the lunate and triquetrum, it usually will interfere with wrist extension. Staples measuring 13 mm wide and 10 mm deep are normally chosen.

Screw Fixation

The development of headless compression screws has facilitated internal fixation of carpal bones by the ability to bury the screw within the carpus. Options include a cannulated mini-Acutrak with a variable-pitched headless screw (Acumed, Beaverton, OR), cannulated AO screw (Synthes, Paoli, PA), or a cannulated Herbert-Whipple screw (Zimmer, Warsaw, IN). Screw fixation affords the opportunity for initiation of earlier range of motion, because more reliable and rigid fixation can be achieved.

Because of the dorsal curvature of the capitate screw, fixation from the capitate to the lunate is somewhat difficult. Usually, one screw is inserted between the lunate into the capitate and a second screw inserted from the lunate into the hamate. It is usually easier to place two screws through and recessed below the articular surface of the lunate into the capitate. Once provisional fixation of the midcarpal fusion site has been obtained, the wrist is flexed to gain access to the proximal articular surface of the lunate. This usually requires significant flexion of the CL unit. To do so, more extensive exposure is required, reflecting the second dorsal compartment radially off the radius and the fourth compartment ulnarly off the radius. A provisional pin is inserted through the proximal articular surface of the lunate and advanced

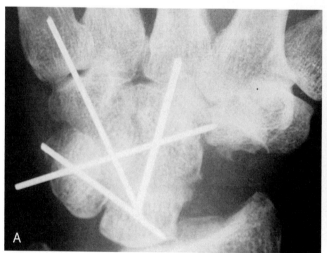
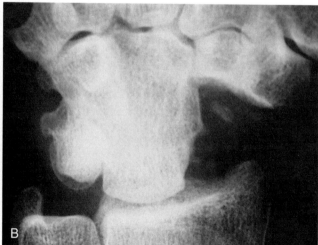

FIGURE 13-22. SLAC wrist reconstruction. **A,** Postoperative radiographic examination 6 weeks after SLAC reconstruction with limited wrist arthrodesis and scaphoid excision demonstrates typical pin placement and adequate bony consolidation. **B,** Six months after SLAC reconstruction, the arthrodesis is radiographically solid and the radiolunate joint well preserved. Note the ulnar displacement of the capitate on the lunate, which tightens the radioscaphocapitate ligament and prevents ulnar translation.

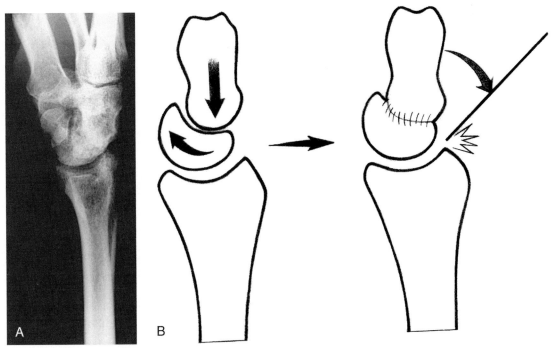

FIGURE 13-23. Capitolunate malalignment after SLAC reconstruction. **A,** Suboptimal capitolunate alignment within the fusion block. The lunate remains in approximately 30 degrees of extension (dorsal intercalated segment instability [DISI]), and the capitate is dorsally displaced. **B,** Resultant impingement of the proximal capitate on the dorsal radius restricts range of motion postoperatively. (From Ashmead D, Watson HK: SLAC wrist reconstruction. *In* Gelberman R [ed]: The Wrist. New York, Raven Press, 1994, pp 319-330. Illustrations by Kate Sweeney.)

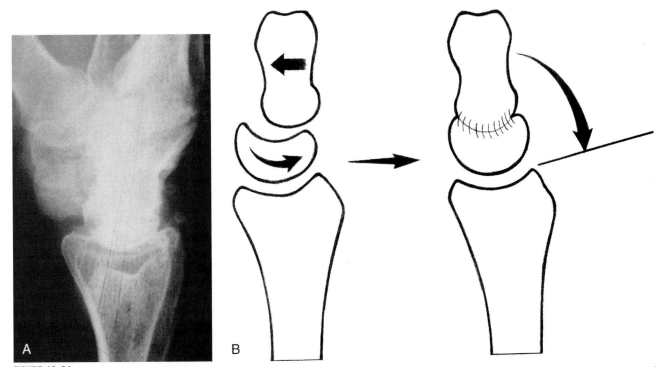

FIGURE 13-24. Capitolunate coaxial alignment after SLAC reconstruction. **A,** Optimal alignment of the capitate and lunate maximizes preservation of carpal height and avoids a dorsal impingement phenomenon. **B,** The extension arc is improved and lunate dorsal intercalated segment instability corrected by displacing the capitate forward on the lunate at the time the pins are placed. (From Ashmead D, Watson HK: SLAC wrist reconstruction. *In* Gelberman R [ed]: The Wrist. New York, Raven Press, 1994, pp 319-330. Illustrations by Kate Sweeney.)

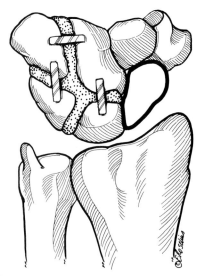

FIGURE 13-25. Depiction of four-corner fusion with power-inserted staples.

into the capitate. A second guide pin is similarly placed from the lunate into the hamate. A cannulated drill is passed over these guide pins and an appropriate-length cannulated headless screw inserted. The guide pins are removed. A third screw is inserted from the ulnar triquetrum across the hamate and into the capitate, passing dorsal to the initial two screws.

Plate Fixation–Spider Plate Fixation (Kinetikos Medical Inc., San Diego, CA)[106]

The surgical approach is as described in the preceding technique. The scaphoid is excised in piecemeal fashion and the tip of the radial styloid excised, preserving the volar ligaments. After exposure of the capitate, hamate, lunate, and triquetrum, any instability is reduced and the bones provisionally held by Kirschner wires across the volar aspect of the four bones. A small rongeur is used to remove cartilage between the four bones. A Spider rasp is centered over the fusion area and advanced by power or hand to a point flush or below the dorsal surface of the carpal bones. This opens up good cancellous surfaces and provides further visualization for additional removal of cartilage between the four bones.

Autogenous cancellous bone graft is packed between each of the four bones and juncture of the four at the bottom of the rasped defect. The Spider plate is aligned to allow maximum screw placement in each of the four bones. If the plate is properly aligned, two screws can be placed in each bone. A holder/drill guide is used to maintain proper alignment of the plate, and a 1.5-mm drill is passed into the capitate. A self-tapping, 2.4-mm screw is placed. In a similar manner, one screw is placed in each of the other bones. Tightening of the screws imparts radial compression to the four bones. An additional screw is placed in each of the bones as space allows. Proper placement is assessed by intraoperative fluoroscopy and standard AP and lateral radiographs. Finally, additional bone graft is packed within the center portion of the four-corner region through the plate.

The capsule and retinaculum are closed with 4-0 absorbable sutures. After skin closure a short-arm bulky dressing and splint is applied, leaving the digits free for motion.

Postoperative Management

At 1 week, sutures are removed and a removable splint is applied to allow for early active range-of-motion exercises. Alternatively, a short-arm cast can be used for an additional 3 to 4 weeks of protection. Radiographs are obtained on a sequential basis until fusion is confirmed and normal activities are allowed.

Scaphoid Excision With Capitolunate Arthrodesis

Stabilization (fusion) of the midcarpal joint in SLAC wrist reconstruction can be obtained either by isolated CL fusion or by four-corner fusion of the capitate, lunate, triquetrum, and hamate. Because there is not a theoretical difference in motion between the two options, four-bone fusion has been recommended to enlarge the fusion surfaces and improve union rate. With the availability of more-rigid methods of fixation, isolated CL fusion has been employed as a simpler procedure requiring only limited bone graft obtainable from the excised scaphoid. Screw fixation permits initiating earlier range of motion.

Technique

The approach to and surgical removal of the scaphoid are performed as listed earlier. The cartilage and subchondral bone of only the capitate and lunate are decorticated, preserving the joint surfaces of the ulnar midcarpal joint. Bone graft is packed into the CL interval to maintain the original carpal height of the capitate and lunate. Failure to do so will lead to increased forces on the triquetral-hamate joint.

A 0.062-inch Kirschner wire is inserted dorsally into the lunate and used as a joystick to reduce the lunate to the capitate. The lunate is provisionally fixed to the capitate with Kirschner wires. Definitive fixation is obtained using two cannulated mini-Acutrak screws or two 3.0-mm cannulated

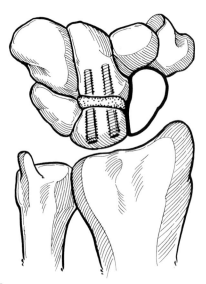

FIGURE 13-26. Capitolunate fusion with excision of the scaphoid. Fixation depicted with two mini-Acutrak screws from lunate to capitate buried below the subchondral surface of the lunate.

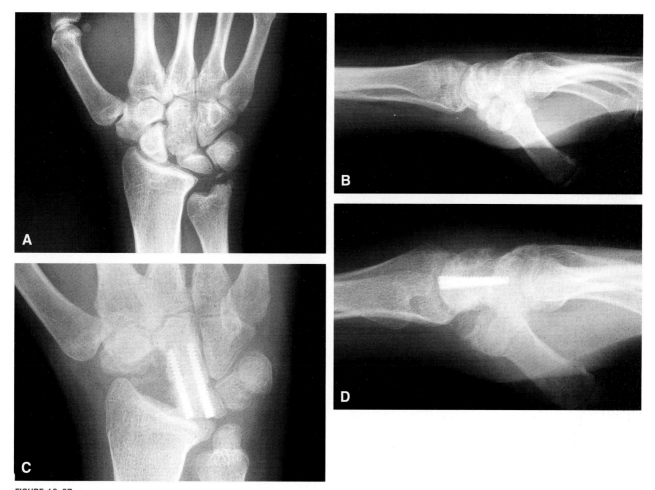

FIGURE 13-27. **A,** AP radiograph of wrist after failed treatment for scapholunate instability associated with distal radius and ulnar deformity. **B,** Lateral radiograph shows static rotatory subluxation of scaphoid.**C,** Postoperative AP radiograph after scaphoid excision and isolated capitolunate fusion with mini-Acutrak screws. **D,** Lateral radiograph after scaphoid excision and isolated capitolunate fusion.

AO screws. Proper screw placement requires flexion of the CL unit to expose the central lunate articular surface. This usually requires elevation of the second and fourth dorsal compartments from the radius. One screw is placed through the radial lunate articular surface and advanced into the capitate. A second screw is placed through the ulnar central lunate surface and directed into the capitate. Both screws are buried to just below the subchondral bone level (Fig. 13-26).

The capsule is closed with 3-0 monofilament nylon and the skin is closed with a subcuticular 3-0 monofilament nylon suture followed by Steri-Strips. A short-arm bulky dressing and splint are applied. At 10 days the sutures are removed and a short-arm thumb spica cast applied. Active range-of-motion of digits is encouraged. Radiographs are checked at 6 weeks and, if fusion is progressing, active range of motion with interval splint protection is initiated. At 10 weeks radiographs are checked and, if fusion is solid, passive range-of-motion and strengthening exercises are allowed.

Case Study (Fig. 13-27)
This 19-year-old man failed treatment for scapholunate instability associated with a high-energy distal radius fracture.

He presented with static rotatory subluxation of the scaphoid and traumatic changes of the proximal capitate. SLAC wrist reconstruction was accomplished with scaphoid excision and isolated CL arthrodesis using two mini-Acutrak screws. Range of motion remained limited, with extension of 20 degrees and flexion of 55 degrees. Grip strength was 50%.

Author's Preferred Method of Treatment for Capitolunate Arthrodesis

Isolated CL fusion can also be performed with excision of both the scaphoid and triquetrum. Because wrist function after CL fusion depends mainly on the RL joint, preservation of the triquetrum is not necessary. Its removal allows for safe shortening and compression of the CL joint and avoids the need for significant interposed graft.[17]

A longitudinal incision is made, starting 3 cm proximal to Lister's tubercle and extending distally to the base of the metacarpals. The third dorsal compartment is opened and the EPL reflected radially. Both the second dorsal and fourth dorsal compartments are subperiosteally elevated from the radius to facilitate wrist flexion and radial and ulnar carpal exposure. The capsule is transversely excised over the CL joint. The capsular incision is extended over to the ECRB. The ECRB is retracted ulnarly, and the ECRL is retracted radially to allow for extension of the transverse capsular incision over the scaphoid. The capsule is reflected off of the lunate to expose the RL joint and confirm that it is intact and free of degenerative disease. If there is degenerative disease, an arthroplasty or total wrist arthrodesis is indicated.

A rongeur is used to remove the scaphoid in piecemeal fashion. A large curet is used to dissect between the scaphoid and volar distal ligaments for excision of the scaphoid distal pole. The radioscaphocapitate and long RL ligaments are carefully preserved. The triquetrum is removed by scalpel dissection.

The midcarpal joint is decorticated by removal of the adjacent cartilaginous surfaces of the capitate and lunate with a rongeur. Cancellous bone graft is not usually needed. If it is required, it is harvested through a drill hole made in the distal radius just proximal to Lister's tubercle between the second and third dorsal compartments.

A 0.062-inch Kirschner wire is inserted into the dorsal lunate to use as a joystick for reduction. The 0.054-inch Kirschner wires are prepositioned for provisional fixation of the capitate to the lunate. One will pass from the dorsal central capitate into the volar lunate. The second will pass from the most ulnar lunate into the capitate. The lunate is flexed back to neutral position. The capitate is translated palmarly and ulnarly with respect to the lunate, and the pre-positioned Kirschner wires are advanced from the capitate into the volar lunate and from the ulnar lunate into the capitate. Reduction and Kirschner wire placements are confirmed with fluoroscopy.

With the wrist flexed, a cannulated guide wire for a mini-Acutrak screw is passed from the radial central surface of the lunate and advanced into the distal capitate. A depth guide is inserted over the guide pin to measure screw length. A screw 4 mm shorter than measured is chosen to provide for recession below the articular surface. A cannulated drill is advanced over the guide pin out to a level coinciding with the proper screw length as measured just below the lunate subchondral bony surface. A mini-Acutrak screw is inserted to the point where its head lies just below the subchondral lunate surface. The guide pin is removed. A second screw is similarly placed through the more ulnar lunate into the capitate (Fig. 13-28). The first screw provides sufficient stability that the ulnar provisional Kirschner wire can be removed if needed before screw placement. The provisional Kirschner wires are removed and fusion checked by fluoroscopy.

Additional cancellous bone harvested from the excised carpal bones is packed into the remaining dorsal recess of the fusion mass.

The capsule is closed with 3-0 braided nylon suture, and the skin is closed with 4-0 or 5-0 monofilament nylon. A short-arm bulky dressing and protective splint is applied.

At 10 days, sutures are removed and a short-arm thumb spica cast applied. All digits are left free for range of motion.

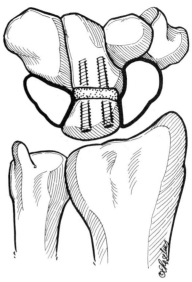

FIGURE 13-28. Capitolunate fusion with excision of the scaphoid and triquetrum. Excision of both scaphoid and triquetrum with capitolunate fusion by Acutrak screw fixation allows for the capitolunate joint to be compressed without requirement that normal height be maintained.

At 6 weeks postoperatively the cast is removed to check radiographs and confirm progressing union. Active range of motion is initiated. A removable short-arm splint is worn between exercises for an additional 2 weeks. At 8 weeks, strengthening is begun. Unrestricted use is allowed after 12 weeks postoperatively.

Pitfalls

Dorsal wrist motion will be limited and RS impingement will occur if the lunate is not adequately reduced from its dorsiflexed position. The most common complication is failure to adequately reduce the lunate from its dorsiflexion deformity. The lunate must be realigned to a neutral position.

Postoperative Expectations of SLAC Reconstruction

It is expected that patients will regain approximately 60% of normal motion. Strength will never equalize and by 1 year usually approaches 80% that of the opposite wrist. In a series of 252 SLAC wrist reconstructions reported by Ashmead and coworkers,[8] union was obtained in 97% of cases, with 91% of patients reporting that pain was diminished or markedly diminished. Mean flexion and extension was 53% of the opposite side, and ulnar deviation was 59% of the opposite side. Mean grip strength was 80%. No secondary degenerative changes were noted in serial follow-up radiographs. In a series of nine SLAC wrist reconstructions reported by Tomaino and associates,[117] flexion/extension averaged 52 degrees, with extension of 22 degrees, flexion of 30 degrees, radial deviation of 9 degrees, and ulnar deviation of 13 degrees. It was judged that six of the nine patients had incomplete reduction of the lunate, leading to diminished extension. Twenty-three patients reported by Cohen and Kozin[25] achieved average extension of 49 degrees, flexion of 31 degrees, radial deviation of 23 degrees, and ulnar deviation of 30 degrees. This represented 58% of the comparison side. Grip strength averaged 79% of the opposite side. Minimal differences in results were seen between treatment by proximal row carpectomy versus scaphoid excision with four-corner fusion when analyzed by range of motion, grip strength, short form-36 health status, and visual analogue scores.[25] Seventeen patients reported by Wyrick and colleagues[146] achieved a 95-degree arc of motion, representing 47% of the opposite side, with extension of 36 degrees, flexion of 31 degrees, radial deviation of 4 degrees, and ulnar deviation of 22 degrees. In both series, radial and ulnar deviation were higher after SLAC wrist reconstruction with four-corner fusion than after proximal carpectomy.

CL fusion with screw fixation offers the ability to simplify the surgery and the fusion mass. Screw fixation can allow for rigid fixation and earlier initiation of range of motion. Kirschner wires alone are probably not sufficient for successful isolated CL fusion. In a series of 18 patients reported by Kirschenbaum and coworkers,[54] there were 6 who developed pseudarthrosis and 5 who had persistent pain. Excision of both the scaphoid and triquetrum theoretically diminishes postoperative flexion and extension influences on the lunate. In a two-center outcome study of isolated CL fusion with excision of the scaphoid and triquetrum, Calandruccio and associates[17] reported an 86% union rate (12 of 14 patients). Two patients with nonunion remained in pain with screws loosening, penetrating, and adversely affecting the RL joint.

At an average 28-month follow-up, postoperative extension was 52% and flexion was 45% of the comparison side. Grip strength averaged 71% of the comparison side. Average time to radiographic fusion was 16 weeks.

What I Tell My Patients

Patients are advised that they will maintain approximately 50% of their normal wrist motion. Grip strength will approximate 70% to 80% of the opposite side. I anticipate 70% of patients will have good relief of pain and maintain a functional, but not normal, arc of motion. I advise patients that surgery is successful most of the time but there is a 30% risk of complications such as residual pain or problems in healing the fusion. There is a small but unlikely chance a second surgery might be needed for conversion to a total wrist fusion.

Scaphoid Stabilization–STT Arthrodesis*

STT arthrodesis (called triscaphe arthrodesis by Watson) is indicated for dynamic or static rotatory subluxation of the

———

*This section is from the chapter on intercarpal arthrodesis in the previous edition of this book, authored by H. Kirk Watson and Jeffrey Weinzweig.

CRITICAL POINTS: SLAC RECONSTRUCTION

INDICATIONS

- Stage III SLAC wrist
- Selected cases of stage II SLAC wrist (e.g., patients involved in heavy labor)
- Scaphoid nonunion and Preiser's disease that have led to SLAC wrist

PREOPERATIVE EVALUATION

- Rule out more generalized inflammatory arthropathy as the cause of the SLAC wrist.
- Evaluate the CL joint. If it is preserved, proximal row carpectomy is an alternative option.

PEARLS

- CL reduction is facilitated by a 0.062-mm Kirschner wire inserted into the central dorsal lunate.
- Palmar and ulnar translation of the capitate will rotate the lunate out of dorsal intercalary segment instability (DISI) deformity.
- Ulnar translation of the capitate onto the lunate will maximize contact and tighten the radial carpal ligaments.
- A large curet is used to dissect between volar wrist ligaments and the distal pole of scaphoid.
- Cup and cone shaping of fusion surfaces enhances cancellous contact area.

TECHNICAL POINTS

- Preserve the volar extrinsic ligaments.

- Confirm proper CL provisional reduction and fixation by fluoroscopy before definitive fixation.
- There must be good apposition of CL joint surfaces.

PITFALL

- Residual dorsiflexion of the lunate may lead to impingement and diminished extension.

POSTOPERATIVE CARE

- Apply noncompressive bulky thumb spica dressing and splint for first 10 days.
- At 10 days convert to short-arm thumb spica cast to be worn for additional 4 weeks.
- Usually active range of motion can be initiated by 6 weeks postoperatively.
- Heavy unrestricted use is deferred until 12 weeks.

ATHLETIC PARTICIPATION

- No athletic use of the involved extremity is allowed for at least 6 weeks. Although screw fixation theoretically may allow for earlier return to full use, persistent reported nonunion rates still suggest wise protection until at least 12 weeks. A cast will not provide for any additional stability beyond that of the screws. It merely limits extremity use and thereby forces experienced by the fusion area.

scaphoid (RSS), persistent symptomatic predynamic RSS with instability, degenerative disease of the STT joint, nonunion of the scaphoid, Kienböck's disease, SL dissociation, midcarpal instability, and congenital synchondrosis of the STT joint.[6,122,125,128,130,134,135,140]

Contraindications

Contraindications primarily include abnormalities of the RS joint, which with increased loading after STT joint fusion will become increasing degenerative and symptomatic. Relative contraindications include STT arthritis without SL instability, more simply treated by excision of the distal 25% of the scaphoid.[36]

Technique

The triscaphe joint is approached through a 4-cm transverse dorsal wrist incision just distal to the radial styloid. Spreading technique is used to preserve dorsal veins and branches of the superficial branch of the radial nerve. The radial styloid is exposed through an incision in the capsule overlying the radial styloid-scaphoid junction, and the distal 5 mm of the styloid is removed with a rongeur, sloping volarly from distal to proximal. A transverse incision in the dorsal capsule is then made, and the RS joint is inspected. If significant degenerative disease is found here, despite the absence of radiographic evidence preoperatively, the procedure of choice is proximal row carpectomy (if the capitate

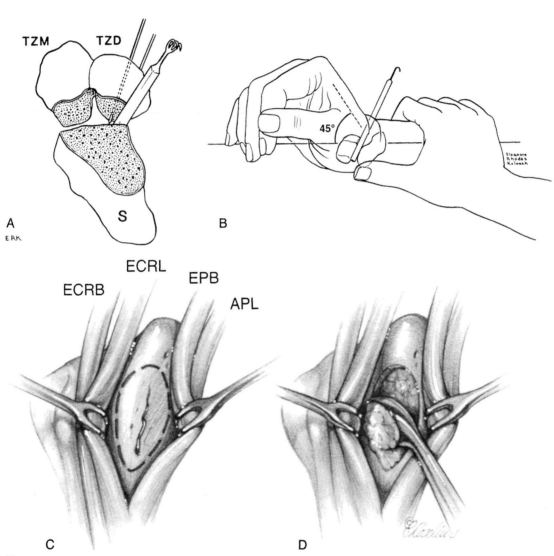

FIGURE 13-29. Triscaphe (STT) arthrodesis. **A,** After removal of articular cartilage from the scaphoid, trapezium, and trapezoid, a spacer is inserted in the triscaphe joint. The normal external dimensions of the joint must be maintained. The pins are preset percutaneously into the trapezoid and driven up to the proximal fusion site. TZM, trapezium; TZD, trapezoid; S, scaphoid. **B,** With the spacer in place, 45 degrees of extension and full radial deviation will prevent overcorrection of the scaphoid. The surgeon's thumb maintains scaphoid reduction within these restraints as the pins are driven. **C,** To harvest bone graft from the distal radius, the first and second dorsal compartment tendons are retracted. A constant small periosteal artery is used as a landmark for the periosteal incision. A teardrop-shaped cortical window is then removed. ECRB, extensor carpi radialis brevis; ECRL, extensor carpi radialis longus; EPB, extensor pollicis brevis; APL, abductor pollicis longus. **D,** Cancellous bone is harvested with a curet, and the cortical window is usually replaced.

has a healthy articular surface) or SLAC reconstruction (if both scaphoid fossa and head of capitate show degenerative wear) rather than triscaphe arthrodesis. The distal aspect of the extensor retinaculum is then opened along the EPL and the triscaphe joint approached through a transverse capsular incision between the ECRL and ECRB tendons.

The entire articular surfaces of the scaphoid, trapezium, and trapezoid are then removed with a rongeur, taking care to remove the proximal half of the trapezium-trapezoid articulation only (Fig. 13-29A). It is mandatory that the subchondral hard cancellous bone also be removed and the softer cancellous surfaces exposed. The cortex dorsal to the articular cartilage on the trapezium and trapezoid is also removed to broaden the surface area for grafting. The volar lip of the scaphoid is rongeured by inserting a dental rongeur deep in the joint and levering the handle distally. Cancellous bone graft is then harvested from the distal radius (see Fig. 13-29C and D).

Two 0.045-inch Kirschner wires are then driven percutaneously in preset fashion from the distal aspect of the dorsal trapezoid proximally. The first, radially positioned Kirschner wire is passed to the point of just touching the surface of the scaphoid. The second, ulnarly positioned Kirschner wire is passed proximally to the point of entering the ST space. In large individuals, one of these Kirschner wires may be a 0.062-inch wire. The wrist is then placed in full radial deviation and 45 degrees of dorsiflexion while the scaphoid tuberosity is reduced by the surgeon's thumb to prevent scaphoid overcorrection (see Fig. 13-29B). A 5-mm spacer, usually the handle of a small hook, is placed into the scaphotrapezoid space to maintain the original external dimensions of the triscaphe joint, and then the radial Kirschner wire is driven into the scaphoid, avoiding placement into the RS joint. The spacer is then removed, and the ulnar Kirschner wire is similarly driven into the scaphoid. Care must be taken when the pins are driven proximally into the scaphoid to avoid placement of the Kirschner wires into the RS joint space or the radius itself. After pinning, the scaphoid should lie at approximately 55 degrees of palmar flexion relative to the long axis of the radius when seen from the lateral view. This ensures optimal RS congruity and maximizes postoperative range of motion. It is not necessary to correct any abnormal rotation of the lunate. The scaphoid should not be overcorrected by placing its long axis in line with the forearm and, thus, markedly decreasing the SL angle. This will limit the motion obtained after surgery.

Cancellous bone is then densely packed into the spaces between the scaphoid, trapezium, and trapezoid using a dental amalgam tamp. Maintenance of the original external dimensions of the triscaphe joint usually translates to a 4- to 8-mm gap between the three bones, which is filled with the cancellous bone graft. The pins are cut beneath the skin level, and the skin incisions are closed with a single-layer subcuticular monofilament suture. The wrist capsule and extensor retinaculum are simply realigned without suturing.

The postoperative dressing consists of a bulky noncompressive wrap incorporating a long-arm plaster splint. The hand is placed in a protected position with the wrist in slight extension and radial deviation, the forearm neutral, and the elbow at 90 degrees.

Postoperative Management*

Maximum initial immobilization is mandatory for these small bone fusions. Three to 5 days after surgery, the bulky dressing is removed and a long-arm thumb spica cast applied.

The proximal carpal row is easily immobilized by casting the forearm and arm, but it is difficult to adequately maintain the position of the distal carpal row. Therefore, the MP joints of the index and middle fingers are flexed to 80 to 90 degrees and included in the long-arm cast while the interphalangeal joints are left free. The index and middle metacarpals are mortised into the carpals as the "fixed unit" of the hand. Thus, their immobilization tends to maintain the position of the distal carpal row. Because there is relatively free motion at the base of the metacarpals of the ring and little fingers, they are not included in the cast.

Four weeks postoperatively, the long-arm cast and intracuticular sutures are removed. A short-arm thumb spica cast is applied for an additional 2 to 3 weeks. Only the thumb is included in this cast. In patients older than age 55 years, 3 weeks in a long-arm cast followed by 3 weeks in a short-arm cast is sufficient.

Six weeks postoperatively, the short-arm cast is removed and radiographs are obtained (Fig. 13-30). If radiographic evidence of union is seen, the pins are removed in the office and the patient is referred for hand therapy for full wrist mobilization. A splint may occasionally be used for an additional 1 or 2 weeks if there is any doubt as to the status of bone healing.

Alternative Techniques
Staples

Power-inserted staples can simplify the fixation process and prevent complications related to Kirschner wire irritation and possible infection. Graft interposition and STT reduction and provisional Kirschner wire fixation are accomplished as described earlier. Definitive fixation is obtained with 13- or 15-mm by 10-mm staples driven by power across the scaphotrapezial and scaphotrapezoid joints. The provisional Kirschner wires can then be removed. Postoperative care is as outlined earlier.

Screw Fixation

Screw fixation is more difficult to apply. Commonly chosen implants include Herbert or cannulated Herbert-Whipple screws, mini-Acutrak screws, and 3.0-mm cannulated or 2.7-mm noncannulated AO screws. Unless a compression-resistant interposed graft is used, it is not advisable to use a technique that will compress or shorten the normal STT joint dimensions. The STT joint should be reduced and provisionally held by Kirschner wires. A 1.1-mm AO guide wire is introduced through the dorsal distal trapezium and advanced into the scaphoid. Its position is checked under fluoroscopy. A second wire is similarly placed from dorsal distal trapezoid and advanced into the scaphoid. Length is measured and an appropriate-length 3.0-mm AO self-drilling, self-tapping cannulated screw is inserted over each

---

*This section is from the chapter on intercarpal arthrodesis in the previous edition of this book, authored by H. Kirk Watson and Jeffrey Weinzweig.

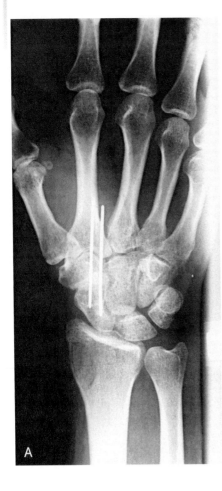

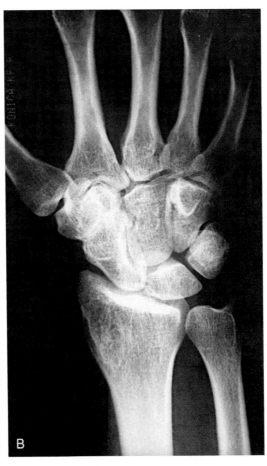

FIGURE 13-30. Triscaphe arthrodesis. **A,** Postoperative radiographic examination 6 weeks after triscaphe arthrodesis demonstrates typical pin placement and adequate bony consolidation. **B,** Three months after triscaphe fusion, the arthrodesis is radiographically solid.

wire. The guide wires are then removed. Postoperative care is as outlined earlier.

Postoperative Expectations

Watson has reported excellent functional results and pain-free, stable wrists after triscaphe limited wrist arthrodesis. After 4 to 6 weeks of hand therapy, the average range of motion is usually 50% to 70% of that of the contralateral normal wrist, increasing to an average of 80% by 1 year after surgery. Grip strength has averaged 90% of that of the unaffected wrist. Long-term radiographic follow-up has revealed only rare instances of progressive RS or intercarpal degenerative change, and only in those patients who had some evidence of disease in these joints at the time of original surgery.[130]

Author's Preferred Method of Treatment for STT Arthrodesis

When there is an equivalent choice of performing either STT fusion or SC arthrodesis, I choose SC arthrodesis. STT fusion can cause significant loss of motion at the basilar thumb joint compared with SC fusion.[76] When fusing the STT joint, I use power-inserted staples as described earlier, which avoid soft tissue–related complications of Kirschner wires and provide at least equal, if not better, immobilization.

Scaphocapitate Arthrodesis

Indications

SC fusion is considered a relatively equal alternative to STT fusion for stabilization of the scaphoid. Accordingly, indications include those of dynamic or rotatory subluxation of the scaphoid (RSS), persistent symptomatic predynamic instability, nonunion of the scaphoid, Kienböck's disease, SC dissociation, and midcarpal instability. There is a particular advantage with chronic scaphoid nonunions in addressing the instability as well as expanding the area of bone healing from distal to proximal scaphoid to capitate.

Most authors believe there are not significant loading differences between SC and STT fusion. Watson believes that better motion is obtained with STT fusion than by SC fusion. Laboratory study by Meyerdierks and colleagues[72] revealed less loss of flexion/extension after SC fusion (19%) than after STT fusion (23%). Another study simulating limited intercarpal arthrodesis by Douglas and associates[28] found no significant difference. After both STT and SC fusions there is diminished joint reactive force at the RL and CL joints. Motion loss does very much depend on proper reduction of the scaphoid to the position between 30 and 57 degrees of flexion with respect to the radius.[77]

Contraindications

Contraindications as in STT fusion include any abnormality of the RS joint that would be susceptible to increased degeneration and symptoms after the altered or increased loading through the RS joint after SC fusion.

Technique

A longitudinal incision from Lister's tubercle is made to the base of the index metacarpal. The dorsal sensory radial nerve branches are identified and protected. The capsule between the ECRB and ECRL is approached. A "T" incision into the capsule is created to expose the adjacent scaphoid and capitate. The midcarpal joint is inspected to confirm that the RS joint has normal cartilage.

Reduction of the scaphoid is required when instability of the scaphoid exists. It usually is not required in most patients with Kienböck's disease. For reduction, the proximal pole is palpably depressed and the distal pole of scaphoid elevated with a 0.062-inch Kirschner wire inserted into the scaphoid or a large skin hook applied around the distal scaphoid. The scaphoid is provisionally fixed to the capitate with Kirschner wires, preserving its normal relationship.

The adjacent cartilage and subchondral surfaces of the scaphoid and capitate are decorticated, with care being taken not to violate the proximal capitolunate joint. Bone graft is harvested from the distal radius proximal Lister's tubercle between the second and third dorsal compartments. A bone graft is packed into the scaphocapitate joint.

Fixation can be accomplished using Kirschner wires, staples, screws, or plate and screws. Safe hardware insertion requires exposure and protection of the radial artery and the dorsal sensory radial nerve branches. If a compressive-resistant bone graft is used, compression screws may be used between the scaphoid and capitate to hold the scaphoid in a 50-degree RS angle.

Author's Preferred Method of Treatment for Scaphocapitate Arthrodesis

The wrist is exposed through a longitudinal incision from Lister's tubercle to the base of the index metacarpal. The dorsal sensory radial nerve branches are protected. The capsule is exposed between the ECRB and ECRL tendons and opened in a "T" fashion. Both the RS and CL joints are inspected.

Provisional Kirschner wires are preplaced into the distal scaphoid and advanced to the scaphocapitate joint surface using a drill guide to protect the radial artery and the dorsal sensory radial nerve branches from being caught up in the Kirschner wire rotation. A 0.062-inch Kirschner wire is placed into the distal dorsal scaphoid to use as a joystick for reduction. The scaphoid is reduced by 45 degrees of wrist dorsiflexion and neutral or slight ulnar deviation. The 0.062-inch Kirschner wire is used to de-rotate the scaphoid into good apposition with the corresponding capitate joint surface. The provisional Kirschner wires are advanced into the capitate, and reduction to a 50-degree RS angle is confirmed by fluo-

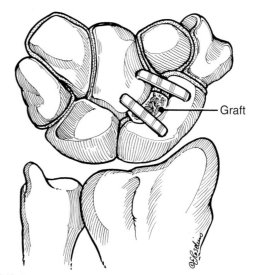

FIGURE 13-31.   Scaphocapitate fusion with staples. Normal space between the scaphoid and capitate is maintained by preservation of the volarmost 20% or 30% cartilage articulation. Decortication is accomplished and graft packed between the scaphoid and capitate, maintaining normal dimensional relationships.

roscopy. It is easier to obtain proper reduction before decortication of the joint surfaces. The dorsal 80% of the SC joint is decorticated down to cancellous bone, including the dorsal apposing edges. Cancellous bone graft is harvested through a drill hole made dorsally just proximal to Lister's tubercle and packed into the fusion space.

Two staples 15 mm wide and 10 or 13 mm deep are inserted by power across the SC joint (Fig. 13-31). The provisional Kirschner wires are removed and the capsule closed with 3-0 braided nylon. The skin is closed with subcuticular 3-0 monofilament nylon followed by Steri-Strips. The hand and wrist are immobilized with a noncompressive short-arm bulky dressing and thumb spica splint.

Postoperative Management

At 10 days, sutures are removed and a short-arm thumb spica cast is applied. At 8 weeks, radiographs are checked and, if satisfactory, a short-arm wrist splint is applied for intermittent protection. Active range of motion is initiated. Strengthening is usually deferred until 10 to 12 weeks postoperatively.

Postoperative Expectations

Range of motion should approximate 50% to 60% of the opposite side. While SC fusion in the laboratory decreases flexion/extension motion by 12.8%[35] to 18%,[28] greater losses are seen clinically. Sennwald and Ufenast[104] reported a flexion/extension arc of 62 degrees. Viegas and associates[123] reported range of motion 50% of the opposite side. Grip strength will approximate 80% of the opposite side, with Pisano and coworkers[91] reporting it at 74% of the opposite side and Sennwald 83% of the opposite side.[104]

Nonunion rates should be similar between STT and SC fusion. Combining results of several series of SC fusion, a 13% to 18% incidence of nonunion has been seen.[59] By meta-analysis of the literature, a 6% to 28% incidence of nonunion can be expected with a 95% confidence interval.

CRITICAL POINTS: SC ARTHRODESIS

INDICATIONS

- Dynamic or static rotatory subluxation of the scaphoid
- Chronic scaphoid nonunion
- Kienböck's disease

PREOPERATIVE EVALUATION

- Evaluate scaphoid stability by Watson's scaphoid shift test.
- Obtain supinated AP radiograph to evaluate SL joint for increased gap and to be sure RS joint is free of degenerative changes.
- Obtain lateral radiograph to evaluate scapholunate angle.
- Obtain hyperpronated AP radiograph to evaluate STT joint.

PEARLS

- Preserve volarmost cartilage surfaces between scaphoid to lunate to maintain normal anatomic relationships.
- It is easier to reduce the scaphoid before decortication.

TECHNICAL POINTS

- Protect radial sensory nerve branches and radial artery by using a small drill guide during Kirschner wire placement.

- Confirm by fluoroscopy or radiograph the proper reduction of the scaphoid to a 50-degree RS angle.
- Separate lunate reduction is not required.

PITFALL

- Avoid over-reduction of the scaphoid, which will limit motion. The scaphoid should be reduced to a 47-degree RS angle.

POSTOPERATIVE CARE

- Initial dressing should be bulky but noncompressive to avoid postoperative pain. Apply short-arm thumb spica splint.
- At 10 days, apply well-molded short-arm thumb spica cast.
- At 8 weeks, check radiographs and initiate active range-of-motion exercises.

ATHLETIC PARTICIPATION

- Use of the involved extremity is precluded for at least 8 weeks. Nonloaded use is allowed at 8 weeks. Full use and any exposure to sudden force should be avoided for at least 10 weeks after surgery. Patients should not expect strong, relatively symptom-free wrist performance until at least 4 months after surgery.

What I Tell My Patients

Patients are advised that they will lose 40% to 50% of wrist motion but should still have a very functional arc. It is possible they may experience postoperative transient tingling over the dorsoradial wrist or hand, which will resolve over time. While the wrist will never feel "normal," almost all patients will feel improvement and will regain 70% to 80% of grip strength. Patients are advised to discontinue smoking preoperatively. Nonunion is unlikely but can occur in 15% of cases, particularly in patients who smoke.

Distal Row: Triquetral Hamate Fusion

Indications

Triquetral hamate fusion is most commonly indicated in the treatment of symptomatic ulnar carpal instability (carpal instability nondissociative [CIND]). It is also indicated for LT instability combined with VISI deformity, resultant from complete tear of the LT interosseous and palmar ligaments along with disruption of the dorsal radiocarpal ligaments.

Triquetral hamate fusion significantly alters wrist motion, removing midcarpal motion and relying on radiocarpal motion. Ulnar midcarpal fusion is contraindicated in the presence of any significant degeneration or pathology of the radiocarpal joint. Isolated triquetral hamate fusion is rarely

indicated because it is easier to obtain adequate fusion by incorporation of the lunate, triquetrum, capitate, and hamate, with no theoretical difference in postoperative range of motion.

Techniques

See four-corner fusion technique under SLAC wrist reconstruction on page 506.

Pearls

Because the CL joint contributes more motion to extension than flexion, the midcarpal joint is positioned in extension to better facilitate activities of daily living (slight lunate palmar flexion).

Total Wrist Arthrodesis

Indications

Indications for total wrist arthrodesis[22,57,73,85,98,103] include the following:

1. Post-traumatic osteoarthrosis of the radiocarpal and midcarpal joints as commonly seen after chronic SL dissociation complex fractures[42,43]
2. A failed, previous, more limited arthrodesis[42]

3. A failed total-joint or previous arthroplasty of the radio-carpal joint
4. Paralysis of the wrist and hand with potential for reconstruction involving the use of wrist or finger motions for tendon transfer
5. Reconstruction after segmental tumor resection, infection, or traumatic segmental bone loss of the distal radius and carpus[42,44]
6. Adolescent spastic hemiplegia with wrist flexion deformity
7. Rheumatoid arthritis[19,22,70]

Contraindications

Contraindications for wrist arthrodesis include:

1. An open epiphyseal plate in the distal radius
2. The nondominant hand in older patients with light work occupations in which an arthroplasty would be more suitable
3. Quadriplegic patients who use their motors for modified grasp and transfer techniques
4. Neurologic diseases or injury causing major sensory deprivation in the hand
5. Advanced rheumatoid disease where "stabilization" techniques are more suitable than formal arthrodesis. (Specialized arthrodesis and stabilization procedures for the rheumatoid wrist[29,70,74] are discussed in Chapter 59.)

Types of Operations

Surgical Approach

Most of the surgical methods previously described use a dorsal approach. The lateral (ulnar) approach advocated by Smith-Petersen[109] has not gained wide acceptance, but the radial approach described by Haddad and Riordan[40] has certain advantages.

Dorsal Approach

The dorsal approach follows a straight incision beginning at the distal third of the index-middle interosseous space, proceeding across Lister's tubercle, and ending over the radius at the proximal border of the abductor pollicis longus (APL) muscle.[43] A flap consisting of radial skin and subcutaneous tissue is carefully elevated off the radial extensor retinaculum. The dorsal sensory branches of the radial nerve are contained within this flap and do not require dissection, except in the most distal part of the incision, where at times small terminal branches may cross the incision.

Most authors recommend an extracompartmental approach for deeper exposure by opening the interval between the third (EPL) and fourth (extensor digitorum communis [EDC]) extensor compartments.[1,19,81] Others prefer the creation of a long, ulnarly based retinacular flap that on closure can be transposed deep in the tendons of the third and fourth dorsal compartments.[61] A radially based flap with an incision into the fourth or sixth extensor compartments is useful when excision of the distal ulna is required.[78] In post-traumatic cases, Hastings and associates[42,44] recommend a transcompartmental approach through the third dorsal compartment with radial transposition of the EPL tendon. This provides for the radial and ulnar margins of the released third compartment to be safely sutured back together on closure without risk of interfering with the tendons of the fourth compartment.

Most authors incise the dorsal capsule in a longitudinal fashion.[42,43,94,102] Mannerfelt[69] created a distally based capsular flap. Millender and colleagues[74-76] incised the capsule in a transverse fashion. Abbott and associates[1] and Carroll and Dick[19] adopted the method of Albert Key,[1] who described development of an osteoperiosteal flap containing the dorsal capsule and thin sections of dorsal cortex from the scaphoid, lunate, and capitate.

Radial Approach

In 1967 Haddad and Riordan[40] described fusion through a radial approach in which a curved "J"-shaped skin incision starts 3 to 4 cm proximal to the radial styloid and extends to a point dorsal and distal to the bases of the second metacarpal. The dorsal sensory branches of the radial nerve are identified and protected, usually to the volar side.

The capsule is incised longitudinally between the first and second dorsal compartments, and the ECRL tendon is transected just proximal to its attachment at the base of the second metacarpal. This leaves a short stump to later be reattached at completion of the procedure. The radial artery is mobilized for protection. Its dorsal branch to the dorsal carpal arch may need to be transected and ligated.

With the wrist in 15-degree extension, a slot is cut in the distal end of the radius, the intercarpal joints, and the second and third CMC joints with a power saw for later insertion of a corticocancellous bone graft.

Ulnar Approach

In 1940 Smith-Petersen[109] described the use of an ulnar approach to the wrist combined with resection of the distal ulna. Other than Lenoble and colleagues,[62] few surgeons have adopted this approach. An incision is started 5 to 6 cm proximal to the ulnar styloid, extends longitudinally to the end of the styloid, and curves anteriorly to the ulnar base of the fifth metacarpal and then distally along the axis of the fifth metacarpal. The distal ulna is exposed subperiosteally, and the distal 2.5 cm is removed by oblique osteotomy. The capsule is reflected from the distal radius and carpus. Slots are cut in the radius and carpus for anchoring of an interposed graft.

Method of Decortication

Most authors remove up to half of the dorsal portion of the carpal bones by using an osteotome or oscillating saw to expose broad cancellous surfaces.[42,62,144] Almost all methods advise decortication of the articular surfaces of each carpal bone, distal radius, and base of the third and/or second metacarpals.[18,42,44,141] Inlay techniques require the creation of a trough cut between the distal radius and either the carpus or second and third metacarpals.[19,40,62,81,109] Campbell and Keokarn recommended complete en bloc resection of part of the carpus and replacement by a thick corticocancellous bone graft block.[18] Some authors recommend excision of the proximal carpal row to simplify correction of the deformity[62,68] or decrease the number of joints to be fused[12,68] by creation of a radiocapitohamate fusion.

Joints to Be Included in the Arthrodesis

In all instances total wrist fusion involves fusion of the radiocarpal and midcarpal joints. This always includes the RS, RL, and CL joints.[1,19,42,43,80,94,102,141] There is no consensus regarding these joints or whether additional joints should be included. Abbott and associates[1] recommended inclusion of the scaphoid and often the trapezoid. Hastings and colleagues[42,43,141] recommended inclusion of the ulnar midcarpal joints (capitohamate, triquetral lunate, and triquetral hamate) only in rheumatoid patients and post-traumatic cases with radiographic or symptomatic involvement of the ulnar midcarpal joint.

Total wrist fusion can be performed along with proximal row carpectomy (capitate-radius arthrodesis), simplifying the number of joints to be fused and limiting the need for bone graft.[12,68]

Abbott and associates[1] advised against incorporation of the CMC joints because of the importance of CMC flexion and rotation in power grip. Brittain[13] contradicted this theory and found no adverse effect on digital flexion and power grip after inclusion of the CMC joint in wrist fusion. Haddad and Riordan[40] recommended incorporation of the second and third CMC joints, as did Rayan,[94] Sagerman and Palmer,[102] and Bolano and Green.[12] Both Bolano and Green[12] and Louis and coworkers[68] noted subsequent symptomatic degenerative changes at the second and third CMC joints when these joints were not initially incorporated in the fusion. Hastings recommends incorporation of the third CMC joint when plate fixation to the third metacarpal is used without plans for subsequent implant removal. Larsson[60] does not recommend incorporation of the third CMC joint and in all cases plans on implant removal. Nagy and Büchler have noted painful nonunions of formerly incorporated third CMC joints and prefer to spare this joint.[82]

Type of Bone Graft

Although fusion in rheumatoid cases can be readily achieved without the use of a bone graft,[74-76] almost all surgeons advise bone grafting in post-traumatic cases. The use of rib grafts was reported by Colonna[26] in 1944 and by Wickstrom in 1954.[143] Brittain used a bone graft from the tibia.[13] Mittal and Jain[78] and Smith-Petersen[109] described the use of the distal ulna.

Until recently, most methods of fusion have used corticocancellous iliac crest bone as onlay or inlay grafts.[18,19,40,94] The cancellous portion encourages incorporation into exposed carpal surfaces, whereas the cortical element lends stability. Abbott and associates[1] advised the use of multiple long strips of cancellous bone. With the advent of plate stabilization in wrist fusion, the implant replaced the need for a cortical element.[42,43,141] In plate arthrodesis, the use of cancellous iliac crest bone graft has provided union rates equivalent to those obtained with corticocancellous iliac grafts.[43] Cancellous iliac crest donor grafts carry a reduced donor morbidity rate when compared with corticocancellous grafts.[43]

The use of a local bone graft, initially devised by Gill,[111] involved a turnabout corticocancellous graft from the distal dorsal radius. Larsson reported successful fusion with a plate and distal ulna bone graft in six nonrheumatoid patients.[60] Weiss and Hastings[141] reported a 100% union rate in 28 cases of plate arthrodesis incorporating a cancellous bone graft from the distal radius and carpus.

Position of Fusion

There is no ideal position for wrist arthrodesis. Several authors have studied the amount of wrist motion required to perform activities of daily living. Most of the studies measured what was "used" in activity as opposed to what

was "required." Swanson and associates[113] suggested an arc between 10 degrees of extension and 10 degrees of flexion. Brumfield and Champoux[14] studied 19 normal volunteers and found that 10 degrees of flexion to 35 degrees of extension were used in 14 activities of daily living. Palmer and coworkers[87] determined that functional motion required an arc between 10 degrees of flexion and 30 degrees of extension and between 10 degrees of radial deviation and 15 degrees of ulnar deviation. Ryu and colleagues[101] found that the majority of activities of daily living could be accomplished with wrist motion between 40 degrees of flexion and 40 degrees of extension and between 10 degrees of radial deviation and 30 degrees of ulnar deviation. In an evaluation of wrist fusion patients by the Jebsen hand function test, 64% of the tasks could be completed within 2 standard deviations of published norms with a fused wrist as compared with 78% with a nonfused wrist.[142]

Pryce[92] and Colonna[26] found that power grip was maximally accomplished in slight extension and ulnar deviation. Brumfield and Champoux[14] recommended 10 degrees of extension. Weiss and Hastings[42,141] recommended 10 to 15 degrees of extension. Kraft and Detels[55] demonstrated equivalent grip strengths in positions varying from neutral to 30 degrees of extension and recommend avoiding fusion in flexion in cases in which it is found to be diminished. Although radiocapitohamate fusion results in twice as much shortening as the AO technique, grip strength is similar.[12]

Resection of Distal Ulna

Abbott and associates[1] and most authors since have recommended preservation of the distal ulna to maintain stability at the DRUJ. If the ulna impinges against the triquetrum, I prefer to remove the triquetrum rather than resect the distal ulna. Excision of the triquetrum corrects the ulnocarpal impingement without creating unnecessary distal instability. Resection is indicated only when the DRUJ is degenerative, unstable, or ankylosed.

Method of Stabilization and Immobilization

Most non-AO methods of fusion require prolonged postoperative immobilization. Abbott recommended the use of a long-arm cast incorporating the digits for 3 weeks, followed by a short-arm cast with the digits free for an average immobilization time of 10 weeks. Campbell and Keokarn[18] used en bloc corticocancellous grafts occasionally supplemented by Kirschner wires and recommended immobilization with a long-arm cast for 3 months. Carroll and Dick[19] used a long-arm cast for 6 weeks followed by a short-arm cast for an additional 6 weeks. Haddad and Riordan,[40] who used a corticocancellous graft and at times a supplemental Kirschner wire, recommended 3 months of long-arm cast immobilization.

AO methods of fusion do not require postoperative immobilization.[42,43,60,141]

Surgical Methods
Dorsal Approach (Carroll and Dick)

Technique.[*]   The dorsal approach usually follows a curvilinear skin incision with the apex at the DRUJ (Fig. 13-32A).

---

[*]This detailed description was provided by Harold M. Dick, MD, in a previous edition.

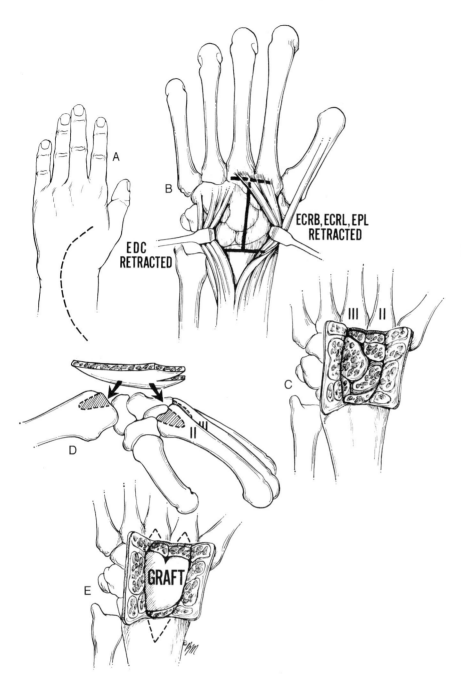

FIGURE 13-32. Dorsal approach to wrist arthrodesis (technique of Carroll and Dick). **A,** Curved incision from the second and third metacarpals to a point 2 cm proximal to Lister's tubercle. **B,** Retraction of the wrist extensors and the extensor digitorum communis (EDC). ECRB, extensor carpi radialis brevis; ECRL, extensor carpi radialis longus; EPL, extensor pollicis longus. **C,** Osteoperiosteal flaps developed. **D,** The corticocancellous inlay graft. The wrist is flexed and distracted to facilitate insertion of the graft. Great care must be taken at this point to not fracture the graft. **E,** Closure of the osteoperiosteal flap over the graft.

The incision begins at a point near the midshafts of the second and third metacarpals and ends 2 cm proximal to Lister's tubercle of the radius. The dorsal skin flap is carefully dissected to protect the branches of the radial sensory nerve. A longitudinal incision is made in the interval between the EPL and the EDC (see Fig. 13-32A). The extensor retinaculum is usually narrowed to 2 cm at this level and in some cases of rheumatoid arthritis is preserved to reinforce the diseased radiocarpal dorsal capsule.

The wrist extensors are retracted to the radial side. They may be divided if necessary for exposure. The EDC is carefully retracted to the ulnar side. The EPL and the wrist extensors are retracted to the radial side of the wound (see Fig. 13-32B). The joint capsule is incised in an "I" fashion between the CMC joints and the radiocarpal level, with care

taken to preserve the two laterally based flaps for later closure (see Fig. 13-32C).

It is helpful to develop an osteoperiosteal flap to keep the integrity of the dorsal capsule intact (see Fig. 13-32C). A thin osteotome is used to remove a thin layer of carpal cortex along with the periosteum and joint capsule as a confluent flap. This procedure is particularly important in a rheumatoid wrist to lessen postoperative extensor tendon adhesions. Intramedullary excavation of the bases of the second and third metacarpals and the radius is then performed, along with removal of the dorsal half of the intervening carpal bones. Rongeurs and bone biters are used for this purpose, along with power drills if desired.

Care is taken to avoid the scaphotrapezial joint. The lateral margin of the graft bed should be in line with the fourth

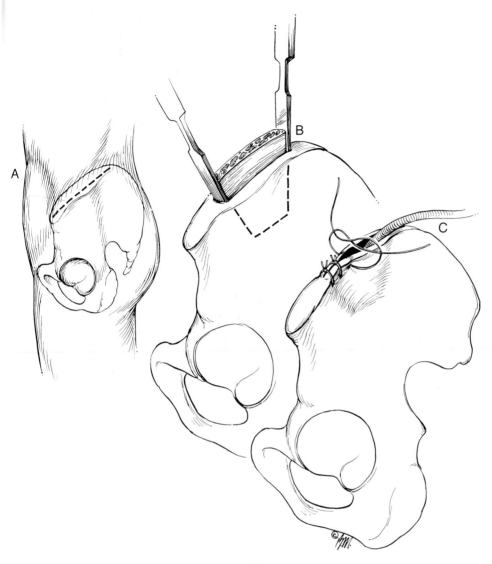

FIGURE 13-33. **A** to **C,** Removal of a corticocancellous graft from the iliac crest site. The graft includes the outer cortex of the ilium. Careful closure of the crest and suction drainage are recommended.

metacarpal base and the ulnar border of the radius; the radial margin is just radial to the second metacarpal.

The dorsal cortex is preserved to provide better stability of the graft (see Fig. 13-32D) and to allow smoother extensor tendon gliding after healing, which is also enhanced by the osteoperiosteal flap.

The iliac graft donor site is exposed by an oblique 6- to 8-cm incision 2 cm distal and parallel to the iliac crest (Fig. 13-33). Care should be taken to avoid branches of the lateral femoral cutaneous nerves of the thigh that emerge medial to the anterior superior iliac spine of the iliac crest. When the plane between the rectus abdominis and hip abductors is found, a broad osteotome is used to develop an osteoperiosteal flap along the crest of the ilium. This greatly facilitates adequate closure of the donor site. Subperiosteal dissection of the ilium is performed on both sides of the crest. When this is accomplished, a corticocancellous graft of appropriate size can be measured (usually 3 to 5 cm). This graft is removed in a single piece from the outer side of the iliac wing. Extra cancellous strips may be removed if desired or needed. The wound is then coagulated as needed; suction drainage is recommended. Closure is performed by simply closing the osteoperiosteal sleeves. The skin is closed with a subcuticular suture.

Carroll and Dick recommended arthrodesis in 15 to 20 degrees of extension and alignment of the second and third metacarpals in the longitudinal axis of the radius. The flare of the radius allows 5 to 7 degrees of ulnar deviation by placement of the graft in this fluted segment of the distal radius. In a spastic patient, 0 degrees extension is preferred. In the rare situation of bilateral wrist arthrodesis, Carroll and Dick also recommend 20 degrees of extension in the dominant wrist and 0 degrees extension on the nondominant side.

The graft is trimmed to a rectangular shape or "rabbit ears" configuration (see Fig. 13-32D) to fit the metacarpal bases and the distal radius. A lock fit is accomplished by traction-reduction of the graft into the medullary canal of the radius proximally and the second and third metacarpals distally. This can usually be accomplished by strong longitudinal traction and flexion on the hand by an assistant while the surgeon works the graft into the medullary canals. Great care must be taken to avoid breaking the "rabbit ears."

Often a good fit of the graft itself will produce a stable enough fit to obviate the need for internal fixation; this occurs in about 50% of cases (see Fig. 13-32E). If necessary, Kirschner wires through the graft and into the radius, either in the medullary canal or as crossed pins, will stabilize the

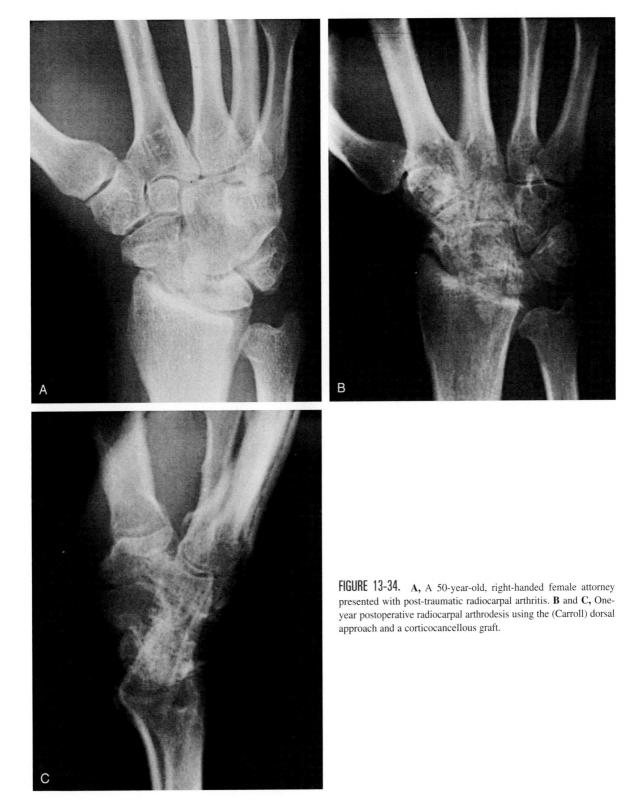

FIGURE 13-34. A, A 50-year-old, right-handed female attorney presented with post-traumatic radiocarpal arthritis. **B** and **C,** One-year postoperative radiocarpal arthrodesis using the (Carroll) dorsal approach and a corticocancellous graft.

graft. Smaller corticocancellous graft pieces are packed along the side of the bridge graft. It is important to close the wrist joint capsule (osteoperiosteal flaps) carefully but to allow for bone bleeding. The dorsal retinaculum is available for reinforcement or replacement. The skin is closed with widely spaced interrupted sutures. A suction catheter drain is optional but probably advisable.

A long-arm plaster cast is applied in the operating room from the fingertips to a position above the elbow. A dorsal wedge of plaster is removed to allow for postoperative swelling.

Postoperative Management. The consensus of most authors[19,26,29,31,84,98] is that a 12-week period is necessary for solid fusion (Fig. 13-34). Usually the first 6 weeks are in a long-arm, well-fitted plaster cast and the final 6 weeks in a short-arm cast. The thumb and distal interphalangeal joints should be free for active motion. When a DRUJ synostosis is planned, the procedure is performed in the final healing period to save the patient a repeat period of immobilization. This is generally done 6 weeks after wrist fusion, so both procedures are complete 12 weeks after wrist arthrodesis surgery.

Dorsal Approach: Capitate-Radius

Technique. Louis and associates[68] described a technique for radiocapitate arthrodesis that is combined with a proximal row carpectomy (Fig. 13-35). In their series of 11 carefully selected patients (5 with spastic upper extremities), there were no nonunions, but 1 patient later required an arthrodesis of the second and third CMC joints because of degenerative changes that subsequently developed in these joints.

The procedure is done through a dorsal longitudinal approach. The proximal 80% of the scaphoid, the entire lunate, the entire triquetrum, and a small portion of the hamate are excised. Twenty percent of the distal scaphoid and most of the hamate are preserved to prevent distal carpal row migration. Articular cartilage is removed from the capitate, and a "reciprocal portal" is prepared in the distal radius. Kirschner wires or staples can be used to stabilize the fusion if necessary. No bone graft is used. Immobilization is continued for 12 to 16 weeks until the fusion is clinically and radiographically solid.

Radial Approach: Haddad-Riordan

Technique. In 1967, Haddad and Riordan,[40] believing that the dorsal approach increases the formation of scarring,

which may limit subsequent tendon gliding, described a radial approach to arthrodesis of the wrist. Their technique used a rectangular corticocancellous graft taken from the inner aspect of the ilium to span the entire distance from the distal radius to the bases of the second and third metacarpals (Fig. 13-36).

A curved "J"-shaped skin incision is begun 3 to 4 cm above the radial styloid in the midlateral aspect of the forearm and extended distally to curve dorsally just distal to the second metacarpal base. The superficial branch of radial nerve is identified and carefully retracted, usually to the volar side. The wrist capsule is exposed between the first and second dorsal compartments, incised longitudinally, and left attached to the volar aspect of the radius. The APL, extensor pollicis brevis, and wrist and finger extensors are mobilized subperiosteally and retracted. The ECRL is transected just proximal to its attachment at the base of the second metacarpal, and a short stump is left so that it can be reattached at the completion of the procedure. The capsule is then removed from the radiocarpal, intercarpal, and second metacarpal joints. The dorsal branch of the radial artery is identified in the anatomic snuff box; its dorsal branch to the dorsal carpal arch may need to be transected and ligated. The radiocarpal joint is then denuded of articular cartilage.

These authors preferred a graft taken from the inner aspect of the ilium because of its concave cortical surface and convex cancellous surface. A graft measuring approximately 3 cm long and 2.5 cm wide is removed with a power saw. Abundant cancellous bone is included.

With the wrist in 15 degrees of extension, a slot is cut in the distal end of the radius, the intercarpal joints, and the second and third CMC joints with a power saw. To prevent injury to the DRUJ, care should be taken to avoid penetration of the saw into the medial cortex of the radius. The graft is then trimmed to fit and impacted solidly into the slot. Often the graft alone will afford adequate stability, but if

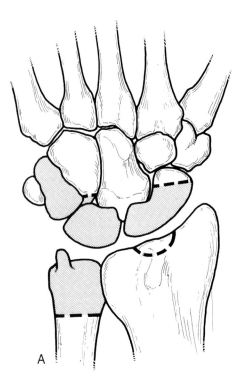
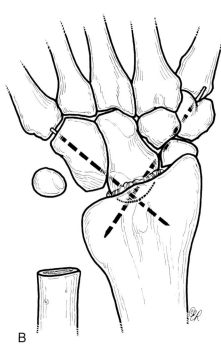

FIGURE 13-35. **A,** Capitate-radius arthrodesis. This method is particularly useful when it is necessary to correct a flexion contracture of the wrist. **B,** The shaded areas indicate the extent of bone resection. (From Louis DS, Hankin FM, Bowers WH: Capitate-radius arthrodesis: An alternative method of radiocarpal arthrodesis. J Hand Surg [Am] 9:365-369, 1984.)

A   B

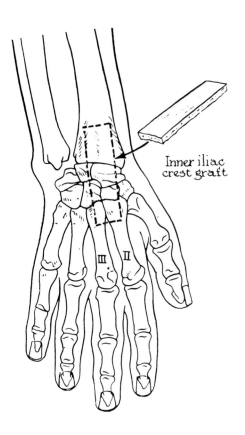

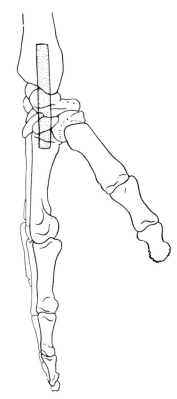

Inner iliac crest graft

FIGURE 13-36. Radial approach to wrist arthrodesis (see text). (From Haddad RJ, Riordan DC: Arthrodesis of the wrist: A surgical technique. J Bone Joint Surg Am 49:950-954, 1967.)

additional stability is required, a smooth Kirschner wire is introduced either longitudinally or obliquely; the pin is cut off beneath the surface and removed 6 to 8 weeks postoperatively. The optimal position is 10 to 15 degrees of extension and slight ulnar deviation (obtained by aligning the second metacarpal with the radius).

The dorsal retinaculum is resutured over the raw bone surface, beneath the abductor pollicis brevis. Immobilization in a long-arm cast is continued until there is radiographic evidence of union, usually at 12 weeks.

Arthrodesis of the Rheumatoid Wrist: Steinmann Pin[21,70,74]

Indications

Arthrodesis of the rheumatoid wrist is frequently required for the correction of pain deformity and instability due to pancarpal arthritis. Correction of radial deviation and supination deformity is essential for proper alignment about MP joint reconstruction or replacement.

Contraindications

Total arthrodesis may be relatively contraindicated in earlier disease when the midcarpal joint is still well preserved and stabilization and alignment can still be achieved by RL fusion. A stable, well-aligned, and arthritic wrist may not need formal arthrodesis if it is not painful. In selected cases of bilateral wrist involvement or limited elbow motion, wrist replacement may be preferred.

Techniques

The patient with rheumatoid arthritic wrist involvement often presents with partial or complete carpal coalescence. Often only minimal efforts and stabilization are needed to properly align and complete the evolving fusion. Arthrodesis is frequently performed at the same stage as hand reconstruction, necessitating an expedient technique. The current techniques have evolved from that described by Clayton[21] and Mannerfelt and Malmsten[70] and popularized by Millender and Nalebuff,[74] utilizing a large Steinmann pin for fixation. Further modification of this method has been described by Feldon, as is described in detail in Chapter 59.

Millender and Nalebuff Technique

The wrist is exposed through a relatively straight dorsal incision. A retinacular flap is elevated from the sixth to first dorsal compartments. Extensor tenosynovectomy is performed. The distal ulna is excised or reconstructed (see Chapter 15) to avoid painful rotation and impingement with the carpus after fusion. The wrist capsule is opened with a transverse incision. With traction and flexion the joint surfaces for fusion are exposed and decorticated to create matching cancellous surfaces.

The medullary canal of the radius is entered with a pointed awl and the largest Steinmann pin chosen that the radius will accept. The Steinmann pin is then drilled distally through the carpus to exit between the second and third metacarpals. The wrist is reduced into neutral alignment and the Steinmann pin tapped into the radius until countersunk into the intermetacarpal space (Fig. 13-37). In cases of marked bone loss additional fixation to prevent rotation may be necessary. This is achieved by a medium-sized Kirschner wire drilled from the fourth or fifth metacarpals into the radius or by one or two power-inserted staples across the radiocarpal joint.

Bone graft from the ulnar head resection is packed into the fusion area. The capsule is closed and extensor retinacu-

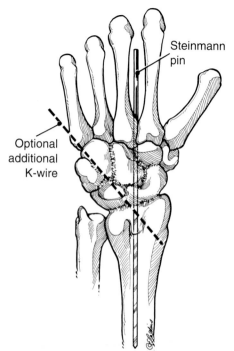

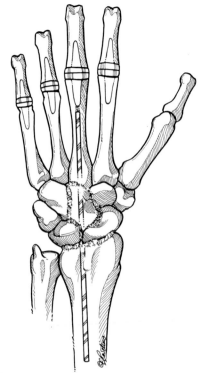

FIGURE 13-37. The Millender-Nalebuff fusion with Steinmann pin recessed within the second web space. An optional Kirschner wire or staple can be used if there is still any rotational instability.

FIGURE 13-38. Modification of the Millender-Nalebuff fusion with the Steinmann pin placed down through the third metacarpal at the same time as metacarpophalangeal implant arthroplasty.

lum transposed and sutured back ulnarly deep to the extensor tendons. A bulky dressing and short-arm splint is applied.

Postoperative Management

The wound is checked and sutures removed at 2 weeks. Usually a short-arm splint suffices for immobilization until healing is confirmed radiographically at 8 weeks. In the case of adjunctive, simultaneously performed reconstructive procedures the splint is modified to incorporate more distal digital dynamic or static splinting.

Author's Preferred Method of Treatment for Wrist Arthrodesis in the Rheumatoid Patient

When performed as an isolated procedure, I have come to prefer plate fixation, as listed in the next section. It offers surprisingly good fixation even in soft, rheumatoid bone and is nearly as expedient to apply. Plate fixation provides for more reproducible fixation in slight extension and does not interfere with the intramedullary spaces.

When the carpus has already partially fused itself and MP joint replacement is to be accomplished at the same time, I will occasionally choose fixation by an intramedullary Steinmann pin. In this instance it is convenient to insert the pin through the distal third metacarpal head after removing the head during MP implant arthroplasty (Fig. 13-38).

A straight, longitudinal incision is made over the dorsal wrist and extended out to the second web space. (Exposure for MP replacement of the index and middle digits is accomplished through the distal aspect of this incision and for the ring and small digits through a second longitudinal incision across the dorsal fourth web space.) The extensor wrist retinaculum is elevated and reflected from the sixth dorsal compartment over to the first compartment. Extensor synovium is excised. The EPL and radial wrist extensor tendons are retracted to the radial side, and the EDC, extensor digiti minimi, and extensor carpi ulnaris tendons are retracted to the ulnar side. The capsule is opened transversely to expose the remaining carpal joints that have not fused. These are decorticated down to cancellous bone. The head of the distal ulna is excised (see Chapter 15).

After excision of the third metacarpal head and preparation of the canal for MP replacement, the largest Steinmann pin that will fit down the diaphysis of the third metacarpal is chosen. An awl is used to gain entrance into the distal radius between the scaphoid and lunate fossae. The Steinmann pin is measured for required length for radius fixation. To do so, the pin is gently tapped proximally into the radius separate from the carpus just until it starts to become snug. An equal-length pin is placed next to the protruding portion and the remaining difference in pin lengths is measured. From this measurement, the length of the MP implant stem is subtracted. This difference will equal that required for intramedullary radius fixation. The MP implant is positioned over the dorsal metacarpal to identify where its proximal tip will lie when implanted. The distance from this point to the proximal edge of carpus is then measured and added to the intramedullary radial length needed. A Danek rod cutter (Medtronic Sofamor Danek, Memphis, TN), a shearing type of pin cutter, is used to cut the Steinmann pin to the measured length, leaving a flat surface. The prepared Steinmann pin is inserted into the distal metacarpal canal and tapped proximally through the metacarpal and carpus until it protrudes from the proximal carpal surface. The wrist fusion surface is reduced and the pin advanced across into the radius. Final tamping of the pin down the metacarpal canal is facilitated by a center punch or by using the discarded portion of the flat cut Steinmann pin. Additional fixation is accomplished by one or two staples power inserted across the radiocarpal joint.

The capsule is closed with 3-0 braided nylon. The extensor retinaculum is transposed deep to the extensors and sutured back ulnarly. The skin is closed with 5-0 monofilament nylon. A noncompressive bulky dressing is applied along with a short-arm splint.

Postoperative Management

Sutures are removed at 10 to 14 days. The wrist is protected with a removable short-arm splint. The splint may incorporate distal splinting according to what distal simultaneous reconstructive procedures have been performed. Splinting is discontinued at 6 weeks.

Author's Preferred Technique For Wrist Fusion (Method of the AO Hand Study Group)

In 1974 the AO manual recommended dorsal compression plate fixation of the radiocarpal joint with iliac bone grafting to achieve wrist arthrodesis. This was updated in 1982 by Heim and Pfeiffer[45,46] and recommended by Wright and McMurtry in 1983.[145] The technique was further modified and an integrated implant system developed by the AO Hand Study Group.*

A straight, longitudinal incision is begun in the mid-metacarpal area and centered between the second and third metacarpals. The incision passes across Lister's tubercle and ends over the dorsum of the distal radius just proximal to the muscle belly of the APL (Fig. 13-39). The radial side of the incision is raised as a flap directly off the dorsal surface of the retinaculum and contains the superficial branch of radial nerve. The dorsum of the retinaculum is opened by incising directly into the third compartment (EPL). The EPL is mobilized from the compartment and transposed radially (Fig. 13-40). Full transposition requires release of the sheath distal to the retinaculum.

The distal radius is exposed subperiosteally, and the longitudinal incision in the periosteum is extended distally through the capsule out to the radial base of the third metacarpal. The insertion of the ECRB is subperiosteally elevated by scalpel dissection and reflected radially. An incision is made

*Drs. Jurg Breenwald, Ueli Büchler, Jesse Jupiter, and Hill Hastings II.

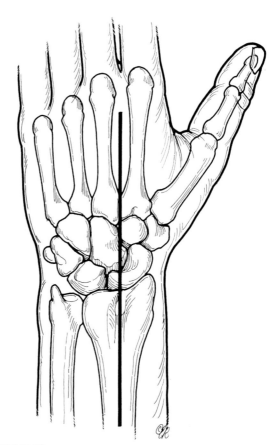

FIGURE 13-39.   The skin incision for an AO wrist fusion starts at the second to third intermetacarpal space distally and proceeds proximally over Lister's tubercle.

in the interosseous fascia on the radial side of the third metacarpal. The dorsal surface of the third metacarpal is exposed without disturbance of the intrinsic musculature on either side. A scalpel blade is used to elevate the two flaps of capsule from the carpus. The second dorsal compartment is elevated subperiosteally from the radius and reflected radially with its underlying capsule. The fourth extensor compartment is elevated subperiosteally from the radius and reflected with its underlying capsule ulnarly over to the DRUJ. The second and fourth dorsal tendinous compartments are not entered. The DRUJ is left undisturbed unless distal ulnar resection is needed.

To allow for flat apposition of the plate on the radius, Lister's tubercle is removed with an osteotome (Fig. 13-41). The dorsal cortices of the base of the third metacarpal and the carpal bones are removed to give excellent visual access to all the joints to be included in the fusion. In most all instances I now perform total wrist fusion with proximal row carpectomy, accomplishing a radiocapitate-metacarpal fusion (Fig. 13-42). This simplifies the fusion, minimizes the need for graft, and avoids potential ulnocarpal impingement. The proximal carpal row is excised, and these bones are morselized for bone graft. The articular cartilage and subchondral bone are removed down to cancellous bone from the distal radius, capitate, proximal hamate, and third CMC joints (Fig. 13-43A and B).

Traditionally, a large corticocancellous bone graft has been used with the AO technique.[45,46] No doubt this stems

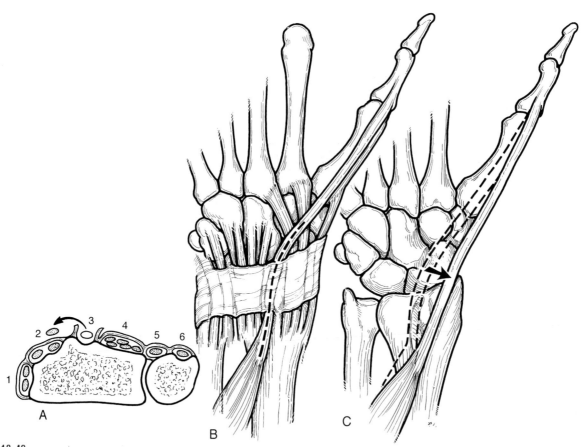

FIGURE 13-40. **A** and **B,** The third dorsal retinacular compartment containing the extensor pollicis longus (EPL) is opened longitudinally. The dorsal, distal forearm fascia over the muscular origin of the EPL is also opened. **C,** The EPL tendon is withdrawn from the compartment and transposed radially.

from older forms of wrist arthrodesis in which a bone graft was relied on to provide stability as well as osteogenesis. Cortical bone is not necessary when an AO plate is used and, when used, compromises the low-contour fit of the plate. A purely cancellous graft is incorporated faster and has been shown to have lower donor site morbidity.[43] Additional cancellous bone can be harvested from within the distal radius through a cortical window made radial to the intended plate position and 1.5 to 2 cm proximal to the wrist joint (Fig. 13-44). In those rare instances in which local bone graft is judged inadequate, I prefer cancellous bone harvested from the olecranon or from a window in the superior aspect of the iliac crest without stripping it of its musculature (Fig. 13-45).

A titanium low-contact dynamic compression plate (LC-DCP) has been designed by the AO Hand Study Group and produced by Synthes (Paoli, PA) to facilitate fusion. The

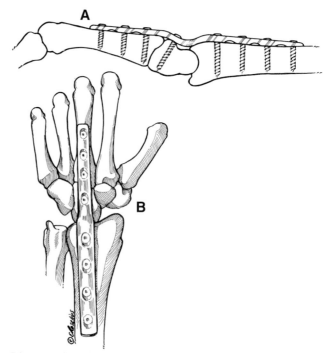

FIGURE 13-42. Radiocapitate-metacarpal fusion. **A** and **B,** Excision of the proximal carpal row allows the capitate to be inset into the radius, simplifying the fusion construct. There is minimal need for graft. Excision of the triquetrum avoids problems with obtaining ulnar midcarpal fusion. It also eliminates the potential for ulnotriquetral impingement.

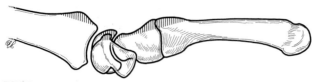

FIGURE 13-41. The dorsal distal aspect of the radius is osteotomized to remove Lister's tubercle. The third carpometacarpal joint is exposed by osteotomy of the dorsal distal portion of the capitate and the dorsal proximal aspect of the third metacarpal.

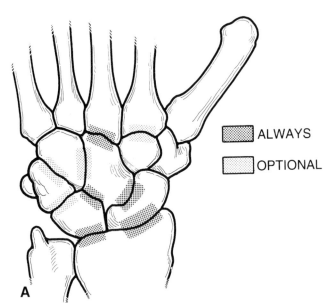

ALWAYS

OPTIONAL

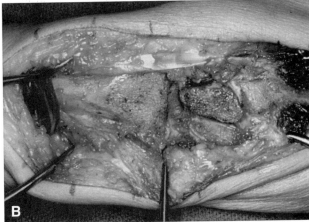

FIGURE 13-43. **A,** Joints always included in the fusion are the radioscaphoid, scapholunate, scaphocapitate, lunocapitate, and capitate–third metacarpal. If the relationships of the ulnar midcarpal joint are disturbed, the joint surfaces between the capitate and hamate, triquetrum and hamate, and lunate and triquetrum are included. The second carpometacarpal joint is rarely included. **B,** Appearance of the dorsal fusion area after decortication of the radioscaphoid, radiolunate, capitolunate, third carpometacarpal, scaphocapitate, capitohamate, and triquetrohamate joints.

edges are tapered to avoid prominence and the screw heads recessed. The surgeon chooses one of three versions (Fig. 13-46). A precontoured version with a short carpal bend is used in most all cases and has been designed to fit with proximal row carpectomy. A longer carpal bend may be used in larger wrists. The plate contour anticipates using the dorsal distal radius as a source of bone graft and requires partial excision of its dorsum. A straight version is used when large segmental carpal traumatic or tumor defects require corticocancellous intercalary graft replacement. These plates require no contouring and provide for an automatic 10 degrees of extension. Each plate uses three self-tapping 2.7-mm screws in the metacarpal, one self-tapping 2.7-mm screw in the capitate, and four self-tapping 3.5-mm screws in the radius.

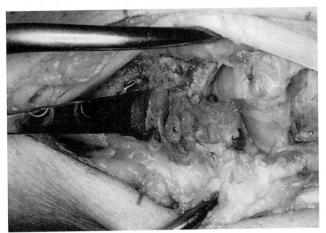

FIGURE 13-44. The dorsal distal aspect of the radius is partially excised by serial osteotome cuts to provide cancellous bone strips that can be used as bone graft material.

In the absence of these wrist fusion plates, a straight plate is chosen and similarly contoured to follow the dorsal radius, carpal sulcus, and dorsal third metacarpal. In small individuals a 9-hole, 3.5-mm reconstruction plate is chosen. In persons with extremely small hands, a 2.7-mm reconstruction or 2.7-mm semitubular plate is chosen. In large individuals, a 3.5-mm LC-DCP is used. The larger size at the metacarpal level may require elective removal after fusion is obtained.

All joints to be fused are packed with cancellous bone before plate fixation. The plate is centered directly over the dorsal aspect of the third metacarpal so that three screws will be placed into the metacarpal (one metaphyseal and two diaphyseal). A marking pen is used to mark the position of the most distal hole. The plate is removed, and a 2.0-mm drill hole is made in a dorsal-to-volar direction under direct vision precisely in the midline of the metacarpal. This is the most critical screw hole because the metacarpal is narrow at this point. If the hole does not pass in a direct dorsal-to-volar direction, the plate will lie somewhat oblique to the frontal plane and potentially rotate the metacarpal when subsequently fixed to the radius. The distal hole is then measured for depth with the plate repositioned and an appropriate-length 2.7-mm self-tapping cortical screw applied.

With the plate thus aligned over the third metacarpal, the most proximal of the three screws in the metacarpal is drilled in neutral mode with a 2.0-mm drill, the depth is measured, and a 2.7-mm screw is inserted. The position of this second screw is also critical because it determines the angle at which the plate will overlie the distal radius. The central of the three metacarpal screws is then inserted. Next, a 2.7-mm cancellous screw is placed in the capitate (Figs. 13-47 and 13-48).

The hand is finally aligned with the forearm, and the capitate is manually compressed into the decorticated distal radius. With the plate aligned over the radius and the hand properly oriented, the second most distal screw in the radius

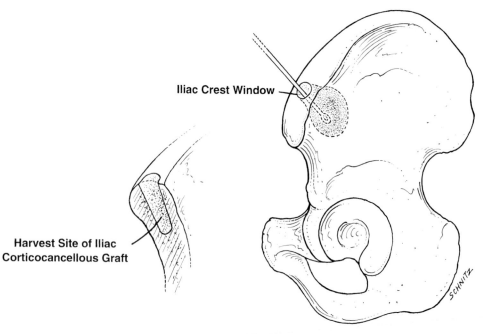

Iliac Crest Window

Harvest Site of Iliac
Corticocancellous Graft

FIGURE 13-45. Harvesting of cancellous bone graft through a small window in the top of the iliac crest without stripping of the muscular origins.

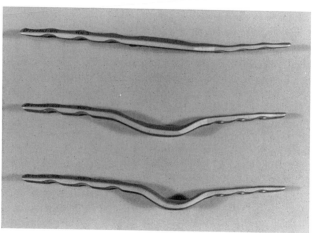

FIGURE 13-46. Three versions of AO wrist fusion plates: short carpal bend, long carpal bend, and straight plate. All use three 2.7-mm metacarpal screws, a 2.7-mm capitate screw, and four 3.5-mm radius screws.

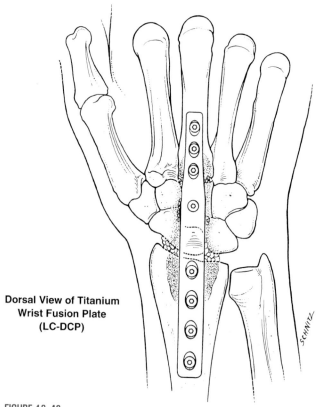

Dorsal View of Titanium
Wrist Fusion Plate
(LC-DCP)

FIGURE 13-48. Dorsal view of wrist fusion with an AO arthrodesis plate. LC-DCP, low-contact dynamic compression plate.

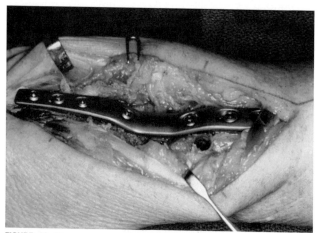

FIGURE 13-47. Position of wrist fusion after plate fixation. Additional cancellous bone graft has been harvested from the metaphysis radial to the plate and proximal to the radioscaphoid joint.

(chosen because it lies in cortical bone) is drilled with a 2.5-mm drill in compression mode and a 3.5-mm cortical screw inserted. The remaining radius holes are fixed with cortical screws.

Finally, if the plate lies in direct contact with the dorsal aspect of the capitate, the screw length is chosen as measured. If there is space between the capitate and the plate, the capitate can be lagged up to the plate and therefore a shorter screw than measured is needed to avoid volar screw penetration through the capitate into the carpal canal.

Closure.   A small suction drain is routinely used and brought out proximally. The retained radial and ulnar leaves of the previously opened third (EPL) compartment are used to close the capsule over the plate as completely as possible. The EPL is left transposed radially out of Lister's canal, slightly elevating the tendon off the radius so that it is supported by the closed second compartment. The EPL tendon does not touch the plate except sometimes at its proximal origin (Fig. 13-49).

Postoperative Management

A bulky short-arm dressing incorporating a volar plaster splint is applied. At 1 week this is converted to a light compressive dressing or sleeve, and the wrist is supported with

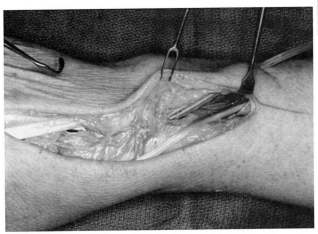

FIGURE 13-49.   Appearance after closure of the third dorsal compartment retinaculum and radial transposition of the extensor pollicis longus tendon.

CRITICAL POINTS: AO WRIST ARTHRODESIS

INDICATIONS

- Pancarpal arthrosis of radiocarpal and midcarpal joints
- Failed past limited arthrodesis
- Failed total-joint or previous arthroplasty
- Paralysis of the wrist and hand with potential for reconstruction involving the use of wrist or finger motions for tendon transfer
- Reconstruction after segmental tumor resection, infection, or traumatic segmental bone loss of the distal radius and carpus[42,44]
- Rheumatoid wrist arthritis/deformity[19,22,70]

PEARLS

- Carefully assess preoperative carpal tunnel symptoms and do concomitant release even for mild symptoms.
- Decorticate dorsal 80% of third CMC joint.
- Remove dorsal distal radius for plate to fit. It is designed to do so for additional source of graft.
- Removal of proximal row simplifies fusion and avoids ulnocarpal impingement.
- In rheumatoid arthritis with ulnar translation, remove part of radial styloid to facilitate realignment of the wrist.

TECHNICAL POINTS

- Transpose EPL.
- Excise proximal row.
- Decorticate third CMC joint, capitate, proximal hamate, and distal radius.
- Place graft in third CMC joint.
- Fix plate to metacarpal first through most distal screw hole.

- Align plate with metacarpal and fix first metacarpal screw hole.
- Fix central hole in metacarpal portion of plate.
- Fix capitate.
- Reduce wrist and fix plate to radius.
- Add additional graft from dorsal distal radius and excised carpal bones to fusion area.

PITFALLS

- Drill hole through metacarpal portion of plate must be in sagittal plane. If not, plate will lie rotated on metacarpal. Subsequent radius fixation will cause rotational deformity to third metacarpal.
- If capitate does not contact undersurface of plate and is lagged up to plate, the screw may end up too long and protrude into the carpal canal.
- If nonself-tapping screws are used, be careful to avoid excessive penetration of the tap through the metacarpal, which may injure the deep motor branch of the ulnar nerve as it crosses radially.

POSTOPERATIVE CARE

- Immobilize the hand and wrist in a bulky dressing and splint for 10 days.
- Then protect against excessive use with a removable short-arm splint until 6 weeks postoperative.
- At 6 weeks discontinue splint.
- At 8 weeks begin strengthening.
- Allow full use at 10 weeks.

ATHLETIC PARTICIPATION

- Patients are given a 5-pound weight limit for the first 8 weeks.
- Full use is allowed after 10 weeks as symptoms allow.

a wrist immobilization splint, which serves to remind the patient and others that a surgical procedure has been done; it does not support or protect the plate. Full active use of the hand and digits is allowed within the range of 1-kg grasp and lifting restrictions. The splint is discontinued at 6 weeks. Full use of the hand is allowed by the 10th week. Radiographic healing is to be expected by 8 to 10 weeks (Fig. 13-50).

Case Study (Fig. 13-51)

This 46-year-old heavy-duty equipment mechanic presented with bilateral Kienböck's disease. Radial shortening osteotomy and Hori pedicle grafting to the lunate was successful on the left side but failed on the right side, with subsequent lunate fragmentation. Wrist fusion was accomplished with proximal row carpectomy technique and AO plate fixation. The splint was discontinued at 5 weeks postoperatively. At 11 weeks

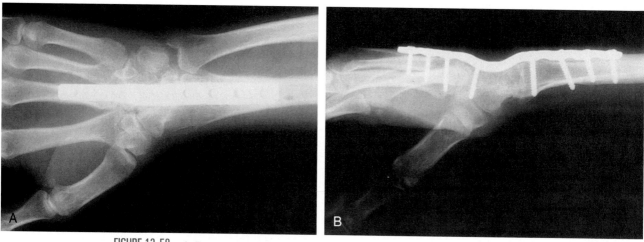

FIGURE 13-50. **A,** Posteroanterior radiograph. **B,** Lateral radiograph showing solidly healed fusion.

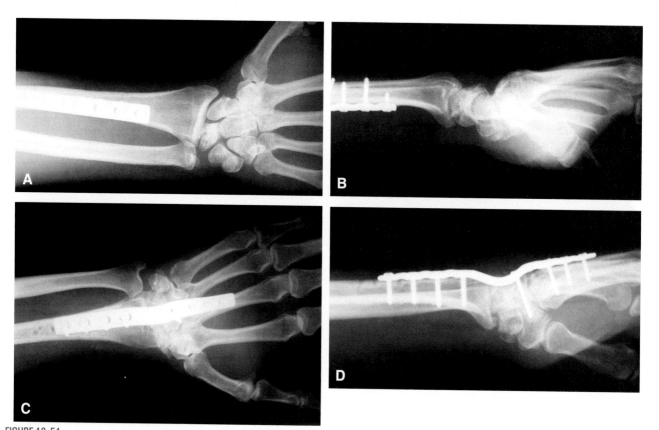

FIGURE 13-51. **A,** AP radiograph shows severe fragmentation of the lunate and failure of healing despite radial shortening osteoplasty. **B,** Lateral radiograph depicting the lunate with Kienböck's osteonecrosis. **C,** Zero-rotation radiograph after radiocapitate-metacarpal fusion with AO titanium wrist fusion plate. **D,** Lateral radiograph of wrist after radiocapitate-metacarpal fusion.

he was working without restrictions on the operative side, including using air-impact tools.

Postoperative Expectations

Most patients experience significant swelling requiring bed rest and careful hand elevation. Fusion should be relatively secure by 6 weeks. A union rate of nearly 100% can be expected with AO wrist fusion with local bone graft alone. Field and associates[33] reported a 0% nonunion rate in 20 cases of plate fusion. Larsson[60] reported a 0% rate in 23 cases, and Weiss and Hastings[141] also had a 0% nonunion rate in 28 patients with a plate and local bone graft. With respect to the predictable fusion rate, the AO method is unrivaled. When nonunion has been seen it most commonly occurs at the third CMC joint. With stabilization of the radiocarpal and midcarpal joints, stress is concentrated distally, and micromotion over a short interval can lead to fibrous union. Prevention depends on careful and complete decortication of the dorsal 80% of the third CMC joint down to cancellous bone. Although some authors have advised against attempts to formally include the third CMC joint in the fusion,[82] not including that joint obligates the surgeon to later removal of the plate to prevent its subsequent loosening or failure by fatigue fracture. When not included, the second and third CMC joints may be at risk of symptomatic degenerative changes developing later.[12,69]

Standard 3.5-mm AO plates have been symptomatic in 19% of cases, the majority at the metacarpal level. The incidence of plate removal for tenderness has been 12%.[42] The lower-profile AO wrist fusion plate uses smaller 2.7-mm screws distally at the metacarpal level and has tapered edges, and the screws are recessed flush with the dorsal plate surface. With use of this lower-profile plate symptoms requiring implant removal are rare.

The incidence of carpal tunnel syndrome after AO plate fusion is between 3.6%[144] (1 in 28 cases) and 10.5%[43] (6 in 57 cases). The surgeon must carefully rule out preoperative carpal tunnel symptoms that might go unrecognized and later become symptomatic after fusion-related swelling or distortion of carpal anatomy. Ideally, the three-dimensional architecture of the carpal canal should not be altered significantly by fusion. The plate should follow the dorsal contour of the carpus. When a space exists between the capitate and the plate, the surgeon should avoid overtightening of this screw, which will lead to abnormal displacement of the capitate toward the plate and distortion of the carpal canal. Postoperative carpal tunnel syndrome in two thirds of the cases will require carpal tunnel release.[43]

Although primary wrist fusion is very predictable in providing pain relief at times, unexplained pain can persist despite successful fusion. This is most commonly seen in patients who have previously undergone multiple failed surgical procedures. When this is the case, selective wrist nerve blocks may be indicated to determine whether wrist denervation is needed.[15]

A 0% to 3.5% incidence of DRUJ pain can be seen after fusion.[43,141] In a series of 85 AO plate wrist fusions, new pain at the DRUJ was seen in only one case and resolved after injection of the joint with 1 mL of betamethasone.

Plate fixation of the radius to the third metacarpal usually "radializes" the wrist and protects against impingement of the distal end of the ulna and carpus. Ulnocarpal abutment can occur when there is a discrepancy between the combined heights of the radius and radial carpus and that of the ulna and ulnar part of the carpus.[119] When the surgeon chooses to maintain and incorporate the proximal row into the fusion, he or she must be sure by visual and radiographic means that the triquetrum does not interfere with the distal ulna. When insufficient space exists between the distal ulna and the triquetrum, the triquetrum should be excised. This is totally avoided by my recommended technique employing excision of the proximal row.

Grip strength will take a year to plateau and will approximate 72% of normal.[42] Bolano and Green[12] found no significant difference in grip strength between fusion with retention of the proximal row and with excision of the proximal row.

Patients should expect a 6-month learning/adaptation period to the fusion. Ninety-two percent of tasks will be performed in a normal manner without undue delay. The greatest functional problems will be perineal care and horizontal use of a screwdriver.

What I Tell My Patients

I tell my patients they will be immobilized in a bulky dressing for 10 days followed by a removable splint until 6 weeks postoperatively. They can expect a 98.5% union rate. Although full use is allowed at 10 weeks they will not feel really adapted until 6 months after surgery. Complete pain relief cannot be guaranteed if they have had multiple previous surgeries. Grip strength will not plateau until 1 year out. With the new AO plate design the chance is minimal that it will require removal.

ANNOTATED REFERENCES

1. Abbott LC, Saunders JBM, Bost FC: Arthrodesis of the wrist with the use of grafts of cancellous bone. J Bone Joint Surg 24:883-898, 1942.

   Before plate fixation, this classic article served as the basis for wrist fusion methods for the next four decades. It described a technique for corticocancellous strut grafting with the cancellous bone facilitating fusion and the cortical aspect providing stability. This technique was the gold standard for a long time until plate fixation replaced it.

19. Carroll RE, Dick HM: Arthrodesis of the wrist for rheumatoid arthritis. J Bone Joint Surg Am 53:1365-1369, 1971.

    This classic article modified the Abbott technique for use in rheumatoid arthritis, describing a rabbit-ears graft, tailored with one portion of the corticocancellous graft inset into the radius and two distal ears into the index and middle metacarpals. This method was the standard used by most hand surgeons until it was supplanted by the AO technique.

20. Chamay A, Della Santa D, Vilaseca A: Radiolunate arthrodesis factor of stability for the rheumatoid wrist. Ann Chir Main 2:5-17, 1983.

    The observant recognition of spontaneous radiolunate arthrodesis by these authors led to the creation of a procedure, radiolunate arthrodesis, which has remained one of the cornerstones for stabilization of the rheumatoid wrist.

28. Douglas DP, Peimer CA, Koniuch MP: Motion of the wrist after simulated limited intercarpal arthrodesis: An experimental study. J Bone Joint Surg Am 69:1413-1418, 1987.

    This was one of the first articles to side-by-side compare different combinations of limited wrist arthrodesis and their effects on overall wrist range of motion. It found that arthrodesis of the scaphoid-trapezium-trapezoid (STT), scaphoid-capitate (SC) and scaphoid-lunate (SL) resulted in same reduction of individual and total motions of the wrist.

40. Haddad RJ, Riordan DC: Arthrodesis of the wrist: A surgical technique. J Bone Joint Surg Am 49:950-954, 1967.

This classic article described the radial approach to wrist fusion to avoid problems with the extensor mechanism and the appearance of thickening of the dorsal wrist. It emphasized the importance of inclusion of the second and third carpal-metacarpal joints into the wrist fusion.

43. Hastings H II, Weiss APC, Quenzer D, et al: Arthrodesis of the wrist for post-traumatic disorders. J Bone Joint Surg Am 78:897-902, 1996.

This paper sealed the replacement of previous corticocancellous bone grafting techniques by plate fixation techniques. It found a 98% union rate with plate fixation compared with 82% by nonplate techniques. It also underscored a significant decreased complication rate with plate fixation as compared with arthrodesis by alternate methods of fixation.

59. Larsen CF, Jacoby RA, McCabe SJ: Nonunion rates of limited carpal arthrodesis: A meta-analysis of the literature. J Hand Surg [Am] 22:66-73, 1997.

This paper addresses one of the biggest problems in evaluating intercarpal arthrodesis—the fact that there are few, if any, serious, reasonable-sized and reliable assessments of nonunion rates. It applies meta-analysis of the literature to predict nonunion rates for the most popular methods of limited arthrodesis. It attempts to remove the relative influence of chance and assessment of nonunion rates by combining multiple papers and applying meta-analysis to their results.

60. Larsson SE: Compression arthrodesis of the wrist: A consecutive series of 23 cases. Clin Orthop 99:146-153, 1974.

This is one of the first articles of a good size to describe the then "new" method of wrist fusion by AO plate fixation in 23 cases.

70. Mannerfelt L, Malmsten M: Arthrodesis of the wrist in rheumatoid arthritis: A technique without external fixation. Scand J Plast Reconstr Surg 5:124-130, 1971.

This classic article employed the use of a Rush pin and staples for simple and expedient wrist fusion in the rheumatoid patient.

74. Millender LH, Nalebuff EA: Arthrodesis of the rheumatoid wrist: An evaluation of sixty patients and a description of a different surgical technique. J Bone Joint Surg Am 55:1026-1034, 1973.

Whereas Steinmann pin fixation was previously described by Clayton, Mannerfelt, and Malmsten, this was the first article to really set it on the map for wrist fusion in rheumatoid arthritis. Over the years, this technique has proven the test of time.

83. Nagy L, Büchler U: Long-term results of radioscapholunate fusion following fractures of the distal radius. J Hand Surg [Br] 22:705-710, 1997.

Very few articles have addressed the problem of radioscapholunate fusion. This is the first study to underscore problems with obtaining radioscapholunate fusion and led to the concept of excising the distal scaphoid to enhance union rate and prevent midcarpal degenerative changes.

87. Palmer AK, Werner FW, Murphy D, Glisson R: Functional wrist motion: A biomechanical study. J Hand Surg [Am] 10:39-46, 1985.

This often-quoted article evaluated functional wrist motion by a triaxial electrogoniometer applied to 52 standardized tasks. "Normal" functional wrist range of motion in these tasks ranged from 5 degrees of flexion to 30 degrees of extension and from 10 degrees of radial deviation to 15 degrees of ulnar deviation. It provided objective evidence that limited wrist motion was not necessarily functionally detrimental.

90. Pin P, Young V, Gilula L, Weeks P: Management of chronic lunotriquetral ligament tears. J Hand Surg [Am] 14:77-83, 1989.

This article calls attention to the important differentiation of isolated LT ligament tear versus LT tear combined with ulnocarpal impaction syndrome. It underscores the importance of this distinction and the need to simultaneously correct ulnar impaction when it is present.

127. Watson HK, Ballet FL: The SLAC wrist: Scapholunate advanced collapse pattern of degenerative arthritis. J Hand Surg [Am] 9:358-365, 1984.

This classic article reviewed 4,000 wrist films to describe and present the most common form of wrist arthritis: Periscaphoid arthritis. It introduced surgeons to the concept of SLAC wrist reconstruction.

129. Watson HK, Goodman ML, Johnson TR: Limited wrist arthrodesis: II. Intercarpal and radiocarpal combinations. J Hand Surg [Am] 6:223-232, 1981.

130. Watson HK, Hempton RE: Limited wrist arthrodesis: I. The triscaphoid joint. J Hand Surg [Am] 5:320-327, 1980.

These two articles set the stage for treatment of scapholunate instability by STT fusion in a technique that has remained unchanged for the past 20-plus years. Part II described various additional combinations of limited wrist arthrodesis.

141. Weiss APC, Hastings H: Wrist arthrodesis for traumatic conditions: A study of plate and local bone graft application. J Hand Surg [Am] 20:50-56, 1995.

The AO Hand Study wrist fusion plate has opened up the door to simplification of wrist fusion and greatly diminished morbidity. This paper documented successful total wrist arthrodesis with 100% union rate and the majority of patients treated on an outpatient surgery basis. It underscores that bone graft other than local carpal or distal radius source is not needed for successful fusion.

142. Weiss APC, Wiedeman G, Quenzer D, et al: Upper extremity function after wrist arthrodesis. J Hand Surg [Am] 20:813-817, 1995.

Although a number of papers have attempted to define what normal wrist motion is required to perform activities of daily living, this is the first paper to analyze in detail patients with wrist fusion from a functional basis. It challenges the concept that motion used in activities of daily living is actually needed to perform those same activities. Patients were evaluated by Jebsen hand function test, activities of daily living test, and Buck-Gramcko-Lohmann scores. Maximum improvement after wrist arthrodesis required an average of 14.5 months, with patients requiring 3 to 6 months to adjust to the fusion of their wrists. Ninety-two percent of activities of daily living could be accomplished in a normal manner without undue delay. The greatest difficulty was experienced using the hand and wrist in a limited space where compensatory motion of the shoulder and elbow was not possible and in activities requiring forced pronation and supination with strong grip.

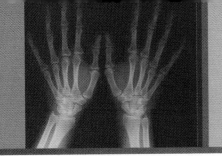

CHAPTER 14

Carpal Instability

Marc Garcia-Elias • William B. Geissler

W rist dysfunction, whether the result of bone fractures or carpal ligament injuries, has long interested the specialist in reconstructive surgery of the hand.[130] In the past three decades much has been unveiled about this subject through widespread laboratory and clinical research. Yet, many aspects of these intriguing conditions remain poorly understood if not totally unknown. There are types of carpal dysfunction that have been only partially explored, most of their treatments being recommended based on intuitions, without adequately controlled trials. On the other hand, these are problems not devoid of adverse social consequences both in terms of disability (longer time off work than scaphoid fractures[366]) and morbidity (frequent development of osteoarthritis[616]) if not properly addressed. Indeed, finding reliable ways to solve carpal dysfunction still is an open challenge.

Since the fourth edition of this book, the number of publications about carpal instabilities has grown exponentially. Many new ideas have been raised that made obsolete some of the concepts discussed not long ago. Consequently, this chapter has been extensively rewritten to include the latest developments in the diagnosis and treatment of carpal instabilities.

By definition, the term *carpal instability* is a synonym of *carpal dysfunction*.[18,174,176] Consequently, understanding carpal anatomy and mechanics is important for a proper treatment of these conditions. This is the reason for starting this chapter with an updated section on normal form and function of the wrist, certainly one of the most complex joints of the human body. The terminology utilized throughout this work is in accordance with the suggestions published by the International Wrist Investigators Workshop.[263]

ANATOMY AND FUNCTION

Osseous Anatomy

The wrist is the link between the forearm and the hand. It involves the distal ends of the radius and ulna, the two carpal rows (proximal and distal), and the bases of the five metacarpal bones (Fig. 14-1). The proximal row consists of the scaphoid, lunate, and triquetrum. The distal row contains the trapezium, trapezoid, capitate, and hamate bones. The

pisiform, despite being a true carpal bone, functions as a sesamoid, providing a lever arm for the flexor carpi ulnaris tendon and having its own pathology.[74,186,379,437] Accessory carpal bones exist in less than 2% of the population, the os centrale being one of the most common. This ossicle, located between the scaphoid, capitate, and trapezoid, has been implicated as an unusual cause of painful "clicking" of the wrist.[484] For those interested in the evolution of the carpal bone nomenclature, the well-documented study by Johnson[270] is recommended.

The radiocarpal joint consists of the antebrachial glenoid, formed by the distal articular surface of the radius in conjunction with the triangular fibrocartilage, and the proximal convexities of the carpal bones.[44,63,562] The distal articular surface of the radius is biconcave and tilted in two planes. In the sagittal plane there is an average 10 degrees of tilt, and in the frontal plane there is an ulnar inclination averaging 24 degrees.[44,149,507] The proximal joint surface of the scaphoid is more curved than that of the lunate.[58] To ensure articular congruency, the radius has two separated articular facets (the scaphoid and lunate fossas), separated by a cartilaginous sagittal ridge, called the interfacet prominence.[46] The biconcave scaphoid fossa is triangular or oval and has a smaller radius of curvature than that of the lunate fossa.[58] The latter is more or less rectangular and also biconcave but shallower and less inclined toward the ulnar side than the scaphoid fossa.[44,58]

The midcarpal joint is a combination of three different types of articulation. Laterally, the convex distal surface of the scaphoid articulates with the concavity formed by the trapezium and trapezoid (scaphotrapezoid-trapezial [STT] joint) and lateral aspect of the capitate (scaphocapitate [SC] joint).[136,150,381,383] The central portion of the midcarpal joint is concave proximally (scaphoid and lunate) and convex distally (head of the capitate) (lunocapitate [LC] joint).[278,279] The medial hamate-triquetral articulation is ovoid or slightly helicoid (triquetrohamate [TqH] joint).[395,396,629,630] The anatomic variations of the midcarpal joint are numerous, the most frequent involving the distal surface of the lunate, which may have one (lunate type I) or two facets (lunate type II) to receive the capitate and proximal pole of the hamate (lunohamate [LH] joint).[73,150,396,597,601]

In the horizontal plane, the bones of the carpus are situated in an arciform manner with a palmar concavity.[312] This arch is closed palmarly by the transverse carpal

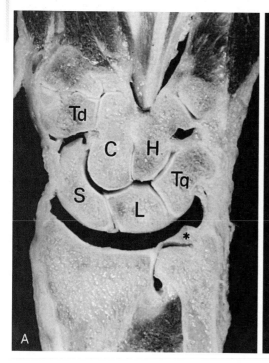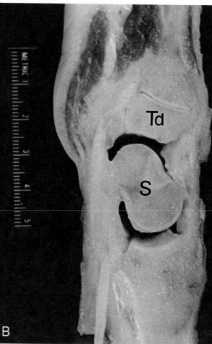

FIGURE 14-1. **A,** Frontal section of a wrist specimen, demonstrating the proximal row of the carpus intercalated between the distal row and the two forearm bones. Td, trapezoid; C, capitate; H, hamate; S, scaphoid; L, lunate; Tq, triquetrum. The triangular fibrocartilage *(asterisk)* is interposed between the radiocarpal joint space and that of the distal radioulnar joint. **B,** Sagittal section of the wrist along the lateral column. The scaphoid (S) appears obliquely oriented relative to the long axis of the forearm. Because of this configuration, when the axially loaded trapezoid (Td) migrates proximally, the scaphoid tends to rotate into flexion.

ligament (flexor retinaculum) constituting the carpal tunnel, the narrowest portion of which is located at the level of the distal carpal row.[44,179,312]

Ligamentous Anatomy

The anatomy of the carpal ligaments is complex and somewhat confusing when descriptions from different articles or textbooks are compared.[44,63,314,347,562] The existence of frequent anatomic variations in ligament size and shape makes things even more complicated.[151,152] Fortunately, several investigators have analyzed a large number of cadaver dissections aiming to produce a more statistically accurate depiction of the diversity of ligament arrangements.[41,151,152,239,369,383,396,597,605] What follows is a general description of the most common pattern of carpal ligament anatomy.

Wrist ligaments are either intracapsular or intra-articular, except for the transverse carpal ligament and the two distal connections of the pisiform to the hamate and the base of the fifth metacarpal, which are located outside the wrist capsule.[63,312,347,379,437,558] The intracapsular ligaments are contained within capsular sheaths of loose connective tissue, making their recognition difficult when surgically approaching the joint.[151,152] By contrast, when observed with an arthroscope from inside the joint, both the intra-articular (scapholunate [SL] and lunotriquetral [LTq] proximal membranes) and the intracapsular ligaments can be clearly identified, the latter under a thin synovial sheath.[108,513]

Agreement exists in defining two categories of intracapsular ligaments: extrinsic and intrinsic (Fig. 14-2).[109,559,562] Extrinsic ligaments are those that connect the forearm bones with the carpus, and intrinsic ligaments are those that have both origin and insertion within the carpus. Anatomic, histologic, and biochemical differences exist between the two types.[45,273,464,605] The extrinsic ligaments are stiffer but with lower yield strength than the intrinsic ligaments. The latter, however, have a relatively larger area of insertion into

cartilage than into bone and much less content of elastic fibers when compared with the extrinsic ligaments. This implies a different mode of failure under stress: the extrinsic ligaments tend to suffer mid-substance ruptures, and the intrinsic ligaments appear to be more frequently avulsed than ruptured.[324]

Extrinsic Carpal Ligaments
Extrinsic ligaments may be subdivided into three major groups: palmar radiocarpal, palmar ulnocarpal, and dorsal radiocarpal ligaments.[40,41,44,46,47,151,152] There are no dorsal ligaments between the ulna and the carpus.

Palmar Radiocarpal Ligaments
Four palmar ligaments connect the radius to the carpus: the radioscaphoid (RS), radioscapho-capitate (RSC), long radiolunate (long RL) and short radiolunate (short RL) ligaments.[41,47,526] The first three originate from the lateral third of the palmar margin of the distal radius and take an oblique course to insert into the scaphoid tuberosity (RS), the palmar aspect of the capitate (RC), and the lunate (long RL). The short RL ligament originates from the medial anterior edge of the radius and has a vertical direction until it inserts into the palmar aspect of the lunate, becoming an important stabilizing structure that prevents this bone from dislocating dorsally in hyperextension injuries.[36,41,344]

The RSC ligament courses around the palmar concavity of the scaphoid, forming a fulcrum over which the scaphoid rotates.[150,321,562] Between the two diverging RSC and long RL ligaments there is the so-called interligamentous sulcus. Its medial prolongation forms the so-called space of Poirier, which represents a relatively weak zone through which perilunate dislocations frequently occur.[345,562] In many instances, the long RL ligament appears to be in continuity with the intrinsic palmar LTq interosseous ligament.[151,347]

The so-called radioscapholunate (RSL) ligament, although long considered a deep intracapsular ligament,[559]

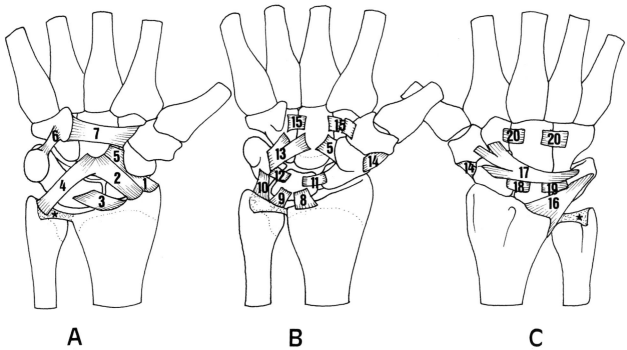

A   **B**   **C**

FIGURE 14-2. Schematic representation of the most consistently present wrist ligaments. These drawings do not aim to replicate the exact shape and dimensions of the actual ligaments, nor their frequent anatomic variations. **A,** Palmar superficial ligaments: (1) radioscaphoid, (2) radioscapho-capitate, (3) long radiolunate, (4) ulnocapitate, (5) scaphocapitate, (6) pisohamate, and (7) flexor retinaculum or transverse carpal ligament. **B,** Palmar deep ligaments: (8) short radiolunate; (9) ulnolunate; (10) ulnotriquetral; (11) palmar scapholunate; (12) palmar lunotriquetral; (13) triquetral-hamate-capitate, also known as the ulnar limb of the arcuate ligament; (14) dorsolateral scaphotrapezial; and (15) palmar transverse interosseous ligaments of the distal row. **C,** Dorsal ligaments: (16) radiotriquetral; (17) triquetrum-scaphoid-trapezium-trapezoid, also known as the dorsal intercarpal ligament; (18) dorsal scapholunate; (19) dorsal lunotriquetral; and (20) dorsal transverse interosseous ligaments of the distal row.

may not be a true ligament because it is formed by loose connective tissue containing a neurovascular bundle supplying the SL interosseous membrane and adjacent osseous structures.[46,236]

Palmar Ulnocarpal Ligaments
Arising from the fovea of the ulna, there is a superficial extrinsic ligament, called the ulnocapitate (UC) ligament, which courses obliquely to attach to the neck of the capitate.[15,44,150,151,175,239] The distal insertions of the UC and RC ligaments form the so-called "distal V ligament."[558] Underneath the UC ligament, arising from the triangular fibrocartilage, are the ulnotriquetral (UTq) and ulnolunate (UL) deep extrinsic ligaments that run vertically toward their distal insertion into the anterior aspect of the lunate and triquetrum. These and the superficial UC ligament form the so-called ulnocarpal ligamentous complex.[44,150,175,239]

Dorsal Radiocarpal Ligaments
The only dorsal extrinsic radiocarpal ligament is the dorsal radiotriquetral (RTq) ligament, a wide, fan-shaped ligament that connects the dorsal edge of the distal articular surface of the radius to the dorsal rim of the triquetrum, with some deep fibers inserting also onto the lunate, and rarely onto the scaphoid.[151,369,558,605]

Intrinsic Carpal Ligaments
Intrinsic carpal ligaments are collections of relatively short fibers either connecting transversely the bones of the proxi-

mal and distal carpal bones (palmar and dorsal interosseous ligaments) or linking the two rows to each other.

Scapholunate Interosseous Ligaments
The SL linkage consists of three distinct structures: the two SL ligaments (palmar and dorsal) and the proximal fibrocartilaginous membrane.[40,45,540] The latter follows the arc of the proximal edges of the two bones from dorsal to palmar, separating the radiocarpal and midcarpal joint spaces.[38,426] The dorsal SL ligament is located in the depth of the dorsal capsule and connects the dorsal aspects of the scaphoid and lunate bones. It is formed by thick and stout collection of fibers, slightly obliquely oriented, with a key role in SL stability.[290,524,525] Its anterior counterpart, the palmar SL ligament, has longer, more obliquely oriented fibers, allowing substantial sagittal rotation of the scaphoid relative to the lunate[279,503] while playing a lesser role in carpal stability.[57,290] The dorsal SL ligament has the greatest yield strength (260 Newtons [N] average), followed by the palmar SL ligament (118 N) and the proximal membrane (63 N).[45] The proximal portion of the membrane often appears perforated in older individuals, which does not necessarily indicate increased instability.[40,597]

Lunotriquetral Interosseous Ligaments
The LTq joint is also constrained by two interosseous ligaments (palmar and dorsal) formed by stout transverse fibers connecting the palmar and dorsal aspects of the two bones.[454] In between the two a fibrocartilaginous membrane closes the joint proximally.[419] Unlike the SL ligaments, the

palmar LTq ligament is stronger than the dorsal one (average yield strengths: 301 N and 121 N, respectively) with the proximal portion the weakest (64 N). Unless perforated by age[597] or injury,[423] this proximal membrane prevents communication between the radiocarpal and midcarpal joint spaces.[38,43,426] The fibers of the two interosseous LTq ligaments are more taut through all ranges of motion than those of the SL ligaments, making for a closer kinematic relationship.[241,479]

The most distal fibers of both palmar and dorsal LTq ligaments are often connected to the distal fibers of the SL joint, forming the so-called palmar and dorsal scaphotriquetral (STq) ligaments.[516,540] These structures may contribute to the stability of the LC joint by providing some enhancement to the depth of the midcarpal fossa.

Midcarpal Ligaments

The only dorsal midpalmar crossing ligament is the so-called dorsal intercarpal ligament. It arises from the dorsal ridge of the triquetrum, courses transversely along the distal edge of the lunate, and fans out to insert on the dorsal rim of the scaphoid, the trapezium, and the trapezoid bones.[151,369,558,605] Often undistinguishable from the dorsal STq ligament, this structure contributes to increase the depth of the midcarpal socket, thus having a stabilizing role to the LC joint.[540]

On the palmar side, the midcarpal joint is crossed by a number of ligaments. Medially, there is a group of fan-shaped fibers that connect the triquetrum to the hamate and capitate.[151,314,316,395,580] This triquetral-hamate-capitate (TqHC) ligamentous complex varies substantially according to the type of lunate (I or II),[395] and, together with the UC extrinsic ligament, it appears essential in ensuring a stable motion to the proximal carpal row.[173,503,628]

Laterally, the scaphoid tuberosity is linked to the distal row by two groups of fascicles, the anteromedial SC ligament and the dorsolateral STT ligament.[121,342] These ligaments are very important in the stabilization of the scaphoid.[173,524]

There is no ligament, palmar or dorsal, between the lunate and the capitate.[21,63] Neither true radial nor ulnar collateral ligaments of the wrist exist.[312,558] Because the wrist is not a true hinge joint, vertically oriented collateral ligaments should not be expected to be present. Their absence is functionally substituted by the structure and actions of the extensor carpi ulnaris tendon medially[669] and the abductor pollicis longus tendon laterally.[279]

Distal Carpal Row Interosseous Ligaments

Connecting transversely, the distal carpal row bones have numerous strong and taut interosseous ligaments (dorsal, palmar, and deep intra-articular).[179,463,479] Recent investigations have found that variations in the palmar capitate-trapezium ligament are implicated in the development of osteoarthritis at the STT joint.[381,383]

BIOMECHANICS

To facilitate positioning of the hand to manipulate objects, lift loads, or perform specific tasks of daily living, the wrist needs to be highly mobile and yet be able to sustain sub-stantial forces and torques without yielding. This can only be achieved through a perfect interaction between wrist motor tendons, joint surfaces, and soft tissue constraints. In the past, different theories have been proposed to explain the intricate mechanism of the wrist (Table 14-1). What follows is a succinct review of wrist biomechanics, based on the more recent findings on both normal carpal motion (kinematics) and force transmission across the wrist (carpal kinetics).

Carpal Kinematics

The wrist can be moved passively by an external force or actively by contracting the muscles with a tendon crossing the joint.[5] The function and efficacy of muscles' contraction depend on their location and distance (moment arm) relative to the instantaneous center of rotation of the carpus at any given wrist position.[321,667]

Except for the pisiform, the proximal carpal row has no direct tendinous attachments. Hence, the moments generated by muscle contraction result in rotational motion starting always at the distal carpal row.[479,667] The bones of the proximal row start moving later, when tension of the ligaments crossing the midcarpal joint reaches a certain level.[494,628]

In normal wrists, very little motion exists between the bones of the distal carpal row.[463,479] Indeed, the distal carpal row is quite rigid,[179,187] and it can be considered one functional unit. During unconstrained flexion of the wrist, the distal row synchronously rotates into flexion but also into some degree of ulnar deviation. In contrast, during wrist extension, the tendency of all distal carpal bones is to rotate into extension and a slight radial deviation. This so-called "physiologic flexion-extension" mostly occurs at the midcarpal joint.[259,381]

The bones of the proximal carpal row appear to be less tightly bound to one another than the bones of the distal carpal row.[278,279,479,517] Although moving synergistically (in similar directions), considerable differences in direction and amount of rotation exist among the scaphoid, lunate, and triquetrum. As demonstrated both in cadaver[291,479,517,640] and in vivo studies,[116,406,430,654,656] when wrist flexion-extension is constrained along the sagittal plane, the scaphoid has a larger amount of rotation (average 90% of the total arc of motion) than the lunate (50%) and the triquetrum (65%).[377,640,654] The average SL angle in full wrist flexion is 76 degrees; it reduces to 35 degrees in full extension.[398,491,503]

During radioulnar deviation of the wrist, the three proximal carpal bones move synergistically from a flexed position in radial deviation to an extended position in ulnar deviation (Fig. 14-4).[113,241,278,414,479] The magnitude of such an out-of-plane motion varies substantially from one individual to another. In some individuals the proximal carpal row rotates basically around the flexion-extension axis during radioulnar deviation (the so-called column wrists), whereas in others the proximal row rotates almost entirely around the radioulnar deviation axis (the so-called row wrists).[113,185,378] In between the two extremes, there is a spectrum of combined behavior depending on a number of individual variables, including wrist laxity,[185] shape of the capitate-hamate proximal surface,[73,381] or type of lunate.[395] The aim of such complex rotations is to maintain the articular

Table 14-1
THEORIES OF WRIST BIOMECHANICS

How the Wrist Moves (Carpal Kinematics)

- *Johnston* (1907)[130]: The carpal bones are arranged into two carpal rows (proximal and distal), each moving as a rigid functional unit about two transverse joints (radiocarpal and midcarpal).
- *Navarro* (1935)[404]: The carpal bones are arranged into three vertical, interdependent columns: (1) the central column (lunate, capitate, and hamate) controls flexion-extension of the wrist; (2) the lateral column (scaphoid, trapezium, and trapezoid) controls load transfer across the wrist; and (3) the medial or rotational column (triquetrum and pisiform) controls pronosupination.
- *Taleisnik* (1978)[559]: Modification of the columnar theory. The pisiform does not function as a carpal bone because it is excluded from the model. Trapezium and trapezoid are part of the central column.
- *Weber* (1980)[629,630]: Two columns: the load-bearing column (capitate, trapezoid, scaphoid, and lunate) and the control column (triquetrum and hamate). Key importance is the helicoidal joint between the triquetrum and hamate.
- *Lichtman, et al.* (1981)[7,316]: The carpus functions as an oval ring formed by four interdependent elements (distal row, scaphoid, lunate, and triquetrum) connected to the adjacent segments by ligamentous links (see Fig. 14-3).
- *Craigen and Stanley* (1995)[113]: Two patterns of motion during radioulnar deviation: the proximal row rotates mostly along the frontal plane (row pattern) or mostly along the sagittal plane (column pattern).

How the Wrist Sustains Load Without Yielding (Carpal Kinetics)

- *Gilford, et al.* (1943)[198]: The scaphoid, as an intercalated bridge between the proximal and distal rows, prevents these to collapse under load.
- *Landsmeer* (1961)[301]: The proximal row, as an intercalated segment between the distal row and the carpus, undergoes a "zigzag" collapse, unless constrained by the obliquely oriented scaphoid.
- *Fisk* (1970)[162]: Introduces the concept of the "concertina" deformity.
- *Linscheid, et al.* (1972)[325]: The scaphoid provides stability as a slider-crank mechanism (three-bar linkage) owing to its oblique placement between the radius and the distal row.
- *Kauer* (1974)[278]: Under load, the obliquely oriented scaphoid tends to rotate into flexion. The lunate, owing to its palmar wedge-shaped configuration, tends to rotate into extension. If the scapholunate ligaments are intact, the two opposite tendencies reach a stable equilibrium.
- *Weber* (1980)[629,630]: The helicoidal shape of the triquetrohamate joint as a factor ensuring stability to the proximal carpal row.

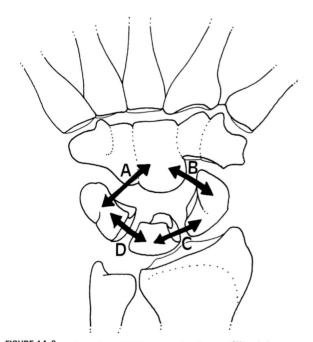

FIGURE 14-3. Adaptation of Lichtman and colleagues'[316] oval ring concept of the wrist. The distal carpal row, as a fixed unit, is connected medially to the triquetrum (link A) and laterally to the scaphoid (link B). In turn, these two bones are connected to the lunate by means of two more links (C and D). Failure of any one of these four ligamentous links is likely to result in an alteration of motion and/or load transfer coordination. (Adapted from Lichtman DM, Schneider JR, Swafford AR, Mack GR: Ulnar midcarpal instability—clinical and laboratory analysis. J Hand Surg [Am] 6:515-523, 1981, with permission.)

congruency between the radius and the distal row in all wrist positions.[8,65] For those interested in carpal kinematics, the literature review published by Moojen and associates[377] is strongly recommended.

Force Transmission Across the Wrist

When the hand is grasping or pinching an object, the joints of the wrist need to be ready to sustain considerable compressive and shear forces.[17,109,173,506] Such loads are not only the result of the external force being applied but also from contraction of the different muscles necessary to ensure finger stability.[107] Studies on force transmission have disclosed that compressive forces at the carpometacarpal (CMC) joints may be as high as 1.5 to 4.2 times the applied force.[17] According to this, the total force being transmitted by all the metacarpals to the distal carpal row can reach values greater than 10 times the applied force at the tip of the fingers.[173] Therefore, if we consider that the average maximum grip strength is 52 kg for a male subject and 31 kg for a female,[222] we can estimate that the wrist may bear loads as high as 520 kg in males or 310 kg in females.

Within the wrist, such loads are distributed following specific patterns, depending on a number of factors: magnitude, direction, and point of application of these loads; orientation and shape of the different articular surfaces; elastic properties of the constraining ligaments; and so forth. According to the latest studies, at the midcarpal level, about 60% of the load borne by the distal row is transmitted across the capitate-scaphoid-lunate (CSL) joint.[505,601] More

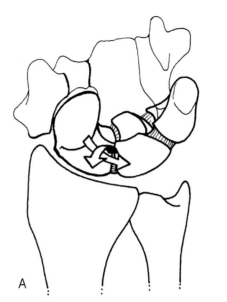 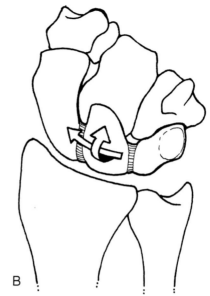

FIGURE 14-4. Schematic representation of the direction of rotation of the proximal carpal row during lateral deviations of the wrist *(arrows)*. **A,** From neutral to radial deviation of the wrist the three bones of the proximal row flex and slightly deviate. **B,** During ulnar deviation there is extension, ulnar deviation, and slight pronation. The amounts of rotation, however, differ from one individual bone to another.

proximally, the forces distribute as follows: RS joint, 50% to 56% of the total load; RL joint, 29% to 35%; and UL joint, 10% to 21%.[57,195,220,505,603] These figures vary substantially with wrist position: the lunate fossa is increasingly loaded with ulnar deviation, and the scaphoid fossa is overloaded with radial deviation.[220] The so-called functional position, which involves slight extension and radial deviation, results in an increased force through the lunate.[195]

Stabilizing Mechanisms of the Wrist

Carpal stability depends on a combination of factors: normal bone geometry, adequate tensioning of ligaments under load, and proper contraction of specific stabilizing muscles. Adequate proprioception is necessary for a proper control of all these factors. Undoubtedly, future research will clarify the distribution and function of the different intracapsular mechanoreceptors and their role in the control of specific muscles, truly the ultimate carpal stabilizers. From a mechanical viewpoint, at least four stabilizing mechanisms have been identified.[173] They can be summarized as follows.

Stabilizing Mechanism of the Distal Row
Tendons included in the carpal tunnel have divergent directions once they emerge in the palm. If their corresponding muscles contract, the flexor tendons of the little finger generate a compressive force to the hook of the hamate. This force would be opposite in direction to the force that is expected to generate the flexor pollicis longus to the inner surface of the trapezium. Such opposite forces would tend to open the palmar carpal concavity (the trapezium toward the radial side, the hamate toward the ulnar side) for both the flexor retinaculum and the strong and taut transverse

intercarpal ligaments.[179,463] Their annular disposition appears essential to maintain the adequate transverse stability to the carpal arch. Failure of any one of these structures is likely to create a particular type of instability, called "axial" or "longitudinal," with the tunnel splitting into two or more unstable columns and displacing in divergent directions.[182]

Stabilizing Mechanism of the Midcarpal Joint
Under axial load, the distal carpal row exerts an axial compressive force onto the proximal row bones. Because of its oblique orientation relative to the long axis of the forearm, the loaded scaphoid tends to rotate into flexion and pronation.[173,292] If the interosseous ligaments connecting transversely the bones of the proximal row are intact, the flexion and pronation moment exhibited by the scaphoid is transmitted to the lunate and the triquetrum. As a consequence, the unconstrained proximal row would rotate into flexion and pronation if not for the presence of the midcarpal crossing ligaments. Especially important midcarpal stabilizers are the palmar TqHC ligament (the so-called ulnar leg of the arcuate ligament), the dorsolateral STT ligaments, the dorsal intercarpal ligament, and the SC ligaments.[173] Failure of these ligaments results in a typical carpal collapse characterized by abnormal flexion of the unconstrained proximal row, a fairly typical pattern of carpal malalignment, known as volar intercalated segment instability (VISI) (Fig. 14-5).[313,325]

Stabilizing Mechanism of the Proximal Row
When axially loaded, the three proximal bones are not equally constrained by the palmar-crossing midcarpal ligaments. In fact, because of the peculiar arrangement of the STT and SC ligaments, the scaphoid is allowed larger

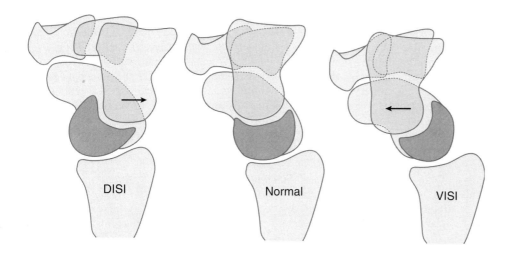

FIGURE 14-5. The two major patterns of sagittal malalignment as described by Dobyns and associates[131] and Linscheid and coworkers.[326] In dorsal intercalated segment instability (DISI) and volar intercalated segment instability (VISI, also known as PISI, for palmar) a midcarpal subluxation is possible *(arrows).*

rotation into flexion and pronation than the lunate, whereas the triquetrum is the most tightly constrained bone of the proximal row.[173,292] If both palmar and dorsal SL and LTq ligaments are intact, such differences in angular rotation are likely to generate increasing torque and intercarpal coaptation of the two SL and LTq joints, further contributing to their stability. Based on this, if the SL ligaments are completely torn, the scaphoid no longer appears constrained by the rest of the proximal row and tends to collapse into an abnormally flexed and pronated posture (the so-called rotatory subluxation of the scaphoid), whereas the lunate and triquetrum, under the influence of the ulnar part of the arcuate ligament, appear to be pulled into an abnormal extension, known as a dorsal intercalated segment instability (DISI).[325] If instead of the SL, the LTq ligaments are the ones that fail, the scaphoid and lunate tend to adopt an abnormal flexed posture (VISI), whereas the triquetrum remains solidly linked to the distal row.[241,465]

Stabilizing Mechanism of the Radiocarpal Joint

The proximal convexities of the scaphoid, lunate, and triquetrum are interconnected by fibrocartilaginous tissue (SL and LTq interosseous membranes), forming what has been called the carpal condyle. Such a biconvex structure does not articulate to a horizontal, flat surface but to an ulnarly and palmarly inclined antebrachial glenoid, formed by the distal articular surfaces of the radius and the triangular fibrocartilage complex (TFCC). In such circumstances, the loaded carpal condyle has an inherent tendency to slide down ulnarly and palmarly.[453] Such a tendency is effectively constrained by both palmar and dorsal radiocarpal ligaments, an oblique orientation that appears ideal to resist such an ulnar and palmar translation tendency. Obviously, failure of these obliquely oriented ligaments is likely to result in a very dysfunctional ulnar and palmar translocation of the carpus relative to the radius.[374,434,453,467,559,562,602,646]

In global terms, all these stabilizing mechanisms are based on the general principle according to which, under load, all carpal bones tend to rotate into specific directions depending on a number of factors: position of the wrist, direction of the load, articular surface geometry, and quality of the capsule and ligaments linking the bone to the surrounding structures. Such reactive displacements are guided by the shape of the involved articular surfaces and neutral-

ized by specific ligaments, the orientation and strength of which allow reestablishing a new equilibrium. The position of the carpal bones will be maintained until the load is discontinued, at which point the original equilibrium is reestablished, with the bones returning to their initial position and orientation. Any injury or disease modifying bone geometry, articular inclination, and/or ligament integrity may prevent the equilibrium to be achieved, in which case a carpal instability appears. Knowledge of the different stabilizing mechanisms is crucial to fully understand and eventually successfully treat this still intriguing problem.[173]

PATHOMECHANICS OF CARPAL LIGAMENT INJURIES

Two mechanisms of injury may result in a carpal ligament injury: direct and indirect. In the first, the force is spent directly from the injury-causing object to the dislocating bone, whereas in indirect mechanisms, the deforming load is initially applied at a distance from the injured joint.[182,368,380] In the latter, the tensile forces are usually transmitted by ligaments[628] and compressive forces are transferred by the adjacent articular surfaces.[173]

Direct Mechanisms

One of the most common direct mechanisms occurs when the wrist is trapped by a power press or a wringer-type machine. Its carpal concavity is suddenly crushed, and the bones dissociate following an axial pattern of dislocation.[182] Laboratory investigations about the energy necessary to produce this form of dislocation and the influence of specific ligaments in its prevention have been published by the senior author and his coworkers.[179] A similar pattern of carpal derangement can be seen after a blast. In all these cases, the dislocating force is applied over a wide surface area of the wrist, creating a global dislocation. By contrast, when the dislocating force is exerted over a small area of the wrist, a localized fracture-dislocation of a carpal bone may occur.*

---

*See references 51, 59, 90, 164, 170, 203, 204, 249, 309, 443, and 529.

Indirect Mechanisms

Most dorsal perilunate dislocations are the result of an indirect mechanism of injury, usually consisting of an extreme extension of the wrist, associated with variable degree of ulnar deviation and radiocarpal/midcarpal supination, often owing to violent trauma such as that sustained in falls from heights or in motorcycle accidents.[344,346] Hyperextension has also been linked to other wrist injuries, such as distal radial fractures or scaphoid fractures.[13,110,629] Although radial fractures may appear associated to a perilunate dislocation,[33] such a combination is not common. Many factors may explain the occurrence of one or another type of injury: age-related differences in bone stock, differences in direction and magnitude of the deforming forces, differences in position of the wrist at the time of impact, and so forth.

In an effort to ascertain both the sequence of injury and the progression of ligamentous damage, Mayfield and colleagues[347] undertook several cadaver studies. Their findings confirmed what Wagner[609,610] had previously suggested: that most carpal dislocations around the lunate (a broad spectrum of injuries ranging from minor SL sprains to a complete palmar dislocation of the lunate) are the consequence of a similar pathomechanic event, the so-called progressive perilunate instability (PLI). Four stages of progressive carpal destabilization have been identified (Fig 14-6).

Stage I: Scapholunate Dissociation/Scaphoid Fracture

As the distal carpal row is extended by the external force, the palmar midcarpal ligaments connecting this to the scaphoid become increasingly taut.[628] This creates a

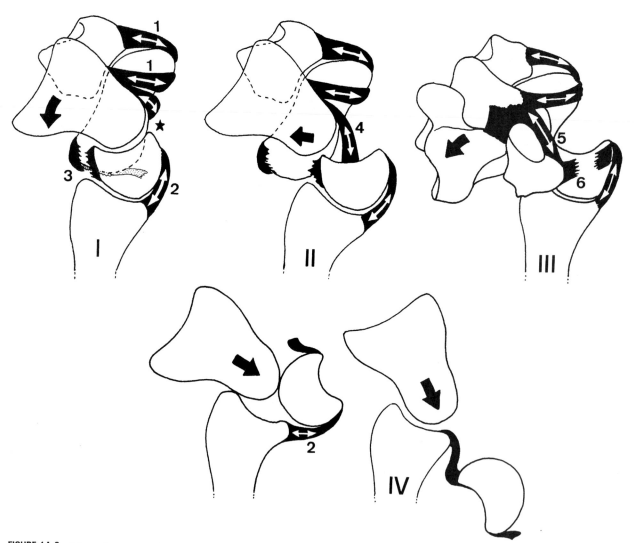

FIGURE 14-6. Schematic representation of the four stages of perilunate instability, viewed from the ulnar side. Stage I: As the distal carpal row is forced into hyperextension *(black arrows)*, the scapho-trapezio-capitate ligaments (1) pull the scaphoid into extension, thus opening the space of Poirier *(asterisk)*. The lunate cannot extend as much as the scaphoid, as it is directly constrained by the short RL ligament (2). When the SL torque reaches a certain value, the SL ligaments may fail, usually from palmar to dorsal. A complete SLD is defined by the rupture of the dorsal SL ligament (3). Stage II: Once dissociated from the lunate, the scaphoid-distal row complex may dislocate dorsally relative to the lunate *(black arrow)*. The limit of such dorsal translation is determined by the RSC ligament (4). Stage III: If hyperextension persists, the ulnar limb of the arcuate ligament (5) may pull the triquetrum into an abnormal extension, thus causing failure of the LTq ligaments (6). Stage IV: Finally, the capitate may be forced by the still intact RSC ligament (4) to edge into the radiocarpal space and push the lunate palmarward until it dislocates into the carpal canal in a rotatory fashion. (Modified from Mayfield JK, Johnson RP, Kilcoyne RK: Carpal dislocations: Pathomechanics and progressive perilunar instability. J Hand Surg [Am] 5:226-241, 1980, with permission.)

progressive extension moment to the scaphoid, which is transmitted to the lunate via the SL ligaments. The lunate, however, is closely constrained by the long and short RL ligaments. As a consequence, there may be a progressive tearing of the SL interosseous membrane and ligaments, from palmar to dorsal, eventually leading to a complete scapholunate dissociation (SLD). If the same process occurs when the wrist is somewhat radially deviated, not only the lunate but also the proximal pole of the scaphoid is strongly constrained by the RSC ligaments.[629] In such circumstances, instead of an SLD, a fracture of the scaphoid is likely. Rarely, hyperextension does not result in scaphoid fracture nor SLD but creates a more distal dissociation at the scaphoid-trapezium level.[30,197,219] In the case of progression, these unusual cases may end up as palmar dislocations of the scaphoid and lunate as a unit.[95,99,286,296,490,566]

Stage II: Lunocapitate Dislocation
Once the SL joint is disrupted or the scaphoid fractured, if wrist extension increases, the distal row may translate dorsally and dislocate relative to the lunate. This may be associated with a detachment of the RSC ligament off the radial styloid. As a consequence of the dislocation a curved capsular rent across the space of Poirier appears, through which the midcarpal joint is exposed palmarly.

Stage III: Lunotriquetral Disruption/Triquetrum Fracture
As the capitate displaces dorsally, the triquetrum-capitate (TqC) ligaments become extremely tensed, creating both an extension moment and a dorsal translation vector to the triquetrum. Such forces may result either in the separation of the triquetrum from the lunate, owing to tearing of the LTq ligaments, or in a sagittal fracture of the triquetrum. In rare instances, neither the triquetrum nor the LTq ligaments fail under such stresses, and carpal derangement progresses in a medial direction, producing a hamate-triquetrum derangement.[62,166,476] This would be more likely in the presence of a congenital LTq coalition.[351]

Stage IV: Lunate Dislocation
When all perilunate ligaments are torn, only the dorsal capsule and palmar RL ligaments can hold the lunate in place. In such circumstances, the dorsally displaced capitate may exert a palmar translation force to the dorsum of the lunate, resulting in a palmar lunate extrusion. Such dislocation is often associated with a variable degree of palmar rotation into the carpal tunnel. Depending on the amount of lunate rotation, stage IV has been subdivided into three categories:[183,230,231]

Lunate dislocation type 1: where the lunate exhibits a minor rotation (less than 90 degrees)

Lunate dislocation type 2: lunate is rotated more than 90 degrees around an intact, nondisrupted, palmar capsule (short RL ligament)

Lunate dislocation type 3: complete enucleation of the lunate with rupture of the palmar capsule

The concept of PLI offers a rational explanation for instabilities on the radial side of the carpus, but it does not offer much help in explaining the ulnar carpal instabilities. In fact, Mayfield and colleagues[344,345,348] did not see any

ulnar perilunate instability without a radial component in their experimental studies. LTq injury may represent a PLI stage III but also may be the result of a "reversed PLI," as suggested by Reagan and coworkers[454] and others.[314,561,599] Indeed, if the wrist is forcefully twisted into extension and radial deviation instead of ulnar deviation, tensile loads are likely to concentrate on the TqHC ligaments. If, in addition, the wrist is hyperpronated at the time of the injury and an external force is applied on the hypothenar area (as when falling backward on the outstretched, internally rotated hand), the triquetrum may be forced by the pisiform to displace dorsally relative to the lunate.[15] This would be the beginning of a reversed destabilization pattern of the wrist in which the LTq dissociation would be stage I; the lunocapitate dislocation, stage II; and the SLD, stage III.[599] This alternative mechanism, although thought to be likely by different authors,[314,454,599] has not yet been confirmed by any laboratory investigation.

DIAGNOSIS OF CARPAL DISORDERS

When dealing with post-traumatic carpal disorders, two clinical situations can be found. At one extreme is the patient who presents after violent trauma, such as a fall from a height, a motorcycle accident, or a crush injury to the wrist who is likely to have a major dislocation. At the other extreme is the patient who may or may not recall a specific traumatic event and presents with a symptomatic wrist. In the former patient the diagnosis of a major carpal derangement may be obvious, but in the latter the identification of a precise carpal dysfunction is often difficult.[32,91,546,563] In this section, the essential clinical and radiologic examinations of carpal instabilities, either acute or chronic, are discussed. Supplemental information on the peculiar features of each entity is provided separately under each specific heading.

Clinical Examination

Physical examination always needs to be preceded by a thorough investigation of the patient's history, with special emphasis on the mechanism of injury. The patient should also be encouraged to provide details about the location, duration, and characteristics of pain; about aggravating and relieving factors; and about previous treatments, if any.[32,91,615] With chronic problems, it is also important to inquire about the patient's job and whether there has been exposure to repetitive stress, vibrating tools, or other potential offending agents.[368]

Except in the case of open dislocations resulting from crush or blast mechanisms, the external appearance of most wrist instabilities may not be particularly dramatic. Not infrequently, major dislocations are missed at presentation owing to a lack of obvious deformity.[183,230] Swelling is generally moderate, and bone displacements may be evident if the patient is seen early after trauma. By contrast, if there has been a delay since the accident, swelling may have increased significantly, making visualization of the displaced segments rather difficult. When present, skin abrasions, contusions, or ecchymosed areas may be helpful in determining the mechanism of injury, as well as potential areas of damage.

Palpation for areas of maximal tenderness is one of the most useful tools in the diagnosis of wrist pathology, especially in patients with chronic instability.[91,563] In acute dislocations, because of extensive soft tissue damage, tenderness is seldom elicited in specific points but rather in a diffuse pattern. Nonetheless, it should always be done, and we recommend its performance in an orderly manner.

In acute cases, range of motion is usually limited by pain, whereas it may be normal in chronic cases. In the latter, joint manipulation is valuable not only in determining the presence of abnormal motion or crepitus but also, and most importantly, in reproducing the patient's pain. Grip and pinch strength also need to be investigated in chronic instabilities to uncover underlying pathology. This can be reduced by actual loss of strength or by inhibition caused by pain. In the latter case, a local lidocaine injection should normalize the dynamometer readings.

A careful assessment of the neurovascular status is imperative, with particular attention to the median and ulnar nerves, which may be injured by direct contusion at the moment of impact, compression by displaced bones, or subsequent swelling in the carpal canal. Moreover, associated soft tissue, bone, and joint injuries known to be caused by a similar mechanism (CMC dislocation, radioulnar joint dislocation, radial head fracture, and elbow dislocation) should be specifically sought as well.

Radiographic Examination

Routine Views

The initial routine radiographic examination in a patient with a suspected carpal injury should include at least four views of the wrist: posteroanterior (PA), lateral, scaphoid (PA in ulnar deviation), and 45-degree semipronated oblique.[36,199,431,456] If some of these projections are omitted, or if their quality is inadequate, the chances of missing important information are high. The PA film should be made with the patient's shoulder abducted 90 degrees, the elbow flexed 90 degrees, and the forearm in neutral rotation (Fig 14-7).[221,425] The lateral view must be a true lateral taken with the elbow adducted to the patient's side, with the wrist in neutral rotation. The dorsal surfaces of the metacarpals, radius, and ulna should be straight to demonstrate any possible alteration of the alignment of the carpal bones. In a true lateral projection, the palmar surface of the pisiform should lie between (and equidistant to) the palmar surfaces of the distal scaphoid tuberosity and the capitate head.[468,662] The PA ulnar-deviated projection must be centered on the scaphoid, and the 45-degree semipronated view should profile the dorsoulnar and radiopalmar aspects of the carpus.

In the PA view without wrist radial or ulnar deviation, three fairly smooth radiographic arcs (Gilula's lines[201]) can be drawn to define normal carpal relationships (Fig. 14-8). A stepoff in the continuity of any of these arcs indicates a displaced intercarpal derangement at the site where the arc is broken.[319,431,470] Furthermore, articulating bones normally have parallel apposing surfaces separated by 2 mm or less. Any overlap between well-profiled cortices of carpal bones or any joint width exceeding significantly that found in the contralateral normal wrist strongly suggests a carpal joint abnormality.

In the PA view of a neutral positioned wrist, the normal lunate has a trapezoidal configuration. It has long been taught that a triangular or wedge-shaped lunate is diagnostic of lunate dislocation (Fig. 14-9). However, when the lunate tilts abnormally in either direction (flexion or extension), it also projects a more triangular shape.[537] Therefore, in neutral position, a triangular lunate does not necessarily mean dislocation but it does imply a tilted lunate, which may or may not be dislocated. It is possible to differentiate a flexed from an extended lunate on a PA view based on the shape of the lunate contour: in DISI (dorsal tilting of the lunate) the lunate is a triangular wedge shape; in VISI (palmar tilting of the lunate) it has a typical moonlike configuration.[84]

Curtis and colleagues[120] and Terry and Ramin[571] have emphasized the importance of soft tissue changes in the evaluation of carpal bone injuries, noting that obliteration or bulging of the fat stripe situated on the radial aspect of the scaphoid is suggestive of injury to this bone. Focal swelling

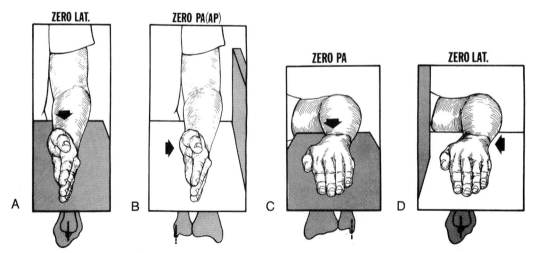

FIGURE 14-7. Taleisnik has illustrated two methods of taking standardized neutral PA and lateral radiographs of the wrist. The arrows indicate the direction of the x-ray beam, which is centered directly over the radiocarpal joint. Palmer and colleagues[425] suggested **A** and **C** as the most adequate to measure ulnar variance. However, in the presence of shoulder stiffness, **A** and **B** may be the only way to obtain correct projections. (From Taleisnik J: The Wrist. New York, Churchill Livingstone, 1985, with permission.)

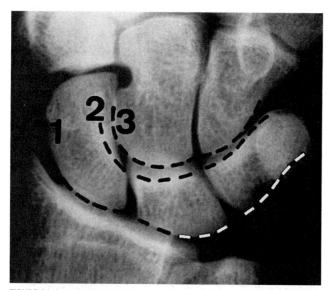

FIGURE 14-8. Gilula and associates[199,201] defined three smooth, curved lines joining the proximal and distal cortical surfaces of the carpal bones that help assess normal carpal relationships. A disruption or stepoff in any one of these lines may indicate a major carpal derangement.

at any place around the wrist deserves closer examination of the bones underlying the swelling to exclude osseous abnormality at that level.

Additional Views

When the initial radiographic evaluation of a patient with a suspected carpal dysfunction does not confirm the diagnosis and clinical suspicion exists, additional views are recommended.[431] Their purpose is to evaluate specific areas of tenderness and swelling and to clarify subtle changes seen in the routine views. In the literature, many projections have been suggested. The following are the most commonly used:

1. Anteroposterior (AP, palm up) view with clenched fist.[131] Axial compression of the carpus by having the patient make a fist or by applying a longitudinal compression force on the wrist may accentuate SLD (Fig. 14-10). It is preferable to obtain this view without extension or flexion of the wrist to enable evaluation of the midportion of the SL joint, as the dorsal and palmar portions of this joint are normally wider than its midportion. Correct positioning of the wrist can be objectively evaluated by looking at the third CMC joint. This joint should be in clear profile when the wrist is not extended or flexed.

2. PA (palm down) view with 10 degrees of tube angulation from the ulna toward the radius.[281,372] This view best demonstrates the SL interval. Measurement of its separation (SL gap) is to be made at the midportion of the joint where its anatomy is more consistent (Fig. 14-11).[501]

3. Oblique view at 20 degrees of pronation off lateral position. This view is used to visualize the dorsum of the triquetrum, where avulsion fractures frequently occur,[199,298] as well as to evaluate the distal pole and the waist of the scaphoid. This view also demonstrates fracture-subluxations of the fifth CMC joint.

4. Oblique view at 30 degrees of supination off the lateral position. The pisotriquetral relationship and hook of the hamate are seen in this view.[199]

5. Lateral view with the wrist radially deviated. The hamate hook can be fairly well profiled on a lateral view with the wrist radially deviated and the first metacarpal palmarly displaced from the other metacarpals as with spreading the metacarpals at the first web space. This places the hamate hook between the bases of the first metacarpal and the other metacarpals.[31]

6. Carpal tunnel view. By profiling the carpal concavity of the wrist, a clearer sight of the hook of the hamate, the pisiform, and the palmar ridge of the trapezium may be obtained.[199,647] In patients with acute injuries, however, pain produced by extending the wrist may not allow this projection to be taken.

7. Static "motion" views. Several authors have suggested a routine "motion" series for any patient in whom there is a suggestion of carpal instability.[319,500,647] This series includes PA and AP views in radial deviation and ulnar deviation, plus additional lateral views in extension and flexion.

Measurement of Carpal Bone Alignment

The amount of carpal malalignment has traditionally been determined measuring specific distances and angles on PA or lateral radiographs.[201,325,491] The angles more frequently used are the capitolunate (CL), SL, and RL, and are based

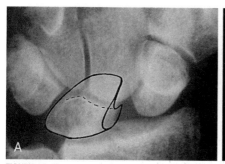
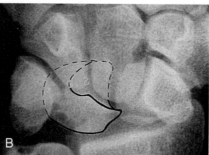
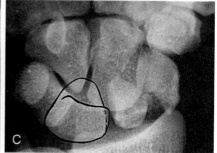

FIGURE 14-9. The shape of the lunate on a PA view may help differentiate a dislocated from a malaligned lunate. **A,** The lunate in a DISI position tends to have an obliquely oriented ovoid configuration, with a prominent wedge-shaped ulnar corner pointing toward the medial aspect of the wrist. **B,** The lunate in VISI has a "C"-shaped or moonlike appearance. **C,** In dorsal perilunate dislocations, minor palmar rotation of the lunate gives this bone the appearance of an isosceles triangle pointing distally.

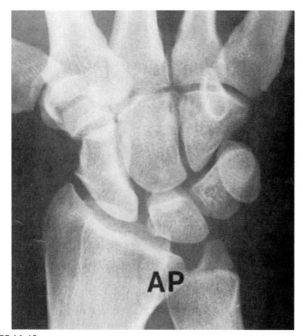

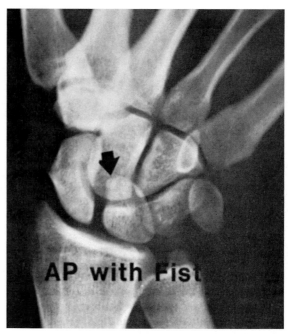

FIGURE 14-10. Dobyns and coworkers[131] suggested that compression of the carpus by having the patient make a fist may accentuate the SLD, as illustrated in these radiographs.

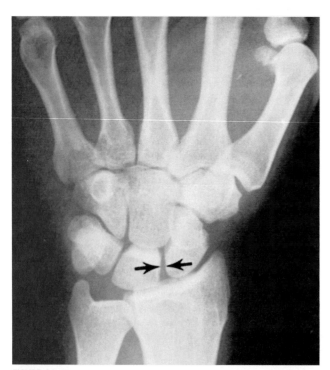

FIGURE 14-11. Kindynis and associates[281] suggested that the SL space is most clearly demonstrated in a PA view with the tube angled 10 degrees from the ulnar side. They also recommended that the gap be measured in its midportion, the landmark being the middle of the flat medial facet of the scaphoid *(arrows)*.

on axes traced on lateral radiographs as shown in Figure 14-12. The more commonly used distances, measured on a PA projection of the neutral-positioned wrist, are ulnar variance, carpal height ratio, capitate-radius index, and ulnar translocation ratio. When interpreting these data, however, one must be aware that the normal ranges of all

these parameters are quite wide,[149,150,319,398] that the reproducibility of these measurements is low,[178,304] and that small errors in rotational positioning of the hand at the time of x-ray exposure may result in substantial variation in angle determinations.[469]

Capitolunate Angle

Despite the fact that the long axes of the radius, lunate, capitate, and third metacarpal are co-linear in less than 11% of normal subjects,[491] the CL angle continues to be helpful, especially when quantifying midcarpal malalignment.[658] The standard method of defining the line representing the lunate is to draw a line perpendicular to a line connecting the palmar and dorsal tips of the lunate.[178,201] The capitate axis is identified by connecting a point in the center of the convexity of the head to a point at the center of its distal articular surface with the third metacarpal. Theoretically, the normal CL axis should be 0 degrees with the wrist in neutral, but the range of normal is ± 15 degrees.[398,491] An alternative method to assess the alignment of the CL joint has been proposed by Loewen and colleagues.[327] According to this method, the ratio between the distances that separate the palmar and dorsal tips of the lunate and the point where the axis of the third metacarpal crosses the CMC joint is 0.74 ± 0.07 in normal wrists (Fig. 14-13).

Scapholunate Angle

According to the tangential method, the scaphoid is represented by a line tangential to the two proximal and distal convexities of the palmar aspect of the bone.[178,201] The angle formed by this line and that of the lunate has been quoted extensively in the literature as one of the major determinants of SLD.[201,325,560] Normal values range from 30 to 60 degrees, with an average of 47 degrees.[325] Although angles greater than 80 degrees indicate an SLD, smaller readings do not necessarily rule out this pathology. Values less than 30

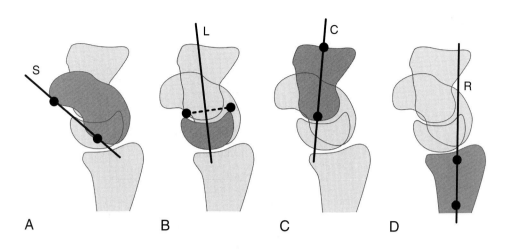

FIGURE 14-12. Carpal angle determination is based on tracing axes to the carpal bones on true lateral radiographs. According to different studies,[178,304] the most reproducible methods of axis determination are as follows: (**a**) the scaphoid (S) is represented by a tangential line that connects the two palmar convexities of the bone; (**b**) the lunate (L) axis is perpendicular to a line that joins the two distal horns of the bone; (**c**) the capitate (C) axis is determined by the center of the two proximal and distal articular surfaces; and (**d**) the axis of the radius is obtained by tracing perpendicular lines to its distal third and connecting the center of these lines.

Ulnar Variance

The relative lengths of the radius and ulna, so-called ulnar variance, and the possible effects of this parameter on various carpal disorders have long been investigated. Ulnar variance needs to be measured on standard PA radiographs, obtained with the shoulder 90 degrees abducted, the elbow 90 degrees flexed, the wrist in the neutral position, and the central x-ray beam centered directly over the wrist.[145,425] One may objectively determine that a PA radiograph was obtained correctly when the extensor carpi ulnaris groove is projected radial to the midportion of the ulnar styloid.[311] Steyers and Blair[552] compared three methods of measuring ulnar variance and concluded that, although all are highly reliable, the method of perpendiculars is the most precise for both interobserver and intraobserver error, compared with the project-a-line or concentric circles techniques. Two studies, by Voorhees and associates[606] and Czitrom and colleagues,[121] showed a higher incidence of ulnar-minus variance among patients with carpal instabilities compared with the normal population. A conclusive explanation for this has not yet been provided.

Carpal Height Ratio

Another helpful parameter in the evaluation of progression of carpal collapse is the so-called carpal height ratio (CHR).[353,667] The term *carpal height* designates the distance between the base of the third metacarpal and the distal articular surface of the radius measured along the proximal projection of the axis of the third metacarpal (Fig. 14-14). Stahelin and coworkers[545] described a more precise method of selecting the points of reference for defining the length of the metacarpal and the height of the carpus. The CHR (carpal height divided by length of the third metacarpal) was found to be 0.54 ± 0.03 in normal wrists.[353,667] Because wrist radiographs often fail to include the entire third metacarpal, some authors[64] have proposed using the length of the capitate instead of the third metacarpal (carpal height divided by capitate length; normal range: 1.57 ± 0.05). According to Bouman and colleagues,[64] this method has greater accuracy than the original method of Youm and McMurtry.[353,570]

Capitate-Radius Index

When carpal collapse affects only one side, it may be monitored by comparing the closest capitate-radius distance

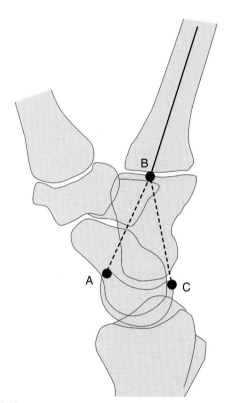

FIGURE 14-13. The alignment of the CL joint can also be assessed, as proposed by Loewen and coworkers.[327] According to this method, the ratio between the distances that separate the palmar and dorsal tips of the lunate and the point where the axis of the third metacarpal crosses the CMC joint is 0.74 ± 0.07 in normal wrists.

degrees are said to suggest a VISI pattern of malalignment,[201] although they are not unusual in patients with STT osteoarthritis.

Radiolunate Angle

The RL angle gives objective evidence of the dorsal tilt of the lunate if the angle is greater than 15 degrees.[325] Nakamura and coworkers[398] suggested this angle as the best estimate of DISI and VISI deformities.

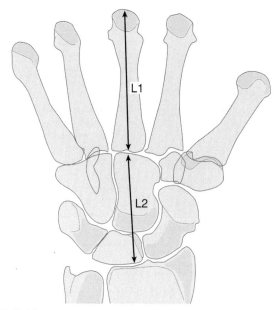

FIGURE 14-14. The carpal height ratio is calculated by dividing the carpal height (L2) by the length of the third metacarpal (L1). The normal is 0.54 ± 0.03. (Redrawn from Youm Y, McMurtry RY, Flatt AE, Gillespie TE: Kinematics of the wrist: I. An experimental study of radial-ulnar deviation and flexion-extension. J Bone Joint Surg Am 60:423-431, 1978, with permission.)

to the contralateral normal side. As demonstrated by Zdravkovic and Sennwald, the left/right capitate-radius index has higher diagnostic accuracy than all other methods of CHR determination.[671]

Ulnar Translation Ratio

In some instability conditions there is an ulnar shift of the carpal bones. The amount of translation can be quantified using different techniques.[88,129,319,353] The more commonly used is the method described by Chamay and colleagues,[88] which measures the perpendicular distance from the center of the head of the capitate to a line from the radial styloid that extends distally and parallel to the longitudinal axis of the radius (Fig. 14-15). The carpal translocation ratio (calculated as the ratio of this distance to the length of the third metacarpal) in normal wrists is 0.28 ± 0.03. Other similar methods use the axis of the ulna[353] or that of the radius[129] as a reference. Their accuracy, however, may not be as high as that of the former method.[441] Finally, there is the method suggested by Bouman and associates,[64] based on the ratio between the length of the radial articular surface and the distance from the radial styloid process to the ulnar corner of the lunate. In normal wrists, this ratio is 0.87 ± 0.04.

Tomography

In the past decade, the use of conventional (linear or poly-directional) tomograms[444] in carpal pathology has been replaced by computed tomography (CT).[449] In the wrist, CT scans are usually taken at 2-mm intervals, along the axial, sagittal, coronal, or any other plane in which the structure of interest can be better visualized.[553] CT has the added advantage of allowing computer manipulation to obtain the

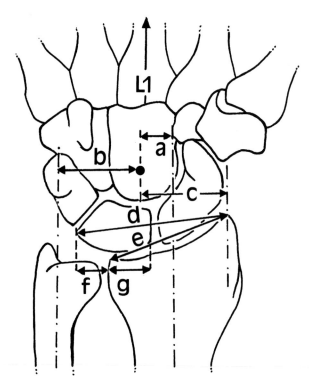

FIGURE 14-15. Ulnar translation of the carpus can be monitored according to different methods. McMurtry and colleagues[353] suggested using the axis of the ulna as a reference to determine if there is an ulnar shift of the center of the capitate head. In normally positioned wrists, the distance b divided by the length of the third metacarpal (L1) should equal 0.3 ± 0.003. According to Chamay and coworkers[88] a vertical line extending distally from the radial styloid offers a more reliable reference to measure the ulnar shift of the capitate. Normal values for the distance c divided by L1 are 0.28 ± 0.03. A similar method was described by DiBenedetto and colleagues[129] by using the longitudinal axis of the radius as a reference. The distance a divided by L1 should be 0.015 ± 0.024. The so-called lunate uncovering index has been suggested by Linn and colleagues[319] as another method to determine the relative position of the lunate with respect to the radius. According to Schuind and associates[507] the ratio between the length of uncovered lunate (f) and the maximal transverse width of this bone ($f + g$) should equal 32.6 ± 11. To measure lunate translocation, Bouman and associates[64] found it more reproducible to use the ratio e/d, which in normal wrists equals 0.87 ± 0.04. The last two methods are more likely to detect ulnar translocations of the lunate than the first three methods, at the expense of being strongly dependent on the wrist being precisely positioned in neutral. Indeed, even minor degrees of radial or ulnar deviation may significantly alter the results.

ideal visualization of the structure to be analyzed. Sanders[489] and Bush and associates[76] showed that a CT scan oriented along the true axis of the scaphoid (i.e., at approximately 45 degrees to the long axis of the radius) is an ideal way to demonstrate the amount of collapse in the "humpback" scaphoid deformity (Fig. 14-16). CT is also useful in evaluating union after intercarpal fusion,[76,169,541] although in many instances the image is compromised by the presence of retained hardware. As with other image techniques,[431] the use of CT with a tailored approach for each individual case is always recommended.[553]

CT has the added benefit of allowing obtention of three-dimensional images of the carpal bones.[37,399,631] This technique contributes enormously to the understanding of specific carpal deformities. When surgery is planned on a

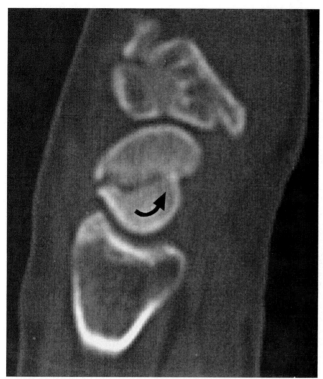

FIGURE 14-16. Computed tomography is useful in the evaluation of carpal collapse secondary to an angulated scaphoid fracture. The amount of proximal fragment rotation *(arrow)* and scaphoid malalignment can be measured using different techniques, as discussed by Smith and associates.[538]

malunited scaphoid or on a complex carpal dislocation, a three-dimensional reconstruction provides excellent visual information about the amount and direction of the displacement. Also, since three-dimensional imaging reconstructs smooth bone surfaces, subtle defects, such as hairline fractures, may be discovered. It is important to remember, however, that all the information provided by a three-dimensional reconstruction was already present on the original CT images.

Distraction Views

In patients with acute fracture-dislocations, the four routine views described earlier are sufficient to establish the diagnosis. Sometimes, however, these are difficult to interpret because of overlapping of the displaced carpal bones.[285] To further investigate these injuries, AP and lateral radiographs with the hand suspended in fingertraps are recommended (Fig. 14-17).[211,212] When using these distraction views, it is not unusual to discover new injuries or a larger extent of bony damage than seen on routine films. In less severe clinical situations, distraction views may also be helpful, such as in identifying dynamic dissociations in the form of stepoff deformities of the SL[660] or LTq joints that are only evident under traction. However, it should be recognized that offset or breaking of "Gilula's lines" may take place at the SL and LTq joints with traction in hyperlax individuals.[431a]

Stress Views

In some instances, dynamic instabilities cannot be diagnosed with a motion series but require stressing a specific joint in different directions to visualize the abnormality. A fairly common technique for investigating midcarpal instabilities involves a dorsopalmar translation of the distal carpal row relative to the radius ("drawer" test).[418,429] Less commonly used, yet productive in terms of discovering abnormal behavior of the radial column, are the views of the wrist in maximal passive ulnar deviation (Fig. 14-18).

Cineradiographs or Fluoroscopy With Videotape

Cineradiography or videotaping a fluoroscopic examination of the wrist provides considerable information in the evaluation of a patient who has a painful snapping or "clunking" wrist in whom routine and special views do not demonstrate the underlying pathology.[264,658] These are patients in whom an abnormal gap and stepoff from joint subluxation appears only under certain loading conditions, the plain films (including fist compression views) being normal.[22,409,448] In these cases, cineradiography is recommended.[448] Alternatively, active motion can be studied by the use of fluoro-

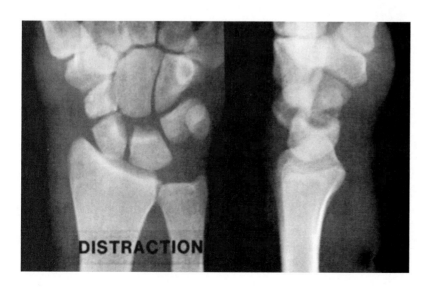

FIGURE 14-17. AP and lateral radiographs taken with the fingers suspended in fingertraps to show the carpus distracted often provide additional information not well visualized in the initial injury films, such as the osteochondral fragments seen here in the CL joint.

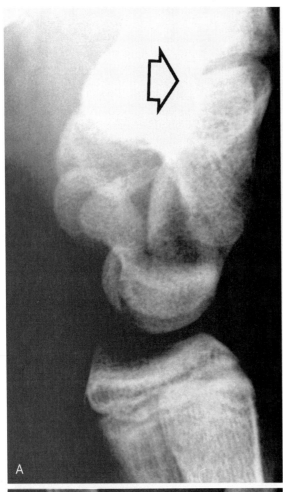

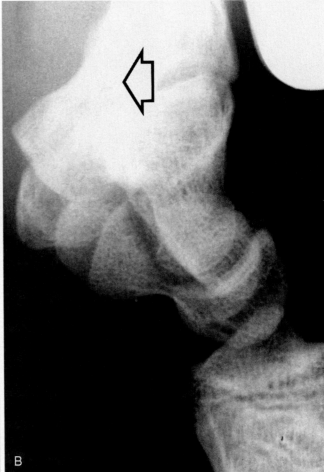

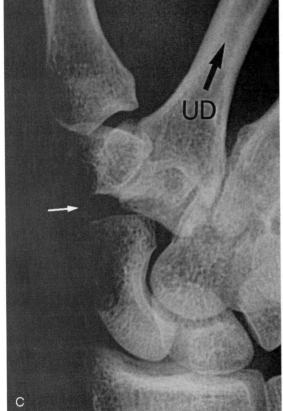

FIGURE 14-18. Stress views are particularly important to assess dynamic instabilities. **A,** In this 15-year-old girl with hyperlax wrists, dorsal stress demonstrates that both the radiocarpal and midcarpal joints are subluxable. **B,** A palmarly directed force, by contrast, appears to be better tolerated, without any noticeable subluxation. **C,** In another, 23-year-old patient, a combination of traction *(black arrows)* and ulnar deviation (UD) demonstrated an increased scaphotrapezial gap *(white arrow),* not present on the contralateral side. Because this finding coincided with the location of major tenderness, a ligament injury was suspected and treated nonoperatively.

scopy connected to a videotape. Fluoroscopy alone is insufficient, because it does not provide a permanent record allowing detailed study of the carpal kinematics.

Routinely, cineradiography includes observation of active movement from radial to ulnar deviation in both AP and PA views, flexion and extension in the lateral view, and radial and ulnar deviation in the lateral view. If the patient has a painful clunk, it is important for that to be reproduced during the examination. Sometimes the patient can reproduce this with active motion, and sometimes provocative stress (passive) maneuvers are required by the radiographer.

Arthrography

Although long considered the gold standard in the assessment of intracarpal derangements,[38,200,360,376,404,426] wrist arthrography has seen a substantial reduction of its indications. The technique was originally introduced based on the assumption that any flow of intra-articularly injected contrast agent from the radiocarpal to the midcarpal space or vice versa is to be interpreted as pathologic. With time we have learned this to be an overstatement, especially in older patients, in whom asymptomatic degenerative, often bilateral perforations are not unusual.[597,665] Furthermore, Belsole and coworkers[38] noted poor correlation between the site of symptoms and the defects seen on arthrography. Herbert and associates[226] performed bilateral arthrograms and found that 74% of their patients had abnormal findings in the opposite, asymptomatic wrist. Yin and associates[666] showed that surgeons performed less aggressive treatments in patients with bilateral symmetric defects shown at arthrography. Cooney[105] found that the arthrographic findings were confirmed by arthroscopic examination in only 12 of 20 consecutive cases. Weiss and colleagues,[637] using triple-injection cinearthrography, found improved accuracy of the technique (60%), yet when it was compared with arthroscopy, the sensitivity was 56% and the specificity was 83% in detecting carpal ligament tears. With new refinements, however, arthrography still has some potential. Particularly in association with high-resolution tomography (arthroscan) or CT the technique appears more accurate than magnetic resonance imaging (MRI) in the assessment of cartilage and ligament status.[43,53,485.572] When injecting the joint it is imperative to watch both the pattern and location of the dye flow. This provides additional data, allowing better detection and estimation of the size of communication defects[318] while detecting unidirectional communications due to valvular effect of the ligament remnants.[338]

Isotope Bone Scans

A technetium Tc 99m isotope bone scan of the wrist is a useful tool when there is a strong suspicion of an obscure intraosseous abnormality, such as infection, tumor, unrecognized osteochondral fracture, or other cause of localized synovitis, and no other method has been able to demonstrate its presence. Obviously, bone scans are of no particular use in detecting carpal dislocations. The bone scan is a nonspecific test[547]; it does not tell us what is wrong, but it can be very useful in pinpointing where the problem is located, particularly when the corresponding images of bone scan and radiographs are superimposed.[370] The use of the bone scan may be most helpful to exclude any osteochondral abnormality in a patient with nonfocal or vague tenderness.

Magnetic Resonance Imaging

Conventional MRI seldom allows clear recognition of subtle ligament injuries.[384] As compared with arthroscopy, MRI without dedicated wrist coils has shown a sensitivity and specificity of 63% and 86%, respectively, in the diagnosis of SL ligament injury, a modest result that does not improve with the use of intravenous contrast medium.[496,613] MRI combined with directly injected intra-articular MRI contrast is being used with increasing frequency throughout the world. There is a general feeling that this technique will be able to show ligament disruptions better than intravenous MRI contrast medium. Also, MR-arthrography can provide additional information about the status of marrow in adjacent bones and the status of surrounding soft tissues. Extensive research, particularly in the development of surface coils, is ongoing, which, doubtless, will improve the accuracy of MRI, facilitating full incorporation of this noninvasive, powerful tool in clinical practice.[293] With the current technology, MRI appears ideal in the diagnosis of carpal dysfunctions secondary to extra-articular soft tissue disease, as well as to help in defining the vascular status of portions of bones at risk for avascular necrosis after trauma, demonstrating subtle fractures and bone marrow edema and some adjacent soft tissue diseases.

Arthroscopy

Wrist arthroscopy has revolutionized the practice of orthopedics by providing the technical capabilities to examine and treat intra-articular abnormalities.[94,108,419,607,637,643] Aside from allowing direct visualization of the cartilage surfaces, synovial tissue, and particularly the interosseous ligaments, under bright illumination and magnification, arthroscopy has proved to be a useful adjunct in the management of both acute and chronic lesions of the interosseous ligaments.

Both the radiocarpal and midcarpal spaces must be evaluated arthroscopically when carpal instability is suspected. Wrist arthroscopy is not considered complete if the midcarpal space has not been examined, particularly when carpal instability is a potential diagnosis.

The proximal fibrocartilaginous portion of the SL and LTq joints (hereafter referred to as SL and LTq membranes) should have a concave appearance, as seen from the radiocarpal space (Fig. 14-19). The SL membrane is best seen from the radiocarpal space in the 3-4 portal. The LTq membrane is usually best visualized with the arthroscope in the 4-5 or 6-R portals because of the oblique relationship within the proximal carpal row, particularly in small wrists (Fig. 14-20).

In the midcarpal space, the SL interval should be tight and congruent without stepoff (Fig. 14-21). Similarly, the LTq interval should be congruent. While occasionally a 1-mm stepoff, which is normal, is seen from the midcarpal space, there is normally slight motion between the lunate and triquetrum visualized from the midcarpal space, which is not seen between the scaphoid and lunate (Fig. 14-22).

When the interosseous membranes are injured, the normal concave appearance between the carpal bones becomes

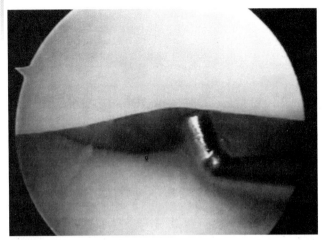

FIGURE 14-19. Arthroscopic view of the normal concave appearance of the SL proximal membrane as seen from the radiocarpal space with the arthroscope in the 3-4 portal.

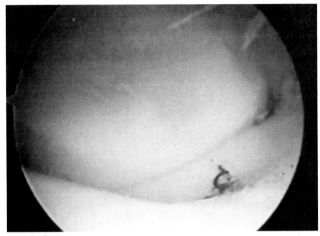

FIGURE 14-22. Arthroscopic view of the normal LTq interval as seen from the midcarpal space with the arthroscope in the radial midcarpal portal.

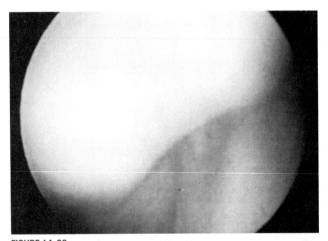

FIGURE 14-20. Arthroscopic view of the normal concave appearance of the LTq proximal membrane as seen from the radiocarpal space with the arthroscope in the 6-R portal.

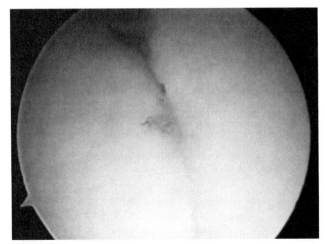

FIGURE 14-21. Arthroscopic view of the tight congruent SL interval as seen from the midcarpal space with the arthroscope in the radial midcarpal portal.

convex. The torn membrane hangs down and blocks visualization with the arthroscope in the radiocarpal space. The degree of rotation of the carpal bones and any abnormal motion are best appreciated from the unrestricted view available in the midcarpal space.

A limited type of intraoperative arthrogram (poor man's arthrogram) may be performed for the evaluation of carpal instability. After the radiocarpal space has been examined, the inflow cannula, which is usually in the 6-U portal, is left in the radiocarpal space. An 18-gauge needle is then placed in either the radial or ulnar midcarpal portal. A tear of the interosseous membrane is suspected if a free flow of irrigation fluid is seen through the needle.

CARPAL INSTABILITY

Definition

Injuries to the wrist resulting in sporadic or permanent carpal malalignment have long been recognized in the medical literature.[127,128,589] The term *instability,* however, was not used until 1967 by Dobyns and Perkins.[132] The landmark papers by Fisk[162] and Linscheid and coworkers[325] helped popularize this term. The true meaning of it, however, has been controversial.[18,263]

Initially, the term *instability* was considered synonymous with *malalignment.*[111,308,325,478] A wrist was said to be unstable when there was a substantial alteration in the sagittal and/or frontal alignment of the carpal bones beyond the limits of what was considered normal. From that viewpoint, instability could always be diagnosed using plain radiographs.[131,201]

Such a concept of instability, however, was soon criticized by different authors,[500,670] who claimed that an alteration of the carpal alignment cannot always be considered pathologic. Congenital hyperlax wrists, for instance, often appear grossly malaligned, yet they frequently remain asymptomatic, are able to handle most activities of daily living, and seldom require treatment. Other wrists, by contrast, remain asymptomatic most of the time, are well aligned, are able to sustain physiologic loads, and become painful only when performing specific tasks (e.g., opening a jar, lifting heavy objects). It is obvious, therefore, that the term *instability* cannot be used as a synonym for *malalignment*.[174]

From a biomechanical point of view, *stability* is defined as the ability of a joint to maintain a normal balance between the articulating bones under physiologic loads throughout its range of motion.[18,75,174,176] According to this definition, a wrist joint should be considered unstable when it is not capable of preserving a normal kinematic and kinetic relationship between the radius, carpal bones, and metacarpals. Hence, stability implies both the ability to transfer functional loads without yielding or losing its internal joint congruency[57,173,558] and the capacity to maintain motion throughout its range without sudden alterations of intercarpal alignment.[290,479]

When a stable wrist is progressively loaded, the joint contact forces should increase smoothly and synchronously, without unexpected changes in direction, magnitude, or location of contact.[600] When a stable wrist moves, no sudden changes in carpal alignment should appear throughout the entire range of motion.[478] Consequently, the term *instability* should be associated not only with the concept of abnormal transfer of loads (dyskinetics) but also with the concept of abnormal motion (dyskinematics).[18,75,174,176]

From this point of view, a grossly malaligned wrist with degeneration of the articular cartilages may be able to bear substantial loads[146]; however, because it cannot experience smooth, painless motion without producing sudden changes of stress on specific areas of cartilage,[596] it fulfills the criteria of a true carpal instability. Similarly, a wrist with a ligament disruption may have a completely normal carpal alignment when unloaded; however, if it is incapable of sustaining functional stress without experiencing abrupt changes in the alignment of the carpal bones, it must be regarded as an unstable wrist.

Based on this definition, carpal instability may result from a wide spectrum of injuries or diseases. Congenital anomalies such as Madelung's deformity,[242,433] scaphoid hypoplasia,[579] or carpal synostosis[213,532] may create abnormal conditions of carpal instability that eventually require specific treatment. Similarly, avascular necrosis,[314,408] infections,[393] inflammatory arthritis,[531] or any other process modifying the shape of the carpal bones may also alter the

necessary interaction between carpal bones and result in instability. Management of these nontraumatic carpal instabilities is discussed elsewhere. This chapter covers only trauma-related carpal instabilities.

Classification

Carpal instability is a syndrome difficult to classify.[212,486] Many diverse clinical conditions may result in an unstable wrist for which different classifications have been suggested.[12,108,212,314,325,546,559,620] Some are based on the location of the major ligamentous injury.[314,559] Others emphasize the direction of the abnormal alignment.[325] Others classify instability according to its severity.[320,620] Unfortunately, none of these classifications is exhaustive to allow categorization of all types of carpal instability yet simple enough to be easily remembered and used clinically.

It is our opinion that the controversy about which classification is best is meaningless, because none can be ideal. Instead, more effort should be spent in providing tools to help the clinician interpret the particular features of each individual case. With this in mind, Larsen and coworkers[237,302] developed an analytical scheme that appears useful in the diagnosis of carpal instability. According to this scheme, to characterize any carpal instability, the following six features need to be investigated (Table 14-2):

1. *Chronicity:* Traditionally, ligament injuries have been classified depending on the time elapsed from injury to diagnosis into three categories: acute, subacute, and chronic. When the injury is diagnosed soon after the accident (acute injury), the ligament healing potential is likely to be optimal. Between 1 and 6 weeks (subacute injury), the deformity is still easily reducible, but the ligaments may have reduced healing potential owing to retraction and/or necrosis of ligament remnants. After 6 weeks (chronic cases), the possibility of achieving an acceptable reduction and primary ligament healing, although possible,[305] is very unlikely. The exception would be ligament avulsions. There are instances where the ligament is detached, but not ruptured, and remains capable of being repaired, with good healing potential,

Table 14-2
ANALYSIS OF CARPAL INSTABILITY

Category I Chronicity	Category II Constancy	Category III Etiology	Category IV Location	Category V Direction	Category VI Pattern
Acute < 1 week (Maximum primary healing potential)	Predynamic Dynamic Static reducible	Congenital Traumatic Inflammatory	Radiocarpal Proximal intercarpal Midcarpal	VISI rotation DISI rotation Ulnar translation	Carpal instability dissociative (CID)
Subacute 1-6 weeks (some healing potential)	Static irreducible	Neoplastic Iatrogenic Miscellaneous	Distal intercarpal Carpometacarpal Specific bones	Carpal instability Dorsal translation Other	Carpal instability non-dissociative (CIND)
Chronic					Carpal instability complex (CIC)
>6 weeks (little healing potential)					Carpal instability adaptive (CIA)

Modified from Larsen CF, Amadio PC, Gilula LA, Hodge JC: Analysis of carpal instability: I. Description of the scheme. J Hand Surg [Am] 20:757-764, 1995, with permission.

beyond the time limit expressed for mid-substance ligament ruptures. In short, it is not the time from injury itself that counts but the fact that time implies a progressive loss of the healing potential of the damaged ligaments.

2. *Severity:* Any carpal instability can be analyzed according to the severity of the resulting subluxation. If carpal malalignment appears only under high stress in specific wrist positions, the case is less severe than if it is permanently present. Based on this, three groups of conditions exist: (1) predynamic instabilities (partial ligament tears with no malalignment under stress), (2) dynamic instabilities (complete ruptures exhibiting carpal malalignment only under certain loading conditions), and (3) static instabilities (complete ruptures with permanent alteration of the carpal alignment).[620]

3. *Etiology:* Most instability problems are caused by trauma. However, certain diseases may also be responsible for a similar type of disorder.[134,393,456,531] In trauma cases, especially if diagnosed early, good repair of the ruptured ligaments can be obtained. By contrast, if ligament rupture results from rheumatoid arthritis, normal healing is unlikely.

4. *Location:* It is important to investigate the location of major dysfunction. This may or may not coincide with the location of the initial injury. Also important is to review whether there is a single problem affecting only one joint or a multilevel dysfunction exists.

5. *Direction:* When present, the magnitude and direction of the carpal malalignment needs to be monitored. Several patterns of carpal malalignment have been recognized[9,131,301,326]; the most common are: (a) dorsal intercalated segment instability (DISI), when the lunate, regarded as an intercalated segment, appears abnormally extended relative to its proximal and distal links; (b) volar intercalated segment instability (VISI), when the lunate appears abnormally flexed; (c) ulnar translocation, when a portion of or the entire proximal row is (or can be passively) displaced ulnarly beyond normal limits; (d) radial translocation, when the proximal row can be passively displaced radially beyond normal, and (e) dorsal translocation, when the carpal condyle, often as a result of a dorsally malunited fracture of the radius, is or can be passively subluxed or dislocated in a dorsal direction (see Fig. 14-5).

6. *Pattern:* There are four major patterns of carpal instability[12,108,324,658]: (a) carpal instability dissociative (CID), when there is a major derangement (fracture and/or ligament avulsion) within or between bones of the same carpal row; (b) carpal instability nondissociative (CIND), when no disruption exists between bones of the same row, yet there is dysfunction between the radius and the proximal row and/or between the proximal and distal rows; (c) carpal instability complex (CIC), when there are features of both CID and CIND types; and (d) carpal instability adaptive (CIA), where the reason for the malalignment is not located within the wrist but proximal or distal to it.

Perilunate dislocations are a good example of a complex (CIC) pattern, as in them coexists a ligament injury at both radiocarpal and intercarpal levels, often resulting in SL and/or LTq dissociation and an ulnar translation of the lunate. The carpal malalignment often seen as an adaptation of an otherwise normal carpus to a malunited distal radius fracture is a good example of a CIA pattern.[567]

CARPAL INSTABILITY DISSOCIATIVE

When a carpal instability is caused by disease or injury resulting in a major malfunction of a joint between bones of the same row, the case is classified as a carpal instability dissociative (CID).[12,108] Dissociative instabilities are common and may result from a variety of conditions, including SLDs, LTq dissociations, unstable scaphoid fractures, nonunions, or malunions, and advanced Kienböck's disease.

Scapholunate Dissociation

The term *scapholunate dissociation* has long been utilized to describe the symptomatic dysfunction that results from rupture of the mechanical linkage between the scaphoid and lunate, with or without carpal malalignment. Despite the fact that the condition was first discussed by Destot,[127,128] and published repeated times as case reports,[24,86,117,132,483,589] it was not until 1972 that the clinical features of SLD were broadly publicized by Linscheid and associates.[325] SLD is probably the most frequent CID problem and may appear either as an isolated injury or associated with other local injuries, such as distal radial fractures[189,367,386,485,613,652] or displaced scaphoid fractures.[52,254,589,595] Although the condition is commonly found among adults, it has also been well documented in skeletally immature wrists.[104,123,672]

Not infrequently, the term *rotary subluxation of the scaphoid* (RSS) has been used as a synonym of SLD.[55,177,620] This is not always appropriate. RSS should be used to describe only those cases in an advanced stage of the injury, in which the ligaments attached to both ends of the scaphoid have failed and the bone has collapsed into flexion and pronation. In less advanced cases, in which only the proximal ligaments are disrupted, the scaphoid may remain normally attached to the distal row preventing a rotatory collapse of the bone.[320] In between the two extremes, there is a broad spectrum of pathology that may or may not exhibit carpal malalignment.[620]

Pathomechanics

As stated earlier, most SLDs are the first stage of progressive carpal destabilization around the lunate, resulting from an indirect mechanism of injury involving wrist hyperextension, ulnar deviation, and midcarpal supination.[344,346,347] There is a spectrum of injuries, from minor SL sprains to complete perilunar dislocations, all being different stages of the same progressive perilunar destabilization process.

The kinematic and kinetic consequences of the loss of the SL ligaments have been investigated by different authors.[57,71,290,354,478,524,525,604] If only the palmar SL ligament and the proximal membrane are sectioned, only minor kinematic alterations are created (predynamic instability).[290,478] These may be sufficient to promote a symptomatic synovitis and require medical attention.

Complete sectioning of the SL membrane and ligaments in cadaver specimens results in substantial alterations of both kinematic and force transmission parameters but not necessarily a permanent carpal malalignment.[57,290,478,604] The scaphoid becomes proximally unconstrained and RS motion increases, whereas RL motion decreases.

Permanent carpal malalignment has never been observed unless there is a concomitant failure of the secondary scaphoid stabilizers, namely the palmar-distal STT and SC ligaments.[342,524] This may occur either acutely, as a result of the hyperextension stress, or secondarily, as a progressive stretching of these structures. In such conditions, the loaded lunate and triquetrum rotate into an abnormal extension (DISI), supination, and radial deviation, while the scaphoid rotates around the RSC ligament into an abnormal flexion, ulnar deviation, and pronation posture (Fig. 14-23).[290,564,604]

The reason for these bones to dissociate in such consistent directions remains controversial.[173,217,279] According to Kauer,[278] the unconstrained lunate has a natural tendency toward displacing into extension owing to its palmar wedge-shaped configuration. Watson and coworkers,[625] however, found that 23% of examined lunates had a reversed dorsal wedge-shaped configuration and suggested that in those cases SLD would induce a VISI rather than a DISI deformity. Weber,[630] by contrast, believes that, once free from the scaphoid influence, the lunate tends to follow the triquetrum toward extension under the influence of the helicoidally shaped TqH joint surfaces.

When the SL joint has been completely dissociated, with the proximal pole of the scaphoid being subluxed dorsoradially, the forces crossing the wrist cannot be distributed normally. An increased compressive and shear stress appears on the dorsal and lateral aspect of the RS fossa,[57,71,604] a

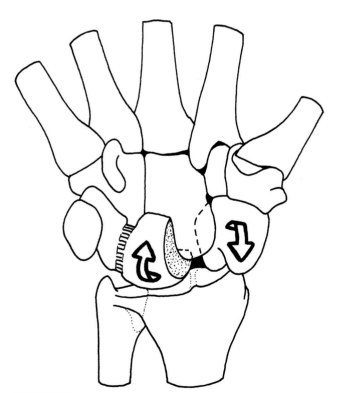

FIGURE 14-23. Schematic representation of the typical displacements that occur in static SLDs. The scaphoid tends to rotate into flexion and slight pronation, whereas the unconstrained triquetrum and lunate supinate and extend into a DISI pattern of malalignment.

situation that Watson and associates[616,621] compared with two spoons sitting one on the other while the handles are not aligned. Such peripheral contact may explain the frequent development of long-term degenerative changes at the dorsolateral edge of the RS joint. The lunate, by contrast, appears rotated into extension but still in contact with normal cartilage thanks to the constraining action of the short RL ligament. This may explain why the RL joint seldom is affected by the degeneration process. The term *scapholunate advanced collapse* (SLAC) has been proposed by Watson and Ballet[616] to refer to the clinical condition in which there has been a progression of degenerative changes from an isolated radial styloid-scaphoid impingement (stage 1), to complete RS osteoarthritis (stage 2) or even midcarpal arthritis (stage 3).

Clinical Forms

Owing to the progression of perilunate destabilization and joint degeneration that follows the untreated instability, different clinical forms of SLD have been recognized.[403,624,652] Depending on the degree of ligament rupture, their healing potential, reducibility, and the presence or absence of cartilage defects, five clinical forms of SLD exist.

Predynamic SLD

When the SL membrane is only stretched or partially ruptured, the resulting instability is called predynamic[620] or also occult.[403] The degree of SL ligament incompetence varies from a minimal distention (grade I, according to Geissler and colleagues' classification[189]) to a partial rupture of the proximal membrane without gross instability (grades II or III) (Table 14-3). At this stage, wrists do not exhibit malalignment nor may any form of stress radiographically show a substantially increased widening of the SL joint space. Dysfunction basically derives from an increased motion between the two bones, generating shear stress, hence the local synovitis, pain, and discomfort.

Dynamic SLD

This clinical form of SLD is characterized by (1) complete disruption of all SL connections including the dorsal ligament, (2) the ligaments are still reparable, not yet retracted or necrotic, with good healing potential, (3) the secondary distal scaphoid stabilizers[524] are still intact or only minimally insufficient, and (4) no cartilage damage, traumatic or degenerative, exists. No permanent malalignment exists at this stage; only under specific loading conditions an increased SL gap may appear. Yet, the wrist may yield or give way when attempting specific tasks in specific wrist positions.[290,478,604] Arthroscopically, gross instability may be observed by displacing the carpal bones with the probe. In Geissler's grade IV, the arthroscope inserted into the radiocarpal joint may be passed through the gap between carpals and allow visualization of the midcarpal joint (see Table 14-3).

Static Reducible SLD

The third, more evolved clinical form is when the injury has not been solved in the acute phase. In many cases, the ligament remnants may have degenerated to a point that cannot be repaired. The resultant malalignment, owing to failure of the secondary stabilizers, is permanent (static

Table 14-3

ARTHROSCOPIC CLASSIFICATION OF CARPAL INTEROSSEOUS LIGAMENT TEARS

Grade	Description
I	Attenuation/hemorrhage of interosseous ligament as seen from the radiocarpal joint. There is no incongruency of carpal alignment in the midcarpal space.
II	Attenuation/hemorrhage of interosseous ligament as seen from the radiocarpal joint. Incongruency/stepoff as seen from midcarpal space. A slight gap (less than the width of a probe) between carpals may be present.
III	Incongruency/stepoff of carpal alignment is seen in both the radiocarpal and midcarpal space. The probe may be passed through the gap between carpals.
IV	Incongruency/stepoff of carpal alignment is seen in both the radiocarpal and midcarpal space. Gross instability with manipulation is noted. A 2.7-mm arthroscope may be passed through the gap between the carpals.

Data from Geissler WB, Freeland AE, Savoie FH, et al: Intracarpal soft tissue lesions associated with an intra-articular fracture of the distal end of the radius. J Bone Joint Surg Am 78:357-365, 1996.

instability) but reducible, and no cartilage defect has appeared yet. Snapping due to self-reduction of the subluxation is a quite common finding.[264]

Static Fixed SLD

Chronic rupture or insufficiency of both primary and secondary SL ligament stabilizers may result in the formation of fibrosis within the surrounding capsule and spaces that appear between the scaphoid and surrounding bones. In such instances carpal malalignment is hardly reducible. If there is no substantial cartilage degeneration, the case fulfills the criteria of static fixed SLD.

Osteoarthritis Secondary to SLD (SLAC Wrist)

Long-lasting carpal malalignment with irreducible subluxation of the scaphoid induces degenerative osteoarthritis that obviously cannot be treated the same as when the cartilage still is in an acceptable condition. It is the so-called SLAC wrist, the treatment of which consists of relieving pain and accepting some functional loss.

Diagnosis

SLD is frequently missed at presentation, especially when the injury is isolated (predynamic or dynamic) or masked by other more obvious injuries.[91,275,564] However, when SLD is static or results from a perilunate dislocation, the problem is more often recognized.[164]

A history of a fall on the outstretched hand should warn the clinician about the possibility of a SL injury, even if there is a distal radial fracture[189,386] or a scaphoid fracture.[52,591] In fact, a substantial amount of distal radial fractures (30% according to Geissler and colleagues[189]) are associated with variable degrees of carpal ligament disrup-

tions. Aside from wrist trauma, SLD may also result from a fall on the elbow,[380] an excessive capsular excision when removing dorsal ganglia,[114,139] joint deterioration in different rheumatoid and congenital diseases,[134,433,456,531] and infection.[393] In children, although SLD is very uncommon, the diagnosis is even more difficult.[104,123,196,672] A high index of suspicion is recommended in order not to miss this injury.

The symptoms of SLD vary markedly, depending on the magnitude and extent of the associated injuries, as well as on the time since the accident.[320] Weakness of grasp, limited motion, dorsoradial swelling, and point tenderness over the dorsal aspect of the SL interval are frequent findings.[209,308,477,564] Pain is common and may be aggravated by heavy use, sometimes coinciding with a snapping or clicking sensation with movement.[264]

Physical Examination

The external appearance of SL instabilities may not be particularly dramatic. Even in the acute phase, swelling may be moderate. Palpation for areas of maximal tenderness is one of the most useful tools in the diagnosis of wrist pathology, especially in patients with chronic SL instability.[91,563] By flexing the wrist and palpating the dorsum of the capsule distal to Lister's tubercle, one can obtain important information about the SL joint. If sharp pain is elicited by pressing this area, the probability of either a recent injury or a chronic localized synovitis is high.[615] Most of these patients also have tenderness in the anatomical snuffbox and over the palmar scaphoid tuberosity.[209] In acute cases range of motion is usually limited by pain, whereas it may be normal in chronic cases.

Scaphoid Shift Test. Passive mobilization of the dysfunctional SL joint is valuable not only in determining the presence of abnormal RS subluxation but also in reproducing the patient's pain. A positive scaphoid shift test, as described by Watson and associates,[615] is said to be diagnostic of SLD (Fig. 14-24). The examiner places four fingers behind the radius. The thumb is placed on the tuberosity (distal pole) of the scaphoid, and the other hand is used to move the wrist passively from ulnar to radial deviation. In ulnar deviation, the scaphoid is extended and assumes a position more in line with the forearm. In radial deviation, the scaphoid is flexed. Pressure on the tuberosity while the wrist is moved from ulnar deviation to radial deviation prevents the scaphoid from flexing. In such circumstances, if the SL ligaments are completely insufficient or torn, the proximal pole will subluxate dorsally out of the radius, inducing pain on the dorsoradial aspect of the wrist. When pressure is released, a typical snapping may occur, indicating self-reduction of the scaphoid over the dorsal rim of the radius. When performing the scaphoid shift test, however, one should be aware of its low specificity.[653,655] Indeed, if the SL ligaments are intact but there are other local problems inducing local synovitis (occult ganglion or dorsal RS impingement), this test may also provoke sharp pain, and it is difficult to discern whether there is an abnormally subluxable proximal scaphoid. Comparison of the two sides is important, although sometimes the opposite "asymptomatic" wrist has a painful scaphoid shift test as well.[141,653] Experience with this test is necessary before it can be evaluated with confidence.

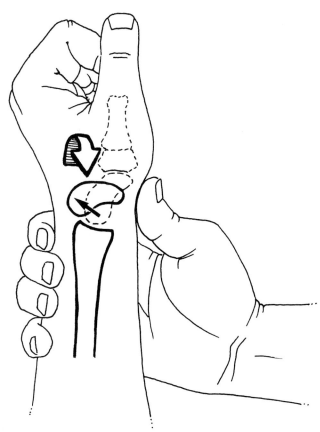

FIGURE 14-24. Watson's[615] scaphoid shift test. Firm pressure is applied to the palmar tuberosity of the scaphoid while the wrist is moved from ulnar to radial deviation *(white arrow)*. In normal wrists, the scaphoid cannot flex because of the external pressure by the examiner's thumb. This may produce pain on the dorsal aspect of the SL interval owing to synovial irritation. A "positive" test is seen in a patient with an SL tear or in lax patients; the scaphoid is no longer constrained proximally and will subluxate out of the scaphoid fossa *(black arrow)*. When pressure on the scaphoid is removed, the scaphoid goes back into position, and a typical snapping occurs.

Resisted Finger Extension Test. The ability of the proximal pole of the scaphoid to carry load without producing pain can be explored by asking the patient to fully extend the index and middle fingers against resistance with the wrist partially flexed.[653] In the presence of an injury or insufficiency of the dorsal SL ligament, sharp pain is elicited at the SL area. Again, this maneuver is not specific but is quite sensitive.

Scapholunate Ballottement Test. The lunate is firmly stabilized with the thumb and index finger of one hand while the scaphoid, held with the other hand (thumb on the palmar tuberosity and index on the dorsal proximal pole), is displaced dorsally and palmarly with the other hand. A positive result elicits pain, crepitus, and excessive displaceability of the joint.

Radiographic Examination

SLD can be suspected by the presence of one or more of the following radiographic features on standard radiographs. Dynamic instabilities require special projections or loading conditions for these features to be observed.

1. *Increased SL joint space.* The so-called Terry Thomas sign[167] (named after the famous English film comedian's dental diastema) is considered positive when the space between the scaphoid and lunate appears abnormally widened as compared with the contralateral side (Fig. 14-25). The SL gap should be measured in the middle of the flat medial facet of the scaphoid.[281,501] Any asymmetrical SL gap greater than 5 mm is said to be diagnostic of SLD, although controversy exists about the value of this parameter.[85,356] If there is no history of a specific traumatic episode, either recent or remote, and yet there is obvious SL diastasis, one must consider either a congenitally increased SL gap (probably bilateral) with or without hyperlax ligaments[500,586] or other less common causes of SLD, including rheumatoid arthritis,[455,531] gout, and calcium pyrophosphate deposition disease.[134,456,511]

2. *"Scaphoid ring" sign.* When the scaphoid has collapsed into flexion (RS subluxation), it has a foreshortened appearance in the AP view. In such circumstances, the scaphoid tuberosity is projected in the coronal plane in the form of a radiodense circle or ring over the distal two thirds of the scaphoid (see Fig. 14-25). This so-called ring sign is present in all cases in which the scaphoid is abnormally flexed, regardless of the cause.[85,262,477,562] The presence of this sign, therefore, does not always indicate SLD, nor does its absence eliminate the possibility of this problem.

3. *"Ring pole" sign.* Blatt[54] noted that in cases of RS subluxation resulting from SLD or any other cause, the shortest distance from the ring sign to the proximal pole of scaphoid is reduced in comparison with the opposite wrist.[85]

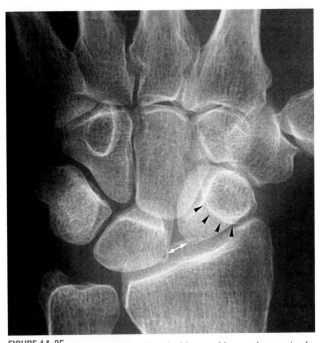

FIGURE 14-25. PA view of the wrist of a 35-year-old man who sustained a hyperextension injury 4 months before seeking medical attention. Note the foreshortened scaphoid with the ring sign *(black arrows)*, representing the frontal projection of the palmar tuberosity, and the increased SL joint space *(white arrow)*, indicating the presence of an SLD with rotatory subluxation of the scaphoid.

4. *Lack of parallelism.* In the normal wrist, when the SL joint is carefully profiled by orienting the x-ray beam properly, the two apposing articular surfaces are flat and parallel.[36,111,372,647] Lack of parallelism in a patient with other supporting findings may indicate the presence of SLD.

5. *Increased SL angle.* In the lateral view, when the scaphoid lies more perpendicular to the long axis of the radius and the lunate appears normally aligned or abnormally extended (DISI), SLD should be suspected (Fig. 14-26).[201,325] In such circumstances, the SL angle is greater than its usual 45 to 60 degrees, with higher angles being seen when there is an accompanying DISI.

6. *Taleisnik's "V" sign.* In the lateral view of a normal wrist, a wide "C"-shaped line can be drawn by uniting the palmar margins of the scaphoid and radius.[559] When the scaphoid is abnormally flexed, the palmar outline of the scaphoid intersects the palmar margin of the radial styloid at an acute angle, forming a sharper, "V"-shaped pattern.

Cineradiography. Even in static SLD, in which the diagnosis can be made on standard radiographs, obtaining further information using cineradiographs is recommended.[264,409,448] They show not only abnormal movement between the scaphoid and lunate but also substantial changes in the movement of the midcarpal joint. For example, the hamate-triquetrum relationship normally changes from full engagement in ulnar deviation to complete disengagement in radial deviation; in SLD patients, this joint remains permanently engaged.[562]

Arthrography. Arthrography may be useful in further defining partial tears of the SL ligaments, as well as in discovering other local problems such as radiocarpal septa, osteochondral defects, or capsular ligament ruptures.[172,632,633] When interpreting arthrograms, however, care must be taken not to confuse degenerative perforations of the central portion of the SL membrane with true ligament ruptures.[356] One must also be aware that arthrographic abnormalities are bilateral in a high percentage of patients, with only one side being symptomatic.[226] Because of these limitations, the use of arthrography has diminished substantially in favor of arthroscopy.[105,607,637]

Arthroscopy. Regarded by most authors as the gold standard technique in the diagnosis of intracarpal derangements, arthroscopy has also been found useful in describing the degree of injury to the interosseous ligaments. The box on page 560 provides some technical tips for a correct arthroscopic diagnosis of SLD dissociation.

According to Geissler and coworkers (see Table 14-3), in grade I injuries, there is loss of the normal concave appearance of the proximal membrane between the scaphoid and lunate.[189] The interosseous structure bulges with a convex appearance as the membrane has become attenuated. (Fig. 14-27). Evaluation from the midcarpal space, however, shows the carpal bones still to be congruent without any increased gap or stepoff. These mild grade I injuries usually resolve with a short period of immobilization. In grade II injuries the interosseous membrane bulges similar in appearance to grade I injuries, as seen from the radiocarpal space. However, in the midcarpal space the involved carpal bones are no longer congruent (Fig. 14-28). In a grade II SL interosseous ligament injury, slight palmar flexion of the scaphoid is observed from the midcarpal space. The dorsal edge of the scaphoid is now palmarly flexed and no longer congruent with the lunate. In grade III injuries, the interosseous space starts to separate and a gap is seen between the involved carpals both from the radiocarpal and midcarpal spaces (Fig. 14-29). A 1-mm probe may be

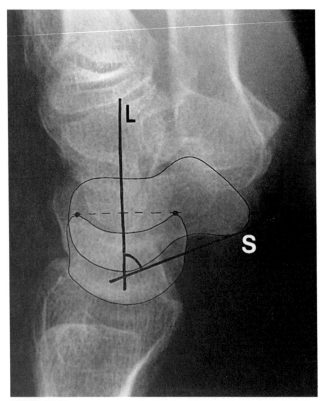

FIGURE 14-26. Lateral view of the same patient as in Figure 14-25. The outlined scaphoid appears abnormally flexed, resulting in an increased SL angle despite the normal alignment of the lunate relative to the radius. S, scaphoid axis; L, lunate axis.

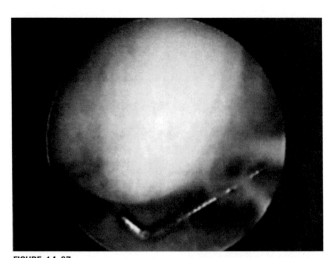

FIGURE 14-27. Arthroscopic view of a Geissler grade I SL interosseous ligament injury as seen from the radiocarpal space with the arthroscope in the 3-4 portal. Note the bulging convex appearance of the ligament. The ligament is attenuated and has stretched, but no gap exists between the carpal bones.

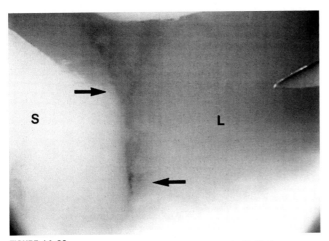

FIGURE 14-28. Arthroscopic view of a Geissler grade II SL interosseous ligament injury as seen from the midcarpal space with the arthroscope in the radial midcarpal portal. Note the palmar flexion of the dorsal edge of the scaphoid and the carpals are no longer congruent *(arrows)*. S, scaphoid; L, lunate.

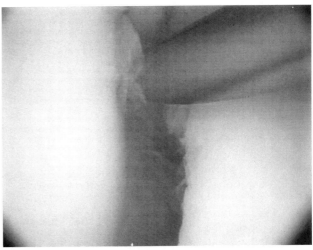

FIGURE 14-30. Arthroscopic view of a Geissler grade III SL interosseous ligament injury as seen from the midcarpal space with the arthroscope in the radial midcarpal portal. Note the SL interval can be opened by twisting the probe. The joint is obviously incongruent *(arrows)*. S, scaphoid; L, lunate.

passed and twisted through the interosseous ligament tear between the involved carpal bones (Fig. 14-30). A portion of the interosseous ligament is still intact. In grade IV injuries, the interosseous membrane and both palmar and dorsal SL ligaments are completely torn and/or detached. A 2.7-mm arthroscope may be passed freely from the midcarpal space to the radial carpal space between the involved carpals (Fig. 14-31).

Treatment

Treatment of SLD is difficult, not always predictable, and seldom entirely satisfactory.[131,324,424] A number of factors may explain this. When the initial injury is a partial SL ligament derangement, it often exhibits normal radiographs for it is frequently missed at presentation. But even if diagnosed early, the ligament remnants are short, making difficult their repair. On the other hand, because these ligaments

are exposed to considerable tensions and torsions, it is not unusual to find successful repairs to deteriorate with time. Certainly, there is no guarantee for an early diagnosed and properly treated SL ligament injury to regain good functional strength and adequate stabilizing capability.

Most commonly, the SLD is discovered when the derangement is evident on plain radiographs. This occurs because the progressive instability has deteriorated the secondary stabilizers, particularly the palmar-distal connections of the scaphoid to the distal row. At this stage, the underlying pathology no longer involves one single structure but consists of a complex multilevel ligament injury, with some ligament remnants retracted or necrotic while others are stretched out, becoming insufficient to stabilize the joint.

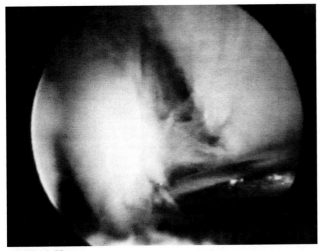

FIGURE 14-29. Arthroscopic view of a Geissler grade III SL interosseous ligament injury as seen from the radiocarpal space with the arthroscope in the 3-4 portal. In grade III SLDs the SL interosseous membrane starts to tear from palmar to dorsal and a gap is seen between the carpal bones. The dorsal SL ligament is still intact.

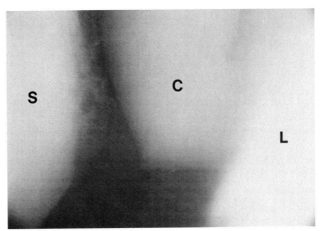

FIGURE 14-31. Arthroscopic view of a Geissler grade IV SL interosseous ligament injury as seen from the radiocarpal space with the arthroscope in the 3-4 portal. The arthroscope can be easily passed between the scaphoid and lunate through the gap. Note the head of the capitate is seen between the carpals. S, scaphoid; L, lunate; C, capitate.

CRITICAL POINTS: DIAGNOSTIC ARTHROSCOPY OF SCAPHOLUNATE DISSOCIATIONS

TECHNICAL POINTS

- After adequate anesthesia, suspend the wrist in a traction tower (4 to 5 kg of traction).
- Pad the traction tower so that the skin of the forearm does not make contact with the tower. This is particularly important if the tower has been used repeatedly throughout the day, because it may retain heat from the stabilization process and could potentially cause a burn to the skin.
- Provide inflow through the 6-U portal, and introduce the arthroscope with a blunt trocar through the 3-4 portal. This is the most ideal portal for visualization of the SL interosseous ligament.
- Make a working 4-5 or 6-R portal, and evaluate the wrist systemically with a probe from radial to ulnar.
- Débride torn fibers of the SL interosseous ligament with the arthroscope in the 6-R portal and insert a shaver in the 3-4 portal.
- Evaluate the SL interval with the probe. Occasionally a gap exists, but it is not initially visualized until the scaphoid and/or lunate are pushed away from each other (Fig. 14-32).
- Place the arthroscope in the radial midcarpal portal, and evaluate the SL interval from the midcarpal space. Close attention is paid to any rotational displacement of the scaphoid with the dorsal lip being rotated distally to that of the lunate. Also, any gap where either the probe or arthroscope can be passed is identified.
- A probe or a needle is inserted through the ulnar midcarpal portal to palpate the SL interval. This also improves visualization.

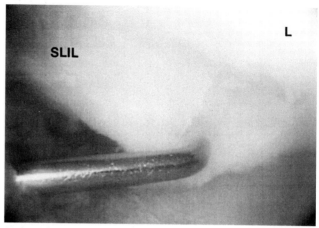

FIGURE 14-32. Arthroscopic view of a partial tear of the SL interosseous ligament as seen from the radiocarpal space with the arthroscope in the 6-R portal. The tear was not readily identifiable until palpated with a probe.

Furthermore, if substantial time has elapsed from the initial injury, degenerative arthritis secondary to wrist malfunction may have appeared, making even more difficult an acceptable outcome. Certainly, treating the injury in the acute phase, when at its best in healing potential, is always more rewarding than having to deal with old unsolved injuries. Indeed, the need for a high index of suspicion in the earliest stage of the disease will never be overemphasized.

In this section, the treatment alternatives proposed for the different clinical forms of SLD are discussed. Patient selection is very important when deciding which treatment is most appropriate. The patient's age, occupation, recreational demands, and level of symptoms must all be considered.

Predynamic (Occult) Scapholunate Dissociation

As stated earlier, an SLD is considered predynamic or occult when the SL ligament injury is not complete, with a normal radiographic appearance throughout the entire range of motion or under stress. The most frequent scenario involves a disruption of the palmar and proximal connections of the SL joint but not the dorsal ligament. Occasionally, the dorsal ligament may have failed first, the palmar ligament retaining some stability to the joint. In both circumstances, a painful dysfunction due to increased shear stress at the SL level may appear. Arthrography may suggest this diagnosis, but most commonly this is made arthroscopically. If the condition is diagnosed in the acute phase, when the healing potential of the disrupted ligaments is at its best, a percutaneous or arthroscopically guided Kirschner wire fixation is recommended. In the chronic predynamic instability, three different approaches have been proposed: (1) proprioception reeducation of the flexor carpi radialis muscle, (2) arthroscopic débridement alone of the torn ligament edges, and (3) electrothermal ligament shrinkage.

Percutaneous Kirschner Wire Fixation of the SL Joint. For acute partial ruptures of the SL ligaments without carpal malalignment, pinning the joint with Kirschner wires may obtain good ligament healing and excellent results.[320,417,560] Image intensification may help to obtain correct alignment of the scaphoid and the lunate. Reduction of the displaced bones can be facilitated by placing two Kirschner wires percutaneously into the dorsal aspects of both scaphoid and lunate to be used as "joysticks" to facilitate reduction. If there is no soft tissue interposition, by pulling the scaphoid wire proximally and ulnarly while the lunate wire is directed distally and radially, the slight displacement may be reduced. A small incision is then made distal to the radial styloid, and blunt dissection is continued with a hemostat so that a soft tissue protector can be placed directly on the scaphoid to avoid injury to the dorsal sensory branches of the radial nerve. Two or more 1.2-mm Kirschner wires are inserted across the SL joint to keep the two bones together during the ligament healing process. To ensure maximal stability, some authors recommend transfixing the SC joint with an additional wire.[417] The wrist is immobilized in a below-elbow cast, and the pin tracts are evaluated every 2 weeks. The wires are usually left in place for 8 to 10 weeks with protection in a removable splint for an additional 4 weeks after motion is begun. Physical therapy for range-of-motion exercises of the fingers is initiated immediately. Range of motion and grip strength of the wrist is begun at 3 months. Strenuous activities are discouraged for the first 6 months.[320]

Arthroscopically Guided Kirschner Wire Fixation of the SL Joint. To improve the quality of the reduction and pin fixation, many authors have suggested direct arthroscopic visualization as an adjuvant technique in Geissler's grade II and III stages of SLD.[480,643] The arthroscope is placed in the 3-4 portal. The Kirschner wires are inserted using a soft tissue protector through the anatomical snuffbox as indicated earlier. The wire can be seen as it enters into the scaphoid with the arthroscope looking down the radial gutter. The goal is to aim the guide wire through the scaphoid into the lunate. By using a skin marker, a line can be drawn on the dorsum of the hand from the proposed location of the lunate and scaphoid. This can help align the pin as it is inserted through the scaphoid into the lunate. In an alternative and easier technique, the wrist can be taken out of traction and under fluoroscopic control the surgeon can then begin inserting the Kirschner wire into the scaphoid aiming toward the lunate. The arthroscope is placed in the ulnar midcarpal portal as the Kirschner wire has been started in the scaphoid. Rotation is best judged in the wrist by looking across the wrist. A probe may be inserted through the radial midcarpal space to control the palmar flexion of the scaphoid. Occasionally, Kirschner wire joysticks are inserted as mentioned earlier to control rotation. This is particularly useful in grade III injuries where a gap exists between the scaphoid and lunate. The surgeon then advances the Kirschner wire across the SL interval aiming for the lunate after the interval has been anatomically reduced under direct vision across the midcarpal space. Fat droplets are frequently seen exiting between the scaphoid and lunate in the midcarpal space as the wire is driven across the interval (Fig. 14-33). Additional wires are then inserted under fluoroscopic control after the first Kirschner wire that controls rotation is placed. Three or four Kirschner wires are normally placed and left in position (Fig. 14-34).

Whipple[643] reviewed the results of arthroscopic management of SL instability utilizing this technique. Forty patients were followed for 1 to 3 years. In his review, patients were classified into two distinct groups according to the duration of symptoms and the radiographic side-to-side SL gap. Eighty-three percent of patients who had a history of instability of 3 months or less and had less than 3 mm of side-to-side difference in the SL interval had maintenance of the reduction and symptomatic relief. Only 53% of patients who had symptoms for more than 3 months and more than 3 mm of side-to-side SL gap had symptomatic relief. This report emphasized the need for early diagnosis and intervention before the onset of fixed carpal alignment and the diminished capacity for ligamentous healing. Similar conclusions have been published by Schädel-Höpfner and colleagues[497] and Ruch and Smith.[481]

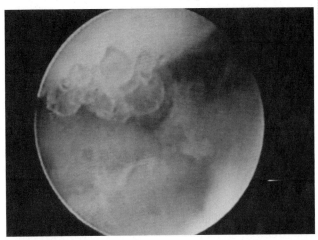

FIGURE 14-33. Arthroscopic view of the SL interval from the midcarpal space with the arthroscope in the ulnar midcarpal portal. Note the fat droplets exiting between the scaphoid and lunate as the Kirschner wires are being driven across the interval.

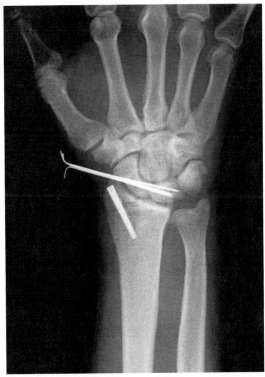

FIGURE 14-34. AP radiographic view of a reduced radial styloid fracture associated with an SL interosseous ligament injury. The ligament injury was discovered during arthroscopic reduction of the fracture and was not apparent on preoperative radiographs.

Re-education of Wrist Proprioception. The role of proprioception re-education in the treatment of mild SL instability should not be underestimated.[307] Particularly in partial SL injuries, when the dorsal SL ligament is intact, optimization of the time response of flexor carpi radialis muscle to wrist loading may play an important role in reestablishing the necessary equilibrium for adequate transfer of loads. Because the flexor carpi radialis uses the scaphoid tuberosity as a hinge toward its distal insertion into the second metacarpal base, it may act as a "dynamic" scaphoid stabilizer. Its contraction generates a beneficial extension moment to the unstable scaphoid, provided the dorsal RS capsule and dorsal SL ligament are intact (Fig. 14-35).[265] Such a stabilizing capability may be enhanced through the flexor carpi radialis muscle strengthening exercises and proprioception training of the wrist. As in other joints where mild instability tends to respond well to proper proprioception training,[307] predynamic SL instabilities may also benefit from this approach. Flexor carpi radialis strengthening exercises are totally contraindicated when the dorsal SL ligament is torn. In such circumstances, the dorsally directed vector produced by the muscle would not extend the bone but it would induce a scaphoid dorsal translation with subluxation of its proximal pole. Adequate evaluation of the extent of ligament damage is, thus, a prerequisite for this type of approach.

Arthroscopic Débridement. With the assumption that in partial ligament injuries discomfort results not from the instability itself but from joint irritation by the ligament remnants, arthroscopic débridement of partial chronic interosseous ligament tears has been often recommended. The technique is relatively straightforward. The grade of the interosseous ligament tear is assessed from the radiocarpal and midcarpal spaces. After the degree of tearing to the SL interosseous ligament is assessed, the arthroscope is placed in the 4-5 or 6-R portal. A shaver is brought into the 3-4 portal to débride the torn fibers of the SL membrane. The goal of management is to débride the unstable tissue flaps back to stable tissue, similar to débridement of the articular disk of the TFCC.

Weiss and associates[638] examined the role of arthroscopic débridement alone for management of complete and partial tears to the interosseous ligaments of the wrist. At an average 27 months after the procedure, 31 of 36 patients who had a partial tear had complete resolution of their symptoms with a grip strength improving an average of 23%. Complete SL tears had a modest outcome, however. The long-term efficacy of this technique to prevent progression of the instability has yet to be determined.

Electrothermal Shrinkage. Electrothermal shrinkage of insufficient or stretched ligaments has been shown to be beneficial in the stabilization of other joints, particularly in the shoulder. The technique should be considered investigational at this time and is based on the theory that by heating the collagen matrix, a shrinkage of the collagen results as the structure denatures. Fibroblasts then grow into the shrunken tissues. Whether the shrunken tissue will act similar to normal tissue or whether the results hold up over time remains unanswered.

The technique is relatively easy. A monopolar or bipolar thermal probe is used. The electrothermal probe is inserted through the 3-4 portal with the arthroscope in the 4-5 or 6-R portal. After mechanical débridement of the disrupted portion of the SL membrane, the electrothermal probe is used to shrink the remaining portion. This involves primarily the membranous portion, but the probe contacts the dorsal SL ligament and capsule (Fig. 14-36). It is important that the probe is continuously moving so as not to concentrate all the heat in one particular space. Also, the entire dorsal capsule should not be painted with the probe. Strips of contracture should be made leaving normal capsule in between to help vascularize and heal the contracted areas. The arthroscope is then placed back in the radial midcarpal space to evaluate the stability of the SL interval after shrinkage. Generally, less motion or gap is observed in the SL interval after electrothermal shrinkage as seen from the midcarpal space.

Burns are a possible complication with electrothermal shrinkage. The wrist is a very small joint and the irrigation fluid in the wrist may be heated up quite quickly. To avoid this, a separate increased inflow from the 6-U portal is utilized and outflow through the arthroscope sheath is continuous to help dissipate the heat. Also, the temperature of the irrigation fluid as it leaves the arthroscope cannula is continuously monitored to make sure it is not becoming too hot. The temperature of the probe is constantly monitored as the tissue is being shrunk so as not to go over 68°C.

Postoperative management of electrothermal shrinkage for chronic partial interosseous ligament tears is controversial. There are limited protocols available. Some authors believe immobilization alone is sufficient. Others believe

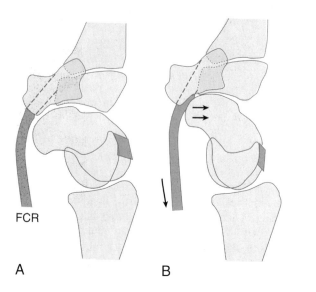

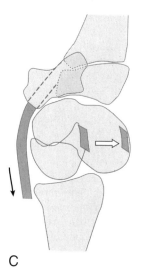

A   B   C

FIGURE 14-35. The direct relationship that exists between the flexor carpi radialis (FCR) tendon and the scaphoid tuberosity (**A**) makes this tendon an important dynamic stabilizer of the wrist, as long as the dorsal SL ligament and dorsal RS capsule are intact. In that circumstance, contraction of the FCR induces an extension moment to the scaphoid (*arrows*) that counteracts the inherent flexion tendency of this bone (**B**). By contrast, if the dorsal SL ligament is disrupted, the dorsally directed vector induced by the FCR results in a dorsal scaphoid subluxation (**C**). Indeed, re-education of the FCR is recommended only in partial SL tears, when the dorsal scaphoid stabilizers are intact.

FCR

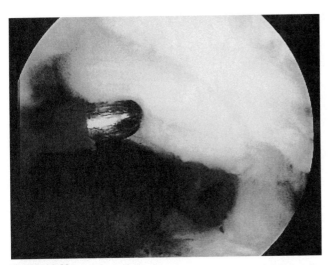

FIGURE 14-36. Arthroscopic view during electrothermal shrinkage of a chronic partial tear of the SL interosseous ligament. Multiple transverse passes are made across the interosseous ligament and dorsal capsule. It is important to increase the flow of irrigation and to monitor the temperature of the outflow fluid to minimize the risk of thermal injury.

temporary Kirschner wire stabilization of the carpus while the collagen shrinkage matures is indicated. Patients typically are immobilized from 6 to 8 weeks after electrothermal shrinkage. Range of motion, grip strength, and physical therapy are initiated similar to the protocol after pinning of acute tears of the SL interosseous ligaments.

Most studies have quite short follow-up. Geissler and Haley[190] reviewed the results in 19 patients with isolated chronic (more than 6 months) SL ligament tears to the wrist. At an average follow-up of 8 months, and utilizing a modified Mayo wrist score, 8 of the 10 patients with shrinkage of a complete SL tear had excellent or good result, as did 7 of 9 patients with shrinkage of a partial tear. Grade II tears to the SL interosseous ligament did significantly better as compared with grade III tears. Of the four patients with a grade III tear to the SL ligament, only one patient had an excellent result. Despite such promising results, the use of electrothermal shrinkage is quite preliminary and further study is required.

Dynamic Scapholunate Dissociation
Dynamic SLDs are characterized by a complete disruption of all SL ligaments (including the dorsal ligament) and by preservation of the secondary scaphoid stabilizers (STT and RSC ligaments[524]). By definition, carpal malalignment in dynamic SLD only appears under specific loading conditions (e.g., clenched fist, loaded ulnar deviation). Yet, there is substantial kinematic dysfunction with inability to sustain full load in most wrist positions.

If the healing potential of the injured ligaments is optimal, without retraction and correct vascularization of the ligament stumps, a direct repair of the dorsal SL ligament is recommended. This, obviously, needs to be associated with a percutaneous SL joint fixation.

Not infrequently, there is no ligament rupture but an avulsion from one end of the SL ligamentous complex (usually the scaphoid).[324] Sometimes this involves a small piece of bone. In these cases, a successful repair can be expected

beyond the time limits of what could be expected from a ligament substance rupture.

Unfortunately, when disrupted through their midsubstance, intrinsic ligaments tend to degenerate quite rapidly, in less than 2 weeks, after which chances for a successful repair diminish exponentially. If the dorsal ligament cannot be repaired, one alternative is to re-create the ligament by using either local tissues from adjacent ligaments or utilize a bone-ligament-bone autograft. Another alternative, in fact one of the most commonly utilized by most hand surgeons, is to perform a dorsal RS capsulodesis.

Only under exceptional circumstances a closed reduction and cast immobilization is an acceptable approach to these patients.[165,568] Despite the reports by King[282] and others[33] in which a complete SLD was successfully treated by immobilization in the "wine waiter's position" (full supination, mid extension, and ulnar deviation), there are no long-term data to sustain this.

Open Reduction, Internal Fixation, and Repair of the Dorsal SL Ligament. Direct ligament repair is only recommended when the dorsal SL ligament has good healing potential, the secondary scaphoid stabilizers are still intact, and there is no cartilage damage (traumatic or degenerative). This approach offers the same advantages as found when treating acute ligament injuries in other joints: (1) assurance that the subluxation is reduced, (2) visualization and treatment of any associated osteochondral damage, and (3) direct repair of torn ligaments.[329] The drawbacks explaining most failures are the high forces transferred by the capitate, tending to disrupt the repair; the poor healing potential in a frequently devascularized area; and the prolonged immobilization required after surgery. Despite these inconveniences, and considering the drawbacks of other alternatives, many authors still believe that there is a place for primary repair.[49,69,97,103,305,329,508,659]

In the past, some authors advocated repairing only the palmar SL ligament or both the palmar and dorsal SL ligaments through a double palmar and dorsal approach.[103,163,164] Certainly, a complete repair would be ideal, but the difficulties of approaching the palmar component without damaging the palmar extrinsic ligaments have led to abandoning this idea. In any case, recent biomechanical research concluded that only the dorsal SL ligament needs to be repaired to achieve relatively normal carpal kinematics in cadaveric specimens.[290]

Dorsal ligament repair is performed as follows. The incision may be longitudinal, "Z"-shaped, or transverse, the latter resulting in a more aesthetic scar at the expense of a less adequate exposure.[329] A dorsal approach to the wrist capsule between the third and fourth extensor compartments, as suggested by Weil and Ruby[634] and others,[417,445] is recommended.

Frequently, when operating early on a torn dorsal SL ligament, there is sufficient ligamentous tissue to permit a reasonable repair. If the ligament is not ruptured but avulsed (sometimes with a small osteochondral fragment), the repair is more effective and consists of reattaching the avulsed ligament to the freshened dorsal edge of the scaphoid or lunate by using transosseous sutures, as described by Linscheid[320] and Lavernia and colleagues (Fig. 14-37),[305] or by using tag suture anchors.[49,421,659] When there is a bone

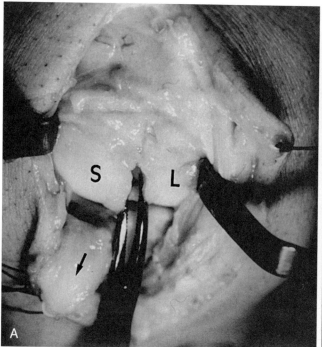

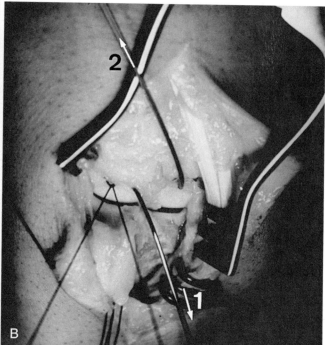

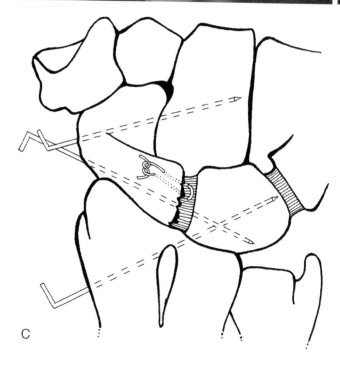

FIGURE 14-37. Open reduction and SL ligament repair in a 27-year-old man who sustained an SLD 6 weeks before surgery. **A,** Through a dorsal approach, a proximally based capsular flap is created *(black arrow)* for later capsulodesis, according to Blatt.[55] With forceps, the SL interval is opened, allowing inspection of the anterior aspect of the joint. **B,** Method of reduction of the joint using two Kirschner wires as joysticks. By pulling the wire inserted into the scaphoid (S) (1) proximally and ulnarly, while the wire in the lunate (L) (2) is held distally and radially, the joint usually becomes anatomically reduced. **C,** At this point, the transosseous sutures previously placed as suggested by Linscheid[320] are tied, and then Kirschner wires securing the reduced carpal bones are inserted.

fragment attached to the ligament, this can be tacked back down into its bed. The repair is to be protected by transfixing both the SL and SC joints with Kirschner wires. In many instances this is supplemented with a dorsal capsulodesis, as described later.[97,305,617] The wires are maintained for a period of 8 to 10 weeks with protection in a removable splint for an additional 4 weeks.

Several series of patients with SLD treated by means of direct repair have been published.[49,305,487,508,659] By combining the data from all those studies (100 patients in total), at an average follow-up of 37 months, pain was absent or significantly reduced in 72% of the patients, with an 87% grip strength and 78% wrist motion as compared with the

contralateral side. Radiographs demonstrated only minimal degenerative changes in less than a third of the patients, and the condition had not progressed to an advanced collapse pattern in the vast majority. Based on their experience, all authors agree that this approach should be considered as the treatment of choice for these patients.[97,305]

Dorsal Radioscaphoid Capsulodesis. Either as an isolated gesture in dynamic SL instability or to protect a direct repair of the dorsal SL ligament, dorsal capsulodesis of the RS joint is nowadays one of the most commonly utilized techniques in the treatment of carpal instability. Popularized by Blatt,[54,55] it consists of tightening the dorsal capsule between the radius and scaphoid to prevent the latter from excessive rotation into flexion. A capsular checkrein is created by raising a 1-cm-wide dorsal capsular flap, leaving its proximal edge attached to the dorsal rim of the radius. Once the scaphoid is reduced by manipulation and maintained with a single Kirschner wire passed obliquely from the distal pole of the scaphoid into the capitate, the flap is tightly inserted into a notch created on the dorsum of the scaphoid at a point distal to the axis of rotation of the scaphoid (scaphoid neck) (Fig. 14-38). Anchor sutures are ideal for this matter.[584] Postoperatively, these patients wear a thumb spica cast for 2 months, after which active range-of-motion exercises are begun. The Kirschner wire may be left in place for an additional month; then it is removed, allowing intercarpal motion to begin 3 months postoperatively.

Different modifications of Blatt's technique have been published. Herbert and coworkers[228] used a reversed capsular flap, leaving its distal end attached to the distal and lateral aspect of the scaphoid and tightly reinserting its proximal end into Lister's tubercle and the floor of the second extensor compartment. A similar procedure was recommended by Linscheid and Dobyns[324,613] in which one half of the dorsal STq ligament is released from the triquetrum, freed from the dorsal rim of the lunate, inverted, and pulled to the dorsum of the radius, where it is strongly anchored. Still another option, defended by Slater and coworkers[533,534] and Szabo and colleagues,[556] is to advance the scaphoid insertion of the dorsal intercarpal ligament from its dorsal ridge to a more distal position at the scaphoid neck to control both flexion and pronation deformities.

Corroborating the positive predictions made in the laboratory,[122] a number of clinical series have reported good results with these procedures.[77,126,206,388,556,584,649] They all agree in that tensioning or augmenting the dorsal RS capsule offers less surgical morbidity than other alternatives. At an average 2 years of follow-up, these studies found absence of symptoms in two thirds of patients, with 75% grip strength as compared with the contralateral side.[77,126,206,556,584,649] When examined with MRI, these patients demonstrate an increased capsular thickening that prevents scaphoid rotary subluxation at the expense of limiting wrist flexion an average of 20 degrees.[55] The long-term stabilizing efficacy of

this capsule has yet to be determined. These methods can be used successfully in the skeletally immature carpus, without adverse effects on growth.[104,672]

Soft Tissue Reconstruction of the Dorsal SL Ligament. Recent publications have reported acceptable results in the treatment of dynamic SL instabilities by replacing the dorsal SL ligament that cannot be repaired with a strip of either the dorsal intercarpal ligament[605] or the dorsal RTq ligament.[142] Both methods involve using a portion of dense connective tissue with a triquetral attachment. That attachment is left intact while the other end is tightly reinserted onto the dorsoulnar corner of the proximal scaphoid. The method uses anchor sutures to facilitate incorporation of the ligament into the previously denuded dorsal and distal cortices of the scaphoid and lunate. Both propositions appear very interesting for their simplicity and low local morbidity. Their early results are said to be most satisfying; yet these techniques are to be considered experimental, until further clinical research and long-term results are presented.

Bone-Ligament-Bone Grafts. Based on the proven success of replacing knee ligaments with bone-ligament-bone grafts, several investigators addressed the in vitro feasibility of using allografts to replace a dorsal SL ligament.[96,118,223,238,523] Schuind[504] suggested the use of a vascularized portion of the radioulnar interosseous membrane. Weiss reported transferring a bone-retinaculum-bone autograft harvested from the region of Lister's tubercle.[636] Harvey and Hanel advocated the use of the third metacarpal-capitate ligament.[224] The surgical approach is identical as for a direct repair. Once the two bones are reduced and transfixed by Kirschner wires, a deep trough is carved at both sides where the bone-ligament-bone graft will be buried and fixed with either mini screws or small wires, or alternatively, by interference fit of the impacted bone fragments.

In theory, by providing tissue with similar elasticity and strength as the original structure, there is a better chance of achieving a more adequate SL linkage. Several potential problems may arise: (1) because the proximal scaphoid is a vascularly compromised area, consolidation of the graft may not be easily achieved; (2) after a long period of immo-

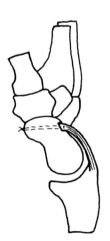 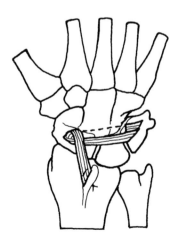 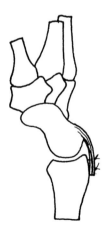

FIGURE 14-38. During the surgical approach to treat rotatory subluxation of the scaphoid, a dorsal capsulodesis of the RS joint may be created and later used to help prevent recurrence of the scaphoid flexion tendency. The first and most popular method was described by Blatt,[55] which uses a proximally based capsular flap. Linscheid and Dobyns[324] preferred using a strip of the dorsal intercarpal ligament, whereas a distally based capsular flap was suggested by Herbert and colleagues.[228]

BLATT 1987   **LINSCHEID 1992**   **HERBERT 1996**

bilization the mechanical properties of the graft may deteriorate and subsequently fail under the amount of stress that will be exerted on it; and (3) reconstructing the dorsal SL ligament alone does not solve the palmar-distal ligament insufficiency that exists by definition in static SL instabilities. The early clinical results by Schuind,[504] Weiss,[636] and Harvey and Hanel[224] are encouraging in the cases in which the secondary stabilizers are still functional (dynamic instabilities). The index of failures of this technique in static instabilities still is unacceptable.[636] As is said for the other types of soft tissue reconstruction, further research is needed before these techniques can be recommended for wide use.

Static Reducible Scapholunate Dissociation

An SLD is considered "reducible static" when (1) the ligament rupture has not been solved in the acute phase, its remnants having degenerated into a retracted, disorganized fibrous stump, precluding a strong direct repair; (2) the secondary stabilizers (STT and SC ligaments[524]) have failed, and a permanent (static) malalignment has appeared; (3) carpal subluxation still is reducible; and (4) no cartilage deterioration has appeared yet.

In rare cases, if the ligament has avulsed cleanly off the scaphoid or the lunate, with or without an attached piece of bone, some authors suggest that ligament repair can still be performed, provided the repair is augmented with a dorsal capsulodesis to compensate for the loss of the secondary stabilizers.[305,652] Others contend that these repairs are associated with an unacceptable rate of attenuation and failure.[659]

For these patients, two different strategies have been proposed: tendon reconstructions and the so-called RASL procedure (reduction-association of the SL joint).[206,305,324]

Tendon Reconstructions. The use of tendon grafts to reconstruct the SL ligaments has evolved considerably since first introduced in 1975 by Dobyns and coworkers.[131] The initial idea was to pass a strip of tendon through holes in the scaphoid and lunate to provide immediate stability by tightly looping the tendon graft around the joint. Unfortunately, the method was based on creating large drill holes in vascular compromised areas, interfering with blood supply, thus resulting in fractures and/or joint degeneration. Poor long-term results followed,[424] for the method fell out of favor. In the 1980s, partial fusions became popular as an alternative solution with apparently excellent short-term results.[202,279,582,618] In the 1990s, however, partial arthrodesis crossing the midcarpal joint showed not to be as benign a procedure as initially thought,[171,260,289] for new alternatives using tendon grafts were sought again. Numerous options have been suggested since.

Almquist and associates[10] reported good results with the use of the so-called four-bone ligament reconstruction. The joint is approached dorsally and palmarly. Holes are made in the capitate, scaphoid, and lunate; and the tendon, the distal end of which is left attached to the third metacarpal, is passed through the holes to reproduce the transverse direction of the dorsal SL ligament (Fig. 14-39). The SL joint is further stabilized with a wire loop, and the wrist is protected with splints for 16 weeks. Thirty-one of 36 patients treated

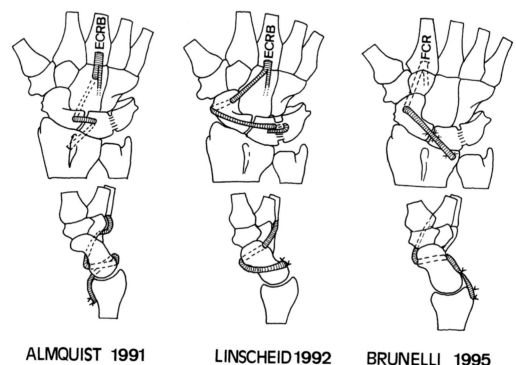

ALMQUIST 1991   **LINSCHEID 1992**   **BRUNELLI 1995**

FIGURE 14-39. Despite the initial discouraging results obtained after the first attempts to reconstruct the SL linkage using tendons, reports suggest that there may still be a role for this type of procedure. An ideal indication would be a subacute, reducible SLD in which ligaments cannot be optimally repaired. Three methods have been described by Almquist and associates,[10] Linscheid and Dobyns,[324] and Brunelli.[69] The last two base their effectiveness on the stabilization of both the proximal and the distal ends of the subluxating scaphoid, without creating bone holes in the vicinity of the vascularly compromised SL joint. ECRB, extensor carpi radialis brevis; FCR, flexor carpi radialis.

with this method returned to work. A biomechanical analysis by Augsburger and associates[28] suggested this method to produce a more physiologic function than the one resulting from an STT partial fusion. Full motion, however, is not expected to be regained, as the tendon graft is set in a way that creates a vertical tether between the capitate and lunate palmarly. As with most modalities of SL ligament reconstruction, long-term results have not been published.

Another option was proposed by Linscheid and Dobyns.[324] A strip of the extensor carpi radialis longus tendon is used to tether the distal scaphoid to prevent its flexion deformity while reconstructing the transverse course of both the dorsal SL and triquetrum-scaphoid ligaments (see Fig. 14-39). Two transverse incisions are used: one short palmar incision over the scaphoid tuberosity and one wide transverse incision on the dorsum of the wrist. The freed strip of tendon is left attached distally and passed through a drill hole made from the dorsal aspect of the distal scaphoid to the tuberosity. The tendon is then passed intra-articularly around the scaphoid waist to emerge in the dorsal incision. The strip of tendon is passed under the dorsal fibers of the LTq ligament, looped around itself, and pulled taut distally to maintain the lunate reduced.

Brunelli and Brunelli[69,70] advocated the use of a strip of the FCR tendon to address both the proximal and distal aspects of the instability that is present in the rotatory subluxation of the scaphoid. Two small transverse palmar incisions are made to identify and obtain a strip of FCR tendon that is left attached distally. Through a separate dorsal incision, all scar tissue formed between the two bones is removed, as well as that formed between the scaphoid, trapezium, and trapezoid. With this, the scaphoid subluxation should be easily reduced. The split tendon is then passed through a drill hole made across the distal scaphoid. According to the initial technique, the split tendon that emerges off the scaphoid hole is sutured to the remnants of the dorsal SL ligament before being pulled taut proximally and anchored to the dorsoulnar corner of the distal radius by transosseous sutures (see Fig. 14-39). This method was subsequently modified by Van den Abbeele and associates,[585] who suggested not to cross the radiocarpal joint but to use the dorsal RTq ligament as a solid anchoring point to the tendon graft (Fig. 14-40). The overall early results

of Brunelli's procedure are very encouraging, with most patients having returned to their previous occupation with complete relief of pain, excellent grip strength, and an average 45 degrees loss of flexion as compared with the opposite hand.[70,585] Until long-term results are available, however, these techniques are to be considered experimental.

The differences between the old and these new methods of tendon reconstruction are substantial. Not only is the SL joint instability addressed but also, and most importantly, the distal palmar component of the scaphoid instability is controlled. Furthermore, the drill holes are not in the vicinity of the SL joint but in an area of the scaphoid with better vascularization, so that the weakening effect is minimal.

Reduction-Association of the SL Joint (RASL Procedure). Based on the observation that failed SL fusions tend to do clinically better than those that achieve fusion, Herbert and colleagues[228] proposed a novel approach to static SL instabilities. This innovative method consists of an open reduction, repair of the ligament remnants, and protection of the repair by internally blocking the SL joint with a transverse Herbert screw for 12 months or more. The goal is to obtain enough intercarpal fibrosis as to allow full loading of these two bones without yielding or losing their connection. Rosenwasser and colleagues[472] reported surprisingly good results using this approach. At an average follow-up of 54 months, 20 treated patients with a static SLD exhibited 91% of their normal wrist motion and 87% grip strength. Somewhat inferior results, but still quite acceptable, were published by Filan and Herbert.[161] Whether these excellent results will deteriorate with time remains unknown.

Static Irreducible Scapholunate Dissociation (Without Arthrosis)

Chronic rupture or insufficiency of both primary and secondary SL ligament stabilizers results in the formation of fibrosis within the empty spaces that appear between the scaphoid and surrounding bones. With time, subluxed joint surfaces tend to deform, making the carpal malalignment even more irreducible. If despite this, there is still not substantial cartilage degeneration, the case fulfils the criteria of an irreducible static SLD.

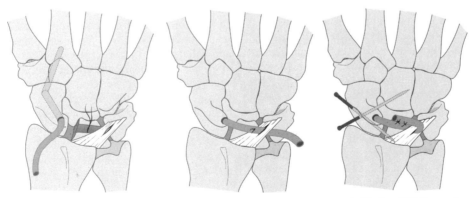

FIGURE 14-40. Schematic representation of the modified Brunelli technique to reconstruct the unrepairable dorsal SL ligament, as proposed by Van den Abbeele and associates.[585] **A,** The FCR tendon is passed obliquely from the palmar scaphoid tuberosity to the dorsal ridge of the scaphoid where the dorsal SL ligament inserts. **B,** The tendon is then buried in a trough created on the dorsum of the lunate by means of an anchor suture. To adjust the tension of the graft a slit in the distal portion of the dorsal RTq ligament is made through which the tendon is looped around and sutured onto itself. **C,** Unlike the original Brunelli method, this method does not attempt to cross the radiocarpal joint with the graft.

The most frequently recommended treatment for the symptomatic, irreducible carpal malalignment secondary to an SLD is a partial fusion. As compared with total wrist fusion, the advantages of arthrodesing only the diseased joint were recognized as early as 1924 by Thornton.[574] Since then, different types of limited intercarpal arthrodeses have been described.* In the laboratory, a number of experimental models have been devised to compare these various types of fusion.[181,193,357,598] Despite controversies about their use in less developed instabilities,[28,206,617] the utility of these procedures is unquestionable in these advanced stages of SLD. The following are the techniques most commonly used.

Scaphotrapezoid-Trapezial Arthrodesis. In the 1980s, STT arthrodesis, also known as "triskaphe" fusion,[617,619] became a popular method of treatment for chronic SLD.[287,288,622] The goal of the procedure is to realign the proximal pole of the scaphoid relative to the scaphoid fossa, so that the RS congruency is restored and the chance of developing later degenerative changes is reduced. When planning such a procedure, it is important that the external dimensions and alignment of the resultant fused block are the same as the external dimensions of the bones in the normal wrist.[16] This means that after the articular cartilage and subchondral bone are removed, the gap remaining between the bones must be filled with cancellous bone graft and the bones must not be pressed together.

Watson, probably one of the most experienced surgeons in this particular field,[617-620,622,623] recommends to proceed as follows. All articular cartilage and subchondral bone is to be excised through a dorsal transverse incision. By placing the wrist extended 25 degrees and radially deviated 20 degrees, the ST joint is transfixed with two parallel Kirschner wires entered from the dorsal aspect of the trapezoid into the scaphoid. During wire insertion, an approximately 5-mm gap between the two bones is maintained by placing a thin metallic spacer in the joint. This defect is later tightly filled with cancellous bone obtained from the distal radial metaphysis. The wrist is immobilized for 3 weeks in a long-arm cast, including the metacarpophalangeal joints of the thumb, index, and middle fingers, followed by 3 more weeks in a short-arm cast. To avoid the problem of having the wires interfere with the insertion of the grafts, Kleinman[287-289] initiates the procedure by fixing the scaphoid to the capitate with two Kirschner wires and then removes the articular cartilage and subchondral bone, fills the space with bone graft, and finally inserts the wires across the joints to be fused.

Another important point is to achieve correct alignment of the scaphoid. According to Minamikawa and associates,[365] the ideal RS angle for maximal wrist motion is from 41 to 60 degrees. Even with direct visualization, however, ideal alignment is not always easy to achieve, with the scaphoid positioned either over-reduced or under-reduced relative to the radius. Under-reduction (scaphoid flexed) fails to close the SL gap correctly, and over-reduction (scaphoid extended) may result in more restricted motion and more severe RS impingement postoperatively.[16,365] Given the choice, under-reduction is probably preferable; it may provide relief of symptoms despite a persistent radiographic

SL gap,[289] whereas over-reduction leads to RS cartilage degeneration.

As experience with STT fusion has accumulated,[276,623] complications and long-term effects have been reported.[171,260,289] Although Watson and associates[623] reported a nonunion rate of 4%, the average rate of nonunion among all the reported series (385 cases) is 14%.[303,527] Range of motion and strength are frequently decreased postoperatively,[143,171] and the results in terms of pain relief are not uniformly predictable. Painful RS impingement is a frequent problem, owing to the fact that in radial deviation the distally fused scaphoid can no longer rotate into flexion, resulting in an increased pressure on the scaphoid fossa.[181,623] To solve this problem, Rogers and Watson[471] recommend incorporating a dorsolateral styloidectomy as a routine part of the STT fusion; this is likely to prevent peripheral (not central) impingement. In fact, some authors[289,623] consider any preexisting cartilage degeneration between the scaphoid and radius to be a contraindication to STT fusion.

SL Arthrodesis. Once believed to be the ideal method of treating SLD, fusion of the SL joint has proved to be one of the less reliable treatments for this condition.[240,527] The small articular surfaces in contact and the magnitude of forces by the capitate tending to separate the two bones, combine to make this fusion difficult to achieve. Furthermore, after this intervention, the mutual shift between the two bones is no longer possible.[517] This results in increased demands on the arthrodesis site, predisposing the fusion to refracture. The proponents of this intervention[11,103] acknowledge that bony union occurs in only about 50% of the cases but claim that the resulting fibrous link between the scaphoid and lunate is often strong enough to significantly decrease the patient's symptoms. In contrast, Hom and Ruby[240] concluded from their poor results in seven patients that SL arthrodesis is not a predictable method for treating SLD.

SC Arthrodesis. SC arthrodesis was first described in 1946 by Sutro[555] for scaphoid nonunion. More recently, it has been applied to the treatment of SLD.[442,473,515] In theory, this operation should have consequences similar to the STT fusion. In the laboratory, Douglas and colleagues[135] showed no difference in total range of motion between the two procedures. The kinematic and kinetic carpal behavior after both types of fusion are also similar,[181,598] both causing abnormal transfer of load and significant loss of midcarpal joint motion, especially in radial and ulnar deviation. Watson and colleagues,[622] however, found less reduction of motion after an STT fusion than after an SC fusion, probably because of the adaptive motion occurring at the trapezoid-capitate level. Yet, the long-term results of this procedure, as recently published by Szalay and Peimer,[668] are quite acceptable, with more than two thirds of patients being satisfied, with minimal disability. At 76 months of follow-up the SC fused wrists exhibited an average 77% grip strength and a 33% reduction in flexion and 46% in radial deviation.

Scaphoid-Lunate-Capitate (SLC) Arthrodesis. Adding the lunate to the SC fusion offers a method of controlling both the scaphoid and the lunate misalignment (Fig. 14-41). The consequence of this is approximately a 50% reduction of wrist motion.[528] It is indicated in a patient with severe

---

*See references 48, 81, 208, 225, 240, 272, 436, 442, 582, 618, and 650.

fixed instability without degenerative changes on the proximal pole of the scaphoid and apposing articular surface of the radius. Rotman and associates[474] reported a series of 17 cases of chronic incompetence of the SL ligaments treated by this method, with an average follow-up of 28 months. They claimed a significant reduction of pain, enabling maintenance of sufficient motion for daily activities and return to heavy work in the majority of patients.

Siegel and Ruby,[527] however, reported that 4 of 11 patients treated with SLC fusion later required total wrist fusion owing to continuous pain.

Radio-Scapho-Lunate Fusion Plus Distal Scaphoidectomy. As already stated in the biomechanics section of this chapter, most activities of daily living involve motion along the so-called dart-throwing or physiologic flexion-

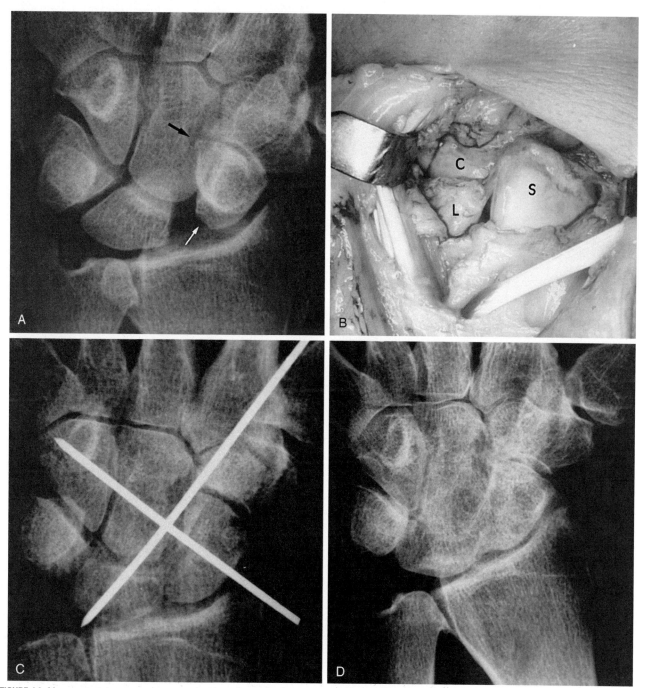

FIGURE 14-41. A 56-year-old man presented with a complaint of pain, lack of strength, and mild reduction of motion 1 year after a twisting injury to his right wrist. **A,** PA view disclosed the presence of static SLD. Slight resorption of the proximal edge of the scaphoid *(white arrow)* and a small osteophyte at its distal and medial edge *(black arrow)* are both indications of the chronicity of the case. **B,** A dorsal approach demonstrated the lack of ligament remnants but no radiocarpal cartilage damage. Note the stepoff between the distal edges of the proximal pole of the scaphoid (S) and lunate (L) proximal to the capitate (C). **C,** Owing to difficulties encountered in properly reducing the carpal bones, a midcarpal fusion was done. **D,** PA view obtained 19 months after surgery. There is a 60% reduction of motion. Other than that, the wrist is again strong, with only some discomfort between the radial styloid and the scaphoid. A radial styloidectomy has been planned. (Courtesy of A. Lluch, Barcelona.)

extension plane, from extension-radial deviation to flexion-ulnar deviation. Such a motion occurs mostly at the midcarpal joint.[259,380] Consequently, if the fixed malalignment of the scaphoid and lunate needs an arthrodesis and the midcarpal joint is unaffected, it is reasonable to fuse the RC rather than the midcarpal joint. If aside from the dissociation, there are abnormalities in the RC joint but the midcarpal articulation is normal, an arthrodesis of the RSL joint is the best choice.[29,515,575] Fusing the RC joint eliminates pain induced by local synovitis while stabilizing the proximal component (the SL acetabulum) of the midcarpal joint.[618] Bach and coworkers[29] used this technique in 21 patients with chronic SLD, 13 of whom returned to their previous employment with an average 48 degrees of flexion-extension and 70% of grip strength.

When fusing the RSL joint, however, the STT joint may become symptomatic and degenerate with time as the consequence of the inability of the scaphoid to flex during wrist flexion and/or radial deviation, creating a local impingement.[394] To avoid such a complication, and to increase the resultant motion, excision of the distal third of the scaphoid is recommended. With this modified technique, the midcarpal "ball-and-socket" articulation is freed from its lateral constraint[350] and allows more than 50% of the overall wrist motion. The early results published so far are very encouraging.[184,337]

Wrist Arthrosis Secondary to SLD (SLAC Wrist)

Long-standing SLDs progressively deteriorate the adjacent joint cartilages following a specific pattern of osteoarthritis, the so-called SLAC wrist.[71,272,511,616,621] According to Watson and Ryu,[621] the cartilage wear initiates between the tip of the radial styloid and the distal scaphoid and progresses proximally until the entire RS joint is involved. At a later stage, the midcarpal joint may also degenerate, usually starting at the lunocapitate interval. In advanced cases, the rest of the carpus may be involved, with the exception of the RL joint, which typically is spared from this degenerative process (Fig. 14-42).

SLAC wrists are not necessarily symptomatic.[146] When they are, soft tissue procedures are not likely to relieve pain. In fact, many authors consider these operations contraindicated in the presence of joint arthrosis. The problem is that all the other alternatives have relative disadvantages. Details of these procedures are described in Chapter 13. The following are some points to be considered when using these techniques in patients with SLD.

Arthroscopy. Wrist arthroscopy plays a limited salvage role in patients with a SLAC wrist. It can be used to evaluate the degree and extent of articular degeneration to determine which salvage procedure is best for the case. Particularly in the decision-making process between a four-corner fusion or proximal row carpectomy, wrist arthroscopy can be a valuable adjunct in determining the status of the articular cartilage in relation to the capitate and the distal radius.

Radial Styloidectomy. Radial styloidectomy is one of the oldest interventions used to relieve wrist pain caused by an impingement between the tip of the radial styloid and a malpositioned distal scaphoid. Obviously, by removing the osteophytic radial styloid process, the cause of the scaphoid

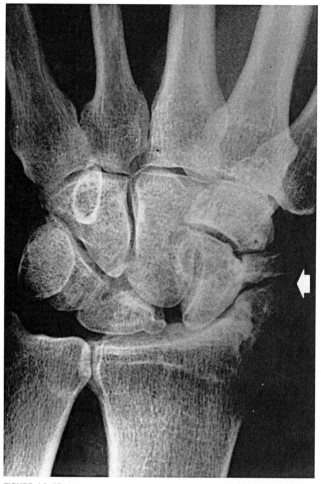

FIGURE 14-42. A typical scapholunate advanced collapse (SLAC wrist). Note the osteophyte formation at the radial styloid-scaphoid articulation *(arrow)*, which is probably an attempt by the joint to stop the destabilization process.

malalignment (nonunion, SLD, STT fusion) is not solved, and recurrence is always possible. When performing a radial styloidectomy through an open lateral approach, caution is required to protect the dorsolateral branches of the radial nerve and not to detach excessively the insertion of the radiocarpal ligaments, which would lead to further instability.[526]

In individuals who desire minimal surgical intervention, arthroscopic débridement and radial styloidectomy may be an option. A working 1-2 portal is made along the dorsal portion of the "snuff box" to protect the radial artery and nerves. Dissection with a hemostat is made to the level of the capsule. An arthroscopic bur is inserted through the 1-2 portal with the arthroscope in the 3-4 portal or occasionally in the 4-5 portal. The tip of the radial styloid is then burred down to the level of the RSC ligament insertion to the distal radius. The area of cartilage degeneration demarcates the area for the bone to be removed.

One advantage of arthroscopic radial styloidectomy is the precise assessment of articular cartilage degeneration and the amount of bone to be removed. The origin of the RSC and long RL ligaments is maintained as the bone is burred. A fluoroscopic unit is essential to assess the amount of bone that has been resected. It is easy to be fooled into thinking a large amount of the radial styloid has been excised as viewed arthroscopically, but in reality under fluoroscopy a minimal amount of bone has been removed.

Scaphoid Replacement Arthroplasty. Replacement of the scaphoid with a silicone or metallic implant is seldom indicated. Many long-term complications, including the devastating particulate synovitis,[432,539] have been reported, precluding its use. Furthermore, it is difficult, if not impossible, to maintain the implant in adequate alignment in a wrist where the loss of periscaphoid ligaments inevitably leads to a midcarpal instability. To prevent such a complication Watson and coworkers[622] initially recommended protecting the implant by fusing the midcarpal (capitate-lunate-triquetrum-hamate) joint. The good results obtained by this technique, however, were thought to be unrelated to the implant,[284] so the use of scaphoid implants was discontinued.

SLAC Wrist Operation. Popularized by Watson and Ballet,[616] the so-called SLAC procedure (scaphoid excision plus a capitate-lunate-triquetrum-hamate fusion, also known as "four corner" fusion) has gained an excellent reputation for the treatment of chronic SLD.[26,492,578] For the operation to be a success, however, a good articular cartilage at the RL level is required. A frequent complication (12% according to Ashmead and associates[26]) is the development of dorsal impingement between the dorsal edge of the radius and the capitate. An important step to avoid this is to fully correct the DISI deformity before placing the Kirschner wires across the LC joint. To regain a normal carpal height, some authors recommend placement of an intercalary graft.[492] Particularly useful is the recently available "spider" plate, a low-profile circular plate designed specifically to be countersunk on the intersection of the four bones so that dorsal impingement is avoided.[652] In selected cases, fusion is limited to the LC joint, particularly in ulnar-plus wrists where an excessively rigid triquetrum could precipitate an ulnocarpal abutment[284] Another alternative, particularly useful in cases with chronic SL and LTq instability (perilunate instability), is to excise both scaphoid and triquetrum before fusing the LC joint.[80]

Proximal Row Carpectomy. Proximal row carpectomy is a controversial salvage operation consisting of the entire excision of scaphoid, lunate, and capitate, thus creating a neoarticulation between the capitate and the lunate fossa of the radius. Although usually performed through a dorsal approach, it can also be done through a palmar capsulotomy, an alternative proposed by Luchetti and coworkers[331] that appears to have several advantages, including an earlier mobilization and preservation of the extensor compartments. In most series, the procedure has proved to be surprisingly good in terms of pain relief and restoration of functional wrist motion and grip strength, with high overall patient satisfaction.[112,210,246,248,331,407] In mechanical terms, this operation converts a complex composite articulation into a single ball-and-socket joint with nonmatching articular surfaces. The wrist can only adjust to such an incongruity if there is good articular cartilage on both the proximal pole of the capitate and in the lunate fossa of the radius. Compared with the SLAC procedure, this technique avoids long immobilization and the risk of nonunion.[578] It

has the added advantage of being convertible to a wrist arthrodesis or arthroplasty if at a later date it evolves into a painful osteoarthritis. Long-term radiocapitate degeneration, although often asymptomatic, is present in about 10% of the patients with more than 10 years of follow-up.[246]

Total Wrist Arthroplasty. Recent advances in total joint replacement of the wrist have made this option a reasonable treatment for the patient who places low demands on the wrist. Unfortunately, most patients with late post-traumatic instability are young individuals engaged in heavy labor to whom a prosthesis is seldom an acceptable choice.

Total Wrist Arthrodesis. Although many surgeons believe that a total wrist arthrodesis should rarely be considered in a heavy laborer with post-traumatic unstable osteoarthritis of the wrist, arthrodesis may be the procedure of choice. According to Hastings and Silver,[225] total pain relief is expected in 85% of wrist fusion patients, with 65% returning to their former occupations. As demonstrated in many clinical series, most patients with a total wrist fusion are able to accomplish all daily tasks by learning to compensate for the loss of wrist motion.[267]

Authors' Preferred Methods of Treatment: SLD

Partial ruptures of the SL ligamentous complex (predynamic, occult SLD) are best treated arthroscopically. Particularly promising are the results obtained by one of us (WG) in the treatment of partial tears (grades I to II) by electrothermal shrinkage of the distended proximal membrane. In more advanced stages, we both believe in débriding the unstable remnants of disrupted membrane, plus reduction and percutaneous pinning of the SL joint with two or more Kirschner wires for 8 weeks. It is always important to check for the integrity of the dorsal SL ligament. If insufficient or torn (dynamic SLD), and yet repairable, we prefer the open technique of joint reduction, ligament repair, and dorsal capsulodesis as proposed by Taleisnik and others.[97,305] Although recognizing its potential future use, we have little experience in the reconstruction of the dorsal SL ligament with bone-ligament-bone grafts, a technique that should be considered experimental at this time.

We no longer consider SL ligament repair, even if reparable, when there is already some malalignment present. We believe that the presence of a DISI indicates a more global problem that can hardly be solved by only addressing the dorsal SL ligament. If the subluxation is easily correctable (reducible static SLD) and no cartilage defect exists, we are having excellent results with the modified Brunelli tendon reconstruction technique as described by Van den Abbeele and colleagues[585] with the following modifications: (1) a trough on the dorsal surface of the lunate is created so that the tendon graft is placed in full contact with cancellous bone, (2) an anchor suture is used to coapt the tendon graft against the lunate, and (3) to get the right tension to the tenodesis, the distal portion of the RTq ligament is used as a pulley around which the tendon is looped and sutured onto itself. This later modification has shown to be beneficial because it pulls the ulnar-side carpus toward the scaphoid, thus helping in the closure of the SL gap (Fig. 14-43).

When the malalignment is irreducible (fixed static SLD) but no cartilage damage is present, one of us (MG-E) has had some success by carefully removing all interposed fibrosis that prevents reduction, followed by the modified Brunelli procedure. If the malalignment is found definitively irreducible, good results have been obtained by fusing the radiocarpal joint and excising the distal third of the scaphoid. In our hands, most midcarpal-crossing arthrodeses provided excellent short-term results but poor long-term outcomes.

When both the RS and the midcarpal joints are involved by the arthritic process (advanced SLAC wrist), we prefer a total scaphoidectomy plus a midcarpal fusion.[492] Being skeptical of the long-term viability of a joint with mismatched articular surfaces, we only occasionally perform proximal row carpectomies.

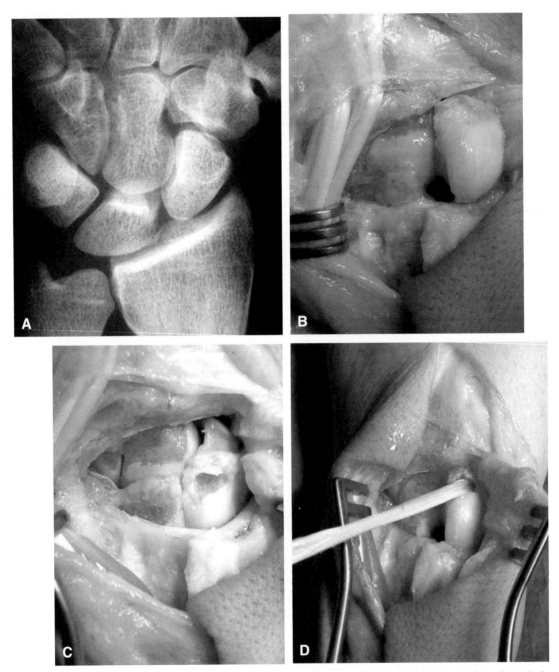

Figure 14-43. A 32-year-old lawyer who sustained an injury to his left wrist 8 months before while playing soccer. **A,** PA radiograph demonstrates a relatively shortened scaphoid with mildly increased SL interval. **B,** The scaphoid viewed from the dorsum could easily sublux, because the entire SL ligamentous complex was ruptured and could not be repaired (static reducible SLD). **C,** A transverse trough was created on the dorsal aspect of the lunate. To ensure that the tendon will be permanently in contact with the lunate cancellous bone an anchor suture was placed in the trough. **D,** A strip of flexor carpi radialis was harvested at the palmar side but left attached distally. Its proximal end was passed through a tunnel emerging at the distal-medial corner of the scaphoid.

Continued

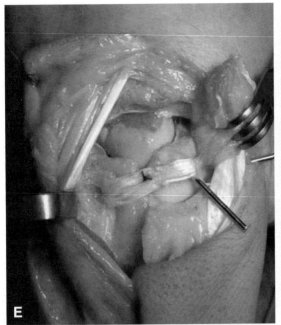

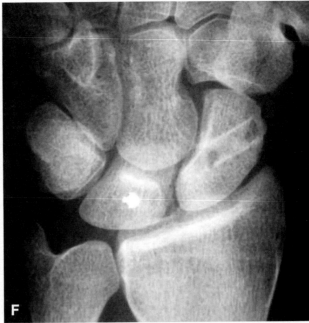

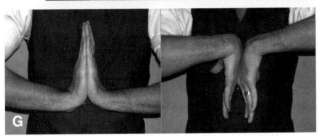

Figure 14-43—cont'd. E, The tendon used the dorsal RTq ligament as an anchor point for adequate tension before being sutured onto itself. Two Kirschner wires were used to immobilize the reconstructed ligament for 6 weeks, plus 4 more weeks in a removable splint. **F,** PA view obtained 8 months post operation. The patient had resumed his former sport activities at 6 months. **G,** At 18 months the wrist remained stable and free of pain with 90% grip strength and 85% motion as compared with the contralateral side.

CRITICAL POINTS: SCAPHOLUNATE STABILIZATION (MODIFIED BRUNELLI AND BRUNELLI[70] TENODESIS)

INDICATIONS

- Dynamic SLD, reducible, with normal cartilage
- Static SLD, reducible, with normal cartilage

PREOPERATIVE EVALUATION

- Perform routine radiographic examination.
- Use clenched-fist view.
- Obtain fluoroscopic evaluation of abnormal carpal motion.
- Obtain MRI to check integrity of flexor carpi radialis tendon.
- Use arthroscopy to rule out cartilage degeneration and/or LTq injury.

TECHNICAL POINTS

- Use a dorsal (zigzag, lazy "S," or longitudinal) approach centered at Lister's tubercle.

- Section the extensor retinaculum along the third compartment.
- Open the septa between II-III, III-IV, and IV-V. Coagulate intraseptal arteries.
- Perform a dorsal capsulotomy following the "fiber splitting" technique, according to Berger and Bishop.[42] (See Fig. 14-43B.)
- Check reducibility by traction or by direct manipulation with Kirschner wires as joysticks.
- Drill a 3.2-mm hole into the scaphoid at the point of insertion of the dorsal SL ligament. (See Fig. 14-43C.)
- Direct the drill hole along the axis of the scaphoid aiming at the palmar tuberosity.
- Make a 1-cm palmar incision over the scaphoid tuberosity and open the flexor carpi radialis tendon sheath.
- Obtain a distally based 8-cm strip of tendon (approximately 3 mm in diameter).

Continued

CRITICAL POINTS: SCAPHOLUNATE STABILIZATION (MODIFIED BRUNELLI AND BRUNELLI[70] TENODESIS)—cont'd

- Retrieve from the dorsum the tendon strip using a wire or a tendon passer (see Fig. 14-43D).
- Carve a transverse trough over the dorsum of the lunate with a rongeur.
- Insert a 1.8-mm anchor suture (Mitek Mini QuickAnchor or similar) into the lunate.
- Localize the distal end of the dorsal RTq ligament and loop the tendon strip around it.
- While tensioning the tendon using the RTq ligament as a pulley, transfix the SL and SC joints (usually two 1.5-mm Kirschner wires are used; sometimes three) (see Fig. 14-43E).
- Without releasing the tendon tension, use the anchor suture to bury the tendon against the lunate cancellous bone in the previously created trough.
- Suture the tendon loop onto itself.

- Carefully close the capsule over the tendon strip.
- Reconstruct the extensor retinaculum.

POSTOPERATIVE CARE

- Apply a short-arm/thumb spica cast for 6 weeks, which is changed at 10 days for stitch removal and radiographs.
- Remove wires at 6 weeks and protect the area in a removable splint for an additional 4 weeks.
- Begin rehabilitation after cast removal to regain motion and grip strength.
- Do not allow contact sports until 6 months after the surgery.
- Probable outcome: a painless wrist with 20 degrees loss of flexion and 75% grip strength.

Lunotriquetral Dissociation

Symptomatic disruption of the LTq supporting ligaments, from either traumatic or degenerative etiology, is not unusual. Yet, the literature concerning these problems is scarce and often misleading in terms of pathogenesis, diagnosis, and treatment. Furthermore, the general awareness of this problem is often poor, which explains why many LTq dissociations still are currently missed or confused with other ulnar-sided wrist problems, such as midcarpal instabilities or TFCC injuries.[15,561]

Although the first case of LTq dissociation was graphically represented by Chaput and Vaillant[89] in 1913, it was not until the detailed descriptions by Linscheid and associates,[325] Dobyns and colleagues,[131] and Taleisnik[559] that wide attention was focused on this pathologic process. Since then, new information has been added that helps to differentiate this problem from similar entities and achieve better results from treatment.*

Pathomechanics

According to the "progressive perilunar instability" theory by Mayfield and associates,[345,346,348] injury to the LTq ligaments occurs in stage III, following rupture of the SL ligaments (stage I) and lunocapitate dislocation (stage II) (see Fig. 14-6). If the SL problem heals spontaneously or with intervention, and the LTq problem remains unresolved, symptoms from the ulnar-side instability may predominate.[125,438]

In other circumstances, an isolated LTq dissociation may result from a reverse pattern of injury originating on the ulnar side of the wrist.[599] Although no laboratory studies have confirmed this mechanism, it seems likely that a fall on the outstretched hand with the wrist positioned in radial deviation and midcarpal pronation is able to tighten the ulnocarpal ligamentous complex to a point where an isolated LTq dissociation may occur.[68] In this situation, the dorsally applied reaction force by the radius on the central column may explain the failure of the LTq fibers and the sparing of the radiocarpal ligaments.[34,454]

Also, a similar instability pattern may appear as the consequence of an ulnar-plus variant, resulting in degeneration of the proximal (fibrocartilaginous) portion of the LTq interosseous membrane by a wear mechanism.[439]

In the laboratory, several attempts to ascertain the consequences of LTq ligament disruptions have been made.[241,465,599] When both the LTq and dorsal RTq ligaments were experimentally sectioned in axially loaded cadaver wrists, the flexion moment by the scaphoid became unconstrained, inducing a conjoint rotation in flexion of the scaphoid and lunate, with subsequent anterior subluxation of the capitate (Fig. 14-44). This, of course, would represent the more advanced stage of the disease, resulting in a static VISI pattern of instability.[12] In less advanced ligament sectioning, when only the palmar and dorsal LTq ligaments were sectioned, increased mobility of the LTq joint was detected (dynamic instability), but not a complete destabilization of the carpus.[241,465] Viegas and colleagues,[599] using intra-articular pressure-sensitive film, did not find any significant change in force transmission across the radiocarpal joint, as compared with the normal wrist, after complete LTq ligament sectioning. These findings may explain the relatively low incidence of radiocarpal arthrosis in late static LTq dissociations.

Diagnosis

LTq dissociation may present as a spectrum of clinical conditions, ranging from asymptomatic partial tears to painful complete dissociation with static collapse, causing a forklike deformity and prominence of the distal ulna.[78,419,599] Some patients describe painful crepitus as they ulnarly

---

*See references 16, 68, 78, 241, 315, 405, 419, 439, 520, and 522.

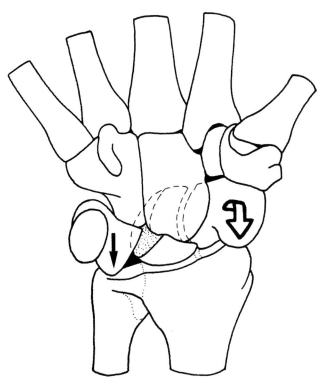

FIGURE 14-44. Schematic representation of the typical carpal bone displacement that occurs when both the extrinsic and intrinsic LTq supporting ligaments have failed. The scaphoid and lunate as a unit fall into flexion (CID-VISI) *(white arrow),* and the unconstrained triquetrum migrates proximally, especially in ulnar deviation *(black arrow).*

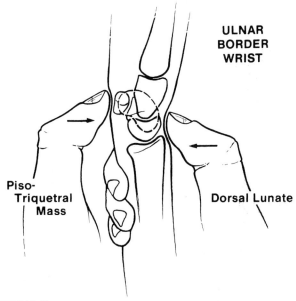

FIGURE 14-45. The "shear test" as described by Kleinman is similar to the ballottement test described by Reagan and coworkers.[454] This test is painful for a patient with a sprain or instability in the LTq joint. (Courtesy of William B. Kleinman, Indianapolis, IN.)

deviate the hand.[439,561] Symptomatic injuries invariably exhibit point tenderness directly over the dorsal aspect of the joint.[454] Pain is usually aggravated with ulnar deviation and supination.[92] Wrist motion is seldom diminished except in the more advanced cases with static carpal collapse. A frequent complaint is weakness or a sensation of instability or giving way. Some patients may have ulnar nerve paresthesias.

A helpful finding is a positive *ballottement test,* as described by Reagan and associates.[454] The lunate is firmly stabilized with the thumb and index finger of one hand while the triquetrum and pisiform are displaced dorsally and palmarly with the other hand. A positive result elicits pain, crepitus, and excessive displaceability of the joint.

A modification of the ballottement test is the *shear test* attributed to Kleinman and mentioned by Ambrose and associates (Fig. 14-45).[16] By stabilizing the dorsal aspect of the lunate, just beyond the medial edge of the distal radius, the pisiform is loaded in a dorsal direction, creating a shear force at the LTq joint that causes pain in the patient.

A variation of the shear test is the *derby test* reported by Christodoulou and colleagues.[92] It involves loading dorsally the pisiform while the patient rotates the wrist along the "dart-throwing" plane (from extension-radial deviation to flexion-ulnar deviation). This provokes reduction of the subluxed LTq joint, by which the feeling of instability disappears and grip strength increases as long as pressure over the pisiform is maintained. This test appears to be very sensitive in the diagnosis of the unstable LTq joint.[92]

A further screening test is the *ulnar snuff box* test described by Ambrose and associates.[16] It involves applying a lateral pressure over the medial aspect of the triquetrum, just palmar to the extensor carpi ulnaris, while the wrist is radially deviated. If this reproduces the patient's symptoms, either an LTq injury or an ulnar styloid-triquetrum impingement syndrome should be suspected. When this test is positive, the possibility of a TFCC problem is less likely.

Unfortunately, most of these provocative maneuvers are very sensitive but poorly specific. A positive response to intra-articular injection of lidocaine does not differentiate LTq tears from other local problems. There are many possible causes of pain on the ulnar side of the wrist, several of which are likely to elicit a painful response to most of these tests. The more frequent include symptomatic LTq synchondrosis secondary to an incomplete congenital coalition,[213,466] degenerative changes on the proximal pole of the hamate secondary to either a long-standing midcarpal instability or a triquetrum-hamate impingement,[73,402] avulsion fractures of the dorsum of the triquetrum,[298,563] pisotriquetral arthropathies,[74] traumatic or degenerative tears of the TFCC,[423] ulnocarpal impaction syndrome (ulnar-plus variance),[93] extensor carpi ulnaris tenosynovitis,[91] and entrapment of the dorsal branch of the ulnar nerve.

Radiographic Examination

Standard wrist views appear normal in most patients with recent dynamic instability caused by a partial tear. Occasionally, in chronic dynamic instabilities, a slight narrowing of the LTq joint with subchondral cyst formation on the apposing sides of the joint may appear. This, however, should not be confused with similar findings in patients with incomplete coalition.[213,466]

When there is complete rupture or attenuation of both intrinsic and extrinsic LTq supporting ligaments, resulting in a static VISI pattern of malalignment, certain radiographic

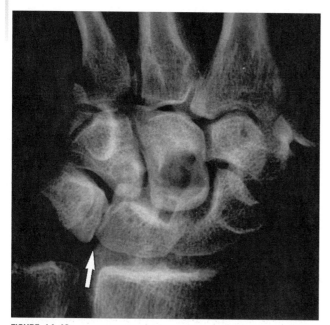

FIGURE 14-46. Late degenerative changes of a static LTq dissociation. Note the typical stepoff in the LTq interval, a break in Gilula's line *(arrow)*, and the midcarpal (hamate-lunate) articular deterioration involving cystic formation within the head of the capitate. The RSL joints are usually spared.

changes are obvious. Most characteristic is the disruption of the normal convex arc of the proximal carpal row (Gilula's line; Fig. 14-46).[16,426,454] This is visualized as a stepoff between the lunate and the triquetrum and a shallow-appearing outline on a PA radiograph. Rarely, there is an increased gap between the two dissociated bones.

If the carpus has collapsed into a static VISI, one can be confused and suspect an SLD, because of the presence of a slightly increased SL gap and a positive ring sign of the flexed scaphoid.[36] The first does not necessarily represent a rupture but an axial load being applied to the most palmar

SL ligament fibers, which, as demonstrated by Kauer,[278,279] are longer and obliquely oriented, allowing an increased, but normal, separation of the two bones.

In static VISI the lunate has a triangular (moonlike) appearance, such that its dorsal pole is superimposed on the mid to distal part of the capitate, obviously implying an abnormal flexion of the SL complex (Fig. 14-47). This appearance does not change in ulnar-deviated views, except for the increased proximal displacement of the triquetrum relative to the rest of the proximal carpal row (Fig. 14-48). In collapsed cases, the carpal height ratio may be abnormal.

In the lateral projection, aside from the VISI pattern of malalignment, it is sometimes possible to find a decreased LTq angle (normal average of 14 degrees, according to Reagan and coworkers[454]) (Fig. 14-49). Assessment of this angular measurement, however, requires films of excellent quality and considerable practice, and even then its determination is often not possible.

Bone scans are a particularly useful tool where doubt exists about the presence of a chronic LTq tear being secondary or not to an ulnocarpal abutment. If the injury is due to a chronic ulnocarpal impingement, the bone scan frequently shows an area of increased uptake in the lunate.[547] In pure LTq instabilities the scan is seldom positive.[283]

Arthrography may demonstrate a communication of dye between the radiocarpal and midcarpal joints.[7] It is important to bear in mind, however, that an arthrographic communication may indicate a traumatic injury, a chronic age-related perforation,[597] or ligament degeneration caused by an ulnocarpal impaction syndrome.[93] Shigematsu and associates[519] found a 100% incidence of LTq perforations in wrists with ulnar-positive variance. Herbert and colleagues[226] showed a high incidence of positive arthrograms in asymptomatic wrists. By contrast, Reagan and coworkers[454] had three negative studies in 16 surgically demonstrated LTq tears.

Cineradiography may be helpful and is always recommended. In static VISI deformities, as the wrist moves from radial to ulnar deviation, in the frontal plane, the TqH joint is always engaged (in the "low" position, as pointed out by

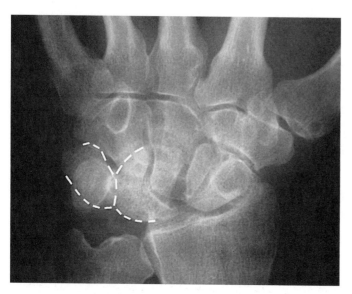

FIGURE 14-47. PA view of static LTq dissociation in a 48-year-old man whose left wrist had been injured in a motor vehicle accident 3 years before this radiograph was taken. The initial radiographs had been normal. One year after the accident, a minor sprain initiated a process of progressive weakness and increasingly painful snapping during lateral deviations. Note the moonlike configuration of the lunate in VISI and "shallow"-appearing outlines of both the proximal and distal LTq borders *(dashed lines)*. The SL joint space is somewhat widened anteriorly. This probably represents attenuation rather then rupture, the consequence of the palmar fibers of this joint being longer than the dorsal ones.

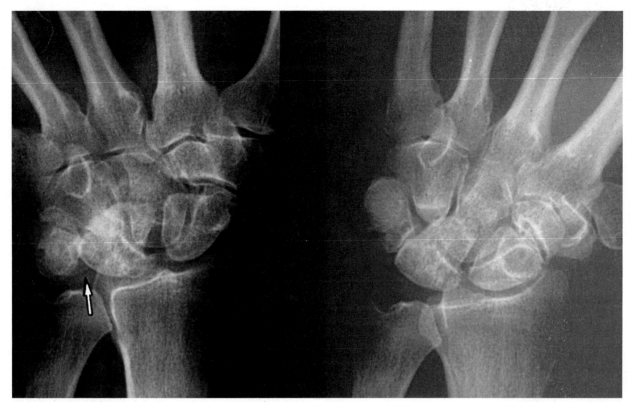

FIGURE 14-48. Dynamic radiographs of static LTq dissociation. During radial deviation *(right)*, both the scaphoid and the lunate are abnormally palmarflexed but the triquetrum is normally aligned relative to the lunate. During ulnar deviation *(left)*, by contrast, there is a significant stepoff between the lunate and triquetrum *(arrow)*.

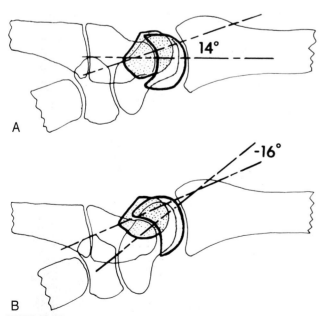

FIGURE 14-49. The LTq angle may be difficult to measure in the lateral radiograph but the angle has been shown by Reagan and coworkers to be decreased in a patient with LTq static VISI. (From Reagan DS, Linscheid RL, Dobyns JH: Lunotriquetral sprains. J Hand Surg [Am] 9:502-514, 1984, with permission.)

Taleisnik[562]) and the SL complex experiences little extension in ulnar deviation (see Fig. 14-48). In the sagittal plane, when the patient attempts to flex, the LC joint hardly rotates but hyperflexes the RC joint.

Arthroscopy has become an increasingly important diagnostic and therapeutic tool for the evaluation of lesions on the ulnar side of the carpus[419] and may also identify previously unrecognized types of ligamentous disruptions.[363] In LTq (Geissler's grade II) interosseous ligament injuries there is slightly increased play between the triquetrum and lunate, with the first being more distal in relation to the lunate (Fig. 14-50). Bulging of the LTq interosseous ligament from the RC space is another sign indicating abnormal stretching of the LTq membrane. In LTq grade III, the interosseous space can be opened with the probe and a gap is seen between the involved carpals both from the RC and midcarpal space (Fig. 14-51). As always, correlation of these findings with those of the patient's clinical examination is important.

Treatment of the Different Forms of LTq Dissociation

The heterogeneity of clinical conditions presenting with substantial damage of the LTq linkage is such that finding a classification where each group could be assigned one specific treatment is difficult. Although conceptually interesting, most previous attempts to classify LTq dissocia-

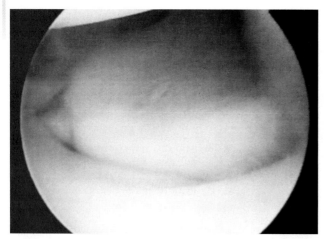

FIGURE 14-50. Arthroscopic view of a Geissler grade II LTq interosseous ligament injury as seen from the midcarpal space with the arthroscope in the radial midcarpal portal. Note the slight distal orientation of the triquetrum. There would be more "play" of the triquetrum than normal when palpated with a probe.

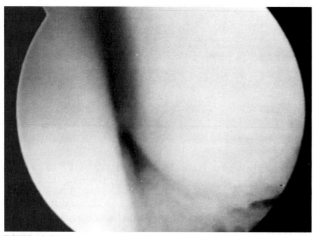

FIGURE 14-51. Arthroscopic view of a Geissler grade III LTq interosseous ligament tear as seen from the radiocarpal space with the arthroscope in the 6-R portal. Note the gap between the carpal bones.

tions[419,454,480,599] failed to cope with the complexity of the issue, either being too simple or poorly clinically useful. To improve its use, we have modified Seidman and Osterman's[419] classification, recognizing six different types of LTq injury with each group having its own prognosis and treatment. Based on this, all cases in the same group would be candidates for a similar treatment. This, of course, does not negate the general principle according to which all treatments need to be individualized according to the patient's age, occupation, recreational demands, and intensity of symptoms.

LTq Dissociation, Type 1 (Acute, Dynamic)

This group is formed by the acute, isolated, partial or complete disruption of the LTq ligaments, without radiographic evidence of malalignment. For a case to be included into this group: (1) the diagnosis has to have been made early, when the healing capacity of the disrupted ligaments is optimal, (2) there must be complete disruption of the intrinsic liga-

ments, and (3) all secondary constraints (extrinsic ligaments) must be intact and competent.

In the past, most authors agreed in that acute LTq injuries causing a dynamic instability were to be treated conservatively, in a carefully molded cast or splint, with a pad beneath the pisiform and over the dorsum of the distal radius to maintain optimal alignment.[283,343,405,439,454] Failures from that approach, however, were not unusual, with some cases progressing toward a static VISI type of carpal instability. Failures were mostly due to lack of ligament healing and the subsequent attenuation of the secondary constraints. In fact, unless pronosupination is blocked by including the elbow in the cast, the amount of motion that occurs in the LTq joint during forearm rotation is substantial owing to the "pistonage" effect of the ulna against the carpus through the TFCC. Such micro-motion prevents proper connective tissue formation at the repair site. Conservative treatment, therefore, is only exceptionally recommended, in which case an above-elbow cast is required.

The introduction of arthroscopy as a routine exploration in wrist trauma allowed much better and earlier recognition of the extent of these lesions (often larger than expected), resulting in an increased awareness of these injuries' potential risk.[468,639] This, and the occasional poor results obtained by conservative means, induced many authors to recommend multiple percutaneous pinning of the joint as the gold standard in the treatment of the early dynamic LTq instability.[283] Osterman and Seidman[419] realized an 80% success rate with this treatment strategy.

The arthroscopic technique for reduction and pinning of acute tears of the LTq ligaments is similar to that for SL injuries. Initially, the radiocarpal space is evaluated with the arthroscope in the 3-4 portal. A working portal is made in the 6-R or 4-5 portal. The tension of the articular disk is carefully probed through the 6-R portal to rule out a peripheral tear of the TFCC. The arthroscope is then transferred to the 6-R portal to better visualize the LTq proximal membrane. The LTq interval can be found by following the lunate distally and ulnarly and looking for a shallow concavity in the sagittal plane. For a better visualization the arthroscope is to be pulled dorsally just before it exits the capsule. The LTq interval should also be evaluated from the midcarpal space through the radial midcarpal portal. A needle or probe can be inserted to the ulnar midcarpal space to evaluate any potential gap and the amount of play between the lunate and triquetrum. It is important to remember that a small amount of play between the lunate and triquetrum is normal. When this occurs, the stepoff is even and the triquetrum is not rotated. Unfortunately, to define the amount of motion that is normal versus abnormal can only be gained through experience.

Arthroscopic pinning of acute LTq ligament injuries may be performed for Geissler's grades II, III and IV injuries. It is easiest to take the wrist out of the traction tower and to insert the Kirschner wires into the triquetrum under fluoroscopy control. It is important to use a soft tissue protector or a 14-gauge needle to protect the dorsal sensory branches of the ulnar nerve. Once the wires are in the triquetrum, the wrist is placed back in traction. With the arthroscope in the radial midcarpal portal, rotation of the LTq joint is controlled using the Kirschner wires as joysticks while the other wires are advanced into the lunate. Three or four Kirschner wires are utilized. The position of the wires is then evaluated under fluoroscopy in the AP and lateral planes. Fat droplets will usually be seen as the wires pass across the triquetrum into the lunate.

Postoperative management is similar to arthroscopic pinning of the SL joint. The patient is placed in a short-arm splint or cast. The Kirschner wires are then removed at 4 weeks, and the wrist is splinted for an additional 4 weeks. Range of motion and strengthening exercises are initiated at 3 months postoperatively. The 80% success rate obtained by Osterman and Seidman[419] supports this strategy.

LTq Dissociation, Type 2 (Chronic, Dynamic)

A ligament rupture is considered chronic when, being underestimated, missed, or left untreated, its two ends have degenerated, diminishing the chances for a successful repair. In such circumstances, a more aggressive approach is necessary to reestablish the synchronicity of motions between the triquetrum and lunate. Different strategies have been proposed: simple arthroscopic débridement, electrothermal shrinkage, ligament reconstruction using a strip of the extensor carpi ulnaris tendon,[522] or LTq intercarpal arthrodesis.[214] No approach has enjoyed consistent success in these chronic injuries.

The technique for arthroscopic débridement of a chronic tear to the LTq interosseous ligament is relatively straightforward. The arthroscope is initially placed in the 3-4 portal and a mechanical débrider is brought in through the 6-R portal. Whereas the normal concave appearance of the LTq interval is not well visualized with the arthroscope in the 3-4 portal, when the membrane is torn its fibers hang down and this can be better seen. With a shaver in the 6-R portal, the torn fibers hanging down are débrided back to a stable surface. The arthroscope is then placed in the 6-R portal to evaluate the final arthroscopic débridement (Fig. 14-52).

Weiss[638] reviewed his results in arthroscopic débridement in partial and complete tears of the LTq interosseous ligament at an average of 27 months after the procedure. Twenty-six of 33 patients who had a complete tear of the LTq interosseous ligament and all the 43 patients who had a partial tear had complete resolution or decrease in symptoms. Patients tolerated débridement of the LTq interosseous ligament better than the SL interosseous ligament in his series, possibly owing to the lower stress that is placed on the ulnar side of the wrist. Débridement of complete LT ligament tears does not address any component of joint instability, and long-term evaluation of this approach is needed.

Tolan and coworkers[576] suggested to treat chronic LTq instabilities by pinning the LTq joint with Kirschner wires while closing the interval between the UL and UTq ligaments with PDS sutures under arthroscopic control. Moskal and colleagues reviewed 20 patients treated with this technique, reporting 13 excellent, 5 good, and 2 fair results, according to the modified Mayo wrist score. Four minor complications were reported.

Tendon reconstruction of complete disruption of the LTq ligaments associated with chronic instability is another alternative.[454,522] The technique consists of reconstructing the LTq linkage with a strip of extensor carpi ulnaris, left attached distally and passed through holes in the lunate and triquetrum. By tightly looping the tendon graft around the LTq joint, immediate stability is achieved. The reconstruction is secured by transfixing the joint with Kirschner wires for 8 weeks, followed by 4 more weeks of protective splint.

Fusing the unstable LTq joint is another alternative.[7,283,405,439] The procedure has met with variable success, a relatively high nonunion rate, and considerable complications.[514] According to Guidera and colleagues,[214] most complications of LTq fusion result from either a poor indication or technical problems. By using cancellous bone graft to fill a biconcave space created in the adjoining bones and stabilizing the joint with multiple Kirschner wires (Fig. 14-53), these authors reported a 100% consolidation in an average of 50 days. In their series of 26 wrists, postoperative flexion-extension averaged 78% of the range measured at the contralateral side, with good or excellent pain relief in 83% of the cases and with 88% of patients returning to their previous occupations. Similar results had been previously published by Kirschenbaum and associates.[283] Yet, a meta-analysis of 143 LTq fusions showed this intervention not to be devoid of problems when incorrectly planned and/or executed: a nonunion rate of 26% and a complication rate of 43% mostly in the form of persistent pain.[343,514,527,588] Indeed, as stated by Sennwald and associates,[514] LTq arthrodesis still is a controversial procedure. Particular care should be taken to differentiate symptomatic LTq tears from ulnar impaction syndrome; in the latter, simple ulnar shortening can simultaneously address both the lunate impaction and the resultant LTq tear.

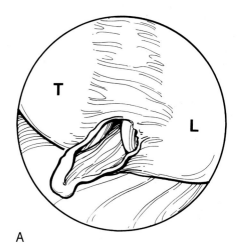
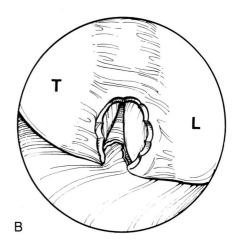

A

B

FIGURE 14-52. A, An idealized drawing to show a tear of the central fibrocartilaginous portion of the lunotriquetral (L, T) interosseous ligament. **B,** Post-débridement view demonstrating intact palmar and dorsal segments of the ligament.

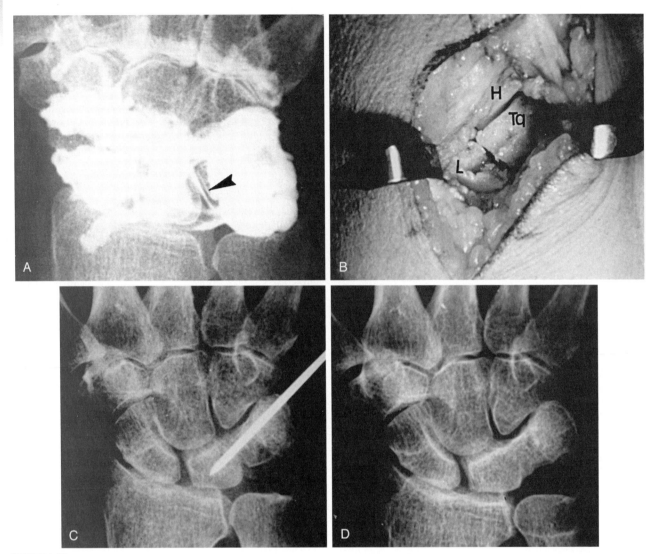

FIGURE 14-53. Chronic ulnar-side wrist pain in a 36-year-old woman who could not recall any traumatic event. **A,** Arthrography demonstrated the presence of dye leakage *(arrow)* between the radiocarpal and midcarpal joints (via the LTq joint), whereas the TFCC was normal. **B,** Increased hypermobility and complete rupture of the LTq interosseous ligaments were demonstrated at operation, so a local fusion was done. A procedure similar to the Russe inlay bone graft of the scaphoid was utilized. H, hamate; Tq, triquetrum; L, lunate. **C,** A single Kirschner wire was used in this patient to secure the joint during the healing process. Currently, after the publications by Nelson and colleagues[405] and Kirschenbaum and associates,[283] we tend to use multiple wires and/or a Herbert screw to improve the chances of healing. **D,** Fifteen months after surgery the fusion was solid but some tenderness persisted. Later studies showed this to be the consequence of an ulnocarpal impaction problem, which was solved by an ulnar-shortening procedure.

The only series of patients comparing ligament reconstruction versus LTq fusion has been reported by Shin and associates.[454,522] It consisted of 57 patients treated for an isolated traumatic tear of the LTq joint and retrospectively reviewed with an average follow-up of 9.5 years. The authors demonstrated a dramatic difference between the two treatment methods, with a 41% nonunion rate and a high reoperation rate for ulnar impaction in the arthrodesis group. Patients who underwent tendon reconstruction of the LTq ligaments had higher subjective and objective outcomes and a much lower complication rate than the arthrodesis.[522]

LTq Dissociation, Type 3 (Static)

This group is formed by cases with complete disruption of the intrinsic LTq ligaments with attenuation of the secondary extrinsic stabilizing ligaments (dorsal and palmar radiocarpal ligaments[241,465]). As a result of such a global ligament insufficiency the carpus collapses into a VISI pattern of malalignment. Because the underlying pathology is both intrinsic and extrinsic, it is not surprising that localized fusions of the LTq joint could not achieve proper control of the malalignment. Indeed, isolated fusion of the LTq joint is bound to fail in this type of instability, and a more extended intercarpal arthrodesis is recommended.[419]

Taleisnik[565] suggested adding an RL fusion to the LTq fusion. As an alternative, the ulnar midcarpal joint may be included in the fusion site. No ligament reconstruction has been found to reliably correct such a complex unstable condition.

LTq + SLD, Type 4 (Acute Perilunate Instability)

By definition, perilunate instabilities, stages III and IV, involve an association of injuries around the lunate including complete rupture of both the SL and LTq interosseous ligaments. The prognosis of the injury, if unsolved, is worse than in the isolated LTq injury: stability is at a higher risk, hence the necessity of a more aggressive approach. Owing to its inherent instability, these conditions are to be treated surgically, most commonly through a double palmar-dorsal approach, emphasizing anatomic reduction of the proximal row, direct ligament repair (particularly its most important palmar LTq component[464,465]), and percutaneous Kirschner wire fixation. If the SL injury has healed correctly but the LTq joint remains unstable, a symptomatic carpal collapse in the form of VISI is likely. By contrast, if both SL and LTq levels remain unconstrained the wrist collapses most commonly in the form of DISI. A more detailed discussion of how to treat perilunate dislocations is provided later in this chapter.

LTq + SLD, Type 5 (Chronic Perilunate Instability)

When not adequately addressed, most perilunate injuries evolve into a state of permanent subluxation (carpal collapse into either a VISI or DISI) with reduction of mobility and grip strength and eventually joint degeneration and the subsequent synovitis and pain. Dealing with chronic bipolar instability is difficult and results obtained through soft tissue reconstructions are seldom acceptable. In the literature there is little information about this specific problem. In general, when the proximal row presents a combined SL and LTq dissociation most authors recommend a proximal row carpectomy.[112,210,246,248,331,407] Alternatively, excision of both scaphoid and lunate while fusing the LC joint may also produce good results.[80] Long-term results of those approaches, however, are not yet available.

LTq Dissociation, Type 6 (Degenerative Ulnocarpal Abutment)

The presence of a positive ulnar variance (ulna plus) is often linked with an increased ulnocarpal pressure that may, with time and repetitive use, provoke a degenerative defect in the proximal portion of the LTq interosseous membrane, eventually destabilizing the joint. Such a defect should not be interpreted (or treated) as if it was a primary injury of the LTq joint but as a secondary feature of an ulnar abutment syndrome. In fact, most failures of LTq fusions appear to be linked to an undetected ulnocarpal impaction.[658] In 1989, Palmer[423] proposed a classification system for tears of the TFCC, which basically divides these injuries into two categories: traumatic (class I) and degenerative (class II) lesions. Perforation of the LTq interosseous ligament occurs in class II-D and II-E degenerative tears. Treatment of class II-D and II-E symptomatic lesions includes arthroscopic débridement and ulnar shortening, if the patient has an ulnar-positive wrist with ulnocarpal impaction.[642] The ulnar head may be shortened arthroscopically or by means of open ulnar-shortening osteotomy. For the arthroscopic technique, the scope is inserted into the 3-4 portal and a bur is placed in the 6-R portal. The ulnar dome is excised through the defect of the torn articular disk. The forearm is rotated to gain access to the peripheral margins of the ulnar head. The bur may be placed proximal to the articular disk through a separate distal radioulnar joint portal for improved access to the ulnar head. Under normal conditions, up to 4 mm of bone may be resected. Fluoroscopy should be used to monitor the resection because magnification makes it

difficult to judge arthroscopically the amount of bone being excised. Care should be taken not to remove too much articular cartilage from the distal radioulnar joint. The surgeon should ensure the preservation of the stability of the distal radioulnar joint by not removing the origins of the distal radioulnar and ulnocarpal ligaments. Electrothermal shrinkage of the ulnocarpal ligaments may be an option when an arthroscopic "wafer" procedure is performed, to increase tension of the ulnar carpal ligaments and potentially decrease the LTq instability secondary to the interosseous ligament tear. Eventually, the procedure is supplemented by a transient fixation of the LTq joint with Kirschner wires, aiming to stabilize the joint by fibrous tissue. Ulnar shortening, however, is contraindicated in the more unstable cases with a static VISI, because it would inevitably tighten the palmar ulnocarpal ligaments and therefore increase the already malaligned lunate.

Authors' Preferred Methods of Treatment: LTQ Dissociation

We do not treat conservatively acute tears of the LTq ligamentous complex (type 1). The morbidity of percutaneous fixation is minimal compared with the benefits of a good ligament healing. Furthermore, by ensuring complete immobilization of the joint with wires, the wrist can be mobilized earlier (at 4 weeks), which allows a much faster recovery of motion. We also strongly recommend repairing the palmar LTq ligament rupture in acute perilunate dislocations (type 4), as it will be emphasized later in this chapter. Trying to repair the dorsal component is seldom successful, owing to the small size and thickness of this ligament, hence the need for a prolonged Kirschner wire fixation. We have little experience with the extensor carpi ulnaris tendon reconstruction suggested by Shin and Bishop,[522] an option that appears as a promising solution for chronic, dynamic LTq dissociations (type 2). It is an anatomically sound intervention, because it replaces the most important stabilizer of the joint, the palmar LTq ligament. Despite criticisms, however, one of us (MG-E) is still happy with LTq fusions, using cancellous bone from the distal radius and multiple Kirschner wires, as recently described by Guidera and associates.[214] It is important to emphasize, however, that in the UC impaction syndrome, no fusion will be successful unless associated with a "wafer" procedure (open or arthroscopic) or with a formal ulnar shortening, our preferred technique.[93,439] One of the advantages of the latter procedure is that, after the ulnar osteotomy is done, the distal ulna can be swung out, allowing exploration of the undersurface of the perforated TFCC, and through it the LTq joint can be débrided and grafted without opening the RC capsule. We do not recommend a localized fusion if there is already a VISI carpal malalignment (type 3) or a bipolar chronic SL and LTq dissociation (type 5). In the first case, we tend to fuse the RL joint together with the LTq joint, whereas in the second case a proximal row carpectomy is preferred.

CRITICAL POINTS: LUNOTRIQUETRAL ARTHRODESIS

INDICATIONS

- Dynamic LTq instability secondary to complete intrinsic ligament rupture, in the absence of an ulnocarpal abutment syndrome (normal TFCC) and normal midcarpal joint
- Perilunar SL and LTq instability

PREOPERATIVE EVALUATION

- Obtain a positive LTq ballottement test.
- Perform fluoroscopic evaluation of abnormal proximodistal shift of triquetrum during radioulnar deviations.
- Perform arthroscopy to rule out TFCC degeneration and/or TqH impingement.

TECHNICAL POINTS

- Use a dorsal (zigzag, lazy "S," or longitudinal) incision centered at the IV-V septum.
- Section the extensor retinaculum along the fifth compartment.
- Open the septum between IV and V. Coagulate the intraseptal artery.
- Perform a "Z" capsulotomy creating two flaps following the "fiber splitting" concept.
- Perform a complete section of the remnants of the LTq ligaments.
- Open the LTq as a book, and remove the adjacent articular surfaces with a dental rongeur to expose cancellous bone. Do not excise the rim of the opposing cortical edges to preserve the normal interosseous separation.
- Harvest cancellous bone from the radius through a window created at the floor of the IV compartment.
- Preset two 1.5-mm nonparallel Kirschner wires in the ulnar aspect of the triquetrum.
- Densely pack cancellous bone graft in the biconcave cavity.
- Reduce the joint and drive the two Kirschner wires into the lunate; verify their position, and cut below the skin surface.
- Use a standard capsular and retinacular closure.

POSTOPERATIVE CARE

- Apply a short-arm/thumb spica cast for 6 weeks, changed at 10 days for stitch removal and radiographs.
- At 6 weeks, remove cast, evaluate with radiographs, and apply a new cast.
- Obtain radiographs out of cast every 2 weeks until healing is obvious, at which point remove the wires using local anesthesia.
- Begin rehabilitation after cast removal to regain motion and grip strength.
- Do not allow contact sports until 6 months after surgery.
- Probable outcome: 75% of patients will have a painless wrist with 80% of global motion and 75% grip strength.

Carpal Instability Secondary to Scaphoid Disorders

The scaphoid has long been recognized as the key element in the maintenance of an adequate relationship between the proximal and distal rows.[198] As an intercalated segment, when the wrist is axially loaded, the scaphoid prevents what Fisk[162] termed the *concertina deformity,* that is, carpal collapse. Not only is its integrity and correct alignment important, but its own geometry needs to be normal so as not to create a global carpal destabilization. If the scaphoid has fractured into two or more unstable fragments, the distal portion has a tendency to follow the motion of the distal row and the proximal fragment acts in concert with the proximal row. In such circumstances, control of the overall carpal motion is no longer possible, resulting in an obvious dyskinematic behavior of the midcarpal joint.[39,536] Furthermore, when fractured, the scaphoid cannot transfer load normally, acting as an imperfect kinetic linkage between the two rows.[596] Under load, its proximal part tends to follow the unconstrained lunate and triquetrum by rotating into extension, while the distal fragment is forced into flexion by the axial force exerted by the trapezoid and trapezium.[39,381,536] Alternatively, if the fracture is obliquely inclined dorsally, the distal portion may displace along the fracture surface, resulting in scaphoid shortening and dorsal RS impingement.[382]

If not properly reduced and stabilized, the fractured scaphoid tends to develop a pseudarthrosis.[110] Stable nonunions rarely have global mechanical consequences. However, if the nonunion is unstable and substantial motion occurs at the nonunion site, the scaphoid frequently undergoes severe deterioration of its palmar cortex, with the subsequent loss of bone stock.[110,192,322,382] In these instances, the so-called humpback deformity often appears: the two scaphoid fragments become malrotated and angulated into flexion and ulnar deviation (dorsolateral convexity) (Fig. 14-54). The resultant carpal instability can be categorized as a proximal CID, because the disruption occurs within the proximal row and typically progresses into a DISI pattern of carpal malalignment. In the presence of a scaphoid fracture, therefore, a dorsal tilting of the lunate (DISI configuration) should be regarded as an indirect sign of scaphoid fracture displacement (see Fig. 14-16).[162-164,537]

If the scaphoid fracture finally heals but in a deformed palmar-flexed posture, its external dimensions will not be normal and the orientation and congruency of its articular facets will be inadequate to cope with its important stabi-

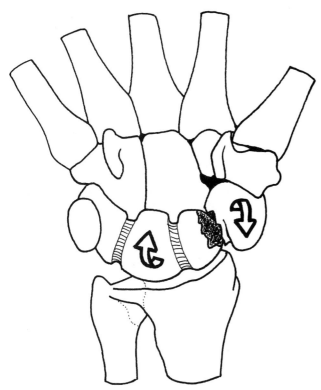

FIGURE 14-54. Schematic representation of the moments *(white arrows)* involved in the displacement of an unstable scaphoid fracture. The distal fragment tends to flex while the proximal fragment follows the lunate and triquetrum into an extended position (DISI configuration).

lizing role.[400] Scaphoid malunions can also be the source of instability and thus of pain, weak grip strength, and reduced motion, especially wrist extension.[72,110,157,159,332,400]

Treatment

Surgery of the unstable scaphoid is technically demanding.[110,164,352,391,577] It requires a high level of expertise and a perfect understanding of the anatomy of the bone, particularly its three-dimensional alignment.[191] The surgeon must be aware of the necessity of obtaining fracture consolidation and, most importantly, of reestablishing the normal length and shape of the scaphoid, so that the anatomic relationship between the bone and the rest of the carpus is normalized.[110,155,397,460,581,664] A thorough description of the techniques to achieve these goals is provided in Chapter 21.

Authors' Preferred Method of Treatment: Unstable Scaphoid Fractures

In acute, potentially unstable fractures (vertical, comminuted), where the risk of developing secondary carpal instability is high, we prefer early open reduction, excision of comminuted fragments, corticocancellous bone grafting, and Kirschner wire fixation. If there is no comminution, arthroscopically guided reduction and percutaneous fixation

is becoming our gold standard of treatment. In any case, displaced fractures are only exceptionally treated conservatively because, indeed, the possibility of a progressive loss of reduction is always substantial. To evaluate intrascaphoid angulation, we prefer the CT technique described by Sanders[489] and the so-called cortical method of determining intraosseous alignment of fragments as described by Smith and associates.[538] If grafting is believed to be necessary, the scaphoid is approached through an anterior Russe incision.[482] In all other cases, the dorsal approach is preferred, because it provides the best anatomic reference to correct any rotational deformity: the articular surface to the capitate.

Carpal Instability in Kienböck's Disease

Although Kienböck's disease is fully covered elsewhere in this book (Chapter 21), it is appropriate to make a brief comment about the peculiar features of the carpal instability that appears when the diseased lunate has collapsed. In fact, one of the prognostic factors of Kienböck's disease, according to the Stahl-Lichtman[314] staging system, is the absence (stage IIIa) or presence (stage IIIb) of a rotatory subluxation of the scaphoid. In stage IIIa the carpus remains relatively stable, whereas in stage IIIb it has collapsed. Indeed, fragmentation of the lunate results not only in loss of the mechanical strength of the central column but also in disruption of the kinematic linkage of the proximal row, owing to failure of both SL and LTq ligament attachments. In such circumstances, the loaded scaphoid tends to follow its natural tendency and progressively collapses into flexion, while the triquetrum migrates proximally. Conceptually, the resultant instability would be categorized as a CID pattern; and, depending on which part of the lunate is most involved (palmar or dorsal), the carpal malalignment may be VISI, DISI, or none if there is a global fragmentation with proximal migration of the capitate.

In the past few years, a number of limited intercarpal arthrodeses have been found beneficial in the treatment of Kienböck's disease. Some of them, especially those eliminating motion between the scaphoid and the distal carpal row (STT and SC), are said to be effective lunate unloading procedures.[442,619] Despite controversies about their lunate decompressive effects, these interventions have proved valuable in preserving carpal stability by preventing scaphoid rotary subluxation.

Our preferred method of treatment for Kienböck's disease, stage IIIb, consists of (1) a 5- to 10-degree lateral closing wedge osteotomy, with or without radial shortening, depending on ulnar variance; (2) removal of any extruded or unstable fragment of the lunate; and (3) SC arthrodesis. The main objective of the fusion is not to decompress the lunate but to stabilize the scaphoid and allow for a better functional outcome. At this stage, any attempt to revascularize the fragmented avascular (dead) bone is likely to fail.

CARPAL INSTABILITY NONDISSOCIATIVE (CIND)

When there is a major carpal dysfunction occurring between the radius and the proximal row and/or between the proximal and distal rows, and yet a relatively normal relationship between the bones of the proximal and distal rows is maintained, the case is considered a nondissociative pattern of carpal instability.[12,658] Depending on which joint is mostly affected, CIND problems can be further subdivided into radiocarpal and midcarpal.

Radiocarpal CIND

Included in this group are patients with insufficiency or rupture of the obliquely oriented radiocarpal ligaments, whose carpus has displaced down the slope of the radius and appears ulnarly translocated.[453] The laboratory investigations by Viegas and colleagues,[602] Ritt and associates,[467] and Wiesner and coworkers[646] determined the importance of specific ligaments in preventing this type of problem. The condition is more commonly seen in rheumatoid patients,[531] in developmental deformities such as Madelung's,[242] after excessive excisions of the distal ulna,[325] and, more rarely, after pure radiocarpal dislocations.[137] In the first group, ligament insufficiency results from the attritional effects of chronic synovitis. In Madelung's deformity, the ligaments fail owing to fatigue, because they must constrain excessive shear forces. Pure traumatic dislocations are very rare, but they frequently result in chronic radiocarpal instability.[137,138]

Ulnar Translocation

The first traumatic ulnar translation of the carpus owing to complete disruption of ligaments was described in 1975 by Dobyns and colleagues.[131] In partial injuries, the carpus may translate palmarly rather than ulnarly in a radiocarpal supinated subluxation, as reported by Bellinghausen and colleagues.[35]

Taleisnik[559,562] pointed out that there are two distinct types of ulnar translation: In type I, the entire carpus, including the scaphoid, is displaced and the distance between the radial styloid process and the scaphoid is widened (Fig. 14-55). In type II, the relationship between the distal row, the scaphoid, and the radius remains normal; the SL space is widened; and the LTq complex is ulnarly translocated. This is an important distinction to make for different reasons. Conceptually, type I is a true CIND instability, whereas type II has features of both CIND (ulnar translocation of the lunate and triquetrum) and CID (SLD), and this, according to the Mayo classification,[12] makes it a CIC pattern of instability. In practice, distinction between the two patterns is useful, because there is completely different ligament involvement, each requiring distinct treatment: type I injuries result from failure of all the radiocarpal ligaments, including the RS and RSC, whereas in type II injuries, neither the RSC nor the RS ligaments are ruptured but there is complete SL disruption. When presented with a widened SL joint (Terry Thomas sign[167]), it is important to bear in mind the possibility of an ulnar translation of the LTq complex (type II injury) and avoid an erroneous diagnosis. Indeed, if a type II ulnar translocation is treated only by stabilizing the apparent SLD, the underlying radiocarpal instability will remain unresolved.

As described in the discussion of the radiographic examination of carpal instabilities, different methods of assessing ulnar translation have been reported (see Fig. 14-15).[441] The two indices using the center of the capitate head as a carpal reference (Chamay and coworkers[88] and McMurtry and associates[353]) should not be used in type II injuries, for in these cases, only the LTq complex is significantly displaced. By contrast, when using the lunate as a reference,[64,319] if the

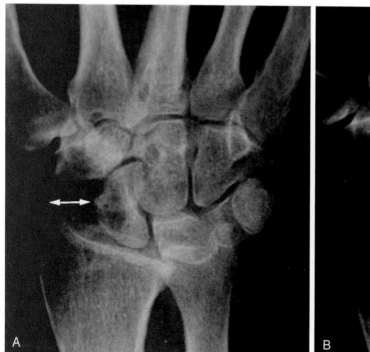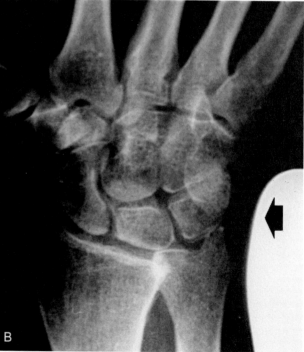

FIGURE 14-55. Ulnar translocation (Taleisnik's type 1[559,562]) in a 50-year-old woman with rheumatoid arthritis. **A,** Note the widened radial styloid-scaphoid space *(white arrow)* and how this unstable situation can be easily reduced (**B**) by laterally directed pressure *(black arrow).*

wrist is slightly radially or ulnarly deviated, the measurements may not be reliable.

A single series of eight patients with traumatic ulnar translation of the carpus was reported by Rayhack and colleagues.[453] Their experience indicates that this is a difficult problem to treat effectively. They had rather disappointing results with delayed ligament repairs and suggested that, in these patients, RL fusion, as reported by Chamay and coworkers[88] and Linscheid and Dobyns[323] for the treatment of ulnar translocation in rheumatoid patients, is probably the only reliable alternative. Penny and Greene,[434] however, reported one such patient who had a satisfactory result after early open reduction and extensive repair of the ligamentous damage through both dorsal and palmar approaches.

Radial Translocation

The so-called radial translocation instability usually appears in badly malunited distal radial fractures where the distal surface healed slightly radially inclined. If in such circumstances both the short RL and UC ligaments are attenuated, ruptured, or avulsed, the loaded carpus may sublux in a radial direction, causing substantial discomfort, reduced grip strength, and a giving-way sensation when the patient attempts to lift a weight.[9] The condition may also appear after an excessive radial styloidectomy.[401] More unusually, ulnar-side ligament support may generate a dynamic radial translation instability even if the radius is normally inclined. In such cases the lateral RC subluxation is visible only when the wrist is stressed in a radial direction. According to Allieu and Garcia-Elias,[9] these conditions are probably not as infrequent as previously thought, responding well to corrective osteotomy of the radius and surgical reattachment of the UC ligaments.

Pure Radiocarpal Dislocation

According to Dumontier and coworkers[137,138] there are two types of RC dislocation. Type 1 includes patients with a pure RC dislocation, without an associated fracture of the distal radius. Type 2 involves an RC dislocation with an avulsion fracture of the radial styloid process containing the origin of the palmar RS and RSC ligaments. The first type is exceedingly rare with no more than 20 cases being reported.[138,147,168,328,374,434] Usually, they are the result of severe shear and rotational injury in young subjects. Associated neurovascular damage is not unusual. Reduction is easy by manipulation, but this is always unstable, owing to the loss of radiocarpal ligament attachments.[147,374] Type 2 RC dislocations with an associated avulsion fracture of the radial styloid have been more frequently reported.[137,138,168,306,387,415] These, however, represent a completely different injury, with a much better prognosis provided that the styloid fracture, which contains the avulsed radiocarpal ligaments, is correctly reduced and fixed.

Midcarpal CIND

The term *midcarpal instability* is commonly used to describe a group of diverse conditions in which there is no dissociation between bones of the proximal carpal row but a dysfunction of both RC and midcarpal joints, the latter tending to predominate. Probably the term *instability of the proximal carpal row*, as suggested by Wright and coworkers,[658] would have been more appropriate, because most of these conditions have abnormalities of both midcarpal and RC levels.[21] For historic reasons, however, and to avoid further confusion, we will keep using the term *midcarpal instability*. Although the literature concerning these conditions is scarce (Table 14-4), substantial contributions have been made[21,148,450,658,669] that will provide a better understanding of one of the most intriguing dysfunctions of the wrist.

Pathomechanics

As discussed in the biomechanics section of this chapter, under axial compressive load the proximal row tends to rotate into flexion and pronation, a tendency that appears to

---

Table 14-4
MIDCARPAL INSTABILITY: IMPORTANT CONTRIBUTIONS

- *Mouchet and Belot* (1934)[385]: First description of a "snapping wrist," diagnosed as "anterior midcarpal subluxation."
- *Sutro* (1946)[554]: Report of two patients with symptomatic clunking of their wrists, one of whom was cured by fusing the midcarpal joint.
- *Linscheid, et al.* (1972)[325]: Description of five patients with a palmar flexion instability, two of whom could voluntarily subluxate their wrists, "to the amusement of friends and the consternation of their doctors." Suggested etiology: congenital or sequel of ligamentous laxity.
- *Lichtman, et al.* (1981)[316]: First description of the so-called ulnar midcarpal instability as a characteristic pattern of radiologic signs (VISI pattern of malalignment) and symptoms (painful, spontaneous wrist click with ulnar deviation) related to failure of the ulnar limb of the palmar arcuate ligament.
- *Taleisnik and Watson* (1984)[567]: Introduction of the term *extrinsic midcarpal instability*, referring to a painful snapping of the midcarpal joint secondary to injuries outside the midcarpal joint, most commonly a distal radial malunion.

- *Louis, et al.* (1984)[329,645]: Description of the so-called capitate-lunate instability pattern (CLIP syndrome), which combines both a midcarpal and a radiocarpal instability. The authors suggested establishing this diagnosis with the aid of fluoroscopy by applying traction and palmar-dorsal translation and observing the increased displaceability of both radiolunate and lunocapitate joints.
- *Lichtman, et al.* (1993)[313]: Identification of four different groups of patients with clinical midcarpal instability
- *Wright, et al.* (1994)[658]: The largest series of soft tissue reconstruction in carpal instability nondissociative (CIND) problems (34 reviewed patients). In a 5- to 8-year follow-up, there was no significant difference between those treated operatively and nonoperatively.
- *Apergis* (1996)[21]: Emphasis on the frequent involvement of both radiocarpal and midcarpal ligaments in most midcarpal instabilities.
- *Feinstein, et al.* (1999)[148]: Quantitative assessment of the midcarpal shift test, allowing grading of the severity of midcarpal ligament insufficiency

be counteracted by the palmar midcarpal crossing ligaments. Especially important stabilizers are the palmar TqHC ligament, the dorsolateral STT ligament, and the SC ligaments.[34,173,316] These ligaments not only play a key kinetic role in preventing midcarpal collapse but also are essential to ensure a smooth, progressive transition of the proximal row from flexion to extension as the wrist deviates ulnarly. Because the proximal bundles of the TqHC ligament are proximally located relative to the axis of ulnar deviation, they pull the triquetrum into extension as the wrist ulnarly deviates (Fig. 14-56). Similarly, the SC ligament is likely to contribute by dragging the scaphoid into extension as the capitate rotates ulnarly.

Of course, one should not forget the influence of the TqH joint in the induction of such rotation.[630] This, however, is not fully effective until the wrist is already somewhat ulnarly deviated and the two bones (triquetrum and hamate) are fully engaged. Consequently, any injury resulting in increased laxity of the TqHC and SC ligaments is likely to have two consequences: (1) the loss of the ability to transfer loads adequately without collapsing into a nondissociative VISI deformity and (2) the rotation of the proximal row from flexion to extension that cannot be smooth and progressive but is sudden and sometimes painful when the wrist reaches a certain amount of ulnar deviation and the TqH joint takes control of the proximal row motion.

In the laboratory, several investigations have addressed the intricate mechanism of midcarpal stabilization.[316,381,383,396,580,599] The consequences of sectioning the midcarpal crossing ligaments are better understood, but still little is known about under what sort of stresses these ligaments fail.

Classification

In 1993, Lichtman and coworkers,[313] based on previous reports in the literature and on their own experience, identified four different groups of patients with clinical midcarpal instability (MCI). With slight modifications, the four groups can be defined as follows (Fig. 14-57):

1. *Palmar MCI.* This group is formed by patients with an acute or chronic nondissociative VISI malalignment, complaining of a painful clunking in the wrist, secondary to attenuation or rupture of the palmar midcarpal crossing ligaments. This group can be divided into two

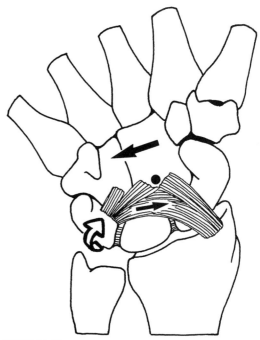

FIGURE 14-56. Suggested mechanism of action of the triquetrum-hamate ligaments during wrist ulnar deviation. As demonstrated by Youm and associates,[667] the center of rotation of the wrist during radioulnar inclinations lies about the center of the head of the capitate. All ligament fibers inserted proximal to it are likely to increase in tension (*small black arrow*) as the wrist ulnarly deviates (*large black arrow*). These fibers play a role in the initiation of the progressive extension of the triquetrum relative to the radius (*white arrow*). When these fibers fail, the proximal row will not extend until a more advanced ulnar deviation is achieved and the hamate-triquetrum articular surfaces become fully in contact, forcing sudden extension of the triquetrum.

subgroups depending on which of the two midcarpal ligament complexes (medial or lateral) is primarily affected. If there is a predominant TqH dysfunction (injury to the TqHC ligament) the case is commonly referred to as "ulnar MCI" as opposed to "radial MCI" where there is a predominant STT dysfunction due to injury of the STT and SC ligaments.[313]

2. *Dorsal MCI.* This variety of MCI is usually formed by young patients with bilateral hypermobile wrists who, as

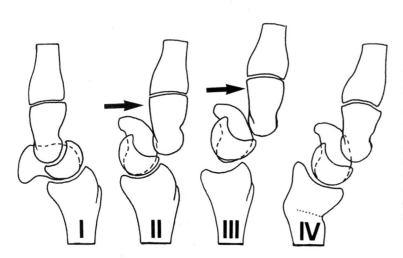

FIGURE 14-57. Lichtman's[313] classification of midcarpal instabilities (MCIs). Type I (palmar MCI): the whole proximal row appears abnormally flexed in the lateral view. Type II (dorsal MCI): normal alignment in standard radiographs, but abnormal midcarpal subluxation when a dorsally directed force (*black arrow*) is applied. Type III (dorsal and palmar MCI): both midcarpal and radiocarpal joints are abnormally subluxable in a palmar and dorsal direction, usually the consequence of increased global laxity. Type IV (extrinsic MCI): the midcarpal dysfunction is the consequence of an extracarpal problem, usually a malunited distal radius as shown here.

a result of either excessive overload or trauma, present with chronic unilateral wrist pain, snapping, and a positive dorsal displacement test. Symptoms in these patients are believed to be secondary to further attenuation or disruption of the RSC ligament. There is no static malalignment of the carpus in this condition. Included in this group are the so-called CLIP wrists reported by Louis and colleagues[329] and the CL instabilities described by Johnson and Carrera.[271]

3. *Dorsal and palmar MCI.* Combination of dorsal and palmar instability, owing to laxity of both midcarpal and radiocarpal ligaments, not infrequently associated with ulnar-minus variance and an increased slope of the distal radius (Fig. 14-58).[21] Included in this group would be the so-called proximal carpal row instabilities reported by Wright and coworkers.[658]

4. *Extrinsic MCI.* Patients with a chronic dorsally malunited radius may develop progressive stretching of the RSC and UC ligaments, thus reproducing the typical symptoms of a dorsal MCI. In palmar malunited fractures, a nondissociative VISI pattern of MCI may appear. According to Allieu and associates,[8,65] these types of problems should not be categorized as true carpal instabilities but as a carpal adaptation to an external problem. In this chapter, carpal instabilities of an extrinsic origin are discussed separately.

Diagnosis

MCI patients typically present with a painful clunk during activities, especially those involving ulnar deviation and pronation in the wrist.[67,148,271,316,561] Except for extrinsic MCIs, rarely is there a specific traumatic event that can clearly explain the onset of symptoms. Instead, most patients have congenital laxity,[188,499] suffer from some sort of repetitive stress[67,115] or chronic use of corticoids,[34] or have sustained mild trauma initiating their wrist pain.[148,499] There

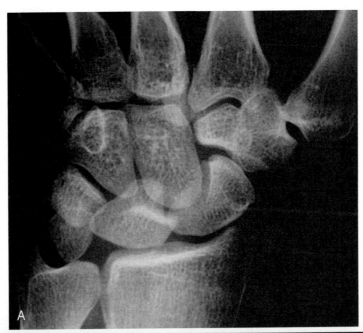

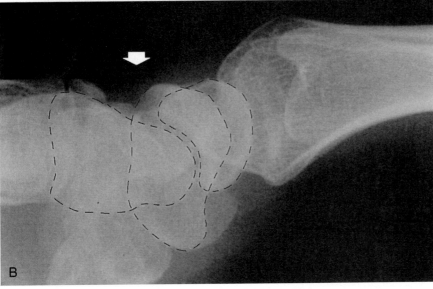

FIGURE 14-58. A, Type III midcarpal instability in a hyperlax 23-year-old woman who became symptomatic (painful catch-up clunk) soon after starting a new job in a meat processing plant. **B,** Note the palmar sag *(white arrow)* owing to the carpal malalignment. Conservative treatment and activity modification yielded good results.

may be an obvious sag in the palmar direction of the mid-carpal joint, actually the consequence of a palmar translation plus supination deformity of the distal row relative to the two forearm bones,[316,467,561,646] or else the joint is normally aligned with the subluxation only appearing under specific loading conditions. Most patients (91% in Wright's series[658]) have evidence of a painful snapping (the so-called catch-up clunk) as the palmar sag is corrected in ulnar deviation. Wrist motion may be reduced, and grip strength is usually impaired.

Differential clinical diagnosis between LTq disruption and palmar MCI can be established by using the LTq ballottement[454] and shear[15] maneuvers (see Fig. 14-45). Both tests are negative in palmar MCIs but induce sharp pain and increased mobility in LTq dissociations.

A useful maneuver to determine the amount of MC joint laxity is the so-called midcarpal shift test, described by Lichtman.[148,316] It consists of reproducing the painful clunk by passively palmar translating and ulnar deviating the wrist in pronation. Based on how much resistance is necessary to maintain the wrist palmarly subluxed in ulnar deviation, wrists are classified into five grades. The more severe MCI is the one in which subluxation is so easily achieved that it can be spontaneously reproduced without assistance from the examiner.[148]

Except for patients with dorsal MCI, radiographs demonstrate the typical VISI deformity, especially on unsupported lateral views compared with the opposite wrist. In the PA view, the scaphoid is foreshortened and exhibits the typical ring sign while the lunate has the typical "moonlike" appearance. A relatively widened SL space is often seen, although this should not be interpreted as a sign of rupture. Indeed, the palmar SL ligament, the one bearing most of the load when the joint is in flexion, is much longer than its dorsal counterpart, allowing a wider (yet normal) separation of the joint. Because the transverse relationship between the three proximal row bones is not violated, both Gilula's lines[431] and SL and LTq angles should be normal. The RL and LC angles, by contrast, are altered in palmar MCI. It is important to obtain comparable views of the opposite wrist for comparison.

Stress views are very useful to demonstrate the type of MCI, particularly the dorsopalmar capitate-displacement test (see Fig. 14-58).[271,418,499] Malalignment, however, is seldom as severe as for static LTq dissociations. By definition, arthrograms should always be negative.[313,658]

Cineradiography and fluoroscopy are the most helpful tools for the diagnosis of these problems.[7,264,448] In the normal wrist, one can recognize synchronized movement of the proximal carpal row from flexion to extension as the wrist ulnar deviates. In MCI, the proximal carpal row remains flexed throughout the entire range of motion except when the wrist reaches a certain ulnar-deviated position when it suddenly snaps into an extended position, often with a quite dramatic, sometimes audible clunk (Fig. 14-59). There may be a contralateral laxity of the wrist, but typically this is not associated with pain. In flexion-extension the study tends to be normal.

The role of arthroscopy in the diagnosis of midcarpal instability is minimal. Under traction, the elongated palmar capsule allows larger than normal separation of the joint with apparently normal palmar ligaments. In long-standing

cases, recurrent subluxation may have caused degenerative changes on the palmar aspect of the lunate or on the proximal pole of the hamate.

Treatment

These patients should always be initially treated with a period of nonoperative therapy, including some type of immobilization, typically splinting, anti-inflammatory medication, and activity modification.[329,645,658] Especially important is to reestablish adequate proprioceptive control of the proximal row by the flexor carpi ulnaris/hypothenar muscles complex. In mild MCIs, isometric contraction of these muscles generates a dorsally directed force onto the triquetrum, via the pisiform, which may diminish the clunking and help in the resolution of symptoms. Failing this, three major options exist: extra-articular procedures (radioulnar joint leveling procedures),[658] soft tissue reconstructions combining both a palmar and a dorsal approach,[219,271,313,658] and limited intercarpal fusions.[188,313,561]

In some patients with ulnar-minus variance, some sort of radioulnar leveling procedure (e.g., radial shortening, ulnar lengthening) has been used.[658] The rationale of this is to provide support to the ulnar side of the wrist by gently pushing the TFCC against the triquetrum and ulnar aspect of the lunate. This appears to inhibit the rotational snap of the proximal row. Out of six patients with a combined palmar and dorsal MCI problem, the authors reported five good or excellent wrist scores. Some of the patients, however, also had some sort of soft tissue reconstruction.

In 1993, Lichtman and coworkers[313] presented a 48-month average follow-up on palmar MCI patients treated by either soft tissue reconstruction (nine patients) or limited carpal fusions, either triquetrum-hamate or four-corner fusions (six patients). They considered six of the reconstructions and none of the fusions to be failures, based on the patients' ability to return to their activities. Loss of motion was 28% in the reconstructed patients and 50% in the fusion group. Other proponents of fusing the midcarpal joint are Garth and colleagues[188] and Rao and Culver.[450] Although in most series about 50% of the patients remained symptomatic, clinically all felt improved. The reported nonunion rate for this arthrodesis is low[527] (see Fig. 14-59).

The option of ligamentous repair has been evaluated by different authors. Johnson and colleagues[271] operated on 11 patients with dorsal MCI with the goal of suture imbrication of the space of Poirier. Over a 4-year follow-up, 9 patients had good or excellent results, with little loss of motion, especially in extension. In 1983, Gibson[197] described a patient with post-traumatic MCI, characterized by a non-dissociative VISI deformity secondary to rupture of the palmar STT ligaments, who had successful surgical ligamentous repair. Two similar cases were reported in 1988 by Hankin and coworkers.[219] Zancolli[669] recommended capsular augmentation of the ulnar-dorsal corner of the TqH joint with a strip of ECU tendon, a technique that was found successful in 16 patients with a localized laxity of the dorsoulnar corner of the TqH joint.

The largest series of soft tissue reconstruction in CIND problems was reported by Wright and coworkers.[658] Sixty-eight percent of the 34 reviewed patients had evidence of a congenitally increased laxity. In a 5- to 8-year follow-up, there was no significant difference between those treated

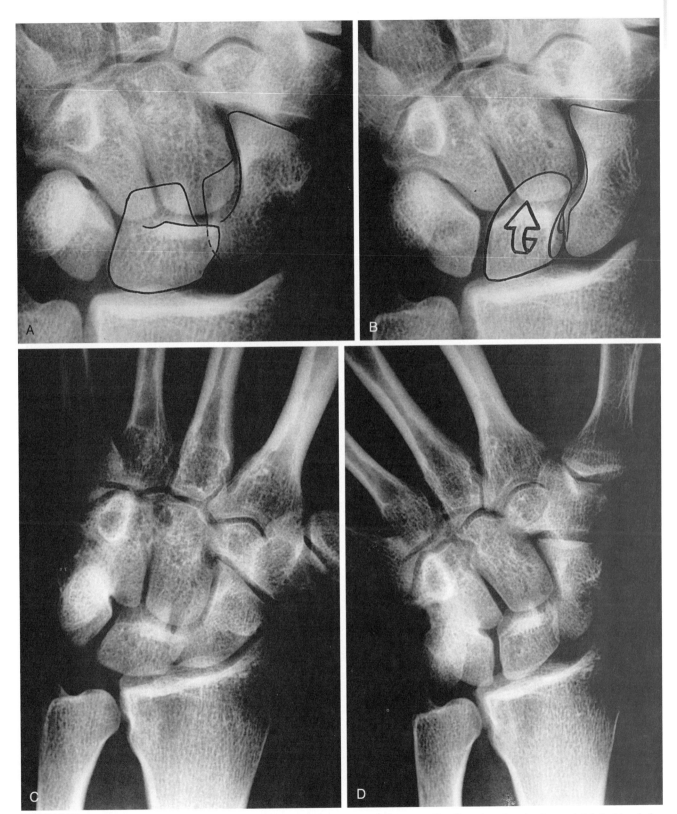

FIGURE 14-59. A 21-year-old man sustained a hyperextension injury to his right wrist 2 years earlier. Since then, there has been painful clunking during radioulnar deviations. Dynamic radiographs demonstrated a sudden shift *(white arrow)* of the lunate and scaphoid from a flexed (**A**) to an extended position (**B**) as the wrist reached a certain degree of ulnar deviation. Conservative treatment did not succeed in relieving his symptoms, and a TqH fusion was performed. Four months after surgery the patient was back to his former occupation, without any complaint. At 18 months of follow-up the clunking had not recurred but an obviously altered carpal kinematics was evident. From radial (**C**) to ulnar deviation (**D**), little midcarpal motion exists. Whether such increased radiocarpal shear will result in early degeneration is unknown but is certainly a good possibility. (Courtesy of J. Aragon, Santa Coloma, Spain.)

operatively and nonoperatively. However, in those patients whose problem was found to depend solely on the insufficiency of one specific ligament, a direct augmentation of that structure tended to have a better result. As always, the more precise the diagnosis, the more specific the treatment can be and the better the chances for success.

Authors' Preferred Method of Treatment: Midcarpal Instability

The dorsopalmar capitate-displacement test[418] is our preferred test to identify which of the four MCI groups the patient is in and what treatment strategy is best for each patient. In general, most midcarpal dysfunctions are initially treated conservatively. Splinting and avoidance of activities reproducing the painful snapping are helpful measures but should always be associated with a program designed to maximize the ability of the flexor carpi ulnaris to become a dynamic stabilizer of the joint. Indeed, this muscle may actively constrain the tendency of the proximal row to collapse into flexion in the absence of palmar midcarpal ligaments. Certainly, muscle-strengthening exercises can resolve the symptoms in most hyperlax teenagers, a group of patients who, in our experience, should very seldom be treated surgically. Recurrence of a painful dysfunction may occur, however, in which case either an arthroscopic palmar midcarpal capsular shrinkage can be attempted (we have not much experience yet, but it looks promising) or a more complex surgical treatment can be considered.

Palmar MCI

In the past, most patients with palmar MCI and normal scaphotrapezial and radiocarpal joints were treated by fusing the TqH joint. Unfortunately, we failed to reproduce the encouraging results reported by others.[188,313,450] Some of our patients kept complaining of RS impingement pain, whereas others disliked not being able to move the hand in a more natural way. Indeed, midcarpal fusion prevents the most useful "dart-throwing" motion (see Fig. 14-59). To find an alternative, one of us (MG-E) started a prospective study of patients having the tenodesis procedure shown in Figure 14-60. Two longitudinal incisions (dorsal and palmar) are used. Two drill holes 3.2 mm in diameter are made: one from the dorsal aspect of the capitate into the carpal canal and another from the anterior aspect of the triquetrum to its dorsal ridge. A strip of extensor carpi radialis brevis tendon is passed through the capitate hole, retrieved palmarly, and passed again through the triquetrum hole to reconstruct the palmar TqC fascicle. The tendon is pulled taut, and sutures reinforcing the remnants of the palmar TqHC ligament are placed. Once back on the dorsum, the tendon is tightly sutured on the origin of the dorsal RTq ligament. Initially we used Kirschner wires to further stabilize the construct. In the latest cases we believed this not to be necessary for we immobilize the wrist in a short spica cast for 8 weeks. The results obtained in seven consecutive cases, with an average

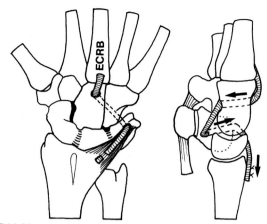

FIGURE 14-60. The authors' preferred tenodesis procedure to reinforce the two major ligament problems in type I palmar MCI. A distally attached strip of the extensor carpi radialis brevis (ECRB) is raised and passed through holes in the capitate and triquetrum to re-create both the ulnar limb of the arcuate ligament (triquetrum-capitate fascicles) and the dorsal RTq ligament.

follow-up of 26 months (14 to 84 months) have been very promising, with minimal discomfort, excellent grip strength, and minimal loss of motion. All patients returned to their occupations without clunking.

Dorsal MCI

When surgery is required for dorsal MCI, which in our experience is very seldom (usually they are hyperlax teenagers responding well to physiotherapy), we are pleased with the method described by Johnson and Carrera.[271] Through an extended anterior approach to the carpal tunnel, the radial and ulnar sides of the space of Poirier are obliterated with 3-0 nonabsorbable sutures to reinforce both the TqHC and the RSC ligaments.[516]

Combined Palmar and Dorsal MCI

In our opinion, there is rarely an indication for surgery in combined dorsal and palmar MCI. As demonstrated by Wright and coworkers,[658] the results of surgery in such multidirectional instabilities are no better than the ones obtained without surgery. In our experience, when all conservative measures failed, these patients respond very well to an RL fusion, a procedure suggested by Taleisnik.[218,565] By fusing the lunate to the radius, the keystone of the carpus is placed in an aligned and stable position, allowing good recovery of grip strength, with excellent pain relief, often with a surprisingly minimal loss of range of motion.

CARPAL INSTABILITY ADAPTIVE (CIA)

Although carpal malalignment secondary to malunited distal radial fractures was already recognized by Dobyns and associates[131] in 1975, the concept of adaptive instability was not introduced until 1982 by Allieu and colleagues,[8,65] who proposed that the intrinsic carpal architecture was not altered by malunited fractures of the distal radius. Therefore, by correcting the underlying pathology, the altered carpal alignment should take care of itself and not require further treatment.[13] In 1984, Taleisnik and Watson[567] confirmed these ideas when they reported on 13 patients with dorsally malunited distal radial fractures and secondary midcarpal dysfunction and malalignment. They used the term *extrinsic midcarpal instability* to differentiate these cases from those with intercarpal instability patterns. In a patient with a dorsal malunited distal radius fracture, the lunate adopts a DISI configuration relative to the capitate, the axis of which becomes dorsal to the long axis of the radius. The condition leads to progressive pain, tenderness to palpation at the midcarpal joint, and occasionally a painful, audible snap. In Taleisnik and Watson's series,[567] a corrective osteotomy consistently resulted in excellent relief of pain and resolution of the carpal instability. A detailed description of the surgical methods to correct these deformities is given in Chapter 16.

This particular pathology, however, should not be confused with those conditions where the distal radius fracture is concomitantly associated with an intracarpal ligament injury.[189] Unless properly recognized and treated, such ligament injuries may evolve into a dissociative instability, which will result in progressive carpal dysfunction long after the distal radius fracture has healed. For a diagnosis of adaptive carpus to be made, it is important to rule out the existence of any significant intracarpal ligament injury.

CARPAL INSTABILITY COMPLEX (CIC)

When the carpal derangement has impaired both the relationship between bones within the same row (CID features) and between rows (CIND features), the resultant dysfunction is categorized as a carpal instability complex (CIC).[12,658] Except for pure radiocarpal dislocations, which are classified with the nondissociative instabilities, all other carpal dislocations are complex and fulfill the criteria of CIC. Within this category of injuries, five groups of carpal dislocations have been identified:

  I. Dorsal perilunate dislocations (lesser arc)
 II. Dorsal perilunate fracture-dislocations (greater arc)
III. Palmar perilunate dislocations (lesser or greater arc)
 IV. Axial dislocations
  V. Isolated carpal bone dislocations

The first two groups have in common a carpal derangement occurring around the lunate—the first as a pure ligament disruption problem, the second involving fracture of the adjacent bones. The third group, although perilunate, results from a different mechanism producing a palmar displacement of the distal row relative to the lunate. The fourth and fifth groups represent a variety of nonperilunate dislocations, usually the result of high-energy trauma.

Dorsal Perilunate Dislocations (Lesser Arc Injuries)

Under the diagnosis of dorsal perilunate dislocation, also known as retrolunate dislocation,[27] different forms of displaced carpal derangement exist. They can be pure ligamentous injuries or fracture-dislocations. Johnson[269] pointed out that most dislocations in the carpus are confined to a relatively vulnerable area around the lunate, including the proximal portions of the scaphoid, capitate, and triquetrum. Based on this, he suggested using the term "lesser arc" injuries to refer to pure perilunate dislocations, as opposed to "greater arc" injuries when one or several bones around the lunate have a concomitant fracture. This section focuses on the lesser arc injury, that is, the dorsally displaced perilunate dislocation without an associated fracture.

Throughout the literature, there has been a tendency to consider dorsal perilunate and palmar lunate dislocations as separate and distinct entities. In reality, as discussed in the pathomechanics section of this chapter, the two conditions represent different stages of the same pathomechanic process, the so-called progressive perilunate instability pattern.[344-346,348] In fact, when one attempts to surgically reduce a palmarly dislocated lunate, a dorsal perilunate dislocation can be easily reproduced. In other words, the position of the bones when the patient is seen in the emergency room does not necessarily reflect the degree of instability or the full extent of the ligamentous damage. Perilunate and lunate dislocations, therefore, are pathogenically equivalent lesions, and their management is almost identical (Fig. 14-61).

Another frequent misconception is that when the lunocapitate joint dislocates (Mayfield's[344] stage II), the scaphoid has either fractured or torn its ligamentous attachments to the lunate. In the literature, however, a number of perilunate dislocations with simultaneous scaphoid fracture and SLD have been reported,[498,595] demonstrating that the two lesions are not mutually exclusive. In fact, most experimentally produced scaphoid fractures have an associated partial SL interosseous ligament failure.[348,498] Herzberg and colleagues,[230] in a multicenter study of 166 perilunate dislocations, found six cases (3.8%) with a concomitant scaphoid fracture and SLD.

Treatment
In the literature, three major methods of treating carpal dislocations have been suggested: closed reduction and cast immobilization, closed reduction and percutaneous pinning, and open reduction and internal fixation.[295]

Closed Reduction and Cast Immobilization
During the 1920s, when case reports of lunate dislocations began to appear, many methods were suggested for closed reduction.[98,205,286,411] Davis,[124] in 1923, recommended using a broomstick as a fulcrum on the palmar surface of the wrist to push the lunate back up into position while simultaneous traction was applied to increase the space between the radius and capitate and make enough room for the lunate. Conwell[102] advocated the broomstick technique but recommended using the fluoroscope to check reduction. Adams[1] advised against the use of a hard surface, which he thought might damage the flexor tendons, suggesting that only the surgeon's fingers should be used as a fulcrum. MacConaill[334] advocated a slightly different method of reduction, employing a flexion maneuver to lock the capitate into the distal concavity of the lunate and then reducing the capitate and lunate together as a unit by extending the wrist. Tanz[569] advocated pronation of the hand relative to the forearm in addition to traction for reduction of a perilunate dislocation. Böhler[60] emphasized the necessity of continuous traction, without manipulation, as the only means of reducing the dislocation. Stevenson[551] recommended sustained traction

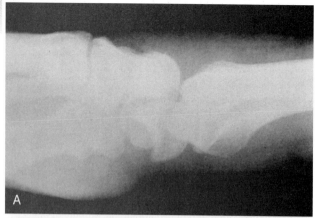

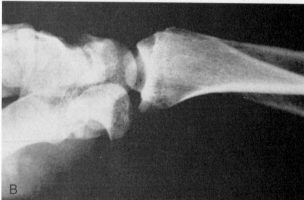

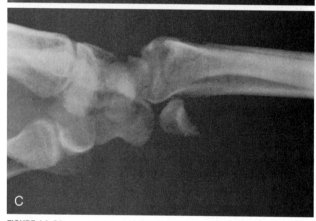

FIGURE 14-61. Carpal dislocations constitute a spectrum of injury, and the initial lateral radiograph in a patient with a carpal dislocation may depict a configuration at any point on that spectrum. **A,** A "pure" dorsal perilunate dislocation. **B,** An intermediate stage. **C,** A "pure" volar lunate dislocation.

with a skeletal distraction device for up to 3 days in long-standing cases in which manual traction was unsuccessful. More recently, an external fixator spanning the wrist has been used successfully by Fernandez[156,158] and Sousa and colleagues[544] as a means of obtaining an indirect reduction through ligamentotaxis and neutralizing the axial forces during the healing process.

Technique of Closed Reduction
Complete muscle relaxation is essential for an atraumatic reduction of a carpal dislocation. General anesthesia, axillary block, and intravenous regional anesthesia (Bier block) are all satisfactory; local infiltration anesthesia is not. An

initial period of 10 minutes of uninterrupted traction with the elbow flexed 90 degrees is helpful before reduction (Fig. 14-62). During traction, PA and lateral radiographs with the carpus distracted are obtained (see Fig. 14-17). These films are of great value in delineating the full extent of carpal damage.[211] Once the wrist has been distracted for 10 minutes, traction is released and the method of reduction described by Tavernier[570] and popularized by Watson-Jones[626,627] is attempted as follows.

With one hand, the patient's wrist is extended (maintaining longitudinal traction), while the thumb of the other hand stabilizes the lunate on the palmar aspect of the wrist. Gradual flexion of the wrist then allows the capitate to snap back into the concavity of the lunate (Fig. 14-63). According to Green and O'Brien,[211,212] reduction of the LC articulation occurs very rapidly as the capitate is brought over into flexion. To facilitate this, the operator's thumb stabilizes the lunate to prevent its being displaced forward by the capitate. Once the LC joint is reduced, and without releasing traction, the wrist is extended gradually while the lunate is pushed dorsally with the thumb, and a full reduction is usually achieved. Obviously, the sooner after injury this is performed, the easier is the reduction.

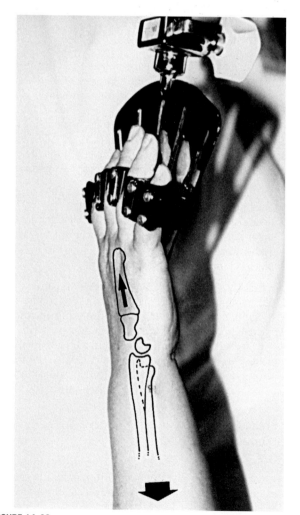

FIGURE 14-62. Before any attempt at closed reduction it is useful to apply 10 minutes of continuous axial traction to stretch out contracted muscle.

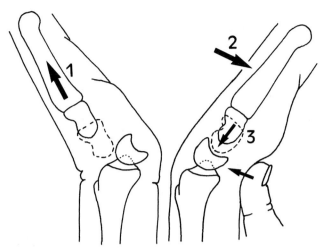

FIGURE 14-63. Schematic representation of Tavernier's[570] method of reduction of dorsal perilunate dislocations. (1) With the wrist slightly extended, gentle manual traction is applied. (2) Without releasing such traction, and while the lunate is stabilized palmarly by the surgeon's thumb, the wrist is flexed, until a snap occurs. This indicates that the proximal pole of the capitate has overcome the dorsal limp of the lunate. (3) At this point, traction is released and the wrist is brought back to neutral.

Few authors still advocate immobilization as definitive treatment for these severe injuries. The many different recommended positions of closed immobilization advocated in the literature include full wrist flexion,[626] slight flexion,[86,102,234,335,483] neutral,[277] and mild extension,[1,334,335] attesting to the fact that this technique does not produce consistently reliable results. Russell[483] and Watson-Jones[627] suggested only 1 week in flexion, followed by 2 weeks in neutral position. Green and O'Brien[211] prefer to initially immobilize the wrist with a dorsal short-arm/thumb spica plaster splint with the wrist in neutral or slight flexion.

Postreduction radiographs are then taken. It is imperative to take enough different views and assess "very critically"[211] the relationship of the capitate and lunate and the position of the scaphoid. An SL angle greater than 80 degrees and an SL gap greater than 3 mm have both been shown to indicate poor prognosis if not corrected.[363,452]

The period of plaster immobilization has also been a subject of considerable controversy in the literature. Several authors favor early mobilization: Adams[1] at 48 hours, Conwell[102] at 5 days, and Cave[87] at 1 week. Most[480,622] advocate 3 weeks of immobilization, although MacAusland[333] and Kaplan[277] recommend 6 weeks. Green and O'Brien,[211] in the few cases in which they considered closed reduction alone to be indicated, recommended 12 weeks of immobilization, with an admonition to weekly reassess the reduction radiographically for at least the first 3 weeks, because gradual loss of reduction occurs in more than two thirds of the cases (Fig. 14-64).[2]

Closed Reduction and Percutaneous Fixation

Because of the inherent instability of the scaphoid after closed reduction of perilunate dislocations, some authors favor percutaneous pin fixation.[643] This is an acceptable method of treatment only if anatomic reduction of all the perilunate joints has been achieved by closed manipulation. Most of what has been said about closed reduction and percutaneous pin fixation of SL and LTq dissociations also applies here.

Technique of Closed Reduction and Percutaneous Fixation

The hand is prepped with a standard surgical prep. The image intensifier or, alternatively, arthroscopic direct vision[643] is essential in this technique. Once reduction has been achieved, or if the surgeon considers it necessary to insert Kirschner wires to manipulate the bones to improve the reduction, the upper extremity is given a standard surgical prep. While the pins are inserted, the wrist is held in the reduced position by a knowledgeable assistant. Using a power drill, two Kirschner wires are inserted from the dorsum into the lunate and scaphoid. With them, under fluoroscopy, the lunate is first reduced relative to the radius and

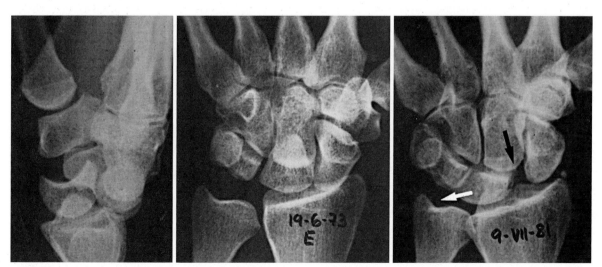

FIGURE 14-64. Nonoperative treatment of this dorsal perilunate dislocation, which consisted of reduction, cast immobilization for 7 weeks, and physical rehabilitation, was considered successful, until the patient was assessed 8 years after the injury. Chronic SLD (*black arrow*) associated with a type II ulnar translation of the lunate (*white arrow*) was the result of this suboptimal reduction.

a 1.2- or 1.5-mm oblique pin from the lateral aspect of the radial metaphysis is inserted across the RL and LTq joints. By manipulating the scaphoid joystick wire, the SL joint is reduced and a second pin is inserted transversely from the anatomical snuff box across the SL joint. Two slightly divergent pins are preferred for adequate fixation across this critical joint. At this point, traction is released and the normal congruency of the LC joint is inspected. If this is thought to be satisfactory, a third pin is passed across the SC joint. To avoid the radial artery and the superficial branch of the radial nerve, a small transverse incision just distal to the radial styloid process is used, followed by blunt dissection to identify and protect these structures before introducing the pins. A small drill guide or angiocatheter sleeve is helpful to avoid soft tissue injury from the drill torque.

The Kirschner wires are either left protruding through the skin, bent at right angles, or cut just under the skin to facilitate later removal. A padded thumb spica splint is applied immediately after the final radiographs have been obtained. This is converted to a thumb spica cast at 7 to 10 days after swelling has subsided and the pin tracts are seen to be free of infection. Radiographs are taken in the new cast to ensure proper maintenance of reduction. The cast and pins are removed at 8 weeks, and immobilization in a dorsal splint is continued for an additional 4 weeks, for a total of 12 weeks after reduction. There is a paucity of long-term results available to adequately critique this technique.

Open Reduction, Internal Fixation, and Ligament Repair

In the literature, there is ample evidence to discourage acceptance of suboptimal reductions of perilunate dislocations.[22,56,183,233,250,258,363,452,542] These, inevitably, lead to poor long-term results. Closed treatment should be continued only when a strictly anatomic reduction has been achieved or when other medical reasons contraindicate surgical intervention. Even when an acceptable restoration of the anatomy has been obtained, one must consider the benefits of an open procedure to avoid the frequently missed osteochondral defects and loose intra-articular bodies that can cause a poor result. In general, open surgery of any carpal dislocation is likely to achieve better results than closed treatment because it allows (1) a more complete recognition of damage, (2) removal of any intra-articularly interposed soft tissue, (3) removal or synthesis of any unstable chondral fragment, (4) a more accurate reduction of bone displacements, and (5) suture of any reparable ligament.[22,230,233,250,258,542] Minami and Kaneda[361] demonstrated that results of these injuries were improved when direct repair of the SL ligament was performed at the time of open surgical reduction.

Many of the early reports suggesting surgery for an irreducible palmarly dislocated lunate (perilunate dislocations were not considered an indication) advocated a dorsal approach, fearing further vascular damage to the lunate from the palmar side.[87,280,335,626] In 1923, Davis[124] devised a "lunate skid" that was designed to facilitate repositioning of the displaced lunate from the dorsum. Subsequent authors[60,69,234,335] have preferred the palmar approach. Böhler's[60] palmar approach was used in conjunction with skeletal traction to open up the RC space.

In 1964, Campbell and colleagues[82] reported on open reduction using a dorsal approach in nine patients and a palmar approach in four. They noted no avascular necrosis after surgery in any of the four patients in whom a palmar approach had been used. Yet in a subsequent article,[83] these authors recommended the dorsal approach because it allows better visualization of the LC joint and correction of the scaphoid subluxation; only if the lunate was greatly displaced or if decompression of the median nerve was necessary would a palmar approach be added.

In 1973, Dobyns and Swanson[133] advocated combining dorsal and palmar approaches to allow the surgeon to assess and repair the palmar capsular rent while controlling from the dorsum the accuracy of the reduction and also repairing the dorsal SL and LTq ligaments. A similar double approach has also been recommended by Meyrueis and associates,[359] Sotereanos and colleagues,[542] and Blazar and Murray.[56]

Taleisnik[559] recommended that these injuries always be exposed from the palmar approach, because this is the site of major ligamentous damage. Adkison and Chapman,[2] by contrast, recommended a dorsal approach only and reported good results by reducing and pinning these joints, without the need for individual ligament repair or augmentation procedures.

Currently, most authors strongly advocate open reduction and ligament repair as the treatment of choice for perilunate dislocations.* Fernandez[156,158] and Sousa and coworkers[544] further suggest the use of external fixation concomitantly with open reduction, because it facilitates exposure and protects the repair. Viegas[594] uses a reduction clamp to approximate the dissociated bones and facilitate a more reliable ligament repair.

Not infrequently, during the first months after reduction, the lunate bone may show increased radiodensity.[428,644] This, however, should not be interpreted as post-traumatic Kienböck's disease, because it tends to progress toward slow recovery without bone collapse in most cases. In the literature, very few cases of lunate fragmentation and collapse after carpal dislocations have been published.[194,388]

According to a multicenter study by Herzberg and colleagues,[230] the average wrist functional score (modified from Green and O'Brien[212]) of 10 acute perilunate dislocations that underwent open reduction and internal fixation was 86 points in Mayfield's stage II or III and 79 points in stage IV (normal score: 100 points). Similar results have been published by Inoue and Kuwahata,[250] Lacour and coworkers,[299] and Minami and Kaneda.[361]

Authors' Preferred Method of Treatment: Perilunate Dislocations

One of us (MG-E) strongly recommends early open reduction, ligament repair, and Kirschner wire fixation in all dorsal perilunate dislocations, regardless of the quality of

---

*See references 22, 56, 183, 230, 233, 250, 258, 363, 452, and 542.

CRITICAL POINTS: PERILUNATE DISLOCATIONS (TECHNIQUE FOR OPEN REDUCTION AND KIRSCHNER WIRE FIXATION: COMBINED DORSAL AND PALMAR APPROACH)

INDICATION

- All perilunate dislocations unless unstable medical condition contraindicates surgery

PREOPERATIVE EVALUATION

- Under axillary block, reduce the dislocation as soon as possible (Tavernier's maneuver).
- During reduction, obtain traction views.
- Place the forearm in elevation in a well-padded above-elbow cast until definitive surgery is possible.

TECHNICAL POINTS

- Center a dorsal 6-cm straight incision on Lister's tubercle.
- Open the extensor retinaculum along the III compartment and expose II to IV compartments. Elective neurectomy is performed on the posterior interosseous nerve.
- Extend a palmar carpal tunnel incision proximally across the wrist in a zigzag fashion. Flexor tendons and the median nerve are retracted radially.
- Search for the dorsal capsule, which is usually found avulsed off the radius. If the dislocation has not been reduced, an obvious empty space between the capitate and radius appears.
- Note that exploration of the palmar capsule will reveal a consistent arciform rent, coinciding with the space of Poirier, coursing along the sulcus between the RSC and long RL ligaments while ulnarly curving across the palmar LTq ligament. If the dislocation is unreduced, through this rent one can see the distal articular surface of the lunate.
- Reduce the lunate under direct vision by manually pushing it back in between the capitate and radius while applying gentle longitudinal traction on the hand.
- Repair the ulnar portion of the capsular rent (in fact, the disrupted palmar LTq ligament) with 3-0 nonabsorbable sutures.
- Note that the lateral portion of the palmar capsular derangement need not be repaired because it is, in fact, an anatomic defect: the interligamentous sulcus between the long RL ligament and the RSC ligament (Fig. 14-65).
- Through the dorsal approach, perform reduction and Kirschner wire fixation of the RL joint.

- Perform reduction and Kirschner wire stabilization of the LTq joint, plus repair of the dorsal ligaments.
- Perform reduction, stabilization, and careful repair of the dorsal SL ligament.
- Stabilize the lunocapitate joint with two crossed Kirschner wires, one through the scaphoid and the other across the triquetrum.
- Obtain radiographs to assess the quality of reduction and the purchase of the pins.
- Except for the flexor retinaculum, close all anatomic planes with sutures, leaving drains.

PEARLS AND PITFALLS

- Even if damage of the dorsal ligaments is not possible, their remnants should be tacked back into position. Suboptimal repairs may still result in acceptable function.
- Make sure that no osteochondral fragments are left inside the articulation.
- If there is substantial damage of the cartilage of the lunate, proximal row carpectomy may be a perfectly acceptable solution.[458]
- When present, radial styloid fractures should be reduced anatomically and held with additional Kirschner wires or screw fixation. If the fracture is comminuted, do not excise the unstable fragments in order not to destabilize the radiocarpal ligaments. Molding the fragments back into place as anatomically as possible is recommended.

POSTOPERATIVE CARE

- Apply a short-arm/thumb spica cast.
- Change the cast at 10 days for stitch removal and radiographs.
- At 8 weeks, remove cast and wires and begin rehabilitation to regain motion and grip strength. A protective removable splint is used between sessions.
- Note that most of these patients will have some permanent limitation of motion and that several months of rehabilitation will be required to regain range of motion and grip strength.

RETURN TO ACTIVITIES

- Return to heavy labor is rarely possible before 6 months and more commonly requires up to 12 months.[230,258,542]

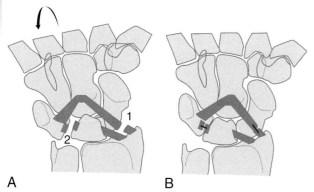

FIGURE 14-65. A, Schematic representation of the two levels of ligament disruption that need to be addressed when approaching palmarly a perilunate dislocation: (1) the origin of the RSC ligament may have avulsed off the radial styloid, and (2) the palmar LTq ligament often is disrupted through its mid substance and only occasionally shows an avulsion type of rupture. **B,** Once properly reduced, the two ligament injuries need to be repaired with mattress sutures *(black lines).* The apparent rent that exists between the avulsed RSC ligament and the long RL ligament needs no repair because it is an anatomic sulcus (space of Poirier).

reduction obtained by closed means. Obviously, this does not apply to those cases in which an unstable medical condition contraindicates surgery, in which case the dislocation is reduced under an axillary block and the operation is delayed. If the patient is reluctant to allow open surgical treatment or if an unstable medical condition is likely to persist for more than 1 week, closed reduction and percutaneous fixation are considered. Operative treatment for dorsal perilunate (Mayfield's[345] stage II or III) and palmar lunate (stage IV) dislocations is identical and differs only slightly from the already described surgical treatment of acute SLD (stage I).

Dorsal Perilunate Dislocations (Greater Arc Injuries)

Strictly speaking, only a trans-scaphoid, transcapitate, transtriquetral perilunate dislocation should truly be called a greater arc injury. This modality, however, is extremely unusual, with only two cases being reported in the English literature.[339,641] All other perilunate fracture-dislocations combine ligament ruptures, bone avulsions, and fractures in a variety of clinical forms. The most frequent is the dorsal trans-scaphoid perilunate dislocation.[229,231,373] Much less common, but interesting from a pathomechanic and surgical point of view, are dislocations involving displaced fracture of the capitate[153,587] and those with displaced fracture of the triquetrum in the sagittal plane.[212,269,413]

Trans-scaphoid Perilunate Dislocations

According to the three largest series of patients,[183,230,299] approximately 60% of perilunate dislocations present with a displaced scaphoid fracture, with most of them (72%) transverse and located in the middle third. Usually, the proximal fragment remains normally connected to the lunate, even if this has undergone a palmar dislocation (stage IV; 16% of all perilunate injuries, according to Herzberg and associates[230]). The exceptions are rare instances in which there is a concomitant SLD, with the proximal scaphoid being extruded dorsally.[253,258,299,498]

The initial management of trans-scaphoid perilunate dislocation, including the need for adequate anesthesia and preliminary traction, is identical to that described for dorsal perilunate dislocations. Radiographs taken with the hand suspended in fingertraps are particularly helpful in the assessment of bone damage and should be obtained routinely. Alternative methods of treatment are as follows.

Closed Reduction and Cast Immobilization

Although rarely recommended, the technique for closed reduction is the same regardless of whether the lunate is palmarly displaced or normally aligned and is almost identical to that described for lesser arc injuries. While maintaining some longitudinal traction, the surgeon stabilizes the lunate by pressing the palmar aspect of the wrist with the thumb.[570,626] From extension, the wrist is gradually flexed. Unless there is some soft tissue interposition, this maneuver brings the capitate back into the concavity of the lunate, sometimes with a snap. The wrist is then held in slight flexion and radial deviation, and a padded thumb spica cast is applied. At this point, it is important to take enough radiographic views to assess the scaphoid fracture reduction. Not only must the scaphoid be anatomically reduced, but the DISI deformity has to be corrected also. If one of these two factors is not completely solved (usually because of capsular interposition between the two scaphoid fragments[266,648]), reduction should be reattempted or, preferably, open treatment performed.

It is essential to have weekly radiographic evaluation of the scaphoid alignment for at least 3 weeks. If at this time the reduction is still acceptable, the wrist is brought from flexion to neutral and immobilized in a short-arm/thumb spica cast until the scaphoid fracture is healed. According to Cooney and colleagues,[110] the healing time reported for this type of fractures averages 16 weeks. Unfortunately, the rate of nonunion after nonoperative treatment approaches 50%.[192,535]

Closed Reduction and Percutaneous Fixation

If surgery is contraindicated or the patient refuses open treatment, once the dislocation has been acceptably reduced by closed means, an alternative to avoid progressive loss of reduction is to place two or more percutaneous Kirschner wires across the fracture and two additional ones stabilizing the SC and LTq joints. Another alternative is to place a trapeziolunate external fixator.[215] If available, arthroscopically guided percutaneous fixation tends to achieve more anatomic reductions than if only the fluoroscope is used.[191] No long-term results have been published using these techniques, however.

Open Reduction and Internal Fixation

By far, this is the most reasonable alternative for achieving anatomic reduction of the many structures that need to be repaired.[212,229,231,298,317,375,657] The same dorsal approach used in lesser arc injuries is recommended (Fig 14-66).[634] Palmarly, the Russe[482] approach as described for grafting scaphoid nonunions is adequate. This approach is mostly used to free the scaphoid fracture from interposed soft tissue,[266,648] to apply bone graft if indicated owing to palmar comminution,[440] and to repair the anterior capsular rent that typically coincides with the scaphoid fracture.[131] The sequence of

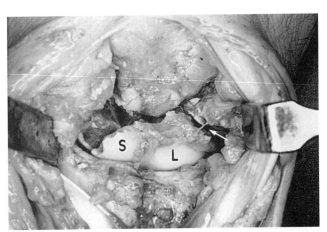

FIGURE 14-66. A dorsal approach for a trans-scaphoid perilunate dislocation provides excellent visualization of the different perilunate structures involved: the lunate (L)-scaphoid (S) fracture, lunocapitate joint, and LTq ligaments. Disruption with a small fragment avulsion *(arrow)* needs to be carefully repaired, as emphasized by Labbé and coworkers.[298] (Courtesy of A. Lluch, Barcelona, Spain.)

joint reduction is identical to that described earlier. Usually, bone reduction is better controlled from the dorsum by using Kirschner wires as joysticks. If the fracture is to be stabilized with a Herbert[227,256,595] or Acutrak[4] screw, this can be done from either approach. Free-hand insertion (without the jig) from the dorsal aspect of the proximal pole aiming at the palmar-distal scaphoid tuberosity is a option preferred by many.

Different outcome studies using this open approach have been published.[230,231,233,542] According to Herzberg and Forissier,[231] the average Mayo wrist function score obtained at 8 years follow-up in 14 trans-scaphoid perilunate dislocations treated with early surgery was 79 points, which is considered a good outcome. Most authors agree that this approach allows recovery of about 110 degrees of active flexion-extension and 75% of grip strength. Most reports, however, emphasize that fixation of the scaphoid alone is not sufficient. Very often, the bad results come from not having stabilized an LTq dissociation or from an ulnar translation of the carpus. Not surprisingly, the worst results are found among the more severely displaced dislocations (stage IV), especially if treatment was delayed for any reason.

Late Treatment of Unreduced Fracture-Dislocations

Despite increased awareness of their clinical and radiologic features, diagnosis of perilunate dislocation is still frequently missed at presentation (in 16% to 25% of the cases, according to different series[183,230,530]) resulting in chronic wrist dysfunction. Delay in treatment has repeatedly been found to be an important factor influencing the long-term outcome of these patients.[183] Yet, as pointed out by Howard and Dell,[243] "all efforts should be made to obtain a reduction in the old dislocation." It is not clear, however, how late an open reduction can be accomplished, although successful cases have been reported up to 35 weeks after injury.[530,635] This generally requires both dorsal and palmar approaches.[106,542] The use of wrist distraction with an external fixator for a period of 1 week before surgery appears to

facilitate open reduction of old dislocations.[544,590] If the bones can be reduced and fixed anatomically, satisfactory results can be expected.[194,530] However, if reduction cannot be accomplished or if there is significant cartilage damage, either a proximal row carpectomy[252,255,458] or a total wrist arthrodesis[225] is indicated. In Siegert and associates'[530] series, the results of isolated excision of only the scaphoid or the lunate were uniformly poor.

Trans-scaphoid, Trans-capitate Perilunate Dislocations

Since the landmark paper by Fenton[153] in 1956, more than 60 cases of the so-called scaphocapitate syndrome have been reported.* The injury consists of a variation of a greater arc dislocation in which both the scaphoid and the capitate are fractured, the latter being displaced with the proximal pole rotating 90 or 180 degrees. Although not yet fully understood, the capitate fracture appears to be produced by direct impact of the bone against the dorsal lip of the radius with the wrist hyperextended and ulnarly deviated.[371,548] Rotation of the proximal fragment appears to occur secondarily, forced by the distal fragment as this returns to neutral position (Fig 14-67).

Because radiographic interpretation of this injury may be confusing, films with the hand suspended in fingertrap traction should be obtained routinely. The squared-off end of the proximal capitate is easily seen in this view. Yet, according to the comprehensive review of the literature by Boisgard and coworkers,[61] of 26 cases with complete information, 8 were unrecognized at presentation.

Fenton[153] advocated excision of the proximal pole of the capitate as primary treatment, because he believed that avascular necrosis and nonunion were inevitable. Although

---

*See references 3, 61, 66, 144, 257, 258, 274, 300, 427, 435, 457, 475, 495, 548, 587, 641, and 651.

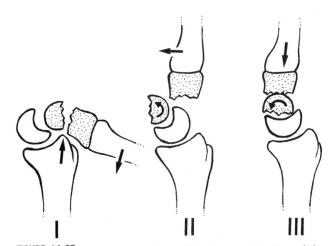

FIGURE 14-67. Probable mechanism of the fracture-dislocation of the capitate as part of the so-called scaphocapitate syndrome, popularized by Fenton.[153] (I) Extreme wrist hyperextension may result in impaction of the neck of the capitate against the dorsal lip of the radius, causing its fracture. (II) When the wrist is brought back into neutral position, the roughed surface of the fracture may contribute to further displacement of the unconstrained proximal pole of the capitate in a rotatory fashion. (III) In some cases, the subsequent axial compression may further displace the proximal fragment, which now appears fully (180 degrees) rotated.

two cases[3,274] have been described in which the fragment healed in its malrotated position, four necroses and two capitate nonunions have been reported in patients treated conservatively.[61,339] By contrast, all 10 cases treated by open reduction through a dorsal approach and internal fixation with Kirschner wires or screws healed uneventfully from 2 to 6 months after surgery.[61,257,427,587] In comminuted cases, primary bone grafting may be indicated.[641] Vance and associates[587] recognized six forms of displacement and recommended that the first step in operative treatment be reduction and fixation of the capitate fracture. If this is not done, the distal fragment of the scaphoid tends to migrate medially, making its reduction and stabilization difficult. It is equally important to achieve anatomic reduction and stabilization of the scaphoid and lunate using the techniques previously described. Transient avascular changes in the proximal pole of the capitate are common, but healing usually occurs. The overall long-term results after open reduction and internal fixation have invariably been good, whereas poor outcomes have been reported with other methods of treatment.[61]

Transtriquetral Perilunate Dislocations

As previously explained, the third stage of Mayfield's[348] "progressive perilunate instability" is defined by the occurrence of LTq dissociation. The lunate is being constrained by the two strong RL ligaments (long and short), and a sudden extension moment is exerted by the dislocating distal row via the TqHC ligaments. Such opposite forces usually result in rupture or avulsion, from palmar to dorsal, of the LTq ligaments. According to the senior author and his colleagues,[183] however, in about a fourth of patients, instead of ligament derangement there is either a sagittal fracture of the body of the triquetrum or a proximal pole avulsion fracture, representing a ligament detachment (Fig. 14-68). During the open procedure, this fragment should not be excised but replaced carefully in its original position to ensure correct ligament stability.[258,298,549]

Palmar Perilunate Dislocations

Palmarly displaced LC dislocations are very infrequent, representing less than 3% of all perilunate injuries.[6,154,330,446,493,509,651] The dislocation may occur in association with a fracture of the lunate in the frontal plane[341,410,593] or as a result of a progressive perilunate instability probably induced by a combination of forced hyperflexion and supination of the wrist relative to the radius.[6,212] In the first case, the capitate subluxation is mild, mostly the consequence of a dorsally displaced lunate fracture.[101,593] In these circumstances, closed treatment is seldom effective, owing to the inherent instability of the fracture. Open reduction using both palmar and dorsal approaches and internal fixation with wires or screws is the method of choice (Fig. 14-69) In palmarly displaced perilunate dislocations without lunate fracture, either SLD or scaphoid fracture is usually present.[202,330,493] The scaphoid fracture typically has a very unstable vertical orientation in the frontal plane, making its recognition difficult on a standard PA view. Klein and Webb[285] described the "crowded carpal sign" or overlap of the proximal and distal rows. The diagnosis is most easily made on the lateral view. Reported cases[362,368,510] with concomitant rupture of extensor tendons suggest that the mechanism of injury is rather violent trauma. In acute injuries, closed reduction using fingertrap traction should be the initial step in management. Although successful treatment has been reported with closed reduction alone,[154,340] these are exceedingly unstable injuries[261,446]; and, in most cases, the only reliable way to realign and stabilize the scaphoid and perilunate injury is operative treatment.[420,509,651]

Axial Fracture-Dislocations of the Carpus

When the palmar concavity of the carpus is involved in a high-energy dorsopalmar compression (crush mechanism), longitudinal disruption of the carpal arch may occur.[182,254] In most instances, the wrist splits into two axial columns, one remaining normally aligned with the radius and the other becoming unstable and displacing in a radial or ulnar direction. The metacarpals usually follow the displacement of their corresponding carpal bones, causing an intermetacarpal derangement (Fig. 14-70). As the carpal arch flattens, the flexor retinaculum may either disrupt or avulse from its lateral insertions. Because carpal derangement appears more or less parallel to the long axis of the forearm, Cooney and colleagues[106] coined the term *axial-loading dislocation* to describe these injuries. Obviously, other

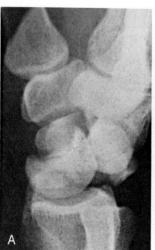
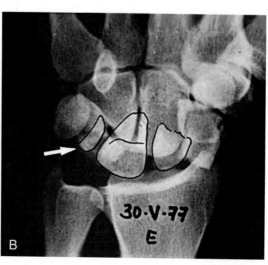

FIGURE 14-68. A trans-scaphoid, transtriquetral, perilunate dislocation. In this case there is a sagittal fracture of the triquetrum *(arrow)*. Therefore the interosseous LTq ligaments are probably intact.

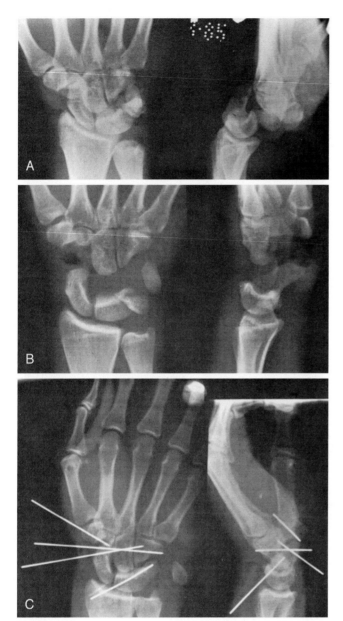

FIGURE 14-69. An example of the rare volar perilunate dislocation (note the incidental finding of a congenital LTq carpal coalition). **A,** The initial injury films. **B,** Distraction films demonstrating gross instability and an associated fracture of the triquetrum not well seen on the initial films. **C,** Films taken in the operating room after open reduction and internal fixation.

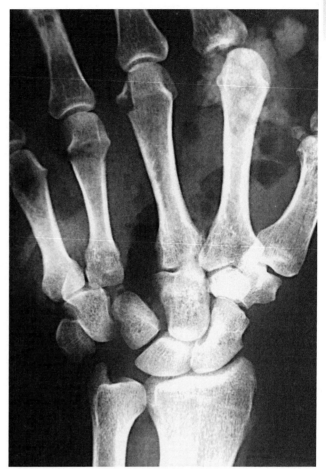

FIGURE 14-70. A peri-hamate, peri-pisiform axial-ulnar dislocation. Note that the vertical disruption involves both the distal carpal row and the base of the third and fourth metacarpals. The pisiform is ulnarly displaced as it remains attached to the flexor carpi ulnaris tendon complex.

descriptive terms such as *longitudinal disruption, sagittal splitting,* or *intercarpal diastasis* may also be appropriate.[390,412,447,451] The first radiologic report of an axial disruption of the carpus was published by Oberst[416] in 1901. Since then, more than 50 cases have been reported, most of these as case reports.[182]

Axial dislocations are probably more common than previously thought. This is especially true in developing countries, where safety measures for wringer-type machines, roller presses, molding presses, and so forth are lacking. Because of the high energy involved in its production, most patients present with severe associated damage to the soft tissue, including disruption of the flexor retinaculum, with resulting traumatic decompression of the carpal tunnel.

In reviewing the bony structures involved, the senior author and his colleagues[182] identified two major groups of injuries (Fig. 14-71): axial-ulnar dislocations, in which the carpus splits into two columns, with the radial column stable with respect to the radius and the ulnar column displacing proximally and ulnarly,[254,412,447,614] and axial-radial dislocations, in which the ulnar part of the carpus remains normally aligned with the radius and the radial aspect of the carpus displaces.[258,355,550,557]

When dealing with these complex fracture-dislocations, a careful assessment of the associated neurovascular and musculotendinous injury is necessary. A radical débridement of damaged muscle, subcutaneous tissue, and skin is preferable to timid débridement. Closed reduction and percutaneous fixation of the displaced bones may be successful,[182] but open reduction and Kirschner wire or screw fixation has yielded more reliable results. Both a dorsal approach to control bone reduction and an extended palmar approach to assess the associated soft tissue injuries are usually required. Because of lack of solid ligamentous remnants, repair of the damaged intercarpal ligaments is seldom possible. In many instances, decompression of the carpal tunnel is not necessary, because the flexor retinaculum has been already disrupted or avulsed extensively by the trauma. In case of doubt, however, inspection of the

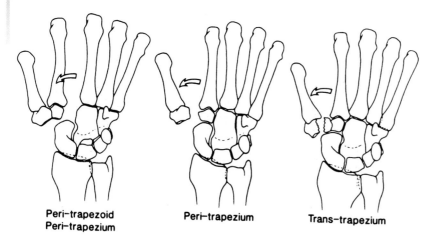

Peri-trapezoid
Peri-trapezium

Peri-trapezium

Trans-trapezium

FIGURE 14-71. Schematic representation of the most frequently reported axial fracture-dislocations. In axial-radial dislocations *(top)* there is an unstable segment displacing in a radial direction, whereas the opposite instability is seen among the axial-ulnar derangements *(bottom)*. (From Garcia-Elias M, Dobyns JH, Cooney WP III, Linscheid RL: Traumatic axial dislocations of the carpus. J Hand Surg [Am] 14:446-457, 1989.)

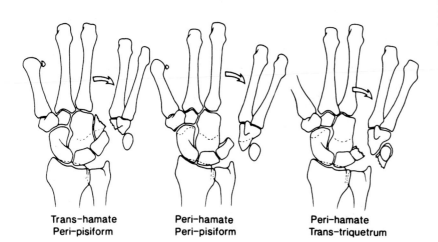

Trans-hamate
Peri-pisiform

Peri-hamate
Peri-pisiform

Peri-hamate
Trans-triquetrum

carpal tunnel is recommended. Immobilization in a cast for 6 to 8 weeks, depending on the extent of injury is advisable. Early intensive physical therapy and later functional therapy facilitate rehabilitation. The long-term results are not particularly good, mostly because of sequelae from the associated tendon and neurovascular involvement.[182]

In less severe dorsopalmar compressions of the carpal concavity, complete rupture of the transverse intercarpal ligaments between bones of the distal row may occur. If not properly healed, these patients may complain of localized discomfort and lack of stability at the dissociated site. These cases have been categorized as dynamic axial instabilities[521] and usually respond well to a localized partial intercarpal fusion.

Isolated Carpal Bone Dislocations

When a localized force, direct or indirect, is concentrated over a single bone of the wrist, the resulting pressure may be sufficient to cause a localized fracture-dislocation. Although rare, all carpal bones have been found to be occasionally dislocated. Unlike axial disruptions, isolated carpal bone dislocations do not necessarily imply a global carpal derangement. Actually, except for the lunate and scaphoid, the carpal dysfunction created by removing the enucleated

bone appears to be quite well tolerated. What follows is a review of the special features of each individual carpal bone dislocation.

Dislocation of the Scaphoid

Palmar dislocation of the scaphoid is a rare injury, with fewer than 30 cases having been completely detailed in the literature.[90,309,443] Two clinical forms have been reported: isolated anterolateral dislocation of the proximal pole of the scaphoid (type I) and scaphoid dislocation associated with an axial derangement of the capitate-hamate joint (type II). An extensive search in the literature in 1995 by Polveche and colleagues[443] identified 14 isolated scaphoid dislocations (type I)* and 11 type II injuries.[19,69,100,140,232, 483,611] Since then, further observations have been published of both types I[20,30,90,309] and II (Fig. 14-72).[488,661]

The most probable mechanism of type I injuries involves a violent hyperpronation injury to the extended and ulnarly deviated wrist, causing SLD first, followed by the enucleation of the proximal pole of the scaphoid around the RSC ligament.[100,336] These injuries also could be the result of

---

*See references 14, 232, 251, 297, 336, 392, 443, 461, 462, 502, 573, and 608.

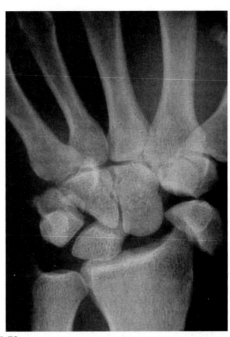

FIGURE 14-72. Anterolateral dislocation of the scaphoid, type I (without concomitant hamate-capitate axial-ulnar dislocation. (Courtesy of F. Urraza, Rosario, Argentina.)

a self-reduced palmar perilunate dislocation, the scaphoid having been left unreduced by capsular interposition. Aside from this, type II injuries also require a high-energy axial compressive load along the third and fourth metacarpals, creating enough shear stress to the capitate-hamate joint to disrupt its strong ligament attachments.[182,463] None of these mechanisms, however, has been proved.

Diagnosis of the condition is straightforward. An abnormal bony prominence adjacent to the radial styloid has frequently been described. In both PA and lateral views, the proximal scaphoid appears enucleated forward and outward, while its distal end remains attached to the trapezium. In type II dislocations there is also a proximal migration of the capitate and an obvious derangement of the capitate-hamate joint.

Closed reduction has been easily accomplished by traction and direct manual pressure in most cases with an early diagnosis, all obtaining good results.[69,100,297,334,461,483,502,573,608] Recent publications, however, have advocated an open reduction through a dorsal approach.[14,20,232,392,611] No avascular necrosis of the scaphoid has ever been reported, and only one case of residual instability has been mentioned, that by Murakami.[392]

Dislocation of the Lunate

As indicated earlier, most palmar dislocations of the lunate are not isolated injuries but the final stage of dorsal perilunate dislocation. Bjerregaard and Holst-Nielsen,[51] Foster,[165] and Schwartz and associates,[510] however, reported on dorsally dislocated lunates. Whether those were the end stage of a palmar perilunate dislocation or the result of a different mechanism was not known. The cases were treated by a partial arthrodesis[51] or carpal bone excision,[165,510] with acceptable results.

Dislocation of the Triquetrum

Only four cases of triquetrum dislocation have been reported, two palmar[170,543] and two dorsal.[50,203] The mechanism of injury was unclear in one case[50]; in two there was a direct crushing mechanism,[170,203] and in one[543] there was a fall onto the extended and ulnarly deviated wrist. In all cases the diagnosis was delayed; yet in all a tender, prominent mass was present. Both patients with palmar dislocation had transient median nerve symptoms. Two cases were treated with excision of the triquetrum,[203,543] one with open reduction and internal fixation,[50] and one with open reduction without fixation.[203] All four patients had reasonably good results.

Dislocation of the Pisiform

Because of its tendinous attachments, for a pisiform dislocation to occur a massive disruption of the flexor carpi ulnaris tendinous complex is needed. This has been rarely reported and is the result of a violent contraction of that muscle with the wrist fixed. If tendon rupture occurs proximal to the pisiform, a distal dislocation of the pisiform may appear.[247,310,364,518] Conversely, if both the pisohamate and pisometacarpal ligaments fail, a proximal dislocation of the pisiform may occur.[25,349] In the case reported by the senior author and his colleagues,[186] failure occurred at its most distal level and the pisiform dislocation was associated with an avulsion fracture of the hook of the hamate and palmar dislocation of the fifth CMC joint. Tendon reattachment is the most appropriate treatment. However, in practice, a pisiformectomy plus repair of the tendon continuity, if correctly executed, is perfectly well tolerated.[25,310]

Dislocation of the Trapezium

Most reported cases of trapezium dislocation could actually be described as peritrapezium axial-radial dislocations,[182,355,550] that is, the trapezium appears displaced together with the first metacarpal (Fig. 14-73). Complete enucleations, by contrast, with proximal and distal joint disruption, are rare, with only six cases reported.[59,204,245,512,529,592] All were palmarly displaced, the result of a blow to the dorsolateral aspect of the wrist or the consequence of a hyperextension-supination injury to the radial-deviated wrist. In four instances, the bone was openly reduced, and in one it was excised. All patients were satisfied with their treatment and able to return to work.

Dislocation of the Trapezoid

Most trapezoid dislocations described in the literature presented with a concomitant displacement of the second metacarpal.[119,180] According to a literature review by Inoue and Inagaki,[249] only 20 complete dislocations of the trapezoid have been reported, 13 of which were isolated extrusions of the bone without other associated fractures or dislocations of adjacent bones. Five of these[207,249,294,459,663] were palmar dislocations, with one[249] having caused an attritional rupture of flexor tendons. There is no clear explanation as to how a wedge-shaped bone (wider dorsally) dislocates palmarly. Probably a direct mechanism associated with hyperextension of the midcarpal joint is involved. Successful closed reduction of the dislocated bone was achieved only in dorsal dislocations.[358] Bone excision has been attempted on three occasions,[207,249,459] all resulting in

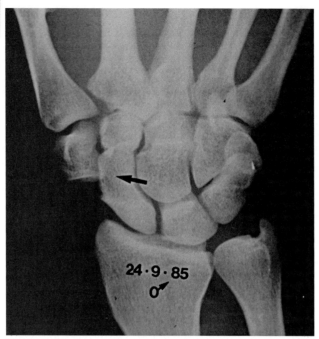

FIGURE 14-73. Dislocation of the trapezium *(arrow)* is often incomplete, and it remains attached to the base of the first metacarpal. When this occurs, the case should be categorized as a peri-trapezium axial-radial dislocation.

proximal migration of the second metacarpal. In three patients,[294,459,663] open reduction and fixation were chosen, resulting in avascular changes of the bone in one case. None of these complications precluded an acceptable outcome.

Dislocation of the Capitate

Three dislocations of the capitate have been reported in the literature. The case reported by Lowrey and associates[330] consisted of complete palmar extrusion of the capitate associated with other carpal injuries as a result of a motorcycle accident. The cases reported by Uhl and Wickline[583] and by Hirata and colleagues[235] have in common the fact of presenting a palmar dislocation of the distal capitate relative to the corresponding metacarpals as well as relative to the hamate. In both instances the bone was found protruding distally into the carpal tunnel, its proximal end being still normally articulated to the lunate. The case reported by Walker and Pradhan,[612] by contrast, was a dorsal dislocation of the capitate and third metacarpal relative to the lunate and hamate. All four cases were treated successfully by open reduction and Kirschner wire fixation, without long-term consequences.

Dislocation of the Hamate

In 1985, Gunn[216] reported on palmar enucleation of the hamate bone in a man who was injured in a traffic accident. According to the author, 10 previous cases had been published. Eight of them, however, could not be categorized as true isolated hamate dislocations but rather were axial-ulnar derangements, with the hamate displacing along with the fourth and fifth metacarpals.[180] The other two, reported by Johansson[268] and Ferraro,[160] were hamate extrusions caused by the direct impact of a sharp tool penetrating the wrist. Dislocations may be palmar or dorsal, and the treatment

alternatives include excision and open reduction and fixation, all of them apparently giving good results.

ACKNOWLEDGMENTS

The authors want to express their gratitude to all who helped in the preparation of this manuscript (Drs. Sergio Barcia, Ilaria Papini, Donna Smith, and Fabian Urraza) and particularly to Dr. Louis Gilula for his careful review of the radiology section of this chapter.

ANNOTATED REFERENCES

18. Anatomy and Biomechanics Committee of the IFSSH: Position Statement: Definition of Carpal Instability. J Hand Surg [Am] 24:866-867, 1999.

Terms such as *carpal instability* and *carpal malalignment* often are used as if they were synonyms. Yet, there are unstable normally aligned wrists and wrists badly misaligned without any functional consequence. This consensus document was published under the auspices of the International Federation of Societies for Surgery of the Hand to clarify this and to avoid future misunderstandings. Certainly, the use of a correct terminology following the guidelines proposed in this document is recommended. Another important terminology essay can be found at IWIW Terminology Committee: Wrist. Terminology and Definitions. J Bone Joint Surg Am 84(Suppl 1):1-69, 2002.

41. Berger RA: The ligaments of the wrist: A current overview of anatomy with considerations of their potential functions. Hand Clin 13:63-82, 1997.

Carpal instability cannot be fully understood without a thorough knowledge of the functional anatomy of the different carpal ligaments. This paper, written by one of the best anatomy and biomechanic researchers of the wrist, updates this subject based on the latest findings in the field. Truly, this is one of the most complete reviews of carpal ligaments ever published.

55. Blatt G: Dorsal capsulodesis for rotatory subluxation of the scaphoid. *In* Gelberman RH (ed): Master Techniques in Orthopedic Surgery: The Wrist. New York, Raven Press, 1994, pp 147-166.

Dorsal capsulodesis is one of the most frequently performed operations in wrist instability surgery. Although apparently simple, obtaining the right tension to the capsular flap to control scaphoid subluxation without stiffening the wrist too much is not as simple as it could seem. In this paper, this technically demanding procedure is analyzed step-by-step by one of its first promoters, Dr. Gerald Blatt.

70. Brunelli GA, Brunelli GR: A new technique to correct carpal instability with scaphoid rotary subluxation: A preliminary report. J Hand Surg [Am] 20:S82-S85, 1995.

When the SL linkage is lost, and the secondary scaphoid constraints are insufficient to control carpal stability, one valid option is the tenodesis procedure described in this paper by Dr. Giorgio Brunelli. If properly executed, this technique may regain scaphoid stability without the adverse consequences of other alternatives such as partial fusions or proximal row carpectomy. In our opinion, this surgical technique is here to stay.

97. Cohen MS, Taleisnik J: Direct ligamentous repair of scapholunate dissociation with capsulodesis augmentation. Tech Hand Upper Extrem Surg 2:18-24, 1998.

In theory, the best way to prevent carpal instability is to repair all acute ruptures of the dorsal SL ligament, certainly the most powerful SL joint stabilizer. In practice, this is not a simple procedure. The experience gained by Dr. Taleisnik, truly one of the best wrist surgeons in the world, is distilled in this nice publication. All those involved in this kind of surgery should carefully read and digest this truly remarkable paper.

130. Dobyns JH, Linscheid RL: A short history of the wrist joint. Hand Clin 13:1-12, 1997.

This paper reviews the history of our understanding of wrist problems. Aside from being an excellent review of the contributions made in the past by a number of hand experts, this paper has the added value of being written by two of the most outstanding protagonists of this fascinating history. Indeed, if Prof. Destot, from Lyon, France, is to be considered the grandfather of the modern "carpology," Drs. Dobyns and Linscheid, together with Drs. Gilford, Fisk, and Taleisnik are truly the fathers, or at least the ones who started the engine that took us where we are now.

138. Dumontier C, Meyer zu Reckendorf G, Sautel A, et al: Radiocarpal dislocations: Classification and proposal for treatment: A review of twenty-seven cases. J Bone Joint Surg Am 83:212-218, 2001.

Pure RC dislocations cannot be treated the same as dislocations that appear associated with a radial styloid fracture. Apparently similar, these two conditions are to be differentiated both in terms of pathomechanics and prognosis. This paper, based on an accurate review of the literature and on the largest series of patients ever reported, classifies and discusses the management of these two types of injury. Certainly, this paper is an important contribution to the understanding of wrist problems.

148. Feinstein WK, Lichtman DM, Noble PC, et al: Quantitative assessment of the midcarpal shift test. J Hand Surg [Am] 24:977-983, 1999.

With a lifelong experience in the study of midcarpal instabilities, Dr. Lichtman's team has, once again, made a great contribution in the field. In this paper the so-called midcarpal shift test is thoroughly investigated and its clinical use well established. When presented with a clunking wrist, the hand surgeon should be aware of the contents of this paper. It will help in deciding how to manage the condition, in which case another paper by the same group is also recommended (Lichtman DM, Bruckner JD, Culp RW, Alexander CE: Palmar midcarpal instability: Results of surgical reconstruction. J Hand Surg [Am] 18:307-315, 1993).

151. Feipel V, Rooze M: The capsular ligaments of the wrist. Eur J Morphol 35:87-94, 1997.

The existence of anatomic variations in the arrangement of carpal ligaments has always been known. Never before, however, has this been so thoroughly investigated and quantified as in this fine investigation. This paper is strongly recommended to those interested in wrist anatomy.

189. Geissler WB, Freeland AE, Savoie FH, et al: Intracarpal soft-tissue lesions associated with an intra-articular fracture of the distal end of the radius. J Bone Joint Surg Am 78:357-365, 1996.

Until the introduction of arthroscopy in the diagnosis of wrist problems, the true incidence of carpal derangements in association with distal radial fractures was underestimated. This paper, later validated by other similar studies, established a basis to the understanding of this important aspect of wrist instability.

211. Green DP, O'Brien ET: Open reduction of carpal dislo-

cations: Indications and operative techniques. J Hand Surg [Am] 3:250-265, 1978.

Very little of what was stated in 1978 by Drs. Green and O'Brien about the management of perilunate dislocations has subsequently required revision. Indeed, that paper elegantly delineated the different varieties of dislocation and their specific management. Most of what is now defended in the present edition of this book emanates from the teachings of these two fine hand surgeons. This paper and others that soon followed from the same group (see Green DP, O'Brien ET: Classification and management of carpal dislocations. Clin Orthop 149:55-72, 1980) are worth an attentive reading.

214. Guidera PM, Watson HK, Dwyer TA, et al: Lunotriquetral arthrodesis using cancellous bone graft. J Hand Surg [Am] 26:422-427, 2001.

Defying the general pessimistic consensus according to which LTq fusions are unreliable, this group of surgeons defends this controversial procedure by reporting 100% union rates and a high index of good functional results. According to these authors, fusing the LTq joint is a technically demanding procedure with a very precise indication. All those attempting this type of surgery should read and learn from these authors' experience.

218. Halikis MN, Colello-Abraham K, Taleisnik J: Radiolunate fusion: The forgotten partial arthrodesis. Clin Orthop 341:30-35, 1997.

The so-called dart-throwing motion, one of the most frequently performed wrist rotations in activities of daily living, mostly occurs at the midcarpal level. Fusing any portion of this joint, therefore, has a substantial impact on the way these activities are done. By contrast, it is not surprising to find patients with an RL fusion who claim to have a "normal" wrist. Indeed, RL fusion may solve a variety of unstable conditions with little disturbance of the most useful midcarpal motion. As emphasized very pertinently in this paper, this partial fusion should not be forgotten as an option in many dysfunctional wrists.

231. Herzberg G, Forissier D: Acute dorsal trans-scaphoid perilunate fracture-dislocations: Medium-term results. J Hand Surg [Br] 27:498-502, 2002.

This paper represents a good example of what can be obtained in patients with a trans-scaphoid perilunate dislocation. Fourteen consecutive patients (more than two thirds of the cases) with an average 8 years' follow-up reported this treatment to provide good functional recovery. Probably this is the best we can expect after such a severe condition. Similar experiences have been published by others (see Sotereanos DG, Mitsionis GJ, Giannakopoulos PN, et al: Perilunate dislocation and fracture-dislocation: A critical analysis of the volar-dorsal approach. J Hand Surg [Am] 22:49-56, 1997).

279. Kauer JMG: The mechanism of the carpal joint. Clin Orthop 202:16-26, 1986.

This paper, written by a renowned professor of anatomy and world expert in wrist biomechanics, still is one of the best analyses of carpal mechanics ever published. In a very didactic way, the interactions between the different bone structures in the wrist are explained both in terms of ability to move as well as capacity to bear loads.

302. Larsen CF, Amadio PC, Gilula LA, Hodge JC: Analysis of carpal instability: I. Description of the scheme. J Hand Surg [Am] 20:757-764, 1995.

This paper was written to help those having trouble analyzing carpal instabilities. Based on their long experience dealing with these conditions, the authors propose a quite useful scheme that allows differentiation of all carpal instabilities according to their etiology, severity, chronicity, and so on. Truly this has been one of the best contributions to modern "carpology" in the past decade.

325. Linscheid RL, Dobyns JH, Beabout JW, Bryan RS: Traumatic instability of the wrist: Diagnosis, classification, and pathomechanics. J Bone Joint Surg Am 54:1612-1632, 1972.

Despite being published more than 30 years ago, most statements made in this paper are still valid; most uncertainties then still remain controversial or unsolved today. That paper was, and still is, a thought-provoking publication, truly a classic that everybody interested in the wrist should revisit from time to time.

348. Mayfield JK, Johnson RP, Kilcoyne RK: Carpal dislocations: Pathomechanics and progressive perilunar instability. J Hand Surg [Am] 5:226-241, 1980.

Studying carpal pathomechanics is not a meaningless intellectual exercise. In fact, knowing wrist mechanics may have great impact on the way we treat patients. A clear example of this can be found in the present study. Dr. Mayfield and associates conclusively demonstrated that there is a pattern of progressive perilunar destabilization when the wrist is exposed to a particular type of hyperextension/ulnar-deviation stress. From that study, we learned that entities as dissimilar as palmar lunate dislocations and dorsal perilunate dislocations are to be treated following the same principles. This classic study still remains unchallenged.

377. Moojen TM, Snel JG, Ritt MJPF, et al: In vivo analysis of carpal kinematics and comparative review of the literature. J Hand Surg [Am] 28:81-87, 2003.

This paper is a good summary of all data published in the past about carpal kinematics, from both in vitro and in vivo studies. Interestingly enough, the results produced by this team are almost identical to the ones reported by other groups (see also Crisco JJ, Wolfe SW, Neu CP, Pike S: Advances in the in vivo measurement of normal and abnormal carpal kinematics. Orthop Clin North Am 30:219-231, 2001).

424. Palmer AK, Dobyns JH, Linscheid RL: Management of post-traumatic instability of the wrist secondary to ligament rupture. J Hand Surg [Am] 3:507-532, 1978.

The history of ligament reconstruction using tendons or bone-ligament-bone grafts is not devoid of failures. If those failures had remained unpublished there would be the risk of somebody repeating such negative experiences. This is why we consider this paper so important. It comes from the Mayo Clinic, from surgeons who have the world's largest experience in soft tissue reconstruction of the wrist. It is a very honest account of what happens when tenodeses go wrong. Indeed, the learning curve was not an easy one for these authors. Learning from their experience will prevent us from embarking on certain adventures already tested in the past and found unreliable.

520. Shin AY, Battaglia MJ, Bishop AT: Lunotriquetral instability: Diagnosis and treatment. J Am Acad Orthop Surg 8:170-179, 2000.

This is another important contribution from the Mayo Clinic, the team who has the longest experience in the treatment of LTq dissociations. This intriguing condition is analyzed both from a pathomechanical and a therapeutic perspective. Particularly interesting is the comparison made between three different treatment modalities: fusion, repair, and tenodesis, the last tending to produce better results.

524. Short WH, Werner FW, Green JK, Masaoka S: Biomechanical evaluation of ligamentous stabilizers of the scaphoid and lunate. J Hand Surg [Am] 27:991-1002, 2002.

This publication is one of the many examples of the excellent work done during the past 20 years by the group of investigators led by Drs. Palmer and Werner, from Syracuse, New York, in the field of wrist mechanics. A sophisticated experimental cadaver model allowing real-time detection of force transmission and carpal kinematic analysis during simulated physiologic motion is presented. This elegant study allowed the authors to demonstrate the stabilizing role of the dorsal SL ligament and that of the secondary constraints, the distal STT and SC ligaments. Truly, this is a great contribution to the understanding of wrist instabilities.

587. Vance RM, Gelberman RH, Evans EF: Scaphocapitate fractures: Patterns of dislocation, mechanisms of injury, and preliminary results of treatment. J Bone Joint Surg Am 62:271-276, 1980.

The different clinical forms of the so-called SC syndrome, each with their peculiarities, are discussed in this paper. Based on an exhaustive literature review, the treatment and expected results of this condition are discussed. Although 25 years have passed since this paper was published, most of what was said then is still valid today. The many publications that subsequently appeared added little to the substance of this already "classic" paper.

623. Watson HK, Weinzweig J, Guidera PM, et al: One thousand intercarpal arthrodeses. J Hand Surg [Br] 24:307-315, 1999.

Dr. Watson and his team probably have the world's largest experience in the use of partial carpal fusions for the treatment of a variety of wrist conditions. This paper can be considered a summary of their huge experience. The results they obtained are remarkable, certainly due to very accurate technique. When in front of a patient requiring a partial fusion, a look into these authors' suggestions is recommended.

658. Wright TW, Dobyns JH, Linscheid RL, et al: Carpal instability non-dissociative. J Hand Surg [Br] 19:763-773, 1994.

Not all clunking wrists are the result of an isolated localized midcarpal ligament injury. In fact, very often the condition involves a multilevel radiocarpal and midcarpal dysfunction. This paper reviews one of the longest experiences in dealing with this puzzling problem. Different surgical alternatives are discussed, none being, unfortunately, universally successful. All those interested in embarking on the adventure of finding a solution for this condition should have a careful look at this honest account of successes and failures. Truly, this is a publication worth reading.

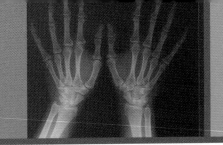

CHAPTER 15

Distal Radioulnar Joint Instability

Brian D. Adams

The distal radioulnar joint (DRUJ) is a diarthrodial, trochoid articulation that provides the distal link between the radius and ulna and a pivot for pronation-supination (Fig. 15-1). Because its articulation is incongruent, the soft tissues play a substantial role in guiding and restraining the joint. During forearm motion, the DRUJ moves synchronously with the proximal radioulnar joint and thus any injury or deformity involving the radius or ulna can alter the function of both joints. The distal radioulnar and ulnocarpal joints are also anatomically and functionally integrated, so that both are affected by traumatic and arthritic conditions. Because of these interdependencies, evaluation and treatment of the DRUJ is challenging. In this chapter, I will attempt to present the relationships between anatomy, function, injury, and disease affecting the DRUJ, along with the rationale and technique of the different treatment options.

ANATOMY AND BIOMECHANICS

The normal arc of pronation and supination ranges among individuals from 150 to 180 degrees. Additional rotation, up to 30 degrees, occurs through the radiocarpal joint. The axis of forearm motion varies during rotation, especially under load, but generally passes near the cross-sectional centers of the radial head proximally and ulnar head distally. At the level of the DRUJ, the axis of motion shifts slightly dorsally with pronation and slightly palmarly with supination. During forearm rotation, translation occurs between the ulnar head and sigmoid notch, resulting in a combination of rolling and sliding movements at the articular surface. The ulnar head slides dorsally in pronation and palmarly in supination. The overall dimensions of the sigmoid notch average 15 mm in the transverse plane and 10 mm in the coronal plane. Total dorsopalmar translation with the forearm in neutral rotation was measured at 8 to 9 mm in normal cadaveric joints subjected to externally applied forces,[144] although recent in vivo studies suggest that the actual amount of translation may be considerably less.[122] Nonetheless, when the forearm is in the neutral position, articular contact is maximal, reaching 60% of the available surface area. At the extremes of pronation and supination

there may be as little as 2 mm of articular contact at the rims of the notch (less than 10% of the articular surface area).[8] Translation can occur because the sigmoid notch is shallow and its radius of curvature is 50% to 100% greater than that of the ulnar head. In anatomic studies, the sigmoid notch's radius of curvature averaged 15 to 19 mm, as compared with only 10 mm for the ulnar head. Despite the notch being shallow, its dorsal and palmar rims contribute substantially to DRUJ stability. The dorsal bony rim is typically acutely angled, whereas the palmar rim is more rounded. However, the palmar rim is augmented by a cartilaginous lip, which is prominent in 80% and more subtle in 18% (Fig. 15-2). The importance of these rims has been shown clinically and in biomechanical investigations, in which post-traumatic deficiencies substantially reduce joint stability.[3,175,184,200]

The articular shape of the DRUJ varies considerably in both the coronal and transverse planes. In the coronal plane, the slopes of the opposing articular surfaces of the notch and ulnar head may be parallel (55%), oblique (33%), or reverse oblique (33%) relative to the long axis of the radius and ulna.[184] Although the slope has no proven impact on joint function in its natural state, acquired changes in lengths of

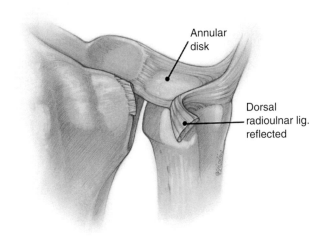

FIGURE 15-1. Distal radioulnar joint with triangular fibrocartilage complex.

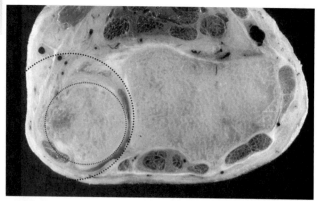

FIGURE 15-2. Cross section through the DRUJ in a cadaver. Note the rims of the sigmoid notch are augmented by fibrocartilaginous lips. The sigmoid notch is shallow and its radius at curvature is substantially larger than at the ulnar head.

the radius or ulna may alter peak articular pressures. For example, a shortening osteotomy through the ulnar shaft for the treatment of ulnar impaction syndrome in a patient with a reverse oblique slope of the DRUJ may concentrate and increase articular pressures at the proximal edge of the notch and the opposing surface of the ulnar head.[158] In the transverse plane, the sigmoid notch subtends an arc of approximately 50 degrees (see Fig. 15-2). Based on an anatomic study of 50 cadavers, four different sigmoid notch shapes were found: flat face (42%), ski slope (14%), "C" type (30%), and "S" type (14%) (Fig. 15-3).[184] The shape has potential implications for risk of traumatic instability and its treatment alternatives. A flat sigmoid notch may be more prone to instability and less responsive to treatment by soft tissue repair alone.[184]

The ulna is the stable unit of the forearm and thus supports loads from the radius and carpus. The ulnar head serves as the articular *seat* for the sigmoid notch around which the radius rotates. The surface of the ulnar head that faces the sigmoid notch forms a slightly asymmetrical, partial cylinder of about a 130-degree arc. The amount of articular cartilage that covers this arc ranges from as little as

50 degrees to as much as 130 degrees.[8,57] Because its curvature is slightly asymmetrical, there is a small "cam effect" at the DRUJ during forearm rotation. The articular surface is generally inclined and shaped to match the slope of the sigmoid notch, but a radiographically appearing mismatch is not uncommon. In a radiographic study, the mean inclination of the sigmoid notch was found to be 8 degrees, ranging from −24 degrees to 27 degrees, whereas the inclination of the opposing ulnar head surface averaged 21 degrees, ranging from −14 degrees to 41 degrees.[158] These differences in inclinations may contribute to explain why symptomatic articular incongruity can develop after ulnar shortening.[158]

The distal articular surface, also called the *dome* or *pole* of the ulna, varies in shape from a partial sphere to nearly flat. A semilunar distribution of cartilage covers much of the dome, which articulates with the articular disk of the triangular fibrocartilage complex (TFCC). At the base of the styloid and encompassing the geometric center of the head is a shallow concavity called the fovea that is devoid of cartilage and replete with vascular foramina that supply vessels to the TFCC (Fig. 15-4). The fovea is the primary attachment site for the radioulnar and ulnocarpal ligaments. The ulnar styloid is a continuation of the subcutaneous ridge of the ulna, projecting 2 to 6 mm distally. It provides an increased area for soft tissue attachments, including the extensor carpi ulnaris (ECU) tendon sheath and the secondary attachments of the radioulnar ligaments. The dorsal (nonarticular) aspect of the head has a groove for the ECU tendon.

Ulnar variance is the term used to relate the difference in lengths of the radius and ulna. *Ulna plus (or positive)* and *ulna minus (or negative)* describe the ulna as longer or shorter, respectively, than the radius. In a radiographic study of 120 normal white subjects, ulnar variance averaged −0.9 mm, ranging from −4.2 mm to 2.3 mm with no differences between genders.[168]

The TFCC, named by Palmer and Werner, is the most commonly used term for the interconnected soft tissues that span and support the DRUJ and ulnocarpal articulations.[137] The term *TFCC* is inclusive of other terms that have been

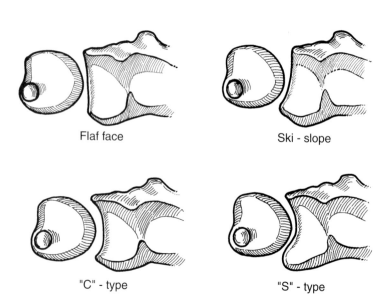

Flaf face

Ski - slope

"C" - type

"S" - type

FIGURE 15-3. Different shapes of the articular surfaces of the DRUJ exist in the transverse plane. The shapes influence DRUJ stability. (Redrawn from Tolat AR, Stanley JK, Trail IA: A cadaveric study of the anatomy and stability of the distal radioulnar joint in the coronal and transverse planes. J Hand Surg [Br] 21:587-594, 1996.)

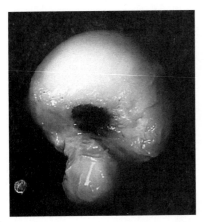

FIGURE 15-4. View of dome of ulnar head. Note the area called the fovea marked in black that lies between the articular surface and the base of the ulnar styloid.

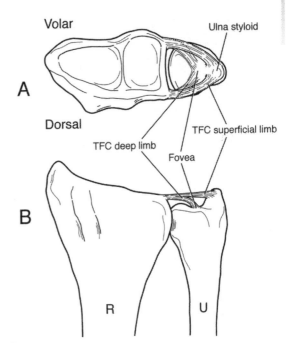

Figure 15-5. Normal division of the dorsal and palmar radioulnar ligaments into superficial (distal) limbs that attach to the ulnar styloid and deep (proximal) limbs that attach at the fovea of the ulnar head. (From Adams B: Distal radioulnar joint. *In* Trumble TE [ed]: Hand Surgery Update 3: Hand, Elbow, and Shoulder. Rosemont, IL, American Society for Surgery of the Hand, 2003, pp 147-157.)

used to emphasize either its fibrocartilage component (e.g., triangular cartilage, articular disk) or its ligament components (e.g., triangular ligament, ulnocarpal ligament complex). The TFCC has several components that are anatomically confluent yet distinct in function.[137] The primary functions of the TFCC are to (1) extend the articular surface of the distal radius to cover the ulna head, (2) transmit axial force across the ulnocarpal joint while partially absorbing the load, (3) provide a strong but flexible connection between the distal radius and ulna that allows forearm rotation, and (4) support the ulnar portion of the carpus through connections to both the ulna and radius. Its anatomic complexity and multiple functions place it at substantial risk for injury and degeneration.

The radioulnar ligaments are the principal stabilizers of the DRUJ. The palmar and dorsal radioulnar ligaments are located at the common juncture of the articular disk, DRUJ capsule, and ulnocarpal capsule. These ligaments are composed of longitudinally oriented lamellar collagen to resist tensile loads and have a rich vascular supply to allow healing. The ligaments extend from the palmar and dorsal distal margins of the sigmoid notch and converge to attach to the ulna in a triangular configuration. As each radioulnar ligament extends ulnarly, it divides in the coronal plane into two limbs. The deep or proximal limb attaches to the fovea, and the superficial or distal limb attaches to the base and midportion of the ulnar styloid (Fig. 15-5). The space between the limbs near the ulnar styloid contains richly vascularized loose connective tissue. This tissue is sometimes called the *ligamentum subcruetum,* which is a confusing term because it has neither the histologic nor mechanical features of a ligament. The diverging fiber arrangement of the radioulnar ligaments has clinical implications, especially as it relates to ulnar styloid fracture. A basilar styloid fracture imparts mechanical discontinuity to the superficial limbs and signifies potential disruption of the deep limbs because of its proximity to their foveal attachments.

The articular disk extends from the ulnar edge of the lunate fossa at the distal rim of the sigmoid notch and blends peripherally with the radioulnar ligaments. There is an inverse relationship between central disk thickness and ulnar variance.[134,181] The disk is composed of fibrocartilage, and the interweaving and obliquely oriented fibers are arranged to bear compressive loads through its central portion (Fig. 15-6).[29] In biomechanical cadaveric studies, approximately 20% of the load transmitted through the wrist passed through the ulna.[138,171] The transmitted force varied with wrist position and increased with ulnar deviation and pronation by up to 150%.[10] Changes in ulnar variance and the presence of the TFCC disk also affect load transmission. Shortening the ulna by 2.5 mm decreased the ulnar load to 4%, whereas increasing ulnar length by 2.5 mm increased the load to 42%. Removal of two thirds or more of the disk reduced the ulnar load to as little as 3%.[139]

Although the disk transmits and absorbs compressive forces, it provides minimal constraint to DRUJ translation.[4] The compression borne by the disk is partially converted to tensile forces that splay the TFCC.[167] This tendency is resisted by the radioulnar ligaments. The disk undergoes substantial deformation during forearm rotation. Increased strains are concentrated in its radial portion during wrist loading, especially in pronation.[4] This region corresponds to the junction of the radially oriented collagen fibers and the obliquely arranged fibers in the central region.[27] These mechanical and histologic findings explain the frequency of traumatic tears near the disk's radial attachment.

The ECU sheath is a stout structure that extends from the dorsal groove in the ulnar head and the dorsal radioulnar ligament to the carpus. It augments the dorsal capsule and provides its own stabilizing effect separate from the ECU tendon. There are three palmar ulnocarpal ligaments that are part of the TFCC. The ulnotriquetral and ulnolunate ligaments originate from the palmar radioulnar ligament and insert on their respective carpal bones. The ulnocapitate

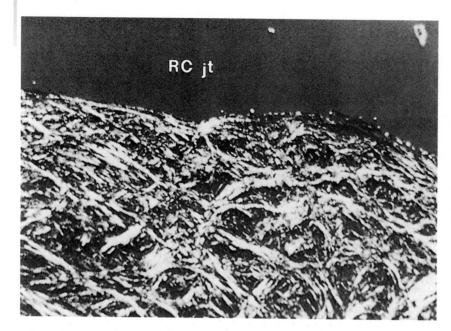

FIGURE 15-6. Collagen fiber orientation varies through the disk of the TFCC depending on the imposed stresses. Its central portion has interweaving and obliquely oriented fibers to bear compressive loads. RC jt, radiocarpal joint. (From Chidgey LK, Dell PC, Bittar ES, Spanier SS: Histologic anatomy of the triangular fibrocartilage. J Hand Surg [Am] 16:1084-1100, 1991.)

ligament, which lies palmar to the other ulnocarpal ligaments, originates directly from the fovea and inserts on the capitate. The contribution of the ulnocarpal ligaments to DRUJ stability is controversial.[44,64] However, because these ligaments have a common origin, injuries or disease affecting soft tissue attachments at the fovea may affect both DRUJ and ulnocarpal stability. This is commonly seen in inflammatory conditions such as rheumatoid arthritis, in which synovitis around the fovea results in dorsal subluxation of the ulna and supination of the carpus.

The soft tissue that variably fills the space between the ulnar capsule, disk, and the proximal aspect of the triquetrum has often been referred to as the meniscus homologue (Fig. 15-7).[137,178] Although its function has not been precisely defined, it consists of well-vascularized loose connective tissue that is likely derived from synovium. The size, shape, and distal insertion of the meniscus homologue varies. In 10% it has a broad distal insertion on the triquetrum and lunotriquetral ligament that obscures arthroscopic visualization of the lunotriquetral interosseous ligament. If torn, it may be a source of pain from repeated irritation.

Because its skeletal architecture imparts minimal stability to the DRUJ, the soft tissues are the prime stabilizers. Several soft tissue structures contribute to DRUJ stability, including the pronator quadratus, ECU, interosseous membrane (IOM), DRUJ capsule, the articular disk, and the palmar and dorsal radioulnar ligaments.[86] The relative contributions of these structures to joint stability are controversial, but there is common agreement that gross instability requires disruption of multiple structures.[86,175] The pronator quadratus and ECU musculotendinous unit provide dynamic stability. The pronator quadratus coapts the joint during active pronation and passive supination. In pronation, ECU contraction elevates the ulnar carpus dorsally and depresses the ulnar head palmarly. The IOM contributes substantially to the mechanical integrity of the forearm. Complete radioulnar dissociation at the DRUJ does not occur unless

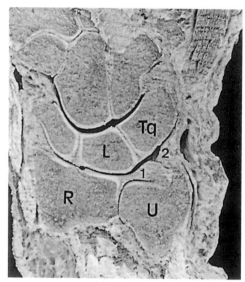

FIGURE 15-7. Meniscus homologue is an irregularly shaped soft tissue structure that variably fills the space between the ulnar capsule, disk, and proximal aspect of the triquetrum. R, radius; U, ulna; Tq, triquetrum; L, lunate; 1, articular disk of the TFC; 2, meniscus homologue. (From Garcia-Elias M: Soft-tissue anatomy and relationships about the distal ulna. Hand Clin 14:165-176, 1998.)

the IOM is incompetent. The central band of the IOM is its strongest portion, providing 71% of the soft tissue contribution to longitudinal forearm stiffness and thus the main structure that resists proximal migration of the radius when the radial head is removed. The TFCC has a lesser role in axial forearm stability. The DRUJ capsule has traditionally been considered too redundant and weak to provide effective joint stabilization. Although biomechanical studies have not emphasized the contribution of the capsule,[202] histologic studies demonstrate a well-defined fiber orientation and suggest a potential stabilizing role of the capsule.[89] The palmar capsule has a prominent redundant fold extending from the inferior radial aspect to the distal ulna border, which forms a pocket for the ulnar head in supination and helps to limit translation. The dorsal capsule is thinner and homogeneous with a transverse orientation indicating less potential to provide stability. Although multiple structures contribute to DRUJ stability, the TFCC is generally accepted as the primary static stabilizer in the transverse plane. Its anatomic organization is mechanically suited to stabilize the joint and yet allow a large arc of forearm rotation.

The precise roles of the radioulnar ligaments have been debated. There are two clinically relevant themes concerning their stabilizing functions.[6,166] First, the ligaments act in concert with the rims of the sigmoid notch to constrain the joint. Second, both ligaments are necessary for normal stability in either direction.[86,175,202] Ligament tension peaks at the extremes of translation and rotation as the ulnar head simultaneously compresses against a rim of the notch creating an interactive, combined tether and buttress to dislocation. In one view of the functions of these ligaments, the dorsal ligament restrains the ulna from dorsal displacement during pronation and the palmar ligament prevents palmar displacement during supination. Supporters of this theory tested the joint with a passive rotation force applied to the joint and measured strain within the ligaments. The major restraining ligament was deemed the one with the greatest strain.[4,86,101,166,195,202] In the opposing view, the palmar ligament prevents dorsal displacement in pronation and the dorsal ligament restrains palmar displacement in supination. These results were found by testing the joint with a passive translation force and observing bone displacements.[8,21,175] Both theories have merit in the clinical management of instability, and the discrepancy can likely be resolved by appreciating the dual insertions of each ligament on the fovea and ulnar styloid. Despite one ligament possibly providing the dominant restraint under a specific condition, the other ligament provides a secondary restraint and both must be injured to allow complete dislocation.[86,202] Thus, in patients with bidirectional or severe unidirectional instability, both ligaments should be suspected of injury.

The vascular supply to the articular disk is variable and plays a central role in its healing potential and the treatment options. Its vascular supply is primarily via the anterior interosseous artery and ulnar artery.[14,108,182] The anterior interosseous artery provides the palmar and dorsal branches to the DRUJ. The dorsal branch supplies most of the dorsal periphery, and the palmar branch supplies the volar periphery near the radius. Dorsal and palmar branches of the ulnar artery supply the styloid area and ulnar part of the volar periphery. Vascular penetration into the disk extends only to its outer 15%, leaving the central portion essentially avascular.[14,27,29,108,109] (Fig. 15-8). With aging, the vascular supply of the peripheral disk decreases.[110] Based on these findings, the central disk has little or no possibility to heal while the periphery of the disk has good potential. Similar to its vascularity, the neural supply of the TFCC excludes the central portion of the disk.[65,130] The volar and ulnar portions of the TFCC receive innervation from the ulnar nerve, and the dorsal portion from the posterior interosseous nerve. The dorsal sensory branch has a variable supply to all portions of the TFCC.

PHYSICAL EXAMINATION

Because the DRUJ, ulnocarpal joint, lunotriquetral joint, and proximal radioulnar joint are closely linked anatomically and functionally, an examination of all joints and structures is essential to ensure that symptoms are being attributed to the correct source. Most symptoms are due to either instability or degeneration, and thus the examination is directed toward these two possibilities. The examiner should inspect the DRUJ, wrist, and forearm both volarly and dorsally for swelling and for differences with the other side. A single palpating fingertip is used to elicit tenderness to best identify potential sites of pathology. Tenderness in the soft depression between the flexor carpi ulnaris (FCU) tendon, ulnar styloid, and triquetrum is evidence of a TFCC injury.

Active and passive motion of the wrist and DRUJ are measured and compared with the opposite side. Decreased motion and crepitus during pronation/supination are signs of DRUJ arthritis, which may be accentuated by manually compressing the joint. ECU tendinitis and lunotriquetral ligament tears can mimic DRUJ symptoms. ECU subluxation is most apparent in supination and ulnar deviation. The lunotriquetral joint is assessed with the shear or ballottement test. In this test, the examiner stabilizes the lunate between the thumb and index finger of one hand while manually shearing the triquetrum against the lunate articular surface in a dorsopalmar direction with the thumb and index finger of the other hand. Pressing and manipulating the pisiform will elicit pain and crepitus in pisotriquetral arthritis.

Increased anteroposterior translation of the ulna on the radius during passive manipulation is evidence of DRUJ instability. Because joint translation varies with forearm position and among individuals, the test must be done in all forearm positions and compared with the opposite side.[124]

To reproduce symptoms caused by disk tears or ulnocarpal degeneration, the ulnocarpal stress test is useful. With the forearm vertical on the examination table, the examiner grasps the hand and applies an axial load through the wrist. The wrist is passively moved through radial and ulnar deviation while simultaneously ranged through pronation and supination.[51,126] I have also found it useful to range the wrist through flexion and extension in different forearm positions while maintaining an ulnar deviation posture under axial load. More central loading of the disk and ulnar dome during the maneuver is obtained by simultaneously depressing the ulnar head volarly with the index and long fingers and pushing the pisiform dorsally (pisiform boost) with the thumb on its palmar surface. Dynamic loading of the ulnocarpal joint by the patient can be done using the press test.[95] In this test, the patient grasps the arm of the chairs and pushes up toward a standing position. A positive test is provocation of symptomatic focal ulnar wrist pain, but the test is not overly specific for a particular process.

IMAGING

Radiography

Radiographic evaluation of the DRUJ should begin with standard posteroanterior (PA) and lateral views. Proper limb positioning and special views may improve the accuracy

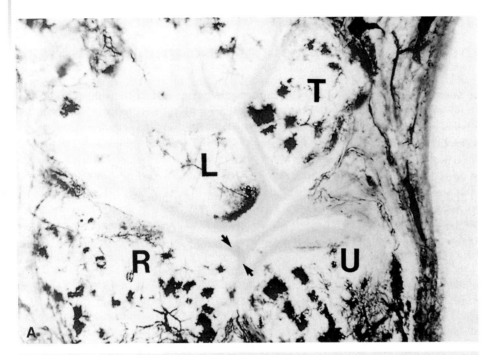

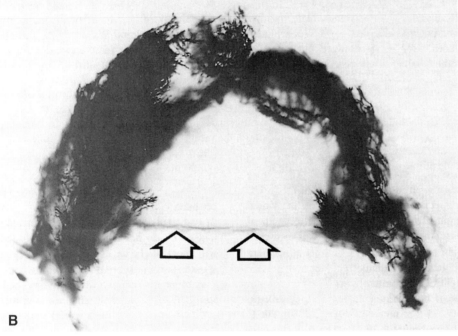

FIGURE 15-8. **A** and **B,** The TFCC is well vascularized in its periphery while only the outer 15% of the disk has vascular penetration. Arrows in both figures identify avascular regions of the TFCC at its attachment to the radius. **A,** Coronal section through the wrist. **B,** Axial view of the TFCC, R, radius; U, ulna; T, triquetrum; L, lunate. (From Bednar MS, Arnoczky SP, Weiland AJ: The microvasculature of the triangular fibrocartilage complex: Its clinical significance. J Hand Surg [Am] 16:1101-1105, 1991.)

and usefulness of radiographs. A standard PA radiograph (neutral forearm rotation) is taken with the shoulder abducted 90 degrees, the elbow flexed 90 degrees, the forearm and palm flat on the cassette, and the wrist in neutral flexion-extension and neutral radial-ulnar deviation. The position of the ECU groove can be used to determine if the PA view is acceptable. When the cortical outline of the groove's concavity is radial to the ulnar styloid's long axis, the PA view is acceptable for measuring ulnar variance.[96] A neutral rotation position has been recommended to standardize ulnar variance measurement, but a recent study found minimal change in ulnar variance throughout the range of forearm rotation, differing only 0.6 mm between pronation and supination.[216] Although changes in variance may be subtle, a PA view with the forearm pronated,[46] or with the patient making a power grip,[52] or with combined pronation and grip may demonstrate dynamic positive ulnar variance.[185] Several techniques have been described to measure ulnar variance on the PA view.[91,133] In a study comparing three commonly used methods, differences were very small and not likely to be of clinical importance.[174] The method of perpendiculars is the most popular. In this method, a line is drawn through the volar sclerotic line of the distal radius perpendicular to its longitudinal axis. The distance between this line and the distal cortical rim of the ulnar dome is measured (Fig. 15-9).

The standard lateral radiograph is taken with the shoulder at the patient's side (0 degrees abduction), the elbow flexed

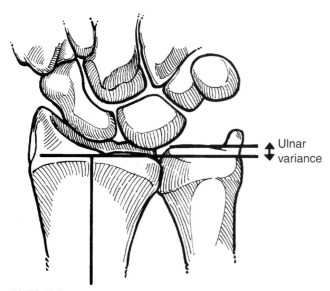

FIGURE 15-9. Ulnar variance is measured by drawing a line through the volar sclerotic line of the distal radius perpendicular to its longitudinal axis. Variance is the distance between this line and the distal cortical rim of the ulnar dome.

⇕ Ulnar variance

90 degrees, and the wrist in a neutral position. An accurate view is marked by the pisiform palmar surface visualized midway between the palmar surfaces of the distal pole of the scaphoid and the capitate (the so-called SPC lateral).[215] Other evidence of correct alignment includes superimpositions of the lesser four metacarpals, the proximal pole of the scaphoid on the lunate and the radial styloid on the center of the lunate. Despite attention to detail of positioning, the lateral view is imprecise for the diagnosis of DRUJ subluxation. Mino and colleagues demonstrated that with as little as 10 degrees of supination from the neutral position, dorsal dislocation appeared only subluxated and dorsal subluxation appeared reduced. Palmar dislocation could be determined, but palmar subluxation could not. With 10 degrees of pronation, dorsal dislocation was not interpretable and dorsal subluxation appeared dislocated.[119,120] Evidence of DRUJ instability can be accentuated in a lateral stress view in which the patient holds a 5-lb weight with the forearm in pronation and the x-ray beam is directed "cross-table."[163]

Semi-supinated and semi-pronated views will better demonstrate the rims of the sigmoid notch and the dorsal and volar aspects of the ulnar head and are thus useful to evaluate for fractures and arthritis. Osteophyte formation at the proximal margin of the ulnar head is a typical early sign of arthritis.

Arthrography

Wrist arthrography once had an important role in assessing lesions of the TFCC[111,135,148,149,155] but was subsequently criticized because its findings showed poor clinical correlation.[107,147] A high incidence of perforations is detected in asymptomatic wrists, including young adults.[24,70,88,111] Conversely, arthrography has also been criticized for low sensitivity compared with arthroscopy.[24,32,34,70,88,111,151,210] Therefore, the clinical implications of the results are unclear. With the increasing application of noninvasive

magnetic resonance imaging (MRI) and arthroscopy, arthrography is used much less frequently. Despite these limitations, a negative arthrogram can be a useful as a screening tool. In a retrospective study of patients with ulnar-sided wrist pain who had an inconclusive physical examination, normal standard radiographs, and a negative wrist arthrogram, most of the patients improved over time and few had persistent substantial disability.[76]

Computed Tomography

Computed tomography (CT) is a valuable tool for evaluating fractures, developmental deformities of the sigmoid notch and ulnar head, and degenerative arthritis. Rozental and associates evaluated a series of distal radius fractures with CT and identified displacement of sigmoid notch fractures that were not recognized on standard radiographs.[155] This radiographic study did not correlate radiographic findings with patient outcome to determine clinical significance of the findings.

CT has become the standard method of imaging for DRUJ instability. To be a valuable study, both wrists must be evaluated in identical forearm positions. It is important to align the forearms in the axis of the gantry and to image in neutral, supination, and pronation. Several measurement methods have been used to assess subtle DRUJ instability. These include the use of dorsal and palmar radioulnar lines described by Mino and associates,[120] the epicenter and congruency methods proposed by Wechsler and colleagues,[208] and, more recently, the radioulnar ratio described by Lo and coworkers (Fig. 15-10).[102] Wechsler and colleagues found the congruency and epicenter methods to be more sensitive and accurate than the radioulnar lines method. Lo and coworkers claimed that all three of these methods both overestimated and underestimated the extent of subluxation.[102] They found the congruency method to be simple and easy but highly subjective, with 90% of cases deemed subluxated whether in a normal or abnormal wrist. The radioulnar ratio method was more reliable but thought to be too cumbersome in the clinical setting, and its use was recommended when subluxation was not clearly evident on side-to-side visual comparison with the unaffected wrist. Pirela-Cruz and colleagues found applied stress to the DRUJ during CT could identify subtle signs of instability.[144]

Magnetic Resonance Imaging

MRI is used to diagnose TFCC tears, but its sensitivity, specificity, and accuracy vary widely among reports (Fig. 15-11) (see Chapter 18).[18,38,66] Similar to CT, MRI can be used to make anatomic measurements to assess instability. Dynamic imaging may become an important tool to identify lesions and instability of the ulnocarpal joint and DRUJ.[56]

Scintigraphy

Scintigraphy has a limited role in assessing the DRUJ but may be useful when the diagnosis is in question or other concurrent problems are suspected. In ulnar impaction syndrome, the ulnar head, lunate, and triquetrum will show increased uptake consistent with chronic inflammation in the bone and soft tissues.

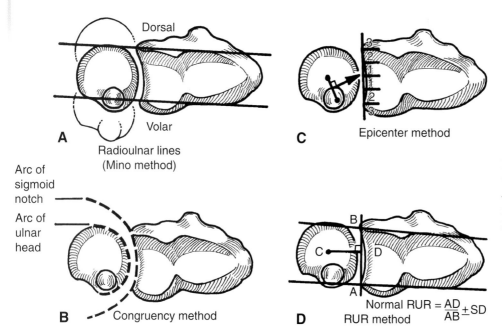

FIGURE 15-10. Measurement methods for assessing DRUJ instability on axial CT images. **A,** Radioulnar lines. **B,** Congruency. **C,** Epicenter. **D,** Radioulnar ratio (RUR). (Redrawn from Adams BD: Distal radioulnar joint instability. *In* Berger RA, Weiss APC [eds]: Hand Surgery, vol 1. Philadelphia, Lippincott Williams & Wilkins, 2004, pp 337-354.)

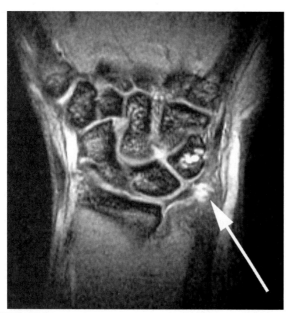

FIGURE 15-11. MR image of an ulnar-peripheral tear of the TFCC demonstrated by a high intensity signal on a T2-weighted image *(arrow).* (From Adams B: Distal radioulnar joint. *In* Trumble TE [ed]: Hand Surgery Update 3: Hand, Elbow, and Shoulder. Rosemont, IL, American Society for Surgery of the Hand, 2003, pp 147-157.)

Arthroscopy

Arthroscopy is sensitive for identifying TFCC tears or degeneration in the central portion of the disk, chondromalacia, and ulnocarpal ligament injuries. In several studies, arthroscopy was more sensitive and accurate than noninvasive imaging modalities.[34,141,151,152] However, incomplete peripheral TFCC tears are more difficult to detect and to judge their severity. Scar and vascular invasion along the TFCC periphery and tears of the lunotriquetral interosseous

ligament or ECU sheath are evidence of injury. A lax or hypermobile TFCC under direct probing, the so-called trampoline effect, is indicative of an unstable TFCC (Fig. 15-12).[71] Reduced tension in the TFCC does not, however, establish the diagnosis of DRUJ instability. In the assessment of DRUJ instability, arthroscopy is most useful to evaluate symptoms that are inconsistent with instability or if other injuries are suspected of contributing to the complaints, especially if these can be treated by débridement alone. The value of DRUJ arthroscopy is limited because visualization is often poor. Wrist arthroscopy is fully presented in Chapters 18 and 19.

TRIANGULAR FIBROCARTILAGE COMPLEX LESIONS

Palmer's classification is the most recognized scheme; it divides TFCC lesions into two broad categories: traumatic and degenerative (see table, Palmer's classification of TFCC Lesions, on next page and Fig. 15-13).[132] Traumatic TFCC injuries are further classified according to location of the tear. Most traumatic tears result from an acute rotational injury to the forearm, a combined axial load and distraction injury to the ulnar border of the forearm, or a fall on the pronated outstretched hand. Although Palmer's classification provides an accurate anatomic description of traumatic tears, it does not guide treatment or indicate prognosis. In addition, the scheme implies that each type occurs in isolation, whereas clinical studies have found that multiple components of the TFCC may tear in the same injury.[106] Most acute, isolated TFCC tears do not require early treatment. The incidence of TFCC injuries associated with distal radius fractures is estimated between 13% and 60% using imaging methods and surgical inspection.[58-60,121]

The necessity of treatment for TFCC tears depends on the presence of associated fractures or malunions and

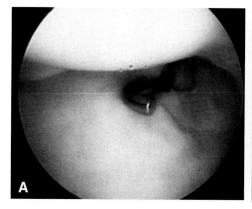
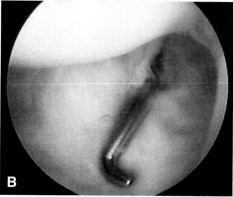

FIGURE 15-12. A and **B,** Normal resiliency of the TFCC to pressure by an arthroscopic probe is reduced with a peripheral tear of its ulnar attachments.

whether there is instability of the DRUJ. Isolated traumatic TFCC injuries are presented separately from those with associated injuries or DRUJ instability.

Degenerative TFCC tears can result from chronic, excessive loading through the ulnocarpal joint and are a component of ulnar impaction syndrome. It is important to recognize, however, that natural degeneration of the ulnocarpal joint structures is very common. In cadaveric examinations, TFCC perforations and chondromalacia of the ulnar head, lunate, and triquetrum were found in 30% to 70% of specimens.[110,137,193,198] Specimens with ulnar-negative variance had fewer degenerative changes.[137] Palmer classified degenerative lesions by the location and severity of degeneration involving the TFCC, ulnar head, and carpus. Treatment of degenerative TFCC lesions is directed toward débridement of the joint and reduction of load across the ulnocarpal joint. Options depend on associated degeneration in the DRUJ and carpus and whether developmental or acquired skeletal deformities coexist (see later section on ulnar impaction).

Palmer's Classifications of TFCC Lesions

Class 1: Traumatic
   A. Central perforation
   B. Ulnar avulsion
      With styloid fracture
      Without styloid fracture
   C. Distal avulsion (from carpus)
   D. Radial avulsion
      With sigmoid notch fracture
      Without sigmoid notch fracture
Class 2: Degenerative (Ulnar Impaction Syndrome)
   A. TFCC wear
   B. TFCC wear
      + lunate and/or ulnar head chondromalacia
   C. TFCC perforation
      + lunate and/or ulnar head chondromalacia
   D. TFCC perforation
      + lunate and/or ulnar head chondromalacia
      + lunotriquetral ligament perforation
   E. TFCC perforation
      + lunate and/or ulnar head chondromalacia
      + lunotriquetral ligament perforation
      + Ulnocarpal arthritis

Class 1A Tear

A class 1A tear typically presents as ulnar-sided wrist pain that is aggravated by power grip, especially with ulnar deviation. This tear is confined to the disk, located 2 to 3 mm ulnar to its radial attachment, and oriented anterior to dorsal. It is a relatively common injury that produces pain and clicking but does not cause DRUJ instability and does not require acute treatment. These tears should initially be managed conservatively by rest, immobilization, anti-inflammatory medications, and corticosteroid injection, but patients with ulnar-positive and ulnar-neutral wrists may be less likely to respond to conservative management.[131]

Arthroscopic débridement is the preferred treatment for traumatic TFCC tears when symptoms persist and is discussed in Chapter 19. If a disk tear is identified during an open DRUJ procedure for another reason, it should be débrided to a clean and stable edge. It is important that the peripheral 1 to 2 mm should be left intact to avoid injuring the radioulnar ligaments. Some authors have described débriding the radial remnant of the disk and repairing it to the edge of the radius. This technique is discussed later for the class 1D tear. Because the results of simple arthroscopic débridement are good, the benefits of this more complex treatment are controversial.

Class 1B Tear

A class 1B injury is a partial or complete avulsion of the TFCC from its ulnar attachments, with or without an ulnar styloid fracture. DRUJ instability may or may not be present. The majority of ulnar styloid fractures do not cause DRUJ instability, which is partly related to the dual ulnar attachments of the TFCC. The styloid shaft provides attachments for portions of the ulnocarpal ligaments, ECU tendon sheath, and superficial limbs of the radioulnar ligaments while the deep limbs insert on the fovea of the ulnar head. The styloid tip is devoid of soft tissue attachments. Thus, a fracture through the base of the styloid is more predictive of a TFCC tear and DRUJ instability than the more common fracture through the shaft or tip.[69] It is important to keep in mind that a complete avulsion of the radioulnar ligaments and gross instability can occur without a styloid fracture.[5,106] Occasionally, a small fleck of bone is avulsed from the fovea indicating disruption of the deep limbs of the radioulnar ligaments. These variations of injury must be recognized to avoid insufficient treatment. Fixation of an ulnar styloid

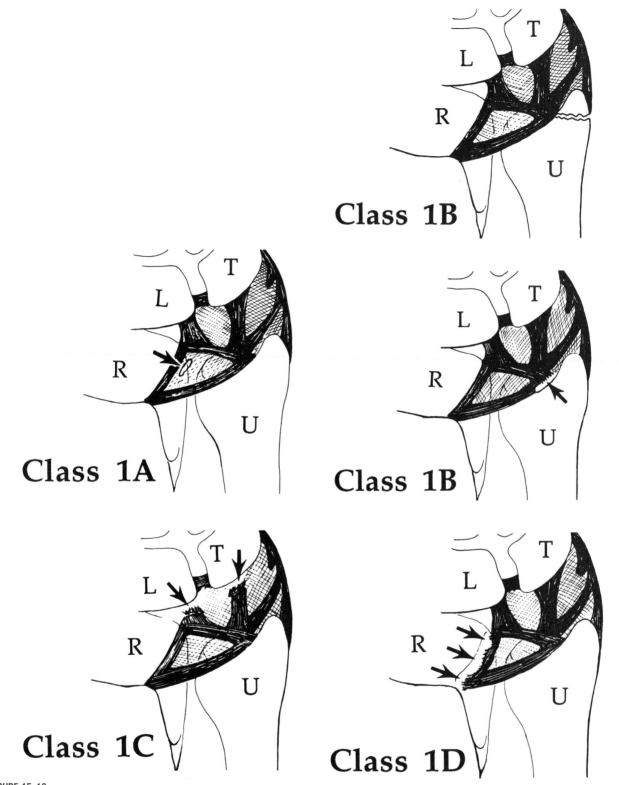

FIGURE 15-13. Palmer's classification separates TFCC lesions into two broad categories: acute and degenerative. See text for descriptions. (From Palmer AK: Triangular fibrocartilage complex lesions: A classification. J Hand Surg [Am] 14:594-606, 1989.)

Continued

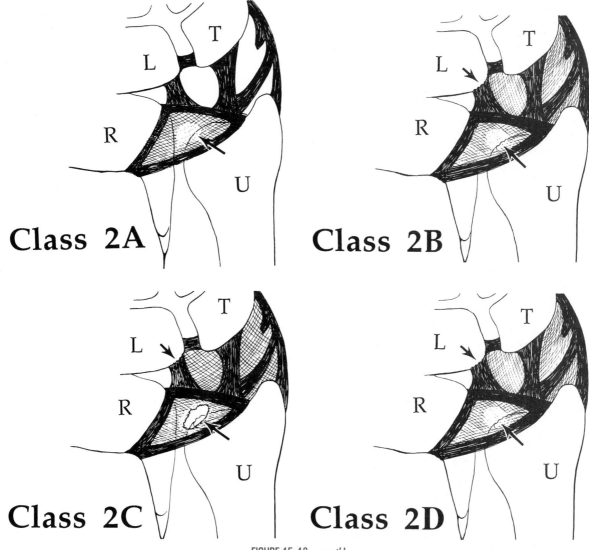

Class 2A

Class 2B

Class 2C

Class 2D

FIGURE 15-13—cont'd.

fracture alone will not be sufficient if the integrity of the radioulnar ligaments is not restored.

Symptoms and physical findings from a class 1B tear are similar to those with a class 1A tear, but a click is usually absent and tenderness is more ulnar, with point tenderness directly over the ulnar fovea (fovea sign). Stressing the joint by passive dorsal and volar translation is likely to produce pain even if the DRUJ is stable.

Because these tears may progress to a potentially destabilizing injury of the TFCC and DRUJ, they should be treated initially by immobilization for 4 to 6 weeks. Subsequent hand therapy is directed toward gradual recovery of motion and strength. Most of these injuries will respond to conservative measures, with surgery indicated for persistent symptoms or onset of DRUJ instability. Arthroscopic treatment of peripheral TFCC tears has evolved rapidly over the past few years. Symptomatic complete tears can be sutured to the capsule using a variety of arthroscopic techniques (see Chapter 19).[189] Because arthroscopic techniques do not repair the TFCC to its anatomic insertion, their indications for DRUJ instability are not well defined. An open repair is considered in chronic injuries especially if

there is an ulnar styloid nonunion (see section on acute DRUJ instability).

Class 1C Tear

A class 1C injury is a partial or complete tear of the ulnocarpal ligaments, either in their mid substance or at their attachments to the lunate and triquetrum. These injuries can occur in combination with class 1B tears and/or lunotriquetral ligament tears.[106] They are reported much less frequently than other TFCC injuries, probably because they are more difficult to diagnose and perhaps because they heal more reliably owing to their good vascular supply. The contribution of the ulnocarpal ligaments to DRUJ stability is unclear.[44,64] The most obvious sign of injury is a volar "sag" of the carpus relative to the ulnar head, analogous to the "caput ulnae" syndrome in rheumatoid arthritis. There is little published literature concerning treatment of these injuries. In general, these injuries should be managed conservatively unless mechanical instability is present. Open repair has been reported in a few cases.[36] Arthroscopic techniques have been described for suture repair or thermal capsular shrinkage, but experience is limited.

Class 1D Tear

According to Palmer's description, a class 1D tear is a partial or complete traumatic avulsion of the TFCC from the radius, with or without a bone fragment. The tear typically may involve one or both radioulnar ligaments. Some reports have confused class 1A and 1D repairs; it is important to reserve the class 1D lesion for true radial detachments. Class 1D injuries are frequently associated with a distal radius fracture and usually respond to accurate fracture reduction of the radius. Only rarely is DRUJ instability caused by a class 1D tear. In the absence of DRUJ instability, symptoms and physical findings are similar to other traumatic TFCC injury types.

Repair of the torn disk to the rim of the radius has been described using open and arthroscopic techniques. A crucial concept underlying success of this repair is to provide a better biologic environment for healing by promoting vascular invasion from the bony rim. Cooney performed a suture repair using an open technique through a dorsal approach; most of the patients achieved good results (Fig. 15-14).[36] Subsequently, a variety of arthroscopic techniques have been described, including the use of specialized jigs.[13,49,77,157,170,189]

Open repair is indicated for large displaced avulsion fractures of the radius involving the rim of the sigmoid notch, because the bony and ligament restraints are both lost. Loss of the buttressing effect of the volar rim can be particularly destabilizing to the DRUJ. In most cases, these injuries are components of a more extensive distal radius fracture and are stabilized by fracture reduction and fixation. Special attention is warranted if DRUJ widening or substantial instability persists after the reduction.

Author's Preferred Technique: Open TFCC Repair for Class 1B Tear

A 5-cm skin incision is made between the fifth and sixth extensor compartments and centered over the ulnar head (Fig. 15-15). The extensor digiti quinti (EDQ) sheath is opened and the tendon is retracted. The DRUJ is exposed through a proximally based "L"-shaped capsulotomy. The longitudinal limb begins at the ulnar neck and extends to the distal edge of the sigmoid notch. Care is taken to preserve the origin of the dorsal radioulnar ligament from the sigmoid notch. The transverse limb is made along the proximal edge of the dorsal radioulnar ligament and extends to the radial margin of the ECU sheath. The capsule is elevated

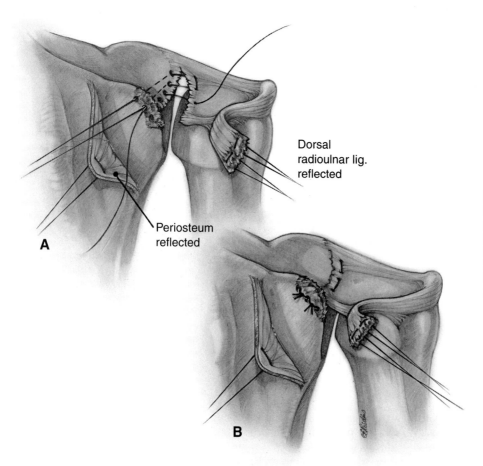

Dorsal radioulnar lig. reflected

Periosteum reflected

A

B

FIGURE 15-14. A and **B,** A Class 1D injury involving the dorsal radioulnar ligament can be repaired by an open technique using transosseous sutures. (Redrawn from Cooney WP, Linscheid RL, Dobyns JH: Triangular fibrocartilage tears. J Hand Surg [Am] 19:143-154, 1994.)

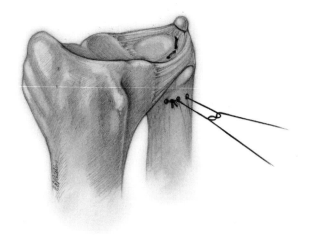

FIGURE 15-15. Open repair of a class IB tear is performed through a dorsal approach with horizontal mattress transosseous sutures through the ulnar neck.

and retracted proximally to expose the ulnar head and neck. The proximal surface of the TFCC is inspected for injury, especially at its attachment to the fovea. Fibrosis is typically present. If the TFCC is suitable for repair, its distal surface is exposed through a transverse ulnocarpal capsulotomy made along the distal edge of the dorsal radioulnar ligament. With the use of a 0.045-inch Kirschner wire, three holes are created in the distal ulna extending from the dorsal aspect of the ulnar neck to the fovea. This site for the holes reduces the irritation from the suture knots compared with the subcutaneous ulnar border. Two horizontal mattress sutures (2-0 absorbable monofilament) are passed from distal to proximal through the ulnar periphery of the TFCC, which lies near the fovea, by entering through the ulnocarpal capsulotomy and exiting through the DRUJ capsulotomy. With the use of a straight needle or a small suture passer, the sutures are passed through the bone holes, with one limb of each suture sharing the center hole. The sutures are tied over the ulnar neck with the joint reduced and the forearm in

CRITICAL POINTS: TFCC OPEN REPAIR OF ULNAR PERIPHERAL TEAR

INDICATIONS

- Palmer's class 1B TFCC tear with unstable DRUJ.
- Consider arthroscopic repair if the DRUJ is stable.

CONTRAINDICATIONS

- Chronic severe instability
- Malunion of the radius or ulna
- Arthritis of the DRUJ

PEARLS

- Begin DRUJ capsulotomy proximally to avoid cutting the dorsal radioulnar ligament.
- Palpate the dorsal radioulnar ligament before making the ulnocarpal capsulotomy.
- Identify and expose the fovea well to accurately place sutures.

TECHNICAL POINTS

- Expose the DRUJ through the fifth extensor compartment.
- Create an "L"-shaped DRUJ capsulotomy.
- Make a transverse ulnocarpal capsulotomy.
- Identify and débride the fovea.
- Remove the ulnar styloid if it is a small fragment.
- Create three transosseous tunnels from the ulnar neck to the fovea.
- Place two horizontal mattress sutures (2-0 absorbable monofilament) in the periphery of the TFCC and through the bone tunnels.

- Tie sutures over the ulnar neck with the forearm in neutral rotation.
- Close the capsulotomies.

PITFALLS

- Avoid cutting the dorsal radioulnar ligament.
- Minimize elevation of the ECU sheath at the ulnar groove.
- Ensure competency of the TFCC for repair.
- Do not place sutures through the disk proper.
- Avoid excessive imbrication when closing the capsule to avoid stiffness.

POSTOPERATIVE CARE

- Initially use a long-arm splint with the forearm rotated 45 degrees toward the most stable position.
- Convert to a long-arm cast for 4 weeks.
- Apply a well-molded short-arm cast for an additional 2 to 3 weeks.
- Use a removable splint for 4 weeks while motion is regained.

RETURN TO ACTIVITIES

- Strengthening and stressful activities are delayed until near-painless motion is recovered.

neutral rotation. The dorsal DRUJ capsule is closed but should not be imbricated, because loss of pronation may result. If the capsule is attenuated, it can be reinforced with a strip of the extensor retinaculum. The extensor digiti minimi is transposed superficial to the retinaculum. A long-arm splint is applied with the forearm rotated 45 degrees toward the most stable joint position (e.g., supination for dorsal instability). At 2 weeks, the splint is converted to a long-arm cast for 4 weeks, followed by a well-molded short-arm cast for an additional 2 to 3 weeks. A removable splint is then used for 4 weeks while motion is regained. Strengthening and resumption of activities is delayed until near-painless motion is recovered.

Outcome

The results reported by Hermansdorfer and Kleinman for open TFCC repair and excision of an ulnar styloid nonunion were generally good. Patients with degenerative changes of the ulnocarpal joint responded less favorably.[71] In patients with concomitant ulnar-positive variance, ulnar-shortening osteotomy should be considered. Cooney and colleagues reported satisfactory results after open TFCC repair, with some patients also undergoing simultaneous ulnar-shortening osteotomy.[36,189] In selected pediatric patients with TFCC injuries, generally good results from TFCC repair have been reported, although few studies are available.[180]

ACUTE DRUJ INSTABILITY

Although the radius together with the carpus make up the mobile unit of the DRUJ, by convention DRUJ dislocation or instability is described by the position of the ulnar head relative to the distal radius. The general classification of acute DRUJ instability that I use is based on anatomic sites

of injury or deformity and is useful in guiding treatment. Discussions of chronic instability due to ligament injury and established skeletal deformity are presented in later sections.

Most isolated DRUJ dislocations are dorsal and are caused by hyperpronation and wrist extension, as occurs in a fall on the outstretched hand. Conversely, volar dislocations occur in the supinated forearm or from a direct blow to the ulnar aspect of the forearm (Fig. 15-16). Although the most common cause for DRUJ instability is a distal radius fracture, instability after accurate reduction and fixation of the distal radius is relatively uncommon. From a prognostic perspective, initial wide displacement of the DRUJ and severe radial shortening are the most important risk factors for persistent DRUJ instability. The radioulnar ligaments can tolerate no more than 5 to 7 mm of radial shortening before one or both ligaments tear.[1] The TFCC typically tears at its ulnar attachments.[106] In most cases, the secondary stabilizers of the DRUJ, including the IOM, ECU subsheath, ulnocarpal ligaments, and lunotriquetral interosseous ligament, maintain sufficient stability during healing to result in a stable joint.[140] As the severity of injury increases, the secondary stabilizers are progressively injured, resulting in increasing instability of the joint. Fracture reduction and maintenance of alignment of the radius are the most important factors to allow stable healing of the disrupted DRUJ. In one series the results of closed reduction and long-arm casting alone were equivalent to concurrently performing a TFCC repair or ulnar styloid fixation.[9] However, in a series of articles evaluating young patients with distal radius fractures, unrepaired peripheral tears of the TFCC were a common cause of persistent symptomatic instability.[97-100] It is important to critically evaluate DRUJ stability after treatment of a distal radius fracture. If instability persists after initial treatment, one option is to pin the ulna to the radius proximal to the DRUJ. Another option, particularly when treating open radius fractures with concomitant DRUJ insta-

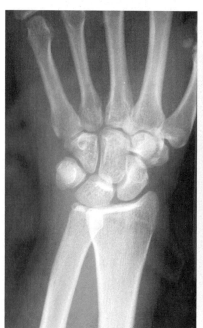 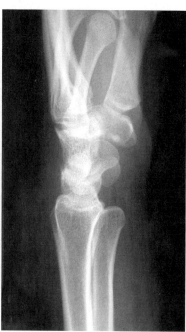

A   B

FIGURE 15-16. Volar dislocation of the DRUJ shows overlap of the ulnar head and sigmoid notch on the posteroanterior view (**A**) and volar displacement of the ulnar head on the lateral view (**B**).

bility, is external fixation of the wrist with an outrigger fixing the distal third of the ulna. When severe or bidirectional instability exists, ulnar styloid fixation, open repair of the TFCC, or ligament reconstruction should be considered.

Ulnar head fractures and sigmoid notch fractures with or without an extensive distal radius fracture pose additional challenges. Although distal radius fractures are known to frequently involve the sigmoid notch, especially the dorsal rim, the extent of involvement is probably underestimated on standard radiographs and better shown by CT.[155] The clinical implication of residual incongruity of the sigmoid notch has not been well studied. Anatomic and biomechanical studies and case reports[200] suggest that the rims of the sigmoid notch play important stabilizing roles for the joint.

In Galeazzi fracture-dislocations of the forearm, a class 1B TFCC injury is almost inevitably present, although there is a spectrum of DRUJ instability that may be associated (Fig. 15-17).[123] In one study, a more distal fracture of the radial shaft was associated with a higher risk of DRUJ instability than a midshaft fracture.[150]

Evaluation

An acute dislocation usually produces an obvious deformity with the ulnar head locked over a rim of the sigmoid notch. Local tenderness, swelling, and limited motion are the characteristic findings on presentation. Deep tenderness along the IOM and swelling or pain at the proximal radioulnar joint may indicate a concomitant Essex-Lopresti injury. Instability following reduction is marked by increased translation of the ulnar head in neutral forearm rotation and may persist in supination or pronation depending on the injured soft tissue stabilizers. Accurate assessment of a DRUJ injury associated with a shaft fracture of the radius or ulna is much more difficult and is usually not possible until the fracture is reduced and stabilized. Radiographs may show subluxation

of the ulnar head on the lateral view and/or partial overlap of the radius and ulna on the PA view. CT is useful to identify avulsion fractures of the rim of the sigmoid notch or to assess the adequacy of DRUJ reduction and can be obtained through plaster.

Simple Dislocations

Isolated dorsal DRUJ dislocation is more common than palmar dislocation. When a DRUJ dislocation is recognized acutely, reduction is easily accomplished unless there is interposed soft tissue, such as the ECU tendon. Under appropriate anesthesia, gentle pressure is applied over the ulnar head while the radius is rotated toward the prominent ulna. After reduction, the joint should be tested over the full range of forearm rotation to determine the stable arc. Typically, a dorsal dislocation is most stable in supination, and a palmar dislocation in pronation. If the joint is only stable in extreme pronation or supination, additional treatment should be considered, such as radial-ulnar pinning in the position of greatest stability or TFCC repair. The TFCC is nearly always ruptured from the ulna.[5,71,106] If the joint is stable in an acceptable position of forearm rotation, it is treated by long-arm casting in this position for 3 to 4 weeks followed by use of a well-molded short-arm cast for 2 to 3 weeks.

TFCC Repair (Class 1B Injury)

Peripheral TFCC tears can be diagnosed and sutured to the capsule using arthroscopic-assisted techniques; however, the indications for this technique in the treatment of DRUJ instability are not defined.[189] Because the arthroscopic repair does not reattach the TFCC to its anatomic attachments on the fovea or the ulnar styloid, it may not be as effective as an open repair in this situation. My preference is to perform an open repair of the TFCC for DRUJ instability. Some authors

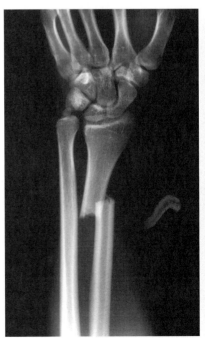
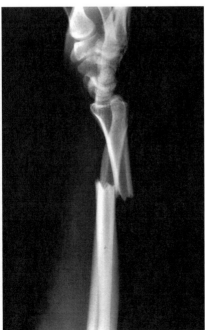

A

B

FIGURE 15-17. A and **B,** A Galeazzi fracture disrupts the DRUJ to varying degrees. After anatomic reduction of the radius, DRUJ stability is assessed and treated if necessary.

have advocated an ulnar-shortening osteotomy in conjunction with either an open or arthroscopic TFCC repair to reduce the loads on the TFCC, especially in patients with positive ulnar variance.[36,189]

Ulnar Styloid Fractures and Nonunions

In his classic article, Frykman reported that ulnar styloid fractures occurred in approximately 61% of distal radius fractures.[54] Few of these fractures are associated with DRUJ instability or continued symptoms. Fractures through the tip of the styloid do not require intervention because they do not cause DRUJ instability and are associated with a good prognosis.[59] Fractures through the styloid base, especially when displaced, are associated with a higher risk of DRUJ instability.[69,112] Fixation of the styloid will restore DRUJ stability provided the TFCC is not otherwise damaged. A variety of methods have been described to fix fractures of the ulnar styloid, including Kirschner wires, tension band wiring, compression screw, variable-pitch headless screws, mini-fragment plates, and suture anchors (Fig. 15-18). The size of the fragment often dictates the fixation options. Hardware irritation with need for hardware removal is not uncommon owing to its subcutaneous location on the ulnar border of the wrist.

In the surgical approach to the styloid, the sensory branch of the ulnar nerve is protected and the ECU sheath is

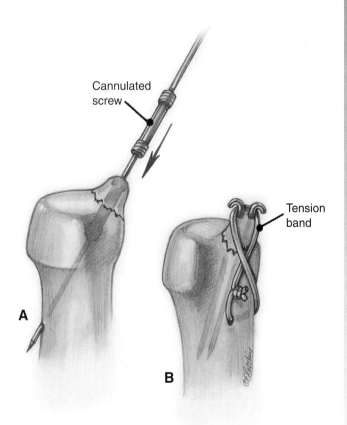

Cannulated screw

Tension band

A

B

FIGURE 15-18. **A** and **B,** Several methods are available to fix an ulnar styloid fracture depending partly on the size of the styloid fragment. (Redrawn from Trumble TE, Culp R, Hanel DP, et al: Intra-articular fractures of the distal aspect of the radius. J Bone Joint Surg Am 80:595, 1998.)

CRITICAL POINTS: ULNAR STYLOID FRACTURE REPAIR

INDICATIONS

- Isolated displaced fracture through base of styloid associated with unstable DRUJ
- Persistent DRUJ instability after accurate reduction of a radius fracture

CONTRAINDICATIONS

- Small fragment through its tip
- Nondisplaced fracture without DRUJ instability

PEARLS

- Minimize irritating hardware whenever possible.
- Use sutures around the fragment if it is small.
- A stable fibrous union in good position is an acceptable result.

TECHNICAL POINTS

- Expose fracture via subcutaneous border of ulna.
- Protect the dorsal sensory branch of the ulnar nerve.
- Base the method of fixation on fragment size and surgeon choice (see text).
- Confirm hardware position, fracture reduction, and DRUJ alignment with fluoroscopy.

PITFALLS

- Do not injure the ulnar nerve sensory branch.
- Avoid splitting the styloid fragment with excessive hardware.
- Do not detach the TFCC attachments to the styloid.
- Avoid opening or elevating the ECU subsheath.

POSTOPERATIVE CARE

- Initially apply a long-arm splint with the forearm rotated 45 degrees toward the most stable position.
- Convert to a long-arm cast for 4 weeks postoperatively.
- Use a well-molded short-arm cast for an additional 2 weeks.
- Use a removable splint for 4 weeks while motion is regained.

RETURN TO ACTIVITIES

- Strengthening and stressful activities are delayed until fracture site is minimally tender.

preserved. The styloid can be exposed through a dorsal incision if necessary for treatment of other injuries, but the preferred approach to the styloid is located just palmar and parallel to the ECU tendon. After passing one or two oblique Kirschner wire(s) through the tip of the ulnar styloid, a 24-gauge tension band is passed around the tip(s) of the wire(s) and through a hole in the ulnar neck in a figure-of-eight fashion (Fig. 15-18). Multiple Kirschner wires or a screw can be used for larger fragments. I prefer to use suture anchor fixation to avoid irritating hardware. In this technique, a bone anchor is inserted through the fracture site and seated below the fracture line into the ulnar neck. The attached sutures are passed through drill holes in the styloid fragment if it is large or passed around a small fragment. The sutures are then crossed over the subcutaneous surface of the ulna and one end is passed through a transverse drill hole made in the ulnar neck to create a figure-of-eight. When the suture ends are tied it creates combined interosseous compression and a tension band. Stability is adequate to allow gentle early motion when allowed by the other injuries.

Symptomatic nonunion of the ulnar styloid is an uncommon problem that is usually best treated by simple subperiosteal excision. If the fragment is large and the TFCC is unstable, the periphery of the TFCC is repaired to the styloid base after fragment excision with transosseous sutures.[69] Alternatively, the nonunion can be repaired, although the benefit of this approach has not been demonstrated.

Outcome

The size and degree of displacement of the ulnar styloid fracture fragment are good predictors of DRUJ stability.[104,112] Although fracture union is not consistently achieved with any technique, sound fibrous healing in a good position is generally compatible with resolution of symptoms and DRUJ stability.[112] In my experience, ulnar styloid nonunion is rarely symptomatic unless the fragment is displaced or associated with DRUJ instability. Independent of the presence and treatment of ulna and TFCC injuries, proper reduction and stability of the radius fracture are essential to achieve good DRUJ function.

POST-TRAUMATIC (CHRONIC) DRUJ INSTABILITY

Symptomatic dysfunction of the DRUJ after wrist injury, and especially after a distal radius malunion, is not uncommon. Residual dorsal angulation of the radius of greater than 20 to 30 degrees is associated with increased loading of the distal ulna, radioulnar incongruity, TFCC distortion, and palmar DRUJ instability.[1,85]

DRUJ instability after a distal radius or forearm malunion usually presents as loss of forearm rotation, prominence of the ulnar head, and ulnar-sided wrist pain. Complaints are caused by a combination of effects of the malunion on the radiocarpal, ulnocarpal, and distal radioulnar joints. Loss of radial length in isolation is rarely associated with substantial loss of rotation or instability but causes a proportionate increase in ulnar load and symptoms of ulnar impaction. Conversely, angular deformities of the distal radius or forearm are more likely to cause gross instability and unidi-

rectional loss of motion. Chronic length discrepancies due to skeletal deficiencies in the proximal forearm, such as an Essex-Lopresti injury, are associated with IOM injuries and produce symptoms of the entire forearm axis. Developmental skeletal deformities, such as Madelung's deformity, behave similar to their post-traumatic counterparts; however, the symptoms typically progress more slowly.

Chronic DRUJ instability can occur in the absence of a distal radius fracture. The most common history is a traumatic event involving a fall on the outstretched hand or an unexpected forcible rotation of the wrist (e.g., a jammed power drill). The injury is followed by ulnar-sided wrist swelling and pain that is aggravated by forearm and wrist motion. If the injury is left untreated, rest pain and swelling typically improve but activity pain, weakness, and mechanical symptoms persist. The distal ulna may remain tender and appear prominent. In mild instability, pain and weakness occur only with activities that require powerful rotation of the forearm during hand grip, such as turning a screwdriver. In more severe cases, a palpable and painful clunk may occur with wrist torsion and loss of rotation may occur from chronic subluxation. Chronic instability rarely improves spontaneously, and it is not known whether instability predisposes to arthritis.

DRUJ instability in children is usually associated with a previous fracture of the distal radius or forearm and often presents late, sometimes years after the fracture. Fracture remodeling may make it difficult to accurately characterize a malunion in children. Loss of forearm motion varies, but the instability is often obvious. An angular deformity of the radius or ulna is typically easily identified on radiographs. A rotational malunion is much more difficult to diagnose but can have equally damaging effects on forearm rotation, leading to chronic ligament attenuation and instability.

Evaluation

A chronically unstable DRUJ causes reproducible clunks that are visible and palpable as the ulnar head dislocates and reduces in the sigmoid notch during active or passive forearm rotation. Passive manipulation of the joint is occasionally necessary to complete the dislocation, and compression across the joint may accentuate the clunk. Subtle degrees of DRUJ subluxation may be more difficult to detect. In palmar subluxation, a slight prominence of the ulnar head is seen on the palmar aspect of the wrist and a depression on the dorsal side. Tenderness is present diffusely about the distal ulna but particularly over the fovea of the ulnar head, which is located in the depression between the FCU tendon and ulnar styloid. Increased translation with passive force is nearly always present in at least one position of forearm rotation. Passive laxity should be assessed with the forearm in neutral, supination, and pronation. Laxity is normally more pronounced in the neutral position than in either pronation or supination. It is essential to compare findings to the contralateral extremity because the normal range of motion and laxity of the DRUJ vary considerably among individuals. Resisted forearm rotation, especially at the extremes of pronation and supination, is often painful. A modification of the press test,[95] originally described to diagnose TFCC tears, is useful for evaluating suspected DRUJ instability.[3] In this modified test, the patient raises from a chair using the hands for assistance by pushing against a tabletop located to his or her front. Instability is shown by greater "depression" of the ulnar head on the affected side and is often associated with pain. Tenderness over the ulnar styloid may signify an unstable nonunion. In a dorsally angulated malunion of the distal radius, the ulnar head is prominent volarly, especially with supination. Children are unlikely to have rest pain and are more likely to complain of pain and popping in the wrist that interferes with recreational activities.

The most specific radiographic signs of instability include a widened DRUJ and prominence of the ulnar head volar or dorsal to the radius. Indirect radiographic signs include a malunited distal radius, deformities of the radial or ulnar shafts, displaced basilar fracture of the ulnar styloid, and a displaced fleck fracture from the fovea. CT is the most accurate imaging modality to evaluate the DRUJ for fractures, arthritis, sigmoid notch incongruity, and instability.

Treatment

Nonoperative management of severe, chronic DRUJ instability usually fails unless the individual is willing to use a splint that restricts forearm rotation. A 4-week trial of forearm splinting or long-arm casting and anti-inflammatory medications is indicated for mild instability, particularly in the low-demand patient.[114] Coexistent conditions, such as ECU tendinitis or ulnar impaction syndrome, should be identified and treated accordingly. Special consideration is given to patients with symptoms of instability who have a flat sigmoid notch and bilateral DRUJ hypermobility, because these patients respond less predictably to reconstructive surgery. A strengthening program for the forearm and wrist should be attempted along with a soft brace or supportive taping during activities. Recurrent dislocations may cause further attenuation of the soft tissue restraints and predispose to degeneration of the rims of the sigmoid notch. In young patients, it may be appropriate to accept intermittent dislocations and follow these patients regularly until skeletal maturity to avoid the potential for iatrogenic physeal injury with reconstructive surgery.

Restoration of stability and a full, painless arc of motion are the goals of surgical treatment for the post-traumatic unstable DRUJ. The anatomic derangements underlying the instability must be correctly identified; causes can be bony deformity, ligament injury, or a combination. Soft tissue repair or reconstruction in the presence of marked bony deformity will fail. In established DRUJ instability without malunion or arthritis, the ideal surgical option is late repair of the TFCC, with the goal of restoration of the mechanical integrity of the detached radioulnar ligaments.[71]

It is critical to evaluate the integrity of the opposing articular surfaces, because unrecognized joint incongruity or arthritis will degrade the surgical outcome. However, it should not be assumed that the articular surfaces have deteriorated or the soft tissues are irreparable in long-standing instability.

A soft tissue reconstructive procedure is indicated when the TFCC is irreparable and the sigmoid notch is competent. Fixation of a basilar fracture of the ulnar styloid alone in chronic instability is usually ineffective because the soft tissues are attenuated. Reconstructive techniques can be classified into three categories: (1) a direct radioulnar tether

that is extrinsic to the joint,[55] (2) an indirect radioulnar link via an ulnocarpal sling or a tenodesis,[23,55,73,191] or (3) reconstruction of the distal radioulnar ligaments.[3,80,163] The techniques in the first two categories may improve symptoms but are not anatomic and do not restore normal joint stability or mechanics in laboratory studies.[142] Nonetheless, these reconstructions may be the only option in some cases and are occasionally used in conjunction with a Darrach excision of the distal ulna or to stabilize a previously resected distal ulna. The techniques described by Boyes and Bunnell[22] (Fig. 15-19) and by Hui and Linscheid[73] (Fig. 15-20) reconstruct the volar ulnocarpal ligaments using a distally based strip of the FCU tendon. These techniques are particularly applicable when ulnocarpal instability is the primary problem and DRUJ instability is a lesser concern. Reconstruction of the distal radioulnar ligaments is the most anatomic approach and has the potential to restore stability without substantial loss of rotation or strength. The procedure is dependent on a mechanically competent sigmoid notch to provide a buttress effect for proper ligament function. If the notch is not competent, either an osteoplasty (described later) must be done concurrently or another surgical option is considered.

Scheker and associates described a technique for reconstruction of the dorsal radioulnar ligament using a tendon graft.[163] Three drill holes are placed in both the distal radius and ulna, and the graft is then woven and tied onto itself. Johnston Jones and Sanders described a technique for reconstruction of both radioulnar ligaments with a palmaris tendon graft.[80] A technique I developed reconstructs the

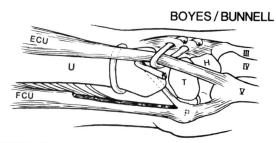

FIGURE 15-19. Technique described by Boyes and Bunnell for chronic DRUJ instability reconstructs the volar ulnocarpal ligaments and creates a tether between the distal radius and ulna. (From Petersen MS, Adams BD: Biomechanical evaluation of distal radioulnar reconstructions. J Hand Surg [Am] 18:328-334, 1993.)

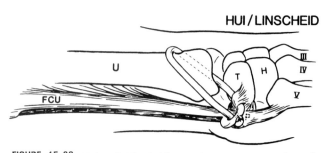

FIGURE 15-20. Hui and Linscheid procedure reconstructs the volar ulnocarpal ligament using a strip of FCU tendon. It is particularly useful for primary ulnocarpal instability and secondary DRUJ instability. (From Petersen MS, Adams BD: Biomechanical evaluation of distal radioulnar reconstructions. J Hand Surg [Am] 18:328-334, 1993.)

anatomic origin and insertion of the palmar and dorsal radioulnar ligaments and is presented here (see Fig. 15-2).[2,3]

Author's Preferred Technique: Chronic DRUJ Instability

A 5-cm incision is made between the fifth and sixth extensor compartments over the DRUJ. The fifth compartment is opened over the radioulnar joint, and the extensor digiti minimi tendon is retracted. An "L"-shaped DRUJ capsulotomy is made with one limb along the dorsal rim of the sigmoid notch and the other just proximal to the dorsal radioulnar ligament (Fig. 15-22). The ECU sheath is not opened or dissected from the ulnar groove during the procedure. If the TFCC is irreparable, then radioulnar ligament reconstruction is performed. Scar is débrided from the fovea, but the functioning remnants of the TFCC are retained. If an ulnar styloid nonunion is present, the fragment is resected subperiosteally through the same incision.

A palmaris longus or plantaris tendon graft is harvested. The periosteum beneath the fourth dorsal extensor compartment is elevated from the dorsal margin of the sigmoid

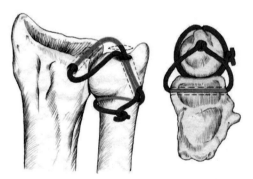

FIGURE 15-21. A method of reconstruction of both distal radioulnar ligaments is shown that uses a palmaris longus tendon graft passed through bone tunnels in the distal radius and ulnar head. Location of bone tunnels and route of tendon graft are shown.

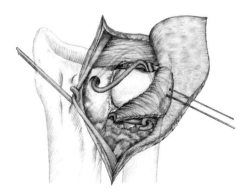

FIGURE 15-22. Dorsal exposure of DRUJ for TFCC repair or ligament reconstruction is obtained by incising the fifth compartment and raising a triangular capsular flap. Ligament reconstruction is shown.

notch. A guide wire for a 3.5-mm cannulated drill bit is driven through the radius several millimeters proximal to the lunate fossa and approximately 5 mm radial to the articular surface of the sigmoid notch. A tunnel is made parallel to the articular surfaces of the lunate fossa and the sigmoid notch. The tunnel site is chosen so that it can be enlarged if necessary to accommodate the graft without disrupting the subchondral bone of the lunate fossa or sigmoid notch. Fluoroscopic views confirm proper guide wire position, and the tunnel is made with a cannulated drill. If a corrective osteotomy for a distal radius malunion is planned in conjunction with the ligament reconstruction, it is easier to create the tunnel before performing the osteotomy; however, tendon graft insertion and tensioning should not be done until the bony correction is completed.

A tunnel is created in the distal ulna between the fovea and ulnar neck. A 4- to 5-mm drill hole is made in the ulnar neck at its subcutaneous border. A guide wire is inserted in the hole and driven through the fovea. Alternatively, the wrist is flexed and the guide wire may be driven through the fovea and out the ulnar neck. A 3.5-mm cannulated drill bit is used to create the tunnel. If necessary, the tunnel may be further enlarged with larger drill bits or gouges to accommodate both limbs of the graft.

The palmar opening of the radius tunnel is exposed through a 3- to 4-cm longitudinal incision extending proximally from the proximal wrist crease between the ulnar neurovascular bundle and finger flexor tendons. A suture retriever is passed through the radius tunnel from dorsal to palmar, and one end of the graft is pulled back through the tunnel. A hemostat is passed over the ulnar head but proximal to the remaining TFCC and pushed through the palmar DRUJ capsule. The other end of the graft is grasped with the hemostat and pulled back along this tract. Both graft limbs are then passed through the ulnar tunnel to exit the ulnar neck. The limbs are passed in opposite directions around the ulnar neck, one passing deep to the ECU sheath. With the forearm in neutral rotation and the DRUJ manually compressed, the limbs are pulled taut, tied together, and secured with sutures. The dorsal DRUJ capsule and extensor retinaculum are closed in layers with 3-0 sutures, leaving the EDQ subcutaneous. The extremity is immobilized in a long-arm cast with the forearm in neutral rotation for 4 weeks, followed by use of a short-arm cast for 2 weeks. A wrist splint is used while motion and strength are gradually recovered. Near full activity is usually permitted after 4 months, but heavy lifting and impact loading are discouraged for another 2 months.

Outcome

Scheker and associates reported complete resolution of pain in 12 of 14 patients at an average follow-up of 1.5 years with his technique.[163] Near full range of rotation was restored postoperatively. There was a 76% increase in grip strength, and all 14 patients were satisfied with their outcome. Johnston Jones and Sanders reported 13 of 14 patients were satisfied at an average follow-up of 26 months.[80] Twelve of these patients returned to their previous occupations and showed no evidence of recurrence. Two patients had early failure of stability. No patient had loss of motion greater than 10 degrees of supination or pronation.

CRITICAL POINTS: RADIOULNAR LIGAMENT RECONSTRUCTION FOR POST-TRAUMATIC DRUJ INSTABILITY

INDICATIONS

- Isolated DRUJ instability with an irreparable TFCC
- In conjunction with a corrective osteotomy of the radius or ulna

PEARLS

- Harvest graft early to determine proper size for bone tunnels.
- Use suture passer for ease of passing graft.
- Ensure position of guide wires using fluoroscopy.
- When performing a corrective osteotomy, make bone tunnels first.

TECHNICAL POINTS

- Expose the DRUJ through the fifth extensor compartment.
- Make an "L"-shaped DRUJ capsulotomy.
- Elevate the fourth extensor compartment from the rim of the sigmoid notch.
- Create a tunnel in the radius using a cannulated drill system.
- Drill a hole in the subcutaneous border of the ulnar neck.
- Insert a guide wire into the hole and through the fovea.
- Create a tunnel in the ulna with a cannulated drill and enlarge it as necessary.
- Expose the volar DRUJ capsule through an incision in the distal forearm.

- From volar to dorsal, pass one graft limb through the radius tunnel using suture passer.
- Pass other limb from volar to dorsal through a puncture in the volar DRUJ capsule.
- Pass both limbs through the ulna tunnel and around the ulnar neck in opposite directions.
- Tie graft limbs together under high tension with forearm in neutral rotation.
- Secure graft with sutures and close the dorsal capsule.

PITFALLS

- Failure to recognize malunion of radius or ulna.
- A flat or deficient sigmoid notch should be augmented by a sigmoid notch osteoplasty.
- Preexisting DRUJ arthritis will be a source of persistent pain.

POSTOPERATIVE CARE

- Initially use a long-arm splint with the forearm rotated 45 degrees toward the most stable position.
- Convert to a long-arm cast for 4 weeks.
- Use a well-molded short-arm cast for an additional 2 to 3 weeks.
- Use a removable splint for 4 weeks while motion is regained.

RETURN TO ACTIVITIES

- Strengthening exercises and stressful activities are delayed until near-painless motion is recovered.

Adams and Berger reported restoration of stability in 12 of 14 patients and resumption of previous work, sports, and avocations without limitations.[3] Recovery of strength and motion averaged 85%. Recurrent palmar instability occurred in 1 patient who had a post-traumatic defect in the palmar rim of the sigmoid notch and in another with persistent ulnocarpal instability. The authors concluded that the procedure is effective for DRUJ instability but requires a competent sigmoid notch and does not fully correct ulnocarpal instability. If the notch is deficient, a sigmoid notch osteoplasty should be considered in conjunction with ligament reconstruction.

Osteoplasty of the Sigmoid Notch and Ulna

CT is helpful to evaluate the sigmoid notch in patients with a history of a fracture involving the sigmoid notch or a suspected deformity of the DRUJ. To improve the mechanical buttressing effect of the sigmoid notch's rim, an osteoplasty can be considered as an isolated procedure or to complement a ligament reconstruction. In the procedure described by Wallwork and colleagues, parallel osteotomies are made, with one just proximal to the lunate fossa and the other at the proximal margin of the sigmoid notch (Fig. 15-23).[200] A third osteotomy is made in the coronal plane 5 mm from the articular surface of the notch and between the first two cuts. The osteotome is carefully advanced, and at each increment it is levered in an ulnar direction to produce a thin, curved, osteocartilaginous flap. The wedge-shaped defect is filled with a bone graft harvested from the distal radius and fixed as necessary with Kirschner wires or sutures. When performed in conjunction with a ligament reconstruction, the tendon graft passes over the osteotomy site and bone graft, which also stabilizes the graft. Because the osteotomies are proximal to the radioulnar ligament, ligament tension is increased, providing additional joint stability. Published results of the procedure are limited, but the concept appears sound. It produced a good result when used as a sole procedure to treat palmar instability in a patient with a flat sigmoid notch.[200] I use the procedure in conjunction with a radioulnar ligament

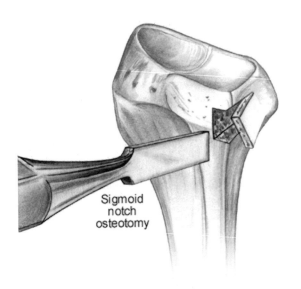

FIGURE 15-23. Sigmoid notch osteoplasty used for DRUJ instability that is caused in part by deficiency of a rim of the notch. A bone graft is inserted beneath the osteochondral flap. (From Adams B: Distal radioulnar joint. *In* Trumble TE [ed]: Hand Surgery Update 3: Hand, Elbow, and Shoulder. Rosemont, IL, American Society for Surgery of the Hand, 2003, pp 147-157.)

reconstruction when the sigmoid notch is relatively flat and have found good results.

An alternative osteoplasty is an angular osteotomy of the ulna. A closing wedge osteotomy is made in the distal third of the ulna to tilt the ulna toward the sigmoid notch with the forearm in the position of instability. The osteotomy is fixed with a compression plate. Preoperative planning, patient selection, and intraoperative assessment must be accurate to achieve a good result with this technique.[28] I have used this procedure only if an ulnar deformity preexisted.

DISTAL RADIUS AND FOREARM MALUNIONS

In evaluating a patient with a distal radius malunion, both the radiocarpal joint and the DRUJ must be considered. Biomechanical studies have shown multiple effects of malunion on DRUJ function, with angulation and shortening of the radius more problematic than displacement or loss of radial inclination.[1,44,64,72,85,122,171,211] Isolated soft tissue reconstruction for instability will fail when there is significant radial deformity. Similarly, a Darrach resection of the distal ulna may result in instability of the residual ulnar stump if performed in the presence of a significant radial malunion.

CRITICAL POINTS: OSTEOPLASTY FOR DEFICIENCY OF THE SIGMOID NOTCH

INDICATIONS

- Developmental or acquired deficiency of sigmoid notch associated with DRUJ instability
- Used in conjunction with distal radioulnar ligament reconstruction or TFCC repair

PEARLS

- When used with a distal radioulnar ligament reconstruction, make the radius bone tunnel first and then create the osteotomy.
- For a volar rim osteoplasty, identify the osteotomy site by palpation and fluoroscopy rather than via a DRUJ capsulotomy.
- When indicated, a ligament reconstruction will help to stabilize the bone graft.

TECHNICAL POINTS

- Make a longitudinal incision over the DRUJ.
- Identify the deficient rim of the sigmoid notch.
- Create two transverse, parallel osteotomies using an osteotome at proximal and distal margins of notch.
- Make the longitudinal osteotomy and lever the rim into position.

- Insert the bone graft and stabilize with sutures.
- Complete other soft tissue repairs or reconstructions.

PITFALLS

- Avoid breaking through the cartilage when levering the rim into place.
- Make the osteochondral flap broad enough but do not violate the lunate fossa.

POSTOPERATIVE CARE

- Initially use a long-arm splint.
- Convert to a long-arm cast for a minimum of 4 weeks to promote bony union.
- Further care depends on concurrent soft tissue procedures performed (see those sections).
- Monitor bone healing with radiographs.

RETURN TO ACTIVITIES

- Unrestricted activities are delayed until near-painless motion is recovered.

An osteotomy to correct angular deformity of the radius will usually restore DRUJ stability; however, radioulnar length discrepancy must also be addressed to improve carpal position and to prevent later development of an ulnar impaction syndrome. A trapezoidal graft to the radius can correct both angulation and length discrepancy simultaneously.[203] In malunions with severe length discrepancy, this approach can be difficult because of the need for a large intercalated bone graft and the potential for delayed union. As an alternative, leveling of the joint can be accomplished with a concurrent ulnar shaft shortening osteotomy. If radial shortening is the only substantial deformity and articular alignment of the radius and carpus is satisfactory, an ulnar shortening via a shaft osteotomy is effective (Fig. 15-24). When bony realignment does not restore stability through a full arc of forearm rotation tested during surgery, a TFCC repair or soft tissue stabilization procedure will be necessary (Fig. 15-25). If DRUJ arthritis is present, one of the arthroplasty procedures described later in this chapter can be performed; however, radioulnar length discrepancy must still be corrected to prevent impingement between the ulnar styloid and the carpus.[20]

Forearm malunion can cause DRUJ instability in addition to loss of rotation.[21,179] The deformity may initially manifest as limited forearm rotation, and instability may develop later as the soft tissues stretch. Soft tissue stabilizing procedures alone will fail in the presence of a forearm malunion. Conversely, corrective osteotomy with plate fixation will often be sufficient to restore stability; TFCC repair or a reconstructive procedure is usually unnecessary.[188] The deformity may involve both the radius and ulna and require osteotomy of both bones. Angulation is corrected through the site of malunion when possible to attain anatomic alignment. A rotational deformity can be corrected simultaneously when an angular deformity is treated. Unless there is DRUJ arthritis, resection of the distal ulna should be avoided. Preoperative planning is important to estimate the desired correction, but the final determination must be made

intraoperatively. Temporary bony fixation can be used to assess the effect of the correction. If stability is not restored through a full arc of forearm rotation, a soft tissue stabilization procedure or DRUJ salvage procedure must be combined with the corrective osteotomy. Operative techniques for correction of malunions are discussed in Chapter 16.

ULNAR IMPACTION SYNDROME

The ulnocarpal joint transmits a substantial load through a relatively small contact area and is thus at high risk for articular degeneration. This degenerative process is commonly called "ulnar impaction syndrome" or "ulnocarpal abutment," which implies that chronic compressive overloading is the primary cause. Shear forces over the articular surfaces and tensile forces through the soft tissues undoubtedly contribute. *Ulnar impingement syndrome* is a term that should be reserved for painful convergence of a resected ulnar stump against the distal radial metaphysis.

Acquired ulnar-positive variance is a known risk factor for ulnar impaction syndrome because of the associated increase in ulnocarpal loading. A 2.5-mm increase in ulnar variance increased ulnocarpal loading by 42% in a cadaver study.[138] In a similar study, changing the tilt of the distal radius from normal to 40 degrees of dorsal tilt increased the ulnar load from 21% to 65%.[171] Common causes of acquired positive variance include radial shortening from a distal radius fracture, Essex-Lopresti injury, and acute or chronic physeal injury (Fig. 15-26).[183] Although biomechanical studies have not shown increased load transmission through the ulnocarpal joint in developmentally ulnar-positive wrists, these wrists can still develop ulnar impaction syndrome for other reasons. In a cadaver study, 73% of ulnar-neutral or ulnar-positive wrists had TFCC perforations, whereas only 17% of ulnar-negative wrists had perforations.[137] The thickness of the disk may play a role, because there is an inverse relationship between ulnar variance and

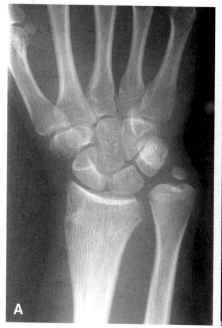
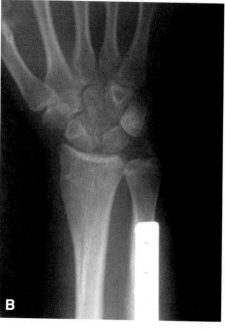

FIGURE 15-24. A and **B,** Radial shortening with disruption of the DRUJ can be effectively treated by ulnar shortening alone if joint widening is not present.

A

B

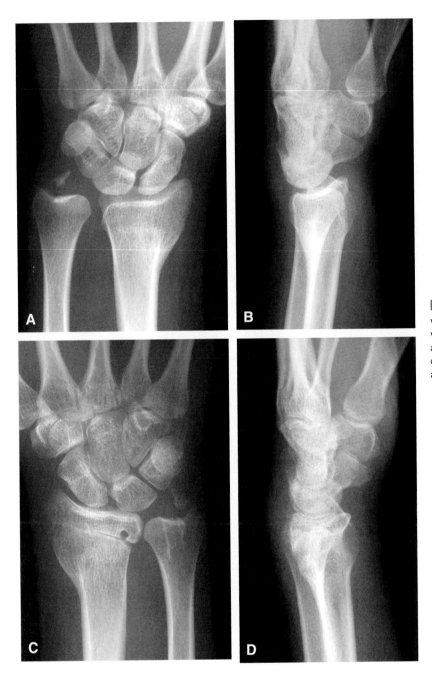

FIGURE 15-25. **A** and **B,** Views of distal radius malunion with DRUJ instability (angulation of the radius, DRUJ widening, and displaced fleck fracture from fovea are seen). **C** and **D,** Treatment was by distal radius osteotomy and distal radioulnar ligament reconstruction as shown in Figure 15-21.

disk thickness; ulnar-positive wrists are associated with a thinner disk that may be more susceptible to perforation.[134] In addition, physiologic increases in ulnar variance of up to 2 mm can occur during power grip, especially when the forearm is pronated. Palmer identified several additional structures at risk for degeneration in this process, including the ulnar head, lunate, triquetrum, and lunotriquetral interosseous ligament.[132]

Evaluation

Ulnar impaction syndrome is characterized by ulnar wrist pain, localized swelling, and occasional limitation of motion. The history and physical findings are similar to those of an acute TFCC tear. Pain is exacerbated most by ulnar devia-

tion during power grip, especially when combined with active pronation and supination. There is tenderness about the volar and dorsal aspects of the ulnar head and the triquetrum. Passive and active ulnar deviation produces pain, which is exacerbated by the examiner simultaneously depressing the ulnar head and elevating the ulnar carpus (pisiform boost). This maneuver better reproduces the joint reaction forces during power grip activities, which load the more central portions of the ulnar dome, TFCC disk, lunate, and triquetrum. While the wrist is loaded in this manner, the forearm can be manually rotated to add a shear force to the joint, which may further exacerbate pain and occasionally produces crepitus. The examiner must consider other diagnoses involving the ulnar side of the wrist that can present with similar findings or coexist, particularly arthritis of the DRUJ.

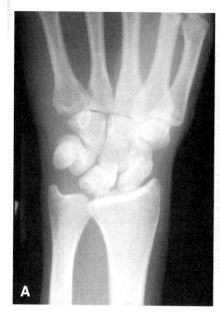
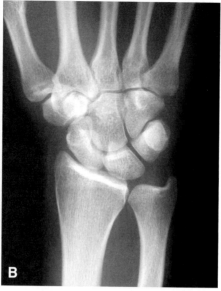

FIGURE 15-26. Comparison radiographs showing positive ulnar variance with ulnar impaction syndrome (note cystic lesions in lunate) caused by premature physeal closure of the distal radius (**A**) and the opposite unaffected wrist (**B**). (From Adams B: Distal radioulnar joint. *In* Trumble TE [ed]: Hand Surgery Update 3: Hand, Elbow, and Shoulder. Rosemont, IL, American Society for Surgery of the Hand, 2003, pp 147-157.)

Standard wrist radiographs are obtained to assess for arthritis involving the carpus and DRUJ and to measure ulnar variance. Because ulnar variance is dynamic, stress PA views can help. A pronated view,[46,133] a grip view,[52] or a view with combined pronation and grip[185] may reproduce dynamic increases in ulnar variance. In a study of 22 patients who presented with ulnar wrist pain, the pronated grip view resulted in statistically significant increases in ulnar variance with an average of 2.5 mm.[185]

Treatment

In treating ulnar-sided wrist pain, it is imperative to remember that degeneration is a common and natural occurrence in the ulnocarpal joint. Several months of conservative management should be tried before proceeding to surgery. Options include modification of activities to avoid repetitive loading with the wrist in ulnar deviation, anti-inflammatory medications, wrist splinting, and corticosteroid injection. Surgery is indicated for patients with clinical and radiographic evidence of ulnocarpal impaction without DRUJ arthritis who do not respond to these measures. The goal of surgery is to reduce ulnocarpal loading.

In a patient with negative or neutral ulnar variance, arthroscopic débridement of the articular disk, chondral surfaces, and lunotriquetral interosseous ligament can be effective. When static or dynamic ulnar-positive variance is present, decreased ulnar loading can be accomplished by a shaft osteotomy or a partial distal ulnar resection. Arthroscopic distal ulnar resection is preferred by some over open procedures because it avoids the potential for hardware irritation and the risk of nonunion (see Chapter 19). Ulnar-shortening osteotomy has the advantage of preservation of the ulnar dome articular cartilage and does not violate the DRUJ or ulnocarpal joint. In cases of post-traumatic ulnar-positive variance, DRUJ congruity is restored by shaft osteotomy, which may improve forearm rotation and reduce the risk of arthritis. Furthermore, the ulnocarpal ligaments are tightened by the procedure, and this may have a salutary effect on associated lunotriquetral or DRUJ instability.

Possible adverse affects should be recognized when considering a shortening osteotomy. Although the articular surfaces of the native DRUJ are not fully congruent and usually tolerate some change in joint alignment, radiographic and cadaver studies have shown that as little as 2 mm of shortening decreases joint contact area and increases pressures in the DRUJ regardless of its shape and inclination.[40,158,184,212] Some DRUJ types may be more susceptible to develop problematic incongruity after ulnar shortening.[158] A joint with a reverse oblique inclination in the coronal plane or a substantial articular mismatch between the sigmoid notch and ulnar head develops the greatest incongruities, with joint contact concentrated at the proximal margin of the notch. Similar changes occur in a joint with a deep sigmoid notch. Predicting the clinical outcome of surgically created DRUJ incongruity is difficult, because it may either stimulate DRUJ remodeling or cause arthritis.

Ulnar-Shortening Osteotomy

Ulnar shortening was originally described by Milch in 1941 for the treatment of ulnar-positive variance after radial shortening from a Colles fracture.[113] Milch used a wire suture to fix the osteotomy. Although the principle remains the same, newer methods include the use of an oblique osteotomy[53] and modern techniques of osseous compression, with or without the use of special compression devices[26,209] or custom plates.[146] An oblique osteotomy allows for an interfragmentary screw, which increases stability and may improve bone healing.[31,92]

Author's Preferred Technique: Ulnar-Shortening Osteotomy

I prefer the technique described by Chun and Palmer (Fig. 15-27). For patients with ulnar-positive variance, the amount of bone to be resected to obtain a final ulnar vari-

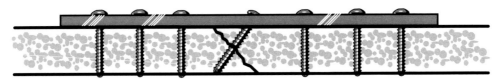

FIGURE 15-27. Ulnar-shortening osteotomy through the shaft is shown using an oblique skeletal cut, a compression plate, and an interfragmentary screw.

ance of 0 or −1 mm is determined on the PA radiograph. A 2- to 3-mm shortening is planned for patients with ulnar-neutral wrists. A skin incision is made along the subcutaneous border of the ulna extending proximally from its neck for 10 cm. The fascia is incised between the ECU and the FCU. The dorsal sensory branch of the ulnar nerve typically lies volar and distal to the exposure. Minimal subperiosteal elevation is performed, so as not to strip the limited blood supply of the distal ulna. A six- or seven-hole 3.5-mm dynamic compression plate is contoured and applied over the ulna's dorsal surface, with its distal edge about 1 cm proximal to the sigmoid notch. The two most distal screws are inserted in the neutral mode. Electrocautery is used to make a mark on the ulna at the osteotomy site, which should lie opposite the third or fourth hole in the plate. A longitudinal mark is also made to ensure proper rotational alignment after the osteotomy. After the most distal screw is loosened and the other screw is removed, the plate is swung away from the ulna. At 45 degrees to the coronal plane, an oblique cut is made through 75% of the ulna. A complete second cut is made parallel to the first. The kerf of the saw blade (width of bone it removes) is accounted for when making the second cut. The first cut is then completed and the resected bone removed. The plate is swung back in place, and the previously inserted screws are replaced and tightened. Axial compression is applied manually to the ulna to oppose the osteotomy, and the plate is clamped to the ulna

proximally. In completing the plate fixation, one or two of the proximal screws are inserted eccentrically in the dynamic compression mode. At the osteotomy site, a compression screw is inserted through a gliding hole and across the oblique osteotomy using a standard interfragmentary compression technique. An ulnar gutter splint is applied for 2 weeks. A removable splint is used with early forearm, wrist, and digital motion, but strenuous activity is restricted until bony union.

Outcome

Several studies have reported a high percentage of success with ulnar-shortening osteotomy. Combining the results using standard technique and equipment, 79 of 90 (88%) patients achieved good or excellent results regarding pain relief and recovery of function with only one nonunion (1%).[26,31,37,209] Delayed union and hardware irritation leading to plate removal are the most common problems. Ulnar shortening has been used in conjunction with delayed repairs of traumatic TFCC injuries[189] and after failed arthroscopic débridement of central disk tears and incomplete avulsions of the TFCC.[74] The concept is to reduce the load on the injured TFCC. Ulnar shortening is also reported as an effective treatment for Madelung's deformity; remodeling of the joint may still occur even when performed in adolescence.[159]

CRITICAL POINTS: ULNAR-SHORTENING OSTEOTOMY

INDICATIONS

- Ulnar impaction syndrome due to developmental or acquired ulnar-positive variance
- DRUJ incongruity from post-traumatic shortening of the radius

PEARLS

- Dorsal plating causes less hardware irritation.
- An oblique osteotomy with lag screw fixation may heal more reliably.

TECHNICAL POINTS

- Make a longitudinal incision over the subcutaneous border of the ulna.
- Subperiosteally expose the dorsal ulnar surface over the planned site of plating.
- Circumferentially expose the osteotomy site.

PITFALLS

- Avoid wide circumferential stripping of the ulna to reduce risk of nonunion.
- DRUJ incongruity may be created if the sigmoid notch has a reverse slope.

POSTOPERATIVE CARE

- Use a wrist splint for protection during stressful activities until bone unites.
- Begin early range-of-motion exercises and allow light use of the hand.

RETURN TO ACTIVITIES

- Await bone union before returning to full activities.

Partial Distal Ulnar Resection ("Wafer" Procedure)

Another treatment option for ulnar impaction syndrome is the so-called wafer procedure, described by Feldon and colleagues in 1992, in which the distal 2 to 4 mm of the ulnar head is excised.[47,48] Although described as an open procedure, it is now commonly performed arthroscopically (see Chapter 19). The procedure is designed to retain the ulnar styloid and foveal attachments of the TFCC. Because it is intended not to disrupt the articular surfaces of the DRUJ, no more than 3 to 4 mm should be resected.

Author's Preferred Technique: Partial Distal Ulnar Resection ("Wafer" Procedure)

A dorsal approach to the DRUJ is used as described for distal radioulnar ligament reconstruction (Fig. 15-28). The distal 2 to 4 mm of the ulnar dome is resected with an osteotome or oscillating saw, with care to preserve the ulnar attachments of the TFCC. If the TFCC becomes detached at the fovea, it is repaired via transosseous sutures as described for TFCC repair. The proximal surface of the disk is inspected and tears are débrided. The dorsal capsule is repaired but not imbricated to avoid stiffness. A sugar tong splint is applied, with conversion to a removable wrist splint at the first postoperative visit. Wrist and forearm motion are begun early, but full activity is not recommended until 8 weeks.

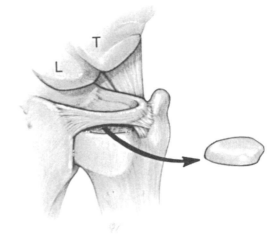

FIGURE 15-28. Resection of the distal dome of the ulnar head ("wafer procedure") decompresses the ulnocarpal joint for ulnar impaction syndrome.

Outcome

In a retrospective review of 13 cases by Feldon and associates, all achieved good or excellent results and none required secondary procedures.[47] In a separate series of 26 patients, 23 were completely satisfied and obtained improved grip with this procedure.[187] Two other smaller studies also reported good results.[16,169] Despite these good final results, the procedure is commonly mired by a long recovery time. In a comparison study of ulnar-shortening osteotomy and the wafer procedure, outcomes were nearly

---

CRITICAL POINTS: PARTIAL RESECTION OF ULNAR DOME ("WAFER PROCEDURE")

INDICATIONS

- Ulnar impaction syndrome, especially in ulnar-neutral or minimally ulnar-positive variance
- The procedure is usually performed arthroscopically.

PEARLS

- Maximum allowed resection is 4 mm.
- It is not necessary to expose the ulnocarpal joint.

TECHNICAL POINTS

- Plan the amount of resection from preoperative radiographs.
- Expose the DRUJ though the fifth extensor compartment.
- Make an "L"-shaped capsulotomy proximal to the TFCC.
- Resect the dome of the ulnar head using an osteotome or small saw.
- Débride the TFCC disk if necessary.
- Close the capsule without imbrication.

PITFALLS

- Avoid cutting the dorsal distal radioulnar ligament during capsulotomy.
- Do not release the ligament attachments at the fovea.
- Excessive resection will damage the DRUJ.

POSTOPERATIVE CARE

- Use a removable wrist splint for comfort.
- Gentle active motion is encouraged early.

RETURN TO ACTIVITIES

- Full activities are allowed at 8 weeks.

identical but reoperation, primarily for plate removal, was more frequent in the osteotomy group.[33]

DRUJ ARTHRITIS

Degeneration of the DRUJ can be caused by post-traumatic arthritis, inflammatory arthritis, osteoarthritis, or, rarely, long-standing DRUJ instability. Differentiating DRUJ arthritis and ulnocarpal impaction syndrome is important in treating degenerative conditions of the ulnar wrist. In some cases, both conditions are present and both require treatment to relieve symptoms. Pain and swelling, decreased grip strength, and stiffness are the most common symptoms. Point tenderness is elicited directly over the DRUJ. Pain is exacerbated by forearm rotation, especially when the joint is manually compressed.

Early radiographic signs of degenerative arthritis of the DRUJ typically occur in the proximal portion of the joint. Osteophyte formation is seen along the proximal margin of the ulnar head, whereas the sigmoid notch is often spared. Based on these findings of localized articular involvement, nonablative procedures have been described. Ulnar shortening, which shifts the proximal margin of the ulnar head out of the sigmoid notch, was reported to relieve symptoms in early DRUJ post-traumatic arthritis.[164] Open surgical resection of the proximal one third of the ulna's articular surface around its entire circumference and 2 to 3 mm deep has also been used.[204] The procedure, called modified arthroplasty, was reported to relieve pain while preserving motion and stability in 10 of 11 patients. Although experience with these procedures is limited, similar approaches have been used successfully in other joints.

In more advanced arthritis, surgical treatments are designed to eliminate the articulation between the distal ulna and radius by resecting all or a portion of the distal ulna, fusing the joint, or replacing the distal ulna. Each of the many described techniques has advantages and disadvantages that should be considered in selecting treatment. Surgical options include the Darrach procedure, the Sauvé-Kapandji operation, hemiresection arthroplasty, implant arthroplasty, wide distal ulnar resection, and one-bone forearm. The last two options are reserved for ultimate salvage, particularly for the failed distal ulnar resection. Because these procedures do not restore normal anatomy, some compromise of function and incomplete pain relief should be expected.

Hemiresection-Interposition Arthroplasty

Because instability is occasionally associated with the Darrach procedure, Bowers designed a surgical procedure that removes the articular surface of the ulnar head and retains the ulnar attachments of the TFCC. The procedure, which Bowers called the hemiresection interposition technique (HIT), was derived from Dingman,[43] who found the best clinical results of the Darrach procedure occurred in patients who had minimal distal ulnar resection that was followed by regeneration within the retained periosteal sleeve. The primary indication for the HIT is post-traumatic or degenerative arthritis of the DRUJ. It may also be useful in patients with severe DRUJ contractures complicated by articular degeneration, which may not be discovered until

the surgical release. Use of the procedure in the treatment of combined DRUJ instability and arthritis warrants caution because the instability will likely be exacerbated. Resection procedures in younger patients are less reliable, because the procedure may help to relieve pain but may result in loss of support for the ulnar carpus over time. Because some convergence of the radius and ulna will occur after partial resection of the ulnar head, ulnar-positive variance is a relative contraindication because it increases the likelihood of impingement between the ulnar styloid and triquetrum. Ulnar carpal translation is also a contraindication to partial or complete excision of the ulnar head because the resection may exacerbate the translation. Irreparable damage to the TFCC is a relative contraindication because the HIT would provide no theoretical benefit over a Darrach procedure. In his original and modified techniques, Bowers created several retinacular flaps for reconstruction of the capsule and ECU stabilization.[19,20] Interposition may be augmented with a ball of tendon or muscle when local soft tissue is insufficient. The matched distal ulnar resection described by Watson and Gabuzda is a similar alternative but does not stress preservation of the TFCC and ulnocarpal ligaments.[206] The concept is to remove all of the articular cartilage and subchondral bone on the radial and dorsal margins of the distal ulna so as to prevent radioulnar impingement during forearm rotation. An intact periosteal sleeve is preserved to maintain continuity with the ulnar carpus, and the exposed cancellous bone encourages strong healing to the surrounding soft tissue sleeve.

Author's Preferred Technique: Hemiresection-Interposition Arthroplasty

I prefer a slight modification of Bowers' procedure, in which the bony resection is less and the soft tissue reconstruction is simpler (Fig. 15-29). It is designed to reduce the tendency for postoperative radioulnar convergence without the need for a tendon graft interposition. Although interposition of autograft or allograft has been advocated to maintain the distal radioulnar space, the space tends to decrease with time and the procedure may be complicated by arthrofibrosis or impingement. By resecting less ulnar head, the amount of radioulnar convergence that can occur is reduced. The seemingly increased risk of developing distal radioulnar bony contact is offset by the increased stability imparted from capturing a larger circumference of the distal ulna with a large capsular-retinacular flap, and it does not preclude adding free soft tissue for added interposition when desired.

The DRUJ is approached dorsally through the fifth extensor compartment in a manner similar to that described earlier for TFCC repair and distal radioulnar ligament reconstruction. The dorsal capsule is raised as a large rectangular flap, with its base extending from the radial edge of the ECU sheath (the ECU sheath is not opened in this procedure). The flap begins over the ulnar neck, continues along the rim of the sigmoid notch, and courses ulnarward just proximal to

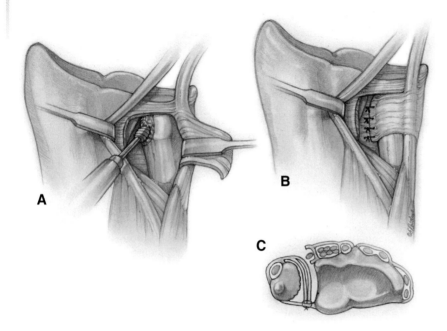

FIGURE 15-29. **A** to **C,** Hemiresection arthroplasty of the distal ulna with soft tissue interposition for arthritis of the DRUJ. In this modification of the procedure described by Bowers, a single, broad dorsal flap composed of extensor retinaculum and dorsal DRUJ capsule is used for interposition and stabilization (see text).

the dorsal radioulnar ligament. Care is taken not to cut the dorsal radioulnar ligament. There is no need to expose the distal surface of the TFCC or carpus unless symptomatic pathology is suspected. Small rongeurs and a bur are used to resect the surface of the ulnar head that articulates with the sigmoid notch to a depth of 3 to 7 mm, with the depth depending on the size of the ulnar head. The head is shaped to resemble a dowel with approximately the same diameter as the ulnar neck. Slight distal tapering is done, but the fovea is not violated so as to avoid detaching the TFCC. To reach the volar portion of the head, the radius and ulna are spread with firm retraction or a laminar spreader is placed proximal

CRITICAL POINTS: HEMIRESECTION-INTERPOSITION ARTHROPLASTY OF THE DISTAL ULNA

INDICATION

- DRUJ arthritis (osteoarthritis, post-traumatic arthritis, early rheumatoid arthritis)

PEARLS

- Avoid excessive resection of the ulnar head.
- To reach the volar portion of the head, use a self-retaining retractor to spread the radius from the ulna.
- The resected surface of the distal ulnar is most easily covered and stabilized by a single large dorsal flap.

TECHNICAL POINTS

- Open the fifth extensor compartment of the DRUJ.
- Create an ulnar-based retinacular flap extending to the radial edge of the ECU sheath.
- Make an ulnar-based, rectangular capsulotomy just proximal to the TFCC.
- Shape the distal ulna to match the diameter of the ulnar shaft.
- Débride the TFCC disk if necessary.
- Shorten the distal ulna if necessary.

- Suture the ulnar edges of both dorsal flaps to the volar DRUJ capsule to cover the resected surface.

PITFALLS

- Untreated ulnar-positive variance may lead to stylocarpal impingement.
- Accentuation of preexisting DRUJ instability is possible, but pain is usually reduced.
- Avoid detaching the foveal attachments of the TFCC or elevating and releasing the ECU sheath.
- Ensure the volar portion of the head is shaped equally.

POSTOPERATIVE CARE

- Immobilize in a long-arm splint or cast in neutral forearm rotation for 3 weeks.
- Use a well-molded short-arm cast that allows some forearm rotation for 3 weeks.
- Advance motion and strengthening gradually.

RETURN TO ACTIVITIES

- Full activities are not allowed for a minimum of 3 months.

to the DRUJ. The proximal surface of the TFCC and the remaining ulnar dome are inspected for degeneration and débrided if necessary.

At this point, a decision about ulnar shortening is made. No more than 2 to 3 mm of ulnar-positive variance is usually accepted to avoid impingement between the triquetrum and the residual ulnar head or styloid. Similarly, in rare instances an unusually long styloid may cause stylocarpal impingement.[186] An assessment for impingement is also done intraoperatively by compressing the radius and ulna while rotating the forearm with the wrist ulnarly deviated. If shortening is necessary, it can be done through the ulnar shaft, the base of the styloid, or the distal ulna. The goal is to create 1 to 2 mm of ulnar-negative variance. If styloid shortening is done, particular care is required not to cut the TFCC foveal attachment or release the TFCC from the styloid. The fragment can be fixed with wire or heavy nonabsorbable suture using a figure-of-eight tension band or an interosseous compression loop. I prefer to shorten the ulna through the midportion of the residual ulnar head because it can be done through the same incision, avoids the risk of injuring the TFCC foveal attachment, requires minimal fixation, and is at a site with good bone-healing potential. In this technique, a slice is removed with an oscillating saw at its midportion. The osteotomy can be fixed using a standard tension band technique with two parallel 0.045-inch Kirschner wires passed obliquely across the osteotomy and a figure-of-eight wire suture. The Kirschner wires are bent over and tapped into the bone. Because the wires often create irritation and require removal, I prefer to fix the osteotomy using a large suture anchor inserted deeply into the ulnar neck as described earlier for fixation of ulnar styloid fractures.

Outcome

Bowers reported on 38 patients, most of whom had rheumatoid arthritis. The results were generally good for pain relief and motion.[20] Results were very good in patients with degenerative or post-traumatic arthritis. Failures were often related to residual ulnocarpal impaction. Bowers now recommends this procedure only in the early stages of rheumatoid arthritis when the stabilizing soft tissues are still effective. He believes the procedure is particularly valuable in post-traumatic and osteoarthritis if ulnocarpal impaction is avoided. Fernandez found the procedure effective when used in conjunction with a radial osteotomy for malunited distal radius fractures.[50] It has also been reported to be successful in conjunction with repairs of the TFCC in patients with ulnar-positive variance.[116] Other authors have reported varied results.

Sauvé-Kapandji Procedure

In 1936, Sauvé[161] and, later, Kapandji[81] described a procedure consisting of a radioulnar joint fusion and creation of a pseudarthrosis proximal to the fusion (Fig. 15-30). The procedure was developed as an alternative to resection of the distal ulna. Indications are similar to those for the Darrach procedure, including post-traumatic DRUJ arthritis, either rheumatoid arthritis, and osteoarthritis. It has an advantage over a distal ulnar resection in patients with rheumatoid

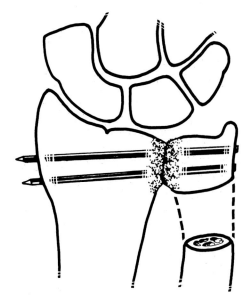

FIGURE 15-30. Sauvé Kapandji procedure forms a fusion between the ulnar head and sigmoid notch and creates a pseudarthrosis through the ulnar neck. One or two cannulated screws are used instead of Kirschner wires if bone stock is adequate.

arthritis because it retains support for the ulnar carpus and thus reduces the risk of ulnar translation.

Some authors have suggested that it may be a better procedure for the treatment of post-traumatic arthritis in young active patients.[62,81,82,199] Potential complications include instability of the ulnar stump and regeneration of the resected segment resulting in loss of motion.

 ## Author's Preferred Technique: Sauvé-Kapandji Procedure

To better visualize the articular surfaces of the DRUJ and to avoid levering out the head fragment, I prefer a dorsal exposure. Others prefer an ulnar approach. A longitudinal incision is made over the sixth extensor compartment extending from the level of the ulnar styloid proximally for 6 cm. The fifth compartment is opened, and the EDQ tendon is extracted. The extensor retinaculum and DRUJ capsule are raised as an ulnar-based flap. The choice of fixation depends on the size and quality of the bone. If it is sufficient, cannulated screw fixation is planned. Two parallel guide wires are inserted into the head just beneath the ECU sheath. The periosteum is excised around the ulnar neck and 1 cm of the neck is resected with an oscillating saw. If there is ulnar-positive variance, a correspondingly greater segment of ulna is removed so that when the head is recessed to neutral variance the resulting gap will be 1 cm. The opposing articular surfaces of the ulnar head and sigmoid notch are denuded to cancellous bone. The ulnar head is held against the sigmoid notch in neutral rotation and at the proper longitudinal position. The wires are driven into the radius and the position is checked with fluoroscopy. One or two 3.5-mm cannulated screws are inserted using a lag technique to gain compression, but tilting of the head must be avoided. If two screws cannot fit, one of the guide wires is retained for additional fixation. The cancellous portion of the resected bone is placed at the fusion site. The pronator quadratus muscle is detached from its ulnar insertion and advanced into the osteotomy site and sutured in place to the ECU sheath, followed by closure in layers. To gain additional stability of the proximal ulnar stump in the young patient with post-traumatic arthritis, I use the FCU tenodesis technique described by Lamey and Fernandez.[50] A distally based strip of FCU tendon is raised and passed into the exposed medullary canal of the ulnar stump and out through a drilled hole in the stump. It is sutured back onto itself under tension. The pronator quadratus is then brought into the gap and sutured in place. A long-arm splint is used for 2 weeks, followed by a short-arm cast until there is radiographic evidence of fusion.

Outcome

Goncalves reported that in 22 patients the results were "consistently better" than historical results with the Darrach procedure.[62] Taleisnik reported elimination of pain, restoration of forearm rotation, and few complications in 24 patients with a minimum 1-year follow-up.[177] The theoret-ically predictable complications of an unstable proximal ulnar stump were observed in only 3 of the 24 patients. Others have found instability of the ulnar stump more common, although not always symptomatic.[199] Many others have expressed general satisfaction with the procedure.*

Distal Ulnar Resection (The Darrach Procedure)

Although Darrach's name has become synonymous with resection of the distal ulna, the technique was described by several others before him.[11,39,93,104,112,196] The general indication for a distal ulnar resection is any condition that causes incongruity or arthritis of the DRUJ, with resultant pain or stiffness. The procedure is particularly effective in a low-demand patient with an incongruous or degenerative sigmoid notch due to the sequelae of an intra-articular fracture. The procedure is also widely used in rheumatoid arthritis, but it has been reported to increase the risk for ulnar translation of the carpus.

Probably more has been written about the Darrach procedure than any other operation concerning the DRUJ, with a wide variation of technical modifications, results,

---

*See references 50, 63, 78, 81, 82, 115, 118, 127, 153, and 160.

CRITICAL POINTS: SAUVÉ-KAPANDJI PROCEDURE

INDICATIONS

- DRUJ arthritis (osteoarthritis, post-traumatic arthritis, rheumatoid arthritis)
- Ulnar translation of the carpus in rheumatoid arthritis

PEARLS

- A cannulated screw system improves the efficiency of the procedure.
- Insert guide wires before resecting the joint surfaces or ulnar neck.
- Fixation with two screws is optimal.
- Recess ulnar head to create slight ulnar-negative variance.
- Perform a tenodesis of the stump if there is evidence of instability.

TECHNICAL POINTS

- Make an incision over the sixth extensor compartment.
- Open the fifth extensor compartment and retract the EDQ.
- Make an "L"-shaped capsulotomy proximal to the TFCC.
- Insert two guide wires into the ulnar head from its ulnar border.
- Excise the periosteum around the ulnar neck.
- Resect 1 cm of the ulnar neck.
- Denude the articular surfaces of the DRUJ.
- Débride the TFCC disk if necessary.
- Align the ulnar head to the sigmoid notch and advance guide wires.
- Insert two cannulated compression screws or one screw and leave the remaining guide wire for fixation.
- Perform an FCU tenodesis stabilization if needed.
- Close the capsule.

PITFALLS

- Stylocarpal impingement can be produced by excessive articular resection.
- Recognize the potential need to stabilize the ulnar stump.

POSTOPERATIVE CARE

- A long-arm splint is used for 2 weeks followed by a short-arm cast until there is radiographic evidence of fusion.

RETURN TO ACTIVITIES

- Full activities are allowed once bony union has occurred.

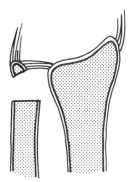

FIGURE 15-31. Darrach procedure resects the distal ulna through the ulnar neck. The ulnar styloid and its attachments can be retained. A variety of techniques have been described to help stabilize the ulnar stump. (Adapted from Dingman P: Resection of the distal end of the ulna (Darrach operation): An end result study of twenty-four cases. J Bone Joint Surg Am 34:893-900, 1952.)

and opinions (Fig. 15-31). Dingman[43] and, more recently, DiBenedetto,[41] Nolan and Eaton,[128] and Tulipan and colleagues[192] have reviewed the procedure with regard to the technical points of extraperiosteal or subperiosteal resection, the obliquity of the cut, whether to remove the styloid, and the amount of bone to be resected. Dingman's study suggested that none of these factors other than the amount of bone resection correlated with the result. He recommended that only the ulna adjacent to the sigmoid notch be resected and that it be done in a subperiosteal fashion because those patients in whom regeneration had occurred appeared to have had better results. He also preferred to retain the ulnar styloid.

Although controversial, many would recommend that the procedure be combined with a soft tissue stabilization technique.

Author's Preferred Technique: Distal Ulnar Resection

An incision is extended proximally from the ulnar styloid process. The bone is approached just volar to the ECU sheath, with care taken to avoid the dorsal cutaneous branch of the ulnar nerve. The periosteum is incised and reflected from the distal 3 cm of the ulna, but the attachments to the ulnar styloid are left intact. An osteotomy is made at the level of the proximal margin of the sigmoid notch. The distal fragment is dissected free, and the ulnar styloid process is osteotomized at its base and left in situ. The periosteal sleeve is closed to provide a firm attachment for the styloid and to help stabilize the ulnar stump. I nearly always perform a soft tissue stabilization procedure as an adjunct to the resection (see next section). The wound is closed in layers. Darrach did not use a splint and allowed active motion within 24 hours. I prefer to use a short-arm splint to support the wrist to prevent full forearm rotation for 2 to 4 weeks until the patient has recovered good digital motion and pain is minimal.

CRITICAL POINTS: DISTAL ULNAR RESECTION (THE DARRACH PROCEDURE)

INDICATIONS

- DRUJ arthritis in the elderly (post-traumatic arthritis or osteoarthritis)
- Post-traumatic DRUJ incongruity due to malunion of radius or ulna in the elderly
- Rheumatoid arthritis involving the DRUJ

PEARLS

- Retain the ulnar styloid and its attachments.
- Resect the distal ulna subperiosteally (partial regrowth of ulna is associated with equal or improved results).
- Interpose soft tissue or the pronator quadratus between the radius and ulna.
- Perform a soft tissue stabilization procedure for the ulnar stump.

TECHNICAL POINTS

- Make an incision extending proximally from the ulnar styloid.
- Incise the periosteum volar to the ECU sheath, and reflect it from the distal 3 cm of the ulna.
- Cut the ulna at the base of the ulnar styloid and at the proximal margin of the sigmoid notch.
- Remove the ulnar segment, and close the periosteal sleeve.
- Perform a soft tissue stabilization of the stump as a routine (see other sections for techniques).

PITFALLS

- Weakness is a common complaint in younger or active patients.
- Ulnar stump instability and radioulnar convergence are potentially serious problems.

POSTOPERATIVE CARE

- A short-arm splint is used for 2 to 4 weeks for support and to prevent full forearm rotation.
- Early digital motion and light hand use are encouraged early.

RETURN TO ACTIVITIES

- Full activities as tolerated are begun at 6 weeks.

Outcome

Regardless of the diagnosis, most patients achieve satisfactory relief of pain and restoration of function.[15] Unfortunately, instability of the ulnar stump in both anteroposterior and coronal planes can develop and produce substantial weakness and pain. Convergence of the proximal ulnar stump can develop into radioulnar impingement and painful crepitus.[68] The amount of instability and impingement is more common with increasing amounts of bony resection. The results are generally worse in patients with higher demands.[7,15,20,68,117,206] In rheumatoid patients, especially those with active synovitis and wrist laxity, there is a risk of developing progressive ulnar translation of the carpus from loss of support by the head of the ulna.

For these reasons the Darrach procedure should be used selectively. It may be useful in patients with low demands with severe DRUJ incongruity, arthritis, or ulnar impaction syndrome when an ulnar-shortening osteotomy or hemi-resection arthroplasty is unlikely to be successful. In patients with rheumatoid arthritis, consideration should be given to concomitant partial or complete wrist fusion.

Stabilization of the Resected Distal Ulna

To reduce the instability created by the Darrach excision, a variety of soft tissue stabilization techniques are used. Blatt and Ashworth sutured a flap of the volar capsule to the dorsal aspect of the ulnar stump.[17] Leslie and associates,[94] O'Donovan and Ruby,[129] and Webber and Maser[207] have tethered the stump with a distally based strip of ECU tendon. Spinner and Kaplan transposed the ECU over the dorsum of the ulnar stump using a flap of retinaculum.[173] Kessler and Hecht created a dynamic sling for the ulnar stump by looping a strip of tendon around the distal ulnar stump and the ECU.[84] Goldner and Hayes formalized these recommendations by passing a proximally based strip of the ECU through a drill hole in the ulnar stump with the forearm in supination.[61] Breen and Jupiter used a combination of

half FCU and half ECU, both threaded into the stump's medullary canal.[23] Tsai and coworkers used a distally based portion of the FCU tendon to stabilize the ulnar stump and looped this tendon over the ulnar stump also to stabilize the ECU.[190] Tsai and Stilwell reported using the ECU in a similar manner.[191] Hunter and Kirkpatrick used Mersilene tape to bind the radius and ulna together.[75] Watson and colleagues lengthened the short ulnar stump to approximate the appearance of a successfully done partial ulnar resection.[205] Advancement and dorsal redirection of the pronator quadratus was used by Johnson as a soft tissue interposition and a dynamic stabilizer to the stump.[79] Ruby and coworkers described a similar use of the pronator quadratus.[156] Kleinman and Greenberg combined ECU tenodesis and pronator quadratus transfer with radioulnar temporary pinning.[90] Insertion of soft tissue allograft with suture fixation to the ulna and radius was reported by Sotereanos.[172]

Author's Preferred Technique: Stabilization of the Resected Distal Ulna

In an elderly, low-demand, or rheumatoid patient, I prefer to stabilize the ulnar stump with a broad flap created from the palmar, ulnocarpal capsule. The flap is transferred to the dorsum of the ulna and attached with sutures through drill holes in the dorsal cortex. The ECU tendon is positioned

---

CRITICAL POINTS: TENODESIS STABILIZATION OF THE RESECTED DISTAL ULNA

INDICATIONS

- Primarily an adjunct to distal ulnar resection
- Instability of previously resected distal ulna

PEARLS

- Transfer the pronator quadratus to augment ulnar stability and reduce radioulnar impingement.

TECHNICAL POINTS

- Incise the skin proximally from the triquetrum.
- Expose the ECU and FCU tendons.
- Create a distally based strip of FCU tendon extending from the pisiform.
- Create a proximally based strip of ECU tendon.
- Resect the distal ulna if not already done.
- Drill a bone hole in the ulnar stump about 1.5 cm from its cut end.
- Pass the FCU strip into the canal and out through the hole dorsally.
- Pass the ECU strip through the hole in the stump from dorsal to volar.

- Both strips are passed around the stump and tied to each other.
- Release and transfer the pronator quadratus through the radioulnar interval and reattach to the dorsum of the ulna.

PITFALLS

- It does not reliably correct or control radioulnar impingement.
- Excessive tightening of the tendon strips will reduce radial deviation.

POSTOPERATIVE CARE

- Immobilize in a long-arm splint with the forearm in neutral rotation for 4 weeks.
- Use a well-molded short-arm cast for 2 weeks.
- Convert to a wrist splint and advance activities gradually.

RETURN TO ACTIVITIES

- Use of a removable wrist splint is encouraged for many months.

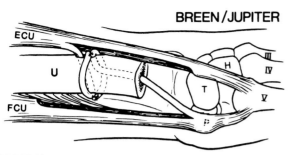

BREEN / JUPITER

FIGURE 15-32. Tenodesis for stabilization of the resected distal ulna using strips of the FCU and ECU tendons as described by Breen and Jupiter. (From Petersen MS, Adams BD: Biomechanical evaluation of distal radioulnar reconstructions. J Hand Surg [Am] 18:328-334, 1993.)

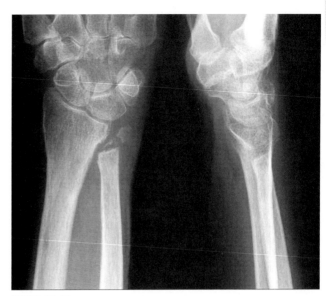

FIGURE 15-33. Radiograph showing excessive excision and consequent radioulnar impingement after a Darrach procedure. Note the remodeling of the radius at the site of impingement.

over the dorsum of the ulna using a sling made from the retinaculum, as described in the section on ECU tendon instability.

In patients with higher demands or those presenting with an unstable previously resected distal ulna, I prefer to stabilize the ulnar stump with a tenodesis using the technique described by Breen and Jupiter because it offers theoretical bidirectional control of the ulnar stump (Fig. 15-32).[23] In this technique, a distally based strip of the FCU is passed into the canal of the ulna stump and out through a prepared bone hole in the ulnar shaft. A proximally based ECU strip is passed through the same bone hole and both strips are wrapped around the shaft and sutured to each other. If the pronator quadratus has not been previously damaged, I will transfer it to augment the stabilization, and it also provides soft tissue interposition to reduce radioulnar impingement. The muscle is detached from the palmar aspect of the ulna, routed through the radioulnar space, and attached to the dorsum of the distal ulna.[79] All of these procedures have been successful in reducing symptoms in small numbers of patients. However, it is rare to completely relieve pain or restore full function.

FAILED DISTAL ULNAR RESECTION

Instability of the distal ulna after a resection may develop early or late. Weakness and pain are associated with excessive dorsopalmar translation and radioulnar convergence. Convergence can progress to impingement of the ulnar stump against the radius, producing crepitus and pain with forearm rotation (Fig. 15-33).[105] Although severe instability of the distal ulna is most commonly associated with the Darrach procedure, it can occur after hemiresection or the Sauvé-Kapandji procedure. A history of painful crepitus about the distal ulna can typically be reproduced during the physical examination by manually compressing the radius against the ulna while passively rotating the forearm. A PA radiograph demonstrates the distal ulna to abut against the radius, which can be accentuated by having the patient hold a weight with the forearm in neutral rotation while the radiograph is taken in a "cross-table" direction.

Treatment of radioulnar impingement is extremely difficult. Bieber and coworkers reported that patients failing a Darrach procedure continued to do poorly despite up to seven additional operations.[15] Several of the ligament reconstructions described earlier have been used with varying success, but the techniques may need modification to produce a better mechanism to prevent recurrent impingement. If a tenodesis or soft tissue interposition was not used in the primary procedure, a revision using one or a combination of these techniques can be effective. A careful review of the patient's previous operation record provides important information regarding available tissues such as the volar DRUJ capsule, pronator quadratus, ECU, and FCU.

In a modestly active patient with adequate soft tissues and proper motivation for rehabilitation, my preferred technique is ulnar head implant arthroplasty. This procedure is presented in the next section. When implant arthroplasty is contraindicated, I prefer to use the method of Breen and Jupiter combined with soft tissue interposition using the pronator quadratus when available or Achilles tendon allograft. For patients who have had repeated failed surgery, either wide ulnar resection or creating a one-bone forearm are alternatives, but these procedures should be used with caution.

Extensive resection of the distal ulna is usually reserved for the treatment of tumors, but one study reported generally favorable results in patients after failed DRUJ reconstructions. Range of motion and grip strength averaged 75% to 90%, but radioulnar instability and convergence led to failure in two cases.[35,214] Radiocarpal instability and ulnar carpal translocation were rare. The surgical approach is straightforward; the ulna is exposed along its subcutaneous border and subperiosteal resection of 25% to 30% of the ulnar length is recommended. Previous traumatic disruption of the interosseous membrane is an absolute contraindication to the procedure.[214]

Creating a one-bone forearm through a radioulnar fusion is the ultimate salvage for the dysfunctional forearm. Complete loss of forearm motion is the sacrifice to alleviate pain and restore forearm stability. A preoperative test of immobilization in different positions of forearm rotation will allow the patient to decide if the procedure is appropriate, as well as the optimal position for fusion. One study of 30 normal subjects determined that 63% of individuals preferred a neutral forearm position for activities of daily living.[201] The procedure is indicated for end-stage radioulnar instability that is recalcitrant to surgical stabilization, paralytic instability, and, rarely, spastic contractures. The fusion can be accomplished by making osteotomies through the radial and ulnar shafts, discarding the proximal radius and the distal ulna, and transposition of the radius to the ulna with plate fixation. Alternatively, the radius and ulna can be collapsed against each other and fixed together with lag screws or a bridging plate. Iliac crest bone graft is recommended. The osteotomy is typically fixed with the forearm in neutral or slight pronation. Successful fusion was achieved in one series with a distal radioulnar fusion fixed with dual lag screws in 60 of 65 cases.[165]

Complications are common, and the nonunion rate in one series was 32%.[143]

DISTAL ULNAR HEAD IMPLANT ARTHROPLASTY

Normal stability and function of the forearm axis require an ulnar head, making implant arthroplasty an attractive concept for the treatment of ulnar head deficiencies and posttraumatic arthritis. Treatment of the unstable resected distal ulna by soft tissue stabilization procedures is unpredictable. A functional ulnar head replacement arthroplasty would function to alleviate radioulnar impingement and restore load transmission. Although a silicone implant combined with soft tissue reconstruction temporarily relieved symptoms and restored stability,[176] inevitable failure of the implant led to recurrence of symptoms and frequent silicone synovitis.[213] Silicone ulnar head implants have since been abandoned.

Van Schoonhoven and associates reported on the use of a ceramic head fixed to a porous-coated titanium stem inserted in the ulnar medullary canal.[197] The head is spherical in the transverse plane and features a concave distal surface to decrease pressure across the ulnocarpal joint. Modularity with three different head and collar sizes accommodated anatomic variations and a variety of bony defects. They treated 23 patients with chronic painful instability following ulnar head resection after an average of 3 previous operations. Symptoms were significantly improved in all patients. Stability was achieved initially in all cases, but two developed recurrence. Both were treated successfully by revising the implant. Slight remoduling of the sigmoid notch and 1 to 2 mm of resorption beneath the collar occurred in all patients but was not progressive. These authors were cautiously optimistic with the short-term results.

A metallic ulnar head implant with a modular head and stem, and including an extended collar for ulnar neck deficiencies, has been developed.[103,162] The implant is indicated for use in acute ulnar head fractures, posttraumatic DRUJ arthritis, rheumatoid arthritis, and failed previous partial or complete resections of the distal ulna, including

---

CRITICAL POINTS: DISTAL ULNAR HEAD IMPLANT ARTHROPLASTY

INDICATIONS

- Radioulnar impingement after partial or complete distal ulnar resection
- Arthritis of the DRUJ (osteoarthritis or post-traumatic arthritis)

PEARLS

- Either a dorsal or ulnar approach is acceptable.
- Deepen and shape a deficient sigmoid notch to improve stability.
- Augment the capsule if necessary with a broad flap of retinaculum.

TECHNICAL POINTS

- When approaching the joint dorsally, raise broad ulnarly based flaps of retinaculum and capsule.
- Carefully release all remaining soft tissue attachments from the bone.
- Maintain the integrity of the ECU sheath when possible by subperiosteal elevation.
- Cut the ulna at the level determined from preoperative templates and operative inspection.
- Deepen and shape the sigmoid notch if necessary.
- Ream the ulnar canal and insert the trial stem.

- Apply the trial ulnar head component and test stability.
- Insert the final implants and retest stability.
- Suture the TFCC and ECU sheath to the implant if appropriate.
- Close the flaps over the implant to create a complete capsule.

PITFALLS

- An unrecognized deficient rim of the sigmoid notch may lead to instability.
- Overzealous soft tissue attachment to the implant may cause stiffness or joint subluxation.

POSTOPERATIVE CARE

- Immobilize in a long-arm splint for 2 weeks followed by a wrist splint for a minimum of 4 weeks.
- Begin strengthening but avoid forceful pronation and supination for another month.

RETURN TO ACTIVITIES

- Gradual return to activities is necessary, especially if there is a tendency for instability or the sigmoid notch required reshaping.

failed silicone implants. The implant head has a site for reattachment of the TFCC, ECU sheath, and ulnocarpal ligaments to help stabilize the DRUJ. Cement fixation of the stem is not typically necessary. Clinical results have not yet been published.

Scheker designed an implant that replaces both the ulnar head and the sigmoid notch, which he considers a total replacement of the DRUJ.[162] It is a ball-and-socket concept that allows axial displacement of the radial component on the ulnar component to accommodate changes in ulnar variance during forearm rotation. The sigmoid notch component consists of a plate with a socket attached to its distal end and fixed to the distal radius by a peg and screws. The ulnar component is a polyethylene ball fitted on a peg that extends from a stem fixed into the ulnar medullary canal. The ball can freely slide axially on the peg but cannot translate. The purpose of this more complex implant is to stabilize the distal radioulnar relationship in cases with loss of both skeletal and ligament support. The prosthesis was used in patients who had partial or complete destruction of the DRUJ, including loss from gunshots, motor vehicle accidents, and excessive surgical resection of the distal ulna for posttraumatic arthritis. A dorsal surgical approach is used and release of the distal IOM may be necessary to achieve proper motion. Immobilization in a long arm splint is used for 3 weeks, after which active range of motion is begun. Twenty-three patients who had at least one previous surgery with partial or complete distal ulna resection were treated.[162] Mean follow-up was 15 months, with a maximum of 40 months. Complete pain relief was reported for all patients and lifting capacity ranged from 2 to 50 lb with an average of 14 lb; however, a 25-lb lifting limit was recommended to reduce the risk of loosening. Normal pronation and supination were observed. The authors reported no complications; however, one prosthesis was removed for suspected infection. While the prosthesis appears to have been successful in treating very difficult problems, the long-term results are unknown. Because it does not provide for the normal translational motion of the DRUJ during forearm rotation, I am concerned that high implant and bone stresses with resultant loosening may become a problem with longer follow-up. As many of these conditions have been treated successfully with an ulnar head implant and soft tissue reconstruction alone, the indications for a sigmoid notch implant remain unclear.

Surgical Technique

Through a dorsal approach, an ulnarly based flap, including the capsule and retinaculum flap, is raised from the ulnar head with care to preserve the integrity of the ECU sheath. The prosthetic head size is chosen to properly tension the soft tissues. In the presence of a malunited radius, a corrective osteotomy is recommended to achieve stability. It is important to surgically contour the sigmoid notch when misshapen by trauma or arthritis. The retinacular flap is advanced on the radius as necessary during closure to create prosthetic stability. A long arm splint is used for 2 weeks, followed by a removable splint for another 4 weeks.

Alternatively, an ulnar surgical approach between the flexor carpi ulnaris (FCU) and ECU is preferred for ease of implantation and to best preserve the capsule. The ECU

sheath is elevated subperiosteally from the distal ulna along with the TFCC and ulnocarpal ligament. The TFCC, ECU sheath, and ulnar wrist capsule are secured with sutures placed through holes in the implant. The forearm is immobilized in mid-rotation with a long arm splint for 3 weeks. A removable splint is used for an additional 3 weeks during which gentle exercises are performed. Strengthening and activities are advanced as wrist and forearm motion recover. In patients with rheumatoid arthritis, longer immobilization may be required for soft-tissue healing.

Outcome

Experience with distal ulna implants is gradually increasing. Biomechanical testing shows the implants nearly restore normal DRUJ kinematics.[103] These implants are particularly attractive for use in patients with radioulnar impingement following a failed partial or complete distal ulnar resection. In my limited experience, pain and instability are improved but not completely corrected. Achieving a good, well-balanced soft tissue envelope around the implant can be challenging in the multiply operated patient. In addition, to properly seat the implant it may be necessary to contour and deepen the deformed sigmoid notch. Despite these concerns, I have found implant arthroplasty to have less morbidity and to be more predictable in short-term follow-up than other surgical options for radioulnar impingement (Fig. 15-34). Longer follow-up studies will be needed to assess its full value.

DRUJ CONTRACTURE

Acquired contractures of the DRUJ may result from trauma, arthritis, or spasticity. Conditions that mimic DRUJ contractures include forearm synostosis, radial head dislocation, and dysplastic congenital conditions. Post-traumatic contractures of the DRUJ capsule are common, especially loss of supination after a distal radius fracture. Physical therapy, including a splinting program, should be used for a period of at least 6 months before considering surgery. Arthritis and DRUJ subluxation are contraindications to surgical release. CT should be done if standard radiographs are inconclusive.

Post-traumatic DRUJ stiffness results from fibrosis and contracture of the capsule. The volar capsule normally has a redundant oblique fold that opens and forms a pocket to accept the ulnar head in supination.[89] After trauma and immobilization in pronation, the fold can become thickened, adherent, and shortened and result in restriction of supination. Contracture of the pronator quadratus from immobilization or injury can also contribute to a pronation contracture. The dorsal capsule is normally much thinner and homogeneous, with transversely oriented fibers. It is much less likely to impede pronation after trauma or prolonged immobilization and more likely to respond to therapy when contracted.

Operative Technique

Dorsal Capsulectomy

A dorsal exposure of the DRUJ is made as described earlier for radioulnar ligament reconstruction. The entire dorsal

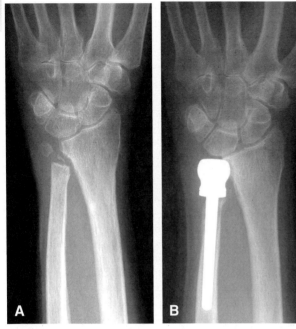

FIGURE 15-34. **A** and **B,** Radiograph of a distal ulna implant arthroplasty (uHead, Avanta Orthopedics, San Diego, CA) for the treatment of radioulnar impingement. Note restoration of radioulnar alignment.

capsule is excised with care not to damage the dorsal radioulnar ligament or ECU sheath. The joint is inspected for injury or arthritis and carefully débrided if necessary. The forearm is gently manipulated into maximum allowable pronation. A long-arm or sugar-tong plaster splint is applied with the forearm in full but not forced pronation and maintained for 2 to 3 weeks. A removable pronation splint is used at night and intermittently during the day for 1 month. Dynamic splinting is used only if the original improvements in motion are not being maintained.

Volar Capsulectomy

A longitudinal incision is made radial to the FCU, extending proximal from the wrist crease. The ulnar neurovascular bundle is retracted ulnarly to expose the pronator quadratus. The distal half of the muscle is raised subperiosteally from the ulna. The palmar radioulnar ligament is palpated, and an "L"-shaped capsulotomy is made, with the transverse limb parallel and just proximal to the ligament. The longitudinal limb is made parallel to the capsule's attachment at the sigmoid notch. The entire volar capsule is excised with care not to damage the palmar radioulnar ligament. If the gain in supination is not adequate after gentle manipulation, the pronator quadratus is completely released or excised.

A long-arm or sugar-tong plaster splint is applied with the forearm in full but not forced supination and maintained for 2 weeks. A removable supination splint is used at night and intermittently during the day for 1 month. Dynamic splinting is used only if losing the original gains in motion.

Outcome

In a report on a small series of patients, improvement in forearm motion was universal, with an average increase in supination of 51 degrees and in pronation of 28 degrees. There were no complications, including no iatrogenic cases of DRUJ instability.[89] In my experience, contracture release is a gratifying procedure for loss of supination after a distal radius fracture when the DRUJ is well aligned and not arthritic. A release in the presence of a subluxated stiff DRUJ is likely to result in a painful joint.

CRITICAL POINTS: CAPSULECTOMY FOR CONTRACTURE

INDICATION

■ Post-traumatic forearm stiffness without DRUJ arthritis, especially loss of supination

PEARLS

■ The volar capsule can be exposed and excised without releasing the pronator quadratus when appropriate.

TECHNICAL POINTS

■ For loss of supination, approach the volar capsule between the ulnar neurovascular bundle and the finger flexor tendons.
■ Retract the pronator quadratus proximally and excise the volar capsule proximal to the TFCC.
■ Release or excise the pronator quadratus if necessary from the ulna.
■ Test DRUJ motion and stability.

■ For loss of pronation, approach the dorsal capsule through the fifth extensor compartment.
■ Excise the capsule proximal to the TFCC.
■ Repair the retinaculum.

PITFALLS

■ Avoid injury to the TFCC.
■ Maximize motion during operative procedure but avoid creating instability.

POSTOPERATIVE CARE

■ Allow immediate and regular range-of-motion exercises under routine supervision.
■ Passive motion with use of static progressive or dynamic splinting may be needed.

RETURN TO ACTIVITIES

■ Early return to full activities is encouraged.

EXTENSOR CARPI ULNARIS TENOSYNOVITIS AND SUBULUXATION

The ECU tendon takes an angular path across the ulnar head to its insertion on the fifth metacarpal base when the forearm is supinated, which is further accentuated by ulnar deviation of the wrist (Fig. 15-35). The ECU tendon is normally held within the groove of the ulnar head by a deep retinaculum, often referred to as the subsheath, which must resist the natural tendency for the tendon to subluxate.[83,136,173,178] The true extensor retinaculum passes over the subsheath without an attachment to the ulna and inserts on the pisiform, triquetrum, fifth metacarpal, and volar soft tissues. Repetitive stress on the subsheath can result in a stenosing tenosynovitis from fibrosis.[42,67,87,125] The tendon can become unstable and dislocated from attenuation or tearing of its sheath.[25,45,154] Recurrent subluxation over the ulnar ridge of the groove can produce a partial tendon rupture.[30]

Volar subluxation of the ECU is a common finding in rheumatoid arthritis and nearly always accompanies the caput ulna syndrome of dorsal ulnar and ulnocarpal subluxation.[12] Although it is rarely symptomatic in these patients, repositioning the tendon to the dorsal aspect of the ulna reduces its deforming force on the wrist and may help stabilize the distal ulna; thus it should be considered whenever performing an isolated ECU tenosynovectomy, a complete extensor tenosynovectomy, DRUJ synovectomy, or distal ulnar resection.

Although ECU stenosing tenosynovitis and instability would appear to be different, their presentations and treatments are quite similar. The patient can typically reproduce the pain or snapping by combined supination and ulnar deviation against resistance. Acute conditions can be treated by rest, immobilization with the forearm in pronation and the wrist in neutral, and anti-inflammatory medications. Although snapping may not resolve, pain is often relieved. Stenosing tenosynovitis can also be treated by corticosteroid injection into the sheath. Surgery is reserved for recalcitrant symptoms.

Sixth Dorsal Compartment Release

A longitudinal incision is made over the sixth compartment. The retinaculum and subsheath are divided. The tendon is inspected and trimmed if frayed. A tenosynovectomy is performed when needed. The groove is inspected for spurs and prominent ridges, which should be trimmed. The retinaculum can be left open or repaired beneath the tendon when the groove has spurs or ridges. Ligament reconstruction (see later) to stabilize the tendon is not typically done, but it should be considered if there is a visible snapping during passive forearm rotation.[87] The patient is immobilized with a plaster wrist splint for 2 weeks followed by return to activities over several weeks.

ECU Tendon Stabilization

A longitudinal incision is made between the fifth and sixth compartments. A volar skin flap is raised while protecting the dorsal branch of the ulnar nerve. The extensor retinaculum is incised at the volar margin of the sixth compartment. The ECU subsheath is opened longitudinally in its midline. The tendon and groove are inspected, and bony spurs are débrided. At this point, a decision is made as to imbrication or performance of a ligament reconstruction. The decision depends on the quality of subsheath tissue and condition of the groove. In more acute cases (less than 6 months), I prefer a repair if the tendon has minimal fraying and the groove is smooth. The sheath is not overtightened; placing a pediatric feeding tube next to the tendon during suturing will reduce this risk. The extensor retinaculum is repaired anatomically.

When the groove is rough or the subsheath is badly damaged, or in chronic cases, a ligament reconstruction to stabilize the tendon is preferred. Spinner and Kaplan use a ½- to 1-inch rectangular flap of retinaculum, with the septum between the fourth and fifth compartments its base.[173] It is raised to Lister's tubercle, folded back, and passed under the ECU tendon. The flap is then brought back over the tendon and sutured to itself, which places the retinaculum's deep surface against the tendon. The previously released retinaculum over the sixth compartment is repaired.

I prefer to create a flap from the retinaculum that had already been partially raised for the tendon exposure

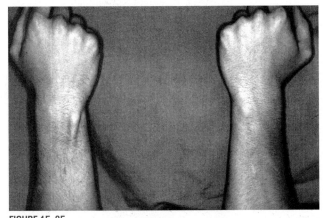

FIGURE 15-35. Subluxation of the ECU tendon from the groove in the ulnar head is shown with the wrist in supination.

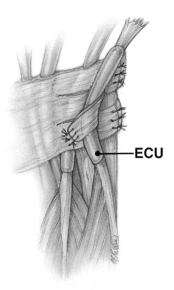

FIGURE 15-36. ECU stabilized by a sling created from the extensor retinaculum.

CRITICAL POINTS: ECU TENDON STABILIZATION

INDICATION

- Symptomatic instability of the ECU tendon at the ulnar groove

PEARLS

- ECU subsheath repair should be considered before creating a retinacular sling.
- If the ulnar groove is shallow, a retinacular sling is usually required.

TECHNICAL POINTS

- Make the skin incision directly over the sixth extensor tendon compartment.
- Incise the retinaculum along the volar edge of the sixth compartment.
- Reflect the retinaculum radially and inspect the ECU subsheath.
- Open the subsheath, retract the tendon, and inspect the groove.
- Débride the groove if necessary and assess the height of its rims.

- Repair the subsheath if its integrity is substantial, and repair the retinaculum.
- If the subsheath is inadequate, raise a radially based strip of the central third of the retinaculum.
- Pass the strip over the ECU tendon and suture it to the proximal third of the retinaculum to create an obliquely oriented sling for the ECU.

PITFALLS

- Avoid injury to the dorsal sensory branch of the ulnar nerve.
- Remove osteophytes and roughness that may cause tendinitis.
- Do not make the sling so tight that it will restrict tendon glide.

POSTOPERATIVE CARE

- Immobilize in a long-arm splint or cast in the position of greatest tendon stability for 4 weeks.

RETURN TO ACTIVITIES

- Full activity is not allowed for 3 to 4 months.

(Fig. 15-36). The retinaculum's central third is raised using two parallel incisions extending from its divided ulnar edge to the septum between the fourth and fifth compartments. The flap is passed under the ECU and then back over the tendon. The flap is sutured to the more proximal portion of the retinaculum rather than itself. This creates a loose sling rather than a noose. The remainder of the retinaculum is repaired anatomically. This technique is easier and requires less exposure than that described by Spinner and Kaplan, but it places the superficial surface of the retinaculum against the tendon. The patient is immobilized for 3 weeks in a short-arm cast, followed by a wrist splint for 2 weeks. After this time, activities are resumed as tolerated.

Outcome

A few case reports and two larger series have reported good results for pain relief with both conservative and surgical treatment for stenosing tenosynovitis.[42,67,87,125] These authors reported no ECU instability by palpation or from passive or active wrist and forearm motion. Surgical failures were often attributed to incorrect diagnosis, with DRUJ arthritis being the most common. ECU tendon stabilization has been successful with good relief of pain and few recurrent subluxations.[25,45,154,173]

ANNOTATED REFERENCES

3. Adams BD, Berger RA: An anatomic reconstruction of the distal radioulnar ligaments for posttraumatic distal radioulnar joint instability. J Hand Surg [Am] 2002;27:243-251.

A technique for anatomic reconstruction of the distal radioulnar ligaments using a palmaris longus graft is described. The procedure is effective for the unstable DRUJ when its articular surfaces are intact and the ulnocarpal ligaments are functional. It can be used in combination with a distal radius corrective osteotomy.

8. af Ekenstam F, Hagert CG: Anatomical studies on the geometry and stability of the distal radioulnar joint. Scand J Plast Reconstr Surg 1985;19:17-25.

A concise and clear anatomic presentation of DRUJ anatomy shows the important interaction between the articular geometry and ligaments in producing joint stability at the extremes of motion.

14. Bednar MS, Arnoczky SP, et al. The microvasculature of the triangular fibrocartilage complex: its clinical significance. J Hand Surg [Am] 1991;16:1101-1105.

Using specialized histological techniques, only the peripheral 10% to 40% of the TFCC was shown to be penetrated by vessels; the center and radial portion of the disk are avascular. This finding shows the poor healing potential of tears in these regions of the disk.

20. Bowers WH: Distal radioulnar joint arthroplasty: The hemiresection-interposition technique. J Hand Surg [Am] 1985;10:169-178.

This classic article describes partial removal of the ulnar head for arthrosis of the DRUJ that preserves some attachments of the TFCC, thus improving stability of the distal ulna and ulnocarpal joint. Results are less predictable in rheumatoid arthritis and if DRUJ instability is present.

23. Breen TF, Jupiter JB: Extensor carpi ulnaris and flexor carpi ulnaris tenodesis of the unstable distal ulna. J Hand Surg [Am] 1989;14:612-617.

A tenodesis procedure for stabilizing the resected distal ulna using a distally based slip of FCU and a proximally based slip of ECU is described. It may be used as a primary procedure or for a failed Darrach procedure due to radioulnar impingement.

31. Chun S, Palmer AK: The ulnar impaction syndrome: Follow-up of ulnar shortening osteotomy. J Hand Surg [Am] 1993;18:46-53.

   The results of ulnar-shortening osteotomy for the treatment of ulnar impaction syndrome using a dynamic compression plate were retrospectively reviewed. Long-term follow-up showed good results with reliable healing and good pain relief.

33. Constantine KJ, Tomaino MM, et al: Comparison of ulnar shortening osteotomy and the wafer resection procedure as treatment for ulnar impaction syndrome. J Hand Surg [Am] 2000;25:55-60.

   The wafer procedure and ulnar-shortening osteotomy were compared in a clinical series for the treatment of ulnar impaction syndrome. The wafer procedure produced equivalent results but without the potential for nonunion or hardware removal.

36. Cooney WP, Linscheid RL, et al: Triangular fibrocartilage tears. J Hand Surg [Am] 1994;19:143-154.

   Using a dorsal approach, open repair of radial and ulnar peripheral tears of the TFCC produced generally good results in patients without DRUJ instability. Ulnar recession improved surgical exposure and corrected ulnar variance.

47. Feldon P, Terrono AL, et al: Wafer distal ulna resection for triangular fibrocartilage tears and/or ulna impaction syndrome. J Hand Surg [Am] 1992;17:731-737.

   Feldon describes partial resection (distal 2 to 4 mm) of the ulnar dome (wafer resection) for symptomatic tears of the triangular fibrocartilage complex or mild ulna impaction syndrome. The triangular fibrocartilage is débrided, repaired, or partially excised, but the ulnar styloid and attached ligaments attached are preserved. The procedure is contraindicated in the presence of DRUJ instability or arthrosis, carpal instability, or substantial positive ulnar variance.

68. Hartz CR, Beckenbaugh RD: Long-term results of resection of the distal ulna for post-traumatic conditions. J Trauma 1979;19:219-226.

   Complete resection of the ulnar head in a large number of patients to treat pain or increase motion were reviewed. Neither pseudoarticulation nor regrowth of the distal ulna was clinically symptomatic. Primary gains were pain relief, increased supination, and increased strength.

71. Hermansdorfer JD, Kleinman WB: Management of chronic peripheral tears of the triangular fibrocartilage complex. J Hand Surg [Am] 1991;16:340-346.

   Open repair of traumatic ulnar-peripheral tears of the TFCC to the fovea of the ulnar head is described. Results were good if no other pathologic conditions coexisted.

73. Hui FC, Linscheid RL: Ulnotriquetral augmentation tenodesis: A reconstructive procedure for dorsal subluxation of the distal radioulnar joint. J Hand Surg [Am] 1982;7:230-236.

   A tenodesing procedure using a slip of flexor carpi ulnaris is described to treat post-traumatic dorsal DRUJ instability. Since its conception the procedure has become recognized as much or more for the treatment of ulnocarpal instability because it augments the palmar ulnocarpal capsule.

89. Kleinman WB, Graham TJ: The distal radioulnar joint capsule: Clinical anatomy and role in post-traumatic limitation of forearm rotation. J Hand Surg 1998;23:588-599.

   Detailed anatomy of the DRUJ capsule and its unique components that contribute to joint stability and those commonly affected by fibrosis causing contracture is presented.

A clinical series showed good improvement in forearm motion when a proper capsulectomy was performed.

102. Lo IK, MacDermid JC, et al: The radioulnar ratio: A new method of quantifying distal radioulnar joint subluxation. J Hand Surg [Am] 2001;26:236-243.

   Four measurement schemes that are used to interpret CT scans for DRUJ instability were compared: Mino, epicenter, congruency, and radioulnar ratio (RUR). RUR was accurate and consistent, whereas the other methods had poor correlations in diagnosing DRUJ subluxation.

106. Melone CP Jr, Nathan R: Traumatic disruption of the triangular fibrocartilage complex: Pathoanatomy. Clin Orthop 1992;(275):65-73.

   In a series of destabilizing traumatic TFCC tears, there was a spectrum of associated injuries involving the extensor carpi ulnaris sheath, ulnocarpal ligaments, and the peritriquetral ligaments. Some of these injuries are amenable to repair when surgery is undertaken for the TFCC.

120. Mino DE, Palmer AK, et al: Radiography and computerized tomography in the diagnosis of incongruity of the distal radio-ulnar joint: A prospective study. J Bone Joint Surg Am 1985;67:247-252.

   Diagnosis of DRUJ subluxation or dislocation using routine radiographs was shown to require a true lateral view, which was often compromised in the clinical setting. CT gave a more accurate determination of joint congruency.

137. Palmer AK, Werner FW: The triangular fibrocartilage complex of the wrist—anatomy and function. J Hand Surg [Am] 1981;6:153-162.

   This now classic work describes the anatomy and function of the TFCC through anatomic dissections and biomechanical testing of cadavers. The TFCC is a confluence of several structures including the articular disc, dorsal and volar radioulnar ligaments, meniscus homologue, and extensor carpi ulnaris sheath. Signs of ulnocarpal impaction syndrome are described. Biomechanical studies demonstrated its role in ulnocarpal joint load transmission and DRUJ stability. The findings argue against complete TFCC excision.

142. Petersen MS, Adams BD: Biomechanical evaluation of distal radioulnar reconstructions. J Hand Surg [Am] 1993;18:328-334.

   A biomechanical study compared three basic design types of nonanatomic reconstructive procedures for DRUJ instability. None restored natural joint stability. Of these extra-articular reconstructions, a radioulnar sling was the most effective.

143. Peterson CA 2nd, Maki S, et al: Clinical results of the one-bone forearm. J Hand Surg [Am] 1995;20:609-618.

   Creation of a one-bone forearm for radioulnar instability secondary to trauma, tumor resection, or congenital deformity was reviewed ("type 2" patients). Results were variable with poor results associated with previous trauma, infection, severe nerve injury, and multiple previous surgical procedures. Significant complications were noted in half.

155. Rozental TD, Bozentka DJ, et al: Evaluation of the sigmoid notch with computed tomography following intra-articular distal radius fracture. J Hand Surg [Am] 2001;26:244-251.

   Patterns of the sigmoid notch fracture associated with distal radius fractures were compared using CT scans and plain radiographs. Plain radiography failed to detect the presence of a fracture in one third and routinely underestimated severity of step-off and articular gapping.

174. Steyers CM, Blair WF: Measuring ulnar variance: A comparison of techniques. J Hand Surg [Am] 1989;14:607-612.

Three commonly used methods for measuring ulnar variance were compared: project-a-line, concentric circles, and perpendicular lines. All methods were highly reliable and thus clinically appropriate.

175. Stuart PR, Berger RA, et al: The dorsopalmar stability of the distal radioulnar joint. J Hand Surg [Am] 2000;25:689-699.

A specialized testing machine analyzed the stabilizing structures of the DRUJ in a cadaveric study. The major constraint to dorsal translation of the ulna was the palmar radioulnar ligament, whereas palmar translation was constrained primarily by the dorsal radioulnar ligament, with secondary constraint provided by the palmar radioulnar ligament and interosseous membrane. The ulnocarpal ligaments and extensor carpi ulnaris subsheath did not contribute significantly. Twenty percent of DRUJ constraint is provided by the articular contact of DRUJ.

184. Tolat AR, Stanley JK, Trail IA: A cadaveric study of the anatomy and stability of the distal radioulnar joint in the coronal and transverse planes. J Hand Surg [Br] 1996; 21:587-594.

The anatomic configuration of the DRUJ was shown to vary in the transverse and midcoronal planes. Disparate radii of curvatures of the sigmoid notch and ulnar head in the transverse plane were confirmed. The palmar rim of the sigmoid notch is augmented by a osteocartilaginous lip. A flat-faced sigmoid notch is considered more prone to instability.

197. van Schoonhoven J, Fernandez DL, et al: Salvage of failed resection arthroplasties of the distal radioulnar joint using a new ulnar head prosthesis. J Hand Surg [Am] 2000;25:438-446.

An ulnar head prosthesis was used to treat painful instability after failed total or partial resection of the ulnar head due to radioulnar impingement. Stability and marked symptomatic improvement were routinely achieved.

200. Wallwork NA, Bain GI: Sigmoid notch osteoplasty for chronic volar instability of the distal radioulnar joint: a case report. J Hand Surg [Am] 2001;26:454-459.

A method is described to augment the palmar rim of the sigmoid notch by creating an osteocartilaginous flap supported by an underlying bone graft. The technique is considered for DRUJ instability when the sigmoid notch is developmentally flat or deficient from trauma.

214. Wolfe SW, Mih AD, et al: Wide excision of the distal ulna: a multicenter case study. J Hand Surg [Am] 1998;23:222-228.

Wide excision of the distal ulna (25% to 50% of its length) used for a variety of diagnoses in 12 patients was reviewed. The authors concluded it is a satisfactory alternative for neoplasms of the distal ulna or salvage of a failed DRUJ reconstruction but not if there is incompetency of the interosseous membrane.

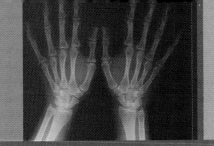

CHAPTER 16

Distal Radius Fractures

Diego L. Fernandez and Scott W. Wolfe

Beginning with Pouteau (1783), Colles (1814), and Dupuytren (1847), the early reports of fractures of the distal radius considered these a group of injuries with a relatively good prognosis irrespective of the treatment given.[46,47,75,115, 208-211] Since then, many have recognized more complexity of the injury and variable outcome.*

As specialization has evolved, orthopedic and hand surgeons have identified and reported more subtle, late problems that limit function and cause pain. These problems include midcarpal instability, incongruity or instability of the distal radioulnar joint (DRUJ), the ulnar impaction syndrome, and pain secondary to small degrees of radial malalignment or intracarpal ligament disruption. The associated complications such as complex regional pain and nerve and tendon injury are covered more completely in other chapters.

We review the several classifications and treatments, as well as our preferred method for treating these fractures and their associated complications, both acute and late, in the adult and pediatric population. Because our goal in treating patients with distal radial fractures is anatomic reduction and optimal restoration of wrist function, a thorough understanding of normal wrist anatomy is an appropriate place to begin.

 Anatomy

The distal radius functions as an articular plateau on which the carpus rests (Figs. 16-1 and 16-2) and from which the radially based supporting ligaments of the wrist arise (Fig. 16-3).[23,29,67,134,166,205,206] The hand and radius, as a unit, articulate with and rotate about the ulnar head via the sigmoid notch of the radius (Fig. 16-4).[1,23] This latter relationship is maintained primarily by the ulnar-based sup-

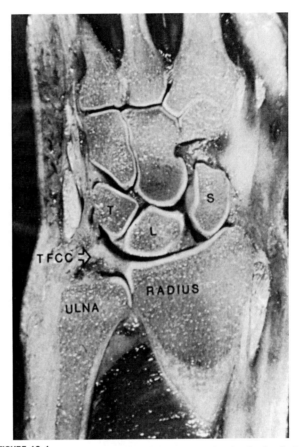

FIGURE 16-1. The scaphoid and lunate articulate with the distal articular surface of the radius and the ulnar head articulates with the sigmoid notch. The triangular fibrocartilage complex (TFCC) is interposed between the ulnar carpus and the ulnar head. S, scaphoid; L, lunate; T, triquetrum.

porting ligaments of the wrist: the triangular fibrocartilage complex (TFCC).[23,205,206,264]

The distal radius has three concave articular surfaces—the scaphoid fossa, the lunate fossa, and the sigmoid notch—for articulation with the scaphoid, lunate, and ulnar head, respectively (Figs. 16-5 and 16-6).[67,166] The sigmoid notch is concave, with a poorly defined proximal margin and well-defined dorsal, palmar, and distal margins (see Fig. 16-6).[1,67]

---

*See references 6, 9-14, 17-20, 22, 25, 26, 31-34, 37, 39-42, 45, 48-51, 53-56, 66, 70, 71, 73, 74, 91, 99, 101, 103, 105, 109-113, 126, 146, 147, 154, 155, 159, 163, 164, 168, 180-182, 188, 200, 201, 203, 217, 219, 220, 231, 234, 236, 238, 240, 244, 253, 254, 258, 265, 266, 268, and 275.

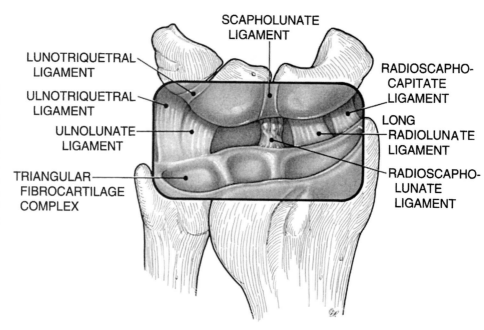

FIGURE 16-2. Arthroscopic anatomy of the radiocarpal joint. Pictured are the articular surfaces of the scaphoid, lunate, triquetrum radius, and triangular fibrocartilage complex. The major extrinsic—radioscaphocapitate, long radiolunate ligament, radioscapholunate, ulnolunate, and lunotriquetral—ligaments of the wrist are shown. The very important intrinsic ligaments of the wrist—the scapholunate ligament and lunotriquetral ligaments—are also shown.

The distal articular surface of the radius has a radial inclination or slope averaging 22 degrees and tilts palmarly an average of 11 degrees (Fig. 16-7).[67,71,186,187,194,245,247,269,272] Radial inclination is measured by the angle formed by a line drawn tangential to the distal radial articular surface on a posteroanterior radiograph and one perpendicular to the shaft of the radius. Palmar tilt is measured by the angle between the plane of the distal articular surface as seen on the lateral radiograph and the plane perpendicular to the longitudinal axis of the radius. The sigmoid notch angles distally and medially an average of 22 degrees to form the "seat" for the ulnar head (see Fig. 16-4).[1,23,203]

The dorsal aspect of the distal radius is somewhat convex and acts as a fulcrum for extensor tendon function (see Fig. 16-5). The radial styloid area may have a groove for the tendon of the first dorsal compartment, and ulnar to this is a dorsal longitudinal prominence, Lister's tubercle, which acts as a fulcrum for the extensor pollicis longus tendon.

CLASSIFICATIONS AND NOMENCLATURE

The nature of many of the classifications mentioned below have been analyzed, examining both the interobserver and intraobserver reliability and reproducibility.[8] We believe that the ideal fracture classification should provide reproducible diagnoses and prognostic considerations, assess the associated soft tissue lesions, and suggest treatment recommendations. Physicians dealing with distal radius fractures should adopt an appropriate classification that fulfills their own needs for clinical and scientific purposes. However, difficulties arise when multicenter studies are undertaken. In these situations a higher degree of reproducibility becomes increasingly necessary.

Beginning with the classic clinical description by Abraham Colles in 1814, numerous authors have attempted to classify these injuries.[17,46,47,57,58,64,65,208-211] There are few areas of skeletal trauma in which eponymic descriptions are so commonly used; however, contemporary authors have purposely avoided assigning their name to one particular configuration and instead have preferred to classify fractures based on a variety of measurements, observations, and characteristics of the injury. Instead of a single position or fracture carrying the name of the author, the classification scheme often bears the author's name or institution.*

Commonly Used Eponyms

Colles' Fracture[46,47]
Figure 16-8 illustrates the typical features of a Colles' fracture, that is, a distal radius fracture with dorsal comminution, dorsal angulation, dorsal displacement, and radial shortening.

Barton's Fracture[17]
Barton's fracture is a displaced, unstable articular fracture-subluxation of the distal radius with displacement of the carpus along with the articular fracture fragment. Barton's fracture may be either dorsal or volar, as shown in Figure 16-9.

Smith's Fracture[210]
Figure 16-9 illustrates three types of fractures of the distal radius with volar displacement, classified as Smith's types I, II, and III by Thomas in 1957.[267]

Chauffeur's or Backfire Fracture[78-80,169]
Figure 16-10 illustrates a chauffeur's fracture with displacement of the carpus and attached radial styloid avulsion.

Lunate Load, Die-Punch, or Medial Cuneiform Fracture
Figure 16-11 illustrates this fracture, which usually represents a depression of the dorsal aspect of the lunate fossa.

_____
*See references 9, 28, 38, 39, 51, 78, 80, 81, 97, 100, 115, 181-183, 185, 213, 214, 219, 220, 252, and 283.

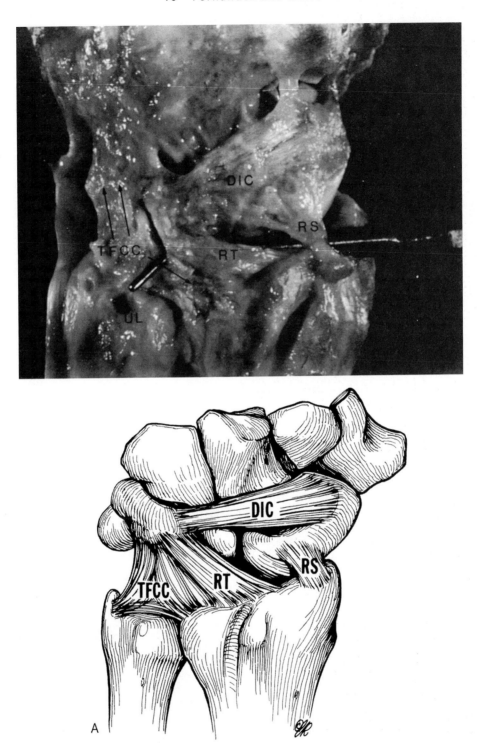

FIGURE 16-3. Dissection and illustration composite showing the dorsal ligaments of the wrist. DIC, dorsal intercarpal ligaments; RS, radioscaphoid; RT, radiotriquetral; TFCC, triangular fibrocartilage complex.

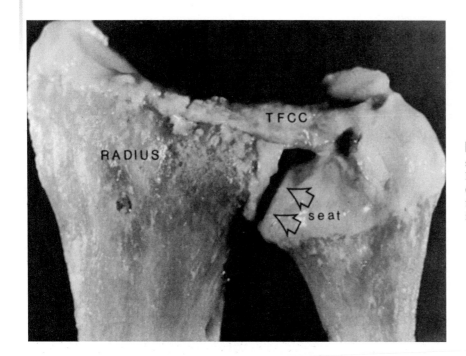

FIGURE 16-4. The ulnar head articulates with the sigmoid notch of the radius at the "seat" of the DRUJ. The triangular fibrocartilage complex (TFCC), the distal restraint of the DRUJ, arises from the most ulnar border of the radius and inserts into the base of the ulnar styloid process.

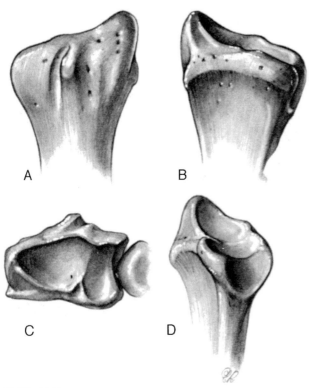

FIGURE 16-5. Artist's drawing of the distal radius. **A,** Dorsal view illustrating Lister's tubercle. **B,** Palmar view showing the scaphoid and lunate fossae distally, as well as the sigmoid notch ulnarly. Vascular foramina can be noted on the palmar and dorsal aspects of the distal radius. **C,** An end-on view of the distal radius and radioulnar joint showing the scaphoid fossa, lunate fossa, and ulnar head resting in the sigmoid notch. **D,** A view of the sigmoid notch from the ulnar aspect.

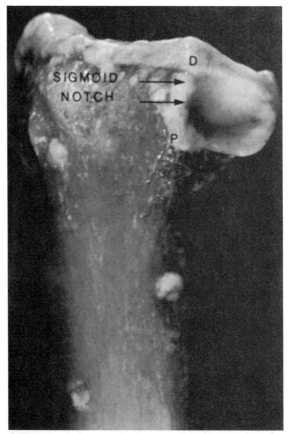

FIGURE 16-6. The sigmoid notch showing distinct dorsal, palmar, and distal borders and an indistinct proximal border. D, distal; P, proximal.

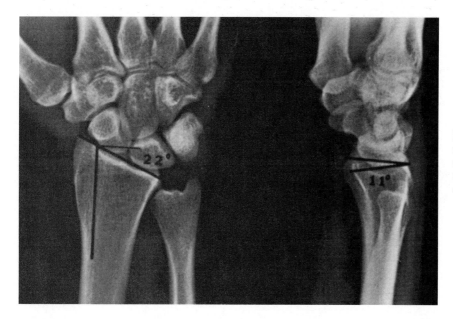

FIGURE 16-7. The anteroposterior radiograph on the left illustrates normal radial inclination of approximately 22 degrees. The lateral radiograph on the right illustrates normal volar tilt of the distal articular surface of approximately 11 degrees.

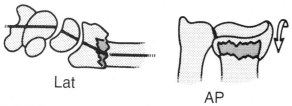

FIGURE 16-8. Diagrammatic representation of the typical deformity seen in a Colles fracture. Dorsal comminution and displacement with shortening of the radius relative to the ulna are present. AP, anteroposterior; Lat, lateral.

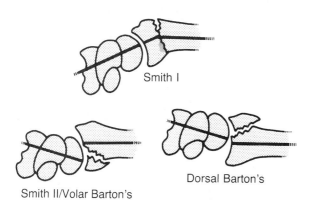

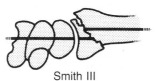

FIGURE 16-9. Thomas' classification of Smith's fractures. Type I Smith fracture: extra-articular fracture with palmar angulation and displacement of the distal fragment. Type II Smith fracture: intra-articular fracture with volar and proximal displacement of the distal fragment along with the carpus. Type III Smith fracture: extra-articular fracture with volar displacement of the distal fragment and carpus. (In type III the fracture line is more oblique than in a type I fracture.) A Smith type II fracture is essentially a volar Barton fracture. A dorsal Barton fracture, illustrated for comparison, shows the dorsal and proximal displacement of the carpus and distal fragment on the radial shaft.

Classifications

Frykman's Classification
In 1967, Frykman prepared a classification that distinguished between extra-articular and intra-articular fractures of the distal radius and the presence or absence of an associated distal ulnar fracture.[100]

Melone's Classification
In 1984, Charles P. Melone, Jr., introduced a classification of distal radial fractures in which he identified four major components of the distal radius: (1) the shaft, (2) the radial styloid area, (3) the dorsal medial facet, and (4) the volar medial facet (Fig. 16-12).[181,182] This classification has drawn very much needed attention to the importance of the medial (lunate) facet of the distal radius (i.e., the "medial complex").

The AO Classification
In 1986 the Swiss Association for the Study of Internal Fixation (ASIF/AO)* accepted a new classification of fractures that was further revised in 1990.[197] In this classification

---

*ASIF (Association for the Study of Internal Fixation) is the English translation of AO (Arbeitsgemeinschaft für Osteosynthesefragen).

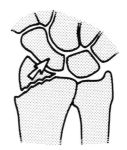
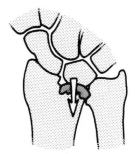

FIGURE 16-10. A chauffeur's fracture is illustrated with the carpus displaced ulnarly by the radial styloid fracture. A lunate load (die-punch) fracture is shown with a depression of the lunate fossa of the radius that allows proximal migration of the lunate and/or proximal carpal row.

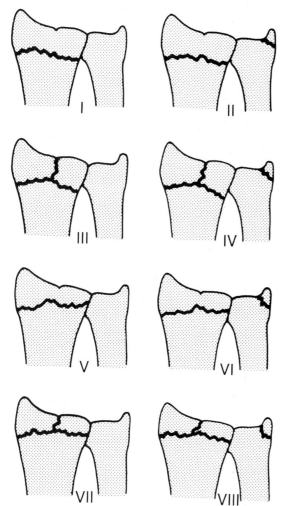

FIGURE 16-11. Frykman's classification of distal radius fractures. Types I, III, V, and VII do not have an associated fracture of the distal ulna. Fractures III through VIII are intra-articular fractures. Higher classification fractures have worse prognoses.

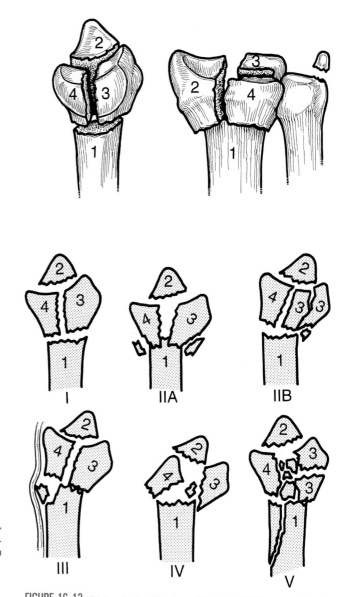

FIGURE 16-12. Melone's classification of distal radial fractures. The four major fragments are (1) the radial shaft, (2) the radial styloid region, (3) the dorsal medial facet, and (4) the volar medial facet. The major fragment of this four-part fracture is the medial facet (i.e., fragments 3 and 4). Types 1 to 4 represent increasingly comminuted fractures, with type 5 being an extremely comminuted, unstable fracture without large identifiable facet fragments.

system, applicable to all long bones, different fractures are broken down into three major types: type A (extra-articular), type B (partial articular), and type C (complete articular) (Fig. 16-13).[122,196,217] The three basic types are further subdivided into groups and subgroups to ultimately produce 27 different fracture patterns at the distal end of the forearm. There is less interobserver agreement when the subdivisions are made. This classification considers the severity of the fracture according to the extent of intra-articular involvement and metaphyseal comminution.

Rayhack's Classification

In 1990 John Rayhack introduced a simple, yet very inclusive classification system of distal radial fractures that categorizes fractures as extra-articular or intra-articular and as stable or unstable (Fig. 16-14).[219,220]

Mayo Clinic Classification

The classification system advocated by and presently used by the Mayo Clinic group is similar to the Rayhack classification (Fig. 16-15).[25,51] Both the Rayhack and the Mayo classification systems allow for subclassification within

types 1 to 4 based on whether the fracture is reducible or nonreducible with ligamentotaxis (external fixation).

"Fragment-Specific" Classification[286-288]

Robert Medoff divides intra-articular fractures of the radius into five major fragments, including the radial styloid, ulnar corner, dorsal wall, articular surface, and volar lip fragments (Fig. 16-16). This classification is treatment oriented, because specific fixation with modular implants for each fracture component are recommended.

Limitations of Classifications

Despite the possibilities offered by the aforementioned classifications, one of the authors (DLF) became increasingly interested in basing classification of distal radius frac-

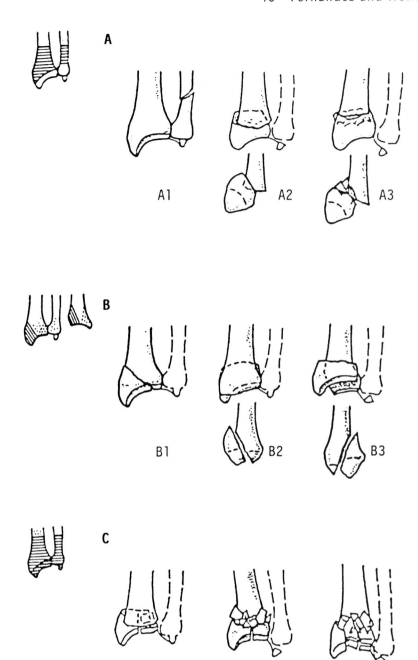

FIGURE 16-13. The comprehensive classification of fractures (AO). **A,** Extra-articular: fractures affect neither the articular surface of the radiocarpal nor the radioulnar joints. A1, extra-articular fracture of the ulna with the radius intact; A2, extra-articular fracture of the radius, simple and impacted; A3, extra-articular fracture of the radius, multifragmentary. **B,** Partial articular: fracture affects a portion of the articular surface, but the continuity of the metaphysis and epiphysis is intact. B1, partial articular fracture of the radius, sagittal; B2, partial articular fracture of the radius, dorsal rim (Barton); B3, partial articular fracture of the radius, volar rim (reverse Barton, Goyrand-Smith II). **C,** Complete articular: fracture affects the joint surfaces (radioulnar and/or radiocarpal) and the metaphyseal area. C1, complete articular fracture of the radius, articular simple and metaphyseal simple; C2, complete articular fracture of the radius, articular simple and metaphyseal multifragmentary; C3, complete articular fracture of the radius, multifragmentary.

tures on the mechanism of injury. As hand surgeons we are confronted not only with management of acute fractures but even more with the associated soft tissue lesions (ligaments, tendons, nerves, and open wounds), as well as the late complications after distal radius fractures, especially those affecting the radiocarpal joint and, perhaps more importantly, the DRUJ. For this reason an effort to include the possible incidence of associated lesions in order of severity was undertaken and published in 1993.[88] Furthermore, the associated DRUJ lesions proposed by one of us (DLF) for the AO classification in 1986 was subsequently simplified in 1992 and revised in 1995.[90]

As noted earlier, studies have analyzed the consistency of the AO classification of distal radius fractures[158] as well as the interobserver and intraobserver reliability and repro-

ducibility of the Frykman, Melone, Mayo, and AO classifications.[8] Observer agreement was considered adequate for the main types of the AO classification in both studies but became more difficult when analyzing the groups and subgroups. Interobserver agreement was rated moderate for the Mayo and fair for the Frykman, Melone, and AO classifications. Both studies concluded that in their present form, these classifications lack the capacity of outcome prediction or comparison of results among different studies.

Fernandez' Classification (Fig. 16-17)

A classification based on the *mechanism of injury* is preferred because the associated ligamentous lesions, subluxations, and fractures of the neighboring carpal bones, as well as concomitant soft tissue damage, are directly related to the

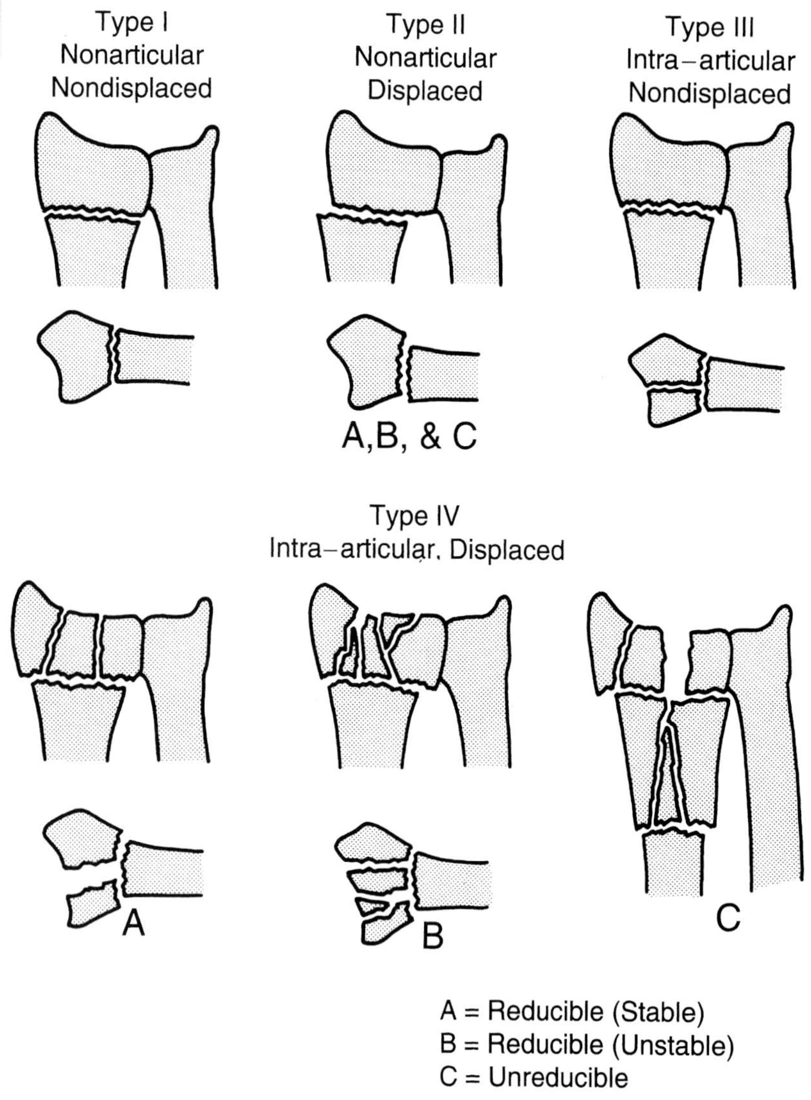

Type I
Nonarticular
Nondisplaced

Type II
Nonarticular
Displaced

Type III
Intra–articular
Nondisplaced

A,B, & C

Type IV
Intra–articular, Displaced

A

B

C

A = Reducible (Stable)
B = Reducible (Unstable)
C = Unreducible

FIGURE 16-14. Rayhack's classification of distal radial fractures. Types 1 to 3 represent noncomminuted fractures, whereas type 4 represents three different classes of comminuted intra-articular displaced fractures.

quality and degree of violence sustained. In addition, knowledge of the mechanism of injury facilitates manual reduction through the application of a force opposite to the one that produced the injury. The biomechanical characteristics of each fracture depend strictly on the mechanism of injury, and, for this reason, fractures of the distal radius may be divided into the following five types:

Type I fractures are *bending fractures of the metaphysis* in which one cortex fails to tensile stresses and the opposite one undergoes a certain degree of comminution (extra-articular Colles' or Smith's fractures).

Type II fractures are *shearing fractures of the joint surface* (Barton's, reversed Barton's, and radial styloid fractures).

Type III fractures are *compression fractures of the joint surface* with impaction of the subchondral and metaphyseal cancellous bone. Current terms used for this type are intra-articular comminuted fractures, complex articular fractures, and pilon radial fractures.

Type IV, avulsion fractures of ligament attachments, includes ulnar and radial styloid fractures associated with radiocarpal fracture-dislocations.

Type V fractures are *high-velocity injuries* that involve combinations of bending, compression, shearing, and avulsion mechanisms or bone loss.

These five basic groups can easily be recognized with standard anteroposterior and lateral radiographs of the wrist. However, special imaging techniques, such as traction views after reduction, tomograms, or a computed tomographic (CT) scan provide a more accurate diagnosis of the displacement pattern, number of fragments, and degree of joint involvement at both the radiocarpal and radioulnar levels (see Fig. 16-17A).

This classification further provides the pediatric fracture equivalent, the probable incidence of associated soft tissue lesions and carpal disruption, and the recommended treatment for each type. From a biomechanical standpoint, this classification scheme points out the ideal method of fixation for each basic type. Type I bending fractures are best treated by a counterforce that will exert tension on the concave side of the angulation. In cases with adequate bone quality and absence of metaphyseal comminution, this force can be applied with a well-molded, three-point contact cast.

Mayo Classification

Extra–articular
- Nondisplaced
- Displaced
  - Stable
  - Unstable

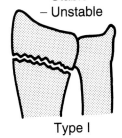

Type I

FIGURE 16-15. Mayo Clinic classification of distal radial fractures. Type 1 is an extra-articular fracture, and types 2 to 4 are intra-articular fractures. Emphasis is given to whether the fracture is displaced or nondisplaced and reducible or irreducible.

Intra–articular
- Nondisplaced
- Displaced (Reducible)
- Displaced (Unreducible)
- Complex

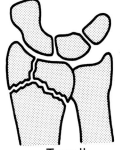

Type II
Radioscaphoid Joint

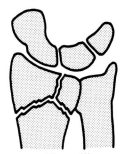

Type III
Radiolunate Joint

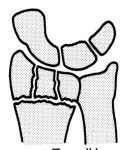

Type IV
Radioscapholunate

Type II shearing fractures usually occur in dense cancellous bone. They are extremely unstable because of the obliquity of the fracture line and are therefore suitable for internal fixation with buttress plates. Restoration of the joint surface in type III compression fractures can be achieved in most cases by applying tension to the joint capsule with fingertraps, external fixators, or pins and plaster techniques. In a number of cases, however, disimpaction of cartilage-

bearing fragments may require limited or extensile open reduction and filling of the cancellous defect with a bone graft. Type IV avulsion fractures are a constant component of radiocarpal dislocations caused by a serious wrist sprain in which rotational forces were part of the mechanism of injury. If such fractures remain displaced, tension wiring or screw fixation is the method of choice. Finally, in the type V combined fracture or high-velocity injury, the fracture may be characterized by one or more of the aforementioned features and a combined method of fixation should be selected for treatment. This classification also may provide prognostic information because the complexity of the bony lesions and the probability of associated soft tissue disruption increase consistently from type I through type V fracture.

Classification of Associated DRUJ Injuries

Figure 16-17B provides a prognostic and treatment-oriented classification of associated DRUJ lesions. Because the final outcome once the fracture has healed depends primarily on *residual joint stability* and/or *post-traumatic arthritic changes*, the classification parameters used are the presence or absence of (1) DRUJ subluxation or dislocation of the ulnar head as a result of a severe concomitant rupture of the

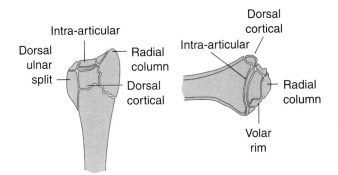

FIGURE 16-16. Fragment-Specific classification (see text).

FRACTURE TYPES (ADULTS) BASED ON THE MECHANISM OF INJURY	CHILDREN FRACTURE EQUIVALENT	STABILITY/ INSTABILITY: high risk of secondary displacement after initial adequate reduction	DISPLACEMENT PATTERN	NUMBER OF FRAGMENTS	ASSOCIATED LESIONS carpal ligament, fractures, median, ulnar nerve, tendons, ipsilat. fx upper extremity, compartment syndrome	RECOMMENDED TREATMENT
TYPE I BENDING FRACTURE OF THE METAPHYSIS 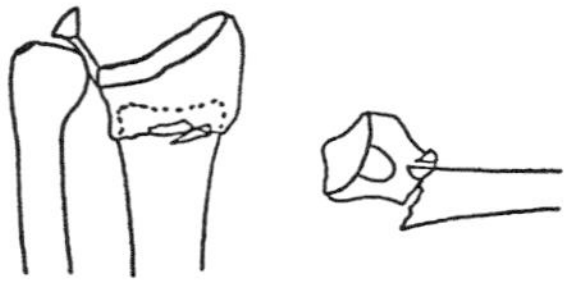	DISTAL FOREARM FRACTURE SALTER II	STABLE UNSTABLE	NON-DISPLACED DORSALLY Colles VOLARLY Smith PROXIMAL COMBINED	ALWAYS 2 MAIN FRAGMENTS + VARYING DEGREE OF METAPHYSEAL COMMINUTION (instability)	UNCOMMON	CONSERVATIVE (stable fxs) PERCUTANEOUS PINNING (extra- or intrafocal) EXTERNAL FIXATION (exceptionally BONE GRAFT)
TYPE II SHEARING FRACTURE OF THE JOINT SURFACE 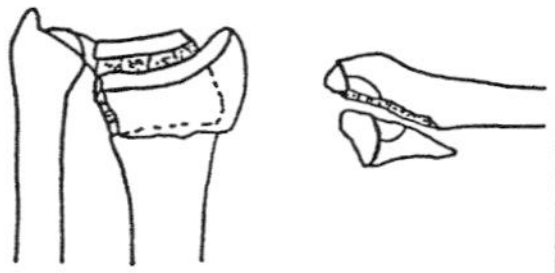	SALTER IV	UNSTABLE	DORSAL Barton RADIAL Chauffeur VOLAR rev. Barton COMBINED	TWO-PART THREE-PART COMMINUTED	LESS UNCOMMON	OPEN REDUCTION SCREW-/PLATE FIXATION
TYPE III COMPRESSION FRACTURE OF THE JOINT SURFACE 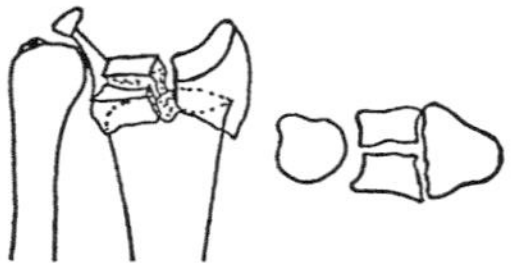	SALTER III, IV, V	STABLE UNSTABLE	NON-DISPLACED DORSAL RADIAL VOLAR PROXIMAL COMBINED	TWO-PART THREE-PART FOUR-PART COMMINUTED	COMMON	CONSERVATIVE CLOSED, LIMITED, ARTHROSCOPIC ASSISTED OR EXTENSILE OPEN REDUCTION PERCUTANEOUS PINS EXTERNAL FIXATION INTERNAL FIXATION PLATE, BONE GRAFT
TYPE IV AVULSION FRACTURES, RADIO CARPAL FRACTURE DISLOCATION 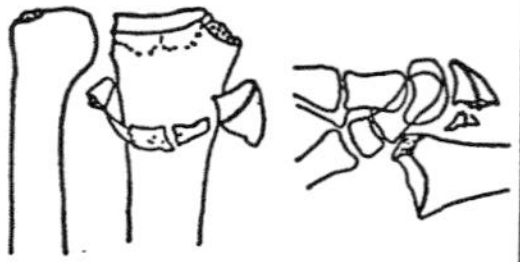	VERY RARE	UNSTABLE	DORSAL RADIAL VOLAR PROXIMAL COMBINED	TWO-PART (radial styloid ulnar styloid) THREE-PART (volar, dorsal margin) COMMINUTED	FREQUENT	CLOSED OR OPEN REDUCTION PIN OR SCREW FIXATION TENSION WIRING
TYPE V COMBINED FRACTURES (I - II - III - IV) HIGH VELOCITY INJURY 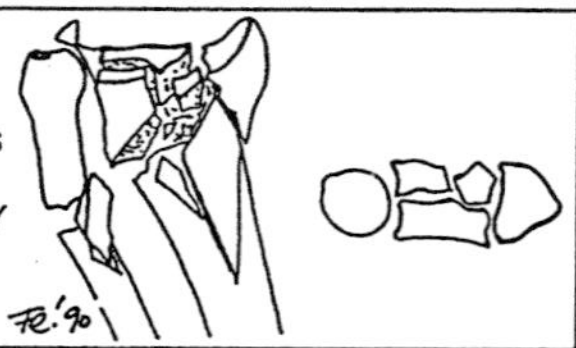	VERY RARE	UNSTABLE	DORSAL RADIAL VOLAR PROXIMAL COMBINED	COMMINUTED and/or BONE LOSS (frequently intra-articular, open, seldom extra-articular)	ALWAYS PRESENT	COMBINED METHOD

A

FIGURE 16-17. A and **B,** The Fernandez classification of distal radius fractures and associated DRUJ lesions.

	PATHOANATOMY OF THE LESION	JOINT SURFACE INVOLVEMENT	PROGNOSIS	RECOMMENDED TREATMENT
TYPE I **STABLE** (following reduction of the distal radioulnar joint is congruous and stable)	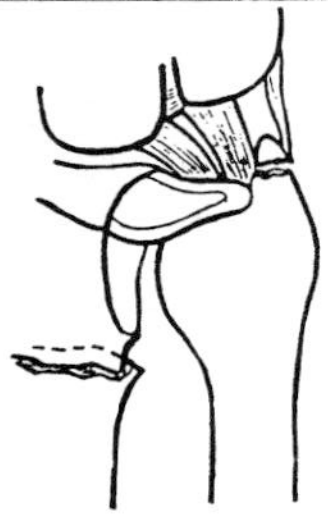 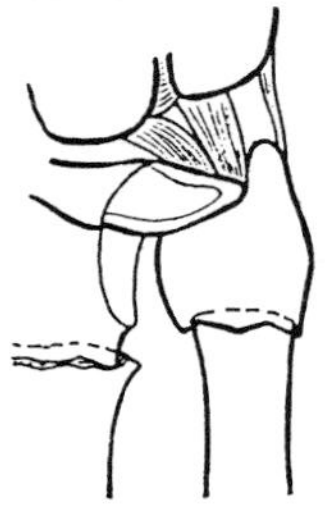 A FRACTURE TIP ULNAR STYLOID B STABLE FRACTURE ULNAR NECK	NONE	GOOD	A + B FUNCTIONAL AFTERTREATMENT ENCOURAGE EARLY PRONATION-SUPINATION EXERCISES NOTE: EXTRA-ARTICULAR UNSTABLE FRACTURES OF THE ULNA AT THE METAPHYSEAL LEVEL OR DISTAL SHAFT REQUIRE STABLE PLATE FIXATION
TYPE II **UNSTABLE** (subluxation or dislocation of the ulnar head present)	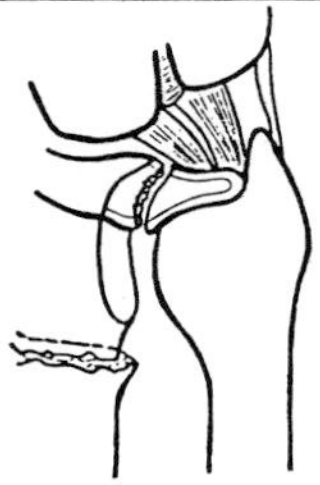 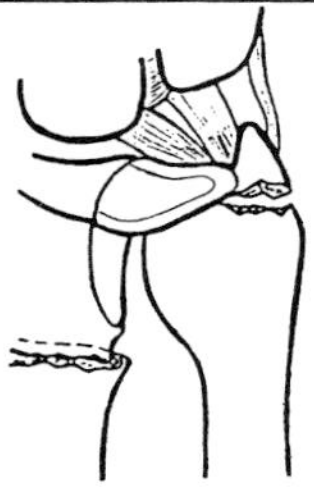 A TEAR OF TRIANGULAR FIBROCARTILAGE COMPLEX AND/OR PALMAR AND DORSAL CAPSULAR LIGAMENTS B AVULSION FRACTURE BASE OF THE ULNAR STYLOID	NONE	- CHRONIC INSTABILITY - PAINFUL LIMITATION OF SUPINATION IF LEFT UNREDUCED - POSSIBLE LATE ARTHRITIC CHANGES	A <u>CLOSED TREATMENT</u> REDUCE SUBLUXATION, SUGAR TONG SPLINT IN 45° SUPINATION 4 TO 6 WEEKS A + B <u>OPERATIVE TREATMENT</u> REPAIR TRIANGULAR FIBROCARTILAGE COMPLEX OR FIX ULNAR STYLOID WITH TENSION BAND WIRING IMMOBILIZE WRIST AND ELBOW IN SUPINATION (CAST) OR TRANSFIX ULNA/RADIUS WITH K-WIRE AND FOREARM CAST
TYPE III **POTENTIALLY UNSTABLE** (subluxation possible)	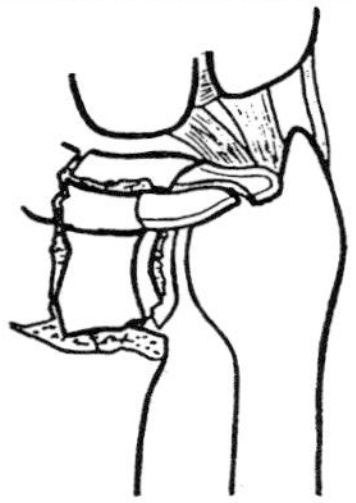 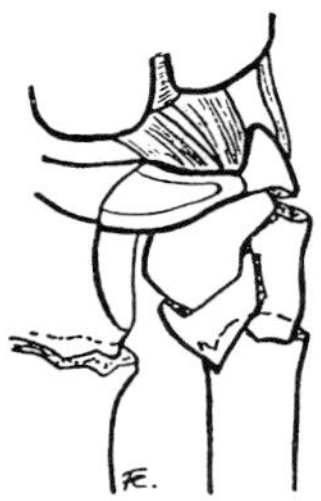 A INTRA-ARTICULAR FRACTURE OF THE SIGMOID NOTCH B INTRA-ARTICULAR FRACTURE OF THE ULNAR HEAD	PRESENT	- DORSAL SUBLUXATION POSSIBLE TOGETHER WITH DORSALLY DISPLACED DIE PUNCH OR DORSOULNAR FRAGMENT - RISK OF EARLY DEGENERATIVE CHANGES AND SEVERE LIMITATION OF FOREARM ROTATION IF LEFT UNREDUCED	A ANATOMIC REDUCTION OF PALMAR AND DORSAL SIGMOID NOTCH FRAGMENTS. IF RESIDUAL SUBLUXATION TENDENCY PRESENT IMMOBILIZE AS IN TYPE II INJURY B FUNCTIONAL AFTERTREATMENT TO ENHANCE REMODELLING OF ULNAR HEAD. IF DISTAL RADIOULNAR JOINT REMAINS PAINFUL: PARTIAL ULNAR RESECTION, DARRACH, SAUVE-KAPANDJI PROCEDURE, OR ULNAR HEAD PROSTHESIS AT A LATER DATE

FIGURE 16-17—cont'd. **B,** DRUJ injury classification.

B

TFCC and secondary stabilizers and (2) the degree of joint surface involvement (intra-articular fracture of the sigmoid notch and/or ulnar head).

The possible associated DRUJ lesions of the DRUJ are classified into *three types* depending on the *residual stability* of the DRUJ after the distal radius fracture has been adequately reduced and stabilized. This implies that the anatomic relationships of the *sigmoid notch* to the *ulnar head* have been re-established through adequate restoration of radial length and sagittal and frontal tilt of the distal fragment.

Type I are *stable DRUJ lesions,* which means that the joint is clinically stable and the radiograph shows articular congruity. These include (1) avulsion of the tip of the ulnar styloid and (2) a stable fracture of the neck of the ulna. In both, the primary stabilizers of the joint (TFCC and capsular ligament) are intact.

Type II are *unstable DRUJ lesions* with clinical and radiographic evidence of subluxation and/or dislocation of the ulnar head as a result of (1) a massive substance tear of the TFCC or (2) an avulsion fracture of the base of the ulnar styloid.

Type III are *potentially unstable lesions* caused by skeletal disruption of the joint surface at (1) the sigmoid notch (four-part distal radius fractures) or (2) the ulnar head.

The pathoanatomy of the lesions, prognosis, and recommended treatment are outlined in Figure 16-17B.

TREATMENT OF ACUTE FRACTURES IN ADULTS

For treatment purposes, we have divided fractures by (1) their radiographic appearance into nondisplaced or displaced fractures, further subdividing displaced fractures into stable and unstable fractures and (2) whether the fracture is open or closed. Furthermore, we have found it helpful for treatment purposes to divide adult patients with distal radial fractures into two groups: the physiologically young and/or active (group I) and the physiologically old and/or inactive (group II) (Fig. 16-18). The treating physician must always bear in mind that with age, bone mass is lost, especially in women.[68] The bone of the distal radius in the elderly is

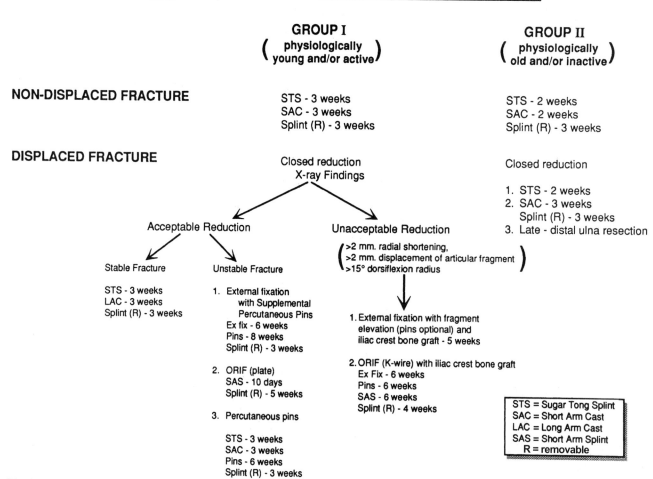

FIGURE 16-18. Our protocol for the treatment of nondisplaced and displaced distal radial fractures in the physiologically young and/or active (group I) and the physiologically old and/or inactive (group II). Nondisplaced fractures require only immobilization in both groups. Displaced fractures require reduction in both groups, but only in group I do we recommend further treatment. Based on the reduction and whether the fracture is stable or not, immobilization is recommended with or without operative treatment. Fractures in which the reduction is unacceptable require reduction of the fragments with external fixation and/or internal fixation and bone grafting.

weaker and thus not only more likely to fracture but also more likely to collapse with plaster immobilization. Yet, the operative aggressiveness with which we approach the fracture must be tempered by the patient's age, functional limits, and general medical condition.

The history and physical examination should include age, handedness, occupation, daily activity level, and general medical condition. The wrist should be inspected for wounds, tendon and nerve function, with special attention to the function of the median nerve.

Nondisplaced Distal Radius Fractures

Nondisplaced distal radius fractures should be treated with a splint or cast of the wrist, leaving the elbow, fingers, and thumb free to avoid stiffness.

Authors' Preferred Method of Treatment: Nondisplaced and Stable Fractures

Group I (Active and Physiologically Young)
We usually apply a splint ("sugar tong") to permit swelling for 3 weeks and then a short-arm cast for 3 weeks, until the fracture is healed both clinically and radiographically. A simple removable splint may be needed for comfort and support by the patient (see Fig. 16-18) for 3 additional weeks.

Group II (Low Activity and Elderly)
This group of patients is better treated with a sugar tong splint for 2 weeks, followed by a short-arm cast for 3 weeks and then a 3-week period of intermittent use of the splint.

We recommend that all patients with distal radius fractures wear a removable prefabricated splint (Fig. 16-19) after immobilization, whether they had a nondisplaced fracture requiring a minimal degree of immobilization or a markedly displaced fracture requiring open reduction. The splint is removed for bathing and range-of-motion exercises daily. Patients are asked to gradually wean themselves from the splint over a 2- to 3-week period. We have found this policy to be extremely helpful for our patients. After plaster immobilization, patients seem concerned that they will fall and refracture the wrist. By providing them with a removable splint that they can wean themselves from as they regain wrist motion and upper extremity strength, much of this anxiety is relieved and their rehabilitation process is shortened.

Minimizing Hand and Shoulder Stiffness
During the period of immobilization and weaning from the splint, all patients are instructed to keep their fingers and shoulder mobile. The "six-pack" exercises are an example of hand exercises popularized by Dobyns and are illustrated in Figure 16-20.[203] In general, motion should be encouraged at least three times a day. Some patients benefit from supervised hand therapy as well as a home program under

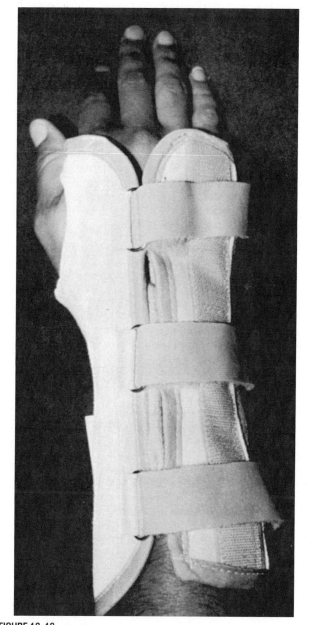

FIGURE 16-19. A prefabricated splint is recommended after discontinuation of plaster immobilization. Many types are commercially available.

the guidance of a hand therapist. Shoulder and elbow motion should also be encouraged and maintained during healing, especially in the elderly.

Displaced Distal Radius Fractures

Abraham Colles, in discussing treatment of the fracture that now bears his name, suggested that closed reduction of a distal radius fracture is usually easily accomplished but that "the distortion of the limb instantly returns on the extension being removed." This historical statement may reflect both a reluctance to treat and very few options for treatment, either open or closed, at the time.

If substantial displacement is present, defined as intra-articular displacement greater than 2 mm, metaphyseal

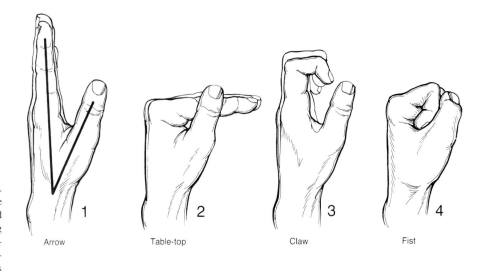

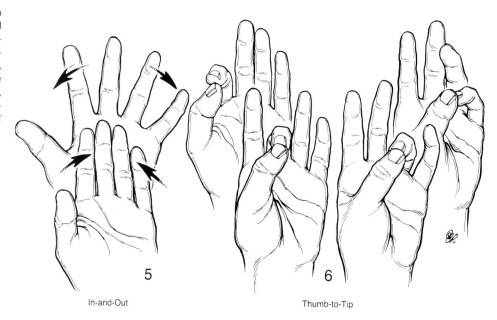

FIGURE 16-20. "Six-pack" exercises. Drawings 1 through 6 illustrate the position that the patient's hand should assume when performing these exercises. It is helpful to illustrate to the patient that full metacarpophalangeal (MP) extension makes the hand look like an arrow, full MP flexion makes the hand look like a tabletop, full MP extension combined with proximal and distal interphalangeal flexion creates a claw, complete finger flexion creates a fist, abduction and adduction of the fingers create an in-and-out motion, and, finally, to complete the exercises, the individual touches the tip of the thumb to the tip of each finger.

1 Arrow 2 Table-top 3 Claw 4 Fist 5 In-and-Out 6 Thumb-to-Tip

angulation greater than 20 degrees, or metaphyseal shortening from collapse greater than 3 mm, we believe that active and physiologically young patients (group I) will experience a suboptimal outcome and sequelae. These include decreased range of motion, wrist pain, subluxation of the DRUJ, midcarpal instability, and post-traumatic arthritis. Of the many complications associated with distal radial fractures, post-traumatic arthritis is perhaps the most serious and disabling to the patient.[54,139,215,247,248,276] Ghormley and Mroz stated, in 1932, that "any injury to the articular surface of the radius is bound to set up active traumatic arthritis in the radiocarpal joint."[109] Frykman showed this to be true not only for the radiocarpal but also for the DRUJ.[100] Knirk and Jupiter found that intra-articular distal radius fractures that healed with depression of an articular component of greater than 2 mm resulted in radiographic evidence of post-traumatic arthritis in more than 90% of the patients reviewed.[154] They did not report the patients' function or have a record of their strength or functional capacity.

Based on the large body of clinical and experimental evidence, we believe that an attempt at anatomic reduction of most distal radius fractures is warranted. Again, the patient's functional demands and general medical condition, however, must always be considered when developing a treatment program for distal radius fractures.

Closed Reduction Techniques

In the 1920s, Böhler introduced the concept of manual traction being applied to the limb and countertraction being applied to the arm.[17,30]

Principles of Closed Reduction and Maintenance of Position

The greatest challenge of closed treatment of the dorsally angulated fracture is to reduce the fracture and maintain the position without excessive flexion of the wrist joint. Even fractures with initially acceptable closed reductions may redisplace and shorten. Although *extreme* palmar flexion and ulnar deviation (the Cotton-Loder position) is mechanically effective in restoring volar tilt, this position cannot be maintained because the fully flexed wrist causes excessive and dangerous median nerve compression.

Palmar Translation in Cast

Agee[2] introduced the concept of multiplanar ligamentotaxis using external fixation, in which longitudinal traction is combined with palmar and also radioulnar translation of the hand on the forearm. Palmar translation creates a sagittal moment of force that moves the capitate, which in turn rotates the lunate palmarly. This produces a rotatory force that effectively tilts the distal radial fragment volarly. A similar observation was reported by Gupta using plaster immobilization in 1991,[114] who reported better reduction results in comminuted fractures when the wrist was immobilized in extension, a position in which the strong volar carpal ligaments (radioscaphocapitate and radiolunate) are under tension and tend to pull the distal fragment anteriorly. Agee[2] further advocated radioulnar translation to realign the distal fragments with the radial shaft in the frontal plane. This is controlled by tension on the soft tissue hinge of the first and second dorsal compartments. Adequate reduction in the frontal plane is important for restoring the anatomic relationship of the sigmoid notch and ulnar head. The application of a dorsopalmar reduction force to restore volar tilt should be utilized because the wrist joint can then be placed in neutral or slight extension in cast. The digits and resting tension of the flexor and extensor tendons are then in a more physiologic position for rehabilitation.

Authors' Preferred Method of Closed Reduction

In dealing with displaced acute fractures of the distal radius, our first step is a gentle, sterile, 5-minute surgical prep of the fracture area. The hematoma associated with the fracture is then infiltrated with 1% lidocaine without epinephrine,[33, 44] and the anesthetic is allowed to diffuse about the fracture site for approximately 5 minutes. If the fracture is seen late and there is significant soft tissue swelling, a regional nerve block (axillary) or general anesthesia is preferred. The arm is gently suspended with fingertraps attached to the thumb and index and long fingers (Fig. 16-21), with 5 to 10 lb of countertraction across the upper arm.

The patient is asked to relax. After allowing the arm to hang from the fingertraps for 5 to 10 minutes, pressure is applied by the treating physician's thumb to the distal fracture fragment in a direction that will reduce the displacement (see Fig. 16-21D). For a displaced Colles fracture, the distal fragment is manipulated with the treating physician's thumb into a minimally flexed to neutral, palmarly translocated and pronated position on the radial shaft. With the hand still suspended from the fingertraps, a radiograph is taken to evaluate the reduction obtained with or without plaster applied, depending on the momentary stability.

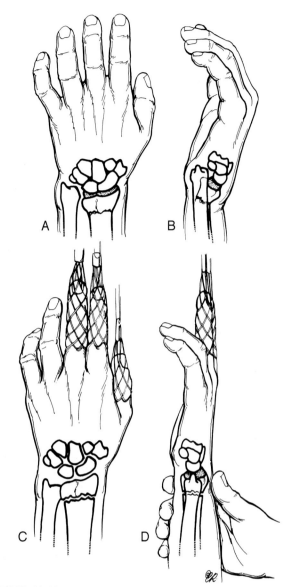

FIGURE 16-21. **A** and **B,** Distal radius (Colles') fracture. **C** and **D,** Our recommended reduction of this fracture. After suspending the arm from fingertraps and allowing for fracture disimpaction, pressure is applied with the thumb over the distal fragment.

Authors' Preferred Position for Plaster Immobilization

Our recommended position of immobilization for a dorsally angulated metaphyseal fracture is that of neutral to slight flexion, ulnar deviation, and neutral forearm rotation (Fig. 16-22).[114] Although theoretic arguments can be made for immobilization of Colles'-type fractures in full supination or full pronation, we favor neutral forearm rotation because it seems to lead to fewer long-term problems in regaining forearm rotation while still maintaining fracture reduction. For patients with radioulnar joint instability, supination may be required. For extra-articular Smith's fractures, in which a pronatory rotational deformity of the distal fragment is always present, immobilization in extension and supination (45 to 60 degrees) in a sugar tong splint or long-arm cast is mandatory for the first 4 weeks, followed by a short-arm cast for an additional 2 weeks.

We prefer to immobilize all acute distal radial fractures in a sugar tong splint[203] (Fig. 16-23). This splint is applied while the arm is suspended from fingertraps after the reduction. As the plaster dries, the fracture is manipulated into the desired position. This splint allows for some swelling while maintaining good maintenance of reduction. As the swelling decreases, the splint can be tightened by simply over-wrapping it with a 4-inch Kling bandage, thus eliminating the need for a cast change and possible associated loss of fracture reduction.

The sugar tong splint can be changed to a short-arm cast or long-arm cast at 2 or 3 weeks, depending on the severity of the fracture and the patient's physiologic status. Care must be taken to check the position of the fracture by radiography 1 week after injury and warn the patient that loss of reduction may occur. Repeat radiographs over the course of healing as well as weekly cast checks may be

needed in those fractures in which displacement in cast is likely. If displacement in cast or splint occurs, skeletal fixation should be strongly considered.

Treatment of Unstable Fractures: Skeletal Fixation

Fractures are judged to be unstable if there is substantial comminution, displacement, or acute instability or for those that collapse and displace during the course of closed treatment.

Closed Reduction and Percutaneous Pin Fixation

Because many unstable fractures of the distal radius have a tendency to become redisplaced in plaster, percutaneous pinning is a relatively simple and effective method of fixation that is recommended for reducible extra-articular fractures and simple intra-articular fractures without metaphyseal comminution but with good bone quality.

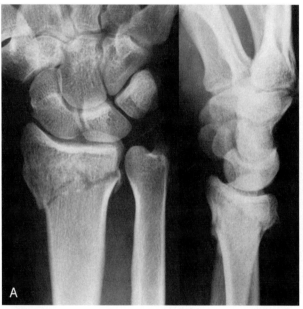

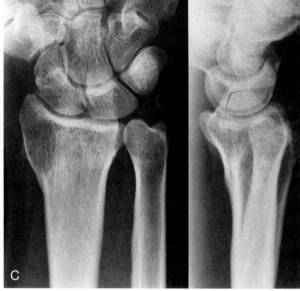

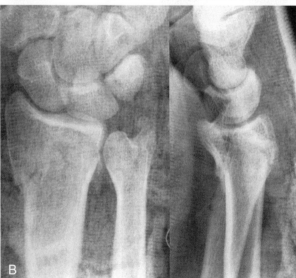

FIGURE 16-22. **A,** Typical radiographic appearance of a Colles' fracture in a young adult. **B,** The fracture was manually reduced and held in slight flexion, ulnar deviation, and slight pronation in a sugar tong splint for 3 weeks, followed by a short-arm cast for another 3 weeks. **C,** Follow-up radiographs at 1 year reveal loss of 2 mm of length but maintenance of normal volar and ulnar tilt. Notice the asymptomatic nonunion of the tip of the ulnar styloid.

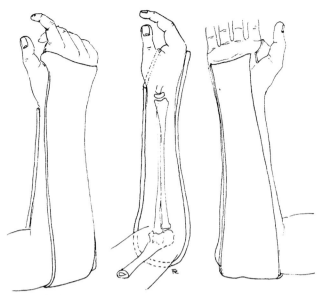

FIGURE 16-23. Sugar tong splint for a distal radius fracture. This splint controls forearm rotation while allowing for some elbow flexion. The palmar crease should be free to allow full metacarpophalangeal flexion.

A variety of different techniques have been described in the literature, and the most commonly used methods are shown in Figure 16-24. These include pins placed through the radial styloid,[162,281] two crossed pins,[41,258] intrafocal pinning *within* the fracture site,[72,144-146] transulnar oblique pinning without transfixation of the DRUJ,[66] one radial styloid pin and a second across the DRUJ,[193] and multiple transulnar-to-radius pins, including the DRUJ.[219,220]

Kapandji has popularized the technique of "double intrafocal wire fixation" to both reduce and maintain distal radial fractures (Fig. 16-25).[146] We believe that this technique is best reserved for noncomminuted extra-articular fractures, although newer refinements of the technique with so-called arum pins (conical nuts) have shown improved results for not only extra-articular fractures but also for certain cases of articular fractures.[129,144,145] The procedure is done in the operating room, usually under brachial block anesthesia. A pneumatic tourniquet is not necessary, but an image intensifier greatly facilitates and shortens the time required for the procedure. After a satisfactory level of anesthesia has been achieved, the hand is prepped and sterile fingertraps applied. The affected hand is then suspended in fingertraps as previously described, with 5 to 10 lb of countertraction applied across the upper arm. Closed reduction is performed in the same manner described on page 659 and the adequacy of reduction confirmed radiographically. Pinning of the fracture is done with the hand suspended in fingertraps or with horizontal fingertrap traction on the operating table. The 1.6-mm (0.0625-inch) Kirschner wires are preferred because these can be inserted with a mini-driver by using only one hand so that the surgeon's other hand is left free to stabilize the fracture.

Under fluoroscopic guidance, one Kirschner wire is inserted into the fracture site in a radial-to-ulnar direction until the ulnar cortex of the radius is felt (see Fig. 16-25A). The wire driver and wire are then moved distally to "lever" the distal radial fragment to regain normal radial inclination. The wire is then advanced through the ulnar cortex. A

second wire is next inserted into the fracture 90 degrees to the first wire in a dorsal-to-palmar direction (see Fig. 16-25B). The wire is advanced until the palmar cortex of the radius is contacted. Next the wire and wire driver are moved distally to "lever" the fragment into its normal position of 12 to 15 degrees of palmar inclination. This second wire is then advanced through the palmar cortex of the radius (see Fig. 16-25C and D).

The fingertraps and countertraction are then removed. If radiographs reveal a stable fracture, the pins are bent and cut off 1 cm above the skin and pin caps applied. If radiographs reveal that the fracture is not adequately stabilized, additional pins (piercing both fragments) are introduced.

Generous incisions are made in the skin around the pins to prevent skin tethering. Care is taken to avoid injury to the cutaneous nerves. A well-padded sugar tong splint is applied for 3 weeks, followed by a short-arm cast for an additional 3 weeks. Full forearm rotation is allowed after 2 weeks. The cast and pins are removed 5 weeks after reduction (Fig. 16-26).

External Fixation for Distal Radial Fractures

Since the original idea of Roger Anderson[9] of using skeletal traction in a "portable" external fixation device for the treatment of comminuted distal radial fractures, there has been constant evolution in both technique and design technology. One of the two most important developments has been the recognition that excessive distraction was harmful to the hand and median nerve and created stiffness. The second development was that distraction alone (ligamento-taxis) could not reduce displaced fractures, especially those with intra-articular fragments and comminution.[12,91,243,273] Several authors have advocated limited open reduction, pin fixation, and replacement of the cancellous bone defect with an autogenous iliac graft after having achieved partial articular reduction, metaphyseal alignment, and radial length with the fixator in place.[91,164,243,244]

Finally, the problem of residual wrist stiffness related to the long period of immobilization of complex fractures with static fixation of the wrist has been addressed by earlier removal of the device, provided that bone grafting has been done to accelerate bone healing[52,87,164] and/or supplemented with internal or Kirschner wire fixation techniques. Early controlled motion of the wrist is sometimes possible between 3 and 5 weeks after the injury without danger of secondary displacement of the fracture if secondary stabilization is used. The theoretical benefit of early motion to reduce the final amount of joint stiffness must be balanced by the concern for loss of reduction, malunion, and early arthritis.

External and Open Reduction With Internal Fixation

Because long-term follow-up studies have demonstrated a correlation between wrist disability and post-traumatic deformity,* there is increasing interest in restoring the best possible anatomy with combined internal fixation, bone grafting, and/or external fixation techniques. Several studies have demonstrated the effectiveness of these combined

---

*See references 37, 54, 100, 104, 154, 173, 179, 236, and 248.

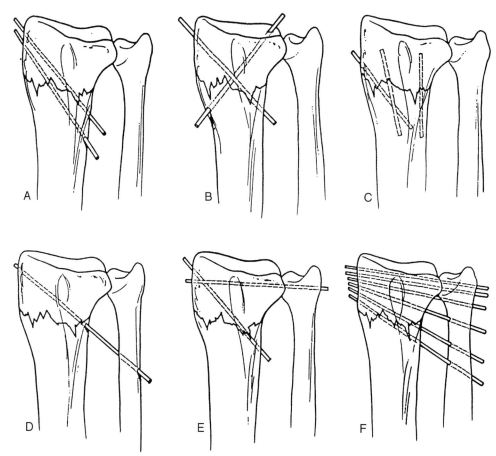

FIGURE 16-24. Several different techniques of percutaneous pinning of unstable bending fractures have been described. **A,** Pins placed primarily through the radial styloid. **B,** Crossing pins from the radial and ulnar sides of the distal fragment into the distal shaft. **C,** The intrafocal technique advocated by Kapandji. **D,** Ulnar-to-radius pinning without transfixation of the DRUJ. **E,** A radial styloid pin and one across the DRUJ. **F,** Multiple pins from the ulna to the radius, including transfixation of the DRUJ.

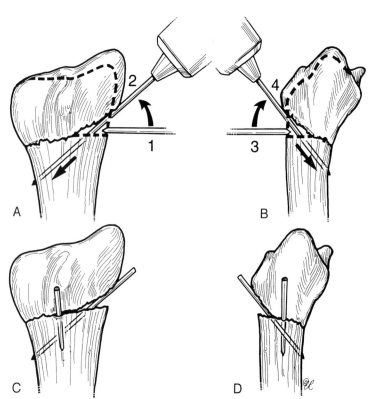

FIGURE 16-25. Kapandji technique of "double intrafocal wire fixation" to reduce and maintain distal radial fractures. A 0.045- or 0.0625-inch Kirschner wire is introduced into the fracture in a radial-to-ulnar direction. When the wire reaches the ulnar cortex of the radius, the wire is used to elevate the radial fragment and re-create the radial inclination. This wire is then introduced into the proximal ulnar cortex of the radius for stability. A second wire is introduced at 90 degrees to the first in a similar manner to restore and maintain volar tilt.

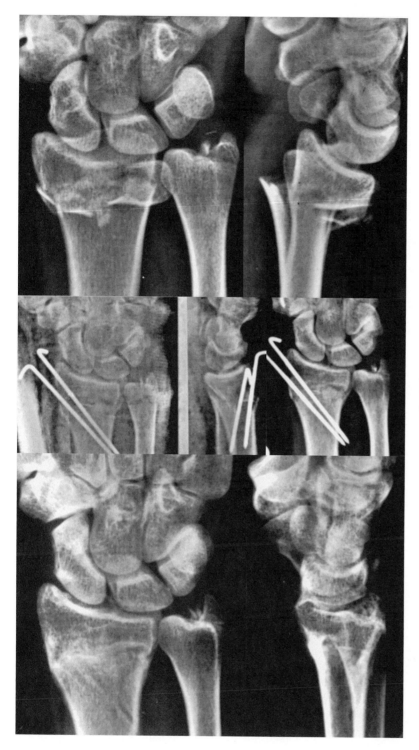

FIGURE 16-26. Unstable dorsally displaced fracture associated with a dorsal die-punch fragment treated by closed manipulation, intrafocal pinning, and cast fixation for 5 weeks. Follow-up radiographs at 6 months reveal an anatomic result.

procedures. Seitz and colleagues[243] reported satisfactory results in 92% of 51 patients with an average age of 50 years. Edwards and Clayton[77] achieved a 96% rate of good or excellent results with external fixation alone, and Jakim and coworkers[138] produced excellent results in 83% of a series of 132 cases with a combination of external fixation, image intensification, local open reduction, and internal fixation with Kirschner wires. Leung and associates[164] combined external fixation with iliac bone grafting in 100

fractures, thus permitting removal of the frame as early as 3 weeks after the operation, followed by functional bracing for another 3 weeks (Fig. 16-27). The overall results in this series were rated good or excellent in nearly all cases. In a number of recent articles reporting the use of combined techniques and a relative short period of static external fixation, final wrist motion averaged 120 degrees for flexion-extension and 140 to 150 degrees of forearm rotation.[91,119,218] Increasing clinical expertise with nonbridging

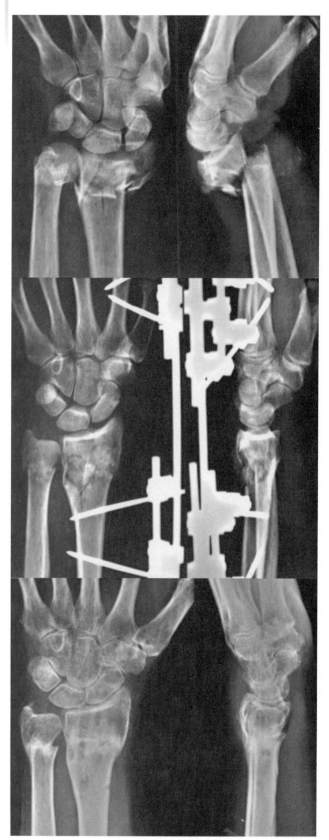

FIGURE 16-27. Comminuted unstable distal forearm fracture *(top)* treated by external fixation and primary autogenous iliac bone grafting *(middle).* The frame was removed at 5 weeks and the wrist protected with a removable wrist splint for another 3 weeks. Follow-up radiographs *(bottom)* demonstrate uneventful healing and satisfactory joint alignment.

fixation for both extra-articular and simple articular fractures, a method that permits early wrist motion, may be applicable in some fractures and may offer a reduction of post-fracture wrist stiffness.[287-289]

Technique of External Fixation

Under brachial block or general anesthesia, the anesthetized upper extremity is sterilely prepped in the operating room from the fingertips to the lower part of the arm, just below a pneumatic tourniquet that has been applied to the arm. Sterile fingertraps are applied to the thumb and index and long fingers. The arm is abducted from the side, the hand suspended in fingertraps, and 5 lb of countertraction applied to the arm. The arm is then draped and the tourniquet inflated. Alternatively, horizontal fingertrap traction with a pulley device attached to a radiolucent hand table may also be used.

Anteroposterior and lateral radiographs of the wrist are then obtained. We have found the use of a sterilely draped C-arm most helpful in evaluating fracture reduction and placement of pins for external fixation. The time taken in draping the C-arm and obtaining the radiographs is usually long enough to allow the fracture fragments to disimpact. If necessary, however, the wrist is gently flexed and extended to disimpact the fracture fragments. Manual reduction is then accomplished by applying pressure in the appropriate direction to restore normal anatomy (see Fig. 16-21). In this manner it should be possible to restore radial inclination and length. The dorsal tilt, however, can usually only be reduced to neutral. If the WristJack (Hand Biomechanics Lab, Sacramento, CA) (Fig. 16-28) external fixator is used, the reduction can be obtained grossly with use of fingertraps and then "fine-tuned" under fluoroscopic control after the fixator has been applied. This device allows for independent palmar carpal translation, with which the volar tilt can be adequately restored.

Two 1-cm-long incisions are made over the dorsal radial aspect of the second metacarpal base and radial shaft. Blunt dissection with scissors exposes the metacarpal. A 3.2-mm tissue protector is then placed on the metacarpal, and 3-mm self-tapping half-pins are inserted at a 30- to 45-degree angle dorsal to the frontal plane of the hand and forearm. The pins should exit the ulnar border of the second metacarpal but not enter the third. Next, through a 4-cm skin incision 8 to 12 cm proximal to the wrist joint, blunt dissection is carried down to the radius (Fig. 16-29). The radial nerve is always visualized and protected. Two 3-mm half-pins (1.5 cm apart) are then introduced through the tissue protector in the space between the tendons of the extensor carpi radialis longus and brevis at a 30-degree angle dorsal to the frontal plane of the forearm. The pins should perforate the medial cortex of the radius but not protrude excessively into the interosseous membrane region. Pin placement should be confirmed fluoroscopically. The proximal wound is closed with 4-0 nylon sutures and the appropriate frame is applied. For relatively stable fractures, a simple frame with a single distraction rod is used. For comminuted unstable fractures, a complex external fixation frame is applied (Fig. 16-30). If the WristJack is used, it is imperative that the metacarpal and radius pins be in the same plane.

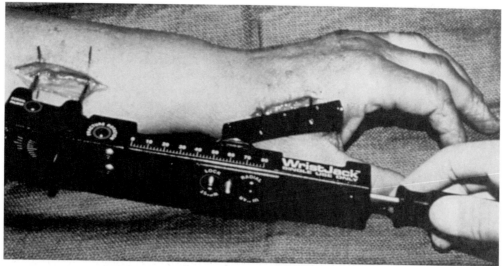

FIGURE 16-28. The WristJack external fixation device has a worm gear to allow multiplanar adjustment of the fracture after the fixation device has been applied.

If nonbridging fixation is selected, proximal pin insertion remains identical while distal pins are now introduced in the distal fragment. A radial-sided pin is placed through a small dorsoradial incision between the wrist extensors in the radial half of the distal fragment. Its direction is dorsopalmar, parallel to the joint surface in the sagittal plane. A second pin is placed in the ulnar aspect of the distal frag-

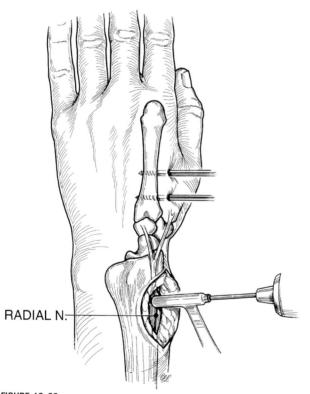

RADIAL N.

FIGURE 16-29. An external fixation device being applied after two 3-mm half-pins have already been introduced into the base of the second metacarpal. Two 3-mm half-pins are then introduced into the distal radius via direct exposure of the radius. The radial nerve is protected by directly identifying the nerve and then inserting the half-pin through a tissue protector that is placed directly on the radius.

ment through a limited incision between the fourth and fifth extensor compartment. Its direction is also dorsopalmar but aimed slightly obliquely from ulnar to radial to engage the palmoulnar cortex of the distal fragment. Having securely fixed the distal pins, a closed reduction is performed using the distal pins as "joysticks" to restore the volar tilt.[290-292] The pins are assembled with separate clamps and rods to create a triangular frame (Fig. 16-31).

Postoperatively, a light bandage that includes a palmar fiberglass or plaster splint is applied. The splint, which provides additional stability to the fracture construct, is optional. We discontinue the splint at the first dressing change (5 days) if a complex frame has been applied and, in the case of a simple frame, at 3 weeks. The frame is removed at 6 weeks. It is recommended that the patient clean the cutaneous/pin interface with peroxide once or twice daily until the wounds have sealed to help prevent pin tract infection. Active and passive finger motion is begun as soon as the anesthetic wears off and is encouraged for the entire time the frame is in place.

Technique of Using External Fixation with Supplemental Percutaneous Pins

After application of either the simple or complex external fixation construct under fluoroscopic control, as just described, 0.045-inch or 0.0625-inch Kirschner wires are introduced into the fracture fragments and fixed to the proximal radial shaft. *One or two* pins driven through the radial styloid fragment and one through the dorsal medial fragment into the radial shaft *combine to produce maximum additional stability.*[289] The pins should pierce the proximal cortex but not penetrate into the ulnar shaft as previously advocated by DePalma.[66]

The pins are cut off 1 cm external to the skin margin and caps applied. A light bandage and palmar splint are applied as previously described with the routine application of an external fixator.

These principles of closed fracture reduction, however, apply only to reducible fractures. Impacted and severely displaced fragments that do not respond to ligamentotaxis or external reduction maneuvers require additional limited open reduction.

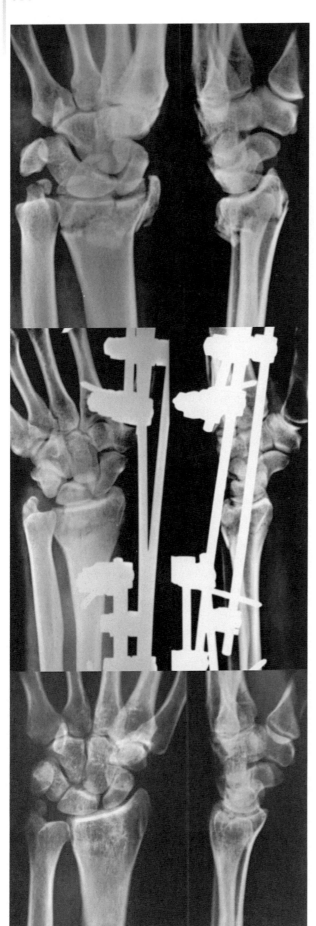

FIGURE 16-30. A complex intra-articular fracture anatomically reduced with ligamentotaxis alone for a period of 6 weeks. Follow-up films at 3 years show excellent articular and metaphyseal alignment.

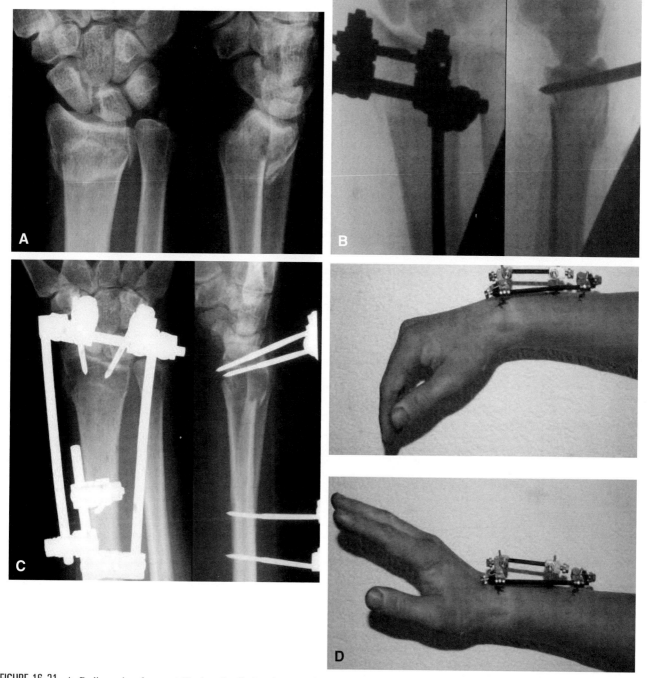

FIGURE 16-31. **A,** Radiographs of an unstable dorsally displaced extra-articular fracture of the distal radius. **B,** Fluoroscopic control of the nonbridging fixator. Notice the converging position of the distal pins in the frontal plane and parallel to the joint surface in the sagittal plane. **C,** Control radiographs 10 days after injury with well-maintained reduction. **D,** Early motion of the wrist is allowed as soon as swelling has subsided.   *Continued*

Technique of External Fixation Combined With Open Reduction, Kirschner Wire, Internal Fixation, and Bone Grafting

Under tourniquet control with the arm resting on a hand table, an external fixation device using a single distraction rod is applied as described earlier after manual or fingertrap reduction of the fracture (Fig. 16-32A). The wrist joint is then approached through a dorsal longitudinal midline incision (see Fig. 16-32B). The skin flaps are elevated and retracted radialward and ulnarward. The extensor retinaculum is then opened over Lister's tubercle and the extensor

pollicis longus retracted radialward. Dissection is carried out sharply beneath the fourth dorsal compartment, leaving a portion of the wrist capsule with the common extensor tendons and a portion of the capsule intact. The same plane of dissection is accomplished beneath the radial wrist extensors. Removal of a segment of the posterior interosseous nerve in the base of the fourth extensor compartment may be done at this time at the discretion of the surgeon. The wrist extensors and extensor pollicis longus are retracted radialward and the finger extensors ulnarward (see Fig. 16-32C). The wrist joint capsule may be opened transversely at

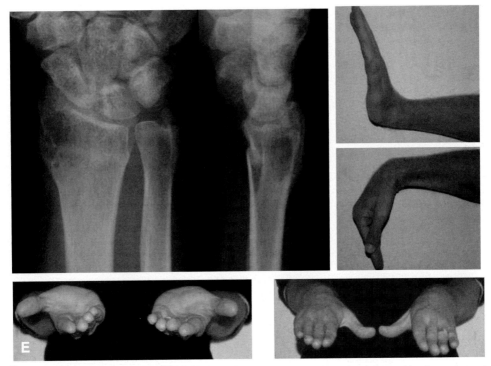

FIGURE 16-31—cont'd. E, Radiographs at 3 months. The fracture has healed without displacement and correlates with a free wrist motion and restoration of complete forearm rotation.

the level of the radiocarpal joint *if necessary* to assess the adequacy of articular reduction. Next, the fragment that involves the radial styloid is stabilized with two Kirschner wires that can be inserted across the radial styloid into the ulnar cortex of the radial metaphysis (Fig. 16-33). The fragments affecting the lunate fossa are manually elevated with a Freer elevator or a pointed awl and percutaneously fixed with 1.2-mm Kirschner wires introduced from the radial aspect of the wrist. The wires usually pass through the radial styloid, pass directly beneath the subchondral bone of the scaphoid and lunate facets and into the elevated fragment, but do not enter the DRUJ (see Fig. 16-32D and E). If there is joint incongruity involving the sigmoid notch of the radius, every attempt is made to achieve anatomic reduction there also. If the volar ulnar fragment remains displaced, reduction through a limited volar approach must be performed to prevent subsequent volar displacement of the carpus (see the section on Limited Open Reduction).

The wound is closed by reapproximating the wrist capsule and extensor retinaculum. We have found it helpful post-operatively to immobilize the forearm in a sugar tong splint for 3 weeks. After 4 to 6 weeks, the external fixator can be safely removed, a removable wrist splint applied, and gentle wrist motion begun. Percutaneous pins may be left in place for 2 to 3 additional weeks at the discretion of the surgeon.

Secondary displacement of distal radius fractures and shortening are due to settling of the distal fragments in the cancellous defect or void at the metaphyseal area. We now routinely perform bone grafting for all subchondral bone defects regardless of the size of the defect if the articular surface has been elevated. The bone graft provides mechanical buttressing of small cartilage-bearing fragments and may accelerate fracture healing by providing additional osteogenic potential. Autogenous bone graft is readily available and has

theoretical advantages over each of the graft alternatives available.[83] Donor site morbidity may be reduced by using trephines or specially designed bone-harvesting devices. For cases in which a greater amount of bone is needed for bicortical grafts for corrective osteotomies, the following open technique is preferred.

Technique of Harvesting Iliac Bone Graft

After a rolled towel has been placed under the ipsilateral sacroiliac joint, the iliac crest region is sterilely prepped and draped. A 5-cm-long incision is made over the iliac crest beginning 2 cm posterior to the anterior-superior iliac spine and coursing posteriorly. With an osteotome a section of the iliac crest, 3 cm in length and 1 cm thick, is reflected on its medial periosteum. This exposes an abundant area of cancellous bone between the two cortical wings. Cancellous bone is harvested. The flap of iliac crest is then turned back down into its bed and sutured in place. (This technique leaves virtually no cosmetic defect to either the eye or touch along the iliac crest.) The wound is then closed in layers over a suction catheter drain.

Bone graft substitutes may be used in combination with external fixation as an alternative to the harvesting of autogenous bone.[342,345] For acute fractures, the need for structural support of the elevated articular surface generally outweighs the need for osteogenic stimulation of healing. The intact radial metaphysis is normally a potent source of osteogenic cells, growth factors, and osteoinductive cancellous bone; and fractures through this area have a strikingly low rate of delayed or nonunion. The ability to further enhance fracture healing by the addition of biologic products has not been demonstrated, except in the situations in which healing potential has been compromised by disease or tobacco use.[335] Thus, bone graft substitutes that demon-

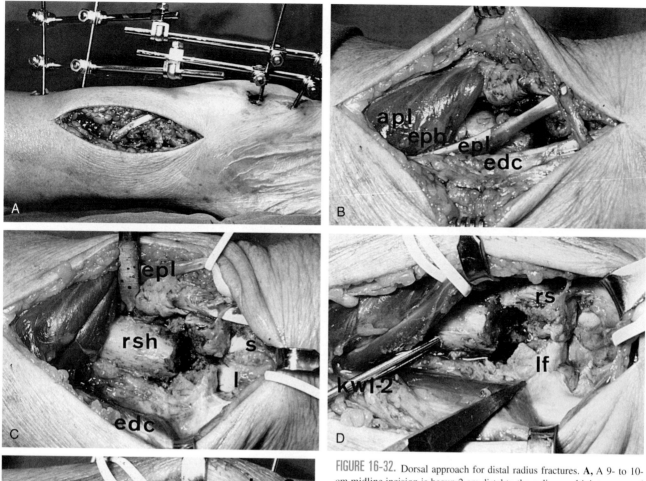

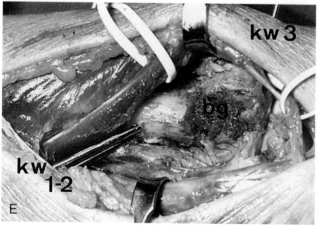

FIGURE 16-32. Dorsal approach for distal radius fractures. **A,** A 9- to 10-cm midline incision is begun 2 cm distal to the radiocarpal joint space and carried proximally to the distal end of the forearm. The extensor pollicis longus is identified by opening the extensor retinaculum and then dissected out of its sheath. Usually Lister's tubercle is contained in one of the metaphyseal fragments of the dorsal comminuted area. **B,** The space between the extensor pollicis longus (epl), abductor pollicis longus (apl), and extensor pollicis brevis (epb) is developed radially to expose the radial shaft (rsh). The ulnar aspect of the distal radius is exposed by elevating the extensor digitorum communis (edc) subperiostally. **C,** The thumb (epl) and wrist extensors are retracted radially and the fourth compartment ulnarly (edc). A transverse wrist capsulotomy exposes the radiocarpal joint, the proximal pole of the scaphoid (s), and the lunate (l). Notice the intra-articular disruption of the fracture and the metaphyseal bone defect. **D,** The radial styloid (rs) fragment has been stabilized with two 1.6-mm Kirschner wires (kw 1-2) inserted obliquely across the shaft fragment into the radial styloid. The die-punch fragment involving the lunate fossa (lf) is being reduced against the lunate and radial styloid fragment with a pointed awl. **E,** Both articular fragments have been stabilized with a transverse Kirschner wire (kw 3) passing across the radial styloid into the die-punch fragment. The metaphyseal defect has been packed with cancellous iliac bone graft (bg).

strate compressive properties equal to or greater than cancellous bone are of greater utility in management of comminuted articular fractures than the purely osteogenic or the combination osteogenic-moldable putty formulations (Fig. 16-34).[331] For unstable Colles' fractures in elderly or osteoporotic patients, the use of methylmethacrylate bone cement[151,156,237] has been recommended by some, but its use has not been widely accepted because of methylmethacrylate's brittle mechanical profile and its exothermic properties. Several

prospective studies support the use of an injectable calcium phosphate cement as an adjunct to percutaneous fixation of distal radius fractures and have documented favorable outcomes in comparison to conventional treatment with autogenous bone or cast treatment alone.[325,343,346] Mechanical and clinical studies demonstrate the limitations of injectable cements as stand-alone fixation and strongly recommend the use of percutaneous wires, screws, or external fixation when considering the use of injectable bone

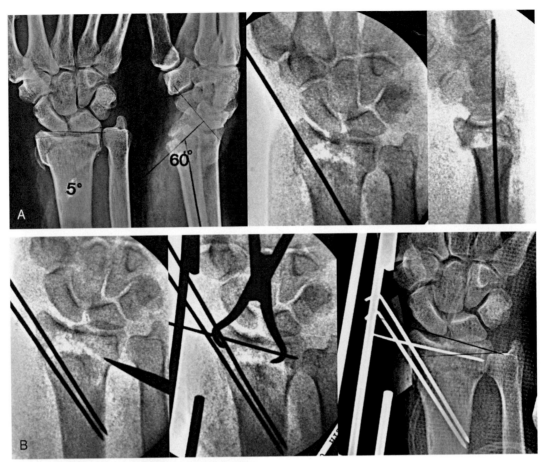

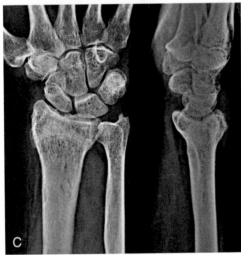

FIGURE 16-33. **A,** Severely displaced four-part intra-articular fracture with 60 degrees of dorsal displacement and 5 degrees of ulnar tilt. After manual reduction and pinning of the radial styloid, intraoperative fluoroscopy shows insufficient reduction of the ulnar fragment and the large size of the metaphyseal bone defect. **B,** After the application of an external fixator, anatomic reduction of the joint surface is achieved through a dorsal approach (see Fig. 16-32); while the sagittal fracture gap is maintained with a pointed clamp, a third Kirschner wire is driven across both articular fragments and the defect grafted. **C,** The pins and fixator were removed at 5 weeks. A follow-up radiograph at 9 months shows a well-preserved joint space and overall adequate fracture alignment.

cements.[332,334] The specific advantages and disadvantages of current bone graft alternatives are presented in Table 16-1.

Articular Fractures: Arthroscopic-Assisted Reduction, Limited Open Reduction, Fragment-Specific Fixation, and Extensive Open Reduction

Indications and Contraindications

Open reduction of articular fractures of the distal radius is indicated in manually active patients with good bone quality and no preexisting wrist pathology when anatomic restora-

tion of the joint surface cannot be achieved by closed manipulation, ligamentotaxis, or percutaneous reduction maneuvers. Delayed open reduction may be indicated for secondary intra-articular displacement if the reduction is lost after a trial of closed reduction and plaster fixation. Articular fractures in elderly, inactive patients and in those with massive osteoporosis have traditionally been considered a contraindication to open reduction because in these patients there is a risk of complications, including failure of fixation devices, iatrogenic nonunion, and reflex sympathetic dystrophy. However, since the recent introduction of "fixed angle" internal fixation devices, both extra-articular and

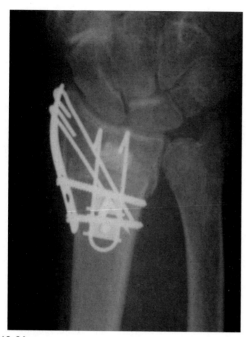

FIGURE 16-34. Posteroanterior radiograph of healed fracture, demonstrating a block of coralline hydroxyapatite bone graft substitute to support the reduced articular surface.

simple intra-articular fractures in elderly, active, osteoporotic patients are now amenable to open reduction and internal fixation. Subchondral buttressing of fixed angle pins or screws attached to the distal part of the plate reduce the incidence of settling or secondary articular displacement by virtue of the "internal fixator" function of the device.[108,293-295]

General factors limiting surgical reconstruction of the articular surface include the number of fragments, their size, the amount of cancellous bone impaction, and associated primary lesions of the articular cartilage. Exact anatomic restoration should not be pursued if articular comminution exceeds more than four to five fairly sizable fragments. If more than that number of fragments is present, the chance of obtaining perfect anatomic reduction of the joint surface and reducing the incidence of post-traumatic arthrosis is not good. However, this statement does not preclude the necessity of improving extra-articular and intra-articular alignment and restoration of radial length with external fixation techniques. In these cases every effort should be made to improve the anatomic relationship of the radius and ulna and ensure normal alignment of the hand and carpus with the long axis of the forearm. If secondary radiocarpal arthritic changes occur, the absence of metaphyseal malunion and shortening will greatly facilitate the performance of secondary reconstructive procedures.

Algorithm for Management of Articular Fractures of the Distal Radius

If the fracture is characterized by a simple intra-articular component (not more than two fragments) and is without significant metaphyseal comminution, closed, arthroscopically assisted, or percutaneous reduction is generally sufficient. In *percutaneous reduction*, the cartilage-bearing fragments are manipulated with an awl or a periosteal elevator through a small skin incision under fluoroscopic and/or

arthroscopic guidance, with a minimum of soft tissue dissection. Many of these cases may be stabilized with percutaneously inserted implants, such as Kirschner wires and/or cannulated screws, as outlined in the preceding sections, provided there is good bone quality (absence of osteoporosis). If the fracture has a simple intra-articular component and extensive metaphyseal-diaphyseal comminution, external fixation, and/or internal fixation with a "fixed angle" device are the methods of choice to restore radial length and metaphyseal alignment. If articular congruity cannot be adequately restored by closed maneuvers or ligamentotaxis after application of an external fixator, a *percutaneous or limited open reduction* in combination with bone grafting is advocated. If the fracture has more than two articular fragments, with increasing metaphyseal or even diaphyseal comminution, *extensive open reduction* and bone grafting become progressively more necessary because joint distraction with horizontal fingertrap traction or external fixation is not capable of disimpaction and realignment of small cartilage-bearing fragments, nor can it accomplish reduction of severely rotated volar lip and ulnar corner fragments.[323]

Arthroscopic Treatment of Distal Radial Fractures

Diagnostic and therapeutic wrist arthroscopy is widely used by many practicing hand surgeons. Its use in conjunction with percutaneous means of fracture fixation offers several advantages in the management of articular fractures of the distal radius.[329,330,337,339] Arthroscopy presents a minimally invasive means to monitor articular reduction, without the additional ligamentous and capsular damage that is inherent in an open inspection of the articular surface. In addition, the arthroscope affords an unparalleled diagnostic view of the interosseous carpal ligaments, the carpal articular surfaces, and the TFCC.[60,106,225,280,282] If indicated, arthroscopic or limited open management of concomitant soft tissue injuries of the carpus or DRUJ may be undertaken simultaneously.

Doi and associates demonstrated improvements in range of motion and fracture reduction in a prospective cohort of patients treated with arthroscopic-assisted percutaneous fixation when compared with a group treated by conventional open reduction and internal fixation for displaced intra-articular fractures of the distal radius.[327] None of the fractures treated in the arthroscopic group required fluoroscopic confirmation of articular reduction. Several authors have recommended routine arthroscopic confirmation of articular surface reduction after demonstrating a high rate of inaccuracy using fluoroscopy alone.[321,328] Concomitant grade III or IV injuries of the scapholunate or lunotriquetral interosseous ligaments have been identified in up to 40% of patients and can usually be adequately treated by temporary Kirschner wire fixation for 6 to 8 weeks.[340]

Operative Technique: Arthroscopic Reduction and Pinning

If considering arthroscopic-assisted reduction and fixation of an intra-articular distal radius fracture, it is prudent to reduce and stabilize the fracture in plaster for at least 72 hours before surgery (Fig. 16-35). The optimum time for arthroscopic reduction is between 3 and 7 days after the injury. Fractures treated acutely by arthroscopic means may have marked extravasation of fluid into the soft tissue, thus creating the possibility of the development of a compartment

Table 16-1
ALTERNATIVES TO AUTOGENOUS BONE GRAFT FOR DISTAL RADIUS FRACTURE MANAGEMENT

Type	Formulation	Application	Indications	Advantages	Disadvantages
Allograft					
Demineralized bone matrix	Amorphous, powder, gel, strips, putty, combinations	Manual insertion	Compromised host, impaired healing, nonunion	Osteoinductive and limited osteogenic potential	Variable osteogenic capability depending on composition and formulation; marginal to no structural support
Cancellous chips	5- to 7-mm freeze-dried cancellous chips	Manual packing	Metaphyseal void, elevated articular surface	Some structural support; osteoconductive and limited osteoinductive	Variable osteoinductive capability; limited structural support
Fresh frozen	Corticocancellous bone segments	Cut to shape, internal fixation	Segmental defect	Customized to defect, high structural support, osteoinductive	Rarely indicated for distal radius fractures; disease potential; immunogenicity; slow incorporation
Cancellous Substitutes					
Tricalcium phosphate combinations	Mixed with hydroxyapatite, collagen, marrow aspirate; available in strips, granules	Manual insertion	Metaphyseal void, elevated articular surface	Osteogenic and inductive when mixed with marrow aspirate	Minimal to no structural support, variable resorption rates
Calcium sulfate	Pellets, paste, putty	Manual or injectable; may harden to block form	Metaphyseal void, elevated articular surface	Resorbable defect filler, replaced by bone; injectable through minimal incision; may be combined with antibiotics	Minimal to no structural support, water-soluble, rapidly resorbed
Nano-particulate b-tricalcium phosphate	Blocks or granular, mixed with marrow	Manual or injectable	Metaphyseal void, elevated articular surface	Resorbable, injectable, porous; moderate compressive strength	Osteogenic and osteoinductive only if mixed with marrow
Coralline hydroxy-apatite	Blocks, granules	Trimmed to shape defect	Metaphyseal void, elevated articular surface	Osteoconductive and porous; compressive strength equal to or exceeding cancellous bone; can shape to fit defect	Slow resorption; radiopacity may obscure healing
Bovine cancellous bone	Block form	Manual, trim to defect	Metaphyseal void, elevated articular surface	Osteoconductive, moderate structural support	Immunogenicity, variable osteoinductivity; not approved for use in United States
Cements					
Calcium phosphate	Mixed components, hardens with time	Injectable, putty or block	Metaphyseal void, elevated articular surface	Can be injected percutaneously; animal models demonstrate resorption/ remodeling; high compressive strength	Not osteoconductive or inductive; slow to remodel and reabsorb; lacks shear or tensile strength

Table continued on following page

Table 16-1

ALTERNATIVES TO AUTOGENOUS BONE GRAFT FOR DISTAL RADIUS FRACTURE MANAGEMENT—cont'd

Type	Formulation	Application	Indications	Advantages	Disadvantages
Cements—cont'd PMMA	Mixed components, hardens in minutes	Injectable	Bone defect, metaphyseal void; augment ORIF in osteopenic bone	Can be injected percutaneously; high compressive strength	Not osteoconductive or inductive; Exothermic; may cause thermal necrosis; brittle, poor shear or tensile strength; limited indications for distal radius
Biologics Recombinant BMP	Powder, strips putty	Manual, injectable	Compromised host or tissue bed, nonunion or delayed union	Osteoinductive; may accelerate healing	Limited indications for distal radius application; dosage and timing not yet clarified

BMP, bone morphogenetic protein; ORIF, open reduction and internal fixation; PMMA, polymethylmethacrylate.

syndrome. After 7 days, however, it becomes difficult to disimpact articular fragments without a formal open reduction.

The arm is sterilely prepped and draped in the usual manner and suspended from sterile fingertraps on the index and long fingers. The hand is then wrapped from the level of the MP joints proximally to the base of the metacarpals and the forearm from just proximal to the wrist up to the elbow with Coban tape to prevent fluid extravasation into the soft tissues. The fracture is next evaluated radiographically with the "C"-arm. A determination is made whether to treat the fracture with percutaneous or internal fixation. If the fracture will require open reduction and internal fixation, arthroscopy is not performed; instead, the arm is removed from the fingertrap distraction mode and placed on a standard arm table and the procedure accomplished. If external fixation either with or without pins is to be used, the fixation device may be applied before the wrist is scoped, obviating the need for a separate traction device.[282,344]

The scope is inserted through the 3-4 portal, and an outflow portal is established either in the 4-5 or 6U portal. Immediate and copious irrigation is critical to clear clot and debris and improve visualization (see Fig. 16-35B). Once this is done, continuous irrigation is maintained through the 6U portal and working portals may be established in the 1-2 and/or 4-5 portals. Doi and associates demonstrated the additional utility of a volar-radial portal, created by means of a limited open incision over the flexor carpi radialis tendon.[327] The 0.0625-inch Kirschner wires are useful as percutaneous "joysticks" when placed into the radial styloid and other large articular fragments (see Fig. 16-35A). Fragment reduction is then accomplished with the joysticks under fluoroscopic control and the reduction stabilized with either 0.045- or 0.0625-inch Kirschner wires (see Fig. 16-35C and D). Pin fixation is augmented with a plaster cast or an external fixator placed in neutralization mode, and pins are left in place for 6 to 8 weeks until healing (see Fig. 16-18).

Concomitant complete tears of the scapholunate or lunotriquetral ligaments should be reduced anatomically and pinned or treated with limited open reduction and repair. A minimum of two divergent pins should cross the affected proximal row of carpal bones, and one or two additional pins should be placed to temporarily stabilize the proximal row to the distal carpal row across the midcarpal joint. Intercarpal pins are left in place for at least 8 weeks, and a slowly graduated program of range-of-motion and resistive exercises begun thereafter. Complete peripheral detachment of the articular disc of the TFCC can also be treated with arthroscopic-guided suture placement at the time of fracture reduction.[320]

Limited Open Reduction

The concept of limited open reduction is defined as the selective surgical exposure of articular fragments that still remain displaced after closed manipulation, fingertrap traction, or ligamentotaxis with external fixation. The main objective of this technique is to achieve anatomic reduction with limited exposure and to minimize the use of implants in an effort to preserve ligament attachments, thereby minimizing iatrogenic soft tissue disruption and preserving the vascular supply of the fragments. This technique is particularly useful for intra-articular four-part fractures of the distal radius without metaphyseal comminution. Metaphyseal alignment, radial length, and reduction of the radial styloid fragment can usually be easily achieved with classic closed reduction maneuvers alone or combined with longitudinal traction. However, the dorsoulnar and volar ulnar fragments that disrupt the lunate fossa and the sigmoid notch may remain displaced because of either impaction in the metaphyseal subchondral bone or soft tissue interposition (Fig. 16-36). The technique of limited open reduction addresses the anatomic restoration of such fragments after percutaneous fixation of the radial styloid fragment.

The choice of surgical approach depends on the location of the displaced fragment. If the volar ulnar fragment is severely rotated, a palmar approach is selected. Because only the volar aspect of the DRUJ and the ulnar corner of the

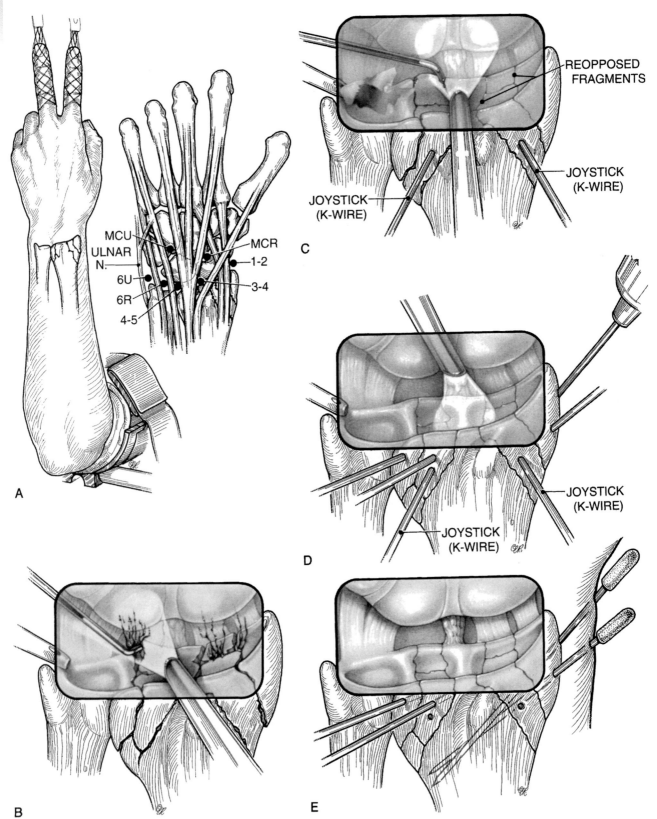

FIGURE 16-35. Operative technique: arthroscopic reduction and pinning of distal radial fractures. **A,** The arm is suspended from fingertraps on the index and long fingers. The following anatomic landmarks are identified: arthroscopic portals 1-2, 3-4, 4-5, 6R (radial), 6U (ulnar), MCR (midcarpal radial), and MCU (midcarpal ulnar). The dorsal sensory branch of the ulnar nerve is noted. **B,** The arthroscope is introduced through the 3-4 or 4-5 portal, and with a probe through the 6R portal the comminuted distal radial fracture is visualized. Clot and hemorrhage extrude from the fracture fragments. **C,** Joysticks (0.0625-inch Kirschner wires) are introduced into the major fragments percutaneously to elevate the fracture fragments into an anatomic position. **D,** Additional Kirschner wires are then introduced percutaneously into the fracture. **E,** The joysticks are then removed, the fixation pins are cut off outside the skin, and caps are applied.

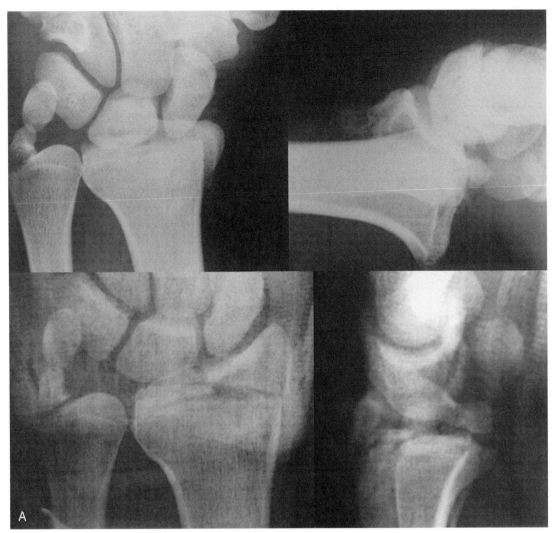

FIGURE 16-36. **A,** After closed reduction of what was thought to be a "simple" Colles fracture, postreduction radiographs show a four-part intra-articular fracture with unacceptable joint stepoffs of the lunate fossa both dorsally and palmarly.   *Continued*

radius need to be visualized, a limited incision that parallels the flexor carpi ulnaris tendon just proximal to the transverse wrist crease provides sufficient exposure. Surgical release of the transverse carpal ligament can be performed if needed by extending the incision in a zigzag fashion across the wrist crease and into the palm. The interval between the flexor tendons and the ulnar artery and nerve is developed, through which the pronator quadratus and volar wrist capsule are exposed. Usually the distal border of the pronator quadratus has been disrupted by the fracture; this allows easy visualization of the metaphyseal fracture line and displaced volar ulnar fragments with minimal soft tissue dissection. If intact, the pronator quadratus is partially released from its ulnar insertion and retracted radially and proximally to expose the fracture site. Extreme care must be taken to avoid injury to the volar arm of the radioulnar ligamentous complex. The volar ulnar fracture fragment is then carefully reduced to restore continuity of the palmar cortex at the metaphyseal area by applying a dorsally directed force with an awl or periosteal elevator. Depending on its size, the fragment may be fixed with a Kirschner wire introduced obliquely in a palmodorsal direction (see

Fig. 16-36B). The wire is retrieved through the dorsal skin while making sure that its palmar end lies flush with the cortical level of the fragment to avoid impingement of the flexor tendons. The wire may be augmented with a suture or additional wire placed through the proximal metaphyseal cortex in a tension band configuration.[324] For larger fragments, a small buttress plate may be applied. This restores palmar stability of the fracture and provides a solid base on which the overlying dorsoulnar or "die-punch" fragment can be reduced.

For limited open reduction of the dorsoulnar fragment, a longitudinal incision through the fifth dorsal compartments is used (Fig. 16-37). Care should be taken when using this approach to preserve the important dorsal radioulnar ligament of the TFCC. With the use of a Kirschner wire as a joystick, or a small elevator, the dorsoulnar fragment is elevated to restore the articular surface. It is important that all traction be relieved during this maneuver so that the lunate can act as a template for the smooth restoration of the lunate facet of the distal radius. A transverse dorsal capsulotomy can be performed if necessary to directly visualize the joint surface and assess the quality of articular congruity

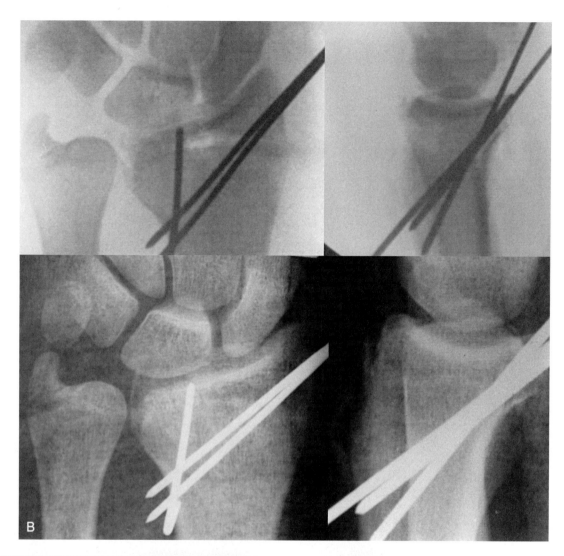

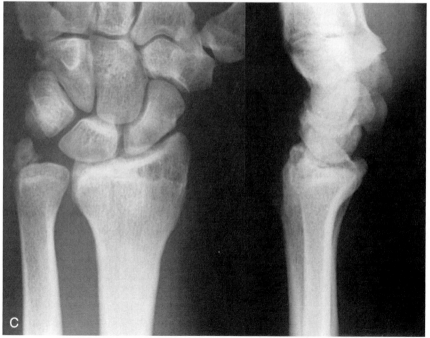

FIGURE 16-36—cont'd. **B,** The radial styloid fragment was pinned percutaneously with two 1.6-mm Kirschner wires. The volar ulnar fragment was reduced through an extended carpal tunnel incision and pinned in a volar-to-dorsal direction. The dorsal die-punch fragment was elevated against the lunate through a small incision between the fourth and fifth compartments. **C,** Postoperatively, a sugar tong splint was applied for 2 weeks, followed by a short-arm cast for another 3 weeks. At 5 weeks the pins and cast were removed. Follow-up films at 2 years show an anatomic result and an asymptomatic fibrous union of the ulnar styloid without DRUJ instability.

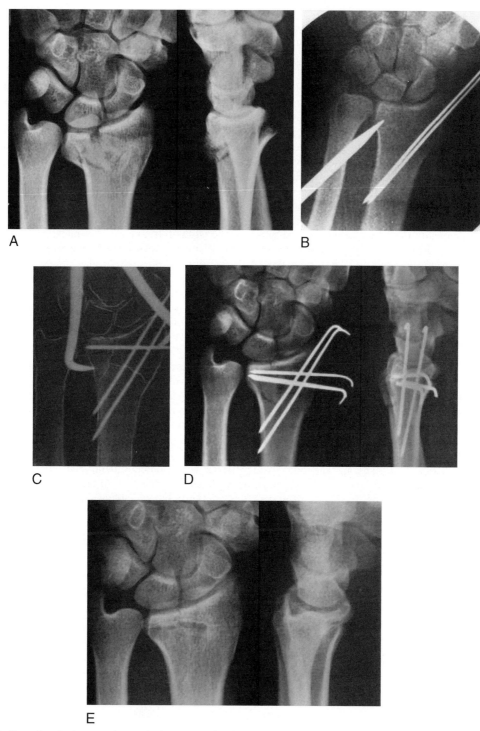

FIGURE 16-37. A, Radiographs of a three-part intra-articular compression fracture of the distal radius treated with a combination of percutaneous pinning and limited open reduction of the ulnar facet fragment. **B,** After closed reduction and insertion of two Kirschner wires through the radial styloid, the ulnar fragment is elevated against the lunate with an awl. **C,** The sagittal gap is reduced with a pointed clamp. **D,** Two 1.2-mm Kirschner wires are driven transversely through both joint fragments. **E,** Radiographs 1.5 years after injury reveal an anatomic restoration of the joint surface and maintained radial length.

of the lunate fossa. If both the palmar and dorsal fragments are anatomically reduced, this implies that articular congruency of the horizontal fracture line that enters the sigmoid notch has been achieved. Thereafter, under fluoroscopic control, the fragment is pinned either with a transversely inserted Kirschner wire across the radial styloid fragment (taking care to not enter the radioulnar joint) or with a Kirschner wire passed obliquely from the dorsoulnar corner of the fragment into the proximal fragment in a volar-radial direction. In those instances in which the fracture gap between the die-punch fragment and the radial styloid remains slightly open, a pointed fracture reduction or tenaculum clamp can be applied between the fragment and the radial styloid to close the articular gap and improve reduction.

Fragment-Specific Fixation

In an attempt to minimize the morbidity of extensive surgical dissections and rigid plate fixation of distal radius fractures, Robert Medoff devised a hybrid technique of percutaneous wire and plate fixation, designed to fix individual fracture fragments through several small incisions.[322,336,338] The technique involves the use of ultra-thin modular implants that can be shaped to customize fixation for different fragment configurations, and the placement of these implants strategically along the lateral and intermediate columns of the radial metaphysis to maximize construct rigidity.[333] A key component of these implant systems is the so-called pin plate that combines the versatility of a Kirschner wire with the rigidity of plate and screw fixation. The bending stiffness of conventional Kirschner wire fixation is dramatically increased by passing the wire through the free end of a plate secured proximally to the radial shaft, creating a pin-plate hybrid with a rigid three-point fixation. Mechanical studies, using an unstable metaphyseal fracture model, have demonstrated that dual 2.0-mm plates, when placed at 50- to 90-degree angles to each other in the axial plane, provide statistically superior fixation to either Kirschner wire–augmented external fixation or a traditional 3.5-mm "T"-plate dorsal plate.[326,341] Fragment-specific fixation is indicated for most unstable and intra-articular fractures of the distal radius and is generally contraindicated in fractures with substantial metaphyseal-diaphyseal extension or severe osteoporosis.

The radial styloid is regarded as the keystone of reduction and stability of intra-articular fractures of the distal radius and is therefore addressed first in the sequence of fragment-specific reduction and fixation. The other key fragments to be considered include the volar lip fragment, the dorsal and volar components of the lunate facet and sigmoid notch, and the impacted articular fragments (see Fig. 16-16). Five to 10 pounds of traction is helpful to grossly align the fragments, applied via fingertraps to the index and long fingers, or through the use of a formal traction table. The radial styloid is approached through a novel 4- to 5-cm incision on the volar radial aspect of the metaphyseal flare, just radial to the radial artery and palmar to the first dorsal compartment tendons.[322] Superficial branches of the radial sensory and antebrachial cutaneous nerves are retracted in the skin flaps, and the first dorsal compartment is opened to expose and retract its tendons. The brachioradialis tendon is split longitudinally and the tendon and periosteum elevated in a dorsal and palmar plane to expose the radius (Fig. 16-38). Complete palmar exposure of the radius is accomplished by elevating the pronator quadratus in continuity with the palmar margin of the brachioradialis and exposing the entire radial styloid by dorsal elevation beneath the second dorsal compartment. The styloid fragment is reduced anatomically and fixed provisionally with a 0.045-inch Kirschner wire. At this time, attention is directed to the intermediate column of the radius, for reduction and fixation of the lunate facet and impacted articular fragments.

Small volar fragments can be approached and reduced via the limited volar-ulnar incision described earlier. The volar-ulnar fragment is readily stabilized with a volar buttress pin "wireform" implant (TriMed, Inc., Valencia, CA), to provide rigid fixation and directly buttress the fractured articular surface of the lunate facet. Larger volar shear fragments are stabilized with a volar buttress L-plate, generally placed through the volar-radial incision described previously.

Dorsal metaphyseal fragments can be exposed through a 4- to 5-cm universal dorsal subperiosteal exposure over the third dorsal compartment. The extensor pollicis longus is isolated and primarily transposed out of its compartment, and the radial metaphysis can be widely exposed by elevating the second and/or fourth compartments in a subperiosteal fashion. It is not generally necessary to open the dorsal capsule to directly inspect the articular surface, and

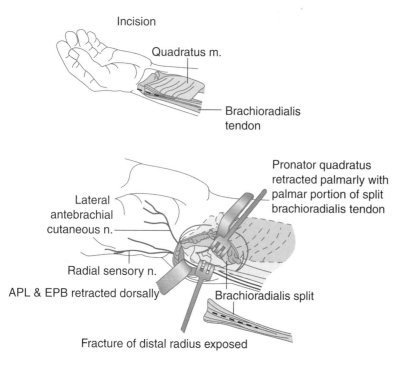

FIGURE 16-38. Volar-radial approach to the distal radius. The brachioradialis tendon is split and elevated subperiosteally to expose the radial column and the volar aspect of the distal radius. APL, abductor pollicis longus; EPB, extensor pollicis brevis. (Copyright © 2001, Virginia Ferrante.)

fluoroscopy is used to document reduction of the fracture fragments and articular surface. Isolated dorsoulnar fragments can be approached through a 2-cm limited incision over the fifth dorsal compartment, but the incision is not extensile and cannot be readily enlarged to gain access to larger metaphyseal and impacted articular fragments.

Dorsal intermediate column fragments are directly reduced and then fixed in position with 2.0-mm miniplates and screws or with any of a series of wireform implants that capture and hold small periarticular fragments (Fig. 16-39). Use of autogenous bone graft or a suitable structural bone graft substitute (see Table 16-1) is recommended to augment and hold reduction of impacted articular fragments. The construct is completed by returning to the radial styloid to complete the fixation with a 2.0-mm radial pin-plate and screws (Fig. 16-40). It is important to place the radial styloid implant in a plane 50 to 90 degrees apart from the plane of fixation for the intermediate column to maximize stability of the fixation construct. The wounds are closed by reapproximation of periosteum over the dorsal and radial implants. The brachioradialis tendon can be closed with a single running suture to provide soft tissue interposition between the implant and the overlying first dorsal compartment tendons. The extensor pollicis longus is primarily transposed

out of its compartment by closing the extensor retinaculum between the second and fourth extensor compartments. The DRUJ is then carefully assessed for stability, and appropriate treatment is rendered for residual instability. The wrist and forearm are temporarily immobilized in a sugar tong plaster splint in slight supination for 5 to 10 days to allow soft tissue healing.

Rehabilitation is predicated on the strength of fracture fixation, but generally patients can be started on a program of active, unresisted motion exercises within a week of surgery. Strengthening exercises are begun after radiographic evidence of fracture consolidation, generally at 6 to 8 weeks postoperatively.

Extensive or Formal Open Reduction

The concept of formal open reduction and stable internal fixation implies the surgical exposure of all fracture components (metaphyseal and articular), usually through a more extensive surgical approach. This is indicated in the following situations: (1) irreducible extra-articular bending fractures of the metaphysis, (2) shearing marginal fractures of the joint surface, (3) irreducible intra-articular fractures, (4) radiocarpal fracture-dislocations, (5) early loss of frac-

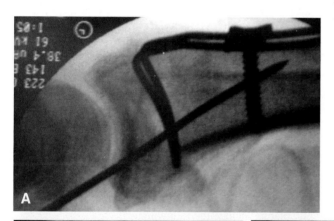

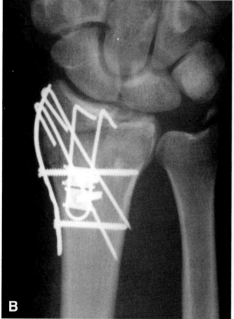

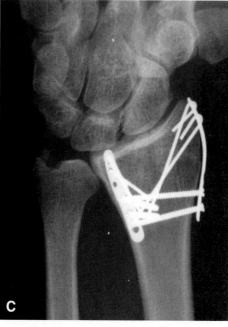

FIGURE 16-39. A, Intraoperative fluoroscopy demonstrating subchondral support for the articular surface and fixation of the comminuted dorsal cortex with a dorsal wireform implant. **B,** Posteroanterior view of wireform implant used to secure shear type fracture of the articular surface. **C,** A dorsal 2.0-mm miniplate used to secure an unstable dorsal-ulnar corner fragment. Note all dorsal implants are supplemented with a radial column implant placed in an orthogonal (90-90) relationship.

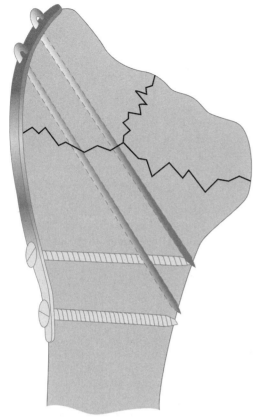

FIGURE 16-40. A 2.0-mm radial pin-plate incorporates 0.045-inch Kirschner wires and two bicortical screws in a tension-band configuration to capture unstable radial styloid fracture fragments.

ture reduction or "nascent malunions" (articular or metaphyseal), (6) fractures associated with carpal injury or soft tissue lesions (nerves, vessels, tendons, or compartment syndrome), and (7) distal radial fractures associated with ipsilateral fractures of the forearm and elbow.

The choice of surgical approach depends on the location and direction of displacement of the fracture fragments. Thus, dorsally or radially displaced fractures have been classically approached through dorsal incisions, whereas volarly displaced fractures (Smith's and reversed Barton's) are approached through palmar exposures. There has been increased interest in the management of dorsally displaced extra- and intra-articular fractures with volar plate fixation, in an attempt to decrease the incidence of extensor tendon irritation associated with dorsally applied implants.[296] Palmar incisions are also appropriate for primary repair of a torn wrist capsule in radiocarpal fracture-dislocations and whenever primary median nerve decompression or flexor compartment fasciotomy is indicated. On the rare occasion when palmar and dorsal articular fragment displacement is present, a combined dorsal and volar exposure may also be used.

Dorsal Plate Fixation

Although overall satisfactory outcomes have been reported with dorsal plating systems, the incidence of extensor tendon complications including irritation, synovitis attrition, and rupture due to direct contact of these structures with dorsal plates is not negligible.[13,222,297,298] To prevent these problems, the use of a retinaculum flap to cover the implant has been recommended but may not always prevent complications.[299]

If a single dorsal plate is used to stabilize an unstable distal radius fracture, the authors highly recommend that the surgeons inform the patient of the possibility of implant removal and attempt to use a retinacular flap or other soft tissue to cover the implant distally. The ulnarly based retinacular flap is begun just radial to the second compartment and elevated to expose the extensor pollicis longus and the radial half of the fourth compartment. After application of the plate, part of the implant comes to lie underneath the fourth compartment and the rest under the second and third compartments. During closure, the retinacular flap is used to cover the plate radially and the extensor pollicis longus tendon is primarily transposed to a subcutaneous position.

When performing conventional dorsal plate fixation of the distal radius, use of autogenous iliac bone graft or an appropriate structural bone graft substitute for the metaphyseal and subchondral defects is important. Bone grafting provides mechanical internal support (buttress effect) for small cartilage-bearing fragments, accelerates bone healing, and provides osteogenic potential to a bone that has been at least partially stripped from the overlying soft tissues. Bone grafting biologically compensates for the relatively extensive exposure required for application of the plate. If fixed angle devices with subchondral buttressing are used, the need of bone grafting is considerably reduced because the chances of secondary displacement of articular fragments are lessened.

Volar Plate Fixation

Regardless of the displacement of the distal fragment (dorsal, volar, radial), volar plating of extra-articular fractures is an effective fixation method that may reduce some of the soft tissue complications associated with dorsal plating.[291,293] The advantages of the palmar exposure and volar plating include the following:

- The simplicity of reduction of dorsally displaced fractures is beneficial because the volar cortex is usually disrupted by a simple transverse fracture line.
- Anatomic reduction of the volar cortex facilitates restoration of radial length, ulnar inclination, and volar tilt.
- The avoidance of additional surgical dissection in the dorsally comminuted area and the maintenance of the anatomical integrity of extensor tendon sheaths, periosteum, and dorsal retinaculum help to preserve the vascular supply of the dorsal fragments.
- Because the volar anatomy of the wrist has a greater cross-sectional space and the implant is separated from the flexor tendons by the pronator quadratus, the incidence of flexor tendon complications is lessened.
- When stabilized with a fixed angle internal fixation device that employs subchondral pegs or screws, control of shortening and secondary displacement of articular fragments is improved and the need for bone grafting is reduced (Fig. 16-41).

Fractures are exposed through the distal part of the Henry approach between the flexor carpi radialis and radial artery

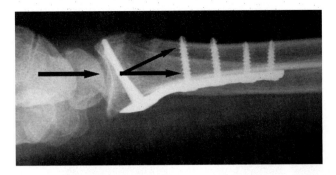

FIGURE 16-41. Ideal positioning of a volar fixed angle plate. Notice subchondral positioning of the distal fixed angle pegs, by virtue of which axial loading is transmitted to the pegs and the volar plate to the radial shaft. The dorsal comminuted area has not been grafted in this case.

through an 8- to 9-cm longitudinal incision directly over the distal course of the flexor carpi radialis tendon (the FCR approach). The virtual space beneath the flexor tendons is developed and the flexor carpi radialis and flexor tendons are retracted ulnarly, thus protecting the median nerve. The radial artery and veins are retracted radially and an "L"-shaped incision in the most radial attachment of the pronator quadratus is then performed and elevated from the volar aspect of the radius and retracted ulnarly. Reduction of dorsally displaced extra-articular fractures is then obtained by disimpacting the volar cortex of the distal fragment with hyperextension of the wrist over a rolled towel, using a small periosteal elevator as a lever, and then flexing the wrist to obtain an anatomic reduction of the volar cortex. While the fracture is temporarily fixed with an oblique Kirschner wire inserted percutaneously through the radial styloid into the proximal fragment, a fixed angle volar plate for dorsally displaced fractures is applied (Fig. 16-42).

The plate is applied to the volar aspect of the radius, and its position is monitored with fluoroscopy. A centrally positioned screw in the oval hole of the shaft is inserted to permit distal or proximal displacement of the plate for ideal placement of the distal edge of the plate. Distal fixation is obtained inserting "fixed angle" smooth pins or screws that are screwed to the transverse part of the plate. Precise drilling with special drill guides that are screwed to the distal holes is mandatory when using fixed angle devices to guarantee perfect engagement of the threaded heads on the plate. A "facet" lateral fluoroscopic view is performed by directing the fluoroscopic beam 20 to 30 degrees distal-to-proximal for optimal visualization of the drill bit for peg or screw placement in the most distal subchondral position. This is particularly important when dealing with osteoporotic bone, because subchondral buttressing will effectively control fracture settling, provided that the pegs are placed immediately below the subchondral plate. The subchondral plate retains greater loading capacity than does the soft osteopenic cancellous bone of the metaphyseal area. After completion of the shaft fixation with self-tapping screws, the implant is covered by suturing the pronator quadratus to the edge of the brachioradialis, and the wound is closed over suction drainage. A plaster splint is worn until suture removal, followed by a removable wrist brace for comfort. Patients are encouraged to mobilize their wrist actively, and functional use of the hand is permitted for light activities. For elderly patients with osteoporotic bone, the postoperative regimen is judged according to the purchase of the implants in bone during surgery. If insufficient screw purchase is present, a light forearm cast is applied after suture removal for a total of 5 weeks after surgery.

CRITICAL POINTS: VOLAR FIXED ANGLE PLATE FIXATION

INDICATIONS

- Extra-articular fractures of the distal radius (including osteoporotic bone)
- Nascent and established distal radius malunion
- Intra-articular fracture

TECHNICAL POINTS

- Make longitudinal incision along the flexor carpi radialis tendon.
- Expose the pronator quadratus between the flexor carpi radialis and the radial artery.
- Detach pronator quadratus with an "L"-shaped incision.
- Reduce fracture by disimpacting the volar cortex.
- Provide temporary fracture fixation with oblique Kirschner wire inserted through radial styloid.
- Apply plate volarly and fix to shaft through oval hole.
- Determine ideal plate position with fluoroscopy.
- Insert fixed-angle smooth pins in subchondral position.
- Use facet lateral fluoroscopic view to control drilling and pin insertion.
- Complete fixation of the plate to the shaft.

For malunions and irreducible intra-articular fractures an extended FCR approach is recommended:

- Tenotomy of the brachioradialis tendon.
- Release the first dorsal compartment.
- Pronation of the proximal fragment is optional.

POSTOPERATIVE CARE

- Apply palmar splint for 14 days, until suture removal.
- If functional after treatment, begin strengthening exercises.
- Evaluate radiographically 4 to 6 weeks postoperatively.

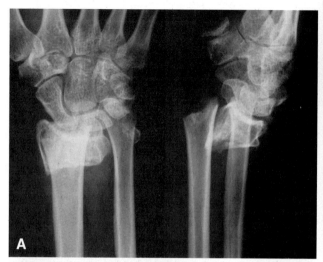

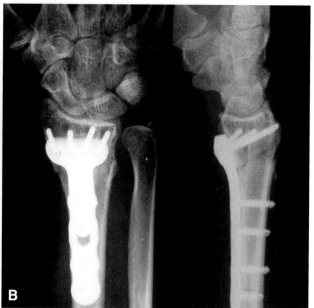

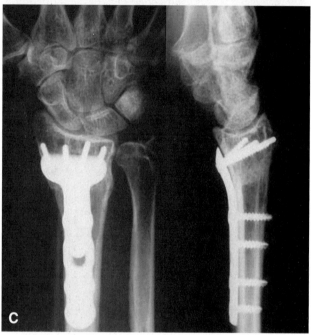

FIGURE 16-42. **A,** Radiographs of a severely displaced irreducible extra-articular fracture of the distal radius in a young woman. **B,** Postoperative radiographs after open reduction and internal fixation with a fixed-angle volar plate. Notice that the dorsal comminuted area has not been grafted. **C,** Radiographs 1 year after injury showing an anatomic result and no evidence of shortening. *Continued*

COMMON FRACTURE VARIANTS

The basic feature common to *shearing marginal fractures of the joint surface* is that a portion of the metaphyseal and epiphyseal areas of the distal radius is intact and in continuity with the unaffected area of the joint surface. The ultimate prognosis of these fractures is good because the displaced articular fragment can be exactly reduced and solidly fixed to the intact distal column of the radius. Furthermore, fractures with a distinct shearing component usually occur in young adults, whose firm cancellous bone offers ideal holding power for internal fixation material.

Fractures of the radial styloid are ideally treated by closed manipulation and percutaneous pinning. However, if anatomic reduction cannot be accomplished because of interposed comminuted joint fragments, open reduction is

performed through a dorsoradial approach. Care must be taken to protect the superficial radial nerve, the radial artery, and the extensor pollicis tendon at the anatomic snuff-box level. The fragment is secured with either Kirschner wires, a pin plate (Fig. 16-43), or a cannulated lag screw (Fig. 16-44). Perilunate carpal disruption may be associated with fractures of the radial styloid, especially when the fragment is small, but more commonly this fragment dislocates with the intact carpus attached to the radial collateral and radiocapitate ligaments. It is frequently associated with a shearing fracture of the dorsal rim of the radius. If the radial styloid fragment shows major proximal and radial displacement and the fracture line enters the joint at the level of the ridge between the scaphoid and lunate fossae, there is a strong possibility of an associated tear of the scapholunate ligament. The scaphoid displaces proximally with the radial

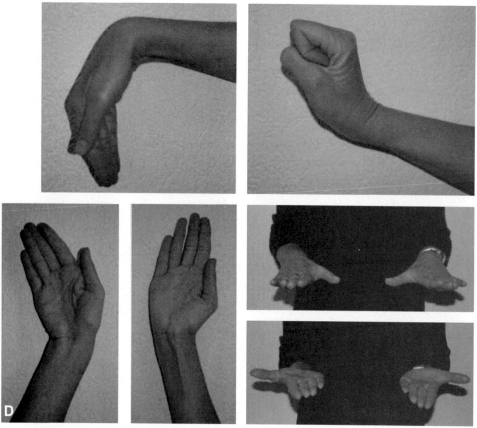

FIGURE 16-42—cont'd. D, The radiographic result correlates with an excellent function of the wrist.

fragment, whereas the lunate remains in its anatomic position. In these instances, careful fluoroscopic or arthroscopic assessment of the scapholunate junction after reduction is imperative. Whenever open reduction is performed, direct inspection of the scapholunate ligament through a limited dorsal arthrotomy is recommended.

Isolated dorsal shearing fractures (dorsal Barton's fractures) are rare but can be stabilized by buttress plate or dorsal buttress wireform fixation, with functional aftercare

started 2 or 3 weeks postoperatively. An alternative method would be the use of an external fixator with the wrist in slight palmar flexion to provide tension on the dorsal radiocarpal ligaments to hold the dorsal fragment in place.

The combination of a *dorsal marginal fracture together with a radial styloid fracture* occurs much more frequently. The intact volar ulnar aspect of the joint surface is clearly seen on the lateral radiograph (Fig. 16-45), and these fractures are commonly misdiagnosed as Colles' fractures

Type II shearing fracture (radial styloid)

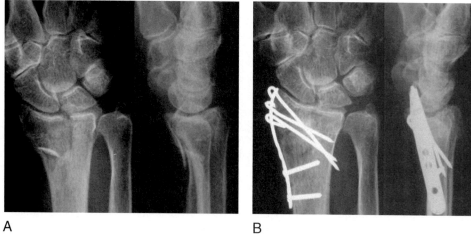

A   B

FIGURE 16-43. A, Intra-articular shearing fracture of the radial styloid with volar displacement in a 66-year-old woman. **B,** Anatomic result 7 months after fixation with a radial pin-plate.

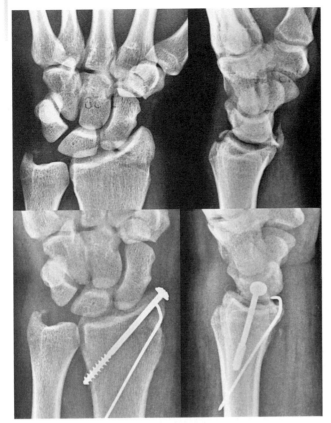

FIGURE 16-44. Radial styloid fracture associated with a displaced intra-articular fragment affecting the palmar radial aspect of the joint margin. Open reduction and anatomic reduction of both fragments were achieved through a radial approach.

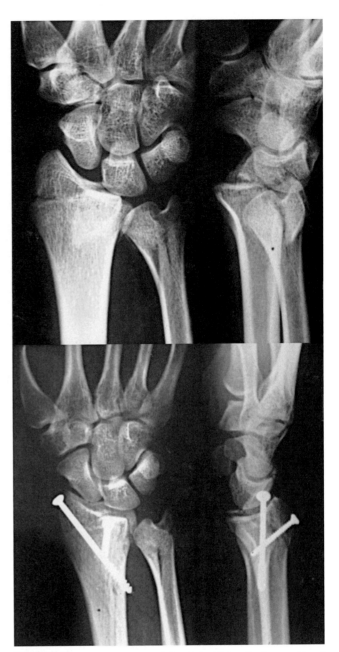

FIGURE 16-45. Combined radial styloid and dorsal shearing fracture (dorsal Barton's) in a 23-year-old woman. Notice the intact volar ulnar portion of the joint surface in the lateral view. Both fragments were securely stabilized with lag screws, which permitted early wrist motion after suture removal.

because the two are similar in appearance. If closed manipulation and percutaneous pinning fail to provide anatomic congruity of the joint surface, open reduction should be carried out. These fractures are exposed through a dorsal longitudinal approach between the second and fourth compartments, with care taken to elevate and mobilize the extensor pollicis longus tendon. First, the radial styloid fragment is carefully reduced, checked for proper realignment at the metaphyseal level, and pinned obliquely to the proximal fragment. Then the dorsal lip fragment is reduced against the scaphoid and lunate, and dorsal subluxation of the carpus is corrected. Intra-articular congruity is visualized directly via a dorsal transverse arthrotomy or with the image intensifier. Articular fragments can then be pinned to the intact volar ulnar corner of the radius. Depending on the size of the dorsal rim fracture, either small "T" or "L" plates or screws may be used for fixation (see Fig. 16-45). Subchondral cancellous bone defects should be grafted with cancellous bone chips taken from the iliac crest.

Fractures of the volar margin of the radius (volar Barton's fractures) are much more common than dorsal rim fractures and are usually caused by a massive hyperextension injury of the wrist joint or through axial compression of the slightly volarly flexed hand. The obliquity of the fracture line and loss of palmar support of the carpus make these fractures inherently unstable. Shortening and palmar displacement of the fragment are always associated with volar subluxation of the carpus. This fracture may affect only the most radial aspect of the palmar articular surface, or it may extend ulnarly into the sigmoid notch. Depending on the quality of bone and the severity of the impact, a variable amount of comminution of the volar fragment may be present. In these cases, lateral tomograms or CT scans of the wrist are helpful in identifying small impacted articular fragments. If the volar lip fragment and the carpus are severely displaced palmarly and radially, the fracture is frequently associated with avulsion of the ulnar styloid or a tear in the TFCC. The widely accepted method of treatment is open reduction and internal fixation by means of a volar buttressing plate.* This method restores articular congruity, and the buttressing effect of the plate that supports the fragment in the reduced position closes the articular gap by direct compression of the fragment against the intact dorsal column of the radius. Fragment-specific fixation with a volar buttress wireform implant is also an acceptable alternative for these unstable fracture fragments.

The fracture can be exposed between the flexor carpi radialis tendon and the radial artery, with radial detachment of the pronator quadratus muscle.[95,124] Other authors[118] prefer the interval between the ulnar artery and nerve and the common flexor tendons, with extension of the incision distally into the palm and primary carpal tunnel release. In our experience, the approach between the radial artery and the flexor carpi radialis provides enough exposure for the treatment of most volar marginal fractures.[141] In the event of primary median nerve symptoms associated with a volar Barton's fracture, carpal tunnel release is performed through a separate small incision because extension of the volar radial approach into the palm can damage the palmar cutaneous branch of the median nerve. After careful exposure of the fracture surface and cleaning out of the fracture hematoma, reduction is obtained by hyperextending the wrist over a rolled towel with the forearm in maximal supination. Fracture reduction can be maintained temporarily with Kirschner wires, but it must be ensured that their point of entry will not jeopardize the application of a small "T" plate. The plate is pre-bent in such a way that there is still a small space between the midportion of the plate and the area just proximal to the fracture site. After checking the definitive position of the plate, the most proximal screw is inserted. Introduction of the second screw firmly compresses the plate against the radial shaft and provides a buttress effect over the distal fragment (Fig. 16-46). The most common pitfall when dealing with volar marginal fractures is failure to stabilize all the fracture components, including the most ulnar volar corner (lunate facet fragment). Care has to be taken to buttress this fragment under the most ulnar edge of the plate, otherwise secondary displacement with volar subluxation of the entire carpus is inevitable (Fig. 16-47).

The buttressing effect of the plate without additional screw fixation through the distal part of the plate may suffice for a single fragment of the volar lip (Fig 16-48). If absolute stability is not achieved with the buttress plate alone, two or three screws may be inserted through the distal holes. After careful hemostasis, the pronator quadratus is reattached over suction drainage. A volar plaster splint with the wrist in neutral position is worn for 14 days, followed by a removable wrist splint for about 2 weeks. The patient is encouraged to use the hand for activities of daily living, but heavy manual work or sports are forbidden for 5 to 6 weeks after surgery, at which time fracture healing is complete.

COMPLEX DISTAL RADIAL FRACTURES

In the group of complex distal radial fractures are those fractures that present a difficult therapeutic challenge because of one or more of the following factors:

- The severity of articular disruption
- An increasing amount of metaphyseal comminution
- Inherent instability and irreducibility
- Segmental bone loss in the distal part of the forearm (gunshot wound, open wounds, crush injuries)
- Association with carpal disruption
- Presence of concomitant ipsilateral fracture and/or dislocation in the upper extremity

These fractures fall into types III, IV, and V of our classification and are injuries that by virtue of their complexity are currently managed by hand or upper extremity specialists. We firmly believe, however, that the choice of skeletal fixation method must be open to a wide range of flexibility and should be adapted to the particular fracture pattern characteristics and the local soft tissue condition. In general, these fracture types will require a combination of (1) longitudinal traction or multiplanar ligamentotaxis for reduction of the metaphyseal fracture, (2) open reduction for restoration of joint congruity, (3) bone grafting of the defect, and (4) some form of internal fixation. Most of these fractures can be treated with a combination of an external fixator, bone grafting, and additional Kirschner wire fixation, as described on page 667. New implant technology, including the fixed-angle devices and fragment-specific fixation techniques described earlier, have enabled stable internal fixation of these complex injuries and may reduce the need for combined internal and external fixation. The use of fixed angle plate designs avoids screw loosening in the distal fragment owing to a "toggling effect" and thus reduces the danger of secondary displacement. Subchondral placement of smooth pegs is useful to buttress small articular fragments and successfully control shortening and angular displacement, especially in osteoporotic bone. Use of these devices to this point has been limited with no distinct advantage over other available methods.

Management of complex articular fractures through a traditional dorsal approach and dorsal single or double plate fixation enables reduction of the radial styloid, central joint impaction, proximal carpal row, and the dorsal die-punch fragment.[13,25,222,300-302] Although it may be utilized in four-part fractures with a nondisplaced volar-ulnar fragment, the risk of iatrogenic displacement is relatively high. The major disadvantage of the dorsal exposure is its inability to permit direct control and manipulation of the volar-ulnar fragment, which is the *keystone* of the distal radial articular surface. Failure to restore the anatomy of the volar-ulnar corner, the concavity of the lunate fossa, and the corresponding area of the sigmoid notch gravely compromises both the radiocarpal and DRUJ. Furthermore, in spite of newer low profile designs, implants placed under the extensor tendons have a substantial incidence of irritation, attrition tendonitis, and late tendon rupture.

Reduction and fixation of compression fractures of the articular surface through a volar approach is also possible.[303] This implies the use of an extended Henry approach, including a release of the radial septum (brachioradialis insertion and palmar sheath of the first extensor compartment), to facilitate reduction of the radial styloid fragment. To visualize the dorsal die-punch and centrally impacted fragments through the fracture plane (intrafocal exposure), the proximal shaft fragment must be pronated with a bone clamp.

*See references 65, 81, 84, 95, 102, 141, 148, 207, 249, and 250.

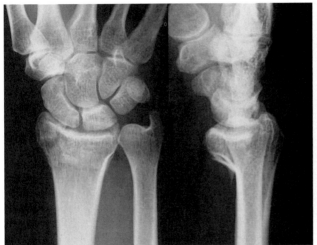

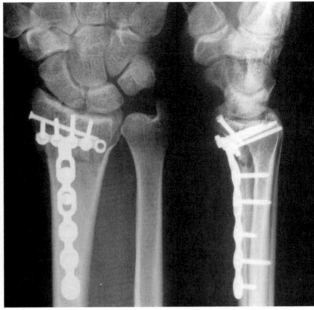

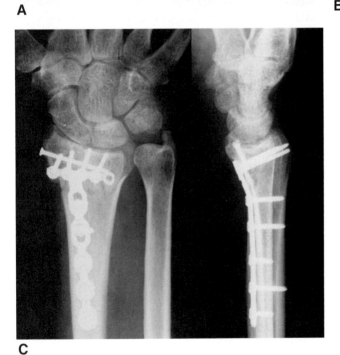

FIGURE 16-46. A, Radiographs of a reversed Barton fracture with comminuted styloid fragment. **B,** Postoperative radiographs after fixation with a volar fixed angle T-plate. Notice additional screw fixation of the radial styloid fragment. **C,** Six months after injury fracture healed in adequate position with well-maintained joint space.

Having pronated the proximal fragment "out of the way," free access to the articular fragments is achieved, and these fragments can be manipulated into a reduced position against the proximal carpal row. Thereafter the proximal fragment is supinated back in place and the fracture fixed with a volar "T"-shaped fixed-angle plate. The volar and dorsal ulnar fragments are stabilized with a screw through the plate. The major advantage of this technique is the preservation of the extensor tendon sleeve and reduction in related tendon complications. Furthermore, a single implant controls stability of both the radial and intermediate columns and provides subchondral buttressing beneath the articular fragments. Indirect reduction of the dorsal

comminuted area and preservation of vascularity accounts for the rapid healing of the dorsal cortex, therefore reducing the need of bone grafting significantly.

Finally, for the more *complex fracture patterns,* such as type IV radiocarpal fracture dislocation[304] and type V or C$_{3-3}$ fractures (combined injuries, high energy trauma), no single implant or technique is appropriate to solve all the components of the fracture and the soft tissue injuries. Usually a combined dorsal and volar exposure with compartment and median nerve release, autologous cancellous bone grafting of the metaphyseal defect, and a combination of external and internal or fragment-specific fixation is required (Fig. 16-49).

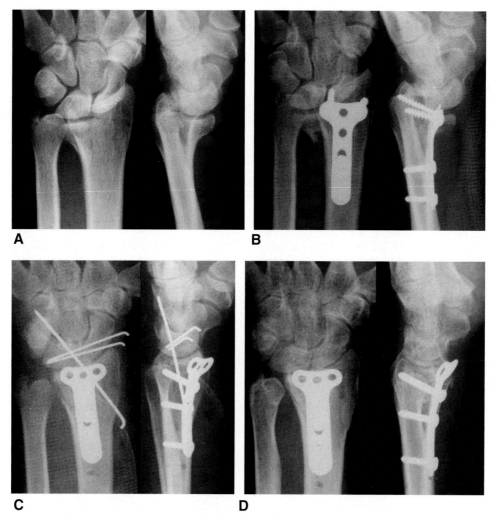

FIGURE 16-47. **A,** Radiographs of a Barton fracture with subluxation of the carpus. **B,** The volar ulnar fragment has not been securely fixed by the T-plate, resulting in further proximal and volar displacement of the ulnar volar fragment and the whole carpus. **C,** Radiographs after reoperation during which a nondiagnosed nondissociative scapholunate dissociation was found. The ulnar volar fragment is buttressed with the T-plate and Kirschner wire fixation to control volar displacement of the carpus, and stabilization of the scapholunate injury was provided with two additional Kirschner wires. **D,** Radiographic appearance of the wrist 1.2 years after reoperation.

ASSOCIATED INJURIES

Distal radius fractures are usually the result of significant trauma to the entire upper extremity.* Because of this, when evaluating a patient with an acute distal radius fracture or a patient with a problem after a distal radial fracture, a complete examination of the entire upper extremity should always be undertaken. One must not overlook associated injuries such as shoulder dislocation, elbow fracture or dislocation, carpal or metacarpal fracture, median nerve injury, or vascular injury.† The associated injuries often lead to more problems than the distal radius fracture itself. Once the other problems have been dealt with, the physician's attention may be directed to the distal radius fracture.

Open Fractures

Most fractures of the distal radius are closed injuries, but we consider any fracture that communicates with the external environment to be an open fracture. The associated skin injury may be massive, or it may be a pinpoint, with the only real indication that the wound communicates with the fracture being a small amount of fatty fluid exuding from the wound. All open fractures should be treated as surgical emergencies. Our treatment plan for open distal radius fractures calls for clinical and radiologic evaluation in the emergency department followed by wound culture. Appropriate intravenous antibiotics are then begun while the patient is prepped for the operating room. As soon as possible, the patient is transported to the operating room, where a general or regional anesthetic is administered. The open wound is enlarged, the wound margins and fracture margins débrided, and the wound irrigated with abundant quantities of saline solution. The question of immobilizing the fracture itself is

*See references 5, 80, 82, 128, 132, 167, 239, 255, 263, and 279.

†See references 13, 17, 19, 48, 59, 68, 122, 140, 147, 171, 199, 209, and 251.

then dealt with. If the wound has been suitably cleaned and the fracture is unstable, we prefer to stabilize the fracture with a plate or a combination of internal fixation with Kirschner wires and an external fixator. If the fracture is stable, the wound is simply closed and the fracture immobilized in a cast. If the wound cannot be suitably cleaned or if the wound has been open for more than 12 hours, the wound is left open and closed secondarily at 48 hours, either directly or with a split-thickness skin graft, with definitive bone care left until the wound has healed.

Associated Median Nerve Injury

Patients with acute distal radial fractures quite frequently have neurovascular compromise (i.e., median nerve symptoms) to a greater or lesser extent. Our treatment plan for such individuals calls for closed reduction of the fracture in the emergency department. If satisfactory reduction is obtained, the nerve compression syndrome is treated with observation alone. In most instances, if the reduction can be maintained, the nerve compression syndrome will resolve or at least improve substantially over the subsequent 24 to 48 hours. If the neurologic symptoms worsen or show little or no sign of improvement over the first 24 to 48 hours after reduction or if the reduction cannot be obtained or maintained in the presence of median nerve compression, we favor early open reduction, carpal tunnel release, and, if necessary, skeletal stabilization of the fracture. Carpal tunnel release is not routinely performed at the time of open reduction of a distal radius fracture unless significant median nerve symptoms were present preoperatively.

Associated DRUJ Lesions

The most common cause of residual disability after fractures of the distal radius continues to be the DRUJ. Therefore this

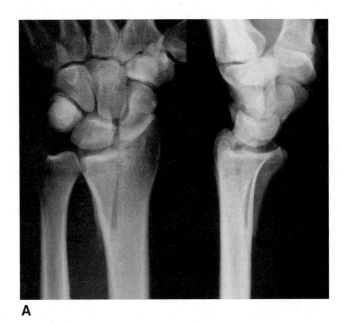

A

Postop x-rays

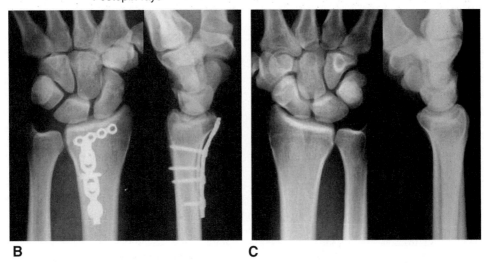

B   **C**

FIGURE 16-48. **A,** Radiographs of an isolated volar shearing fracture of the radiolunate facet. **B** and **C,** Postoperative and comparative radiographs of both wrists showing anatomic reduction of the fracture stabilized with a contoured T-plate and a separate lag screw. *Continued*

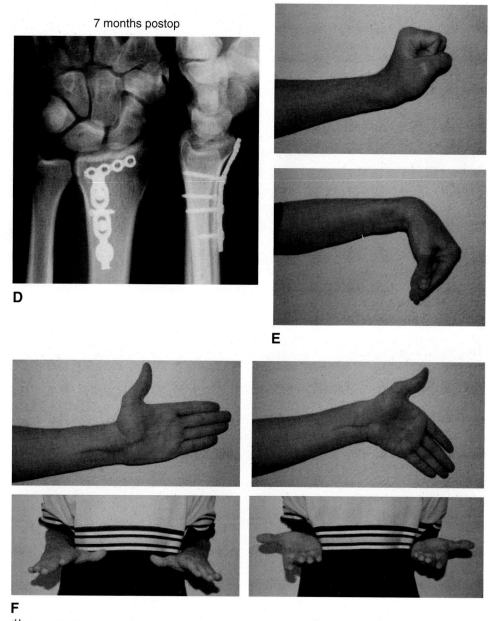

FIGURE 16-48—cont'd. D and **E,** Six months after injury, the fracture has healed in anatomic position with free range of flexion-extension. **F,** Radioulnar deviation and forearm rotation.

joint deserves as thorough an evaluation in the acute stage as the distal radial fracture itself to address these injuries at an early stage and achieve anatomic restoration.

To assess the involvement of the DRUJ in acute distal radial fractures, the following issues should be analyzed: intra-articular incongruity (sigmoid notch, ulnar head), subluxation caused by inadequate reduction of the radius, TFCC tears, capsular soft tissue injury, and ulnar styloid avulsion with DRUJ subluxation in spite of adequate restoration of the anatomy of the distal radius. Acute ulnocarpal abutment caused by massive initial shortening must also be assessed. Some element of DRUJ instability is present in every displaced radius fracture. The key to a successful result depends on exact restoration of the anatomic relationships of the joint (bone, articular surfaces, ligaments), which must be maintained during the first 6 weeks after injury.

The associated DRUJ lesions are classified into three types depending on the stability of the DRUJ after the distal radius fracture has been reduced and stabilized. This implies that the anatomic relationships of the sigmoid notch to the ulnar head have been reestablished through adequate restoration of radial length and sagittal and frontal tilt of the distal fragment (see Fig. 16-17B).

Type I includes *stable* DRUJ lesions, which means that (1) the joint is clinically stable and the radiograph shows articular congruity (these lesions would include minimally displaced avulsion fractures of the tip of the ulnar styloid and stable fractures of the neck of the ulna) and (2) the primary stabilizers of the TFCC and capsular ligament are intact or minimally disrupted.

Type II consists of *unstable* DRUJ lesions with (1) clinical and radiographic evidence of subluxation and/or

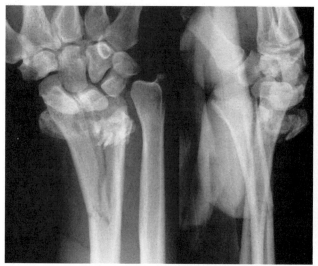

A

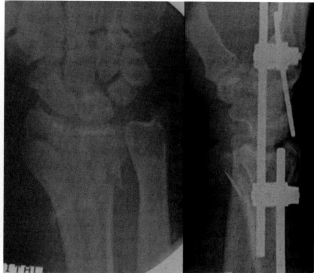

B Initial closed reduction, external fixation and open management of transverse wound over the ulnar head. Additional sensory ulnar nerve neurapraxia was present.

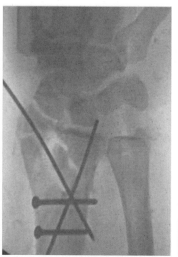
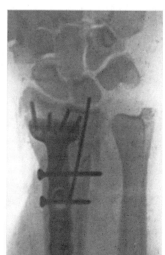
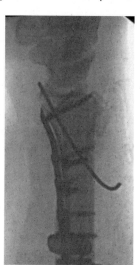

C

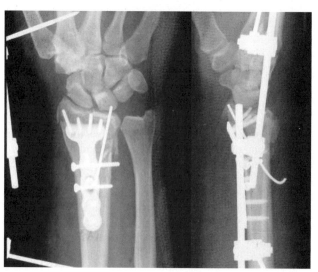

D

FIGURE 16-49. **A,** Radiographs of a severely displaced type V complex distal radial fracture with intra-articular and metaphyseal comminution. **B,** Partial insufficient reduction obtained with application of an external fixator. **C,** Intraoperative fluoroscopic views showing reconstruction of the metaphyseal fracture with two transverse lag screws, provisional fixation of the radial and ulnar fragments with Kirschner wires, and application of a volar fixed angle device (DVR plate). An oblique from palmar to dorsal inserted Kirschner wire has been applied to the volar ulnar fragment. **D,** Postoperative radiographs showing an acceptable reduction and restoration of radial length. The fixator was maintained for 3 weeks. *Continued*

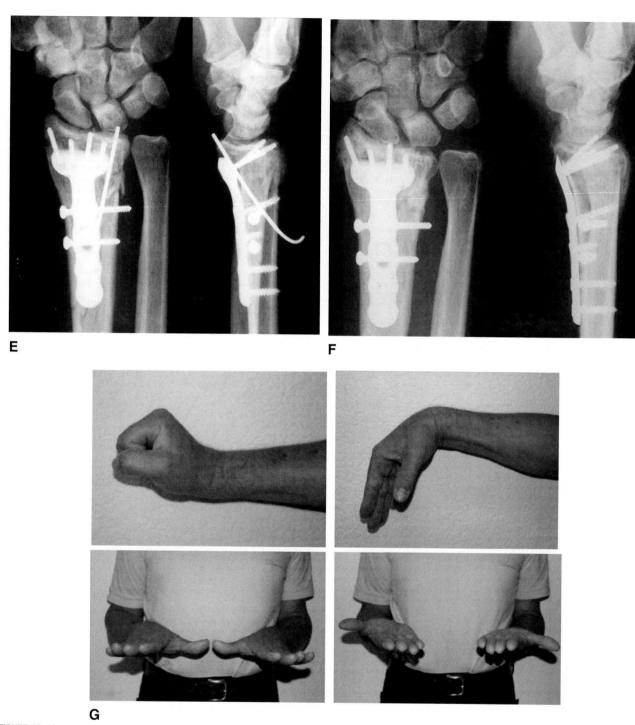

E

F

G

FIGURE 16-49—cont'd. **E,** Fracture healed at 6 weeks after surgery. Notice healing of the dorsal and ulnar comminuted area. At this time the additional Kirschner wire was removed. **F,** Radiographs at 1 year show a good restoration of the joint surface and a well-remodeled distal radius. **G,** Patient restored an adequate arc of flexion and extension and free forearm rotation.

dislocation of the ulnar head because of a massive tear of the TFCC and/or secondary DRUJ stabilizers or (2) an avulsion fracture of the base of the ulnar styloid.

Type III lesions are *potentially unstable* lesions caused by skeletal disruption of the joint surface at the sigmoid notch (four-part fracture of the distal radius) or the ulnar head. In certain instances, combined lesions such as a fracture of the ulnar styloid and a fracture of the sigmoid notch may occur simultaneously.

This classification offers the possibility of assessment of the lesion by clinical examination and simple radiographs of the wrist. If arthroscopic evaluation is performed, more accurate documentation of TFCC ruptures may be obtained by using the classification system devised by Palmer.[204]

Class I lesions are traumatic tears of the TFCC according to this classification. Type A lesions have a central perforation, type B lesions involve peripheral ulnar tears, type C lesions are distal tears, and type D lesions are radial tears of the TFCC from the radius (along the sigmoid notch).

Treatment Options for DRUJ Lesions

As outlined in Figure 16-17B, three treatment options are possible: (1) early mobilization, (2) closed treatment and cast immobilization with or without radioulnar pinning, and (3) operative management, including open and arthroscopic techniques. *Functional aftercare* with early active forearm rotation exercises and no additional external support is recommended for type I stable injuries and also for those fractures of the distal end of the ulna that have been rigidly fixed with plates and in which the screws have adequate holding power. Early motion is also recommended for type III comminuted fractures of the ulnar head to allow for fracture remodeling. *Closed treatment* includes careful physical assessment of DRUJ disruption after reduction and stabilization of the radius fracture. Anatomic reduction of the radius usually results in relocation of the ulnar head in the sigmoid notch, as in Galeazzi fractures of the distal shaft. Dislocation of the DRUJ requires disruption of at least one margin of the TFCC, the ulnar insertion being more common than detachments from the radius. Most DRUJ dislocations are successfully treated by 6 weeks of cast immobilization with the forearm in neutral rotation.[271] However, a grossly unstable DRUJ dislocation may require reduction in 45 degrees of supination or percutaneous transfixation of the ulna to the radial shaft with dual 0.062-inch Kirschner wires. The Kirschner wires are placed just proximal to the joint so that the articular cartilage is not violated. It is helpful to leave the tip of the wires protruding through bone on both the radial and ulnar ends, in case wire breakage occurs in the interosseous space.

Surgical intervention is often required for type II unstable DRUJ lesions. When the ulnar styloid fragment is avulsed at the base or is significantly displaced in association with an unstable DRUJ, open reduction and internal fixation should be considered. The joint is exposed between the extensor digiti quinti and the extensor carpi ulnaris to view the styloid fragment. Care is taken to prevent injury to the dorsal sensory branch of the ulnar nerve. Tension band or interosseous wiring is the technique most frequently used because the ulnar styloid fragment is usually too small for a compression screw. A 24-gauge wire is passed either around or preferably through the styloid fragment and through the ulna at the axilla of the shaft and the articular surface and tied with the forearm in neutral rotation. Alternatively, the fragment is stabilized with two Kirschner wires and a tension band wire passed proximally through the ulnar shaft (Fig. 16-50). It is important to preserve or reconstruct the tendon sheath of the extensor carpi ulnaris. The forearm is immobilized in neutral rotation for 6 weeks. With the advent of the ultra-thin "pin plates," basilar styloid fractures can be rigidly fixed with two Kirschner wires and a contoured ulnar pin plate to the ulnar shaft. This may be performed through a 3-cm incision between the flexor carpi ulnaris and extensor carpi ulnaris tendons with minimal additional soft tissue disruption (Fig. 16-51). Immediate stability of the

DRUJ is restored, and protective forearm rotation can be initiated within 7 to 10 days of surgery.

Alternatively, depending on the surgeon's skill, TFCC lesions may also be treated with arthroscopic repair by using 2-0 PDS sutures[107] that are tied over the floor of the extensor carpi ulnaris sheath with the forearm in supination. Arthroscopy also provides information regarding indications for fixation of the ulnar styloid fragment. The articular disc is palpated when an ulnar styloid fragment is present. The disc should be taut and have a trampoline effect when palpated. When the articular disc is taut by palpation, the ulnar styloid fragment does not need to be stabilized because the majority of the TFCC is still attached to the ulna. When the articular disc has lost its tension, a peripheral tear of the TFCC is suspected. Repair of the peripheral tear restores the tension of the TFCC and enhances stability of the DRUJ. Repair should include reapproximation of the ulnar styloid if it is displaced. Stabilization of the ulnar styloid fragment should also be considered when the articular disc is lax to palpation and a peripheral tear is not present. When DRUJ instability is associated with a dorsally displaced dorsoulnar fragment of the distal radius as in type III lesions, exact anatomic reduction of the sigmoid notch is imperative to restore stability. Associated TFCC lesions should be addressed simultaneously as described previously.

Associated Carpal Ligament Injuries

Carpal ligament disruption coexists with both intra-articular and extra-articular fractures of the distal radius. Certain fracture patterns, such as radiocarpal fracture-dislocations and severely displaced radial styloid fractures entering the ridge between the scaphoid and lunate fossae, have well-defined obligatory concomitant intrinsic or extrinsic ligament disruptions in the carpus. The incidence of associated carpal ligament disruption with fractures of the distal radius has been documented with both arthrographic[98,127] and arthroscopic[106,116,225,305] evaluation of the wrist. The incidence of scapholunate tears in conjunction with distal radius fractures is approximately 30% and for lunotriquetral tears it is approximately 15%.

Theories on the pathomechanics and the possible mechanism of injury of carpal ligament disruption in distal radial fractures have been analyzed and reported by Saffar[229] and by Mugdal and Hastings.[195] Tensile stresses in ulnar deviation after a fall on an outstretched hand would explain avulsion of the radial styloid and perilunate disruption of the intrinsic ligaments as formerly reproduced experimentally by Mayfield and coworkers.[176] Axial or compression loading associated with shearing fractures of the radial styloid occurs when the wrist is loaded in radial deviation and extension.[229] This produces a scapholunate tear, especially when the radial fracture enters the joint at the ridge between the lunate and scaphoid fossae (Fig. 16-52A). Similarly, impaction of the lunate in a die-punch fracture would produce a shearing stress at the scapholunate junction and a tear of the scapholunate ligament (see Fig. 16-52B).[92]

In fractures with severe shortening and complete DRUJ disruption, the head of the ulna impacts on the triquetrum while the scaphoid and lunate are driven proximally by axial

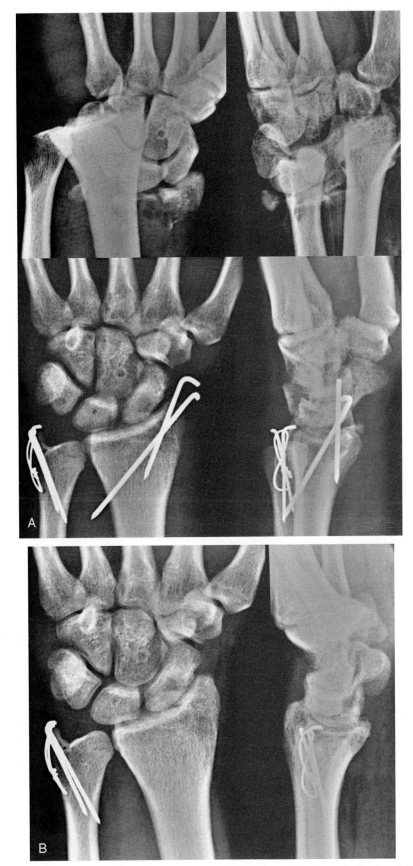

FIGURE 16-50. **A,** Severely displaced radiocarpal fracture-dislocation. After open reduction and Kirschner wire fixation of the radial styloid, the DRUJ was grossly unstable. The bony avulsion of the triangular fibrocartilage complex was treated with tension band wiring. **B,** Follow-up radiographs at 2 years show a congruent DRUJ.

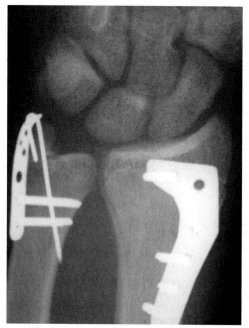

FIGURE 16-51. A 2.0-mm ulnar pin plate can be applied over a percutaneous Kirschner wire to rigidly fix unstable basilar ulnar styloid fractures with two proximal screws.

compression loading. This results in combined lunotriquetral and TFCC disruption (see Fig. 16-52C). Although certain fracture types have a distinct associated capsuloligamentous lesion, wrist arthroscopy could not provide a clear correlation between fracture patterns and the extent or location of intercarpal tears.[106,225] Dissociative lesions require aggressive operative treatment. Open repair of the lesion is recommended after reduction and fixation of the distal radial fracture. This includes reduction of carpal subluxation, restoration of normal alignment, Kirschner wire stabilization, and ligament repair using intraosseous suture

techniques. If external fixation is used for immobilization, care is taken to use the frame in a neutralization fashion to prevent carpal loading of the radial articular surface while simultaneously avoiding overdistraction and malalignment of the carpus. Arthroscopic pinning may be used alternatively,[106,306] especially for reducible lesions. Partial nondissociative lesions, on the other hand, may heal uneventfully in the period of immobilization required for consolidation of the distal radial fracture.

Authors' Preferred Method of Treatment: Displaced Fractures

A summary of the indications for our preferred methods is shown in Figure 16-17 on pages 654 and 655.

Elderly and Infirm Patients
In sedentary, ill, or inactive patients, we favor closed reduction and a sugar tong splint for 2 weeks followed by a short-arm cast for 3 weeks and then a removable splint for an additional 3 weeks (see Fig. 16-18). If the fracture settles and/or shortens in this group of patients, we do not recommend more aggressive treatment, but instead favor late reconstruction such as a distal ulna resection if the patient continues to be symptomatic.

COMPLICATIONS

Although it was once believed by many that all patients with distal radius fractures did relatively well, regardless of the treatment, it is now well recognized that distal radius fractures are associated with a high complication rate and

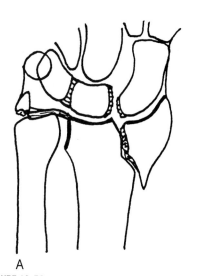
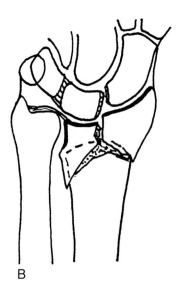
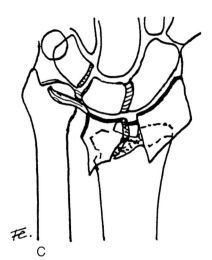

FIGURE 16-52. Mechanism of injury of intercarpal ligament disruption. **A,** Extension and radial deviation produce a proximally displaced shearing fracture of the radial styloid, scapholunate dissociation, and an avulsion fracture of the ulnar styloid. **B,** Axial compression with severe impaction of the lunate fossa accounts for shearing loading of the scapholunate junction and ligament tear at this level. **C,** Axial compression and ulnar deviation with severe radial shortening produce acute ulnocarpal abutment and disruption of the lunotriquetral and triangular ligaments.

frequently poor results. Fractures involving the radiocarpal or distal radioulnar articular surface are especially prone to complications.

Cooney and coworkers, in an excellent review of 565 fractures, found a complication rate of 31%.[54] Gartland and Werley, in reporting "surprisingly good results," found unsatisfactory results in 31.7% of their patients.[104] Bacorn and Kurtzke reported a series of 2132 cases of Colles' fracture recorded by the New York Compensation Board. Only 2.9% were judged to have no permanent disability, and the average disability regardless of age, adequacy of treatment, or severity of fracture was 24% permanent loss of function of the hand.[14]

The complications associated with Colles' fracture that result in these surprisingly high unsatisfactory results are persistent neuropathy, radiocarpal or radioulnar arthrosis, malposition/malunion, nonunion, tendon ruptures, reflex sympathetic dystrophy, finger stiffness, and Volkmann's ischemia.* An understanding that these problems exist and are relatively common sequelae of distal radial fractures should lead us to be more aggressive in the original care of such fractures.

Reflex Sympathetic Dystrophy

Although full-blown reflex sympathetic dystrophy is a relatively uncommon problem, milder variants are surprisingly common in conjunction with distal radius fractures. Early attention to patients with an inordinate amount of pain, finger stiffness, or paresthesias may prevent many of the problems of this serious complication. Early splinting or immobilization to alleviate pain, removal or splitting of a dressing or cast to relieve pressure, elevation of an edematous hand, and intensive hand therapy are frequently very helpful in preventing the development of full reflex sympathetic dystrophy.[143] Recognition and treatment of acute median nerve compression may also abort the development of dystrophy. For patients who do not respond to early local measures, sympathetic blocks, even while the cast is in place, should be considered (see Chapter 57).

Nonunion

Nonunions of distal radius fractures are extremely rare, but they do occur and are usually symptomatic.[117,141] In contrast, nonunions of ulnar styloid process fractures in conjunction with distal radius fractures are quite common and yet are rarely symptomatic.[70] Treatment of distal radius nonunions must be individualized and based on the patient's symptoms, functional deficit, and bony substance. Basically, however, one should strive to achieve union with rigid internal fixation and iliac crest bone grafting.[307] Symptomatic nonunions of the ulnar styloid are best treated with styloid excision unless the ulnar styloid fragment is quite large, in which case the fragment should be treated with open reduction and internal fixation.[120] If the styloid nonunion is accompanied by distal ulnar instability, the TFCC should be reattached to the fovea at the time of fragment excision or fixation.

Malunion

Reduction and maintenance of reduction of the fracture remain the single most important factors in the overall outcome of a distal radius fracture. Malunions of distal radius fractures, as one might expect, are quite common. Based on comments in the literature, one would not expect that many of these malunions would be symptomatic, but in our experience they are frequently found to cause significant symptoms. Malunions result in wrist pain (radiocarpal, radioulnar, and/or ulnocarpal), decreased range of motion, and/or midcarpal instability.[32,86,87,128,155,186,262] Recognition of associated carpal malalignment and DRUJ derangement is mandatory to decide whether additional procedures together with radial osteotomy are necessary to guarantee a good result. Assessment of carpal malalignment with malunited Colles' fractures includes the recognition of (1) dorsal subluxation of the entire carpus, (2) adaptive type I dorsiflexed intercalated segment instability or midcarpal flexion deformity that is *lax* and corrected by radial osteotomy (Fig. 16-53), and (3) a type II or *fixed* dorsiflexed intercalated segment instability malalignment, which does not improve after radial osteotomy and represents a chronic stage of scapholunate instability not diagnosed at the time of initial injury. Spontaneous realignment of an adaptive dorsiflexed intercalated segmental instability is demonstrated with a lateral radiograph of the wrist taken in the same amount of extension as the dorsal angulation of the distal radius.[89,308] Depending on whether the malunion is extra-articular, intra-articular (affecting both the radiocarpal and radioulnar joints), or complex (metaphyseal and articular deformity), post-traumatic wrist deformity can be corrected with extra-articular osteotomies, intra-articular osteotomies, or a combination of both. The decision to do a simultaneous procedure at the DRUJ depends on the amount of radial shortening and the presence of osteoarthritic changes or instability of the joint.[89] Usually instability and ulnocarpal impingement as a result of shortening, angulation, or malrotation of the distal end of the radius with no degenerative changes can be corrected by restoration of the radial deformity alone. Optimally, an osteotomy should be performed as soon as the soft tissues demonstrate an absence of trophic changes, radiographs reveal limited or no osteoporosis, and wrist mobility is adequate. Early correction provides easier radial and DRUJ realignment owing to the absence of soft tissue and capsular contractures and results in a considerable decrease of total disability and an earlier return to work.[42]

Operative Technique: Extra-articular Radial Osteotomy

The aims of radial osteotomy are to restore function and improve the appearance of the wrist by correcting the deformity at the level of the old fracture site. The osteotomy should reorient the joint surface to guarantee normal load distribution, reestablish the mechanical balance of the midcarpal joint, and restore the anatomic relationships of the DRUJ. Because radial shortening is a constant component of the deformity, both in malunited Colles' and Smith's

---

*See references 6, 10, 37, 40, 51, 53, 54, 70, 139, 153-155,165, 168, 170, 184, 188, 190-192, 198, 226, 227, 246, 256, 260, 262, 269, 270, 276, 278, 284, and 285.

Malunited Colles' fracture with Type 1 adaptive DISI

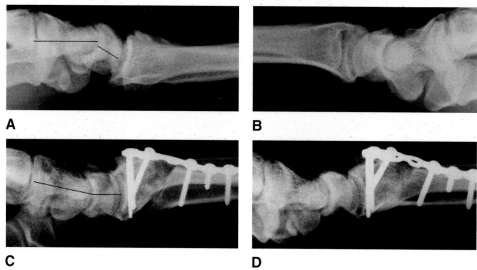

A **B**

C **D**

FIGURE 16-53. A, Type I adaptive DISI deformity of the carpus in a malunited Colles fracture. **B,** Comparative radiographs of the opposite wrist showing a normal alignment. **C,** Restoration of normal carpal alignment after radial osteotomy. **D,** Carpal alignment is maintained 1 year after osteotomy.

fractures, an opening wedge osteotomy that is transverse in the frontal plane and oblique (parallel to the joint surface) in the sagittal plane is used to permit radial lengthening. This osteotomy allows:

- Radial lengthening of up to 10 to 12 mm
- Correction of volar tilt in the sagittal plane
- Correction of ulnar tilt in the frontal plane
- Correction of rotational deformity in the horizontal plane

It is important that the osteotomy be parallel to the articular surface. If it is parallel to the long axis of the radius, a secondary deformity will be created when the osteotomy is opened (Fig 16-54B).

A corticocancellous bone graft from the iliac crest is cut to fit the bone defect created by the osteotomy. If a partial or complete resection of the distal end of the ulna is performed simultaneously, the resected ulnar head can also be used to fill the radial defect. Preoperative planning and the use of

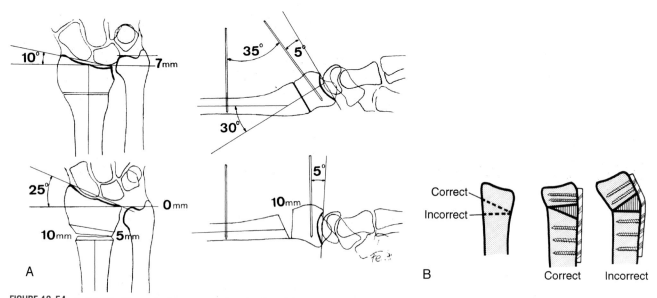

A **B** Correct Incorrect

FIGURE 16-54. A, Distal radius malunion: preoperative planning of the osteotomy. *Top left,* For correction in the frontal plane, the amount of shortening (7 mm in this patient) is measured between the head of the ulna and the ulnar corner of the radius on the anteroposterior radiograph. The lines for the measurement are perpendicular to the long axis of the radius. The preoperative ulnar tilt was reduced to 10 degrees in this patient. *Bottom left,* To restore the ulnar tilt to normal (average, 25 degrees), the osteotomy is opened more on the dorsoradial side than on the dorsoulnar side. *Top right,* For correction in the sagittal plane, the dorsal tilt (30 degrees in this patient) is measured between the perpendicular to the joint surface and the long axis of the radius on the lateral radiograph. The Kirschner wires are introduced so that they subtend the angle that corresponds to the dorsal tilt plus 5 degrees of volar tilt (30 degrees + 5 degrees = 35 degrees in this patient). *Bottom right,* After opening the osteotomy by the correct amount, the Kirschner wires lie parallel to each other. **B,** It is imperative that the osteotomy be parallel to the articular surface to avoid creating a secondary deformity.

Kirschner wires to mark the angle of deformity are mandatory to guarantee accurate angular correction, simplify the procedure, and diminish the need for intraoperative radiographic control. Radiographs of the uninjured wrist are useful to determine the physiologic ulnar variance for each particular patient and should be used to calculate restoration of radial length (see Fig. 16-54A).

Nonstructural grafts such as morcellized cancellous grafts can be used only in combination with an implant that maintains a stable correction of the distal fragment throughout the time required for bony healing. *Corticocancellous grafts* shaped and interposed in the defect restore cortical continuity, increase intrinsic stability, and reduce the need for stronger implants, provided that bone quality (no osteoporosis) is adequate. *Fixed angle plates or external fixators* are ideal for corrective osteotomies in osteopenic bone or nascent malunions).[309]

Technique: Osteotomy for Malunited Colles' Fracture

Malunions of Colles' fractures are exposed through a dorsal incision, as described for open reduction of complex fractures, between the third and fourth extensor compartments (see page 671). About 1 inch proximal to the wrist joint the osteotomy site is marked with an osteotome. If T-plate fixation of the osteotomy is planned, Lister's tubercle should be removed with an osteotome to provide a flat surface on which to apply the plate. If Kirschner wire fixation of the osteotomy is used, Lister's tubercle should be left in place because it is a useful point of entry for dorsopalmar wire fixation. To be sure that the osteotomy, as seen in the sagittal plane, is parallel to the joint surface, a fine Kirschner wire

is introduced through the dorsal part of the capsule into the radiocarpal joint and along the articular surface of the radius. In accordance with the preoperative plan, two 2.5-mm Kirschner wires with threaded tips are inserted so that the angle of correction in the sagittal plane is subtended on both sides of the future osteotomy (Fig. 16-55). These wires not only control intraoperative angular correction but also help manipulate and maintain the distal fragment in the corrected position with a small external fixator bar until the graft is inserted in the defect. The osteotomy is performed with an oscillating saw, with care taken not to osteotomize the volar cortex completely. It is then opened dorsally and radially by manipulating the wrist into flexion, by applying a laminar spreader dorsally, or by using 2.5-mm Kirschner wires as joysticks. The osteotomy is opened until both wires are parallel in the sagittal plane.

A small external fixator bar with two clamps is attached between both Kirschner wires to maintain reduction of the distal fragment. Opening up the osteotomy on the radial side can be difficult, but sometimes this can be facilitated with a small laminar spreader while allowing the distal fragment to rotate along the long axis of the distal threaded Kirschner wire. Complete tenotomy of the brachioradialis tendon is recommended to facilitate alignment of malunions with severe radial deviation and shortening. For such cases, two additional Kirschner wires with threaded tips may be used between both fragments and a distraction device applied temporarily.

The iliac bone graft is shaped to conform to the dorsoradial bone defect and is inserted while making sure that the fit is snug. At this point, a 1.6- or 2.0-mm Kirschner wire is

---

CRITICAL POINTS: RADIAL OSTEOTOMY FOR MALUNITED COLLES' FRACTURE

INDICATIONS

- Symptomatic malunion (pain, weakness, cosmetic disturbance)
- Limited palmar flexion
- DRUJ incongruency, limited forearm rotation
- Adaptive carpal instability

TECHNICAL POINTS

- Use dorsal approach with incision centered on Lister's tubercle 6 to 7 cm long.
- Expose distal radius between third and fourth compartment.
- Mobilize extensor pollicis longus tendon.
- Mark osteotomy 2 cm proximal to the joint.
- Use Kirschner wires to determine the angle of correction (these may also be used as joysticks).
- Perform osteotomy parallel to joint surface in the sagittal plane and transverse in the frontal plane.
- Open osteotomy dorsally until Kirschner wires are parallel (use laminar spreader or temporary external fixator).

- Fill defect with preshaped corticocancellous bone graft (iliac crest).
- Morcellized cancellous grafts or bone substitutes can be alternatively used in combination with fixed-angle devices.
- Use temporary Kirschner wire fixation and fluoroscopic control (for position of the distal fragment and DRUJ congruency).
- Perform internal fixation of osteotomy (2.7 condylar plate or radial pin plate and a fixed angle buttress pin).

POSTOPERATIVE CARE

- Apply palmar splint for 14 days, until suture removal.
- If functional after treatment, begin strengthening exercises.
- Evaluate radiographically at 6 to 8 weeks postoperatively.
- Dorsal implants that produce tendon irritation should routinely be removed at a later date.

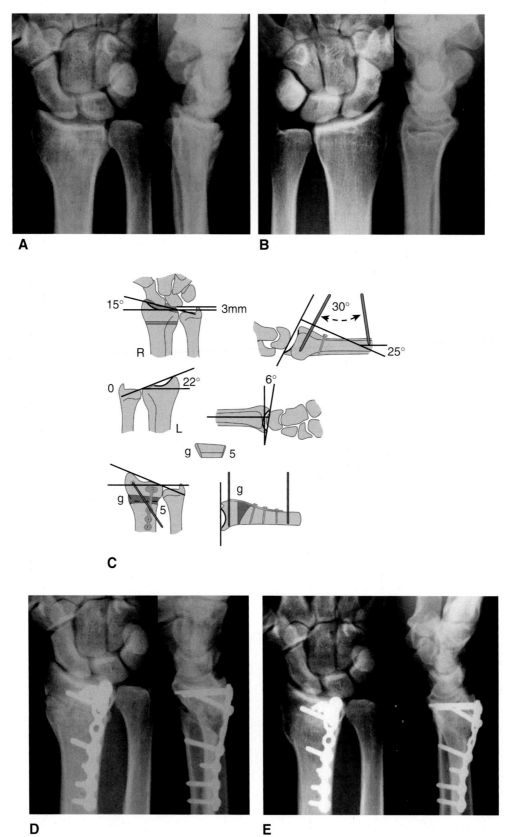

FIGURE 16-55. **A,** Radiographs of a malunited Colles' fracture with 30 degrees of dorsal tilt, 15 degrees of ulnar inclination, and an ulnar-plus-variance of 3 mm. **B,** Comparative radiographs for preoperative planning. **C,** Preoperative planning of the open wedge dorsal osteotomy and fixation with the mini-condylar plate. Immediate postoperative radiographs (**D**) and 1.5 years after osteotomy with anatomic restoration of wrist anatomy and carpal alignment (**E**).

driven obliquely from the radial styloid across the graft and into the proximal fragment, after which the threaded wires and the external fixator bar may be removed. Then, with the elbow in 90 degrees of flexion, intraoperative forearm rotation and wrist motion are checked. Radiographic control with the image intensifier may be advisable at this point to assess the quality of correction and radial lengthening before definitive internal fixation of the osteotomy. The osteotomy can be stabilized by a variety of methods. In young adults with good bone quality and especially when the volar cortex is not disrupted, simple Kirschner wire fixation (one through the radial styloid and one through Lister's tubercle in an oblique dorsopalmar direction) offers adequate stability. However, this method requires protection in a short-arm cast for 4 to 6 weeks.

Rigid fixation with plates may be used alternatively; they offer the advantage of early wrist rehabilitation after suture removal, usually 2 weeks after surgery. The use of lower profile implants has helped to diminish extensor tendon irritation. The senior author (DLF) uses a 2.7-mm condylar plate underneath the fourth compartment (see Fig. 16-55).[310]

The other prefers the use of a radial pin plate and a fixed-angle "buttress-pin" wireform implant that spans the opening wedge osteotomy and provides rigid fixation when combined with corticocancellous graft (Fig. 16-56). An external fixator applied dorsally with two threaded pins in both main fragments can also be selected as a means of skeletal fixation.[212]

Alternatively, malunited dorsally angulated fractures can be corrected through a volar approach to avoid the extensor tendon irritation that is characteristically associated with dorsal plate fixation.[311,312] Precise placement of fixed-angle volar "T" plates anatomically designed to adapt to the volar radial surface facilitates restoration of the position of the distal fragment after introduction of bone graft in the dorsal defect (Fig. 16-57). The presence of severe degenerative changes in the DRUJ mandates resection of the distal ulna or prosthetic replacement of the joint. In this situation, a closing wedge palmar osteotomy is a technically simpler procedure and can be accompanied by a primary prosthetic ulnar head replacement with restoration of a 0-mm ulnar variance.

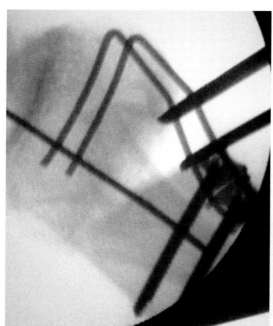

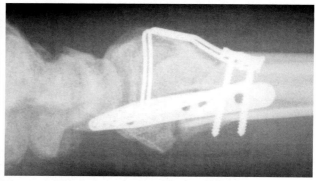

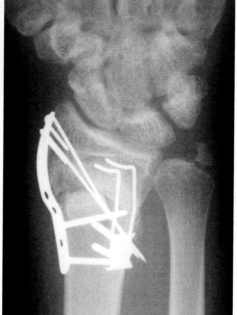

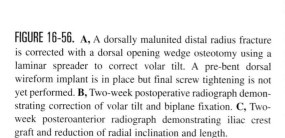

FIGURE 16-56. **A,** A dorsally malunited distal radius fracture is corrected with a dorsal opening wedge osteotomy using a laminar spreader to correct volar tilt. A pre-bent dorsal wireform implant is in place but final screw tightening is not yet performed. **B,** Two-week postoperative radiograph demonstrating correction of volar tilt and biplane fixation. **C,** Two-week posteroanterior radiograph demonstrating iliac crest graft and reduction of radial inclination and length.

A

B

C

Dynamic mid-carpel instability in a malunited fracture
with 10° of dorsal tilt. Painful "clicking" on ulnar deviation

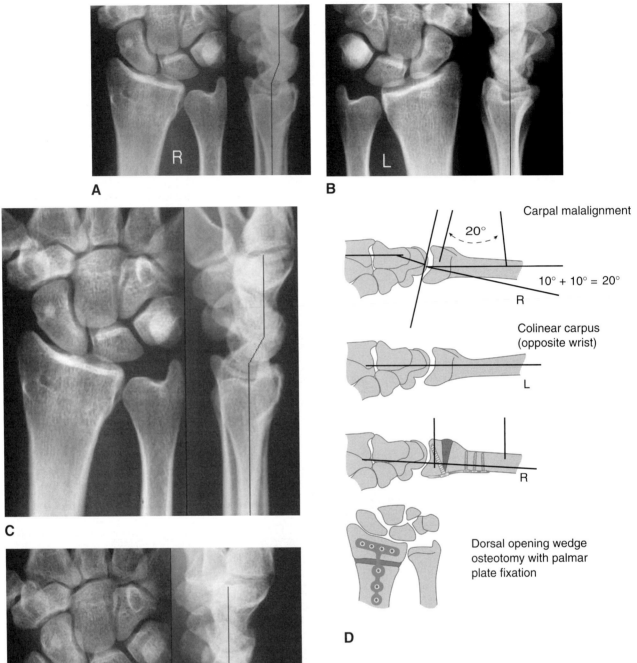

Carpal malalignment

20°

10° + 10° = 20°

R

Colinear carpus
(opposite wrist)

L

R

Dorsal opening wedge
osteotomy with palmar
plate fixation

D

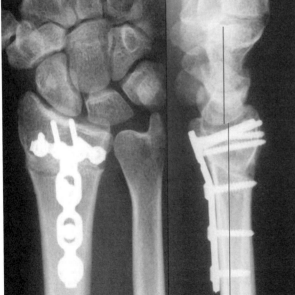

E

FIGURE 16-57. **A,** Dynamic midcarpal instability in a malunited Colles'
fracture with 10 degrees of dorsal tilt. The patient has a painful clicking on
ulnar deviation. **B,** Comparative radiographs of the left wrist showing a
normal carpal alignment. **C** and **D,** Preoperative radiographs and planning:
The open wedge osteotomy was performed through a volar approach
and fixed with a fixed angle plate and morcellized cancellous bone.
E, Realignment of the distal radius with restoration of a 10-degree volar tilt,
improved carpal alignment, and controlled instability. Notice subchondral
positioning of central fixed angle pegs.

If length discrepancy between the ulna and the radius is more than 12 mm, a combined radial osteotomy and simultaneous ulnar shortening is preferred. Tricortical grafts with separate screw fixation to the main fragments and volar plate fixation are recommended. If radial shortening is more than 2 to 3 cm, progressive lengthening with distraction osteogenesis techniques is recommended to prevent nerve and tendon dysfunction.

Watson's Trapezoidal Osteotomy

In 1988, Watson and Castle described the technique of biplanar osteotomy plus a trapezoidal distal radial local autogenous bone graft for the treatment of malunion of the distal radius (Fig. 16-58).[276] These authors recommend

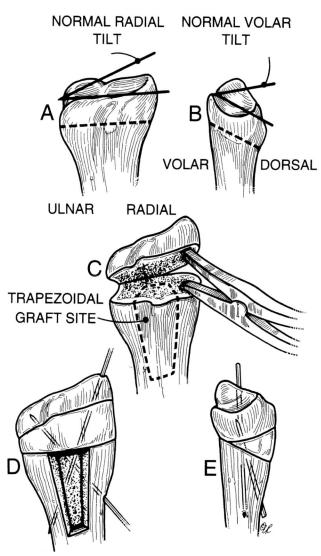

FIGURE 16-58. The operative technique of trapezoidal osteotomy for the treatment of malunion of the distal radius, as described by Watson,[276] uses distal radial bone. **A** and **B,** The osteotomy is made 1 cm proximal to the articular surface parallel with the articular surface. **C,** With a lamina spreader, the distal fragment is elevated and displaced to produce a biplanar osteotomy. An appropriate section of distal radial bone is then outlined on the dorsal aspect of the distal radius. **D** and **E,** The bone graft is harvested, rotated 90 degrees, packed into the biplanar osteotomy site, and fixed with two Kirschner wires.

exposure of the distal radius through a transverse dorsal incision, although a standard longitudinal approach may also be used. The articular surface of the radius is visualized, and the osteotomy is made parallel with the articular surface approximately 1 cm proximal to it. In a biplanar mode, to correct the loss of radial tilt and volar inclination, the osteotomy is opened and held in position with a laminar spreader while a radiograph is obtained. If the correct amount of tilt has been produced to restore normal radial inclination and volar tilt, a trapezoidal corticocancellous graft is obtained from the radius just proximal to the osteotomy site dorsally. The bone graft is removed from the radius, rotated 90 degrees, and then reinserted into the osteotomy site. If correction of the volar tilt is insufficient, it is increased by volarly flexing the wrist while the graft is wedged deeper into the osteotomy space. The osteotomy and graft are secured with two crossed 0.0625-inch Kirschner wires and protected in a cast for 4 to 6 weeks. This technique has the advantage of using a local graft, so it can be performed with the use of regional anesthesia. We would, however, not recommend it whenever severe shortening is present and disruption of the volar cortex is necessary to restore length. In this case, larger grafts from the iliac crest are more suitable.

Malunited Smith's Fractures

The classic symptoms of malunion after volarly displaced fractures include decreased wrist extension, ulnar deviation, and supination. Because of the tendency for Smith's fractures to heal with a pronation deformity of the distal radius, the lack of supination may be especially troublesome for the patient. These malunions are exposed through the distal part of the classic volar Henry approach between the flexor carpi radialis and the radial artery, with radial detachment of the pronator quadratus muscle and partial disinsertion of the flexor pollicis longus from the radial shaft. Two Kirschner wires are inserted on the volar aspect to mark the angle of correction, as shown in Figure 16-59. The palmar opening wedge osteotomy, grafting, and plating are then carried out as for the Colles' deformity but in a reversed manner from the volar side. Care must be taken to not overcorrect the physiologic palmar tilt of 10 degrees when manipulating the distal fragment into dorsiflexion. The application of a volar "T" plate automatically derotates the pronation deformity of the distal fragment by virtue of the flat surface of the plate. Plate fixation is strongly recommended because practically all malunited Smith's fractures have a pronation deformity of the distal fragment and an apparent dorsal subluxation of the distal ulna.[313] Dorsiflexion of the distal fragment and derotation, as well as lengthening, reorient the sigmoid notch of the radius with respect to the ulnar head (Fig. 16-60).

Intra-articular Osteotomies

The role of osteotomy in correcting an intra-articular malunion of the radiocarpal joint after a distal radius fracture is limited by both chronology and the type of injury.[174, 228] The osteotomy should be done as early as possible after fracture, and the fracture plane can be readily identified upward of 8 to 12 weeks after injury. Preoperative wrist arthroscopy plays a valuable role in evaluating the amount of cartilage damage and intra-articular incongruence. The presence of bare subchondral bone areas represents a formal contraindication for osteotomy. Tomograms, CT scans, and

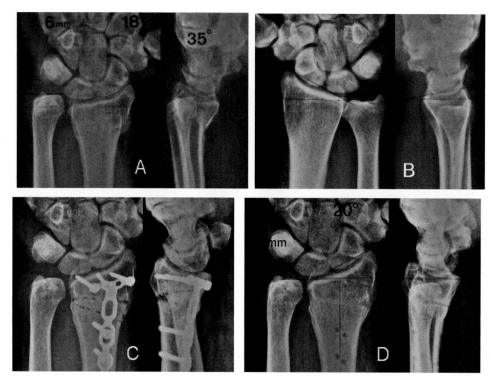

FIGURE 16-59. **A,** Radiographs of a malunited Smith fracture with 35 degrees of increased volar tilt, pronational malalignment, 18 degrees of ulnar inclination, and 6 mm of ulnar plus. **B,** Comparative radiographs of the opposite wrist for preoperative planning. **C,** Immediate postoperative radiographs showing palmar open wedge and derotation osteotomy. Notice palmarly inserted trapezoidal bone graft and a volar T-plate. **D,** radiographs 1.5 years after operation and after removal of hardware. Volar tilt was restored to 10 degrees, ulnar inclination to 20 degrees, and there was 0 degrees of ulnar variance.

three-dimensional computer-generated bone models may be useful to plan the operation. In addition, it is preferable to reserve such a procedure for those malunited fractures that have a relatively simple intra-articular component. Such fractures include malunited radial styloid fractures, volar or dorsal shearing (Barton's) fractures, and dorsal die-punch fractures. The choice of surgical approach is as indicated for the fracture scenario in the acute stage.

DRUJ Procedures

The most common cause of residual wrist disability after fracture of the distal radius is the DRUJ. The three basic conditions responsible for pain associated with limitation of forearm rotation are incongruency, impaction, and instability of the joint. Less frequent findings are the painful nonunion of the ulnar styloid, the palmar capsular contracture of the joint, and radioulnar impingement (after distal ulnar resections or Sauvé-Kapandji procedures). Depending on each particular post-traumatic scenario, these findings may present isolated or combined. Incongruency of the DRUJ may be due to (1) extra-articular deformity of the radius or ulna, which leads to an abnormal orientation of the joint surfaces (sigmoid notch-ulnar head) in space; (2) intra-articular joint surface disruption by the fracture affecting the sigmoid notch and/or the ulnar head; (3) extra- and intra-articular factors combined. Impaction, defined as the abnormal contact of two bony surfaces, occurs at the ulnocarpal level as a result of post-traumatic radial shorten-

ing (*synonyms:* abutment or impingement syndrome). With continuing impaction of the ulnar head against the carpus, progressive traumatic changes follow, such as attenuation and tears of the TFCC, chondromalacia (ulnar head, lunate, triquetrum), attenuation and tears of the triquetrolunate ligament, and, finally, ulnocarpal osteoarthritis. Instability is the result of loss of ligament support due to rupture or avulsion of the triangular ligament. Additional lesions of secondary joint stabilizers (capsular ligaments, sheath of the extensor carpi ulnaris, interosseous membrane, pronator quadratus) or intra-articular bony disruption of the joint surface may aggravate the degree of laxity.

If the patient's main complaints are localized to the DRUJ (pain associated with limitation of forearm rotation) and the angulation of the joint surface in the sagittal and frontal planes is less than 10 degrees, a reconstructive procedure at the distal radioulnar level is indicated, without a radial osteotomy. However, if significant radial deformity is clearly associated with identifiable DRUJ problems, radial osteotomy and the appropriate DRUJ procedure are performed simultaneously.

For radial shortening and ulnocarpal impaction with acceptable congruency of the sigmoid notch and the ulna, as demonstrated by CT, a shortening osteotomy of the ulna is the procedure of choice. Ulnar shortening decompresses the ulnar compartment of the wrist, reestablishes DRUJ congruity, and tightens the TFCC, which exerts a stabilizing effect on the distal ulna. A transverse or oblique[40a] osteotomy

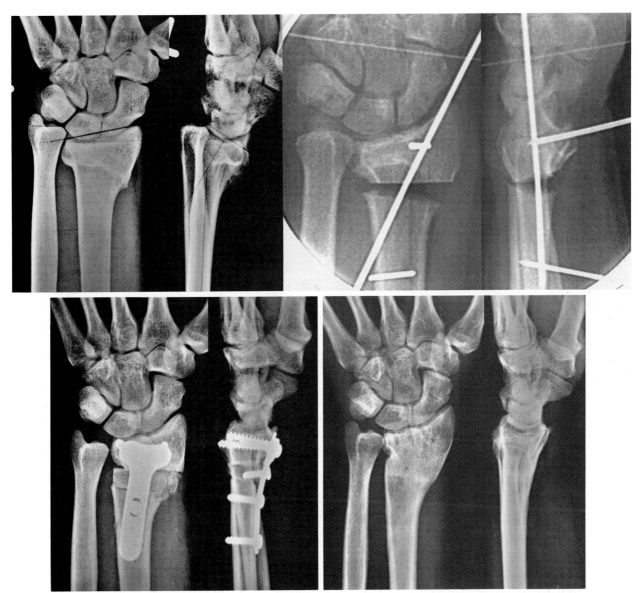

FIGURE 16-60. **Top,** Malunited Smith's fracture with palmar and pronatory displacement of the distal fragment resulting in marked limitation of supination. Intraoperative Fluoroscan views show the opening palmar wedge-shaped osteotomy with the Kirschner wires used for determination of the angle of correction. **Bottom left,** Postoperative radiographs show massive graft interposition and solid plate fixation with restoration of length and frontal and sagittal inclination of the joint surface. **Bottom right,** Three years' follow-up radiographs show restoration of DRUJ congruity and forearm rotation.

with resection of a bony segment and rigid fixation with a compression plate is recommended (Fig. 16-61).

If associated instability of the DRUJ is present, transosseous reattachment of the TFCC is performed simultaneously with the radial osteotomy.[107] If the triangular ligament is in continuity with an ulnar styloid fragment, bony reattachment with proximal displacement via a tension band wiring technique is preferred.[89] An additional ulnar sling capsulorrhaphy with an ulnarly based extensor retinaculum flap as described by Stanley and Herbert[257] is advisable.

If plain radiographs or CT scans demonstrate post-traumatic incongruity or degenerative changes of the radio-

ulnar joint, either a resection arthroplasty, an ulnar head prosthetic replacement (Fig. 16-62), or a DRUJ arthrodesis is required to alleviate pain.[314] The advantages of partial ulnar head resection[15,24,69,277] over complete resection of the ulnar head are that the ulnocarpal ligaments and the TFCC remain in continuity with the distal ulnar stump. Partial ulnar resection does not alter the ulnar variance, and therefore additional ulnar shortening, either at the styloid level or at the ulnar shaft, should be performed to prevent stylo-carpal impingement. The disadvantages of the Darrach procedure, such as loss of grip strength, loss of ulnar support of the carpus, and instability of the distal ulnar stump, are well known,[177] but the most common cause of failure is due

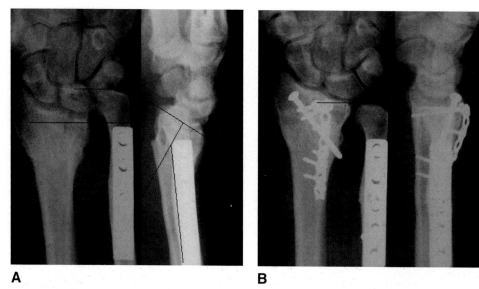

FIGURE 16-61. A, A malunited distal radius fracture with associated fracture of the distal ulna. Notice radial shortening of more than 12 mm associated with a dorsal tilt of 30 degrees of dorsal carpal subluxation. **B,** Radiographs 12 months after corrective osteotomy of the distal radius combined with a shortening osteotomy of the ulna simultaneously.

to excessive resection of the distal ulna. Primary tenodesis of the ulnar stump with a tendon sling of both the extensor and flexor carpi ulnaris tendons as described by Breen and Jupiter[27] or with extensor carpi ulnaris and pronator quadratus interposition[152] may reduce the potential instability and radioulnar impingement problems associated with this procedure. Our observation has been that ulnar stump tenodesis stretches out with time, so that currently we prefer to treat radioulnar impingement with an ulnar head prosthesis based on the acceptable mid-term results reported with this procedure.[315,316] Table 16-2 summarizes one of the authors' (DLF's) algorithms for DRUJ problems after distal radius fractures. The Darrach procedure[62] still has a place in the treatment of distal ulnar derangement or osteoarthritis after Colles' fracture in elderly patients, or it can be used as a salvage procedure for failed reconstructive procedures of the radioulnar joint.

DRUJ arthrodesis with the creation of a proximal pseudarthrosis[235,317] preserves both the ulnocarpal ligaments and the bony support of the carpus. This operation is extremely useful for restoration of free forearm rotation in cases with fixed DRUJ subluxation after articular fractures of the distal radius and severe destruction of the joint.

Capsular contraction of the DRUJ may be responsible for limitation of forearm rotation, especially supination after distal radius fractures. Having ruled out joint incongruity, subluxation, radioulnar synchondrosis, interosseous membrane contracture, or derangement of the proximal radioulnar joint as other possible causes of limitation of forearm rotation, surgical release is helpful if the condition does not improve after a trial of physiotherapy. The volar aspect of the joint is exposed through a longitudinal incision just ulnar to the flexor carpi ulnaris tendon. Having exposed and protected the dorsal cutaneous branch of the ulnar nerve, the flexor carpi ulnaris tendon and the ulnar neurovascular

bundle are retracted radially. Next the pronator quadratus is sectioned longitudinally 5 mm radially to its ulnar insertion. The contracted palmar capsule is exposed, retracting the pronator quadratus radially. A longitudinal capsulotomy proximal to the volar edge of the TFCC (volar radioulnar ligament) close to the sigmoid notch is begun and continued proximally to the neck of the ulna, and passive supination is then tested. If capsular section does not restore full supination, a total palmar capsulectomy is performed.[318] In the authors' experience, longitudinal capsulotomy and pronator quadratus release alone has proved to be sufficient in the vast majority of patients with pronatory contracture of the DRUJ. Postoperatively the wrist is maintained in full supination for 2 weeks in a sugar tong splint, followed by physiotherapy and dynamic supination bracing if necessary.[319] For accurate descriptions of these procedures, see Chapter 15.

TREATMENT OF DISTAL RADIUS FRACTURES IN CHILDREN

Distal radial epiphyseal injuries are the most common epiphyseal injury and account for about 50% of all epiphyseal injuries.[3,4,36,130,171,230,261] They usually occur in children between the ages of 6 and 10. The physeal injury is usually a type II fracture in the Salter-Harris classification (Fig. 16-63).[3,4,230] Treatment consists of a gentle attempt at closed reduction followed by immobilization in a long-arm cast for 4 to 6 weeks.[130]

Repeated attempts at reduction should be avoided, for even if the reduction is poor, remodeling is usually such that no functional deficit is noted. As with all epiphyseal fractures, occasionally what appears to be a type II or type III fracture is really a type V fracture, which is a crushing injury of the germinal cells of the epiphysis. When this happens,

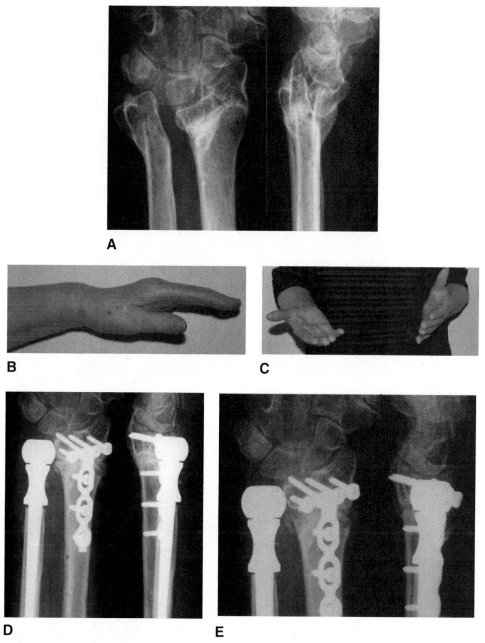

FIGURE 16-62. A, A severely malunited distal radial fracture with malunion and dissociation of the DRUJ. **B** and **C,** Notice deformity in the sagittal plane and massive limitation of supination. **D** and **E,** Immediate postoperative radiographs: the radial deformity was corrected through a volar approach, the distal ulna was used as an interposed graft, and the distal ulna was primarily replaced with a Herbert ulnar head revision prosthesis.   *Continued*

premature closure of all or part of the epiphyseal plate results and deformity of the distal radius develops as the patient grows (Fig. 16-64).

A number of individuals come to the clinician's office with chronic ulnar wrist pain in their teenage years and no history of previous trauma. A radiograph of the wrist in these individuals may very possibly reveal positive ulnar overgrowth with premature distal radial physeal closure (Fig. 16-65). This entity (i.e., epiphyseal closure as a result of repetitive load) has been described in gymnasts but probably also occurs in an individual who has had repetitive high-load stress on the wrist for a considerable period of time, such as a competitive teenage tennis player.[4] A radiograph of the opposite wrist usually reveals open epiphyses and normal ulnar variance.

The treatment of choice for premature epiphyseal closure must be individualized. Treatment options include epiphysiodesis of the distal ulnar epiphysis, distal radial osteotomy, ulnar shortening, epiphyseal bar resection, and insertion of a spacer such as fat or a combination thereof (Figs. 16-66 and 16-67). All treatment decisions should be predicated not only on the patient's cosmetic and functional desires but also on any future deformities that might develop as a result of abnormal epiphyseal growth.

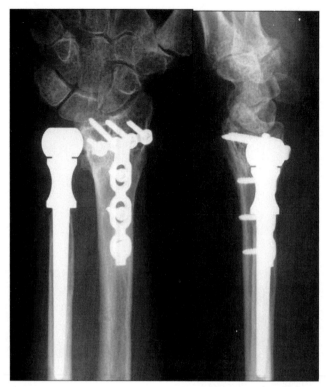

F

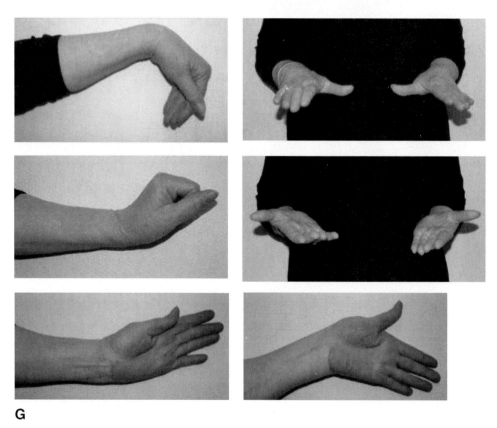

G

FIGURE 16-62—cont'd. F, Appearance 2.5 years after surgery: the wrist is perfectly aligned with remodeling of the sigmoid notch, and the noncemented prosthesis is perfectly incorporated. **G,** The patient had adequate functional range of motion. Notice massive improvement of the limited supination.

Table 16-2

MANAGEMENT ALGORITHM FOR DISTAL RADIOULNAR JOINT (DRUJ) DISORDERS AFTER DISTAL RADIUS FRACTURE

Disorder	Management
DRUJ incongruity	
Extra-articular	Reorient sigmoid notch with radial osteotomy
Intra-articular (post-traumatic arthrosis)	Depending on severity of degenerative changes, age, dominance, and occupation, resection arthroplasty, Sauvé-Kapandji procedure, or prosthetic replacement
Combined	Radial osteotomy and DRUJ procedure as for intra-articular disorder
DRUJ instability	Reattachment of triangular fibrocartilage complex (open/arthroscopic) Proximal reinsertion of ulnar styloid nonunion Capsulodesis (ulnar sling procedure—Herbert) Shortening osteotomy of the ulna Other ligament reconstructions
Ulnocarpal abutment (impaction)	Restore radioulnar index or ulnar variance to normal Ulnar shortening osteotomy Wafer procedure (Feldon) Radial lengthening osteotomy Combined radius-ulna osteotomies Epiphysiodesis; distraction-osteogenesis techniques in growing skeleton
Symptomatic (painful) nonunion of ulnar styloid	Simple excision
Capsular retraction	Capsulotomy
Pronatory contracture of the DRUJ	Pronator quadratus release and palmar capsulotomy
Radioulnar impingement Painful radioulnar contact after resection of the distal ulna or unstable stump after Sauvé-Kapandji procedures	Ulnar head prosthesis

Note: If these conditions present associated, two or more procedures may need to be combined. A classic example is malunited Colles' fracture and degenerative changes in the DRUJ.

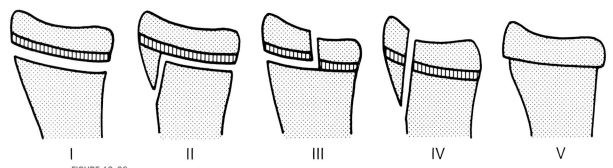

FIGURE 16-63. Salter-Harris classification of distal radial epiphyseal fractures in children. Type V is a crush injury.

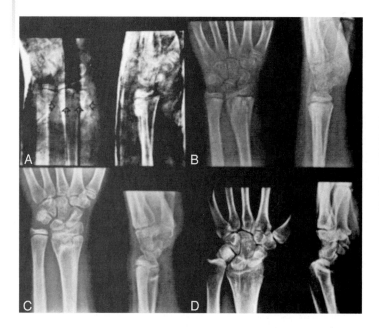

FIGURE 16-64. **A,** Radiographs illustrate a type II epiphyseal fracture of the distal radius as seen through plaster at age 10. **B,** Early healing of the fracture. **C,** Partial epiphyseal closure at age 13, with some early ulnar overgrowth and increased volar tilt of the distal radius. **D,** Radiographs at age 22 reveal marked ulnar overgrowth and volar tilt of the radius 12 years after this type II fracture of the distal radius with partial epiphyseal closure.

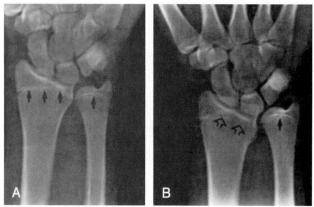

FIGURE 16-65. **A,** Radiographs of the wrist of a 14-year-old asymptomatic gymnast with an ulnar neutral variant. **B,** The symptomatic wrist of that same gymnast with a marked ulnar-plus variant and a closed distal radial epiphyseal plate.

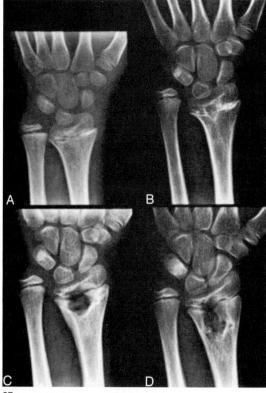

FIGURE 16-67. **A,** Early distal radial epiphyseal closure 1 year after a type II fracture (partial type V) of the distal radius. **B,** Ulnar overgrowth 2 years later is revealed as a result of partial distal radial epiphyseal closure. **C,** The same wrist 3 months after resection of the distal radial epiphyseal bar and insertion of an abdominal fat graft. **D,** The same wrist 1.5 years later with the distal radial epiphysis completely open, the fat still in place, and some partial correction of the discrepancy in relative radioulnar lengths.

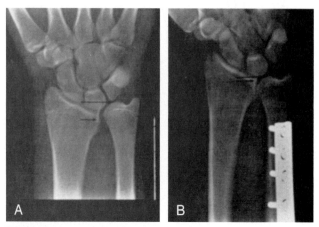

FIGURE 16-66. **A,** Preoperative radiographs of a symptomatic patient with ulnar impaction secondary to premature distal radial epiphyseal closure. **B,** The same wrist after an ulnar shortening osteotomy.

ANNOTATED REFERENCES

289. Wolfe SW, Swigart CR, Grauer J, et al: Augmented external fixation of distal radius fractures. J Hand Surg [Am] 23:127-134, 1998.

   The authors created a reproducible model of an unstable extra-articular radius fracture and measured precise motion of the fracture fragments during physiologic load application to the wrist muscles. They provide a mechanical rationale for the use of direct fragment fixation with percutaneous Kirschner wires to augment the stability of external fixation.

290. Fischer T, Koch P, Saager C, Kohut GN: The radio-radial external fixator in the treatment of fractures of the distal radius. J Hand Surg [Br] 24:604-609, 1999.

   The technique of non-spanning external fixation is reviewed in a single cohort study of 15 extra-articular fractures and two intra-articular fractures. The authors advocate splint wear to augment the fixation and begin gentle wrist motion at 2 weeks postoperatively. The fixator was left in place for an average of 6.5 weeks, and excellent maintenance of length and alignment was documented.

293. Jupiter JB, Ring D, Weitzel PP: Surgical treatment of re-displaced fractures of the distal radius in patients older than 60 years. J Hand Surg 27A:714-723, 2002.

   The authors provide rationale and supportive patient-derived outcome validation for early operative treatment of failed closed reductions in patients aged 60 or greater. Half of the fractures were palmar-displaced, underscoring the inherent instability of this fracture type.

294. Orbay JL, Fernandez DL: Volar fixation for dorsally displaced fractures of the distal radius: A preliminary report. J Hand Surg [Am] 27:205-215, 2002.

   This paper challenges conventional wisdom by demonstrating excellent results in 31 dorsally displaced fractures treated with a fixed-angle device applied through a volar approach to the distal radius. For articular comminution, the authors describe an extended volar incision that reflects the proximal radius to allow articular restitution prior to placement of the volar plate.

302. Jakob M, Rikli DA, Regazzoni P: Fractures of the distal radius treated by internal fixation and early function. J Bone Joint Surg Br 82:340-344, 2000.

   A consecutive series of 74 fractures treated by internal fixation with 2.0-mm mini-plates and early wrist range of motion demonstrated good or excellent results and minimal loss of fracture alignment at 1 year follow-up. The authors provide compelling clinical evidence to support the concept of columnar fixation using ultra low-profile implants positioned in two planes to maximize stability and minimize soft tissue disruption.

304. Dumontier C, Meyer zu Ruckendorf G, Sautet A, et al: Radiocarpal dislocations: Classification and proposal for treatment: A review of twenty seven cases. J Bone Joint Surg Am 83:212-218, 2001.

   Outcomes are presented for 27 patients treated for radiocarpal dislocation, as well as a useful classification and treatment scheme based on the presence or absence of a large radial styloid fragment. The high incidence of degenerative arthritis and ulnar translocation underscores the generally poor prognosis associated with this severe injury.

305. Lindau T, Arner M, Hagberg L: Intra-articular lesions in distal fractures of the radius in young adults. J Hand Surg [Br] 22:638-643, 1997.

   Arthroscopic inspection of 35 intra-articular and 15 extra-articular fractures demonstrated an unusually high rate of associated soft tissue (98%) and chondral lesions (32%). The authors question the advisability of instituting early range of motion after internal fixation of distal radius fractures given the high incidence of ligament injury and caution against the sustained application of traction when immobilization with external fixation is chosen.

306. Smith DW, Henry MK: Comprehensive management of soft-tissue injuries associated with distal radius fractures. J ASSH 3:153-164, 2002.

   A variety of serious soft-tissue injuries can accompany fractures of the distal radius and should be aggressively identified and treated to restore optimal outcome. The authors advocate a volar approach for fixation, combined with arthroscopic and limited open diagnosis and treatment of associated nerve compression and ligament injuries.

307. Fernandez DL, Ring D, Jupiter JB: Surgical management of delayed union and non-union of distal radius fractures. J Hand Surg [Am] 26:201-209, 2001.

   Eight surgically treated and two non–surgically treated fractures of the distal radius that went on to symptomatic delayed or nonunion were treated with internal fixation and autogenous bone graft, with progression to union and salvage of the radiocarpal joint in all cases. The authors advocate early intervention to restore radioulnar and radiocarpal function and stress the importance of biplanar fixation using fixed angle implants when disuse or advanced age have led to osteoporotic bone.

308. Park MJ, Cooney WP, Hahn ME, et al: The effects of dorsally angulated distal radius fractures on carpal kinematics. J Hand Surg [Am] 27:223-232, 2002.

   In addition to the alterations in radioulnar and ulnocarpal relationships that occur with dorsal malunions of the distal radius, the authors confirmed changes in radiocarpal and midcarpal posture and kinematics with progressive degrees of abnormal radial tilt in a cadaveric malunion model. Those wrists that displayed adaptive midcarpal flexion deformities (DISI) had more severe detrimental effects on carpal motion, and the authors make recommendations to help guide the decision for corrective osteotomy.

312. Prommersberger KJ, van Schoonhoven J, Lanz UB: Outcome after corrective osteotomy for malunited fractures of the distal end of the radius. J Hand Surg [Br] 27:1:55-60, 2002.

   A large series of corrective osteotomy for dorsal (n = 29) and palmar (n = 20) malunited distal radius fractures is presented, together with objective follow-up data at 18 months. The authors conclude that function is correlated with restoration of alignment, and patients with multiplanar preoperative deformities fare less well after surgical correction.

313. Shea K, Fernandez DL, Jupiter JB, Martin C Jr: Corrective osteotomy for malunited, volarly displaced fractures of the distal end of the radius. J Bone Joint Surg [Am] 79:1816-1826, 1997.

   The importance of attainment and maintenance of acceptable alignment during healing of distal radius fractures is reinforced by this 5-year retrospective study of 25 symptomatic patients who underwent corrective osteotomy for volar malunion. Although the procedure resulted in marked improvements in motion, strength, and pain, the authors performed additional surgery in 11 of 25 individuals and found significant residual distal radioulnar joint symptoms in over half of this cohort.

315. van Schoonhoven J, Fernandez DL, Bowers WH, Herbert TJ: Salvage of failed resection arthroplasties of the distal radioulnar joint using a new ulnar head prosthesis. J Hand Surg [Am] 25:438-446, 2000.

Two-year data are presented for 27 patients after prosthetic ceramic radioulnar arthroplasty and soft tissue stabilization for failed radioulnar joint resection arthroplasty. The authors conclude that this is a safe and reliable procedure to salvage stability and improve symptoms after unsuccessful resection arthroplasty of this important joint.

338. Medoff RJ, Kopylov P: Immediate internal fixation and motion of comminuted distal radius fractures using a new fragment specific system. Orthop Trans 22:165, 1998.

A novel fixation system is introduced based on the concept of "fragment-specific fixation," wherein individual fragments are identified and fixed with modular wireform devices and miniature pin-plates. Secure fixation of comminuted fractures using a biplanar configuration enables immediate resumption of range of motion and very satisfactory results in this preliminary cohort of patients.

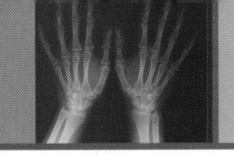

CHAPTER 17

Fractures of the Carpal Bones

Peter C. Amadio and Steven L. Moran

ractures of the carpal bones are common and typically a consequence of a fall on an outstretched hand. The specific injury—to the carpus, radius, elbow, shoulder, or a combination of joints—depends on load and joint positioning at the moment of impact.[71,175,682] The complex arrangement and kinematics of the carpal bones may make a systematic approach daunting, but there are three general groups: perilunate pattern injuries, axial pattern injuries, and local impaction/avulsion injuries.[175] In their complete form, perilunate and axial pattern injuries are classified under carpal instabilities and are discussed in Chapter 14. In their incomplete forms, these patterns help explain the anatomy of many common carpal fractures and point the way to a better understanding of associated injuries.

Perilunate pattern injuries include the most common carpal fracture, that of the scaphoid, as well as most capitate and some triquetral fractures.[125] As the name implies, these injuries occur in an arc around the lunate. A fracture to any one of these bones, particularly if the line of injury conforms to a perilunate arc, mandates a search for possible related injuries to other bones and joints along the perilunate injury pathway, even if a true perilunate fracture-dislocation has not occurred.

Axial pattern injuries[288] are typically the result of powerful anteroposterior compression forces, as may occur in an explosion injury or severe crush. Again, although details of this instability problem are covered elsewhere, it is important for the sake of carpal fracture analysis to know that the injury propagates in both the radial and ulnar directions, generally separating the carpus on either side of the capitate. As with perilunate pattern injuries, axial pattern fractures are by definition unstable and usually require surgical treatment.

The third main category consists of isolated carpal bone injuries that occur due to localized force concentration. These injuries include dorsal chip fractures of the triquetrum,[214] trapezial ridge fractures,[473] pisiform fractures, and hamate hook[55] fractures. Avascular necrosis of carpal bones can be either a cause or a consequence of carpal fractures.[17] Kienböck's disease,[42] Preiser's disease,[658] as well

as avascular necrosis of the pisiform and capitate are discussed in this chapter.

The frequency of carpal fractures has been reported in several large series.[344,504,612] Scaphoid injuries are the most common (Table 17-1), followed in frequency by triquetral fractures. Trapezoid fractures are the least common.

FRACTURES OF THE SCAPHOID

In the upper extremity, the incidence of fractures of the scaphoid is second only to that of fractures of the distal radius.[45,46,56,62,122,579-581] Like distal radius fractures, scaphoid fractures usually result from a fall on the extended wrist. In an epidemiologic study from Norway it was found that 82% of scaphoid fractures occurred in males, with the highest incidence occurring between the ages of 20 and 30 years. Fractures of the scaphoid accounted for 11% of hand fractures and 60% of carpal fractures.[272] Seventy to 80 percent of scaphoid fractures occur at the waist or midportion,

Table 17-1
INCIDENCE OF CARPAL FRACTURES

Bone	Number	% of Total
Scaphoid	5036	78.8
Triquetrum	880	13.8
Trapezium	144	2.3
Hamate	95	1.5
Lunate	92	1.4
Pisiform	67	1.0
Capitate	61	1.0
Trapezoid	15	0.2
	6390	

Data from references 571, 662, and 686.

We wish to acknowledge the contributions of **Julio Taleisnik, MD,** to preceding editions of this chapter.

whereas 10% to 20% occur at the proximal pole.[69,374,513] Scaphoid fractures are rare in children and occur most frequently in the distal third.[169,628,698] Symptoms may be minimal, and the injury may often be missed, being dismissed as "just a sprain," except for the persistence of symptoms (pain and swelling) in the anatomical snuff-box area.

Mechanism of Injury

Fractures of the scaphoid have been explained as a failure of bone caused by a compressive or tension load.[552] Todd[627] referred to the "snapped waist" fracture as a response similar to a sugar lump subjected to sudden tension load. Cobey and White[113] suggested that the scaphoid actually breaks because of compression rather than tension loads, the compression being exerted against its concave surface by the head of the capitate. The position of radial or ulnar deviation was thought to determine whether the scaphoid would break at its waist or more proximally or distally.[154] Horii has also postulated that the mechanism of fracture may be secondary to the concentration of external forces through the second metacarpal. The force is then dispersed to the trapezium and trapezoid, which induce a shear stress at the scaphoid waist.[270] The degree of wrist extension at impact is also important in determining whether the fracture occurs in the forearm, the distal radius, or the carpus. Frykman[204] subjected cadaver wrists to static loading and observed that greater extension of the wrist resulted in more distal fractures. Extension of 35 degrees or less resulted in fractures of the forearm. Extension of 90 degrees or more resulted in injury to the carpal bones. Fractures of the scaphoid were produced consistently after radial deviation was added. An additional factor is the point of application of the ground force at impact.[151,153] This was confirmed by Weber and Chao on fresh cadaver specimens.[682] With the wrist in 95 to 100 degrees of extension *and* the load applied concentrated on the radial half of the palm, these authors demonstrated

that a fracture of the scaphoid could consistently be reproduced in the laboratory (Fig. 17-1).

The combination of radial deviation and wrist extension beyond 95 degrees tends to lock the scaphoid within the scaphoid fossa. At this point, the palmar ligaments, particularly the radioscaphocapitate ligament, act as a fulcrum on which the distal pole may flex palmarly, resulting in a waist fracture.[336,374] Torsion forces may also be considered an important factor in producing this fracture.[190,191,193,227] More proximal fractures are thought to be the result of initial dorsal subluxation of the scaphoid before forced supination.[402] In general, the principal vector for scaphoid fractures is extension, whereas scapholunate injuries tend to occur when ulnar deviation and intercarpal supination occur concomitantly. Concurrent scaphoid fractures and scapholunate tears are uncommon but must be included in the differential diagnosis.[402]

Anatomy

The scaphoid has five articulating surfaces and is almost entirely covered by cartilage.[307] It contacts the radius, lunate, capitate, trapezium, and trapezoid. The scaphoid is a mechanical link between the proximal and distal carpal rows.[371,659] The shape of the scaphoid is such that the center of the distal articular surface is palmar to the proximal articular surface. This results in the production of a flexion moment on the scaphoid with axial loading of the wrist (Fig. 17-2).[48]

There are multiple ligamentous attachments to the scaphoid. The scapholunate interosseous ligament inserts

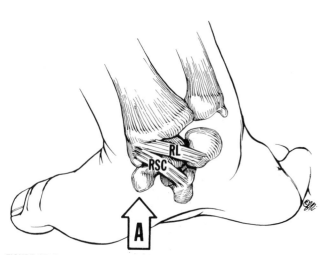

FIGURE 17-1. Mechanism of fracture of the scaphoid according to Weber and Chao. Force applied to the radial half of the palm *(arrow A)* with the wrist in 95 to 100 degrees of dorsiflexion produces bending loads on the unprotected distal half of the scaphoid. The proximal half is protected between the radius and the palmar radiocarpal ligaments. RL, radiolunate ligament; RSC, radioscaphocapitate ligament. (From Taleisnik J: The Wrist. New York, Churchill Livingstone, 1985.)

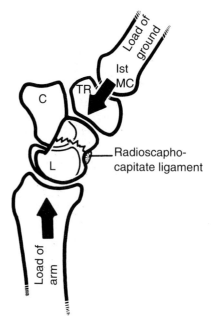

FIGURE 17-2. With axial loading of the wrist a flexion moment arm is produced over the distal pole of the scaphoid. The scaphoid tends to fracture at the waist at the level of the radioscaphocapitate ligament. C, capitate; L, lunate; TR, trapezium; 1st MC, metacarpal.

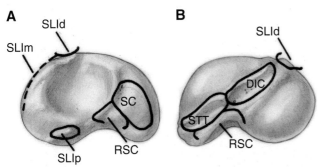

FIGURE 17-3. Ligamentous attachments to the radial and ulnar aspects of the scaphoid. **A,** Medial surface of a right scaphoid demonstrating the attachment zones of the scaphocapitate ligament (SC), radioscaphocapitate ligament (RSC), and the dorsal (SLId), membranous (SLIm), and palmar (SLIp) regions of the scapholunate interosseous ligament. **B,** Right scaphoid from a dorsoradial perspective demonstrating the attachment zones of the scaphotrapezial-trapezoid ligament (STT), radioscaphocapitate ligament (RSC), dorsal intercarpal ligament (DIC), and the dorsal region of the scapholunate interosseous ligament (SLId).

into the proximal, dorsal, and palmar edges of the proximal pole. The radioscaphocapitate ligament has radial attachments to the lateral palmar surface of the scaphoid waist, and its central portion surrounds and inserts on the proximal surface of the distal pole. The scaphotrapezium ligament attaches to the lateral surface of the distal pole, and the proximal half of the dorsal intercarpal ligament inserts dorsally and laterally.[52,164,661] The scaphocapitate ligament attaches to the palmar and lateral nonarticular surface of the distal pole of the scaphoid (Fig. 17-3).[48]

Because of the bending moment on the scaphoid, fracture forces tend to produce a compressive force on the volar cortex and tension on the dorsal cortex. When fractures occur proximal to the waist of the scaphoid there is a high incidence of displacement because of the opposing forces between the proximal and distal ligaments.[50,332,333] The persistent flexion force on the distal pole and the extension moment on the proximal pole account for the characteristic "humpback" deformity that is seen with chronic scaphoid malunions.[47]

Blood Supply of the Scaphoid

The scaphoid receives its blood supply through ligamentous attachments. The studies of Grettve,[240] Minne and colleagues,[424] and Taleisnik and Kelly[607] described three principal arterial groups supplying the scaphoid. Because of their spatial relationship to the scaphoid, these groups were named lateral volar, dorsal, and distal (Fig. 17-4).[464,607] In a more recent investigation, Gelberman and Menon[224] described two instead of three vascular systems: the first entering dorsally and the second from the volar side and limited to the tubercle.

All these studies consistently demonstrated poor blood supply to the proximal pole, particularly in comparison with the abundant supply to the distal two thirds of the scaphoid. The proximal pole is an intra-articular structure completely covered with hyaline cartilage that has a single ligamentous attachment (the deep radioscapholunate ligament) and is dependent on an intraosseous blood supply. The limited vascular supply at the proximal pole is similar to that at the head of the femur: when fracture occurs through the body of the scaphoid (or neck of the femur), vascularity of the isolated fragment is jeopardized. In their study of vascular foramina in dried scaphoids, Obletz and Halbstein[464] found 13% without vascular perforations and 20% with only a single small foramen proximal to the waist. Therefore, in

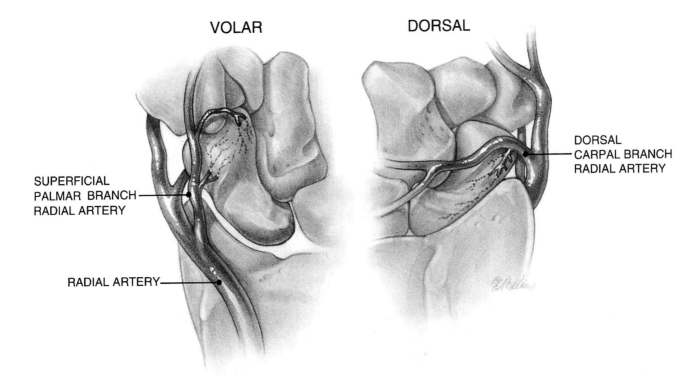

FIGURE 17-4. Schematic representation of the blood supply of the scaphoid.

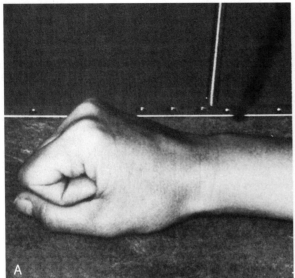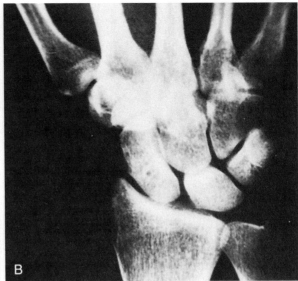

FIGURE 17-5. **A,** Positioning for a posteroanterior radiograph obtained with the fingers flexed into a fist. **B,** Slight dorsiflexion is produced to place the longitudinal axis of the scaphoid in a plane more nearly parallel to that of the film.

their opinion, 30% of middle third fractures could be expected to interfere with the blood supply to the proximal fragment and lead to avascular necrosis or nonunion. This potential is greater in more proximal fractures. There is sufficient experimental data to explain the high incidence of nonunions and avascular necrosis of the proximal fragment among fractures of the proximal third of the scaphoid.[376] Fractures in this location take an average of 6 to 11 weeks longer to heal than those in the middle third[154,529,594] and have demonstrated an incidence of avascular necrosis of 14% to 39%.[122,483,529] There is no evidence that any meaningful blood supply enters the scaphoid from the scapholunate ligament.

Diagnosis

The diagnosis of a fracture of the scaphoid is suggested by the patient's age, the mechanism of injury, and the initial signs and symptoms, but it is confirmed only by radiographic examination. Tenderness with palpation over the scaphoid tubercle and anatomical snuff-box and tenderness with longitudinal compression are physical findings that have been shown to have a diagnostic sensitivity of 100% during the initial evaluation of scaphoid fractures.[202,241,480] The presence of tenderness over the anatomical snuff-box without deformity should suggest a fracture of the scaphoid, and a complete set of radiographs should be obtained.[680] As many as 18 views have been proposed for an exhaustive study of the injured wrist,[235] but only 4 must be included in the initial routine examination: one posteroanterior, one lateral, and two oblique projections.

For the posteroanterior study it is best to position the hand with the fingers flexed into a fist (Fig. 17-5).[485,529,551,590] This produces slight extension and ulnar deviation and places the longitudinal axis of the scaphoid in a plane more closely parallel with that of the film. This will also accentuate a scapholunate gap, which is important in the differential diagnosis of a scapholunate injury.[621] Ulnar deviation

(Fig. 17-6) improves visualization of the fracture by placing the scaphoid waist in profile.[255,404,551,581] The lateral projection is helpful for evaluation of carpal alignment and determination of carpal instability (Figs. 17-7 and 17-8).

The incidence of false-negative initial radiographs for scaphoid fracture has been reported to be between 2% to 25%.[155,360,480,619,668,669] If initial studies are nonconfirmatory and clinical examination points to a scaphoid fracture, traditional teaching has recommended immobilizing the wrist in a splint and repeating radiographs in 1 to 3 weeks.* Resorption around the fracture line during this period of immobilization will allow identification on repeat radiographs. The disadvantage of this protocol is that it delays diagnosis, inconveniences the patient, and adds cost in terms of repeat evaluation, splint material, and additional radiographs.[294]

Other diagnostic features and tests have been suggested to make this period of immobilization unnecessary. Terry and Ramin[615] have called attention to a small radiolucent area normally present next to the scaphoid in anteroposterior radiographs that they named the navicular fat stripe. The fat stripe is a linear collection of fat between the radiocollateral ligament and the tendon sheaths of the abductor pollicis longus and extensor pollicis brevis,[18,130,444] and a fracture on the radial side of the wrist can either displace or obliterate this line (Fig. 17-9). Banerjee documented low accuracy of this sign in a blinded radiologic review of 40 scaphoid fractures and 40 control cases and concluded that the scaphoid fat pad sign is a poor predictor of scaphoid fracture.[34] Carver and Barrington[102] suggested that soft tissue swelling on the dorsum of the wrist is a more reliable radiologic sign than displacement of the fat stripe.

Other imaging techniques have been proposed for detection of suspected fractures, including ultrasound[139,408,443] isotope scanning,[306,447,521,622] carpal box radiographs,[520,522,523]

---

*See references 25, 89, 90, 138, 263, 404, 529, 578, 580, 582, and 631.

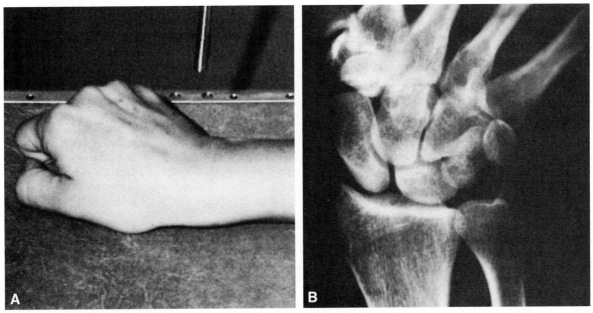

FIGURE 17-6. A better profile of the entire scaphoid is obtained in the posteroanterior view with the fingers flexed into a fist and the wrist in ulnar deviation.

trispiral tomography,[51,128,373,572] computed tomography (CT),[355,539] and magnetic resonance imaging (MRI; Fig. 17-10)).[78,162,200,211,279,358,617] The multiplicity of approaches highlights the difficulties encountered in evaluating a patient with a suspected scaphoid fracture.[428] The navicular fat stripe,[34] carpal box views,[520] and ultrasound[443] may aid in the clinical diagnosis but cannot be relied on to exclude a fracture. Several studies have demonstrated the sensitivity of a bone scan to be 100%[213,306,595] with a positive predictive value of 93%[620] and a specificity of 98%.[618] Thus, a negative isotope scan virtually excludes the presence of fracture.[697] Increased focal activity soon after trauma, although not specific for fracture, suggests scaphoid injury or possible scapholunate ligament tear, even if radiographs and CT scans fail to demonstrate a fracture.[305,470,595] Scintigraphic studies can be positive as early as 7 to 24 hours after fracture; however, optimal imaging is obtained after 48 hours. Premature imaging may show only diffuse hyperemia due to traumatic synovitis, which can obscure uptake at the fracture site.[444]

A negative isotope scan obtained within 2 weeks of the injury should exclude a fracture. If the scan is positive, even with negative radiographs a fracture or ligamentous injury must be strongly suspected, and further imaging should be obtained or the wrist should be immobilized for 2 to 3 weeks, followed by repeat radiographs.[595,622] Trispiral tomography or CT scans of areas of increased isotope uptake are often useful to visualize small, minimally displaced fractures.[539] If tomographic studies are negative but symptoms persist, the possibility of a scapholunate injury should be more strongly considered.[621]

Teil-van Buul and associates[622] studied the cost-effectiveness of diagnostic strategies for suspected scaphoid fractures. The most sensitive method in this study was initial radiographs, followed by a bone scan at 2 weeks if the patient is still symptomatic without evidence of fracture. Although slightly more expensive than simply repeating radiographs, this strategy identified more fractures and thus saved the considerable long-term costs of initial under-treatment and nonunion. Zarnett and coworkers recommended simply treating all equivocal cases as fractures.[710] Although the simplicity of this approach is appealing, the consequences of overtreatment must be considered, because less than 15% of suspected scaphoid fractures are ultimately confirmed as fractured.[4,7,8]

MRI has become increasingly useful in the evaluation of acute and occult fractures. Previously, MRI was primarily used to predict the vascular status of the proximal fragment in cases of scaphoid nonunions.[134,347,484,537,636] Normal marrow elements produce high-intensity signals on T1-weighted images. Avascularity or marrow edema will lead to alterations in these signals.

Early comparative studies by Tiel-van Buul and colleagues suggested that MRI was less sensitive and more expensive when compared with bone scintigraphy. MRI was

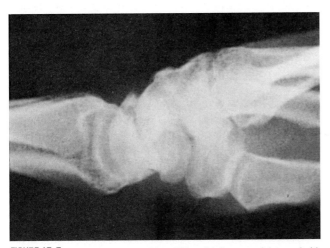

FIGURE 17-7. Severe dorsal carpal instability after fracture of the scaphoid.

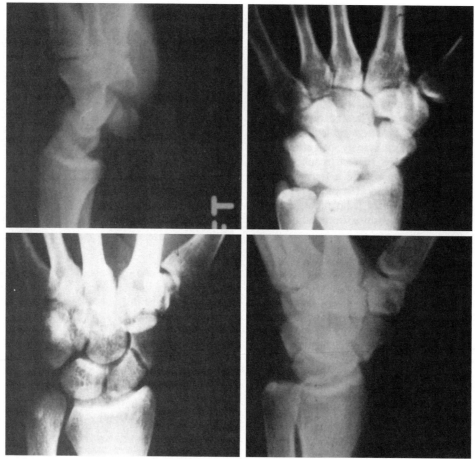

FIGURE 17-8. Less frequent volar carpal instability after a displaced fracture of the middle third of the scaphoid.

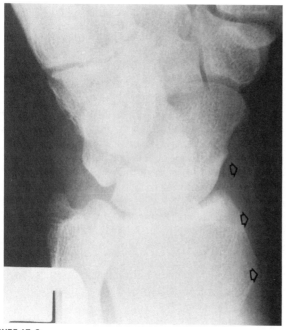

FIGURE 17-9. Scaphoid ("navicular") fat stripe *(arrows)* seen in an oblique projection. (From Taleisnik J: The Wrist. New York, Churchill Livingstone, 1985.)

also associated with a 16% noncompliance rate owing to the development of claustrophobia in several patients.[523,617,623] More recent studies, however, have found up to 100% sensitivity and specificity for identifying acute scaphoid fractures.[77,78,211,495] Gaebler and colleagues performed a prospective blinded study of 32 patients in whom a scaphoid fracture was suspected. MRI was performed at an average of 2.8 days after trauma, with a sensitivity and specificity of 100%.[211] False-positive results have been found in some studies due to MRI's sensitivity to marrow edema.[276] Other prospective studies have shown MRI to be more sensitive and specific in the diagnosis of occult scaphoid fractures and soft tissue wrist injuries when compared with bone scintigraphy.[78,162,200,210,211,495,616] In Breitenseher's report, occult fractures of the capitate, trapezium, and distal radius were identified with MRI during the course of study period; this reminds us to include these fractures in our differential when evaluating any patient with acute wrist pain.[77,495] Most recently, Dorsay has shown that immediate MRI of suspected scaphoid fractures provides a cost benefit when compared with splinting and repeat radiographs (see Fig. 17-10).[162,346]

Our protocol for diagnosis consists of plain radiographs, followed by immediate MRI if radiographs are equivocal and there is high clinical suspicion of fracture. If centers are

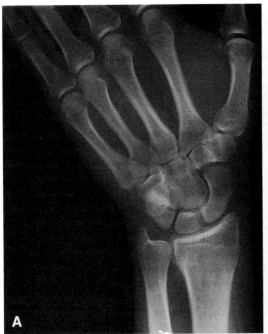

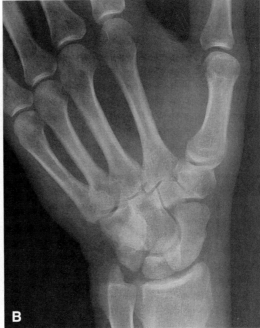

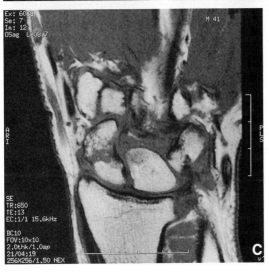

FIGURE 17-10. A and **B,** A 35-year-old man presented with persistent snuff-box tenderness and negative radiographs at 1 week post injury. **C,** Occult nondisplaced scaphoid fracture was detected with MRI.

CRITICAL POINTS: EVALUATION OF SUSPECTED SCAPHOID FRACTURE

- Obtain neutral posteroanterior, oblique, and lateral radiographs, with addition of radial and ulnar deviation and clenched fist view if necessary.
- Perform MRI for clinically suspected cases with normal radiographs or bone scan at 72 hours from injury.
- If MRI or bone scan is negative, no fracture is assumed.
- If bone scan positive but cannot delineate fracture location on radiographs, obtain CT or MRI.

not equipped with a dedicated extremity MR unit, then a bone scan should be obtained within 48 to 72 hours to evaluate the wrist.

Classification and Assessment of Fracture Stability

Determining optimal treatment depends on accurate diagnosis and fracture classification. This is especially true for acute fractures because improper early treatment may increase the risk of nonunion or the need for surgery. Displacement of the fracture has been shown to be a predictor for delayed or failed union.[169] Thus the ability to distinguish between unstable and stable fractures helps determine treatment options.

Herbert has devised an alphanumeric classification system that combines fracture anatomy, stability, and chronicity of injury (Fig. 17-11).[257] Russe[529] classified scaphoid fractures into three types according to the relationship of the

TYPE A:
STABLE ACUTE FRACTURES

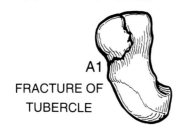

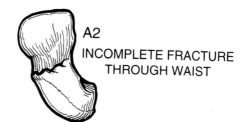

A1
FRACTURE OF
TUBERCLE

A2
INCOMPLETE FRACTURE
THROUGH WAIST

TYPE B:
UNSTABLE ACUTE FRACTURES

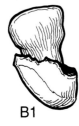

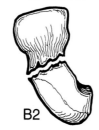

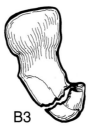

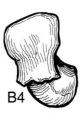

B1
DISTAL OBLIQUE
FRACTURE

B2
COMPLETE FRACTURE
OF WAIST

B3
PROXIMAL POLE
FRACTURE

B4
TRANS-SCAPHOID-
PERILUNATE
FRACTURE DISLOCATION
OF CARPUS

TYPE C:
DELAYED UNION

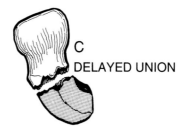

C
DELAYED UNION

TYPE D:
ESTABLISHED NONUNION

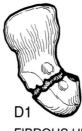

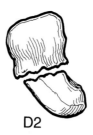

D1
FIBROUS UNION

D2
PSEUDARTHROSIS

FIGURE 17-11. Herbert has devised an alphanumeric classification system that may have prognostic significance.[257]

fracture line to the long axis of the scaphoid (Fig. 17-12). Horizontal oblique and transverse fractures were described as stable and expected to heal after immobilization for 6 to 12 weeks. Vertical oblique fractures were said to have a high longitudinal shear component and require longer immobilization owing to inherent instability. Desai found that, in reviewing 151 acute scaphoid fractures, interobserver and intraobserver reproducibility of the Herbert and Russe classification system with radiographs was fair. In addition, radiographic assessment of fracture level, comminution, and

displacement did not consistently predict fracture healing.[117,149] We emphasize duration, stability, and displacement to guide our treatment of scaphoid fractures (see Authors' Preferred Method of Treatment).

Nondisplaced fractures are stable and usually heal with a high rate of union and return of function. When a fracture is angulated or displaced, regardless of the direction of the fracture line, the fracture is unstable and will likely require operative management. Carpal instability should be suspected in all displaced fractures.[681] Diastasis of the scapho-

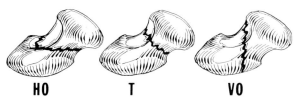

FIGURE 17-12. Classification of fractures of the scaphoid (Russe). HO, horizontal oblique; T, transverse; VO, vertical oblique. (From Taleisnik J: The Wrist. New York, Churchill Livingstone, 1985. © 1985, Elizabeth Roselius.)

lunate interval or lunate extension may suggest associated scapholunate instability.[118,193,435]

Accurate evaluation of displacement, rotation, and stability may be difficult with plain radiographs. Loss of carpal height can be a tipoff to significant fracture angulation. Questions with regard to fracture displacement may be answered with CT[545] and trispiral tomography.[373,517,545,572] CT has the advantage of permitting analysis and reconstruction in various planes such as the long axis of the scaphoid[376]; even three-dimensional reconstruction is possible and may be of use, particularly in chronic nonunions with loss of bony substance (Fig. 17-13).[43,455,683]

Management of Acute Scaphoid Fractures (Middle Third)

Middle third fractures are the most common fractures of the scaphoid and, like all scaphoid fractures, share a high rate of delayed union and nonunion. A delay in treatment, either because of the patient's failure to seek treatment after a seemingly trivial injury or because of a missed diagnosis, can adversely affect union.[36,353,405,657]

Factors that affect acute fracture stability include the degree of initial displacement, fracture comminution, and associated carpal instability. A failure to recognize concomitant carpal instability may lead to a high rate of complications of treatment.[57,75,193,435] Gross fracture malalignment or scapholunate dissociation[57,132,684] leads to a loss of scaphoid support for the proximal and distal carpal rows[351,571] and distorts load-bearing characteristics.[701] Most frequently, the lunate becomes extended and the carpus collapses into a "concertina"[193] or dorsal intercalated segment instability (DISI)[372] deformity. Less frequently, the lunate rotates into flexion, a volar intercalated segment instability (VISI) pattern. Carpal malalignment cannot occur unless either the scaphoid fracture is significantly angulated, there is a concomitant major capsular injury, or both. Any degree of carpal malalignment must therefore be considered an indication for detailed analysis including CT or MRI[211,616] (see Chapter 14 for further discussion of carpal instability).

Nonoperative Treatment of Acute Scaphoid Waist Fractures

If the fracture is stable it may be treated with immobilization. Historically there have been three main areas of disagreement in nonoperative treatment of acute fractures of the scaphoid: (1) the position of the wrist in plaster, (2) the need to include joints other than the wrist in the cast, and (3) the duration of immobilization. For nonoperative treatment to be successful, immobilization must remain effective until

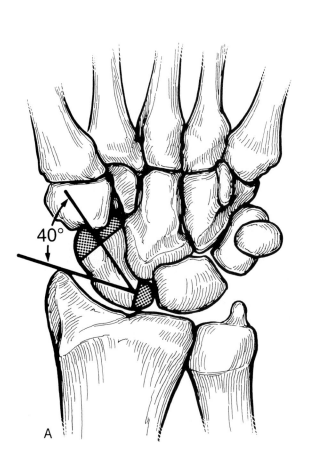

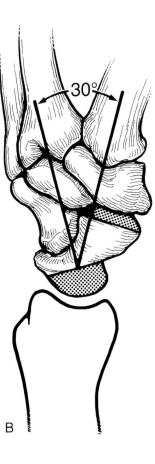

FIGURE 17-13. A, Normal anteroposterior anatomy of the scaphoid perpendicular to the proximal and distal articular surfaces forms an intersection at a mean angle, as shown here, of 40 ± 4 degrees. Examiner error is roughly ± 5 degrees. **B,** The normal lateral intra-articular angle is 24 ± 5 degrees. The example shown here measures 30 degrees. (Redrawn from Amadio PC, Berquist TH, Smith DK, et al: Scaphoid malunion. J Hand Surg [Am] 14:679-687, 1989.)

union of the fracture. It is important to allow the hand to function, because this seems to enhance the healing potential and reduce atrophy. However, sweat and regular wear tend to soften plaster casts and thin the underlying padding. Fiberglass, now the present standard for cast material, is more durable and remains snug for a longer period of time.[22]

Position of Immobilization: Wrist

The optimal position of casting has been investigated intensely, but there is virtually no consensus.[378] In general, displaced or angulated fractures usually require operative treatment, so by default a fracture being treated by closed means will be undisplaced and probably stable. Such fractures require protection rather than reduction, and this probably explains why wrist position has little effect on union rates in practice. Experimental data[329] based on Squire's concepts of mechanics[583] support immobilization of even "problem" fractures of the scaphoid (involving the proximal pole, displaced or nonunited) with the wrist in full ulnar deviation and some extension and the forearm supinated. Ulnar deviation and extension align the scaphoid with the long axis of the forearm and tighten the radial-sided wrist ligaments, supporting the scaphoid between the trapezium and radius. Supination is believed to shift the lunate radially and support the scaphoid against the radius. O'Brien, however, believed that wrist *flexion* and *radial deviation* would produce better apposition of the fracture fragments.[126,465] Despite these views, in a randomized prospective study, Hambidge found that the position of wrist immobilization (20 degrees of flexion or 20 degrees of extension) had no significant impact on fracture healing. The wrists, however, that had been immobilized in flexion were found to have a greater restriction of extension at 6-month follow-up.[247] Wrist position should be such that radiographs taken after the cast is applied show anatomic coaptation of the fragments and normal alignment of the carpus. However, if reduction is required, surgical fixation is far more secure than any cast and is preferred.

Type of Cast: Which Joints to Immobilize

The second point of contention is the immobilization of joints other than the wrist. It is most common to include the thumb in a position of opposition. This effectively eliminates any potential disruptive action, particularly from the abductor pollicis longus[594] and brevis.[577,578] However, some authors, including Böhler,[62] Herbert,[257] Hambidge,[247] and Clay and colleagues,[111] have not found the nonunion risk to be increased with below-elbow casting and the thumb left free. Clay and colleagues found, in a study of 292 randomized patients treated with wrist immobilization and followed for 6 months, that there was no benefit to additional immobilization of the thumb. Union occurred in 78% of the thumb-spica group and 77% of the thumb-free group.[111]

Inclusion of the elbow in the scaphoid cast was first suggested by Grace in 1929[233] and again by Verdan[656] in 1954. Verdan placed great emphasis on eliminating the action of the volar radiocarpal ligament on the scaphoid during pronation and supination.[657] In the same year, Stewart[594] reported 436 fractures treated in the U.S. Army Medical Corps in a short-arm/thumb spica cast with a union rate of 95%. More recently, Dickson and Leslie[155] reported a 95% union rate and a mean time to union of 75 days in 222 fractures treated with a short-arm/thumb spica cast. Experimental studies[179,345,519] have shown that forearm rotation does not induce intercarpal motion, provided that the wrist and thumb are immobilized.

Others have disagreed with these findings. Broomé and coworkers[79] and Gellman and associates[225] both reported a statistically significant reduction in the time needed for fracture healing when long-arm casting was used, in comparable series treated with and without elbow immobilization.[329] Three-dimensional motion analyses, performed by Kaneshiro, has shown that with forearm rotation and short-cast immobilization there is displacement between the proximal and distal portions of a scaphoid osteotomy. A mean displacement of 3.4 mm was found to occur as the forearm rotated between 60 degrees of supination and 60 degrees of pronation.[313]

Historically, some have advised complete immobilization of the fingers in a fist cast[506] or three-digit cast[146] during the initial period of fracture healing, but there is no compelling evidence to suggest that this degree of immobilization has a positive effect on healing. Surgery for unstable fractures is preferable to a course of protracted and extensive limb and digit immobilization.

We conclude that the use of a long-arm cast is probably not justified in all scaphoid waist fractures but should be strongly considered for the initial period of immobilization. Inclusion of the elbow is not usually a problem as far as late stiffness is concerned. Should there be a strenuous objection from the patient or a contraindication to elbow immobilization, an epicondylar bearing (Munster type) cast may be applied to restrict pronation-supination while allowing some flexion-extension of the elbow.[413]

Duration of Immobilization

The duration of immobilization for scaphoid waist fractures was rather brief in early reports.[148,382] As experience accumulated, it became clear that longer periods of immobilization produced higher rates of union. Assessment of union is impossible by physical examination alone.[87] Reliance on radiographs alone may also be unreliable. Dias has shown that intraobserver and interobserver reliability in evaluating union at 12 weeks is poor.[153] CT is a more reliable imaging modality to identify trabecular bridging after 12 weeks of immobilization.[32] MRI has also been shown to provide useful information in verifying fracture union, as evident by a return of normal marrow signal across the fracture line.[412]

Once union has been verified and the cast removed, recovery of motion in uninvolved joints is usually prompt. Wrist motion can return to nearly normal in 1 to 5 weeks.[62,169,594] Even so, the long period of casting and the potential for economic hardship in young, active adults prompted Russe[529] to comment: "since the period of immobilization may, in some cases, require many months, operative treatment by an experienced surgeon may be considered preferable." Some have argued that young men who suffer scaphoid fractures may be prone to noncompliance[325] with casting, perhaps because of psychological factors. An extensive study of 92 patients by Ryley, however, showed that the personality profile of scaphoid fracture patients was not different from that of age-matched controls. If anything, noncompliance seemed to be related to dissatisfaction with long waiting times in hospital clinics and protracted periods of cast immobilization.[533] The availability of more consistently successful surgical techniques has led many to recommend surgery not only for ununited scaphoid fractures but also for delayed unions* and some acute fractures, whether displaced or nondisplaced.

There is a growing movement toward surgical intervention for the fixation of nondisplaced acute scaphoid fractures[4,64,246,284,509,511,534,566-568] Early rigid fixation may allow for early active motion, earlier return to sports and work, and higher patient satisfaction.[246,511,611] In a recent study from the Netherlands, average time away from work for scaphoid fractures treated with cast immobilization averaged approximately 4.5 months.[649] In a prospective randomized study with 12-year follow-up comparing early open operative treatment and cast immobilization, Saeden found that return to work was quicker in manual laborers treated operatively. There were, however, no significant differences in long-term functional results between the two groups.[534]

Arthroscopic-assisted or percutaneous fixation of fractures may avoid the potential problems associated with long-

term cast immobilization and avoid the problems associated with formal open repair.[566,692] Open repairs can injure the volar carpal ligaments and have the potential to create carpal instability.[260] With the advent of cannulated screws and intraoperative radiographic monitoring, percutaneous or minimally invasive fixation is now the approach of choice for several surgeons and published reports site union rates as high as 100%.[246,284,566-568,706] Some surgeons allow their patients to move immediately after surgery.[246,284,706] Prospective trials support the use of percutaneous scaphoid fixation techniques as an alternative for the treatment of nondisplaced scaphoid fractures (Fig. 17-14).[4,64] Bond has shown that the use of screw fixation allows patients to return to work at an average of 7 weeks earlier and a decrease in time to union of 5 weeks.[64] Other studies have found no difference in the time to bony union.[4]

In general, most nondisplaced fractures of the scaphoid will heal if immobilized. Percutaneous screw placement can be associated with technical problems in inexperienced and even in experienced hands. Wires may break, and the margin for error is small. Exposed threads within the radiocarpal or midcarpal joint will certainly lead to arthritis. We believe percutaneous fixation is an excellent option for the young athlete who wishes to return to sports earlier and in the person who wants to avoid long cast wear, but only after a thorough discussion of the risks of screw placement.

*See references 89, 113, 122, 142, 160, 169, 263, 411, 634, and 646.

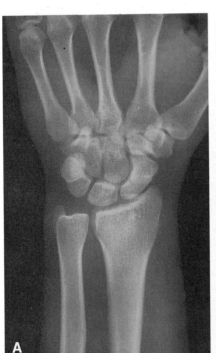
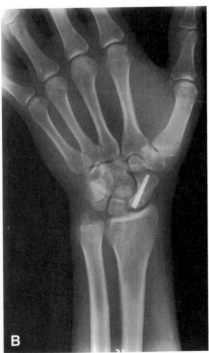

FIGURE 17-14. A, A 24-year-old football player suffered a nondisplaced scaphoid fracture midseason. **B** and **C,** A compression screw was placed percutaneously, and the patient returned to practice at 6 weeks.

Authors' Preferred Method of Treatment: Acute Scaphoid Waist Fractures

Immobilization of Acute Scaphoid Fractures

There is universal agreement that the vast majority of acute nondisplaced scaphoid fractures will heal if immobilized properly and for a long enough period.* Both Cooney and coworkers[126] and Herbert[256] use a radiographic assessment of fracture stability to guide their treatment protocols. Stable fractures (no displacement or angulation) are treated in a below-elbow thumb spica cast. The wrist may be positioned in slight wrist extension.[307] Unstable fractures are those showing displacement of 1 mm or more between fragments, fragment angulation, or abnormal carpal alignment. If nonoperative treatment is elected for an unstable fracture, the surgeon must ensure that carpal and scaphoid alignment can be restored by manipulation or positioning. The absolute requisite is to accept nothing less than anatomic alignment; an above-elbow cast is required in such cases. If anatomic alignment cannot be achieved or maintained, one should proceed to open reduction and internal fixation. With the advent of cannulated screw systems, which can be used percutaneously under arthroscopic or fluoroscopic control, we are much more aggressive in performing operative reduction for fractures with any signs of instability. In general our indications for casting are (1) nondisplaced waist fractures and (2) distal pole fractures in good position (to be discussed later).[307]

Nondisplaced fractures that present later than 4 weeks after injury are at increased risk of nonunion and require longer periods of immobilization to achieve union.[386] If nonoperative treatment is chosen for these fractures, we prefer initial immobilization for 2 to 3 weeks in an above-elbow cast, followed by a short-arm cast until CT-confirmed healing.

Operative Management of Acute Scaphoid Fractures

Acute fractures with displacement, angulation, or carpal malalignment should be treated with open reduction and internal fixation. Multiple methods of internal fixation have been described, including Kirschner wire, compression screw,[†] staple fixation,[95,136,334,437,705] and even plate fixation.[277] Unless comminution is present, bone grafts are not necessary for acute injuries.

Kirschner Wires. Kirschner wires can be inserted percutaneously or through any surgical exposure. They are versatile, are easy to insert and remove, do not require a radial styloidectomy or extended approaches to facilitate exposure, and provide satisfactory stability. They can be clipped flush with the bone as permanent implants or, more frequently, left prominent beneath the skin or protruding through the skin for later removal. Fixation may not be as stable as with screws, however, and if the pins protrude or erode through the skin, pin tract infection may occur. Nonetheless, because of their versatility, Kirschner wires should remain an important part of the tool kit for any surgeon treating scaphoid fractures or nonunion.

Staples. Staple fixation for scaphoid fractures was popular in the 1980s but has been all but eclipsed by newer methods of screw fixation.[95,334,335] Satisfactory results were reported in 85% to 90% of cases. The technique is demanding inasmuch as fracture reduction is dependent on accurate placement of the staple.[335] Recently, operative fixation with shape memory staples, made of a nickel-titanium alloy that is malleable when cold but rigid at body temperature, have been recommended.[136,437,705] Cugola and Testoni[136] have used shape memory staples in eight cases with good results, but we believe that these limited, preliminary results are insufficient to recommend shape memory staples at this time.

Compression Screw. Screw fixation was proposed by McLaughlin[410] in 1954 and is now favored by many authors.[‡] The technique of compression screw osteosynthesis should be meticulous to avoid unwanted complications such as delayed union or nonunion caused by imprecise screw insertion.[123,170,252,637] Leyshon and coworkers[366] have had a satisfactory experience in treating acute and ununited fractures with a scaphoid lag screw inserted through an extended lateral or volar bayonet-shaped incision. A radial styloidectomy was not required, and screw insertion could be accomplished under direct vision. They advised against disturbing the fracture site or using bone grafts in conjunction with screw fixation. Fernandez has also used a compression screw successfully.[185] Trumble and associates[637] emphasized the importance of screw placement in the central axis of the scaphoid, which may be more easily accomplished by the use of the newer cannulated screws and intraoperative fluoroscopy. A recent modification of screw fixation involves the use of a two-piece screw.[352] The proximal part of the screw tip is hollow and threaded; the head has threads that fit into the threaded portion. Tightening the screw head on the screw tip creates compression. The advantage of this type of screw is that length (and compression) can be adjusted after placement of the screw tip. The screw tip can be placed precisely in subcortical bone in the proximal scaphoid fragment; the head of the screw is then inserted and compression achieved without fear of disturbing screw tip placement. Reported experience with this device is limited, however.

Headless Compression Screws. In 1984 Herbert and Fisher[259] published their experience with the use of a double-threaded bone screw and special instrumentation for scaphoid fractures and nonunions. The screw lacks a head and instead uses two separate thread diameters and pitch to engage both fracture fragments and simultaneously compress the bone fragments during insertion (Fig. 17-15). It does not require removal and may be used for small fragments and with bone grafts. Because there is no screw head, both ends of the screw remain buried under cartilage and consequently do not interfere with attempts at early motion. A specially designed compression jig holds the fragments aligned and in apposition before inserting the screw

---

*See references 62, 155, 165, 169, 379, 448, 449, 471, 501, 518, 551, 576, 577, and 594.

†See references 189, 191, 256, 372, 401, 411, 510, 638, 657, and 681.

‡See references 68, 79, 80, 127, 185, 193, 253, 256, 283, 404, 454, 499, 515, 637, and 692.

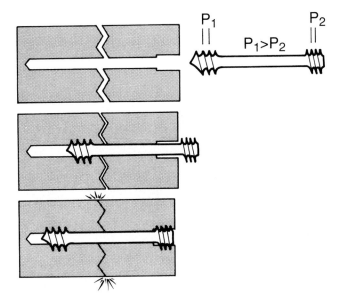

FIGURE 17-15. The difference in pitch between the leading thread (P1) and the trailing thread (P2) of the Herbert screw governs the rate of "take-up" or drawing together of the two bone fragments to produce compression. (Redrawn from Herbert TJ, Fisher WE: Management of the fractured scaphoid using a new bone screw. J Bone Joint Surg Br 66:114-123, 1984.)

and provides guidance for both the direction and the depth of insertion. The amount of compression provided by the differential pitch mechanism has been reported to be minimal,[499] and most of the compression is provided by the compression jig or manually during screw insertion. Disadvantages of this technique include the technical difficulty of accurate screw placement,[582] but attention to operative detail can be rewarded with good results.[86,188,196,505]

To minimize exposure requirements, Whipple[692] described a cannulated variant of the Herbert screw that can be inserted under fluoroscopic or arthroscopic control. Several variations of cannulated screws are available. These screws allow for substantial compression while limiting incisions and disruption of carpal ligaments.[246,260,284,566-568,706] High union rates have been reported when using these screws for both acute fractures and nonunions.[64,246,282,284,566,568,616] Although laboratory studies have shown the Herbert screw constructs to have less strength or ability to compress the fracture fragments than other devices,[318,556] the main complications have related more to poor screw placement[68,131,454,515,637] than to screw failure.

Comparisons Between Screw Types. Since Herbert and Fisher's initial report in 1984[259] there have been several technical advancements in screw design. Many surgeons now favor cannulated screws over the original Herbert design, primarily for their technical ease in placement. Biomechanical reports have attempted to examine the benefits of one screw type over another. Shaw found that the compression provided by the ASIF 4.0- and 3.5-mm cancellous bone screw was greater than that of the Herbert screw.[556,557] Similar findings were confirmed by Rankin.[499] Reports indicate that larger-diameter screws may be beneficial in resisting repetitive compressive loads across the scaphoid. Toby found that the ASIF, Acutrak, and

Herbert-Whipple screws demonstrated superior resistance to cyclical bending loads when compared with the Herbert screw.[625]

Several studies have attempted to show benefit of one type of screw over another.[625,638] Though compression does appear to enhance healing, it is not clear if the increased compression provided by one type of screw in a cadaveric study translates to improved clinical or radiographic outcomes.[180] In a study by Christodoulou, only 55% of nonunions treated with Kirschner wires attained union whereas 85% of ASIF screws and 77% of Herbert screws united.[109] In a clinical comparison by Trumble there were no differences between the Herbert-Whipple screw and AO/ASIF screw in terms of fracture healing or ease in placement.[638] These authors demonstrated that accurate placement of the screw was more important than the type of screw utilized and that time to healing was shorter when screw position was in the central third of the scaphoid.[637] Central screw placement was more consistent when a cannulated screw was used. The majority of these screws are manufactured of titanium, and their use does not preclude the use of MRI in subsequent evaluations of healing or vascularity.[212]

Long-term studies need to be performed to determine whether screw placement may lead to degenerative changes in neighboring joints. Scaphotrapezial-trapezoid (STT) arthritis has been reported after both Herbert screw and AO/ASIF screw placement.[94,534,563,642,706]

Technique of Screw Osteosynthesis (Herbert and Fisher).[259] Use of the Herbert screw is difficult, with a very narrow margin for error. Herbert's precise instructions should be studied carefully and the operation practiced on a cadaver wrist before attempting it on a patient. The approach is similar to Russe's: a palmar "hockey stick" incision is made superficial to the distal flexor carpi radialis tendon and angled distally onto the base of the thenar eminence to fully expose the distal end of the scaphoid. The volar carpal ligaments are divided and tagged for later reapproximation. Displaced fractures are reduced manually or with the assistance of Kirschner wire "joysticks." The scaphotrapezial joint is opened and a portion of the trapezium excised to enable positioning of the screw in the central third of the scaphoid. The Huene alignment jig is positioned with its tip hooked around the proximal pole at its dorsal margin, and the drill guide is firmly clamped against the tubercle to provide compression at the fracture site. The length of the screw is read directly off the calibrated guide. A series of two drills are used, followed by a tap for the leading threads. The screw is inserted below until the head is flush with the subchondral bone and the jig removed. Radiography or fluoroscopy should be used in the operating room to confirm satisfactory position of the screw. Careful repair and immobilization of the volar carpal ligaments must be performed to avoid late instability (Fig. 17-16). A conforming dressing and a thumb-spica splint is applied. Immobilization is maintained for at least 4 weeks to protect the volar ligament repair. Some authors advocate active range-of-motion exercises from the beginning in acute fractures when a limited operative exposure has been performed; when a bone graft is required, more prolonged cast immobilization is advised, usually for 4 to 6 weeks.

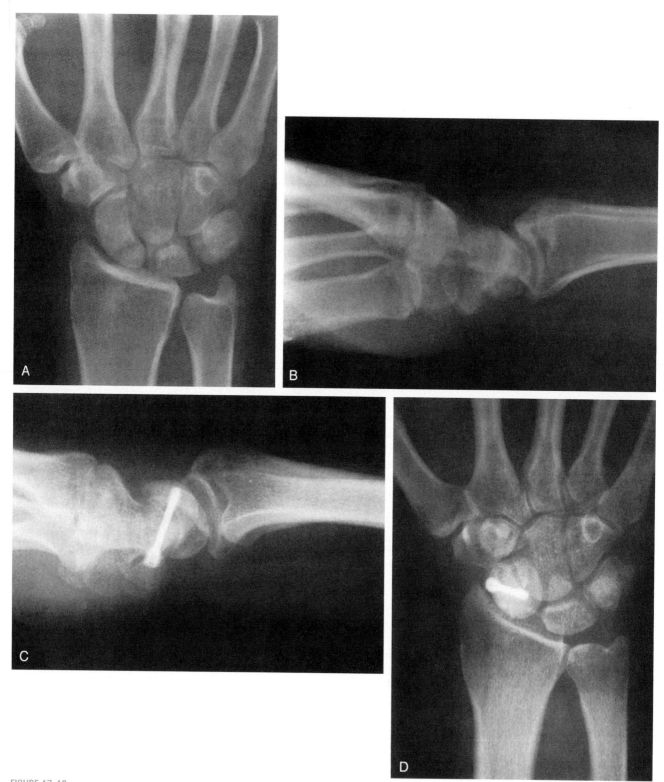

FIGURE 17-16. Preoperative anteroposterior (**A**) and lateral (**B**) radiographs of a proximal pole fracture. **C,** Postoperatively the scaphoid is well fixed with a Herbert screw, but the anteroposterior radiograph (**D**) shows that the scaphoid has been destabilized by rotation and foreshortening.

Botte and Gelberman[72] have described a technique of intraoperative radiographic control that may make insertion more predictable. In this technique the fracture is provisionally fixed with a 1.2-mm (0.045-inch) Kirschner wire. The jig is then applied, and a second 1.2-mm Kirschner wire is inserted down the barrel of the jig. A radiograph confirms fracture reduction, jig location, and approximate future screw position. If all is satisfactory, the Kirschner wire is removed from the barrel of the jig and the Herbert screw inserted in the usual way. Alternatively, the guide wire can be left in place and a cannulated screw inserted. Either an AO 3.5-mm cannulated screw[637] or a cannulated Herbert-Whipple screw may be used.[692]

Percutaneous Screw Fixation. Percutaneous compression screws can be inserted through both palmar and dorsal approaches. For the dorsal approach, a 0.045-inch guide wire is placed into the proximal pole of the scaphoid. Position is verified with a fluoroscopy unit. If there is any question about position, a small incision can be made approximately 1 cm proximal and ulnar to Lister's tubercle. The hand is then pronated and flexed until the scaphoid appears as a cylinder under fluoroscopy. The center of the cylinder roughly corresponds with the central axis of the scaphoid. The wire is placed through the central axis of the scaphoid and advanced distally to exit the skin on the thenar eminence. Before extending the wrist to check wire placement, the wire must be advanced until the trailing end clears the radiocarpal joint. Failing to perform this step can lead to bending or breakage of the wire. Once the wire is in position, the wrist can be flexed again and a parallel wire is placed to prevent fragment rotation during screw placement. The central wire is withdrawn dorsally to correct position and measured for screw length (before reaming). A reamer is then passed over the guide wire, and hand or power drilling is used to prepare the scaphoid for the screw. Reaming is stopped short of the opposite cortex. Care must be taken to prevent wire pullout during the reaming step. Screw length is then measured from a screw guide placed over the guide wire or with a second Kirschner wire placed at the base of the scaphoid next to the primary guide wire. The difference in length between the two wires is the length of the screw. We usually subtract 3 to 5 mm from the measured length so that the screw may be safely countersunk and to prevent unwanted distraction at the fracture site. Newer screws allow one to separately apply compression after the screw is countersunk within the bone. Arthroscopy can be used as an adjunct to perform or verify fracture reduction and confirm that the screw is completely seated within the scaphoid.[568]

When using the volar approach for screw placement, the hand is placed on a folded towel with the wrist in extension. We have found it helpful to place the hand directly onto a covered fluoroscopy unit, which then serves as the operative table. This simplifies imaging as the wire is placed into the scaphoid. An alternative approach is to place the thumb into a traction tower during guide wire placement[250]; this ensures ulnar deviation of the wrist and uncovers the tubercle of the scaphoid. The guide wire is started at the distal radial pole of the scaphoid, and this occasionally requires the wire to pass through the trapezium. The wire is then advanced dorsally and ulnarly, aiming toward the dorsal and proximal

pole of the scaphoid. A small incision facilitates use of the cannulated reamer from the palmar direction. Screw placement then proceeds in a similar manner to the dorsal approach.

The key to these techniques relies on the accurate placement of the Kirschner wire before screw placement. This technique should only be used for nondisplaced fractures or for fractures that can be anatomically reduced with closed or arthroscopic manipulation.[567] If fracture reduction cannot be verified arthroscopically or fluoroscopically, then conversion to an open procedure should be performed.[692] The tech-

---

CRITICAL POINTS: PERCUTANEOUS SCAPHOID FIXATION

INDICATION

- Acute nondisplaced or minimally displaced fractures

TECHNICAL POINTS

- Either dorsal or volar approach may be used.
- Central position of the guide wire is crucial.
- Reduction and wire placement is verified with fluoroscopy.
- An antirotational wire may be placed before reaming.
- Reaming is stopped short of the far cortex.
- Screw length is determined with the use of a depth gauge or parallel wire. Screw length should be 3 to 5 mm shorter than measured length to prevent protrusion of the screw into the radiocarpal or STT joint.

PEARLS

- Placement of the guide wire when using the dorsal approach is aided by pronation and flexion of the wrist.
- The scaphoid can then be visualized as a cylinder aiding in the central placement of the guide wire.
- The volar approach is aided by making a small incision and bluntly dissecting down to trapezium.

PITFALLS

- Poor placement of guide wire
- Wires breaking within scaphoid

POSTOPERATIVE CARE

- Splint and early range-of-motion exercises

SPECIAL CONSIDERATIONS

- Consider for athletes.

niques are not appropriate for severely comminuted fractures or those that require bone grafting for restoration of length.[258]

Fractures of the Proximal Pole of the Scaphoid

Treatment of proximal third scaphoid fractures depends on the size and vascularity of the fragment and the age of the fracture. Fresh injuries may heal after prolonged immobilization, although the peculiar blood supply of the scaphoid renders these fractures particularly vulnerable to avascular necrosis and nonunion.[507] Unfortunately, imaging studies such as gadolinium-enhanced MRI are not able to predict which of these fractures may heal without surgery. In a study by Dawson, 32 fractures were assessed with dynamic gadolinium-enhanced MRI 1 to 2 weeks after injury. Their results showed that poor proximal vascularity was not a consistent predictor of scaphoid nonunion.[143]

There is a growing sentiment that most proximal pole fractures should be treated operatively, because of their high propensity for nonunion and the increased duration of immobilization required for nonoperative management. Modern techniques of internal and percutaneous fixation have increased healing rates and tipped the scale in favor of early operative treatment for these injuries, particularly for the young and active. For those proximal third fractures that fail to unite after 6 months of nonoperative treatment, particularly when the fragments are smaller than 30% of the scaphoid, vascularized bone grafting has added a viable surgical treatment.[186,321,477,709] In our opinion, acute proximal pole fractures should be treated operatively to (1) provide complete immobilization to optimize revascularization and (2) avoid lengthy plaster immobilization and high risks of nonunion.[339,513]

If the proximal fragment is large enough to accommodate the trailing end of a headless compression screw, attempts at dorsal fixation should be considered. DeMaagd and Engber used a Herbert screw inserted freehand from the dorsal approach[148] and reported success in 11 of their 12 patients. Retting and Raskin also used the dorsal approach and a Herbert compression screw acutely on 17 proximal pole fractures and obtained 100% union (Fig. 17-17).[513] If the fragment is too small, Kirschner wires can be used. After the union is solid, the Kirschner wires or staples should be removed, while screws can generally be left in place.

Fractures of the Distal Third of the Scaphoid

Fractures of the scaphoid distal pole are infrequent.[154,263,483,491] They may be limited to the scaphoid tuberosity or may involve the entire distal third of the bone. Prosser and asso-

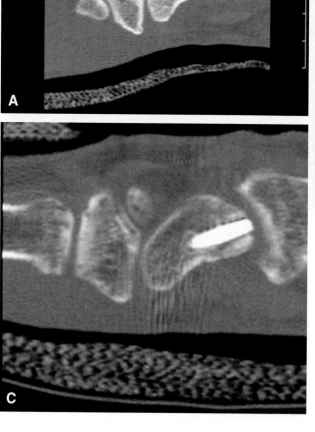

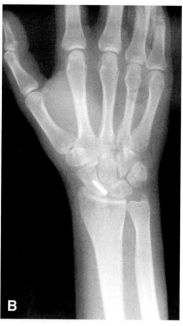

FIGURE 17-17. **A** and **B,** A proximal pole fracture in a 32-year-old man was treated acutely with a mini-compression screw placed from a limited dorsal approach. **C,** Union was verified with a CT scan at 6 months.

ciates[491] reviewed 37 cases of scaphoid distal pole fractures and proposed a classification in three groups: type I, tuberosity fractures; type II, distal intra-articular fractures; and type III, osteochondral fractures. In Russe's classification,[529] fractures of the distal third were commonly of the transverse, stable type and in his experience united rapidly, usually after 4 to 8 weeks in a short-arm/thumb spica cast.

Fractures of the tuberosity are extra-articular and usually stable, with a generous blood supply.[177,376,464,607] They tend to heal promptly and are best treated in a short-arm/thumb spica cast for 3 to 6 weeks. Vertical fractures into the STT joint, Prosser's type II, may be difficult to detect[128] and may require special diagnostic views and imaging techniques. Plaster immobilization is usually successful for distal fractures (Fig. 17-18). Just as for other intra-articular injuries, open reduction and internal fixation should be considered when the fracture fragments are unacceptably displaced or offset.

Nonunion of the Scaphoid

In most instances, nonunions of the scaphoid are treated by surgical means. Previous reports suggested that established nonunions, particularly if stable and without carpal collapse,[193] may not require treatment because they might remain essentially symptom free.[154,378,404,405] However, it has become clear from a growing number of publications that ununited fractures or fracture malunions, if left untreated, will progress to osteoarthritis and impaired wrist motion.[65,307,313,384,393,418,527,654]

Published studies concerning the "natural history" of scaphoid nonunion may be flawed because they are retrospective and not population based.[322] It is possible that their findings simply reflect selection or referral bias. Nonetheless, it is logical to assume that the severity of osteoarthritis and the rapidity of its progression are greater for displaced fractures and in the presence of coexistent carpal instability.

Few nonunions remain stable, undisplaced, or free of arthritis after 10 years. Long-standing scaphoid nonunion leads to a pattern of arthritis originally described by Watson and Ballet.[676,679] It is described in a four-stage progression, similar to that seen with scapholunate dissociation. Stage I is characterized by arthritic changes and osteophyte formation at the radial styloid. Stage II patients have developed arthritis at the radioscaphoid joint. Stage III patients have arthritic involvement of the midcarpal joint (capitolunate and scaphocapitate joints). Stage IV patients have arthritis involving all but the radiolunate joint. This progression has been termed as *scaphoid nonunion advanced collapse* or SNAC wrist.[679] Frequently, the scaphoid proximal pole escapes degenerative change in this collapse pattern, behaving kinematically like its tightly bound lunate. When unrestrained by the distal scaphoid the lunate assumes an extended posture because of the unchecked extension force of the lunotriquetral ligament. Over time this can result in a DISI deformity that may lead to abnormal capitate wear and eventual midcarpal arthritis. Because of the propensity for degenerative progression, even asymptomatic patients with stable undisplaced nonunions should be advised of the probablility of late degenerative changes. Mack and coworkers[384] recommend that all displaced nonunited scaphoid fractures be reduced and grafted, regardless of symptoms, before the onset of osteoarthritis. For stable, undisplaced nonunion, prolonged immobilization may lead to union in some patients, but this treatment is not recommended because it may produce permanent wrist impairment and the risk that reconstructive surgery will be necessary after 4 to 6 months of immobilization.[62,594]

Avascular necrosis of the proximal pole is an additional factor that renders the scaphoid fracture resistant to healing with both nonoperative and operative methods. Proximal pole vascularity cannot be determined from plain radiographs, because increased radiographic density of the proximal fragment correlates poorly with the presence of avascular necrosis.[236] Trumble[636] has shown that MRI appearance is a more reliable indicator of avascular necrosis, as determined by histologic analysis of biopsy specimens. Green[236] recommended direct scrutiny of the fracture surfaces for punctate bleeding points at the time of surgical excavation as the best method to determine scaphoid vascularity.

Electrical and Ultrasound Stimulation of Nonunions
Although the mechanism of action in tissues is not fully understood, electrical stimulation has been used for the treatment of fracture nonunions. Electrical currents may be delivered directly to a fracture, either through surgical implantation of an anode, cathode, and battery (the "invasive" method)[696] or through percutaneous placement of the cathode, with skin surface attachment of the anode (the "semi-invasive" method).[29,67] By contrast, "noninvasive" methods create an electromagnetic field around the fracture by incorporation of electric coils in a plaster cast at the fracture site. Pulsed electromagnetic field treatment is pain free and noninvasive and may be used in the presence of infection.[606] Frykman and associates[205] reported their initial experience in treating 44 chronic (> 6 months) scaphoid nonunions by noninvasive, pulsed electromagnetic field (PEMF) therapy. Thirty-five (80%) were reported to have

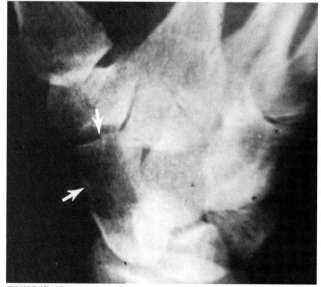

FIGURE 17-18. Vertical fracture of the distal pole of the scaphoid *(arrows)*.

healed after a mean of 4.3 months of combined PEMF and plaster immobilization. However, when Adams and associates updated the series, they found that several of the fractures that had appeared to be healed were in fact still ununited.[1] The technique was far less effective for avascular and proximal pole nonunions. Results suggest that PEMF is not as effective as bone grafting techniques, and its use should be considered only for patients when surgery is not an option.[1,41,156,205] Pulsed electromagnetic field treatment is not inexpensive and requires a high level of patient compliance. It is absolutely contraindicated for fractures with SNAC arthritis, carpal instability, or synovial pseudarthrosis.[156]

Ultrasound also has been used in an attempt at promoting bony healing. The mechanism of action may be related to alterations in cellular calcium metabolism.[479,532] It also has been shown to upregulate the gene expression of aggrecan and platelet-derived growth factor.[290,702] In addition, it increases blood flow to the fracture site even after removal of the ultrasound device.[156]

The use of ultrasound to accelerate healing in acute fractures has been examined by Mayr and others.[342,403] Mayr studied its use for 30 acute scaphoid waist fractures and documented CT-confirmed healing at an average of 62 days in the control group and 43 days in the ultrasound group. Examination at 6 weeks showed that 55% of the control group was healed, compared with 81% of the ultrasound group.[403] Nolte reported its use in the treatment of four scaphoid nonunions.[463] Three of four patients healed after 6 months of immobilization and ultrasound use; the one failure occurred in a proximal pole nonunion.

The early data suggest a possible role for ultrasound to accelerate scaphoid fracture healing, but its use in established nonunions requires further study. Long-term evaluation and further randomized prospective trials are required to fully delineate the roles of both ultrasound and electrical stimulation in the treatment of acute and nonunited scaphoid fractures.

Operative Treatment of Scaphoid Nonunion

Surgical treatment is indicated for established scaphoid nonunions and those fractures that have failed to heal after nonoperative management. The presence of degenerative, avascular, or cystic changes should not preclude operative treatment but will clearly affect the choice of procedure. In their evaluation of treatment of nonunions of the scaphoid, the Pennsylvania Orthopedic Society[483] concluded that "no one method of treatment can be used for all types of disability caused by an ununited fracture of the carpal navicular." It was further stated that "a well-stocked surgical armamentarium ready for any contingency does exist." This statement, written in 1962, is even more appropriate today with the addition of new forms of treatment such as percutaneous fixation[136,437,705] and vascularized bone grafts.[186,244,321,709] The choice of procedure will vary with the surgeon's preference and experience, the type of fracture, the patient's age, and the presence of periscaphoid arthrosis. Jupiter and colleagues suggested that nonunions can be divided into three major groups: (1) an established nonunion without secondary degenerative arthritis, (2) a nonunion with radiocarpal degenerative changes, and (3) scaphoid nonunion with advanced degenerative changes throughout the wrist.[307]

For group 1 patients, obtaining anatomic bony union is the major goal. For group 2, bony union will need to be combined with additional procedures to palliate local arthritic changes. Group 3 patients will usually require some type of salvage operation.

The following is a discussion of frequently used surgical techniques for the operative treatment of scaphoid nonunions. Salvage procedures such as partial or total arthrodesis and arthroplasty for the treatment of nonunions of the scaphoid are briefly reviewed; the techniques for these procedures are discussed in detail elsewhere.

Bone Graft Procedures

Bone grafts for scaphoid fractures were first advocated by Adams[2] in 1928. In subsequent years other authors[448,449] reported their experience with the use of cortical grafts. In 1937, Matti[400] showed that fracture healing can also be achieved by cancellous bone chips packed into an excavated nonunion using a dorsal approach. This technique was modified by Russe,[529] who used a volar approach to create and fill an egg-shaped cavity within the scaphoid fracture site with an oblong cancellous bone peg and additional cancellous bone chips. In 1980, Russe reported a modification of his original technique,[530] and the technique was published in the English literature in 1985 by Green.[236] This involved insertion of two corticocancellous grafts into the scaphoid excavation with their cancellous sides facing each other.[40,160,165,169,411,440,634,646,658] The remainder of the cavity is filled with 2-mm cancellous chips (Fig. 17-19).

Russe[236,529,530] and others[274] favor the iliac crest as the source of graft because they believe that this source of bone has a higher osteogenic potential.[236,529,530] However, others have used local bone graft from the radial metaphysis.[82,236,273] A simultaneous dorsoradial approach to the nonunion site and radial styloidectomy[35,82] provides adequate exposure and a volume of 1 to 1.5 mL of cancellous graft.[236] Recently there has been an interest in the use of trephine bone grafting for the treatment of scaphoid nonunions. A cylindrical bone graft is harvested from the iliac crest using bone trephine

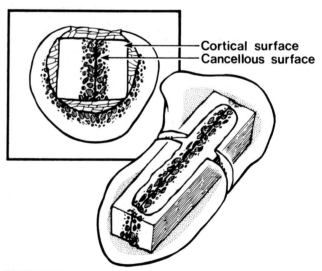

Cortical surface
Cancellous surface

FIGURE 17-19. Modern Russe technique using two corticocancellous bone grafts. (From Green DP: The effect of a vascular necrosis on Russe bone grafting for scaphoid nonunion. J Hand Surg [Am] 10:597-605, 1985.)

biopsy forceps. This results in decreased morbidity at the iliac crest donor site and more rapid harvest of graft. The scaphoid nonunion site can be resected with the same trephine, so little time is spent contouring the bone graft. Proponents of the technique believe the bone dowel is more stable than conventional grafts, and the technique is technically simplified.[363,394]

The Russe procedure may be effective in achieving union in angulated scaphoid malunions, but it is difficult to correct significant DISI deformity with this procedure. This technique is indicated for symptomatic, established nonunions and delayed unions without osteoarthritis or carpal malalignment. The presence of a collapsed scaphoid nonunion with dorsal carpal instability will reduce union rates.[99,131,435,549] Russe grafts may be performed in the presence of cystic changes[440]; however, the procedure is not as reliable in cases of avascular necrosis.[125] Long-term (3 to 10 years) clinical results of Russe grafting are satisfactory, but post-traumatic arthritis can occur in up to 50% of patients.[266,370,586] Barton recently demonstrated improved rates of union with inter-

calated corticocancellous grafting and screw fixation when compared with the Russe technique.[38]

Intercalated "Wedge" Bone Graft. In 1970, Fisk[193] observed that in chronic scaphoid nonunions that have progressed to carpal collapse, realignment of the scaphoid fragments creates an anterior wedge-shaped defect that can best be corrected by an anterior wedge-shaped bone graft (Fig. 17-20). Fisk showed that this procedure will correct the abnormal extension of the lunate and restore carpal alignment while simultaneously correcting scaphoid anatomy. Fisk proposed a lateral approach for this operation and concurrent radial styloidectomy; the radial styloid was used as the source of the wedge graft, and natural compressive forces were relied on for stabilization.[192,194] Fernandez[184,185] modified Fisk's technique by inserting a carefully measured wedge-shaped or trapezoidal iliac bone graft through a volar approach and recommended internal fixation. Wedge grafting can be successful even after previous failed bone graft attempts. Daly reported 95% union rates in 26 patients

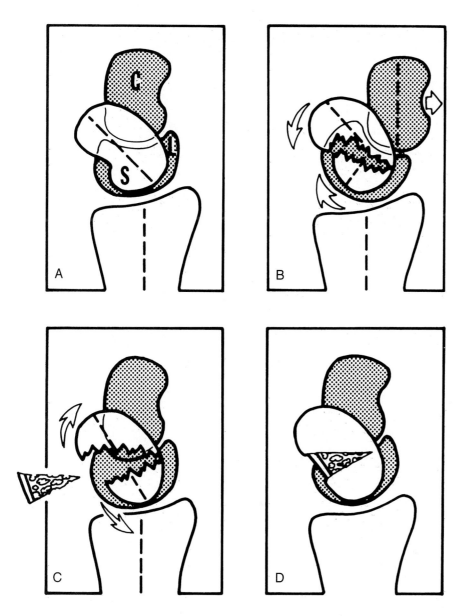

FIGURE 17-20. **A,** Schematic representation of normal alignment of the scaphoid (S), lunate (L), and capitate (C). **B,** Nonunion of a fracture of the scaphoid with palmar flexion of the distal fragment and a dorsal intercalated segment instability pattern. **C,** The scaphoid alignment is corrected. **D,** It is maintained by the insertion of a palmar wedge-shaped bone graft. (From Taleisnik J: The Wrist. New York, Churchill Livingstone, 1985.)

using this technique, including 11 patients who had failed previous bone graft surgery.[140] Del Pinal recommended the use of a combined volar wedge graft in conjunction with a dorsal retrograde compression screw in cases of proximal pole nonunions with DISI deformity.[147]

The results reported by Fernandez[184,185] and others[127,671] show slightly lower union rates than those reported by Russe with his technique, but an opening wedge graft is indicated in situations in which a Russe graft would lead to inadequate correction and nonunion or malunion.[127,452,586] Thus, it may be inappropriate to base a comparison of intercalated wedge grafting and Russe grafting on union rates alone. In a review of 150 united scaphoid fractures treated over a 24-year period, Barton found that the wedge graft with Herbert screw fixation produced the highest rates of union; however,

clinical and radiologic success did not always correlate. The best clinical results in this study were obtained with those who had successful unions using the modified Russe approach.[38] In a quantitative meta-analysis of the literature, Merrell and colleagues found that, in unstable nonunions, screw fixation of intercalated wedge grafts was superior to use of Kirschner wire fixation, with a 94% union rate compared with a 77% union rate.[415]

Bone Graft Technique (Original Russe Method)[529]

A 4- to 5-cm longitudinal incision is made along the radial border of the flexor carpi radialis tendon (Fig. 17-21A), centered at a level even with the tip of the radial styloid, which usually corresponds to the level of the fracture itself. The capsule is divided longitudinally (see Fig. 17-21B), and

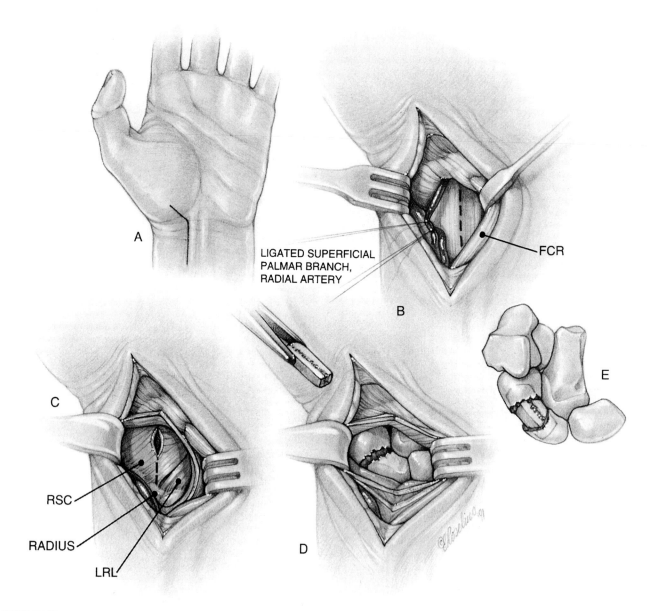

FIGURE 17-21. Original Russe bone graft technique. **A,** The incision. **B,** The flexor carpi radialis tendon (FCR) is retracted to expose the volar capsule. **C,** The volar capsule is divided longitudinally to expose the radioscaphocapitate (RSC) and long radiolunate (LRL) ligaments. Care should be taken to minimize ligament injury. **D,** An egg-shaped cavity is created distal and proximal to the fracture line. A corticocancellous bone graft, usually obtained from the ipsilateral iliac crest, is fashioned to fit snugly into this cavity. **E,** The corticocancellous bone graft has been wedged into the cavity of the scaphoid. The stability of the graft and the fracture fragments should be satisfactory. If not, additional fixation with one or two Kirschner wires is recommended.

the underlying deep volar radiocarpal ligaments are either divided partially and retracted or completely severed and tagged for later repair (see Fig. 17-21C and D). An egg-shaped cavity is created well into both fracture fragments without using power tools. A cancellous bone graft is then obtained from the ipsilateral iliac crest and fashioned into an ovoid plug large enough to fit snugly into the scaphoid cavity (see Fig. 17-21E). The graft is impacted into both fragments as these are forcibly distracted. Once the graft is in place, both fragments and the graft itself are manually compressed to produce a satisfactory degree of stability. Internal fixation is reserved only for situations in which instability persists after the bone graft is in place. In such cases, Kirschner wires are inserted parallel to each other and to the longitudinal axis of the scaphoid. The radiocarpal ligaments are repaired, and the hand and wrist are immobilized in a compression-type dressing incorporated into a long-arm cast. This is changed to a long-arm/thumb spica cast at 5 to 7 days and to a short-arm/thumb spica cast at 6 weeks postoperatively. If the intraoperative construct is very stable or if internal fixation was used, a short-arm/thumb spica cast may be used from the outset. The total immobilization time for this procedure averages 4 months. Union rates of 90% or better have been reported in some series.[236,530]

Volar Wedge Bone Graft Technique (Fisk-Fernandez)[184,192]

Preoperatively, radiographs are obtained of the injured and normal scaphoid, and tracings are performed to plan the resection, as well as the size and shape of the bone graft (Fig. 17-22). The surgical approach is similar to that used for a Russe bone graft. The resection is carried out with an oscillating saw. The resulting surfaces can be freshened with a rongeur or curet. Fernandez advocates repeated drilling of the proximal fragment, should this be sclerotic. A tricortical corticocancellous bone graft is obtained from the iliac crest. The scaphoid fragments are then distracted to correct flexion and length while at the same time an assistant tips the lunate and, with it, the proximal fragment of the scaphoid into satisfactory alignment. A 0.045-inch Kirschner wire may be drilled into the lunate for use as a joystick to aid reduction. Wrist extension or ulnar deviation helps hold the scaphoid defect open. A wedge-shaped or, more commonly, trapezoidal graft is fashioned from the iliac bone. It is helpful to use small osteotomes as sizers to accurately measure the wedge-shaped defect of the scaphoid and assist in designing the graft insert. The cortical margin corresponding to the inner table of the iliac crest is positioned ulnarly at its articulation with the capitate and the rounded cortical surface corresponding to the crest of the ilium facing palmarward. Protruding portions are trimmed flush. Two 0.045-inch Kirschner wires are then introduced from the palmar aspect of the distal fragment, through the graft and into the dorsal aspect of the proximal fragment. A compression screw may also be used.[185,256,259,451] Intraoperative radiographs or an image intensifier is used to ensure satisfactory correction and placement of the internal fixation. Because of the considerable change in scaphoid dimensions, capsular closure may be difficult. In these cases repair may be aided by using a portion of the flexor carpi radialis sheath to cover the capsular defect.[314] If Kirschner wires are used, Fernandez proposes postoperative immobi-

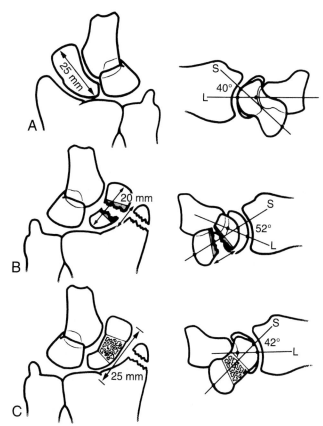

FIGURE 17-22. Preoperative planning for insertion of a wedge-shaped graft. **A,** Tracing of the opposite uninjured wrist and measurement of scaphoid length and scapholunate angle. **B,** Calculation of size, resection area, and form of graft. **C,** Definitive diagram of the operation. (Redrawn from Fernandez DL: A technique for anterior wedge-shaped grafts for scaphoid nonunions with carpal instability. J Hand Surg [Am] 9:733-737, 1984.)

lization in a below-elbow cast for 8 weeks, followed by removable splinting until healing is confirmed with tomograms or CT. Kirschner wires are removed at this point, an average of 10 to 11 weeks postoperatively. If screw fixation is elected and is stable, both Fernandez[185] and Herbert[256,257] permit mobilization as early as 2 weeks postoperatively. Even with ideal planning, a properly sized and shaped wedge graft may not completely correct an established collapse deformity. In such cases the problem rests not only in the abnormal scaphoid anatomy but also in the separate attenuation or contracture of the capsular ligaments. When preoperative templating identifies pronounced collapse and lunate dorsal tilt, it is advisable to intraoperatively correct the lunate tilt before resection and grafting of the scaphoid.[629] This can be performed indirectly under fluoroscopic control by maximally flexing the wrist and directing a 0.062-inch Kirschner wire across the radial styloid and into the lunate to hold it in a slightly overcorrecting posture of flexion. This simultaneously restores the scaphoid proximal pole to proper alignment and facilitates resection and sizing of the graft. The Kirschner wire can be removed in the office at 4 to 6 weeks postoperatively.

Vascularized Bone Grafting of Scaphoid Nonunion

Surgical techniques and the relevant anatomy of vascularized bone grafting are covered in detail in Chapter 50.

This section will focus on the indications and results of vascularized bone grafting for scaphoid nonunions.

In 1983, Braun reported 100% healing rate with the pronator pedicle vascularized bone graft from the distal radius for the treatment of 8 patients with Kienböck's disease, 1 with Preiser's disease, and 5 with scaphoid delayed union.[76] Kawai and Yamamoto,[320] Kuhlmann and associates,[345] and Papp and colleagues[477] also reported 100% union rates in a total of 37 additional patients with scaphoid nonunions that ranged in duration from 4 to 196 months. Pechlaner and coworkers[481] reported 25 successful procedures using a free vascularized iliac crest graft for scaphoid nonunion. Subsequently, other forms of vascularized bone grafting have been advised for scaphoid nonunions and, in particular, for the avascular or proximal pole variants. Fernandez and Eggli[186] have advised implantation of the second intermetacarpal vascular bundle into a drill hole in the proximal pole of resistant scaphoid nonunions. They reported success in 10 of 11 patients with avascular nonunions of the scaphoid when this procedure was combined with inlay corticocancellous bone graft and internal fixation. Six of their 11 patients had undergone previous surgery with conventional grafting techniques.

Zaidemberg and colleagues[709] and later Sheetz and associates[559,561] described a versatile set of vascular pedicles on the dorsum of the wrist that can be used to provide vascularized distal radius bone to a variety of sites in the carpus. Laboratory studies using canine models have shown that these pedicled vascularized grafts will increase bone blood flow to an avascular segment and increase the levels of osteoid and osteoblastic activity.[598] Reports of these procedures, whether pedicled from the palmar carpal artery,[398] dorsal metacarpal arteries,[388,397,708] distal radius,[390,645] or harvested as free vascularized bone,[158,209,249] demonstrate union rates of 80% to 100%. We believe the 1,2 intercompartmental supraretinacular artery (1,2 ICSRA) graft is the most useful for scaphoid nonunions.[561] Excellent results have been reported by several authors, even for difficult fractures involving the proximal pole.[709] Steinmann and others have emphasized that, despite high union rates with vascularized grafts, preoperative radiocarpal arthritis usually correlates with poor clinical outcome.[397,592]

Indications for vascularized grafting of a scaphoid nonunion include management of nonunions with failed prior surgery, particularly in cases with osteonecrosis of the proximal pole. There is no consensus as to the indications for its use as a primary procedure in difficult waist fractures or acute proximal pole fractures.

Technique of Pronator Pedicle Graft[320]

The scaphoid is exposed and prepared as for Russe bone grafting. The incision is extended proximally so that the pronator quadratus is also exposed. A block of radius of appropriate size (usually 15 to 20 mm long, 8 to 10 mm wide, and 5 to 6 mm deep) is outlined at the level of the distal pronator quadratus insertion (Fig. 17-23). A fine

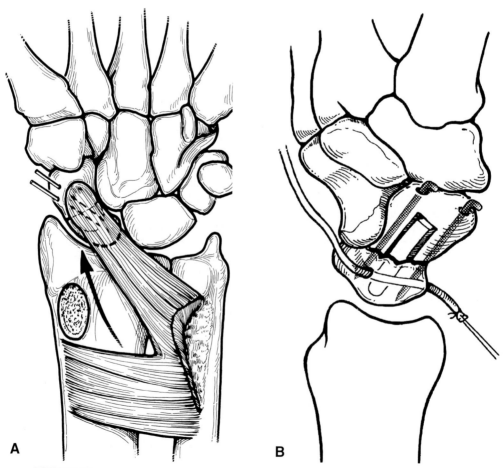

FIGURE 17-23. A, Pronator pedicle bone graft. **B,** Second intermetacarpal vascular bundle implantation.[186]

osteotome is used to elevate the bone block in continuity with the distal 15 to 20 mm of pronator quadratus fibers. The muscle fibers attached to the bone block are carefully freed by blunt dissection from the remaining proximal portion of the pronator quadratus so that the graft can be rotated distally on a pedicle based on the ulnar attachment of the distal muscle fibers. If the graft will not reach easily, a separate incision can be made over the ulna and the pronator quadratus freed subperiosteally to permit additional advancement. The graft is inserted into the scaphoid defect and fixed with two longitudinal Kirschner wires.

Technique for Dorsal Distal Radius Vascularized Bone Graft (1,2 ICSRA Graft)

The extremity is elevated for exsanguination and a tourniquet inflated. Esmarch bandage application makes the vessel identification more difficult. A gentle curvilinear dorsal radial incision is used to expose the scaphoid and bone graft donor site (Fig. 17-24A). Branches of the superficial radial nerve are identified and retracted. Subcutaneous tissues are gently retracted, and the 1,2 ICSRA and venae comitantes are visualized on the surface of the retinaculum between the first and second extensor tendon compartments (see Fig. 17-24B). The vessels are dissected toward their distal anastomosis with the radial artery (toward the anatomical snuff-box). The first and second dorsal extensor compartments are opened at the level of the bone graft site to create a cuff of retinaculum containing the vessels and their nutrient arteries to bone (see Fig. 17-24C). The graft is centered approximately 1.5 cm proximal to the radiocarpal joint to include the nutrient vessels. Before elevation of the bone graft, a transverse dorsal-radial capsulotomy is made to expose the scaphoid nonunion site (see Fig. 17-24D).

In proximal pole fracture nonunions, a dorsal inlay graft is most appropriate. Curets are used to remove any fibrous tissue from the nonunion site. Osteotomes or high speed burs are used to prepare a slot that spans the fracture site to receive the bone graft (see Fig. 17-24E). If the proximal pole fragment is too small to create a slot, the graft is shaped to lie within the concavity of the proximal pole. After preparation of the nonunion site, the graft is elevated. The center of the graft is placed approximately 1.5 cm from the radiocarpal joint. Graft elevation begins with ligation of the 1,2 ICSRA and accompanying veins proximal to the graft. The vessels are mobilized distal to the graft to separate them from the radius and joint capsule but leaving them applied to the graft itself. Sharp osteotomes create the radial, ulnar, and proximal osteotomies of the graft. The distal osteotomy is performed in two stages, moving the pedicle radial then ulnarward to prevent injury to the pedicle. The graft is then gently levered out to create a distally based pedicle (see Fig. 17-24F).

The graft is resized as needed using bone cutters and transposed beneath the radial wrist extensors. It is gently press-fit into the prepared slot in the nonunion site (see Fig. 17-24G and H). Supplemental internal fixation with Kirschner wires or scaphoid screws may be safely placed without jeopardy to the pedicle. If cannulated screw fixation is chosen, it may be advantageous to place the screw before final sizing and insetting of the vascular graft. The wrist capsule and extensor retinaculum are reapproximated. A bulky long-arm/thumb plaster spica splint is then applied.

Vascularized Interpositional Wedge Graft for Scaphoid Nonunion

In the event that scaphoid foreshortening and angular deformity requires an interpositional bone graft, a vascularized wedge graft may be placed through a dorsoradial approach. In this case, the scaphoid is prepared before graft elevation (Fig. 17-25A). The dimensions of the palmar cortical defect, internal defect, width, and depth are noted. When a wedge graft is used, the vessels are placed palmarly to allow a palmar cortical strut for stability (see Fig. 17-25B). A graft sufficiently large to fill the internal scaphoid defect is harvested as previously described (see Fig. 17-25C). The graft is carefully trimmed to match the dimensions of the defect, such that it will be used as a volar cortical strut. The graft is then inserted into the defect with the vascular pedicle placed palmarly and is secured with Kirschner wires or compression screw fixation (see Fig 17-25D), and the wound is closed as previously described.

Proximal Pole Nonunions

When considering treatment for a delayed union or nonunion of a proximal pole fracture, the size and vascularity of the proximal fragment must be assessed. The vascular status of the proximal fragment has a major impact on nonunion outcome, but it is difficult to evaluate proximal pole vascularity preoperatively.[74,85,596] Increased radiographic density of the proximal pole correlates poorly with proximal pole blood flow when correlated with MRI or surgical findings.[163,438,484] An MRI interpretation of vascular status cannot be relied on to consistently predict which proximal pole fracture will heal.[245] A better assessment of proximal pole vascularity is provided with dynamic, gadolinium-enhanced MRI, which has 83% accuracy when correlated with intraoperative punctate bleeding.[104] Although not extensively investigated, serial MRI may also prove helpful to assess the progression of scaphoid healing. A revascularization front has been found to develop within the distal fragment, which progresses at an average of 0.7 mm/wk. If this front is able to proceed within 2 mm of the fracture line within 8 weeks, fracture healing will generally occur.[347]

If the fragment is a full third of the scaphoid, a bone graft using Russe's technique may be successful (Fig. 17-26). For viable proximal pole fragments, Matti's technique,[400,634] in which cancellous bone chips are packed tightly into the fracture from a dorsal approach, may be considered. Kirschner wire or headless screw fixation can be performed using a freehand or cannulated technique. Inoue reported 80% successful union with cancellous bone grafting and Herbert screw placement through a dorsal approach.[286] Another option is a vascularized graft from the distal radius.[512,559] Some authors have advocated inclusion of the lunate in the fixation construct, using staples, Kirschner wires, or a screw inserted in a proximal-to-distal direction,[15,334,377] to increase stability. For small or avascular fragments, simple excision, with or without a soft tissue spacer,[35,45,46,263,392,578,594] costochondral graft,[146,478,540] or allograft,[103] has been used with variable success.

Revision of Failed Bone Graft

Data suggest that up to 95% of scaphoid bone grafts will heal.[140,185] Despite this, a small percentage may fail to unite. Whether to repeat the same procedure, try a different graft-

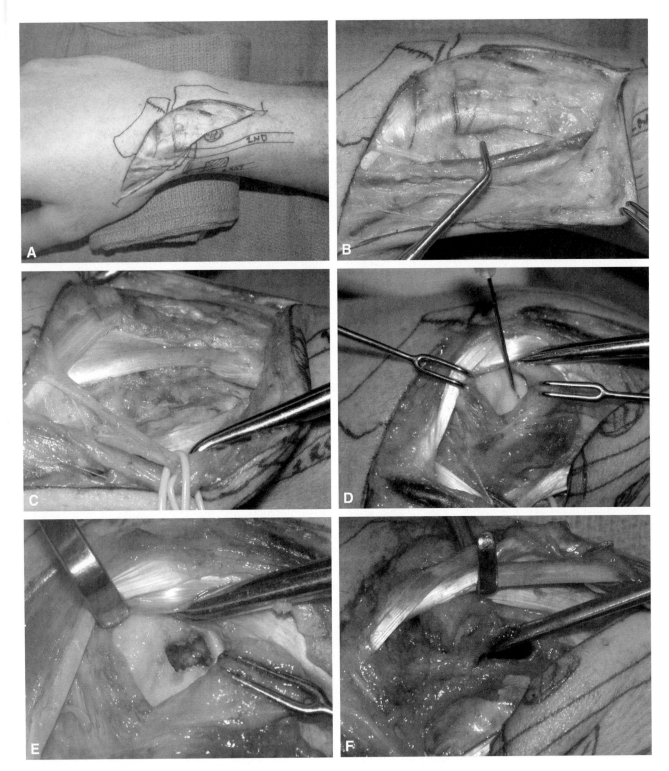

FIGURE 17-24. A, Standard incision for use of the 1,2 ICSRA graft. **B,** Vessel is visualized between the first and second dorsal compartments. **C,** The first and second dorsal compartments are opened and a cuff of retinaculum is left with the vessel overlying the bone. **D,** Scaphoid is exposed through a transverse radial capsulotomy. Nonunion site identified with needle. **E,** A slot is burred into the scaphoid. The graft will span the fracture site. **F,** The graft is elevated using osteotomes, taking care to protect the nutrient vessel.

Continued

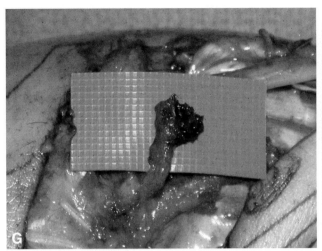
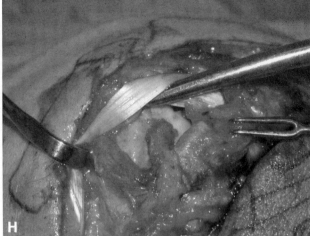

Figure 17-24—cont'd. G and **H,** The graft is trimmed to fit the slot at the nonunion site and gently press-fit into the defect. The graft may be held in place with a single temporary Kirschner wire if the graft fit is difficult.

ing operation, perform a salvage procedure, or do nothing is therefore a common clinical conundrum. Inoue reported 8 patients with persistent nonunions after failed Herbert screw fixation. All patients underwent bone grafting with repeat screw insertion. Union was obtained in 75% of patients.[282] Smith and Cooney[569] reviewed 25 patients with repeat bone grafting to a nonunited scaphoid and specifically addressed four types of revision procedures: repeat Russe grafting, Maltese cross graft (Fig. 17-27), interpositional wedge graft, and vascularized bone graft. Twenty-two of their 25 fractures united, but clinical outcomes were less impressive, with only eight excellent or good functional results. Most of the poor results were attributed to persistent carpal instability, multiple surgeries, or prolonged immobilization. Based on their results, Smith and Cooney proposed a treatment algorithm for failed scaphoid grafts. If there are midcarpal degenerative changes, a salvage procedure should be done. If degenerative changes are limited to the radial styloid, osteosynthesis may be attempted but a radial styloidectomy should be included. If there are large cysts in the scaphoid, these should be excised by curet and a Maltese cross graft inserted. If the proximal pole is avascular, a vascularized bone graft should be used. If neither cysts nor avascularity is present but carpal malalignment and/or humpback deformity is, a Fisk-Fernandez-type wedge graft may be used. Finally, if none of these situations applies, a standard Russe graft may be used.[124] Although we generally concur with these recommendations, we prefer a vascularized bone graft to manage a failed, properly performed Russe graft regardless of the location of the nonunion. Preoperative imaging studies are very helpful for surgical planning, to better understand the fracture fragment alignment and vascularity.

Prognosis for Scaphoid Nonunion Surgery

Several recent papers have discussed prognostic factors for the healing of scaphoid nonunions after reconstructive surgery. In a multicenter study by Schuind and colleagues of 138 patients, prognostic risk factors for surgical failure included heavy laborers, chronic nonunions (>5 years), degenerative change requiring a concomitant radial styloid-

ectomy, and a short duration of postoperative immobilization.[547] Other authors have similarly documented a decreased success rate with increasing duration of nonunion.[285,553] In a study by Shah and Jones, union rates were 80% if the nonunion was treated within 5 years but dropped to 50% if the nonunion had been present for more than 5 years. Additional factors associated with lower healing rates included the presence of avascular necrosis and previous scaphoid surgery. In a quantitative meta-analysis of the literature, Merrell and colleagues found that for avascular proximal pole fractures, union was achieved in 88% of those patients with a vascular graft versus 47% with a screw and wedge fixation.[415]

Scaphoid Malunion

Although scaphoid nonunion is more common, scaphoid malunion does occur.[301,343] Identification of malalignment after union was first described through evidence of carpal collapse[118,193,457] and later by direct measurement of the intrascaphoid alignment.[16,539,572] The typical lateral appearance of the malunited scaphoid has prompted the name "humpback scaphoid" to describe the deformity (Fig. 17-28),[16,127,572] which results from flexion angulation between the proximal and distal poles. Scaphoid malunion has been shown experimentally[88,571] to result in altered carpal mechanics and clinically to result in pain, weakness, limited motion (especially extension), and degenerative changes.[16,452]

Malunions have been described as early (<6 months post injury) and late (>1 year after injury). Whereas a few authors have advocated corrective osteotomy be attempted, no comparative studies have been performed to document a significant improvement in hand function. In a study by Jiranek and associates, presence of an increased lateral intrascaphoid angle or "humpback" deformity after scaphoid nonunion surgery was not predictive of subjective satisfaction or functional abilities.[301] The same study documented significant differences in objective measures of degenerative change, correlated with the degree of malunion. It is possible that correction of the malunion may delay or prevent the development of significant radiocarpal arthritis.[187,383]

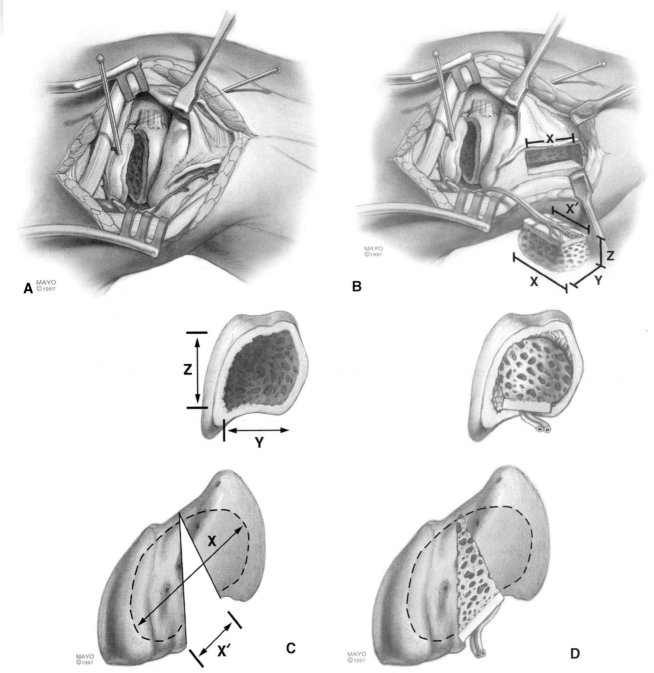

FIGURE 17-25. Use of a dorsal radius vascularized graft in cases of malunion or humpback deformity. **A,** The scaphoid is prepared before graft elevation. **B,** A large graft is harvested that can then be shaped into a wedge. **C** and **D,** The graft is then trimmed to fit the defect dimensions and used as a volar strut. (By permission of Mayo Foundation for Medical Education and Research. All rights reserved.)

Lynch and Linscheid reported their series of five patients who presented with DISI deformity and scaphoid malunion. All patients underwent corrective osteotomy. Follow-up averaged 9 years, and all patients had improvement in range of motion, grip strength, and Mayo wrist scores.[383] These authors have emphasized the importance of correcting the radiolunate angle, thus reducing the DISI deformity, before bone grafting.[383,629] Fernandez has emphasized the importance of correcting the pronatory rotational malalignment of the distal fragment as well.[187] Preoperative CT evalua-

tion is crucial to determine size and shape of graft for these cases.

The literature is confusing in this regard; many "corrective osteotomies" are found, on careful review, to be either through relatively recent unions (i.e., <6 months post injury) or through fibrous nonunions.[54] Such early cases may be treated with a Fisk/Fernandez opening wedge bone grafting; the results of such treatment have been rewarding.[16,54,452] Those solidly united fractures, seen 1 year or more after union, present a more difficult picture.[16] Often, degenerative

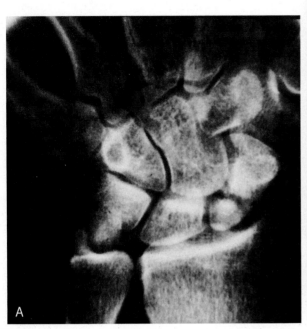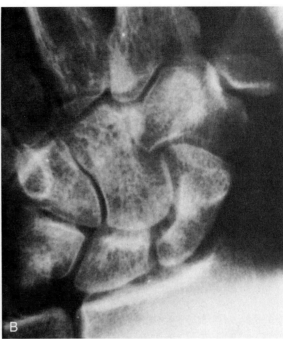

FIGURE 17-26. **A,** Preoperative radiograph of a fracture of the proximal third of the scaphoid. **B,** Postoperative appearance 5 months after a volar bone graft procedure (Russe).

changes are already present. For such cases, treatment guidelines have been suggested.[16] If intrascaphoid angulation is 20 degrees or less (in comparison to normal), the long-term results are similar to those of anatomic union and nothing should be done. More severe degrees of malunion can be managed by either corrective osteotomy or cheilec-

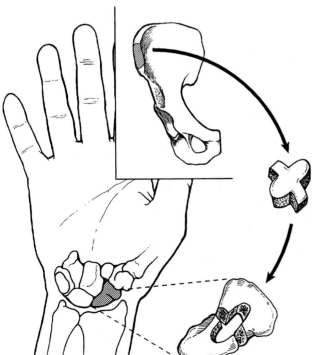

FIGURE 17-27. Maltese cross graft.

tomy (excision of the scaphoid "hump" and any impinging dorsal osteophytes).[16,383,629] Salvage procedures can be approached as for symptomatic nonunion and based on the degree of pain and arthrosis present.

Salvage and Palliative Procedures

Salvage procedures are required if the proximal or distal scaphoid poles are fragmented or collapsed or midcarpal degenerative changes have developed.

Radial Styloidectomy

Radial styloidectomy is performed subperiosteally through the anatomical snuff-box. Care must be taken to preserve the important volar radial ligament attachments; if more than 1 cm of styloid is removed, the radioscaphocapitate ligament origin will be significantly compromised (Fig. 17-29).[564] The radial styloid fragment may be used as a bone graft.[35,82] As an isolated procedure for SNAC arthritis, styloidectomies have been unsatisfactory,[404,483] but they have enjoyed success when combined with bone grafts, with or without internal fixation.[35,122,404,483] Although some authors consider styloidectomy to be an essential part of the treatment of nonunions,[581] the procedure does consistently improve on the results of bone grafting alone.

Bentzon's Procedure

This operation was initially used by Bentzon in 1939 and was first reported in 1941.[44] The concept is to convert a painful nonunion into a pain-free pseudarthrosis by introducing a soft tissue flap between the fracture fragments. In spite of its attractive simplicity,[81,500] Bentzon's procedure has failed to become popular outside of Scandinavia.[6,500] A long-term review showed persistent good results 22 to 39

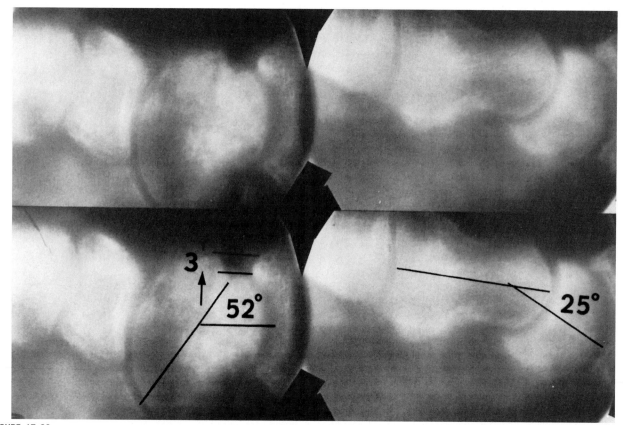

FIGURE 17-28. Scaphoid malunion. A tomogram shows scaphoid foreshortening and dorsal intercalated segment instability deformity with a 3-mm humpback, 52-degree internal angle (normal is 24 degrees), and 25-degree capitolunate angle.

years after Bentzon's operation in selected patients. Carpal collapse, found in 15 of 26 patients, and osteoarthritis, present in 7, did not result in clinical disability.[61] Bentzon's arthroplasty may still be considered a satisfactory alternative when prolonged immobilization is contraindicated and after bone graft procedures have failed.

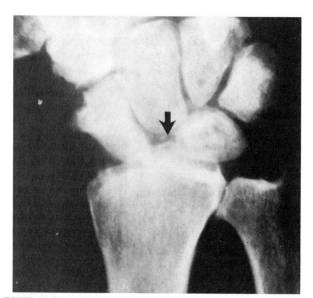

FIGURE 17-29. An excessively generous radial styloidectomy may be a factor in carpal instability *(arrow)*, as shown here.

Distal Scaphoid Resection

Excision of the distal scaphoid has been recommended for degenerative arthritis and pain in long-standing non-unions.[389,528] This procedure is not appropriate for patients with ongoing capitolunate arthritis. This procedure may be performed through a volar, lateral, or arthroscopic approach. This procedure may be used as an alternative for patients unwilling to consider partial wrist arthrodesis (Fig. 17-30).

Proximal Row Carpectomy

Proximal row carpectomy has also been advocated for the treatment of ununited fractures of the scaphoid. Although Hill[263] found the procedure indicated in older patients with symptomatic nonunion who did not wish to accept a long period of immobilization, others[24,133,280,306] have used this treatment for younger, active, heavy workers with very good functional and clinical results. Proximal row carpectomy may be preferable to fusion in cases where motion is preferred, but it is contraindicated in the presence of midcarpal arthrosis. Krakauer and coworkers[338] have compared proximal row carpectomy with intercarpal fusion. They found that carpectomy preserved better motion, an average arc of 71 degrees versus 54 degrees for limited arthrodesis. Both types of procedure preserved reasonable strength and reduced pain. A recent dual cohort study by Cohen and Kozin compared the two procedures and found no significant differences in range of motion or strength and recommended both as motion-preserving procedures for scapholunate advanced collapse (SLAC) and SNAC arthritis.[115]

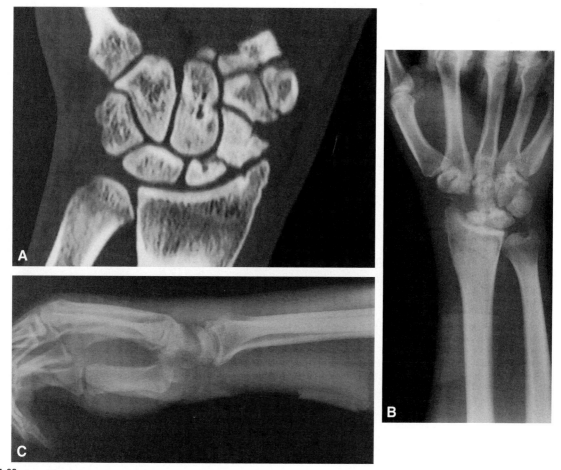

FIGURE 17-30. **A,** A 30-year-old man presented with a 10-year history of scaphoid nonunion. **B,** Distal scaphoid resection was performed through a limited dorsal incision. **C,** At 6 months the wrist shows little evidence for DISI deformity.

Technique of Proximal Row Carpectomy

Either a transverse or longitudinal dorsal wrist incision can be utilized, depending on surgeon preference (Fig. 17-31). Flaps are raised at the level of the extensor retinaculum to elevate and protect the cutaneous branches of the ulnar and radial nerves. The extensor retinaculum is incised over the extensor pollicis longus and the tendon retracted out of its compartment. The retinaculum and the contents of the fourth dorsal compartment can be reflected to the ulnar side for additional exposure. We routinely excise the terminal portion of the posterior interosseous nerve just proximal to the wrist because entrapment of this purely sensory portion of the nerve (to the wrist capsule) has been implicated as a possible cause of postoperative pain. The procedure is simple, quick, and without morbidity. The nerve can be found at the most radial margin of the fourth dorsal compartment, just deep to the extensor digitorum communis (EDC) tendons and alongside the 3-4 intercompartmental septum. A 2- to 3-cm segment is removed just proximal to the articular surface of the radius. The wrist capsule is then incised longitudinally, along the third metacarpal axis; alternatively, a ligament splitting approach may be employed.[49] The lunate and triquetrum are removed, usually in this order. The scaphoid can be excised in its entirety, although we prefer to leave its distal third attached to the

trapezium and trapezoid for additional support of the thumb ray. Carpal impingement on the radial styloid in radial deviation can be managed by limited styloidectomy, but it is important not to destabilize the wrist by removing the radioscaphocapitate ligament in continuity with the resected styloid. The proximal pole of the capitate is seated into the lunate concavity of the radius; if stability is questionable, a temporary Kirschner wire may be used for 3 to 4 weeks to maintain this position. The pisiform is not excised. Closure is performed in layers and includes the extensor retinaculum. The wrist is immobilized in a bulky conforming plaster dressing for 4 to 6 days and then converted to a short-arm cast for 3 to 5 weeks. Gradual increased motion is permitted using a removable splint for 2 to 4 weeks, or until the patient is capable of free use of the wrist.

Partial Arthrodesis

In 1946, Sutro[599] and, in 1952, Helfet[254] proposed to treat nonunions of the scaphoid by arthrodesing both fragments to the capitate when there was extensive sclerosis, resorption of the fragments, or degenerative changes between the scaphoid and capitate. When the radiocarpal joint is involved with osteoarthritis and the scaphocapitate joint is satisfactory, some have suggested fusion of both scaphoid fragments and the attached lunate to the radius instead.[231]

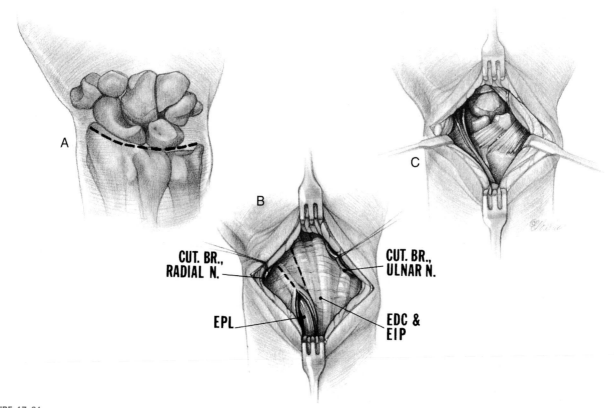

FIGURE 17-31. Dorsal approach to the wrist with a transverse incision. **A,** Incision. **B,** The extensor pollicis longus (EPL) is exposed. EDC, extensor digitorum communis; EIP, extensor indicis proprius. **C,** Subcapsular and subperiosteal exposure of the joint through a longitudinal retinacular and capsular incision between the third and fourth dorsal extensor compartments. (From Taleisnik J: The Wrist. New York, Churchill Livingstone, 1985.)

Other types of limited arthrodesis have been proposed.[234] In our opinion the vast majority of nonunions of the scaphoid may be satisfactorily treated with techniques other than limited arthrodesis. However, scaphoid excision and limited intercarpal fusion should be considered as a salvage procedure, particularly when extensive midcarpal degenerative changes have occurred or after repeated failures of bone grafting.[385,676] Although the "four-corner" fusion or SLAC wrist procedure was initially proposed to be used with a silicone scaphoid implant, the silicone implant is now contraindicated (Fig. 17-32).[168,626,660] The techniques of limited wrist arthrodesis are described in Chapter 13.

Scaphoid Replacement and Silicone Particulate Synovitis

Silicone synovitis is the term given to an inflammatory arthropathy seen in some patients after silicone implant arthroplasty, particularly of the wrist or carpal bones (Fig. 17-33).[100,232,482,524,570,574,695] The pathophysiology appears to relate to microparticulate fragmentation of the implant. All silicone polymers fragment when abraded; this is a particular risk in load-bearing implants such as those of the wrist. Clinically, the manifestations are those of an inflammatory synovitis around the implant; radiographically, osteopenia and later cyst formation are noted. On surgical exploration, a proliferative synovitis is demonstrated, often with bony invasion. Histologically, the synovitis is characterized by macrophages, which can be shown to have engulfed silicone particles. Only particles of a certain size

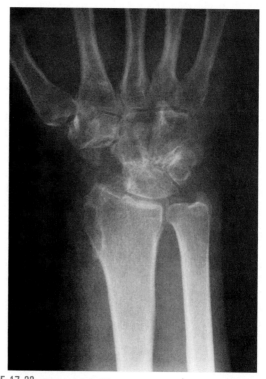

FIGURE 17-32. When scaphoid nonunion is associated with capitolunate and radioscaphoid arthritis, pain can be reduced and motion can be preserved with a procedure combining midcarpal arthrodesis with scaphoid excision, as shown here.

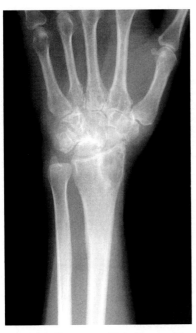

FIGURE 17-33. Advanced silicone synovitis in 52-year-old woman who had undergone silicone scaphoid replacement 20 years ago.

induce the phenomenon.[482] Particles too large to be engulfed by a single cell tend to become encapsulated instead and do not induce as much inflammation. Smaller fragments, of macromolecular size, may induce an immune reaction.[570] Fragments larger than molecular size but still small enough to be engulfed by cells seem to be those implicated in most cases of silicone synovitis. It has been suggested that the high-performance silicone polymer, developed because of its superior tear resistance, may be more likely to abrade into the smaller particles characteristic of silicone synovitis than the "old style" softer silicone. Regardless, the problem was increasingly reported as longer-term follow-up of silicone implants of carpal bones and wrists became available. Most early proponents of silicone implant arthroplasty have reversed their support of the procedure.[8]

Silicone synovitis is treated by removal of the implant and curettage of the reactive bone cysts. Large cysts may require bone grafting. For severe cases involving scaphoid or lunate implants, proximal row carpectomy or wrist arthrodesis may be indicated.

All patients with silicone implants in place should be advised of the possibility of silicone synovitis. For patients with implants in place without evidence of silicone synovitis, regular follow-up, on an annual or biannual basis, is advisable.

Authors' Preferred Methods of Treatment: Scaphoid Fractures (Summary)

SCAPHOID FRACTURES: MIDDLE THIRD FRACTURES

- *Fresh stable, undisplaced:* Short-arm/thumb spica cast or percutaneous compression screw.

- *Fresh undisplaced but potentially unstable (vertical oblique or reduced trans-scaphoid dislocations) and previously untreated stable fractures older than 3 weeks:* Percutaneous compression screw fixation or long-arm/thumb spica cast.

- *Fresh displaced or angulated:* Open reduction and internal fixation (Kirschner wires or Herbert screw).

- *Nonunions, asymptomatic, stable:* Russe-type graft or vascularized graft. Because of a strong likelihood of late osteoarthritis; patients should know that symptoms and functional results are less predictable in the long term than are radiographic results.

- *Symptomatic nonunions without osteoarthritis, definitive avascular necrosis, or carpal collapse:* Vascularized graft with addition of compression screw or Russe-type graft.

- *Nonunions with carpal collapse (DISI) without osteoarthritis or definitive avascular necrosis:* Anterior wedge bone graft with internal fixation (Kirschner wires or Herbert screw) or vascularized graft.

- *Nonunions with limited radioscaphoid osteoarthritis, without avascular necrosis:* Bone graft and limited styloidectomy or scaphoid excision and midcarpal arthrodesis, particularly if carpal alignment is suggestive of midcarpal (lunocapitate) instability or collapse. If nonunion is present for 5 to 10 years, consider distal pole excision with styloidectomy.

- *Nonunions with definitive avascular necrosis:* Vascularized bone graft or replacement of the proximal fragment with soft tissue or scaphoid excision and midcarpal arthrodesis.

- *Nonunions with more extensive osteoarthritis:* Excision of the scaphoid with midcarpal arthrodesis or total wrist arthrodesis.

SCAPHOID FRACTURES: PROXIMAL THIRD FRACTURES

■ *Acute, full third fractures:* Retrograde fixation from a dorsal approach using a short Herbert screw is our procedure of choice. If surgery cannot be performed or is rejected by the patient or if the fragment is not amenable to this type of fixation, a long-arm/thumb spica cast, followed by a short-arm/thumb spica cast, can be used.

■ *Delayed or nonunion, full third fragment:* Open fixation with vascularized bone graft; ultrasound treatment in a long-arm/thumb spica cast, followed by a short-arm/thumb spica cast, is an option for patients who are not surgical candidates.

■ *Persistent nonunion, full third, no avascular necrosis:* Matti or Russe bone graft and internal fixation across both fragments.

■ *Nonunion after failed treatment or with an avascular fragment and for very small proximal pole fractures:* Excision of the fragment with soft tissue interposition.

SCAPHOID FRACTURES: DISTAL THIRD FRACTURES

■ *Fractures of the tuberosity:* Short-arm/thumb spica cast.

■ *Fractures of the distal third:* Short-arm/thumb spica cast.

■ *Intra-articular displaced:* Open reduction and internal fixation.

■ *Nonunions:* Very rare, amenable to Russe bone graft.

SCAPHOID FRACTURES: MULTIPLY OPERATED NONUNIONS

■ *No arthritis, avascular necrosis, cysts, or collapse:* Russe graft, vascularized graft, or ultrasound.

■ *Collapse, no arthritis, no avascular necrosis:* Fisk-Fernandez graft; if large cysts are present, consider a Maltese cross graft. If an adequate bone grafting procedure has already been performed, strong consideration must be given to the use of a vascularized bone graft.

■ *Any arthritis:* Scaphoid excision/midcarpal fusion.

Scaphoid Fractures in Children

There are several series documenting scaphoid fractures in children.[7,37,108,121,238,242] Scaphoid fractures are the most common pediatric carpal fracture but represent only 0.34% of fractures in children and 0.45% of children's upper limb fractures.[108,357] The scaphoid ossifies eccentrically, with the distal pole ossifying first. Because of this, fractures in the pediatric population tend to occur in the distal third of the scaphoid.[369] Adolescents tend to demonstrate fracture patterns that are similar to adults.[369]

Christodoulou and Colton[108] reviewed 77 children between the ages of 8 and 14 years who had had a scaphoid fracture. One third were distal tubercle fractures and another 26% were in the distal third. Only 38% were mid-third fractures, and only two involved the proximal pole. Nearly one fourth of the fractures involved only a single cortex, and only five of the fractures were displaced. Wulff[703] also reported a series of 33 children with scaphoid fractures: 97.3% of these fractures were apparent on initial radiographs, and 64% of fractures occurred in the distal third. There was one nonunion in a distal third fracture in Christodoulou's series and one nonunion of the scaphoid waist in Wulff's series. Other nonunions have been reported.[356,698] Scaphoid fractures in children are often associated with fractures of the distal radius[7,239,262] and may represent a component of a greater arc injury. Careful examination of the carpus should rule out a nondisplaced fracture of the capitate or scaphocapitate syndrome.[544]

Occult fractures can also occur in children. MRI has been shown to be very valuable in detecting these fractures early in the pediatric population.[121,302] Avascular necrosis of an unossified proximal pole has also been reported in children.[356] This can manifest early as a delay in the appearance of the proximal part of the scaphoid ossification center. Treatment of scaphoid fractures in children should generally be nonoperative, although Toh and colleagues[628] reported good results with Herbert screw fixation in 25 adolescents. Attempts at surgical repair should probably be deferred until skeletal maturity to allow the proximal fragment to ossify.[356] Even carpal malalignment from malunion can respond to the effects of continued growth; Suzuki and Herbert[600] reported 2 boys, aged 9 and 10, with initial post-fracture DISI that resolved spontaneously over a period of 4 years. Mintzer reported their result with operative treatment of 13 pediatric scaphoid nonunions. Four of the nonunions were treated with a Matti-Russe procedure and nine were treated with Herbert screw fixation and iliac crest bone grafting. All patients went on to union with excellent clinical results.[425] Most recently, Waters has reported the use of vascularized bone grafts for the treatment of three scaphoid nonunions in adolescents. All fractures healed at a mean of 3.4 months. At a mean follow-up of 5.5 years no patient had developed radiocarpal arthritis and there was no evidence of scapholunate dissociation.[674]

Preiser's Disease

In 1910 Preiser described a rarefying osteitis of the scaphoid that he distinguished from a scaphoid fracture.[490] He compared the condition with Kienböck's disease and thought that the etiologies were similar. Since Preiser's time, both whole bone and proximal pole avascular necrosis of the scaphoid have been described.[11,183,243,647,652,658] The etiology has been variously related to collagen vascular disease, steroid therapy, repetitive trauma, or idiopathic causes.[145] Clinical findings are related to local pain and tenderness. Radiographically, involved areas are typically sclerotic and often there is fragmentation of the proximal articular surfaces (Fig. 17-34A and B).[261] CT and MRI may be helpful to define the changes (see Fig. 17-34C). This condition can present in children.[299]

Treatment of Preiser's disease has not been standardized. Nonoperative symptomatic management, joint débridement, silicone replacement arthroplasty, and electrical stimulation have all been tried, with mixed results.[11,183,243,650,658] Kawanishi and colleagues[321] reported two cases of vascularized bundle implantation with good results. Vascularized bone graft may also be considered.[76] The success of scaphoid-preserving procedures may be compromised by chronic degenerative changes that are often present in the carpus at the time of reconstruction, particularly at the radial styloid and radioscaphoid articulation; this makes pain free motion after successful salvage difficult. Furthermore, there is often a lack of satisfactory cortical bone into which a graft can be inserted, as the surface is too fragmented. Therefore, if revascularization is to be considered, the patient should also consent to scaphoid excision and midcarpal arthrodesis should vascularized grafting prove technically impossible. If revascularization is attempted and proves unsuccessful, scaphoid excision combined with either midcarpal arthrodesis or proximal row carpectomy may be appropriate for

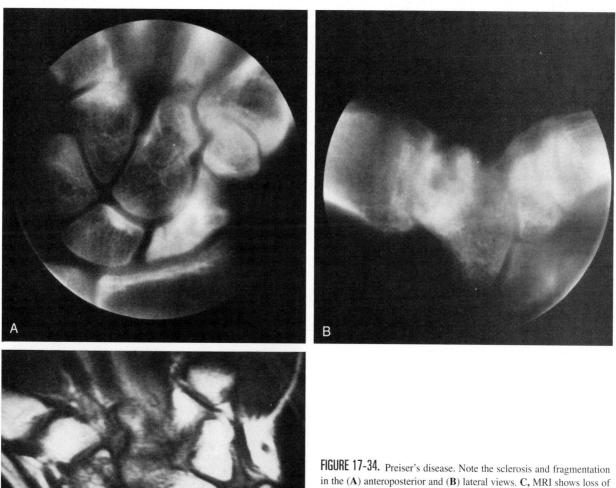

FIGURE 17-34. Preiser's disease. Note the sclerosis and fragmentation in the (**A**) anteroposterior and (**B**) lateral views. **C,** MRI shows loss of signal in the scaphoid.

persistently symptomatic cases. De Smet has reported satisfactory results with proximal row carpectomy.[145] Given the lack of reliable treatment options, in the absence of severe pain and disability a conservative approach is probably warranted and should be discussed with the patient.[414]

FRACTURES OF THE LUNATE

Acute Fractures of the Lunate

Fractures of the lunate, as distinguished from Kienböck's disease, are rare.[344,504,541,612] Teisen and Hjarbaek[612] have divided these injuries into five groups based on a review of 17 cases collected over a period of 31 years, during which time 93 cases of Kienböck's disease were also seen at the same institution. Group 1 fractures, affecting the volar pole, were by far the most common, and included 9 of the 17 cases (Fig. 17-35). There were four group 2 fractures, defined as small marginal chip fractures. Group 3, of which there were two examples, were of the dorsal pole. Groups 4 and 5, with single examples each, represented sagittal and transverse fractures, respectively (Fig. 17-36). Eleven of the 17 patients were monitored for periods ranging from 4 to 31 years, and in none did the progressive sclerosis and collapse typical of Kienböck's disease develop.

Because important stabilizing ligaments and nutrient vessels are attached to the palmar pole of the lunate, displaced group 1 and 5 fractures should be fixed with Kirschner wires or cannulated screws to decrease the risk of wrist instability and to minimize the chances of osteonecrosis.[120,215,219] Sagittal, marginal, and distal pole fractures are less likely by location to be unstable and thus may be more appropriately treated by nonsurgical means.

Kienböck's Disease

In 1910, Robert Kienböck[323] published his classic description of lunatomalacia. Although the etiology of lunatomalacia may be related to avascular necrosis, as Kienböck suspected, the actual cause leading to the loss of blood supply has remained elusive. Considerable progress has been made, however, in understanding the pathomechanics and biomechanics of lunate collapse and in evaluating the longer-term clinical results of treatment.

Etiology

The blood supply of the lunate arises from both dorsal and palmar vessels.[222,223] Internal anastomoses are present, so both dorsal and palmar flow must be occluded for the lunate to lose circulation; fractures that split the bone into dorsal and palmar halves or dislocations that leave a capsular hinge intact should not be expected to result in avascular necrosis and, indeed, clinically do not appear to do so. Thus, one must consider other factors to determine the etiology of Kienböck's disease.

The loss of blood supply to the lunate has been attributed to primary circulatory problems,[31,359] to traumatic interference with circulation, to ligament injury with subsequent degeneration and collapse,[161,323,391] and to single or multiple fractures resulting in secondary vascular impairment.* Although fracture-dislocations or dislocations of the carpus may result in increased radiodensity of the lunate, this is a transient phenomenon that should not be confused with the progressive changes that characterize Kienböck's disease.[693] Whether fractures or fissures precede the avascular changes or occur secondarily in an already weakened bone has not been satisfactorily established.[17,606] It is likely that both mechanisms occur.[17] Elevated intraosseous pressure from altered carpal mechanics may be the most likely common pathway.[298,548] Schiltenwulf and associates[548] have shown that the intraosseous pressure of the normal lunate is greater in wrist extension than in the neutral position and that the difference, 40 mm Hg, is far greater than the difference seen in the normal capitate (7 mm Hg). This rise in intraosseous pressure may help explain the lunate's predisposition for osteonecrosis. This mechanism may also explain the increased prevalence of Kienböck's disease in patients with spastic hemiplegia.[303]

In 1928, Hultén[275] published a study of the distal radioulnar relationship in normal wrists and in patients with Kienböck's disease. In 51% of the normal individuals the distal articular surfaces of the radius and ulna were found to be at the same level (ulnar neutral), and 23% were found to be ulnar minus, with the ulna proximal to the radius. In contrast to this normal proportion, the majority of patients with Kienböck's disease (18 of 23) showed an ulnar-minus

---

*See references 58, 103, 157, 230, 315, 439, 451, 485, 584, and 624.

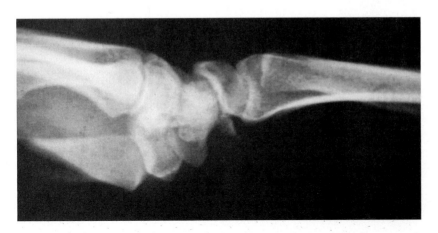

FIGURE 17-35. This proximal pole fracture of the lunate requires open reduction and internal fixation. (From Failla JM, Amadio PC: Recognition and treatment of uncommon carpal fractures. Hand Clin 4:469-476, 1988.)

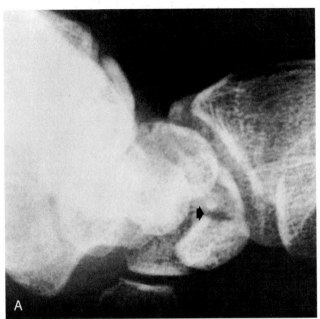

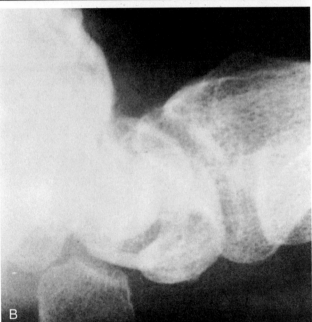

FIGURE 17-36. **A,** A lunate fracture *(arrow)* following a fall on the hand with the wrist in dorsiflexion was successfully treated by immobilization and the application of pulsing electromagnetic field treatment. **B,** Appearance after 5 months of treatment. (From Taleisnik J: The Wrist. New York, Churchill Livingstone, 1985.)

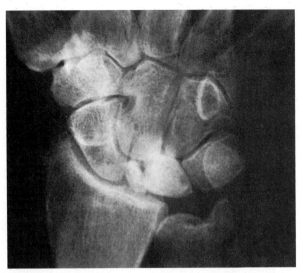

FIGURE 17-37. Fragmented, avascular lunate. Note the ulnar-minus variant.

variant (Fig. 17-37); only five cases showed a neutral or zero variant (Fig. 17-38). The ulnar-plus relationship was not present in any patient in this group with Kienböck's disease. Although no simple etiologic factor could be verified for this disease in Axelsson's extensive review,[30] enough objective data were found to support Hultén's minus variant theory. Gelberman and colleagues[222] also found a statistically significant relationship between the negative ulnar variant and Kienböck's disease, although it was not considered a primary etiologic association. Stahl and Reis[585] observed the development of typical Kienböck's disease in the ipsilateral wrist of a patient with a preexistent unilateral

post-traumatic ulnar-minus deformity. They believed this to be additional evidence in favor of the etiologic relationship between lunatomalacia and ulnar-minus variance. In contrast to these studies, D'Hoore examined 125 normal wrists and 52 wrists of patients with Kienbock's disease and found no statistical difference in ulnar variance.[152] If the cause of Kienböck's disease was solely due to the mechanical differences or variance in load in the "ulnar-minus" state, it would seem that Kienböck's disease would be more widespread in patients who have undergone Darrach procedures or ulnar shortenings (see Chapter 15). In addition, Kristensen and coworkers[340] have reported that at least some of the relative shortening of the ulna might actually represent new bone formation on the ulnar margin of the radius, a form of acquired ulnar-minus variance (Fig. 17-39). Finally, the association between ulnar variance and Kienböck's disease may share an interrelationship with ethnicity; although the association is fairly common in European populations,[30,222,275] it is less so in Japan.[310,330] Nakamura's study noted that a negative ulnar variance occurs with equal frequency in the general population and Kienbock's patients.[458]

In 1966, Antuña Zapico[22] observed a relationship between the shape of the lunate and the length of the ulna (Fig. 17-40). He described a type I lunate, seen in ulnar-minus wrists, as having a proximal apex or crest (see Fig. 17-40A). Types II and III were more rectangular or square and coexisted with zero and plus variants (see Fig. 17-40B and C). In Antuña Zapico's opinion, the trabecular pattern in type I was the weakest (see Fig. 17-40D), with a greater potential for bone fatigue and stress fracture under loads. Fragmentation was more frequent in ulnar-minus variants with type I lunates. Razemon[503] pointed out that in addition, ulnar-minus wrists provided poor coverage for the lunate; in these cases there is a large portion of the lunate that is not covered by the radius, which creates uneven stress under loads, with the radial half being the most susceptible to compression. A study of load stresses on the lunate[315] supported Hultén's theory by showing concentration of forces on the lunate during extension and ulnar deviation and tensile forces on the distal surface of the lunate, predisposing it to fracture. Armistead and associates[26] suggested

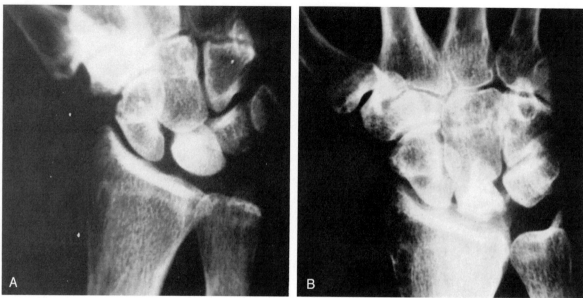

FIGURE 17-38. A, Lunatomalacia in a wrist with a zero-variant radioulnar relationship. **B,** Late lunate collapse and fragmentation in the same patient.

that in extreme extension the volar radiolunate and lunotri-quetral ligaments become tense. This tension is transmitted to the volar pole of the lunate. The triquetrum is able to shift proximally on the more compliant ulnocarpal complex, but the lunate is subjected to both tension and the nutcracker effect between the capitate and radius (Fig. 17-41), and failure occurs most frequently between the anterior and middle thirds of the lunate.

Finally, Mirabello[427] and Werner and Palmer[689] both pointed out that radial slope in the anteroposterior projection can have a significant effect on both the forces transmitted to the lunate and the age at onset of Kienböck's disease.

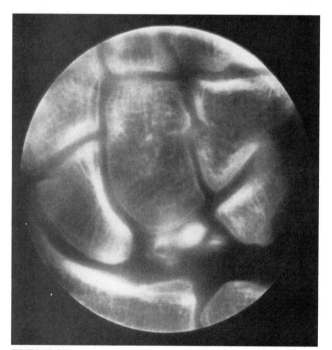

FIGURE 17-39. New bone formation after joint leveling is on the radius, not the lunate.

Tsuge found that radial inclination was decreased in patients with Kienböck's disease.[640]

There are multiple case reports associating Kienböck's disease with disease processes such as lupus, scleroderma, carpal coalition, sickle cell, and corticosteroid use.[137,312,354,399,434] These case reports fail to establish a consistent correlation between any specific disease process and the development of Kienböck's disease. Until the true etiology of Kienböck's disease is elucidated, routine screening for specific medical diseases is not indicated.[10]

It is obvious that no single factor can be cited for the development of Kienböck's disease. In all likelihood, the genesis of lunatomalacia requires some combination of load (repeated compression strains, a single severe compression force, or tension on the concave distal surface of the lunate), vascular risk,[171,222] and mechanical predisposition.[17,22] Synovitis, intra-articular effusion,[451] and the unavoidable continuous stress of normal function on this "carpal key-stone"[391] interfere with attempts at healing. This insidious combination of factors may render the lunate susceptible to a nutcracker effect between a prominent radius and the head of the capitate, thus setting up a self-perpetuating mechanism of progressive lunate collapse.

Diagnosis

The diagnosis of Kienböck's disease is usually made by radiographs. The condition tends to occur in young adults. The presenting signs and symptoms include pain and stiffness in the wrist and some swelling and tenderness localized to the area of the lunate dorsally. The history of a specific traumatic event predating the onset of symptoms is frequently absent, although some form of injury is described by a significant number of patients. There is limitation of motion and a striking weakness of grip for the relative paucity of clinical findings. Extensor tendon rupture, although rare, has been reported as an initial presenting sign.[281,446,497] Symptoms of carpal tunnel syndrome have also been reported.[42,606] Radiographs may appear normal in the early stages of the disease, except for the ulnar-minus

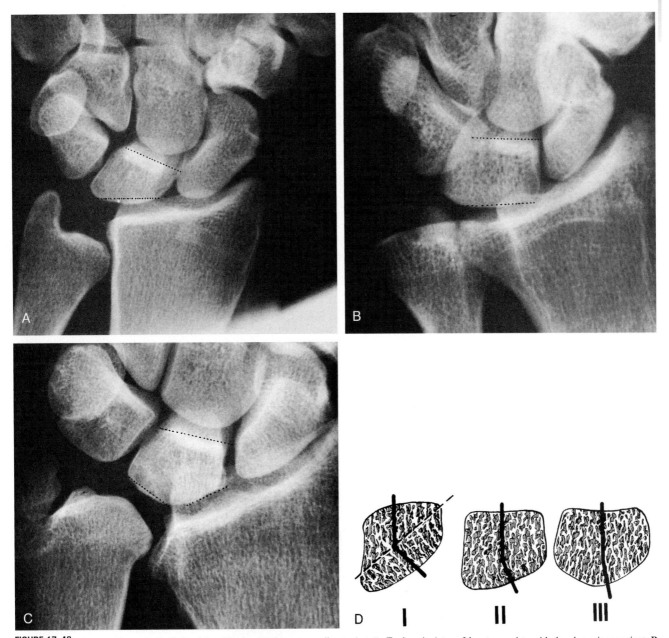

FIGURE 17-40. Types of lunate and relationship with ulnar variance according to Antuña Zapico. **A,** A type I lunate coexists with the ulna-minus variant. **B** and **C,** Type II and III lunates coexist with zero and ulna-plus variants. **D,** Trabecular patterns for type I, II, and III lunates. (From Taleisnik J: The Wrist. New York, Churchill Livingstone, 1985.)

variant and a type I lunate. If strongly suspected, one should proceed to CT[494] or MRI.[17,134,278,508,639] Care must be taken when interpreting MR images of the lunate; we have seen cases in which the subchondral inflammatory changes and edema associated with ulnolunate impaction have produced signal changes similar to those seen in Kienböck's disease. Typically, in such cases the changes are limited to the ulnar side of the lunate and are seen in the context of an ulnar-plus variant.

Bone scintigraphy may also show abnormally high uptake by the lunate in early Kienböck's disease.[17] During the ensuing weeks, the typical radiographic findings of lunate sclerosis and progressive loss of lunate height help establish the diagnosis (see Fig. 17-38). Later, fragmentation of the lunate results in dissociation within the proximal

carpal row and allows the scaphoid and triquetrum to rotate in opposite directions: the scaphoid rotates into palmar flexion and the triquetrum rotates into extension (Fig. 17-42). The net effect is one of progressive loss of carpal height.[606] Eventually, degenerative joint changes develop primarily as the result of carpal collapse and scaphoid rotation (Fig. 17-43).[10,292]

Clinical Staging

We usually use a staging system originally proposed by Stahl[584] and later popularized by Lichtman,[367,368] although its reproducibility has been called into question by some[295,300] (Fig. 17-44). We find the staging system to be useful in both discussing treatment options and charting disease progression (or regression) after intervention, because it is based on

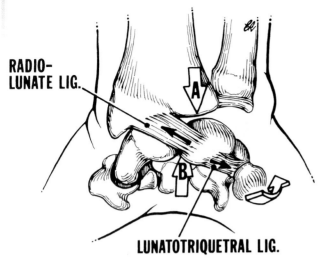

**RADIO-
LUNATE LIG.**

LUNATOTRIQUETRAL LIG.

FIGURE 17-41. In extreme dorsiflexion, the radiolunate and lunotriquetral ligaments become tense and produce equal forces in opposite directions acting on the lunate *(black arrows).* The triquetrum is more likely to shift dorsally and proximally on the more compliant ulnocarpal cartilaginous complex *(right arrow).* Added compression from the radius *(arrow A)* and capitate *(arrow B)* results in lunate failure (see Arner and Hagberg[27]). (From Taleisnik J: The Wrist. New York, Churchill Livingstone, 1985. © 1985, Elizabeth Roselius.)

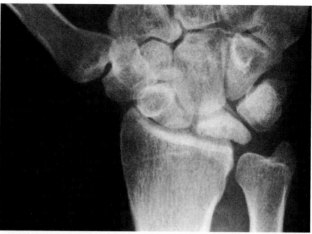

FIGURE 17-42. Collapse and flattening of the lunate with radiographic evidence of opposite rotations of the scaphoid (palmar flexed) and triquetrum (dorsiflexed). (From Taleisnik J: The Wrist. New York, Churchill Livingstone, 1985.)

the appearance of the lunate on plain radiographs. In stage I there is a linear or compression fracture but otherwise normal architecture and density. In stage II, density is abnormal, without lunate or carpal collapse. Lunate collapse is present in stage III. Stage III is often separated into stage IIIA, without carpal collapse (i.e., carpal height is normal,

radioscaphoid angle is less than 60 degrees), and stage IIIB, with carpal collapse (diminished carpal height, radioscaphoid angle greater than 60 degrees).[229] In stage IV, extensive osteoarthritic changes are present. With the advent of bone scans and MRI it has been possible to identify changes that precede radiographic stage I. The identification of an abnormal MRI or bone scan with negative wrist radiographs has been called "stage 0" Kienböck's disease.[17,134] Because of the additional sensitivity that bone scans and MRI provide in the diagnosis of Kienböck's disease, they should be considered part of the evaluation of patients with

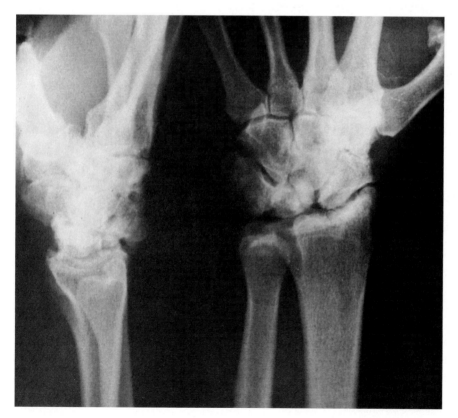

FIGURE 17-43. Carpal collapse and degenerative changes 27 years after the onset of Kienböck's disease.

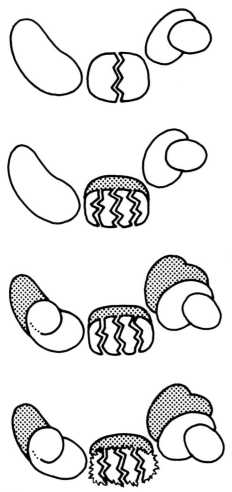

FIGURE 17-44. Diagrammatic representation of the stages of progression of lunatomalacia *(from top to bottom).* (1) The lunate is not collapsed. Carpal alignment is normal. There is no osteoarthritis. (2) Lunate fragmentation and initial lunate collapse. Carpal height is normal. There is no osteoarthritis. (3) Lunate fragmentation and collapse with carpal shortening and instability. There is no evidence of osteoarthritis. (4) The last stage, when perilunate osteoarthritic changes are present. (From Taleisnik J: The Wrist. New York, Churchill Livingstone, 1985.)

wrist pain localized to the region of the lunate, particularly if an ulnar-minus variant is present. It is also important to remember that tomographic staging typically results in identification of a worse grade of Kienböck's disease than that suspected on routine radiographs.[494] This is particularly true in stages I to III. As noted earlier, stages IIIa and IIIb are determined by the absence or presence of collapse, which often can be judged only by additional imaging studies. Condit and colleagues have shown that patients with Kienböck's disease and preoperative carpal collapse are unlikely to have good or excellent clinical results, regardless of the treatment.[119]

Treatment

There are many treatment options for Kienböck's disease, ranging from observation to complex surgical reconstruction. The search for a universally acceptable treatment plan continues some 80 years after Kienböck's description. A review of the literature shows that many different surgical procedures have been proposed to correct any of the multiple factors that may lead to lunate collapse or to treat the collapsed lunate itself.*

Nonoperative Treatment

Stahl[585] recommended prolonged immobilization as the treatment of choice for Kienböck's disease. Evidence has been presented that suggests that patients not subjected to operative treatment rarely change their occupations whereas different surgical procedures result in an inability to resume occupations in nearly half of all cases.[536] Tajima surveyed 80 wrists with Kienböck's disease seen during a 42-year period and noted no appreciable difference in the end results of nonoperative versus surgical treatment.[604] Kristensen and coworkers monitored 46 nonsurgical patients for a minimum of 5 years and a mean of 20 years; although two thirds had arthritic changes in the wrist at follow-up, only a fourth had significant pain.[341] Evans and associates[173] also found satisfactory wrist function in long-term follow-up of patients treated nonsurgically. Taniguchi and colleagues[610] reported radiographic worsening in 70% of the 20 patients they monitored for 35 years, but only 20% of their patients had disabling symptoms. Fujisawa and associates[207] reported four patients observed over 15 years whose radiographic appearance actually improved without treatment. Other long-term follow-up studies, however, have shown failure rates from nonoperative treatment to approach 80%[42,416] and inferior results when compared with radial shortening procedures.[538]

There are only a few studies reporting the outcome of incidentally diagnosed Kienböck's disease in the literature. Taniguchi reported 14 patients who had the diagnosis of Kienböck's disease made on hand radiographs taken for other hand problems.[609] All patients had stage IV disease. The average age at diagnosis was 67 years. Patients were all judged to have good to excellent hand function based on Dornan's criteria.[161]

It appears that nonoperative management is associated with a progression in radiographic lunate deformity and carpal collapse.[416] The severity of radiographic findings does not always correlate with clinical complaints,[427] a situation similar to asymptomatic scaphoid nonunion. This radiographic certainty/symptomatic uncertainty disjunction is what makes prognostication and treatment decisions difficult. Pain may not necessarily increase with nonsurgical treatment, but it is unlikely to decrease; therefore, we believe that surgical intervention is appropriate for patients with symptomatic Kienböck's disease.

Operative Treatment

Intracarpal Procedures

Lunate Excision. Although several authors have reported good results after simple excision of the lunate,[59,103,161,228,391,525] others have called this procedure a "crippling" or a "mutilating" operation[584] and a useless procedure.[59] In an effort to prevent shift of the remaining carpal bones after

---

*See references 5, 110, 133, 161, 234, 275, 328, 359, 376, 456, 486, and 602.

excision of the lunate, implants of Vitallium,[375] acrylic,[5,141] Silastic,[408] and biologic tissues[167,288,317,319,643] have been proposed. Vitallium and acrylic prostheses have had only limited clinical trials, without widespread acceptance. A Silastic implant has been used extensively in the past, but problems with silicone synovitis have sharply reduced acceptance of this implant.*

A review of the literature suggests that the clinical results of most soft tissue lunate replacement procedures[288,317,319,643] are similar to those of silicone implants.[8,317,367,368,589,603] Lunate replacement will not prevent carpal collapse[97,252,317,588]; however, some studies have reported long-term satisfactory results with fascial replacement.[98] Ueba[644] reported on 15 patients followed for over 16 years who underwent resection of the lunate and interposition arthroplasty using palmaris or plantaris tendon. Care was taken to preserve the palmar ligaments, and patients were maintained in an external fixator for 4 weeks. All 15 patients were pain free with good to excellent results despite a progression in carpal collapse. Indications for lunate excision and arthroplasty should probably be confined to stage III patients until further long-term studies are available.

Smith and associates[574] theorized that reducing compression loads on the implants by intercarpal arthrodesis might reduce implant deformation, fibrillation, and synovitis. They also suggested that after intercarpal arthrodesis, the implant may serve little purpose. Several authors have proposed that there may be no need to remove or replace the lunate if considering intercarpal arthrodesis.[8,12,173,179,234,664,678,686]

Capitate-Hamate Arthrodesis. Chuinard and Zeman[110] recommend that the capitate be fused to the hamate to prevent proximal migration of the capitate-third metacarpal axis into the defect that is created by gradual collapse of the lunate. According to these authors, this procedure should remove the distal pressure by the capitate on the lunate and allow revascularization. Oishi and associates reported a series of 45 patients in which 93% reported improvement in pain, improvement in grip strength, and no significant loss of motion during a 32-month follow-up.[468] Recent biomechanical studies by Iwasaki and associates and others, however, show that capitate-hamate fusion does not significantly alter lunate compressive loads.[269,291,635] In the normal wrist, the capitate and hamate are already firmly bound by short, stout ligaments, and motion between them is close to nil. Collapse of the lunate and its fragmentation allows collapse of the entire proximal carpal row through foreshortening of the scaphoid and distal migration of the triquetrum on the hamate[606]; the capitohamate relationship should have no effect on this phenomenon.[269]

Capitate-hamate arthrodesis has also been proposed in conjunction with shortening of the capitate.[13] A recent biomechanical study by Viola and associates showed that capitate shortening in conjunction with capitohamate fusion significantly decreased the load across the radiolunate articulation while increasing mean radioscaphoid pressure.[663] When performing this procedure, it is important to ensure that the hamate does not impinge on the lunate; if it does, removal of the proximal tip of the hamate is advised.[248]

Scaphotrapezial-Trapezoid Arthrodesis. Only a fusion designed to cross the midcarpal joint, such as between the scaphoid, trapezium, and trapezoid or the scaphoid and capitate,[12,675,678] could theoretically succeed in preventing carpal shortening. STT arthrodesis is a commonly performed procedure, and reported results are similar with or without concomitant lunate excision.[12,543,678] However, because STT arthrodesis and the presence of an abnormal or absent lunate have the effect of concentrating load on the radioscaphoid articulation,[269,291,292] there is a risk that ultimately this procedure may result in progressive degeneration between the radius and scaphoid.[198,291,331] Minami stated that the main negative factor influencing clinical outcome after STT fusion was the progression of osteoarthritis at the radioscaphoid joint.[420] Recent in vivo biomechanical studies by Iwasaki suggest that with the progression of the disease from stage IIIa to IIIb there is a natural increase in load distribution through the radioscaphoid joint.[292] Iwasaki suggests that limited joint fusion may overload an already damaged joint and that procedures such as joint leveling, which tend to load the ulnolunate articulation,[689] may be preferable. The technique of STT arthrodesis is discussed in Chapter 13. Other types of arthrodesis for the midcarpal joint, such as scaphocapitate fusion,[550] appear to be similarly effective from a clinical and biomechanical point of view.[269,291]

Capitate Shortening. Almquist and colleagues[13] described capitate shortening with or without concomitant capitohamate arthrodesis as an option for the treatment of Kienböck's disease, especially for wrists with ulnar-plus variance. He reported good results in 17 cases, but the follow-up period was not specified. Horii and associates[269] have shown that capitate shortening decreases the load on the lunate by 66%, but at the cost of a 150% increase in scaphotrapezial load. Although avascular necrosis of the proximal capitate pole has not been reported as a complication of capitate shortening, it must certainly be a concern because all of the blood supply to the head of the capitate enters distally.

Joint-Leveling Procedures. The joint-leveling operations include ulnar lengthening† and radial shortening.‡ Radial shortening has become the mainstay for treatment of Kienböck's disease in the ulnar-minus wrist, in all but the most advanced (stage IV) cases. The success of this procedure is explained on the basis of postoperative changes in the ulnolunate relationship, which appears to unload the lunate.[395]

Of the two procedures, shortening of the radius may be easier to perform than ulnar lengthening, with less potential for postoperative pseudarthrosis and a more direct approach to decompressing the lunate. Ulnar lengthening works by advancement of the triangular fibrocartilage complex ahead of the lengthened ulna. Disruption of distal radioulnar joint (DRUJ) function is not usually a problem, but, experimentally, DRUJ pressures do increase with joint leveling unless the radius is translated laterally at the same time.[687] This

---

*See references 8, 100, 232, 308, 365, 482, 524, 574, 662, 666, and 693.

†See references 26, 30, 150, 173, 486, 546, 576, 624, and 655.

‡See references 14, 171, 432, 456, 472, 493, 503, 546, 565, 686, and 699.

represents another argument in favor of radial shortening over ulnar lengthening.[456,686] This situation may be further aggravated if the DRUJ is not parallel to the axis of shortening. Often in severely ulnar-minus wrists the distal radius will actually overhang the head of the ulna distally so that either radial shortening or ulnar lengthening will produce impingement and joint incongruity.[197] In such cases, ulnar lengthening is probably contraindicated. If joint leveling is elected, correction should be made through the radius, by which means the distal radial fragment can be translated to maintain congruity of the DRUJ.[456,686] In our experience these are extremely rare, and postoperative symptoms arising from the DRUJ are usually transient.

Although partial denervation of the wrist after radial leveling procedures may occur, this alone does not fully explain the long-lasting benefit obtained. Armistead and colleagues[26] have shown increased radiolunate distance after ulnar lengthening in intraoperative arthrograms obtained before and after ulnar lengthening. Trumble and coworkers[635] monitored lunate strain with electronic strain gauges and found that bone-leveling procedures were as effective as STT fusions in relieving lunate loading through a functional range of wrist and forearm motion. Their study revealed that only 2 mm of shortening of the radius, or lengthening of the ulna, was required to maximize lunate decompression. This, of course, would greatly reduce the danger of postoperative radioulnar disruption and eliminate the need to exactly make up the radioulnar length discrepancy when the discrepancy is more than 2 mm.

Clinical outcomes are generally favorable after radial shortening procedures. Quenzer reported on 68 patients who underwent radial shortening. Ninety-three percent had significant improvement in pain at an average follow-up of 52 months. Grip strength improved in 74% of patients and motion improved in 52%.[493] In a long-term outcome study of 88 patients, Wintman and colleagues found that after radial shortening there were significant improvements in motion and grip strength. In addition, only 3 of the 34 patients employed outside the home were unable to return to their original occupations.[699] Salmon and associates found that patients with radial shortening procedures tended to have less pain, better grip strength, and a slower progression of their disease process when compared with patients treated conservatively[538]; however, other reports have failed to show any change in the natural history of lunate collapse (see Fig. 17-38).[293,546,686,699] Although there is some evidence that new bone is formed at the distal radius (see Fig. 17-39),[633] this new bone is of unknown clinical significance. The main attraction of "leveling" techniques is that the carpus is left undisturbed. The procedure is indicated primarily in patients with ulnar-minus variance, maintenance of lunate architecture,[526] preservation of the lunocapitate joint,[26] and absence of degenerative changes (Lichtman stages I to IIIA).

Technique of Radial Shortening.   Almquist and Burns[14] recommend a longitudinal radiopalmar approach to the distal radius. Dissection proceeds ulnar to the radial artery. The pronator quadratus and the origin of the flexor pollicis are exposed, the periosteum incised along the brachioradialis and flexor pollicis longus insertion, and the radius exposed subperiosteally. An osteotomy is performed using an oscillating saw and a wafer of radius removed that is equivalent to the desired amount of shortening—at least 2 mm and no more than 4 mm. The wafer can be morselized and used as a graft. Fixation is provided with a volar "T"-plate (Fig. 17-45). Alternatively, the osteotomy can be placed more proximally in the diaphysis and a dynamic compression plate used. Care must be taken to ensure good apposition of the dorsal cortex; gapping may lead to delayed union (Fig. 17-46). An oblique metaphyseal osteotomy has the advantage of permitting a lag compression screw across the osteotomy site, but it is technically more demanding.

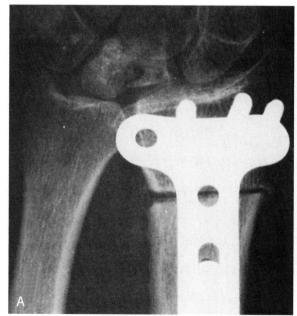 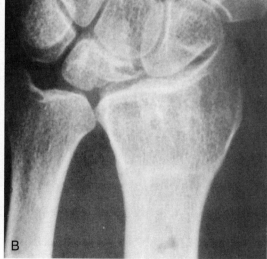

FIGURE 17-45. Radial shortening for the treatment of Kienböck's disease. **A,** Initial postoperative radiograph. **B,** Late (2 year) postoperative radiograph. The patient is free of symptoms. The appearance of the lunate is improved. (From Taleisnik J: The Wrist. New York, Churchill Livingstone, 1985.)

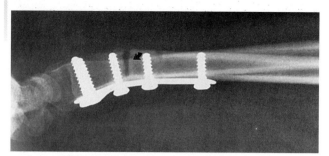

FIGURE 17-46. Gapping may lead to delayed union.

Botelheiro has shown that distal metaphyseal osteotomies produce fewer complications, in terms of nonunion and delayed union, when compared with distal diaphyseal osteotomies.[70] As with ulnar lengthening, rotation needs to be checked; if blockage occurs, radial translation of the distal fragment will usually correct the situation. Closure is performed in layers. Immediate postoperative immobilization with a conforming dressing and a sugar tong splint is changed at the time of suture removal for a long-arm cast. At 4 weeks, a short-arm cast is used until bony union.

Some surgeons prefer a dorsal approach for radial shortening.[546] Exposure is easier, and posterior interosseous neurectomy can be performed at the discretion of the surgeon. However, a dorsal plate is more prominent and may require removal at a second operation.

Angular Osteotomy of the Distal Radius. Watanabe, Nakamura, and associates[459,641,672] have proposed a radial closing wedge osteotomy (Fig. 17-47) as an option, particularly for patients with ulnar-neutral wrists. The procedure is based on a two-dimensional model of wrist forces that predicts reduced loading on the lunate with decreased radioulnar inclination of the distal radial articular surface.[672] This experimental evidence has had some clinical corroboration by Mir and coworkers.[426] They showed that patients with Kienböck's disease are more likely than unaffected individuals to have ulnar inclination of the distal radius exceeding 25 degrees. Tsuge and Nakamura also showed that patients with Kienböck's disease had more radial inclination than did those with unaffected wrists.[640] Garcia-Elias found a significant positive correlation between functional improvement and the percent reduction in calculated peak radiolunate pressures.[216] The greatest clinical and biomechanical improvements were found with closing wedge osteotomies of 5 to 10 degrees. Interestingly, Werner and Palmer[689] found in an in vitro model that a radial *closing* wedge osteotomy increased pressure on the lunate whereas a radial *opening* wedge osteotomy lowered lunate forces. Kam has also shown that a radial opening wedge osteotomy was more effective than a radial closing wedge osteotomy in diminishing lunate strain.[309]

There are several clinical series that support the use of closing wedge osteotomies for the treatment of Kienbock's disease.[350,429,575,641] Wada reviewed the results of 13 patients after radial closing wedge osteotomy at 14 years and found good long-term results. A radial shift of the carpal bones was present on postoperative radiographs that resulted in an increased lunate-covering ratio.[667] Lamas performed a biplanar dorsolateral radial closing osteotomy in 26 patients with stage II and III disease. The biplanar osteotomy not only corrected radial inclination but also normalized the palmar tilt of the radial surface. Follow-up MRI obtained at an average of 3.5 years postoperatively showed improvement in T1- and T2-weighted images, suggestive of revascularization, in all patients.[350]

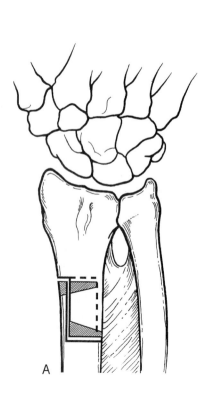

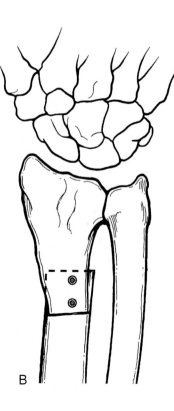

FIGURE 17-47. A and **B,** Radial closing wedge osteotomy.

A

B

The biomechanical data surrounding angular osteotomies for the radius are conflicting. Some studies suggest that there is continuation of carpal collapse and a progression of osteoarthritis with these procedures.[673] In addition, there are little data concerning the long-term effects that these osteotomies may produce at the DRUJ. Closing wedge osteotomies can be considered for patients with stage II or III Kienböck's disease, but further long-term studies are required before they can be advocated for all ulnar-neutral or ulnar-plus patients.

Metaphyseal Decompression. The majority of surgical procedures for Kienbock's disease will produce some hyperemia within the wrist. In addition, most procedures require some period of extended immobilization. These factors alone may help produce some improvement in patient's symptoms and may help to explain the often conflicting clinical and biomechanical data surrounding the many different types of osteotomies described for the treatment of Kienbock's disease. Illarramendi's report of radial and ulnar metaphyseal decompression for Kienböck's disease supports this theory.[277] Twenty-two patients were followed for an average of 10 years after radial and ulnar metaphyseal decompression. Sixteen patients were pain free, whereas four noted only occasional pain. Motion returned to 77% of the contralateral wrist, and grip strength was 75%. Although no comparison group was studied, these results are comparable to those reported for joint-leveling procedures. The main benefits of this procedure are its technical simplicity and the avoidance of the potential complications of nonunion, DRUJ incongruency, and ulnocarpal abutment.[14,26,460,493,667]

Vascularized Bone Graft for Kienböck's Disease. In 1979, Hori and colleagues[268] reported their experience with implantation of a dorsal metacarpal arteriovenous pedicle into the lunate as treatment for Kienböck's disease and scaphoid nonunion. Nine cases of vascular bundle implantation for Kienböck's disease were reported, with improvement in eight. Other reports have followed.[199] Domoter, in 1974,[159] Saffar,[535] in 1982, and Brüser,[83] in 1986, reported their experiences in replacing the necrotic lunate with the pisiform on a vascular pedicle. Good results were reported at relatively short (<2 years) follow-up. Bochud and Büchler reported 32 patients monitored for a minimum of 2 years and an average of 6.7 years after vascular pedicle implantation and bone grafting for Kienböck's disease.[60] Initial restoration of lunate anatomy was good in 95% of their patients; at final follow-up, however, only a third had retained any correction and nearly half the long-term results were fair or poor. Tamai and colleagues have reported similar results.[608] Gabl has advocated the use of a free vascularized tricortical iliac bone graft for stage III disease to prevent further lunate collapse.[208] Satisfactory results have also been reported with pronator pedicle grafting.[76,362] Moran and coworkers have reviewed the results of vascularized bone grafting for the treatment of Kienböck's disease.[436] In a study of 48 patients over a 10-year period, 98% of patients experienced significant pain relief. Grip strength was improved whereas flexion extension arc did not change. Postoperative MRI showed evidence for revascularization in 60% of the lunates. Evidence for revascular-

ization was associated with significant improvements in Mayo wrist scores after surgery. To protect the lunate during the early period of revascularization, temporary unloading of the lunate with an external fixator or scaphocapitate pinning for 8 to 12 weeks was recommended for all of these bone-grafting procedures.[105,208,562,704]

Revascularization of the lunate, whether by dorsal or volar pedicle grafting, seems a reasonable adjunct to joint-leveling or other lunate-sparing surgery, but there has not yet been convincing demonstration of an additional benefit such as long-term restoration of carpal height or arrest of disease progression. From a technical perspective, the use of a dorsal distal radius pedicled vascularized bone graft has the advantages of a shared incision for harvesting and placement of the graft and one that avoids the risk of injury to the palmar carpal ligaments.[560,562]

Technique for Dorsal Radial Vascularized Bone Graft for Revascularization of the Lunate. The anatomy for this procedure is based on the work of Sheetz.[559] We have found the fourth and fifth extensor compartment artery (ECA) graft to be best in the treatment of Kienböck's disease. Although the distal fourth ECA can be used as its pedicle, the fifth ECA is preferred, connected to the fourth ECA via their common origin (Fig. 17-48A, B). This combined fourth and fifth ECA pedicle is ideal, owing to the large diameter of the fifth ECA and the great length of the combined pedicle, which can reach anywhere in the carpus. Additionally, the ulnar location of the fifth ECA affords protection to the pedicle during the wrist capsulotomy.

Harvesting of the fourth ECA plus fifth ECA graft requires identification of the fifth ECA by opening of the fifth dorsal extensor compartment. The fifth ECA and venae comitantes are visualized on the radial aspect of the compartment, lying adjacent to or partially within the septum separating the fourth and fifth extensor compartments. The fifth ECA is traced proximally to its origin from the anterior interosseous artery, where the fourth ECA is also identified and distally traced. A bone graft centered 11 mm proximal to the radiocarpal joint and overlying the fourth ECA that includes the nutrient vessels is outlined (see Fig. 17-48C). Once the graft is marked, a capsulotomy is performed to expose the joint. A dorsal ligament–sparing capsulotomy is preferred.

The lunate is then inspected. If the cartilage shell of lunate is not compromised or fragmented, vascularized bone grafting is feasible. Necrotic bone is removed with a bur or curets, using both direct visualization and an image intensifier, leaving a shell of intact cartilage and subchondral bone through a dorsal opening. The lunate is gently expanded to normal dimensions if collapsed using a small blunt-ended spreader (see Fig. 17-48D). The anterior interosseous artery is ligated proximal to the fourth and fifth ECA. Graft elevation is completed, and the tourniquet is deflated to verify blood flow to the graft (see Fig. 17-48E). Cancellous bone graft is packed into the lunate followed by insertion of the vascularized bone graft, orienting the pedicle vertically with the cortical surface arranged in a proximodistal orientation to maintain lunate height during revascularization (see Fig. 17-48F). No internal fixation is necessary provided the lunate is not fractured, and the graft is carefully shaped and impacted into the bone.

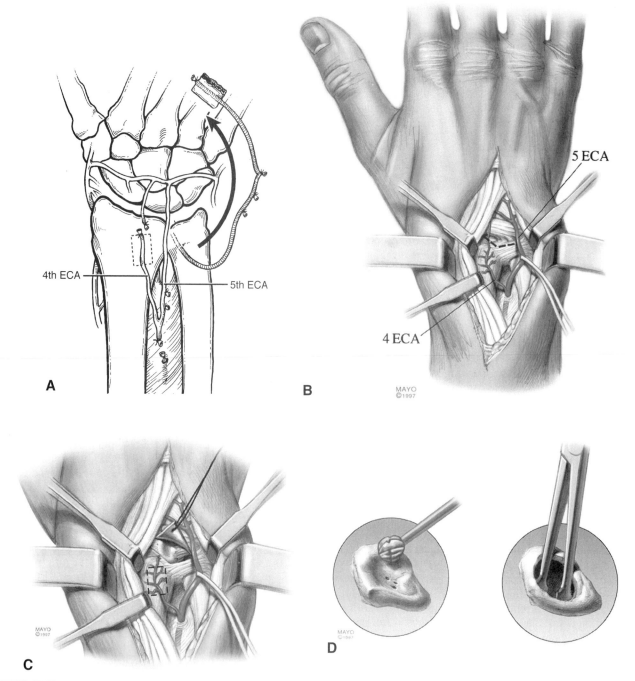

A

B

C

D

FIGURE 17-48. Technique of 4+5 ECA (extensor compartment artery) pedicled graft for Kienböck's disease. **A,** Schematic depicting the mobility of the harvested graft for use throughout the carpus. **B,** The location of the fourth and fifth ECA pedicles. Harvesting of the fourth ECA + fifth ECA graft requires identification of the fifth ECA by opening of the fifth dorsal extensor compartment. The fifth ECA is traced proximally to its origin from the anterior interosseous artery, where the fourth ECA is also identified and distally traced. **C,** A bone graft centered 11 mm proximal to the radiocarpal joint and overlying the fourth ECA that includes the nutrient vessels is outlined. Once the graft is marked, a capsulotomy is performed to expose the joint. **D,** Necrotic bone is removed with a bur or curets, leaving a shell of intact cartilage and subchondral bone through a dorsal opening. The lunate is gently expanded to normal. (By permission of Mayo Foundation for Medical Education and Research. All rights reserved.)

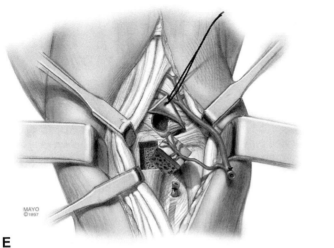
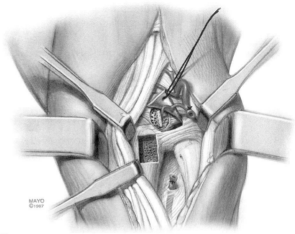

E   **F**

FIGURE 17-48—cont'd. **E,** The anterior interosseous artery is ligated proximal to the fourth and fifth ECA. Graft elevation is completed, and the tourniquet is deflated to verify blood flow to the graft. **F,** Cancellous bone graft is packed into the lunate followed by insertion of the vascularized bone graft. (Copyright Mayo Foundation. All rights reserved.)

To unload the lunate postoperatively during the revascularization process we prefer scaphocapitate pinning with two percutaneously placed 0.0625-inch Kirshner wires for 8 to 12 weeks. A layered closure of the wrist capsule and extensor retinaculum is performed with nonabsorbable sutures, and a bulky hand dressing is applied.

External Fixation and Direct Lunate Unloading. This procedure has been recommended for early-stage Kienbock's disease with and without bone grafting.[337,711] Theoretically this procedure unloads the lunate, which may facilitate revascularization and healing. This procedure may provide some benefit in stage 0 or stage I Kienbock's disease,[337] but its utility in the presence of substantial lunate collapse has yet to be proven.

Salvage Procedures

Wrist Arthrodesis. Radiocarpal fusion is indicated for patients with stage IV Kienbock's disease and for patients who fail to improve after other surgical procedures. Reports indicate that pain relief is adequate after this procedure, but most patients will continue to have some pain despite total wrist fusion.[542]

Proximal Row Carpectomy.[133,280,305] The indications for proximal row carpectomy are more limited than those for radiocarpal fusion, and its use for Kienbock's disease has been rather infrequent. A recent comparison between STT fusion and proximal row carpectomy in advanced Kienbock's disease found no significant difference between either procedure when comparing postoperative grip strength, pain relief, or range of motion.[453] Provided that the head of the capitate and the lunate facet of the radius are relatively preserved, proximal row carpectomy is probably best indicated for stage IIIB Kienbock's disease, especially in an ulnar-neutral wrist.[43,614]

Denervation of the Wrist. Wrist denervation has been advocated for the management of advanced Kienbock's disease.[172] The results have been unpredictable, however,

with pain relief at 4 years in only half the patients reported by Ekerot and colleagues.[172,685]

Kienböck's Disease in Children

Kienböck's disease is rare in children. Until recently, only single case reports had been published; these suggested that a nonoperative approach might benefit children more than adults. Recently, Kim and coworkers[324] reported seven children aged 9 to 15 with Kienböck's disease. All were initially treated nonoperatively. The three patients younger than 12 years of age all healed with nonoperative treatment; all others required surgery, either capitate shortening or radial shortening. Based on this information, it would seem reasonable to manage children with Kienböck's disease who were younger than 12 with 6 to 12 weeks of cast immobilization. This approach also may be tried in older children, but it seems likely that children age 12 or older will respond more like adults.

Authors' Preferred Method of Treatment: Kienböck's Disease

In general, there are four factors to consider when deciding on treatment for Kienböck's disease[606]: (1) the stage of involvement, (2) ulnar variance, (3) the patient's age and functional level, and (4) the presence or absence of arthritis. Given the volume of clinical and experimental evidence available, it seems reasonable to approach the ulnar-neutral or ulnar-minus variants in skeletally mature individuals in stages I through III with joint-leveling osteotomies; of these we prefer *radial shortening*. For a patient with an ulnar-positive variance, a midcarpal approach appears to us to be more reasonable, either in the form of STT fusion, scaphocapitate fusion, or capitate shortening. Each of these procedures could be augmented with the use of a vascularized graft. For stage IV, a complete wrist fusion, or proximal row carpectomy (if the capitate and radial surfaces permit), should be considered. In children older than 12, there may be a place for direct vascular implantation and bone grafting.[17] A supplemental temporary external fixator may be helpful to unload the lunate as it revascularizes in such cases.

ISOLATED FRACTURES OF OTHER CARPAL BONES

Fractures of the remaining carpal bones represent less than 40% of carpal fractures.[271,272] Although less common than scaphoid fractures, these injuries can also lead to long-term wrist morbidity if improperly treated. Many of these fractures require specialized radiographic views to identify, and the physician must often initially rely on physical examination to make the diagnosis. Because of this, these fractures may be missed on initial presentation.[215] In addition, these fractures are often associated with ligamentous disruption and with axial or perilunate type injury patterns, making the potential for secondary carpal instability significant.[215,554,573]

Fractures of the Triquetrum

Fractures of the triquetrum are reported to represent the second[28,39,62,545,551,554] or third[84,700] most common group of carpal bone fractures. Triquetral fractures are also the second most common carpal fracture in children.[361] They are commonly associated with other carpal injuries (Fig. 17-49) and may be seen with both perilunate and axial pattern fracture-dislocations.[125,288,593] The mechanism of injury may be a rotation or twisting motion,[39,545] a shear force applied by impingement of the hamate on the posteroradial projection of the triquetrum,[84] a fall with the wrist in extension and ulnar deviation,[84,151,157,214,551] direct impaction by the ulnar styloid,[173,196,203] or a direct blow to the dorsum of the carpus.[39,264] Skaters appear to be particularly prone to this injury.[221]

CRITICAL POINTS: OPERATIVE TREATMENT OF KIENBÖCK'S DISEASE

INDICATIONS

- Depends on stage and ulnar variance

Variance	Stage 1	Stage 2	Stage 3A	Stage 3B	Stage 4
Minus	Radial shortening; consider revascularization	Radial shortening; consider revascularization	Radial shortening	STT arthrodesis or capitate shortening or proximal row carpectomy	Wrist arthrodesis
Neutral	Revascularization or radial shortening or metaphyseal decompression	Revascularization or radial shortening	Radial shortening	STT arthrodesis or capitate shortening or proximal row carpectomy	Wrist arthrodesis
Positive	STT or SC arthrodesis or capitate shortening	STT or SC arthrodesis or capitate shortening	STT or SC arthrodesis or capitate shortening	STT arthrodesis or capitate shortening or proximal row carpectomy	Wrist arthrodesis

PEARLS

- Because many different treatments seem to be effective, keep it simple!

TECHNICAL POINT

- Consider palmar approach for radial shortening and dorsal approach for the others.

PITFALLS

- Failing to unload the lunate during the initial revascularization period may lead to further lunate collapse.

- The lunate fossa should be free of arthritis if one chooses to perform a proximal row carpectomy.

POSTOPERATIVE CARE

- Cast until bony healing (usually 4 to 8 weeks).

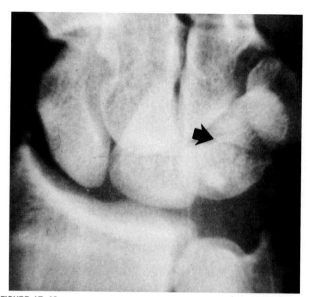

FIGURE 17-49. Dorsal perilunate transtriquetral dislocation. *Arrow* points to a fracture in the body of the triquetrum.

These fractures often become asymptomatic despite dorsal cortical fragments that may remain ununited. Occasionally, a tender fragment may require excision.[84] Avulsion fractures may, however, include the site of attachment of the dorsal intercarpal and radiotriquetral ligaments; as such, an avulsion fracture may represent a *forme fruste* of a reverse perilunate injury. Usually, however, such fractures cause little morbidity and can be treated by 6 weeks of immobilization in a cast or splint.[71,144,175,264]

The second type of fracture involves the main body of the triquetrum[39] (see Fig. 17-50B). This type occurs less frequently than a dorsal cortical fracture and, if isolated, is usually undisplaced. Rarely, triquetral body fractures are seen in conjunction with a perilunate fracture-dislocation, and treatment is predicated by the particular combination of bone and ligamentous injuries. Isolated triquetral body fractures can generally be treated successfully by cast immobilization for 4 to 6 weeks. CT or scintigraphy may be necessary to make the diagnosis.[39,175] Nonunion of triquetral body fractures can occur,[166] but they are exceedingly rare. Isolated dislocation of the triquetrum is very rare and should be reduced by closed or open means, as necessary.[114,606]

The third type of triquetral fracture is an avulsion fracture off the volar aspect.[66,84,364,573] The condition is not common but can be a sign of carpal instability because it usually represents an avulsion of the palmar ulnar triquetral ligaments and possibly the intercarpal lunotriquetral ligament.[573] This fracture is often missed on initial radiographs because the fragment may be hidden behind the hamate or the remaining portion of the triquetrum. Radial deviation views aid in identification of the fragment as will physical examination in localizing pain over the palmar aspect of the

There are three main types of triquetral fractures. Dorsal cortical fractures (Fig. 17-50A) are produced by avulsion,[39,91,548,551] shear forces,[84] or impaction.[176,214,364] Impaction is probably the most common mechanism.[176,201] In a study in which 76 patients with triquetral fractures were compared with 100 uninjured patients, Garcia-Elias[214] found that the mean size of the ulnar styloid was significantly ($P < .0001$) longer in the fracture patients. Triquetral impaction fractures are better visualized on oblique and lateral radiographs.[71,91,504]

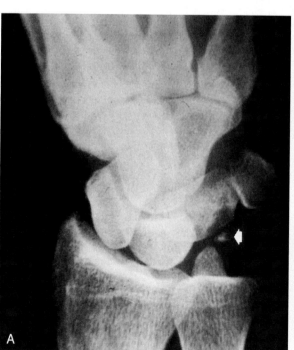

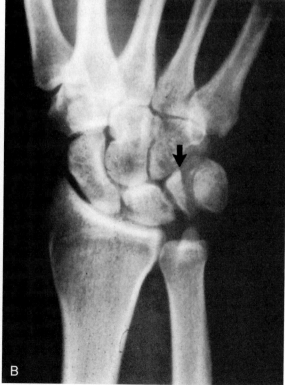

FIGURE 17-50. Fractures of the triquetrum. **A,** Dorsal cortical fracture *(arrow).* **B,** Fracture of the body of the triquetrum *(arrow).*

triquetrum.[573] CT or MRI can delineate the fracture if suspected. Ideal treatment for this fracture type has not been established, and treatment should be focused on restoration of carpal stability.

A final rare mechanism of triquetral fracture has been reported in association with dislocation of the pisiform.[387,487,601] The mechanism of fracture is thought to be due to shear force produced by pisiform subluxation. Fractures tend to occur at the distal ulnar surface within the pisotriquetral joint and may be treated with osteochondral resection of the fragment in combination with pisiform resection.[616]

Fractures of the Pisiform

The pisiform is an uncommonly fractured carpal bone, because pisiform fractures represent only 1% of carpal fractures.[39,504,653] The most common mechanism of injury for pisiform fracture is probably a direct blow to the hypothenar eminence,[195,653] but repetitive trauma has also been implicated.[289] The pisiform becomes fixed at the pisotriquetral joint as the hand moves into extension. Forceful contraction of the flexor carpi ulnaris as the hand strikes the ground usually produces a transverse avulsion fracture.[554] Parasagittal and comminuted fracture patterns are also reported.[215] Approximately half of all pisiform fractures occur in association with other upper extremity injuries; consequently, the diagnosis may be overlooked initially.[175,195,653] Pisiform fractures are also missed because they are difficult to see on routine radiographs of the wrist.[71,175,195,653] Special views such as supination oblique and carpal tunnel views or special techniques such as scintigraphy or CT are often needed to make the diagnosis.[175,195,349] The blood supply of the pisiform is robust, but avascular necrosis has been reported.[396,665] Careful examination of the ulnar nerve is mandatory because of the pisiform's close proximity to Guyon's canal.[96]

The pisiform ossifies between the ages of 8 and 12 and is the last carpal bone to ossify. There may be multiple centers of ossification, giving it a fragmented appearance before the age of 12. This normal variant must be distinguished from a fracture in children.[195,349]

Cast treatment of acute pisiform fractures has been recommended,[195] but there is no evidence that this alters the natural history of the injury. Pisiform fractures may result in nonunion[39] or post-traumatic pisotriquetral arthritis.[175,195,474,653] These late sequelae may or may not be symptomatic; if disabling symptoms do occur, pisiform excision is usually successful in reducing pain and improving function.[27,474] Pisiform excision appears to have little effect on the strength of wrist flexion.[27] Complications of pisiform excision are rarely reported but may include tendon or ulnar nerve injury.[387,423,442,487]

Technique of Pisiform Excision

The recommended technique is similar to that described by Palmieri.[474] An anterior approach is used, with a gently curved or zigzag incision slightly radial to the palpable pisiform. The ulnar nerve is exposed and the pisohamate ligament divided to decompress Guyon's canal. This maneuver reduces the risk of intraoperative nerve injury and prevents the development of secondary compression in Guyon's canal postoperatively. If the fracture is old and the flexor carpi ulnaris tendon is intact, a longitudinal incision

is made in the tendon and periosteum and the pisiform is shelled out. The tendon and skin are then closed and a soft dressing applied. Because the flexor carpi ulnaris is left functionally intact, motion may begin as soon as the patient is comfortable; typically, full activities can be resumed within a few weeks to months.[474] If the injury has resulted in a transverse fracture with a wide diastasis, the flexor carpi ulnaris will not be intact; in such cases the transverse rent in the tendon is used to visualize and shell out the two halves of the pisiform. The tendon is then repaired. A postoperative dressing is applied, with the wrist immobilized in slight flexion and ulnar deviation to protect the tendon repair. Wrist motion exercises are begun 3 to 4 weeks postoperatively.

Fractures of the Trapezium

Isolated injuries of the trapezium are infrequent and comprise approximately 3% of carpal fractures.[271,554] Fractures are usually associated with fractures of other bones, typically the first metacarpal and the radius.[129,409,433,531] The mechanism of injury may be direct or indirect. Trapezial ridge fractures may be secondary to direct injury or may occur indirectly by avulsion of the flexor retinaculum.[467,473,488] Trapezial body fractures may occur either in association with a longitudinal impact from the thumb metacarpal[237,288,327,488] or as a result of thumb hyperextension. In the latter scenario, the trapezium is thought to lever against the scaphoid[19] or the tip of the radial styloid.[287,297] Cyclists appear to be particularly prone to trapezial body fractures.[409,488]

There are three main types of fractures: fractures of the body, marginal trapeziometacarpal injuries, and fractures of the trapezial ridge. The diagnosis may be suspected by the presence of localized tenderness and swelling after injury. Fractures of the ridge present with localized tenderness immediately distal to the tuberosity of the scaphoid. Fractures of the trapezial ridge are of two types (Fig. 17-51).[473] Type I injuries occur at the base and usually heal with immobilization. Type II fractures, those of the tip, are much less likely to heal with immobilization; symptomatic nonunions are generally treated by surgical excision of the ununited fragment through a palmar approach. The diagnosis of trapezial ridge fractures is verified only by adequate radiographic examination, including Bett's view,[606] which is obtained with the elbow raised from the cassette, the thumb extended and abducted, the hand somewhat pronated, and the hypothenar eminence resting on the plate. The center beam is directed to the STT joint. A carpal tunnel view is mandatory when a fracture of the trapezial ridge is suspected. Occasionally, fractures of the trapezial ridge may result in symptoms of median nerve compression.[407,473]

Body fractures are typically tender just anterior or dorsal to the tendon of the abductor pollicis longus, approximately 1 cm distal to the tip of the radial styloid. Thumb motion may be painless, but pinch between the thumb and fingers is weak. Undisplaced body and marginal trapeziometacarpal fractures can usually be treated with plaster immobilization in a thumb spica cast for 4 weeks, followed by intermittent protective splinting and gradual mobilization. Displaced body fractures usually have an intra-articular extension into the trapeziometacarpal joint. The fracture line runs from this articulation to the dorsal and lateral surfaces of the trape-

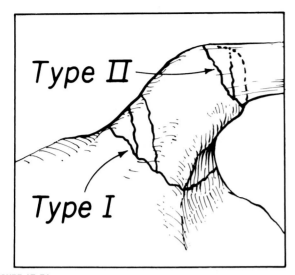

FIGURE 17-51. Trapezial ridge fractures. Type I, base; Type II, tip. (From Palmer AK: Trapezial ridge fractures. J Hand Surg [Am] 6:561-564, 1981.)

zium and may[265] spare the scaphotrapezial joint.[269,304] CT may be very helpful in delineating the anatomy of the fracture lines. Characteristically, the major fragment displaces dorsally and proximally with the first metacarpal.[304] These fractures must be exposed surgically, reduced accurately, and internally fixed with screws[201,265] or with Kirschner wires[129,409] to prevent long-term instability and pain. The radial artery can be distorted by fracture swelling, and its course should be identified during open reduction to prevent iatrogenic injury.[106] Aching pain and weakness may persist after intra-articular fractures have healed, and unreduced fractures or malunions may progress to degenerative arthritis of the trapeziometacarpal joint. For disabling degenerative arthritis, either trapeziometacarpal arthrodesis or excisional arthroplasty of the trapezium can afford satisfactory relief.

For acute dislocations of the trapezium, closed reduction should be attempted. When this is unsuccessful, open reduction with temporary fixation for 3 to 4 weeks by Kirschner wires is the procedure of choice.

Fractures of the Trapezoid

Isolated trapezoid fractures are rare.[39,430,492,504] The trapezoid is well protected by the strong ligaments that bind it to the trapezium, capitate, and index metacarpal and by the bony geometry of its carpometacarpal articulation. Typically, trapezoid fractures are the result of indirect force application along the axis of the index metacarpal. Trapezoid fractures are often associated with dorsal dislocation of the trapezoid or the index metacarpal[71,175,218] as a component of carpometacarpal or axial pattern dislocations.[217,218] Palmar dislocations and fracture-dislocations of the trapezoid may also occur.[514] As with many carpal injuries, routine radiographs often fail to demonstrate trapezoid fractures.[175,504] Diagnosis and analysis are usually best achieved with the aid of computed or complex motion tomography.

Isolated fractures of the trapezoid without displacement may be treated nonoperatively.[504] Fractures with displacement should be reduced and stabilized.[71,91] If the fracture fragment is small, closed reduction and cast protection may be sufficient.[71] Larger fragments may require open reduction

with internal fixation.[91] Chronic injuries are probably best treated by a combination of open reduction, bone grafting, and carpometacarpal arthrodesis.[217,492] Trapezoid excision is not advised[71,175] because of the theoretical risk of proximal metacarpal migration and carpometacarpal instability. However, a single case of trapezoid excision has been reported,[365] and that patient had a satisfactory result at 3 years' follow-up.

Fractures of the Capitate

Fractures of the capitate may be identified in combination with other major carpal fractures or as isolated injuries. They are reported to comprise 1% of all carpal fractures.[92,271] Bizarro[56] included six "incomplete" fractures of the capitate in his series of carpal injuries, of which at least five were located in the body. In Böhler's review of 826 carpal injuries from 1926 to 1936,[62] only seven fractures of the capitate were found, a frequency of 0.8%. However, in 1962, Adler and Shaftan[3] reviewed 79 cases found in the literature and added 12 of their own. Forty-eight of these cases were isolated body fractures, 11 were the so-called scaphocapitate syndrome, and 32 accompanied other carpal injuries. Rand and associates[498] added 13 more cases: 3 were isolated fractures, 8 were associated with scaphoid fractures, and 2 were associated with other carpal injuries. With the advent of MRI, more nondisplaced capitate fractures have been identified when searching for occult scaphoid fractures.[92]

Isolated capitate fractures are often undisplaced. However, because the proximal pole of the capitate is entirely intra-articular, waist fractures may result in avascular necrosis.[3,326,498] Nonunions are common without treatment and frequently require reconstruction in the form of midcarpal arthrodesis,[3] bone grafting,[688] or excision arthroplasty.[326] Residual symptoms are the rule, but usually these are not usually disabling.[3,498]

The diagnosis of capitate fractures depends on a high degree of suspicion, particularly when one is evaluating a potential scaphoid fracture. Although scintigraphy may be helpful,[267] diagnosis will often require CT or MRI.[92,498,688] Approximately 50% of capitate fractures will be associated with concomitant ligamentous and bony injures; thus a thorough evaluation of the wrist is warranted in all patients.[554] Dorsal distal articular margin fractures can be associated with fracture-dislocations of the third and fourth carpometacarpal joints.[217,554]

Treatment of Capitate Fractures

Treatment of capitate fractures if undisplaced and without evidence of avascularity may be with cast immobilization. Displaced fractures are usually part of a greater arc injury or the scaphocapitate syndrome (below), and this injury pattern should be ruled out before proceeding with surgical intervention. For displaced or unstable fractures, Kirschner wire fixation or compression screw fixation may be used.[707] If open reduction is required, a dorsal approach is the most efficacious.

Scaphocapitate Syndrome

The scaphocapitate syndrome consists of fracture of the neck of the capitate and concomitant fracture of the scaphoid waist, with malrotation of the proximal capitate fragment

(Fig. 17-52). It represents a variant of the perilunate pattern of injury. The mechanism of injury may involve a direct blow to the dorsum of the wrist while flexed[84,182,651] or, more frequently, a fall on the outstretched hand with the wrist in extension.[591] Fenton[181] postulated that extension is accompanied by radial deviation, which causes the waist of the scaphoid to be struck by the radial styloid. According to Fenton, the scaphoid fracture occurs first; when the injury force is not fully dissipated on the scaphoid, fracture of the neck of the capitate takes place. The malrotation of the proximal fragment was thought to take place consequent to a continuation of the initial thrust. Stein and Siegel[591] demonstrated in cadaver specimens that fracture of the capitate could be produced in forced extension by the dorsal lip of the radius striking the capitate whereas the scaphoid fractured in tension created at the midcarpal joint level by the forced extension. This mechanism of capitate fracture had similarly been suggested by Destot.[151] With the loss of stability across the midcarpus secondary to this double fracture, an abnormal range of angulation in extension becomes possible. The head of the capitate rotates together with the proximal fragment of the scaphoid. Several radiographic patterns may be identified[651]; most commonly,

this is an isolated scaphocapitate fracture and, less frequently, it is one that accompanies a dorsal perilunate dislocation (Fig. 17-53). The diagnosis is based entirely on careful radiographic evaluation and can be missed. The injury may be labeled an isolated fracture of the scaphoid or a typical trans-scaphoid perilunate fracture-dislocation and the lesion of the capitate overlooked.[23,476] This injury pattern has been reported in children.[406]

In patients with scaphocapitate syndrome, persistent displacement of the head of the capitate can remain after overall carpal alignment is restored by closed means. Case reports have documented union of the fractured scaphoid with persistent displacement and nonunion of the capitate head that demonstrated a pain-free wrist with minimal loss of function.[3,651] More commonly, symptoms persist; and for this reason treatment is usually advised. Excision of the head of the capitate may be considered,[181,182,381] but most authors[71,91,175,498,504,651] favor anatomic surgical reduction and fixation. The reduction should be done as soon as possible after injury, but certainly within the initial 3 to 4 weeks after injury. Even with ideal treatment, complications are common. Nonunion, avascular necrosis, and functional limitations are more the rule than the exception.[3,203,498] Initial

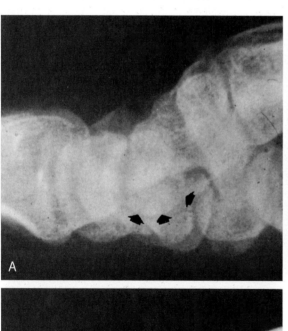

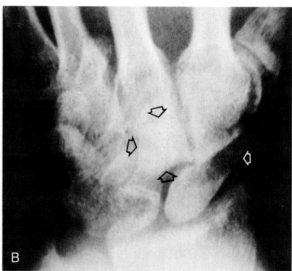

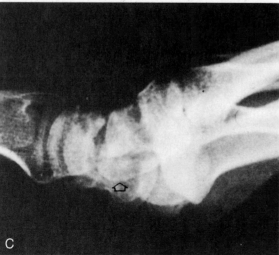

FIGURE 17-52. Scaphocapitate fracture syndrome. **A,** Initial lateral radiograph. The head of the capitate is rotated 90 degrees and lies volar to the body *(arrows)*. **B,** Initial posteroanterior radiograph. *Arrows* point to fractures in the head of capitate and scaphoid. **C,** Two-year follow-up. The scaphoid fracture is healed, but the head of the capitate remains displaced and ununited *(arrow).* The patient is symptom free. Wrist motion and strength are nearly normal.

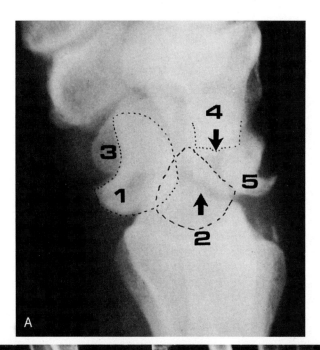

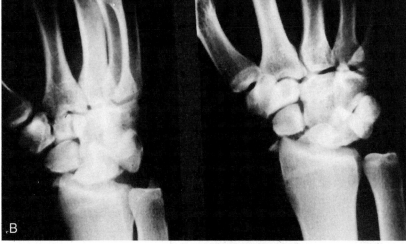

FIGURE 17-53. Complex comminuted transscaphoid, transcapitate dorsal perilunate fracture-dislocation. **A,** Lateral radiograph. 1, lunate; 2, proximal scaphoid fragment; 3, distal scaphoid fragment; 4, neck of capitate; 5, head of capitate. **B,** Posteroanterior radiographs.

Continued

bone grafting procedures may be required for fractures with severe comminution[498,690] and secondary bone grafts used for delayed unions and nonunions.[203,498] If the head of the capitate is avascular or surrounded by poor articular surfaces, it may require excision and/or scaphocapitolunate arthrodesis. Both Fenton and Rosen[182] and Kimmel and O'Brien[326] have reported excision of an avascular head of the capitate and its replacement with an anchovy-type fascial graft, with satisfactory results at follow-up ranging from 6 months to 3 years.

Treatment of Scaphocapitate Syndrome

If scaphocapitate syndrome is diagnosed within 3 or 4 weeks of injury, open reduction is carried out using a dorsal approach, with internal or Kirschner wire fixation of the fractures. Apergis, in a series of six patients, believed this lesion was always part of a greater arc injury and recommended evaluation and additional repair of the lunotriquetral component of the injury.[23,441] Cast immobilization was continued until both fractures healed. For late diagnosis,

treatment becomes a matter of judgment. If the scaphoid has healed or is healing in a satisfactory position, observation may be appropriate because some patients will remain relatively symptom free for many years despite significant capitate head displacement.[3,498] If bone vascularity is intact and avascular necrosis is absent, capitate and scaphoid fixation can be performed with Kirschner wires or compression screw fixation. Symptomatic patients seen late with evidence of radioscaphoid or midcarpal arthritis are probably best treated by a salvage procedure such as a four-corner fusion.

Avascular Necrosis of the Capitate

The capitate is at particular risk of avascular necrosis because the proximal pole is entirely intra-articular. By necessity, the blood supply must enter entirely from a proximal pedicle.[223,475,653] Both dorsal and palmar vessels are typically present, but the relative contribution of each to the proximal pole varies considerably.[475,652] In addition to trauma, the etiology of capitate avascular necrosis has been ascribed to

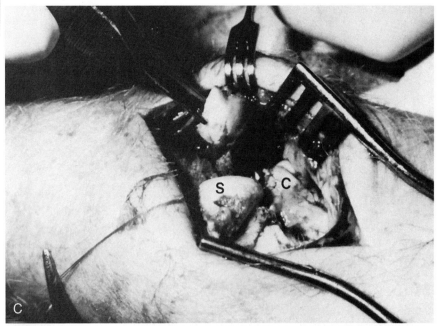

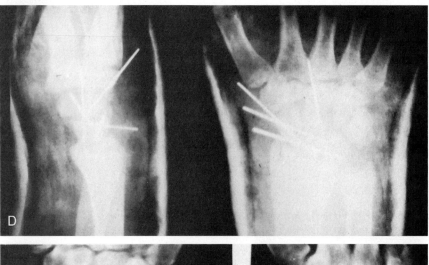

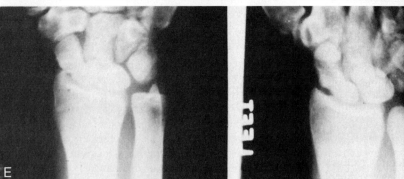

FIGURE 17-53—cont'd. **C,** Appearance at surgery, dorsal approach. The head of the capitate is held by forceps. S, scaphoid fragment; C, body of capitate. **D,** Radiographic appearance after open reduction and internal fixation. **E,** Appearance 6 months postoperatively.

ligamentous laxity,[461] vibration,[226,296] steroid use,[316] repetitive wrist extension,[63,496] and idiopathic causes.[348,694] The natural history appears to be one of progressive collapse with variable symptoms (Fig. 17-54). Verification of vascular status may be made with MRI.[215,445]

Milliez and coworkers[419] have summarized the literature and added three cases of their own. They classified involvement as proximal involvement (type I), distal or body involvement (type II), and total bone involvement (type III). Type I appears to be most common. Five of six cases

observed for more than 2 years had arthritic changes, most frequently at the scaphocapitate joint. Attempts to promote revascularization by bone grafting have met with mixed success.[296,419,498,652] Other treatment options include nonoperative management,[380,419,461,496] bone grafting,[502,516] midcarpal arthroplasty,[63,326,419] midcarpal arthrodesis,[296,380,419] and capitohamate arthrodesis.[445] At short-term follow-up, results are reported to be satisfactory with each of these options. No long-term follow-up reports on capitate avascular necrosis are available.

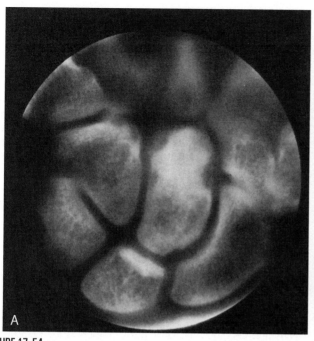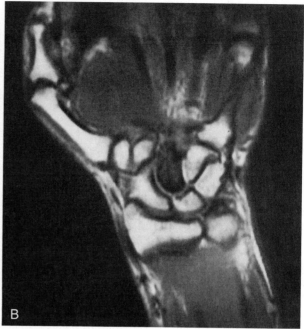

FIGURE 17-54. Avascular necrosis of the capitate. This 30-year-old man gave a long history of exposure to vibration in his occupation as a tool grinder. Note the (**A**) sclerosis and fragmentation of the proximal articular surface with a "crescent sign" (subchondral fracture typical of osteonecrosis) in the scaphocapitate articulation. **B,** MRI shows complete loss of signal in the capitate.

 ## Authors' Preferred Method of Treatment: Avascular Necrosis of the Capitate

Given the limited information available, it is reasonable to treat capitate avascular necrosis symptomatically. If symptoms are minor, observation seems appropriate. Persistent symptoms may require either midcarpal arthrodesis (see Chapter 13 for technique) or capitate head resection arthroplasty with fascial "anchovy" interposition.

Fractures of the Hamate

There are two main varieties of hamate fractures: those involving the body and those localized to the hamular process (hook).[417] From a clinical standpoint, these two fracture types may present with similar findings, and, on occasion, the two may occur simultaneously. There is generally pain on the ulnar half of the wrist, localizing swelling, and tenderness, usually over the dorsoulnar projection of the body of the hamate.[55,101,588]

CRITICAL POINTS: CAPITATE HEAD RESECTION ARTHROPLASTY

INDICATION

- Persistent and disabling pain, not controlled by simpler means, associated with capitate head avascular necrosis

PEARLS

- Infrequently indicated

TECHNICAL POINT

- Dorsal approach; remove necrotic capitate with rongeur down to bleeding bone. Fill space with either fascia lata autograft, Gelfoam, or similar filler.

PITFALL

- If there is significant midcarpal degenerative change, consider midcarpal arthrodesis. Fill space of capitate head with fresh cancellous autograft.

POSTOPERATIVE CARE

- Cast for 3 to 4 weeks, then splint and encourage wrist motion. Two to 3 months needed for recovery.

Fractures of the Body of the Hamate

Detection of fractures of the body of the hamate requires careful radiographic examination, often including several oblique projections until the plane of the fracture can be clearly seen (Fig. 17-55). The fracture line is usually oblique, either ulnar or, more frequently, radial to the radiographic projection of the hook.[417] Tomography or CT may also be of help in detection. The injury may also occur as a component of a greater arc injury.[554] Subtle findings on radiographs may include loss of the normal cascade of the metacarpal heads and widening of the intermetacarpal space between the middle and ring metacarpals.[107] Associated injuries include fracture or fracture-dislocation of the ring and little finger metacarpal bases, axial carpal instability, hamate dislocation, ulnar nerve palsy, and compartment syndrome.[9,33,178,217,311,555]

Isolated body fractures are generally stable injuries and become asymptomatic after a period of immobilization of 4 to 6 weeks, even if fibrous union is present. This may occur because the fracture line remains entirely extra-articular or, if it enters the carpometacarpal joint, it does so between the facets for the articulation of the fourth and fifth metacarpals. If the fracture fragments are displaced or if carpometacarpal instability is present, open reduction and internal fixation with Kirschner wires should be done.[73,466,605] Avascular necrosis of the intra-articular proximal pole of the hamate may develop in proximal fractures.[648]

Fractures of the Hook of the Hamate

Fractures of the hook of the hamate may be missed even when they are clinically suspected.[489] This injury should be strongly suspected when a deep, ill-defined pain is described on the ulnar half of the wrist, particularly in golfers,[101,450,462,595,630] but also in tennis, baseball, and squash players.[101,450,462,595,630] Symptoms are aggravated when attempting to swing a golf club, tennis racquet, or baseball bat. Tenderness may be elicited by deep palpation over the

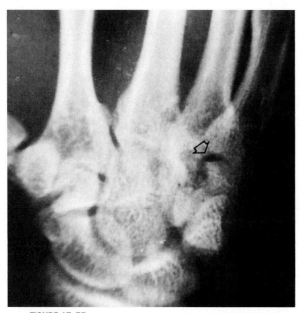

FIGURE 17-55. Fracture of the body of the hamate *(arrow).*

tip of the hook of the hamate in the palm and by pressure on the dorsal ulnar aspect of this bone.[101,588] Lateral movements or flexion of the little finger against resistance increases the discomfort, especially when the wrist is ulnarly deviated. This is because the hook serves as a pulley for the flexor tendons in ulnar deviation and with power grip.[670] Associated ulnar and median nerve symptoms have been reported[118,558,597] and attributed to hemorrhage within and around Guyon's canal.[273,462,558] Flexor tendon ruptures may also occur by attrition against the roughened edges of the fracture fragments.[112,135,251,421,469,613] Other injuries associated with hook of hamate fractures include fourth and fifth carpometacarpal (CMC) joint injuries[220] and transverse carpal ligament avulsions of the the hamulus and trapezial ridge.[632]

Fracture of the hamulus is most likely secondary to a direct blow produced by the butt end of a golf club, baseball bat, or tennis racquet or after a fall striking the base of the hypothenar area.[55,93,101,462,586,588,630,677] Hamulus fractures may be suspected on the basis of an abnormal bone scan,[55,489] but the diagnosis is confirmed by radiographic demonstration of the fracture. The carpal tunnel profile view described by Hart and Gaynor[250] is particularly helpful (Fig. 17-56). An oblique projection obtained with the hand in 45 degrees of supination and the wrist in radial deviation[21] and an extension or lateral view with thumb abducted and the wrist radially deviated are also useful (Fig. 17-57).[53,462] In both these projections, demonstration of the hamulus may require several radiographs in slightly different degrees of rotation until a satisfactory profile of the hook is obtained. Complex motion tomography[373] and CT[489,586] are also excellent techniques for visualization of the hamulus.[2] The superiority of CT compared with conventional radiographs has been demonstrated by Andresen. In this study, CT was compared with conventional posteroanterior, lateral, and fluoroscopically positioned oblique films. CT was found to have a sensitivity of 100%, specificity of 94%, and 97.2% accuracy in identifying hook fractures whereas radiographs had only a 72% sensitivity, 88% sensitivity, and accuracy of 80.5%.[20]

Hamulus fractures typically progress to nonunion if left untreated. This has been ascribed to its poor blood supply[475,677] and to the mechanical forces of the flexor tendons in the carpal tunnel, which tend to displace the fracture fragment ulnarly with grip.[677] Failla[174] studied the vascular supply of the hamulus and described a variable pattern. All hamates have a nutrient vessel that enters at the radial base of the hamulus, but only 71% have a nutrient vessel entering its tip. Thus, 29% of the population are at risk for osteonecrosis of the hamulus with fracture distal to the basal nutrient artery.

Fractures diagnosed early may heal with cast immobilization.[55,691] For those diagnosed late, most authors advise excision of the hook of the hamate fragment (see Fig. 17-56B), even in fractures through the base of the hamulus.[55,417,630,677] Ultrasound has been proposed as an option for hamulus nonunions.[206]

The reported results of hamulus excision are generally good.[55,101,587,588] Some pain and weakness persist, but most patients are able to return to full athletic and occupational activities. Osteosynthesis can yield excellent results,[55,677] but the technique is demanding and failures can occur.[55]

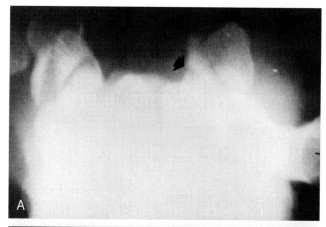

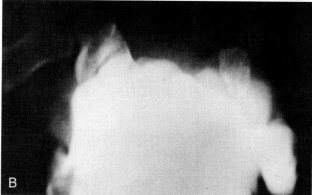

FIGURE 17-56. **A,** Fracture at the base of the hook of the hamate *(arrow)* in a carpal tunnel projection. **B,** Postoperative appearance. The hook of the hamate has been excised.

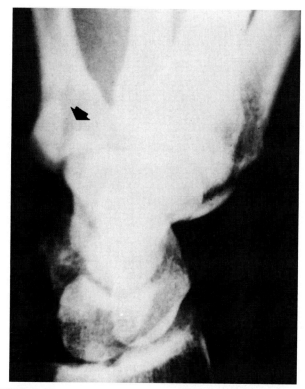

FIGURE 17-57. A fracture of the hook of the hamate *(arrow)* is seen in an oblique radiograph obtained in 45 degrees of supination, slight radial deviation, and dorsiflexion.

Authors' Preferred Method of Treatment: Hook of Hamate Fractures

If a fractured hook of the hamate is diagnosed acutely, cast immobilization should be tried, as described by Bishop and Beckenbaugh.[55] For hamulus fractures diagnosed more than a few weeks after injury, excision of the fragment with periosteal repair through an anterior approach is preferred for most patients. Osteosynthesis may be considered for delayed union and nonunion in a high-performance athlete such as a professional golfer or baseball player, but in our experience this has little to offer over excision in terms of functional outcome.

Technique of Excision of the Hook of the Hamate

Mizuseki and coworkers[431] proposed a medial approach centered at the fifth carpometacarpal joint and dorsal to the abductor digiti minimi. Other authors[55,677] approach the tip of the hamulus through a short palmar incision overlying the projection of the hook. Care should be taken to preserve the integrity of the motor branch of the ulnar nerve, which is in close proximity to the hamular process. In some patients there may be difficulty localizing the fracture site, but subperiosteal dissection and gentle manipulation of the tip

of the hamulus should lead to the site of nonunion. The fracture fragment is excised and the base of the hook of the hamate is rasped smooth and covered by careful repair of the overlying periosteum. Postoperative immobilization is required only until acute tenderness subsides, after which a gradual return to full activities is allowed.

Technique of Bone Grafting for Hamulus Nonunions[677]

Exposure is the same as for excision of the hamulus. The hamulus is progressively reamed to accommodate a matching cylindrical corticocancellous graft, which may be obtained most conveniently from the distal radius. Care is taken to preserve the cortical walls of the hamulus and the hamate body. The graft is impacted across the nonunion site. Supplemental fixation may be provided by a Kirschner wire, if desired. A long-arm cast including the ring and little fingers is maintained for 3 weeks postoperatively. A short-arm cast is continued until union is achieved. Vigorous activity should be avoided for 3 months.

FRACTURES OF CARPAL BONES, BESIDES THE SCAPHOID, IN CHILDREN

With the exception of the scaphoid and triquetrum, carpal bone fractures in children are uncommon.[361] Case reports exist of greater arc injuries in children, presenting with nondisplaced triquetral, capitate, and scaphoid fractures diagnosed late and progressing to nonunion.[116,406] One should always be cognizant of perilunate or axial injury

CRITICAL POINTS: HOOK OF HAMATE FRACTURES: EXCISION

INDICATION

▨ Acute fracture or nonunion

PEARLS

▨ Use part of palmar incision that would be used for carpal tunnel release, because it is extensile and can be used for subsequent palmar surgery if needed.

TECHNICAL POINTS

▨ Palmar approach.

▨ Identify and excise hamulus.

▨ Rasp base.

▨ Close skin only.

PITFALL

▨ Motor branch of ulnar nerve loops around hamulus: BEWARE.

POSTOPERATIVE CARE

▨ Splint until comfortable; then encourage motion and function.

SPECIAL CONSIDERATIONS

▨ Consider open reduction and internal fixation in athletes.

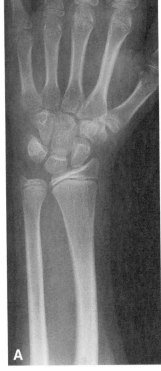
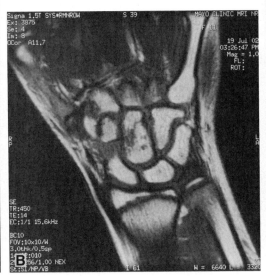
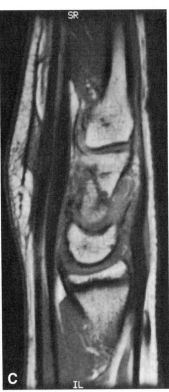

FIGURE 17-58. **A** to **C,** Occult fracture of the capitate in a 13-year-old hockey player. MRI reveals an oblique nondisplaced fracture of the body of the capitate.

patterns even in children. Finally, isolated capitate fractures can also occur in children, as reported by Minami.[422] Complaints in children after trauma should be taken seriously, and a thorough evaluation should be performed to rule out fracture. We have found MRI to be very helpful in the diagnosis of fractures in the immature wrist (Fig. 17-58).

ANNOTATED REFERENCES

Scaphoid Fractures

16. Amadio PC, Berquist TH, Smith DK, et al: Scaphoid malunion. J Hand Surg [Am] 14:679-687, 1989.

Forty-six scaphoid fractures were evaluated at 6 months after union. Twenty had a normal scaphoid alignment with lateral intrascaphoid angles less than 35 degrees. A lateral intrascaphoid angle greater than 45 degrees was identified as a predictor of poor outcome. This article establishes the measurements for the intrascaphoid angles used when evaluating malunions but now also applied to any displaced fracture.

153. Dias JJ, Taylor M, Thompson J, et al: Radiographic signs of union of scaphoid fractures: An analysis of interobserver agreement and reproducibility. J Bone Joint Surg Br 70:299–301, 1988.

Interobserver agreement and reproducibility of opinion were assessed for the radiographic diagnosis of union of scaphoid fractures on films taken 12 weeks after injury. There was poor agreement on whether trabeculae crossed the fracture line, whether there was sclerosis at or near the fracture, and whether the proximal part of the scaphoid was avascular. Scaphoid union should be evaluated with the use of postoperative CT at 6 months after injury to ensure there is no evidence of nonunion, sclerosis, or avascualr necrosis. Radiographs taken 12 weeks after a scaphoid fracture do not provide reliable and reproducible evidence of healing.

188. Filan SL, Herbert TJ: Herbert screw fixation of scaphoid fractures. J Bone Joint Surg Br 78:519-529, 1996.

The senior author reports his massive experience with 431 patients. Interesting findings included the high percentage of patients who had soft tissue interposed at the fracture site observed during open repair. Hypertrophic scarring was a common postoperative complication. After screw placement, some STT joint changes were seen radiographically but were not believed to be symptomatic.

224. Gelberman RH, Menon J: The vascularity of the scaphoid bone. J Hand Surg [Am] 5:508-513, 1980.

One of the three classic articles describing the precarious blood supply to the scaphoid. Fifteen cadavers were studied using injection techniques. Seventy to 80 percent of the scaphoid's intraosseous vascularity can be derived from the radial branch entering the scaphoid's dorsal ridge. A volar approach to the scaphoid is recommended as the least disruptive to the proximal pole blood supply.

236. Green DP: The effect of avascular necrosis on Russe bone grafting for scaphoid nonunion. J Hand Surg [Am] 10:597-605, 1985.

Defines the gold standard for determining the vascularity of the proximal pole—lack of punctate bleeding. Forty-five patients were treated for scaphoid nonunions using the Russe bone graft. All patients with absence of punctate bleeding from the proximal pole failed to obtain union.

513. Retting ME, Raskin KB: Retrograde compression screw fixation of acute proximal pole fractures. J Hand Surg [Am] 24:1206-1210, 1999.

Seventeen patients with acute proximal pole fractures were examined. All patients were treated with a retrograde Herbert screw placed through a limited dorsal approach. Union was obtained at an average of 13 weeks. This article strongly supports the belief that all proximal pole fractures should be immediately treated with internal fixation.

529. Russe O: Fracture of the carpal navicular: Diagnosis, non-operative treatment and operative treatment. J Bone Joint Surg Am 42:759-768, 1960.

The author outlines his operative technique for scaphoid nonunions. A union rate of 90% was achieved with this technique.

567. Slade JF, Gutow AP, Geissler WB: Percutaneous internal fixation of scaphoid fractures via an arthroscopically assisted dorsal approach. J Bone Joint Surg Am 84(Suppl 2):21-36, 2002.

This article beautifully illustrates the dorsal percutaneous technique, with excellent intraoperative images.

569. Smith BS, Cooney WP: Revision of failed bone grafting for nonunion of the scaphoid. Clin Orthop Rel Res 327:98-109, 1996.

This article reports the results of 25 patients who developed secondary nonunion of the scaphoid. Nineteen of these patients were treated with a secondary bone graft. The article provides a treatment algorithm with emphasis on correcting carpal instability.

709. Zaidemberg C, Siebert JW, Angrigiani C: A new vascularized bone graft for scaphoid nonunion. J Hand Surg [Am] 16:474-478, 1991.

This is the article that started the recent movement to vascularized grafts and stimulated Bishop to further evaluate the anatomy of the dorsal blood supply to the radius. Eleven patients with scaphoid nonunions were treated, and all achieved union at an average of 6.2 weeks.

Kienböck's Disease

14. Almquist EE, Burns JF Jr: Radial shortening for the treatment of Kienbock's disease: A 5- to 10-year follow-up. J Hand Surg [Am] 7:348-352, 1982.

This article establishes radial shortening as a reliable treatment option for patients with Kienbock's disease who have an ulnar-positive wrist. The study examines 12 patients with early-stage Kienbock's disease and an ulnar-minus variant treated with radial shortening osteotomies. Eleven of the 13 patients showed functional improvement and were satisfied with the surgery. Patients were able to return to normal activity.

208. Gabl M, Lutz M, Reinhart C, et al: Stage 3 Kienbock's disease: Reconstruction of the fractured lunate using a free vascularized iliac bone graft and external fixation. J Hand Surg [Br] 27:369-373, 2002.

This article presents another option for the treatment of Kienbock's disease utilizing a free vascularized bone graft. This is a rather extensive operation, but this technique does allow for the placement of a firm cortical strut within the lunate that may help support the dorsal cortex and prevent further collapse.

223. Gelberman RH, Gross MS: The vascularity of the wrist: Identification of arterial patterns at risk. Clin Orthop 202:40-49, 1986.

A dye injection technique was used to examine 75 cadaver limbs. Eight percent of lunates were found to have a single intraosseous vessel or large areas of bone dependent on a single vessel. The majority of lunates had an excellent blood supply.

248. Hanel DP, Hunt TR: Captitate shortening osteotomy: Kienbock's disease. Atlas Hand Clin 4:45-58, 1999.

Explains the technique for capitate shortening osteotomy, which is one of the few operations that truly "unloads the lunate."

275. Hultén O: Uber anatomische Variationen den Handgelenkknochen. Acta Radiol Scand 9:155-168, 1928.

The wrists of 23 patients with Kienbock's disease were compared with 400 normal wrists. The majority (61%) of normal wrists were ulnar neutral, 16% were ulnar positive, and 23% were ulnar negative. Seventy-four percent of the wrists of the Kienböck's disease patients were greater than 1 mm ulnar negative. An association was made between ulnar-negative variance and Kienböck's disease.

277. Illarramendi AA, Schulz CC, De Carli P: The surgical treatment of Kienböck's disease by radius and ulna

metaphyseal core decompression. J Hand Surg [Am] 26:252-260, 2001.

Illarramendi and colleagues noted spontaneous resolution in symptoms of Kienbock's disease in a patient who suffered a distal radius fracture. This led to the theory that local hyperemia after any type of osteotomy may resolve or improve the vascularity within the lunate. The authors have obtained excellent results with their localized corticotomy procedure and have avoided the morbidity associated with radial shortening and other intercarpal procedures.

323. Kienbock R: Uber traumatische Malazie des mondbeins und ihre Folgenzustande: Entartungsformen und kompressionsfracturen. Fortsch Geb Roentgen 16:77-103, 1910-1911.

Learn German or read the classic reprint in Kienbock R, Peltier L (trans-ed): Concerning traumatic malacia of the lunate and its consequences: Degeneration and compression fractures [classic reprint]. Clin Orthop 149: 4-8, 1980. This article describes the clinical and radiographic findings in patients with lunatomalacia.

368. Lichtman DM, Mack GR, MacDonald RI, et al: Kienbock's disease: The role of silicone replacement arthroplasty. J Bone Joint Surg Am 59:899-908, 1977.

The article contains the modification of Stahl's classification scheme breaking Kienbock's disease into four major stages.

635. Trumble T, Glisson RR, Seaber AV, Urbaniak JR: A biomechanical comparision of the methods for treating Kienbock's disease. J Hand Surg [Am] 11:88-93, 1986.

Lunate strain was examined as a measure of the axial load on the lunate. STT fusion, radial shortening osteotomies, and ulnar lengthening osteotomies were successful in relieving the load on the lunate. Capitohamate fusions were found to be ineffective. Length changes of 2 mm in the radius or ulna resulted in the lunate decompression without significantly increasing the risk of distal radioulnar joint derangement.

676a. Watson HK, Monacelli DM, Milford RS, Ashmead D IV: Treatment of Kienbock's disease with scaphotrapezial arthrodesis. J Hand Surg [Am] 21:9-15, 1996.

The results of STT arthrodesis in 28 patients with Kienböck's disease were studied with an average of 4.5 years of follow-up. Seventy-seven percent of patients obtained good to excellent results. Wrist extension and wrist flexion each averaged approximately 50 degrees.

Carpal Fractures

84. Bryan RS, Dobyns JH: Fractures of the carpal bones other than the lunate and navicular. Clin Orthop 149:107-111, 1980.

The authors describe the triquetrum as the third most common carpal bone fractured. The two major patterns of triquetral fractures are described. Pisiform fracture patterns and hamate fractures are also described in detail. This article notes complications associated with hamate hook fractures, including tendon rupture and ulnar neuropathy.

217. Garcia-Elias M, Bishop AT, Dobyns JH, et al: Transcarpal carpometacarpal dislocations, excluding the thumb. J Hand Surg [Am] 15:531-540, 1990.

Thirteen patients with major fractures of bones of the distal carpal row were examined. All patients had evidence of carpometacarpal instability. Diagnosis of the injury was made early in only eight patients. Delay in diagnosis was associated with poor outcome. At initial presentation, symptoms included pain, loss of grip strength, and mild limitation of finger motion. In three patients an acute carpal tunnel syndrome developed a few days after the accident. This article emphasizes the importance of looking for associated fractures when presented with carpometacarpal dislocations.

348. Kutty S, Curtin J: Idiopathic avascular necrosis of the capitate. J Hand Surg 20:402-404, 1995.

Chronic wrist pain can be due to multiple problems. This paper emphasizes the importance of a broad differential. Clinical and standard radiologic examinations were initially inconclusive, whereas MRI was diagnostic. Midcarpal arthrodesis gave a satisfactory short-term result.

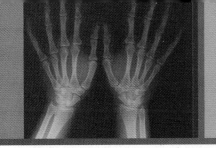

CHAPTER 18

Wrist Arthroscopy: Anatomy and Diagnosis

David S. Ruch and Gary G. Poehling

Although diagnostic arthroscopy of the wrist was first reported by Chen in 1979,[12] it was not until 1986 that Roth and colleagues[31,32] published a series of cases that served to define the role of arthroscopic surgery of the wrist. In the ensuing years, wrist arthroscopy has become the gold standard in evaluating and treating chronic wrist pain.[3,23,35] Multiple authors have compared the diagnostic ability of arthroscopy to arthrography and arthrotomy. Arthroscopy was found to more accurately identify and define ligamentous and triangular fibrocartilage injuries in the wrist and is now the benchmark for evaluation of the accuracy of other imaging modalities, including computed tomography and magnetic resonance imaging (MRI).[11,39]

In recent years, arthroscopy has advanced from a diagnostic modality to a therapeutic tool that permits surgical management of intra-articular lesions without the morbidity associated with arthrotomy. Arthroscopy has been successfully used for procedures, such as débridement and repair of triangular fibrocartilage complex (TFCC) tears, repair of partial and complete interosseus ligament injuries, resection of ganglia, synovectomy, débridement of articular defects, loose body removal, and as an adjunct in the treatment of distal radius fractures.*

ARTHROSCOPY AS AN IMAGING MODALITY

The value of arthroscopy as an imaging modality has grown since the original work of Roth and colleagues. Although high-resolution MRI using dedicated wrist coils has been demonstrated to be a highly accurate and noninvasive method for diagnosis and localization of TFCC disruptions,[30] arthroscopy has been found to be superior to conventional MRI, particularly with post-traumatic ulnar-sided peripheral tears in a younger patient population.[22,27] In fact, two studies have documented 100% sensitivity with accuracy of 79% to 97% in the diagnosis of TFCC tears.[22,30]

INDICATIONS

Arthroscopy of the wrist is indicated for (1) diagnosis of unresolved wrist pain after 3 months of conservative management; (2) treatment of mechanical symptoms, secondary to triangular fibrocartilage tears and interosseus ligament injuries; (3) débridement of loose bodies, osteochondritic lesions, and synovitis; (4) assistance in anatomic reduction and fixation of intra-articular fractures or acute perilunate instabilities; (5) treatment of ulnar impaction syndrome, including débridement of the lunotriquetral ligament triangular fibrocartilage perforations and distal ulnar resection (wafer procedure); and (6) resection of dorsal ganglia off of the scapholunate ligament.†

Anatomy

Arthroscopic portals are defined by their relationship to the extensor compartments on the dorsum of the wrist (Fig. 18-1). There are 10 described dorsal portals for the wrist: 5 at the radiocarpal joint, 2 at the midcarpal joint, 1 at the scaphotrapeziotrapezoid (STT) joint, and 2 at the distal radioulnar joint (DRUJ).

Palmar portals have been documented to be safe while allowing visualization of the dorsal ligaments and dorsal rim of the radius.[18] One cadaver study documented the relationship of the palmar radial portal to the adjacent neurovascular structures.[34] The palmar portal lies over 3 mm from the radial artery and the palmar cutaneous branch of the median nerve. The portal permitted visualization of the palmar portion of the scapholunate interosseous ligament (SLIO) and the dorsal capsular ligaments. Establishment of the palmar portal was demonstrated to facilitate arthroscopic-assisted reduction of distal radial fractures.[18] In one clinical series of 30 patients, there were no adverse findings associated with its use.

---

*See references 5, 6, 19, 25, 26, 29, 28, 33, 32, and 38.

†See references 1-6, 9, 13, 14, 19, 23, 25, 26, 28, 29, 31-33, and 35.

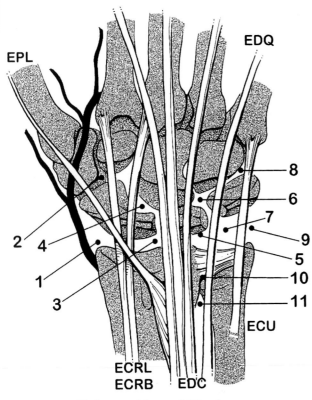

EPL

EDQ

8
6
7
9
5
10
11

ECU

2 4
1
3

ECRL
ECRB   EDC

External Land Marks

1. 6R portal
2. STT portal
3. 3-4 portal
4. RMC portal
5. 4-5 portal
6. UMC portal
7. 6R
8. Triquetral hamate
9. 6U
10. DRUJ distal
11. DRUJ proximal

FIGURE 18-1. Diagram illustrating the six dorsal compartments of the wrist and their relationship to the underlying carpal bones and the extensor compartments. EPL, extensor pollicis longus; EDQ, extensor digiti quinti; ECU, extensor carpi ulnaris; ECRL, extensor carpi radialis longus; ECRB, extensor carpi radialis brevis; EDC, extensor digitorum communis; STT, scaphotrapeziotrapezoid; RMC, radial midcarpal; UMC, ulnar midcarpal; DRUJ, distal radioulnar joint.

RADIOCARPAL PORTALS

The 1-2 Portal

The 1-2 portal lies in the anatomical snuffbox between the tendons of the extensor pollicis brevis (EPB) and the extensor carpi radialis longus (ECRL). The extensor pollicis longus (EPL) tendon is distal to the portal. Passing superficially through the anatomical snuffbox are branches of both the lateral antebrachial cutaneous nerve and the radial nerve (Fig. 18-2). Deep to the nerves, and just distal to the optimal portal location, lies the deep branch of the radial artery. A cadaveric study has shown that creation of this portal places the trocar within a mean distance of 3 mm from both the radial sensory nerve and the radial artery, thereby limiting the utility of this portal.[1] If the portal is necessary, care should be taken to use careful blunt dissection through a limited incision before use of the trocar.

The 1-2 portal allows visualization of the distal scaphoid, radial styloid, and the radial-sided ligaments. The first ligament visualized off the radial styloid is the thick large

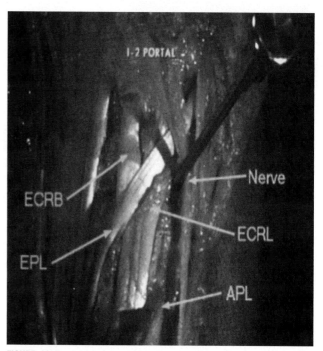

FIGURE 18-2. Cadaveric wrist demonstrating the relationship of the 1-2 portal to the radial artery and superficial radial nerve. ECRB, extensor carpi radialis brevis; EPL, extensor pollicis longus; ECRL, extensor carpi radialis longus; APL, abductor pollicis longus.

radioscaphocapitate (RSC). Just ulnar to the RSC ligament and separated by a well-defined sulcus is the long radiolunate (LRL) and the adjacent short radiolunate (SRL) (Fig. 18-3). Between these two ligaments lies the radioscapholunate ligament (RSL), otherwise known as the ligament of Kuenz and Testut. Although the RSL ligament itself is quite small, it possesses a thick tuft of fat and synovial tissue that increases its prominence at the base of the radial ridge and

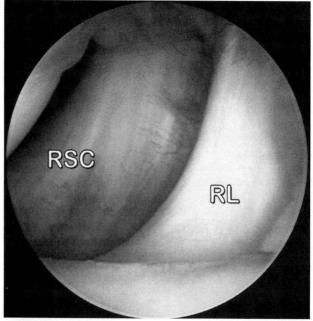

FIGURE 18-3. Arthroscopic view demonstrating the radioscaphocapitate ligament (RSC) and the long portion of the radiolunate ligament (RL).

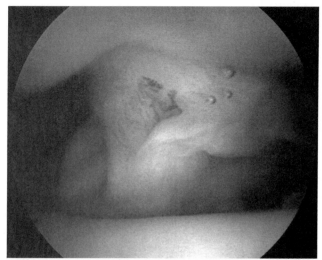

FIGURE 18-4. Synovial tuft overlying the RSL ligament. Note the cleft of the SLIO ligament directly above the synovial tuft.

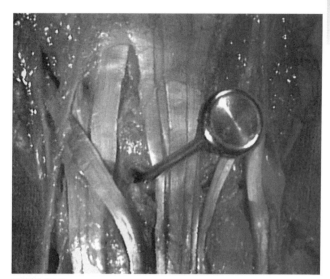

FIGURE 18-6. The 3-4 portal located between the EPL radially and EDC dorsally.

below the SLIO (Fig. 18-4). The RSL embryologically provides a neurovascular bundle to the SLIO.[8]

Following the RSL up from the palmar margin of the radius leads to the convex central, or membranous, portion of the SLIO (Fig. 18-5). Histologically, this ligament consists of thick volar and dorsal collagenous segments and a central fibrocartilaginous portion. This central portion provides a smooth articulation with the radius but does not provide mechanical stability to the scapholunate articulation.[7]

Although the 1-2 portal allows visualization of the radial styloid and scaphoid, the arthroscope passes down the 22-degree inclination of the distal radius and under the lunate only with difficulty. It is for this reason that the majority of radial-sided procedures make use of the 3-4 portal.

The 3-4 Portal

The 3-4 portal lies between the EPL and the extensor digitorum communis (EDC) tendons and is a relatively safe portal

with no underlying vessels or nerves (Fig. 18-6). This portal is located 1 cm distal to Lister's tubercle between the scaphoid and the lunate. Entry into this portal demonstrates the RSL at the palmar margin of the articular surface with the SLIO directly in front of the arthroscope. The articular surfaces of the radius and the proximal carpal row can be fully appreciated through this portal. Furthermore, all of the palmar extrinsic ligaments and the articular disk of the TFCC are easily appreciated (Fig. 18-7). The arthroscope may also be partially withdrawn and directed distally and dorsally to visualize the dorsal capsular attachment to the scaphoid and the SLIO.

The 4-5 Portal

The 4-5 portal lies between the EDC and the extensor digitorum quinti (EDQ) immediately distal to the insertion of the TFCC on the ulnar margin of the radius. Entry into this

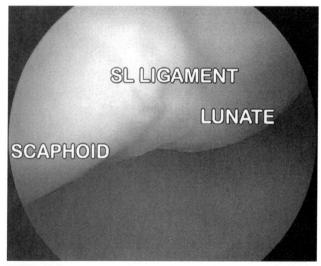

FIGURE 18-5. The SLIO ligament. Note the smooth contour of the scapholunate interval and the matching congruity of the distal radius.

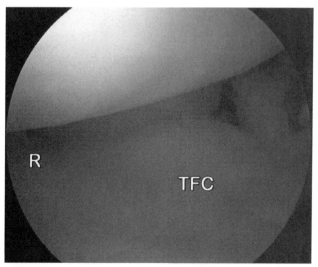

FIGURE 18-7. The articular disk of the TFCC (TFC) with its attachment to the margin of the radius (R).

portal positions the arthroscope with the TFCC articular disk below, the lunotriquetral interosseus ligament above, and the ulnolunate and ulnotriquetral ligaments directly in front (Fig. 18-8). The lunotriquetral articulation is directed vertically away from the plane of the distal radius. Therefore, the arthroscope must be directed ulnarly and distally to fully evaluate the articular surface of the triquetrum and the lunotriquetral interosseus ligament, which are not adequately visualized from either the 1-2 or the 3-4 portal. To demonstrate the ulnar-sided attachment of the triangular fibrocartilage, the arthroscope may be directed ulnarly.

The 6-R and 6-U Portals

The 6-R and 6-U portals are named by their relationship to the extensor carpi ulnaris (ECU) tendon. The 6-U portal lies ulnar to the ECU, close to the dorsal branch of the ulnar nerve. The ulnar nerve typically gives rise to two to three branches, which pierce the capsule of the ulnocarpal joint, making the nerve particularly vulnerable to injury while creating the 6-U portal.[10] The 6-R portal lies immediately radial to the tendon between the EDQ and the ECU (Fig. 18-9). The dorsal branch of the ulnar nerve is usually ulnar to this portal; however, branches of this nerve may lie directly over the portal, again necessitating careful blunt dissection before creation of the portal.[1]

Entry into the 6-R portal places the arthroscope immediately above the ulnar insertion of the triangular fibrocartilage with the ulnotriquetral ligament directly in front of the scope. The triquetrum lies above, as does the synovial-lined pisotriquetral recess just to the ulnar side of the ulnotriquetral ligament. The prestyloid recess may be visualized at the far ulnar side of the articular disk. This recess may be distinguished from an avulsion of the articular disk by its synovial lining. Furthermore, the disk should still have a taut, trampoline-like nature (Fig. 18-10).

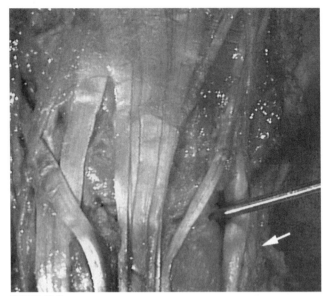

FIGURE 18-9. Trocar in the 6-R portal adjacent to the dorsal sensory branch of the ulnar nerve.

MIDCARPAL PORTALS

Midcarpal arthroscopy is invaluable in the visualization of scapholunate and lunotriquetral congruity and may confirm extrinsic ligamentous injury.[21] The midcarpal radial portal is located 1 cm distal to the 3-4 portal, in line with the radial margin of the third metacarpal. Entry into this portal places the scope between the concave surface of the scaphoid and the proximal radial pole of the capitate (Fig. 18-11). The radial midcarpal portal allows excellent visualization of the distal pole of the scaphoid, proximal pole of the capitate, and scapholunate articulation (Fig. 18-12). Conversely, volar ligamentous anatomy is poorly appreciated because of the restricted access of this joint; however, it may be possi-

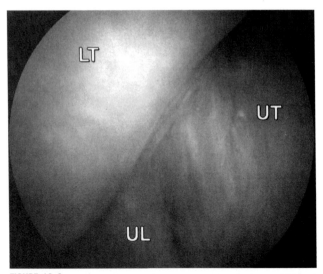

FIGURE 18-8. Arthroscopic view demonstrating the ulnolunate (UL) and the ulnotriquetral (UT) ligaments as well as the lunotriquetral (LT) interval.

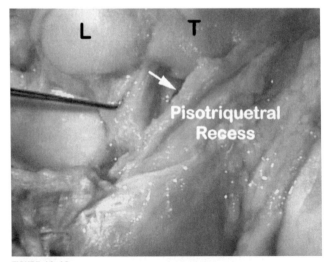

FIGURE 18-10. Cadaveric dissection showing the probe on the ulnocarpal ligaments and the pisotriquetral recess immediately adjacent to them and below the triquetrum (T). L, lunate.

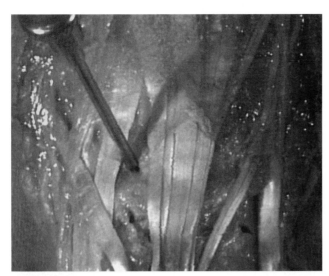

FIGURE 18-11. Cadaveric specimen with the trocar in the midcarpal radial portal.

ble in lax wrists to pass the arthroscope sufficiently palmarly to visualize both the continuation of the RSC and the palmar ligament between the scaphoid tuberosity and the trapezial ridge.

The midcarpal ulnar portal is located approximately 1 cm distal to the 4-5 portal immediately in line with the fourth metacarpal. The portal is located at the intersection of the lunotriquetral articulation and the capitate hamate joint. Viegas has demonstrated that approximately 65% of patients have a type II, or hamate, facet of the lunate that may be visualized through this portal.[36,37] The midcarpal ulnar portal allows visualization of the lunotriquetral joint, triquetral hamate articulation, and ulnar margin of the capitate (Fig. 18-13). In particularly lax wrists, the triquetrocapitate ligament and triquetrohamate ligaments may also be visualized palmarly.

The STT portal is located at the ulnar margin of the EPL tendon between the ECRL, the extensor carpi radialis brevis (ECRB), and the distal pole of the scaphoid. At this level,

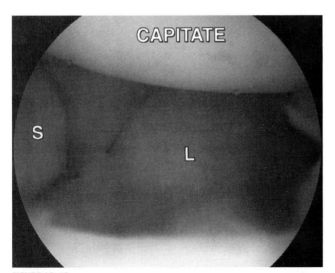

FIGURE 18-12. View through the midcarpal radial portal demonstrating the congruity of the scaphoid (S) and lunate (L) from the midcarpal joint.

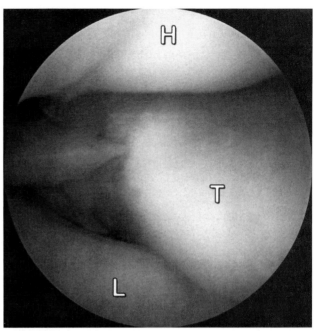

FIGURE 18-13. View from the midcarpal radial portal demonstrating the lunotriquetral articulation from the midcarpal joint. H, hamate; T, triquetrum; L, lunate.

the radial artery lies radial to the EPL and the ECRL; however, this portal is located in close proximity to the terminal branches of the radial sensory nerve. Entry into the STT joint positions the scope so that the trapezoid is dorsal and ulnar, the trapezium is palmar and radial, and the distal pole of the scaphoid is proximal. Although the articular surfaces of these carpal bones are well visualized, appreciation of the palmar ligaments remains difficult, even with distraction on the thumb. Instrumentation of this joint may be accomplished using the arthroscope in the midcarpal radial portal and the STT joint (Fig. 18-14).

DISTAL RADIOULNAR JOINT PORTALS

The DRUJ may be entered through a portal situated either proximal or distal to the ulnar head. The proximal DRUJ portal is located proximal to the sigmoid notch of the radius and ulnar metaphysis. The arthroscope is directed slightly distally, and it is possible to injure a small articular branch of the posterior interosseus nerve that passes in the ulnar margin of the distal radius. The distal DRUJ portal is located between the ulnar head and the TFCC. Additional traction may help to avoid injury to the articular margin of the distal ulna and to the attachments of the articular disk.

PALMAR PORTAL

The palmar portal enters the joint in the interval between the RSC and the LRL ligaments. The portal allows visualization of the dorsal radial styloid and the dorsal radiocarpal ligament while also enabling superior visualization of the palmar SLIO (Fig. 18-15). Ulnar passage of the scope remains difficult owing to the proximity of the lunate.

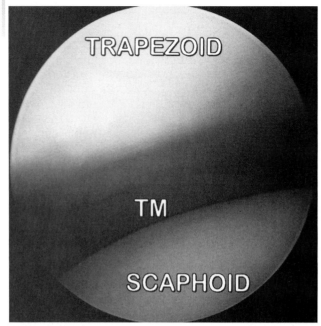

FIGURE 18-14. View from the STT portal demonstrating the scaphoid below, the trapezoid above, and the trapezium (TM) distally.

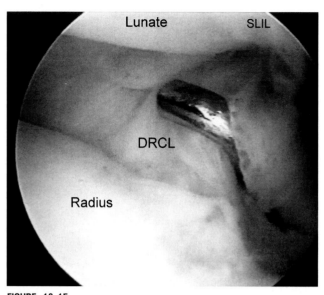

FIGURE 18-15. View through the palmar radiocarpal portal allowing visualization of the dorsal radiocarpal ligament (DRCL). The probe is in the 3-4 portal. (Courtesy of David Slutsky, MD, Torrance, CA.)

TECHNIQUE OF DIAGNOSTIC ARTHROSCOPY

The patient is positioned supine on the operating room table after induction of regional or general anesthesia. The shoulder is in 90 degrees of abduction with the upper extremity on an arm board. The elbow is flexed 90 degrees, and the digits are placed in fingertraps. Distraction may be provided using an overhead traction apparatus or a free-standing portable sterile traction apparatus (Fig. 18-16). Traction is adjusted to 7 to 10 pounds, and the wrist is positioned in 15 to 20 degrees of palmar flexion. An 18-gauge needle is then introduced into the 3-4 portal. The needle should follow the anatomical 12-degree palmar tilt of the distal radius. The joint is then insufflated using 5 to 7 mL of lactated Ringer's solution or until complete joint distention with easy back flow is established. If 10 mL or greater is able to be easily injected, it is likely that the fluid is flowing into the midcarpal joint or into the radioulnar joint. The 3-4 portal is then created 1 cm distal to Lister's tubercle. Of the many available techniques, the authors prefer to use a No. 11 blade to cut only the skin. The arthroscopic sheath and blunt trocar are then gently inserted, again approximating the radio-

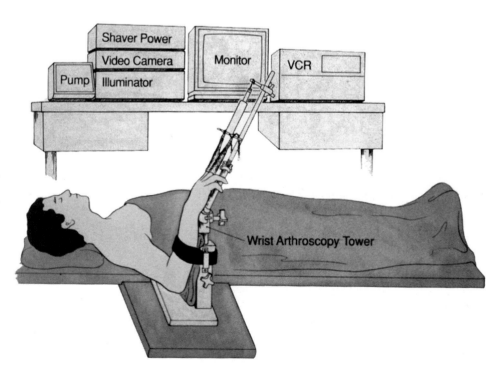

FIGURE 18-16. Position of the patient supine with the upper extremity on an arm table and the wrist distracted using a sterile distraction apparatus.

carpal tilt. The trocar is withdrawn and the camera is inserted. A small joint arthroscope (1.7 to 3.0 mm in diameter) with a 30-degree viewing angle is the standard for use in wrist arthroscopy.

A variety of irrigation systems may be used. Gravity inflow may be utilized, allowing hydrostatic force to distend the wrist capsule. The inflow may be directed through a 6-R portal, or it may be passed through the arthroscopic sheath with the outflow established at a 6-R or 6-U portal. A simple modification of gravity inflow involves the use of intravenous tubing with a small polyethylene pouch and a one-way valve. This allows for the assistant to manually pump fluid into the wrist and allows for greater distention than might otherwise be obtained using gravity.

The authors routinely make use of a pump to maintain distention of the capsule (3M, Minneapolis, MN). The pump permits constant regulation of pressure and can help to control bleeding in procedures such as synovectomy. Caution must be exercised when making use of the pump with distal radius fractures because it permits some extravasation to occur through the damaged capsule. The authors have made use of a pump system for approximately 8 years and have not experienced any complications with its use. There are no case reports of compartment syndrome in the upper extremity after wrist arthroscopy.

The 3-4 portal permits visualization of approximately 70% of the radiocarpal joint. The surgeon should evaluate both the bony anatomy and extrinsic radiocarpal ligaments. The telescope can then be directed dorsally at the capsular insertion on the scapholunate ligament, then ulnarly to better visualize the central portion of the TFCC. The ulnolunate and ulnotriquetral ligaments are more difficult to appreciate from this portal.

Diagnostic arthroscopy of the radiocarpal joint requires the creation of an ulnar-sided portal to evaluate the remainder of the wrist. The 6-R portal is created by inserting a needle immediately radial to the ECU tendon while visualizing its position with the arthroscope. The arthroscopic view permits evaluation of the angle of the portal and prevents injury to the TFCC during insertion of the cannula. Outflow cannulas may be placed in the 6-R portal initially while radial-sided arthroscopy is being performed, and then the arthroscope may be switched to this portal. The 6-R portal allows visualization of the bony structures including the articular surfaces of the lunate, the triquetrum, and the lunotriquetral interosseus ligament. It also permits evaluation of the peripheral margin of the TFCC, including both the radial and ulnar attachment of the articular disk and ulnolunate and ulnotriquetral ligaments. The presty-loid recess and pisotriquetral space may also be visualized from this portal by rotating the scope at a 30-degree angle.

The 4-5 portal serves as an alternative to the 6-R portal to allow evaluation of the ulnar-sided structures. The portal is also invaluable in the débridement of the free margin of the TFCC or lunotriquetral ligaments. A full radius synovial resector or suction punch can be inserted into this portal while the arthroscope is maintained in the 6-R portal. The portal may also accommodate the arthroscope when débridement of either the scapholunate ligament (through the 3-4 portal) or the lunotriquetral ligament (through the 6-R portal) is required.

DIAGNOSTIC MIDCARPAL ARTHROSCOPY

Diagnostic arthroscopy of the wrist should not be considered complete until the midcarpal joint is assessed. Arthroscopy of the midcarpal joint may be accomplished through either the midcarpal radial portal or the midcarpal ulnar portal. For the midcarpal radial portal, an 18-gauge needle is placed 1 cm distal to the 3-4 portal in line with the radial margin of the third metacarpal.

Normally there is no communication between the radiocarpal and midcarpal spaces and the portal will accommodate only 3 to 5 mL of fluid to distend the joint. The trocar is directed at a slight palmar tilt between the capitate and the scaphoid. The usual diameter is between 1.7 and 2.7 mm. This diagnostic examination is performed by directing the scope radially to the STT joint to allow visualization of any degenerative changes in the distal pole of the scaphoid, the trapezoid (dorsal), and the trapezium (palmar). Débridement of this joint may require placement of the STT portal for insertion of a shaver.

After evaluation of the STT joint, the scapholunate articulation is first visualized, followed by the proximal pole of the capitate and the scaphocapitate joint. It is often easier to assess congruity of the scapholunate joint from this portal. If a question arises, the scapholunate interval may be stressed by inserting a probe in the radiocarpal joint while the arthroscope is in the midcarpal portal. Specifically, one should examine the tilt of the lunate and the congruity of the concave surfaces of the scaphoid and the lunate. A scaphoid shift (Watson test) can be performed while visualizing the scapholunate articulation through the midcarpal joint to directly assess its dynamic stability.

To completely evaluate the triquetral hamate joint or débride the lunotriquetral joint, an ulnar midcarpal portal may be created. Again, it is useful to identify the optimal placement of the portal by first placing an 18-gauge needle approximately 1 cm distal to the 4-5 portal, in line with the fourth metacarpal. Care should be taken to examine the type II, or hamate, facet of the lunate[36] for degenerative changes in unexplained causes of dorsal ulnar pain.

DIAGNOSTIC ARTHROSCOPY OF THE DISTAL RADIOULNAR JOINT

The DRUJ portals allow visualization of the undersurface of the TFCC complex and condition of the ulnar head. Visualization of the DRUJ may prove advantageous when evaluating for ulnar impaction syndrome in the absence of complete TFCC perforation. The primary portal for arthroscopy of the DRUJ is the proximal portal, located immediately proximal to the sigmoid notch of the radius. To relax the dorsal capsule, the wrist should be placed in supination. This can be achieved by releasing the positioning straps so that the forearm may be supinated while maintaining distraction with fingertraps. The sigmoid notch, ulnar head, and thickened margins of the TFCC may be evaluated peripherally. To accurately assess the undersurface of the TFCC, the distal DRUJ portal must be created. This portal is best created by pre-placement of an 18-gauge needle to avoid damage to the dorsal attachment of the TFCC. The undersurface of the TFCC, origin of the ulnocarpal ligaments, and articular surface of the ulna may then be examined. The ultra-thin 2-mm arthroscope may facilitate access to the distal radioulnar joint.

PALMAR PORTAL ARTHROSCOPY

The palmar portal may be created both from an inside-out technique or using the relative safe zone afforded by the flexor carpi radialis (FCR) sheath. If the inside-out technique is used, the switching stick or blunt trocar is passed in the interval between the RSC and the LRL ligaments. Care should be exercised to verify that the blunt trocar or switching stick is emerging radial to the FCR to avoid injury to the median nerve. A second technique described by Slutsky is to make a transverse incision radial to the FCR and to retract the tendon ulnarly to place the trocar through the floor of the FCR sheath.[34] Care must be taken to avoid the palmar cutaneous branch of the median nerve. Visualization of the dorsal capsule and the dorsal radiocarpal ligament insertion on the radius is usually excellent. It may be useful to place a probe from the 4-5 portal dorsally to sweep the capsule away from the arthroscope to visualize the dorsal portion of the scapholunate ligament.

POSTOPERATIVE CARE

The wrist is removed from the fingertraps. The authors do not routinely suture the portals closed but rather allow them to drain. They are covered with sterile gauze dressings, and a wrist splint is applied with the wrist in 20 degrees of extension and the metacarpophalangeal joints of the digits free. The forearm is placed at neutral rotation and neutral deviation.

The splint is removed at the first postoperative visit, and range-of-motion exercises are initiated. The authors do not routinely make use of occupational therapy after this procedure. The majority of patients have only a mild swelling at their first postoperative visit and are able to perform range-of-motion exercises on their own. A splint may be used for strenuous activity for approximately 4 weeks; after that, patients are encouraged to remove it. The majority of patients are able to perform activities of daily living by 2 weeks after diagnostic arthroscopy. Full recovery is anticipated by 6 weeks postoperatively.

COMPLICATIONS

Arthroscopy of the wrist remains a superior method of visualizing intra-articular pathology when compared with arthrotomy, yet complications have been reported in the literature.[15,16,20] After a review of the complications reported in the literature, De Smet estimated a 2% complication rate, of which most were related to the size of the instrumentation relative to the intrinsic tightness of the joints. Despite the relatively well-documented portal anatomy, injuries to the extensor tendons, radial artery, and the superficial branches of the radial and ulnar nerves have all been described.[16] The tendon most at risk for arthroscopy is the EPL. Both acute and late rupture of this tendon have been reported. Neurovascular complications are related to the more ulnar portals.

The majority of these complications may be minimized by careful creation of the portals, the use of blunt instruments in creating the arthrotomy, and care when placing pins. The 1-2 portal is in close proximity to the S_2 and S_3 branches of the radial sensory nerve as well as the radial artery. Despite the cadaveric data describing the proximity of the 6-R portal to transverse radioulnar branches, there are no reports of complications associated with the use of that portal. The 6-U portal is in close proximity to dorsal branches of the ulnar nerve, and, in particular, the transverse radioulnar sensory branch. This nerve has been shown to be within 2.9 mm of suture passers used in repair of peripheral TFCC tears.[24] The 4-5 portal lies distal to the terminal branch of the posterior interosseous nerve and avulsion of this branch has been reported after arthroscopy.[17]

CRITICAL POINTS: DIAGNOSTIC ARTHROSCOPY

INDICATIONS

- Grading of intercarpal ligament injuries
- Assessment of ulnar-sided wrist pain
- Assistance in reduction of intra-articular fractures
- Visualization of soft tissue and cartilaginous lesions

PITFALLS

- 1-2 portal → radial artery and superficial radial nerve
- 3-4 portal → EPL tendon
- 6R portal → transverse branch of dorsal branch of ulnar nerve
- 6U portal → dorsal sensory branch of ulnar nerve

TECHNICAL POINTS

- Perform adequate distraction.
- Use blunt dissection for portal placement.
- Include 4-5 or 6-R portal to completely assess the ulnar side.
- Include midcarpal arthroscopy.

POSTOPERATIVE CARE

- Use removable cock-up wrist brace and ice bag.
- Begin range-of-motion exercises by 3-5 days postoperatively.
- Begin strengthening at 3 weeks.

SPECIAL CONSIDERATIONS

- Position of the wrist and forearm and duration of immobilization are determined by the arthroscopic procedure performed.

ANNOTATED REFERENCES

2. Adolfsson L: Arthroscopic diagnosis of ligament lesions of the wrist. J Hand Surg [Br] 19:505-512, 1994.

One hundred forty-four patients with post-traumatic wrist pain but normal standard radiographs were examined by wrist arthroscopy. Ligamentous lesions were observed in 75 patients. TFCC lesions, classified according to the Palmer classification and including lunatotriquetral interosseous ligament lesions, were seen in 61, and SLIO lesions were noted in 14 patients. Degenerative TFCC changes were equally common in patients younger than age 40 years but significantly more common with more than 2 years' duration of symptoms.

3. Adolfsson L: Arthroscopy for the diagnosis of post-traumatic wrist pain. J Hand Surg [Br] 17:46-50, 1992.

Thirty patients with post-traumatic wrist pain were investigated by arthroscopy. The clinical findings and type of injury were compared with the pathologic morphology seen at arthroscopy. In 21 (70%) of patients, arthroscopic findings gave a plausible explanation for the symptoms.

4. Adolfsson L, Jorgsholm P: Arthroscopically-assisted reduction of intra-articular fractures of the distal radius. J Hand Surg [Br] 23:391-395, 1998.

Twenty-seven patients with intra-articular fractures of the distal radius with a step of more than 1 mm in the joint surface after attempted closed reduction were treated by reduction under arthroscopic control and percutaneous fixation. All fractures healed without measurable incongruity of the joint surface and at follow-up 3 to 38 months after surgery 19 patients had excellent and 8 patients had good results according to the Mayo-modified wrist score.

7. Berger RA: The gross and histologic anatomy of the scapholunate interosseous ligament. J Hand Surg [Am] 21:170-178, 1996.

The SLIO was evaluated in transverse, sagittal, and coronal planes in 21 fresh and 16 fixed adult cadaver wrists. This ligament is consistently divisible into three anatomic regions: dorsal, proximal, and palmar. The dorsal region is thick and composed of short, transversely oriented collagen fibers. The proximal region is principally composed of fibrocartilage, with a few superficial, longitudinally oriented collagen fibers. The proximal region may extend distally a few millimeters into the scapholunate joint space, thus resembling a knee meniscus. The RSL ligament separates the proximal and palmar regions of the SLIO, extending distally to cover the dorsal surface of the palmar region of the SLIO. The palmar region is thin and composed of obliquely oriented collagen fascicles, just dorsal to and separate from the LRL ligament.

9. Bienz T, Raphael JS: Arthroscopic resection of the dorsal ganglia of the wrist. Hand Clin 15:429-434, 1999.

Arthroscopic ganglion resection provides a means by which dorsal wrist ganglia may be safely resected while avoiding the requisite scar accompanying open resection. Use of the arthroscope provides a much more complete examination of the wrist, allowing assessment of the cause of the ganglion as well as associated intra-articular problems. In a previous pilot study, 50% of patients demonstrated visible intra-articular abnormalities, including scapholunate ligament laxity and perforations, TFCC tears, or chondral degeneration at the radial and triquetral-hamate joints. Use of the shaver within the joint allows the surgeon to directly address the ganglion's site of capsular origin, ensuring that the "one-way valve" mechanism is resected. The authors' initial experience was that the recurrence rate after arthroscopic resection was equal to or lower than after open resection. There is now some suggestion that resection of only the ganglion stalk, without

removal of the sac, is feasible but may yield slightly higher recurrence rates than formal open resection of the sac and stalk. This may be attributed to cases in which the capsular attachment to the scapholunate ligament is débrided without identification and removal of a true stalk. The recurrence rate of a ganglion that has previously recurred also appears to be higher than that of primary resection. The authors look forward to publishing their completed results of an ongoing follow-up study comparing open, arthroscopic, and recurrent ganglion resections.

11. Cantor RM, Stern PJ, Wyrick JD, Michaels SE: The relevance of ligament tears or perforations in the diagnosis of wrist pain: An arthrographic study. J Hand Surg [Am] 19:945-953, 1994.

This study assessed the clinical significance of arthrographic abnormalities in the ligaments of a painful wrist by comparison arthrography of the asymptomatic wrist. Fifty-six patients with unilateral wrist pain underwent selective bilateral arthrography to assess interruptions of continuity of the triangular fibrocartilage, lunotriquetral, and scapholunate ligaments. In patients with ligament defects in the symptomatic wrist, 88% of defects near the radial attachment of the triangular fibrocartilage, 59% of lunotriquetral defects, and 57% of scapholunate defects were bilateral.

13. Chou CH, Lee TS: Peripheral tears of triangular fibrocartilage complex: Results of primary repair. Int Orthop 25:392-395, 2001.

In 16 patients with ulnar wrist pain, we performed primary arthroscopic or open repair of the peripheral rim tears of the TFCC (14 ulnar, 4 volar, and 3 radial tears). The wrist function was assessed before and 1 year after the repair using the Mayo-modified wrist score. The average pain score improved from 9.1 ± 8.0 to 21.2 ± 6.5, the average functional score from 5.0 ± 8.1 to 20.6 ± 6.3; the average motion score from 4.7 ± 2.8 to 15.6 ± 7.3; and the average grip point from 4.4 ± 3.5 to 15.6 ± 7.7; all with significant differences (*P* < .01). Ten of the 17 cases had instability of the DRUJ, and 5 had recurrent instability after repair.

14. Corso SJ, Savoie FH, Geissler WB, et al: Arthroscopic repair of peripheral avulsions of the triangular fibrocartilage complex of the wrist: A multicenter study. Arthroscopy 13:78-84, 1997.

A multicenter study to assess arthroscopic reconstruction of the peripheral attachment of the TFCC was undertaken. A total of 44 patients (45 wrists) from three institutions were reviewed. Twenty-seven of the 45 wrists had associated injuries, including distal radius fracture (4), partial or complete rupture of the scapholunate (7), lunotriquetral (9), ulnocarpal (2), or radiocarpal (2) ligaments. There were two fractured ulnar styloids and one scapholunate accelerated collapse (SLAC) wrist deformity. The peripheral tears were repaired using a zone-specific repair kit. The patients were immobilized in a munster cast, allowing elbow flexion and extension but no pronation or supination for 4 weeks, followed by 2 to 4 weeks in a short-arm cast or removable wrist splint. All patients were re-examined independently 1 to 3 years postoperatively by a physician, therapist, and registered nurse. The results were graded according to the Mayo-modified wrist score. Twenty-nine of the 45 wrists were rated excellent; 12, good; 1, fair; and 3, poor. Overall, 42 of the 45 patients (93%) rated as satisfactory and returned to sports or work activities.

15. Culp RW: Complications of wrist arthroscopy. Hand Clin 15:529-35, 1999.

Wrist arthroscopy has become an essential tool in the evaluation and treatment of a variety of wrist injuries and disease processes. As such, an understanding of complications related to wrist arthroscopy is critical to overall outcome. Complications are based on the unique anatomy of the wrist, portal locations, surgical technique, and type of procedure performed.

16. De Smet L: Pitfalls in wrist arthroscopy. Acta Orthop Belg 68:325-329, 2002.

The authors estimated the complication rate to be about 2%, of which equipment failure was the most frequent. The authors further document injury of the overlying tendons, nerves, and even the radial artery. They also point out that the anatomy of certain wrists can cause considerable difficulties in obtaining a clear view. Finally, they found that the correlation between the clinical and radiographic findings with arthroscopic findings may be difficult.

17. del Pinal F, Herrero F, Cruz-Camara A, San Jose J: Complete avulsion of the distal posterior interosseous nerve during wrist arthroscopy: A possible cause of persistent pain after arthroscopy. J Hand Surg [Am] 24:240-242, 1999.

A case of avulsion of the distal posterior interosseous nerve during wrist arthroscopy is presented. Surgeons unaware of this entity may attribute persistent mid-dorsal wrist pain to the underlying disease rather than to iatrogenic damage to the distal posterior interosseous nerve.

18. Doi K, Hattori Y, Otsuka K, et al: Intra-articular fractures of the distal aspect of the radius: Arthroscopically assisted reduction compared with open reduction and internal fixation. J Bone Joint Surg Am 81:1093-1110, 1999.

This was a prospective study comparing the results of arthroscopically assisted treatment to conventional treatment of distal radius fractures. Thirty-four fractures were treated with arthroscopically guided reduction with use of one volar and two dorsal arthroscopic portals. The fractures were pinned, and external fixation was used with or without an autogenous bone graft. Intraoperative fluoroscopy was not used. Forty-eight fractures were treated with conventional open reduction and internal fixation (ORIF) with a plate and screws or with pinning, with or without external fixation. The average duration of follow-up for all fractures was 31 months. The arthroscopically assisted group had better outcomes than the group that had had conventional ORIF. The group that had had an arthroscopically assisted procedure also had significantly better ranges of flexion-extension and radioulnar deviation of the wrist and grip strength ($P < .05$). The radiographic results showed that the patients who had had an arthroscopically assisted procedure had better reduction of volar tilt, ulnar variance, and articular (gap) displacement than did those who had been managed with conventional ORIF ($P < .05$ for each comparison).

21. Hofmeister EP, Dao KD, Glowacki KA, Shin AY: The role of midcarpal arthroscopy in the diagnosis of disorders of the wrist. J Hand Surg [Am] 26:407-414, 2001.

The findings of midcarpal versus radiocarpal arthroscopic examinations were compared in the diagnosis of a variety of wrist pathology in 89 patients. In cases of acute wrist instability, arthroscopy added to the radiocarpal diagnosis in 21 of 26 (82%) of the wrists. In cases of chronic wrist instability, midcarpal arthroscopy added to the radiocarpal diagnosis in 46 of 55 (84%) of the wrists. In the distal radius group 5 of 8 wrists had additional pathology on the midcarpal arthroscopy examination, leading to additional surgical intervention. The authors demonstrate that midcarpal arthroscopy added statistically significant information to the radiocarpal examination compared with wrist arthroscopy performed without a midcarpal examination.

22. Kato H, Nakamura R, Shionoya K, et al: Does high-resolution MR imaging have better accuracy than standard MR imaging for evaluation of the triangular fibrocartilage complex? J Hand Surg [Br] 25:487-491, 2000.

The authors compared the findings of high-resolution MRI and standard MRI in the detection of tears of the triangular fibrocartilage in 33 patients with chronic wrist pain on the ulnar side. With arthroscopy as the standard of reference, sensitivity was 100%, specificity was 53%, and accuracy was 79% with the high-resolution MRI, against 83%, 67%, and 76% with the standard MRI, respectively. High-resolution MRI showed a higher sensitivity but a decreased specificity in the assessment of the triangular fibrocartilage.

24. McAdams TR, Hentz VR: Injury to the dorsal sensory branch of the ulnar nerve in the arthroscopic repair of ulnar-sided triangular fibrocartilage tears using an inside-out technique: A cadaver study. J Hand Surg [Am] 27:840-844, 2002.

This anatomic study of the commonly described inside-out Tuohy needle technique was performed to better define the course of needle passage relative to the anatomic structures in this region including the dorsal sensory branch of the ulnar nerve (DBUN) and ECU tendon. Ten fresh-frozen cadaver specimens had arthroscopic-guided passage of a Tuohy needle through the triangular fibrocartilage. Dissection of the ulnar side of the wrist was performed and various measurements were recorded. The average minimum distance between suture A (the suture closest to the nerve) and the DBUN was 1.9 mm. The average minimum distance between suture B and the DBUN was 2.7 mm. The distance between the two sutures at the level of the capsule averaged 6.2 mm. The distance between the DBUN and the ECU averaged 7.2 mm. In 5 of 10 specimens the sutures exited on opposite sides of the DBUN. The DBUN is variable in its course, but in every case it passes in close proximity to the sutures that exit the ulnar side of the wrist in arthroscopic repair of ulnar-sided triangular fibrocartilage tears.

25. Minami A, Ishikawa J, Suenaga N, Kasashima T: Clinical results of treatment of triangular fibrocartilage complex tears by arthroscopic débridement. J Hand Surg [Am] 21:406-411, 1996.

To determine indications for arthroscopic débridement and the management of TFCC tears, we reviewed 16 wrists retrospectively. The mean patient age was 30 years, with a range of 20 to 53 years. The follow-up period averaged 35 months. Two groups were identified: post-traumatic tears (n = 11) and degenerative tears (n = 5). The results of arthroscopic débridement were compared and analyzed based on the preoperative and postoperative evaluation of pain, range of motion, grip strength, return to work, patient acceptance, and complications. Failures were further evaluated to determine identifiable lesions or anatomic defects associated with poor results. Patients with positive ulnar variance and lunotriquetral interosseous ligament tears had a poor clinical outcome. Good results correlated with grip strength; all patients with post-traumatic TFCC tears had excellent results, whereas those with degenerative TFCC tears did poorly.

28. Osterman AL, Raphael J: Arthroscopic resection of dorsal ganglion of the wrist. Hand Clin 11:7-12, 1995.

Arthroscopic resection is a reasonable approach for operative treatment of the dorsal ganglion. Arthroscopy is safe and addresses the key anatomic pathology. Recurrences to date have been equal to or less than with the open technique. Arthroscopic resection minimizes the surgical scar. Arthroscopy also permits evaluation of any intra-articular pathologic condition of either midcarpal or radiocarpal joints. In our series, 42% of patients had intra-articular pathologic conditions. In this study, these findings were recorded but not treated. Symptom resolution, therefore, correlated with ganglion resection and not with intra-articular pathologic conditions.

30. Potter HG, Asnis-Ernberg L, Weiland AJ, et al: The utility of high-resolution magnetic resonance imaging in the evaluation

of the triangular fibrocartilage complex of the wrist. J Bone Joint Surg Am 79:1675-1684, 1997.

This is a prospective study to assess the utility of high-resolution MRI in the detection and specific localization of tears of the TFCC. The study examined 77 patients with wrist pain using a dedicated surface coil and three-dimensional gradient-recalled techniques to assess the cause of the ulnar-sided wrist pain. The findings on the MR images were compared with the arthroscopic findings. Fifty-seven of the 59 tears that were suspected on MR images were confirmed with arthroscopy; the two suspected tears that were not confirmed had been interpreted as small partial tears on the MR images. With use of arthroscopy as the standard, MRI had a sensitivity of 100%, a specificity of 90%, and an accuracy of 97% for the detection of a tear (k = 0.93, *P* < .00001). Fifty-three of the 57 tears were localized correctly with use of MRI. With regard to the location of the tear, MRI had a sensitivity of 100%, a specificity of 75%, and an accuracy of 92% (k = 0.9, *P* < .0001).

33. Ruch DS, Poehling GG: Arthroscopic management of partial scapholunate and lunotriquetral injuries of the wrist. J Hand Surg [Am] 21:412-417, 1996.

Outcome was studied in 14 patients with chronic mechanical (crepitant) wrist pain (symptomatic for more than 6 months) who had undergone arthroscopic débridement and early mobilization for the treatment of isolated partial scapholunate and lunotriquetral ligament injuries. Fourteen patients were available for a minimum 2-year follow-up interview, physical examination, and radiographic evaluation.

Eleven patients had complete relief of symptoms and had returned to work within 7 weeks of surgery. The other 3 (all workers' compensation cases) reported occasional mild wrist pain; two had returned to work a mean of 6.5 weeks after surgery, and the third did not return for 1 year. None of the patients had a statistically significant loss of grip or pinch strength. Radiographs and dynamic examination under fluoroscopy demonstrated no abnormalities. Thirteen of the 14 patients were highly satisfied, although 2 patients still had occasional mild wrist pain. Arthroscopic débridement of partial intrinsic ligament injuries provided excellent relief of painful crepitant symptoms and allowed for early return of wrist function in 13 of 14 cases.

34. Slutsky DJ: Wrist arthroscopy through a volar radial portal. Arthroscopy 18:624-630, 2002.

This study described the neurovascular relationships of a volar radial wrist arthroscopy portal and documented additional pathology of the dorsal capsular structures and the palmar region of the SLIO ligament that was not seen through the dorsal portals. There was a greater than 3-mm safe zone surrounding the portal that was free of any neurovascular structures. Clinically, there were no complications from the use of the portal. Additional pathology that was not visible from a dorsal portal was identified in 10 of 20 cases. This included 1 case of hypertrophic synovitis of the dorsal capsule, 1 patient with an avulsion of the RSL ligament, 1 patient with a tear restricted to the palmar region of the SLIO, and 7 patients with tears of the dorsal radiocarpal ligament.

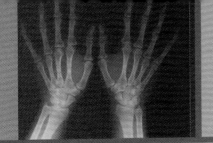

CHAPTER 19

Wrist Arthroscopy: Operative Procedures

Randall W. Culp, A. Lee Osterman, and Robert A. Kaufmann

Over the past 20 years wrist arthroscopy has advanced from a diagnostic to a therapeutic procedure and has replaced, in many cases, open arthrotomy.* As with procedures in larger joints, patients undergoing less invasive surgery may benefit from decreased morbidity and shortened recovery. With continued investigation and honest clinical outcomes assessment, we will be better able to fully evaluate the benefits of arthroscopy. In the past two decades there has been spectacular growth in the use of wrist arthroscopy, and there is no doubt that this trend will continue. Table 19-1 lists specific procedures that can be performed arthroscopically; many of these have been accepted as standard treatment methods.

SYNOVIAL BIOPSY

Synovitis may result from local trauma and internal derangement of the wrist, or it may stem from inflammatory disorders such as rheumatoid arthritis, pigmented villonodular synovitis, infection, or crystal deposition disorders such as gout and pseudogout. In such conditions, normal synovium proliferates within the prestyloid recess, beneath the dorsal capsule, among the volar extrinsic ligaments, and within in the midcarpal joint. The amount and location of hypertrophic synovium and the extent of its inflammation can provide diagnostic clues to the type and significance of wrist pathology. For example, symptomatic tears of the articular disk of the triangular fibrocartilage complex (TFCC) are usually associated with a localized ulnar synovitis. Débridement is necessary to fully evaluate the disruption and is best accomplished by using a powered full-radius resector or a more aggressive synovectomy side-cutting blade (Fig. 19-1). The ideal blade sizes for the wrist range from 2.0 to 4.5 mm. The speed and direction of the blade can be varied, with shaver speeds under 900 rpm being most useful for resecting synovium. Blade oscillation improves

Table 19-1
OPERATIVE WRIST ARTHROSCOPIC PROCEDURES

Arthroscopic reduction and internal fixation

Synovial biopsy

Synovectomy for inflammatory arthritis

Septic wrist débridement

Evaluation and staging of Kienböck's disease

Evaluation and treatment of chondral lesions

Chondroplasty

Loose or foreign body removal

Triangular fibrocartilage lesions

Débridement

Repair of peripheral tears

Arthroscopic wafer

Evaluation and treatment of carpal instability

Arthroscopic reduction and internal fixation

Arthroscopic treatment of fractures
    Distal radius
    Scaphoid

Dorsal ganglion resection

Contracture release

Arthroscopy salvage procedures
    Radial styloidectomy
    Proximal row carpectomy

resection efficiency by clearing debris from the shaver orifice.

The primary role of arthroscopy in inflammatory conditions is diagnostic: it can provide direct assessment of joint involvement as well as be used for synovial biopsy.[102] Diagnostic biopsy is particularly useful for the crystal deposition diseases, sarcoidosis, pigmented villonodular synovitis, and granulomatous infections. Synovectomy shavings

---

*See references 7, 21, 32, 37, 57, 68, 73, 99, 104, 107, 120, 149, 172, and 177.

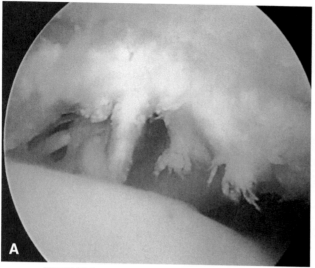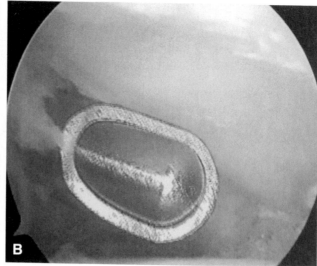

FIGURE 19-1. A, Arthroscopic appearance of pseudogout. **B,** Arthroscopic débridement and biopsy with a 2.7-mm full radius resector.

can be collected from a filter attached to the suction,[126] but it is often more effective to manually harvest synovial pieces with an arthroscopic instrument.

COMPLETE SYNOVECTOMY

In rheumatoid arthritis, the indications for arthroscopic synovectomy are similar to those for open synovectomy (i.e., those patients with a well-preserved wrist joint and active wrist synovitis who have failed medical management). When compared with open arthrotomy, the arthroscopic technique offers superior visualization and easier access to all wrist compartments to effectively remove pathologic synovium.

A complete synovectomy requires the use of multiple portals to access all areas of the radiocarpal and midcarpal joints. It is also important to include the distal radioulnar joint (DRUJ), which is often the site of significant synovial proliferation. Fortunately, in rheumatoid wrists the DRUJ space is distended, allowing for easier access.[75] The distracted wrist is positioned in supination, and the joint is visualized through the proximal DRUJ portal while a distal working portal is established just beneath the TFC.

A contraindication to arthroscopic synovectomy is dorsal tenosynovitis. In this condition, the weakened and displaced extensor tendons are at risk for injury during portal placement. One additional caveat relates to rheumatoid skin, which is more likely to macerate when distraction fingertraps are applied, particularly when the procedure length is greater than an hour.

Adolfsson and Nylander[3] reported pain improvement after arthroscopic wrist synovectomy in 18 of 18 patients with rheumatoid synovitis. Motion increased from 69 to

---

CRITICAL POINTS: COMPLETE SYNOVECTOMY

INDICATIONS

- Rheumatoid arthritis
- Active wrist synovitis that has failed medical management

PREOPERATIVE EVALUATION

- Rule out septic arthritis.
- Rule out dorsal tenosynovitis (portals may injure weakened extensor tendons).

PEARLS

- DRUJ access is easier in rheumatoid arthritis because of joint space distention.
- There is less morbidity (stiffness), shorter rehabilitation, and fewer complications than with open synovectomy.

TECHNICAL POINTS

- Use multiple portals to access all areas of the radiocarpal and midcarpal joints.
- Include the DRUJ (distracted wrist positioned in supination).

PITFALLS

- Whether synovectomy deters long-term progress of arthritis remains questionable.
- Distraction fingertraps may macerate rheumatoid skin.

POSTOPERATIVE CARE

- Begin early active wrist motion without strengthening during first 6 weeks.

90 degrees in the flexion-extension arc, and grip strength peaked at 87% by 6-month follow-up. Their study did not address the DRUJ. Other less detailed reports[42,81,148,157] have suggested similar benefits. Overall, morbidity and complications for arthroscopic synovectomy were reduced, particularly in terms of wrist stiffness and length of rehabilitation, when compared with a historical control using the open procedure. Whether such synovectomy deters the long-term progress of the arthritis could not be answered.[5]

Septic arthritis of the wrist requires prompt decompression. In the knee and shoulder, arthroscopic management has been shown to yield superior or equivalent results to open arthrotomy.[152] No study has systematically addressed the role of arthroscopic management of the septic wrist, although it has been included as an arthroscopic indication by several authors.[7,81,118] We believe its use merits consideration.

Arthroscopy allows for thorough lavage of the joint, as well as biopsy, culture, and synovectomy. Anecdotally, our experience with 14 cases has been very positive. Septic arthritis was caused by organisms that included *Staphylococcus,* *Streptococcus,* and *Neisseria gonorrhoeae,* and all patients were treated within the first week by arthroscopic drainage and appropriate antibiotics. It must be cautioned that until the efficacy of arthroscopic lavage has been fully established, caution in its use must be warranted.

CHONDROPLASTY AND LOOSE BODIES

Articular cartilage damage is a common cause of wrist pain.[72,79,121,135] Although Koman and coworkers[72] noted articular cartilage damage in 62% of 54 patients evaluated arthroscopically for chronic wrist pain, the true incidence remains unknown. The causes for cartilage damage are numerous. Most commonly, it occurs secondary to other wrist pathologic processes, such as ligamentous instability, fracture, or inflammatory arthritis. Impacted shearing loads may cause focal articular damage.[77] The presence of the medial facet of a type II lunate increases the incidence of chondromalacia at the hamate proximal pole.[160-163] Idiopathic chondral defects have been reported as well. Viegas and coworkers[159,162] described a scaphoid cartilaginous lesion with characteristics consistent with osteochondritis dissecans, as seen in other joints. Many of these articular lesions cannot be identified with noninvasive imaging studies. Without high-resolution surface coils, conventional magnetic resonance imaging (MRI) cannot detect 3-mm or smaller defects in the articular surface. Such defects, however, can cause troublesome symptoms and progress in size. Bone scan may be used and has demonstrated modest sensitivity. The value of diagnostic arthroscopy was demonstrated in one series of 68 patients with chronic wrist pain.[184] Arthroscopy revealed 24 primary chondral lesions, of which 17 were located in the midcarpal joint. In these patients a triple-phase bone scan was positive in 66%.

It is important to classify chondral lesions for descriptive, prognostic, and therapeutic reasons. We have modified the system devised by Outerbridge[110] for the patella for use in the wrist. Grade I represents softening of the hyaline surface, as can often be seen in Kienböck's disease. Grade II is used to describe fibrillation and fissuring. In grade III, there is a fibrillated lesion of varying depth in the articular surface

irrespective of size. Grade IV has a full-thickness defect down to bone. Arthroscopic classification helps the surgeon to systematically apply treatment and to recommend appropriate restrictions and activity modification.

Arthroscopic treatment for lesions of grade I to III involves simple débridement of the accompanying synovitis and surface fibrillation. Treatment of grade IV lesions is controversial. There is no confirmed evidence of hyaline cartilage regeneration after chondral abrasion, but the procedure may stimulate the formation of reparative fibrocartilage. The ideal indication for abrasion chondroplasty is a well-circumscribed grade IV lesion. Drilling of the defect to subchondral bleeding bone will produce a clot that fills the defect and, in turn, a fibrocartilaginous patch. The ability of this regenerated fibrocartilage to withstand load over time is questioned, but there is some evidence that it may bind to the adjacent hyaline cartilage and offer protection against defect extension. The majority of experimental clinical work on this subject pertains to knee surgery.[65]

Common sites of grade IV lesions are the proximal pole of the hamate, distal pole of the scaphoid, ulnar side of the lunate, and proximal pole of the scaphoid.[33,48,161] Through appropriate portal selection, a shaver is used to débride the fibrillated cartilage. A small arthroscopy knife can be used to resect the damaged cartilage and create a well-defined crater with vertical walls. A small electric bur is then used to resect 1 to 2 mm of the bone at the base of the crater. With the tourniquet not inflated it is useful to observe the blood clot filling the crater. According to the principles advocated by Salter and associates,[133] early active wrist motion without strengthening is encouraged during the first 6 weeks postoperatively.

Chondroplasty is not helpful if there is global loss of articular cartilage. In this case, arthroscopy can be used to stage the arthritis and select an appropriate salvage treatment. It should also be emphasized that, where possible, the cause of the articular defect must be corrected. For example, a kissing lesion of the lunate and distal ulna secondary to ulnocarpal impaction syndrome would not be improved by chondroplasty and requires a wafer resection or formal ulnar shortening to correct the condition.

Arthroscopy has been used in the evaluation and staging of chondral damage secondary to Preiser's or Kienböck's disease.[86] Articular cartilage softening and fibrillation occurs as early as stage II Kienbock's disease, and arthroscopy will occasionally reveal a fissure fracture of the distal lunate facet or an osteochondral flap off the proximal lunate. Unsuspected tears of the interosseous ligaments are arthroscopically detected in many patients. Watanabe and associates[165] found scapholunate tears in 29% of patients with stage II and 30% with stage III disease. Lunatotriquetral tears were seen in 39% of patients with stage III disease. Currently, we still base our treatment of Kienböck's disease on imaging findings but, in the future, it may prove helpful to assess the joint arthroscopically. One caveat to be mentioned is that if lunate revascularization is planned, the ulnar radiocarpal portals are best avoided so as not to interfere with the fourth or fifth compartment donor blood vessels.

Loose bodies can result from direct injury or sloughing of established cartilage defects and may cause wrist pain and mechanical symptoms such as locking.[181] If a loose body is suspected, double-contrast arthrography or MRI may be

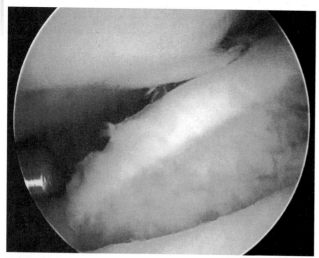

FIGURE 19-2. Arthroscopic chondral lesion of distal radius treated with débridement.

helpful. Arthroscopic removal is the treatment of choice (Fig. 19-2).

ARTHROSCOPY IN THE TREATMENT OF TRIANGULAR FIBROCARTILAGE LESIONS

Injury of the TFCC is frequently implicated as a cause of ulnar wrist pain. Wrist arthroscopy has now become a standard tool in the diagnosis and treatment of these injuries.*

Anatomy

The triangular fibrocartilage complex (TFCC) is a cartilaginous and ligamentous structure interposed between the ulnar carpus and distal ulna.[22,23,67,117] The triangular fibrocartilage (TFC) is composed of a central articular disk and its bordering radioulnar ligaments. The articular disk arises from the articular cartilage on the corner of the sigmoid notch of the radius and inserts into the base of the ulnar styloid. The central disk is made up of interwoven sheets of collagen fibers obliquely oriented to withstand multidirectional stress and is avascular and aneural. The dorsal and volar radioulnar ligaments are the stout, fibrous thickenings along the dorsal and palmar edges of the articular disk that have dual insertions onto the styloid and the basistyloid foveal area of the ulna. They function as a unit to stabilize the DRUJ by limiting rotational and axial migration. On the palmar margin of the TFC is the ulnocarpal ligament complex, formed by the ulnolunate and ulnotriquetral ligaments. These ulnar extrinsic ligaments support the ulnar carpus. On the dorsal roof of the TFCC is the extensor carpi ulnaris (ECU) and its stout subsheath, both stabilizing structures of the ulnar carpus.

The vascularity of the TFC has been carefully studied.[11,23,106,153] The circulation arises from the ulnar artery through its radiocarpal branches and from the anterior interosseous artery through its dorsal and palmar branches. These vessels supply the TFC in a radial fashion. Histologic

---

*See references 7, 10, 27, 32, 38, 49, 69, 84, 92, 97, 103, 109, 112, and 172.

CRITICAL POINTS: CHONDROPLASTY AND LOOSE BODIES

NDICATIONS

- Articular cartilage damage may be secondary to ligamentous instability, fracture, or inflammatory arthritis.
- Ideal indication for abrasion chondroplasty is a well-circumscribed grade IV (full-thickness) lesion.
- Loose bodies can result from direct injury or sloughing of established cartilage defects.

PREOPERATIVE EVALUATION

- Common sites of grade IV lesions:
  - Proximal pole of the hamate
  - Distal pole of scaphoid
  - Ulnar side of lunate
  - Proximal pole of the scaphoid
- Loose bodies may cause wrist pain and locking.

PEARLS

- Type II lunate (medial hamate facet) lesion increases incidence of chondromalacia.
- Defect drilling to subchondral bone produces clot that transforms into fibrocartilaginous patch.

TECHNICAL POINTS

- Use shaver to débride fibrillated cartilage.
- Use small arthroscopy knife for resection of damaged cartilage.
- Use small bur for resection of 1 to 2 mm of bone.
- With tourniquet not inflated, observe blood filling the crater.
- If lunate revascularization is planned, avoid ulnar portals that interfere with donor blood vessels.

PITFALLS

- Chondroplasty is not helpful in global loss of cartilage (need staging procedure to guide salvage treatment).
- Cause of articular defect must be corrected (ulnar shortening or wafer for ulnocarpal impaction syndrome).

POSTOPERATIVE CARE

- Early active wrist motion without strengthening during first 6 weeks

sections demonstrate their penetration to occur only in the peripheral 10% to 40%[11] with the central section and radial portions remaining avascular. In vivo studies using a laser Doppler probe have confirmed these findings[106] and support the concept that peripheral TFC injuries may heal, whereas tears of the avascular central portion cannot.

Biomechanics

The TFCC has several important biomechanical functions. It is a major stabilizer of the DRUJ and a stabilizer of the ulnar carpus.[114,116,117] The amount of load transferred to the distal ulna from the carpus is directly proportional to the ulnar variance. In neutral ulnar variance, approximately 20% of the load is transmitted. With positive ulnar variance there is a correspondingly decreased thickness in the central portion of the disk and the load across the TFC increases.[114] Load transmission also varies with rotation of the forearm. In supination, the radius moves distally on the ulna and creates a relative negative ulnar variance. In pronation, this is reversed. The ulna also moves within the sigmoid notch in a dorsal direction with pronation and volarly with supination.[12] During this translation, the dorsal and volar radioulnar ligamentous portions of the TFCC become tense, befitting their stabilizing role.[70]

Mechanism of Injury

Traumatic injuries of the TFCC result from the application of an extension-pronation force to an axially loaded wrist, such as in a fall on an outstretched hand. These injuries can also occur from a dorsal rotation injury such as when a drill binds and rotates the wrist instead of the bit.[172] Another mechanism of injury may occur from a distraction force applied to the volar forearm or wrist.[83] Finally, tears of the TFC are commonly found in patients with fractures of the distal radius.[30,45,54]

Not all perforations and defects in the TFC are traumatic. Several authors have shown an age-related correlation with lesions in the TFC,[89,161] but many of these defects are asymptomatic. Patients with positive ulnar variance are more susceptible to such attritional lesions.[47] In some instances, an acute injury is superimposed on an otherwise asymptomatic tear.

Classification

Although several classification systems have been described,[15,27,172] we find Palmer's description[111,112,115] to be most useful. He divided TFC injuries into two basic categories: traumatic (type I) and degenerative (type II) (see Chapter 15). Traumatic lesions are classified according to the location of the tear within the TFC. Degenerative lesions are associated with positive ulnar variance and are often associated with damage to surrounding structures such as the lunatotriquetral ligament or articular surfaces of the lunate, triquetrum, and distal ulna.

A type IA lesion represents an isolated tear in the central portion of the TFC disk. The tear usually occurs several millimeters medial to the radial attachment and is oriented in a volar-to-dorsal direction, often resulting in an unstable flap.

Type IB lesions represent a peripheral tear of the TFC from its insertion on the distal ulna. This lesion can occur either with a fracture of the ulnar styloid or as an avulsion from its ulnar-sided attachments. Because the periphery of the TFC is continuous with the floor of the ECU sheath, this type of injury can be associated with concomitant disruption of the ECU sheath and may clinically demonstrate subluxation of the ECU tendon. Type IB injuries may also be associated with clinical instability of the DRUJ.

Type IC lesions represent a disruption of the TFCC from the volar ulnocarpal extrinsic ligaments and may result in a supination deformity of the carpus on the ulna.

Type ID lesions represent avulsions of the TFC from its radial attachment on the sigmoid notch. These are usually linear and oriented in a volar-to-dorsal direction. They occur within 1 to 2 mm of the medial corner of the radius and are often seen with distal radial fractures.

Diagnosis

The clinical symptoms of a TFC injury consist of ulnar-sided wrist pain and often clicking[103,109] occurring after a fall on a pronated wrist or a traction or twisting injury. Symptoms are not generally disabling, are mechanical, and respond to rest.

Physical examination will usually reveal tenderness over the ulnar wrist.[151] The TFC compression test is a provocative maneuver that is positive when it yields a painful response. The examiner axially loads and simultaneously rotates the ulnar-deviated wrist. Often a painful click reproduces the patient's symptoms. As with all provocative maneuvers, it is important to compare the findings with those in the opposite wrist. DRUJ stability should also be assessed. Significant instability will often demonstrate a positive "piano key" sign with prominence of the distal ulna. Gross laxity represents significant disruption of the TFCC. Repair of gross instability is often beyond the scope of arthroscopic intervention, and arthroscopic repairs are most beneficial when instability is mild. The ulnar carpus should be examined for excessive supination on the distal ulna or a "sag" deformity, which is suggestive of type IB or IC lesions. The lunatotriquetral joint should also be examined to rule out a concomitant ligament tear. Examination will usually reveal point tenderness over the lunatotriquetral interval or the ulnar snuffbox. A shuck test or lunatotriquetral ballottement test will often be positive.[125] The patient will often have an associated tendinitis of the ECU tendon. The ECU tendon should be checked for subluxation. Grip strength, measured with a Jamar dynamometer, should demonstrate valid, although weakened, grip strength curves.

In some instances, differential anesthetic injection may be helpful in localizing the symptomatic source. The differential diagnosis for ulnar-sided wrist pain consistent with TFCC injury includes ECU subluxation, lunatotriquetral ligament injury, pisotriquetral arthritis, chondral lesions of the ulnar lunate or midcarpal joint, ulnar artery thrombosis, and ulnar neuropathy at the wrist.

Imaging Studies

Radiologic examination should include plain radiographs with neutral-rotation posteroanterior and lateral views.

These films will allow an assessment of carpal alignment, ulnar styloid morphology, and, most importantly, ulnar variance.[98] Positive ulnar variance may be associated with an impaction-type cystic lesion in the ulnar half of the lunate. The configuration, alignment, and any arthritic change of the DRUJ should be noted. Clenched-fist radiographs in full ulnar deviation and pronation[154] may show evidence of dynamic variance changes.

Advanced Imaging Studies

Advanced imaging techniques include arthrography, computed tomography (CT), triple-phase bone scan, and MRI. The role that each of these studies plays in the work-up of a suspected TFC tear is debated. Imaging studies should never replace a careful history, physical examination, plain radiographs, or a reasoned correlation of signs and symptoms with the reported pathology.

Wrist arthrography can be done as a static single radiocarpal injection or by the preferred triple-injection method described by Zinberg and Palmer.[76,183] The first step in this test involves injection of contrast material into the radiocarpal joint. It is critical to observe the dye during the early flow phase as it is injected. If no dye leakage occurs into the midcarpal joint or DRUJ then additional and separate injections of the midcarpal joint and DRUJ are performed after adequate time has passed to allow absorption of the contrast agent from the first introduction. Midcarpal injection is advantageous for detecting tears of the proximal row interosseous ligaments, and the DRUJ injection is useful for visualizing peripheral TFC tears. Utilizing three injections for wrist arthrography ensures that one-way flaps are not missed. Additional techniques that have been helpful include digital subtraction[12] and the use of a pain marker.

The efficacy of wrist arthrography, although superior to conventional MRI in assessing TFC and intrinsic ligament integrity,[138] is still in question.[18,25,26] A high incidence of symmetrical findings has been reported in the opposite asymptomatic wrist, which led Gilula and colleagues[87,127,180] to conclude that bilateral triple-compartment arthrograms with clinical correlation of asymmetric dye leakage with patient's symptoms is necessary. Furthermore, arthrography cannot determine the tear size, degree of instability, or associated synovitis or chondral change.[129,168]

CT is best reserved when a question of instability or DRUJ incongruency arises. Such a situation occurs very infrequently in the work-up of TFC lesions. CT should be performed in 1-mm contiguous intervals through the DRUJ in supination, pronation, and neutral, using the techniques described by Mino and colleagues.[93]

A triple-phase bone scan has been helpful in identifying inflammation of the wrist. It can be considered a "visual sedimentation rate" of wrist inflammation and as a validity test in patients with poorly localized or excessive symptoms. A symptomatic TFC tear will manifest a mildly increased uptake on both the vascular and bone phases. In our experience, there is a correlation between a positive bone scan ulnarly and a satisfactory outcome after TFC débridement.

MRI has become the most widely used imaging study in the diagnosis of TFC tears.[40,55,56,62,101,141] The importance of using dedicated wrist coils has been emphasized, because conventional MRI without dedicated sequences and small joint wrist coils lacks sufficient sensitivity to detect ulnar-sided TFC avulsions or lunatotriquetral ligament injury.[95] In one study, the use of high-resolution MRI pulsed sequences and dedicated wrist coils increased the sensitivity of TFC diagnosis, as confirmed arthroscopically, to 100%, with an accuracy of 97%.[122] Our own studies and those of others[46,121,155] have shown MRI to be approximately 90% accurate for central and radial tears, a percentage to be approached only in very specialized centers.[16] T2-weighted images in the coronal plane have the greatest diagnostic value. The synovial fluid of the joint appears as a bright image with T2 weighting and outlines the TFC tear similar to that of an arthrogram. Unlike arthrography, MRI can detect marrow changes, thus making it ideal for detecting early avascular necrosis. Many patients with ulnar impaction will have marrow changes on the ulnar side of the lunate, and this should be carefully differentiated from Kienböck's disease.

When compared with other imaging modalities, arthroscopy is highly accurate in diagnosing lesions of the TFC.[119,129,168,184] Arthroscopy can assess the tear size and stability, as well as associated synovitis and chondral or ligament lesions. The finding of ulnar-sided synovitis in association with a tear usually correlates with a clinically significant TFCC tear. Complete diagnostic wrist evaluation must always include a midcarpal arthroscopy. It has been shown to add significant information and is more sensitive than radiocarpal arthroscopy for assessment of scapholunate and lunatotriquetral wrist instability.[61]

INDICATIONS FOR ARTHROSCOPIC TREATMENT

Initial treatment of most *acute* TFC injuries is by immobilization. Care should be taken to rule out any significant instability of the DRUJ, as well as associated injuries such as subluxation of the ECU tendon. If routine radiographs are negative and instability is not present, immobilization for 4 weeks is recommended.[89,90] A peripheral tear would be expected to heal because of its good vascularity. In subacute injuries, judicious use of a corticosteroid injection to quiet down local synovitis or ECU tendinitis, as well as a short course of wrist therapy, may also be helpful.

Many central tears become asymptomatic even though they do not heal. This is particularly true in wrists that have neutral ulnar variance; one study showed no worsening over an average of 9.5 years.[105] By contrast, symptoms from TFC tears associated with positive ulnar variance did worsen with time.

A correlation between patient age and TFC perforations has been made.[71,88,162] Mikic identified no TFC perforations in patients younger than 30 years yet observed a linear progression with age such that 53% of specimens from individuals older than age 50 were found to have a TFC perforation.[88] In contrast, Tan and coworkers[150] described a high incidence of congenital perforations in fetal cadavers, and this supplies support for our belief that central defects may occur without symptoms. It is important to keep both factors in mind before fully attributing a patient's wrist pain to a perforation observed on an imaging study.

Arthroscopic TFC surgery is indicated for patients with a proven or suspected TFC injury and ulnar wrist symptoms sufficient to interfere with activities. Patients should have failed a 3- to 4- month nonoperative treatment program of rest, immobilization, and anti-inflammatory medication. On occasion, we will intervene earlier for the high-performance athlete with a documented unstable TFC tear and disabling pain.[170]

Arthroscopic Treatment

Type I: Traumatic TFC Lesions

Type IA Lesions

Type IA lesions are isolated central tears of the TFC without instability. In patients with neutral or negative ulnar variance who have failed nonoperative treatment, arthroscopic limited débridement of the unstable portion of the tear will give excellent relief of symptoms.[38,49,85,169] (Fig. 19-3). The biomechanical effect of excision of the articular disk has been examined.[2,69,117] Two thirds of the central portion of the TFC may be excised with no demonstrable effect on forearm axial load transmission or stability, as long as the dorsal, volar, radial, ulnar, and ulnocarpal ligaments are maintained. Removal of more than two thirds of the disk or ligamentous disruption will destabilize the DRUJ. Adams[2] has emphasized that the peripheral 2 mm of the TFC must be maintained to avoid such instability problems.

Laser use in wrist arthroscopy has received attention in the literature.[137] The holmium:yttrium-aluminum-garnet laser has been used to resect synovium and the TFC with clinical results comparable to those using conventional techniques.[14,97] The characteristics of this laser are its infrared spectrum, fiberoptic capability, and effectiveness in a liquid medium. Small 70-degree probes are now available that allow variable concentration of the laser energy to efficiently resect tissues ranging from synovium to bone.[96] Potential advantages of this method are enhanced speed, precision, and hemostasis. Concerns about damage to normal articular cartilage have been raised, but the major

limitation to widespread use continues to be its expense. Currently, standard arthroscopic instrumentation can successfully accomplish all therapeutic interventions.

Authors' Preferred Method of Treatment: Type IA Lesions

The patient is given regional anesthesia, and a well-padded tourniquet is placed on the upper arm. After induction of anesthesia, a careful clinical reexamination of the wrist is performed to identify the presence of DRUJ instability, abnormal clicking, or ECU subluxation. The wrist is then placed under traction using a traction tower. Initial placement of the arthroscope is through the 3-4 portal. After systematic examination of the radial side of the wrist, the arthroscope is directed ulnarly. For symptomatic lesions, synovitis is usually observed near the prestyloid recess. An ulnar portal, either at the 4-5 or more commonly 6-R location, is used to insert a 2.0- to 3.0-mm full-radius motorized suction shaver. An 18-gauge needle, placed under direct visualization, may be beneficial for establishing optimal working portal placement. The tourniquet may be inflated as necessary should bleeding be encountered.

After débridement of associated synovitis, a small probe is inserted to assess flap tear stability, TFC tension, ulnar extrinsic ligament integrity, and lunatotriquetral ligament disruption.

When resecting an unstable flap, conventional punches and/or small-joint suction punches are used to excise the bulk of the lesion. A small-joint banana blade is useful for transecting the most ulnar portion of the flap. If this technique is performed, the underlying distal ulna should not be used as a cutting board and only the blade tip is allowed for cutting. The unstable portion is excised as an isolated fragment in a similar fashion to that used in management of bucket handle tears of the knee meniscus. The small-radius resector is ideal for trimming edges. Occasionally it is useful to switch the viewing and working portals and introduce the suction punch or shaver from the radial side to smooth the ulnar remnant. We cannot overemphasize the importance of excising only the unstable portion, taking care to leave the peripheral attachments undisturbed.

Patients with a traumatic central tear associated with positive ulnar variance may sometimes demonstrate chondromalacia and other impaction lesions. These cases are best treated with limited débridement and ulnar recession by an arthroscopic wafer resection or ulnar shortening osteotomy. This procedure is discussed in detail under the treatment of type II degenerative lesions.

After the radiocarpal arthroscopy, the midcarpal joint is always inspected. After arthroscopic procedures, the wrist is again re-examined under anesthesia. Clicks that were generated by the TFC abnormality will generally disappear after débridement. Portal sites are closed with either an adhesive bandage or a 4-0 nylon suture. A splint is worn full time for the first week to support the wrist and extensor tendons. Intermittent splint use continues for 3 weeks with

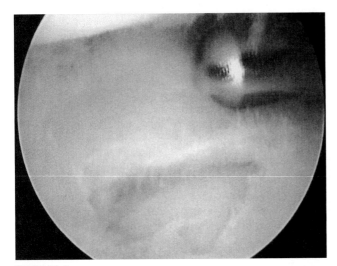

FIGURE 19-3. Limited arthroscopic débridement with 2.7-mm full radius resector.

restrictions placed on forceful grasping and repetitive rotatory activities. In some patients, a supervised therapy program may help achieve the best possible outcome.

The outcomes of type IA débridement have been rewarding, with 80% to 85% of patients requiring no further surgery and having a good to excellent result.[38,49,85,92,176]

Type IB Lesions

The diagnosis of a chronic type IB peripheral tear at the base of the ulnar styloid can be difficult to establish. Clinically, aside from ulnar wrist pain and a possible positive TFC stress test, mild distal radioulnar joint instability may be noted. In an isolated lesion without an ulnar styloid fracture, plain radiographs will be normal. Arthroscopy is ideal for defining peripheral lesions. From a radial-sided viewing, radial portal synovitis and an underlying peripheral tear are noted. The pathognomonic finding is loss of the normal TFC tension as defined by a probe introduced through an ulnar portal. As Hermansdorfer and Kleinman have described,[60] the tension in the TFC should be taut, similar to a drumhead or trampoline. If the probe sinks into the TFC as though into a feather bed, a peripheral tear should be suspected.

One caveat in treating type IB peripheral tears is the realization that these tears can be associated with ECU instability. The floor of the fibrous sheath of the ECU[17] is intimately connected to the periphery of the TFC. With a hypersupination force, both the floor of the ECU sheath and the periphery of the TFC can be torn. In fact, Melone and Nathan[83] have postulated that there is a continuum of injury on the ulnar side of the wrist beginning with the ECU sheath through the peripheral portion of the TFC and continuing on through the ulnar extrinsic and lunatotriquetral ligaments. Thus, ECU subluxation accompanying a peripheral tear represents an early stage of this sequential injury pattern. Treatment of the combined lesion requires not only arthroscopic repair of the peripheral TFC tear but also open reconstruction of the ECU sheath (see Chapter 15).

Several authors[34,94] have reported successful open repair of peripheral TFC lesions. From multiple studies[34,41,152] it is now clear that arthroscopic repair compares favorably with the open technique. Two main techniques share an outside-to-inside suturing method. An alternate approach is the inside-to-outside approach popularized by Poehling and colleagues,[120] in which a Tuohy needle is used to direct the sutures from the radial side of the wrist across the tear. The sutures are retrieved ulnarly and tied. The drawback of this technique is that the counterincision position and the exit points are somewhat difficult to control. Complications relative to irritation of the dorsal ulnar sensory nerve have been reported. Currently, we favor an outside-to-inside technique from the ulnar side as originated by Whipple and Geissler.[176]

Authors' Preferred Method of Treatment: Type IB

A standard arthroscopic setup is used and the scope introduced through the 3-4 portal. After synovectomy, the edges of the tear are débrided with a full-radius shaver to encour-age healing and to stimulate vascular ingrowth. A small 1-cm incision is made just radial to the ECU tendon. The radial aspect of the sheath is opened for approximately 1 cm, with care taken not to disrupt the medial sheath and, thereby, the stability of the ECU. With the ECU retracted ulnarly, two arthroscopic TFC repair needles are passed through the capsule and across the tear under arthroscopic visualization. We find either using the meniscus mender[10] or one of several commercially available TFC repair devices most useful for this. A wire loop is then passed through one needle to retrieve a 2-0 PDS suture that has been passed through the other needle. This allows the passage of a loop-type suture across the tear, which, when drawn tight, will approximate the tear. Two to four sutures may be required. The sutures are tied over the dorsal wrist capsule rather than exteriorized over a button. The forearm is immobilized in a Münster cast for 4 weeks, after which a therapy program is started.

This reparative procedure has enjoyed gratifying outcomes with 85% to 90% achieving good to excellent results at long-term follow-up.[182]

When an unstable peripheral tear is associated with an ununited ulnar styloid fragment, an open procedure must be performed to address the ulnar styloid fragment either through bony reattachment or fragment excision and reattachment of the TFC to the remaining distal ulna.

Type IC Lesions

Type IC lesions involve TFC disruption from the ulnar extrinsic ligament complex. The patient may demonstrate a carpal supination deformity. Imaging techniques are often not useful. For example, wrist arthrography will often show communication to the pisotriquetral joint, but this is a normal variant. Arthroscopically, the diagnosis is made by finding lax ulnar extrinsic ligaments, as well as easy and direct visualization of the pisotriquetral joint through the 6R portal. Ulnar extrinsic attenuation or disruption may require arthroscopic reefing or a tenodesis procedure.

Authors' Preferred Method of Treatment: Type IC

If the defect in the ulnar extrinsic ligaments can be repaired, a small 1-cm incision is made volar to the ECU tendon in the area of the triquetral snuffbox. Care is taken to avoid injury to the dorsal sensory branch of the ulnar nerve or to the volar ulnar neurovascular structures. The technique is similar to the outside-to-inside repair of peripheral TFC lesions. Needles are passed through the capsule in the area of the defect in the ulnar extrinsic ligaments. The looped sutures of 2-0 PDS are then brought out and tied at the capsule level. When this lesion is present and repaired arthroscopically, it is often common to reef the dorsal ulnar portion of the TFC ligament as described for type IB lesions. If the defect is large, an open repair is performed. The type of open repair remains controversial. We favor a volar approach that shortens the ulnar extrinsic ligaments, and we often augment the repair with a distally based strip of flexor carpi ulnaris (FCU) brought dorsally.

Type ID Lesions

Type ID lesions involve radial detachment of the TFC from the sigmoid notch of the distal radius. Although not broken out in Palmer's classification, this lesion could rightly be subdivided into those that occur in isolation and those that occur in association with distal radial fractures. Normally, the articular cartilage of the radius continues around the medial corner and into the sigmoid notch. The TFC originates from this articular location. Given this cartilage barrier, vascular studies suggest that there is poor potential for healing of such radial tears. However, if this cartilage is disrupted mechanically or by fracture and the attachment site occurs on vascularized bone, healing can occur. Cooney and colleagues[28] reported excellent results with open radial-sided TFC repairs. Arthroscopic repair techniques have been described by Sagerman and Short,[132] Jantea and associates,[64] and Trumble and colleagues.[156]

Authors' Preferred Method of Treatment: Type ID

Triangular fibrocartilage tears located within 2 mm of the sigmoid rim and oriented vertically in a volar-to-dorsal direction are amenable to repair. A standard arthroscopic traction setup is used. Once the tear has been identified and determined to be reparable, a small bur is introduced through the 4-5 portal and the attachment site along the sigmoid notch of the radius is abraded to bleeding bone. An alignment guide as described by Jantea and colleagues[64] is used. In the interval between the FCU and ECU tendons, a 0.045-inch Kirschner wire is passed through the capsule to fix the detached TFC to the prepared radius. The jig, which is essentially a wire guide, is then placed over this Kirschner wire to provide alignment of the entry point on the radial side of the wrist.

A small longitudinal skin incision is then made between the first and second extensor compartments. Care is taken to avoid injury to the superficial branch of the radial nerve, the radial artery, and the extensor tendons. The jig and wire are adjusted to make sure that these structures are avoided. The jig is used to create two parallel drill holes exiting at the TFC insertion point on the radius. An 18-gauge spinal needle is then placed in the jig and passed through the distal radius to exit at the prepared bone interface and then passed through the TFC. In a similar fashion, a second 18-gauge spinal needle is introduced parallel to this. The trocars are removed from the 18-gauge needles, and a 2-0 PDS suture is inserted through one needle and retrieved through the opposite needle with a wire loop catcher. The suture is tied down over the radius, and the tension of the TFC is confirmed under arthroscopic visualization. If necessary, a second suture is used. If an alignment jig is not available, an alternative technique described by Trumble and associates in which a cannula and preloaded meniscal repair suture are used is equally effective.[156] The patient is immobilized in a Munster cast for 4 weeks, after which a gradual therapy program is initiated.

When a radial TFC tear is identified during the arthroscopic treatment of a distal radial fracture, the radial portion of the TFC is pinned back to the radius with 0.035-inch Kirschner wires. The TFC fixation pin is left percutaneous and usually removed at 4 weeks. Arthroscopic and/or arthrographic evaluation in several of these patients has confirmed healing of the radial attachment.

Type II: Degenerative TFC Lesions (Ulnocarpal Impaction Syndrome)

Degenerative central tears of the articular disk are seen with increasing frequency with advancing age and in many cases are asymptomatic.[88] Most symptomatic degenerative tears of

---

CRITICAL POINTS: TRAUMATIC TFC REPAIR

INDICATIONS

- TFC tears associated with neutral or negative ulnar variance
- Proven or suspected TFC injury with ulnar wrist symptoms sufficient to interfere with activities
- Failure of nonoperative treatment: rest, immobilization, and anti-inflammatory medication

PREOPERATIVE EVALUATION

- Is there ulnar-sided wrist pain with clicking?
- Is there a history of a fall on a pronated wrist or a twisting injury?
- Have the symptoms lessened with rest?
- Is there tenderness over the ulnar side of the wrist?
- Is there a positive TFC compression test?
- Check for DRUJ, lunatotriquetral, and ECU tendon pathology.

PEARLS

- Excise only unstable central TFCC, leaving peripheral attachments intact.

TECHNICAL POINTS

- Type IA lesions: débride.
- Type IB lesions: repair.
- Type IC lesions: perform type IB repair + ulnar extrinsic ligament capsulodesis or repair.
- Type ID lesions: reattach to sigmoid notch.

PITFALL

- Traumatic central tear and positive ulnar variance may need ulnar shortening.

POSTOPERATIVE CARE

- Begin early motion exercises if TFCC débridement only.
- Use Münster cast for 4 weeks after TFCC repair.

the TFC are related to chronic overloading of the ulnocarpal joint. The primary pathology in these cases is not limited to the TFC itself but also to the sequelae of chronic ulnar impaction, or abutment, between the ulna and the carpus. Ulnar impaction is generally progressive and we recommend surgical correction in sufficiently symptomatic patients.

The causes for ulnar impaction are varied. Primary ulnar impaction syndrome is related to increased ulnar variance. Wrists with neutral or positive ulnar variance have a 73% incidence of tears or perforations as compared with only 17% in specimens with negative ulnar variance.[161] Secondary causes of ulnar impaction syndrome include distal radial fractures that heal with dorsal tilt and radial shortening. Short and associates[139] correlated increases in dorsal tilt of the distal radius with increased forces transmitted to the distal ulna during axial loading. Other secondary causes include distal radial growth arrest after physeal fractures in children and proximal migration of the radius after radial head resection. Ulnar impaction may also be dynamic, occurring only with load activities such as grip or forceful rotation. Thus, a patient with static neutral or even negative ulnar variance may dynamically experience ulnar abutment. Arthroscopy plays a definite role in the treatment of primary ulnar impaction, whereas in secondary abutment, open reconstructive surgery is often required.

In Palmer's classification, the progressive degenerative changes of ulnar impaction are subdivided into five categories:

Type IIA: Wearing of the TFC without perforation or chondromalacia

Type IIB: Wearing of the TFC with chondromalacia of the lunate or ulna

Type IIC: True perforation of the TFC with lunate chondromalacia

Type IID: TFC perforation plus lunate and/or ulnar chondromalacia and lunatotriquetral ligament perforation; no carpal instability patterns such as volar-flexed intercalated segment instability (VISI) are present.

Type IIE: TFC perforation with generalized arthritic changes ulnarly involving the lunate and ulna; there is perforation of the lunatotriquetral ligament and ulnocarpal arthritis.

Diagnosis of a degenerative tear should be suspected in an older patient who complains of nontraumatic ulnar-sided wrist pain. Physical examination will reveal tenderness over the distal ulna that increases with rotatory motion and loading of the wrist. The TFC compression test is often positive. The impaction sign, or pain with forced ulnar deviation, is usually dramatically positive and should be performed in neutral, supination, and pronation. Other provocative maneuvers such as the shuck test should be performed to assess lunatotriquetral ligament stability. The DRUJ compression test may be positive if arthritic changes are present. Measurement of grip strength in pronation and supination may also be helpful.

As mentioned previously, ulnar variance radiographs are critical. The presence of any cystic changes on the ulnar aspect of the lunate or in the ulnar head should be recorded, as well as DRUJ incongruency or arthritis. Arthrography is seldom used, but radiocarpal or radioulnar injection can demonstrate a central TFC tear, and midcarpal injection may show a lunatotriquetral perforation.

MRI has been applied to the diagnosis of ulnar impaction. Symptomatic patients will have focal signal intensity changes in the ulnar part of the lunate that must not be confused with Kienböck's disease. Imaeda and associates[62] noted focal abnormal signal intensity on the ulnar aspect of the lunate in 87% of patients with ulnar impaction; 43% showed similar changes on the triquetrum and 10% had these changes on the radial aspect of the ulnar head. After surgical correction, the signal intensity often returned to normal. MRI can also reveal tears in the TFC with a high degree of accuracy but is less sensitive to detect tears in the lunatotriquetral ligament.

Diagnostic arthroscopy is the best method for staging ulnar impaction progression. Arthroscopy can directly evaluate the chondral surfaces for evidence of fibrillation or more severe chondral changes not visible with current imaging techniques. The TFC lesion is generally central and ragged when compared with the more linear traumatic tear. The lunatotriquetral ligament and lunatotriquetral stability can be assessed from the radiocarpal and midcarpal joints.

Treatment

The primary goal of treatment for degenerative tears of the TFC is to unload or decompress the ulnar carpus and ulnar head. This decompression can be accomplished by ulnar shortening osteotomy, partial ulnar head resection, or ulnar salvage procedures. Ulnar shortening osteotomy was originally described by Milch[91] in 1941. Darrow and colleagues[31] rekindled interest in ulnar recession, and now this procedure has been modified by the use of rigid fixation methods.[13,17,20,24,124,167] Partial ulnar head resection, or so-called *wafer* procedure, leaves the DRUJ intact. In this technique, the distal articular surface of the ulna is removed to bring its length to neutral based on the preoperative findings from a pronated grip radiograph.[155] Feldon and colleagues[43,44] devised the wafer technique as an open procedure, but it is now also performed arthroscopically.[178] Modified Darrach, Sauve-Kapandji, or hemiresection interposition techniques are best reserved for managing distal radioulnar arthritis.

Authors' Preferred Method of Treatment

Types IIA and IIB

Standard arthroscopic evaluation will confirm the presence of chondromalacia and the continuity of the TFC and lunatotriquetral ligament. Any synovial inflammation is débrided. After the arthroscopy, an open ulnar shortening osteotomy is performed.

Type IIC

The ragged central tear is débrided with a suction punch to reveal the radial aspect of the ulna through the margins of the trimmed tear. With the use of a 3-4 viewing portal, a 4-mm bur is introduced through an ulnar portal and the arthroscopic wafer procedure begun. When using the bur it is important to pronate and supinate the wrist so as to evenly level the margins of the distal ulna. The medial corner of the radius serves as an anatomic landmark to assess the level of the resection. The limit of resection that can be accomplished arthroscopically is between 3 and 4 mm.

After the radial third of the ulna has been resected through the tear, an 18-gauge needle is placed in the DRUJ beneath the tear. With this needle used as a marker, an operative portal into the DRUJ is established. Through this portal site a bur or a small ⅛-inch osteotome is inserted to carefully remove the ulnar portion of the distal ulna beneath the remaining TFC. With the use of the bur or osteotome, the distal ulna is leveled to the base of the styloid, taking full advantage of frequent fluoroscopic evaluation in various rotatory positions to confirm accurate resection. The exact amount of cartilage and subcondylar ulnar bone to be resected has been investigated. Wnorowski and colleagues[178]

showed that excision of 3 mm of subcondylar bone decreased the force transmitted across the ulnar head by 50%; further bone resection did little to decrease this force farther. In our experience, arthroscopic resection produces a negative ulnar variance of 2 mm, which is sufficient to unload the ulnar carpus.

Postoperative treatment involves an intermittent short-arm splint for 4 weeks with active range-of-motion exercises for the wrist, followed by a graduated strengthening program at 4 weeks.

Types IID and IIE

These two represent the end stages of ulnar impaction syndrome and are characterized by lunatotriquetral ligament disruption and resultant lunatotriquetral instability. If significant arthritic changes are also noted at the DRUJ, some type of distal ulnar resection is indicated. If no significant DRUJ degeneration is appreciated, arthroscopic débridement of the TFC is performed as described for type IIC lesions, and the lunatotriquetral interval is carefully eval-

---

CRITICAL POINTS: DEGENERATIVE TFC LESIONS (ULNOCARPAL IMPACTION SYNDROME)

INDICATIONS

- Degenerative tears from chronic overloading of the ulnar carpus
- Palmer's classification guides treatment

PREOPERATIVE EVALUATION

- Injury is suspected in older patient with nontraumatic ulnar-sided wrist pain.
- Check for tenderness over distal ulna that increases with rotatory motion and wrist loading.
- Perform shuck test to assess lunatotriquetral ligament stability.
- DRUJ compression test is positive if arthritis is present in this joint.
- Radiographs shows cystic changes on ulnar aspect of lunate or in ulnar head.
- MRI shows focal signal changes in ulnar portion of lunate.

PEARLS

- Neutral or positive ulnar variance has 73% incidence.
- Obtain posteroanterior film with hand in pronated grip to assess dynamic ulnar abutment.
- Earlier intervention is wise because degeneration is progressive.
- Diagnostic arthroscopy is best method for staging ulnar impaction.
- Pronate and supinate the wrist during arthroscopic wafer procedure to evenly level distal ulna.

TECHNICAL POINTS

- Type IIA: Wearing of TFC without perforation or chondromalacia: open ulnar shortening osteotomy.
- Type IIB: Wearing of TFC with chondromalacia of lunate or ulna: open ulnar shortening osteotomy.
- Type IIC: True perforation of TFC with lunate chondromalacia: central tear débrided and arthroscopic wafer procedure or open ulnar shortening.
- Type IID: Type IIC plus/minus ulnar chondromalacia plus lunatotriquetral ligament perforation (no VISI): TFCC débridement and arthroscopic wafer (lunatotriquetral is stable). Open ulnar shortening if LT is unstable.
- Type IIE: Type IID with generalized arthritic changes (VISI is present): ulnar shortening osteotomy with lunatotriquetral débridement (lunatotriquetral pinning if still unstable after ulnar shortening).

PITFALL

- MRI abnormality should not be confused with Kienböck's disease.

POSTOPERATIVE CARE

- Use intermittent short-arm splint for 4 weeks (gentle wrist active range-of-motion exercises) followed by strengthening program.
- If lunatotriquetral was pinned, use short-arm cast for 6 weeks. Remove pins at 6 to 8 weeks. Begin graduated hand therapy.

uated both through radiocarpal and midcarpal joints. If the ligament is frayed but the midcarpal joint demonstrates no significant stepoff at the lunatotriquetral interface and there are no chondromalacic changes on the hamate, an arthroscopic wafer procedure is performed similar to that for type IIC lesions. This approach is particularly applicable to older individuals.

If evidence of lunatotriquetral instability is noted such as fraying of the ulnar extrinsic ligaments, lunatotriquetral interface translation, or hamate chondromalacia, an ulnar shortening osteotomy is preferred. The frayed lunatotriquetral ligament as well as radiocarpal and midcarpal joint synovitis are débrided. A chondroplasty of the hamate may be performed if needed. After the ulnar shortening osteotomy, the lunatotriquetral interval is reassessed arthroscopically. Often improved stability is noted secondary to ulnar extrinsic ligament tightening, and no further treatment is indicated. If there is still significant instability, percutaneous Kirschner wire fixation of the lunatotriquetral interval is performed with two or three 0.045-inch wires. These wires are buried subcutaneously. A short-arm cast is worn for 4 to 8 weeks, with the percutaneous pins removed in the office at 6 to 8 weeks. A graduated therapy program is then begun, with maximum improvement being reached by 4 months.

The outcome of arthroscopic surgery for degenerative type II lesions requires long-term follow-up. Results at 3 to 5 years have yielded good to excellent results in 75% of cases.[97]

ARTHROSCOPY IN THE TREATMENT OF WRIST LIGAMENT INJURIES

Wrist arthroscopy has improved our understanding of the normal and pathologic anatomy of the intrinsic and extrinsic ligaments of the wrist. A thorough discussion of the role of arthroscopy in the management of wrist ligament injuries is presented in Chapter 14.

ARTHROSCOPY IN THE TREATMENT OF DISTAL RADIAL FRACTURES

Increasingly, wrist arthroscopy is seen as a valuable adjunct in the management of intra-articular distal radius fractures.[30,52,54,58,173,179] It allows for visualization of intercarpal soft tissue injury and is superior to C-arm and plain radiographs for assessing the gap between articular fragments.[39] Furthermore, the use of percutaneous pins aids in anatomically restoring and maintaining an articular surface reduction.

Indications

Indications for arthroscopic-assisted reduction and internal fixation (ARIF) include intra-articular distal radial fractures with articular displacement greater than 2 mm after an attempt at closed reduction. It may also be indicated in nondisplaced intra-articular fractures or extra-articular distal radius fractures in which an associated carpal ligamentous

injury is suspected.[1] It can be used in conjunction with various fixation techniques, including percutaneous pinning, external fixation, and open reduction and internal fixation (ORIF).[50] If a significant bone defect is noted as commonly seen after elevation of a die-punch fragment, limited-incision bone grafting is recommended (see also Chapter 16). Contraindications to ARIF include compartment syndrome, severe soft tissue injury, significant median nerve compromise, or an open joint injury.

Arthroscopy is not required in the majority of distal radial fractures. In the past 5 years at our tertiary referral center, only 15% of distal radial fractures required arthroscopy as compared with 60% treated by casting or pin fixation/external fixation and 25% through ORIF.

Authors' Preferred Method of Treatment

The timing of arthroscopic reduction is between 3 and 7 days after fracture. When done acutely, visualization is often obscured by active bleeding. Conversely, if done after 7 days, it is difficult to manipulate the fracture fragments into proper position.

The operating room setup and operative portals are identical to those for elective wrist arthroscopy. Swelling, however, may make it difficult to palpate the extensor tendon intervals. The use of bony landmarks such as the bases of the second and third metacarpals, the radial styloid, and the distal ulna can be helpful. Fluoroscopy may aid in needle placement and portal establishment. Traction is mandatory because ligamentotaxis does help in the reduction of major fracture displacement. This traction can be applied through a standard wrist tower, or more commonly we will keep the wrist horizontal and slightly flexed while applying traction with sterile fingertraps on the thumb, index, and long fingers over the end of an arm table. In cases in which external fixation is necessary to maintain fracture reduction, an easily adjustable external fixator system can be used to generate needed traction.[179] The arthroscopic sheath is usually introduced in the 3-4 portal and an outflow cannula established in the 6-R or 6-U portal. It is important to limit fluid extravasation into the soft tissue. Gravity flow is usually sufficient, and we prefer lactated Ringer's as the irrigating solution because of its easy resorbability. In cases in which an arthroscopic pump is used, care should be taken to accurately record inflow and outflow quantities. The forearm is often wrapped with an Esmarch bandage to prevent fluid migration into the forearm.

The first views obtained are often those of red fibrin clot, which must be lavaged. Through a working portal, a full-radius resector is used to clear the joint of clot and debris. The surgeon must be meticulous in this critical step to ensure adequate visualization and strategically plan articular fragment reduction.

Two-part fractures such as those of the radial styloid are the most amenable to treatment. Two 0.045-inch Kirschner wires are placed in the radial styloid under fluoroscopic guidance. These should be inserted through a 14-gauge needle to protect the radial artery and superficial branch of the radial nerve. The pins can then be used as joysticks to manipulate the radial styloid fragment into place. Rotational malalignment can be prevented by observation of the volar aspect of the fracture line. When the reduction is anatomic, the Kirschner wires are driven across the fracture site. A bone tenaculum, applied percutaneously, may also help compress and hold the fracture fragments during this stage. The Kirschner wires may be left as the definitive fixation, or the surgeon may choose to replace them with a cannulated screw (Fig. 19-4).

In more complex lunate die-punch fractures, preliminary reduction of the radial styloid is performed. A ⁷⁄₆₄-inch Steinmann pin is used to stabilize the radial styloid laterally to the radial shaft. Care should be taken to avoid pinning the unstable die-punch portion of the fracture so as not to impede further reduction efforts. The die-punch fragment is often depressed and may be manipulated with a Freer

periosteal elevator through a small longitudinal incision lying in line with the fourth extensor compartment. The die-punch fragment is elevated and stabilized to the previously pinned radial styloid with a 0.045- or 0.062-inch Kirschner wire. Bone grafting is helpful, and donor bone is harvested from either the iliac crest or the proximal ulna. Bone graft substitutes may also have a role. The majority of three- and four-part fractures also require external fixation, and the use of bone grafting materials allows for removal of the external fixator at 4 to 6 weeks, with the pins left in until about 7 weeks.

Melone four-part fractures[82] usually require open reduction of the volarly displaced lunate fragment. Here again, the reconstruction begins with stabilizing the radial styloid to the radial shaft. Then through a limited open volar incision placed between the finger flexors and the ulnar neurovascular bundle, the volar surface of the radius is exposed. The volar die-punch fragment is manipulated into position and fixed with a small buttress plate, usually a 2.7-mm

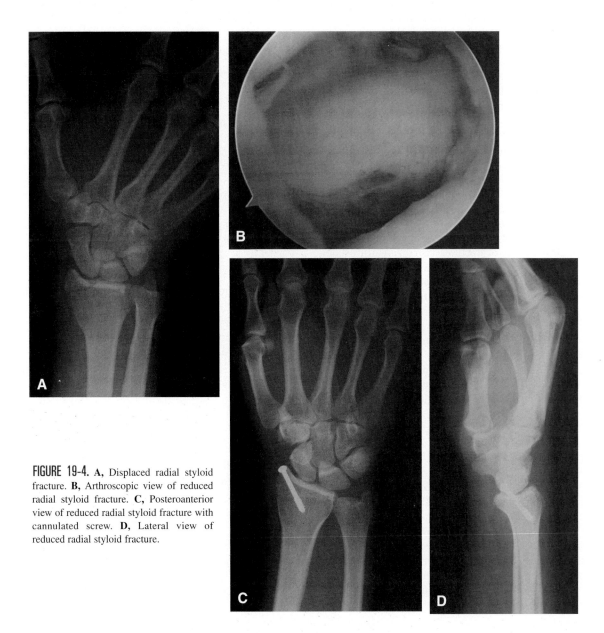

FIGURE 19-4. A, Displaced radial styloid fracture. **B,** Arthroscopic view of reduced radial styloid fracture. **C,** Posteroanterior view of reduced radial styloid fracture with cannulated screw. **D,** Lateral view of reduced radial styloid fracture.

condylar plate. The remaining part of the reduction is done arthroscopically, as for a three-part fracture.

In volarly displaced fractures requiring ORIF with a buttress plate, Levy and Glickel[78] have stressed the importance of arthroscopically ensuring articular congruency after plating.

Assessment and Treatment of Associated Soft Tissue Injuries

Wrist arthroscopy is an invaluable tool for identifying soft tissue injury after distal radial fractures.[30,52,54,58] Many of these lesions are almost impossible to evaluate using noninvasive techniques. Geissler and colleagues[54] evaluated 60 patients with displaced radial fractures and noted soft tissue injuries in 68%, of which 43% were TFC lesions, 32% scapholunate ligament tears, and 15% lunatotriquetral ligament tears, whereas 20% had multiple soft tissue injuries. Chondral lesions of the carpal bones occur with an incidence of 23% to 44%.[30,54]

Complete and partial scapholunate ligament tears are associated with radial styloid and lunate impaction fractures, dorsal displacement of the radius greater than 20 degrees, and static dorsal intercalated segment instability (DISI) on a pre-reduction radiograph. There was no correlation between scapholunate tears and radial shortening or ulnar styloid fractures. When carpal incongruency is apparent through both radiocarpal and midcarpal portals and a probe can be passed from the radiocarpal to the midcarpal joint through the scapholunate ligament, ARIF is indicated. In our series,[30] this occurred in 25% of cases.

Lunatotriquetral tears are less common and may be associated with a basiulnar styloid fracture or VISI pattern on the pre-reduction radiograph. Only 5% were unstable enough to require percutaneous pinning.

Traumatic tears of the TFC are most common and are reported in 20% to 65% of fractures visualized arthroscopically. Such tears are commonly found with radial shortening greater than 4 mm, dorsal displacement greater than 20 degrees, and an impacted lunate die-punch fracture. There is no correlation, however, with the presence of an ulnar styloid fracture or the overall fracture pattern. As for traumatic isolated tears, treatment is dependent on the classification of injury. Central lesions are generally débrided. Peripheral ulnar lesions can be repaired with the method described for type IB tears. The more common radial-sided tear is usually pinned to the radius with one or two small Kirschner wires introduced ulnarly. Unlike isolated radial lesions, the cartilaginous medial corner is disrupted and does not require further surface preparation. These pins are generally removed at 4 weeks.

Complications of ARIF for distal radial fractures have been minimal in our cases, with no infections or secondary carpal tunnel syndromes. Fifteen to 20 percent of patients will have settling of the fracture fragments postoperatively, resulting most commonly in some loss of volar tilt. To counter this, we are now adding one or two dorsal Kapandji intrafocal pins through the fracture site.[66] Five to 10 percent of patients develop complications related to percutaneous pin placement, including loosening, infection, and sensory nerve irritation.

CRITICAL POINTS: DISTAL RADIUS FRACTURES

INDICATIONS

- Intra-articular distal radial fractures with articular displacement greater than 2 mm
- Nondisplaced fractures with suspicion of carpal ligamentous injury

PREOPERATIVE EVALUATION

- Three-day delay allows arthroscopic reduction without obscured visualization from active bleeding.
- Fracture is treated no later than 7 days (difficult to manipulate fragments into position).

PEARLS

- Wrist arthroscopy allows excellent visualization of articular gapping and soft tissue injury.
- Volar lunate fragment (Melone 4-part) should be converted to Melone 3-part through open buttress plating.

TECHNICAL POINTS

- Swelling makes finding portals difficult, and bony landmarks or fluoroscopy may be needed.
- Traction (ligamentotaxis) helps reduce fracture displacement.
- Limit fluid extravasation by wrapping forearm with Esmarch bandage and using gravity flow.
- Use lactated Ringer's as irrigating solution (easy resorption).
- Use fluoroscopic insertion of Kirschner wires through a 14-gauge needle to protect from neurovascular injury.
- Pins can be used as joysticks to manipulate fracture fragments.
- Dorsal die-punch fragment may be elevated through small longitudinal incision.

PITFALLS

- Postoperative loss of volar tilt may be countered by adding dorsal pins through fracture site.
- Radial sensory nerve irritation may occur.
- There may be failure to appreciate concomitant interosseous ligament disruption.

POSTOPERATIVE CARE

- Apply short-arm cast or external fixator for 6 weeks. Pins can be removed at 6 to 8 weeks. Begin graduated hand therapy.

Outcome

Wolfe and associates[179] reported excellent outcomes in a small series of arthroscopically reduced wrist fractures. Our experience over 6 years[30] demonstrates an average flexion-extension loss of 25 degrees and a grip strength loss of 20%. Eighty-five percent achieved good to excellent results using standardized wrist scoring methods. No secondary salvage surgeries were necessary.

ARTHROSCOPIC TREATMENT OF SCAPHOID FRACTURES

Cast immobilization is an accepted standard of care for nondisplaced scaphoid fractures, and internal fixation is recommended for displaced fractures. ARIF represents an alternative to these two methods in selected patients. It is indicated for displaced but reducible scaphoid fractures or for nondisplaced and unstable fractures.[51] Percutaneous rigid internal fixation may also be a desirable alternative for patients who would experience undue psychological or economic hardship with prolonged immobilization.

The technique pioneered by Whipple[175] requires elaborate equipment to facilitate scaphoid fixation and is one of the most demanding arthroscopic procedures. A more recent technique popularized by Slade and associates avoids the use of compression jigs and is facilitated by the use of percutaneous cannulated screw fixation.[142-144] The technique may be applicable to selected scaphoid nonunions as well.[142] In our referral practice with over 100 acute scaphoid fractures per year, fewer than 5% are treated arthroscopically.

Authors' Preferred Method of Treatment

Standard arthroscopic traction is applied. The initial portal is the radial midcarpal, which allows hematoma evacuation and excellent waist fracture visualization. If the fracture is nondisplaced and amenable to arthroscopic fixation, a volar incision is made. If reduction is necessary, direct manipulation of the distal pole and percutaneous manipulation of the proximal pole using a joystick are helpful. Once reduced, a Kirschner wire provisionally stabilizes the reduction.

A 2-cm incision is made radial to the FCR and centered on the scaphotrapezial joint. Blunt spreading down to this joint capsule will protect against injury to the palmar cutaneous nerve or radial artery. The joint capsule is elevated, and the volar tubercle of the trapezium is excised with an osteotome or rongeur. This provides full access to the distal pole of the scaphoid.

CRITICAL POINTS: SCAPHOID FRACTURES

INDICATION

- Displaced scaphoid fracture in patient who does not want cast immobilization

PREOPERATIVE EVALUATION

- Search for displaced but reducible scaphoid fractures or nondisplaced unstable fractures.

PEARLS

- Distal pole is manipulated directly, and proximal pole is manipulated with a percutaneous joystick.

TECHNICAL POINTS

- Standard arthroscopic traction is applied.
- Radial midcarpal portal visualizes waist fracture fragments.
- A volar 2-cm incision is made radial to the FCR (centered on the scaphotrapezial joint).
- Avoid palmar cutaneous nerve and radial artery.
- Kirschner wire provisionally stabilizes reduction.
- Volar tubercle of trapezium is excised with a rongeur, clearing access to distal pole of scaphoid.

- A 4-5 radiocarpal portal and a 1-2 portal are created to introduce a target hook of the Whipple compression jig.
- The hook is seated on the dorsal scaphoid 1 to 2 mm radial to the scapholunate ligament.
- The guide barrel of the jig is slid down to the exposed articular surface of the scaphoid.
- A guide pin is inserted down the center of the barrel jig.
- An accessory pin controls rotation.
- A cannulated drill tap and cortical broach are followed by a cannulated Herbert-Whipple screw.

PITFALL

- This technique is one of the most demanding arthroscopic procedures.

POSTOPERATIVE CARE

- Apply a short-arm/thumb spica splint for 10 days. Begin protected wrist mobilization and active range-of-motion exercises at 2 weeks.

With the arthroscope in the 4-5 radiocarpal portal, a 1-2 portal is created to introduce the target hook of the Whipple compression jig. The visualized hook is seated on the dorsal scaphoid 1 to 2 mm radial to the scapholunate ligament. The guide barrel of the jig is slid down to the exposed articular surface of the scaphoid. The jig is then compressed to maintain the reduction.

A primary guide pin is inserted down the center of the barrel jig and its position confirmed fluoroscopically. If satisfactory, an accessory pin is placed to control rotation. A cannulated drill tap and cortical broach are successively used, followed by an appropriate-length cannulated Herbert-Whipple screw. Accuracy and stability of the fracture are confirmed both arthroscopically and fluoroscopically. After closure of the volar incision, a short-arm/thumb spica splint is applied for 10 days. If the desired stability has been achieved, protected wrist mobilization and activities are permitted by 2 weeks.

For proximal pole fractures, our technique is different in that Kirschner wires replace screw fixation. The initial portal is the ulnar midcarpal, which gives a clearer perspective of the fracture line. Two 0.045-inch Kirschner wires are inserted from the dorsal side of the wrist and passed percutaneously through the small proximal pole and across the fracture site on the wrist. With image and arthroscopic verification of stable anatomic reduction, the pins are cut off beneath the volar skin for later office removal. Initial immobilization is 4 weeks, followed by a similar protocol as for waist fractures.

Outcome

This technique demonstrates healing rates of 95% with a dramatically reduced period of immobilization when compared with patients treated nonoperatively.[104,174]

ARTHROSCOPIC RESECTION OF DORSAL WRIST GANGLIA

Although the cause, natural history, and pathogenesis of dorsal ganglion cysts remain controversial, a correlation with scapholunate ligament injury[123] as well as origination from the dorsal capsule and/or dorsal fibers of the scapholunate ligament has been postulated.[4,19,36,166] Current treatments include benign neglect, aspiration, and surgical excision. Aspiration, with or without cortisone injection, enjoys a success rate of 40%.[128] If aspiration has failed and the cyst remains symptomatic, surgical excision is a reasonable option.[4,19]

The goals of ganglion surgery should be ganglion resection through a cosmetically acceptable scar while maintaining wrist range of motion.[140] Open ganglionectomy has often been described as trading a scar for a lump. Complications such as scar hypertrophy and joint stiffness, particularly with volar flexion loss, have been reported.[80] The goal of arthroscopic resection is to minimize scarring and hopefully avoid capsular stiffness that may occur with open resection. Additionally, any underlying instability of the intrinsic scapholunate ligament, implicated as causative for a dorsal ganglion,[166] will be thoroughly assessed at the time of arthroscopy.

Authors' Preferred Method of Treatment

A standard arthroscopic setup is used. After regional or general anesthesia, a tourniquet is applied and inflated. Before wrist distraction, a thorough wrist examination under anesthesia, including the scaphoid shift test, is performed.

The ganglion and standard portal sites are outlined with a marker. Initial scope placement is through an ulnar portal most commonly at the 6-R location. Alternative portal placement includes the 4-5 or the 1-2 portal. The scope is guided radially and directed to the dorsum of the scapholunate ligament. Approximately two thirds of patients will demonstrate a readily visible pearl-like ganglion stalk. When such a stalk is not seen, the origin is assumed to be from the dorsal capsule, in which case synovitis is usually noted. A needle placed through the skin and extended into the stalk is utilized. A ganglion portal, almost always equivalent to the standard 3-4 portal, is established. A full-radius resector, suction punch, or manual punch instrument is used to resect a 1-cm diameter of dorsal capsule at the ganglion origin (Fig. 19-5). Care should be taken to avoid intrinsic scapholunate ligament injury. Dorsal synovitis, where present, is débrided. In one third of cases, the underlying extensor tendons may be visible. The arthroscopy is completed by systematically examining all radiocarpal and midcarpal structures through the appropriate portals.

The wrist is removed from the traction tower and re-examined. It is important to ensure that the extra-articular portion of the ganglion has been fully ruptured. If not, in cases of bilobed cyst structures, aspiration or manual rupture is required. Portal sites are closed with one suture or adhesive bandages. A volar splint is applied until the first dressing change at 1 week. At that time, all portal sutures are removed and active wrist range-of-motion exercises begun. Normal hand use is permitted as tolerated, but strenuous use of the hand and wrist should be avoided for 6 weeks.

Outcome

In our prospective series,[108] 42% of the patients had articular abnormalities. Most common were problems of the intrinsic ligaments such as perforation of the central portion of the scapholunate ligament, laxity or redundancy of the scapholunate ligament, and small perforations of the TFC. These lesions were catalogued but not treated. No patient had evidence of static carpal instability; and, in those patients who had wrist pain, all but one had relief of their symptoms after ganglion excision. This patient had significant radial chondromalacia, and it remained a source of his symptoms.

To date, there has been only 1 recurrence in more than 150 arthroscopic ganglionectomies (less than 1%). This compares favorably with open ganglionectomy recurrence rates of 2% to 40%. Portal site scars usually blend imperceptibly. No patient in our series has lost significant volar flexion, and no other complications have been observed.

Arthroscopic resection may also play a role in the treatment of occult dorsal ganglia. Sanders and others[134,158] have alluded to the difficulty of making this diagnosis. If a patient has persistent point tenderness over the scapholunate ligament that responds appropriately to immobilization and

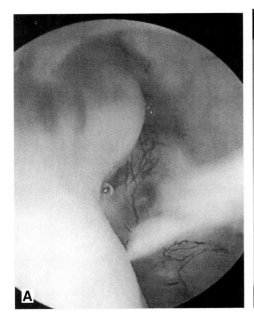
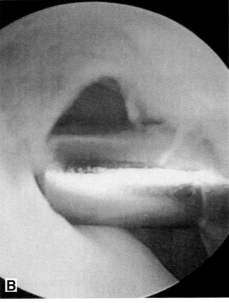

FIGURE 19-5. **A,** Arthroscopic view of dorsal ganglion stalk from 6-R portal *(upper left)*. **B,** Full radius resection removes dorsal stalk with 1-cm diameter of dorsal capsule.

injection, and if other causes of wrist pain have been excluded, arthroscopic resection of a small portion of the dorsal capsule in this area has been helpful in selected cases. Here the intra-articular portion of the arthroscopic examination is normal and a ganglion stock is routinely not seen. The technique of arthroscopic resection is similar to that for a palpable dorsal ganglion.

No arthroscopic technique has been described for volar wrist ganglia, although techniques for volar portal placement have been described for use in other procedures.[145,146]

ARTHROSCOPIC WRIST CONTRACTURE RELEASE

Although many patients will have an element of permanent wrist stiffness after significant injury, frank arthrofibrosis

CRITICAL POINTS: DORSAL GANGLION

INDICATIONS

- Dorsal ganglion cysts
- To minimize scarring and avoid potential capsular stiffness that may occur with open resection
- Suspicion of underlying wrist pathology
- For occult dorsal ganglia

PREOPERATIVE EVALUATION

- Ensure that mass is a ganglion (transillumination).
- Perform provocative wrist tests to assess for wrist instability.

PEARLS

- Dorsal ganglia may represent underlying instability of the intrinsic scapholunate ligament.
- Aspirate or manually rupture bilobed ganglion after resection if mass is still present.

TECHNICAL POINTS

- Outline ganglion with a marker.
- Initial scope placement is in 6-R portal.

- Scope is guided radially and directed to the dorsum of the scapholunate area.
- Ganglion stalk or dorsal synovitis (origin in dorsal capsule) is identified.
- Needle is placed through ganglion (rupturing it) and then extended into stalk.
- Use suction punch through 3-4 portal to resect 1-cm area of dorsal capsule.
- Perform systematic evaluation of potential underlying pathologic process that may have contributed to ganglion.

PITFALL

- Avoid injury to the intrinsic scapholunate ligament.

POSTOPERATIVE CARE

- Apply volar splint for 1 week.
- Begin active wrist range-of-motion exercises at 1 week, and allow normal hand use as tolerated.
- Avoid strenuous activity for 6 weeks.

rarely develops. When it does occur, it is most often associated with a healed distal radial fracture but it can be seen after ganglion resection, after ligamentous injury, or as a late residual of reflex dystrophy. In a patient with full digital motion and radiographically acceptable bony architecture, arthroscopic contracture release is a rewarding procedure.

Authors' Preferred Method of Treatment

A standard arthroscopic setup is used. After regional or general anesthesia, a tourniquet is applied and inflated. The 3-4 and 6-R portals are established and intra-articular adhesions are removed to improve visualization. A Freer elevator or small banana blade is needed to incise the adhesions, which are then removed with a suction punch or power shaver. Usually, a probe or trocar can be manipulated across the radiocarpal joint to further clear a visual path and facilitate triangulation. Partial release of the dorsal capsule is necessary to regain volar flexion, but violation of the volar extrinsic ligaments or the intrinsic ligaments is contraindicated. Gentle passive mobilization of the wrist is then gradually performed to stretch the wrist into maximum extension and flexion. Intensive therapy is begun on the first postoperative day.

Outcome

Unfortunately, the motion gained at surgery is infrequently preserved; however, in a review of 23 patients, all but 2 regained functional motion.[104] Preoperative flexion averaged 9 degrees and extension, 15 degrees. Postoperatively, at a 2-year follow-up, the arc of motion improved to 42 degrees of flexion and 58 degrees of extension.

ARTHROSCOPIC SALVAGE PROCEDURES

Excisional arthroplasties such as radial styloidectomy and proximal row carpectomy can be performed arthroscopically and lend themselves nicely to this approach.[8,130] Anecdotal cases of intercarpal fusion have been performed arthroscopically as well, including scaphotrapezial trapezoid and four-quadrant fusion.

Radial Styloidectomy

Authors' Preferred Method of Treatment

Radial styloidectomy is an early salvage procedure that may provide significant symptomatic benefits to patients with

end-stage arthritis who do not wish a formal reconstructive procedure such as proximal row carpectomy or partial or complete fusion. It is particularly useful in patients with scapholunate or scaphoid nonunion advanced collapse (SNAC) who are symptomatic but have maintained good grip strength and range of motion. Arthroscopic radial styloidectomy allows decompression of radial impingement with minimal morbidity.

A standard arthroscopic setup is used. After regional or general anesthesia, a tourniquet is applied and inflated. Radiocarpal and midcarpal portals are created, followed by synovectomy and débridement of the radiocarpal and midcarpal joints. Attention is turned to the radial styloid, and care is taken to identify the extrinsic radioscaphocapitate and long radiolunate ligaments. Four to 5 millimeters of the styloid is resected, which generally corresponds to the radial border of these ligaments, but this depends on the extent of cartilage wear. While viewing from the 3-4 portal, a 3- to 4-mm covered bur is inserted through the 1-2 portal and the styloidectomy begun (Fig. 19-6). In some cases, a small osteotome will facilitate bone removal. Arthroscopic and fluoroscopic observation confirms the amount of resected styloid. Care is taken to preserve the volar radial extrinsic ligaments. Once completed, the wrist is radially deviated to arthroscopically confirm that all areas of impingement have been decompressed.

After surgery, an intermittent splint is worn for 3 weeks. An early active range-of-motion exercise program is begun after the first week and a graduated strengthening program started during the fourth week.

Arthroscopic Proximal Row Carpectomy

Authors' Preferred Method of Treatment

Proximal row carpectomy is another motion-preserving salvage procedure for wrist arthritis that may be performed arthroscopically.

After arthroscopic confirmation of acceptable articular surfaces on the proximal pole of the capitate and in the lunate fossa, a 4-mm bur is used to begin removing the proximal scaphoid. The space thus created allows improved visualization of the lunate, which is then burred (Fig. 19-7). Throughout this process, iatrogenic injury to the lunate fossa or proximal capitate must be avoided. To accomplish this a Freer elevator is placed in a midcarpal portal while small osteotomes help morcelize the bones and pituitary rongeurs help remove larger fragments. The technique is tedious but not difficult, with operative times between 60 and 90 minutes. When the carpectomy is completed, the preserved radial and ulnar extrinsic ligaments should be clearly visible. Any radial styloid impingement requires concomitant styloidectomy. The capitate should articulate with the lunate fossa. Postoperatively, the wrist is immobilized in a cast or removable splint for 4 weeks, followed by intermittent

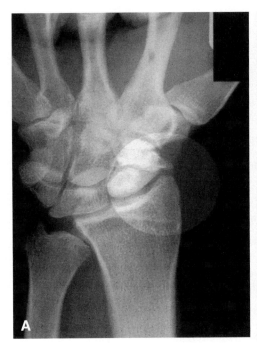

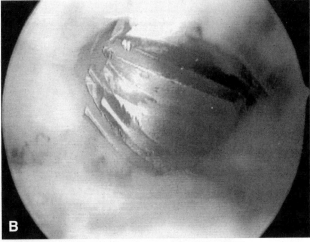

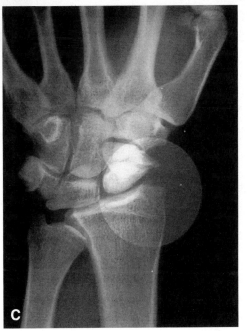

FIGURE 19-6. A, SNAC wrist with radial styloid, distal scaphoid involvement. **B,** Arthroscopic bur to remove radial styloid. **C,** Radiograph demonstrating post removal radial styloid.

CRITICAL POINTS: SALVAGE PROCEDURES

INDICATIONS

Radial Styloidectomy

■ Early salvage procedure if patient does not want formal open reconstructive procedure for scapholunate or scaphoid nonunion advanced collapse.

Proximal Row Carpectomy

■ Motion-preserving salvage procedure for late stage scapholunate or scaphoid nonunion advanced collapse.

PREOPERATIVE EVALUATION

Radial Styloidectomy

■ Look for painful radial deviation and positive Watson test with good grip strength and range of motion.

Proximal Row Carpectomy

■ Similar as above with decreased range of motion and grip.

Continued

CRITICAL POINTS: SALVAGE PROCEDURES—cont'd

PEARLS

Radial Styloidectomy

- Arthroscopic and fluoroscopic observation confirms amount of styloid resected.
- Radially deviate wrist and arthroscopically confirm impingement correction after resection.

Proximal Row Carpectomy

- More than one bur is likely to be needed.
- Preserved radial and ulnar extrinsic ligaments should be clearly visible after procedure.

TECHNICAL POINTS

Radial Styloidectomy

- Arthroscopic synovectomy and débridement of precarpal and midcarpal joints.
- Styloidectomy performed through 1-2 portal using 3- to 4-mm covered bur.
- Radial border of volar extrinsic ligaments is level to which styloid is resected.
- View styloidectomy from 3-4 portal.

Proximal Row Carpectomy

- Confirm acceptable articular surfaces on proximal pole of capitate and lunate fossa.

- Use 4-mm bur to remove proximal scaphoid and then lunate and triquetrum.
- Residual styloid impingement requires concomitant styloidectomy.

PITFALLS

Radial Styloidectomy

- Preserve volar radial extrinsic ligaments.

Proximal Row Carpectomy

- Avoid damage to lunate fossa or proximal capitate (protected with Freer elevator in midcarpal portal).
- Technique is tedious and may require 60 to 90 minutes.

POSTOPERATIVE CARE

Radial Styloidectomy

- Use intermittent splint for 3 weeks with early active range-of-motion exercises at 1 week and graduated strengthening started at 4 weeks.

Proximal Row Carpectomy

- Use short-arm splint for 4 weeks followed by intermittent splinting and wrist exercises. Begin strengthening at 8 weeks.

---

splinting and a wrist rehabilitative program. Strengthening is begun by the eighth week.

SMALL-JOINT ARTHROSCOPY

The success of wrist arthroscopy has stimulated the application of small-joint arthroscopy into other hand areas. Ryu and Fagan[131] have successfully treated thumb metacarpophalangeal ulnar collateral ligament rupture with arthroscopic reduction of the Stener lesion and immobilization. DeClerg and coworkers[35] described an isolated case of arthroscopic synovectomy of the metacarpophalangeal joints.

A number of centers are evaluating the arthroscopic indications for problems of the thumb carpometacarpal joint. Menon[84] performed arthroscopic trapezial resection and tissue resection on 31 patients. No ligament reconstruction was required. Follow-up found relief of pain in 87% and an average pinch strength of 11 lb.

Our current indications for thumb carpometacarpal arthroscopy include intra-articular fractures such as Bennett's fracture, synovitis, or stable degenerative or post-traumatic arthritis.

Authors' Preferred Method of Treatment

Distraction is applied only to the thumb, with a traction tower. Viewing and operative portals are just radial (volar) and just ulnar (dorsal) to the abductor pollicis longus. A needle is used to define the joint space, and 1 to 2 mL of Ringer's lactate is infused. A 2.0- to 2.9-mm scope is inserted through one portal and a 1.9-mm full-radius resector through the other. After the joint is arthroscopically cleared, a systematic examination begins. The base of the first metacarpal is identified by moving the thumb while the trapezium and volarly situated anterior oblique ligament are palpated with a probe. When a fracture is present, reduction is confirmed arthroscopically and the fragments are percutaneously pinned. In arthritic joints, a limited débridement is performed (Fig. 19-8).

COMPLICATIONS OF WRIST ARTHROSCOPY

Complications after arthroscopy are uncommon and based on wrist anatomy, portal location, surgical technique, and

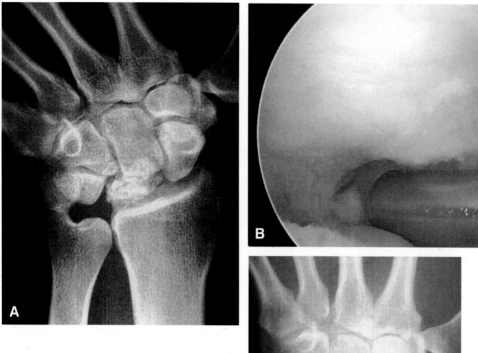

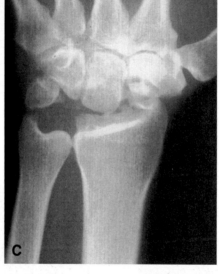

FIGURE 19-7. **A,** Stage III Kienböck's posteroanterior view. **B,** Use of arthroscopic bur to remove proximal carpal row. **C,** Postoperative radiograph of proximal row carpectomy.

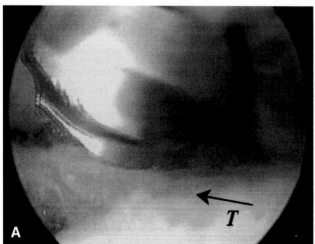

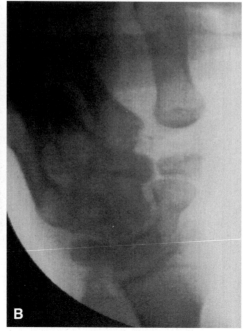

FIGURE 19-8. **A,** Thumb CMC arthroscopy with arthroscopic bur removing portions of trapezium (T). **B,** Radiographs demonstrating hemitrapeziectomy.

type of procedure performed.[29] Potential sources include those related to traction and arm positioning, portal establishment, general arthroscopic complications, and procedure specific pitfalls. Small[147] recorded an incidence of 0.59% in 395,000 procedures. Roth and coworkers[7] identified 17 complications in 214 cases of diagnostic wrist arthroscopy. Reflex sympathetic dystrophy was most common (3.7%), followed by sensory branch neurapraxia (2.3%) and tendon problems (0.9%). All complications resolved with nonoperative treatment.

Fortems and associates[46] identified one case of extensor pollicis longus rupture after arthroscopy. In a review of our 463 therapeutic arthroscopies, the overall complication rate was less than 3%. There were no tendon or nerve lacerations, and the majority of complications related more to pin fixation than to the arthroscopy. The morbidity directly correlated with the difficulty of the procedure, being least for arthroscopic débridement of the TFC and dorsal ganglia and most for the stabilization of fractures and ligaments.

Warhold and Ruth[164] and Whipple[171] have both catalogued a list of potential complications and, more importantly, how to avoid them. A few caveats are worth emphasizing. In certain medical conditions, such as rheumatoid arthritis, the digital skin may be fragile and damaged by standard metal fingertraps. The use of flexible, nylon fingertraps has been advocated. When establishing a portal, always spread down to the wrist capsule with a hemostat, thus protecting the sensory nerves and extensor tendons. Never plunge forcibly into the joint to avoid iatrogenic scuffing of the articular surfaces. Like a name carved in a tree trunk, such effects are permanent and potentially more damaging than the original lesion. Minimize the duration of wrist arthroscopy procedures to avoid metacarpophalangeal joint stiffness and nerve injury from prolonged traction.[29]

ACKNOWLEDGMENTS

We would like to thank Kelly P. Gambino, MSN, CRNP, and Leslie Ristine for their valuable assistance in the preparation of this chapter.

ANNOTATED REFERENCES

11. Bednar MS, Arnoczky SP, Weiland AJ: The microvasculature of the triangular fibrocartilage complex: Its clinical significance. J Hand Surg [Am] 16:1101-1105, 1991.

This study of cadaver wrists, injected with India ink, demonstrates the blood supply of the TFCC to be limited to the periphery. Thus, tears in those areas have the potential for repair. A tear at the radial margin or central portion of the TFCC may have less healing potential and would be best treated by débridement.

18. Canter RM, Stern PJ, Wyrick JD, Michaels SE: The relevance of ligament tear or perforations on the diagnosis of wrist pain: An arthrographic study. J Hand Surg [Am] 19: 945-953, 1994.

This is an excellent paper with important implications for the clinician. Patients who had a positive three-compartment arthrogram on the affected side underwent bilateral arthrography. There was a high prevalence of bilateral symmetric lesions. The results raise uncertainty as to the significance of interrupted ligaments on arthrography to the diagnosis of wrist pain.

24. Chun S, Palmer AK: The ulnar impaction syndrome: Follow up of ulnar shortening osteotomy. J Hand Surg [Am] 18: 46-53, 1993.

Ulnar impaction syndrome, which is often diagnosed arthroscopically, can be treated with ulnar shortening osteotomy. This long-term follow-up study confirms this success. Complications were rare.

25. Chung KC, Zimmerman NB, Travis MT: Wrist arthrography versus arthroscopy: A comparative study of 150 cases. J Hand Surg [Am] 21: 591-594, 1996.

The authors found a significant discrepancy between arthrographic and arthroscopic findings in a comparative study. It confirms the accuracy and efficiency of wrist arthroscopy.

29. Culp R: Complications of wrist arthroscopy. Hand Clin 15:529-535, 1999.

This review article identifies the most common complications of wrist arthroscopy, such as sensory branch neurapraxia or tendon problems. Methods of avoidance are also discussed.

54. Geissler WB, Freeland AE, Savoie FH, et al: Intraarticular soft tissue lesions associated with an intraarticular fracture of the distal end of the radius. J Bone Joint Surg Am 78:357-365, 1996.

This excellent study highlights the usefulness of wrist arthroscopy in evaluating intra-articular distal radius fractures as identified in the high frequency of associated ligamentous injuries. It also offers a useful classification system to assess the severity of the soft tissue ligamentous injuries.

88. Mikic ZD: Age changes in the triangular fibrocartilage of the wrist joint. J Anat 126:367-384, 1978.

A classic study demonstrating age-related perforations or defects in the TFCC. Thus, not all abnormalities of the TFCC are traumatic nor are they symptomatic.

103. Osterman AL: Arthroscopic débridement of triangular fibrocartilage complex tears. Arthroscopy 6:120-124, 1990.

This was one of the earliest studies to document the efficacy of arthroscopic TFCC débridement for central and radial sided tears.

108. Osterman AL, Raphael J: Arthroscopic resection of the dorsal ganglion of the wrist. Hand Clin North Am 11:7-12, 1995.

This article describes the indications, technique, and success rates for arthroscopic excision of dorsal ganglions of the wrist. Since this original article, others have documented the advantages of this technique for the experienced arthroscopist.

111. Palmer AK: Triangular fibrocartilage complex lesions: A classification. J Hand Surg [Am] 14:594-606, 1989.

This article describes a classification for TFCC lesions that is most useful. It divides injuries into two types, traumatic and degenerative. Each category is subdivided by location and associated ligamentous or arthritic conditions. This classification scheme is helpful for treatment planning.

116. Palmer AK, Werner FW: The triangular fibrocartilage complex of the wrist: Anatomy and function. J Hand Surg [Am] 6:153-162, 1981.

This classic article describes the anatomy and function of the TFCC. It was one of the original descriptions of the complex of structures in this area and their purpose.

156. Trumble TE, Gilbert M, Vedder N: Arthroscopic repair of the triangular fibrocartilage complex. Arthroscopy 12:588-597, 1996.

As the technical capability of wrist arthroscopy improves, the ability to repair lesions of the wrist exists. This study confirms that arthroscopic repair of peripheral tears of the TFCC is a valid technique with results equal to, if not better than, open repair.

162. Viegas SF, Patterson RM, Hokanson JA, Davis J: Wrist anatomy: Incidence, distribution and correlation of anatomic variations, tears and arthrosis. J Hand Surg [Am] 18:463-475, 1993.

This excellent cadaver study confirms that pathologic conditions consisting of ligament tears and arthrosis are common in older specimens. Bilateral changes were quite common. This knowledge is imperative in the arthroscopic treatment of wrist pathology.

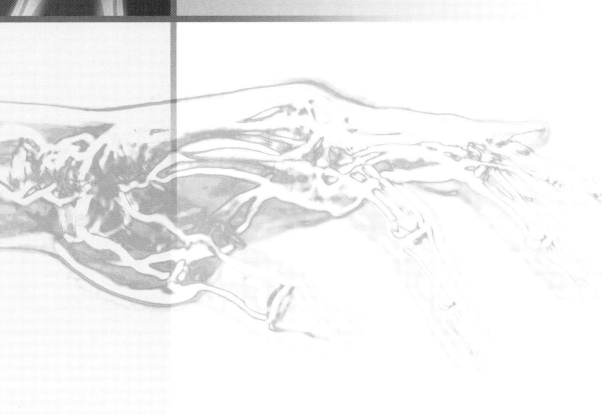

PART IV

Elbow and Forearm

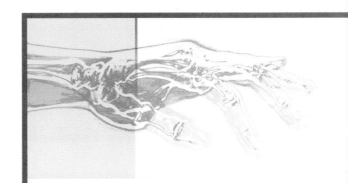

Trauma and Fractures

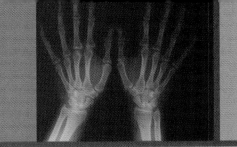

CHAPTER 20

Fractures of the Distal Humerus

David P. Barei and Douglas P. Hanel

Fractures of the distal humerus continue to pose a substantial therapeutic challenge. Because these fractures are relatively rare, the experience of any single surgeon is limited.[50,139] The complexity of the anatomy, the fracture comminution, and the limited points for secure fixation make the task of achieving stable fixation to allow early range of motion challenging, even for experienced surgeons.

Injuries of the distal humerus include extracapsular fractures in the supracondylar region, extra-articular intracapsular (transcondylar) fractures, isolated unicondylar fractures, partial or complete articular fractures, and, the most common pattern, combined supracondylar-intercondylar fractures. We also address the more infrequent patterns, which carry different demands.

PREOPERATIVE EVALUATION

Fractures of the distal humerus occur in distinct patient groups. Those that occur in physiologically young patients are typically the result of high-energy mechanisms, such as motor vehicle collisions or falls from significant heights.[52] Open wounds, other ipsilateral upper limb injuries, and general systemic injury frequently can occur because of the heightened energy of the trauma that occurs.[52] However, as the elderly population increases there is also an increasing incidence of low-energy falls resulting in fractures of the distal humerus. This distinctive version of the fracture is characterized by poor bone quality and may be associated with poor general health or preexisting arthritic changes.[122,123]

History and Physical Examination

The history should focus on the mechanism and time of injury and the identification of other sites of injury. It is also necessary to recognize prior elbow injury or surgery or preexisting conditions of the entire upper extremity. In addition, preexisting medical conditions, medications, and an overall functional assessment are necessary to determine the optimal treatment. An understanding of the patient's

physical demands at work will assist in planning the goals and duration of rehabilitation and the timing and modifications at the workplace.

In addition to a complete physical examination, particularly in the setting of a high-energy mechanism, a detailed and focused examination of the injured extremity should be performed. Inspection of the limb may demonstrate swelling, bruising, and deformity, particularly angulation and shortening. A complete circumferential inspection of the elbow is performed to avoid missing open wounds, which most commonly occur on the posterior aspect.[98] Patients are typically unable to perform any significant elbow range of motion secondary to pain.

The distal vascular status is evaluated by inspecting the color of the distal extremity and by palpation of the radial and ulnar pulses. Poorly palpable pulses are checked using noninvasive Doppler ultrasound studies. If there is a questionable pulse and gross malalignment of the arm, gentle traction can often realign the limb, restoring the distal pulse. Angiography or urgent operative vascular exploration is necessary in those patients who continue to demonstrate an abnormal vascular examination. A detailed neurologic examination of the hand and digits, including motor function, sensation, and two-point discrimination, should be performed and recorded to identify any injury to the median, radial, ulnar, anterior interosseous, or posterior interosseous nerves. These findings, particularly two-point discrimination, should be recorded for later reference should there be a change before or after surgery. At the conclusion of the physical examination, a sterile dressing is placed over any open wounds and a lightweight above-elbow splint is applied.

Radiographic Examination

Standard anteroposterior and lateral radiographs are generally sufficient to make the diagnosis of a fracture of the distal humerus and to provide a reasonable assessment of the fracture pattern. Radiographs of significantly displaced fractures, however, may be incomprehensible because the normal radiographic landmarks become distorted.[167] Gentle traction can substantially improve alignment to provide more understandable images, both anteroposterior and lateral. Some sedation may be needed if this is performed in the emergency department. Alternatively, traction images in the operating room can also be obtained once complete anesthesia has been achieved.[8] Invariably, the previously bizarre appearance of the distal humerus becomes much more understandable (Fig. 20-1). Computed tomography (CT) is helpful for fractures distal to the olecranon fossa or in the coronal plane (Fig. 20-2).[68,96,137] CT may also be useful in older patients to assess the degree of comminution and aid in deciding whether internal fixation should be attempted versus total elbow replacement.

Anatomy

The distal humerus is triangular when viewed from anteriorly or posteriorly. The humeral diaphysis diverges into medial and lateral bony columns in the metaphyseal portion of the distal humerus (Fig. 20-3). These medial and lateral columns form the supracondylar region of the distal humerus and are characterized by sharp, thin ridges on their respective medial and lateral aspects. Suspended between the medial and lateral columns is the transversely oriented trochlea, which represents the most distal portion of the humerus, or base of the triangle. The trochlea (Gr. "pulley") is covered anteriorly, inferiorly, and posteriorly with articular cartilage, creating an arc of approximately 270 degrees.[95] The spatial relationships of the medial column, lateral column, and trochlea are conceptually similar to a spool of thread being held between the thumb and index finger.[70]

The medial column diverges approximately 45 degrees from the humeral diaphysis and is composed mainly of cortical bone. The most distal portion of the medial column ends at the medial epicondyle, located approximately 1 cm proximal to the distal end of the trochlea. The medial epicondyle serves as the origin for the flexor-pronator mus-

cle mass of the forearm and the medial collateral ligament complex. The medial epicondyle also serves as the anterior and superior boundary of the cubital tunnel, through which the ulnar nerve travels. Because of the intimate relationship of the ulnar nerve to the medial epicondyle, any operative approach along the medial column requires identification and protection of the nerve.

The most distal portion of the lateral column extends to the distal aspect of the trochlea and diverges from the humeral diaphysis at approximately a 20-degree angle. The lateral column terminates anteriorly with the capitellum, while the posterior aspect of the lateral column presents a nonarticular, osseous surface. When viewing the distal humerus from its inferior surface, the transition of the lateral column from bone posteriorly to the anterior articular surface of the capitellum occurs at the most distal aspect of the lateral column along a line connecting the medial and lateral epicondyles. The capitellum, therefore, subtends an arc of articular surface of approximately 180 degrees. This distal posterior osseous surface of the lateral column is an important anatomic area. In contrast to the cartilage covered medial column, this posterior surface is available for fixation devices used in the treatment of lateral column and/or capitellar fragments. The capitellum, in addition to its role in elbow stabilization both in motion and resistance to varus and valgus stress, articulates with the radial head, providing a surface for forearm rotation.

The posterior aspect of the lateral column is covered by the distal origin of the medial head of the triceps muscle and, distally, by the origin of the anconeus. The brachioradialis and extensor carpi radialis longus take their origin from the lateral supracondylar ridge. The common extensor mass, consisting of the extensor carpi radialis brevis, extensor digitorum communis, and extensor carpi ulnaris, and the cephalad portion of the anconeus muscle originate from the lateral epicondyle, immediately posterior to the origin of the lateral collateral ligament complex. The lateral collateral ligament complex and the common extensor

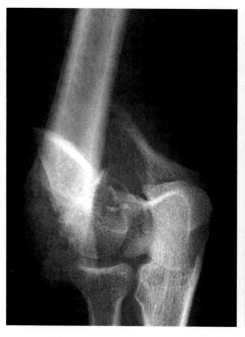
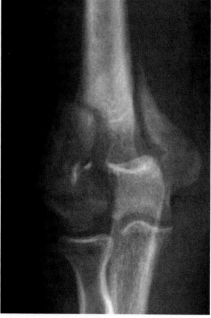

FIGURE 20-1. Anteroposterior (**A**) and lateral (**B**) radiographs of a severely displaced fracture of the humerus.

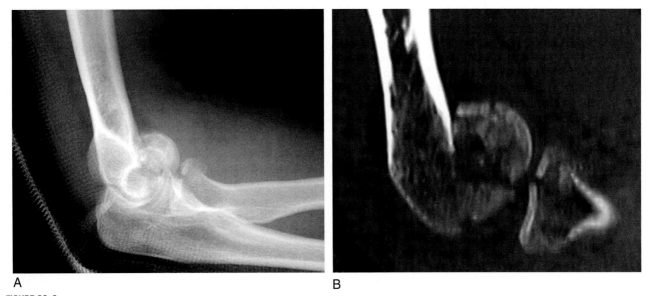

A   B

FIGURE 20-2. A, Lateral radiographic image of a coronal shear variant capitellar fracture. **B,** Sagittal re-formation of the same image more clearly identifies the comminution of the distal portion of the lateral column. The preoperative plan may now require the use of bone graft or changing the anticipated exposure.

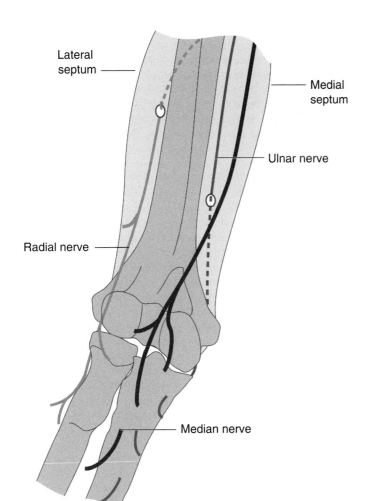

Lateral
septum

Medial
septum

Ulnar nerve

Radial nerve

Median nerve

FIGURE 20-3. Anterior and posterior views of the osseous distal humerus and important bony landmarks.

origin blend together and do not necessarily have discrete origins.[118]

Distally, the medial and lateral columns are separated by the olecranon fossa posteriorly and the coronoid fossa anteriorly. These two structures are immediately adjacent to each other and are separated by a thin intervening bony septum. This septum occasionally has a defect or aperture within it creating a communication between the coronoid and olecranon fossae, a normal anatomic variant.[59] The radial fossa lies immediately lateral to the coronoid fossa and is a component of the lateral column. The olecranon fossa is a thinning of the distal humeral metaphysis that accepts the tip of the olecranon process during extension of the elbow joint. This fossa is filled with fat in the normal state, but it may become filled with fibrous tissue after injury or surgery and is partially responsible for the lack of extension commonly seen after fractures about the elbow. Similarly, the coronoid and radial fossae accept the coronoid process and radial head, respectively, during elbow flexion. An appreciation of these fossae helps one avoid inadvertent placement of screws within these areas and the associated restriction in elbow range of motion.

The majority of surgical exposures of the distal humerus are performed using a posterior approach; therefore, an understanding of the anatomic relationships and paths taken by the ulnar and radial nerves is essential to the safe management of these injuries (Fig. 20-4). In the intact humerus, the radial nerve can be found crossing the posterior aspect of the humeral shaft approximately 20 cm proximal to the medial epicondyle (74% the length of the humerus) to 14 cm proximal to the lateral epicondyle (51% the length of the humerus). At the lateral aspect of the humeral shaft, the radial nerve trifurcates into a branch to the medial head of the triceps, the lower lateral brachial cutaneous nerve, and the continuation of the radial nerve into the forearm (the posterior interosseous nerve and the superficial cutaneous nerve). After the trifurcation, the posterior interosseous continuation of the radial nerve pierces the lateral intermuscular septum approximately 10 cm proximal to the lateral epicondyle (the distal 36% of the humerus) (Fig. 20-5).[39,44,105]

At the level of the distal attachment of the coracobrachialis to the humerus, approximately 10 cm proximal to the medial epicondyle, the ulnar nerve courses from the anterior compartment to the posterior compartment of the arm by piercing the medial intermuscular septum.[23] The nerve then travels along the anteromedial border of the medial head of the triceps along the medial intermuscular septum, ultimately traveling posterior to the medial epicondyle of the distal humerus (Fig. 20-6). In approximately 70% of the population, a thick fascial band (arcade of Struthers) connects the medial head of the triceps to the intermuscular septum crossing the ulnar nerve approximately 8 cm proximal to the medial epicondyle.[150] An anatomic clue to the presence of this fascial band is to identify muscle fibers of the medial head of the triceps crossing superficial to the ulnar nerve.[151] As the nerve passes posterior to the medial epicondyle, it becomes enclosed in a fibrous sheath, the roof of the cubital tunnel. As the nerve exits the cubital tunnel, it courses between the two heads of the flexor carpi ulnaris (FCU), passes beneath the fibrous origin of the flexor digitorum superficialis, and travels distally through the anterior compartment of the forearm on the anterior surface of the flexor digitorum profundus. The first branch of the ulnar nerve provides sensory innervation to the elbow capsule.[75,132,151] After exiting the cubital tunnel, motor branches to the FCU can be identified. The remaining branches of the ulnar nerve are encountered in the distal forearm and hand.

CLASSIFICATION

For decades, fractures of the distal humerus were collectively referred to as "T" or "Y" fractures, when they involved both columns, or as unicondylar fractures, when they involved only one column. With improvements and refinements in operative fracture management over the past 30 years, a greater understanding of the complexity and variability of fracture patterns affecting the distal humerus has occurred. Ideally, classifications of fractures should provide a common basis for reporting results, permitting comparisons between different surgeons and cohorts of patients. In addition, the classification should guide decision making and enable some degree of prognostication for each patient. Finally, the classification system should be easy to use, widely accepted, and reproducible.[90] At this time, there is no fracture classification system for the distal humerus that fulfills these objectives adequately.[161] Suboptimal observer variability has been demonstrated in several independent reports examining numerous classification systems, suggesting that this problem is not unique to classification systems of fractures of the distal humerus.[6,7,11,32,56,65,81] Despite these shortcomings, a review of the relevant classification systems provides insight into the possible fracture patterns of the distal humerus.

Current Classification Systems and Concepts

Comprehensive

Column Concept
Jupiter has recommended that the distal humerus be described as two diverging columns supporting an intercalary articular surface, the trochlea, rather than as rounded projections known as condyles.[70] Conceptualizing the distal humerus as medial and lateral columns more accurately describes the injury patterns and allows consistency in the general fracture categories. The Mehne and Matta classification is based on the surgical anatomy, and the columnar concept[70,101] and helps to formulate an effective preoperative surgical tactic. The basic surgical aim is to restore all three elements of the distal humeral triangle (medial column, lateral column, and intervening trochlea) with enough stability to allow early functional movement. Using this classification system, there are three basic fracture categories: intra-articular, extra-articular intracapsular, and extracapsular. Intra-articular fractures are subclassified as single- or bicolumnar injuries, capitellar fractures, or trochlear fractures. Extra-articular intracapsular fractures traverse both columns of the distal humerus without involving the articular surface and are uncommon fractures more likely to be seen in the pediatric population. Extracapsular fractures are composed of injuries to the medial or lateral epicondyles.

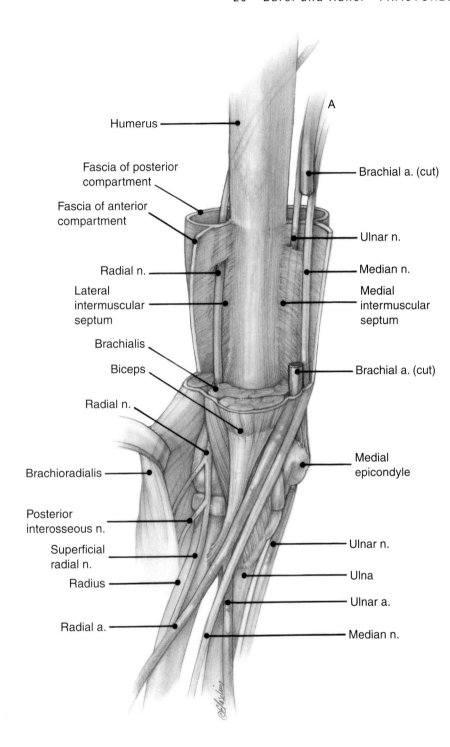

A

Humerus

Fascia of posterior compartment

Fascia of anterior compartment

Radial n.

Lateral intermuscular septum

Brachialis

Biceps

Radial n.

Brachioradialis

Posterior interosseous n.

Superficial radial n.

Radius

Radial a.

Brachial a. (cut)

Ulnar n.

Median n.

Medial intermuscular septum

Brachial a. (cut)

Medial epicondyle

Ulnar n.

Ulna

Ulnar a.

Median n.

FIGURE 20-4. Relationships of the major anatomic structures within the upper extremity. The ulnar nerve travels from the anterior compartment to the posterior compartment, the radial nerve passes from the posterior compartment to the anterior compartment through the lateral intermuscular septum, and the median nerve stays in the anterior compartment between the biceps and the brachialis.

Intra-articular Fractures

Single-Column Fractures. Single-column injuries are uncommon (Fig. 20-7).[76] They are divided into medial or lateral *column* fractures, rather than medial or lateral *condyle* fractures as previously described by Milch.[102] Lateral column fractures are reportedly more common than medial column fractures.[102,116] Rather than emphasizing the involvement of the lateral trochlear ridge, as Milch suggests,[102] this classification system differentiates two types of single-column fractures, namely, "high" fractures

and "low" fractures. "High" fractures have the following characteristics:

- The fractured column contains the bulk of the trochlea.
- The ulna and radius follow the displacement of the fractured column.
- Internal fixation is predictable, because of the size of the fragment.

"Low" single-column fractures have the opposite characteristics for each of the just-mentioned items. Originally, these injuries were believed to be the result of abduction or

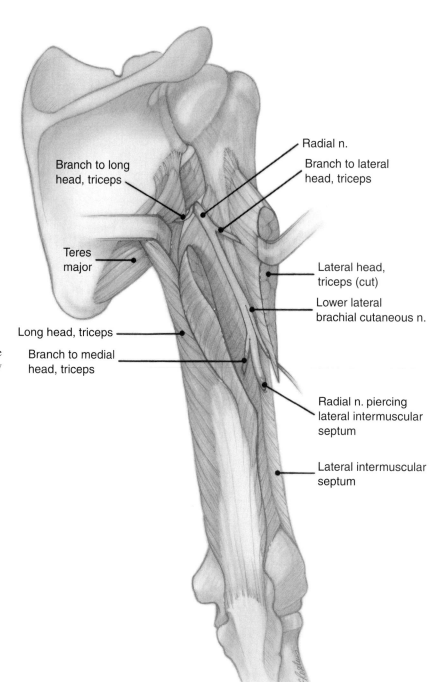

FIGURE 20-5. The posterior view of the humerus focusing on the midshaft to the elbow joint.

adduction forces, with involvement of the lateral trochlear ridge being a major determinant of elbow stability.[102] Jupiter, conversely, suggests that extensive capsular injury and collateral ligament rupture is more likely to be responsible for the ultimate displacement of the fragment than involvement of the lateral trochlear ridge.[16,70]

Bicolumnar Fractures. Fractures that involve both columns comprise the vast majority of injuries to the distal humerus and, by definition, affect all three limbs of the distal humeral triangle. In this classification system, bicolumnar fractures are classified in a descriptive fashion, with comminution being a variant superimposed on the

basic fracture pattern (Fig. 20-8).[70,101] The main patterns include:

1. "T"-pattern, which may be "high" or "low," depending on whether the transverse component of the fracture is above or below the superior limit of the olecranon fossa
2. "Y"-pattern
3. "H"-pattern
4. Lamba pattern, described as medial if the obliquely oriented supracondylar fracture line travels from proximal medial to distal lateral, or as lateral, if the fracture line travels from proximal lateral to distal medial

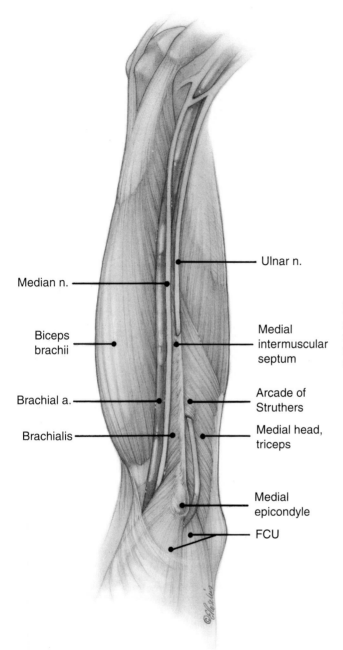

Median n.

Biceps
brachii

Brachial a.

Brachialis

Ulnar n.

Medial
intermuscular
septum

Arcade of
Struthers

Medial head,
triceps

Medial
epicondyle

FCU

FIGURE 20-6. The course of the ulnar nerve as it proceeds through the medial intermuscular septum of the upper extremity as it travels toward the elbow. Note the relationship of the brachial artery to the median nerve.

The value of this classification system is in differentiating fracture patterns that occur at or below the level of the olecranon and coronoid fossae.[135] The more distal fractures produce small articular fragments that challenge secure fixation. The "H"-type injury produces a small trochlear fragment that may be completely devoid of soft tissue attachments. This fragment is frequently difficult to secure, and the potential for avascular necrosis exists.[135]

Extra-articular Intracapsular Fractures. Unlike supracondylar fractures, the transcolumnar fracture lies partially or entirely within the joint capsule of the distal humerus. Transcolumnar fractures display a main fracture line that crosses the distal humerus without involving the distal humeral articular surface. The lack of articular involvement differentiates them from the more common bicolumnar

(intra-articular) patterns. Transcolumnar fractures are distinguished from one another on the basis of the location and orientation of the major fracture line. This gives rise to four basic transcolumnar fracture patterns: high, low, abduction, and adduction (Fig. 20-9). The high and low patterns can be further subdivided into flexion and extension subgroups. These fractures are uncommon in adults, and the literature specifically discussing this injury type is limited.[70,127] Several authors have suggested that this fracture, when encountered, is usually more common in elderly persons with osteopenic bone.[13,59,127] Important surgical considerations for management of this fracture type include:

1. The more distal the fracture is (low types), the more difficult neutralization of the articular fragment becomes.[13] This is worsened in the presence of osteopenic bone.[59]

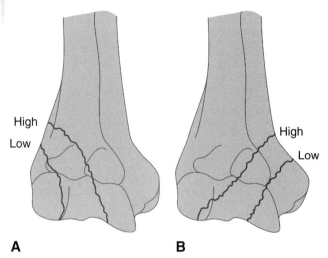

FIGURE 20-7. **A,** Lateral column fracture of the distal humerus. **B,** Medial column fracture of the distal humerus.

2. Those fractures managed nonoperatively or with nonrigid fixation may develop excessive callus formation that obliterates the olecranon, coronoid, and radial fossae, resulting in a loss of motion.[13,59]

AO/ASIF System

The AO/ASIF classification is a comprehensive alphanumeric fracture classification system that distinguishes extra-articular, partial articular (where continuity is maintained between the shaft and a portion of the articular surface), and complete articular injuries.[115] The three main categories, types A, B, and C, group injuries according to increasing severity, intuitively suggesting that a partial articular injury is more severe than an extra-articular injury and that a complete articular injury is more severe than a partial articular injury. Within each type, emphasis is placed on the comminution of the supracondylar metaphysis and/or the articular surface. All three types are extensively subdivided to include most fracture patterns. Type C3 fractures are the most severe, with significant comminution of the articular surface and supracondylar area.

Although involvement of the articular surface is an integral component of most injuries of the distal humerus and a component of the classification systems already described, identification of fracture patterns unique to the articular surface continues to evolve. Conceptually, injuries of the articular surface of the distal humerus may be considered as a spectrum, rather than as discrete entities, because the components of the articular injury may be found in isolation (pure articular injury) or in association with supracondylar injury.

Capitellum

Fractures of the capitellum have been recognized since the mid-19th century (Fig. 20-10).[47] Despite their rarity,[16] two types of fractures have traditionally been described.[4,28,100,147] The type I, or Hahn-Steinthal injury, is a fracture of the capitellum that involves a large portion of the osseous structure of the capitellum.[47,153] The fragment varies in size

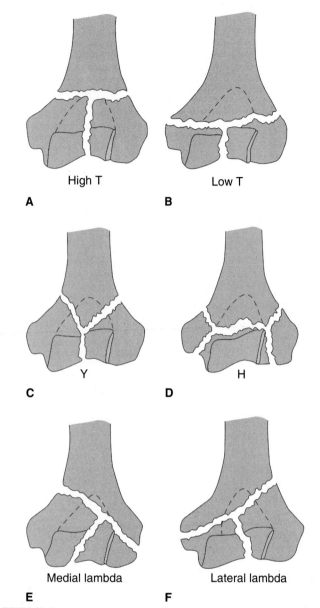

FIGURE 20-8. Bicolumnar fracture classification of fractures of the distal humerus.

and usually contains a part of the adjacent lip of the trochlea.[4] The type II fracture, or Kocher-Lorenz pattern, is superficial and mainly involves the chondral surface of the capitellum with very little bone attached.[78,88] This fracture type essentially results in a shell of capitellar articular cartilage with minimal subchondral bone.[4,28,100,147] More recently, Bryan and Morrey have classified capitellar fractures into three types.[16] Type I fractures are complete fractures of the capitellum (similar to the Hahn-Steinthal lesion), type II fractures are superficial lesions (corresponding to the Kocher-Lorenz pattern), and type III fractures are comminuted patterns. A fourth type of capitellar fracture, described by McKee and associates, is termed the *coronal shear fracture*.[96] This fracture involves the capitellum but also extends beyond the lateral trochlear ridge to include a variable, but significant, portion of the trochlea.

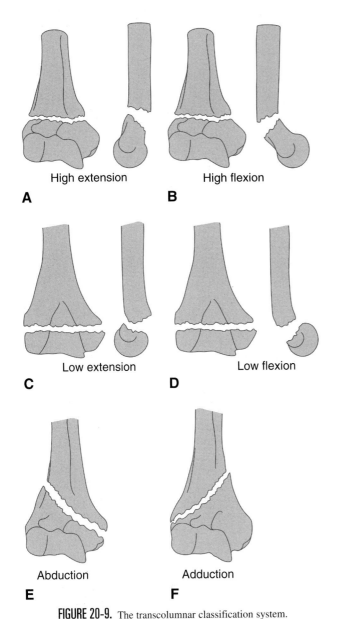

FIGURE 20-9. The transcolumnar classification system.

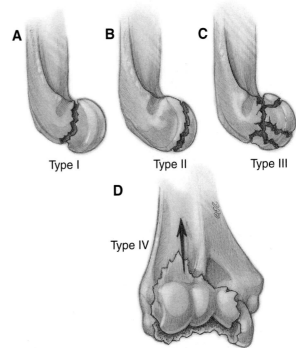

FIGURE 20-10. The four types of capitellum fractures. **A,** Type I fracture is a single fracture line of the capitellum that involves a fair-sized piece of bone as well as the anterior aspect of the joint. **B,** Type II is just a thin fragment, with very little bone attached to the anterior cartilage. Type II fractures have much less bone attached to the cartilage than is seen in type I fractures. **C,** Type III is a fracture of the capitellum that is in multiple fragments. **D,** A type IV fracture includes the capitellum but also extends over medially to take off the lateral trochlear lip.

The radiographic hallmark of the coronal shear fracture pattern is the "double-arc" sign on the lateral radiograph, which represents the subchondral bone of the capitellum and lateral trochlear ridge.[96]

Despite the different fracture patterns and variations that exist, fractures of the capitellum are essentially shearing coronal plane injuries.[95] The mechanism of these fractures appears to be an axial load, with the final fracture configuration determined by the degree of elbow flexion at the time of loading.[16,61,86,96,121,141]

Trochlea

Isolated trochlear fractures are exceedingly rare injuries.[16,59,68] Although a formal classification system has not been developed, the two main patterns are fractures of the entire trochlear process and osteochondral fractures.[42,59,100] Jupiter, and others, have suggested that the rarity of these injuries may be due to the trochlea lying protected within the depth of the semilunar notch of the olecranon, without capsular, muscular, or ligamentous attachments.[13,59,68] The mechanism of injury remains speculative given the rarity of the injury, but it may involve the coronoid acting as a fulcrum when a force is applied to the flexed elbow.[68] The osteochondral patterns, however, may be associated with elbow dislocations, implying the involvement of a shearing force.[13,42]

Other Articular Patterns

Emphasizing the fact that articular fractures of the distal humerus may represent a continuum of injury, Ring and Jupiter evaluated 21 patients with pure articular fractures of the distal humerus.[137] The fracture fragments included and extended beyond the capitellum but did not extend above the base of the olecranon fossa. Five different patterns of injury were identified with increasing involvement of the posterolateral articular surface and medial articular surface (Fig. 20-11). Type 1 injuries are the coronal shear fractures previously described by McKee.[96] Type 2 fractures are type 1 fractures with involvement of the lateral epicondyle. Type 3 fractures have associated impaction of the metaphyseal bone posterior to the capitellum. Type 4 fractures demonstrate the additional feature of a fracture of the posterior aspect of the trochlea. Finally, type 5 fractures are type 4 fractures with a fracture of the medial epicondyle. These specific fracture types represent a progression of injury

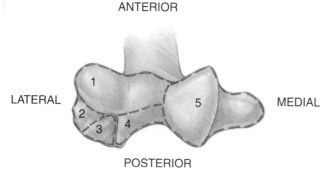

ANTERIOR

LATERAL   MEDIAL

POSTERIOR

FIGURE 20-11. Classification of pure articular injuries of the distal humerus.

severity extending from an isolated articular component displaced in the frontal plane to combinations of shearing and impaction injuries of the capitellum and trochlea with a limited zone of metaphyseal bone support. Because of the difficulty in appreciating some of the potential fracture fragments with standard radiographs, CT scanning with three-dimensional reconstructions may enhance comprehension and preoperative planning.[96,137]

HISTORICAL REVIEW

The history of fracture care was marked by a significant change in management philosophy during the 1960s. The group is known as Arbeitsgemeinschaft für Osteosynthesefragen (AO), or the Association for the Study of Internal Fixation (ASIF) in English-speaking regions. The principles, as originally written, especially apply to fractures of the distal humerus.[114,143]

1. Fracture reduction and fixation to restore anatomic relationships, particularly of the articular surface
2. Stability by fixation or splintage, as the personality of the fracture and injury requires
3. Preservation of the blood supply to soft tissues and bone by careful handling and gentle reduction techniques
4. Early and safe mobilization of the part and the patient

Prior to the AO's development, and before wider acceptance of their principles, strong opposition to operative management of distal humerus fractures existed. Patterson wrote, "Since open operation leaves so much scar tissue and, as a rule, gives no better results than conservative closed methods, an effective means of applying traction to the region of the olecranon is very useful."[124] Reich recognized that open reduction was the only procedure that offered any hope of complete functional restoration.[133] He also recognized that the unsatisfactory results seen with open treatment were due to the "frank exposure" and the difficulty in reducing and maintaining reduction.[133] In the decades preceding the AO advances, numerous publications debated the superiority of results in patients treated with open versus conservative methods.* Numerous closed techniques were described, including manipulation and casting, olecranon traction, cast traction, and condylar reductions using ice tongs or clamps.[54,74,133,139,154] Influential authors such as Watson-Jones and the contradictory views of 1964 and 1966

Instructional Course Lectures from the American Academy of Orthopaedic Surgeons on these fractures continued the controversy.[74,104,163] Although known for their classification system, Riseborough and Radin concluded their article by noting that open reduction and adequate internal fixation is not easy and would seem to offer little chance of a good outcome.[139] The authors believed that open reduction was very rarely indicated. Advocates of either closed or open management recognized that the inability to obtain and maintain a reduction and the subsequent need for rigid immobilization ultimately resulted in poor outcomes (Table 20-1).[2,14,29,57,63]

During the late 1960s and early 1970s an increasing number of publications reported satisfactory results with operative reduction and fixation of distal humerus fractures.† A review of the operative techniques contained in these reports demonstrates an increasing use of plate and screw fixation rather than Kirschner wire fixation and recommendations of early postoperative mobilization. The importance of proper technique was illustrated by Johansson and Olerud,[63] who suggested that, "The osteosynthesis demands as stable fixation as possible, and in our experience this is best obtained by screws, but at the same time exact apposition of the fracture surfaces is required." They further noted that stable osteosynthesis eliminated the need for postoperative immobilization.[63] The 1980 report by Horne underscored the poor results that are obtained when the goals of open reduction and internal fixation (ORIF) are not met.[57] He wrote, "The availability of excellent equipment for the internal fixation of fractures is not an indication for its use," ultimately concluding that, except for simple fractures and unicondylar fractures, conservative management is the recommended treatment.[57] Shortly thereafter, Jupiter published the results of 34 intercondylar fractures of the humerus managed operatively using the techniques advanced by the AO/ASIF.[71] The high proportion of good or excellent results, using a score incorporating range of motion and pain, finally solidified the advantages of ORIF for these fractures.

The last three decades of the 20th century have demonstrated tremendous advances in the understanding of the various fracture patterns, the techniques used to obtain anatomic reduction and fixation, and the evaluation of these results. An improved appreciation of fracture patterns and techniques together with substantial progress in the understanding of surgical anatomy of the elbow has allowed dramatic advances in post-traumatic management of the stiff and/or arthritic elbow. Advances in arthroplasty and newer fixation techniques are both options for the management of comminuted fractures of the physiologically sound but elderly patient. The optimal implant, however, remains unknown. The use of tensioned-wire fixators and allograft materials have permitted salvage of the most challenging acute high-energy injuries in the younger patient. Perhaps most importantly, the development and implementation of limb- and patient-specific outcome scores has allowed investigators to more accurately associate patient satisfaction with objective measures. These scoring systems appear

---

*See references 19, 20, 29, 31, 54, 102, 103, 124, 133, 154, and 157.
†See references 14, 19, 34, 52, 68, 72, 99, 142, 160, and 166.

Table 20-1
CLOSED AND INDIRECT METHODS OF REDUCTION OF DISTAL HUMERUS FRACTURES

Study	Year	Description
Hitzrot[54]	1932	Described 25 patients treated with traction. Based on his results, the author strongly advised against open reduction, stating that anatomic reduction was of secondary importance. Eastwood would later agree, stating that a perfect anatomic reduction is not necessary to obtain a good result. Few agree with this view today.
Patterson[124]	1935	Described a technique of closed reduction, cast immobilization, and pin traction through the cast, rather than the olecranon. The flexion/extension arc was 130 degrees. The arm was noted to be "painless and strong."
Reich[133]	1936	Described a reduction technique using ice tongs to compress the condylar displacement, with portable traction to allow the patient to be ambulatory. The results in 6 patients were noted to be good in 3, fair in 2, and poor in 1. These outcomes were believed to be better than the complications and results demonstrated by ORIF.
Eastwood[29]	1937	Reviewed 14 patients treated with a collar-and-cuff support followed by early elbow mobilization (credited to H. O. Thomas). The results were so satisfactory that the author believed it was unwise to use any other technique and concluded by stating that function is more important than radiographic appearance.
Miller[103]	1939	Described the "blind nailing" technique for intercondylar fractures of the distal humerus. The author surmised that for improved joint function, accurate reduction of joint fractures is important. At the time, it was believed that open techniques created significant additional trauma to uninjured areas of the distal humeral soft tissue envelope. The technique expands on Reich's initial report.
Trynin[154]	1941	Case report of an intercondylar fracture of the distal humerus treated with a carpenter's clamp to reduce the intercondylar fracture. The author summarized the prevailing thinking by stating that, "manipulation and closed reduction are always the method of choice, provided reduction can be obtained by this means." A functional arc of motion with satisfactory union and alignment was obtained.
Watson-Jones[163]	1944	This classic fracture textbook by the influential author concluded that, "Operative reduction and internal fixation is not justified by the results." The surgical dissection, avascularity of fragments, and the use of metallic implants were believed to result in dense adhesions and stiffness. Manipulative reduction, brief casting, and motion were recommended.
Keon-Cohen[74]	1966	The variance of opinion continued as this author wrote "little or nothing is gained by attempting to reassemble the fragments and contain them by some form of internal fixation. Even the classic T and Y fractures are best left alone; the results of operative treatment with internal fixation in perfect anatomical reposition are disappointing almost invariably; in fact, I will go further and say that usually they are extremely bad." He advocated closed reduction and immobilization in the less-comminuted fractures and olecranon pin traction for 3 weeks in the more comminuted types.
Riseborough and Radin[139]	1969	Unveiled the Riseborough-Radin classification system. The authors suggested that this classification allowed therapeutic decision making based on the amount of rotatory deformity and comminution. Despite this therapeutic classification system, they believed that ORIF was rarely indicated. This classification system would be utilized for approximately 2 decades. The best results were obtained in 22 of 29 patients treated with casting or traction.
Brown and Morgan[10]	1971	Described the "bag of bones" technique for closed management of intercondylar "T"-shaped fractures of the distal humerus. The flexion/extension arc in 6 of 10 patients was greater than 105 degrees. Better motion appeared to be obtained in the elderly, with younger adult patients having restricted arcs less than 85 degrees. These results continued to challenge those obtained by proponents of ORIF. The role of the "bag of bones" technique in the elderly was strengthened.
Horne[57]	1980	Review of 50 patients with supracondylar, condylar, and supracondylar/intercondylar fracture patterns. Of the 29 patients treated surgically, 16 had poor results compared with 6 of 21 patients treated with casting. Inadequate internal fixation and prolonged postoperative immobilization were responsible for the poor results. The author recommended conservative treatment for supracondylar/intercondylar distal humerus fractures, particularly when comminuted.

to more closely correlate with the patient's ultimate functional abilities than the more traditional measurement scales, such as range of motion or radiographic appearance. These outcome devices will greatly assist in the assessment of new management techniques in the future (Table 20-2).

OPERATIVE MANAGEMENT

Operative management of specific fractures of the distal humerus requires identification of both fracture and soft tissue particulars, as well as patient characteristics, including age, associated injuries, comorbidities, and functional level before injury. These considerations are then used to determine the reconstructive tactic, including patient positioning, operative approach, and choice of fixation implants. Important preoperative decisions include the following:

- Determination of whether the fracture is reconstructable or if the patient is better served by elbow arthroplasty
- An estimation of the need for visualization of the articular surface to determine the surgical approach and handling of the extensor mechanism
- Identification of a stable fixation construct that will allow early unrestricted range of motion

Table 20-2
OPEN METHODS OF REDUCTION OF DISTAL HUMERUS FRACTURES

Study	Year	Description
Van Gorder[157]	1940	Reported 8 patients with fractures of the distal humerus operatively managed using a posterior "triceps-turndown" approach (credited to Campbell) where an inverted "V" of the triceps aponeurosis is incised and reflected distally to gain exposure. Subsequent authors used it for open reduction of similar fractures.
Cassebaum[20]	1952	Utilized the olecranon osteotomy for management of nine "T" and "Y" fractures of the distal humerus. This appears to be the first report of the trans-olecranon approach for management of distal humerus fractures. The original description was credited to MacAusland in 1915.[89]
Evans[31]	1953	As a way of improving the results of closed treatment and minimizing the complications seen with open treatment, Evans reported on 5 patients treated with limited fixation. A medial or lateral approach was used, depending on the fracture pattern, and reduction and fixation of only the articular surface was performed. The supracondylar component was managed with a brief period of immobilization in flexion, followed by motion.
Milch[102]	1964	Classic early work on isolated fractures of the humeral condyles, their injury mechanism, and their relationship with elbow dislocation. It was hypothesized that involvement of the lateral wall of the trochlea was associated with injuries that also led to elbow dislocation. In those elbows with dislocations, Milch recommended open treatment.
Miller[104]	1964	This Instructional Course Lecture reviewed a 3-year experience of fractures of the distal humerus treated with closed means versus ORIF. In one of the first comparative series of distal humerus fractures, the author noted that the operative group had a substantially greater elbow range of motion than the closed treatment group (111 vs. 47 degrees). This author was convinced that ORIF was the procedure of choice but recognized the following limitation: "If the arm requires immobilization after open reduction and fixation, then the advantage of surgery is lost."
Kelly and Griffin[73]	1969	The authors described 5 patients with "T"-condylar fractures of the distal humerus treated with ORIF using an anterior approach. The focus was on fixation of the articular surface. Rigid fixation of the condyles to the shaft was not performed. There does not appear to be any other report of this approach for these fractures.
Cassebaum[19]	1969	Reports 36 distal humeral "T" and "Y" fractures treated with internal fixation using a trans-olecranon approach. An elbow arc of 50 to 165 degrees was recognized as excellent because the majority of tasks could be completed within this range. The author's range of motion criteria for excellent, good, and fair would be used extensively in subsequent reports.
Muller, et al.[114]	1970	The first English edition of the AO manual was published.
Bryan and Bickel[14]	1971	Reviewed 25 operatively managed distal humerus fractures treated through a posterior approach. The authors preferred screw fixation rather than use of Kirschner wires and recommended early mobilization after secure internal fixation. They suggested that their patients would not have done as well with closed methods but that the open technique should be left to an experienced surgeon. They also warned that on occasion, the difficulties encountered during ORIF of comminuted distal humerus fractures "may be mortifying." This paper was presented during a period when there was no consensus in the literature regarding the best method of treatment for these fractures.

Table 20-2

OPEN METHODS OF REDUCTION OF DISTAL HUMERUS FRACTURES—cont'd

Study	Year	Description
Scharplatz and Allgower[142]	1975	Review of 105 fracture-dislocations of the elbow. The principles of the AO operative treatment of the distal humerus were outlined: reconstruction of the joint surface first, the trochlea being the most important part, then connection to the shaft of the humerus.
Jupiter, et al.[71]	1985	The results of 34 intercondylar fractures of the distal humerus treated with operative fixation using AO techniques. Of 34 patients 27 obtained good to excellent results at a mean of 5.8 years. The ability to achieve improved and more predictable results with operative treatment even in the comminuted fracture was confirmed.
Zagorski, et al.[166]	1986	Compared the results of 42 intra-articular fractures of the distal humerus. Twenty-nine were treated operatively with screws or plate/screw constructs. Thirteen were treated nonoperatively. Seventy-six percent of patients treated with open techniques had a good to excellent result as compared with 8% in the conservatively treated group. The authors believed that final fracture reduction was clearly related to functional end results.
Jupiter, et al.[72]	1988	Twenty-two unicondylar fractures were managed operatively: 18 had good to excellent results. This paper illustrated AO principles applied to unicondylar fractures.
Helfet and Hotchkiss[48]	1990	This biomechanical study evaluated implant configurations and distal humeral fracture stability. The 90-degree orthogonal plate construct was identified and proven to be mechanically superior. The authors could not find a difference between one-third tubular plates, 3.5-mm reconstruction plates, or mixed plates.
John, et al.[64]	1994	The first large series evaluating contemporary ORIF techniques in distal humerus fractures in the elderly. The average age was 80 years, with a range from 75 to 90. Eighty-five percent were believed to have a functional arc of motion (>90 degrees). Sixty-six percent had no pain. Implant failures were related to the use of one-third tubular plates.
Garcia, et al.[37]	2002	Consecutive series of 19 patients, all greater than 60 years old treated with primary total elbow arthroplasty (TEA) for non-reconstructable fracture of the distal humerus. There was no associated inflammatory illness. Three-year follow-up demonstrated 68% with no pain and a mean Mayo score of 93 (excellent). This paper clearly demonstrates the early advantages of TEA in this patient population. Long-term data, however, are lacking. ORIF versus TEA in the elderly population continues to be debated.

Timing of Operative Intervention

Fractures of the distal humerus are best managed early, but as with most complex, intra-articular fractures, definitive treatment should be delayed until optimal surgical resources, personnel, and the necessary implants are available. Preoperative planning is essential and should include imaging studies necessary to request the resources mentioned earlier. Patients with isolated injuries are managed at the discretion of the surgeon, readiness of the operating suite, and the availability of implants. Elderly patients or patients with associated comorbidities must be stabilized before fracture reconstruction. Patients who are managed within 24 hours appear to have fewer complications associated with heterotopic ossification and elbow stiffness and may be more likely to return to work.[82]

Polytrauma

Patients with multiple orthopedic trauma or associated multisystemic trauma are managed according to their overall status and prioritization of their other injuries. This situation may, however, result in a significant delay in definitive management from days to weeks. Such delays ultimately make fracture reduction and fixation more diffi-cult and jeopardize the long-term outcome. Close collaboration with the trauma team leader, general surgeon, or intensivist allows these team members to appreciate the importance and benefits of early fracture fixation. Similarly, the treating orthopedist should be available to proceed with fixation once the patient's condition has been stabilized and he or she has been cleared for surgery.

Open Fractures

Open fractures are managed urgently with irrigation and débridement. Definitive internal fixation should be applied when the wound is free of contamination and the general condition of the patient permits the procedure.[43,113] McKee reviewed the results of 26 open intra-articular supracondylar fractures managed with a posterior exposure and medial and lateral column plating.[98] The overall infection rate in this series was 11% (3 of 26); however, only one patient developed a deep infection requiring surgical débridement.[98] Other authors have noted a deep infection rate of as high as 28% in high-energy fractures.[43] However, a much larger proportion of Gustilo type III fractures[45,46] were noted in the latter study as compared with McKee's report (45% vs. 15.4%) and may account for the apparent discrepancy in infection rates.

Fractures in Physiologically Elderly and Total Elbow Replacement

The management of functional but physiologically elderly patients is individualized because good results have been demonstrated with both ORIF and total elbow arthroplasty (TEA).[21,36,37,64,120,126,131] Unfortunately, there are no randomized controlled trials that compare ORIF and TEA in this patient population. The available literature evaluating elbow arthroplasty in older patients with acute fractures demonstrates excellent early results, with a satisfactory flexion/extension arc of approximately 110 degrees and excellent relief of pain.[21,33,36,37,120,131] Unfortunately, the length of follow-up in these studies is between 2 and 4 years and does not address the long-term concerns of implant loosening, mechanical failure, revision requirements, and functional implications. Long-term results in patients with TEA for inflammatory arthritis appear durable.[40,53,146,165] However, the results of TEA in patients with post-traumatic arthritis show lower patient satisfaction and possibly greater mechanical failure rates than those with inflammatory arthritis.[53,146]

ORIF in elderly patients has also been demonstrated to give satisfactory results. Pereles demonstrated an average arc of motion of 112 degrees, functional Mayo elbow scores, and no difference in SF-36 scores when compared with normal data in 14 patients with distal humerus fractures treated with ORIF.[126] Twelve patients had good or excellent results, but only 25% of patients reported no pain. The mean age in this group was 70 years. John evaluated 49 older patients (mean age 80 years) an average of 18 months after ORIF.[64] Eighty-five percent achieved good or very good results, with 85% having a range of motion of 90 degrees or greater. Sixty-six percent of these patients reported no pain. This group included extra-articular fractures (16%), unicolumnar fractures (27%), and bicolumnar fractures (57%).

Frankle and colleagues compared the results of TEA with ORIF in female patients older than 65 years of age sustaining distal humerus fractures.[33] Patients treated with TEA demonstrated significantly better results using the Mayo Elbow Performance Score than those treated with ORIF. The authors suggest that women older than the age of 65 with significant associated comorbidities (rheumatoid arthritis, osteoporosis, and conditions requiring systemic steroids, among others) and the presence of articular comminution be managed with TEA. Provided that the articular fracture components are large, the authors prefer ORIF as long as the patient's physiologic age is younger than 90 years.

We agree with the findings of Frankle and colleagues that successful management of these patients must take into account the patient's physiologic age, functionality, associated comorbidities, and fracture characteristics. Fracture characteristics in this patient population that are unreliably stabilized with internal fixation include:

- Significant comminution of the trochlea
- Associated coronal plane fracture patterns
- Fractures that occur almost entirely below the olecranon fossa

In these injuries, the small fragments combined with frequently coexisting osteoporosis make total elbow arthroplasty an attractive alternative. CT is particularly useful in assessing the presence of coronal plane fracture fragments.

Patient Position and Anesthesia

Fractures of the distal humerus can be managed with the patient in the supine, lateral, or prone position, with the choice based on the anticipated exposure, the presence of other injuries, and surgeon preference.[50,51,99,117,142] The lateral and prone positions (Fig. 20-12) are most commonly employed when proceeding with posterior exposures of the elbow. The supine position is typically reserved for lateral elbow exposures or for the patient with multisystemic trauma that precludes lateral or prone positions.

ORIF of fractures of the distal humerus is typically a lengthy procedure requiring a general anesthetic. Postoperative pain control may include the use of selective upper extremity nerve blockades; however, the postoperative neurologic examination of the hand will be impaired for the duration of the block. A sterile tourniquet may be employed provided that it can be placed proximal enough on the arm to avoid interference with ORIF of the fracture.

OPERATIVE EXPOSURES

CRITICAL POINTS: OPERATIVE EXPOSURES

PARATRICIPITAL

- It elevates the triceps from posterior aspects of distal humerus and medial and lateral intermuscular septa.
- It can be converted to olecranon osteotomy if needed.
- Laterally, it can be developed into an extensile posterior exposure.
- It offers the least visualization of the articular surface when compared with other exposures.
- It is least disruptive to the extensor mechanism.

Indications

- Supraconodylar and transcondylar fractures
- Bicolumnar fractures with simple articular involvement
- Medial or lateral column only can be developed for treatment of unicolumnar fractures with simple articular involvement.

OLECRANON OSTEOTOMY

- It improves maximal articular surface visualization.
- Osteotomy nonunion rates are approximately 10%.
- Symptoms may occur secondary to prominence from osteotomy fixation implants.

Indications

- Unicolumnar or bicolumnar fractures with articular comminution

CRITICAL POINTS: OPERATIVE EXPOSURES—cont'd

Indications—cont'd

■ Articular fracture variants with significant posterior and/or medial involvement

■ Authors' preferred exposure for fractures of the distal humerus with significant articular displacement or comminution

TRICEPS-SPLITTING

■ Familiar exposure of the distal third of the humeral meta-diaphysis is provided.

■ For adequate articular visualization the triceps insertion is dissected off the proximal one fourth of the ulna medially and laterally.

Indications

■ Supracondylar and transcondylar fractures

■ Bicolumnar fractures with significant disruption of the triceps aponeurosis (i.e., open fractures)

■ Geriatric fractures that may require conversion to TEA

BRYAN-MORREY "TRICEPS-SPARING"

■ Extensor mechanism is reflected off the posterior aspect of the humerus and olecranon from medial to lateral.

Indication

■ Authors' preferred exposure for ORIF of geriatric fractures that may require conversion to TEA

TRICEPS-REFLECTING ANCONEUS PEDICLE (TRAP)

■ It preserves neurovascular supply to anconeus.

■ It allows conversion to TEA if required.

■ Articular visualization is similar to that of both triceps-splitting and triceps-sparing approaches.

Indications

■ Similar to those of triceps-splitting and triceps-sparing approaches

LATERAL

■ Initial dissection should be anterior to the lateral epicondyle, along a line bisecting the capitellum.

■ Medial column articular injuries are not well visualized.

CRITICAL POINTS: OPERATIVE EXPOSURES—cont'd

LATERAL—cont'd

■ Visualization is enhanced by:
  • Elevating the musculature and joint capsule from the anterior aspect of the supracondylar ridge of the distal humerus.
  • Detachment of the lateral ligamentous complex from the lateral epicondylar region.

Indication

■ Isolated lateral column articular injuries (capitellar fractures and variants)

Virtually all fractures of the distal humerus treated operatively can be approached through a midline posterior skin incision (Fig. 20-13). An effort should be made to deviate the incision a full 2 cm away from the tip of the olecranon. Whether one chooses to deviate medial or lateral to the olecranon process is a surgeon preference. The incision is carried through subcutaneous fat and muscle investing the fascia of the triceps. The lateral and medial plane of dissection is directed between the triceps muscle and the muscle-investing fascia. The next step in any exposure of the medial column is identification and protection of the ulnar nerve. The ulnar nerve will be seen as the medial intermuscular septum is approached. The nerve is mobilized and tagged with a Penrose drain secured by a loose knot. Instruments are not attached to the Penrose drain to prevent excessive traction on the nerve. The medial intermuscular septum is incised if fracture management requires exposure of the anteromedial elbow. Similarly, the laterally directed dissection leads to the lateral intermuscular septum. Unfortunately, the course of the radial nerve is less obvious than its medial counterpart, but there are some clues to its identification. First, the nerve crosses through the intermuscular septum approximately halfway along the length of the humerus, or half the distance between the tip of the acromion and the tip of the olecranon. Second, if the dissection is directed from the lateral epicondyle proximally, the cutaneous branches to the posterior lateral arm and forearm will be encountered in the dissection of the lateral intermuscular septum. These cutaneous nerves are branches of the radial nerve, and they can be followed proximally to their origin. Finally, and least reliable, is the fact that the radial nerve travels around the humerus in a bed of fat. Careful proximally directed dissections will lead to this bed of fat and the radial nerve. In the majority of distal humerus fractures treated with open reduction the radial nerve will not need to be exposed. The lateral intermuscular septum, however, will be divided for exposure to the anterolateral elbow region. This approach provides near-circumferential access to both medial and lateral columns.[107] Importantly, this posterior midline approach can be utilized for later reconstructive procedures, obviating the need for multiple skin incisions.

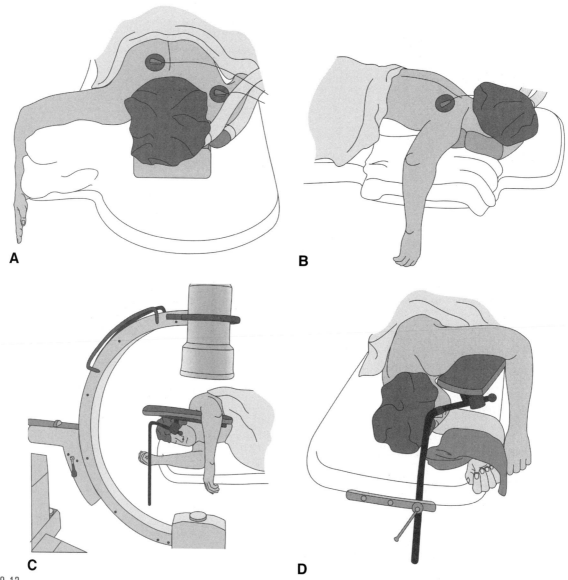

FIGURE 20-12. **A** and **B,** A surgical patient in the prone position before ORIF. **C** and **D,** The same patient in the lateral position. Note the "C"-arm used for anteroposterior radiographs.

How the extensor mechanism of the elbow is subsequently managed is dictated by the fracture personality. For significant intra-articular fractures of the distal humerus requiring direct visualization of the articular surface there are two options for management of the extensor mechanism: an olecranon osteotomy or soft tissue mobilization about the olecranon.

Paratricipital Approach

The least disruptive posterior approach is the paratricipital exposure.[3,145] This dissection entails mobilization of the triceps off the posterior aspect of the medial and lateral intermuscular septa and the posterior aspect of the humerus. Medially, the ulnar nerve is identified and protected. Laterally, the radial nerve is identified and mobilized, allowing the potential to surgically manipulate approximately 95% of the posterior aspect of the humeral shaft.[39] At the

elbow joint, the triceps can be retracted posteriorly and distally, enabling visualization of the posterior aspect of the lateral column and limited visualization of the posterior aspect of the trochlea (Fig. 20-14). Supracondylar fractures, transcondylar fractures, and simple intra-articular fractures (unicolumnar or bicolumnar) without articular comminution are the main injuries that can be managed with this exposure. It is exceedingly difficult to appreciate, let alone secure, comminuted intra-articular fractures of the distal humerus through this exposure.

Olecranon Osteotomy

The olecranon osteotomy is the classic exposure for reduction and fixation of intra-articular fractures of the distal humerus.[19,20,89] As in the paratricipital approach, the triceps muscle is mobilized from the medial and lateral septa and followed distally. The osteotomy is performed at the deepest

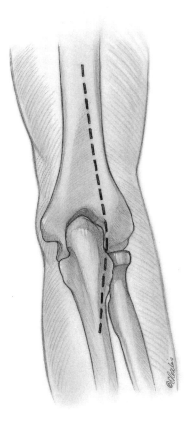

FIGURE 20-13. Posterior view of the upper arm and elbow area showing the location of the skin incision. The ideal surgical incision is a generally straight line that gently curves laterally (or radially) to avoid the tip of the olecranon.

portion of the trochlear notch of the olecranon process and is coincident with an area devoid of articular cartilage, called the "bare area." Transverse and chevron osteotomies have been described, the latter being favored because of its increased postfixation mechanical stability, increased bone surface area, and improved union potential.[35,71] To avoid splitting the proximal olecranon fragment, the apex of the chevron points distally.[95] It is typically initiated with a fine oscillating saw and completed with a thin osteotome. The triceps muscle and the osteotomized proximal half of the olecranon are then reflected superiorly (Fig. 20-15). Techniques of olecranon osteotomy fixation include Kirschner wire/tension band constructs, screw/tension band constructs, and plate fixation.[17,19,20,50-52,71,72] The advantage of the olecranon osteotomy is the excellent and direct visualization of the distal humeral articular surface,[164] enabling anatomic reduction. Complications or disadvantages include osteotomy nonunion, delayed union, and hardware prominence.[52] Increased operative exposure time is a potential drawback of the olecranon osteotomy but may be offset by the visualization afforded for direct articular reduction. The olecranon osteotomy is most commonly used in the management of bicolumnar fractures with articular displacement. However, any articular injury of the distal humerus, including unicondylar fractures, and pure articular fractures extending posterior to the capitellum and/or the posterior aspect of the trochlea are indications for this exposure.[71,137]

Triceps-Splitting Approach

The triceps-splitting approach described by Campbell splits the triceps aponeurosis and medial head in the midline.[18,24,98] Subperiosteal dissection of the distal humerus and proximal ulna is performed both medially and laterally. It is important to understand that this dissection does not cease at the tip of the olecranon but continues along the proximal one fourth of the ulna with dissection of the triceps insertion off the proximal ulna medially and laterally (Fig. 20-16). The joint capsule is divided to allow visualization of the articular surface. At the conclusion of the procedure, the triceps is repaired back to the proximal ulna with interrupted, nonabsorbable suture through osseous drill holes. Advantages of this exposure are its technical ease, the ability to use the trochlear notch as a template against which the distal humerus can be reduced, and the avoidance of hardware about the proximal ulna.[95] A potential complication of this exposure is the loss of strength of elbow extension. McKee and colleagues, however, were unable to demonstrate a difference in elbow extension strength in patients treated with the triceps-splitting approach when compared with patients treated with an olecranon osteotomy, making it a satisfactory alternative to the olecranon osteotomy.[99] The main disadvantage of this exposure is the inability to directly visualize a significant portion of the articular surface. The main indications for this exposure have included bicolumnar intra-articular fractures of the distal humerus and extra-articular supracondylar fractures. This exposure is also indicated when the triceps aponeurosis has been transected by the distal aspect of the humeral diaphysis. When this occurs, the fracture is typically open posteriorly.[98] In this situation, an olecranon osteotomy further disrupts the integrity of the extensor mechanism and is a relative contraindication. McKee and colleagues were able to demonstrate improved results with the triceps-splitting approach in these open injuries when compared with using an olecranon osteotomy.[98]

Bryan-Morrey "Triceps-Sparing" Approach

The Bryan-Morrey "triceps-sparing" approach is commonly used for performing total-elbow arthroplasty procedures,[15] but it may also be used for fixation of fractures of the distal humerus. After a midline posterior skin incision is performed, the ulnar nerve is identified along the medial aspect of the triceps and is elevated from its bed. Dissection carries through the cubital tunnel and fascia over the flexor carpi ulnaris muscle until the first motor branch is identified. Once the ulnar nerve is freed and protected, dissection continues with the elevation of the medial aspect of the triceps off the posterior aspect of the medial intermuscular septum and posterior aspect of the distal humerus. Distally, the fascia over the flexor carpi ulnaris is incised toward the ulna. The triceps insertion is then sharply reflected directly off bone (Fig. 20-17). This medial-to-lateral dissection is continued until the anconeus and triceps can be retracted over the lateral humeral condyle. Because the fascia over the proximal ulna is thin and prone to perforations during its elevation, some authors have described elevation as an osteoperiosteal flap.[125] A small osteotome can be used to elevate the fascia with small petals of bone, which aids in

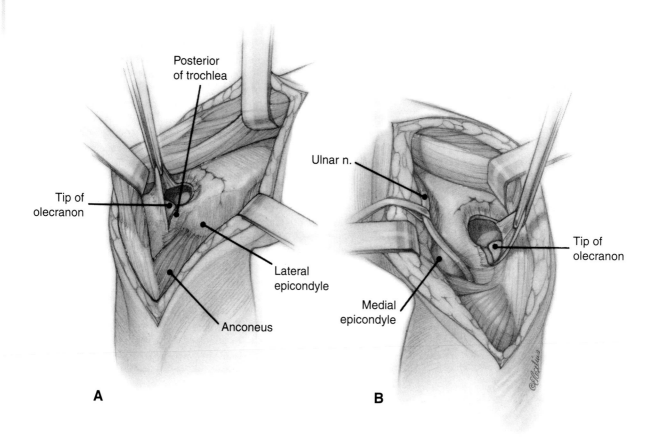

FIGURE 20-14. Paratricipital approach. **A,** Starting at the lateral epicondyle, the triceps is elevated from the posterior aspect of the humerus. A more proximal dissection will reveal the radial nerve crossing the lateral margin of the humerus to enter the anterior compartment of the arm. Through this dissection the lateral column is readily identified. The lateral aspect of the trochlea is appreciated but visualizing the articular surface is difficult. **B,** The medial column and medial aspect of the trochlea are exposed after mobilizing and protecting the ulnar nerve.

FIGURE 20-15. Olecranon osteotomy. The entire posterior aspect of the humerus is exposed and the articular surface visualized after performing an olecranon osteotomy.

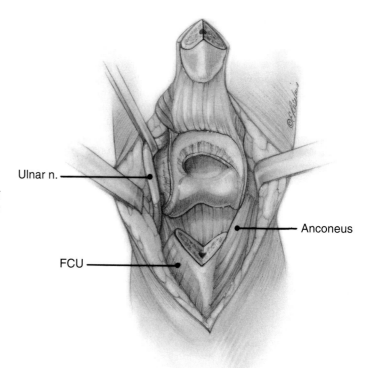

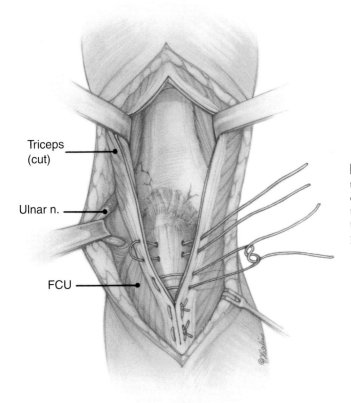

Triceps
(cut)

Ulnar n.

FCU

FIGURE 20-16. Triceps splitting. In this approach, the distal one third of the triceps is simply split longitudinally to the olecranon process. At the olecranon process, the split continues longitudinally, with elevation of the triceps insertion sharply off the bone medially and laterally. The triceps is essentially split into medial and lateral halves and retracted peripherally, allowing visualization of the underlying distal humerus.

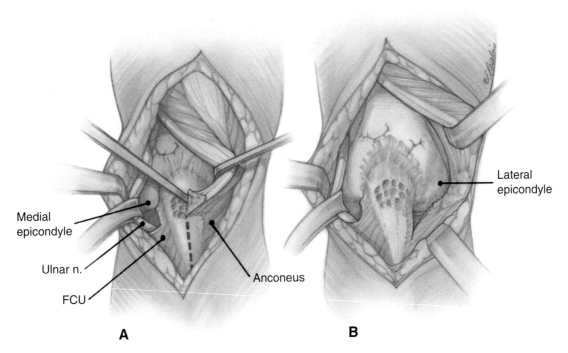

Medial
epicondyle

Ulnar n.

FCU

Anconeus

Lateral
epicondyle

A   **B**

FIGURE 20-17. Bryan-Morrey triceps-sparing approach. **A,** Initiation of the dissection on the medial aspect. **B,** The entire triceps insertion taken off the proximal ulna. Note view of posterior aspect of distal humerus.

repositioning the triceps insertion at the conclusion of the procedure (restoring the normal length-tension relationship) and in healing of the extensor mechanism back to the proximal ulna. The triceps insertion is repaired back to the proximal ulna with nonabsorbable transosseous suture. Advantages and disadvantages of this approach are similar to the triceps-splitting procedure. This exposure is indicated in the older patient undergoing ORIF of a distal humerus fracture that may require intraoperative conversion to a total elbow arthroplasty.

Triceps-Reflecting Anconeus Pedicle Approach

The triceps-reflecting anconeus pedicle (TRAP) approach, as described by O'Driscoll, offers an extensile option for surgical exposure of the distal humerus without the need for an olecranon osteotomy, while preserving the neurovascular supply to the anconeus muscle.[117] After an adequate midline posterior skin incision, the ulnar nerve is identified and protected as in all the previously described procedures. The interval between the anconeus and extensor carpi ulnaris is identified and followed to the lateral border of the ulna. Beginning distally, the anconeus is dissected subperiosteally off the lateral aspect of the ulna and the dissection carried proximally toward the lateral epicondyle and along the lateral supracondylar ridge. Medially, the triceps is mobilized as described in the Bryan-Morrey approach.[15] The dissection medially along the proximal ulna ends 10 cm distal to the olecranon joining with the distal extent of the lateral exposure. The triceps insertion is sharply removed from the olecranon and carried laterally to become confluent with the previous lateral dissection. Ultimately, the distal humerus and proximal ulna are exposed subperiosteally and a triceps and anconeus flap is created and mobilized proximally to allow visualization of the distal humerus

(Fig. 20-18). As with all procedures that sharply detach the triceps insertion from the olecranon, heavy nonabsorbable transosseous suture repair is mandatory to restore extensor mechanism integrity. Similar to the Bryan-Morrey exposure, the exact insertion of the triceps into the olecranon may be identified with the incorporation of a small wafer of bone or a suture to aid in anatomic repair.[15,125] Advantages of this approach include the avoidance of complications of the olecranon osteotomy, preservation of the anconeus as a dynamic stabilizer of the lateral aspect of the elbow and vascular muscle bed for the proximal ulna and lateral elbow, and, similar to the Bryan-Morrey approach, the ability to convert to total elbow arthroplasty should fracture reduction and fixation prove to be unattainable.

Lateral Approach

The lateral approach may be initiated with either a lateral or a posterior skin incision.[26,79,125] The posterior skin incision requires the elevation of a full-thickness lateral cutaneous flap, but it may be preferred should alternate deep dissection be required, such as conversion to an olecranon osteotomy, or if future reconstructive procedures are anticipated. The main indication for this approach, and its extensile variations, is in the management of significant fractures of the capitellum and other articular fracture variants.

In Kocher's lateral approach the dissection is directed through the substance of the anconeus and the lateral capsule and then carried proximally from the exposed radial head. Hotchkiss[58] notes that this exposure disrupts a significant portion of the posterolateral capsular complex. He advocates that a better lateral approach is one that preserves this vital structure by starting proximally at the lateral condyle and proceeding distally. With the use of the skin incisions described earlier, the lateral epicondyle is palpated

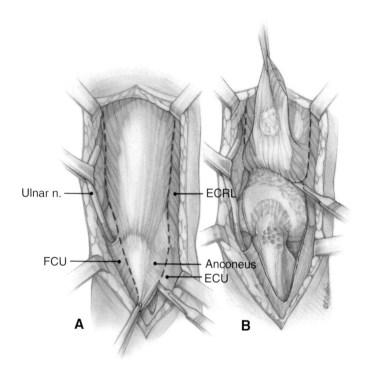

FIGURE 20-18. The TRAP approach. **A,** The posterior view of the distal humerus after the skin incision. Important features here are the ulnar nerve and the dotted lines that indicate where the deep dissections begin. **B,** Illustration of how the triceps insertion and the anconeus are taken off as a single structure from the proximal ulna. The extensor mechanism is reflected cephalad. ECRL, extensor carpi radialis longus; ECU, extensor carpi ulnaris.

and the muscles taking origin from the anterior surface of this ridge are elevated with sharp dissection. The anterior joint capsule is raised and the capitellum is exposed. Attached to the lateral condyle are the fibers of the lateral ligament complex. Hotchkiss suggests that "the articular surface of the capitellum should be bisected as one looks from the vantage point of the lateral aspect of the capitellum" and that all of the capsular structures that run anterior to this imaginary line can be elevated, whereas all of those posterior should be preserved (Fig. 20-19).[58] The anterior capsule is elevated as a single layer to the level of the capitohumeral joint. Further distal joint exposure requires dividing the annular ligament. Still further distal dissection requires entering the common extensor compartment. The most posterior portion of this muscle mass is elevated from the septum separating it from the anconeus. As the common extensor mass is elevated, the intermuscular septum, the anconeus and the posterior lateral ligamentous complex are left intact. This will expose the muscle fibers of the supinator muscle. The supinator muscle can be elevated from the posterior lateral margin on the ulna while holding the forearm in full pronation. This approach protects the posterior interosseous nerve while exposing the head and neck of the radius. Fractures of the lateral column and shearing fractures of the capitellum can be identified and reduced with this approach.

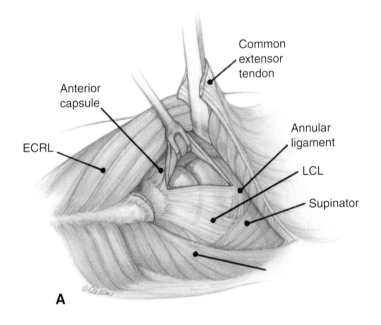

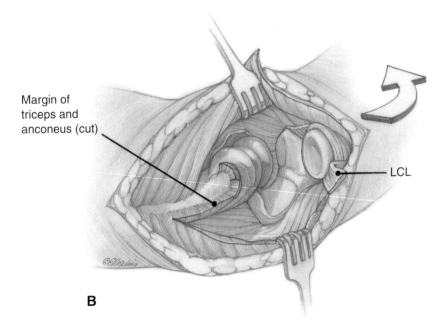

FIGURE 20-19. **A,** The pertinent anatomy of the lateral approach to the distal humerus. **B,** The elbow can be "unhinged" once the lateral collateral ligament (LCL) complex is taken off the lateral epicondyle.

Should the posterior aspect of the lateral column need to be exposed then the triceps muscle is lifted from the posterior face of the lateral column and the medial edge of the triceps followed into the anconeus muscle. The posterior joint capsule can be elevated off of the dorsal aspect of the lateral column, but those joint fibers that are found emanating from the distal lateral aspect of the lateral column should be left intact. They are the posterior lateral ligaments of the elbow.

In those cases in which visualization of the posterior and inferior aspect of the lateral column are still inadequate, the origin of the lateral collateral ligament and the lateral margin of the triceps and anconeus can be elevated from the lateral epicondyle. At this point, the elbow can be hinged open on the intact medial collateral ligament complex (Fig. 20-19B).[107,137] At the conclusion of the procedure, the lateral collateral ligament is returned to its origin and secured to the lateral epicondyle with transosseous nonabsorbable suture or suture anchors.

FIXATION PRINCIPLES

The goal of operative fixation of fractures of the distal humerus is to restore articular congruity, re-establish anatomic mechanical axes, and obtain enough fracture stability to allow early, unrestricted elbow range of motion. A number of factors contribute to making these goals difficult to obtain, including:

1. The relatively small, cancellous distal fragments offer poor fixation potential.
2. The complex osseous anatomy makes plate contouring difficult.
3. Screws that violate the articular surfaces and the olecranon, coronoid, and radial fossae will hamper motion.
4. Osteoporotic bone compromises construct stability.

Despite the numerous fracture patterns possible, several fixation principles will be applicable to all fracture patterns:

1. Kirschner wires are used to provide provisional fixation before definitive plate fixation and should be placed strategically to avoid interference with the application of definitive implants. Common diameter sizes are 0.045-inch (1.14 mm), 0.054-inch (1.37 mm), and 0.062-inch (1.57 mm). When these wires cannot be placed to reliably maintain a provisional reduction, small 2.0-mm plates secured with 2.0-mm screws may be used to secure a critical reduction zone. As with the placement of Kirschner wires, these small temporary plates should not interfere with the definitive fixation.
2. Fixation of the trochlea should achieve interfragmentary compression but avoid stenosis.[67,71] This latter situation may be encountered in patients with central sulcus comminution and functional bone loss (Fig. 20-20). Stenosis results in joint incongruity and altered cartilage loading, leading to decreased range of motion and post-traumatic arthritis.
3. Bicolumnar fractures are managed with medial and lateral column plates. To enhance stability of the fracture, plates should be placed at 90 degrees to each other, typically posterior on the lateral column and medially on the medial column.[48,62] In highly unstable situations, with metaphyseal comminution or bone loss, other authors have recommended medial and lateral plates at 180-degree orientation to improve torsional and bending stiffness.[144]
4. Whenever possible, screws placed into the distal articular segment should be through a plate that is subsequently attached to the diaphysis.[119] Because of the limited space available for fixation devices within the trochlea, placement of screws through the plate allows two functions to be performed with a single implant, namely, neutralization of sagittal fracture lines within the trochlea and attachment of the trochlea to the humeral diaphysis.

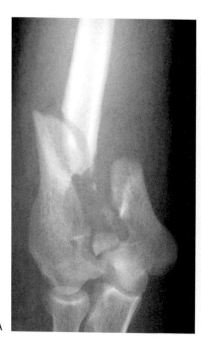
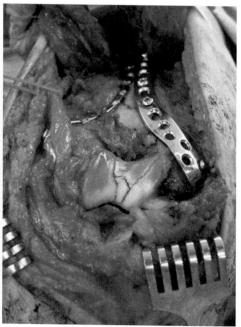

FIGURE 20-20. A, Anteroposterior injury radiograph of a bicolumnar distal humerus fracture. Note the central trochlear comminution. **B,** Intraoperative photograph of the same injury after reduction and definitive stabilization using an olecranon osteotomy exposure. Note the central trochlear comminution has been reduced and stabilized. Failure to reduce this fragment may result in overcompression of the trochlea and, ultimately, ulnotrochlear incongruity.

A

B

5. Smaller articular fragments can be secured with Herbert screws or independent 1.5-, 2.0-, or 2.4-mm screws that are countersunk below the articular surface.[96,137,152] Placement of these implants is typically performed to neutralize coronal plane articular fragments before fixation of the more common sagittally oriented trochlear fragments. These implants need to be strategically placed so as not to interfere with the trochlear fixation coming from the medial and lateral plates.

6. For bicolumnar injuries, the medial plate is typically a reconstruction plate, allowing easier contouring to accommodate the curved medial condyle and epicondyle, while the lateral plate is a dynamic compression plate. The distal portion of the posterolateral dynamic compression plate can be placed almost to the distal extent of the lateral column, allowing screws to be placed anteriorly into the subchondral bone of the capitellum. Both plates are typically small fragment (3.5 mm) implants but may be smaller depending on the size of the patient and the instability of the fracture pattern. Newer precontoured periarticular plates are available that largely eliminate the need for intraoperative plate contouring. The distal portion of these plates allows screw placement along the coronal plane from lateral to medial across the condyles, rather than into the smaller capitellar region, theoretically improving fixation of the distal articular segment. Fixed-angle screw/plate implants are also available that appear to enhance fracture fixation, particularly in osteoporotic bone. These devices, however, have predetermined screw trajectories that may result in suboptimal screw placement or inadvertent intra-articular screw placement and should be used with an understanding of their limitations.

7. Medial column fractures that result in the separation of the trochlea from the medial epicondyle ("H"-pattern) are particularly challenging, because the trochlea has no attachment to the medial or lateral column and may be devoid of soft tissue attachments. In this situation, the medial plate needs to be brought around the medial epicondyle and then distally along the medial wall of the trochlea. The most distal hole of the plate can then be used to additionally secure the trochlea. Plate contouring of this area is quite difficult and can be performed on an anatomic model preoperatively to decrease operative time, or, alternatively, a precontoured periarticular distal humeral plating system can be used. Because of the metallic bulk in this region of the cubital tunnel, the ulnar nerve is routinely transposed.

8. Secure fixation of the reconstructed articular segment to the distal humeral meta-diaphysis can be enhanced with the placement of a screw that begins at the distal portion of either the medial or lateral column plate and travels retrograde within the distal medial or lateral column, engaging the distal humeral diaphyseal cortex. These "column screws" improve the construct rigidity across the distal humeral metaphysis, but they should not jeopardize fixation of the distal articular surface to the medial or lateral plates.

9. Unicondylar fractures may be managed with single-column screw/plate implants, or screw fixation alone, with both options demonstrating satisfactory results.[72] With single-column plating techniques, the plate typically functions as an anti-glide device. In those unicondylar fractures with column comminution in the supracondylar region, the plate acts as a buttress.

Authors' Preferred Method of Treatment

Fracture management requires the surgeon to be prepared with a thorough preoperative plan but versatile enough to modify the initial plan as the reduction and fixation proceeds.[91] Because every fracture is unique, principles, rather than a strict series of steps, should be understood and followed. Common pitfalls should be anticipated before the patient enters the operating room. Conceptually, they may be organized as those related to the fracture pattern or those related to fixation problems.

General Considerations and Potential Pitfalls

Unanticipated fracture lines or comminution can pose significant problems in the execution of a preoperative plan and may require intraoperative modifications, including the conversion of the anticipated operative exposure into another and/or modification of the fracture construct. Fracture patterns that are particularly troublesome are (1) coronal plane fractures of the capitellum and/or trochlea, (2) separation of the medial aspect of the trochlea from the medial column, and (3) "low" (very distal) fracture patterns.

These fracture characteristics can be identified on the plain radiographs, particularly on quality traction films. When the presence of these fractures is suspected, CT may aid in the diagnosis.[96,137] When associated coronal fractures exist, these are reduced and managed before reduction of the remainder of the articular surface. Fracture of the trochlea from the medial column frequently requires distal modification of the medial column plate to ensure rigid fixation of the articular segment to the humeral shaft. Low fracture patterns result in a small distal articular segment that jeopardizes distal fixation. *We believe an olecranon osteotomy is required to adequately manage these fracture patterns* (see later).

Achieving adequate fixation to allow early range of motion is critical for successful management of fractures of the distal humerus. The articular segment is predictably the area where fixation may be suboptimal. When distal fixation is tenuous, several options exist to enhance fixation. By placing several screws through the distal portions of both medial and lateral plates across the distal articular segment, empowered fixation can be achieved through the "interference" of the screws within the segment. The risk in this technique is the loss of reduction as the screws are forced to engage one another. A second option, particularly useful in the elderly, is to shorten the humerus in the metaphyseal fracture area creating enhanced bone contact and a more stable supracondylar construct. Additionally, the use of three or more plates can be used distally to obtain orthogonal fixation within each column. These supplementary plates can provide surprisingly good stability and have been shown to be clinically effective in this setting.[41,67]

Supracondylar and Transcondylar Fractures: Proximal Patterns

Displaced extra-articular fractures of the distal humerus are managed operatively to avoid prolonged immobilization of the elbow joint and resultant stiffness. Patients may be positioned in the lateral or prone position, depending on the presence of other injuries. Because of the distal location of the fracture, stabilization generally requires the application of medial and lateral column plates, and therefore, a paratricipital approach using a posterior skin incision is performed. Given the extra-articular nature of these fractures, an olecranon osteotomy is not indicated. Occasionally, the fracture morphology results in the lateral column extending proximally to a point that sufficient distal fixation may be obtained with a single plate fixed proximally along the posterior aspect of the humeral diaphysis and, distally, along the posterior aspect of the lateral column (e.g., abduction transcondylar variant). In this situation, the extensile exposure described by Gerwin is utilized, without the need for dissection of the medial column.[39] However, if at any point the stability of the fracture is in question, then this approach is easily expanded to the paratricipital exposure, allowing manipulation and stabilization of the medial column.

Bicolumnar Fractures in the Physiologically Active Patient

CRITICAL POINTS: BICOLUMNAR FRACTURES

PREOPERATIVE EVALUATION

- Obtain anteroposterior, lateral, and traction view radiographs.
- Consider CT for:
  - Extreme distal (or "low") fracture patterns in geriatric patients
  - Articular variant patterns

PITFALLS

- Unrecognized articular comminution, particularly in the coronal plane
- Fracture lines that separate the medial trochlea from the medial column
- Unanticipated poor bone quality (osteoporosis)

OPERATIVE EXPOSURE

- Choose the exposure that allows you the ability to reduce and stabilize the articular surface best.
- As patient age increases, choose an exposure that does not compromise TEA.
- The authors prefer an olecranon osteotomy for managing displaced, comminuted fractures involving the articular surface. The Bryan-Morrey "triceps-sparing" approach is preferred for patients who may require conversion to TEA.

TECHNICAL POINTS

- Medial and lateral column fixation provides best fracture stability.
- A medial plate is usually a reconstruction-type implant and is applied directly medially; a lateral implant is frequently stiffer (dynamic compression plate) and is applied to the posterior aspect of the lateral column.
- Medial fixation is typically applied first because it is less likely to be obstructed by temporary Kirschner wires.

- Precontoured periarticular plates are available, but they may still need minor contour adjustments.
- Secure articular fragments with screws that are placed through a plate, whenever possible.
- Consider ulnar nerve transposition.
- Before wound closure the elbow is placed through a range of motion to ensure fracture stability.

POSTOPERATIVE CARE

- The elbow is splinted in extension at the conclusion of the procedure.
- Range-of-motion exercises are begun within 24 to 48 hours postoperatively. The patient must understand that the initial goal of rehabilitation is to obtain motion.
- A prefabricated extension splint is made before discharge from hospital and is used at night.
- Active flexion and passive extension is performed for all exposures, except for the lateral and paratricipital exposures, which are allowed active extension.
- Gentle stretching and active range-of-motion exercises for both extension and flexion are initiated at 6 weeks. Extension splinting is discontinued at this time.
- Resistive and strengthening exercises begin at week 12 and should be commensurate with radiographic consolidation.

ATHLETIC PARTICIPATION/MANUAL LABOR

- Consolidation of fracture lines radiographically is required.
- Strength should be approaching 75% of the contralateral uninjured extremity.

Bicolumnar fractures of the distal humerus are managed operatively with ORIF techniques using a posterior universal midline skin incision. Patients are usually placed prone on a radiolucent table with a Plexiglas platform to support the humerus. This position may be used in the presence of other orthopedic injuries, including the presence of stable or stabilized spine fractures and pelvic external fixators. The prone position is particularly useful for fractures that extend into the humeral diaphysis, allowing easier fluoroscopic imaging. The lateral position is chosen for patients who are otherwise unable to be placed prone. Definitive fixation is with medial and lateral plate and screw implants. Multiple plate constructs are considered for significantly comminuted fractures on a case-by-case basis.

Minimally Comminuted Fractures

Preoperatively, the degree of articular comminution and displacement is assessed. Those fractures with simple articular splits, large condylar fragments, and without major displacement are exposed using the paratricipital approach. If a satisfactory reduction can be obtained along the medial and/or lateral column(s) in the supracondylar region, this reduction is performed first, allowing indirect reduction of the articular surface. The supracondylar reductions are provisionally stabilized with Kirschner wires. The adequacy of articular reduction is mainly confirmed fluoroscopically; but with retraction of the triceps aponeurosis posteriorly and flexion of the elbow, the posterior aspect of the trochlea is also directly visualized and palpated with a small periosteal elevator, confirming or disproving the fluoroscopic images. Adjustment of the articular surface reduction is performed with larger-diameter Kirschner wires placed into the condyles to act as joysticks. Once the articular surface is realigned, a large pointed reduction clamp is placed across the condyles and the articular surface is compressed. The articular reduction is then provisionally maintained with Kirschner wires.

Fractures with significant comminution of the articular surface are treated using an olecranon osteotomy. The reduction sequence is varied, depending on the particular fracture patterns (see later).

Multiplanar Articular Involvement

Fractures that display multiplanar involvement of the articular surface (coronal plane fragmentation) are managed first with reduction and stabilization of the anterior articular components. This is usually accomplished by displacing the sagittal fracture line, allowing access to the medial aspect of the capitellum and the lateral aspect of the trochlea. By allowing the metaphysis to shorten through the supracondylar fracture, visualization of the anterior components of the articular surface is facilitated. The anterior articular surface is typically definitively stabilized at this point with posterior to anterior mini-fragment screws while direct visual confirmation of secure anatomic reduction can still be performed. Once the anterior articular surface is secured, the sagittally oriented fracture(s) (separating the distal articular surface into medial and lateral components) is (are) reduced and provisionally stabilized. The metaphyseal fracture is then reduced, essentially orienting the distal humeral articular segment appropriately beneath the meta-diaphysis. This segment is then provisionally stabilized, and intra-operative fluoroscopy is used to confirm the adequacy of reduction.

Simple Supracondylar Involvement

Intra-articular fractures that demonstrate minimal comminution in the supracondylar region demonstrate long fracture planes in this region that are amenable to anatomic reduction (medial and lateral lambda patterns). When these features are present, the authors prefer to begin the reduction and temporary stabilization sequence in this supracondylar area first. The goal is to reliably restore a segment of the articular surface to the meta-diaphysis and then build the remaining articular surface to this restored column. This sequence is effective provided that the supracondylar area can be reduced and provisionally stabilized reliably.

Combined Articular and Supracondylar Comminution

These fractures are a significant challenge and must be individualized. In fracture patterns in which metaphyseal comminution is extensive, we initially focus on the reduction and temporary stabilization of the articular surface. The distal humeral articular surface is then oriented and provisionally stabilized in the proper transverse, sagittal, and coronal planes relative to the meta-diaphyseal region. In situations with marked metaphyseal comminution, this area is indirectly reduced and fixed with the aid of appropriately contoured or precontoured periarticular plates. This maintains viability of the metaphyseal fragments, allowing predictable union. In the older patient undergoing ORIF, the humerus can be shortened through the comminuted metaphysis to allow intrinsic bone contact and stability of the entire construct. Shortening provides minimal functional deficits, provided the olecranon and coronoid fossae are not obliterated, and offers improved fracture stability and union in the older patient population.

Technique for Olecranon Osteotomy

CRITICAL POINTS: OLECRANON OSTEOTOMY

CREATION

- Preoperatively determine whether a 4.5-mm cortical screw or a 6.5-mm partially threaded screw will be used to secure the osteotomy. This is based on the diameter of the medullary canal.
- Identify the bare area and confirm this with fluoroscopy.
- Predrill the proximal ulna using a 3.2-mm drill bit. This will serve as the thread hole for both 4.5-mm and 6.5-mm screws. If a 4.5-mm screw is anticipated, a 4.5-mm glide hole is created initially.
- A 2.5-mm drill hole is placed through the dorsal surface of the proximal ulna at the anticipated position of the osteotomy apex.

Continued

CRITICAL POINTS: OLECRANON OSTEOTOMY—cont'd

CREATION—cont'd

- An oscillating saw initiates the chevron osteotomy (apex pointing distally) at the bare area. The previously placed 2.5-mm drill hole helps orient the operator.
- A fine osteotome is used to "fracture" the articular surface, completing the osteotomy.

FIXATION

- Place a 3.2-mm drill bit antegrade into the drill hole of the osteotomized fragment. Continue passing the drill bit into the medullary canal of the ulna.
- Medial and lateral pointed bone reduction clamps are placed across the osteotomy. The intramedullary drill bit helps to eliminate translational deformities during this maneuver.
- Kirschner wires are used to secure the osteotomy.
- A transverse drill hole is created in the proximal ulna, distal to the osteotomy.
- Remove the drill bit and insert the intramedullary screw and washer.
- Before final tightening of the screw, cerclage wire is passed beneath the washer and through the transverse hole in the proximal ulna. A figure-of eight pattern is used.
- The cerclage wire is tightened, and the screw is secured.
- Remove Kirschner wires and clamps.
- Place the elbow through a range of motion and ensure stability of the osteotomy.

PITFALLS

- Before performing the osteotomy, the drill bit must be placed at the center of the olecranon and pass smoothly down the medullary canal of the ulna. Eccentric placement of the drill hole in the olecranon may result in translational forces and malreduction of the osteotomy during fixation.
- Osteotomies that are not perpendicular to the intramedullary screw will displace with tightening.
- Long 6.5-mm screws that significantly engage the bow of the ulna may displace the osteotomy. This is less likely to occur with the less stiff 4.5-mm screws.

CRITICAL POINTS: OLECRANON OSTEOTOMY—cont'd

PEARLS

- If poor purchase is obtained with a 4.5-mm screw, the screw length can be increased to engage more of the curved portion of the ulna. Improved distal purchase is obtained as the screw bends to accommodate the medullary canal. If this still fails to give satisfactory purchase, a 6.5-mm screw should be used.
- Osteotomies that remain unstable, or that continually displace with final tightening of the intramedullary screw, are managed with plate stabilization.

For maximum visualization of the articular surface of the distal humerus, we prefer to perform an olecranon osteotomy. At the conclusion of the procedure, the osteotomy is secured with a medullary screw and tension band technique. The screw is placed in a unicortical fashion with distal purchase obtained from the screw threads interacting with the endosteal surface. In most patients, a 4.5-mm screw and washer is used; however, in older patients or those with larger stature, a 6.5-mm screw is occasionally used. The technique for a 4.5-mm screw is described.

Creation of Osteotomy

Visualization of the "bare area" of the olecranon is performed by division and elevation of the medial and lateral capsular attachments along the olecranon process and corresponds to the deepest portion of the semilunar notch. With the use of the lateral fluoroscopic image, the olecranon is predrilled, first with a 4.5-mm glide hole to the level of the anticipated osteotomy. This is followed with a 3.2-mm drill bit. It is imperative to begin the drill hole in the center of the proximal aspect of the olecranon process relative to its medial and lateral surfaces. Once the glide hole in the metaphyseal area of the olecranon is passed, the drill is placed on oscillate to avoid exiting the ulnar diaphysis inadvertently. At the approximate middle and proximal third junction, the ulna curves, presenting a convexity laterally. Drilling is stopped at this curved area, 90 to 120 mm distal to the tip of the olecranon. The length of the anticipated screw is measured, and the proximal ulna is tapped with a 4.5-mm tap. This last step is eliminated if self-tapping screws are used.

A small sponge is placed between the articular surface of the semilunar notch and the fractured articular surface of the distal humerus. This allows an assistant to provide counterpressure on the proximal ulna and to avoid inadvertent injury to the distal humeral articular surface. With the aid of the lateral fluoroscopic image, a 2.5-mm drill is placed in the midline dorsal surface of the olecranon process immediately across from the "bare area." The drill is advanced to the subchondral surface but not through it (Fig. 20-21A). A fine oscillating saw is used to create the osteotomy into, but

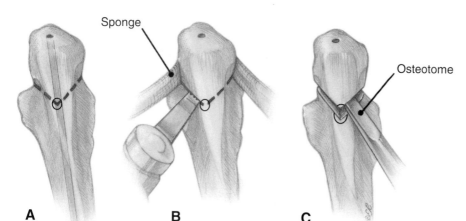

Sponge

Osteotome

FIGURE 20-21. A, The shape of the chevron osteotomy with the apex pointing distally. Note the drill hole at the apex. **B,** Sponge protecting the articular surface of the distal humerus. **C,** Osteotomy with osteotome.

A   **B**   **C**

not through, the subchondral bone (Fig. 20-21B). The osteotomy is created in a chevron pattern, with the apex of the chevron pointing distally (Fig. 20-21A). The 2.5-mm drill hole on the dorsal surface orients the operator and avoids creating an "X" at the apex of the osteotomy. A thin osteotome is inserted into the saw tract and the osteotomy completed by cracking the remaining osteochondral surface (Fig. 20-21C). The tip of the olecranon and triceps is reflected proximally. A suture is used to hold the extensor mechanism to the skin of the proximal arm as a retraction aid. A moistened sponge is draped over the exposed triceps musculature and olecranon. A clinical example is provided in Figure 20-22.

Fixation of Osteotomy

Fixation of the osteotomy is performed immediately before wound closure. The previously placed proximal retraction suture is removed, allowing the extensor mechanism to return to its normal orientation. A 2.5-mm drill bit is used to create a bicortical drill hole from medial to lateral in the ulnar shaft 3 to 4 cm distal to the osteotomy site, in anticipation of the tension band wire. A long 3.2-mm drill bit is placed by hand through the previously created drill hole in the tip of the olecranon process and delivered down the medullary canal of the ulna. This drill bit acts as a guide rail along which the olecranon process can be steered, helping to eliminate translational deformities. Medial and lateral large point-to-point reduction forceps are placed across the osteotomy and are used to fine-tune the reduction and to ultimately compress the osteotomy. Two 0.062-inch Kirschner wires are then placed from the olecranon process, across the reduced osteotomy, and into the dense bone of the coronoid process, providing provisional stability. The 3.2-mm drill bit is removed, and the appropriate-length 4.5-mm screw and washer are placed into the proximal ulna but not fully tightened. A tension band wire, usually 18 gauge, is cut into two segments. One segment is placed through the medial-to-lateral drill hole created distal to the osteotomy site. The second is placed from medial to lateral at the tip of the olecranon process. This second wire is placed deep to the triceps insertion and washer, at the proximal aspect of the screw. The screw is tightened enough to trap the wire beneath the washer but still allow the wire to be manipulated. A figure-of-eight pattern is created with the wire, and

the proximal ends are twisted to the corresponding ends of the distal wire in a double-knot technique. The knots are placed medially and laterally, avoiding the tip of the olecranon, helping to decrease implant prominence. Once the tension band wire has been fully tightened, the screw is finally fully seated and tightened. Temporary clamps and Kirschner wires are removed. The elbow is placed through a range of motion, and a secure osteotomy is ensured. Infrequently, because of inadvertent osteotomy obliquity, comminution, or olecranon fracture, stability of the osteotomy cannot be ensured with the screw/tension band technique. In these situations, the authors proceed with plate osteosynthesis of the osteotomy.

Fixation Sequence

The fixation sequence is varied and depends on the individual fracture characteristics. Because most of the Kirschner wires are placed in a posterior to anterior direction, the medial surface of the distal humerus is usually unobstructed and free of temporary implants, allowing the medial plate to be placed first. This plate is a reconstruction plate applied directly medially with attention paid to ensuring that it is accurately contoured around the medial epicondyle. The first screw inserted is usually at a point immediately proximal to the most proximal fracture line on the medial column. Slight undercontouring of the plate along the medial supracondylar ridge allows a buttressing effect distally as the screw is tightened. The orientation of the plate on the medial column is confirmed on anteroposterior and lateral intraoperative fluoroscopy. Screw fixation proceeds distally with placement of screws across the distal humeral articular surface. Finally, screws are placed in the proximal portion of the plate. Because the medial implant is a malleable reconstruction plate, it tends to be contoured to the bone rather than displacing the provisionally reduced fracture to the plate. Once the medial column plate is secured to the medial column, several redundant Kirschner wires may be removed to decrease interference when the lateral column is subsequently secured. We typically use a stiff precontoured posterolateral periarticular plate to provide rigid lateral column stability while allowing screws to be placed from lateral to medial across the distal humeral articular surface. The distal-lateral portion of the plate is confirmed to be in a

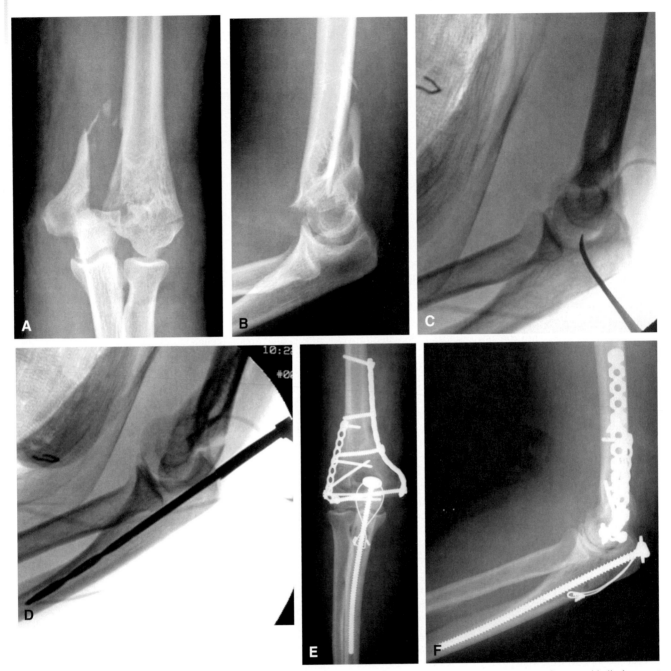

FIGURE 20-22. Anteroposterior (**A**) and lateral (**B**) injury radiographs demonstrate a supracondylar intercondylar distal humerus fracture with displacement of the articular surface and very low injury of the lateral column. To improve visualization of the articular surface, an olecranon osteotomy was chosen as the preferred surgical approach. **C** and **D,** On the intraoperative fluoroscopic images, a small elevator is used to demonstrate the "bare area" of the semilunar notch, and the proximal ulna is predrilled before creation of the osteotomy. **E** and **F,** Final radiographs demonstrate reduction and stabilization of the distal humerus fracture and fixation of the osteotomy using a 4.5-mm screw with washer and tension band wiring.

satisfactory position both clinically and fluoroscopically and is applied closely to the lateral epicondylar region to avoid plate prominence in this area. The plate is maintained in the appropriate position with several Kirschner wires, and screws are strategically inserted beginning distally and working proximally.

Unicolumnar Fractures

The surgical tactic for management of single-column fractures of the distal humerus begins with an assessment of the degree of comminution of the articular surface and a close inspection of the opposite column to rule out subtle fracture lines that change the diagnosis to a bicolumnar injury. Invariably, significantly displaced fractures of the lateral or medial column are approached through a universal posterior skin incision with the patient in the prone or lateral position. Depending on the involved column, the corresponding paratricipital interval is developed. Regardless of which column is fractured, the ulnar nerve is routinely mobilized and protected. If significant articular surface comminution exists, both paratricipital intervals are exposed and an olecranon osteotomy is performed. If the articular surface is not comminuted, the fractured column is mobilized and the triceps is elevated off the posterior aspect of the distal humerus. The fracture is reduced using cortical surfaces "reads", indirectly reducing the articular surface. The olecranon is distracted, and the articular reduction is assessed under direct vision and with palpation with a blunt periosteal elevator. If a satisfactory reduction cannot be obtained, or the articular surface is significantly comminuted, then the authors proceed with an olecranon osteotomy. In significantly displaced, or "high," unicolumnar fractures, the radius and ulna frequently follow the displaced trochlear fragment. In this situation, reduction of the fractured column is quite difficult without the aid of an osteotomy because the weight of the arm continues to act as a displacing force.

Lag screw fixation alone is infrequently used for these injuries, with the authors preferring to supplement stabilization with plating of the injured column.

Capitellar and Articular Variant Fractures

Isolated capitellar fractures and other articular fracture variants are managed operatively in the physiologically active patient. Thin-cut preoperative CT is performed in patients whose fracture patterns demonstrate significant involvement of the posterior aspect of the capitellum or trochlea on plain radiographs. In the physiologically older patient, significant articular comminution and displacement is treated with elbow arthroplasty.

Fractures of the Capitellum

Capitellar fractures and associated variants, including the coronal shear pattern, are managed with the patient in the supine position. The common feature of these fractures is that they are mainly confined to the anterolateral aspect of the distal humerus and are accessible using a Kocher approach.

The patient is placed supine on the operating table, and a radiolucent arm board is used to support the injured extremity. A posterior universal skin incision is made, and the anconeus/extensor carpi ulnaris interval is developed. The joint capsule is incised and the fracture identified, cleansed of its hematoma, and assessed. Simple fractures may be reduced at this point; however, comminuted capitellar fragments, or those that extend beyond the lateral trochlear ridge, require improved visualization. To improve visualization, the proximal interval is extended by detaching the origins of the extensor carpi ulnaris, common extensor tendon, and a portion of the extensor carpi radialis longus from the lateral supracondylar ridge. The origin of the lateral collateral ligament is detached sharply from its origin at the lateral epicondyle, and the elbow joint capsule is incised at its origin on the distal humerus. The capitellar fracture fragments are then reduced with dental picks to the intact distal humerus. Strategic temporary fixation is performed with small Kirschner wires, and the reduction is confirmed under direct vision and with biplanar fluorographic imaging. Definitive fixation is performed with 1.5-, 2.0-, and/or 2.4-mm countersunk screws. Final radiographs are obtained and approved. The lateral collateral ligament is repaired to its origin using suture anchors, and the extensor origins are repaired along the lateral supracondylar ridge.

Articular Fracture Variants

These fracture patterns are considered separately from capitellar fractures because of their potential involvement of the posterior aspect of the capitellum, lateral epicondyle, trochlea, and medial epicondylar region. With increasing involvement of the posterior and medial articular surfaces, visualization, reduction, and stabilization become increasingly difficult. As described by Ring and colleagues, the inability to reduce the anterior capitellar fragments, or a capitellar fracture involving the lateral epicondyle, suggests the presence of this associated posterior injury.[137]

In those patterns that involve the capitellum and the posterior aspect of the lateral column, the posterolateral aspect of the medial head of triceps and the anconeus are elevated. The elbow is hinged open posterolaterally allowing access to the posterior aspect of the lateral column. If the fracture begins to involve the posterior aspect of the trochlea or medial epicondyle, we prefer to use an olecranon osteotomy with a posterior skin incision to more reliably access the components of these challenging fractures. Stabilization is with small or mini-fragment screws. Fractures with significant comminution or impaction may require bone grafting and/or plating to help support articular segments.

Special Situations

Massive Bone Loss

Patients sustaining open injuries with massive bone loss are, fortunately, rarely encountered. The initial focus is on determining if the limb is viable and/or salvageable. A detailed vascular examination of the ipsilateral hand and digits is critical. In situations with a salvageable injury, the open wound is thoroughly irrigated and débrided in the operating room. An intraoperative assessment of the amount of bone loss is performed and correlated with the radiographic assessment. Because of the high-energy involved in the creation of these injuries, patients will frequently have associated polytrauma and/or markedly contaminated wounds about the elbow, and temporary spanning external fixation is performed acutely. This temporary fixation allows the skeleton and soft tissues to be stabilized rapidly and allows other serious injuries to be managed. A simple uniplanar external fixator is applied, with Schanz pins placed into the humeral diaphysis under direct vision (to avoid injury to the radial nerve), and into the ulna. Repeated débridements are performed until all nonviable tissue is excised. Definitive management depends on the type and amount of bone lost.

Nonarticular Bone Loss

Patients with a reconstructable articular surface and supracondylar bone loss are managed with ORIF, shortening of the humerus through the area of bone loss, and placement of antibiotic beads in the region of any residual bone defect. Delayed bone grafting is performed once the soft tissue envelope has stabilized, typically at 6 to 8 weeks. Patients are at high risk for elbow stiffness or ankylosis that may be improved with elbow mobilization procedures once fracture union is confirmed.

Articular Bone Loss

Options for patients presenting with significant articular bone loss include procedures that allow the development of a pseudarthrosis in the region of the distal humerus, elbow fusion, and allograft elbow replacements. In severely contaminated wounds or selected patients, some of these injuries are managed with a brief period of immobilization to allow soft tissue recovery, followed by active range-of-motion exercises. These patients will develop a mobile pseudoarticulation that provides some mobility and function. Elbow fusions are typically reserved for those patients with articular loss, overt infection, and painful, mobile residual articulations not amenable to elbow arthroplasty.[92,130]

In situations with dramatic articular bone loss, the authors prefer allograft replacement.[1,9,25,155,156] This option offers the ability to maintain a mobile, comfortable elbow articulation in the short term and restore bone stock for later elbow arthroplasty if needed.

Ballistic Injuries

Low-energy ballistic injuries usually demonstrate minor to moderate contamination and soft tissue injury and minor to moderate bone comminution. The fracture is managed according to the principles outlined previously.

Conversely, high-energy ballistic injuries are associated with neurovascular injury, large contaminated wounds, and significant skeletal comminution with or without functional bone loss. The management of these injuries is with repeated débridement until a healthy, viable soft tissue envelope is created. Fixation is performed using the principles outlined earlier. The surgeon should anticipate some amount of bone loss (articular and/or nonarticular) when managing these fractures. Some of these injuries have been salvaged with circular tensioned-wire fixators[80,138] or uniplanar external fixation as definitive treatment,[113] but we have little experience with this in the acute setting.

POSTOPERATIVE CARE

At the conclusion of the procedure, the surgical incisions and traumatic wounds are covered with sterile gauze bandages and the extremity is placed into a long-arm plaster splint with the elbow in extension. Once the plaster has hardened, anesthesia is reversed and the patient is awakened and transferred to a hospital bed. Patients are managed with 24 hours of postoperative administration of antibiotics. A suction drain, if utilized, is removed after 24 hours. Approximately 48 hours postoperatively the splint is removed and the surgical incision is inspected. Range-of-motion exercises are begun provided the surgical incision is sealed. Therapy is performed several times per day and consists of active range of motion of the shoulder, forearm, wrist, and fingers. Exercises are initially performed under the supervision of a physical therapist before discharge. Active and active-assisted elbow flexion is permitted for all situations. Patients managed via a paratricipital approach or an olecranon osteotomy are allowed active elbow extension. Those patients treated with the Bryan-Morrey approach perform passive, gravity-assisted elbow extension for 6 weeks. A resting thermoplast extension splint is fabricated before patient discharge, and the patient is instructed to wear the splint at all times when not engaging in therapy, particularly at night. The extension splint is then weaned at the 4- to 6-week mark from daytime wear but is continued at night

for several more weeks. Strengthening exercises, particularly resisted elbow extension, are deferred until radiographic union occurs.

Patients are examined in the outpatient clinic at the following *intervals*:

- Seven to 10 days postoperatively for examination of the surgical incision, suture removal, edema control, and reinforcement of physical therapy regimen. Patients who are unclear regarding the importance, frequency, or timing of physical therapy are seen by a therapist in the outpatient clinic area to review exercises and to arrange outpatient therapy at a convenient location.
- Week 6 for motion evaluation, weaning of extension splinting, and radiographs
- Week 12 for motion evaluation, radiographic assessment, and initiation of strengthening and stretching exercises
- Weeks 20 to 26 for motion evaluation, radiographic assessment, identification of patient concerns, and to discuss return to athletics or heavy labor
- Week 52 and as needed for final radiographic assessment and identification of any patient concerns

EXPECTATIONS

Several parameters exist that are used to assess the outcome of fractures of the distal humerus. Elbow range of motion, forearm rotation, the occurrence and time to union, and complication rates have all been reported in the literature. It is recognized, however, that these parameters may not accurately reflect the patient's perception of satisfaction. For this reason, limb- and disease-specific validated outcome scoring measures have been created in an attempt to more accurately assess outcomes of numerous conditions.

All fractures of the distal humerus will be associated with some degree of measurable loss of range of motion, particularly extension. Despite this absolute loss of "normal" motion, most patients can expect functional results. Those patients with significant associated polytrauma, high-energy injuries, or significant soft tissue injury can be expected to have worse outcomes.

Most activities of daily living require a flexion-extension arc at the elbow of approximately 100 degrees (30 to 130 degrees) and an arc of forearm rotation between 50 degrees of supination to 50 degrees of pronation.[111] In bicolumnar fractures of the distal humerus treated with contemporary techniques, McKee and colleagues have demonstrated a flexion-extension arc of approximately 108 degrees with a mean flexion contracture of approximately 25 degrees.[99] This represents approximately 74% of the motion as compared with the contralateral, uninjured side. Similarly, flexion and extension strength were approximately 75% that of the uninjured side.[99] Other authors have demonstrated similar functional motion arcs and losses of flexion and extension strength.[41,71] These motion and strength limitations may be responsible for the mild impairments identified on standardized outcome scoring systems.[41,99]

Expectations must be tailored to the individual patient, and the data obtained by McKee and associates[98,99] and Gofton and coworkers[41] provide a useful framework for discussion with patients and their families. In patients with isolated, closed fractures of the distal humerus, or those with open fractures without significant contamination or soft tissue destruction, the expected results are similar to those described previously. Patients with sedentary employment are encouraged to return to part-time work when they are feeling systemically stable. Ideally, the workplace should allow for slower completion of tasks, with frequent breaks for rest or periods of physical therapy. Those patients who are engaged in more physical labor are also encouraged to return to the workplace, but clearly in a modified role. Patients who are active in heavy labor are assessed individually. Frequently an independent medical examination or physical capacities review is performed to obtain an objective measure of their ability to return to the same or similar job. These employment issues frequently are foremost on patients' minds, and discussion of the plan to return to work is initiated early in the management phase.

At the authors' institution, a high percentage of these fractures are secondary to high-energy injuries and have associated polytrauma. Patients who sustain significant associated injuries are expected to have a worse outcome in terms of range of motion and strength.[135,138] In the polytraumatized patient in whom the operative delay approaches 7 days, significant stiffness has been noted. In these patients, the authors still strive for anatomic reduction of the articular surface and axial realignment, planning on delayed excision of heterotopic ossification, and/or capsular release. This "staged" approach to an ultimately functional elbow is explained to the family and patient during the early phase of care. In these situations, the ultimate outcome is satisfactory provided the distal humeral articular anatomy is restored at the time of the initial procedure and the patient is able to fully participate in the postsurgical rehabilitation program.[38,93,136,158]

The functional outcome after ORIF of capitellar fractures and the coronal shear variant appears to be very satisfactory,[96,152] with several authors describing near-normal flexion-extension and pronation-supination arcs.[22,60,96,129,152] The majority of patients in these series were managed with screw fixation, with comparatively poorer results noted with Kirschner wire fixation.[83,129] Because of the absence of significant soft tissue attachments to the capitellar fragment, avascular necrosis is a commonly discussed potential complication of this fracture pattern. Avascular necrosis changes noted with plain radiography, however, appear to be relatively infrequent, with an incidence ranging from 0% to 20% in larger series.[85,96,129,152] The clinical sequelae of avascular necrosis appear to be even less frequent than its radiographic incidence.[84,152] With more of the articular surface involved, a decrease in the flexion-extension arc and lower functional outcome scores have been demonstrated.[137]

COMPLICATIONS

Nonunion of Distal Humerus

Nonunion of fractures of the distal humerus has been reported to occur in 2% to 10%, invariably occurring in the meta-diaphyseal region.[2,34,71,106,148,149,160,166] It is primarily the consequence of inadequate fixation[52,66,77,148] that may be the result of other predisposing factors such as high-energy

injuries, extensive comminution, and poor bone quality. Patients are typically significantly disabled secondary to pain and loss of function. The frequent presentation is of a painful, mobile nonunion with significant motion restriction at the ulnohumeral articulation. Associated ulnar neuropathy is not uncommon.[49]

A small number of these nonunions can be treated satisfactorily in a brace, but the majority require operative management to achieve a stable, comfortable, functional elbow. Surgical reconstruction is technically demanding because of the distorted local anatomy, scarring, retained or broken implants, poor bone quality of the articular component, and capsular contracture.[1,49,94] Despite these difficulties, operative reconstruction is the procedure of choice in active individuals. The surgical plan involves a wide posterior surgical exposure incorporating previous skin incisions if possible. The use of an olecranon osteotomy depends on the presence of significant articular malunion or nonunion and the location of the supracondylar nonunion. If an osteotomy is not required, a paratricipital exposure is performed. The ulnar nerve is identified and freed from scar tissue well above and below the medial epicondyle. Substantial perineural fibrosis is often encountered. Posterior capsular adhesions and fibrosis are resected, particularly those crowding the olecranon fossa. Anterior capsular adhesions are released by working through the nonunion site or by elevating the structures from the lateral supracondylar ridge. The lateral collateral ligament origin should be preserved during this exposure, but it may be elevated and subsequently repaired if needed. The nonunion site is cleared of its fibrous material, and the bone ends are resected to healthy, bleeding margins. Intraoperative cultures are routinely obtained. Secure fixation typically entails medial and lateral plate fixation, and bone grafting is invariably required. The elbow is placed through a range of motion, and the stability of the construct is tested. The ulnar nerve is transposed anteriorly. Early motion is initiated once the wound is sealed.

Results of nonunion repair have been satisfactory. Helfet demonstrated satisfactory union in 51 of 52 patients after a single procedure.[49] The average motion arc improved from 71 degrees preoperatively to 94 degrees postoperatively, but it is likely that the preoperative motion was a combination of ulnohumeral and nonunion motion, giving an overestimation of the preoperative motion arc. Similarly, McKee demonstrated an average postoperative arc of motion of 97 degrees with ulnar nerve function improving in all cases.[94] Excellent improvement in pain can be expected, but associated injuries can influence the ultimate functional outcome and significant long-term disability may persist despite bony union.[1,49,69,94]

The use of total elbow replacement in ununited fractures in the elderly has also been described.[106,109,134] This is particularly effective in low-demand patients with poor bone stock. Satisfactory results can be expected provided that septic complications are minimized.[109,110]

Nonunion of Olecranon Osteotomy

Nonunion or delayed union of the olecranon osteotomy has been reported in the literature with rates of up to 10%.[41,51,52,55,71,149] Henley described 3 of 29 (10%) osteotomies that developed delayed union or nonunion.[52] More recently,

Gofton reported 2 of 22 (9%) olecranon osteotomies with nonunions.[41] Several factors, such as lack of inherent fracture interdigitation and suboptimal osteotomy fixation, are believed to be responsible for the development of this complication.[51,52] Furthermore, olecranon osteotomy nonunions have been described with both Kirschner wire and screw fixations.[52,71] The use of a chevron osteotomy, rather than a transverse osteotomy, creates increased surface area for bone union and improved rotational stability of the osteotomy and would be expected to improve union rates.[35] Despite this rationale, Petraco was unable to demonstrate any significant biomechanical differences in the stability of three different osteotomy methods.[128]

To prevent the occurrence of olecranon osteotomy nonunion, we prefer to create a chevron osteotomy. Compressive apposition of the osteotomy surfaces is performed with the application of medial and lateral clamps that are removed once the osteotomy is temporarily secured with Kirschner wires. Medullary screw fixation, rather than Kirschner wires, is used for a secure definitive construct. At the conclusion of the osteotomy fixation, the elbow is placed through a range of motion to assess the stability of the osteotomy. Any significant gapping or instability should be recognized and managed. In those unusual situations where this occurs, we prefer immediate plate fixation to improve osteotomy stability and healing.

Management of an olecranon osteotomy nonunion is with repeat osteosynthesis using plate fixation and autogenous bone grafting (Fig. 20-23). In situations in which the proximal fragment is of insufficient size or quality, the fragment is excised and the triceps tendon is advanced.[95]

Infection

The deep infection rate of surgically managed fractures of the distal humerus is surprisingly low despite the soft tissue dissection, prolonged operative time, and frequency of open injuries. Most deep infection rates reported range from 0% to 9%.[41,50,52,72,98,99] Management of acute postoperative wound infections requires débridement of nonviable tissue and an assessment of fracture stability. If the implants continue to stabilize the fracture, management is with suppressive culture-specific antibiotics until union occurs. In the setting of sepsis with fracture instability, treatment requires débridement and antibiotics with repeat osteosynthesis when the infection is controlled. Late presentations after union respond well to removal of internal fixation and antibiotic therapy.

Ulnar Neuropathy

Symptoms attributable to dysfunction of the ulnar nerve are common after fractures of the distal humerus.[34,50,71,135] Patients presenting with reconstructive issues almost invariably have ulnar nerve symptoms and/or signs, particularly when the nerve has been left in its native position. Factors responsible for postoperative ulnar neuropathy include injury from displaced bone fragments, excessive manipulation and retraction during the surgical procedure, and fibrosis and scarring of the tissues around the nerve in the region of the medial epicondyle and cubital tunnel.[95,135,140]

The authors utilize several techniques to minimize complications attributed to the ulnar nerve. When the posterior

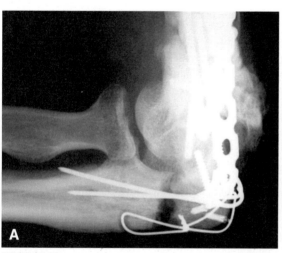
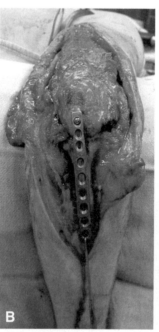
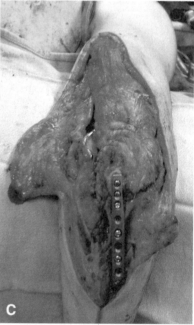

FIGURE 20-23. A, Lateral radiograph of a bicolumnar distal humerus fracture managed using an olecranon osteotomy. The osteotomy was secured with Kirschner wires and figure-of-eight tension band technique. Note the obvious nonunion at the site of the osteotomy. **B,** Intraoperative photograph of the posterior aspect of the right elbow. The hand is located at the bottom of the image. The olecranon nonunion has been débrided to viable bone margins and autogenous bone graft applied. A dynamic compression plate has been applied to the dorsal surface and secured to the proximal fragment. The proximal portion of this plate is narrowed and has a tighter hole spacing to accommodate multiple 2.7-mm screws into the smaller proximal olecranon fragment; the distal aspect of the plate is composed of a standard 3.5-mm plate and hole specifications. The bone hook located at the distal aspect of the plate is used to tension the plate and, therefore, compress the nonunion. **C,** Intraoperative photograph of the posterior aspect of the right elbow demonstrating final screw placement and secure fixation of the nonunion.

approach is used, adequate liberation of the nerve proximally and distally is performed at the beginning of the procedure, with care taken not to devascularize the nerve during mobilization. A broad Penrose drain is used for retraction purposes. To minimize traction injury to the nerve, the ends of the Penrose drain are sutured rather than clamped. At the conclusion of the procedure, anterior subcutaneous transposition of the nerve is performed for most fractures of the distal humerus. Isolated capitellar fractures and variants, lateral condyle fractures, or those fractures managed using Kocher's interval do not require transposition. Using routine transposition, Wang was unable to identify any postoperative ulnar neuropathy in 20 patients treated with dual plating.[162] Other authors have shown similar results with routine anterior ulnar nerve transposition.[30,41]

The successful management of ulnar neuropathy has been demonstrated with ulnar neurolysis and anterior transposition.[94,97,158] Despite the high patient satisfaction and improved objective measures, ulnar nerve function does not appear to normalize, and all efforts at minimizing complications of the ulnar nerve should be taken.[95,97]

Stiffness and Heterotopic Ossification

Most patients who are operatively managed with appropriate internal fixation usually obtain functional flexion/extension arcs. Significant contractures may be encountered in patients who are polytraumatized, undergo a significant delay before definitive management, sustain high-energy injury, or have open fractures (Fig. 20-24).[82,137,158] When

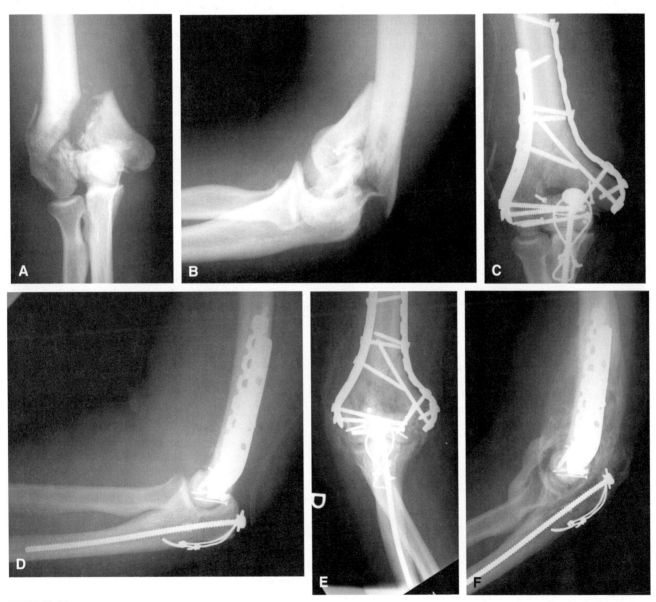

FIGURE 20-24. This 24-year-old man was involved in a high-speed motor vehicle collision. He sustained serious injuries, including severe bilateral pulmonary contusions, a closed head injury, and multiple fractures. **A** and **B,** The injury anteroposterior and lateral radiographs of the right distal humerus show significant displacement and comminution of the articular surface. Because of his other injuries, operative fixation of the distal humerus fracture was performed 8 days after the accident. **C** and **D,** Operative treatment consisted of medial and lateral plate fixation via an olecranon osteotomy. **E** and **F,** Follow-up radiographs demonstrate maintenance of reduction and union of his fracture but also the development of massive periarticular elbow heterotopic ossification resulting in complete ankylosis of the elbow joint.

compared with patients managed within 24 hours of injury, Kundel and coworkers demonstrated significant differences in time to return to work, ultimate range of motion, and incidence of significant heterotopic ossification in patients treated beyond 24 hours.[82] In this same study, the cases of ankylosing heterotopic ossification occurred exclusively in the delayed group. Provided the fracture proceeds to union with satisfactory restoration of the articular surface and mechanical axes, a good result can still be obtained after capsular release and heterotopic ossification excision.

To prevent significant ankylosis, we prefer to manage fractures of the distal humerus as soon as possible, achieving secure fixation that allows early and unrestricted motion. Heterotopic ossification prophylaxis is rarely used, because the authors have found patient compliance with medical prophylaxis exceedingly low.

Management of the stiff elbow after operative fixation of a distal humerus fracture entails removal of internal fixation; capsulectomy; débridement of the olecranon, coronoid, and radial fossae; and excision of ectopic bone if necessary.[12,38,93,108,136,158,159] This is performed after fracture union, typically between 6 and 12 months after injury, and is dependent on complete fracture union and recovery from any other injuries that the patient may have incurred.[158] For a successful outcome, it is vital that the patient be able to devote full attention to the postoperative rehabilitation after contracture release.

ANNOTATED REFERENCES

21. Cobb TK, Morrey BF: Total elbow arthroplasty as primary treatment for distal humeral fractures in elderly patients. J Bone Joint Surg Am 79:826-832, 1997.

In one of the first significant contributions evaluating the effectiveness of total elbow arthroplasty for comminuted fractures of the distal humerus in the elderly, these authors retrospectively reviewed their results of primary total elbow arthroplasty for the treatment of an acute fracture of the distal humerus in 20 consecutive patients (21 elbows). Nine patients (10 elbows) had associated rheumatoid arthritis, and the mean follow-up was 3.3 years. Using the Mayo elbow performance score, 15 elbows had an excellent result and 5 had a good result; there were inadequate data for one elbow. There were no fair or poor results. The mean arc of flexion was 25 to 130 degrees. The results suggest that total elbow arthroplasty can be an alternative form of treatment of a severely comminuted fracture of the distal aspect of the humerus in older patients. The authors also note that this procedure is not an alternative to osteosynthesis in younger patients.

37. Garcia JA, Mykula R, Stanley D: Complex fractures of the distal humerus in the elderly: The role of total elbow replacement as primary treatment. J Bone Joint Surg Br 84:812-816, 2002.

These authors evaluated 19 consecutive elderly patients with distal humerus fractures treated by primary total elbow replacement. The average follow-up was 3 years. Unlike the report from Cobb and Morrey, no patient had inflammatory or degenerative arthritis of the elbow. At follow-up 11 patients (68%) reported no pain, 4 (25%) had mild pain with activity, and 1 had mild pain at rest. The mean flexion arc was 24 degrees to 125 degrees, and the mean Mayo elbow score was 93. The authors concluded that primary total elbow

arthroplasty was an acceptable option for the management of comminuted fractures of the distal humerus in elderly patients.

39. Gerwin M, Hotchkiss RN, Weiland AJ: Alternative operative exposures of the posterior aspect of the humeral diaphysis with reference to the radial nerve. J Bone Joint Surg Am 78:1690-1695, 1996.

This useful cadaveric anatomic study evaluated the course of the radial nerve and described an alternate exposure of the posterior aspect of the humeral diaphysis. The authors use this modified approach with an olecranon osteotomy for displaced intra-articular fractures of the distal humerus with proximal diaphyseal extension.

41. Gofton WT, Macdermid JC, Patterson SD, et al: Functional outcome of AO type C distal humeral fractures. J Hand Surg [Am] 28:294-308, 2003.

This articles reviews 23 patients with bicolumnar distal humerus fractures treated with a posterior approach and orthogonal plating. Twenty-two of 23 patients were managed using an olecranon osteotomy. The excellent functional results are similar to those obtained by McKee and colleagues and can be used as a guideline for expected results. Importantly, they also demonstrate the absence of significant ulnar neuropathy with routine anterior ulnar nerve transposition. The benefits of ulnar nerve transposition at the time of operative fixation are strengthened by this report and confirm those previously described by Wang.

48. Helfet DL, Hotchkiss RN: Internal fixation of the distal humerus: A biomechanical comparison of methods. J Orthop Trauma 4:260-264, 1990.

This important biomechanical publication formally demonstrated the benefits of orthogonal plating of the distal humerus. Although the authors found no significant difference in rigidity or strength testing between using one-third tubular, 3.5 mm reconstruction, or mixed plate constructs, later clinical information would suggest that the one-third tubular construct is associated with implant failure, malunion, and nonunion.

52. Henley MB, Bone LB, Parker B: Operative management of intra-articular fractures of the distal humerus. J Orthop Trauma 1:24-35, 1987.

Thirty-three patients with intra-articular distal humerus fractures were operatively managed. Most were young patients who had sustained high-energy injuries. The authors demonstrated 92% good or excellent results. An important contribution of this paper is that one-third tubular plates were associated with failure and stiffer implants were recommended. Also, they reported a 31% olecranon osteotomy complication rate, mostly with Kirschner wire fixation. This high rate would prompt proponents of the osteotomy to utilize improved fixation, while others would pursue the advantages of triceps-elevating approaches.

68. Jupiter JB, Barnes KA, Goodman LJ, Saldana AE: Multiplane fracture of the distal humerus. J Orthop Trauma 7:216-220, 1993.

This paper describes a unique but complex intra-articular fracture of the distal humerus. The term *multiplane fracture* has been applied to highlight a fracture pattern that features not only the well-recognized "T" fracture lines in the sagittal and horizontal planes but also a coronal fracture of the trochlea. This paper improves the understanding of distal humeral fracture anatomy.

70. Jupiter JB, Mehne DK: Fractures of the distal humerus. Orthopedics 15:825-833, 1992.

This publication reviews the column concept of the distal humerus and the Mehne and Matta classification system. The importance of the column concept and this classification system is that it identifies the interdependence of the medial, lateral, and trochlear components in stabilizing bicolumnar fractures of the distal humerus, allowing the surgeon to formulate a preoperative plan based on the location of the fracture.

71. Jupiter JB, Neff U, Holzach P, Allgower M: Intercondylar fractures of the humerus: An operative approach. J Bone Joint Surg Am 67:226-239, 1985.

   A series of 34 intercondylar fractures of the distal end of the humerus were treated by open reduction over a 10-year period. Using AO/ASIF techniques, 13 results were rated as excellent; 14, as good; 4, as fair; and 3, as poor. The mean follow-up was 5.8 years. This paper confirmed consistent and satisfactory results could be obtained with the proper operative management of these fractures.

72. Jupiter JB, Neff U, Regazzoni P, Allgower M: Unicondylar fractures of the distal humerus: An operative approach. J Orthop Trauma 2:102-109, 1988.

   In one of the few papers evaluating unicolumnar fractures, the authors of this paper demonstrated consistent and satisfactory results in 22 patients treated with modern AO/ASIF techniques. At an average follow-up of 5.9 years, 12 elbows were rated as excellent, 6 as good, and 4 as fair.

96. McKee MD, Jupiter JB, Bamberger HB: Coronal shear fractures of the distal end of the humerus. J Bone Joint Surg Am 78:49-54, 1996.

   The authors of this paper identified a shear fracture of the distal articular surface of the humerus, with anterior and proximal displacement of the capitellum and a portion of the trochlea. The pathognomonic double-arc sign was characterized on the lateral radiograph. The authors detail their surgical approach to this fracture pattern and describe excellent results. This fracture pattern would later be identified as a component of unique injury patterns occurring entirely within the articular segment of the distal humerus.

99. McKee MD, Wilson TL, Winston L, et al: Functional outcome following surgical treatment of intra-articular distal humeral fractures through a posterior approach. J Bone Joint Surg Am 82:1701-1707, 2000.

   Twenty-five patients who had an isolated, closed, displaced, intercondylar, intra-articular fracture of the distal humerus repaired operatively through a posterior approach and modern fixation were identified. All patients completed both limb-specific and general health-status questionnaires, and muscle-strength was objectively tested. This would be the first study to objectively measure flexion/extension strength after ORIF of distal humerus fractures. The authors hypothesized that these objective findings may explain the mild residual physical impairment detected with limb-specific outcome measures and physical function components of general health-status measures. The flexion/extension arc and muscle power end points are useful guidelines when reviewing expected outcomes with patients.

137. Ring D, Jupiter JB, Gulotta L: Articular fractures of the distal part of the humerus. J Bone Joint Surg Am 85:232-238, 2003.

   The importance of this paper is that it continues to define the spectrum of injury that may occur to the articular surface of the distal humerus. Five components of the injury were identified: (1) the capitellum and the lateral aspect of the trochlea, (2) the lateral epicondyle, (3) the posterior aspect of the lateral column, (4) the posterior aspect of the trochlea, and (5) the medial epicondyle. All fractures were reduced and were stabilized with implants buried beneath the articular surface. The average arc of ulnohumeral motion was 96 degrees (range, 55 to 140 degrees). The results according to the Mayo Elbow Performance Index were excellent in 4 patients, good in 12, and fair in 5.

139. Riseborough EJ, Radin EL: Intercondylar T fractures of the humerus in the adult: A comparison of operative and nonoperative treatment in twenty-nine cases. J Bone Joint Surg Am 51:130-141, 1969.

   Classic paper that introduces the Riseborough and Radin distal humerus fractures classification system. The results of 29 patients were reviewed and compared. This paper illustrates that technically poor surgery can lead to results worse than nonoperative care. Approximately one decade after the beginnings of the AO group, the authors conclude that ORIF offers little chance of a good outcome.

162. Wang KC, Shih HN, Hsu KY, Shih CH: Intercondylar fractures of the distal humerus: routine anterior subcutaneous transposition of the ulnar nerve in a posterior operative approach. J Trauma 36:770-773, 1994.

   This paper demonstrates the benefits of routine subcutaneous transposition of the ulnar nerve when operatively managing bicolumnar fractures of the distal humerus with medial and lateral plating techniques. Unlike previously published reports, the authors found no postoperative ulnar neuropathy in their patient group. This would later be supported by Gofton and colleagues.[41]

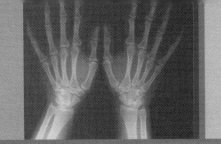

CHAPTER 21

Fractures of the Head of the Radius

Graham J. W. King

Fractures of the head of the radius are the most common fractures of the elbow. The majority occur between the ages of 20 and 60 years of age, with the incidence in females being twice that in males. Whereas nondisplaced fractures typically occur in isolation, displaced fractures are frequently associated with ligament injuries of the medial and lateral collateral ligaments and/or the interosseous ligament. In more severe injuries, dislocations of the elbow and forearm may be associated with fractures of the head of the radius. Fractures of the coronoid, olecranon, and capitellum are commonly seen with fractures of the radial head and further impair elbow stability. The head of the radius is an important stabilizer of the elbow in the setting of these associated bony and ligamentous injuries.

Although minimally displaced fractures of the radial head usually have a favorable functional outcome with nonoperative management, there is little information demonstrating the optimal treatment of patients with displaced and/or comminuted fractures. In 1935, Jones stated, "Fracture of the head or neck of the radius with displacement is a serious injury. While the prognosis is good for recovery of a useful elbow, rarely is it a normal elbow."[95] This statement remains true today. The indications for surgical management of these fractures are not well defined in the literature. Fragment size, number of fragments, degree of displacement, and bone quality influence decision making regarding the optimal management. Associated injuries and a block to motion are also important factors to consider. Good results have been reported after open reduction and internal fixation (ORIF) for selected noncomminuted displaced fractures of the radial head. Excision of fragments, early or delayed excision, and arthroplasty all have a role in the management of these common injuries.

HISTORICAL REVIEW

Paul of Aegina (AD 625-690) was likely the first to report an injury to the proximal radius, as documented by Schwartz and Young in an excellent review of the early history of fractures of the head of the radius.[174] Desault, in 1811, suggested that fractures of the proximal radius were uncommon relative to the middle or distal end and that diagnosis was difficult owing to the surrounding thick muscular covering. In 1897, Helserich described a fracture of the radial head and suggested that resection of the radial head was helpful for late deformity. Subsequently, a number of authors expressed opinions regarding nonoperative treatment, passive manipulation, removal of fractured fragments, and excision of the entire radial head.

In 1910, Hammond stressed the utility of radiology in making the diagnosis of a fracture of the radial head, which he noted to be difficult based on the history and physical examination alone.[74] He also found that marked fracture displacement was a poor prognostic sign for outcome with nonoperative management and recommended excision of the fragments or the radial head. In 1926, Cutler described three types of fractures of the radial head and recommended closed treatment for undisplaced fractures.[39] He recommended surgery if a displaced fragment interfered with full motion, prevented reduction of an elbow dislocation, and in the cases of malunion, caused ankylosis or forearm stiffness.

Watson-Jones reported, in 1930, that only 50% good results could be obtained in the management of displaced fractures of the radial head.[208] He avoided excision of the radial head because of the "inevitable" radial shortening with subluxation or dislocation of the lower end of the ulna. Angulated fractures were stabilized with a sling of kangaroo tendon because he believed that angulation interfered with forearm rotation. In 1935, Jones reported on the outcome of 78 patients with fractures of the radial head and/or neck treated at the Massachusetts General Hospital.[95] He noted good results could be achieved by excising fragments that involve less than one third of the radial head. He reported better results with early versus late excision of the radial head.

In 1940, Murray reported on 459 cases of fractures of the radial head and neck managed at the Liverpool Infirmary over a 10-year period. He recommended early motion for undisplaced fractures, manipulation of displaced fractures, and open reduction as a last resort. Small fragments could be excised, but total excision was recommended for comminuted fractures.[145] In 1950, Carstam reported on a series of 74 patients with a fractured radial head or neck that were treated operatively over a 20-year period and reviewed at an average of 8 years.[29] Carstam considered that most fractures of the radial head were not isolated injuries; most of these patients had an elbow subluxation that had spontaneously reduced. He suggested that ORIF should be considered for marginal fractures with moderate displacement and reported good results. The results of fragment excision and whole-head excision were not appreciably different. He noted changes such as cubitus valgus and proximal migration of the radius were frequent but did not commonly cause symptoms, except in children.

In 1954, Mason reviewed 100 patients who had sustained a fracture of the radial head and described a classification system.[124] He recommended nonoperative treatment for undisplaced type I fractures and reported good results. Type II fractures, which he described as "marginal sector fractures with displacement," had more variable results. He recommended that conservative treatment should be pursued if the fracture fragment did not involve more than one fourth of the articular circumference and was reasonably well aligned. In all other cases, "no matter how minimal the tilting and comminution of the fracture segment" he recommended excision of the radial head. He described the axiom of treatment of a fracture of the radial head as "If in doubt—resect." Type III fractures were comminuted, and he advised primary excision of the radial head and reported good early results. None of the patients in this series was treated with ORIF. In 1962, Johnston added a fourth subtype to the Mason classification, fracture of the radial head associated with an elbow dislocation.[94] He considered that excision of the radial head was not a benign procedure and stated, "If in doubt, treat conservatively."

Subsequent to these papers, there has been an explosion of interest in anatomy of the radial head,[15,26,68,108] biomechanics,* and fracture management.[84] The importance of the radial head to the kinematics and load transfer of the elbow is now better understood, and there is an increasing interest in salvaging the radial head when possible.[†] Advances in screw and plate designs have resulted in increasing utilization of ORIF for displaced fractures of the radial head with excellent results for simple fracture configurations. Whereas long-term follow-up studies suggest that excision of the radial head is generally well tolerated clinically in the absence of associated ligament injuries, the incidence of osteoarthritis has been high.[‡] Implant arthroplasty of the radial head has become popular for the treatment of comminuted displaced fractures where ORIF is less predictable. Speed reported the use of a metallic arthroplasty of the radial head in 1941.[187] Subsequently, acrylic was employed with some early success.[31] Silicone implants gained widespread use in the 1970s and early 1980s.[§] More recently there has been a resurgence of interest in metallic implant arthroplasty, owing to problems with wear and failure of silicone when placed under compressive load.[¶] The success of first-generation metallic implants has resulted in newer modular designs to allow easier implantation and improved sizing options to provide a closer match to patient anatomy.[15,71,108,117]

Anatomy

The anatomy of the radial head is complex and highly variable.[108] The head of the radius consists of a circular concave dish that articulates with the spherical capitellum (Fig. 21-1). The dish has a greater radius of curvature than the capitellum, making this articulation only moderately constrained. The articular dish is variably offset from the axis of the radial neck. The margin of the radial head that articulates with the radial notch of the ulna is slightly elliptical,[11] producing a cam effect during forearm rotation that displaces the radial shaft somewhat radially during pronation.[55] The proximal radioulnar articulation comprises

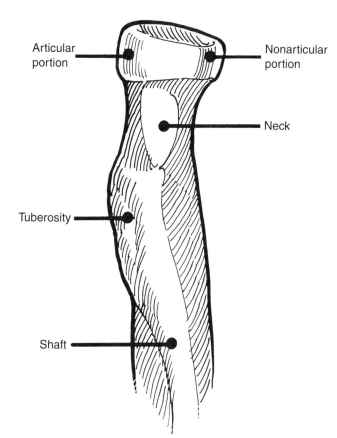

FIGURE 21-1. Anatomy of the proximal radius. The radial head is somewhat elliptical. The concave surface of the radial head that articulates with the capitellum is variably offset in a radial direction from the axis of the radial neck. The portion of the radial head that does not articulate with the radial notch of the ulna is more rounded, whereas the articulating portion is more flattened.

* See references 2, 4-6, 11, 72, 92, 109, 140, 141, 143, 144, 158, 160, 176, 179, and 194.

†See references 7, 19, 23, 49, 53, 54, 58, 62, 63, 79, 84, 102, 106, 114, 128, 154-156, 164, 168, 170, 172, 180, and 203.

‡See references 19, 35, 56, 57, 66, 88, 91, 104, 113, 135, 171, 188, and 206.

§See references 16, 19, 27, 67, 120, 127, 142, 189, 192, 199, 202, and 209.

¶See references 28, 47, 76, 77, 97, 98, 110, 138, 159, 182, and 187.

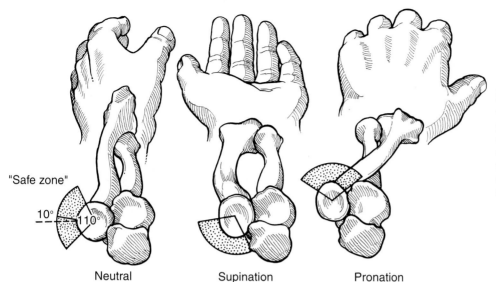

"Safe zone"

10° 110°

Neutral   Supination   Pronation

FIGURE 21-2. Nonarticular portion of the radial head. The nonarticular portion "safe zone" of the radial head can be identified as a 110-degree arc centered on a point 10 degrees anterior to the midpoint of the lateral side of the radial head with the forearm in neutral rotation.

an arc of 60 to 70 degrees and is highly congruous, allowing for minimal translation during forearm rotation. The antero-lateral one third of the articular margin is devoid of cartilage, allowing placement of internal fixation without impinge-ment with the radial notch during forearm rotation. A "safe zone" for internal fixation has been described as a 110-degree arc centered on a point 10 degrees anterior to the midpoint of the lateral side of the radial head as judged with the forearm in neutral rotation (Fig. 21-2).[26,55,184,186] This nonar-ticular portion can also be identified by the rounded shape of its margin relative to the flatter surface that articulates with the proximal radioulnar joint. The rotational interval between Lister's tubercle and the radial styloid of the distal radius is another useful anatomic landmark for the nonartic-ular portion of the radial head. Placement of plates on the nonarticular margin may be required when managing frac-tures involving the radial neck. The radial head is surrounded by the annular ligament; therefore, bulky internal fixation is poorly tolerated. Implants should be low profile to minimize soft tissue adherence that may impede forearm rotation.

The cancellous trabeculae are oriented perpendicular to the surface of the radial head, confirming the load-bearing function of the radial head. It has been suggested that the subchondral bone is weaker in the anterolateral portion of the radial head[11]; however, this is not supported by com-puted tomography (CT)[46] or by a recent biomechanical study that demonstrated that the cancellous bone quality is similar throughout the radial head.[68] These results suggest that the quality of screw fixation should be similar regard-less of the location of screw placement in the radial head.

The blood supply of the radial head comprises both intraosseous and extraosseous sources.[65] Vessels penetrate the radial neck from the periosteum at the head/neck junc-tion; the dorsolateral periosteum is a key area for these branches. Preservation of the periosteal attachment of dis-placed fragments is important during ORIF of fractures of the radial head and neck.[78]

A better understanding of the lateral ligamentous anatomy of the elbow has resulted in improvements in surgical technique during surgery on the head of the radius.

The lateral ulnar collateral ligament is an important stabilizer against posterolateral rotational instability of the elbow (Fig. 21-3).[44,146,148] Conventional surgical approaches to the radial head through Kocher's interval (between the extensor carpi ulnaris and the anconeus) often cause iatro-genic injury to the lateral ulnar collateral ligament unless the dissection is brought more anterior such that the radial collateral and annular ligaments are divided at the mid axis of the radial head. Additionally this approach tends to expose the radial head too posterior to permit internal fixa-tion of the commonly involved anterolateral portion of the radial head. Maintaining the integrity of the lateral ulnar collateral ligament or performing a strong repair to bone is essential to prevent instability, which may be an important cause of failure of internal fixation, late pain, and arthritis. Repair of the fascial interval between the anconeus and extensor carpi ulnaris has also been shown to further aug-ment elbow stability.[33] For isolated fractures of the radial

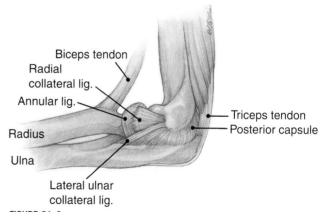

Biceps tendon
Radial collateral lig.
Annular lig.
Radius
Ulna
Triceps tendon
Posterior capsule
Lateral ulnar collateral lig.

FIGURE 21-3. Lateral ligaments of the elbow. The lateral ligaments of the elbow include the radial collateral, lateral ulnar collateral, and annular ligaments. The lateral ulnar collateral ligament is an important stabilizer against posterolateral rotational and varus instability of the elbow. The annular ligament stabilizes the proximal radioulnar joint and contributes to varus and posterolateral rotatory elbow stability by virtue of its attachment to the radial collateral ligament.

head without associated ligamentous or osseous injuries, a more anterior muscle-tendon splitting approach through the common extensor origin at the midportion of the radial head should be considered. This approach allows for good visualization of the radial head and avoids detachment of the lateral ulnar collateral ligament. However, it is less extensile distally, limited by the proximity of the posterior interosseous nerve, which lies on average 33 mm (minimum 22 mm) from the capitellum in supination and 52 mm (minimum 38 mm) in pronation.[41]

Resisted isometric elbow flexion has been estimated to generate forces up to four times body weight across the joint.[4] The radiocapitellar articulation may account for up to 60% of the load transfer across the elbow.[72] In one study it was demonstrated that up to three times body weight can be transmitted to the radiocapitellar joint during strenuous activities.[3,4] Contact forces across this articulation are greatest with the forearm in pronation.[141] Displaced fractures of the radial head result in a decreased residual surface area available for load transfer and therefore increased cartilage contact pressures, which may predispose to arthritis. Excision of the radial head increases the tension in the medial collateral ligament and concentrates the forces acting across the elbow on the lateral aspect of the coronoid. Amis and coworkers estimated that this force may be as high as nine times body weight.[3] Posterolateral rotational instability of the elbow is aggravated by excision of fragments or the entire radial head as a consequence of both the loss of "capture" of the articulating dish of the radial head by the capitellum and a diminished tensioning effect on the lateral collateral ligament.[13,146] Repair or replacement of displaced fractures should be helpful to improve load transfer and improve elbow stability; however, further clinical and biomechanical studies are needed.

The head of the radius is an important valgus stabilizer of the elbow, particularly in the setting of an incompetent medial collateral ligament.[109,140,144,158,173] In-vitro biomechanical studies have shown that the kinematics and stability of the elbow are altered by excision of the radial head, even in the setting of intact collateral ligaments.[92,105] Replacement of the radial head with metallic prostheses has been demonstrated to improve the stability of elbows with intact and deficient medial and/or lateral collateral ligaments.[105,109] Axial forearm stability is also improved by metallic prostheses of the radial head in the setting of an interosseous ligament disruption.[176] Silicone replacements are inferior to metallic implants in restoring both axial and valgus stability.[86,87,109,160,176]

PREOPERATIVE EVALUATION

Clinical Assessment

Inspection may reveal ecchymosis along the forearm and/or medial aspect of the elbow. Careful palpation of the medial collateral ligament of the elbow, the interosseous ligament of the forearm, and the distal radioulnar joint should be performed, because these injuries are often subtle and may not be evident even with a careful physical examination. Because associated injuries of the shoulder, forearm, wrist, and hand are common, these areas should be carefully examined.

Range of motion, including forearm rotation and elbow flexion/extension, should be evaluated. Palpable and auditory crepitus should be noted during forearm rotation. Forearm rotation is generally preserved but may sometimes be limited by pain or a mechanical block. In these circumstances, aspiration of the hemarthrosis and injection of a local anesthetic should be considered, but not before 24 hours so the hemarthrosis does not reaccumulate.[42,83,161,204] With sterile technique and with the forearm in pronation to protect the radial nerve, a needle is introduced into the lateral soft spot located at the center of a triangle formed by the lateral epicondyle, olecranon, and radial head (Fig. 21-4). After the hemarthrosis is aspirated, 10 mL of 1% lidocaine (Xylocaine) is injected. Persistent loss of rotation after pain relief suggests a mechanical block, whereas palpable grating suggests articular incongruity that requires surgical management. Loss of terminal elbow flexion and extension is expected as a consequence of an elbow effusion and does not necessarily indicate a mechanical block requiring surgical treatment.

Imaging

Anteroposterior, lateral, and oblique elbow radiographs usually provide sufficient information for the diagnosis and treatment of fractures of the head of the radius. The x-ray beam must be centered on the radiocapitellar joint to ensure a tangential view of the radial head. Because a hemarthrosis prevents elbow extension, two anteroposterior radiographs

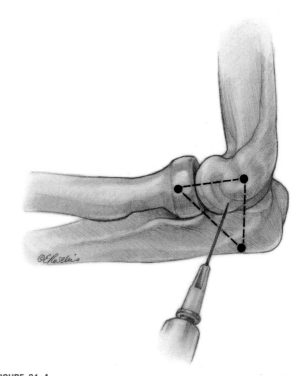

FIGURE 21-4. Aspiration of the elbow. Under sterile technique with the forearm maintained in pronation, a needle is introduced into the center of a triangle formed by the lateral epicondyle, radial head, and tip of the olecranon. The hemarthrosis is aspirated and local anesthetic is injected. An improvement in rotation is suggestive of pain-limiting motion, whereas a persistent restriction of rotation is suggestive of a mechanical block requiring surgical management.

may be required if there is significant loss of extension: anteroposterior views of the distal humerus and the forearm. A radiocapitellar view can be useful because it places the radial head in profile.[69] The elbow is positioned for a lateral radiograph, but the x-ray tube is angled 45 degrees cephalad (Fig. 21-5). In patients with undisplaced fractures of the radial head or neck, plain radiographs may only demonstrate elevation of the anterior or posterior fat pads (sail sign) as a consequence of a hemarthrosis (Fig. 21-6). Bilateral posteroanterior radiographs of both wrists in neutral rotation should be performed to evaluate ulnar variance in patients with wrist discomfort and in those who have a comminuted fracture of the radial head because there is a higher incidence of an associated interosseous ligament injury in these patients.[40] Ultrasound or magnetic resonance imaging may be useful to evaluate the presence of an interosseous ligament tear in suspected cases.[52] Because of the cylindrical shape of the radial head, conventional elbow radiographs often underestimate the degree of articular surface involvement and displacement.[94,106] CT is useful to quantify fracture size, location, displacement, and comminution in cases in which the indications for surgery are less clear. CT may also assist with preoperative planning with respect to the need for specialized equipment for fracture fixation or prosthetic replacement.

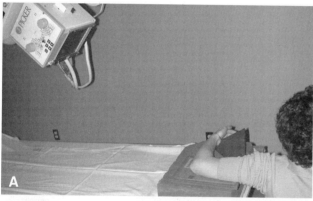

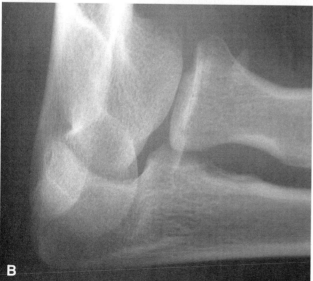

FIGURE 21-5. The radiocapitellar view can be useful because it places the radial head in profile. **A** and **B,** The elbow is positioned for a lateral radiograph, but the x-ray tube is angled 45 degrees cephalad.

Classification

Mason classified fractures of the radial head into three types: type I—fissure or marginal sector fractures without displacement; type II—marginal sector fractures with displacement, and type III—comminuted fractures involving the whole radial head (Fig. 21-7).[124] One study has demonstrated moderate to poor intraobserver and interobserver reproducibility of this classification based on plain radiographs.[137] Other authors have reported that many Mason type II fractures are reclassified to type III during surgery owing to additional fracture segments being found that are not appreciated on plain radiographs.[106] Johnston added a fourth type, fracture of the radial head associated with an elbow dislocation.[94] This additional category does little to direct treatment of fracture of the head of the radius other than to emphasize that excision of the radial head without replacement is contraindicated in the setting of an associated elbow dislocation. Morrey has suggested that fractures that are isolated be referred to as "simple or uncomplicated", whereas those associated with other soft tissue or bony injuries be referred to as "complex or complicated."[139]

More recently, Hotchkiss developed a management-based classification with three types (Table 21-1)[84]:

Type I—undisplaced or minimally displaced (<2 mm) small marginal fracture of the radial head or neck with no mechanical block to motion

Type II—displaced (>2 mm) fracture of the radial head or neck that is reconstructable with ORIF; may have mechanical block or be incongruous; more than a marginal lip fracture

Type III—comminuted fracture of the radial head or neck that is unreconstructable as judged by radiographs or at surgery; usually requires excision for movement

While this latter classification helps to direct treatment, the type of operation needed is less clear because the distinction between type II and III fractures remains problematic. The decision as to what fracture is reconstructable depends on surgeon factors such as experience and implants available, patient factors such as osteoporosis, and fracture factors such as fragment size, comminution, and associated soft tissue injuries. The final decision as to whether a fracture is reconstructable or whether it requires excision and/or replacement of the radial head can often only be decided during surgery. Therefore, this classification, to some extent, may be of more use retrospectively and is less helpful in deciding which type of surgery should be performed.

Associated Injuries

The mechanism of injury is commonly a fall on the outstretched hand. When the radial head fractures under axial or valgus loads, a comminuted head or neck fracture is likely caused by failure in compression (Fig. 21-8). In one cadaveric study, an isolated fracture of the radial head was most likely to occur with an axial load applied between 35 and 80 degrees of flexion.[6] In 1924, Odelberg-Johnson reported that elbow subluxation was an important mechanism of wedge fractures in a series of cadaveric experiments.[149] In the author's experience posterolateral rotatory subluxation of the elbow, the first stage of an elbow dislocation,[148] likely

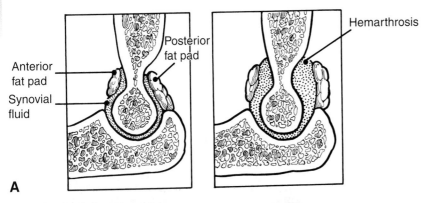

A

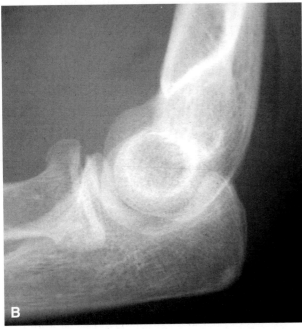

B

FIGURE 21-6. Fat pad sign. **A,** Normal position of fat pads in the elbow and displacement of fat pads induced by an intra-articular effusion. **B,** Lateral radiograph demonstrating anterior and posterior fat pad signs in a patient with an undisplaced fracture of the radial head.

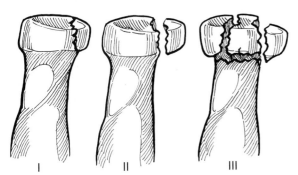

FIGURE 21-7. Mason classification. Mason described three types of fractures of the radial head: type I, undisplaced; type II, displaced wedge fragment(s); and type III, comminuted.

causes many of these anterolateral wedge fractures. This segment of the radial head shears off as the rim of the radial head dish subluxes off the capitellum with the forearm in neutral to supination. In many cases a partial or complete lateral ligament injury is noted in patients undergoing surgery for displaced anterolateral wedge fractures and may require concomitant management.

Displaced fractures of the radial head are commonly associated with disruption of ligaments of the elbow or forearm. In one study, no patient with a minimally or undisplaced fracture had an associated disruption of the medial collateral ligament when stress radiographs were performed.[40] However, 71% of patients with a displaced shear fracture of the radial head or an impacted fracture of the radial neck had a medial collateral ligament injury. All of the patients with a comminuted fracture had disruption of the medial collateral ligament of the elbow or the interosseous ligament of the forearm (91% and 9%, respectively). Johansson, using arthrography, reported medial collateral ligament or capsular disruptions in 4%, 21%, and 85% of Mason type I, II and III fractures, respectively.[93] In one series of patients with Essex-Lopresti injuries presenting for reconstruction, 15 of 20 patients had undergone resection of the radial head without knowledge of the forearm ligamentous injury, suggesting that this uncommon injury may be easily missed in clinical practice.[200] Collectively, these data suggest that minimally displaced fractures have a low incidence of associated soft tissue disruption. More displaced and comminuted fractures are likely of higher energy and therefore have a greater incidence of associated ligamentous injuries.

Table 21-1

HOTCHKISS CLASSIFICATION OF PROXIMAL RADIAL FRACTURES*

Type I

Nondisplaced or minimally displaced fracture of head or neck

No mechanical block to rotation

Displacement less than 2 mm or a marginal lip fracture

Type II

Displaced (usually > 2 mm) fracture of head or neck (angulated)

May have mechanical block to motion or be incongruous

Without severe comminution (technically possible to repair by open reduction and internal fixation)

More than a marginal lip fracture of the radial head

Type III

Severely comminuted fracture of the radial head or neck

Judged not reconstructable on basis of radiographic or intraoperative appearance

Usually requires excision for movement

---

*All of these fractures may have associated injuries such as a coronoid fracture, elbow dislocation, or medial collateral or interosseous ligament tears.

From Hotchkiss RN: Displaced fractures of the radial head: Internal fixation or excision. J Am Acad Orthop Surg 5:1-10, 1997.

Fractures of the capitellum may be seen as chondral injuries[24,78,79] or displaced osteochondral fractures. Ward and Nunley reported that 50% of patients with capitellar fractures had an associated fracture of the radial head, whereas only 1% of fractures of the radial head had a capitellar fracture.[207] For displaced fractures of the radial head treated operatively, the incidence of an associated capitellar fracture was 24%. These injuries may or may not be visible with plain radiographs or CT and are often only diagnosed at surgery. Capitellar fractures may be responsible for a block to elbow or forearm motion in the absence of significant displacement of a fracture of the radial head seen radiographically (Fig. 21-9).

Dislocations of the elbow are seen in 3% to 10% of patients with fractures of the radial head.[94,96,112,166] Patients with an associated elbow subluxation or dislocation may have a fracture of the coronoid as part of a "terrible triad" injury with disruption of one or both collateral ligaments of the elbow.[165] Small coronoid fragments typically present as triangular fragments situated anteriorly in the coronoid fossa and are often mistaken as a fragment of the radial head. Larger coronoid fragments are typically associated with greater instability of the elbow and require specific treatment, as outlined in Chapter 22. Most authors recommend that elbow fracture-dislocations be managed by immediate closed reduction followed by treatment of the radial head as for isolated fractures.[21,56,94,96,156] Whereas some authors recommend urgent operative management of the radial head

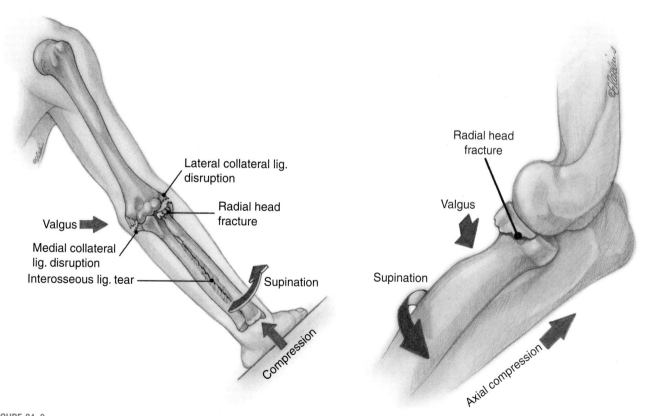

FIGURE 21-8. Mechanism of fracture of the radial head. **A,** Valgus and/or axial loading of the elbow causes failure of the radial head in compression and possible medial collateral ligament or interosseous membrane disruption. **B,** Posterolateral rotatory subluxation of the elbow causes disruption of the lateral ulnar collateral ligament and the anterolateral aspect of the radial head to shear off as it slides off the capitellum with the forearm in supination. This mechanism likely explains the commonly associated lateral ligamentous injuries and chondral damage of the capitellum seen with this fracture pattern. Continued subluxation of the elbow may result in a fracture of the coronoid, disruption of the medial collateral ligament, and a complete dislocation.

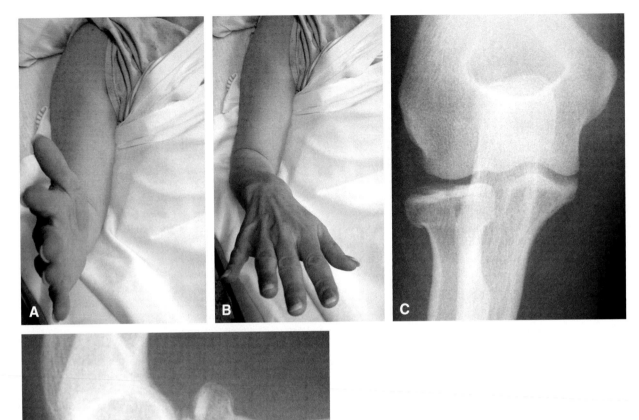

FIGURE 21-9. Capitellar cartilage shear fracture. **A** and **B,** Clinical photographs of a 49-year-old woman with a persistent block to supination 2 weeks after a minimally displaced fracture of the radial head. **C** and **D,** Preoperative anteroposterior and lateral radiographs demonstrating a displaced fracture of the radial head.

Continued

if needed (within 24 hours) to reduce the incidence of heterotopic ossification, this practice remains controversial.[61,94] Early motion seems to improve outcome; therefore, urgent, not emergent, management of the fracture is appropriate. Excision of the radial head without replacement should be avoided in patients with associated dislocations because of a high risk of redislocation and instability.[56,96,171] Fractures of the olecranon or proximal ulna may be seen in association with fractures of the radial head as a variant of the Monteggia fracture, particularly with higher-energy injuries such as those sustained in a motor vehicle accident or a fall from a height.[138,156]

Neurologic injuries are uncommon but may be associated with concomitant injuries or severe fracture displacement.

TREATMENT OPTIONS

Fractures of the head of the radius should be managed based on patient factors such as age, bone quality, associated injuries, and activity level.[73] Fracture factors that influence decision making include fracture size, displacement and location, and the presence of a block to forearm rotation. For example, an older patient with osteoporosis and a comminuted fracture is a poor candidate for internal fixation. Arthroplasty of the radial head is the preferred option for displaced unreconstructable fractures in the setting of an associated injury to the medial collateral or interosseous ligaments because excision further compromises instability.[86,87,105,109,122,158,160,176]

The initial management of a fracture of the radial head associated with an elbow dislocation is a gentle closed reduction of the elbow under intravenous sedation. Repeat radiographs taken after the reduction should be obtained to better evaluate the fracture for further management, either nonoperative or operative. A careful assessment for an associated fracture of the coronoid and/or capitellum is needed in patients with a fracture of the radial head, particularly in patients with a history of an elbow dislocation. The presence of a coronoid fracture suggests an unstable elbow for which

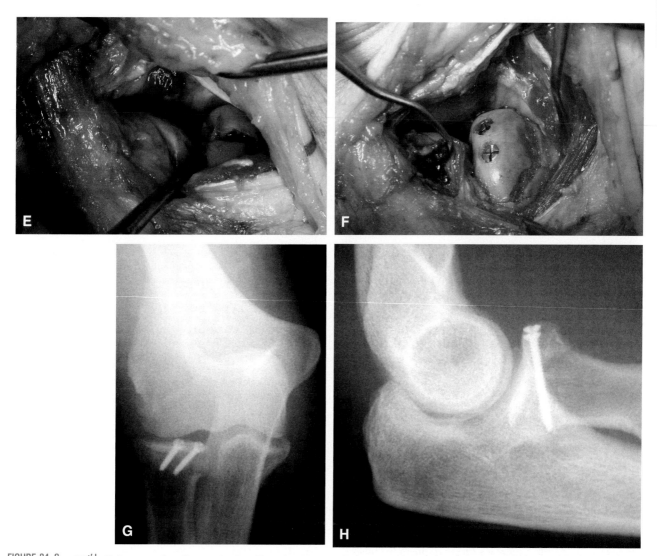

FIGURE 21-9—cont'd. **E,** Intraoperative photograph of cartilage shear fracture. **F,** Intraoperative photograph demonstrating reduction of the fracture with two 2.0-mm screws and cancellous bone grafting of the radial neck from the lateral epicondyle. **G** and **H,** Postoperative anteroposterior and lateral radiographs after ORIF of the radial head and débridement of the capitellum.

operative management may be required to achieve an optimal outcome. The author's recommended management algorithm is shown in Figure 21-10.

Nonoperative Management

Undisplaced or minimally displaced fractures of the radial head and neck and small marginal head fractures, which do not cause a block to forearm rotation, are best treated with early active range-of-motion exercises. Fractures less than one third of the diameter of the radial head that are displaced less than 2 mm are candidates for nonoperative management. Depressed fractures generally do not impede forearm rotation, whereas extruded fragments do, often by virtue of their impingement with the proximal radioulnar joint and annular ligament. Whereas some authors have recommended cast immobilization,[70,126] most studies have supported the concept of early motion.[30,118,125,125,197,201,210] Aspiration of the elbow hemarthrosis and injection of local anesthetic, as previously described, should be considered only if there is sufficient pain to prevent evaluation of

forearm rotation.[42,161] In a prospective randomized clinical trial, aspiration and injection of anesthetic in the absence of a mechanical block to motion were demonstrated not to alter the final outcome.[83]

Active motion should be begun within 1 week, owing to the frequent development of elbow stiffness with longer periods of immobilization. A collar and cuff, or sling, is used for comfort between periods of active motion and discontinued by 4 weeks (Fig. 21-11). The use of a static progressive extension splint should be considered at night if elbow extension does not progressively improve in the first 4 to 6 weeks after the injury. Although these fractures are generally stable and subsequent displacement is uncommon, careful clinical and radiographic follow-up is required. Late displacement may be more common in fractures involving more than one third of the radial head.[124]

Open Reduction and Internal Fixation

The use of ORIF should be considered for noncomminuted fractures that are displaced 2 mm or more and involve a

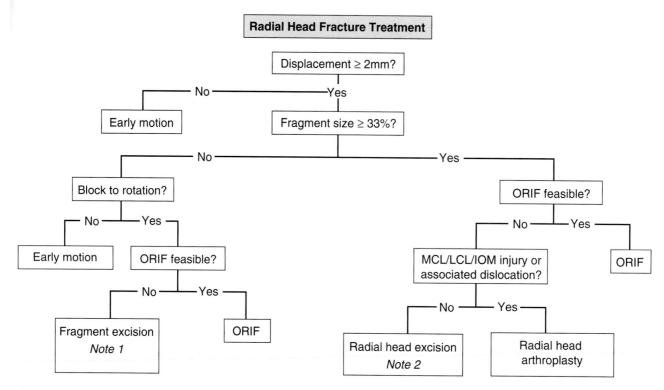

Note 1: Fragments that articulate with the proximal radioulnar joint should not be excised owing to radioulnar incongruity: radial head arthroplasty preferred.

Note 2: The author considers all comminuted radial head fractures that cannot be reconstructed as likely to have an associated ligament injury; therefore, radial head arthroplasty is routinely performed.

FIGURE 21-10. Author's recommended management algorithm for fracture of the head of the radius. MCL, medial collateral ligament; LCL, lateral collateral ligament; IOM, interosseous membrane.

"significant" portion of the radial head. Mason suggested that displaced fractures greater than one fourth of the diameter of the radial head should be treated by excision.[124] Geel and colleagues recommended ORIF of displaced (> 2 mm) fractures involving more than one fourth of the radial head.[63] Radin and Riseborough[163] suggested that displaced fractures greater than one third of the radial head should be managed operatively. Miller and others reported that fragment size had no effect on the outcome of type II fractures.[136] The decision as to the size and displacement of a fracture for which surgery has a better outcome than nonoperative management is unknown, owing to a lack of scientific data directing clinical practice. In one in-vitro biomechanical study a progressive loss in radiocapitellar joint stability was observed with increasing size of wedge defects in the radial head.[13] Wedge defects greater than one third of the radial head did not contribute to stability in this model. These data suggest that, particularly in the setting of elbow instability, fixation of fragments smaller than one third of the radial head may be advantageous. Whereas it seems that most displaced intra-articular fractures in other joints benefit from anatomic reduction, stable fixation, and early motion, displaced fractures of the radial head have historically often been managed nonoperatively if they do not impede joint motion. Persistent articular displacement will result in abnormal joint contact pressures and may predispose to arthritis and pain. Although delayed excision of the radial head is typically helpful in these circumstances, complete relief of symptoms is not assured.[20,57,206] Current thinking is that fractures displaced 2 mm or greater, involving one third

or more of the radial head, should be considered for operative reduction, even if they do not impede joint motion. Fractures with a mechanical block to motion have a clear indication for surgical treatment regardless of their size. Small fragments that are extruded into the proximal radioulnar joint and block forearm rotation are included in this group if stable internal fixation can be achieved.

The degree of displacement of a fracture of the neck of the radius that requires surgery in adults is unknown.[9] Whereas most undisplaced fractures of the radial neck heal when treated with early motion, nonunions do occur.[32,54,134,167] Nonoperative treatment is recommended except in the setting of associated injuries requiring surgical management such as fractures of the coronoid or olecranon. Translation of the radial head on the neck produces a cam effect and often impedes forearm rotation if it is greater than 2 to 3 mm. Neck angulation of more than 20 degrees in adults commonly interferes with forearm rotation owing to altered kinematics with the capitellum and radial notch of the ulna and should be considered for surgical management.[9]

The decision to repair, excise, or replace the radial head can often only be determined intraoperatively. ORIF of multifragmented fractures can be successful if stable internal fixation is achieved so that early motion can be initiated.* One study has reported a high incidence of complications following ORIF of greater than three fragments,

---

*See references 19, 23, 49, 53, 63, 78, 79, 84, 102, 106, 128, 150, 151, 154-156, 164, 168, 170, 172, 180, and 203.

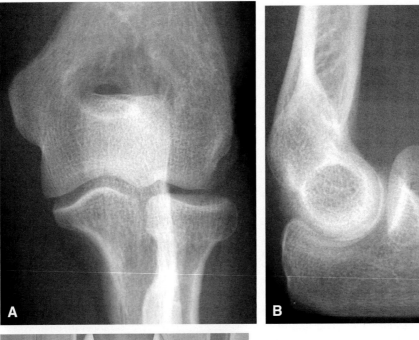

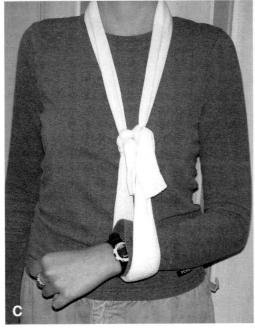

FIGURE 21-11. Hotchkiss type I fracture. Anteroposterior (**A**) and lateral (**B**) radiographs of a 55-year-old woman with an undisplaced fracture of the radial neck. **C,** Management with a collar and cuff sling. The patient had a complete return of motion and no residual pain.

suggesting an alternative treatment method should be considered for more comminuted fractures.[168] Failure to achieve a congruous reduction and rigid fixation owing to comminution or osteoporosis should prompt the surgeon to intraoperatively consider excision of the radial head or replacement. Tenuous fixation in the setting of associated ligamentous injuries should be avoided because minimal residual instability after ligament repair will likely lead to fixation failure.[106,166,168] Failed surgical reconstruction usually leads to articular injury to the capitellum and radial notch of the ulna. Stiffness and pain frequently require further surgery, often with less than satisfactory outcomes. The outcome of patients with failed internal fixation is typically not as successful as those managed initially with excision of the radial head or replacement, suggesting that

intraoperative decision making is critical to optimize treatment outcome.

Reduction and internal fixation of displaced fractures of the radial head using arthroscopy is difficult owing to the inability to distract the radiocapitellar joint to properly evaluate the articular reduction. Furthermore, bleeding often compromises the view such that a 3- to 5-day delay before surgery is recommended. Standard elbow arthroscopic techniques and equipment are employed; however, a 70-degree scope is helpful to better visualize the joint surface. The efficacy and indications for arthroscopic reduction of fractures of the radial head are evolving. Open surgical approaches remain the current standard of care. Although most authors prefer a Kocher approach,[111] some have employed a lateral epicondyle osteotomy.[78]

Fixation is performed using bioabsorbable pins, small threaded wires, headless screws, 1.5-, 2.0-, or 2.7-mm screws and plates, or 3.0-mm cannulated screws depending on fragment size. Smooth Kirschner wires are useful to reduce fragments and provide provisional fixation, but they should not be employed for definitive fixation because of their tendency to migrate during the postoperative period. Threaded Kirschner wires may be useful for small fragments not amenable to screw fixation, but the cut ends of the wires must be burred so that they lie below the articular cartilage. Screws should be placed through the stronger bone of the articular margin and countersunk to prevent impingement with the radial notch and annular ligament.

The use of crossed cannulated 3.0-mm screws has been found to be effective in stabilizing the radial head on the radial neck in the absence of comminution. Intramedullary fixation has also been reported.[100] Plate fixation is employed for comminuted fractures of the radial neck in an effort to stabilize the radial head onto the neck and achieve union.[114] Fixed-angle plate fixation has been demonstrated to be biomechanically superior to the standard "T"-plates.[153] Premolded proximal radial plates are lower in profile and stronger than standard "T"-plates and may yield improved results. Plates should be placed on the nonarticular portion of the radial head. This can easily be determined intraoperatively as the lateral portion of the radial head with the forearm maintained in neutral rotation.[186] If bone grafting is required after elevation of a depressed fragment, the lateral epicondyle is a convenient source.

Excision of Fragments of the Radial Head

Fragment excision is infrequently indicated with the advent of improved fixation systems. Cartilage flaps and small displaced fragments (<33% of the radial head) that block forearm rotation due to extrusion into the proximal radioulnar joint or loose fragments that prevent elbow flexion/extension are treated with open or arthroscopic fragment excision if ORIF is not technically feasible because of small fragment size, comminution, or osteoporosis.[30,95,145,211] Fragments that articulate with the proximal radioulnar joint should not be excised because of interference with forearm rotation. An image intensifier and a pituitary rongeur facilitate fragment excision when using an open approach.

Delayed Excision of the Radial Head

Early motion with delayed excision of the radial head may be considered in patients with displaced fractures who have no mechanical block to forearm or elbow motion. This approach may be useful in elderly low-demand patients with injuries to the medial collateral or interosseous ligaments and in patients with a delayed presentation. The radial head can be excised either open or arthroscopically if the patient remains symptomatic after healing of the fracture and any associated ligamentous injury.[1,20,57] The radial head is excised just distal to the radial notch with careful preservation of the lateral ulnar collateral ligament and repair of the annular ligament if done through an arthrotomy. An image intensifier should be employed intraoperatively to ensure an adequate excision, whether performed open or arthroscopically.

Excision of the Radial Head

Prior to the development of more reliable methods of internal fixation, displaced fractures of the radial head, both simple and comminuted, were commonly treated by open excision of the radial head.* Although less frequently performed today, excision of the radial head is preferable to an unstable or incongruous ORIF.[168] Should radial head reconstruction not be technically possible, associated soft tissue injuries and concomitant fractures should be evaluated because acute excision of the radial head is contraindicated in the setting of concomitant disruption of the medial collateral ligament, interosseous ligament, or an elbow dislocation.[1,94,169]

The radial head can be excised either through an arthrotomy or arthroscopically,[119,132,133] as described earlier. Intraoperative valgus and varus stress views should be obtained with an image intensifier after excision of the radial head to ensure competency of the medial and lateral collateral ligaments of the elbow.[40] Axial stress views to look for an interosseous ligament tear should also be performed by evaluating changes in ulnar variance at the wrist (Fig. 21-12). If these intraoperative stress tests are negative, there was no associated elbow dislocation and there is no clinical suspicion of a ligamentous injury, acute excision of the radial head without implant replacement may be considered. Given the high incidence of associated ligamentous injuries with comminuted fractures, and the difficulty in diagnosing these associated conditions, I perform a metallic arthroplasty for all acute unreconstructable fractures of the radial head. Careful preservation of the lateral ulnar collateral ligament and repair of the annular ligament should be performed if the radial head is excised open. The timing of excision is controversial owing to concerns regarding the potential development of heterotopic ossification, with some authors recommending early excision (<24 hr)[1,61,89,94,196] and others excision within 10 days.[29,90,124] The presence of an associated dislocation and head injury appears to be the risk factor most associated with the development of heterotopic ossification after elbow surgery.[1,60,196]

Arthroplasty of the Radial Head

Replacement arthroplasty is indicated for displaced comminuted fractures of the radial head where an anatomic reduction and stable internal fixation is not achievable and there are, or are likely to be, associated soft tissue or bony injuries. These include soft tissue injuries to the medial or lateral collateral ligaments or the interosseous ligament and/or injury to the triangular fibrocartilage and bony injuries of the coronoid or olecranon. Silicone implants have been employed in the past.[16,19,27,120,142,189,192,209] However, they are biomechanically inferior to metal and have a significant incidence of failure due to fracture and fragmentation with the production of silicone synovitis.[67,109,123,127,160,176,199] Recent clinical series using metallic implants have reported good results relative to earlier reports using silicone.[47,76,77,98,110,138,159,182] To date, most metallic implants that have been developed and used employ a monobloc design, making size

---

*See references 1, 18, 30, 35, 39, 81, 95, 104, 104, 124, 135, 145, 163, 177, 188, 204, and 206.

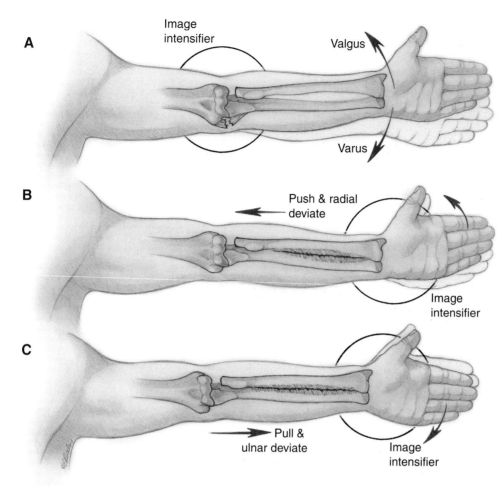

FIGURE 21-12. A, A valgus and varus stress test of the elbow should be performed to evaluate the integrity of the medial and lateral collateral ligaments using an image intensifier before excision of the radial head. **B** and **C,** Similarly, the axial stability of the forearm should be evaluated by alternatively applying axial traction/ulnar deviation and compression/radial deviation to the forearm and wrist while monitoring ulnar variance at the wrist with an image intensifier.

matching suboptimal and implant insertion often difficult owing to the need to subluxate the elbow to allow for insertion of these devices.[71] Recently, modular metallic prostheses of the radial head have become available, with separate heads and stems, allowing improved sizing options and easier implantation. The implantation techniques for the currently available implants vary somewhat; however, most employ a Kocher approach and either preserve or repair the lateral collateral ligament.[111] Currently available devices include spacer implants, press-fit and ingrowth stems, and bipolar and ceramic articulations. There are no reported clinical studies comparing the outcome of different radial head implant designs.

Even with intact ligaments, biomechanical data have demonstrated an alteration in the kinematics and stability of the elbow after excision of the radial head.[92,105] Recent data from the author's laboratory have demonstrated that metallic replacement of the radial head restores the kinematics and stability of the elbow similar to that with a native radial head.[105] On the basis of these in-vitro data and the known high incidence of concomitant ligamentous injuries with comminuted fractures, I routinely replace the radial head in the setting of an unreconstructable fracture. The clinical efficacy of this philosophy, however, remains unproven. Given the variable results of excision of the radial head at long-term follow-up* and the encouraging medium-term

results of metallic arthroplasty,[76,77,110,138,182] this issue clearly requires further study.

Author's Preferred Method

Surgical Approach

The patient is placed in the supine position on the operating table, and a sandbag is placed beneath the ipsilateral scapula to assist in positioning the arm across the chest. Prophylactic intravenous antibiotics are administered. General or regional anesthesia is employed. After prepping and draping, a sterile tourniquet is applied. A midline posterior elbow incision is made just lateral to the tip of the olecranon, and a full-thickness lateral flap is elevated on the deep fascia (Fig. 21-13). This extensile incision decreases the risk of cutaneous nerve injury and provides access to the radial head, coronoid, and medial and lateral collateral ligaments if needed for the management of more complex injuries.[43,152]

*See references 20, 22, 25, 35, 37, 57, 62, 66, 81, 88, 91, 104, 113, 135, 143, and 195.

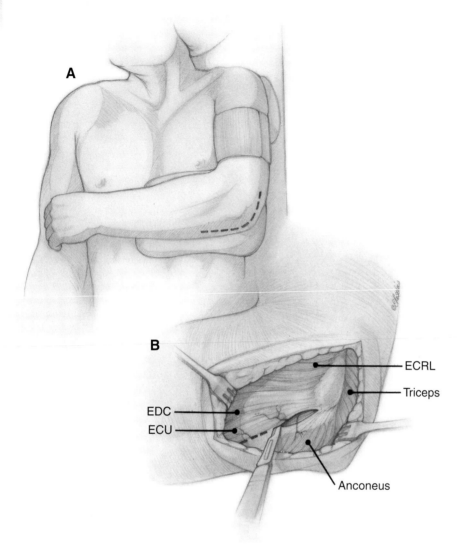

ECRL

Triceps

EDC

ECU

Anconeus

FIGURE 21-13. Posterior skin incision. **A,** Posterior midline skin incision is employed just lateral to the tip of the olecranon. **B,** A full-thickness lateral flap is elevated. The use of this incision allows access to the medial aspect of the elbow (if necessary) to manage associated injuries to the medial collateral ligament, is less obvious due to its location, and has a low incidence of cutaneous nerve injury. ECU, extensor carpi ulnaris; EDC, extensor digitorum communis; ECRL, extensor carpi radialis longus.

The placement of the incision posteriorly is also more cosmetically acceptable than standard laterally placed incisions. The forearm is maintained in pronation to move the posterior interosseous nerve more distal and medial during the surgical approach.[190]

The fascial interval between the anconeus and extensor carpi ulnaris (Kocher's interval)[111] is identified by noting the diverging direction of the muscle groups and small vascular perforators that exit at this interval (Fig. 21-14). After incising this interval, the extensor carpi ulnaris is elevated slightly anteriorly off the underlying lateral collateral ligament, and the radial collateral and annular ligaments are incised longitudinally at the mid axis of the radial head. Dissection should stay anterior to the lateral ulnar collateral ligament to prevent the development of posterolateral rotatory instability. The humeral origin of the radial collateral ligament and the overlying extensor muscles are elevated anteriorly off the lateral epicondyle to better expose the anterior half of the radial head if required. Humeral avulsion of the lateral collateral ligament and common extensor muscles from the lateral epicondyle is commonly noted in

patients after fractures of the head of the radius and is a constant finding in patients with a concomitant elbow dislocation, simplifying surgical exposure of the radial head.[148] In these circumstances the radial head is easily visualized after opening the fascia of the Kocher interval, at which point a bald lateral epicondyle is evident. Posterior dissection should be avoided in the setting of intact ligaments to preserve the integrity of the lateral ulnar collateral ligament and thereby maintain the varus and posterolateral rotatory stability of the elbow.[45,147,148] If further exposure is needed, release of the posterior component of the lateral collateral ligament can be considered, but careful ligament repair is required at the end of the procedure. Dissection distal to the radial tuberosity, although rarely required, is achieved by careful elevation of the supinator and identification of the posterior interosseous nerve.

For patients with isolated simple fractures of the radial head not requiring a more extensive exposure, a muscle-tendon splitting approach can be employed (Fig. 21-15). With a posterior skin incision as outlined earlier, or alternatively, a more classic lateral incision centered over the

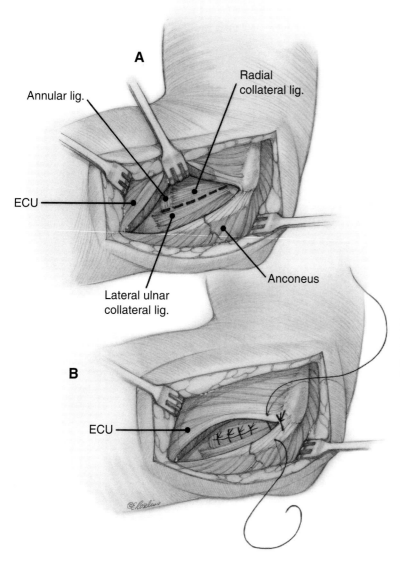

A

Annular lig.

Radial
collateral lig.

ECU

Lateral ulnar
collateral lig.

Anconeus

B

ECU

FIGURE 21-14. Kocher's approach to the radial head. The interval between the anconeus and extensor carpi ulnaris (ECU) is opened as evident by the divergent muscle fibers and vascular perforators that exit this interval (see Fig. 21-13B). **A,** The ECU is elevated anteriorly off the lateral collateral ligament and an arthrotomy is performed at the midportion of the radial head, thereby avoiding detachment of the lateral ulnar collateral ligament. The annular ligament usually needs to be divided to achieve adequate exposure of the fracture. The radial collateral ligament commonly needs to be elevated anteriorly and thereby detached off the lateral epicondyle to achieve visualization of the anterior portion of the radial head. **B,** Closure of the arthrotomy is accomplished by repairing the radial collateral ligament to the intact lateral ulnar collateral ligament. The fascia of the Kocher interval is then repaired. If the lateral ligaments are incompetent either as a result of injury or surgical release, a careful repair is required as outlined in Figure 21-22.

lateral epicondyle, the common extensor muscles and the underlying radial collateral and annular ligaments are divided longitudinally at the middle aspect of the radial head. The forearm is maintained in pronation, and dissection distal to the radial tuberosity is avoided to protect the posterior interosseous nerve. The radial collateral ligament and common extensor muscles are elevated anteriorly off the lateral epicondyle if needed to further improve exposure. As outlined earlier, if further exposure of the radial head is needed, division of the posterior component of the lateral collateral ligament can be considered, but a meticulous ligament repair is required. Extension distal to the proximal aspect of the radial tuberosity requires exposure of the posterior interosseous nerve.

The capitellum is evaluated for chondral injuries or osteochondral fractures. Associated fractures of the coronoid, olecranon, and proximal ulna are managed as indicated. Careful decision making is needed to determine the optimal management of a fracture of the radial head intra-

operatively. The age and expectations of the patient, number of fragments, extent of comminution, quality of bone, and associated ligamentous and osseous injuries are considered before proceeding with management.

Fragment Excision

If a decision can be made preoperatively that a small, displaced fragment cannot be reliably fixed with ORIF, fragment excision can be performed arthroscopically in those experienced with this technique (Fig. 21-16). Localization of the fragment is usually superior to that achieved with a limited arthrotomy, and the morbidity is minimal. Standard elbow arthroscopic techniques as described in Chapter 26 are employed to remove the displaced fragment typically 3 to 5 days after injury to avoid problematic bleeding, which may be evident if surgery is performed too acutely.

The decision as to whether a fracture can be reliably fixed is more commonly made intraoperatively during an

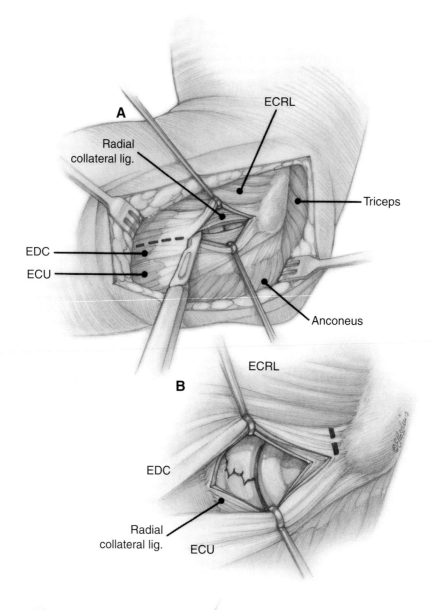

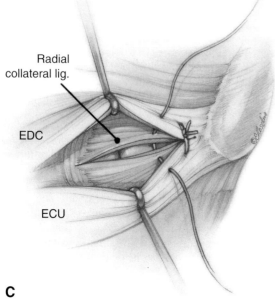

C

FIGURE 21-15. Direct lateral approach to the radial head. **A,** Through either a direct lateral or a posterior midline incision the common extensor origin, the lateral collateral, and the annular ligaments are divided longitudinally at the midportion of the radial head through the extensor digitorum communis (EDC) tendon. The forearm is maintained in pronation to protect the posterior interosseous nerve. The common extensor origin and lateral ligaments are divided as a single layer. **B,** Elevation of the radial collateral ligament and extensor muscles anteriorly off the lateral epicondyle may be needed to provide better access to anterior fragments of the radial head. This approach gives adequate access to manage most displaced wedge fractures of the radial head. **C,** Closure of the muscle/tendon/ligament splitting approach is accomplished with a side-to-side repair. ECRL, extensor carpi radialis longus; ECU, extensor carpi ulnaris.

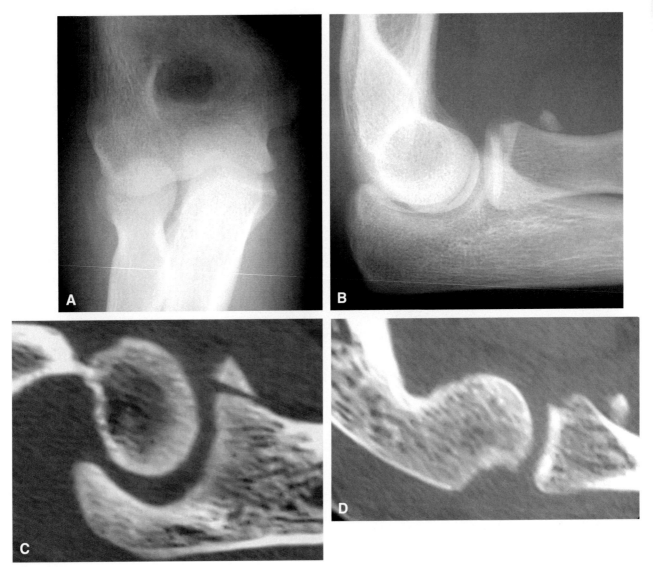

FIGURE 21-16. Excision of fragment of radial head. Anteroposterior (**A**) and lateral (**B**) radiographs of a 32-year-old man who fell while rollerblading. He had limited prosupination. **C** and **D,** CT demonstrated an undisplaced coronoid fracture, a posterior capitellum impression fracture, and a fragment of the radial head anterior to the radial neck.

Continued

CRITICAL POINTS: FRAGMENT EXCISION

INDICATION

- Displaced unreconstructable fragment less than one third of the diameter of the radial head

PEARLS

- Localize fragments with CT preoperatively and image intensifier intraoperatively.
- Compare size of missing section of radial head to removed fragment(s) intraoperatively to determine whether all fragments have been found.

PITFALLS

- Displaced medial fragments may be missed if a lateral surgical approach is used.

TECHNICAL POINTS

- Arthroscopic removal allows complete joint inspection.
- Use an open approach through the common extensor tendon split or Kocher's interval.
- Consider fixation if it is technically possible.
- Use a pituitary rongeur and copious irrigation to remove fragments.

POSTOPERATIVE CARE

- Early range-of-motion exercises are critical to avoid annular ligament adherence to a deficient portion of the radial head.

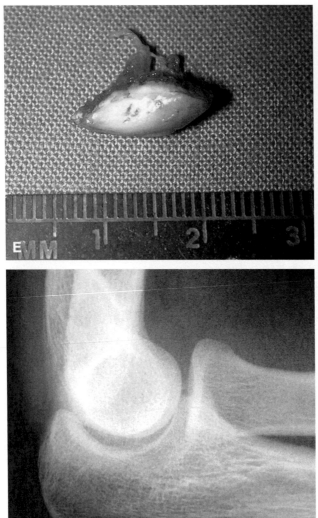

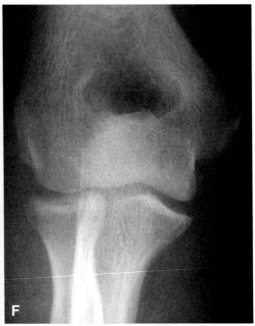

FIGURE 21-16—cont'd. **E,** Attempts to retrieve the fragment arthroscopically failed due to its location distal to the radial head, and an arthrotomy was needed to excise the small fragment. **F** and **G,** After a lateral ligament repair and early range-of-motion exercises the patient recovered a full arc of forearm rotation and a functional arc of elbow motion.

attempted open reduction. An image intensifier, a pituitary rongeur, and copious irrigation are employed to facilitate extraction of small, displaced unreconstructable fragments.[95,211] Inadvertent removal of a coronoid fragment should be avoided by noting its attachment to the anterior capsule. The radial head is evaluated to ensure the deficient portion does not articulate with the radial notch in any position of forearm rotation. Congruent tracking of the residual radial head with the capitellum is checked before careful wound closure with repair of the annular, radial, and lateral ulnar collateral ligaments, as described later. Removal of the anterior rim of the radial head in the setting of a lateral collateral ligament injury may contribute to residual posterolateral rotatory instability. Careful lateral collateral ligament repair and rehabilitation with the forearm in pronation is essential to achieve a successful outcome.[45]

Open Reduction and Internal Fixation

In my experience, arthroscopic reduction and internal fixation of fractures of the radial head has not been rewarding, owing to the difficulty in obtaining a good view of the articular dish, which is obscured by the curvature of the capitellum. The inability to distract the radiocapitellar joint makes visualization of the reduction much more difficult than similar approaches at the wrist or knee. Further complicating arthroscopic reduction and internal fixation is the small working space in which the fragments can be manipulated and limited safe-approach angles for fixation devices.

One of the two open surgical approaches is used, as previously described. Displaced fragments are reduced gently to avoid articular cartilage damage and loss of any residual periosteal attachment with its concomitant blood supply (Fig. 21-17).[65] Smooth Kirschner wires are used as joysticks to elevate depressed fragments and to achieve provisional fixation. Do not use threaded Kirschner wires because they interfere with the tactile control of insertion depth by the surgeon, thereby increasing the probability of penetration of the articular surface on the opposite side. Fragments are fixed using appropriate screws ranging in size from 1.3 to 3.0 mm. Cannulated 3.0-mm screws are employed for larger fragments because they can be quickly placed over the guide wires used for provisional fixation. Smaller screws are inserted through the pin tracts used for the provisional

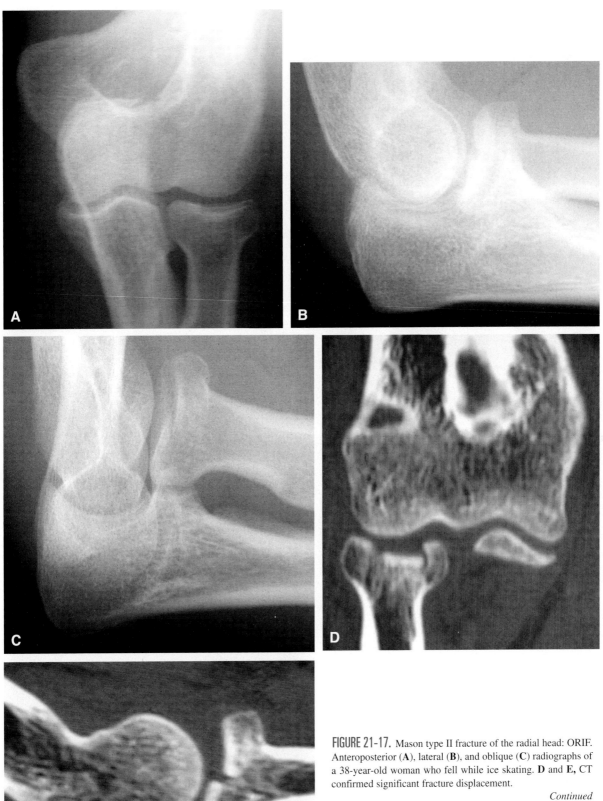

FIGURE 21-17. Mason type II fracture of the radial head: ORIF. Anteroposterior (**A**), lateral (**B**), and oblique (**C**) radiographs of a 38-year-old woman who fell while ice skating. **D** and **E,** CT confirmed significant fracture displacement.

Continued

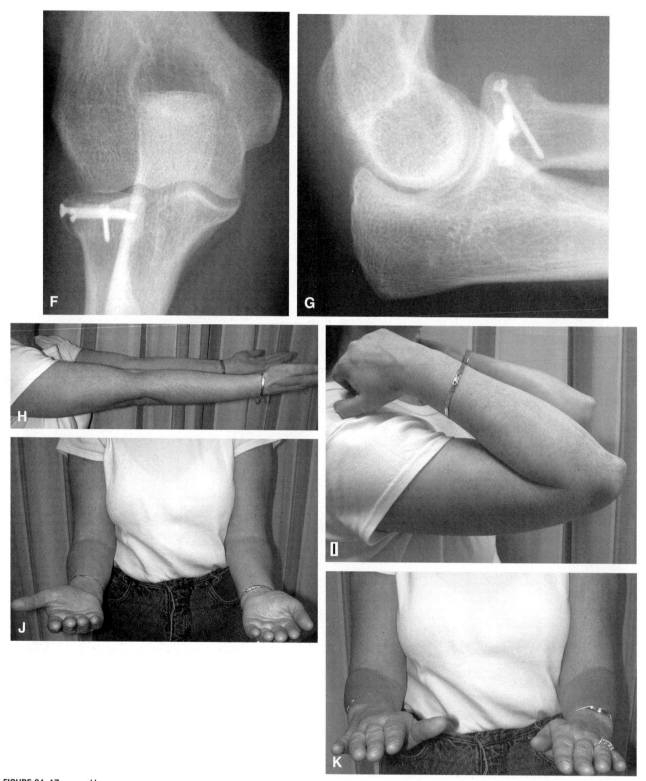

FIGURE 21-17—cont'd. **F** and **G,** The patient underwent ORIF of the radial head with 2.0- and 1.5-mm screws. **H** to **K,** The patient recovered a full arc of elbow and forearm motion and had no pain 6 months after the injury.

fixation. Screws are inserted through the articular margin of the radial head and countersunk to avoid impingement with the annular ligament and radial notch. Screws that are too long should be avoided because they may protrude and interfere with forearm rotation. While drilling, take care to avoid perforation of the far cortex while determining accurate length measurements with a depth gauge.

In comminuted fractures in which the radial head has separated from the neck, the radial head should be assembled on a back table. After rigid fixation of the radial head has been achieved, it is secured to the radial neck using divergent screws or a plate. Noncomminuted fractures are fixed under compression using divergent cannulated 3.0-mm screws (Fig. 21-18). The cannulated feature of the screws prevents the tips from glancing off the cortex when placed at an oblique angle. Comminuted fractures should be fixed with a plate, preferably a fixed-angle device with locking screws or a blade to prevent collapse. Standard 2.7- or 2.0-mm "T"-plates provide less rigid fixation than fixed-angle devices and tend to have a high risk of nonunion and forearm stiffness (Fig. 21-19).[153] New precontoured radial head plates may be superior to previous designs. Plates should be placed on the nonarticular portion "safe zone" of the radial head to prevent interference with the proximal radioulnar joint.[26,184] Gaps between the head and neck should be grafted using cancellous bone obtained from

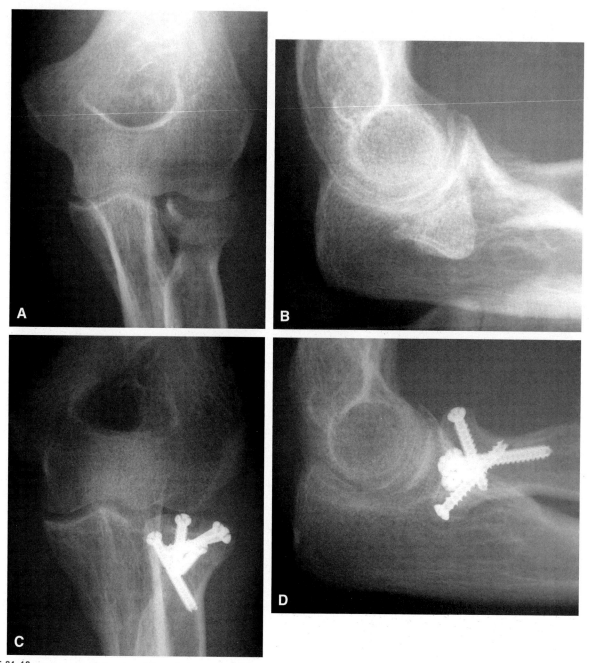

FIGURE 21-18. Mason type II fracture of the radial head and neck: ORIF. Anteroposterior (**A**) and lateral (**B**) radiographs of a 52-year-old woman who slipped and fell and sustained a displaced fracture of the radial head and neck. **C** and **D**, The fracture of the radial head and neck was fixed using cannulated 3.0-mm screws.

Continued

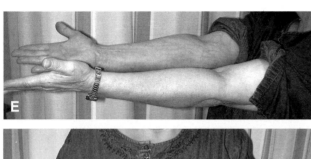

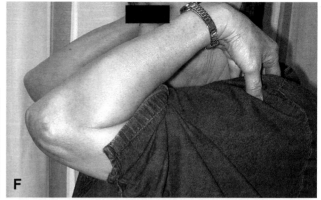

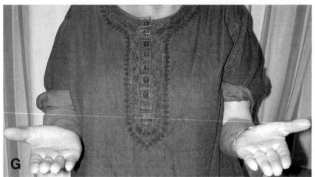

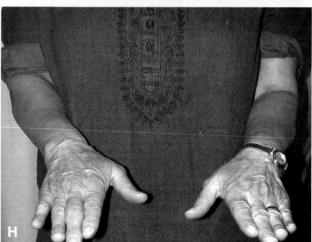

FIGURE 21-18—cont'd. **E** to **H**, An excellent clinical result was achieved with no evidence of avascular necrosis at 6 months.

CRITICAL POINTS: OPEN REDUCTION AND INTERNAL FIXATION

INDICATION

■ Displaced (≥2 mm) reconstructable fragment larger than one third of the diameter of the radial head or smaller extruded fragment interfering with forearm rotation.

PEARLS

■ CT may be helpful in deciding on surgery for borderline displacement.
■ Avoid screw penetration through opposite cortex.
■ Fragments typically are quite anterior; avoid posterior dissection with damage to lateral ulnar collateral ligament.

PITFALLS

■ Minimize hardware impingement with annular ligament.
■ Nonrigid fixation and osteopenia are recipes for failure.
■ Consider radial head arthroplasty if there are more than three fragments, especially in an older patient.

TECHNICAL POINTS

■ Use an open approach through the common extensor tendon split or Kocher's interval.
■ Consider fixation if it is technically possible.
■ Cross-cannulated screws work well for noncomminuted fractures of the radial neck.
■ Fixed angle plate is preferred for comminuted fractures of the radial neck.
■ Nonarticular portion of the radial head presents laterally with forearm in neutral rotation (use the "safe zone" for hardware placement).
■ Careful ligament repair is required to avoid radiocapitellar subluxation with failure of fixation.

POSTOPERATIVE CARE

■ Early range-of-motion exercises are critical to avoid annular ligament adherence to hardware or fracture lines.

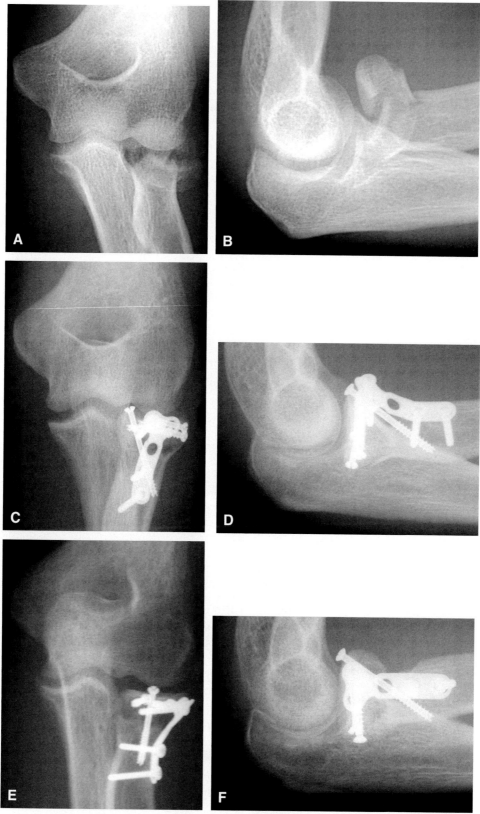

FIGURE 21-19. Mason type III fracture of the radial neck: ORIF. Anteroposterior (**A**) and lateral (**B**) radiographs of a 24-year-old man who fell off a snowmobile, sustaining a comminuted fracture of the radial head and neck. **C** and **D,** The fracture was fixed using a 2.7-mm "T"-plate and cannulated 3.0-mm screws. **E** and **F,** An excellent initial clinical result was achieved; however, at 4 months, the patient developed a symptomatic nonunion and avascular necrosis, requiring further surgery.

the distal humerus through a small hole in the lateral epicondyle, the proximal ulna, or the distal radius.

Hardware placement should be checked with an image intensifier at the completion of the internal fixation to ensure that screw lengths are appropriate. Plain radiographs are insufficient; imaging in multiple positions of forearm rotation is needed to confirm appropriate placement of the hardware. Nonanatomic reduction and poor fixation are recipes for failure, and alternative treatment options should be considered under these circumstances.[106,168]

Excision of the Radial Head

I rarely perform excision without replacement for acute fractures of the radial head. The radial head can be resected through either of the two open surgical approaches described earlier (Fig. 21-20). Complete excision of the radial head is critical to avoid symptoms of internal derangement from a retained fragment. The excised fragments should be reassembled outside the elbow to ensure that all of the radial head has been retrieved. A micro sagittal saw is used to complete the resection until it is just distal to the

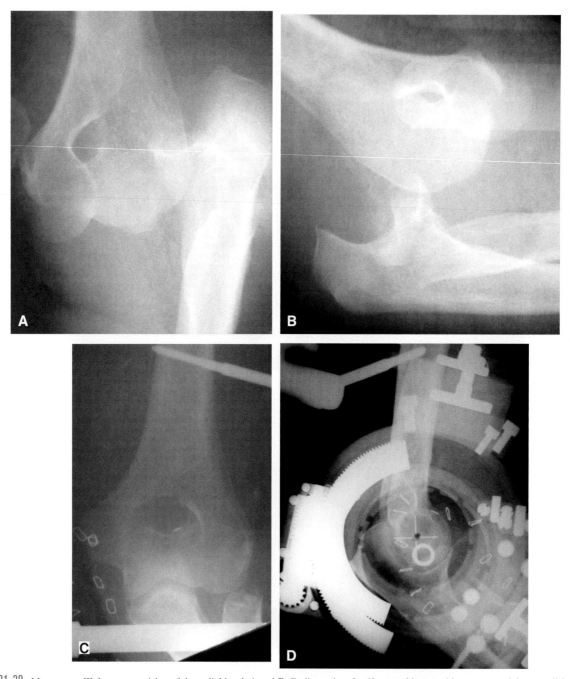

FIGURE 21-20. Mason type III fracture: excision of the radial head. **A** and **B,** Radiographs of a 69-year-old man with a compound fracture-dislocation of the elbow and renal insufficiency. Owing to extensive contamination of the wound, delayed treatment, and chronic immunosuppression he was managed by excision of the radial head without replacement. **C** and **D,** An articulated external fixator (Compass Hinge, Smith and Nephew Richards) was employed to maintain a concentric reduction of the elbow.
Continued

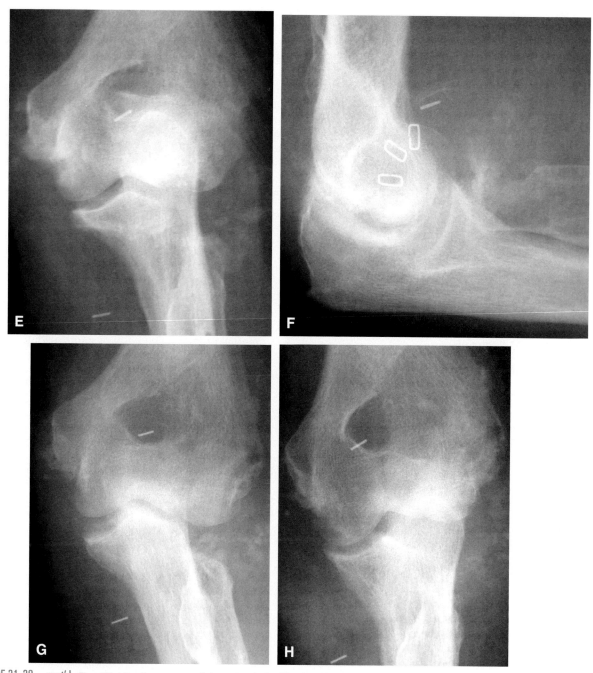

FIGURE 21-20—cont'd. **E** and **F,** After fixator removal the patient had mild pain and a functional arc of motion. Stress testing disclosed significant residual valgus instability (**G**) and varus instability (**H**).

radial notch. Excessive removal of the radial neck should be avoided to prevent radioulnar impingement. After excision of the head of the radius the valgus, varus, axial, and rotational stability of the elbow should be evaluated and a check for residual fragments performed using an image intensifier.[40] If there is any suggestion or suspicion of an associated ligamentous injury (and there usually is as previously described), arthroplasty of the radial head is recommended. The lateral collateral ligament and Kocher's interval are carefully repaired to reduce the residual laxity induced by both the approach and loss of ligament tensioning resulting from excision of the radial head.

I perform arthroscopic excision of the radial head for nonunions, malunions, and post-traumatic arthritis. Resection can be readily accomplished by those experienced with elbow arthroscopy using standard portals and instruments (see Chapter 26).[119,132,133] A high-speed bur, resectors, and pituitary rongeurs are employed to remove the cartilaginous and osseous fragments. A tourniquet and epinephrine-containing irrigation are essential to control bleeding. Just as for open excision of the radial head, imaging is used to ensure that the elbow and forearm are stable, all of the fragments have been removed, and an adequate resection has been accomplished.

CRITICAL POINTS: EXCISION OF THE RADIAL HEAD

INDICATIONS

▪ Rarely employed
▪ Displaced unreconstructable fracture larger than one third of the diameter of the radial head without known associated or probable medial or lateral collateral or interosseous membrane injury

PEARLS

▪ Assemble excised fragments to ensure all are removed; intraoperative fluoroscopy is helpful.

PITFALLS

▪ Avoid unrecognized ligamentous injuries.
▪ Excessive excision of the radial neck causes radioulnar impingement.

TECHNICAL POINTS

▪ Use an open approach through the common extensor tendon split or Kocher's interval.
▪ Excise the radial head just distal to the proximal radioulnar joint.
▪ Use intraoperative fluoroscopy to perform varus, valgus, and axial stress tests.
▪ Carefully perform lateral ligament repair with plication to decrease residual lateral laxity.

POSTOPERATIVE CARE

▪ Early range-of motion exercises are critical to avoid soft tissue adherence to the radial neck.

Implant Arthroplasty of the Radial Head

With the use of a Kocher approach as described earlier, while respecting the lateral ulnar collateral ligament, all fragments of the radial head are removed (Fig. 21-21). The implantation technique will vary slightly depending on the arthroplasty design selected. A minimal amount of radial head is removed at a right angle to the medullary canal of the radial neck to make a smooth surface for seating of the radial head. The appropriate diameter and height of the radial head implant are determined using the reassembled resected head for comparison. Preoperative templating of the contralateral normal radial head should be employed in the setting of a secondary radial head replacement but is not required for a primary replacement for an acute fracture. In the setting of elbow instability, avoid undersizing the diameter of the radial head because a larger-diameter head tends to resist joint subluxation better, thereby preventing edge loading on the articular margin of an undersized device.

Over the past 10 years I have employed a noncemented metallic implant that functions as a spacer while healing of the soft tissue occurs.[76,77,138] Most implants are now modular to facilitate improved matching of size of the native radial head and neck.[108] In addition, modular implants allow easier placement in the setting where the lateral ligaments of the elbow are competent. The radial neck is delivered laterally using a Hohman retractor carefully placed around the posterior aspect of the proximal radial neck. An anteriorly based retractor should be avoided owing to the risk of injury to the posterior interosseous nerve. The medullary canal of the radial neck is reamed using hand reamers until cortical contact is encountered with a goal to achieve a nontight fit

CRITICAL POINTS: IMPLANT ARTHROPLASTY OF THE RADIAL HEAD

INDICATION

▪ Displaced unreconstructable fracture larger than one third of the diameter of the radial head with known associated or probable medial or lateral collateral or interosseous membrane injury

PEARLS

▪ Radial head articular surface should be at level of proximal radioulnar joint.
▪ If radial head does not track on the capitellum, then downsize the stem.
▪ Translate the radial neck laterally to facilitate implant placement.

PITFALLS

▪ Avoid Hohman retractors around the anterior radial neck because of pressure on the posterior interosseous nerve.
▪ Avoid undersizing the diameter of the radial head.
▪ Avoid excessive thickness of the radial head.

TECHNICAL POINTS

▪ Use an open approach through the Kocher interval.
▪ Excise the radial head perpendicular to the radial neck.
▪ Choose an implant thickness to restore radial head height.
▪ Use intraoperative fluoroscopy to check implant thickness by evaluating medial and lateral joint thickness of the ulnohumeral joint, which should be equal.
▪ Careful lateral ligament repair is required.

POSTOPERATIVE CARE

▪ Early range-of-motion exercises are critical to avoid adherence of soft tissue to the radial neck.

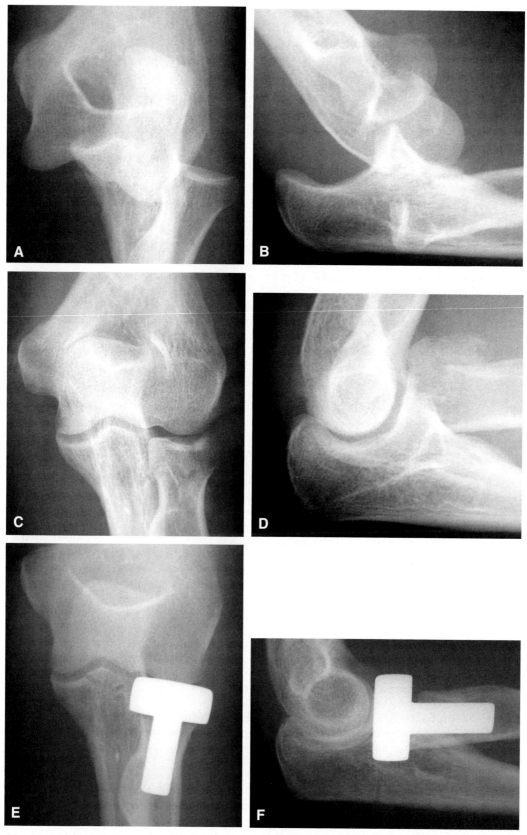

FIGURE 21-21. Mason type III fracture: replacement of the radial head. Anteroposterior (**A**) and lateral radiographs (**B**) of a 52-year-old woman who fell off a tractor sustaining a comminuted fracture of the radial head, a displaced fracture of the coronoid, and an elbow dislocation are noted. **C** and **D,** Post-reduction radiographs demonstrate the comminuted nature of the fracture of the head of the radius. **E** and **F,** After suture repair of the coronoid, a modular arthroplasty was employed (Evolve, Wright Medical Technology, Arlington, TN). The lateral ligaments were repaired using drill holes in the lateral epicondyle, and the elbow was sufficiently stable for early postoperative range-of-motion exercises. A medial collateral ligament repair was not required to allow early motion after repair of the other injured structures. A good functional outcome was achieved.

of the trial stem. A trial head is inserted onto the stem, and the diameter, height, and congruency of the prosthesis are evaluated both visually and with the aid of an image intensifier. The radial head prosthesis should articulate at the same height as the coronoid and radial notch of the ulna. The alignment of the distal radioulnar joint is confirmed by ensuring that the ulnar variance is equivalent to the opposite wrist. The lateral and medial portions of the ulnohumeral joint should be of similar width on an anteroposterior fluoroscopic view, confirming that the prosthesis is neither too thick nor thin, resulting in a varus or valgus alignment of the elbow, respectively. Overstuffing the radiocapitellar joint with a radial head implant that is too thick should be avoided to reduce the risk of cartilage wear on the capitellum from excessive pressure. If the prosthesis is not tracking properly on the capitellum with forearm rotation, a smaller stem size should be placed to ensure that the articulation of the radial head with the capitellum is optimal.

The surgical implantation of a monobloc radial head implant, in which the head is fixed to the stem, may be difficult if the elbow is not grossly unstable, such as after an elbow dislocation. Atraumatic placement of such implants can often be achieved by lateral translation of the proximal radius after division of the annular ligament. In some patients insufficient translation of the proximal radius prevents the insertion of a monobloc or preassembled modular implant. In these circumstances, posterolateral subluxation of the proximal radius will be needed, necessitating division and subsequent repair of the lateral ulnar collateral ligament. Some modular implants allow insertion of the stem first and then placement of the radial head onto the stem with coupling in situ. This feature significantly reduces the exposure needed and, therefore, simplifies the implantation procedure.

Closure

After fragment excision, ORIF, or excision or replacement of the radial head, the lateral collateral ligament and common extensor muscle origins are repaired back to the lateral condyle. If the posterior half of the lateral collateral ligament is still attached to the lateral epicondyle, then the anterior half of the lateral collateral ligament (the annular ligament and radial collateral ligament) is simply repaired to the posterior half using interrupted absorbable sutures. If the lateral collateral ligament and extensor origin have been completely detached either by the injury or surgical exposure, they should be securely repaired using drill holes through bone and nonabsorbable sutures. I prefer drill holes as opposed to suture anchors because the soft tissues can be drawn toward the attachment site, better tensioning the repair (Fig. 21-22). A single hole is drilled at the axis of motion (the center of the arc of curvature of the capitellum) and connected to a hole placed anterior and posterior to the lateral supracondylar ridge. A locking suture technique is employed to gain a secure hold of the lateral collateral ligament and common extensor muscle fascia. The ligament sutures are pulled into the holes drilled in the distal humerus using suture retrievers. The forearm should be pronated, and varus forces avoided, closing the lateral side of the elbow while tensioning the sutures before tying. The knots should be left anterior or posterior to the lateral supracondylar ridge to avoid prominence.

POSTOPERATIVE MANAGEMENT AND EXPECTATIONS

Outcome Data

Nonoperative Management

The outcome of undisplaced fractures of the radial head is generally favorable, with return of function within 6 to 12 weeks. Late displacement is uncommon but has been reported, particularly with fracture fragments that are greater than one third of the diameter of the radial head.[124,163] Careful clinical and radiographic follow-up of these injuries is mandatory. Residual pain is uncommon. Mild residual flexion contractures of 10 to 15 degrees are not infrequent sequelae.[118,124,125,197,201,210] Some patients develop arthrofibrosis and a more severe capsular contracture unresponsive to therapy and splinting requiring arthroscopic or open capsular release (see Chapter 25). Stiffness is more common in patients with associated injuries such as an elbow dislocation, ligamentous injury, or coronoid fracture. Overall, most series report 85% to 95% good results for undisplaced fractures managed with early motion. An initial period of cast immobilization does not appear to be necessary, nor is it advisable, as demonstrated in one prospective randomized trial.[201] Aspiration of the elbow in the absence of a block to forearm rotation does not appear to influence ultimate outcome.[42,83]

Although successful nonoperative management has been reported for displaced fractures of the radial head, the outcome seems to be less reliable.[1,24,102,124,136,163] Mason reported that 9 of 15 patients had some pain at an average of 11 years after nonoperative treatment for fractures involving greater than 25% of the joint surface.[124] He advocated excision of the radial head. Radin and Riseborough reported better motion in patients with displaced fractures managed with excision than that achieved with nonoperative treatment.[163] Burton reported that only 2 of 9 patients with displaced fractures managed nonoperatively had good results; he recommended excision of the radial head in such cases.[24] Khalfayan and coworkers reported on 26 patients with Mason type II fractures at an average of 18 months after either ORIF or nonoperative treatment with early motion.[102] The operatively treated group had 90% good or excellent results, whereas the nonoperatively treated group had 44% good or excellent results. Pain, functional limitations, and osteoarthritis were more frequent in the nonoperatively treated group.

Open Reduction and Internal Fixation

The clinical outcome of ORIF of the radial head has been good when an anatomic reduction and rigid internal fixation has been achieved and early range-of-motion exercises initiated in the postoperative period.* There has been a low incidence of nonunion, avascular necrosis, or stiffness requiring further surgery. For simple partial articular fractures, success rates generally exceed 90%; however, the outcome has been poorer and the complication rate has been higher in patients with more comminuted fractures, partic-

---

*See references 9, 19, 23, 29, 49, 53, 56, 63, 78, 79, 84, 102, 106, 128, 150, 154-156, 164, 168, 170, 172, 180, and 203.

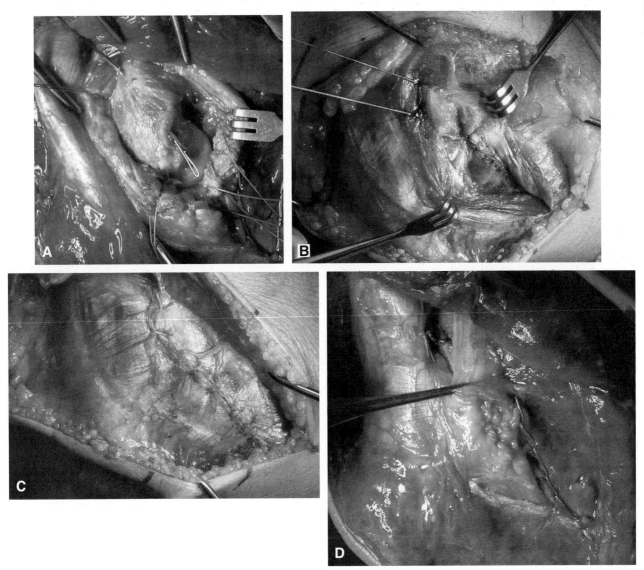

FIGURE 21-22. Lateral ligament repair technique. Method of suture repair of torn or detached lateral collateral ligament complex using sutures through bone tunnels in the lateral epicondyle. **A,** A single hole is drilled at the axis of motion (the center of the arc of curvature of the capitellum) and connected to a hole placed anterior and posterior to the lateral supracondylar ridge. **B,** A locking suture technique is employed to gain a secure hold of the lateral collateral ligament. The interval between the radial and lateral ulnar collateral ligaments and the annular ligament is closed as this suture is brought back to the lateral epicondyle. The ligament sutures are pulled into the holes drilled in the distal humerus while maintaining the forearm in pronation and avoiding varus forces while tying the sutures. **C,** A side-to-side repair of the Kocher interval is used to augment stability. **D,** Alternatively, the fascia of the Kocher interval can be closed as for the ligaments and the repair can be secured to the lateral epicondyle through the aforementioned drill holes.

ularly fractures that completely separate the radial head and neck. King and colleagues reviewed 14 elbows treated with ORIF at an average follow-up of 32 months.[106] Mason type II fractures had 100% good or excellent results. Only 33% of Mason type III fractures treated with ORIF had a good or excellent result. An associated elbow dislocation did not affect the results significantly but was associated with an increased fixed flexion deformity. Fractures were often more comminuted than suggested by plain radiographs. The authors suggested that careful intraoperative decision making is required in deciding between reconstruction or excision of the radial head. Excellent results were obtained provided an anatomic reduction with stable fixation and early range of motion was achieved. If a stable anatomic reduction cannot be obtained, then alternative treatment

methods should be considered. Ring and coworkers reviewed the results of ORIF of fractures of the radial head in 56 patients.[168] The authors recommended ORIF for partial articular fractures consisting of a single fragment and for complete articular fractures with three or fewer fragments. The authors recommended that comminuted fractures were best managed by excision of the radial head or replacement arthroplasty. Concomitant injuries such as dislocations and other fractures increased the failure rate of ORIF of the radial head.

There are no prospective randomized studies comparing ORIF with alternative methods of management. The clinical and radiographic results of nonoperatively treated displaced fractures were inferior to a similar group of patients treated with ORIF as reported by Khalfayan and colleagues.[102]

Boulas and Morrey compared the outcome of 36 patients managed with ORIF, excision, Silastic replacement, and nonoperative management.[19] The best outcome was achieved with ORIF of displaced radial head fractures.

Fragment Excision

Although fragment excision is infrequently indicated with the advent of improved small fragment fixation systems, the outcome can be favorable in carefully selected patients. Fragment excision should be limited to small marginal fragments that are not amenable to ORIF because of comminution or osteopenia. Some authors have reported good results in over 80% of patients, but others have reported less satisfactory results.[95,145,211] Carstam reported that 17 of 33 patients (52%) managed with fragment excision had good or excellent results.[29]

Delayed Excision of the Radial Head

Reports in the literature are conflicting as to the success of delayed excision of the radial head.[1,20,29,57,163] Delayed excision was often employed in the past because of concerns about stiffness and heterotopic ossification with early surgery.[1,20,29,61] Current thinking is that the extent of the initial trauma and the presence of concomitant associated injuries are more important variables in the development of stiffness. Surgical timing is now thought to be less critical, so early excision of the radial head is generally preferred.[21,57,80] Currently delayed excision is employed for late fracture displacement or the development of arthritis. Considerable improvement in pain and motion can be expected, but the pain relief is variable, primarily dependent on whether arthritis has developed in the ulnohumeral joint.[1,20,57,101] Adler and Shaftan reported good results with delayed excision (8 weeks) and recommended against early excision except in the setting of a block to motion.[1] Timing of excision with respect to the development of heterotopic bone was not found to be a significant issue. Broberg and Morrey reported that delayed excision (1 month to 20 years after fracture) improved motion and decreased pain in 81% of the 21 patients reviewed.[20] In 77% of patients there was a good or excellent result. Osteoarthritis was common at follow-up, being mild to moderate in 77%. Fuchs and Chylarecki reported better outcome after early (<2 weeks) versus delayed excision.[57] Sixty-nine percent of patients who underwent early excision were satisfied as compared with 44% with a delayed excision.

Primary Resection of the Radial Head

The outcome after primary resection of the radial head without replacement is controversial in the literature, with some authors reporting good clinical and radiographic results and others reporting a high incidence of pain, valgus and/or axial instability, weakness, and degenerative elbow and/or wrist arthritis, particularly at long-term follow-up.* Morrey and coworkers reported 80% satisfactory results after resection for displaced fractures of the radial head at an average of 20 years of follow-up.[143] Mild ulnohumeral arthritis was common radiographically, but residual symptoms were uncommon and mild. Wrist pain occurred in 15% of patients but was usually mild. Proximal migration averaged 2 mm. Coleman reported good results in 17 patients at a similar duration of follow-up.[35] Fifteen of these patients

had radiographic evidence of arthritis. More advanced arthritis was evident in patients with type III fractures. Fuchs and Chylarecki assessed the outcome of 108 patients after radial head resection at an average of 6 years. Sixty-four percent had an isolated fracture, and 26% had an associated elbow dislocation.[57] Clinical outcome and strength were better for patients treated with a primary versus a secondary resection. Ikeda and Oka reviewed 15 patients treated with early radial head resection for a fracture at an average of 10 years.[88] All patients had reduced elbow power, and only 5 patients were pain free. Janssen and Vetger reported on 21 patients with a Mason type III fracture treated by excision of the radial head at between 16- and 30-year follow-up.[91] Only 4 of their patients had elbow pain. Of the 16 patients who had radiographic follow-up, 11 had degenerative arthritis of the elbow. Berger and coworkers reported good or excellent results in 10 of 30 patients at an average of 5 years.[16] Valgus deformity of the elbow was common. Josefsson and colleagues reported on 23 patients with an elbow dislocation associated with a displaced fracture of the radial head.[96] Nineteen patients had the radial head excised at an average of 2 days after injury. In four elbows with an associated displaced fracture of the coronoid process, redislocation occurred. A follow-up examination performed in 19 patients between 3 and 34 years after the injury demonstrated severe osteoarthritis in 12 elbows. Reduced range of motion was the most common complaint, and reduced extension was the most common finding. To lower the risk and prevent severe instability, the authors recommended that the radial head should be preserved if possible in the setting of an associated elbow dislocation. If the radial head had to be resected, repair of torn ligaments and muscles was considered essential. Mikic and Vukadinovic reported on 58 patients who had been treated with excision of a radial head and who were reviewed at an average of 6.5 years.[135] Osteoarthritis was present in 52%, and residual symptoms were found in 43%. Forearm rotation was limited in 58%. Twenty-five percent had symptomatic proximal migration of the radius with distal radioulnar joint symptoms. Given their 50% fair or poor results, the authors suggested that the indications for excision of the radial head should be relatively limited.

Arthroplasty of the Radial Head

Silicone arthroplasty of the radial head, although initially successful in many patients,[16,19,27,115,120,142,189,192,209] has fallen out of favor because of problems with residual instability and late arthritis. Reports of implant fracture and silicone synovitis due to particulate debris have provided further evidence to support the use of alternative materials.[67,123,127,189,199,202] Whereas the short- and medium-term results of metallic radial head implants are encouraging, the long-term outcome with respect to loosening, capitellar wear, and arthritis has not been reported.* Moro and coworkers reported the functional outcome of 25 patients managed with a metallic arthroplasty of the radial head for unreconstructable fractures at an average follow-up of 3.5 years.[138] The results were rated as 3 poor, 5 fair, and 17 good or excellent. The radial head prosthesis restored elbow stability

---

*See references 28, 47, 76, 77, 98, 110, 138, 159, 182, and 187.

when the fractured radial head occurred in combination with a dislocation of the elbow, rupture of the medial collateral ligament, fracture of the coronoid, or fracture of the proximal ulna. There were mild residual deficits in strength and motion. No patients required removal of the implant. Harrington and coworkers reported their experience with metallic arthroplasty of the radial head in 20 patients at an average follow-up of 12 years.[76] The results were excellent or good in 16 and fair or poor in 4. Four patients had removal of the implant. Knight and colleagues reported on 31 patients with comminuted fractures of the radial head treated by primary replacement with a Vitallium prosthesis at mean follow-up of 4.5 years.[110] There was reliable restoration of stability and prevention of proximal radial migration. There were no dislocations or prosthetic failures, but two implants were removed for loosening. Smets and associates reported the results of a bipolar radial head prosthesis for comminuted fractures of the radial head in 15 patients with a mean follow-up of 25 months.[182] Thirteen prostheses were inserted for acute Mason III fractures, and 2 were inserted for chronic problems after fracture of the radial head. There were 10 excellent or good and 3 fair or poor results in the group with acute fractures. One prosthesis was removed after 8 months for severely decreased elbow function. In the group with chronic problems, there were 2 fair results. There were no dislocations or prosthesis fractures or signs of loosening.

Postoperative Protocol

After fragment excision, ORIF, excision of the radial head, or replacement arthroplasty and lateral soft tissue closure as previously described, the elbow should be placed through an arc of flexion/extension intraoperatively while carefully evaluating for elbow stability in pronation, neutral, and supination.[82] Pronation is generally beneficial if the lateral ligaments are still deficient,[45] supination is helpful if the medial ligaments are deficient,[8] and neutral position is used if both sides have been damaged. In patients who have an associated elbow dislocation, repair of the medial collateral ligament and flexor pronator origin should be performed if the elbow subluxates at 40 degrees or more of flexion after appropriate management of the radial head and lateral ligament as previously described. Management of associated ligamentous injuries and fractures of the coronoid is discussed in Chapter 22.

The elbow with a stable osseous and ligamentous repair should be splinted in extension and elevated for 24 to 48 hours to diminish swelling, decrease tension on the posterior wound, and minimize the tendency to develop a flexion contracture. In the setting of a more tenuous ligamentous repair or the presence of some residual instability at the end of the operative procedure, the elbow should initially be splinted in 60 to 90 degrees of flexion in the optimal position of forearm rotation to maintain stability as outlined earlier.

Indomethacin, 25 mg three times daily for 3 weeks, may be considered in patients undergoing surgery on the radial head to decrease postoperative pain, reduce swelling, and potentially lower the incidence of heterotopic ossification. In patients with a concomitant dislocation, those undergoing delayed or repeat surgery, and those with an associated head injury, the incidence of heterotopic ossification may be increased.[1,196] The efficacy of indomethacin in the prevention of heterotopic ossification of the elbow remains unproven. This medication should be avoided in elderly patients, those with a history of peptic ulcer disease, or those with a known allergy to the drug. Radiation is rarely used in acute injuries but may be considered postoperatively in high-risk patients such as those with both a head injury and a fracture-dislocation, particularly in those with a contraindication to the use of indomethacin. A single focal dose of 500 cGy 1 day postoperatively has been shown to be efficacious in preventing recurrent heterotopic ossification after synostosis takedown and elbow contracture release.[14]

For an isolated fracture of the radial head treated with a lateral ulnar collateral ligament–sparing approach, active range-of-motion exercises should be initiated on the day after surgery. A sling or collar and cuff with the elbow maintained at 90 degrees is employed for comfort between exercises. A static progressive extension splint is fabricated for night-time use (Fig. 21-23). This splint is adjusted weekly as extension improves and is continued for 12 weeks. Strengthening commences once fracture union is secure, typically 6 to 8 weeks postoperatively.

Patients with associated fractures and ligamentous injuries should begin active flexion and extension motion within a safe arc 1 day postoperatively. A resting splint with the elbow maintained at 90 degrees and the forearm in the appropriate position of forearm rotation is employed for 3 to 6 weeks. Active forearm rotation is performed with the elbow in flexion to minimize stress on the medial and/or lateral ligamentous injuries or repairs. A static progressive night extension splinting program is initiated as ligamentous healing progresses and stability improves, usually at 4 to 6 weeks postoperatively. Passive stretching is not permitted for 6 weeks to reduce the incidence of heterotopic ossification. Strengthening exercises are initiated once the fracture and ligament injuries have adequately healed, usually at 8 to 12 weeks postoperatively.

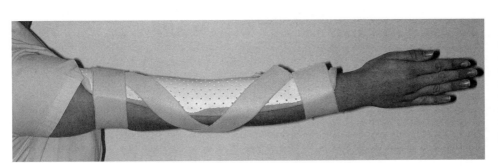

FIGURE 21-23. Static progressive extension splint. An orthosis is molded to the anterior surface of the elbow and forearm to maintain the elbow in comfortable extension. The splint is worn at night and adjusted weekly by a therapist as motion improves.

Complications

Nerve Injury

Posterior interosseous nerve injuries are uncommon but may occur after management of fractures of the head of the radius. Risk factors include dissection distal to the radial tuberosity and placement of retractors around the distal radial neck.[131,190,191,198] Prevention of these injuries can be achieved by maintaining the forearm in pronation while performing the surgical approach.[41] Placement of retractors around the proximal radial neck should be done cautiously and only under direct vision. Retraction should be performed for short periods to prevent a compression neurapraxia. Isolation and protection of the posterior interosseous nerve is recommended if dissection is required greater than 3 cm distal to the radial head with the forearm in supination and 5 cm in pronation.[41] Crawford reported the development of radial tunnel syndrome in two patients after remote excision of the radial head.[37]

Avascular Necrosis

Avascular necrosis is likely common after fractures of the radial head because displaced fragments typically have an absent or precarious blood supply.[65] Fortunately, it is usually asymptomatic, the fragments usually heal if stably fixed and revascularize uneventfully, and late collapse is uncommon. A temporizing approach should be taken. Avascular necrosis of the entire radial head in association with fractures of the radial neck is more problematic because this is often associated with the development of a nonunion and failure of hardware, requiring excision or revision to an arthroplasty (Fig. 21-24).

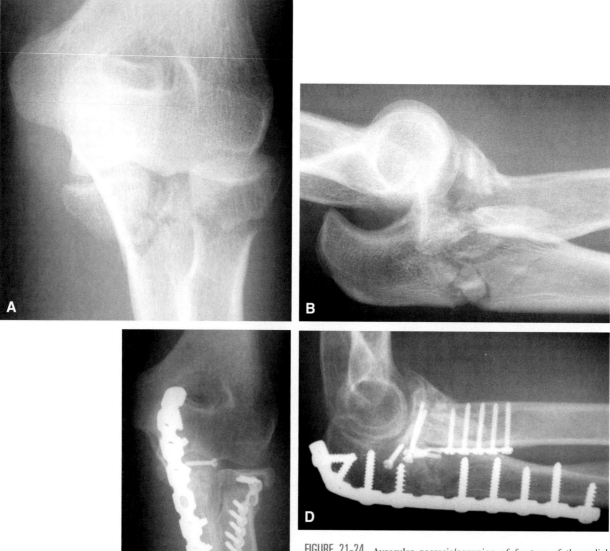

FIGURE 21-24. Avascular necrosis/nonunion of fracture of the radial neck. Anteroposterior (**A**) and lateral (**B**) radiographs demonstrating a comminuted radial head and a proximal ulnar fracture treated with ORIF of the radial head/neck and ulna. **C** and **D,** The patient developed a nonunion of a fracture of the radial neck with associated avascular necrosis and a stiff elbow with limited forearm rotation.

Continued

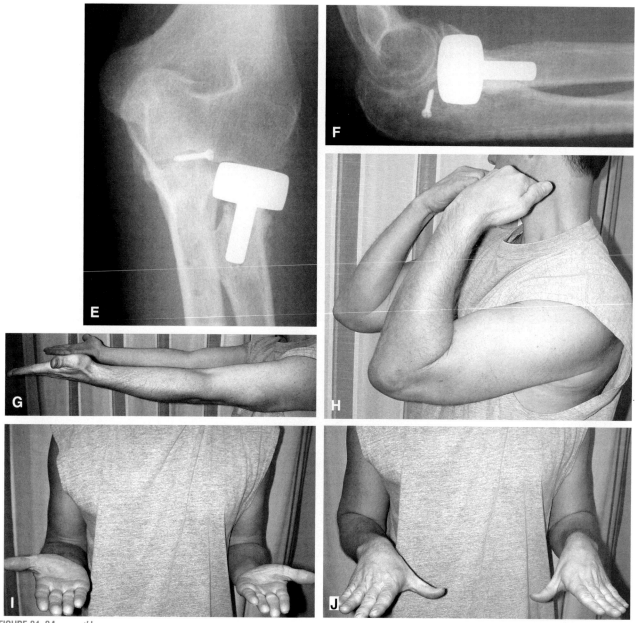

FIGURE 21-24—cont'd. **E** and **F,** The patient was managed with an elbow contracture release, removal of hardware, and an arthroplasty of the radial head. **G** to **J,** An excellent range of motion was achieved postoperatively.

Nonunion

Nonunions are often associated with avascular necrosis and seem to be more common in patients with displaced fractures of the radial neck, particularly if the internal fixation is not secure.[32,54,106,134,167,168] Nonunions should be managed without surgery if they are not symptomatic.[32,167] ORIF with bone grafting or excision or replacement of the radial head may be employed if the nonunion is symptomatic.[134] My experience with attempts to achieve union in this setting has been poor, likely owing to compromised blood supply.

Malunion

Malunions are usually seen as a consequence of inappropriate initial treatment, unstable fracture fixation, or collapse owing to avascular necrosis. Restricted motion, pain, click-

ing, and crepitus are typical clinical features. Extra-articular or intra-articular osteotomies[12] (Fig. 21-25) may be helpful in younger patients, whereas excision or replacement of the radial head should be considered in those who are older and of lower demand. Careful preoperative planning is required if an osteotomy is being considered. If there is significant osteoarthritis of the capitellum, excision of the radial head may be preferable. Preservation of a periosteal sleeve of the elevated fragment should be attempted to avoid problems with avascular necrosis and/or healing. Rigid fixation and bone grafting should be performed to promote union and early postoperative range-of-motion exercises initiated.

Osteoarthritis

Osteoarthritis is seen as a consequence of articular cartilage damage from the initial injury, articular incongruity, or

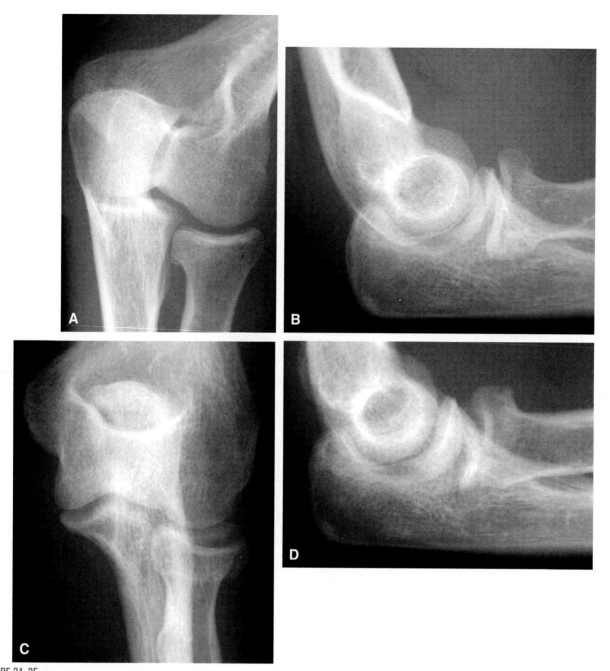

FIGURE 21-25. Malunion of fracture of radial head. Initial anteroposterior (**A**) and lateral (**B**) radiographs of a 39-year-old woman who sustained a fracture of the radial head with early motion. **C** and **D**, She presented 1 year after injury with persistent lateral elbow pain and clicking.   *Continued*

persistent instability. Pain and stiffness develop as the arthritis progresses. Although typically beginning in the radiocapitellar joint, it often progresses to involve the ulnohumeral articulation. Débridement, either open or arthroscopic, can be helpful to manage mechanical symptoms from loose bodies or osteophytes. Radial head arthroplasty can be employed in the early stages when the capitellum is not too severely arthritic (Fig. 21-26). Excision of the radial head, either open or arthroscopically, can be helpful if the ulnohumeral joint is not too involved and there is no residual elbow or forearm instability. Ulnohumeral arthritis tends to progress more rapidly in my experience after excision of the radial head so débridement or replacement is preferred over

excision. Total elbow arthroplasty may be required for more generalized post-traumatic elbow arthritis.

Stiffness and Heterotopic Bone

Stiffness is a common sequela of fractures of the head of the radius and may be due to capsular contracture, heterotopic ossification, impinging hardware, or retained cartilaginous or osseous fragments.[61,106,124,168] Loss of terminal extension is most frequent. Capsular contractures identified at 6 to 8 weeks usually respond to passive stretching under the supervision of a physical therapist.[107] Static progressive splinting using a flexion cuff and/or a resting extension splint may also be helpful in regaining terminal range. A dynamic

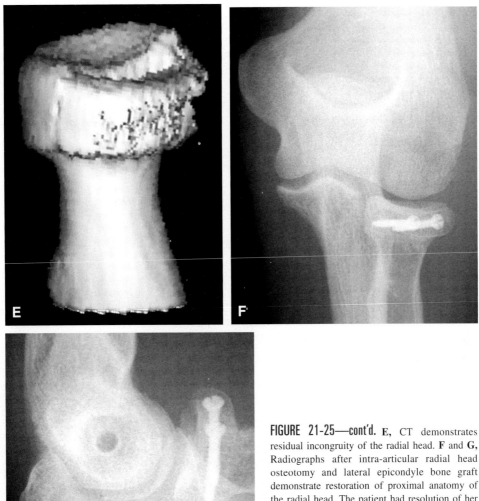

FIGURE 21-25—cont'd. E, CT demonstrates residual incongruity of the radial head. **F** and **G,** Radiographs after intra-articular radial head osteotomy and lateral epicondyle bone graft demonstrate restoration of proximal anatomy of the radial head. The patient had resolution of her pain and clicking.

prosupination splint is employed for patients with loss of forearm rotation.[178] Turnbuckle splinting instituted 12 to 16 weeks postoperatively can be useful to regain flexion or extension in patients refractory to standard therapy.[64]

Patients who fail nonoperative management and who are symptomatic due to residual stiffness can be reliably managed by open or arthroscopic capsular release, which restores a functional arc of motion in most patients.[34,103,121] Loss of forearm rotation tends to be less successfully treated on a delayed basis than loss of flexion-extension, which can be improved even years later. I have had much better results when operating early for loss of rotation that does not respond to therapy, typically at 4 to 6 months postoperatively (Fig. 21-27).[14,99] This may be due to secondary contractures of the interosseous ligament or distal radioulnar joint.

Heterotopic bone can be excised as soon as the cortical margins are well defined and the elbow is noninflam-matory.[129] Bone scans are not useful in directing surgical timing. Patients treated with early excision of heterotopic bone (<6 months) are managed by a single dose of radiation postoperatively to prevent recurrence, typically 500 cGy. Late excision is usually managed using indomethacin, with radiation reserved for those with a contraindication or known intolerance to nonsteroidal anti-inflammatory agents.[107] Patients with residual cognitive deficits after head injuries should also be considered for radiation owing to a higher risk of recurrent heterotopic bone.[59]

Valgus Instability

Late symptomatic valgus instability is uncommon unless the radial head has been excised and not replaced. Prevention is key because late reconstruction often leads to less than satisfactory results. Medial collateral ligament reconstruction has not been reliable in restoring stability in the absence of a radial head replacement, likely owing to attenuation of

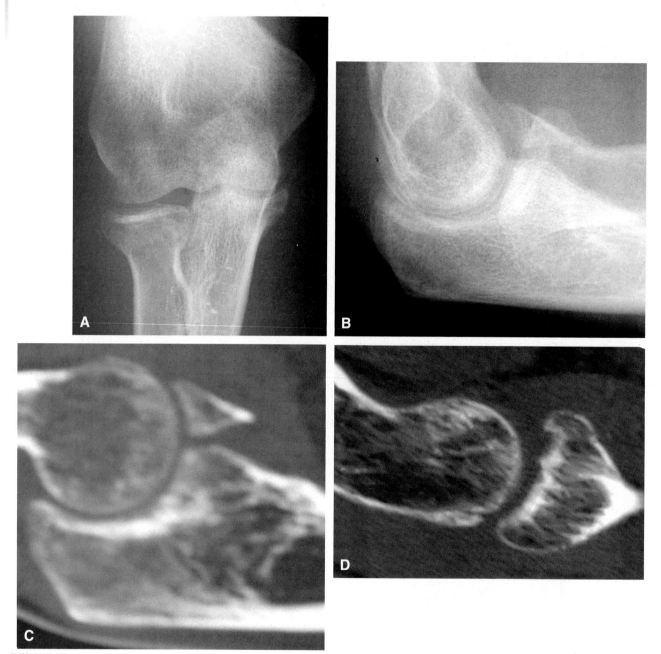

FIGURE 21-26. Osteoarthritis of radial head. Anteroposterior (**A**) and lateral (**B**) radiographs of a 46-year-old construction worker who had Kirschner wire fixation for a comminuted fracture 4 years previously. **C** and **D,** CT confirms an ununited coronoid fracture and incongruity of his radial head.

Continued

the soft tissue repair. Metallic arthroplasty of the radial head may have a role to play in the salvage of these difficult clinical problems provided the capitellar cartilage is not excessively damaged and the proximal radius has not subluxated too far posteriorly such that the radial neck cannot be realigned with the capitellum. Valgus instability can be managed with metallic replacement of the radial head and reconstruction of the medial collateral ligament at the same time.[36,183]

Axial Instability

Morrey and Coleman and their colleagues reported that proximal migration of the radial head averaged 2 mm in patients who had a radial head resection, and most were asymptomatic.[35,143] The incidence and magnitude and symptoms of proximal migration vary considerably from series to series.[130,195] Lewis and Thibodeau reported this phenomenon in 7 of 8 patients who had an excision of the radial head; 2 of their patients were symptomatic.[116] Some patients have greater migration and may develop impingement of the proximal radial stump on the capitellum or the distal ulna on the carpus. True Essex-Lopresti injuries are uncommon[17,38,48,50,75,104,115]; however, they often go unrecognized[51,200] and present as a late problem.[22,25,130,185] If detected early, preservation of the radial head with ORIF or metallic radial head arthroplasty is indicated.[176] Late reconstruction of axial

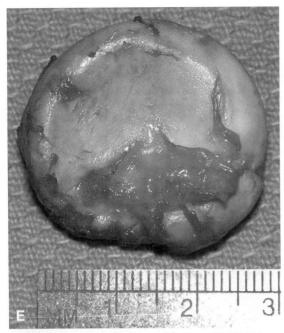

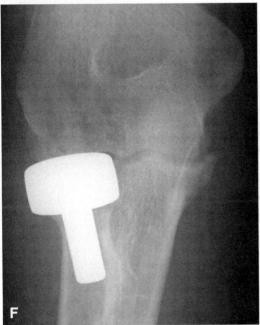

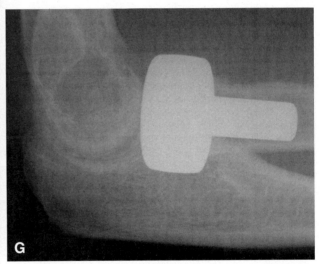

FIGURE 21-26—cont'd. **E** to **G,** Excision of the radial head and metallic arthroplasty improved his pain and allowed him to return to a supervisory position.

forearm instability remains a difficult surgical problem without a definitive solution.[25,86,162,179,185] Whereas a one-bone forearm can solve the instability problem, nonunions and other complications are common.[157] Salvage using allografts of the radial head has been reported; however, increasing experience and longer follow-up suggest a high incidence of complications such as nonunion, collapse, and resorption.[193] Reconstruction of the interosseous membrane has been proposed in biomechanical studies; however, there are no clinical outcome studies available.[85,175,181,205] Ulnar shortening alone is ineffective, because the correction in ulnar variance is commonly not maintained.[185] I prefer to recon-

struct late axial instability in a staged manner using a metallic implant of the radial head. Prerequisites are a proximal radial stump that can be reduced to the capitellum and the absence of significant capitellar arthritis. The metallic arthroplasty of the radial head is performed first, avoiding overstuffing the radiocapitellar joint. Six months later an ulnar shortening osteotomy is performed to restore the normal relationship of the distal radial ulnar joint. This staged reconstruction seems to allow the cartilage and bone of the capitellum to respond to reloading in a more graduated manner and avoids capitellar erosion and pain that has been seen when completing a single-stage reconstruction (Fig. 21-28).

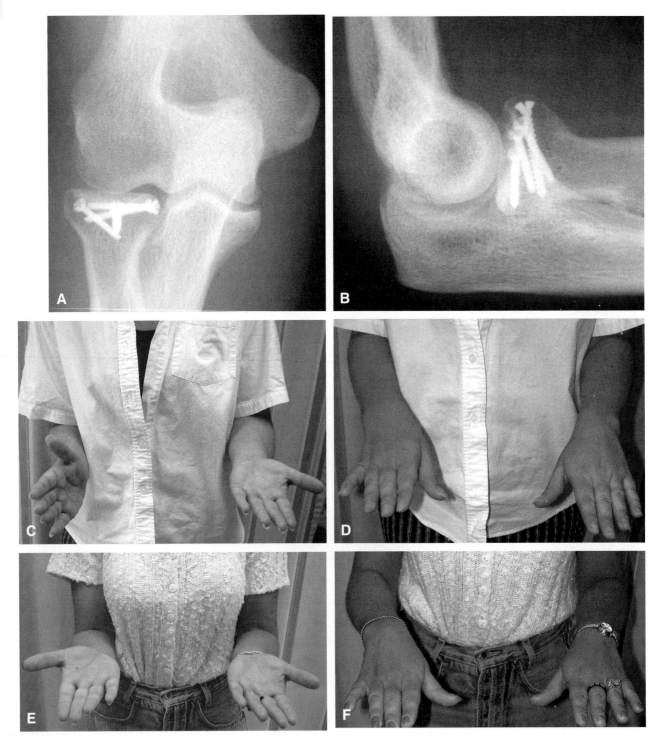

FIGURE 21-27. Arthroscopic release for rotation loss. **A** and **B,** Radiographs of a 36-year-old woman 4 months status post ORIF of a displaced fracture of the radial head. **C** and **D,** Clinical appearance with loss of rotation that had persisted in spite of physiotherapy and splinting. **E** and **F,** At 6 weeks after arthroscopic release of arthrofibrosis there was marked improvement in forearm supination.

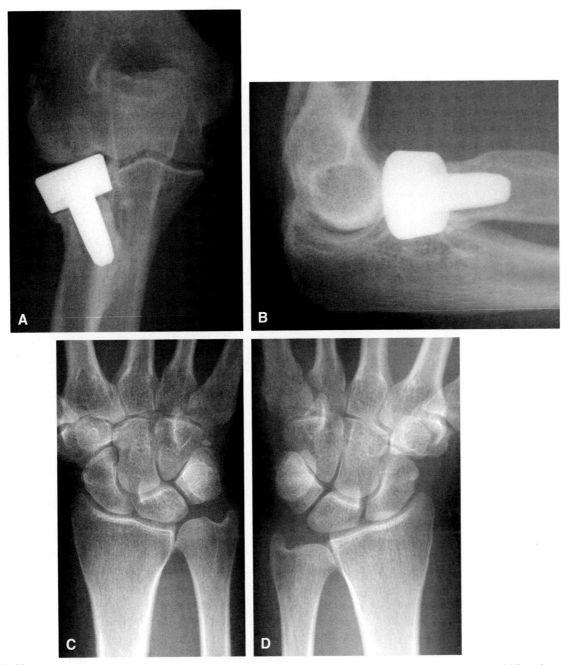

FIGURE 21-28. Essex-Lopresti prosthetic reconstruction. Anteroposterior (**A**) and lateral (**B**) radiographs of the right elbow and bilateral posteroanterior wrist radiographs (**C** and **D**) of a 47-year-old woman who had previously had two Silastic and one metallic arthroplasty for a missed Essex-Lopresti injury initially managed with excision of the radial head. She had persistent pain in both her elbow and wrist.   *Continued*

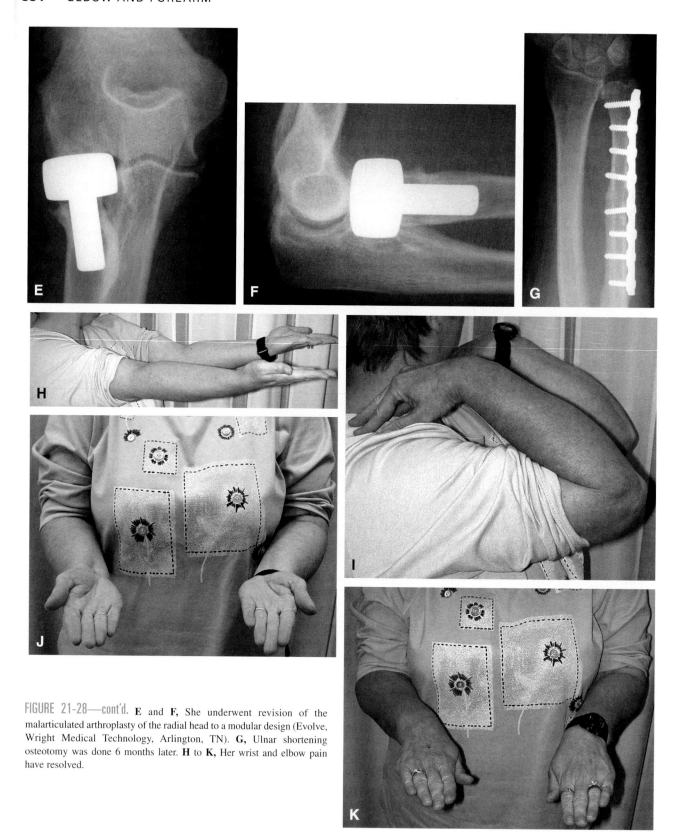

FIGURE 21-28—cont'd. **E** and **F,** She underwent revision of the malarticulated arthroplasty of the radial head to a modular design (Evolve, Wright Medical Technology, Arlington, TN). **G,** Ulnar shortening osteotomy was done 6 months later. **H** to **K,** Her wrist and elbow pain have resolved.

ANNOTATED REFERENCES

8. Armstrong AD, Dunning CE, Faber KJ, et al: Rehabilitation of the medial collateral ligament–deficient elbow: An in vitro biomechanical study. J Hand Surg [Am] 25:1051-1057, 2000.

    In a cadaveric study, muscle activity and forearm supination were demonstrated to improve the stability of the medial collateral ligament–deficient elbow with the arm in the dependent position.

19. Boulas HJ, Morrey BF: Biomechanical evaluation of the elbow following radial head fracture: Comparison of open reduction and internal fixation versus excision, Silastic replacement and nonoperative management. Ann Chir Main 17:314-320, 1998.

    The authors reviewed 36 patients with fractures of the radial head treated with four different techniques. The best outcome was achieved with ORIF of displaced fractures of the radial head.

40. Davidson PA, Moseley JB Jr, Tullos HS: Radial head fracture: A potentially complex injury. Clin Orthop Rel Res 297:224-230, 1993.

    Clinical examination and stress radiographs were performed on 50 patients with a fracture of the radial head. Of the 11 patients with a comminuted fracture, all had valgus or axial instability. Seventeen patients with a displaced vertical shear fracture or impacted fracture of the radial neck had evidence of an injury to the medial collateral ligament. All of the 22 patients with an undisplaced or minimally displaced fracture of the radial head had a stable elbow.

41. Diliberti T, Botte MJ, Abrams RA: Anatomical considerations regarding the posterior interosseous nerve during posterolateral approaches to the proximal part of the radius. J Bone Joint Surg Am 83:809-813, 2000.

    In a cadaveric study, the authors demonstrated that the lateral aspect of the proximal radius is best approached with the forearm maintained in supination to prevent injury to the posterior interosseous nerve. The safe zone was an average of 33 mm (minimum, 22 mm) from the capitellum in supination and 52 mm (minimum, 38 mm) in pronation.

45. Dunning CE, Zarzour ZD, Patterson SD, et al: Muscle forces and pronation stabilize the lateral ligament deficient elbow. Clin Orthop Rel Res 388:118-124, 2001.

    In a cadaveric study, muscle activity and forearm pronation were demonstrated to improve the stability of the lateral collateral ligament–deficient elbow with the arm in the dependent position.

50. Essex-Lopresti P: Fractures of the radial head with distal radio-ulnar dislocation. J Bone Joint Surg Br 33:244-247, 1951.

    The author reports three cases of a comminuted fracture of the radial head associated with a dislocation of the distal radioulnar joint. He advised against excision of the radial head in the setting of these concomitant injuries.

52. Failla JM, Jacobson J, van Holsbeeck M: Ultrasound diagnosis and surgical pathology of the torn interosseous membrane in forearm fractures/dislocations. J Hand Surg [Am] 24:257-266, 1999.

    Ultrasound was used to effectively diagnose and precisely locate a torn interosseous membrane in two forearm fracture-dislocations. The surgical pathology in three forearm fracture-dislocations (2 Galeazzi injuries and 1 Essex-Lopresti injury) shows a longitudinal oblique tear of the interosseous membrane, parallel to its major palmar fibers, oriented from proximal radial to the distal ulnar. The authors demonstrated the feasibility of direct primary repair of the torn interosseous membrane associated with the Essex-Lopresti injury in a clinical case.

57. Fuchs S, Chylarecki C: Do functional deficits result from radial head resection? J Shoulder Elbow Surg 8:247-251, 1999.

    The authors assessed the outcome of 108 patients after resection of the radial head at an average of 6 years. In 64% of the patients only the radial head was fractured. In 26% of the patients the fracture was combined with a dislocation of the elbow. Clinical outcome and strength were better for patients treated with primary resection than for patients treated with secondary resection. Of the patients treated with primary resection 45% had no restrictions in daily life and 64% had no limitations at work.

72. Halls AA, Travill A: Transmission of pressures across the elbow joint. Anat Rec 150:243-247, 1964.

    In a study of seven cadaveric forearms loaded at the wrist, 57% of the forces were transmitted across the radiocapitellar joint and 43% across the ulnohumeral joint.

76. Harrington IJ, Sekyi-Otu A, Barrington TW, et al: The functional outcome with metallic radial head implants in the treatment of unstable elbow fractures: A long-term review. J Trauma 50:46-52, 2001.

    The authors report their experience with metallic arthroplasty of the radial head in 20 patients at an average follow-up of 12 years. The results were excellent or good in 16 and fair or poor in 4. The prosthetic radial head restored elbow stability when the fractured radial head occurred in combination with a dislocation of the elbow, rupture of the medial collateral ligament, fracture of the coronoid, or fracture of the proximal ulna. Four patients had removal of the implant.

87. Hotchkiss RN, Weiland AJ: Valgus stability of the elbow. J Orthop Res 5:372-377, 1987.

    In a cadaveric study, the anterior portion of the medial collateral ligament was demonstrated to be the primary stabilizer of the elbow to valgus stress. The relative contribution of the posterior ligament was minimal. After excision of the radial head alone, the slope of the load-displacement curve decreased an average of 30%. Silicone rubber replacement of the radial head did not significantly improve the stability to valgus stress after excision of the radial head.

88. Ikeda M, Oka Y: Function after early radial head resection for fracture: A retrospective evaluation of 15 patients followed for 3-18 years. Acta Orthop Scand 71:191-194, 2000.

    The authors reviewed 15 patients treated with early resection for a fracture of the radial head at an average of 10 years. All patients had reduced elbow power, and only 5 patients were pain free.

91. Janssen RP, Vegter J: Resection of the radial head after Mason type III fracture of the elbow. J Bone Joint Surg Br 80:231-233, 1998.

    Twenty-one patients with a Mason type III fracture of the radial head treated by excision were evaluated at between 16 and 30 years' follow-up. Only 4 of the patients had elbow pain. Of the 16 patients who had radiographic follow-up, 11 had mild degenerative arthritis of the elbow with joint space narrowing and osteophytes.

92. Jensen SL, Olsen BS, Sojbjerg JO: Elbow joint kinematics after excision of the radial head. J Shoulder Elbow Surg 8:238-241, 1999.

    In a cadaveric study, the authors demonstrated that, even in the setting of intact collateral ligaments, the kinematics and stability of the elbow are altered by excision of the radial head.

94. Johnston GW: A follow-up of one hundred cases of fracture of the head of the radius with a review of the literature. Ulster Med J 1:51-56, 1952.

One hundred fractures of the radial head were reviewed. Type I fractures had good results with nonoperative treatment. The author recommended nonoperative treatment for displaced fractures because excision resulted in wrist pain in 7 of 11 patients. "If in doubt, treat conservatively." He described a type IV fracture of the radial head associated with an elbow dislocation. Treatment of the radial head was as an isolated injury, mostly by delayed excision at 2 to 4 weeks.

96. Josefsson PO, Gentz CF, Johnell O, Wendeberg B: Dislocations of the elbow and intraarticular fractures. Clin Orthop (Sep [246]):126-130, 1989.

Of 23 patients with an elbow dislocation associated with a displaced fracture of the radial head, 19 patients had the radial head excised at an average of 2 days after injury. In 4 elbows with an associated displaced fracture of the coronoid process, redislocation occurred. A follow-up examination performed in 19 patients between 3 and 34 years after the injury demonstrated severe osteoarthritis in 12 elbows. To lower the risk and prevent severe instability, the authors recommend that the radial head should be preserved if possible. If the radial head must be resected, suturing of torn ligaments and muscles at the epicondyles was considered essential.

102. Khalfayan EE, Culp RW, Alexander AH: Mason type II radial head fractures: Operative versus nonoperative treatment. J Orthop Trauma 6:283-289, 1992.

Twenty-six patients with Mason type II fractures of the radial head were evaluated at an average of 18 months after either ORIF or nonoperative treatment with early range of motion. The operatively treated group had 90% good or excellent results whereas the nonoperatively treated group had 44% good or excellent results. Pain, functional limitations, and osteoarthritis were more frequent in the nonoperatively treated group.

106. King GJ, Evans DC, Kellam JF: Open reduction and internal fixation of radial head fractures. J Orthop Trauma 5:21-28, 1991.

ORIF of displaced fractures of the radial head was reviewed in 14 elbows at an average follow-up of 32 months. Mason type II fractures had 100% good or excellent results. Only 33% of Mason type III fractures treated with ORIF had a good or excellent result. Fractures were often more comminuted than suggested by plain radiographs. Excellent results were obtained provided an anatomic reduction with stable fixation and early range of motion were achieved. If a stable anatomic reduction cannot be obtained, then alternative treatment methods should be considered.

109. King GJ, Zarzour ZD, Rath DA, et al: Metallic radial head arthroplasty improves valgus stability of the elbow. Clin Orthop Rel Res 368:114-125, 1999.

In a cadaveric study the authors demonstrated that silicone arthroplasty of the radial head did not improve the valgus stability of the medial collateral ligament–deficient elbow. All three metallic radial head implants conferred stability similar to the native radial head.

110. Knight DJ, Rymaszewski LA, Amis AA, Miller JH: Primary replacement of the fractured radial head with a metal prosthesis. J Bone Joint Surg Br 75:572-576, 1993.

Thirty-one comminuted fractures of the radial head treated by primary replacement with a Vitallium prosthesis were reviewed at mean follow-up of 4.5 years. Twenty-one patients had an associated dislocation or ulnar fracture. There was reliable restoration of stability and prevention of proximal radial migration. There were no dislocations or prosthetic failures, but two implants were removed for loosening. The prosthesis was recommended for use as a spacer to stabilize the elbow after severe injuries while the soft tissues heal.

124. Mason ML: Some observations on fractures of the radial head with a review of one hundred cases. Br J Surg 42:123-132, 1954.

The author reports his results of 100 patients with fractures of the radial head. Undisplaced fissure or marginal fractures without displacement (type I fractures) did well with nonoperative management. Marginal sector fractures (type II) did well with nonoperative treatment if less than one fourth of the radial head was depressed and not tilted. The author recommended early excision of the radial head for all other type II fractures with displacement, comminution, or tilting. Comminuted fractures involving the whole radial head (type III) were managed by early excision. The author's axiom in the treatment of fractures of the radial head was "If in doubt, resect."

138. Moro JK, Werier J, MacDermid JC, et al: Arthroplasty with a metal radial head for unreconstructible fractures of the radial head. J Bone Joint Surg Am 83:1201-1211, 2001.

The authors report the functional outcome of 25 patients managed with a metallic radial head arthroplasty for unreconstructable fractures of the radial head at an average follow-up of 3.5 years. The results were rated as 3 poor, 5 fair, and 17 good or excellent. The radial head prosthesis restored elbow stability when the fractured radial head occurred in combination with a dislocation of the elbow, rupture of the medial collateral ligament, fracture of the coronoid, or fracture of the proximal ulna. There were mild residual deficits in strength and motion. No patients required removal of the implant.

144. Morrey BF, Tanaka S, An KN: Valgus stability of the elbow: A definition of primary and secondary constraints. Clin Orthop Rel Res (Apr [265]):187-195, 1991.

The stabilizing structures of the elbow that resist valgus stress were studied in vitro. In the otherwise intact elbow, absence of the radial head did not significantly alter the three-dimensional characteristics of motion in the elbow joint. Isolated medial collateral release caused an increase in valgus laxity of 6 to 8 degrees. Release of the medial collateral ligament and resection of the radial head resulted in gross valgus laxity and elbow subluxation. This study defines the medial collateral ligament as the primary constraint of the elbow joint to valgus stress and the radial head as a secondary constraint.

168. Ring D, Quintero J, Jupiter JB: Open reduction and internal fixation of fractures of the radial head. J Bone Joint Surg Am 84:1811-1815, 2002.

The authors reviewed the results of ORIF of fractures of the radial head in 56 patients. Unsatisfactory results were noted in 4 of 15 patients with comminuted Mason type II fractures, whereas satisfactory results were achieved in all patients with noncomminuted Mason type II fractures without associated ligamentous injuries or fractures. Their outcome for patients with Mason type III fractures with one or two fragments was satisfactory in 11 of 12 patients, whereas 13 of 14 patients with more than three fragments had an unsatisfactory result. The authors recommend ORIF for partial articular fractures consisting of a single fragment and for complete articular fractures with three or fewer fragments. Comminuted fractures were best managed by excision of the radial head or replacement arthroplasty.

176. Sellman DC, Seitz WH Jr, Postak PD, Greenwald AS: Reconstructive strategies for radioulnar dissociation: A biomechanical study. J Orthop Trauma 6:516-522, 1995.

In a cadaveric study, the authors demonstrate that silicone implants for the radial head did not improve the axial stability of the interosseous ligament–deficient forearm. Metallic implants restored stability similar to the intact radial head. Reconstruction of the interosseous ligament further increased stability.

182. Smets S, Govaers K, Jansen N, et al: The floating radial head prosthesis for comminuted radial head fractures: A multicentric study. Acta Orthop Belg 66:353-358, 2000.

The authors report the results of a floating radial head prosthesis (Judet) for comminuted fractures in 15 patients with a mean follow-up of 25.2 months. Thirteen prostheses were inserted for acute Mason III fractures and 2 were inserted for chronic problems. According to the Mayo Elbow Performance Index there were seven excellent, three good, one fair, and two poor results in the group with acute injuries. One prosthesis was removed after 8 months for severely decreased elbow function. In the group with chronic problems, there were two fair results. There were no dislocations or prosthesis fractures. None of the prostheses showed signs of loosening.

186. Soyer AD, Nowotarski PJ, Kelso TB, Mighell MA: Optimal position for plate fixation of complex fractures of the proximal radius: A cadaveric study. J Orthop Trauma 12:291-293, 1998.

In a cadaveric study, the authors demonstrate that internal fixation of the proximal radius with a "T"-plate should be performed with the forearm in neutral rotation and the hardware placed laterally.

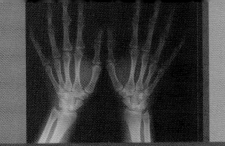

CHAPTER 22

Fractures of the Proximal Ulna

David Ring and Jesse B. Jupiter

Fractures of the proximal ulna comprise olecranon fractures, olecranon fracture-dislocations, Monteggia fractures, and fractures of the coronoid process. Fractures of the proximal ulnas can compromise the function of both the elbow and forearm articulations. The recognition of patterns and common injury characteristics is improving and, in turn, may improve the results of treatment.

PREOPERATIVE EVALUATION

As with other traumatic injuries, the first step in management is to perform a thorough evaluation according to the Advanced Trauma Life Support guidelines. Most of these fractures are associated with low-energy falls in older patients,[54] and these patients should be evaluated for medical conditions that may have contributed to the fall, for injuries related to older age (e.g., other osteoporosis related fractures, subdural hematoma), and for the impact the injury may have on their social situation (i.e., will they be unable to live independently while recovering).

The elbow should be checked for wounds and the neurovascular injury. Anterior and lateral Monteggia fractures can be associated with injury to the posterior interosseous nerve. Fracture-dislocations can injure the ulnar nerve. High-energy, complex fractures of the proximal ulna are occasionally associated with forearm compartment syndrome.

The initial radiographs obtained after the injury are often of limited quality owing to the deformity and pain in the limb. Nevertheless, it is usually possible to discern the overall pattern of the injury, which, in turn, leads one to suspect other injury components that may not be immediately obvious. For example, a posterior olecranon fracture-dislocation is often associated with fractures of the radial head and coronoid process as well as injury to the lateral collateral ligament complex,[54] whereas an anterior fracture-dislocation rarely involves injury to the radial head or collateral ligaments.[53]

Radiographs obtained after manipulative reduction and splint immobilization of the limb (when appropriate) may provide better views of the elbow and additional information about the injury (Fig. 22-1A and B). When additional information about fractures of the radial head or coronoid may influence decision making, computed tomography (CT) is useful (see Fig. 22-1C). In particular, three-dimensional reconstructions with the distal humerus removed can provide a very accurate characterization of the injury (see Fig. 22-1D and E). By using such images, the preoperative planning will be more accurate.

Additional information regarding the character of the injury can be obtained by viewing the elbow under the image intensifier once the patient is anesthetized. For some complex injuries, complete characterization of the injury pattern—and therefore a final treatment plan—can only be made based on operative exposure. The surgeon must therefore be comfortable with extensile exposures providing adequate access to the injury components.

Anatomy

The Trochlear Notch of the Ulna

The trochlear notch of the ulna has a nearly 180-degree circumference, making it one of the most inherently constrained human articulations. Further enhancements to stability include a central longitudinal ridge that interdigitates with a groove in the trochlear articular surface of the distal humerus and a posterior tilt of the articular surface with the angle between the tip of the coronoid and olecranon processes subtending an approximately 30-degree angle with a line parallel to the ulnar shaft[31] (Fig. 22-2A and B).

The articular surface has separate coronoid and olecranon areas separated by a nonarticular transverse groove[30,60] (see Fig. 22-2B). Consequently, the treatment of articular fractures of the trochlear notch should focus primarily on restoration of the proper relationship between the coronoid and olecranon processes, with injury to the region between their articular facets having less impact than similar injuries at other articulations.[53,54]

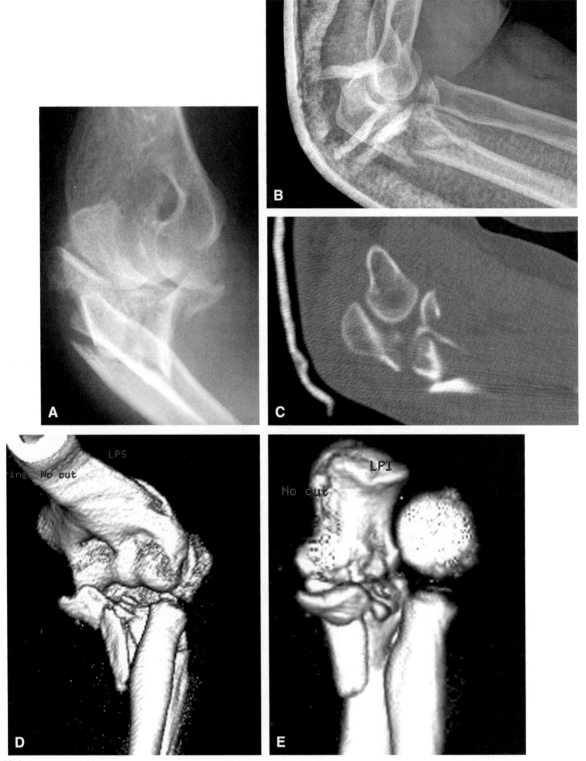

FIGURE 22-1. Imaging of complex proximal ulna fractures. **A,** Radiographs taken immediately after the injury, before manipulative reduction, give important information about the injury pattern and displacement. **B,** After manipulative reduction and splinting, the characteristics of the fractures may be more apparent. **C,** Two-dimensional CT can show greater detail, but it can be difficult to follow specific fracture fragments between images. **D,** Three-dimensional reconstructions of CT images can be easier to interpret, particularly after the distal humerus has been removed from the image (**E**). (Copyright © Massachusetts General Hospital Department of Orthopaedic Surgery.)

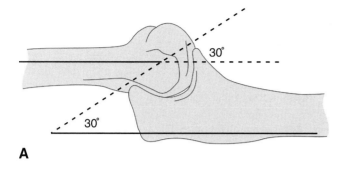

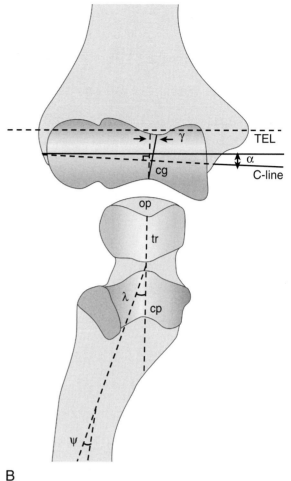

FIGURE 22-2. Anatomy of the trochlear notch. **A,** The trochlear notch of the ulna has a nearly 180-degree circumference that tilts somewhat posteriorly. A line drawn between the tips of the olecranon and coronoid processes should create a 30-degree angle with a line parallel to the ulnar shaft. **B,** The stability of the ulnotrochlear articulation is enhanced by interdigitation of a central ridge in the trochlear notch with a groove in the trochlea. The trochlear notch has separate coronoid and olecranon articular facets with an intervening nonarticular area. (Copyright © Massachusetts General Hospital Department of Orthopaedic Surgery.)

The Coronoid Process

It is useful to consider the following areas of the coronoid articular surface: the anteromedial facet, the lesser sigmoid notch region, the tip, and the base. The anteromedial facet, in particular, is now recognized as a critical stabilizer of the elbow under varus and rotational stress.[51]

The soft tissue attachments to the coronoid also figure prominently in the understanding of proximal ulna fractures (Fig. 22-3). The anterior band of the medial collateral ligament inserts on the base of the coronoid process.[6] Consequently, the anterior band of the medial collateral ligament is likely to be intact in complex fractures associated with large fractures of the coronoid base or anteromedial coronoid fractures, with its function disrupted by the bony injury and restored with stable internal fixation.

The brachialis has a broad insertion that extends distal to the coronoid process.[6] Even with large coronoid fractures, a substantial portion of the brachialis insertion remains on the ulnar shaft.

The lateral collateral ligament complex has a broad insertion on the lateral ulna below the radial head and neck and below the level of most coronoid fractures.[10] Traumatic failure of this complex occurs almost without exception as an avulsion of its origin from the lateral epicondyle and not as an intrasubstance tear or avulsion from the ulna.

The anterior capsule inserts a few millimeters below the tip of the olecranon process.[6] This has been interpreted to

mean that very small coronoid fractures (a simple fleck according to Regan and Morrey) may represent intra-articular free fragments; however, operative treatment of these injuries discloses that coronoid tip fractures are much larger on exposure than might be guessed based on radiographs and that they always include the capsular insertion.[48,49,51,56]

Olecranon

The junction of the olecranon process with the proximal ulnar metaphysis occurs at the transverse groove of the olecranon, which is a nonarticular area with consequently less subchondral bone and is also a relatively narrow area in the sagittal plane. These factors may increase the susceptibility to fracture at this site.[30]

The triceps has a very broad and thick insertion onto the posterior and proximal aspects of the olecranon. This is notable during the application of a plate that contours around this portion of the bone: if the center of the triceps insertion is not split and elevated from the bone, the proximal aspect of the plate will rest well off the bone. For complex olecranon fractures this situation may sometimes be preferable to additional dissection of the soft tissue attachments.

Radial Head

The anatomy of the radial head is difficult to replicate with a prosthesis. It has a slightly elliptical cross section and

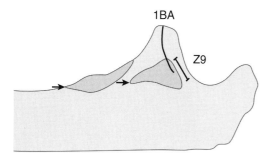

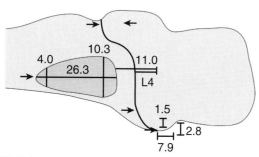

FIGURE 22-3. Soft tissue attachments to the coronoid. The brachialis has a broad and very distal insertion that goes beyond the coronoid and is therefore not disrupted by coronoid fractures. The anterior band of the medial collateral ligament inserts at the base of the coronoid process so that only a very large or medial-sided coronoid fracture will involve the medial collateral ligament insertion. The anterior elbow capsule inserts a few millimeters below the tip of the coronoid process; however, even coronoid fractures that are very small on radiographs nearly always remain attached to the capsule. (Copyright © Massachusetts General Hospital Department of Orthopaedic Surgery.)

interdigitates precisely with both the lesser sigmoid notch and the lateral lip of the trochlea, not to mention the capitellar articular surface.[25] The slight angulation of the proximal radius with respect to the shaft further complicates attempts to reconstruct or replace the radius.

When applying implants, several anatomic features are important. First the posterior interosseous nerve runs deep to the supinator along the lateral aspect of the radial neck and is therefore at risk during operative dissection and implant application. While full pronation provides an average of approximately 5 cm of safe area for dissection and internal fixation,[11] this is not the usual position for internal fixation, and it may be safest to routinely expose the nerve when very distal dissection is needed.[20]

Second, the radial head has a relatively small nonarticular surface and implants placed on the articular surface must be countersunk. This is possible with plates as well as screws.[15] The nonarticular area can be determined as a roughly 90-degree arc with its midpoint directly laterally with the arm in neutral position, with a slightly greater margin anteriorly.[59] As a rough guide to this area, the area between Lister's tubercle and the radial styloid on the distal radius has been suggested.[7]

Finally, the vascular supply to the radial head is limited and tenuous.[61] This may be part of the explanation for the nonunions observed after both operative and nonoperative treatment.[46,57]

The Anatomy of Elbow Stability

Attempts to quantify the contributions of various anatomic structures to elbow stability have suggested that the anterior band of the medial collateral ligament is the most important stabilizer of the elbow under valgus stress[33] and suggest that the radial head is a secondary stabilizer to valgus stress.[34] It may be more useful to consider the roles of the medial collateral ligament and radial head as overlapping and synergistic rather than hierarchical. Throwing a baseball or javelin well probably requires both structures.

Observations of valgus stability have had a strong influence on considerations of elbow stability overall; however, if global elbow stability or the ability to maintain a concentric reduction are considered, then things become more complex. Subluxation or dislocation of the elbow are more directly related to injury to the lateral collateral ligament complex than to the medial collateral ligament.[35,39,48] It is important to understand that complete dislocation of the elbow can occur with the anterior band of the medial collateral ligament intact. Furthermore, the majority of recurrent elbow instability is related to lateral collateral ligament insufficiency.[37] Loss of the radial head, coronoid, or olecranon will exacerbate this posterolateral rotatory instability.[50]

Mechanical studies in cadavers have demonstrated a progressive loss of ulnohumeral stability with greater amounts of olecranon excision, even when all of the ligaments and the radial head are preserved.[1]

Mechanical studies that have been presented but not yet published have found that even small coronoid fractures can have a substantial affect on elbow stability in cadavers.[3,38] In this situation, the importance of the coronoid fracture is probably undervalued given the association of coronoid fractures with patterns of injury that are notoriously unstable and probably reflect greater capsuloligamentous and musculotendinous injury in addition to the loss of bony buttress.[56]

The contribution of the radial head to stability may not be apparent in the laboratory until several soft tissue structures have also been divided, but in the clinical setting, when managing complex trauma of the elbow and forearm, contact between the radial head and capitellum provides substantial stability. Furthermore, some have suggested that the ulnohumeral joint is more susceptible to arthritis in the absence of radiocapitellar contact,[58] although this will be difficult to prove or disprove.

Classification/Patterns of Injury

Monteggia Fractures

Fractures of the proximal ulna that do not involve the trochlear notch often have associated dislocation of the proximal radioulnar joint—the so-called Monteggia lesion.[31,54,55] The most commonly used classification of these injuries is that by Bado, who distinguished four lesions based on the direction of dislocation of the radial head: type 1, anterior; type 2, posterior; type 3, lateral; and type 4, any direction, associated with a diaphyseal fracture of the radius.[2] In practice the most useful distinction is between fractures with anterior or lateral displacement of the radial head and those with posterior displacement. The management of injuries with anterior or lateral displacement centers on stable restoration of the ulnar alignment, which nearly always restores alignment and function of the proximal radioulnar joint.[44,54,55]

The Bado type 2 or posterior Monteggia lesion has long been recognized as a distinct injury that is usually associated with fracture of the radial head and often occurs in the setting of osteoporosis.[23,41,42] There is a spectrum of posterior Monteggia injuries with similar features that vary according to the location of the ulnar fracture.[23] These have been subclassified as type A when the fracture is at the level of the trochlear notch (involving the olecranon and often the coronoid processes); type B, in the metaphysis just distal to the trochlear notch; and type C, in the diaphysis. Type D fractures are multifragmented fractures that involve more than one region[23] (Fig. 22-4). These fractures are inherently unstable by virtue of the associated capsuloligamentous damage, fracture and dislocation of the radial head, and the morphology of the ulnar fracture, which often involves a triangular or quadrangular fragment of the ulna that includes the anterior ulnar cortex and sometimes the coronoid process.

Olecranon Fractures

The Mayo classification of olecranon fractures distinguishes three factors that have a direct influence on treatment: (1) fracture displacement, (2) comminution, and (3) ulnohumeral instability[31] (Fig. 22-5). Type 1 fractures that are nondisplaced or minimally displaced are either noncomminuted (type 1A) or comminuted (type 1B) and are treated nonoperatively. Type II fractures feature displacement of the proximal fragment without elbow instability—these fractures require operative treatment. Type IIA fractures (without comminution) are usually treated with tension band wire fixation. When the fracture is oblique an ancillary interfrag-

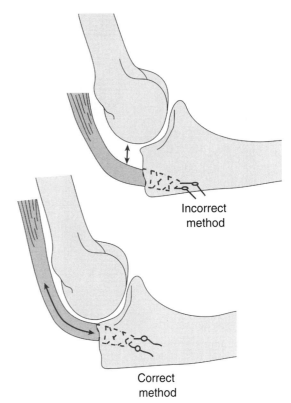

FIGURE 22-5. When the triceps is advanced and reattached to the proximal ulna after olecranon excision, it is better to insert it close to the articular margin. (Copyright © Massachusetts General Hospital Department of Orthopaedic Surgery.)

mentary compression screw can be added. Type IIB fractures are comminuted and require plate fixation. Type III fractures feature instability of the ulnohumeral joint.

Olecranon Fracture-Dislocations

Fractures of the proximal ulna can appear extremely complex. The identification of basic injury patterns can facilitate management. Even a simple fracture pattern of the olecranon can have associated injuries, which the surgeon must be careful not to miss.

Posteromedial varus rotational instability pattern injuries have only recently been recognized and described (Fig. 22-6). The central element of this injury is a fracture of the anteromedial facet of the coronoid process, resulting in varus instability.[51] There is an associated injury of either an avulsion of the lateral collateral ligament complex from the lateral epicondyle or a fracture of the olecranon but rarely both. The radial head is rarely fractured.

On rare occasion, a simple elbow dislocation is associated with a fracture of the olecranon (Fig. 22-7). The pattern of olecranon fracture may represent a bony alternative to rupture of the medial collateral ligament complex.

The majority of olecranon fracture-dislocations occur in either an anterior or a posterior direction.[53,54] Anterior olecranon fracture-dislocations have been described as trans-olecranon fracture-dislocations because the trochlea of the distal humerus implodes through the trochlear notch of the ulna as the forearm translates anteriorly[5,53] (Fig. 22-8A). This pattern can be confused with posterior fracture-dislocations with a similar appearance, so the term *anterior*

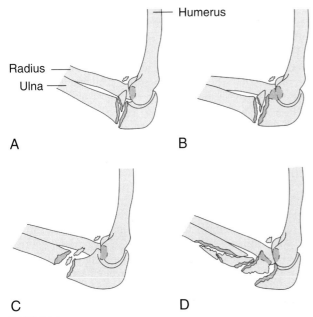

FIGURE 22-4. There is a spectrum of posterior Monteggia injuries starting at the ulnohumeral joint with fractures of the olecranon and coronoid (**A**), the most common location at the proximal ulnar metaphysis (**B**), at the diaphyseal level (**C**), and complex fractures that involve multiple levels (**D**). (Copyright © Massachusetts General Hospital Department of Orthopaedic Surgery.)

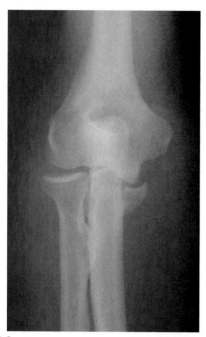

FIGURE 22-6. The posteromedial varus rotational instability pattern injury has only recently been recognized. It is characterized by a fracture of the anteromedial coronoid facet and rupture of the origin of the lateral collateral ligament complex from the lateral epicondyle. (Copyright © Massachusetts General Hospital Department of Orthopaedic Surgery.)

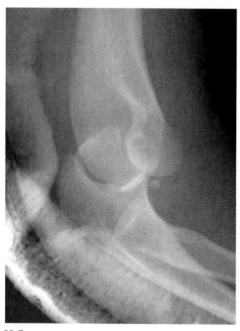

FIGURE 22-7. In this unusual case, a patient has sustained a posterior dislocation of the elbow associated with a fracture of the olecranon process on the medial aspect, essentially avulsing the posterior aspect of the medial collateral ligament complex. (Copyright © Massachusetts General Hospital Department of Orthopaedic Surgery.)

olecranon fracture-dislocation may be preferable. Anterior fracture-dislocations are injuries to the ulnohumeral articulation with the radioulnar relationship relatively preserved and the radial head rarely injured. The fracture of the proximal ulna can be very complex, including fragmentation

of the olecranon, fragmentation extending into the ulnar diaphysis, and fracture of the coronoid. Associated collateral ligament injury is unusual.[5,53]

It is useful to consider posterior fracture-dislocations of the olecranon as the most proximal type of posterior Monteggia injuries.[23] Common factors of posterior Monteggia injuries include an apex posterior fracture of the ulna, posterior translation of the radial head with respect to the capitellum, fracture of the radial head, and frequent injury to the lateral collateral ligament complex. With posterior olecranon fracture-dislocations (or type A posterior Monteggia fractures according to Jupiter and colleagues[23]) the fracture of the ulna occurs at the level of the olecranon and is nearly always associated with a fracture of the coronoid process (Fig. 22-9A). It is important to emphasize that when a complex olecranon fracture-dislocation is identified as being posterior in direction, fractures of the radial head and coronoid and injury to the lateral collateral ligament should be suspected.

HISTORICAL REVIEW

It is notable that Lister selected fracture of the olecranon as the first fracture to undergo internal fixation (with a silver wire) using his antiseptic surgical techniques in 1873.[16] Screws may have been used even earlier.[4] Since that time, attempts to repair fractures of the olecranon with simple wiring techniques or long screws have been associated with problems with loosening and migration—or at least prominence—of implants, leading to secondary surgeries to address symptoms and complications such as infection, malunion, and nonunion.[26] This led to a debate regarding whether to repair these fractures or simply excise them and advance the triceps.[14] With careful consideration of technical aspects of olecranon fixation, the complications have been diminished to the point that excision of the olecranon is used very rarely and usually in a very infirm patient.

The major developments in proximal ulna fractures have related to the recognition of the more complex injury patterns just described. It is now recognized that both simple olecranon fractures associated with other fractures or ligament injuries and comminuted olecranon fractures are better treated with a plate and screws than with simpler techniques intended for simple olecranon fractures. The characterization of anterior and posterior patterns of olecranon fracture-dislocations is not new but is better recognized, and the value of these distinctions in patient management is better understood.

Our understanding of fractures of the coronoid is expanding rapidly. The importance of a separate fracture of the anteromedial facet is evidence that the Regan and Morrey classification[45] may no longer be adequate to describe these injuries. Whereas Regan and Morrey cited large coronoid fractures as more troublesome,[45] recent work has shown that operative fixation of these fractures can be associated with good results[53,54] and that smaller fractures are often associated with more troublesome injury patterns such as the terrible triad.[56] Currently, many surgeons now believe that the majority of coronoid fractures associated with complex injury patterns merit internal fixation; however, the exposures and fixation techniques are still in evolution.[49,51]

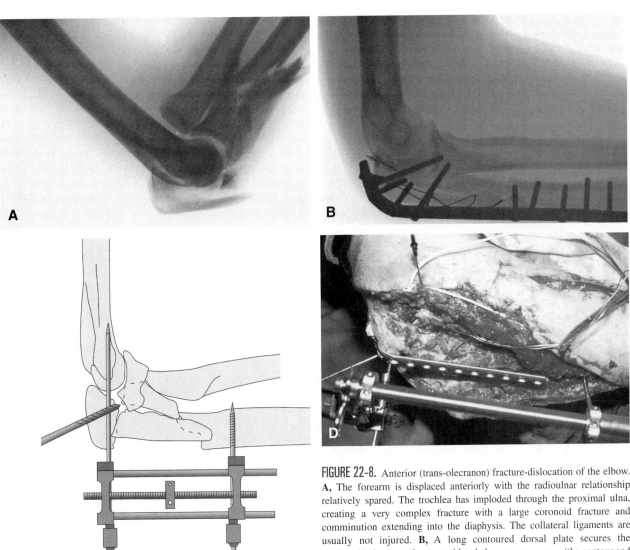

FIGURE 22-8. Anterior (trans-olecranon) fracture-dislocation of the elbow. **A,** The forearm is displaced anteriorly with the radioulnar relationship relatively spared. The trochlea has imploded through the proximal ulna, creating a very complex fracture with a large coronoid fracture and comminution extending into the diaphysis. The collateral ligaments are usually not injured. **B,** A long contoured dorsal plate secures the relationship between the coronoid and olecranon processes (the contour and dimensions of the trochlear notch) and bridges the comminution. A tension wire engages the fragmented olecranon process. **C,** As described by Mast, an external fixator can assist with reduction and provisional fixation. **D,** The olecranon fragment is held to the trochlea with a stout smooth Kirschner wire. Distraction between this wire and a second distal wire helps realign the intervening fragments. (See also Color Figure 22-8D.)(Copyright © Massachusetts General Hospital Department of Orthopaedic Surgery.)

TYPES OF OPERATIONS

Skin Incision

A midline posterior skin incision is used for all complex fractures of the proximal ulna. Traumatic wounds are incorporated. Some surgeons prefer that the incision not pass directly over the olecranon and curve it slightly.[29] A direct midline incision may cut fewer cutaneous nerves.[12]

Excision and Triceps Advancement

The olecranon process is rarely so fragmented that it cannot be repaired. Tension wire techniques can gain fixation of the soft tissue attachments until healing occurs. As a result, excision of the olecranon and triceps advancement is used sparingly for primary treatment of fractures of the olecranon and occasionally for treatment of secondary complications. As primary treatment, excision of the olecranon is best suited to infirm older patients with limited functional demands. The surgeon must be certain that the collateral ligaments, radial head, and coronoid process are intact.

The fragments of the olecranon are excised. Drill holes are made starting from immediately adjacent to the articular margin of the remaining olecranon and exiting the dorsal surface of the ulna. Stout sutures are placed in the triceps using one of a variety of techniques designed to gain hold over a broad portion of the tendon. These are then passed through the drill holes in the ulna, tensioned, and tied.

The elbow is immobilized for 4 weeks, and active motion is allowed thereafter. In low demand individuals, formal therapy is not necessary.

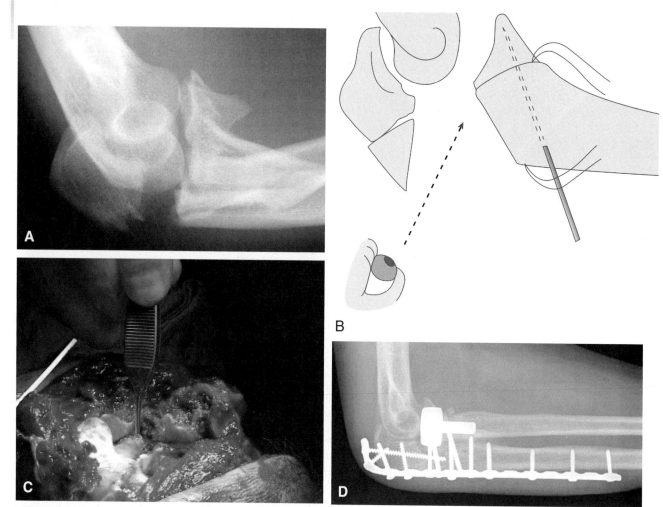

FIGURE 22-9. Posterior olecranon fracture-dislocation (posterior Monteggia fracture type A). **A,** Posterior olecranon fracture-dislocations feature fractures of the coronoid and radial head and frequent injury to the lateral collateral ligament complex. **B,** The coronoid fracture can be visualized and manipulated through the olecranon fracture. **C,** In this patient the coronoid was fractured into three major fragments: anteromedial, central, and lesser sigmoid notch. **D,** Again a contoured dorsal plate is applied with additional screws repairing the coronoid and the radial head replaced with a prosthesis. (See also Color Figure 22-9C.) (Copyright © Massachusetts General Hospital Department of Orthopaedic Surgery.)

CRITICAL POINTS: OLECRANON EXCISION AND ADVANCEMENT OF THE TRICEPS

INDICATIONS

- Comminuted, osteoporotic fracture
- Older, infirm, inactive patient
- No instability or associated fractures
- Salvage of complex cases
- Rarely used today

PREOPERATIVE EVALUATION

- Anteroposterior and lateral radiographs of the elbow
- Evaluation of elbow stability under anesthesia

PEARLS AND PITFALLS

- If the triceps is not advanced to the articular margin of the ulna, this margin may be prominent and grind against the trochlea of the distal humerus.
- Suture anchors cannot be relied on in osteoporotic metaphyseal bone, and the sutures should be passed through drill holes and tied over the dorsum of the ulna.

POSTOPERATIVE CARE

- Cast immobilization for 4 to 6 weeks
- Unrestricted active use of the arm thereafter with selective use of therapy

ATHLETIC PARTICIPATION

- Not applicable

Tension Band Wiring

Tension band wiring is appropriate for relatively simple fractures at the level of the transverse groove of the trochlear notch, without associated ligament injuries or fracture of the coronoid or radial head (Fig. 22-10A). Tension band wire techniques have been described using screws or Kirschner wires. The most common mistake is the failure to distinguish a simple fracture at the transverse groove from a fracture more distal or complex, where a tension band technique will likely fail.

The fracture is opened and hematoma removed to be sure that comminution and articular involvement are limited. Periosteum and muscular attachments are elevated minimally, just enough to ensure accurate reduction of the fragment. A large tenaculum clamp can be used to maintain reduction of the olecranon. A drill hole made in the dorsal surface of the ulna can provide a good anchor point for the distal tine of the clamp.

Kirschner Wire Technique

Two parallel Kirschner wires are drilled across the osteotomy site. The majority of surgeons use 0.062-inch wires, but we use 0.045-inch wires with few problems. The wires are often drilled parallel to the ulnar diaphysis, but we and others favor drilling the wires obliquely so that they pass through the anterior ulnar cortex, just distal to the coronoid process.[9,43] This is intended to limit the potential

for wire migration by anchoring the wires in the anterior ulnar cortex. After exiting the anterior cortex, the wires are retracted between 5 and 10 mm, anticipating subsequent impaction of the wires into the olecranon process proximally.

The extensor carpi ulnaris and flexor carpi ulnaris muscles are partly elevated from the apex of the ulna distal to the osteotomy site to expose the cortex. The appropriate distance between the fracture and this drill hole has been commented on based on mechanical calculations, but the placement of these holes is determined more practically by transition from the flat proximal ulna to the apex posterior triangular shape of the diaphysis. Likewise, the placement of the drill holes in the anteroposterior plane is not critical except that they should not be excessively dorsal as to risk breaking out of the ulna. Large drill holes (2.5 mm) facilitate wire passage.

Many surgeons use a single 18-gauge stainless steel wire for the tension wire, but we prefer to use two 22-gauge stainless steel wires, each passed through its own drill hole distally. The smaller wires are less prominent.

The tension wires are placed in a figure-of-eight over the dorsal ulna. The proximal end of the wire is passed dorsal to the Kirschner wires through the insertion of the triceps using a large-gauge needle. The tension wires are then tensioned on both the medial and lateral sides of the ulna until the wire rests flush with the ulna. Some surgeons prefer to twist the wires until they are very tight, but this cannot be done with

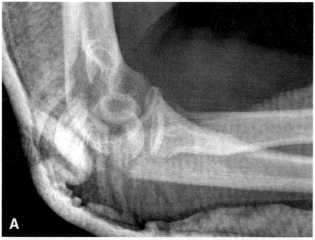

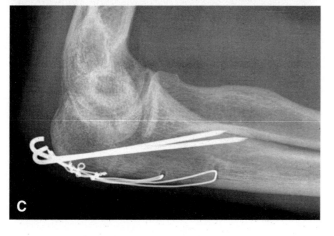

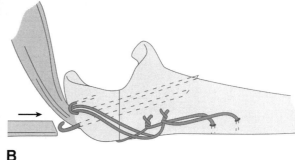

FIGURE 22-10. Tension band wiring. **A,** Tension band wiring is suitable for simple fractures without fracture of the radial head or coronoid or dislocation/subluxation of the ulnohumeral joint. **B,** A technique using anteriorly oriented Kirschner wires, impaction of the proximal ends into the olecranon beneath the triceps insertion, and two small-gauge tension wires can limit hardware-related problems. **C,** Active motion is initiated the morning after surgery. (Copyright © Massachusetts General Hospital Department of Orthopaedic Surgery.)

smaller gauge wires, which will break. The wire does not need to be tight; it is only important to take up all of the slack in the wires. This is done by twisting the wire until it starts to bend over itself. The twisted ends are trimmed and bent into adjacent soft tissues to limit prominence.

The proximal ends of the Kirschner wires are bent 180 degrees and trimmed. The triceps insertion is then incised, and these bent ends are impacted into the proximal olecranon with a bone tamp (see Fig. 22-10B and C). The strength of the fixation can be tested by completely flexing the elbow; the fracture should not separate.

Screw Technique

Some surgeons prefer to use screws instead of Kirschner wires. Some recommend using a very long screw that engages the intramedullary canal of the ulnar diaphysis distally.[21] Others recommend aiming the screw anteriorly to engage the anterior ulnar cortex. An oblique screw is particularly well suited to an oblique fracture. The remaining portion of the technique is as described for the Kirschner wire technique.

A large (6.5 mm) screw, meant to capture the distal canal of the ulna, may cause a fracture of the distal ulna on insertion. If this occurs, the tension band technique must be abandoned for the plate fixation described next.

Plate and Screws

Standard Techniques

A plate and screws are used for comminuted olecranon fractures (Fig. 22-11), Monteggia fractures (Fig. 22-12), and olecranon fracture-dislocations (see Figs. 22-8 and 22-9).

When a plate is applied to the proximal ulna, it should be contoured to wrap around the proximal aspect of the ulna. A straight plate will only have two or three screws in metaphyseal bone proximal to the fracture. Many patients with complex proximal ulna fractures have osteopenic bone, which further compromises the strength of plate and screw fixation. Bending the plate around the proximal aspect of the olecranon provides additional screws in the proximal fragment. In addition, the most proximal screws are oriented orthogonal to more distal screws. Finally, the most proximal screws can be very long screws crossing the fracture line into the distal fragment. In some cases, these screws can be directed to engage one of the cortices of the distal fragment, such as the anterior ulnar cortex.

A plate applied to the dorsal surface of the proximal ulna also has several advantages over plates applied to the medial or lateral aspects of the ulna. Placing the plate along the flat dorsal surface can assist with obtaining and

---

CRITICAL POINTS: TENSION BAND WIRING

INDICATIONS

- Simple, noncomminuted fracture
- No instability or associated fractures
- Location of the fracture must be at or proximal to the midpoint of the olecranon fossae

PREOPERATIVE EVALUATION

- Anteroposterior and lateral radiographs of the elbow

PEARLS

- The use of two smaller-gauge wires can limit the prominence of the knots.
- Kirschner wire engagement of the anterior ulnar cortex and olecranon can limit migration.
- Small implants placed appropriately provide adequate fixation for active motion.

TECHNICAL POINTS

- Fracture site can be opened to evaluate articular surface.
- Dorsoulnar drill hole is used as anchor point for reduction clamp.
- Two 0.045-inch Kirschner wires exit anterior ulnar cortex distal to coronoid process.
- Retract Kirschner wires 5 to 10 mm for later impaction.

- Two 22-gauge stainless steel wires are placed through separate drill holes in the ulnar diaphysis.
- Wires are passed underneath the triceps insertion using a large-bore needle.
- Figure-of-eight wires are tensioned both medial and lateral.
- Bend the Kirschner wires 180 degrees using a wire-bending pliers.
- Impact the cut proximal ends of the Kirschner wires into the olecranon.
- Test security of the fixation through full flexion.

PITFALLS

- Small (22-gauge) wires are easy to break: use tension but do not tighten.
- Wires left above the triceps insertion are prominent when swelling resolves.

POSTOPERATIVE CARE

- Active elbow motion initiated the morning after surgery
- Arm used for light functional activity
- Resistive exercises when early healing established (about 6 weeks)

ATHLETIC PARTICIPATION

- Allowed after healed fracture, normal or near-normal motion, and strength (4 to 6 months)

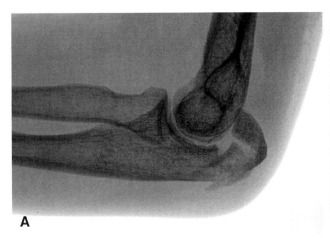

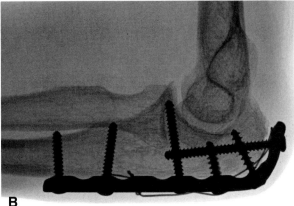

FIGURE 22-11. Plate fixation. **A,** Plate fixation is used for comminuted fractures and fracture-dislocations. **B,** The plate is applied to the dorsal surface of the ulna and contoured around the proximal olecranon. A tension wire engaging the triceps insertion can enhance fixation. (Copyright © Massachusetts General Hospital Department of Orthopaedic Surgery.)

monitoring reduction. The dorsal surface is in the plane of the forces generated by active elbow motion so that the plate functions to a certain extent as a tension band. Finally, dorsal plate placement requires very limited soft tissue stripping.

Exposure of the ulna should preserve periosteal and muscle attachments. A plate contoured to wrap around the proximal ulna can be placed on top of the triceps insertion with few problems. This is particularly useful when the olecranon fragment is small or fragmented. Alternatively, the triceps insertion can be incised longitudinally and partially elevated medial and lateral sufficient to allow direct plate contact with bone.

Distally, a dorsal plate will lie directly on the apex of the ulnar diaphysis. This might seem unsettling to some surgeons but has not been a problem. One advantage of this situation is that the muscle need only be split sufficiently to gain access to this apex: there is no need to elevate the muscle or periosteum off either the medial or lateral flat aspect of the ulna. No attempt is made to precisely realign intervening fragmentation. Once the relationship of the coronoid and olecranon facets is restored and the overall alignment is restored, the remaining fragments are bridged, leaving their soft tissue attachments intact. In spite of extensive fragmentation, bone grafts[22] are rarely necessary if the soft tissue attachments are preserved.[53,54]

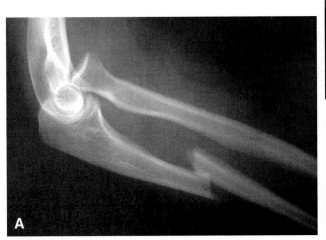

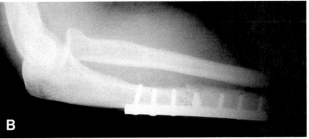

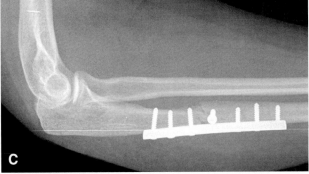

FIGURE 22-12. Anterior (Bado I) Monteggia fracture. **A,** The anterior Monteggia fracture (fracture of the ulnar diaphysis with anterior dislocation of the proximal radioulnar joint) is uncommon in adult patients. **B,** Persistent subluxation of the proximal radioulnar (and radiocapitellar) joints nearly always reflects residual malalignment of the ulna. **C,** Revision of the ulnar fixation achieved better alignment of the forearm. (Copyright © Massachusetts General Hospital Department of Orthopaedic Surgery.)

CRITICAL POINTS: PLATE FIXATION

INDICATIONS

- Comminuted fractures of the olecranon
- Fracture-dislocations of the elbow

PREOPERATIVE EVALUATION

- Anteroposterior and lateral radiographs of the elbow
- CT scan/three-dimensional reconstructions to evaluate coronoid and radial head

PEARLS

- Pattern of injury can indicate injury components/prognosis.
- Medial facet coronoid fractures may need direct medial fixation.
- Ancillary tension wire can enhance fixation of small, comminuted, or osteoporotic olecranon fragments.
- Restoration of the coronoid and olecranon processes is critical.
- If stripping is limited and fixation is secure, the metaphyseal bone will heal without grafting in most cases.

TECHNICAL POINTS

- Dorsal skin incision
- Full-thickness skin flaps

- Access coronoid through olecranon fracture or medial or lateral exposure
- Provisional fixation of articular fragments to distal humerus as needed
- Contoured dorsal plate fixation

PITFALLS

- Third tubular plate may be inadequate; may need dynamic compression plate or equivalent.
- Comminuted coronoid fractures may need to be protected with hinged fixation.

POSTOPERATIVE CARE

- Active elbow motion is initiated the morning after surgery when fixation secure.
- Avoid stressing lateral collateral ligament repair; advise patient not to abduct shoulder.
- Arm is used for light functional activity.
- Arm is protected in a splint or hinged external fixation for complex or tenuous repairs.
- Resistive exercises can begin when early healing is established (about 6 weeks).

ATHLETIC PARTICIPATION

- Allowed after healed fracture, normal or near-normal motion, and strength (minimal 4 to 6 months)

Monteggia Fractures

The majority of anterior and lateral Monteggia lesions feature diaphyseal fractures of the ulna. Standard compression plate techniques with the plate applied to one of the flat surfaces of the ulna should restore forearm alignment.[54] *If the radial head does not align with the capitellum after the ulna is reduced, misalignment of the ulna is the cause until proved otherwise* (see Fig. 22-12). Only on rare occasions is a separate open reduction of the radial head necessary. If a soft tissue block to reduction is present, the posterior interosseous nerve may be entrapped. Therefore, one simply should not divide the tissue without adequate exposure.

Posterior Monteggia injuries that do not involve the ulnohumeral joint most frequently occur at the level of the proximal ulna metaphysis. In this location a dorsally applied plate is preferred[55] (Fig. 22-13). Posterior Monteggia injuries are also associated with radial head fractures and lateral collateral ligament injuries that may need to be addressed.

Fracture-Dislocations

Fractures of the radial head and coronoid process can be evaluated and often definitively treated through the exposure provided by the fracture of the olecranon process. With little additional dissection, the olecranon fragment can be mobilized proximally, providing exposure of the coronoid through the ulnohumeral joint. If the exposure of the radial head through the posterior injury is inadequate, a separate muscle interval (e.g., Kocher's or Kaplan's intervals[29]) accessed by the elevation of a broad lateral skin flap can be used.

If the exposure of the coronoid is inadequate through the straight dorsal skin incision, a separate medial or lateral exposure can be developed. Posterior olecranon fracture-dislocations often require a lateral exposure to address a fracture of the radial head or coronoid or to repair the lateral collateral ligament. When the lateral collateral ligament is injured it is usually avulsed from the lateral epicondyle. This facilitates both exposure and repair. The lateral collateral ligament origin and common extensor musculature can be included in an anterior or posterior flap or mobilized distally.

Improved exposure of the coronoid can be obtained by releasing the origins of the radial wrist extensors from the lateral supracondylar ridge and elevating the brachialis from the anterior humerus and by excising the fractured radial head.[49,51] A medial exposure, between the two heads of the flexor carpi ulnaris, or by splitting the flexor-pronator mass more anteriorly may be needed to address a complex fracture of the coronoid, particularly one that involves the anteromedial facet of the coronoid process (see Fig. 22-6).

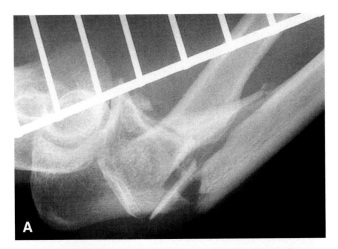

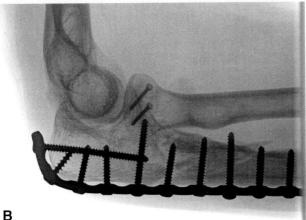

FIGURE 22-13. Metaphyseal posterior Monteggia fracture. **A,** Fractures at the level of the metaphysis often feature a triangular or quadrangular anterior fragment. **B,** Contoured dorsal plate fixation can provide adequate stability to bridge this comminuted area and prevent recurrent apex posterior deformity. (Copyright © Massachusetts General Hospital Department of Orthopaedic Surgery.)

The fracture of the coronoid can often be reduced directly through the elbow joint using the limited access provided by the olecranon fracture[18,19,36] (see Fig. 22-9). Provisional fixation can be obtained using Kirschner wires to attach the fragments either to the metaphyseal or diaphyseal fragments of the ulna or to the trochlea of the distal humerus when there is extensive fragmentation of the proximal ulna.[17,27] An alternative to keep in mind when there is extensive fragmentation of the proximal ulna is the use of a skeletal distractor (a temporary external fixator).[27,53] (See Fig. 22-16.)

External fixation applied between a wire driven through the olecranon fragment and up into the trochlea and a second wire in the distal ulnar diaphysis can often obtain reduction indirectly when distraction is applied between the pins. Definitive fixation can usually be obtained with screws applied under image intensifier guidance. The screws are placed through the plate when there is extensive fragmentation of the proximal ulna. If the coronoid fracture is very comminuted and cannot be securely repaired, the ulnohumeral joint should be protected with temporary hinged or

CRITICAL POINTS: EXTRA-ARTICULAR MONTEGGIA FRACTURES

INDICATIONS

- Anterior or lateral Monteggia fractures
- Extra-articular Monteggia fractures

PREOPERATIVE EVALUATION

- Anteroposterior and lateral radiographs of the elbow

PEARLS

- Residual radiocapitellar malalignment nearly always reflects ulnar malalignment.
- Posterior Monteggia fractures are often associated with radial head fractures and lateral collateral ligament injury (and therefore elbow instability).

TECHNICAL POINTS

- Open reduction of the ulna fracture
- Closed reduction of the proximal radioulnar joint/radiocapitellar relationship
- Plate fixation of the ulna
- Long plate for comminuted fractures
- Contoured dorsal plate for proximal, osteoporotic fractures
- Check forearm and elbow relationships through full motion
- Open reduction and stabilization of radial head rarely necessary

PITFALLS

- Residual malalignment of the ulna
- Ulnohumeral instability after posterior Monteggia fracture owing to inadequate treatment of radial head and lateral collateral ligament
- Early loss of alignment of the ulna owing to inadequate plate—often a plate placed on the medial or lateral surface of the ulna and with too few proximal screws

POSTOPERATIVE CARE

- Active motion the morning after surgery
- Functional use of the arm for light tasks
- Resistive exercises when early healing established (about 6 weeks)

ATHLETIC PARTICIPATION

- Allowed after healed fracture and normal or near-normal motion and strength (4 to 6 months)

static external fixation or with temporary pin fixation of the ulnohumeral joint depending on the equipment and expertise available.

A long plate is contoured to wrap around the proximal olecranon. A very long plate should be considered (between 12 or 16 holes), particularly when there is extensive fragmentation or the bone quality is poor. When the olecranon is fragmented or osteoporotic, a plate and screws alone may not provide reliable fixation. In this situation, it has proved useful to use ancillary tension wire fixation to control the olecranon fragments through the triceps insertion.

Authors' Preferred Method of Treatment

Nondisplaced, Stable Fractures (Type I)
We use cast immobilization for stable, nondisplaced fractures of the olecranon. The elbow is immobilized at 90 degrees of flexion and neutral forearm rotation. The cast is discontinued after 3 or 4 weeks, and active-assisted elbow range-of-motion exercises are initiated. These injuries are rare, and careful surveillance for displacement must be employed.

Displaced Without Comminution and Proximal to the Midpoint of the Olecranon (Type IIa)
For simple, noncomminuted fractures without associated ligament injuries, we use tension band wiring. We use 0.045-inch Kirschner wires directed to engage the anterior ulnar cortex distal to the coronoid and bent 180 degrees and impacted into the olecranon proximally. We use two 22-gauge stainless steel tension wires each passed through its own hole to limit the prominence of the implants.[9]

Displaced With Comminution and/or Dislocation of the Elbow
For comminuted fractures and fracture dislocations we use a dorsal plate and screws contoured to wrap around the proximal ulna.[48,53,54] For some complex fractures we place the proximal aspect of the plate over the triceps insertion, and otherwise we elevate the triceps insertion and place the plate directly on bone. When the proximal olecranon fragment is small, fragmented, or osteopenic, we also use a tension wire that engages the triceps insertion (see Figs. 22-8 and 22-10). In our experience, plates with numerous small screws for the olecranon fragment have not been reliable in this situation. For fracture-dislocations we use the methods described earlier.

Coronoid Fractures
For fractures of the coronoid that involve the anteromedial facet we use a medial plate unless the fragments are large enough to reliably repair with screws.[51] For nonreconstructable or very complex fractures of the coronoid we use 4 to 8 weeks of hinged external fixation to maintain a concentric ulnohumeral reduction and protect the healing coronoid.

POSTOPERATIVE MANAGEMENT AND EXPECTATIONS

Postoperative Protocol

The goal of internal fixation of the proximal ulna is secure fixation allowing active-assisted elbow motion the day after surgery. In the unusual circumstance with more tenuous fixation (usually in an older patient with a complex, osteoporotic fracture) the elbow can be immobilized in a removable elbow splint for 4 weeks before initiating active-assisted elbow motion.

Hand exercises are critical to eliminating hand swelling and preventing hand stiffness. Passive elbow manipulation and joint mobilization are never used. Gravity-assisted and splint-assisted exercises under the control of the patient are very useful. Static progressive splints have been more useful than dynamic splints in our experience.

Resistive exercises and strengthening of the limb are delayed until early healing are established. Full activity is allowed when solid healing is apparent—usually between 3 and 4 months after injury. Plate removal is elective and should be delayed at least 12 to 18 months after injury to avoid the risk of refracture.

Expected Outcome

Intra-articular elbow injuries are commonly associated with some loss of elbow flexion. With very complex injuries the flexion contracture may be as much as 30 to 40 degrees. Near full flexion should be possible in the absence of heterotopic bone or ulnar neuropathy but is also commonly restricted after complex injuries. Forearm rotation is rarely restricted with injury to the olecranon, but posterior fracture-dislocations associated with fracture of the radial head can be associated with diminished forearm rotation.

There is a moderate chance of additional surgery related to prominent or loose implants, elbow contracture with or without heterotopic ossification, or ulnar neuropathy.

Arthrosis is uncommon except after fracture-dislocations, particularly those that involve a coronoid fracture. In spite of arthrosis, the elbow is usually durable if the trochlear notch is restored.

COMPLICATIONS

Early Failure of Fixation

Tension band wire constructs can fail when used for complex fractures or fracture-dislocations (Fig. 22-14), but they rarely fail when used for simple fractures unless the patient returns to forceful activity too soon. Plate loosening is most common in older patients with fracture-dislocations when a noncontoured plate has been placed on either the medial or the lateral side of the proximal ulna (Fig. 22-15).

Failed internal fixation can be salvaged with realignment and repeat internal fixation using a dorsal contoured plate and screws (see Figs. 22-14 and 22-15). If there is a bone defect or delayed union, autogenous cancellous bone graft can be applied to the fracture site.

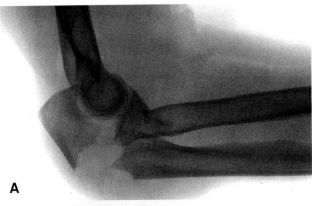

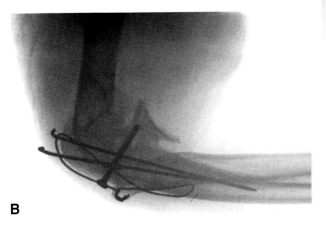

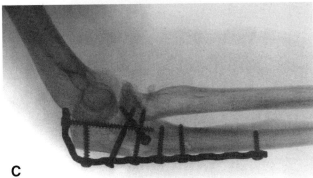

FIGURE 22-14. Failed operative fixation of a posterior olecranon fracture-dislocation. **A,** Type A posterior Monteggia fracture with fractures of the olecranon, coronoid, and radial head. **B,** Internal fixation with a tension band wire construct and a screw proved insufficient. **C,** Revision to a dorsal contoured plate achieved better alignment and more secure fixation. (Copyright © Massachusetts General Hospital Department of Orthopaedic Surgery.)

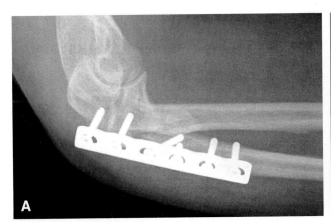

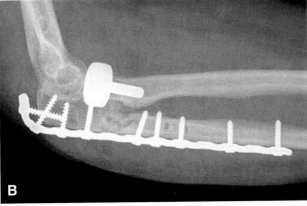

FIGURE 22-15. Plate loosening after operative treatment of a posterior Monteggia fracture. **A,** Posterior Monteggia fractures are common in older, osteoporotic patients. A plate applied to the medial or lateral surface and not contoured around the proximal ulna may have inadequate hold on the proximal metaphyseal segment. **B,** Revision to a long contoured dorsal plate can achieve better fixation and improve elbow and forearm function. (Copyright © Massachusetts General Hospital Department of Orthopaedic Surgery.)

Infection

Infection is unusual after operative treatment of a closed injury and is most often encountered after a complex open injury. In either case, if stable fixation is retained the infection can be treated without implant removal. Adequate soft tissue coverage, serial débridements, and parenteral antibiotics can often eradicate an infection and at a minimum can allow healing to become established before implant removal. For this to be successful, no devitalized tissue can remain in the wound. If there is extensive devitalized tissue, then a more thorough débridement and removal of implants may be necessary.

Instability

Elbow instability can occur after posterior olecranon-fracture dislocations and posterior Monteggia fractures.[50] It can be the result of one or more features including residual posterior angulation of the proximal ulna with posterior subluxation of the radial head with respect to the capitellum;

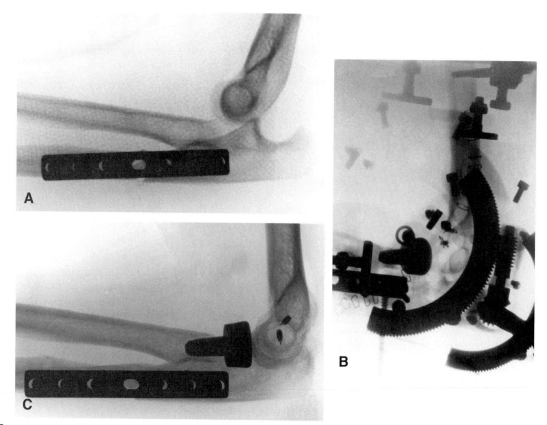

FIGURE 22-16. Ulnohumeral instability after posterior Monteggia fracture. **A,** Surgeons are occasionally surprised by ulnohumeral instability after what was perceived to be a forearm injury; however, posterior Monteggia injuries can include fracture of the radial head and injury to the lateral collateral ligament complex. **B,** Open relocation of the ulnohumeral joint, restoration of radiocapitellar contact with a radial head prosthesis, repair of the lateral collateral ligament complex, and temporary hinged fixation were used to restore stability. **C,** A stable, well-aligned elbow and forearm with good function was achieved. (Copyright © Massachusetts General Hospital Department of Orthopaedic Surgery.)

inadequate restoration of the coronoid or radial head; or lateral collateral ligament injury. Restoration of these factors along with temporary hinged external fixation can usually restore stability and is addressed more completely in Chapter 23 (Fig. 22-16).

Nonunion

Nonunion after simple olecranon fractures is very unusual.[40] Proximal ulna nonunion usually occurs after a fracture-dislocation of the proximal ulna. Union can usually be achieved with contoured dorsal plate fixation and autogenous bone grafting[40,52] (Fig. 22-17).

Ulnar Neuropathy

Ulnar neuropathy is an important and increasingly recognized sequel of complex elbow trauma. Patients who struggle with flexion during the postoperative period and have hypersensitivity or complaints of pain greater than

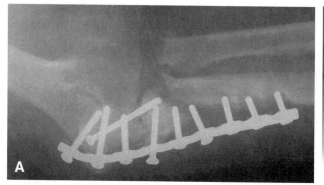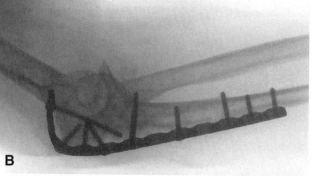

FIGURE 22-17. Nonunion of the proximal ulna. **A,** Nonunion of the proximal ulna is most common after a complex fracture and is uncommon after simple olecranon fracture. This patient has loose internal fixation and a synovial nonunion. **B,** Contoured dorsal plate fixation and autogenous cancellous bone grafting achieved union and improved elbow and forearm function. (Copyright © Massachusetts General Hospital Department of Orthopaedic Surgery.)

expected should be carefully evaluated for symptoms and signs of ulnar neuropathy.

On occasion, a patient who initially is recovering well will lose motion and have increased pain between 4 and 6 weeks after injury concomitant with signs and symptoms of ulnar neuropathy. Patients with this type of subacute ulnar neuropathy might benefit from ulnar nerve release.[13]

Chronic ulnar neuropathy can respond to ulnar nerve release. Even weakness and atrophy can sometimes improve after release, although it may take many years.[28]

Stiffness/Heterotopic Ossification

Stiffness is a very common complication of fractures of the proximal ulna. The ulnar nerve should be carefully evaluated and addressed as just described. If heterotopic ossification is restricting motion, this can be resected as soon as radiographically mature (with 3 to 4 months) as long as the soft tissue envelope is stable and mobile.[24,47] Postoperative radiation can provide useful prophylaxis against recurrent heterotopic bone (see Chapter 25).

In the absence of ulnar neuropathy or heterotopic bone, capsular contracture will usually respond to active-assisted elbow mobility exercises. Dynamic or static-progressive splints are also very useful in this situation. If nonoperative treatment is unsuccessful, then operative capsular excision will restore motion in most patients.

Arthrosis

Severe arthrosis is uncommon after proximal ulna fractures. With lesser grades of arthrosis, the native elbow will function better than a prosthetic or interpositional arthroplasty and should be maintained as long as possible. Older, infirm patients with severe arthrosis can be treated with semi-constrained total elbow arthroplasty.[32] Healthy active patients with stiffness and pain from arthrosis may be better treated by interpositional arthroplasty.[8]

ANNOTATED REFERENCES

5. Biga N, Thomine JM: La luxation trans-olecranienne du coude. Rev Chir Orthop 60:557-567, 1974.

   See the annotation discussing references 5 and 53 after reference 53.

13. Faierman E, Wang J, Jupiter JB: Secondary ulnar nerve palsy in adults after elbow trauma: A report of two cases. J Hand Surg [Am] 26:675-678, 2001.

   Some patients that initially do well after elbow trauma will develop ulnar neuropathy between 4 and 8 weeks after injury (subacute) that may lead to loss of motion and increased pain, limiting hand function.

23. Jupiter JB, Leibovic SJ, Ribbans W, Wilk RM: The posterior Monteggia lesion. J Orthop Trauma 5:395-402, 1991.

   See the annotation discussing references 23, 41, 42, and 54 after reference 54.

24. Jupiter JB, Ring D: Operative treatment of post-traumatic proximal radioulnar synostosis. J Bone Joint Surg Am 80:248-257, 1998.

   See the annotation discussing references 24 and 47 after reference 47.

26. Macko D, Szabo RM: Complications of tension-band wiring of olecranon fractures. J Bone Joint Surg Am 67:1396-1401, 1985.

   The authors carefully evaluated migration of the Kirschner wires used as part of a tension band fixation of the olecranon. Among 15 patients with prominent wires, only 7 were due to actual migration of the wires. The others had been left prominent at the end of the procedure and caused problems when the swelling of the limb decreased. This emphasizes the importance of meticulous and careful technique in the application of tension band fixation of the olecranon.

28. McKee MD, Jupiter JB, Bosse G, Goodman L: Outcome of ulnar neurolysis during post-traumatic reconstruction of the elbow. J Bone Joint Surg Br 80:100-105, 1998.

   The traditional pessimism regarding advanced post-traumatic ulnar neuropathy is brought into question by these data, which show that even muscle atrophy can often improve with long-term follow-up after ulnar neurolysis and transposition.

41. Pavel A, Pittman JM, Lance EM, Wade PA: The posterior Monteggia fracture: A clinical study. J Trauma 5:185-199, 1965.

   See the annotation discussing references 23, 41, 42, and 54 after reference 54.

42. Penrose JH: The Monteggia fracture with posterior dislocation of the radial head. J Bone Joint Surg Br 33:65-73, 1951.

   See the annotation discussing references 23, 41, 42, and 54 after reference 54.

45. Regan W, Morrey BF: Fractures of the coronoid process of the ulna. J Bone Joint Surg Am 71:1348-1354, 1990.

   As virtually the only paper to focus specifically on fractures of the coronoid process of the ulna, this is the classic. The conclusion that larger fractures do worse must be considered in the context of the study. The fractures were classified based on size and concomitant elbow dislocation, and none was treated operatively. More recent work emphasizes that fractures of the coronoid process should be considered in the setting of the overall injury pattern, with larger fractures that are part of an olecranon fracture-dislocation associated with good results with internal fixation and small fractures that are part of a terrible triad or posteromedial varus rotational instability pattern being potentially very troublesome.

47. Ring D, Jupiter J: The operative release of complete ankylosis of the elbow due to heterotopic bone in patients without severe injury of the central nervous system. J Bone Joint Surg Am 85:849-857, 2003.

   The management of heterotopic ossification of the elbow has been based on tradition and the bad experiences of some authors. As the results in these two papers show, successful resection of heterotopic bone can be achieved in a large percentage of cases with substantial improvements in function in most and an acceptable complication rate.

53. Ring D, Jupiter JB, Sanders RW, et al: Trans-olecranon fracture-dislocation of the elbow. J Orthop Trauma 11:545-550, 1997.

   Biga wrote his medical student thesis on fractures of the olecranon with anterior dislocation of the forearm, identifying the characteristic oblique or comminuted fracture patterns with frequent involvement of the coronoid process. We adopted the term *trans-olecranon fracture-dislocation*, reviewing a series of 17 patients. In spite of the complexity of the fractures—including a large fracture of the coronoid in 8 patients and fragmentation extending into the diaphysis in 6 patients—union and good functional results were limited only by associated problems limiting rehabilitation of the limb. The capsuloligamentous structures are relatively spared so that restoration of the normal contour and dimensions of the trochlear notch restores stability. The term *trans-olecranon* has proved insufficient to distinguish this injury from posterior injuries, and we now prefer the terms *anterior and posterior fracture-dislocation of the elbow.*

54. Ring D, Jupiter JB, Simpson NS: Monteggia fractures in adults. J Bone Joint Surg Am 80:1733-1744, 1998.

Pavel and colleagues and Penrose emphasized the unique nature of the posterior Monteggia lesion as being more common in older osteoporotic individuals and often associated with fracture of the radial head. Whereas some authors have specifically excluded very proximal posterior Monteggia injuries in which the proximal radioulnar relationship is relatively spared, Jupiter and colleagues pointed out the common features of posterior Monteggia injuries whether the fracture is at the level of the diaphysis, metaphysis, or elbow joint. By virtue of frequent radial head and lateral collateral ligament injuries, the posterior Monteggia fracture can compromise both forearm and elbow function. In a later paper, we reviewed 10 years' experience with the treatment of Monteggia fractures in adults. Posterior (Bado type 2) fractures predominated by a ratio of greater than 5:1. Sixty percent of patients with posterior fractures were women, and the average age was 58 years. Sixty-eight percent had fracture of the radial head. Twenty-six patients had fracture of the coronoid—all as a single large fragment (Regan and Morrey type III). Patients with Bado type I injuries were younger (average age of 26 years), were more often male (71%), and were often injured in very high-energy accidents with ipsilateral fractures and neurovascular injuries commonplace. Overall, 40 of the 48 patients reviewed ultimately obtained good or excellent function according to the rating of Broberg and Morrey. However, 13 of 26 (50%) patients with a posterior Monteggia fracture associated with fracture of the radial head either required a second operative procedure within the first 4 months of the injury or had an unsatisfactory final result.

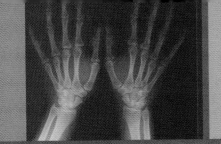

CHAPTER 23

Complex Traumatic Elbow Dislocation

Dean Sotereanos and Robert N. Hotchkiss

One of the most challenging conditions of the elbow to treat is the complex dislocation. This injury pattern has been referred to as the "terrible triad" because the three recognizable features are (1) dislocation of the elbow, (2) fracture of the coronoid (may include the proximal ulna), and (3) fracture of the radial head. It is essential to define and describe this particular condition because the failure to recognize this injury can frequently result in a less than optimal outcome.

A complex dislocation can first be defined as what it is not—a simple dislocation. A simple elbow dislocation is characterized by a posterior dislocation of the elbow without a meaningful associated fracture. Once the elbow joint is gently manipulated and reduced, the joint is stable and does not re-dislocate unless placed in a position of jeopardy of near-full extension and supination. It is helpful to review Chapter 24 in which this aspect of elbow instability is described quite well.

In contrast, the complex dislocation is inherently and immediately unstable unless operative repair is undertaken and attention is paid to protection of those repairs while mobilization is initiated. The immediate danger, after surgical repair, is losing the reduction of the joint (Fig. 23-1). Our goal in this chapter is to discuss the recognition and treatment of this condition and to concentrate on the pitfalls and the need for definitive treatment.

REQUIREMENTS OF A FUNCTIONAL ELBOW

For the elbow to support the hand in lifting objects and move through a useful range of motion, the joint must be stable to varus load and resist the near-constant posterior force that results from pull of the biceps, brachialis, and triceps. The varus load begins to occur as the shoulder is abducted, even to a small degree, and weight is placed in the hand (Fig. 23-2). You can test this yourself. Reach out to pick up a book or glass. As you hold the shoulder in abduction, the stress on the elbow is primarily a varus load, impacting the medial facet of the coronoid/trochlea and tensing the lateral ligament complex (see Chapter 24). Overall stability and

resistance to posterior dislocation comes from both the coronoid and radial head and, to lesser extent, the medial ligament. In this injury, restoration of coronoid function is desirable, especially if more than 50% of the anterior surface is fractured. Radiocapitellar contact widens the articulation of the elbow in concert with the ligaments (see Chapter 21). We agree with most authors[4,7,11,14,16-19,22,23,25] and believe that restoration of radiocapitellar function is not only desirable but often crucial in these injuries, especially when the coronoid is fragmented.

Finally, the medial collateral ligament, the focus of painful instability in the throwing athlete (see Chapter 26), is important for valgus stability but seems to heal with excellent function without direct repair or reconstruction in most acute injuries. For isometric healing to occur, elbow motion in the reduced position is required after injury.[6,23]

Therefore, in order of importance, the structures and surfaces that permit functional joint restoration are coronoid-trochlear contact and load bearing, posterolateral ligament function, radial head and capitellar contact and load bearing, and medial collateral ligament function.

OPTIONS AND OUTCOME AFTER COMPLEX DISLOCATION—THE "COMPLETE" TREATMENT IMPERATIVE

There are two factors that have great impact on outcome and complexity of the surgical procedures and postoperative management: failed previous surgical attempts and delay in treatment.[3,5,7,9,12,13,19-23,26] Obviously other factors also affect the outcome of this injury, such as severity, degree of comminution, and age of the patient. However, these are features that are handed to us on presentation. If, however, we commit the patient to surgery with inadequate or incomplete skills, insufficient equipment, or inattentive surveillance in the postoperative period, the outcome could be dramatically and negatively affected. In other words, an unsuccessful attempt because of inadequate resources often creates stiffness, scarring, and delay that renders the prospect for ultimate success unlikely.

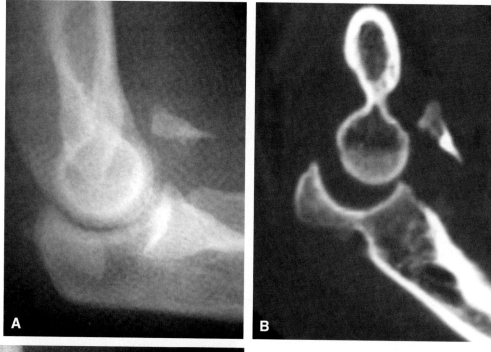

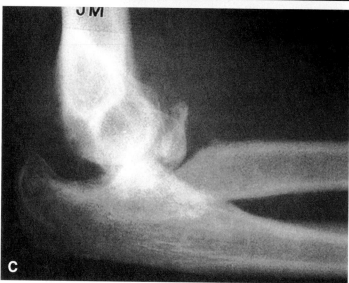

FIGURE 23-1. **A,** Postreduction radiograph in a 45-year-old patient after a complex fracture-dislocation. Note the coronoid fragment, suggestive of a severe injury. **B,** After 3 weeks in a hinged brace, the patient began to lose motion. CT confirmed loss of reduction. **C,** A similar case, 3 months after not recognizing re-dislocation, has occurred. This case becomes a "delayed" treatment case requiring both contracture release and hinged external fixation.

In a rough order of importance, the following are the factors that bear on outcome:

1. Previous failed surgery
2. Delay (>2 weeks) in treatment
3. Comminution of the coronoid and proximal ulna
4. Severity of injury—amount of dislocation and displacement
5. Age of patient*—the older, the poorer the outcome

*This injury is uncommon in older patients (e.g., >60 years). We speculate that these patients will more likely fracture the distal humerus.

MECHANISM OF INJURY

The most common cause of injury is fall from a height—often from a ladder or down a set of steps. Increasingly in an active adult population we see falls from skateboards, in-line skates, and other higher velocity activity. Many can recall landing on an outstretched hand, but it is surprising how frequently a patient cannot recall how he or she impacted the ground.

The fall produces an axial compressive force to the elbow because of the weight of the body. As the fall continues, the body rotates internally, forcing the forearm into external rotation (supination) and the elbow into valgus. The combination of these three forces (axial compression, supination

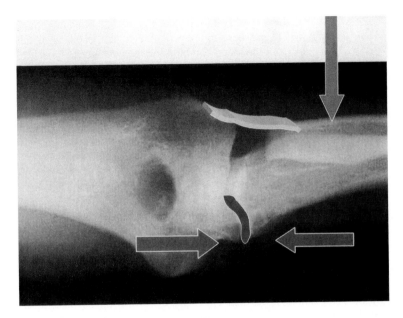

FIGURE 23-2. The elbow joint experiences varus stress when shoulder abduction occurs. The resistance to varus load comes from tension in the posterior lateral collateral ligament and load across medial facet of the coronoid and distal humerus. (Copyright Robert N. Hotchkiss.)

moment, and valgus deformation) explains accurately the mechanism of posterolateral subluxation, which consequently leads to posterior dislocation.[2] Approximately 90% of all dislocations of the elbow occur with posterior or posterolateral displacement of the olecranon.

PREOPERATIVE EVALUATION

Patient Evaluation

Acute Injury

Fracture-dislocations of the elbow usually present as notable pain, swelling, and visible deformity. Physical examination should include neurovascular assessment and evaluation of ipsilateral associated injuries. A concomitant injury of the wrist and shoulder occurs in 10% to 15% of cases. Distal radioulnar joint tenderness may indicate an interosseous ligament rupture (Essex-Lopresti injury). All injuries should be assessed before reduction is attempted. Neurovascular evaluation before and after preliminary reduction should be carefully performed and documented. All three major nerves that cross the elbow require evaluation before treatment, because all three can be injured. The most vulnerable is the ulnar nerve, because it sits directly medial to the joint. These injuries rarely damage the median and radial nerves, but cases of the median nerve trapped in the joint have been reported. Monitoring of the soft tissue swelling is essential in cases of massive soft tissue injury to avoid missing the diagnosis of compartment syndrome.

Delayed Treatment

For patients who present for delayed treatment who may have had previous surgery, a careful assessment of their range of motion, pain, and nerve function should be recorded. Ulnar nerve function may be already diminished without the patient being aware because of the pain and overall impact of the injury at the elbow. Both flexion and extension should be checked as well as forearm rotation.

Patient Expectations and the Preoperative Discussion

The outcome from these injuries is unpredictable, especially when treating those injuries that have previously unsuccessful attempts with weeks or months of delay. It is important to emphasize to the patient that, if left untreated, the dislocated or subluxated elbow will likely deteriorate; that overall function, motion, and strength will likely not improve; and that the main goal is to restore stable, useful motion, not a normal or high-performance elbow. The time to recovery is also measured in months, not weeks. We also remind the patient that the ulnar nerve is quite vulnerable during dissection and surgical repair. It is common that even with minimal symptoms of ulnar nerve dysfunction after surgery, there may be more numbness and weakness for a few days or weeks before recovery.

For patients older than 60 years of age, total elbow replacement should also be discussed as a potential alternative for function and pain relief.

There can also be an accusatory tone to the discussion, reflecting frustration of the patient and family related to the failure of previous care. It is best for the patient and the family to focus on what is needed now for the sake of elbow function and avoid finger-pointing or speculation on previous treatment decisions.

Facility, Equipment, and Treatment Team Evaluation—Preoperative Planning

Most of the acute cases present in a dramatic fashion and provoke a natural impulse to proceed to immediate surgery for needed treatment. However, as noted earlier, an inadequate attempt that results in continued instability, redislocation, and subsequent delay can severely compromise the final result. It is our recommendation that the surgeon carefully consider an inventory of the team, equipment, and combined skills available before proceeding to the operating room. In our own practices we often delay going to surgery

EQUIPMENT*

Internal fixation sets for:
- Radial head fractures
- Coronoid fractures
- Complex proximal ulna fractures

Implants for:
- Radial head replacement

Bone anchors for soft tissue reattachment

Hinged external fixation for the elbow

Imaging: mini-C-arm or regular C-arm

*Individual fracture patterns will dictate which of these is specifically needed.

to make certain that all of these aspects are optimized. We do not prefer to start these difficult cases in the middle of the night with surgical support staff that is unfamiliar with the long list of equipment needed. For the delayed treatment cases, even more contingency planning should be performed.

IMAGING

Acute Injury

Plain radiographs of the elbow before attempted provisional manipulation can be quite helpful in assessing the extent of displacement (Fig. 23-3). Try to imagine the structures that have been compromised and will need either repair, restoration, or protection after injury. The radial head, proximal ulna, coronoid, and distal humerus should be inspected. The relationship of the ulnohumeral joint and radiocapitellar joint may suggest both fracture and dislocation (Fig. 23-4A). Because there are overlapping structures, computed tomography (CT) may also assist in planning and delineating the size and displacement of the fracture fragments (see Fig. 23-1).

Assessment of the adjacent joints, shoulder, and wrist should also be included if the clinical examination suggests injury.

Delayed Treatment and Those Patients With Previous Surgery

In those cases in which the patient has undergone previous treatment but has an elbow that remains either dislocated or unstable, the imaging must be tailored to the individual circumstances. Plain radiographs are mandatory, but because the joint is often stiff and the patient is unable to change its position this situation requires some creativity and collaboration with the radiology staff for nonstandard views. The goal of plain radiographs is to document the integrity and alignment of the articulating surfaces of the distal humerus, radial head, and proximal ulna. Internal fixation and radial head implants can obscure the joint surfaces and alignment. Displaced intra-articular fragments are also difficult to see.

Where there is internal fixation, magnetic resonance imaging (MRI) has been more valuable than CT, because the scatter from the metal can be effectively reduced.

As the images are reviewed, it is helpful to recall the requirements for stability as listed earlier (see "requirements for a functional elbow").

For those patients with recurrent instability who are not resting in a dislocated position, the methods described in Chapter 24 may be helpful.

CLASSIFICATION OF COMPLEX FRACTURE-DISLOCATIONS

As mentioned earlier, the focus of this chapter is the unstable complex fracture-dislocation. This means that a simple closed manipulation may temporarily hold the joint in a more favorable position but stable motion without operative treatment is not possible.

There is no consensus on classification because these injuries are both relatively uncommon and quite individual. There are several versions of radial head fracture classifications that are useful (see Chapter 21). Rather than review these classifications, the purpose here is to provide some guidance in treating the overall injury.

The most important and first distinction can be made between those injuries seen in the acute setting (less than 2 weeks from injury) and those greater than 2 weeks with or without prior surgery. The primary difference in the acute setting is that the dislocated joint is not yet fixed by normal postinjury fibrosis, scar formation, and maturing hematoma. This often permits a less aggressive detachment of soft tissues between the forearm and humerus and reduces the need for hinged external fixation. In patients who have had more than one operation and after several weeks or months have passed with the joint still dislocated or perched, the operation is more complex and results are less predictable. If the articular cartilage of the trochlea has been permanently injured, the chances of achieving a strong, painless, and functional joint are less likely.

Authors' Preferred Treatment

Acute Injuries (<2 Weeks)

For acute injuries, all three components—the ulna, radial head, and posterolateral ligament complex—should be addressed. In general, fractures of the coronoid and proximal ulna should be reduced and held with internal fixation, the radial head should be repaired or replaced, and the posterolateral ligament complex should be repaired.

Position of the Patient

The supine position is usually best for exposure of the lateral and medial aspects of the joint. If the proximal ulna requires internal fixation, a modified lateral position allows a better view of the dorsal surface of the ulna, while still allowing a view of the lateral ligament complex and repair or replacement of the radial head. The application of hinged external fixation in this position is slightly more challenging but doable.

Surgical Exposure

Again, the indication for operative treatment is the inability to achieve and maintain stable reduction with the associated radial head fractures and/or coronoid fractures. The lateral approach to the elbow in most cases is best for open reduction, inspection of the joint, repair or replacement of the radial head, and repair of the posterolateral ligament complex.

The posterior or medial incision is generally not needed, unless hinged fixation or decompression and transposition of the ulnar nerve is needed. The other indication for the medial approach to the joint is for open reduction and internal fixation of the medial facet fracture of the coronoid (see Fig. 23-3).

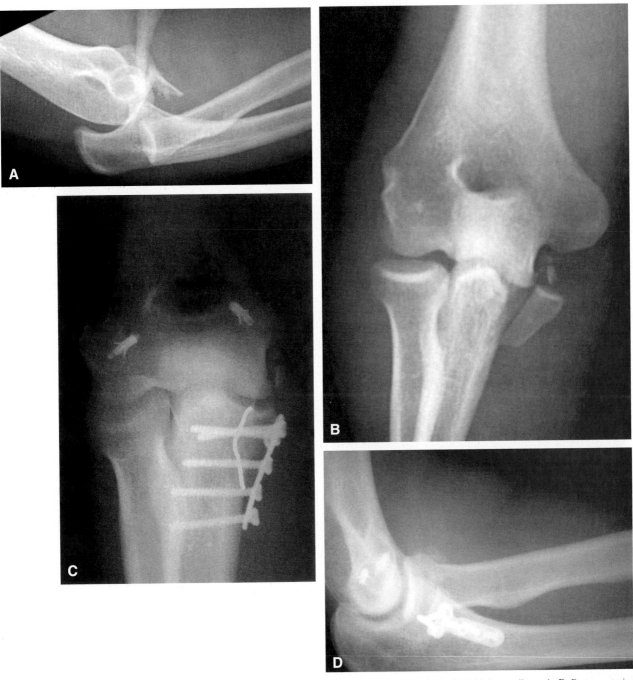

FIGURE 23-3. **A,** Complex fracture-dislocation in a 42-year-old man. Note the degree of displacement in the initial injury radiograph. **B,** Posteroanterior view of same injury. Note the medial facet fracture of the coronoid and the gap between the radial head and the capitellum. **C,** Appearance after buttress plating of the coronoid fragment and the soft tissue was tacked back to bone on the lateral side. The ulnar nerve was transposed for safe exposure of the coronoid fragment. The patient experienced temporary numbness in the distribution of the ulnar nerve. **D,** Lateral view. (**A** to **D,** Copyright Robert N. Hotchkiss.)

Radial Head Fracture

By using the lateral approach the ulnohumeral joint is inspected and any interposed bodies are removed. The fracture of the radial head if reparable is fixed; if it cannot be repaired the radial head is replaced with a metal implant. With the coronoid intact, repair of the anterior capsule is not necessary. We then repair the lateral ligament rupture, which is almost always torn, with the use of suture anchors (usually torn from the humerus origin), and we also repair the origin of the extensor tendons. The stability of the elbow is then tested, and if it is stable we proceed to closure and immobilization in a long-arm splint.

Fractures of Coronoid and Proximal Ulna

Fractures of the coronoid process that involve 50% or more of the coronoid process (type II and III) usually affect the stability of the elbow joint after relocation and have to be fixed. If the radial head is fractured and excised through the lateral approach, the coronoid fracture can be visualized and secured through this view. The fragment can be fixed through a medial approach with the elbow in flexion with the use of a mini cannulated screw, suture anchors, or bone-tunnel and suture technique. The medial approach may also be needed, especially if the medial facet is involved. These fractures represent shear fractures or avulsion fractures of the anterior capsule and not avulsion fractures of the brachialis. If the coronoid is comminuted and the fragments cannot be reapproximated to the ulna, the coronoid process can be shaped from the comminuted radial head or iliac crest bone graft and fixed to the ulna with a screw. However, this anterior buttress is not a perfect match for the surfaces of the trochlea. In some cases even a fracture of less than one third of the coronoid could cause instability, usually when it is associated with ligamentous injuries, whereas in other cases despite the fracture of even 50% of the coronoid processes the elbow joint is stable. This indicates that coronoid fractures should be assessed individually because any type or height involvement can be related to instability. This can be partially explained by the direction of the fracture of the coronoid.

Fractures of the proximal ulna are more completely discussed in Chapter 21. It is worth mentioning that there can be both comminuted fractures of the ulna and ulnohumeral dislocation (Figs. 23-5 and 23-6; see also Fig. 23-4). If only the fracture is addressed, the dislocation will remain untreated.

For fractures of the medial facet of the coronoid, these should be repaired with rigid internal fixation, if possible (see Fig. 23-3). If the fragment is too small, the fracture fragments may be reduced and held in position using a suture or wire, but this fixation cannot be expected to sustain load during rehabilitation (see Fig. 23-5). The use of hinged external fixation may be needed in this setting to protect the reduction and neutralize the forces tending toward re-dislocation.

Lateral Ligament Repair

Direct repair could be done with the use of bony anchors if the ligament is avulsed from the humerus or the ulna. If the ligament has a mid-substance tear after direct repair, passing a No. 2 absorbable suture through the same course as for a ligament reconstruction can augment the ligament. In case of inadequate lateral ligament tissue it can be reconstructed with the use of palmaris longus graft through a lateral approach. Seldom is the tendon graft required for acute injuries.

In our experience, injuries to the medial collateral ligament do not have to be repaired. However, if in the process of repairing the coronoid, transposing the ulnar nerve, or using the medial exposure to visualize the joint there is an opportunity to oppose the soft tissues of the medial side, we will do so.

Contingency After Acute Injury—Hinged External Fixation

The radial head, medial coronoid (proximal ulna), and lateral ligament complex all require direct repair or restoration. The need for hinged external fixation is a contingency decision that should be based on security of the repairs (bony and ligamentous) and immediate stability as judged with the patient on the operating table.

If the fixation of the coronoid is a wire suture or single screw, this should be regarded as tenuous for at least 6 to 8 weeks. Hinged external fixation can be used to neutralize the load on these repairs and to preclude catastrophic re-dislocation and mechanical failure of the repairs.

If the elbow seems unstable and vulnerable to re-dislocation after fixation of the associated fractures and repair of the lateral collateral ligament and anterior capsule, we also recommend the use of an external fixator that will stabilize the joint and allow immediate mobilization. Terminal extension can be limited for the first 2 to 3 weeks if this is necessary. If external fixation is applied, the patient starts moving the elbow from the first postoperative day, gradually increasing the range of motion. The external fixator is removed 8 weeks later and the patient starts strengthening exercises of his arm. The patient returns to his or her previous activities usually 4 to 6 months after the repair when full strength of the arm is regained.

Delayed Treatment With or Without Previous Surgery

In this setting, the challenge is to restore the same key components as described earlier, but in a setting of extensive scar formation, partially or united bone fragments, and a subluxated or dislocated joint (see Figs. 23-1C, 23-4, and 23-6). For patients who are several weeks or months out from the original injury, the difficulty of the case is even more notable because there is often damage to the articular surfaces.

Position of the Patient

The best position for delayed operative treatment may be the prone position (Fig. 23-7). This position permits a simple posterior incision and a wide exposure of the joint. This position also makes application of the hinged fixator somewhat simpler because there is a tendency for the joint to rest in a position of reduction rather than dislocation. The drawbacks of the prone position are that it takes greater preparation to position the patient and that care must be taken to check the legs, back, and head for pressure points. If the members of the anesthesia team have experience with sur-

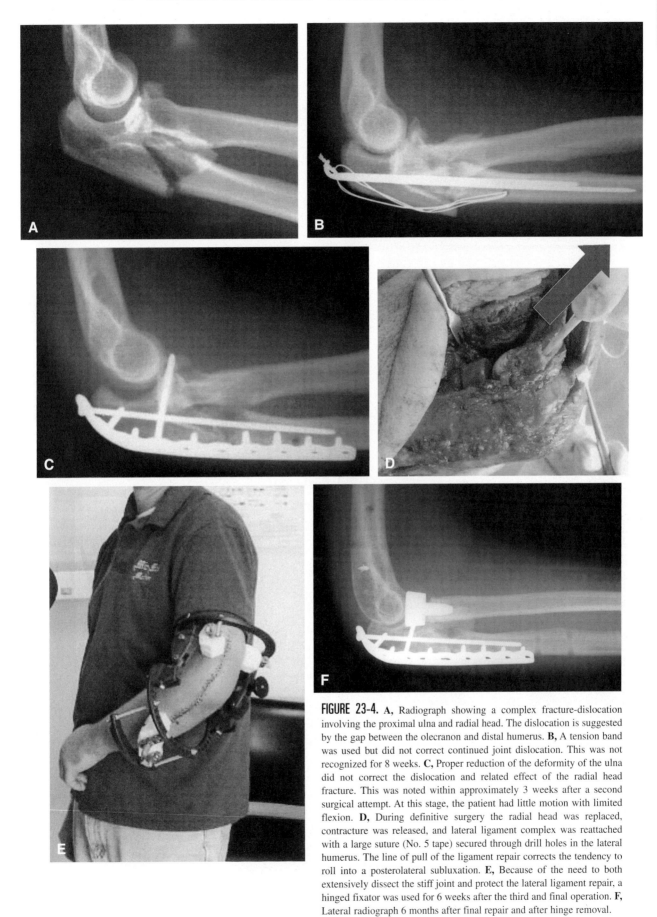

FIGURE 23-4. A, Radiograph showing a complex fracture-dislocation involving the proximal ulna and radial head. The dislocation is suggested by the gap between the olecranon and distal humerus. **B,** A tension band was used but did not correct continued joint dislocation. This was not recognized for 8 weeks. **C,** Proper reduction of the deformity of the ulna did not correct the dislocation and related effect of the radial head fracture. This was noted within approximately 3 weeks after a second surgical attempt. At this stage, the patient had little motion with limited flexion. **D,** During definitive surgery the radial head was replaced, contracture was released, and lateral ligament complex was reattached with a large suture (No. 5 tape) secured through drill holes in the lateral humerus. The line of pull of the ligament repair corrects the tendency to roll into a posterolateral subluxation. **E,** Because of the need to both extensively dissect the stiff joint and protect the lateral ligament repair, a hinged fixator was used for 6 weeks after the third and final operation. **F,** Lateral radiograph 6 months after final repair and after hinge removal.

Continued

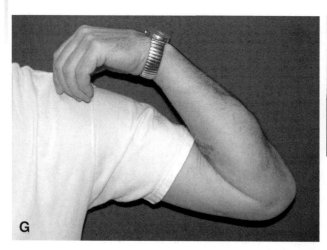

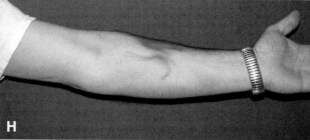

FIGURE 23-4—cont'd. **G** and **H,** Results of treatment 1 year after injury. (**A** to **H,** Copyright Robert N. Hotchkiss.)

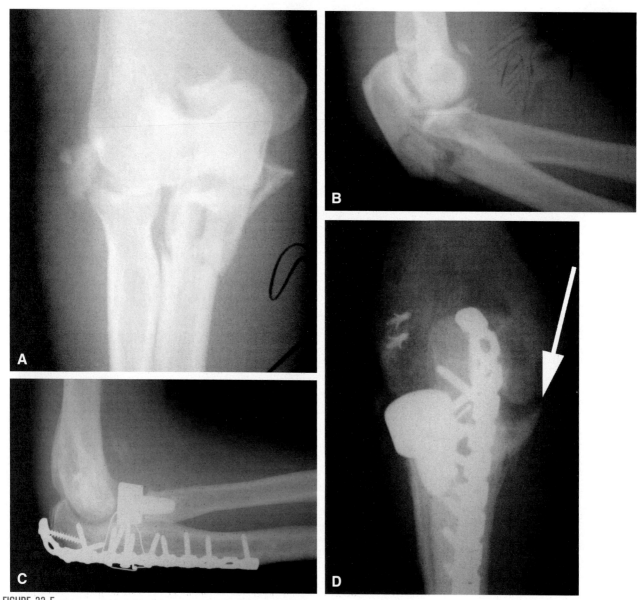

FIGURE 23-5. Posteroanterior (**A**) and lateral (**B**) radiographs of an acute fracture-dislocation in a 22-year old, 3 days after injury. Coronoid is quite fragmented, including the medial facet. Radial head is not reparable. **C** and **D,** Postoperative radiographs after radial head replacement, internal fixation of proximal ulna, and use of hinged external fixation for 6 weeks (approximately 1 year after surgery). Note the use of a single wire to secure a portion of the coronoid. The medial facet of the coronoid (**D,** *arrow*) was held in place using the hinged fixator to neutralize displacement.   *Continued*

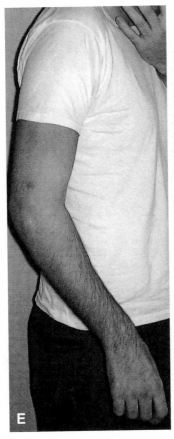

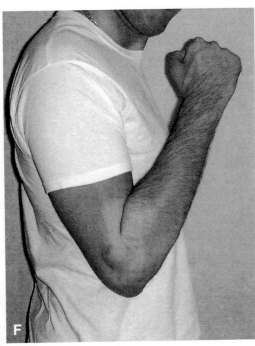

FIGURE 23-5—cont'd. E and **F,** Motion of elbow, approximately 1 year after injury. Note the predictable loss of extension with adequate and useful flexion. (**A** to **F,** Copyright Robert N. Hotchkiss.)

gery of the spine, they can often assist in safely positioning the patient. A Foley catheter should also be placed.

We tend to use the prone position for patients in whom the use of a hinged fixator is likely.

Incisions

The skin incisions are dictated by previous incisions and the particular case. We prefer a posterior skin incision that permits access to the lateral and medial joint surfaces, the ulnar nerve, and the posterior ulna. Although access to the coronoid may seem limited from this approach, once the joint is fully exposed through the lateral and/or medial sides, adequate access can be achieved.

Ulnar Nerve

The first structure that must be identified and protected is the ulnar nerve. Dissection of the nerve must be carefully performed, usually starting proximal to the previous dissection. We do not attempt to dissect into the fascicles but rather free the nerve gently, transposing it to an anterior subcutaneous location with adequate mobilization to perform the open reduction.

Open Reduction of the Joint

Once the nerve is free, the next task is to reduce the joint and expose the fracture fragments for fixation or, in the case of the radial head, excise it for replacement. The thickened capsule both on the anterior and posterior surfaces must be completely excised to permit the joint to be reduced. The posterior olecranon fossa and the coronoid fossa are also gently excavated down to the original surfaces so that the

ulna can track in the trochlear groove. The joint surfaces on both sides of the joint are usually covered with thickened scar tissue, and this layer must be carefully lifted away without damaging the underlying remaining articular cartilage. A small blunt elevator is often useful at this portion of the case. The condition of these surfaces is not predictable, and we have often been surprised by finding extensive delamination and damage. At other times the surfaces have survived and appear relatively healthy.

As this dissection is pursued the lateral ulnocollateral ligament complex should be identified and isolated for later reattachment and repair. We do not routinely repair or reconstruct the medial ligaments; however, if there is tissue that can be approximated on the medial side, after reduction of the joint, it should be prepared for repair.

Bone Repair

Once the joint has been completely dissected free of restraining scar and it can be held in a reduced position through an acceptable range of motion, the bone work can be done. There are occasions in which malunion of the ulna must also be addressed before the joint is stable, and the surgeon should be prepared for these situations. Nonetheless, with the joint now reduced, the radial head can be prepared for replacement. In cases of delayed treatment, we have not found repair to be likely or possible.

Ligament Repair

The lateral ligament complex, as described in Chapter 24, must be reattached to the humerus. An entry drill hole should be placed just anterior to the axis of rotation, and a

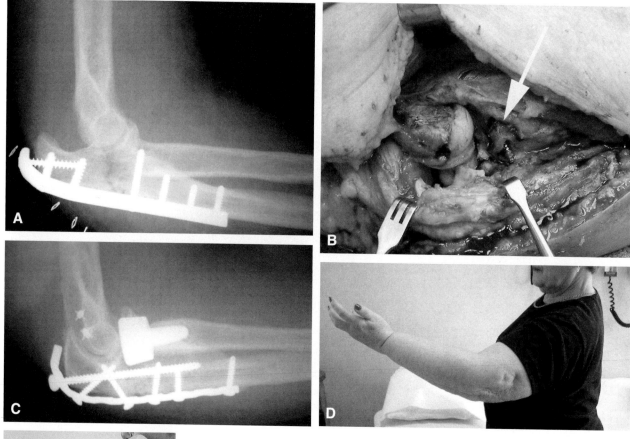

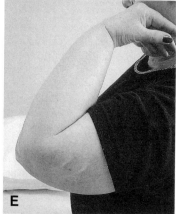

FIGURE 23-6. **A,** Lateral radiograph of 64-year-old patient 3 weeks after initial open treatment of complex fracture-dislocation. Both radial head and coronoid are displaced. **B,** Intraoperative view of displaced coronoid *(arrow)* and proximal ulna fracture with the joint dislocated. Patient required lateral ligament repair, replating the ulna, a radial head implant, and the application of hinged external fixation. **C,** Lateral radiograph showing reduction (6 months after surgery). **D** and **E,** Postoperative motion showing loss of extension (~45 degrees) and adequate flexion (~130 degrees). (**A** to **E,** Copyright Robert N. Hotchkiss.)

heavy suture, usually a No. 2 Fiberwire,* is passed into the hole that exits proximal to the epicondyle. A locking weave using a Krackow-type loop is used to secure the bundle of tissue that once contained the posterolateral ligament complex. A second hole in the bone is used to tie the suture over, once the joint is secured (see Fig. 23-4D). It is important not to tie all of the ligament repairs if a hinged fixator is going to be used. At this stage the joint is grossly unstable, and we prefer to secure the joint into position with hinged fixation and with the sutures in place but not tied. Finally, we tie them securely into place, without fear of dislodging the repair while putting the fixator in place. Additional bone

anchors can be used to secure the posterior tissues to the anterior lateral capsule, further improving the varus stability.

The Use of Hinged External Fixation
There have been many reports about the use of hinged fixation of the elbow to provide temporary stability after fracture-dislocation.[2,3,7,8,10,12,15,17,19,21,22,24,28] The most common theme in these reports is that these devices are complicated to use, difficult to wear, but vital in cases of gross instability. In other words, if all of the steps listed earlier are executed with great skill and the joint re-dislocates or the coronoid fixation fails because of excessive loading, all is lost.[1,20,21,27] In these cases of both delay and previously failed surgical attempts, there is often only one more chance to achieve stable and useful elbow function. If persistent painful dislo-

---

*Before Fiberwire was available, No. 5 Mersilene was used.

CHAPTER 24

Recurrent Instability of the Elbow

Shawn W. O'Driscoll

PREOPERATIVE EVALUATION

Clinical Presentation

It has become apparent that recurrent elbow instability is probably more common than previously thought. Indeed, in two long-term reports, 15% and 35% of patients, respectively, were interpreted to have symptoms of recurrent instability, although the authors could not usually demonstrate the instability on examination.[18,21] This might be related to the fact that physical examination maneuvers permitting the diagnosis of recurrent instability of the elbow have only recently been elucidated.[36]

Presentation and History

Patients typically present with a history of recurrent painful clicking, snapping, clunking, or locking of the elbow, and careful interrogation reveals that this occurs in the extension portion of the arc of motion with the forearm in supination. With a prior history of dislocation, the diagnosis is to be suspected, but it should be considered even when there has been trauma without dislocation or has been surgery for tennis elbow or on the radial head. The most common cause is a dislocation with inadequate ligamentous healing. However, just as there is a spectrum of instability in the shoulder, from subluxation to frank dislocation requiring reduction, there also is a spectrum of instability in the elbow. The presence of recurrent symptomatic subluxation has been confirmed in patients after minor injuries such as "sprains" of the elbow successfully treated by ligament reconstruction. Rarely, severe tissue laxity or chronic overload, such as that seen in crutch-walking patients or connective tissue disorders, can also be responsible for this condition. Postsurgical causes are iatrogenic owing to violation of the ulnar part of the lateral collateral ligament complex with inadequate attention to its repair.[23,28,36] This typically occurs from lateral releases for tennis elbow or after surgery on the radial head.

Physical Examination

The history is characteristic, but the findings on physical examination require expertise to elicit. There are four principal physical examination tests (Figs. 24-1 and 24-2): the postero-lateral rotatory apprehension test, the lateral pivot-shift test, the posterolateral rotatory drawer test, and the push-up test. Whereas the lateral pivot-shift test is challenging to perform, and therefore may give a false-negative result, the postero-lateral rotatory apprehension test is much more sensitive, just as the anterior apprehension test of the shoulder is for a patient with shoulder instability (see Fig. 24-1D). With the patient in the supine position and the affected extremity positioned overhead, the wrist and elbow are grasped as though one might think of holding the ankle and knee when examining the leg. The elbow is supinated with a mild force at the wrist, and a valgus moment and compressive force are applied to the elbow during flexion. This results in a typical apprehension response with reproduction of the patient's symptoms and a sense that the elbow is about to dislocate. Reproducing the actual subluxation, and the clunk that occurs with reduction, can often only be accomplished with the patient under general anesthesia or occasionally after injecting local anesthetic into the elbow joint. The lateral pivot-shift test performed under those circumstances results in subluxation of the radius and ulna away from the humerus, producing a prominence posterolaterally over the radial head and a dimple between the radial head and the capitellum (see Fig. 24-1C). As the elbow is flexed to 40 degrees or more, reduction of the ulna and radius together on the humerus occurs suddenly with a palpable, visible clunk. It is the reduction that is apparent. A lateral stress radiograph taken before the clunk can be helpful to demonstrate the rotatory subluxation (see next section). It is very important to realize that subtle degrees of instability are easily missed and require a high index of suspicion for diagnosis.

A much easier test to perform, but less dramatic than the lateral pivot-shift test, is the posterolateral rotatory drawer test (see Fig. 24-2), which is a rotatory version of the drawer or Lachman test of the knee. During this test the lateral side of the forearm subluxates away from the humerus, pivoting around the medial collateral ligament.[20] The final test is the push-up test noted by Regan (personal communication) in which the patient's symptoms are reproduced as he or she attempts to stand from the sitting position by pushing on the seat with the hand at the side and the elbow fully supinated.

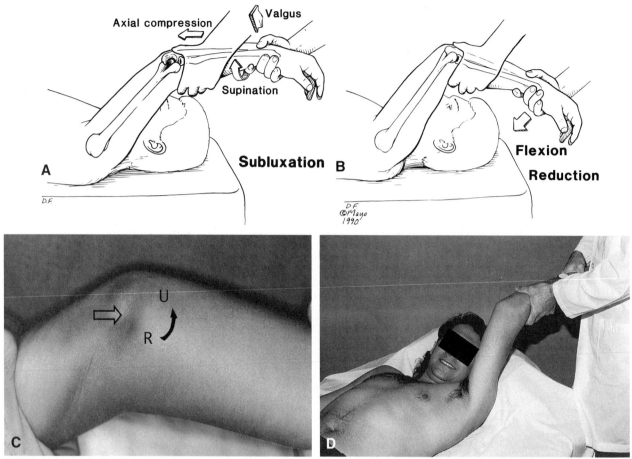

FIGURE 24-1. **A,** The *lateral pivot-shift test* for posterolateral rotatory instability of the elbow is performed with the patient supine and the arm overhead. A supination/valgus moment with axial compression is applied during flexion, causing the elbow to subluxate maximally at 40 to 70 degrees of flexion. **B,** Further flexion produces a palpable visible clunk as the elbow reduces if the patient is able to relax enough to permit that part of the examination. Unfortunately, the subluxation/reduction maneuver is usually not possible in the awake patient. **C,** If the patient is able to relax adequately, or is under general anesthesia, the elbow can be observed to subluxate so that the radius and ulna (R, U) rotate off the humerus *(curved arrow).* The skin is sucked in *(open arrow)* behind the radial head. **D,** This creates apprehension in the patient, who notes the sensation that the elbow is about to dislocate. This posterolateral rotatory apprehension test is highly sensitive, with false-negative findings having been observed only in patients with either profound instability or severe soft tissue laxity. (A and B from O'Driscoll SW, Bell DF, Morrey BF: Posterolateral rotatory instability of the elbow. J Bone Joint Surg Am 73:441, 1991; C and D from O'Driscoll SW: Elbow instability. Hand Clin 10:405-415, 1994. Reproduced with permission from Mayo Foundation.)

Radiographic Features

As part of the preoperative evaluation, plain anteroposterior and lateral radiographs are sometimes adequate but oblique views can be helpful. Impaction fractures of the posterior (nonarticular surface of the) capitellum occur as a result of posterolateral rotatory subluxation of the elbow and are analogous to the Hill-Sachs lesion of the shoulder. CT scans with three-dimensional reconstruction are also very helpful. In one study, nine patients suspected of having posterolateral rotatory instability and nine asymptomatic subjects were imaged by MR and the symptomatic patients explored surgically. Tears of the ulnar part of the lateral collateral ligament were noted in all symptomatic patients. The anterior fibers of the lateral collateral ligament, including the annular ligament, were intact.

Stress radiographs may be necessary to rule out unsuspected instability, especially with anteromedial fractures. Continuous imaging with an image intensifier is preferable, but careful positioning and examination in the radiology suite are satisfactory after some experience has been obtained. A

lateral stress radiograph at the point of maximum rotatory subluxation during the pivot-shift test is useful. To control humeral rotation, and therefore accurately align the elbow with the x-ray beam, the stress radiograph is best obtained by placing the lateral side of the elbow against the x-ray plate with the shoulder and wrist in the same plane as the elbow and then directing the x-ray beam from medial to lateral (Figs. 24-3 and 24-4). Malrotation makes the stress radiograph very difficult to interpret. The anteroposterior radiograph taken during the posterolateral rotatory stress test shows a slight malalignment of the ulnohumeral joint and/or overlap of the radial head and capitellum.

Valgus and varus stability are always assessed as well. It is essential to realize that pseudovalgus instability can exist in the presence of posterolateral rotatory instability. This occurs as the coronoid and radial head slide under the trochlea due to posterolateral rotatory displacement and then permitting valgus angulation to occur by pivoting around the intact medial collateral ligament. A false-positive valgus stress test is most likely to be observed during open radial head excision

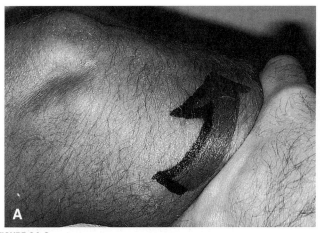

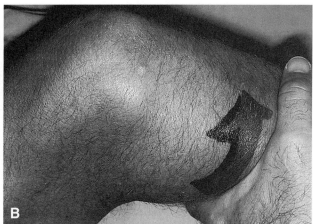

FIGURE 24-2. **A,** An easier, but less dramatic, test to perform than the lateral pivot-shift test is the posterolateral rotatory drawer test, which is similar to the drawer or Lachman tests of the knee. With the arm held in the same overhead position as in Figure 24-1, the lateral side of the forearm is rotated away from the humerus (**A**), pivoting around the medial collateral ligament so that the radius and ulna subluxate away from the humerus, leaving a dimple in the skin behind the radial head. **B,** Reduction occurs with derotation or further flexion. (Reproduced with permission from Mayo Foundation.)

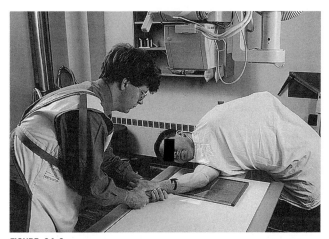

FIGURE 24-3. **A,** Patient positioning for lateral stress radiograph. It is difficult to control humeral rotation adequately when the x-ray beam is directed from lateral to medial. Instead, stress is best obtained by placing the lateral side of the elbow against the x-ray plate with the shoulder and wrist in the same plane as the elbow and then directing the x-ray beam from medial to lateral. (Reproduced with permission from Mayo Foundation.)

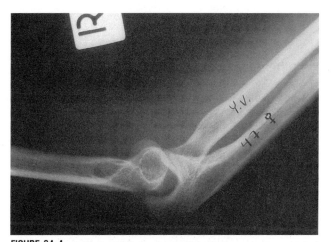

FIGURE 24-4. A 47-year-old woman complained of recurrent mechanical symptoms for several months after having fallen from a horse. She had a positive posterolateral rotatory apprehension test, as in Figure 24-1D. The lateral stress radiograph, taken as illustrated in Figure 24-3, confirmed posterolateral rotatory instability. The radius and ulna subluxate posterolaterally from the humerus, leaving a gap in the ulnohumeral articulation and permitting the radial head to sit posterior to the capitellum. (Reproduced with permission from Mayo Foundation.)

when the lateral collateral ligament complex has been opened and therefore destabilized. To prevent this, valgus instability should always be tested while keeping the forearm fully pronated with a modest force.

Arthroscopic examination will confirm excessive opening of the ulnohumeral articulation and posterior subluxation of the radial head with supination stress applied to the elbow.

 Anatomy

To understand recurrent elbow instability, one must consider the normal ligamentous anatomy of the lateral collateral ligament complex, the bony anatomy of the coronoid

and radial head, and deformity of the distal humerus due to supracondylar malunion.

Lateral Collateral Ligament Complex

The critical ligamentous structure in preventing recurrent instability of the elbow is the ulnar part of the lateral collateral ligament, also known as the lateral ulnar collateral ligament[37,39] (see Fig. 24-18). This is a structural homologue of the anterior band of the medial collateral ligament. Recent publications have discussed the anatomy of the lateral collateral ligament complex. In the case of the lateral collateral ligament of the elbow, the critical component (with reference to posterolateral rotatory instability) is the ulnar part. This thickening of the lateral collateral ligament complex originates on the lateral condyle of the humerus, just anterior to the common extensor origin on the epicondyle, and then passes over and blends with the annular ligament and capsule to insert on the tubercle of the supinator crest of the ulna, just distal to the radial head. Its insertion lies beneath the fascia of the supinator, and so exposure of the ligament at that point requires dissection under the supinator and its fascia. The lateral ulnar collateral ligament is most effectively dissected by starting distally and working proximally. When this dissection is performed by a surgeon with experience doing so, the identity of this ligament is no less convincing that than of the inferior glenohumeral ligament of the shoulder.

Bony Anatomy: Role of the Coronoid and Radial Head

Deficiencies in either or both of the major bony constraints (coronoid and radial head) can predispose to recurrent instability. These can be congenital or acquired.

Role of the Coronoid

Coronoid fractures are most commonly seen in association with radial head fractures as part of the "terrible triad" (coronoid fracture, radial head fracture, elbow dislocation).[12] They typically involve the tip of the coronoid and occur as a result of an elbow subluxation or dislocation, via a posterolateral rotatory displacement of the ulna under the trochlea.[29,35] The mechanism is a fall onto the outstretched hand, with valgus and supination moments applied to the ulna as it flexes on the humerus during axial loading.[36] The implication of these fractures is that the elbow had subluxated or dislocated, just as a bony Bankart lesion of the glenoid does for anterior shoulder instability.[34,35] Their effect on elbow stability is proportionate to the amount of coronoid lost or fractured. Small coronoid tip deficiencies may not need to be reconstructed in all cases of recurrent instability, but larger fragments must be. Until recently our understanding of coronoid fractures has been lacking, and thus there is little written regarding their management.[3-5,30,35,44,45]

Another variety of coronoid fracture has been recognized to involve the anteromedial facet. This injury is a specific pattern of fracture-subluxation that occurs due to posteromedial rotatory instability, as described later. It appears deceptively benign despite its propensity for persistent joint incongruity and premature arthritis. Based on our current understanding, coronoid fractures have been classified into tip, anteromedial, and basal fractures.[32,38] The first two are highly relevant in cases of recurrent elbow instability.

Finally, the coronoid may be congenitally deficient. The deficiency may be gross and obviously involving much of the coronoid process or just the anteromedial facet. In the latter case, which has not yet been reported in the literature, the deficient anteromedial coronoid facet predisposes the elbow to chronic attenuation of the lateral collateral ligament and posteromedial capsule owing to (varus) posteromedial rotatory instability (see later). Importantly, it also puts the elbow more at risk of sustaining a dislocation, which, if treated by lateral collateral ligament reconstruction at a later date for recurrent dislocation, will also, in my experience, increase the risk of failure (unpublished data).

Role of the Radial Head

The radiocapitellar joint functions in load bearing. The radial head acts as a secondary stabilizer of the medial collateral ligament to valgus load,[13,25,27] and together with the coronoid it bears axial load and provides an anterior buttress resisting posterolateral rotatory subluxation of the elbow joint in a secondary capacity.[6,24,36] During strenuous activities, axial force of up to 90% body weight can be transmitted to the radiocapitellar articulation from the hand-forearm unit.[26] Contact forces at this joint are greatest in pronation, which also results in slight anterior translation of the radial head on the capitellum.

The radial head is slightly elliptical with an offset concavity that articulates with the capitellum. The radial head and neck are angulated and offset with respect to the shaft and the neck. The anterolateral one third of the head surface lacks thick articular cartilage and strong subchondral support, making this region more susceptible to fracture. Through the mechanism of concavity-compression against the capitellum, the radial head confers significant stability to the elbow. Thus, even small rim fractures can compromise stability. The same is true for radial neck malunions.

The most critical role of the radial head is that of a secondary constraint to elbow instability. As it has been defined to be secondary constraint,[27] many surgeons have mistakenly interpreted it to be "less important" than the medial collateral ligament or the coronoid. However, it must be recognized that once the coronoid is deficient the radial head becomes a critical determinant of elbow stability. Data from my laboratory show that with as little as 4 to 6 mm of coronoid lost or deficient, the radial head becomes essential for elbow stability.[33]

Deformity Due to Supracondylar Malunion

Recently, long-standing cubitus varus deformities have been documented to lead to tardy posterolateral rotatory instability 2 to 4 decades after a malunion occurred.[1,2,9,14,22,41] Patients complain of lateral elbow pain and symptoms of recurrent instability. The spectrum of cubitus varus and posterolateral rotatory instability may also include dislocation (snapping) of a portion of the medial head of the triceps and ulnar nerve and ulnar neuropathy.[49] The onset may follow a specific traumatic event or surgery (radial head excision or tennis elbow release) or may develop spontaneously. On examination, there is usually tenderness over the lateral collateral ligament complex and common extensor tendon. Positive tests for posterolateral rotatory instability (see earlier) are present. Laxity to varus testing is often evident.

Cubitus varus malalignment secondary to a varus deformity of the distal humerus produces two biomechanical disturbances, which appear to act together to stretch out the lateral collateral ligament complex. First, with varus malalignment the mechanical axis (wrist-to-shoulder) displaces medial to the elbow. The repetitive varus torque caused by this malalignment results in increased tensile stress on the lateral collateral ligament, especially when an axial force is applied to the limb, such as occurs with rising from a chair (Fig. 24-5). This can further alter the mechanical axis.

Second, varus malalignment also displaces the triceps force vector medially to create repetitive external rotatory torque on the ulna. With the elbow flexed to 90 degrees and

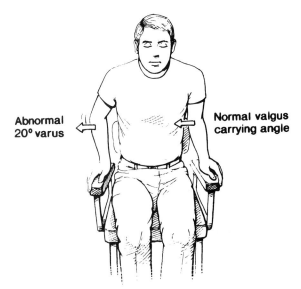

FIGURE 24-5. Varus deformity (right arm) creates repetitive varus torque at the elbow during axial loading and resisted extension, such as occurs when arising from a chair. This can lead to chronic attenuation of the lateral collateral ligament complex. (From O'Driscoll SW, Spinner R, McKee M, et al: Tardy posterolateral rotatory instability of the elbow due to cubitus varus. J Bone Joint Surg Am 83:1358-1369, 2001. Reproduced with permission from Mayo Foundation.)

viewed from the posterior aspect, it is readily apparent that varus deformity at the distal humerus causes medial displacement and external rotation of the ulna along its long axis (Figs. 24-6 and 24-7). As a result of this, the triceps force vector, which can be resolved into two force vectors parallel and perpendicular to the joint surface, has a medial displacement force vector (see Fig. 24-6F2). In addition, the triceps force vector is offset from the center of rotation of the deformity of the distal humerus such that the moment arm creates external rotation torque on the ulna (i.e., supination). These repetitive abnormal torques cause chronic medial overpull of the triceps, which, during childhood growth, can cause medial elongation of the olecranon. Repetitive stress to such a malaligned elbow, as would occur when getting up from a chair, can further exacerbate and precipitate the biomechanical alterations. In addition, the cubitus varus deformity may predispose the elbow to injury during a fall (Fig. 24-8).

Whether the elbow experiences acute trauma or not, these abnormal repetitive varus and external rotation torques combine to cause attenuation of the lateral collateral ligament complex. Such attenuation permits excessive external rotation (supination) of the forearm with respect to the humerus. This represents the first stage of the pattern of posterolateral rotatory instability.[40]

This biomechanical explanation for posterolateral rotatory instability is consistent with and complementary to the previously proposed mechanism (see Fig. 24-8).[36,40] This current description emphasizes the effect of cubitus varus on the triceps in providing an external moment arm. During a fall, the arm is extended at the elbow, and on impact with the ground, the elbow starts to flex.[40] During flexion, the triceps will experience an eccentric load to resist flexion; and in the setting of chronic cubitus varus and attenuation of the lateral

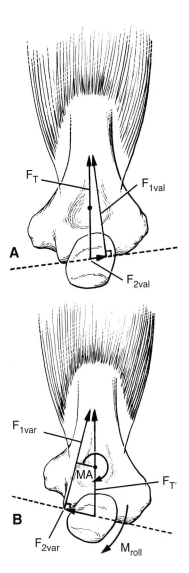

FIGURE 24-6. Biomechanics of the triceps mechanism and its effect on ulnohumeral stability. **A,** Normal alignment with slight valgus carrying angle. The triceps force vector (F_T), which is almost perpendicular to the joint line, can be resolved into two perpendicular vectors. A slight valgus force (F_{2val}) exists. **B,** Cubitus varus. The triceps force vector ($F_{T'}$) can be resolved into two force vectors: F_1, which is perpendicular to the joint surface, and F_2, which is directed medially. This medial force vector causes external rotation of the ulna about its long axis (M_{roll}). The offset between F_1 and the axis of rotation (due to the deformity at the supracondylar level) causes a moment arm (MA) through which external rotation and varus deforming torques occur with triceps contraction. (From O'Driscoll SW, Spinner R, McKee M, et al: Tardy posterolateral rotatory instability of the elbow due to cubitus varus. J Bone Joint Surg Am 83:1358-1369, 2001. Reproduced with permission from Mayo Foundation.)

collateral ligament complex, the eccentric triceps contraction will cause hypersupination of the forearm at the elbow (excessive external rotation), which is the initial component of posterolateral rotatory subluxation. Thus, it is believed that contraction of the displaced medial triceps is important both in the activation of the posterolateral rotatory instability and in the development of the injury (e.g., during a fall).

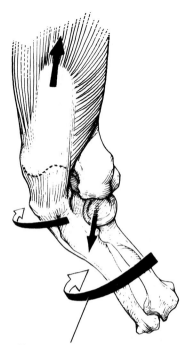

Posterolateral rotatory subluxation

FIGURE 24-7. Mechanism of deforming torsional forces. With active triceps contraction *(solid straight arrow)* while extension is being resisted the deforming forces and moments referred to in Figure 24-5B cause a medial pull and external rotation torsion on the ulna about its long axis *(small curved arrow)*. This not only rotates the ulna into external rotation but also causes the radial head to rotate posterolaterally off the capitellum *(straight dashed arrow)*. These represent the initial kinematic displacements of posterolateral rotatory subluxation *(large curved arrow)*. Over time, these chronic forces cause attenuation of the lateral collateral ligament complex, including the ulnar part, leading to frank posterolateral rotatory subluxation. (From O'Driscoll SW, Spinner R, McKee M, et al: Tardy posterolateral rotatory instability of the elbow due to cubitus varus. J Bone Joint Surg Am 83:1358-1369, 2001. Reproduced with permission from Mayo Foundation.)

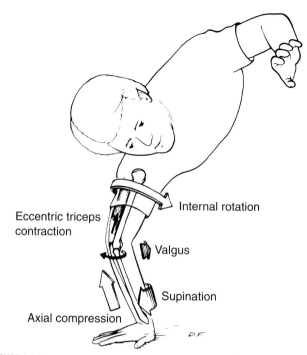

FIGURE 24-8. With a fall on the outstretched arm, the forces and moments in posterolateral rotatory instability are created and the preexistent pathology and abnormal mechanics of the patient with chronic cubitus varus deformity predispose the patient to this injury. These include a supination valgus torque at the elbow (internal rotation of the humerus) while exposing an axial load during flexion. Eccentric triceps contraction rotates the forearm off the humerus in external rotation. Eccentric triceps contraction also causes the elbow to rotate off in a valgus direction, despite the preexisting varus deformity. (From O'Driscoll SW, Spinner R, McKee M, et al: Tardy posterolateral rotatory instability of the elbow due to cubitus varus. J Bone Joint Surg Am 83:1358-1369, 2001. Reproduced with permission from Mayo Foundation.)

Biomechanical disturbance can be confirmed intraoperatively by stimulating the triceps (predominantly the medial head) using a transcutaneous electrical neural stimulation (TENS) unit (FasTens 2220S, Rehabilicare, New Brighton, MN). While preventing the elbow from extending, the combination of varus articular malalignment and medial elongation of the olecranon permits the triceps to roll the ulna into external rotation and to subluxate the elbow posterolaterally (Figs. 24-9 and 24-10).

Internal rotation is also a component of the clinical deformity of post-traumatic supracondylar humeral varus malunions. It is possible that such internal rotation deformity contributes to the instability. Unfortunately, rotational malalignment was recorded in only five of the patients in this series, so it is not possible to know its effect on posterolateral rotatory instability. However, preliminary studies in cadavers and in a mathematical model suggest that the important factors in displacing the triceps are the varus deformity and the location of the triceps insertion on the olecranon, rather than the internal rotation or flexion/extension deformity.[50]

In some patients, ligament reconstruction alone may provide excellent results; these situations include elbows with a small (less than perhaps 15 degrees) varus angulation, instability due to a discrete injury (not instability caused by chronic stretching of the ligament), or low demand, older, or nonathletic individuals. However, ligament reconstruction without osteotomy puts a larger stress on the repair. It is recommended that patients with a varus deformity of 15 degrees or more be treated by both osteotomy and ligament reconstruction (see Figs. 24-9 and 24-10). It appears that corrective osteotomy, which restores a normal valgus alignment, helps to stabilize the ligamentous laxity. In some case, osteotomy alone may be adequate if there is only subtle instability or if the patient places only limited demands on the elbow. For a large deformity, I recommend that osteotomy and ligament reconstruction be combined because I have found that either osteotomy alone or ligament reconstruction alone has a high likelihood of failure in the presence of a large (greater than 15 degrees) bony deformity and high postoperative functional demands. Osteotomies that do not restore a valgus carrying angle seem destined for failure, based on biomechanical principles. Further study and experience with more patients with this problem will be required before definitive surgical recommendations can be defined.

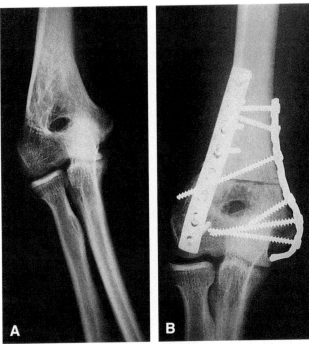

FIGURE 24-9. **A,** Preoperative anteroposterior radiograph of a man presenting with tardy posterolateral rotatory instability 3 decades after having sustained a supracondylar fracture resulting in cubitus varus malunion. He was treated by corrective osteotomy and lateral collateral ligament reconstruction, which restored the normal valgus carrying angle as seen in the postoperative radiograph (**B**). (From O'Driscoll SW, Spinner R, McKee M, et al: Tardy posterolateral rotatory instability of the elbow due to cubitus varus. J Bone Joint Surg Am 83:1358-1369, 2001. Reproduced with permission from Mayo Foundation.)

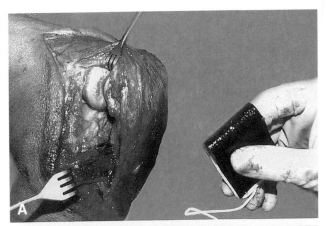

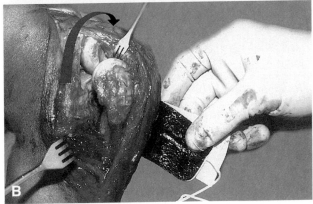

FIGURE 24-10. **A,** Intraoperative oblique view of the right elbow with the joint reduced. **B,** Photograph of the same elbow after stimulation of the triceps muscle with a TENS unit, while extension of the elbow is resisted. Contraction of the triceps (principally the medial head) causes the ulna to rotate externally off the humerus and the forearm to swing around into valgus *(curved arrow)*, re-creating the displacements of posterolateral rotatory instability. (From O'Driscoll SW, Spinner R, McKee M, et al: Tardy posterolateral rotatory instability of the elbow due to cubitus varus. J Bone Joint Surg Am 83:1358-1369, 2001. Reproduced with permission from Mayo Foundation.)

HISTORICAL REVIEW

Mechanism of Dislocation

The traditional teaching that the mechanism of dislocation is hyperextension was unsubstantiated by data.[48] Although the previously proposed mechanism might occur, it is reasonable to consider the following as a unified concept that can be used to explain the full clinical spectrum of acute, chronic, and recurrent elbow instability. This mechanism has now been confirmed in live videos of two patients obtained during the actual dislocations (unpublished data).

Elbow dislocations or subluxations typically occur as a result of falls on the outstretched hand. The elbow experiences an axial compressive force during flexion as the body approaches the ground. As the body "rotates internally" on the elbow (forearm rotates externally on the humerus) a supination moment occurs at the elbow. A valgus moment results from the fact that the mechanical axis passes through the lateral side of the elbow. This combination of valgus and supination with axial compression during flexion is precisely the mechanism that results in a posterolateral rotatory subluxation or dislocation of the elbow and can be reproduced clinically by what is referred to as the "lateral pivot-shift test," which is described later. The pathoanatomy can be thought of as a circle of soft tissue disruption from lateral to medial in three stages (Fig. 24-11). In stage 1 the ulnar part of the

lateral collateral ligament is disrupted (the remainder of the lateral collateral ligament complex may be intact or disrupted). This results in posterolateral rotatory subluxation of the elbow, which reduces spontaneously (Fig. 24-12). With further disruption anteriorly and posteriorly the elbow in stage 2 instability is capable of an incomplete posterolateral dislocation in which the medial edge of the ulna rests on the trochlea such that a lateral radiograph gives one the impression of the coronoid being perched under the trochlea (see Fig. 24-12, 2). This can readily be reduced with minimal force or by the patient manipulating the elbow himself or herself. In stage 3, the coronoid and radial head are fully posterior to the trochlea and capitellum, respectively. Depending on the severity of tissue disruption in stage 3 (a, b, or c), the elbow will be (a) stable in valgus, (b) unstable in valgus, or (c) grossly unstable except when flexed more than 90 degrees after reduction.

Thus, dislocation is the final of three sequential stages of elbow instability resulting from posterolateral ulnohumeral rotatory subluxation, with soft tissue disruption progressing from lateral to medial. In each stage, the pathoanatomy

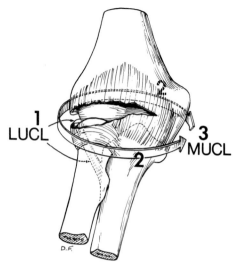

FIGURE 24-11. The "Horii circle" soft tissue injury progresses in a "circle" from lateral to medial in three stages correlating with those in Figure 24-2A. In stage 1, the ulnar part of the lateral collateral ligament, the lateral ulnar collateral ligament (LUCL), is disrupted. In stage 2 the other lateral ligamentous structures and the anterior and posterior capsule are disrupted. Stage 3, disruption of the medial ulnar collateral ligament (MUCL), can be partial, with disruption of the posterior MUCL only (3A), or complete (3B). The common extensor and flexor origins are often disrupted as well. (From O'Driscoll SW, Morrey BF, Korinek S, An KN: Elbow subluxation and dislocation: A spectrum of instability. Clin Orthop 280:186-197, 1992.)

correlates with the pattern and degree of instability. This was confirmed in a cadaver study, in which 12 of 13 elbows could be dislocated posteriorly with the anterior medial collateral ligament intact.[40]

Josefsson and colleagues[15,19] documented that both the medial and lateral collateral ligaments were disrupted in acutely dislocated elbows explored surgically. However, this is entirely compatible with the proposed mechanism of dislocation, as the final stage is disruption of the anterior medial collateral ligament and then the common flexor pronator origin by any continuation of the axial force or external rotatory moment once the coronoid passes behind the trochlea.

Indeed, the observation that the medial collateral ligament is usually torn in simple dislocations (no fractures) and not in fracture-dislocations corroborates this further. When the elbow dislocates without fracturing the coronoid or radial head, the forearm has a tendency to sudden severe displacement once the coronoid and radial head clear the trochlea and capitellum, respectively. Therefore, displacement can be severe enough to cause extensive soft tissue tearing. On the other hand, when the coronoid and radial head are fractured, significant energy is absorbed in a gradual progression by the fractures, thereby dissipating the force that would otherwise have caused sudden severe displacement after the coronoid passes beneath the trochlea.

These pathoanatomic stages all correlate with the clinical degrees of elbow instability. The roles of the flexor/pronator and common extensor tendon origins are not known, but they are probably important secondary stabilizers of the elbow. Certainly, their fibers blend with and augment those of the collateral ligaments with which they are contiguous. In severely unstable elbows that have not sustained any fractures, both tendon origins are usually disrupted.

This posterolateral rotatory mechanism of dislocation results in less soft tissue damage than would a hyperextension or valgus mechanism. The kinetics are clinically relevant and reproducible. They explain the spectrum of instability, from posterolateral rotatory instability to perched dislocation, to posterior dislocation without or with disruption of the anterior medial collateral ligament, which occurs with further posterior displacement. Such a posterolateral rotatory mechanism for dislocation would be compatible with those suggested by Osborne and Cotterill[42] and by Roberts.[47]

For several reasons other mechanisms such as hyperextension need not be implicated to explain the majority of clinical observations (although other mechanisms probably occur in some cases). A posterolateral rotatory mechanism would be consistent with the observation that some patients experience recurrent dislocations requiring reduction and also have a positive lateral pivot-shift test.[36] Furthermore, such patients with recurrent dislocations are successfully treated by surgical reconstruction of the lateral collateral ligament complex alone, without any surgery on the medial side.[8,10,28,36,42,43,51] Together, these suggest that the essential

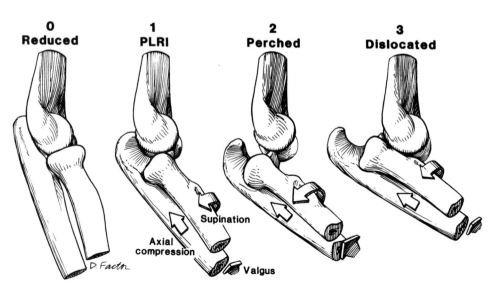

FIGURE 24-12. Elbow instability is a spectrum from subluxation to dislocation. The three stages illustrated here correspond with the pathoanatomic stages of capsuloligamentous disruption in Figure 24-2B. Forces and moments responsible for displacements are illustrated. (From O'Driscoll SW, Morrey BF, Korinek S, An KN: Elbow subluxation and dislocation: A spectrum of instability. Clin Orthop 280:186-197, 1992.)

lesion of such instability is on the lateral side. Finally, it has not been shown that the results of surgical repair of the anterior medial collateral ligament after acute dislocations are superior to those of nonoperative treatment.[15,16]

Spectrum and Patterns of Instability

It is currently recognized that recurrent dislocations of the elbow represent one end of a spectrum of instability that ranges from minimal subluxation to gross dislocation. In most cases, recurrent instability follows a traumatic dislocation as a result of inadequate soft tissue healing and/or bony deficiency involving (typically) the coronoid or radial head. It can result from iatrogenic violation of the lateral collateral ligament complex during surgery for tennis elbow or on the radial head. It can develop as a tardy form of instability, from chronic soft tissue stretching due to connective tissue disorders, or from repetitive overload such as occurs in patients with long-standing cubitus varus deformity from childhood supracondylar malunions. Finally, congenital hypoplasia of the coronoid can also predispose the patient to recurrent instability.

Because of the complex geometry of the elbow, and the high degree of articular congruity of its hinge-like articulation, recurrent instability affecting this joint is usually a coupled three-dimensional abnormal motion pattern that involves not only translation but also varus/valgus and axial rotation of the ulna referable to the humerus. It can present in one of two forms: posterolateral rotatory instability or posteromedial rotatory instability.

Posterolateral Rotatory Instability

This is the most common pattern of elbow instability, particularly that which is recurrent.[28,36] It is discussed in detail in the earlier section on the pathomechanics of elbow instability. It is usually posterolateral rather than direct posterior so that the coronoid can pass inferior to the trochlea. It is three-dimensional displacement of the ulna on the humerus (the radius moving with the ulna) such that the ulna "supinates" (i.e., externally rotates) away from the trochlea (see Figs. 24-1 to 24-4).

Posteromedial Rotatory Instability

Posteromedial rotatory instability has only recently been described in the literature.[31,32] It is a corollary to posterolateral rotatory instability except that there is an obligatory fracture or deficiency of the anteromedial coronoid. This bony component is necessary to permit the coronoid to subluxate beneath the prominent medial trochlea. The mechanism is a varus/posteromedial rotation injury with axial loading. Flexion and abduction torque at the shoulder, while the elbow is flexing under axial load, which causes the elbow to go into varus and forces the medial trochlea to ride up onto the anteromedial coronoid. These forces and displacements disrupt the lateral collateral ligament (usually by avulsion from beneath the common extensor tendon origin), the posterior band of the medial collateral ligament and posteromedial capsule, and the anteromedial coronoid, which is fractured off by a shearing mechanism (Figs. 24-13 and 24-14). The coronoid fracture may be large and comminuted or small and involve only the segment between the tip and sublime tubercle. This condition can masquerade

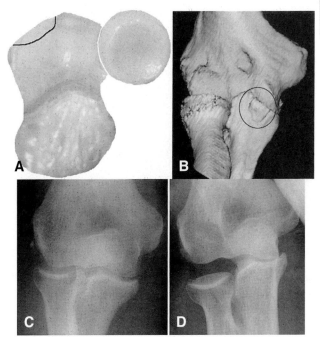

FIGURE 24-13. Anteromedial coronoid fractures occur by a varus posteromedial rotatory displacement pattern, in which the medial trochlea rides up onto the anteromedial coronoid, creating a shear fracture, after the lateral collateral ligament has been disrupted (usually avulsed). **A** and **B,** Location of the anteromedial coronoid fracture fragment shown in a schematic illustration and a three-dimensional CT reconstruction. Fracture fragment is indicated in B by the *small circle.* **C** and **D,** Anteroposterior radiographs with and without a varus/posteromedial rotatory stress applied contrast what initially appears to be almost a normal radiograph revealing significant varus instability and apparent narrowing of the medial ulnohumeral joint. The displacement and mechanism of injury are as described and illustrated in Figure 24-12. (From O'Driscoll SW, et al: Difficult elbow fractures: Pearls and pitfalls. *In* Ferlic DC (ed): Instructional Course Lectures, Volume 52. Rosemont, IL, American Academy of Orthopaedic Surgeons, 2003, pp 113-134. Reproduced with permission from Mayo Foundation.)

as posterolateral rotatory instability because the disrupted lateral collateral ligament permits the elbow to rotate off posterolaterally.

Anteromedial fractures have not been previously addressed in the literature concerning the coronoid. The initial fracture (subtype 1) is located anteromedially, between the tip of the coronoid and the sublime tubercle in an oblique plane, between the coronal and sagittal planes (see Fig. 24-13). Medially, the fracture line usually exits the cortex in the anterior half of the sublime tubercle, that is, in the anterior portion of the anterior bundle of the medial collateral ligament. Laterally, the fracture exits just medial to the tip of the coronoid. Comminution can extend to involve the tip (subtype 2), the sublime tubercle (subtype 3), and the body of the coronoid (see basal fractures below), depending on the energy of the injury.

The significance of this injury is that the elbow has a tendency to articulate incongruently under axial load or gravitational varus stress (Fig. 24-15). On lateral tomograms, the medial trochlea can be seen to articulate with the small coronoid fragment but not the majority of the ulna (see Fig. 24-15B). Instead, there is point loading at the fracture site on the ulna, which causes high stresses on the cartilage of

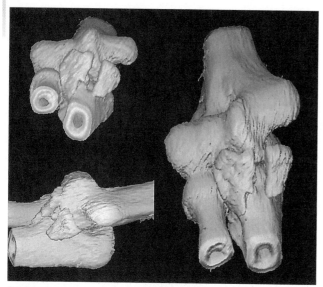

FIGURE 24-14. Mechanism of injury for anteromedial coronoid fractures. In this case an anteromedial subtype 3 coronoid fracture is illustrated, with involvement of not just the anteromedial fragment but the tip and the sublime tubercle as well. Under varus and axial loads, while the elbow is flexing, flexion and abduction torques at the shoulder cause the medial trochlea to ride up onto the anteromedial coronoid, which is fractured off by a shearing mechanism. (Reproduced with permission from Mark Cohen, MD.)

to experience normal gravitational force while being imaged. Closkey and coworkers may have derived a misleading conclusion concerning the effect of coronoid fractures on elbow stability in a recent biomechanical study.[5] They found that a loss of up to 40% of the coronoid did not change the elbow's resistance to direct posterior subluxation. However, they did not evaluate stability with coupled motions in posterolateral or varus-posteromedial rotation. I have verified that simulation of an anteromedial subtype 1 coronoid fracture in a cadaver, in association with lateral collateral ligament detachment, permits varus-posteromedial rotatory instability as seen clinically. Copf and associates found that if the radial head is fractured, even small coronoid tip fractures involving as little as one sixth of the height of the coronoid must be fixed to maintain elbow stability.[7] Several studies have documented the integrity of the coronoid to be the key prognostic factor affecting stability in fracture-dislocations.[11,17,46] The key to considering this diagnosis is to recognize the "isolated" coronoid fracture, that is, a coronoid fracture without a radial head fracture (especially in the absence of apparent dislocation). A deficiency (malunion, nonunion, prior excision) of the anteromedial coronoid may appear benign but predisposes the elbow to persistent and recurrent instability, which can lead to post-traumatic arthritis. Thus, these deficiencies need to be reconstructed (Fig. 24-17).

the medial trochlea. This pattern of fracture-subluxation is somewhat analogous to that of a Bennett fracture-dislocation of the thumb. Joint incongruity such as this naturally can (and does appear to) lead to rapid-onset arthritis within a few years or less (Fig. 24-16). Confirming the incongruity may require lateral tomograms or CT reconstruction. To demonstrate this incongruity, the elbow should be permitted

Author's Preferred Method of Treatment

Surgical reconstruction of the lateral collateral ligament complex is performed by imbricating the ligament and posterolateral capsule and reconstructing the ulnar part of

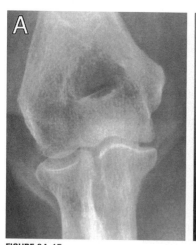 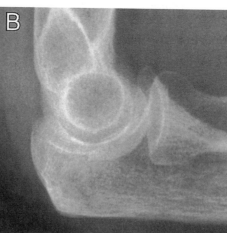 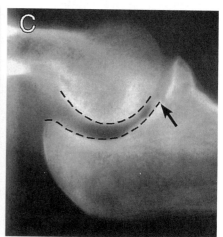

FIGURE 24-15. **A** and **B,** Anteroposterior and lateral radiographs of an anteromedial subtype 2 coronoid fracture, showing what appears to be no significant displacement and anatomic joint alignment. **C,** Lateral trispiral tomogram (taken with slight gravitational varus stress on the elbow) through the medial portion of the ulnohumeral articulation shows an anteromedial subtype 2 fracture (involving the anteromedial coronoid and the tip) with joint incongruity due to varus posteromedial rotatory subluxation. In this case, the medial trochlea has displaced anteriorly and distally along with the anteromedial coronoid fragment, which it displaced and with which it remains congruent. This results in point contact between the medial trochlea and the coronoid at the fracture site *(arrow),* which over the course of a few months leads to medial trochlear erosion. The incongruity is indicated by the ulnohumeral joint being widened posteriorly and converging anteriorly *(indicated by converging dotted lines).* (From O'Driscoll SW, et al: Difficult elbow fractures: Pearls and pitfalls. *In* Ferlic DC (ed): Instructional Course Lectures, Volume 52. Rosemont, IL, American Academy of Orthopaedic Surgeons, 2003, pp 113-134. Reproduced with permission from Mayo Foundation.)

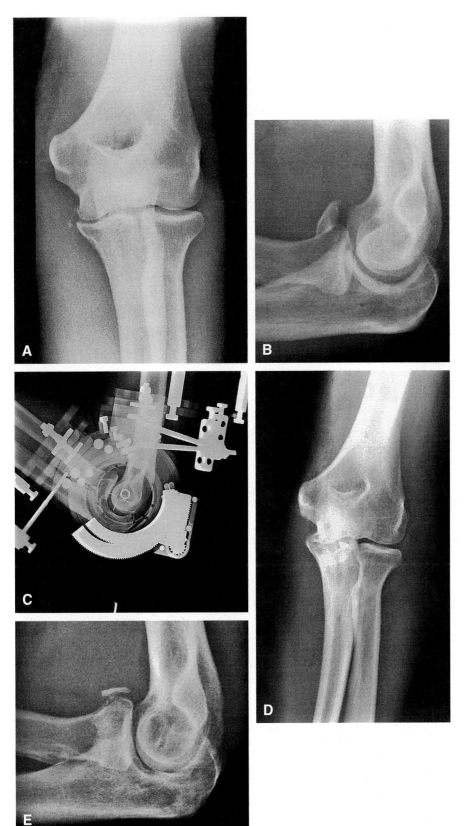

FIGURE 24-16. **A** and **B,** Preoperative antero-posterior and lateral radiographs of an antero-medial subtype 2 coronoid fracture involving the tip and the anteromedial segment over to, but not including, the sublime tubercle. **C,** Postoperative radiograph in a hinged external fixator, after arthroscopic reduction and suture fixation of the fragments, revealing concentric joint alignment and slightly non-anatomic reduction of the fragments. **D** and **E,** Anteroposterior and lateral radiographs taken 1 year after operation showing medial ulno-humeral collapse and early arthritis. (From O'Driscoll SW, et al: Difficult elbow fractures: Pearls and pitfalls. *In* Ferlic DC (ed): Instructional Course Lectures, Volume 52. Rosemont, IL, American Academy of Orthopaedic Surgeons, 2003, pp 113-134. Reproduced with permission from Mayo Foundation.)

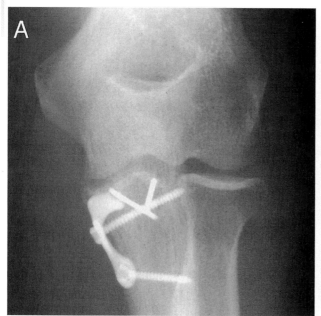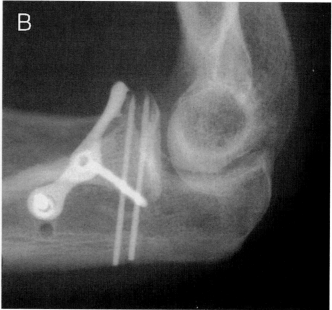

FIGURE 24-17. Anteroposterior and lateral radiographs of an anteromedial coronoid fracture fixed with a congruent plate and two fine, threaded Kirschner wires. (From O'Driscoll SW, et al: Difficult elbow fractures: Pearls and pitfalls. *In* Ferlic DC (ed): Instructional Course Lectures, Volume 52. Rosemont, IL, American Academy of Orthopaedic Surgeons, 2003, pp 113-134. Reproduced with permission from Mayo Foundation.)

the lateral collateral ligament using a plantaris tendon allograft (see Fig. 24-20). The reconstructive technique that is currently employed involves isometric placement of the origin on the lateral epicondyle and fixation to bone at either end.

In cases of recurrent instability involving bony deficiencies, it is my philosophy to reconstruct or replace all constraints. Nonunions involving only the coronoid tip are reduced and fixed with transosseous sutures in combination with threaded Kirschner wires.[30] The sutures are passed over the coronoid fragment, through the attached capsule, and back down through two separate holes in the ulna just proximal to the distal edge of the fracture and tied tightly. If the coronoid tip had previously been excised, the capsule is reattached as described. Nonunions of the anteromedial coronoid are treated by anatomic reduction and by rigid fixation with a precontoured coronoid buttress plate that has prongs to grasp the small coronoid fragment.

Partial radial head deficiencies are reconstructed with a metal radial head prosthesis. I have satisfactory short-term (limited) experience reconstructing these lesions with partial radial head allografts, but long-term follow-up is not yet available.

Technique of Posterolateral Ligament Reconstruction

With the patient supine, the affected limb is prepped and draped from the tourniquet on the upper arm distally to include the hand. If no palmaris longus is present, the leg is prepped and draped to permit access to the knee region for obtaining the semitendinosus tendon. An allograft semitendinosus tendon is kept available. The elbow is operated on with the arm across the patient's chest.

The reconstruction technique, illustrated in Figures 24-18 to 24-20, is intended to re-create the ulnar part of the lateral

collateral ligament complex (Fig. 24-18). Through a 10-cm Kocher-type skin incision the deep fascia is incised along the supracondylar ridge and distally between the anconeus and extensor carpi ulnaris muscles (see Fig. 24-5). The supracondylar ridge is exposed proximally by reflecting the triceps partially off the posterior humerus and the extensor carpi radialis longus partially off the anterior distal humerus. The anconeus is reflected off the lateral side of the ulna and capsule. The common extensor origin is partially reflected to expose the capsule. Attenuation of both the capsule and ligamentous complex should be assessed and laxity confirmed. This is usually proximal to the annular ligament, and the capsular laxity is best appreciated by rotating the ulna externally.

The capsule and common extensor tendon are incised longitudinally, just anterior to the posterior border of the tendon. With a 3-mm bur, the insertion site for the tendon graft is then prepared by creating two holes in the ulna, one near the tubercle on the supinator crest (which is felt by stressing the elbow in varus or supination) and the other 1.25 cm proximally at the base of the annular ligament (Fig. 24-19). A trough joining these two holes is created with a curved awl from the Bankart set of shoulder instruments. A suture is passed through these two holes and tied to it. It is then pulled toward a point just anterior to the lateral epicondyle and grasped with a hemostat at the estimated isometric center of rotation of the elbow. The isometric ligament origin is then determined by flexing and extending the elbow to see if the suture moves. No movement occurs if the suture and hemostat are on the isometric point. This point is usually more anterior than might be thought. The *entry site* for the graft, hole number 3, is then burred into the humerus at that point. Because the hole is bigger than the tip of the hemostat, one should make the hole posterior and proximal to the hemostat point. If it is

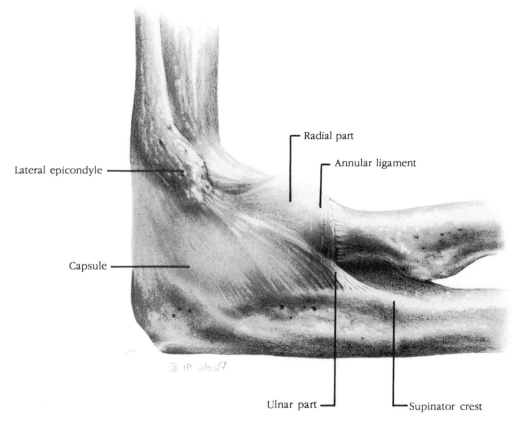

Lateral epicondyle ———

Capsule ———

Radial part
Annular ligament

Ulnar part ———
——— Supinator crest

FIGURE 24-18. Illustration of the lateral collateral ligament complex shows that it is a complex of fibers consisting of the radial part, the ulnar part, and the annular ligament, all of which blend together. Casual observation does not allow appreciation of the components of this complex. The ulnar part is indistinct at its origin on the lateral epicondyle. In fact, the common extensor origin also blends with this but has been excised for the purpose of this illustration. It arches over the annular ligament with which it is closely integrated. It is most distinct along its anterior border as it inserts on the tubercle of the supinator crest. There is an additional fan-shaped insertion posterior to this, along the base of the annular ligament and just proximal to it. This gradually thins out until only the capsule remains.

placed distal or anterior, the tendon graft will be lax in extension and tight in flexion or vice versa. A hole is made on either side of the supracondylar ridge about 1.5 cm proximally and tunnels created with the curved and straight awls between the two holes as well as between each hole and at the isometric origin on the lateral condyle (see Fig. 24-19).

A 15-cm tendon graft is prepared by weaving a running locking Krackow stitch with a 2-0 Ethibond suture through each end. Initially I harvested a palmaris graft, but my current preference is for a plantaris allograft. Other options include a split semitendinosus autograft or allograft or a strip of lateral triceps tendon. The graft is then brought through the first two holes in the ulna, holes 1 and 2 (see Fig. 24-19). It is essential that the capsule be closed under the graft so that it does not rub against the capitellum or radial head. My preferred method for achieving this is to make a small hole in the posterior capsular flap, near the epicondyle, through which both limbs of the graft are passed before entering the humeral tunnels. The more anterior limb of the graft is then passed into the *entry site*, hole number 3, in the lateral epicondyle and out through hole number 4 posteriorly. The more

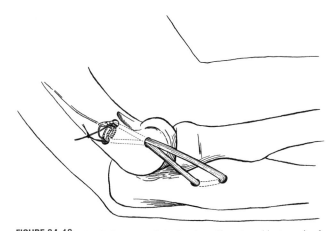

FIGURE 24-19. Two holes are made in the ulna adjacent, and just proximal, to the tubercle on the supinator crest. A 15-cm tendon graft is then passed through the bone tunnels and brought into the humerus at the isometric center of rotation of the elbow to exit through bone tunnels on either side of the supracondylar ridge. The graft is tensioned with the elbow in 40 degrees of flexion and full pronation and then tied around the supracondylar ridge.

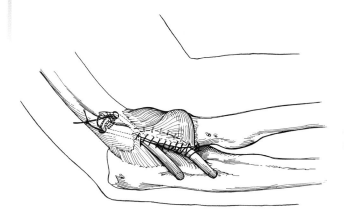

FIGURE 24-20. The capsule is closed and plicated (actually before tensioning the graft), and the original arch of the ulnar part of the lateral collateral ligament is restored by pulling the graft anteriorly and suturing it to the capsule. This also prevents the graft from slipping posterior to the radial head. The capsule must be closed *under* the graft to prevent it from rubbing on the radial head or capitellum.

posterior limb of the graft is passed into the same *entry site*, hole number 3 in the lateral epicondyle, and out through hole number 5 anteriorly (see Fig. 24-19). Both limbs of the graft are then wrapped over the supracondylar ridge and pulled back into the trough joining holes 4 and 5, and the sutures are tied. The tendons are also tied to each other where they overlap on the supracondylar ridge. Before tying the sutures, the graft is tensioned with the elbow in 40 degrees of flexion and full pronation. The reconstruction is augmented by passing a heavy double-stranded No. 1 PDS absorbable suture through the same course as the tendon graft. This suture is woven through the capsule in an arch, which serves two purposes. First, this provides dynamic protection to the reconstruction, because tension on the suture causes it to straighten out before it ruptures. Second, it prevents the suture from slipping deep to the capsule where it can rub on the capitellum or radial head. Before tightening the tendon graft, the capsule is closed and plicated. The capsule must be closed *under* the graft to prevent it from rubbing on the radial head or capitellum. The original arch of the ulnar part of the lateral collateral ligament is restored by pulling the graft anteriorly and suturing it to the capsule (Fig. 24-20). This also prevents the graft from slipping posterior to the radial head. If further tension is desirable, this can be accomplished by closing the distal triangular opening between the two limbs of the graft. During closure, the forearm is held pronated to protect the repair and the arm is no longer held across the chest in a position that is conducive to varus stress.

In children with open epiphyseal plates, the graft would cross the physis so I do not do this operation. Instead, the lateral collateral ligament is elevated from its origin, tightened, and resutured to the isometric point on the lateral epicondyle with heavy sutures that pass through bone but not the physis. The method is similar to that described by Osborne and Cotterill.[42]

Bony Reconstruction of the Coronoid

Congenital or post-traumatic deficiencies of the coronoid may require bony reconstruction in addition to the lateral collateral ligament. This is especially true for recurrent posteromedial rotatory instability. Unfortunately, at this time, our understanding of how to best perform such reconstructions is limited. At my institution, I have utilized a number of approaches, including structural autografts from the tip of the olecranon, from a radial head that had previously been partially resected (and needed to be completely removed and replaced), and bicortical or tricortical iliac crest grafts. I have also employed osteochondral allografts of either coronoid or radial head. Unfortunately, results have been disappointing and unpredictable with each of these methods. In particular, graft resorption has been a problem. Further advances are needed in this area.

POSTOPERATIVE MANAGEMENT AND EXPECTATIONS

There are no rigid protocols that can be applied to postoperative protection of the ligament reconstruction and maintaining motion. Our understanding of the optimal management is still evolving. Traditionally, the elbow has been immobilized in a cast for 3 weeks and then protected in a hinged brace for a further 9 weeks. While contractures are not common, they can occur. Alternative recommendations have included the use of a removable (bivalved) long-arm cast for 6 weeks, permitting the patient to remove the cast for gentle exercises to preserve motion. I have also tried commencing motion in a hinged brace within the first week after surgery but have had some cases of early stretching of the repair, as evidenced by laxity of the elbow at 2 to 4 months postoperatively. My current approach is to immobilize the elbow for 3 weeks in a long-arm cast with the forearm in pronation and then commence active motion in an adjustable locking hinge brace (Aircast, New Jersey) with the forearm still in pronation. The patient comes out of the brace for forearm rotation exercises, which are performed actively in the overhead position. Pronation protects the lateral collateral ligament from gravitational varus stress, as does keeping the elbow in the overhead position. The latter also permits the triceps to function as an elbow stabilizer.

In some patients with severe instability or generalized laxity, or in revision cases, one is concerned about a higher risk of failure. In such patients, as well as in children and in those patients who have previously been in cast immobilization of the elbow for 6 weeks without developing contractures, immobilization is continued for 6 weeks. Alternatively, an extension block is used with the hinged brace.

CRITICAL POINTS: LATERAL COLLATERAL LIGAMENT RECONSTRUCTION

INDICATION

- Posterolateral rotatory instability

PREOPERATIVE EVALUATION

- Lateral pivot-shift apprehension test (posterolateral rotatory apprehension test)
- Lateral pivot-shift test
- Posterolateral rotatory drawer test
- Push-up test
- Examination under anesthesia: lateral pivot-shift test and posterolateral rotatory drawer test
- Lateral stress radiograph

PEARLS AND PITFALLS

- Lateral pivot-shift test is difficult to perform in awake patient (more reliable if examined under anesthesia).
- Posterolateral rotatory drawer test is easiest to demonstrate the instability.
- Posterolateral rotatory apprehension test is most sensitive.
- Posterolateral rotatory instability is difficult to diagnose if the radial head is absent.
- False-negative test results may occur if the medial collateral ligament is deficient.
- Posterolateral rotatory instability may be misdiagnosed as valgus instability at the time of lateral arthrotomy for treatment of radial head fracture.
- If the degree of instability is severe, apprehension may not be present.
- The most important technical part of the procedure is to correctly establish the isometric origin on the humeral condyle. It is more anterior than is obvious.
- The most important postoperative concern is to avoid the varus gravitational stresses that are

applied to the elbow when the forearm is in a plane other than the sagittal plane.

TECHNICAL POINTS

- Two holes are made in the ulna adjacent and just proximal to the tubercle on the supinator crest.
- A suture is passed through the two holes and tied to it. The isometric ligament origin is determined by flexing and extending the elbow while holding the suture against the humerus to identify the point of epicondylar attachment in which the suture does not move.
- Two bone tunnels are then made in the humerus at the common isometric origin.
- The capsule is closed and plicated so that the graft is extra-articular.
- The tendon graft (palmaris longus) is placed through the bone tunnels and tightened with the elbow in 40 degrees of flexion and full pronation.
- The original arch of the ulnar part of the lateral collateral ligament is restored by pulling the graft anteriorly and suturing it to the capsule.
- The reconstruction is augmented with a double-stranded No. 1 PDS suture through the same bone tunnels.

POSTOPERATIVE CARE

- Protect the reconstruction in a pronated position in a cast for 10 to 21 days and then with a hinged brace for 6 weeks.
- Avoid gravitational varus stress.
- Consider using a brace for an additional 6 weeks.
- Perform active range-of-motion exercises with the arm in the overhead position keeping the humerus vertical because triceps contraction stabilizes the elbow.

ANNOTATED REFERENCES

5. Closkey RF, Goode JR, Kirschenbaum D, Cody RP: The role of the coronoid process in elbow stability: A biomechanical analysis of axial loading. J Bone Joint Surg Am 82:1749-1753, 2000.

   The authors found that a loss of up to 40% of the coronoid did not change the elbow's resistance to direct posterior subluxation. However, they did not evaluate stability with coupled motions in posterolateral or varus-posteromedial rotation. Isolated coronoid fractures involving this much of the coronoid are usually anteromedial fracture-subluxations, which are potentially serious injuries. An "isolated" coronoid fracture, that is, a coronoid fracture without a radial head fracture or apparent dislocation, is highly likely to be an anteromedial fracture-subluxation with lateral collateral ligament injury and the potential for joint incongruity.

6. Cohen M, Hastings H: Rotatory instability of the elbow. J Bone Joint Surg Am 79:225-233, 1997.

   Pure rotational laxity was evaluated in cadaver elbows before and after sequential release of the lateral soft tissues. The common extensor tendon and the lateral collateral ligament complex (including the annular ligament) were interdependent in stabilizing the elbow. True posterolateral rotatory instability, a three-dimensional displacement, was not studied in the model.

7. Copf F, Holz U, Schauwecker HH: [Biomechanical problems in elbow joint dislocations with coronoid and capitulum radii fractures (author's transl)]. Langenbecks Arch Chir 350:249-254, 1980.

If the radial head is fractured, even small coronoid tip fractures involving as little as one sixth of the height of the coronoid must be fixed to maintain elbow stability.

11. Heim U: [Combined fractures of the radius and the ulna at the elbow level in the adult. Analysis of 120 cases after more than 1 year]. Rev Chir Orthop Reparatrice Appar Mot 84:142-153, 1998.

Of 120 fracture-dislocations of the elbow, the coronoid was identified as the key component. Good results were rare and arthritis common after trans-olecranon fractures involving both the radial head and the coronoid.

13. Hotchkiss RN, Weiland AJ: Valgus stability of the elbow. J Orthop Res 5:372-377, 1987.

This is a detailed biomechanical study of the constraints to valgus instability in cadaver elbows. It shows that the anterior band of the medial collateral ligament is the primary constraint to valgus instability. The posterior portion is relatively insignificant. The radial head was found to contribute 30% of valgus stability, but this is probably artificially high because the radius and ulna were fixed with respect to each other. A subsequent study by Morrey and coworkers[27]did not confirm this. Replacement of the excised radial head with a Silastic prosthesis did not significantly improve biomechanical stability.

15. Josefsson P, Gentz C, Johnell O, Wendeberg B: Surgical versus non-surgical treatment of ligamentous injuries following dislocation of the elbow joint: A prospective randomized study. J Bone Joint Surg Am 69A:605-608, 1987.

In all cases treated surgically both ligaments were found to be disrupted. The results of the treatment were similar whether they were operated on or treated nonoperatively. However, considering the long-term data of Eygendaal and colleagues (J Bone Joint Surg Am 82:555-560, 2000), instability may be more common, and more serious, than suggested by this article. Also, this study took place before the authors were aware of the most common form of recurrent instability of the elbow or how to diagnose it—posterolateral rotatory instability. Current experience would indicate that virtually all elbow dislocations have posterolateral rotatory instability. Muscle tone is correctly described as an important dynamic stabilizer of the elbow.

17. Josefsson PO, Gentz CF, Johnell O, Wendeberg B: Dislocations of the elbow and intraarticular fractures. Clin Orthop (Sep):126-130, 1989.

Of 19 patients with an elbow dislocation associated with a fracture of the radial head that was treated by radial head excision, 4 had redislocations. All four redislocations were associated with a displaced fracture of the coronoid process.

18. Josefsson PO, Johnell O, Gentz CF: Long-term sequelae of simple dislocation of the elbow. J Bone Joint Surg Am 66: 927-930, 1984.

This is a very long-term follow-up of 52 children and adults with dislocation of the elbow. One third of patients had slight or moderate flexion contractures. Instability was seen in about 15%. However, the study took place before the authors were aware of the most common form of recurrent instability of the elbow or how to diagnose it—posterolateral rotatory instability. This was the most common complication other than ectopic ossification, which was not described to be related to the loss of extension. It was primarily in the collateral ligaments.

21. Melhoff TL, Noble PC, Bennett JB, Tullos HS: Simple dislocation of the elbow in the adult. J Bone Joint Surg Am 70: 244-249, 1988.

This landmark long-term study of 52 elbow dislocations revealed significant concerns. Fifteen percent had significant flexion contractures of 30 degrees or more. Stiffness was proportional to the duration of immobilization. Thirty-five percent had symptoms of instability. This could be interpreted to be due to posterolateral rotatory instability, which had not been described at the time of review of these patients. The results were poor or fair with 4 weeks or more of immobilization. Ectopic ossification was seen in half of the patients but not related to contracture development.

22. Mondoloni P, Vandenbussche E, Peraldi P, Augereau B: [Instability of the elbow after supracondylar humeral non-union in cubitus varus rotation.] Rev Chir Orthop Repartrice Appar Mot 82:757-761, 1996.

The authors describe two patients with recurrent elbow instability resulting from chronic cubitus varus malunions from supracondylar fractures in childhood.

23. Morrey B: Reoperation for failed surgical treatment of refractory lateral epicondylitis. J Shoulder Elbow Surg 1:47-55, 1992.

Tennis elbow is a condition that remains a "thorn in the side" of physicians and surgeons in many ways. Failure of surgical treatment sometimes results in despair. This paper provides a logical and constructive approach to the failed tennis elbow surgery patient. If symptoms remained the same postoperatively, the cause was usually inadequate release or incorrect diagnosis. If the symptoms were different, the cause was usually ligamentous laxity. The real value of this paper is probably in the generic approach to failed surgery for any operation, and we would be well served by carefully studying the philosophy of this approach.

26. Morrey BF, An K-N, Stormont TJ: Force transmission through the radial head. J Bone Joint Surg Am 70:250-256, 1988.

The force across the radiohumeral joint is maximal with the elbow extended and the forearm pronated. This corresponds to the position of loading of the radial head with radial head fractures.

27. Morrey BF, An K-N, Tanaka S: Valgus stability of the elbow: A definition of primary and secondary constraints. Clin Orthop 265:187-195, 1991.

Using sophisticated aerospace technology to map the position and orientation of a body in three-dimensional space using a highly accurate electromagnetic tracking system, the authors' demonstrated with sequential cutting and resection that the anterior band of the medial collateral ligament is the primary constraint to valgus instability and the radial head is a secondary constraint. Minimal instability occurs throughout the arc of motion after radial head excision if the medial collateral ligament is intact. From the data in this paper the indication for radial head replacement is valgus instability due to combined medial collateral ligament laxity and absence of the radial head due to excision. Of course, it is possible that adequate medial collateral ligament repair might obviate the need for radial head replacement.

35. O'Driscoll SW: Elbow instability. Hand Clin 10:405-415, 1994.

An important feature to recognize is that the small (type I) flake fractures of the coronoid are not "avulsion" fractures but shear fractures caused by impaction of the coronoid against the trochlea as the ulna dislocates under the humerus.

36. O'Driscoll SW, Bell DF, Morrey BF: Posterolateral rotatory instability of the elbow. J Bone Joint Surg Am 73:440-446, 1991.

Posterolateral rotatory instability of the elbow is a condition that has not previously been described. The clinical and radiographic characteristics of this condition are described in detail, and this report is the first of a series that describe the anatomy, pathology, kinematics, surgical technique, and results of surgery for this condition. Elbow instability is a spectrum from recurrent subluxation to dislocation, with this posterolateral rotatory pattern of instability being the common denominator.

37. O'Driscoll SW, Horii E, Morrey BF, Carmichael SW: Anatomy of the ulnar part of the lateral collateral ligament of the elbow. Clin Anat 5:296-303, 1992.

   This anatomic study advances and corrects our misunderstanding about the anatomy of the lateral collateral ligament. There is indeed a "true ligament" on the lateral side, the ulnar part of the lateral collateral ligament, which originates isometrically on the lateral epicondyle and inserts on the ulna at the tubercle of the supinator crest just distal to the annular ligament over which it passes. This lateral ulnar collateral ligament is the primary constraint to posterolateral rotatory instability and is analogous to the anterior band of the medial collateral ligament. It has been overlooked in previous studies and surgery because it lies deep to the fascia of the supinator.

40. O'Driscoll SW, Morrey BF, Korinek S, An K-N: Elbow subluxation and dislocation: A spectrum of instability. Clin Orthop 280:186-197, 1992.

   Elbow subluxation and dislocation are part of a spectrum of instability with a common mechanism of posterolateral rotatory displacement. This occurs by a combination of axial load, valgus, and supination moments as the elbow flexes. The "Horii circle" describes the pattern of soft tissue disruption that starts on the lateral side and progresses anteriorly and posteriorly to the medial side in three stages. At each stage of instability, the anatomic, clinical (symptoms and signs), and radiographic features correlate and dictate treatment principles. This applies to acute, recurrent, and chronic instability.

42. Osborne G, Cotterill P: Recurrent dislocation of the elbow. J Bone Joint Surg Br 48:340-346, 1965.

   This classic article describes the presentation, pathology, and treatment of recurrent dislocation of the elbow, documenting that the lateral collateral ligament complex is the location of the pathoanatomy.

46. Ring D, Jupiter JB, Sanders RW, et al: Trans-olecranon fracture-dislocation of the elbow. J Orthop Trauma 11:545-550, 1997.

   Eight patients with trans-olecranon fractures also had large coronoid fragments that were fixed. Comminution of the trochlear notch did not preclude a good result provided that stable, anatomic fixation of large coronoid fragment was achieved.

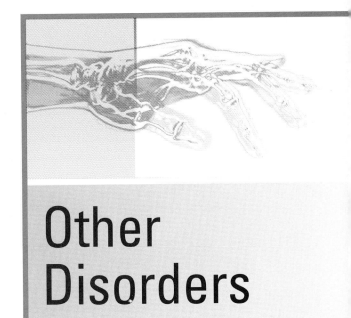

Other Disorders

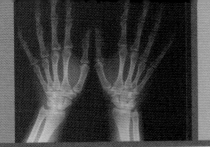

CHAPTER 25

Treatment of the Stiff Elbow

Robert N. Hotchkiss

Although this text carries the title *Operative Hand Surgery* and was originally conceived as a compilation of surgery of the hand, attention to the problem of the stiff elbow is warranted for three reasons. First, loss of motion of the elbow directly restricts the ability to place the hand in space to and from the body, thereby disabling the function of the entire upper limb. Second, surgeons skilled in operations on the hand are increasingly called on to evaluate and treat stiff elbows after trauma, arthritis, and other conditions. Surgical release of a contracted elbow often requires meticulous dissection of neurovascular structures at the elbow, an area of anatomy that usually falls most comfortably under the purview of the hand surgeon. Finally, in the past 10 years, more dependable methods and techniques that make contracture release more reliable and clinically possible have developed.

HISTORY OF TREATMENT OF THE STIFF ELBOW

For many years, the published literature, including textbooks on orthopedics, reflected a general reluctance to treat the stiff elbow surgically. As is the case with most advances in care, the condition was seldom discussed in textbooks, although Wilson[64] was one of the few who wrote about the subject in the 1940s.

Many other authors have written about treatment of the stiff elbow. Because of the constraints of the published literature, these submissions either reflected a single surgical approach,[15] considered treatment of a single etiology,[54] or mixed patients with some requiring interposition arthroplasty.[41] The weakness of this kind of reporting is that the covariables of age, cause of contracture, associated injuries, and location of pathology cannot be easily stratified and the data or methods compared. Even the terms used—*contracture,* stiff elbow,† post-traumatic*, and *arthrolysis* are not applied with enough precision for comparative purposes. Nonetheless, each of these reports has merit, some more than others.

The results reported in the most recent journals reflect a consensus that open capsulectomy, carefully performed

on the willing patient, using both a medial and/or lateral approach to the elbow joint, results in a consistent and notable improvement of motion with small risk of serious complication.[20,26,36,44,61,63] For further reading I recommend the well-written summaries of King,[28] Modabber and Jupiter,[39] and Sojbjerg.[57]

WHO IS TO BLAME FOR THE STIFF AND CONTRACTED ELBOW?

Even with attentive, supervised therapy many patients will not regain their optimal motion after injury. Nonetheless, it is still important to institute active motion with gentle passive assistance as soon as is practical after injury. Unfortunately, it is still common to see active motion started 6 weeks after injury or surgery, which is often too late. Our understanding of what creates a stiff joint is very crude and primitive. We do know that an intra-articular effusion causes the joint to assume a position of flexion to maximize capacity and minimize pressure.[5] This fact may explain the position of flexion assumed for comfort immediately after injury. Once in that position, we have observed that the flexors and extensors tend to co-contract, perhaps to minimize pain, leading to more permanent stiffness. More research is needed to understand this muscular activity after trauma and other conditions.[1,50] In an uninjured joint, the elbow has adequate clearance for full extension and flexion and the capsule is thin and usually transparent. After trauma, the capsule thickens and limits both flexion and extension as both a "block" and a "tether."

After injury, our tools for minimizing the contracture are generally limited to physical therapy and splinting. Manipulation has been reported as useful but should be approached with caution after fracture or in the presence of internal fixation. Undoubtedly, as we begin to understand more about protective or overactive muscle reflexes and pain, as well as the molecular biology of scar formation, we will have better tools to minimize pathologic contractures.

It is helpful to remember a few guidelines when discussing a stiff elbow with a patient and the family, especially after trauma:

1. Unless evidence of gross malpractice exists, the contracture is seldom caused by the method of internal

---

*See references 3, 7, 15, 17, 18, 23-25, 38, 41, 44, 51, 55, 62, and 64-66.
†See references 4, 8, 20, 26, 28, 29, 36, 42, 57, and 61.

fixation or technical performance of the previous surgeon.

2. The therapist has usually not *failed* but rather *not helped to improve* the patient's motion. Many therapists have minimal experience with post-traumatic elbows and are appropriately timid. However, blaming them for using a dynamic splint with little success for 9 months (which is not uncommon) serves no purpose. The therapist is often caught between the frustration of the patient and the hidden worry of the surgeon, both of whom see the failure to regain motion as a defeat.

3. The patient is also usually not at fault. In search of the reasons for failure, it is not uncommon for patients to state that both the surgeon and the therapist say, "I didn't work hard enough. . . ." We all have patients who respond to treatment quite differently. A traumatized elbow demonstrates a wide range of response. It is helpful to listen carefully to the patient and family. Most will tell of weeks and months of visits to the therapist, painful dynamic splints, and, finally, frustration. Any patient on whom you are considering operative treatment must be brought onto the team and made to feel an integral part of the solution.

In summary, there is usually little value in spending time laying blame for a stiff or contracted elbow. More productive use of time can be spent discussing your evaluation and plans to improve the situation and your rationale of treatment.

FEATURES OF THE STIFF ELBOW

Operative treatment of a stiff elbow begins with an understanding of the cause of each patient's contracture and the patient's functional requirements, both vocationally and avocationally. Other factors such as age of the patient and time from injury must be considered, and these are covered in more detail later.

These factors, taken together, determine not only the indications for surgery but also which surgical approach and postoperative treatment are likely to produce a successful result. The following checklist is intended to help guide patient selection, the operative approach, and postoperative rehabilitation, but as with any set of guidelines, the judgment of the treating surgeon and therapist must be used on an ongoing basis and "course corrections" made as the case dictates. The need for mid-course corrections in the operating room and during the postoperative period is a constant and fundamental feature of operative treatment of a stiff elbow. To make these adjustments, the surgeon and therapist must have all of the resources of assessment and treatment available to them.

PREOPERATIVE EVALUATION AND CONSIDERATIONS

Taking the History

Age of the Patient

Decreased motion of the elbow can be present at any age. However, *loss* of motion from injury is the most common complaint. By the time adulthood is reached, patients with congenital deformity and associated limited motion have usually adapted and adjusted their environment. Shoulder and neck movements have generally accommodated, and the need for operative intervention is minimized. This is fortunate inasmuch as the likelihood of increasing motion is often limited because of severely distorted architecture of the joint.

For patients who had a normal elbow before injury, the loss of motion is often quite noticeable, both cosmetically and functionally. Their hope is restoration of full, normal mobility, although this is seldom possible.

The age group with the highest success in my practice is from 18 to 50 years old. These are generally people with high motivation, capable of understanding their disability, and seeking to change it. Lower rates of success are generally achieved with the elderly and, surprisingly, the pediatric population.[36,58] This is not to say that these patients should be eliminated from consideration or represent a contraindication. I have many examples of patients 8 to 15 years old with intra-articular malunions that, once corrected, regained noticeable, even remarkable function. However, a child with post-traumatic stiffness and joint injury with cartilage damage is very challenging and should be approached with great caution.

Surgical treatment should be carefully considered in adolescents, especially those who are in a rebellious phase or lack maturity for cooperation.[2] Occasionally, parents will bring an unwilling and uncooperative teenager for consideration of operative contracture release. This group of patients will generally not participate in the postoperative therapy program and fail to regain motion. Some may even worsen after operative treatment.

Elderly patients with a stiff elbow may have significant associated swelling of the hand and shoulder stiffness, both of which limit the possibility of success and the impact of gained mobility of the elbow. In addition, the quality of the joint may be so poor that the only reasonable option is total elbow replacement. In these cases, the long-standing dysfunction, usually caused by protracted immobilization of the entire limb, makes for prolonged and often incomplete restoration of function.

Duration of Contracture and Timing of Operative Release

There has been much speculation about the timing of contracture release, especially the excision of heterotopic ossification (HO) (Fig. 25-1). Although the use of technetium bone scans was touted in the past to predict the "activity" and therefore the probability of recurrence of HO, this test should be discarded as irrelevant because the scan sometimes remains "hot" for many years.

The optimal timing of intervention depends on the source of the contracture. If the loss of motion is due to a fracture that has fallen apart because of failed internal fixation or a persistently dislocated elbow, waiting serves no purpose.[34] These patients should have the joint surfaces and congruity restored as soon as practical in the hope of preserving some function. These cases are the most difficult and require both contracture release and restoration of the architecture, followed by immediate motion. Often hinged external fixation is required (see Chapter 23).

For patients who have normal or nearly normal articulation, the timing of intervention should be based on documented failure of physical therapy and progressive splinting to improve motion. Although there is increased interest in earlier operative intervention, it is important to be certain that all nonoperative methods have been exhausted. In general, most patients do not improve after 4 to 6 months past injury (except those with pediatric supracondylar fractures). At the 6-month mark, unless there is significant brain injury, the HO has usually matured and can safely be removed without fear of recurrence (see Fig. 25-1). Some have reported that contracture release after more than 1 year after injury has been associated with a lesser gain in motion.[20] For patients who have had a significant loss of motion for more than 10 years, regaining substantial motion may be impossible without humeral shortening and ulnohumeral arthroplasty because of median nerve and brachial artery length.

Pain and the Stiff Elbow

Most uncomplicated post-traumatic contractures are not very painful. There may be some discomfort at end range, but the zone of limited motion is generally comfortable. If not, one should suspect post-traumatic arthrosis or joint incongruity. Patients who have had excessively forceful manipulations or passive mobilization in a misguided attempt to restore motion at a late date may have reactive pain and swelling. However, as scar maturation and tissue equilibrium occur, this inflammatory response usually abates.

Another source of pain may be ulnar nerve entrapment.[11] Patients with a sensitive or trapped ulnar nerve after trauma may not exhibit the usual symptoms and signs of cubital tunnel syndrome. Instead of a definitive loss of sensibility in the distribution of the ulnar nerve, the patients may only exhibit resistance and reluctance to flexion in the first 2 months and tenderness along the medial elbow. As the con-

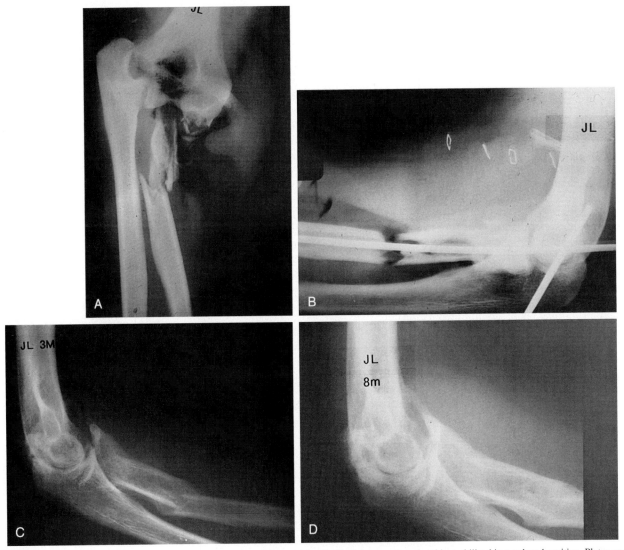

FIGURE 25-1. **A,** Severe open injury caused by a motor boat propeller in a lake. **B,** The joint was pinned and immobilized in a reduced position. Plates were not used for fear of infection and soft tissue stripping. **C,** Three months after the injury, wispy immature heterotopic ossification can be seen forming along the anterior surface of the joint. **D,** At 8 months, both sides of the joint are enveloped by bone. The patient has no motion in the elbow.   *Continued*

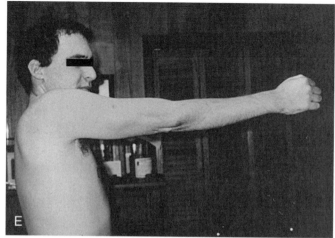

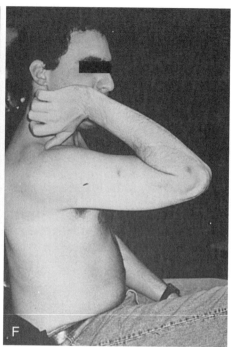

FIGURE 25-1—cont'd. **E** and **F,** Two years after open release and hinged external fixation with a Compass hinge, the patient has nearly full extension and flexion without pain or deterioration of the joint. This excellent result was possible because the initial treating surgeon kept the joint reduced. Despite the ensuing stiffness, the reduced joint protected cartilage and ligaments. (A-F, © Robert N. Hotchkiss.)

tracture matures, the ulnar nerve is not under tension and therefore may not exhibit dysfunction.

In primary arthritis of the elbow associated with anterior and posterior osteophyte formation, pain is usually present at the end range of flexion and extension. The middle range is usually comfortable and without crepitation. However, as the condition progresses and further deterioration of the trochlear surface of the humerus and other cartilage loss occurs, the pain will be more constant, severe, and present in all positions.

Assessment of Motion Loss and the Effect on Function

Morrey and colleagues[45] studied normal subjects by electrogoniometry and determined that most tasks of daily living could be performed in a range of 30 to 130 degrees of flexion and extension. This study was helpful in defining what most normal people use throughout the course of daily activity, but it did not ask the question of *what is required for these tasks.*

With the assistance of our therapy department, my colleagues and I studied 52 patients with decreased elbow motion and recorded the tasks that they could perform with and without specified adaptations. Twenty *elbow-dependent* tasks ranging from buttoning a collar to reaching for a lower drawer were evaluated. The goal was to examine which tasks could be performed and, of those performed, which required a significant postural or spatial adaptation. Without recanting the entire study, suffice it to say that patients lacking flexion of more than 110 degrees were unlikely to be able to button a collar, shave, place an earring, or tie a scarf or necktie. The adaptations possible are limited because flexion of the neck and wrist is of limited help. Lack of extension, however, is much more easily accommodated for. In our study, flexion contracture of greater than 40 degrees required positional adaptation, but the tasks could still be accomplished. Reaching the feet or toes was possible with increased knee, hip, and trunk flexion. For opening low drawers, the patient could kneel to pull them open bimanually. In other words, positioning the hand in space, away from the body or to the feet, is limited with loss of extension, but the patient can accommodate to this by moving the trunk (and hand) more closely to the object of interest. Adaptation is less possible with loss of elbow flexion.

Although loss of flexion is generally ignored in the published literature, every effort should be made to improve flexion when there is less than 105 degrees. In our study, patients could not compensate for loss of flexion. The neck and wrist are limited in their capacity to flex to assist the hand in reaching the neck, face, head, or ears. Lacking elbow flexion limits buttoning a collar, using eating utensils, and self-care of the hair, face, and neck.

An important conclusion from our study was that if improved extension is sought, it should not be obtained at the expense of flexion. This is not a "trade" that patients will want to make.

In preoperative assessment it is helpful for patients to detail what tasks they have difficulty performing because of limitation of motion. Patients may be quite functional with a 40-degree flexion contracture but simply not like the appearance. Given the complexity of the surgery and the postoperative effort usually required, I generally do not recommend contracture release for appearances only.

Elbow motion *must* be carefully documented by goniometry and a standardized technique. I have found the interobserver error in trained personnel to be about ±10 degrees. My own intraobserver error is about 5 degrees when using a special large goniometer. Given these numbers, I doubt the value of reporting elbow measurements in increments of less than 5 degrees. It is important for the surgeon to measure the angles personally and not merely rely on measurements recorded by the therapists.

What Degree of Motion Is Necessary?

It is impossible to set absolute indications for operative contracture release. Generally, any patient with a 40-degree loss of extension or less than 105 degrees of flexion will benefit from improved motion and should be considered for contracture release. It is seldom possible to guarantee full extension, irrespective of the operative approach or postoperative management. This point is especially important to discuss with patients such as gymnasts, who require full extension, even hypertension, to "lock out" during handstands or floor exercises. Occasionally, patients have post-injury contractures of 30 degrees or less and, despite being very functional, seek nearly full extension for sports, especially for the throwing hand. If the contracture is simple and uncomplicated by heterotopic bone formation or joint incongruity, these patients can often be improved by either arthroscopic release or a release from the lateral approach.

Physical Examination of the Ulnar Nerve

The ulnar nerve is very vulnerable to injury, scarring, and dysfunction after trauma, distal humeral internal fixation, and complex dislocations. Because of this vulnerability, very careful preoperative assessment of the nerve is mandatory. In many cases it is not possible to be certain whether the nerve has been transposed. Even if the previous operative note is available and states that a transposition was performed, the nerve may have slipped back into a more posterior position.

If the ulnar nerve is entrapped or shows signs of significant dysfunction, neurolysis and transposition at the time of contracture release can be quite helpful by restoring sensibility and strength in the proximal muscles innervated by the ulnar nerve. The more distal intrinsic muscles of the hand are less likely to recover, although occasionally in younger patients dramatic improvement may be seen.

Most patients with loss of flexion require ulnar nerve transposition at the time of surgery, and this point should be discussed with the patient. Patients with primary osteoarthritis of the elbow often demonstrate osteophytes extending into the cubital tunnel. These patients, usually middle-aged men, may have a very subclinical, indolent course. When carefully examined, the intrinsic wasting may be subtle and the loss of sensibility discovered only with light touch or two-point discrimination. If there is doubt, preoperative electrophysiologic testing, with special attention to electromyography (EMG), should be performed.

Patients may have temporary postoperative ulnar nerve dysfunction, especially if the nerve is already symptomatic. Most improve with neurolysis and transposition, but recovery is often quite slow if the dysfunction has been present for a long time.

Technical Note. When dissecting the ulnar nerve, there is seldom any reason to perform an internal neurolysis or intrafascicular or even epineural dissection. Instead, the goal is to free the nerve from the entrapment posterior to the axis of the joint and to allow it to be transposed to the anterior position. Leaving a cuff of soft tissue, especially in a setting of reoperation, poses less threat to nerve function than trying to strip all soft tissue from the nerve.

Imaging the Stiff Elbow

Many radiologic features need to be assessed before surgery is considered:

- What is the quality of the joint and relative health of the cartilage?
- Where is the hardware and is it impeding motion? (Is removal necessary?)
- Where is the HO?
- Are the fractures healed?

The quality of the articular surfaces in a stiff post-traumatic elbow is of paramount importance. The ulnohumeral joint is probably more important than the radiocapitellar joint, although having both intact and functional is optimal. Assessing this joint and the quality of the cartilage is best done with plain radiographs. If this is insufficient, computed tomographic (CT) scans with thin slices in the sagittal and coronal planes may be needed. Trispiral polytomography is becoming rare as an imaging technique because of scarcity of the equipment. CT with careful orientation and thin-slice technique is an adequate replacement and generally exposes the patient to less radiation.

Ultimately, however, the articular surface must be inspected at the time of surgery to determine whether there is adequate cartilage in the functional zone of motion. If the surface is of poor quality, interposition arthroplasty or, in older patients, total elbow replacement must be strongly considered. In my experience, patients with healthy cartilage have a more predictably successful outcome than do patients who require interposition arthroplasty, even if a hinge distractor is used in otherwise identical situations.

A significant flexion contracture may preclude visualization of the distal humeral articular surface with standard radiographic techniques. Typically the technician places the film plate perpendicular to the joint at mid range. An anteroposterior (AP) view with the distal humerus lying flat on the cassette is a helpful additional view. A true lateral view is also mandatory. In some cases I also obtain true lateral views in maximal active flexion and maximal active extension. Technicians find these difficult at first because the humerus tends to internally or externally rotate at the extremes of position and the "true lateral" view is lost.[32] These additional views may show subtle shifts of the joint, as well as previously unseen projections of heterotopic bone.

For fracture cases, it is sometimes difficult to determine whether union has been achieved, especially when plates and screws overlie the area in question. CT is problematic because of "noise" from the metal. Magnetic resonance imaging (MRI) techniques are improving to better assess fragment healing, viability, and perfusion—even in the presence of metallic hardware.[13,31]

At no time have I used bone scans to assess a contracted elbow, finding them of no use in patients with post-traumatic contracture with or without heterotopic bone.

THE PREOPERATIVE DISCUSSION

Once you have determined that a surgical release *could* be performed, it is important to discuss expectations, the surgery, and the potential complications with the patient.

With this discussion alone, the patient may shy away and appropriately conclude that it is possible to live quite well with the limitation of motion.

Much like rehabilitation after flexor tendon repair, if you do not have the full cooperation and dedication of the patient, you may not succeed. Given the complexity of some cases, the attempted release may worsen motion.

As detailed later, each contracture requires at least two operative plans. If the first approach does not succeed in achieving the expected goal during surgery, the second option should be employed. If you believed that a medial approach to the joint alone would permit a complete capsulectomy but found the lateral structures both limiting and out of safe reach, then the lateral approach should be considered. Likewise, postoperative management varies greatly, depending on each patient's individual response. It is important to explain the variability in response to operative release. Fortunately, most patients with contractures already understand this. They have often already been told that this was in some way their fault or the fault of their "muscles" (see page 939 on "blame"). Some require very little supervised therapy, even little continuous passive motion (CPM); others need serial static bracing (flexion and extension) and occasionally a carefully administered manipulation. For massive HO with long-standing contractures, I also explain the use of dynamic hinged external fixation.*

If during any of this discussion you detect unwillingness or wariness, waiting may be warranted. I also encourage patients to discuss their questions with other patients, and I keep a list of former patients willing to discuss their operative experience.

Patients should also be informed about the possibility of transient, increased ulnar nerve symptoms.

THE OPERATIVE PLAN AND INTRAOPERATIVE "COURSE CORRECTIONS"

The operative tools needed for successful contracture release range from arthroscopy to hinged external fixation to total elbow arthroplasty. Deciding which one you need depends on the age of the patient, cause of the stiffness, quality of the joint, and, in some ways, the quality of the patient. As we have gained experience with both the different causes of contracture and types of patients, we have also had access to new tools and methods of treatment. The best care for a given contracture patient is the minimally necessary surgery, including minimal anatomic exposure, and rehabilitation to achieve the desired result. For instance, a patient with a range of 40 to 105 degrees and HO will usually require exposure of the capsule for complete excision from both the medial and lateral approaches but not necessarily hinged fixation. In this situation, the use of hinged fixation may potentially improve extension (from 20 degrees achieved with capsulectomy alone to perhaps 5 degrees with hinged fixation), but I do not believe that this is worth the cost or aggravation to the patient.

In a different circumstance with more massive HO, hinged external fixation is needed to stabilize the elbow postoperatively and permit immediate motion with intermittent passive stretch.

I set out to perform the operation most likely to achieve the goal, but I am always prepared to raise the level of complexity one notch, and I explain this to the patient preoperatively. In other words, if I think that an arthroscopic release is likely to be sufficient, I also plan for the possibility of an open release if full passive motion is not achieved on the table. In cases in which I am reasonably certain that a dual-approach, anterior/posterior release will suffice, I may plan for hinged fixation in case there is unexpected muscle-tendon tightness and failure to regain extension or flexion on the table or the joint is surprisingly or excessively worn and requires interposition. Having now performed over 100 contracture releases, I have found the need for hinged fixation to be less likely. In older patients with suspected cartilage damage or avascular bone, total elbow replacement should be available and discussed before surgery.

Predicting what you need and what will succeed is an iterative process that comes from your own experience and the seasoned opinions of others. It is important to be prepared to change and not be wedded to any single approach.[28] Orthodoxy here should only be a dedication to optimizing your patient's motion, not to a single exposure, approach, or given device.

Anesthesia for Contracture Release

Regional blocks are preferred[34] and are in fact the only method I have used for contracture release over the past 8 years. The elbow can be somewhat problematic for regional anesthesia. Axillary blocks may leave the upper end of the medial incision with sensibility. A small amount of local anesthetic in this area is usually all that is needed. Occasionally, an axillary and an interscalene block are needed to sufficiently anesthetize the entire region. Both a sensory and complete motor block are needed for effective relaxation and patient comfort. Because some of the procedures can be long, sedation is also helpful and usually required. Long-acting agents are the norm. Bupivacaine may leave the patient blocked for 24 to 48 hours. Although this may cause the surgeon concern, especially being unable to check the status of the nerve, the pain relief and slow return of sensation are helpful as the patient begins motion the next day. My colleagues and I have also begun using a subclavicular brachial plexus catheter for sustained pain relief with some early and promising results.[47]

General anesthesia with endotracheal intubation may always be used if regional blocks are unsuccessful or the anesthesia staff is unwilling to do regional blocks. More narcotics may be needed in the immediate postoperative period.

In children I also use regional blocks combined with general anesthesia. This is the best of both worlds for this challenging age group.

Arthroscopic Release

My personal view of this tool is that it is becoming more applicable as the instruments are improved and experience is gained. This method works best in a young athlete with

---

*As a matter of disclosure, the author helped design and patent the Compass Elbow Hinge (manufactured by Smith & Nephew, UK). Royalties based on sales are received by the author.

loose bodies or a history of a hyperextended elbow and resultant minimal but annoying contracture. The anterior capsule can safely be released under direct arthroscopic visualization.

The other group is typified by a 45- to 55-year old with primary osteoarthritis and simple osteophytes projecting from the coronoid and the tip of the olecranon.[32] In my opinion, arthroscopic release *should not* be performed if the patient requires ulnar nerve transposition or if there are large osteophytes in the posteromedial corner. The posteromedial corner is the floor of the cubital tunnel. I have treated one patient who had the ulnar nerve accidentally débrided with an arthroscopic shaver. Other injuries have also been reported.[19] The surgeon should resist the temptation of using the shaver in this region. In addition, the open techniques are safe and relatively simple and permit visualization of the relevant neurovascular structures if needed. It is my firm belief that one should understand and be able to perform an open capsulectomy (described below) using both approaches before using the arthroscope as the primary tool of visualization and capsulectomy.

OPEN RELEASE

When an open release is planned, the location of the potential pathology and the nature of the contracture should determine the approach to the joint. One should not feel constrained to use one approach over another because of an unfounded allegiance to a given method. If the patient has a simple flexion contracture related to a radial head fracture, the lateral approach is usually sufficient and is relatively simple to perform.[5,6,24,30,35] In more complex cases in which the ulnar nerve requires exposure, I usually begin with the medial "over-the-top" exposure.[27,40,63] I am always prepared to use a supplementary lateral approach in these cases if there is HO located on the lateral side or if I am concerned about the position and safety of the radial nerve. Unless you use an approach that dislocates the joint, such as the Bryan-Morrey exposure, you will undoubtedly encounter situations in which either the lateral approach to the joint is inadequate for a safe, complete release or vice versa. It is therefore important to understand both the medial and lateral approaches and be able to pull them "off the shelf" as needed in the operating room. Both a transhumeral and transolecranon approach have been described, but I have not used either.[21,65] I also no longer use the Outerbridge-Kashiwaga procedure[43] (transhumeral trephination), which is designed to treat patients with primary arthritis of the elbow. If there is a significant lack of flexion (limited to less than 90 degrees), evidence of ulnar nerve dysfunction, or osteophytes in the posterior medial joint line, I prefer the medial "over-the-top" approach. As described in the next section, this approach permits exposure of the ulnar nerve and access to the anterior and posterior osteophytes. If flexion is minimally limited and the ulnar nerve is palpable and mobile, I prefer arthroscopic débridement and contracture release.

Only rarely can contracture be treated with anterior capsulectomy alone. Of the more than 100 contractures that I have treated operatively over the past 10 years, only a handful were adequately freed by incising the anterior cap-

sule alone. In most instances you should always plan to have access to the posterior joint surface, whether from the medial or lateral side of the joint.

The advantage of knowing and using both approaches is that you can protect the anterior medial ligament on the medial side by using the medial "over-the-top" approach. From the lateral exposure, the posterolateral ligaments described as noted by Husband and Hastings and others[5,24,35] can be protected.

MEDIAL "OVER-THE-TOP" APPROACH

The principal advantages of this approach are as follows:

- Allows exposure, protection, and transposition of the ulnar nerve
- Preserves the anterior medial collateral ligament
- Preserves the posterolateral ulnohumeral ligament complex
- Permits both anterior and posterior access to the joint
- Allows access to the coronoid and anterior osteophytes with an intact radial head
- Can be easily converted to the triceps-sparing exposure of Bryan-Morrey, which permits complete dislocation of the joint and a more extensile approach (for total elbow replacement)

The disadvantages are as follows:

- Difficult to remove heterotopic bone on the lateral side of the joint
- Poor access to the radial head

Patient Position and Preparation

The patient is usually supine with the arm supported by a hand table (Fig. 25-2A). It is helpful to bring the patient as far as possible onto the hand table. The patient's head may require support with a small foam ring because a standard pillow projects too far toward the shoulder and impedes the skin prep. Two folded towels should be placed under the ipsilateral scapula to lift the shoulder away from the surgical table. The prep should extend to and include the axilla to allow a sterile tourniquet to be applied after the prep. For the surgeon to visualize the anterior and posterior surface of the distal humerus, the patient should have fairly free external rotation of the shoulder.

Skin Incision and Superficial Exposure

The skin incision for this exposure can vary between the boundaries of a pure posterior skin incision and a midline medial incision (see Fig. 25-2B). The key to this exposure is identification of the *medial supracondylar ridge* of the humerus (see Fig. 25-2C). At this level one can locate the medial intermuscular septum, the origin of the flexor-pronator muscle mass, and the ulnar nerve. This location also serves

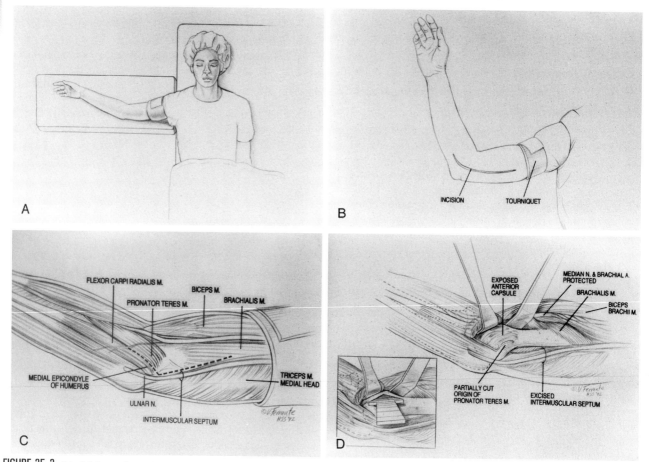

FIGURE 25-2. Medial "over-the-top" approach. **A,** The supine position is the most useful. A folded towel should be placed under the ipsilateral scapula. **B,** The skin incision may vary according to previous incisions. If the incision is made along the posterior surface, larger flaps are needed. **C,** The intermuscular septum should be recognized as a landmark and excised for adequate mobilization of the ulnar nerve. **D,** The anterior capsule is first exposed by splitting fibers between the flexor carpi ulnaris and the pronator. The anterior portion of the medial collateral ligament is protected. *Continued*

as the point to begin the subperiosteal extracapsular dissection of the joint for both the anterior and posterior surfaces.

Once the subcutaneous skin is elevated, the first structure to identify is the medial intermuscular septum. If the skin incision is more posterior, the medial intermuscular septum can be found by locating the aponeurosis of the triceps tendon 2 to 3 cm proximal to the medial epicondyle and gently spreading with scissors anteriorly. Anterior to the septum and running immediately on top of the fascia (and not in the subdermal tissue) is the medial antebrachial cutaneous nerve, which usually has several branches. Generally this nerve can be traced distally and protected in this approach, but the branching pattern varies. It is occasionally necessary to divide this nerve to gain full exposure and adequately mobilize the ulnar nerve, especially in redo surgery. If nerve dissection is required, the nerve should be divided as far proximally as the skin incision will allow while ensuring that the cut nerve end lies in the subcutaneous fat. If the patient has had previous surgery, the ulnar nerve should be identified proximally before proceeding distally. If a previous anterior transposition has been performed, the nerve should be fully identified and mobilized before proceeding. In this setting, the nerve is flattened over the medial flexor-pronator muscle mass. Great care is needed to dissect the nerve in this location.

Once the medial intermuscular septum has been identified proximally, the surface of the origin of the flexor-pronator muscle mass can be found by dissecting at this same level and sweeping the subcutaneous tissue laterally. In most cases the medial antebrachial cutaneous nerve will be in this flap of subcutaneous tissue. The nerve will generally cross to the posterior aspect of the elbow distal to the epicondyle and can be elevated with the flap and retracted out of harm's way.

The medial intermuscular septum can now be excised from its insertion on the supracondylar ridge to the proximal extent of the wound, usually about 5 cm. There are many veins and perforating arteries at the most distal portion that require cautery. The septum can be cleared of muscle by using a small Cobb elevator along the posterior surface above the ulnar nerve.

Anterior Capsular Exposure

The supracondylar ridge is located and the anterior muscle is elevated with a wide Cobb elevator (see Fig. 25-2D). All the anterior structures in the distal humeral region are elevated sufficiently subperiosteally to allow placement of a wide Bennett retractor. The median nerve, brachial vein, and brachial artery are superficial to the brachialis muscle. Once

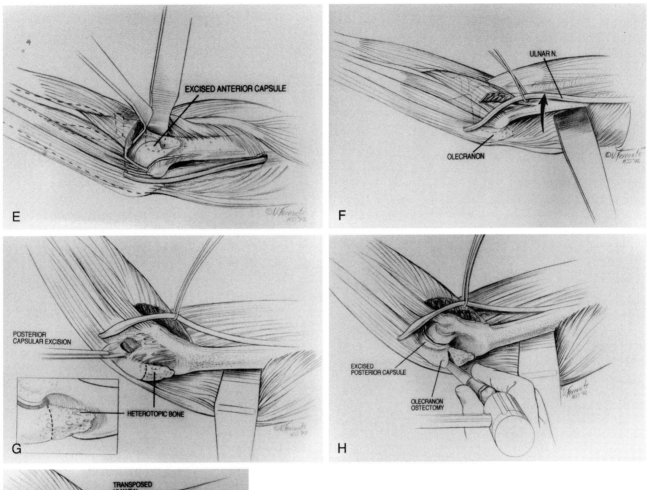

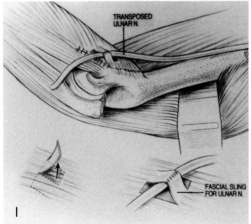

FIGURE 25-2—cont'd. **E,** Once exposed, the capsule is sharply excised. Anterior heterotopic ossification (HO) arising from the coronoid is usually excised at this point. **F,** The ulnar nerve is then carefully mobilized and moved forward. **G,** The posterior surface is now exposed for excision of the capsule and HO. **H,** The tip of the olecranon is removed to clear the posterior fossa. **I,** The ulnar nerve is left in the anteriorly transposed position. A fascial sling or subcutaneous fat sling can be fashioned to hold the nerve anteriorly transposed without constriction.

the septum is excised, the flexor-pronator muscle mass is divided parallel to its fibers, with approximately a 1.5-cm span of flexor carpi ulnaris tendon left attached to the epicondyle. A small cuff of fibrous tissue of the origin can be left on the supracondylar ridge as the muscle is elevated. This facilitates reattachment when closing. A proximal, transverse incision in the lacertus fibrosus may also be needed to adequately mobilize this layer of muscle. The flexor-pronator origin should be dissected down to the level of bone but superficial to joint capsule. As this plane is developed, the brachialis muscle will be encountered from the underside. This muscle should be kept anterior and elevated from the capsule and anterior surface of the distal humerus.

It is often helpful at this point to return to the supracondylar ridge by sharply dissecting down to bone on the medial surface of the humerus. The ulnar nerve should be lying posteriorly. Dissection of the capsule to separate it from the brachialis muscle can proceed both laterally and distally.

At this point it is helpful to feel for the coronoid process by gently flexing and extending the elbow. For the first few times using this approach the coronoid will seem quite deep and distal. A deep, narrow retractor may facilitate exposure of the coronoid. From this vantage and after capsular excision, the radial head and capitellum can be visualized and freed of scar as needed.

In the case of contracture, the capsule, once separated from the overlying brachialis and brachioradialis, can be sharply excised (see Fig. 25-2E). The radial nerve lies between the brachialis and brachioradialis. Care should be taken when elevating over to the lateral side to stay deep to these two muscles. If heterotopic bone or previous surgery has potentially displaced the nerve, it is safer to make a lateral incision at this point and either identify the nerve or convince yourself that you are deep to the nerve with the plane of dissection.

The very anterior medial corner of the exposure deserves special comment. In a contracture release, the anterior medial portion often requires release. To see this area, a small narrow retractor can be inserted to pull the attached flexor carpi ulnaris medially. This will allow visualization of the very anterior medial capsule and also afford protection of the anterior medial collateral ligament.

Posterior Capsular Exposure

The ulnar nerve should now be fully mobilized to permit anterior transposition (see Fig. 25-2F). Because the intermuscular septum has been excised, only the vascular attachments and perineural investments confine the nerve proximally. The ulnar nerve is carefully elevated by using a vessel loop for retraction. The dissection needs to be carried distally enough to allow the nerve to sit in the anterior position without kinking distal to the epicondyle.

The posterior capsule of the joint is exposed in a fashion analogous to that for the anterior capsule. The supracondylar ridge is again identified. With a Cobb elevator the triceps is elevated from the posterior distal surface of the humerus. The exposure should be proximal enough to permit the use of a Bennett retractor.

The posterior capsule can be separated from the triceps as the elevator sweeps in a proximal-to-distal direction. The medial joint line should also be identified (see Fig. 25-2G). In contracture release, the posterior capsule and posteromedial ligaments should be excised. The medial joint line, up to the anterior medial ligament, should also be exposed and the capsule excised. Along this line there is usually heterotopic bone on the olecranon or posterior medial osteophytes. More olecranon needs to be excised than one would expect (see Fig. 25-2H). The posterior fossa must be completely clear of impinging soft tissue or bone. If not, maximal extension will be limited.

Structures That Require Repair

Flexor-Pronator Muscle Origin. The flexor-pronator mass should be reattached to the supracondylar ridge with nonabsorbable braided 1-0 or 0 suture. If enough fibrous tissue was left behind, no holes in bone are needed. If not, drill holes in the edge of the supracondylar ridge can be made to secure the flexor-pronator muscle mass. The lacertus fibrosus often requires release to permit full medial reattachment.

Ulnar Nerve Transposition. After reattachment to the medial supracondylar region, the ulnar nerve should be transposed and secured with a fascial sling to prevent poste-

CRITICAL POINTS: MEDIAL APPROACH

ANTERIOR JOINT

- Center skin incision posterior to medial epicondyle (may be directly posterior).
- Identify and protect all branches of the medial antebrachial cutaneous nerve.
- Identify and dissect ulnar nerve to permit anterior subcutaneous transposition.
- Lift flexor-pronator off medial supracondylar ridge with Cobb elevator.
- Divide flexor carpi ulnaris leaving 1 cm of posterior portion attached to epicondyle.
- Bluntly separate anterior muscle, leaving capsule behind.
- Excise capsule from distal humerus to proximal ulna (coronoid process).
- Continue dissection to lateral edge of joint line.
- Check for areas of remaining taut capsule by gently manipulating into extension and flexion.

POSTERIOR JOINT

- Starting at medial supracondylar ridge, lift triceps off with Cobb elevator.
- Continue dissection distally lifting the triceps tendon, leaving posterior capsule behind.
- Excise the posterior capsule, including the posteromedial corner.
- Remove the posterior olecranon, usually about 1 cm (depends on size of osteophyte).
- Check for posterior impingement.
- Check for areas of remaining taut capsule by gently manipulating into extension and flexion.
- If there are still soft tissue limitations along the lateral joint line, these can be incised, but beware of the radial nerve; if uncertain, approach from the lateral column.

rior subluxation (see Fig. 22-2I). The sling can be fashioned by elevating two overlapping rectangular flaps of fascia. The nerve is then placed under the flaps, and these are approximated with adequate room so that nerve is not compressed, only stabilized. Superficial fat flaps can also be used to maintain the nerve in the anterior position. I use whatever keeps the nerve in an anterior position without tension, compression, or kinks. The joint should be flexed and extended to ensure that the nerve is free to move.

LATERAL APPROACH[5,24,35]

Patient Position and Skin Incision

The patient is usually in the supine position and the arm supported by a hand table. A sterile tourniquet for the upper arm is useful because it permits proximal exposure if needed. The skin incision is centered over the lateral epicondyle. The proximal extent of the skin incision depends on the needs of the case. For contracture release or treatment of fractures of the distal humerus, the skin incision may extend to 4 to 8 cm proximal to the lateral epicondyle, as needed. For simple contracture release, the incision may need to be extended only to the supracondylar ridge. For exposure of the radial head, the proximal extension may need to be only 5 cm. Extension of the exposure to 10 cm proximal to the lateral epicondyle may risk injury to the radial nerve. If proximal extension to 10 cm or more above the lateral epicondyle is planned, the radial nerve should be identified in the interval between the brachioradialis and brachialis.

Skin Incision and Superficial Approach

The skin incision does not need to be over the lateral epicondyle but may also begin in the posterior midline. If this incision is used, a longer skin incision will be needed and larger flaps developed to gain access to the lateral joint.

The anterolateral approach to the elbow remains anterior to the anconeus. Once the full-thickness skin flaps have been elevated, the key to this exposure is identification of the lateral supracondylar ridge of the distal humerus and the posterior border of the wrist extensor muscle mass, the extensor carpi radialis brevis. The flare of the ridge is palpated just superior to the lateral epicondyle, anterior to the triceps and posterior to the brachioradialis. The plane of dissection will continue in the midline of the epicondyle, but specifically not posterior to the epicondyle, especially distally.

Access to the Anterior Capsule

With the retractor in place, sharp division of the more distal capsule, down to bone, will expose the articular portion of the distal humerus. When this exposure is used for contracture release instead of elevating the entire soft tissue envelope as a single layer, an elevator is used to bluntly separate the brachioradialis and the capsule as the dissection proceeds distally. In this interval the radial nerve is more vulnerable because the plane of dissection is more superficial. However, if the elevator is carefully advanced on top of the capsule and the muscle fibers pushed anteriorly, the radial nerve will be protected by muscle. If in doubt, find the nerve between the brachioradialis and brachialis. The capsule should be excised at the level of the joint, across to the medial side.

The joint should be gently manipulated to test whether sufficient release has been achieved. If not, a decision needs to be made about whether to switch to the medial joint exposure or expose the posterior joint from the lateral side and protect the posterolateral ligament complex.

Exposing the Posterior Capsule From the Lateral Side

As described by Husband and Hastings,[5,24,35] the posterior capsule can be safely excised from the lateral side; even HO can be removed from the posterior surface. If the ulnar nerve has not been exposed, remember that it is vulnerable, trapped in scar, and located at the very edge of the posteromedial extent of the exposure, often the most difficult to see.

The posterolateral ligament complex is identified and *not* incised. An elevator is introduced near the supracondylar flare of the distal humerus and swept distally along the posterior surface. It is helpful to leave the capsule attached before excising it. The tip of the olecranon usually requires excision to clear the posterior fossa for adequate extension.

Immediate Postoperative Care

Drains: Closed Suction

Although I have heard on occasion surgeons remark that they do not use closed suction drainage, I believe that this is vital in almost all cases after open release. Occasionally, a simple lateral approach with anterior-only release is associated with minimal postoperative bleeding and drains are not required. However, as the complexity of the surgery and the severity move up the scale, postoperative hematoma must be avoided. Retained blood and hematoma cause pain, inflammation, and occasional temporary nerve dysfunction, all of which retard progress toward improved motion.

If hinged fixation or CPM is planned for the immediate postoperative period, I secure the drains with sutures. Because these drains are left in place for 2 to 3 days after

---

CRITICAL POINTS: TECHNICAL TIPS AND SUGGESTIONS

- Wait to remove hardware until end of release and then after the gentle manipulation needed during the procedure.
- Secure the suction drains with sutures and plan to leave them in place as the postoperative CPM is underway.
- Seldom, if ever, does the range of motion improve from what is gained in the operating room.
- Honestly measure and dictate in the operative note the degree of motion achieved with light pressure applied in both flexion/extension and supination/pronation.
- Splint the patient in the position of greatest "challenge" before beginning CPM. In general, this is in extension.
- If splinting in flexion, inspect the posterior skin over the olecranon. Occasionally this will blanch and lead to skin breakdown if not progressively flexed.

surgery, they can easily be dislodged either during placement of the hinged external fixator or during CPM.

The First 24 Hours

Many authors prefer to begin CPM immediately after surgery. I have tried this and on occasion have been pleased. However, I now use the first 24 hours for rest, ice, and elevation of the extremity. If there is no fixator, I use a sling to hold the entire limb above the heart and pack the elbow in ice. If a hinge fixator is used, the device is set in maximal tolerable extension and ice bags placed around the elbow.

Special Circumstances

Fractures of the Distal Humerus After Open Reduction and Internal Fixation

After fractures of the distal humerus, the stiffness of the joint can come from intra-articular malunion, HO, or capsular contracture. CT is helpful for visualizing the distal humerus and specifically the ulnohumeral joint. In thin patients, the plates on the medial and lateral columns of the distal humerus may feel quite superficial and the patient often requests their removal. The fracture must be solidly healed if the hardware is to be removed. If there is uncertainty, be prepared to plate and bone graft the nonunion on discovery while still performing the contracture release. If the fracture is healed and the hardware is to be removed, the contracture release is done first, followed by hardware removal. If the hardware is removed first, refracture may

occur even with gentle manipulation during the contracture release. This complication can be avoided by releasing the contracture, performing the intraoperative manipulation, and then removing the hardware if indicated.

In elderly patients, if there is a nonunion or if avascular necrosis of the articular surface is suspected, total elbow replacement with a semiconstrained implant is the best option. I prefer the Coonrad-Morrey elbow in this instance (see Chapter 27).

Nonunion of the Distal Humerus

Most nonunions of the distal humerus are associated with joint contracture. This finding is especially true in patients with failed attempts at internal fixation. Once the hardware failure becomes apparent, the elbow is often immobilized in the slim hope that union may occur in the presence of mechanical hardware failure. To treat the nonunion, the elbow joint must be completely relieved of contracture. If not, the newly plated nonunion site will experience continued excessive torque and be prone to another mechanical failure. If the joint contracture is released, stress is minimized at the distal humeral fixation.

Head Trauma and Brain Injury (Fig. 25-3)

Patients with head trauma and associated residual spasticity have two strikes against them.[1,14,49] First, they tend to have exuberant HO and are often prevented from seeking care for excision in the first year. Therefore the ankylosis is usually complete and the surrounding tissue quite thickened and

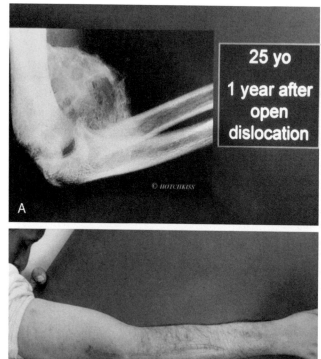

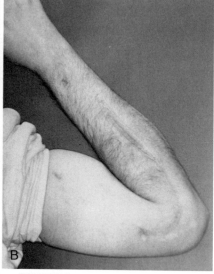

FIGURE 25-3. **A,** A 25-year-old man presented with previous head trauma and open elbow dislocation. He had no permanent spasticity and had complete volitional control. Because of extensive heterotopic ossification, the distal humerus required complete exposure and excision of ligaments. This degree of intraoperative instability requires hinged external fixation. This patient wore the hinge for 10 weeks. **B** and **C,** Three years after surgery he retained excellent motion and strength. (**A-C,** © Robert N. Hotchkiss.)

unyielding. Second, voluntary control of the elbow is difficult to judge. I have tried to assess effective volitional control in these patients after the brain injury has stabilized by both physical examination and surface electromyography. Minimally, patients must be able to fire the biceps and triceps on command before considering release. Unfortunately, the capacity to contract these muscles volitionally while the joint is ankylosed does not guarantee the ability to flex and extend with strength once passive motion is achieved. I have unfortunately seen patients regain remarkable passive motion after the excision of massive HO only to watch them gradually lose mobility over a period of months because of a lack of active strength and effective control over the entire extent of motion. In addition, the hand, wrist, and forearm may also be spastic and of little use beyond simple positioning. The goals and expectations of the patient (and the family) must be carefully weighed before proceeding with contracture release. Nonetheless, this is also a group of patients who are extremely grateful if they can regain some motion for positioning their hands for transfer, the use of motorized devices, and self-care.

It is important to allow the brain injury to recover. This may mean waiting 12 to 24 months. Recovery of volitional muscle control and strength will occur in adjacent muscles and should be viewed as a positive prognosis. During this time, the family and patient will become more realistic about the goals of contracture release. In addition, the patient's capacity for rehabilitation and social setting will generally settle into place, permitting a more reasoned assessment of the patient and family's capacity for postoperative care and rehabilitation.

Hinged Fixation After Contracture Release

Indications for the use of hinged external fixation[12,16,27,48,52,53,55] are (1) instability after contracture release, (2) excessive muscle tendon tightness noted at the time of complete capsular release (dynamic hinged fixation/Compass Elbow Hinge) (Fig. 25-4), and (3) distraction arthroplasty (with or without interposition).[12,16,27-29,41,48,60]

Application of a Hinged Fixator: The Technical Challenge

Each type of hinged fixator requires a detailed understanding of the principles of use, method of application, and the problems that may be encountered. I believe it is essential that the primary surgeon be familiar with one type of fixator and the specific techniques required for successful application. Each of the companies that manufacture these devices provides instructional materials and courses. It may be useful to pay a visit to someone with experience. The assisting surgeon should also be familiar with the device and its application. During placement, one set of eyes is often needed to place a half-pin properly while the primary surgeon makes certain that the overall alignment of the device is maintained.

In addition to the technical challenge, these cases can be of long duration, exceeding 4 hours. In the beginning, a difficult contracture release, requiring extensive dissection with careful protection of all nerves, can be tiring. The application of the hinged fixator cannot be viewed as an afterthought. If the pins are misaligned or care is not taken

to ensure that the joint is completely reduced, then all the work is for naught.

Instability After Release

Instability after release is common and has been noted by many authors, especially in patients with severe joint involvement or those with more massive HO.[14] In these cases the stabilizing ligaments are often trapped in the HO and cannot be protected during release. Even if the ligaments are not completely released, a wide area of capsular excision and stripping is often needed to free the joint. In this circumstance, especially if there has been a long-standing limitation (more than 18 months), the patient has a very difficult time regaining motion and maintaining that motion in the first 8 weeks after surgery. Hinged fixation is used in those settings where acute and gross instability is created after contracture release (Fig. 25-5). In general, as one gains experience, there is less need for the use of hinged fixation after contracture release.

Excessive Muscle Tightness

In a long-standing contracture with excessive muscle tightness, some have recommended lengthening of the biceps, brachialis, or triceps tendons.[8] In my opinion this should be avoided if at all possible. The muscle-tendon unit is undoubtedly shortened in the case of a long-standing contracture, but lengthening these structures in a nonspastic patient risks loss of strength and requires some protection of the repair during rehabilitation.

As we have gained more experience, the need for hinged fixation in cases of muscle tightness is rare. However, when it is needed, I prefer to use the Compass Elbow Hinge in this setting and let the passive worm gear steadily and progressively increase the range of position, much like an Ilizarov lengthening.

Distraction Arthroplasty

For interposition arthroplasty, there are several devices that provide stability and distraction of the joint. The two types of devices can be separated by hinged fixators with and without a passive drive mechanism. The principle of fixator use is based on temporarily stabilizing the joint after resurfacing the joint with fascia or cutis (skin with the epidermal layer removed). The fixator replicates the flexion/extension axis of the elbow permitting motion. The axis of rotation, centered at the distal humerus, is located by several methods, depending on which device is used. External fixation pins, usually two in the humerus and two in the ulna, are then applied. The axis pin is then removed so that there is less chance of infection during the postoperative period. The Compass Elbow Hinge differs in that a passive drive mechanism permits passive mobilization, but it is considered by most to be more complicated to apply. All devices require an understanding of the anatomy and kinematics of the elbow.

If hinged fixation is used, the device must be left on for at least 6 to 8 weeks while maximizing motion and allowing the soft tissues to regain stability. Further information about both of these devices is available from the manufacturers. Familiarity with one or both devices is essential for complex reconstructive surgery on the elbow.

The clinical results from distraction arthroplasty for posttraumatic contracture are not stellar. Often the patient feels

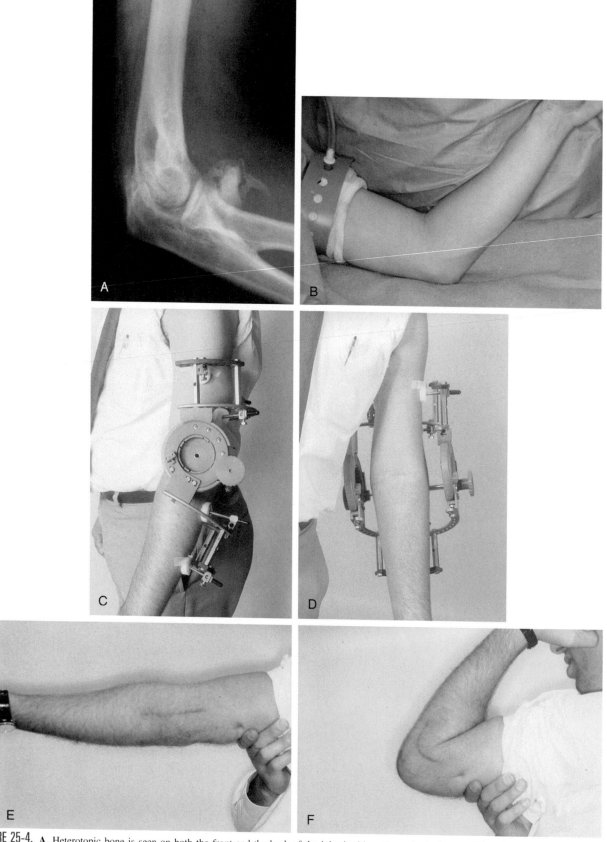

FIGURE 25-4. **A,** Heterotopic bone is seen on both the front and the back of the joint in this radiograph. A fracture-dislocation and previous attempt at contracture release were unsuccessful. **B,** Maximal extension under anesthesia. **C** and **D,** Patient wearing the first Compass Elbow Hinge design. **E** and **F,** Range of motion approximately 2 years after treatment. No degenerative changes developed in the joint. (**A-F,** © Robert N. Hotchkiss.)

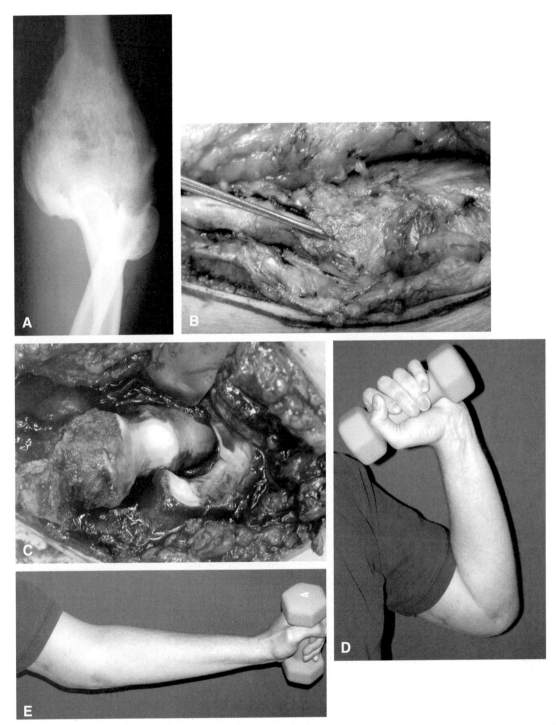

FIGURE 25-5. **A,** An ankylosed elbow after combined head and elbow trauma in a 45-year-old confined to a wheelchair. Note the faint hint of a joint line in the ulnohumeral joint. **B,** The ulnar nerve is covered by bone during neurolysis. (Freer elevator is under shelf of bone.) **C,** Intraoperative instability from radical resection of medial heterotopic ossification that included medial ligaments, requiring the use of hinged fixation. **D** and **E,** At 6 months there is good mobility and he is able to transfer using his left arm. (**A-E,** © Robert N. Hotchkiss.)

instability. The distal humerus may also undergo bony disso-lution over months, resulting in more laxity and instability. I use interposition arthroplasty with hinged fixation very sparingly in the post-traumatic patient. The goals should be limited to some pain relief and a notable gain in motion (espe-cially flexion). Few if any patients achieve a high-performance elbow with heavy lifting capacity and full mobility.

Postoperative Management

Adjuvant Therapy for Heterotopic Ossification
The efficacy of nonsteroidal medication or irradiation for the prevention of HO has not been studied using randomized double-blind trials. Nonetheless, there are numerous reports that support the use of indomethacin or low-dose radiation

for the prevention of recurrent growth of HO.[10,22,26,37,53,56] The use of gentle CPM, passive turnbuckle splinting, or dynamic external hinged fixation has undoubtedly diminished the incidence of HO, irrespective of adjuvant therapy. Jupiter and colleagues reported abandoning the use of any nonsteroidal agents and reported no pathologic recurrence of HO. I am less certain and usually ask patients to take a single daily dose of indomethacin (75 mg slow release) for 6 weeks after release. Some patients are unable to tolerate these medications because of either gastrointestinal symptoms or headache.

In adults who have widespread HO and appear to have a tendency for formation with only minor trauma, I will use radiation therapy. Patients who have undergone major organ transplantation are especially vulnerable to HO formation and usually are not permitted to take oral anti-inflammatory agents.[46]

Physical Therapy and Splinting

Static Splints

A knowledgeable therapy department is a valuable, perhaps crucial asset for success in treating stiff elbows. Each patient, once the contracture is released, may benefit from physical therapy to overcome the spasm and pain associated with immediate motion. As with many conditions, the frequency of visits to the therapist varies from patient to patient. However, the need for splints is nearly universal. Several texts and articles describe the fabrication and use of these devices.[18,23,33,66] Undoubtedly, there will also be continued improvement in the design, comfort, and effectiveness as materials and technology improve. I do not use any dynamic splints, including the Dynasplint, for elbow contractures. I have found that patients do not tolerate these splints and compliance is very low. The splints described in

this text rely instead on intermittent passive positioning. With these splints, an incremental displacement is applied to the joint, followed by stress relaxation of the muscle and soft tissue. For reasons that remain unknown, this approach, much like an Ilizarov lengthening, is more effective with my patients. The constant torque applied by the dynamic splints is less well tolerated, which often lowers compliance.

The splints I use on a regular basis are designed to maintain the gains made in the operating room. Seldom if ever can a surface splint (as opposed to hinged external fixation) increase the motion that was achieved on the table.[17]

Resting Extension Splint. For patients using CPM, my colleagues and I have made use of the resting extension splint, which is fabricated 3 to 4 days postoperatively. The splint is worn to maintain extension after removing the CPM device, usually at night. A slight extension moment applied by tightening the splint's strap is most effective at maintaining the position of the elbow at or near full extension. If the elbow is tending toward a flexion contracture of 30 degrees or more, a turnbuckle should be considered.

Turnbuckle Splint (for Extension or Flexion). The turnbuckle splint (Fig. 25-6), as first reported by Green and McCoy,[9,18] is invaluable in static progressive splinting. In my view, this splint is most helpful for patients with a 25- to 40-degree flexion contracture that requires mechanical assistance to increase extension. The Mayo Clinic has a variation on this theme that has also been used with success.[31]

These splints are generally required for 8 to 12 weeks after surgery. Initially the splints cannot be used because of pain and swelling. As the acute postoperative swelling and pain subside, these are most useful. The duration of wear must be tailored to the individual. Most cannot wear them

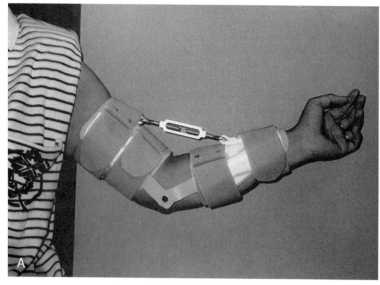

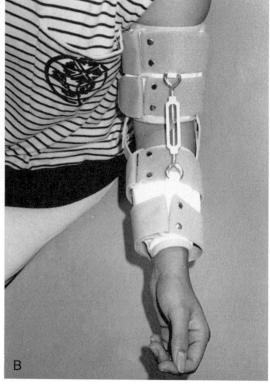

FIGURE 25-6. The turnbuckle splint is especially effective with flexion contractures of more than 40 degrees. Once the patient achieves more extension, other splinting devices may be more effective. (Courtesy of S. Davila, San Antonio, TX.)

all the time, especially when a significant displacement force is applied. However, even if these splints only help maintain the position gained in the operating room during the early phase, they are worth using. Later, the splint will help regain the motion that has been temporarily lost during the acute postoperative pain.

The "Come-Along" Flexion Splint. Improvement in flexion is highly valued by the patient, more so than gains of extension. I have found that a static progressive splint, fabricated from D-rings and straps, is well tolerated and not as limiting or as complicated to construct as a turnbuckle device. The patient simply pulls the straps on either side in a sequential fashion, pulling the elbow into more flexion, as tolerated (Fig. 25-7).

Continuous Passive Motion

CPM devices have been used by many authors and are reported to assist in maintaining the motion gained after surgical release.[15,29]

I use CPM in all patients who have undergone open release but were not fitted with a dynamic hinged fixator. After arthroscopic release, a supervised outpatient program usually suffices with end-range splinting.

CPM is very helpful when used with a different principle in mind than continuous motion. My concept is that the device should be used as *intermittent passive positioning.* Rather than having the device flexing and extending the elbow on a continuous basis, my patients begin CPM the day after release, the first 12 to 24 hours being used for rest and elevation. The CPM is initially set at the maximal tolerable positions of extension and flexion. It is important to remove the bandages in the antecubital fossa because they will block

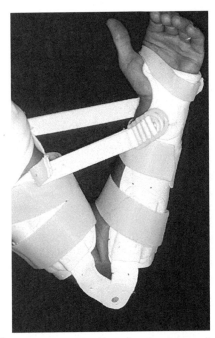

FIGURE 25-7. A "come-along" splint designed to increase flexion of the elbow. The patient advances each successive ring onto a hook placed on both the dorsal and palmar surfaces of the distal portion of the forearm section. Once the soft tissues have relaxed, the next ring is hooked into place. (© Robert N. Hotchkiss.)

flexion. The patient (or parent) is taught to use the button that stops the machine. The rate of displacement is set at the absolute minimum. The patient is then instructed to allow the device to move the elbow to maximal extension and then stop and hold at that position for 20 to 30 minutes. The button is then clicked to resume motion to the point of maximally tolerated flexion. Again, the position is held for 20 to 30 minutes. In this way the joint is held at the extremes of position from the beginning, which is the goal. Cycling the joint faster and more frequently has no advantage and may increase the amount of swelling. If the CPM evokes significant guarding, another nerve block, either axillary or interscalene, is administered. Most patients do not require this, but I do not hesitate to use another nerve block if needed.

Hinged External Fixation With Gear Drive: Passive Motion

When using the Compass Elbow Hinge, passive motion is usually initiated the second postoperative day. The gear mechanism is used to gradually gain extension over the first few days after surgery. Flexion and active motion, while using the unlocked position, are usually started as the swelling diminishes. For a more complete schedule of aftercare, the reader is referred to the technical manual provided by the manufacturer.

EXPECTATIONS AND RESULTS

The results of most reports and my personal experience are gratifying, with significant improvement in over 90% of patients. The published literature, as mentioned in the first section of this chapter, is filled with inconsistent inclusion criteria, different methods of operative exposure, and variance in postoperative management. This lack of standardization reflects the varied nature of the condition, differences among patients, and continued enhancements in surgical technique and postoperative devices and management. As with all complex surgical procedures, there are complications, disappointments, and failures.

For an uncomplicated flexion contracture (<40 degrees), extension will usually improve to 5 to 10 degrees of residual contracture without loss of flexion.

For more complex contractures with well-localized HO and motion limited in both flexion and extension (50 to 105 degrees), a final range of motion of 20 to 130 degrees is a reasonable expectation.

For patients with less than 40 degrees of total motion who require hinged fixation, a reasonable goal is 25 to 130 degrees.

Some patients do surprisingly well and can achieve even better results despite starting with a completely ankylosed joint (see Fig. 25-1).[53]

COMPLICATIONS AND OBSTACLES

Acute Recurrent Stiffness: "Gelling"

In my experience with the last 100 contracture releases, nearly 25% of patients experience a temporary setback in their progress. The primary reason to carefully follow the patients in the first 2 to 3 weeks after surgery is to assess the range of motion. It is critical to record their motion in the operating room and immediately after surgery while in the hospital. Commonly, the patient with preoperative loss of flexion begins to lose the gains made in the operating room in flexion. For me, the critical measure is a *failure to achieve 105 to 110 degrees* of flexion between the second and third week after surgery. If progress has stalled, the patient is taken to the recovery room for a repeat brachial block with as little sedation as possible. A *gentle* manipulation is performed. Often the elbow will be splinted in the flexed position for 12 hours followed by an immediate resumption of therapy and splinting. Less sedation allows the patient to witness and visualize the amount of motion achieved.

It is less common to lose extension in the early recovery phase, but the same level of scrutiny should be applied. Using this approach,* all but 3 of 50 patients were returned to within 15 degrees of the range of motion achieved in the operating room.

Nerve Palsies

The ulnar nerve, as noted earlier, is particularly vulnerable because of entrapment, possible previous injury, and simple need to handle the nerve in most cases. Care must be taken to painstakingly mobilize and protect the nerve during contracture release and if hinged fixation is used. Even with these precautions, I have found that about 10% of patients will have dysfunction of the nerve after release. Most of these resolve over a period of days, weeks, or months. Often there is preoperative ulnar nerve dysfunction that may not be evident. It is therefore important to document ulnar nerve function preoperatively and warn patients that nerve function may temporarily worsen and may not necessarily improve to normal after release. As mentioned earlier, arthroscopic release may pose even greater risk of permanent damage.[19]

The radial nerve is also vulnerable, especially if excessive retraction is applied through the lateral approach. The other point of vulnerability is distally at the level of the posterior interosseous nerve. If there is abundant HO at the lateral joint, the radial nerve should be carefully exposed and protected during excision of the HO. In most cases the HO lifts the nerve and muscle away from the joint. In unreduced dislocations with HO or in more proximal fractures, the radial nerve may be entrapped in bone and require meticulous, painstaking dissection from the surrounding bone. I have had two patients with temporary radial nerve palsies after contracture release. Both palsies resolved completely.

Heterotopic Ossification

Recurrent pathologic HO (i.e., ossification that blocks motion) after contracture release is rare. With the advent of better methods of restoration of motion in the early post-

operative period, this complication rarely occurs. It is not uncommon to see HO along the ligamentous structures or edge of the capsule. As a reflection of the benignity of these flecks of bone, this condition is sometimes referred to as "ectopic calcification" as opposed to HO. This bone usually does not restrict motion. In the more dramatic cases of ankylosis, the use of hinged external fixation has eliminated the need for temporary casting or splinting in a flexed position for instability, surely an invitation to recurrent HO in the past.

Pin Tract Infections

With the use of hinged external fixation, either the Mayo device or the Compass Elbow Hinge, the risk of pin tract infection is significant. I advise each of my patients that there is a 50-50 chance of needing to take oral antibiotics for the duration of treatment. (I also use this same figure for external fixation at the wrist.) The actual incidence of pin redness and erythema is 60% for the elbow. I treat each of these patients with a 5- to 7-day course of an oral cephalosporin. In no patient has pin tract–related osteomyelitis developed.

Joint Infection

A far more worrisome and potentially devastating infection may occur in the joint itself. The most vulnerable patient is one with poor soft tissue coverage and a history of previous infection. Another risk factor is distraction interposition arthroplasty in a patient with poorly vascularized bone. (The majority of infections in my practice have come after this procedure.) In these cases, the distal humerus often has a poor blood supply, and the material inserted as interposition is avascular and a foreign body. Additionally, external pins either at the joint or nearby may act as the nidus for spread into the joint. If these do become infected, the joint should be débrided of all foreign material and stabilized by using different pin sites. Although my experience with these patients is fortunately limited, they often perform surprisingly well despite the travail.

Soft Tissue Deficiencies or Wound Necrosis

Patients with burns or long-standing contractures may lack sufficient soft tissue to permit mobilization or develop skin necrosis over the tip of the olecranon, especially as they attempt to regain flexion.[7,9,53,59] If it is possible to predict the need for additional soft tissue, it is usually better to perform the soft tissue reconstruction as a separate procedure before contracture release. Depending on the amount of tissue needed, the flaps I most commonly use are either a gracilis free flap with split-thickness skin graft or a radial forearm flap as an island pedicle for smaller defects over the olecranon. The radial forearm flap, using the distal skin and fascia at the distal forearm, causes a donor defect that bothers some patients. Nonetheless, the coverage over the olecranon is ideal in thickness and mobility. The delayed recognition of skin loss after contracture release may temporarily stall progress, but acting quickly to cover the wound with sufficient soft tissue will usually rescue the contracture

---

*Reported at the annual meeting of the American Society for Surgery of the Hand, 2001.

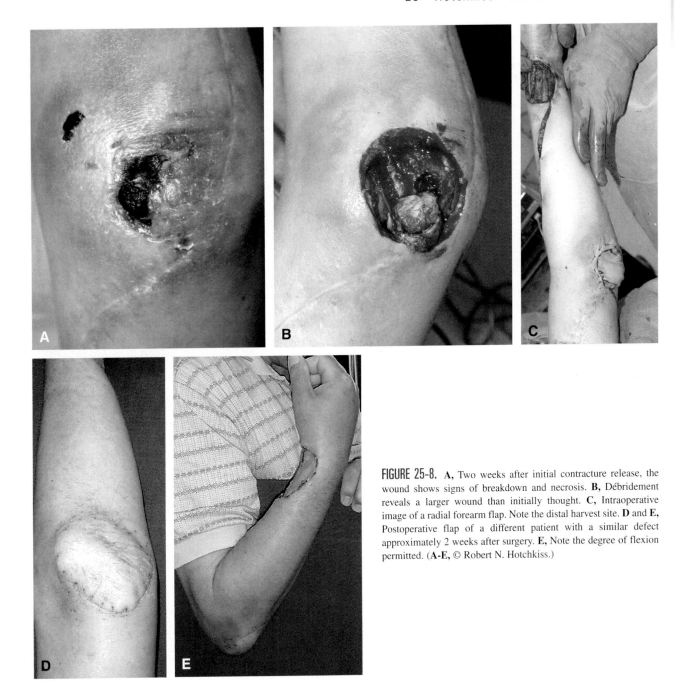

FIGURE 25-8. **A,** Two weeks after initial contracture release, the wound shows signs of breakdown and necrosis. **B,** Débridement reveals a larger wound than initially thought. **C,** Intraoperative image of a radial forearm flap. Note the distal harvest site. **D** and **E,** Postoperative flap of a different patient with a similar defect approximately 2 weeks after surgery. **E,** Note the degree of flexion permitted. (**A-E,** © Robert N. Hotchkiss.)

release and permit the flexion gained in the primary contracture release. In other words, do not sit and hope that the posterior ulceration will simply get better, especially if there is exposed bone (Fig. 25-8). (See Chapter 47 for a more detailed discussion of coverage of elbow defects.)

Complete Failure to Achieve Improved Motion

Three to 8 percent of patients will completely fail to achieve an improvement in motion and sustained painless function with stability. The usual cause of failure is articular surface destruction that is either underappreciated or progressive as motion and use are resumed. Morrey refers to this as intrinsic contracture.[42] The only option here is to resurface the elbow. In older patients, a total elbow arthroplasty is the optimal choice. In the younger patient, distraction interposition arthroplasty may be an option but must be carefully considered.

Finally, a small group of patients, estimated to be 1% to 2%, seem to suffer from a pathologic fibrosis of the joint. Despite careful dissection, relatively routine operative release and attentive rehabilitation fail to avoid re-formation of the contracture without any notable HO. In these rare cases,[2] I have returned to excise the contracted capsule and used hinged fixation with the passive drive (i.e., Compass Elbow Hinge) with success.

ANNOTATED REFERENCES

2. Bae DS, Waters PM: Surgical treatment of posttraumatic elbow contracture in adolescents. J Pediatr Orthop 21:580-584, 2001.

   These authors reported on 13 adolescent patients with very favorable results. The majority of patients underwent a medial approach to the joint.

5. Cohen MS, Hastings H: Post-traumaticc contracture of the elbow: Operative release using a lateral collateral ligament sparing approach. J Bone Joint Surg [Br] 80:805-812, 1998.

   The authors describe a safe method and the important lateral approach that should be understood by surgeons performing contracture release. The importance of sparing the posterolateral ligament complex is emphasized.

26. Jupiter JB, O'Driscoll SW, Cohen MS: The assessment and management of the stiff elbow. Instr Course Lect 52:93-111, 2003.

    This review article provides a useful summary from authors with great experience and expertise.

35. Mansat P, Morrey BF: The column procedure: A limited lateral approach for extrinsic contracture of the elbow. J Bone Joint Surg [Am] 80:1603-1615, 1998.

    These authors report on the results of 38 elbows treated with a lateral approach to the joint. The authors emphasize the utility and safety of the lateral approach for many patients.

38. Mih AD, Wolf FG: Surgical release of elbow-capsular contracture in pediatric patients. J Pediatr Orthop 14:458-461, 1994.

    The authors describe the treatment of nine pediatric patients, with six of the nine from prior trauma. This group of patients is difficult and more unpredictable than the adult patient.

42. Morrey BF: Posttraumatic stiffness: Distraction arthroplasty. Orthopedics 15:863-869, 1992.

    This important article emphasizes the influence of the quality of the articular surface on the outcome of surgical intervention. The indications for distraction interposition arthroplasty with hinged external fixation are also discussed reporting the high rate of complications.

53. Ring D, Jupiter JB: Operative release of complete ankylosis of the elbow due to heterotopic bone in patients without severe injury of the central nervous system. J Bone Joint Surg [Am] 85:849-857, 2003.

    The authors report on eleven patients with complete ankylosis of the elbow, seven from burns and eight after trauma. They describe the added complexity of treating complete ankylosis, including the tactical approach needed for soft-tissue coverage, safe exposure, and postoperative mobilization.

58. Stans AA, Maritz NG, O'Driscoll SW, Morrey BF: Operative treatment of elbow contracture in patients twenty-one years of age or younger. J Bone Joint Surg [Am] 84:382-387, 2002.

    Surgical treatment of the adolescent patient with post-traumatic elbow stiffness can be rewarding, but the authors found the results were less favorable than in a previous adult cohort. Patient selection and understanding the motivation of the family are crucial to success.

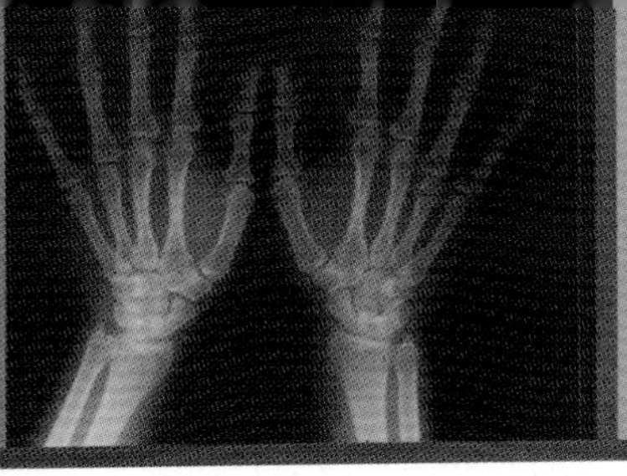

CHAPTER 26

Arthroscopy and the Thrower's Elbow

Struan H. Coleman • David W. Altchek

Arthroscopy of the elbow has emerged as an invaluable tool in both the diagnosis and treatment of pathologic processes specific to the throwing athlete. Arthroscopy is commonly used to remove loose bodies, débride osteophytes, and treat osteochondral lesions. We also believe it should be used to evaluate joint instability and, consequently, assess the need for ligament reconstruction. An understanding of the pathophysiology and natural history of elbow injuries specific to the throwing athlete is essential for effective management, because early intervention can prevent the late sequelae of medial instability.

ANATOMY AND BIOMECHANICS OF THE THROWER'S ELBOW

The elbow is a hinge joint with articulations between the radius, ulna, and humerus (Fig. 26-1). The ulnotrochlear and radiocapitellar articulations have contact through a flexion-extension arc of approximately 135 degrees[11] (Fig. 26-2)

whereas the proximal radioulnar joint, which lies at the base of the olecranon, articulates through a pronation-supination arc of 160 degrees[11] (Fig. 26-3). Elbow flexion is limited by contact of the soft tissue structures of the forearm, particularly the biceps brachii muscles; elbow extension is limited by the contact between the olecranon process of the ulna and the olecranon fossa of the humerus.[46] The ligaments between the ulna and carpal bones limit supination, whereas pronation is limited by the soft tissues on the surface of the radius and ulna.[11]

The articulations of the elbow can be divided into two major compartments: an anterior compartment comprising the anterior radiocapitellar joint laterally and trochlear coronoid medially (Fig. 26-4) and a posterior compartment comprising the posterior radiocapitellar joint laterally, the radioulnar joint centrally, and the olecranon-trochlear articulation medially (Fig. 26-5).

For the throwing athlete, the medial soft tissue structures of the elbow, the medial (ulnar) collateral ligament complex (MCL), the flexor pronator muscle group, and the ulnar

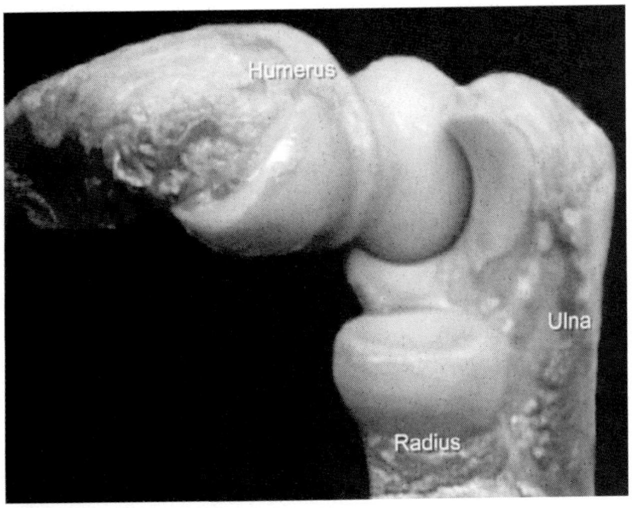

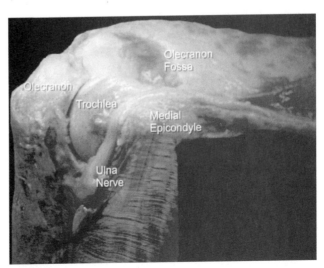

FIGURE 26-1. The elbow joint is a complex of three separate joints: radiocapitellar, olecranon-trochlear, and proximal radioulnar joints. (From Poehling GG, Ruch DS: Bowman Gray Orthopaedic Manual–1996. Winston-Salem, NC, Wake Forest University, 1996.)

FIGURE 26-2. The olecranon-trochlear joint allows flexion and extension. This configuration confers anteroposterior stability. (From Poehling GG, Ruch DS: Bowman Gray Orthopaedic Manual–1996. Winston-Salem, NC, Wake Forest University, 1996.)

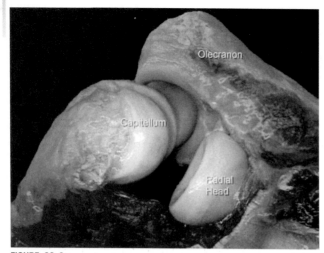

FIGURE 26-3. The radiocapitellar joint allows pronation and supination through the full range of flexion and extension. (From Poehling GG, Ruch DS: Bowman Gray Orthopaedic Manual–1996. Winston-Salem, NC, Wake Forest University, 1996.)

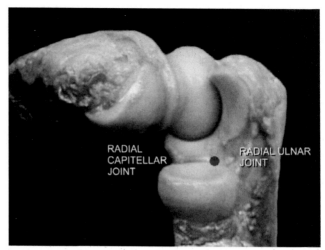

FIGURE 26-5. The posterior compartment: radiocapitellar joint, radioulnar joint. (From Poehling GG, Ruch DS: Bowman Gray Orthopaedic Manual–1996. Winston-Salem, NC, Wake Forest University, 1996.)

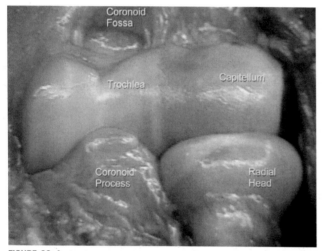

FIGURE 26-4. The anterior compartment. (From Poehling GG, Ruch DS: Bowman Gray Orthopaedic Manual–1996. Winston-Salem, NC, Wake Forest University, 1996.)

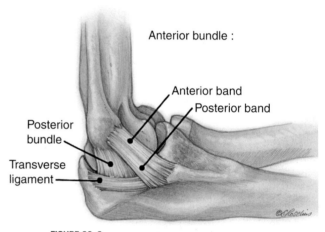

FIGURE 26-6. The anatomy of the MCL of the elbow.

nerve, are commonly injured.[11,21,42] The MCL comprises anterior and posterior bundles (Fig. 26-6).[42] The anterior bundle originates on the inferior aspect of the medial epicondyle of the humerus, inserts onto the sublime tubercle of the ulna, and is eccentrically located with respect to the axis of elbow motion.[42,76] The anterior bundle is further divided into anterior and posterior bands that tighten in reciprocal fashion with elbow flexion: the anterior band tightens with extension and the posterior band tightens with flexion.[17,21] This reciprocal arrangement allows the anterior bundle to remain taut through the full range of elbow flexion. The fan-shaped posterior bundle runs from the medial epicondyle to the medial margin of the semilunar notch and is a secondary stabilizer of the elbow, with flexion angles greater than 90 degrees.[17,21]

The anterior bundle of the MCL is the primary restraint to valgus stress; the radial head is a secondary restraint. Cutting studies demonstrated that the anterior band is the primary restraint to valgus rotation at 30, 60, and 90 degrees of elbow flexion and is a co-primary restraint at 120 degrees of flexion.[17,21] The posterior band is a co-primary restraint at 120 degrees of flexion and is a secondary restraint to valgus load at 30, 60, and 90 degrees of flexion.[17,21] The osseous articulations provide the primary stability to varus and valgus loads at flexion angles of less then 20 degrees and greater than 120 degrees. The posterior bundle is a secondary restraint at 30 degrees of elbow flexion and is not susceptible to valgus load when the anterior bundle is intact.[17]

The flexor-pronator group is composed of the pronator teres, the flexor carpi radialis, the palmaris longus, the flexor digitorum superficialis, and the flexor carpi ulnaris. The flexor pronator group originates from the medial supracondylar ridge and the medial epicondyle of the humerus. The ulnar nerve is also located on the medial elbow and is susceptible to injury in the throwing athlete, particularly as it passes through the cubital tunnel and then between the two heads of the flexor carpi ulnaris (Fig. 26-7).

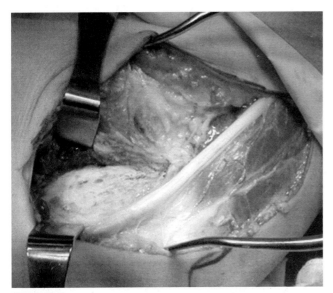

FIGURE 26-7. A dissection of the medial elbow showing the ulnar nerve before it dives between the two heads of the flexor carpi ulnaris.

BIOMECHANICS OF THROWING

The phases of the throwing motion have been described.[21] The transition from late cocking to early acceleration, in which the speed of elbow extension has been estimated to reach 3000 degrees/sec, generates loads on the medial elbow estimated between 100 and 120 Newton meters in the elite pitcher; these loads approach the tensile strength of the MCL.[21,42] The radiocapitellar joint, as a secondary restraint to valgus load, sees compressive and shear loads as forces are transferred across the elbow to the lateral side; these forces can lead to fragmentation of the lateral joint.[11,42,47,56]

During the throwing motion, the flexor-pronator group dynamically facilitates transfer of the loads from the medial elbow distally; however, electromyographic data comparing normal throwers to those with MCL insufficiency demonstrate that the dynamic stabilizers of the flexor pronator group are unable to compensate for MCL laxity, and, in fact, show slightly decreased activity in the setting of injury.[42]

The elbow reaches terminal extension during the follow-through phase, characterized by rapid deceleration and dissipation of the forces across the elbow.

THE THROWING ATHLETE: VALGUS INSTABILITY, EXTENSION OVERLOAD, AND IMPINGEMENT

Repetitive valgus loading of the MCL in the overhead athlete, categorized as an overuse syndrome, can lead to microtears of the ligament and subsequent attenuation.[11,42,47,56] Conway and coauthors reported that 90% of the MCL tears in their group were acute-on-chronic injuries and most commonly occurred in the midsubstance of the anterior bundle.[26] MCL insufficiency in the throwing athlete results in medial instability and abnormal valgus rotation of the elbow; the resulting abnormal mechanics of the elbow is termed *valgus extension overload*.[11,42,47,56] When untreated, valgus extension overload of the elbow has three main consequences, listed in order of chronicity (Fig. 26-8):

1. Increased contact pressures over a decreased area in the posteromedial elbow, particularly between the medial tip of the olecranon and the medial crista of the humeral trochlea
2. Posterior medial and posterior impingement of the elbow, with a wedging of the olecranon into the fossa during acceleration, and the subsequent development of osteophytes and possible loose bodies within the elbow joint
3. Increased compressive forces across the radiocapitellar joint with cartilage injury, lesions of osteochondritis dissecans, and fragmentation

HISTORY OF THE THROWING ATHLTE WITH AN INJURY TO THE MEDIAL SIDE OF THE ELBOW

The majority of throwing athletes with a pathologic process of the elbow will present with a history of episodic medial side and/or posterior pain with late cocking, early acceleration, and follow-through. Throwers with an acute injury to the MCL, although rare, will experience a sudden onset

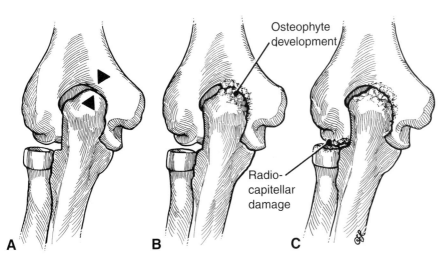

FIGURE 26-8. Drawing depicting the effects of valgus extension overload on the posterior and lateral aspects of the elbow.

of medial pain, with or without a "pop," and an immediate inability to throw. The acute-on-chronic injury to the MCL is characterized by episodic medial pain with one event of sharp pain and the inability to throw. The athlete with MCL attenuation and medial instability may also describe an inability to throw at normal speeds, loss of control, and arm fatigue.

Chronic injury to the MCL often results in ulnar neuritis because inflammation of the ligament produces a secondary irritation of the nerve, as the nerve passes through the cubital tunnel. The incidence of ulnar nerve symptoms in the throwing athlete ranges from 11% to 40% in the literature.[4,11,26,42] Patients will describe pain and numbness around the nerve and into the hand in the ulnar nerve distribution. In the setting of chronic MCL injury and valgus extension overload, athletes may also describe loss of extension secondary to posterior osteophytes, locking from loose bodies, crepitation, and lateral pain from radiocapitellar joint chondromalacia or osteochondritis dissecans.

The history of elbow pain in the throwing athlete should include the following information:

1. The duration of symptoms
2. The phase of the throwing motion that elicits symptoms
3. The location(s) of the pain
4. The presence of ulnar nerve symptoms
5. The level of the athlete's performance (i.e., the speed of the pitch)

PHYSICAL EXAMINATION

Observation of the elbow may reveal an effusion in the setting of acute injury. Fluid in the elbow is usually palpated in the soft triangle formed by the radial head, the lateral epicondyle, and the tip of the olecranon. Next, range of motion is assessed with attention to loss of extension. Flexor-pronator injury is best evaluated with palpation of the tendon with resisted forearm pronation. The medial epicondyle should be palpated to rule out epicondylitis. The ulnar nerve can be palpated directly for irritation and subluxation. Posterior tenderness should alert the examiner to posterior impingement secondary to medial injury and instability.

We do not believe that injury of the MCL can be accurately assessed by direct palpation, owing to the overlying muscle group and the close proximity to the ulnar nerve. Direct testing for MCL injury is performed by placing a valgus load across the elbow at 30 degrees of flexion with the patient lying supine. To apply the valgus load the examiner places one hand on the distal humerus to control rotation and the other hand on the forearm. The forearm is maximally pronated, and the elbow is flexed to 30 degrees during the application of the valgus force (Fig. 26-9). The test is positive when (1) the maneuver reproduces the patient's symptoms of medial elbow pain and (2) some degree of laxity is present. MCL instability is better assessed at higher elbow flexion angles, but it is difficult to stabilize the humerus with more than 30 degrees of flexion.

O'Driscoll[71a] has described a test for MCL injury that he has termed the *moving valgus stress test.* The patient is placed supine, and the shoulder is placed in abduction and

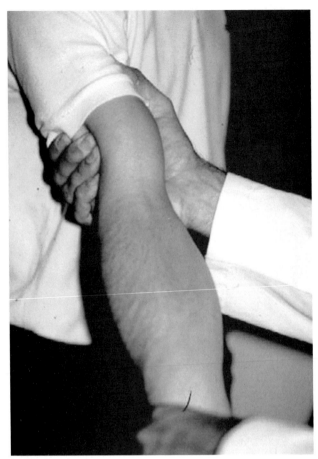

FIGURE 26-9. Physical examination of the elbow depicting a valgus stress test for the evaluation of the MCL.

external rotation. Next, a valgus load is applied to the elbow while the elbow is moved through an arc of flexion-extension. The test is positive for MCL injury when it produces pain localized to the medial elbow. Based on preliminary studies and our own observation this test is sensitive for MCL injury.

IMAGING

Standard radiographs of the elbow are obtained for the throwing athlete with elbow pain. These include anteroposterior, lateral, and axial views. An oblique axial view with the elbow flexed to 110 degrees is sometimes useful for evaluating posteromedial osteophytes.[114]

The standard radiographs of the thrower's elbow may yield the following findings[42]:

- Spurs on the posterior tip of the olecranon, which are usually medial and may be fragmented (Fig. 26-10)
- Calcification within the MCL (Fig. 26-11)
- Medial spurs at the joint line between the humerus and ulna adjacent to the MCL
- Loose bodies, usually located in the olecranon fossa. (Up to 30% of loose bodies are not visualized with plain radiographs.)

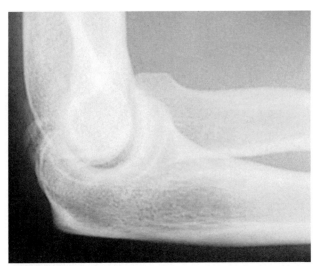

FIGURE 26-10. Radiograph of the elbow depicting a posterior spur with fragmentation.

An additional imaging modality is useful when evaluating elbow pain and dysfunction in the throwing athlete and may be critical when determining the competency of the MCL. A prospective study comparing computed tomographic (CT) arthrography and magnetic resonance imaging (MRI) of the elbow in throwing athletes for the evaluation of

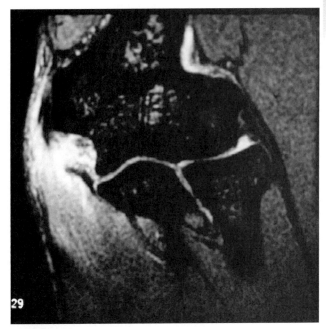

FIGURE 26-12. MR image of the elbow depicting an injury to the MCL.

the MCL reported that CT arthrography has a sensitivity and specificity of 86% and 91%, respectively, whereas MRI is 57% sensitive and 100% specific.[107] Saline- or gadolinium-enhanced MRI improves the sensitivity of diagnosing MCL injury to 92%.

Recent advances in MRI using three-dimensional volumetric gradient-echo techniques with axial and sagittal sections have obviated the need for contrast agents at some institutions, as illustrated in Figure 26-12.[87] In addition to ligament injury, MRI can elucidate cartilage changes in any of the compartments. At the present time we regard MRI in a 1.57-T magnet with an appropriate elbow coil as the "gold standard" for confirming the diagnosis of MCL rupture or for staging the degree of injury.

ELBOW ARTHROSCOPY

Historical Perspective

In 1931, Burman[15] described elbow arthroscopy in cadavers using a 3-mm endoscope. He concluded that arthroscopy of the elbow was not feasible "since the joint space is so narrow for the relatively large needle" and that the anterior approach was "out of the question." In 1932, after he had successfully performed 10 elbow arthroscopies in cadavers, Burman revised his opinion and concluded that the elbow joint "can be visualized directly by means of the arthroscope."[15]

Johnson,[46] in 1981, described a proximal medial portal that Burman alluded to in 1932. In 1985, Watanabe[114] in Japan, Andrews and Carson[2] in the United States, and Guhl[39] in the United States published clinical studies demonstrating the usefulness and the safety of elbow arthroscopy. In 1986, Lynch and colleagues[55] described the neurovascular structures and their relationship to the described portals. The first

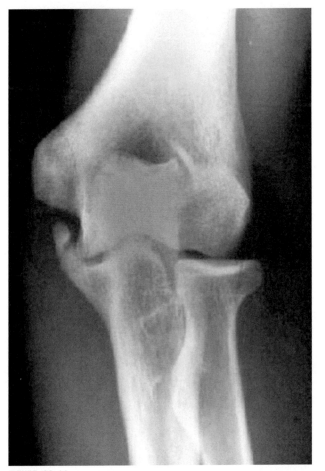

FIGURE 26-11. Radiograph of the elbow depicting calcification of the MCL.

warnings of problems with a distal anterolateral portal came in 1988 with a report by Papilion and coworkers[83] when they presented a case of a radial nerve palsy following the use of this portal. In 1989, Poehling and Whipple[84] described the prone position and the utilization of the proximal medial portal.

In 1990, Lindenfeld[53] and, in 1991, Verhaar[111] both concluded that it is safer to start from the anteromedial portal of the elbow than from the anterolateral portal. In 1993, Stothers and associates[102] accurately described a proximal lateral portal used in the anterior approach to the elbow. In 1994, Field and colleagues[34] described three lateral portals—distal, middle, and proximal—concluding that the distal portal (3 cm distal and 1 cm anterior to the lateral epicondyle) was the most dangerous and that the proximal lateral portal was the safest. In 1995, Stothers and associates[102] confirmed that the proximal lateral portal was safest.

Indications for Elbow Arthroscopy in the Throwing Athlete

The indications for arthroscopy of the elbow in the throwing athlete include evaluation of valgus instability, removal of loose bodies, removal of osteophytes, and treatment of osteochondritis dissecans.

Positioning

Elbow arthroscopy can be performed with the patient supine, prone, or in the lateral decubitus position. Anesthesia can be either general or an axillary block.

Portal Placement

There are seven portals that have been most commonly described for elbow arthroscopy and that can be further divided into anterior and posterior portals. Anterior portals are the proximal medial portal, the anterolateral portal, and the proximal lateral portal. The posterior portals consist of the midlateral (soft spot) portal, the posterior lateral portal, the transtriceps portal, and the accessory lateral portal.

Anterior Portals

The *anterolateral portal* is located 1 cm distal and 1 cm anterior to the lateral epicondyle (Fig. 26-13). It is safest to create this portal with an inside-out technique owing to the proximity of the radial nerve.

The *proximal medial portal* is located 2 cm proximal to the medial epicondyle and anterior to the intermuscular septum and provides visualization of the entire anterior compartment. The portal is created using a blunt trocar and cannula with the elbow flexed to 90 degrees. The septum protects the ulnar nerve while the trocar is advanced into the central portion of the elbow against the anterior margin of the humerus. This places the brachialis muscle between the arthroscope and the brachial artery and median nerve (Fig. 26-14).

The *proximal lateral portal,* as described by Stothers and associates[102] is 2 cm proximal to the lateral epicondyle of the humerus and lies on the anterior margin of the humerus (Fig. 26-15). It is considered safest of all anterior portals.

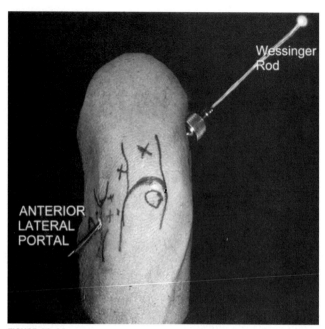

FIGURE 26-13. The anterolateral portal is established using an inside-out technique. (From Poehling GG, Ruch DS: Bowman Gray Orthopaedic Manual–1996. Winston-Salem, NC, Wake Forest University, 1996.)

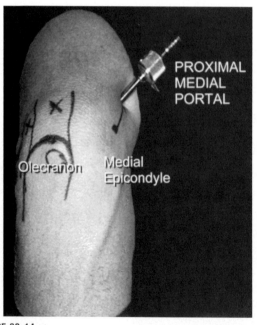

FIGURE 26-14. Establishment of the proximal medial portal is usually the first step. (From Poehling GG, Ruch DS: Bowman Gray Orthopaedic Manual–1996. Winston-Salem, NC, Wake Forest University, 1996.)

Posterior Portals

The *soft spot portal* is located at the center of a triangle bordered by the olecranon, the lateral epicondyle, and the radial head (Fig. 26-16). The soft spot portal is used for insufflation before arthroscopy and for visualization and instrumentation of the inferior radiocapitellar joint and the proximal radioulnar joint (Fig. 26-17).

The *posterolateral portal* is created at the level of the tip of the olecranon and just lateral to the border of the triceps

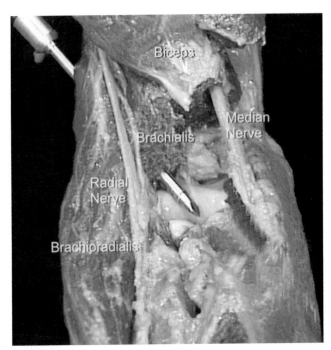

FIGURE 26-15. The proximal lateral portal. (From Poehling GG, Ruch DS: Bowman Gray Orthopaedic Manual–1996. Winston-Salem, NC, Wake Forest University, 1996.)

(Fig. 26-18). The posterior lateral portal is the main viewing portal for the posterior compartment of the elbow.

The *transtriceps portal* is created 3 cm proximal to the tip of the olecranon and is used for visualization and instrumentation of the tip of the olecranon, the humeral fossa, and the humeral trochlea (Fig. 26-19).

The *accessory or adjacent lateral portal* (Fig. 26-20) is made in the area of the soft spot portal and is used for visualization and instrumentation of the radiocapitellar joint, in particular for osseous and chondral procedures related to osteochondritis dissecans of the joint.

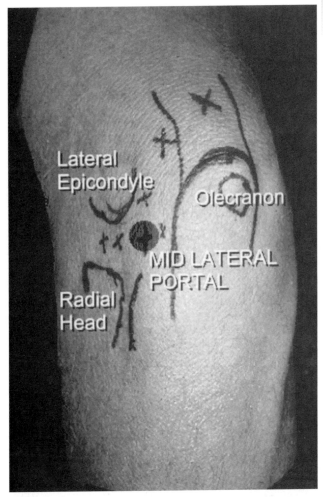

FIGURE 26-16. The midlateral (soft spot) portal. (From Poehling GG, Ruch DS: Bowman Gray Orthopaedic Manual–1996. Winston-Salem, NC, Wake Forest University, 1996.)

 Authors' Preferred Technique

We prefer to position the patient supine because it allows for easy conversion to open MCL reconstruction. We also prefer an axillary block rather than general anesthesia because of safety issues and postoperative pain management. The axillary block is administered, and a nonsterile tourniquet is placed on the upper arm. The arm is then prepped and draped in the usual sterile fashion; the arm is placed in a sterile arm holder and suspended across the chest (Fig. 26-21).

Landmarks, most importantly the course of the ulnar nerve, are drawn on the elbow using a sterile marker (Fig. 26-22). An 18-gauge needle is inserted into the midlateral (soft spot) portal and is used to distend the elbow joint with 30 mL of normal saline (see Fig. 26-17). Most elbow joints will allow a larger expansion of the anterior compartment in 90 degrees of flexion than in extension. The central portion of the capsule is loose, and this distention allows easy access into the joint.

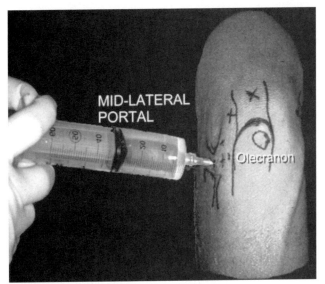

FIGURE 26-17. Elbow joint distention via the midlateral (soft spot) portal. (From Poehling GG, Ruch DS: Bowman Gray Orthopaedic Manual–1996. Winston-Salem, NC, Wake Forest University, 1996.)

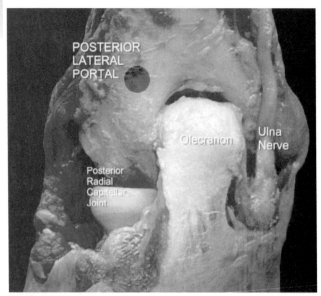

FIGURE 26-18. The posterolateral portal. (From Poehling GG, Ruch DS: Bowman Gray Orthopaedic Manual–1996. Winston-Salem, NC, Wake Forest University, 1996.)

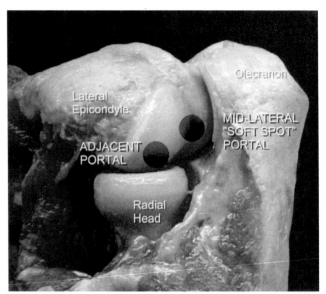

FIGURE 26-20. The adjacent portal. (From Poehling GG, Ruch DS: Bowman Gray Orthopaedic Manual–1996. Winston-Salem, NC, Wake Forest University, 1996.)

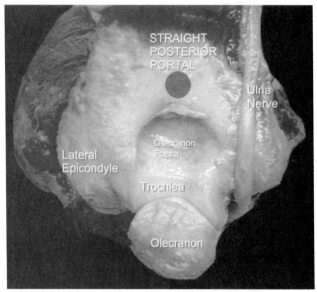

FIGURE 26-19. The straight posterior, or "transtriceps," portal. (From Poehling GG, Ruch DS: Bowman Gray Orthopaedic Manual–1996. Winston-Salem, NC, Wake Forest University, 1996.)

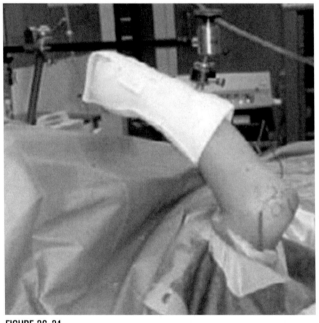

FIGURE 26-21. Author's preferred position for elbow arthroscopy. The arm is placed in an arm holder and positioned across the chest.

Anterior Compartment Arthroscopy and Pathology in the Throwing Athlete

The first portal developed is the proximal lateral portal, followed by the proximal medial portal. The anterior compartment can then be visualized in its entirety from both the lateral and medial portals. From the lateral portal we evaluate the medial capsule, the coronoid process, the medial humerus, and the anterior humeral fossa. From the lateral portal loose bodies present in the humeral fossa can be morselized (Fig. 26-23). In older throwers who have early osteoarthritis and loss of flexion, coronoid spurs are resected

with the arthroscope in the lateral portal and a 3.5-mm shaver in the medial portal (Fig. 26-24).

Medial laxity is evaluated with the arthroscopic valgus stress test. Medial ulnohumeral opening of 1 to 2 cm suggests complete anterior bundle insufficiency (Fig. 26-25); an opening of greater than 4 mm usually indicates complete MCL insufficiency. Timmerman and Andrews[105] report that they are able to visualize 20% to 30% of the anterior band of the MCL through the anterior portals and approximately 50% of the posterior band through the posterior portals. We have reported that while we are able to visualize the entire

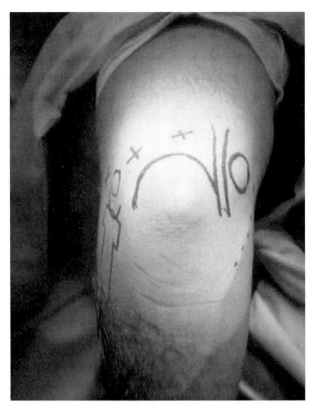

FIGURE 26-22. Landmarks are drawn on the elbow before the start of arthroscopy. Landmarks (in a clockwise direction) include the radial head, lateral epicondyle, olecranon, ulnar nerve, and medial epicondyle.

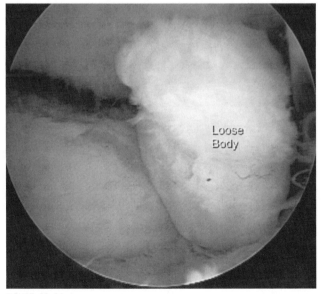

FIGURE 26-23. A loose body in the anterior compartment of the elbow joint. (From Poehling GG, Ruch DS: Bowman Gray Orthopaedic Manual–1996. Winston-Salem, NC, Wake Forest University, 1996.)

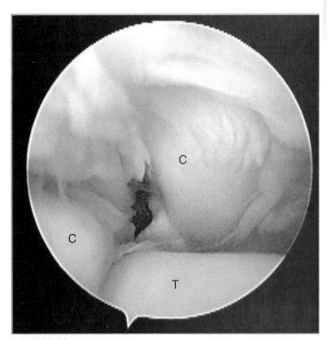

FIGURE 26-24. Arthroscopic photograph showing the coronoid process (C), the olecranon (O), and the trochlea (T).

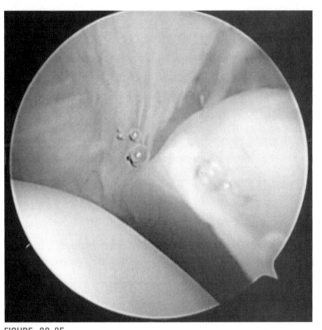

FIGURE 26-25. Arthroscopic photograph depicting an opening of the medial ulnohumeral joint of more than 1 cm.

posterior band of the MCL through a posterior portal, 90% of the time we believe the anterior band is not visible with elbow arthroscopy.[33]

The arthroscopic valgus stress test, in combination with the history, physical examination, and imaging studies, can help the surgeon decide about the need for MCL reconstruction in the throwing athlete. Conversion to open reconstruction from diagnostic arthroscopy is easily achieved. Surgical techniques for MCL reconstruction have been described in the literature.

Posterior Compartment Arthroscopy and Pathology in the Throwing Athlete

Before placing the arthroscope in the posterior compartment we place a large (6.5 mm) inflow cannula into the anterior compartment. Additionally, we use inflow through the

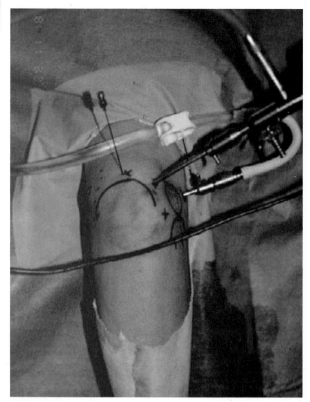

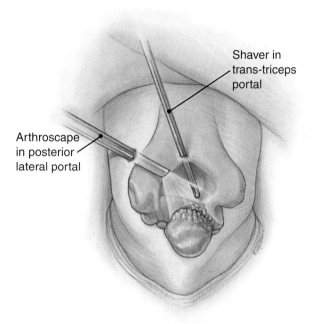

FIGURE 26-27. A drawing depicting the posterolateral portal and its use in reaching pathology located on the medial aspect of the olecranon and humerus.

arthroscope. We begin arthroscopy of the posterior compartment with the posterolateral portal for visualization. The transtriceps portal is then established and becomes the working portal (Fig. 26-26). Arthroscopy of the posterior compartment in the throwing athlete is used to evaluate and resect a posteromedial osteophyte on the olecranon, remove loose bodies, and treat cartilage lesions of the capitellum and radial head.

Posteromedial and Posterior Olecranon

The medial olecranon and medial humerus are visualized by placing the arthroscope in the medial gutter through the posterolateral portal (Fig. 26-27). A fragmented spur of the posteromedial olecranon, if present, is débrided with a 3.5-mm shaver through the transtriceps portal (Fig. 26-28). Chondromalacia of the medial cristae of the humeral trochlea and posteromedial olecranon is often present in the thrower's elbow and is indicative of early MCL insufficiency.[3,11,42] In our experience, 70% of throwers who have chronic MCL insufficiency also have fragmented lesions, particularly posteromedially.

Next, the tip of the olecranon is evaluated for spurring and osteophyte formation (Fig. 26-29). A 3.5-mm shaver is then used to resect the tip of the olecranon (Fig. 26-30). The tip of the olecranon is excised most easily from medial to lateral. Care should be taken to resect a minimal amount of bone and to avoid injury to the triceps insertion. A postresection radiograph can be obtained in the operating room (Fig. 26-31). Loose bodies, when encountered, are removed through the transtriceps portal.

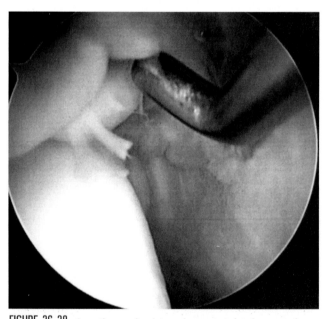

FIGURE 26-28. An arthroscopic picture demonstrated a fragmented spur arising from the posteromedial olecranon. The probe in the picture was introduced through the transtriceps portal.

Lateral and Medial Gutters

To view the lateral gutter the arthroscope is placed in the posterolateral portal (Fig. 26-32). The medial gutter is approached with the arthroscope in the transtriceps portal. Loose bodies are removed from the gutters as indicated.

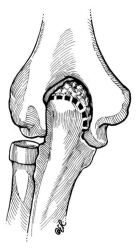

FIGURE 26-29. An illustration depicting an abnormal tip of the olecranon.

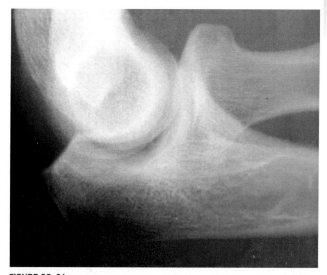

FIGURE 26-31. A radiograph of the elbow after a resection of the tip of the olecranon. Note the squared tip of the bone.

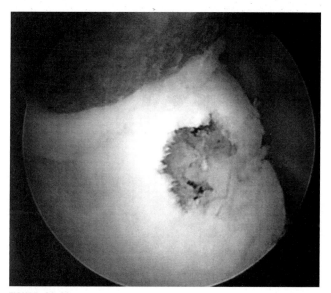

FIGURE 26-30. An arthroscopic photograph showing the tip of the olecranon after resection with a 3.5-mm shaver through the transtriceps portal.

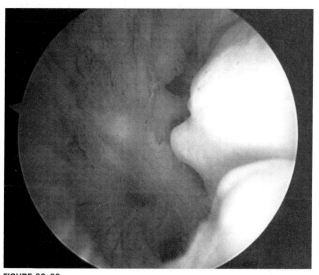

FIGURE 26-32. An arthroscopic view of the lateral gutter. The arthroscope is placed through the posterolateral portal.

Radiocapitellar Joint

The radiocapitellar joint is primarily visualized by directing the arthroscope down the lateral gutter from the postero-lateral portal. The cannula can be directed more anteriorly or posteriorly depending on the location of the pathology. Accessory portals in the radiocapitellar region are used to better visualize lesions of the posterior capitellum.

The capitellum and radial head are evaluated for bony and articular cartilage fragments (Fig. 26-33). All fragments should be removed and the base of the lesion microfractured (Fig. 26-34).

POSTOPERATIVE CARE

Postoperatively patients are placed in a sling and a well-padded dressing. Patients undergoing MCL reconstruction are braced, and motion is restricted to between 45 and 90

degrees of flexion. Motion is advanced to full over a 5-week period. After a strengthening program is instituted patients return to tossing at around 4 months postoperatively.

For patients undergoing débridement alone, postoperative rehabilitation is focused on immediately restoring full motion followed by a strengthening program. A stretching program begins with wrist flexors and extensors followed by elbow flexors and extensors. Low-weight, high-repetitive isometric exercises are incorporated early to improve endurance. Special attention is given to strengthening the flexor carpi radialis and pronator teres, which can become weak with inhibition. Isometric and isokinetic programs are advanced to plyometrics to induce a rapid transition between eccentric and concentric muscle contraction during the throwing motion.

In the early stages of rehabilitation after elbow arthro-scopy, significant time is spent to restore shoulder strength and relieve any posterior shoulder contracture. Strengthen-

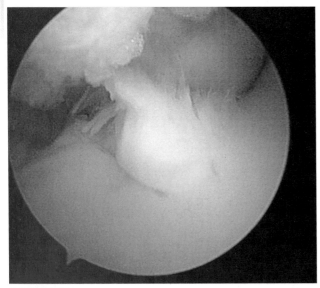

FIGURE 26-33. An arthroscopic picture showing a chondral defect of the capitellum. The camera is introduced through the posterolateral portal and directed down the lateral gutter to visualize the radiocapitellar joint.

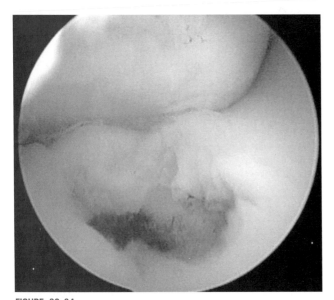

FIGURE 26-34. An arthroscopic picture after treatment for a capitellar lesion with débridement and microfracture.

ing of the rotator cuff and periscapular muscles is instituted early in the postoperative period. Finally, an interval throwing program is introduced as the patient's strength improves. Generally after débridement alone tossing is allowed within 6 to 8 weeks.

OUTCOMES

For throwers who undergo arthroscopic débridement without MCL reconstruction, reoperation rates are high[4,21] and are most often due to unrecognized medial instability. One fourth of baseball players requiring a second surgery required an MCL reconstruction.[107] Other reasons for reoperation in this setting include inadequate initial débride-

ment, particularly of the posterior osteophytes, osteophyte re-formation, and untreated osteochondritis dissecans of the capitellum.

For throwers who undergo MCL reconstruction and débridement, the rates of patients who return to competition at the same level range from 61% to 97%.[11,21,47] The operative technique and the postoperative rehabilitation program appear to be the two most significant predictors of outcome for this group of patients.

For throwing athletes with a stable elbow who undergo arthroscopy for posterior impingement there is a high rate of return to sports at the same level. However, we, along with other authors, have found that the most common cause for posteromedial impingement is partial or complete tears of the MCL. Observation alone in the setting of MCL injury has been shown to have a significant failure rate. We believe that the arthroscopic valgus stress test, along with a careful history, physical examination, and the appropriate imaging studies, is essential when determining medial instability and the need for an MCL reconstruction.

COMPLICATIONS

Careful portal placement during elbow arthroscopy is crucial to avoid neurovascular damage. The literature reports the radial nerve to be injured most commonly; the ulnar median and, in particular, both the posterior and anterior interosseous nerves are also at risk.[96] Savoie and Field report an incidence of complications related to elbow arthroscopy to be approximately 3%, or 16 complications reported from 465 cases of elbow arthroscopy; 7 of these were transient whereas 9 were permanent deficits.[96] Neurovascular structures are particularly at risk during the creation of medial portals as well as during anterior capsular release for flexion contractures. A knowledge of elbow anatomy should help the surgeon to avoid injuring neurovascular structures during arthroscopy of the elbow joint.

CRITICAL POINTS: ELBOW ARTHROSCOPY IN THE THROWING ATHLETE

ETIOLOGY

- Repetitive valgus overload of the MCL
- Attenuation of the MCL
- Results in medial elbow instability
- Abnormal valgus rotation of the elbow
- Increased contact pressures in the posteromedial elbow
- "Valgus extension overload"

PATHOLOGY OF VALGUS EXTENSION OVERLOAD

- Posteromedial and posterior impingement
- Chondromalacia of the medial cristae of the trochlea

CRITICAL POINTS: ELBOW ARTHROSCOPY IN THE THROWING ATHLETE—cont'd

PATHOLOGY OF VALGUS EXTENSION OVERLOAD—cont'd

- Chondromalacia of the posteromedial olecranon
- Osteophytes, spurring, and loose bodies
- Osteochondritis dissecans and fragmentation of the radiocapitellar joint

CLINICAL MANIFESTATIONS

- Medial side and/or posterior pain
- Arm fatigue
- Loss of throwing velocity and control
- Failure of conservative treatment

INDICATIONS

- Evaluation of valgus instability
- Removal of loose bodies
- Removal of osteophytes, spurs
- Treatment of osteochondritis dissecans

TECHNICAL POINTS

- Position patient supine with arm across chest.
- Use an axillary block.
- Apply a nonsterile tourniquet.
- Draw landmarks.
- Distend the elbow with 30 mL of saline through the "soft spot."
- Develop proximal lateral and proximal medial portals.
- Evaluate medial capsule laxity, medial humerus, coronoid, and anterior fossa.
- Remove osteophytes and treat osteochondritis dissecans.
- Place a 6.5-mm inflow cannula into the anterior compartment.
- Establish the posterolateral portal (arthroscope).
- Establish the transtriceps portal (working portal).
- Evaluate and treat posteromedial osteophytes on the olecranon.
- Resect the tip of the olecranon.
- Remove loose bodies.
- Evaluate and treat osteochondritis dissecans of the radiocapitellar joint.

POSTOPERATIVE CARE (DÉBRIDEMENT)

- Apply a well-padded dressing and sling.
- Begin early range-of-motion exercises and strengthening program.

CRITICAL POINTS: ELBOW ARTHROSCOPY IN THE THROWING ATHLETE—cont'd

POSTOPERATIVE CARE (DÉBRIDEMENT)—cont'd

- Begin stretching: wrist then elbow.
- Start endurance training with high-repetition isometrics.
- Strengthen flexor carpi radialis and pronator teres.
- Strength shoulder range of motion.
- Begin tossing at 6 to 8 weeks after surgery.

ANNOTATED REFERENCES

17. Callaway GH, Field LD, Deng XH, et al: Biomechanical evaluation of the medial collateral ligament of the elbow. J Bone Joint Surg Am 79:1223-1231, 1997.

    Elbow instability and pain in throwing athletes can result in large part from injury to the anterior bundle of the MCL. Clinical examination of complete tears is difficult to detect. This paper sought to determine the angle of elbow flexion in which valgus angulation was most pronounced and, therefore, could be detected on manual testing. The anterior and posterior bands of the anterior bundle have been proven to tighten reciprocally. These bands were placed under maximum valgus load to determine their vulnerability to injury.

26. Conway JE, Jobe FW, Glousman RE, Pink M: Medial instability of the elbow in throwing athletes: Treatment by repair or reconstruction of the ulnar collateral ligament. J Bone Joint Surg Am 74:67-83, 1992.

    Overload of elbow ligaments and microtrauma can result in ligament weakness and rupture. This study was designed to assess the results of repair and reconstruction of the MCL in throwing athletes. In addition, factors that affect these results were also discussed.

40. Hamilton CD, Glousman RE, Jobe FW, et al: Dynamic stability of the elbow: Electromyographic analysis of the flexor pronator group and the extensor group in pitchers with valgus instability. J Shoulder Elbow Surg 5:347-354, 1996.

    Fine-wire EMG was used in this study to compare elbow muscle function and stability in baseball pitchers with MCL deficiency and pitchers with normal elbows. The results have shown that both groups displayed similar patterns of muscle activity during the various phases of throwing, but they differed in the level of muscle activity. Maximizing resistance to valgus stress and maintaining normal firing patterns within the flexor pronator group can be bolstered by rehabilitation and strengthening.

69. Mullen DJ, Goradia VK, Parks BG, Matthews LS: A biomechanical study of stability of the elbow to valgus stress before and after reconstruction of the medial collateral ligament. J Shoulder Elbow Surg 11:259-264, 2002.

    The stability of an MCL reconstruction throughout a full arc of elbow flexion was first tested in this study. The results show that reconstruction of the anterior bundle of the MCL using a palmaris tendon autograft provides excellent stability at acute angles of flexion postoperatively.

76. O'Driscoll SW, Jaloszynski R, Morrey BF, An KN: Origin of the medial ulnar collateral ligament. J Hand Surg [Am] 17:164-168, 1992.

Anatomic observation of the elbow has shown that the anterior bundle of the MCL originates as the anterior inferior surface of the medical epicondyle. This study was designed to assess the percentage of medial epicondyle that can be removed without interfering with the MCL. In addition, the question of whether the MCL attaches to both the condyle and epicondyle was also examined.

87. Potter HG: Imaging of post-traumatic and soft tissue dysfunction of the elbow. Clin Orthop 370:9-18, 2000.

Basic radiographic evaluation of elbow trauma continues to use anteroposterior, lateral, and oblique views. However, soft tissue trauma to the ligaments of the elbow can be optimally observed through thin-slice high-resolution MRI. In addition, this paper discusses further methods of diagnostic imaging for the elbow, such as ultrasound and tomography.

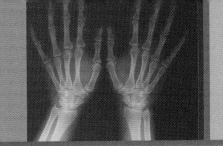

CHAPTER 27

Total Elbow Arthroplasty

Mark S. Cohen • Leonid I. Katolik

Total elbow arthroplasty has become increasingly used for the treatment of debilitating elbow arthropathies. Although clinical outcomes after total elbow arthroplasty were initially disappointing, modifications in surgical technique and implant design have made this an increasingly reliable procedure. Prosthetic replacement of the elbow relieves pain and typically provides a functional arc of motion, thereby allowing patients to better perform activities of daily living. The longevity and durability of the implants still remain in question, especially in patients younger than 70 years of age and with expectations of normal use. Long-term follow-up studies will be available as more of the devices are implanted in a wider range of patients. The high potential for mechanical failure and loosening currently makes this procedure most suitable for older patients with lower demands. Refinements in materials, implant design, and surgical technique may one day extend the suitability of total elbow arthroplasty to a wider array of pathologic processes as well as to a broader demographic spectrum.

PREOPERATIVE EVALUATION

The most common indication for total elbow replacement is arthritis that causes pain, stiffness, and loss of function.[24] The most common group of patients who undergo elbow replacement are those with rheumatoid arthritis. The majority of these patients have bilateral disease and often multiple joint involvement. Post-traumatic arthritis, acute comminuted fractures of the distal humerus, and primary osteoarthritis are less frequent indications. Pain relief is the primary goal of total elbow replacement. Improved function includes enough motion, stability, and strength for the tasks of daily living, but because of current implant designs, high loads or lifting objects greater than 10 pounds is discouraged for fear of more rapid prosthetic failure. Once loss of motion occurs, upper extremity function is significantly impaired. Because elbow motion permits the patient to position the hand in space to and from the body, it is very difficult to compensate for elbow stiffness, particularly loss of flexion. If successful, total elbow replacement can both relieve pain and restore a useful arc of motion for activities of daily living.

Rheumatoid Arthritis

Approximately two thirds of patients with rheumatoid arthritis have arthritic changes in the elbow. Isolated presentation of rheumatoid arthritis of the elbow occurs in less than 10% of patients. As with other major joints affected by rheumatoid arthritis, the elbow undergoes a predictable pattern of intra-articular degeneration of the ulnohumeral and radiocapitellar surfaces, ultimately leading to functional loss in advanced cases. Rheumatoid arthritis is commonly classified into four radiographic stages, based on physical examination and plain radiographs (Fig. 27-1):

Stage 1 reveals osteoporosis and active synovitis with normal radiographs.

Stage 2 demonstrates chronic synovitis with mild arthritic changes and mild loss of joint space.

Stage 3 is characterized by active synovitis with either joint articular destruction (type A) or an advanced loss of subchondral bony architecture (type B).

Stage 4 demonstrates extensive loss of bone and gross instability.

Rheumatoid arthritis of the elbow can also lead to secondary compressive neuropathies of the upper extremity. Antecubital cysts and proliferative synovitis may extend through the joint, producing compression of the posterior interosseous nerve in the region of the proximal radioulnar joint. Similarly, the ulnar nerve lies along the medial ulnohumeral joint and may be compromised by bony deformity, instability, as well as direct soft tissue compression from synovitis.[24,61] A careful neurologic evaluation is thus required in any patient being considered for elbow replacement surgery. The preoperative examination must also include careful assessment of the ipsilateral shoulder, distal radioulnar joint, wrist, and hand.

Patients with rheumatoid arthritis often develop means to effectively compensate for loss of elbow function despite significant joint destruction. These patients typically have multiple joint involvement and lower physical demands. As with other joints affected by rheumatoid arthritis, the function of the upper limb exceeds expectations based on radiographs alone.

The nonsurgical treatment of rheumatoid arthritis of the elbow is similar to the treatment of arthritis in other joints. Nonsteroidal anti-inflammatory medications may decrease

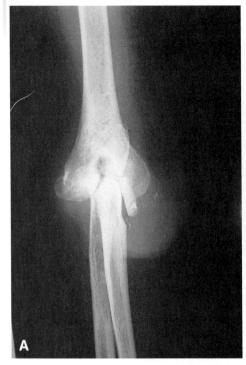

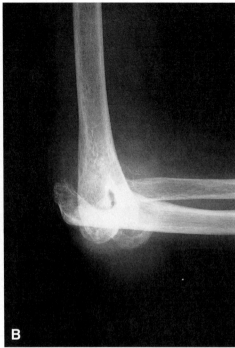

FIGURE 27-1. Anteroposterior (**A**) and lateral (**B**) radiographs of a severe stage 4 rheumatoid elbow. The loss of bone support and ligamentous integrity leads to gross joint instability.

synovial reactivity and alleviate pain and swelling in more mild cases. Immunosuppressive agents, such as gold salts, methotrexate, and antimalarial agents, are used for more aggressive disease, although serious side effects include thrombocytopenia, hepatic or renal insufficiency, and pulmonary toxicity. Newer anti–tumor necrosis factor agents, such as leflunomide or infliximab, may be quite effective but also may reduce the patient's ability to mount a response to infection. Oral corticosteroids are a common adjunct to medical management, and intra-articular corticosteroid injections can be effective for acute episodes of painful synovitis and "flares" about the elbow. These can be combined with a short period of static long-arm splinting in an effort to mollify symptoms.

Post-traumatic Arthritis

The elbow is one of the most intolerant joints in the body to trauma, with a high propensity for stiffness and arthritis. Because of the tightly constrained nature of the joint, articular incongruity is often poorly tolerated and can lead to progressive loss of motion, function, and pain. Post-traumatic arthritis is an increasingly common indication for replacement arthroplasty.[36,58] The treatment of post-traumatic arthritis, however, must take into account the age and activity level of the patient, degree of impairment, and joint pathology involved. Given the limited survivorship of elbow arthroplasty, non-implant techniques such as internal fixation for nonunion and malunion,[9,38,48] joint release and débridement, and interposition arthroplasty should be considered in younger, more active adults. Evaluation of deformity and the quality of the articular surface may require additional radiographic studies in these patients, such as computed tomography. Replacement arthroplasty should be considered when the ulnohumeral joint is no longer

salvageable (Fig. 27-2). This option is typically limited to individuals older than age 60 years with lower physical demands.

Fractures of the Distal Humerus

Total elbow arthroplasty may be indicated for elderly patients with displaced and severely comminuted fractures of the distal humerus.[4,12,13,20,23,49] In the past, the so-called bag-of-bones treatment was recommended because the fracture fragments were too small and the bone too osteoporotic to permit stable internal fixation. However, this treatment of hopeful neglect frequently resulted in significant pain, stiffness, and decreased function of the upper extremity. In the low-demand patient, total elbow replacement after a fracture beyond repair may permit a more rapid return to function. Total elbow replacement should also be considered in patients with preexistent joint destruction and rheumatoid arthritis (Fig. 27-3). Elbow arthroplasty should again be limited to older individuals with lower demands.

Primary Osteoarthritis

Primary osteoarthritis of the elbow is rare in women and affects middle-aged and older individuals. Most cases involve the dominant side in men at or after the fifth decade, and many patients report a lifetime of manual labor. The most common presenting complaint in this population is pain at the extremes of motion with loss of terminal flexion and extension. Loss of forearm rotation is less common. Mechanical symptoms can also be present owing to loose bodies within the joint.

Individuals with primary arthritis of the elbow typically have bony overgrowth and osteophytes at the coronoid and olecranon processes, respectively. Fluffy densities may be

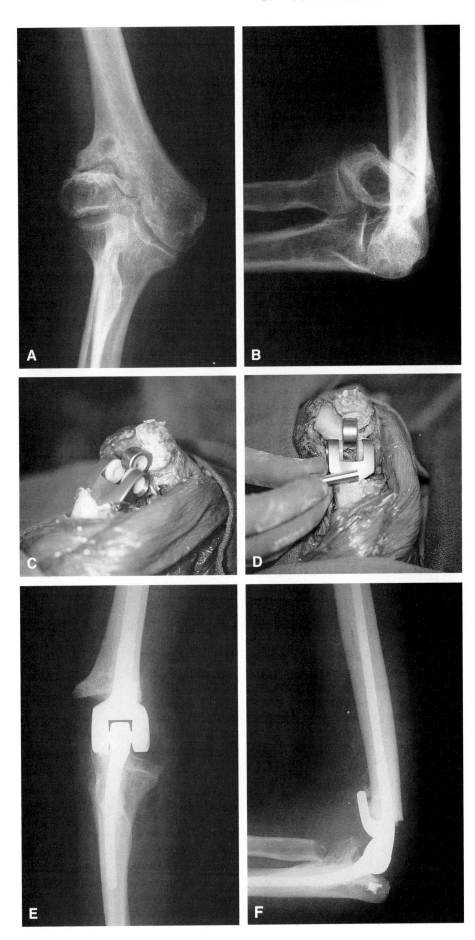

FIGURE 27-2. Anterior (**A**) and lateral (**B**) radiographs depicting post-traumatic arthritis of the elbow in a 66-year-old man with severe deformity and loss of function. **C,** Intraoperative view with triceps reflected showing humeral and ulnar components cemented into place. Remaining humeral condyles have been resected. **D,** Semi-constrained arthroplasty uses axis pin to unite components. Final anteroposterior (**E**) and lateral (**F**) radiographs of total elbow arthroplasty.

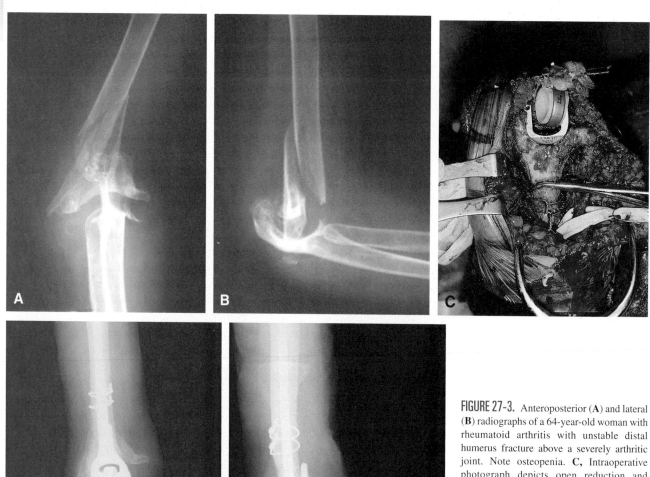

FIGURE 27-3. Anteroposterior (**A**) and lateral (**B**) radiographs of a 64-year-old woman with rheumatoid arthritis with unstable distal humerus fracture above a severely arthritic joint. Note osteopenia. **C,** Intraoperative photograph depicts open reduction and internal fixation of fracture with cerclage wires and cemented arthroplasty components. Postoperative anteroposterior (**D**) and lateral (**E**) radiographs. Note reduction of humerus fracture. *Continued*

observed filling the olecranon and coronoid fossae, and loose bodies can be seen. Narrowing at the radiocapitellar joint is a common finding. This joint may be the "wear generator" in many patients despite a lack of pain specifically during forearm rotation.[24] The central aspect of the ulnohumeral joint is characteristically spared in this patient population. Pain throughout the entire arc of elbow motion usually signifies synovitis or articular cartilage degeneration in the central ulnohumeral articulation. This is rare and only seen in late disease.

Up to 20% of patients with primary osteoarthritis of the elbow will have some degree of ulnar neuropathy. The close association of the nerve to the posteromedial joint capsule leaves it susceptible to impingement from osteophytes or from medial joint synovitis expanding the capsule. Early cubital tunnel syndrome in these patients may often manifest as pain at the medial elbow. It is thus important to

examine these individuals for signs of ulnar nerve irritability and traction.

Initial management of primary elbow arthritis consists of activity modification, anti-inflammatory medication, intra-articular injection, and, occasionally, therapy. When these modalities prove unsuccessful, surgical intervention may be warranted if symptoms persist. Given the generally young age and high functional demand of patients with primary osteoarthritis at the elbow, prosthetic replacement is generally not recommended. Joint débridement and release has traditionally served as the primary surgical option for the treatment of these patients because the central ulnohumeral joint space is typically maintained. Total joint replacement is reserved for individuals with more advanced arthrosis with lower functional demands who are older than 60 to 65 years of age.[27] The mechanical failure of total elbow replacement in this group of patients has been well docu-

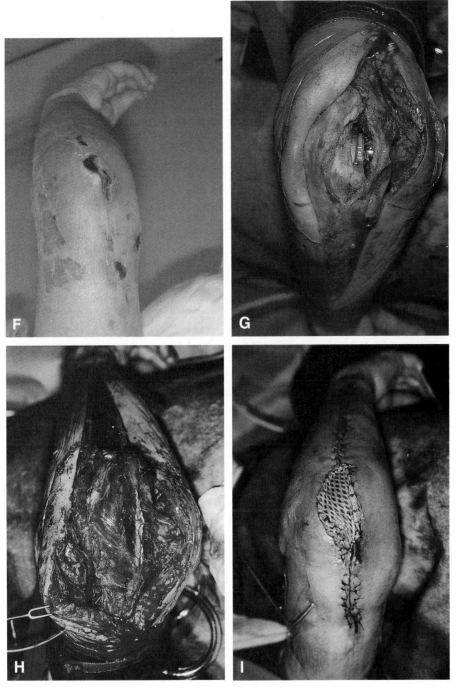

FIGURE 27-3—cont'd. F, Patient unfortunately had a wound dehiscence, which failed local wound care. She was on several immunosuppressive agents. **G,** Intraoperative view once skin is opened. The component is visible and communicates with the wound due to partial triceps subluxation laterally. **H,** Joint and component coverage obtained with flexor carpi ulnaris muscle pedicle flap. **I,** Final coverage with split-thickness skin graft over muscle. The joint cultures grew several organisms. The patient received 6 weeks of intravenous antibiotics and is on chronic oral suppression therapy. She had not had a clinically recurrent infection by the time of her 3-year follow-up.

mented and should be carefully reserved for those patients who can reduce their level of activity.

Hemophilic Arthropathy

Patients with hemophilia may present with severe joint destruction as a result of hemophilic arthropathy. Involvement is commonly multiarticular, affecting shoulders, elbows, hips, knees, and ankles. Potentially severe functional deficits may result. Surgical intervention for hemophilic arthropathy requires a coordinated, multidisciplinary approach. Factor VIII must be supplemented during the perioperative period. Furthermore, the prevalence of human immunodeficiency virus (HIV) infection in this population predisposes patients to considerable risks, which include an increased incidence of secondary infection and a more rapid progression to AIDS in patients with low CD4 counts.[15,26] Whereas prosthetic replacement of affected hips and knees in hemophiliacs is now almost commonplace, reports on results in this population are quite limited.[2,3] Further investigation is needed to define the role of total elbow replacement in treating hemophilic arthropathy.

CONTRAINDICATIONS

There are several absolute and relative contraindications for total elbow arthroplasty:

1. *The presence of infection at the elbow.* Any suspicion of infection in the skin, soft tissue, or bone should cause a postponement of the surgery.[71] Patients with rheumatoid arthritis with poor skin quality and taking immunosuppressive drugs are especially prone to catastrophic postoperative infection. Other sources of bacteria, such as the urinary tract, should also be evaluated. If an attempt at internal fixation for fracture has failed, the site should be suspected for deep infection and cultures obtained with the patient free of any antibiotic treatment. The organisms can be quite indolent, especially *Staphylococcus epidermidis.* Methicillin-resistant *Staphylococcus aureus* has become more common and should also be suspected.

2. *Complete ankylosis or the neuropathic joint.* In patients with complete and painless ankylosis of the elbow, implant arthroplasty may not improve overall function. Although improvement in functional arc of motion has been reported after conversion of elbow arthrodesis to prosthetic replacement,[10,33] the nature of the underlying pathologic process leads to frequent postoperative complications and a less predictable outcome. Total elbow replacement is contraindicated in patients with neuropathic joint destruction owing to the inherent inability of these patients to comply with postoperative restrictions.

3. *Poor quality soft tissue at the elbow.* Severely contracted, scarred, or burned skin needs to be assessed before considering total elbow replacement. For the implant to properly function, the skin and soft tissue needs to be both pliable and permit manipulation for placement of the implant. If there is inadequate soft tissue, a muscle flap should be considered before arthroplasty.

HISTORICAL REVIEW

The earliest successful attempt to replace a portion of the elbow with a metallic bearing surface was reported by Venable in 1952,[68] nearly 2 decades before Dee's report of the first total elbow arthroplasty in 1972.[6,7] In the intervening years we have witnessed ingenious and creative attempts to treat disorders of the elbow for which arthrodesis would have been the only alternative. A variety of bearing surfaces and materials, including acrylic, stainless steel, and nylon, were used to fashion both hemiarthroplasties and custom implants to replace either the distal humeral or proximal ulnar articular surfaces. Most notable were Eaton and Barr's report of endoprosthetic replacement of the distal humerus with a Vitallium component in 1965,[1] and later Johnson and Schlein's custom Vitallium prosthesis for replacement of the proximal ulna.[22]

Joint hemi-articular resurfacing prostheses further sought to provide a durable, less destructive means to restore articular congruity, pain relief, and motion. Examples included the Vitallium ulnar interposition or "saddle" surface replacement by Peterson and Bickel,[46] and the distal humeral resurfacing prosthesis designed by Stevens and Street.[63] Peterson

and Bickel's design, in spite of affording the recipient a limited arc of motion, enjoyed satisfactory relief of pain, stability, and, in many cases, longevity of more than 10 years. The Stevens-Street design showed results to be either poor or unpredictable in patients with inflammatory arthritis or hemophilia. However, success was reported in restoring adequate function in 80% of patients with post-traumatic arthritis.

It became clear that hinged arthroplasty, such as that designed and reported by Dee in 1972, generated large moments at the prosthetic interface and a high rate of implant loosening. The earliest attempts at nonconstrained designs were unstemmed resurfacing arthroplasties, such as the Pritchard,[47] Wadsworth,[55] and Kudo[28] prostheses. Long-term follow-up demonstrated an unacceptably high incidence of component loosening in the Wadsworth design, leading the investigators to conclude in 1984 that "prosthetic replacement of the elbow should be regarded as experimental."[55] The unstemmed Kudo design showed a high incidence (70%) of proximal subsidence of the humeral component, which was often severe enough to cause posterior displacement of the humeral prosthesis.[28] It became accepted that surface replacements should incorporate a stemmed design. Unfortunately, Kudo's stemmed humeral implant (Kudo 3) was plagued by fatigue failure of the stems, particularly in uncemented titanium designs and in patients in whom resorption of the condyles had occurred.[29]

The Souter-Strathclyde implant incorporated flanges projecting into the capitellum and the medial epicondyle to provide improved resistance to torsional forces compared with other unconstrained resurfacing prostheses (Fig. 27-4).[54,65] Long-term survivorship of 69% to 80% has been demonstrated. The Norway prosthesis has used a consistent design since 1982, although its use outside Norway is limited. It incorporates a locking ring into its nonhinged, semiconstrained, cemented design to improve stability if the collateral ligaments are deficient. A failure rate of 3.4% at a mean follow-up of 4.3 years has been reported.[52]

As the tightly constrained, hinged implants failed, second-generation loose or "sloppy" hinged designs were introduced, including the Coonrad-Morrey and Pritchard-Walker II designs. These theoretically allowed a linked prosthesis to act as a semiconstrained implant.[41] Biomechanical evaluation demonstrated that functional laxity after arthroplasty was less than the structural laxity of the implant, suggesting diminished load transfer to the cement-implant interface. To further strengthen the construct of the loosely hinged prosthetic design, an anterior flange was added. The introduction by Gschwend, Scheier, and Bahler of the GSB III semiconstrained prosthesis[17] illustrated these goals. Similarly, the anterior flange Coonrad-Morrey prosthesis significantly reduced the "windshield-wiper" effect of stem loosening in the humeral canal and resisted posteriorly directed forces that occur during elbow motion.

TYPES OF OPERATIONS

At present, two general types of implants currently exist for the arthritic elbow: linked and unlinked. An unlinked or nonconstrained prosthesis relies on adequate bony support

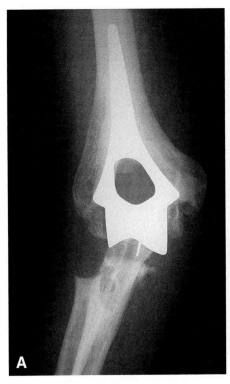
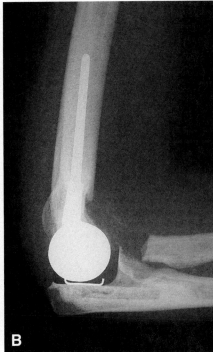

FIGURE 27-4. Anteroposterior (**A**) and lateral (**B**) radiographs of a Souter-Strathclyde nonconstrained implant. The ulnar component consists of polyethylene, which is radiolucent.

and collateral ligaments for stability. This theoretically decreases loosening at the bone-cement interface but carries a greater risk for instability, especially in the rheumatoid population. Currently available unlinked designs include the Souter-Strathclyde (Howmedica, Rutherford, NJ), Kudo (Biomet, Europe), Capitellocondylar (Johnson and Johnson, New Brunswick, NJ), Sorbie-Questor (Wright, Arlington, TN), and ERS (DePuy, Warsaw, IN) implants.

Semi-constrained devices have the advantage over unlinked with respect to stability. However, even with several degrees of varus-valgus laxity, the most popular "sloppy" hinge mechanisms allow only a small area of contact between the humeral and ulnar components, leading to high-contact stresses. Polyethylene wear of the bushing, osteolysis, and subsequent failure remain clinical problems.[21,33] Commonly used semiconstrained designs include the Coonrad-Morrey (Zimmer, Warsaw, IN), GSB III (Sulzer Orthopedics, Austin, TX), Pritchard II (De Puy, Warsaw, IN), and Triaxial (Johnson and Johnson, New Brunswick, NJ).

In practice, reports of pain relief and functional gains appear similar for linked and unlinked designs. Currently, however, the majority of implants used in the United States involve a linked mechanism. In an effort to improve on polyethylene wear, several newer implants have been introduced. Some do not depend on a true hinge for stability and will theoretically lead to decreased wear (Discovery, Biomet, Warsaw, IN). Other prostheses have the capacity to be inserted in an unlinked or a linked fashion (Latitude, Tornier, Saint-Ismier, France; Acclaim, DePuy, Warsaw, IN). No long-term data exist on these newer designs. It is hoped that continued advances in biomaterials and more anatomic designs will lead to improved and more durable implant options.

Authors' Preferred Method

We use a semiconstrained linked prosthesis with either a loose hinge or a spherical articulation[20] for the majority of elbow replacement surgeries. Although the unlinked designs should theoretically have lower loosening rates, this is not proven. The procedure is performed in a laminar flow room. The patient is positioned in a semi-lateral decubitus position on a bean bag, and the affected arm is rested across the chest on a bolster. A sterile tourniquet is applied. A posterior skin incision is utilized and taken down to the fascia, raising full-thickness fasciocutaneous flaps medially and laterally. The ulnar nerve is carefully dissected out and transposed anteriorly into a subcutaneous pocket and protected throughout the procedure.

Several options exist for reflection of the triceps mechanism to expose the joint. The traditional approach is that described by Bryan and Morrey in which the triceps is elevated from medial to lateral in continuity with the anconeus to expose the distal humerus and elbow. We have recently abandoned this approach owing to postoperative triceps insufficiency, presumed to be related to failure of the repair. We now use a straight triceps-splitting approach as described by Gschwend, in which the triceps muscle and tendon are split longitudinally and sharply elevated off the proximal ulna down the midline (Fig. 27-5).[11,17] This allows for a more satisfying repair of the triceps muscle and tendon at the completion of the procedure with less theoretical tendency for the triceps to slide back laterally off of the olecranon process. It is yet to be determined if the rate of triceps insufficiency will be reduced with this method.

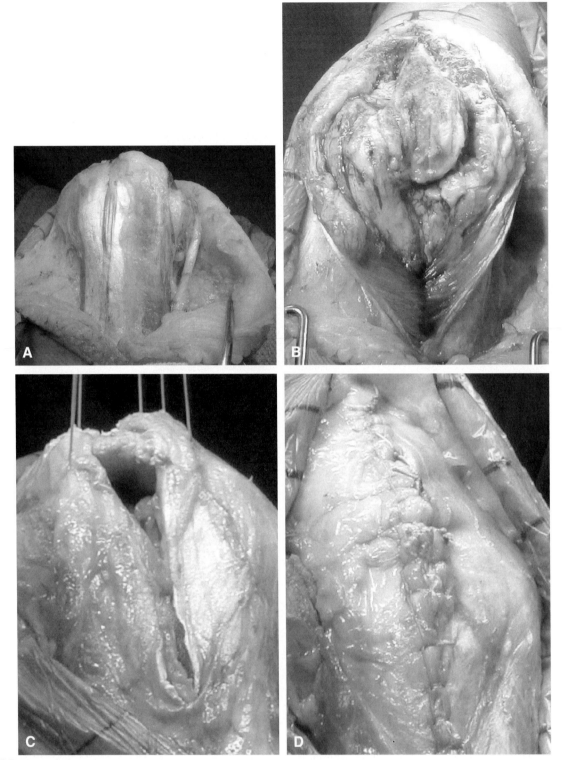

FIGURE 27-5. **A,** Intraoperative view of Gschwend triceps-splitting approach to the elbow. Note the ulnar nerve has been dissected out and protected. Split occurs in the tendinous portion of the triceps. **B,** Joint exposure obtained with full-thickness medial and lateral flaps. **C,** Sutures in place for repair and closure of the split. **D,** Final repair, with several sutures placed through drill holes in the olecranon.

Whichever approach is chosen to reflect the triceps mechanism, it is important to carefully dissect Sharpey's fibers off of the olecranon process in a subperiosteal fashion. This can be very tedious, especially in the rheumatoid population. A knife should be used for this purpose, not a monopolar cautery. The latter can lead to tissue necrosis and may inhibit tendon healing after repair. The insertion point of the triceps on the tip of the olecranon should be tagged to allow for anatomic repair after implantation. This may help decrease triceps dysfunction postoperatively.

In cases with deficient distal humeral columns, including fractures and nonunions, one can use a true triceps-sparing approach. In this way, the distal humerus is excised and one can work through either side of the triceps insertion while preserving its attachment to the olecranon (Fig. 27-6). Because triceps insufficiency is not uncommon after arthroplasty and humeral condylar resection does not affect the ultimate strength or functional outcome when using semi-constrained devices,[34,35] we have been resecting the distal humerus at the proximal aspect of the trochlea in very selected cases (e.g., elderly patients with rheumatoid arthritis). This approach necessitates complete release of the collateral ligaments and flexor-pronator and extensor muscle origins from the humerus. The theoretical disadvantages of muscle origin disruption and loss of bone stock allow one to implant the prosthesis without violating the triceps insertion on the olecranon. Rehabilitation is simplified, and this may improve elbow extension power and control.

Once the joint surfaces are exposed, including the trochlea, humeral columns, and the olecranon process, the bony work is initiated. Exposure is facilitated by hyperflexion and subluxation of the elbow with external rotation of the shoulder. The tip of the olecranon and the tip of the coronoid process are resected to decrease the potential for impingement. Bony impingement of the olecranon or coronoid should be checked both during trial implant insertion and after the permanent implant is seated. Unless the arthritis is limited to the ulnohumeral articulation, the radial head is excised. Care should be taken to place retractors around the neck of the radius to protect the posterior interosseous nerve, which lies just anterior to the radial head outside the elbow capsule. Next, the central aspect of the trochlea is resected and the humeral canal is entered with a bur. The entry point is typically more posterior than initially appreciated. Once the canal is defined, cutting guides are typically used to prepare the distal humerus, and trial implants can be evaluated. Complete seating of the prosthesis can be blocked by the anterior cortex, which occasionally has to be deepened to accept the anterior flange of the implant.

The ulna is more difficult to prepare than the humerus. The ulnar canal is commonly entered with a bur, and the opening is enlarged with a bur and rasps. Care must be taken not to perforate the thin cortices of the proximal ulna, especially in patients with rheumatoid arthritis. If the alignment is in question, an image intensifier may be helpful to confirm the direction of the rasp, bur, and stem. One must appreciate the 4- to 5-degree valgus angulation of the shaft of the ulna relative to the greater sigmoid notch. When there is difficulty seating a rasp, bone at the canal entry is most commonly the limiting factor. A posterior trough is commonly required in the olecranon to avoid placing the ulnar

component in flexion. Once component sizes are chosen, one should insert trial implants to ensure an adequate arc of motion without impingement.

During insertion of the trial components, the range of motion should be carefully examined. Joints that were quite stiff before surgery require a capsular release and may require a more generous resection of the distal humerus to achieve an acceptable position of extension, usually less than a 20-degree flexion contracture.

We use polyethylene cement restrictors in both the humeral and ulnar canals. As the humeral canal gets larger proximally, standard restrictors often do not allow for a seal and umbrella designs are more effective (Tornier, Saint-Ismier, France). The outer diameter of the ulnar restrictor must be trimmed to allow for passage down the shaft. Alternatively, a small piece of cancellous bone may be used in the ulna. The canals are lavaged, dried, and injected with antibiotic-laden cement in a retrograde fashion using a cement gun with thin tubing. It is helpful to cool the cement and inject in a more liquid state because it can become difficult to deliver viscous cement down long, thin tubing. Components are usually cemented individually with pressure maintained on the seated implants until polymerization is complete. Excess cement is removed during this process.

Hemostasis is obtained once the tourniquet is deflated and the triceps mechanism is meticulously repaired. We use a running, locking, Kevlar-reinforced suture passed through drill holes in the olecranon tip for reattachment. This aspect of the procedure is very important, and care must be taken to complete a secure and anatomic repair. Tension after reattachment of the triceps needs to be checked so that full flexion can be achieved without detachment. If the Gschwend splitting approach is chosen, the running, locking stitch can be placed several millimeters away from the tendon edge and additional side-to-side interrupted sutures can be placed centrally. More than one transosseous suture is commonly used with either method. The soft tissues are then closed in a routine fashion and the ulnar nerve is maintained in a subcutaneous position anterior to the epicondyle.

POSTOPERATIVE CARE AND EXPECTATIONS

In rheumatoid patients with thin and friable skin, we often immobilize the elbow for 10 to 14 days to allow for soft tissue healing before motion is instituted.[32] If the triceps was released from the ulna during exposure, the repair must be protected by restricting active extension against resistance for 6 to 8 weeks postoperatively. Initially, we often use a sling during the day with a night-time elbow orthosis in maximum extension to decrease the potential for a flexion contracture postoperatively. At follow-up, patients are counseled on the importance of protecting the joint from excessive loads. Empirically, a limit of 5 lb lifting with the operated arm after surgery is recommended. Yearly clinical and radiographic evaluations are arranged regardless of clinical symptoms.

The expected outcome after uncomplicated surgery is a near-painless and functional arc of elbow motion. Patients commonly do not recover terminal elbow extension but do ultimately regain full flexion within several months. Overall

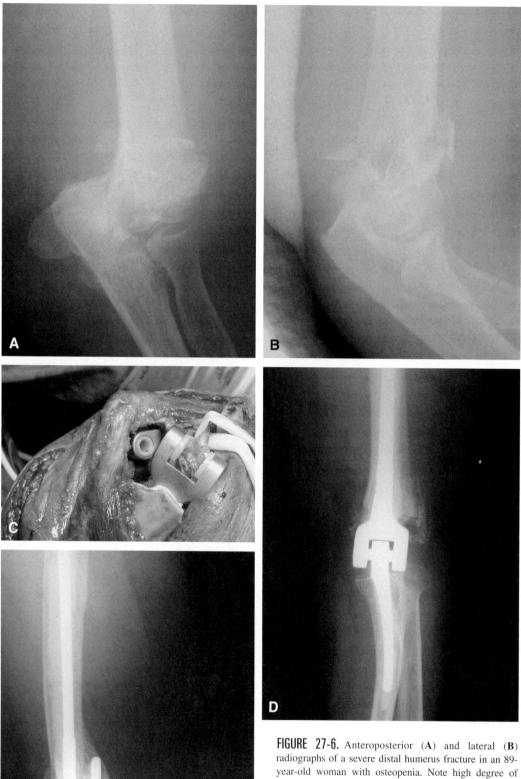

FIGURE 27-6. Anteroposterior (**A**) and lateral (**B**) radiographs of a severe distal humerus fracture in an 89-year-old woman with osteopenia. Note high degree of comminution and osteopenia. **C,** Intraoperative view showing triceps-preserving approach with exposure of the humerus by working on each side of the triceps mechanism without distal detachment. This approach is possible in fractures or nonunions when the distal humerus is resected. Anteroposterior (**D**) and lateral (**E**) radiographs postoperatively with cemented semiconstrained arthroplasty in place. Note condylar resection. (Photo **C,** courtesy of Graham King, MD.)

functional scores and satisfaction are generally higher and long-term complications lower in rheumatoid patients than for those with post-traumatic arthritis.[14] This relates to the lower demands of the rheumatoid population. While pain relief is almost uniformly excellent in rheumatoid individuals, range of motion often improves only modestly. This is especially true in patients with very limited elbow function preoperatively, such as that seen in juvenile rheumatoid disease. The elbows of these individuals often remain quite stiff even after successful arthroplasty.

For post-traumatic arthritis, results are less uniform. One study reported 38 of 41 joints being functional at 5-year follow-up with the use of a semiconstrained prosthesis for post-traumatic dysfunction. Ninety-five percent of these were believed to be satisfactory, with minimal or no elbow pain in 75% of cases. However, 27% of patients had a major complication. These included infection, component fracture, and bushing wear. The authors correlated failure with inability to adhere to the strict lifting requirements postoperatively and excessive preoperative joint deformity.[58]

When arthroplasty is used for acute trauma after distal humerus fracture, successful results can be obtained in selected patients. The largest study reviewed 49 cases with an average follow-up of 7 years. Many of the patients (62%) had coexistent conditions, with nearly 40% suffering from rheumatoid arthritis. It is therefore difficult to generalize to patients with only fractures. Although 93% of patients had a satisfactory outcome, 29% of patients reported complications. These included wound problems, transient nerve dysfunction, component fracture, and component loosening. The authors stressed the need for strict inclusion criteria when using arthroplasty in this setting.[23]

COMPLICATIONS

When the world literature is reviewed, the complication rate of total elbow arthroplasty varies between 20% and 45%.[19] Intraoperatively, fracture of a humeral condyle can be treated with simple excision. Alternatively, if the fragment is large, reduction and internal fixation can be considered (Fig. 27-7). The risk of intraoperative complications due to bone loss is significantly increased in individuals with advanced rheumatoid arthritis.[30] Late humeral condyle fracture can occur, most commonly along the medial column. This typically heals uneventfully with a short-term period of joint protection.

Regardless of the care taken in dissection and transposition of the ulnar nerve, sensory dysfunction is not uncommon after arthroplasty surgery. Ulnar motor weakness is less common. The incidence of postoperative ulnar neuropathy has been reported in up to 25% of patients.[19,40,61] Excessive traction on the nerve perioperatively, hematoma, constricting dressings, thermal damage due to polymerization of methylmethacrylate, and devitalization of the nerve during translocation have all been implicated as causative factors. Whereas incomplete sensory deficits typically improve with time, normal subjective sensation does not return in all cases, especially in the elderly with multiple comorbidities.

Elbow extension weakness after arthroplasty is more common than typically appreciated, especially if the triceps insertion has been detached using the traditional Bryan-Morrey approach.[37,39,45] In one review, mean extension strength was found to be less than 50% of the normal side using standardized testing.[35] Although the etiology of triceps insufficiency is unclear, possible explanations include alteration of the joint level affecting triceps tension and failure of the reattachment with tendon retraction or subluxation. We believe the latter to be more probable and have observed this mode of tendon failure during revision surgery for loosening (see Fig. 27-3). Fortunately, even with detachment of the triceps from its insertion on the olecranon tip, some extensor function typically remains. Because elbow extension weakness is reasonably well tolerated using gravity assistance, there is usually little indication for triceps repair or reconstruction owing to insufficiency after arthroplasty.

Instability after total elbow arthroplasty is largely limited to unlinked designs and is believed to occur with a mean frequency of 7%.[42,51] Prevention of instability with a non-linked prosthesis depends on meticulous technique with restoration of proper tension to the soft tissues after implantation. Ligamentous insufficiency is a relative contraindication for these designs. Furthermore, implants that sacrifice the radial head decrease lateral joint support and impart a greater load to the collateral ligaments. Finally, axial malalignment of either components may compromise stability.[25,62] Limiting elbow extension in the immediate postoperative period may minimize the incidence of dislocation.[60] If a dislocation occurs, immobilization of the elbow at 90 degrees for 3 to 6 weeks is anecdotally recommended. Recurrent symptomatic instability is addressed with soft tissue reconstruction when possible or revision to a linked design.

Disassembly of a linked prosthesis may occur. This was a particular complication in the earlier designs such as the GSB III.[18] It was believed that an overly extensive soft tissue release, as well as component malposition, might lead to a gradual overload of the linkage mechanism until ultimate disassembly.

Mechanical Failure

Mechanical failures, loosening, and osteolysis underscore the fact that arthroplasty is relatively contraindicated in patients who anticipate strenuous physical activity or who are not expected to comply with the postoperative protocol. Arthroplasty candidates must be willing to agree to postoperative limitations of no lifting greater than 5 or 10 pounds and no repetitive lifting of any object greater than 2 to 3 pounds. Optimal cementing technique may help minimize loosening. This includes careful canal preparation, the use of a cement restrictor, and the application of low viscosity cement with pressurization. These methods are thought to improve the initial fixation of the humeral component and perhaps to decrease the incidence of aseptic loosening.[5,8]

Unfortunately, wear debris and osteolysis can be seen relatively early even in individuals with lower demands (Fig. 27-8). This may be secondary to stress concentration and mechanical wear of the bushings in the current semiconstrained designs. Suboptimal positioning of the prosthesis may significantly affect longevity. For example, it has been shown that if the humeral component of the Coonrad-Morrey prosthesis is inserted in more than 10 degrees of malrotation, the varus and valgus laxity during the flexion

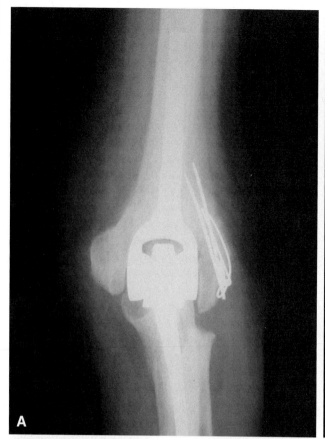

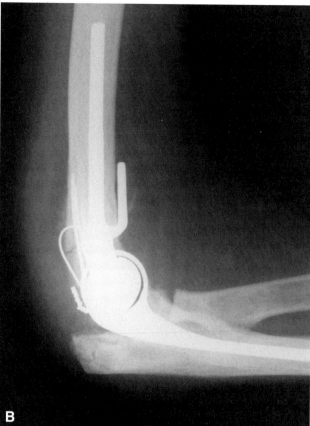

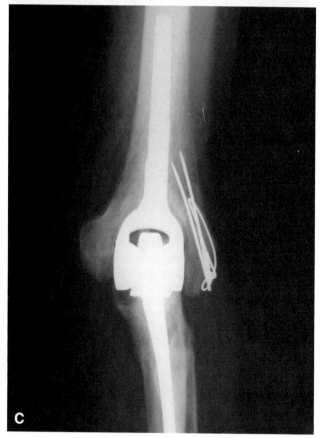

FIGURE 27-7. Anteroposterior (**A**) and lateral (**B**) radiographs depicting tension band wire technique used to repair fracture of the lateral column that occurred intraoperatively. Most commonly these fragments are excised. Internal fixation was chosen due to the patient's young age and the proximal extent of the fracture. This preserves bone stock as well as the extensor muscle origin at the epicondyle. **C,** Healing of fracture at 3-month follow-up.

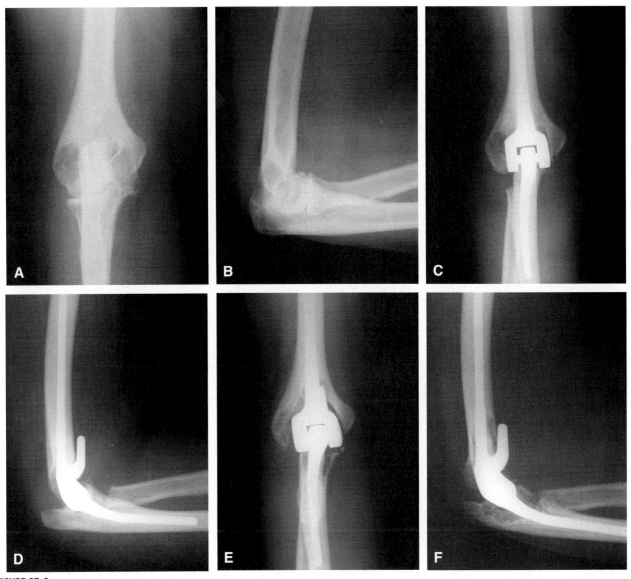

FIGURE 27-8. Anteroposterior (**A**) and lateral (**B**) radiographs of a 57-year-old woman with rheumatoid arthritis and advanced elbow arthritis. She failed conservative measures. Anteroposterior (**C**) and lateral (**D**) radiographs immediately postoperatively depicted a semiconstrained device. Anteroposterior (**E**) and (**F**) lateral films at 3-year follow-up. Note osteolysis involving the distal humerus and the proximal ulna adjacent to the hinge.   *Continued*

and extension arc follows the structural limits of the hinge.[59] This removes the theoretical advantage of the sloppy hinge mechanism and leads to increased stresses on the polyethylene and the bone-cement interface. Excessively tight soft tissues, such as that following inadequate release, may also contribute to wear.

If progressive osteolysis is noted on serial radiographs, even in the absence of symptoms, consideration must be given to revision surgery. If the components are stable and positioned appropriately, débridement, bone grafting, and replacement of the polyethylene bushings may be all that is indicated. Consideration may also be given to oral diphosphonates, which slow osteolytic progression. If the components are found to be loose intraoperatively, implant revision is required.

The potential for component fracture is inherent to any implantable device. For the elbow, a resultant force vector of up to three times body weight is directed anteriorly in

flexion and posteriorly in extension. Approximately 1 million compression-distraction loading cycles are generated per year.[37] In spite of these tremendous stresses, advanced metallurgy and modifications in prosthetic design make ulnar or humeral stem fracture an uncommon event, cited from 0.6%[19] to 12%.[58] The most common cause of implant fracture is periarticular osteolysis, leading to cantilever bending and fatigue fracture of the prosthetic stem (see Fig. 27-8). In this setting, revision surgery is required.

Periprosthetic fractures of the humerus and ulna after total elbow arthroplasty can be very challenging. This can be related to significant trauma to the upper extremity or represent a pathologic fracture from osteolysis and bone loss at the tip of the stem (Figs. 27-9 and 27-10). The incidence is cited as between 3% and 5%.[19,43] These are managed based on location of the fracture, the quality of prosthetic fixation, and the quality of the remaining bone stock. Experience with periprosthetic fractures in the lower

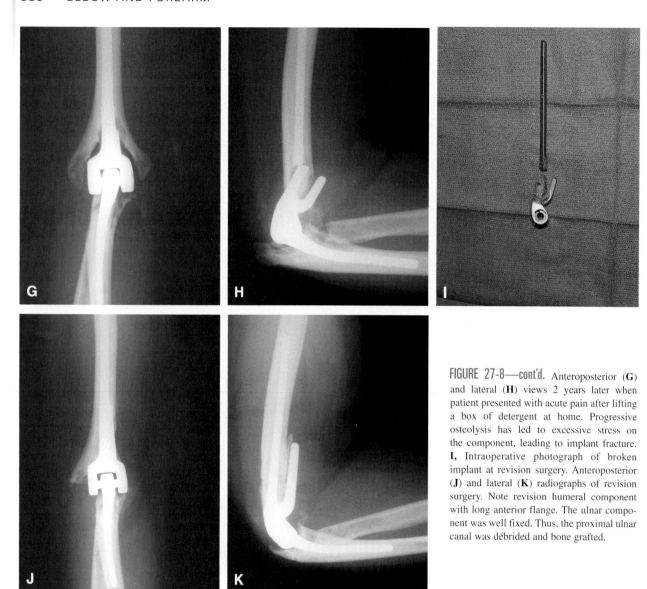

FIGURE 27-8—cont'd. Anteroposterior (**G**) and lateral (**H**) views 2 years later when patient presented with acute pain after lifting a box of detergent at home. Progressive osteolysis has led to excessive stress on the component, leading to implant fracture. **I,** Intraoperative photograph of broken implant at revision surgery. Anteroposterior (**J**) and lateral (**K**) radiographs of revision surgery. Note revision humeral component with long anterior flange. The ulnar component was well fixed. Thus, the proximal ulnar canal was débrided and bone grafted.

extremity[31,53] has been extrapolated and applied to the upper extremity.[43,56] However, noncemented stems, which comprise the bulk of revision fixation options in the lower extremity, are not available in revision total elbow arthroplasty. When the components are stable, standard internal fixation is typically indicated with or without the incorporation of allograft struts (see Fig. 27-9). Periprosthetic fractures around a loose humeral component can be treated with revision cemented arthroplasty using strut allograft augmentation to improve bone stock with predictable union rates.[56]

Infection

Infection is a potentially devastating complication of total elbow arthroplasty.[69] The rate of infection has been reported between 1% and 11% in the literature, with approximately half being superficial infections and half being deep.[19,70,72] Risk factors include immunosuppressive therapy or immune compromise, diabetes mellitus, poor nutrition, obesity, multiple prior surgical interventions, prior infection, and prolonged wound drainage.[67] Infection rates may be lessened

with proper prophylactic measures, such as the use of intravenous antibiotics, antibiotic impregnated cement, care and preservation of a robust soft tissue envelope, laminar flow operating rooms, and exhaust suits.

When a deep infection occurs, a decision has to be made regarding implant preservation. Patient factors, duration of symptoms, bacteriology, quality of component fixation, the presence of a sinus, and a history of preceding bacteremia are important considerations in treatment planning.[64,66,67] Options include surgical débridement (with polyethylene exchange) combined with chronic suppressive antibiotic therapy versus implant removal with or without a second-stage reimplantation. *S. aureus* infections may be more amenable to repeat débridement and component retention.[70] Although less virulent, *S. epidermidis* has an increased propensity for adherence and biofilm formation and has been associated with a high failure rate with attempted prosthetic retention.[16,44,70] Early, multiple irrigations and débridements with component retention may be possible for well-fixed components, a duration of symptoms of less than 30 days, infection with a low-virulence organism, and a

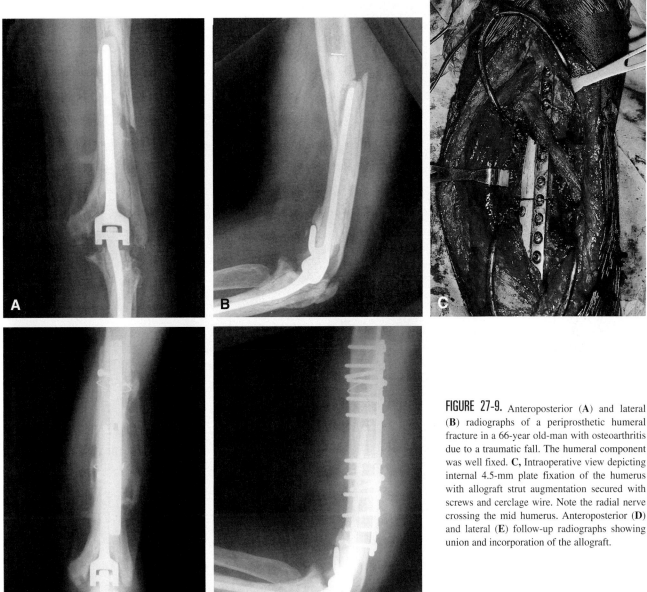

FIGURE 27-9. Anteroposterior (**A**) and lateral (**B**) radiographs of a periprosthetic humeral fracture in a 66-year old-man with osteoarthritis due to a traumatic fall. The humeral component was well fixed. **C,** Intraoperative view depicting internal 4.5-mm plate fixation of the humerus with allograft strut augmentation secured with screws and cerclage wire. Note the radial nerve crossing the mid humerus. Anteroposterior (**D**) and lateral (**E**) follow-up radiographs showing union and incorporation of the allograft.

medically fit patient.[72] A suitable soft tissue envelope is required for healing, and local muscle pedicle flaps are occasionally required to cover and seal the joint (see Fig. 27-3). The overall success of irrigation and débridement ranges from 22% to 70%.[69,70]

Staged exchange presents an alternative for an infected total elbow arthroplasty. Much of the experience of staged exchange is derived from the success described in the lower extremities. In the medically fit patient with a loose component with duration of infection greater than 21 days, this may be a viable option for salvage of a total elbow arthroplasty. It requires meticulous cement removal that may involve extended osteotomies of the ulna and humerus. This is followed by placement of an antibiotic-laden cement spacer, 6 weeks of intravenous antibiotics, and negative tissue biopsy before replantation.

For chronic deep infections after total elbow arthroplasty, resection arthroplasty probably remains the only viable option. It is clearly the treatment of choice for the severely debilitated or medically compromised patient, including patients with HIV infection. If the medial and lateral humeral columns are left intact and contoured to encircle the remaining ulna, the patient will likely be left with reasonable stability and a limited pain-free range of motion. An exception may be considered for elderly, debilitated patients with multiple medical problems and well-fixed components who are asymptomatic and have no systemic signs of infection. These individuals often develop a draining sinus, which serves to decompress the joint. When it is chosen to leave an infected prosthesis in place in this specific clinical setting, chronic oral suppressive antibiotics and local wound care are continued indefinitely.

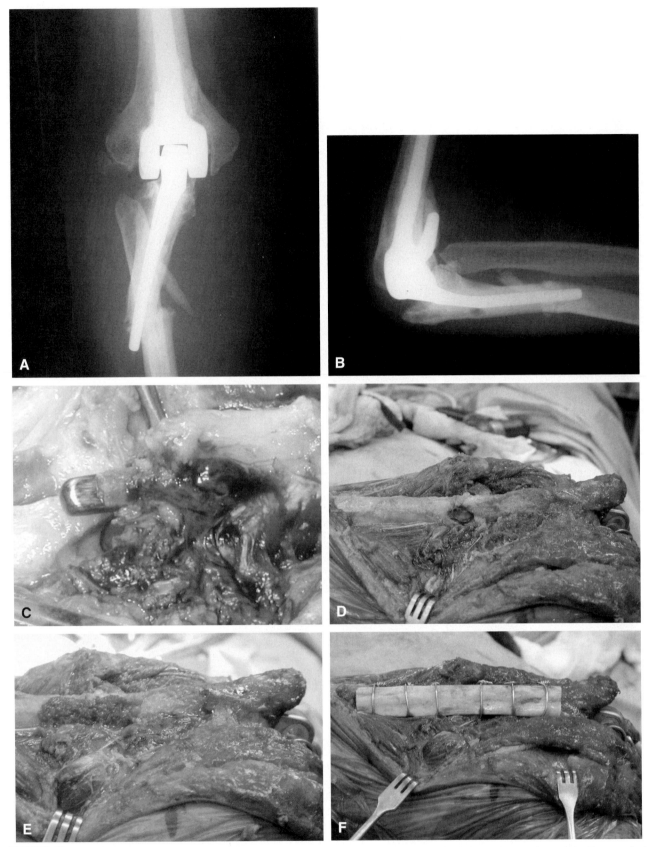

FIGURE 27-10. Anteroposterior (**A**) and lateral (**B**) radiographs of a periprosthetic fracture at the tip of the ulnar stem due to distal osteolysis. Note osteolysis in the ulnar canal on the lateral film. **C,** Intraoperative photograph of ulnar component with black discoloration of surrounding soft tissues characteristic of osteolysis. The ulnar stem was loose. **D,** Long-stem revision component has been cemented in place with ulna reduced. Note the lateral defect in the cortex due to osteolysis, which precipitated the fracture. **E,** Cancellous bone graft applied over defect and along lateral cortex proximal and distal to the fracture.

Continued

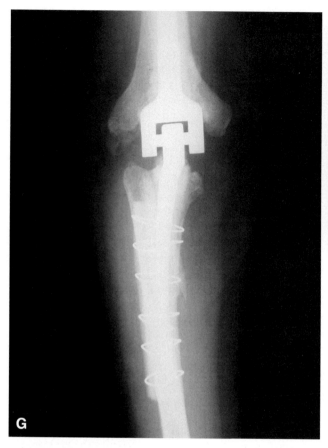

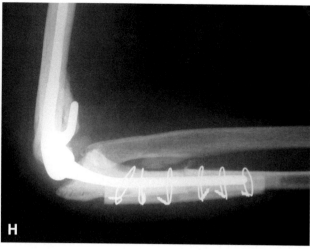

FIGURE 27-10—cont'd. F, Allograft strut wired to the ulna. Follow-up anteroposterior (**G**) and lateral (**H**) radiographs depicting revision prosthesis and allograft incorporation.

CRITICAL POINTS: TOTAL ELBOW ARTHROPLASTY

INDICATIONS

▪ Pain, stiffness, and loss of function associated with:
  • Rheumatoid arthritis
  • Post-traumatic arthritis
  • Primary osteoarthritis
  • Hemophilic arthropathy
  • Comminuted fracture of the distal humerus in the elderly when osteosynthesis not possible

CONTRAINDICATIONS

▪ Neuropathic joint
▪ Poor soft tissue coverage
▪ Presence of infection at the elbow

TECHNICAL POINTS

Exposure Through Full-Thickness Fasciocutaneous Flaps Posteriorly

▪ Transpose ulnar nerve.
▪ Reflect triceps.
  • Carefully dissect Sharpey's fibers off the olecranon in subperiosteal fashion.
  • Bryan and Morrey: Elevate triceps from medial to lateral in continuity with anconeus.

• Gschwend: Split triceps muscle and tendon longitudinally and elevate them off proximal ulna in midline.
• Triceps sparing approach (insertion left intact): Useful in patients with deficient distal humeral columns (fractures, nonunions).

Humeral Preparation

▪ Resect central aspect of the trochlea.
▪ Enter humeral canal with a bur.
▪ Use cutting guides to prepare the distal humerus.
▪ Evaluate trial implants.
▪ May need to deepen anterior cortex to accept the anterior flange of the implant and allow complete seating of the prosthesis.

Ulnar Preparation

▪ Resect tips of olecranon and coronoid process.
▪ Enter canal with a bur and enlarge it with rasps.
▪ Must appreciate 5 degrees of valgus of ulnar shaft relative to sigmoid notch.
▪ Bone at canal entry often limits complete component seating.

Continued

CRITICAL POINTS: TOTAL ELBOW ARTHROPLASTY—cont'd

Trial Components

- Evaluate ROM.
- Use capsular release if needed.

Cement

- Thoroughly lavage and dry canals.
- Restrictors in humerus and ulna
- Use thin flexible tubing for retrograde filling.
- Use low-viscosity cement (consider antibiotic-laden cement).
- Use cement early in polymerization process.

Repair of Extensor Mechanism

- Use multiple transosseous sutures distally.

Closure

- Wound is closed in layers after hemostasis is achieved.
- Ulnar nerve is transposed anteriorly.

- Drains are optional with adequate hemostasis.
- Compressive dressing is applied and arm is splinted in partial extension.

POSTOPERATIVE CARE

- Elevate the elbow and begin intravenous therapy with antibiotics.
- Begin active and gentle passive range-of-motion exercises at 7 to 10 days. (In immunosuppressed or rheumatoid patients with thin, friable skin, the elbow can be immobilized for a longer period to allow soft tissue healing before motion is initiated.)
- Protect triceps if detached for 6 to 8 weeks.
- Use night-time elbow extension splint for sleep in maximum extension to limit potential flexion contracture.
- Limit lifting to 5 lb with operated extremity indefinitely.

ANNOTATED REFERENCES

2a. Bryan RS: Total replacement of the elbow joint. Arch Surg 112:1092-1093, 1977.

Total replacement of the elbow joint has been performed on 86 elbows at the Mayo Clinic, all but 15 in patients with rheumatoid arthritis. The Mayo design, which replaces both radiohumeral and humeroulnar joints, was used in 41 elbows, almost all in rheumatoid patients, with 71% good results. The Coonrad hinge with polyethylene bushings was used in 34 elbows; it was successful in 64% of rheumatoid patients but failed in 46% of post-traumatic patients with bone loss. Previous designs have failed because of humeral loosening. Total elbow replacement is a technique still to be perfected in medical centers before general release.

4a. Connor PM, Morrey BF: Total elbow arthroplasty in patients who have juvenile rheumatoid arthritis. J Bone Joint Surg Am 80:678-688, 1998.

Because there is little information in the literature regarding this procedure, the authors attempted to learn about the long-term results by evaluating 19 patients (24 elbows) with juvenile rheumatoid arthritis who had been managed with total elbow arthroplasty. At an average of 7.4 years (range, 2 to 14 years) after the operation, there was an improvement in the average Mayo elbow performance score from 31 points (range, 5 to 55 points) preoperatively to 90 points (range, 55 to 100 points). Twenty-two (96%) of the 23 elbows available at the most recent follow-up evaluation caused little or no pain, but the improvement in the range of motion was not as reliable. The average arc of flexion improved from only 63 degrees preoperatively to 90 degrees postoperatively; the average postoperative arc of flexion began at 35 degrees, with additional flexion to 125 degrees. There were 13 complications, including one perioperative death, that affected 12 of the 24 elbows. Seven of the nine early complications, including a fracture of the olecranon, subluxation of the prosthesis, stiffness of the elbow, and problems with wound healing, led to an additional operative procedure but did not adversely affect the long-term outcome after appropriate diagnosis and treatment. Late complications (aseptic loosening, instability, and worn bushings) led to three poor results. None of the 18 semiconstrained prostheses had radiographic evidence of loosening at the most recent follow-up evaluation. Of the 23 elbows that had been followed for at least 2 years, 12 (52%) had an excellent result, 8 (35%) had a good result, and 3 (13%) had a poor result.

7a. Dent CM, Hoy G, et al: Revision of failed total elbow arthroplasty. J Bone Joint Surg Br 77:691-695, 1995.

Twenty-five patients with rheumatoid arthritis were reviewed who had failure of 26 primary total elbow arthroplasties causing pain and loss of function. Most revision cases required special custom implants to treat varying bone loss and soft tissue disruption. Assessment showed satisfactory functional results in the patients treated by revision at a mean follow-up period of 35 months. The review suggests that revision surgery produces short- to medium-term pain-free function and is the treatment of choice for a failed total elbow arthroplasty in the absence of infection.

7b. Ewald FC, Jacobs MA: Total elbow arthroplasty. Clin Orthop (182):137-142, 1984.

In the 8-year experience at the authors' institution (1974-1981) with an unlinked resurfacing elbow prosthesis, one failure occurred due to loosening of an ulnar component (1 of 153; 0.6%). The authors concluded that loosening of the prosthetic components in bone is not a serious problem but that other problems remain. Postoperative dislocation continued after a lateral approach was adopted but improved with the use of components of variable sizes. Ulnar nerve palsies are an unsolved problem and require special investigation in the rheumatoid patient. Other soft tissue problems have been relieved by the more physiologic lateral approach. Indications have been expanded to include post-traumatic or osteoarthritic conditions in relatively inactive elderly patients.

10a. Fink B, Krey D, et al: Results of elbow endoprostheses in patients with rheumatoid arthritis in correlation with previous operations. J Shoulder Elbow Surg 11:360-367, 2002.

Fifty-nine patients with rheumatic destruction of the elbow received 20 St. Georg, 20 GSB III, 13 Souter-Strathclyde, and 13 Kudo endoprostheses. Among the various prosthetic categories, 43.9% of the joints had had preceding rheumatoid surgery. Fifty-one patients with 54 prostheses were examined after a mean follow-up of 5.7 ± 4.1 years using the Inglis score and analyzing all radiographs. Complications occurred in 20% to 25% of prostheses. Of the St. Georg prostheses, 6 (30%) had to be exchanged, as well as 4 (20%) of the GSB III prostheses and 4 (30.7%) of the Souter-Strathclyde prostheses. Radiolucent lines greater than 1 mm were observed in 26% of the St. Georg prostheses, 23% of the GSB III prostheses, 27% of the Souter-Strathclyde prostheses, and 9% of the Kudo prostheses. In contrast to the clinical results, the intraoperative and postoperative complications, as well as the rate of failure and radiolucent lines, showed a statistically significant relationship to previous operations of the joints, especially with the resection interposition arthroplasty. It was concluded that resection interposition arthroplasty seems to be associated with complications and failures when a subsequent endoprosthesis is used.

13a. Garcia JA, Mykula R, et al: Complex fractures of the distal humerus in the elderly: The role of total elbow replacement as primary treatment. J Bone Joint Surg Br 84:812-816, 2002.

Between 1995 and 2000, 19 consecutive patients with fractures of the distal humerus were treated by primary total elbow replacement using the Coonrad-Morrey prosthesis. No patient had inflammatory or degenerative arthritis of the elbow. The mean age at the time of injury was 73 years (61 to 95). The mean time to follow-up was 3 years (1 to 5.5). At follow-up 11 patients (68%) reported no pain, 4 (25%) had mild pain with activity, and 1 had mild pain at rest. The mean flexion arc was 24 degrees to 125 degrees. The mean supination was 90 degrees (70 to 100 degrees), and pronation was 70 degrees (50 to 110 degrees). No elbow was unstable. The mean Disabilities of the Arm, Shoulder and Hand score was 23 (0.92 to 63.3), and the mean Mayo elbow performance score was 93 (80 to 100). Of the 16 patients, 15 were satisfied with the outcome. Radiologic evaluation revealed only 1 patient with a radiolucent line at the cement-bone interface. Primary total elbow arthroplasty is an acceptable option for the management of comminuted fractures of the distal humerus in elderly patients when the configuration of the fracture and the quality of the bone make reconstruction difficult.

14. Gill DR, Morrey BF: The Coonrad-Morrey total elbow arthroplasty in patients who have rheumatoid arthritis: A ten to fifteen-year follow-up study. J Bone Joint Surg Am 80:1327-1335, 1998.

Seventy-eight elbows were managed with a Coonrad-Morrey total elbow arthroplasty between 1981 and 1986. Forty-one patients (46 elbows) were alive and had been followed for at least 10 years after the procedure (group 1). The remaining 28 patients (32 elbows) had died or had had a revision less than 10 years after the procedure or had been followed for less than 10 years (group 2). The patients in group 1 had a younger mean age at the time of the procedure, but all other preoperative parameters were similar for both groups. At the latest follow-up evaluation, 97% of the elbows (45 of the 46 in group 1 and 31 of the 32 in group 2) were not painful or were only mildly painful. The mean arc of flexion-extension was 28 to 131 degrees; this represents an increase of 13 degrees compared with the preoperative value. Seventy-six of the 78 elbows had long-term radiographic evaluation. There were two loose ulnar components; one was associated with an

infection. Five bushings were completely worn, and six were partially worn. Complications occurred in 11 elbows and were serious, necessitating reoperation, in 10. Delayed complications included three avulsions of the triceps, two deep infections, two ulnar fractures, and one fracture of an ulnar component. In addition, two elbows were revised because of aseptic loosening. No patient had persistent ulnar neuritis or serious skin complications. At the latest clinical follow-up evaluation, according to the Mayo elbow performance score, 43 of the 78 elbows had an excellent result; 26, a good result; 7, a fair result; and 2 (both in group 2), a poor result. The rate of survival of the prosthesis was 92.4%, with 86% good or excellent and 14% fair or poor results.

16a. Gschwend N: Present state-of-the-art in elbow arthroplasty. Acta Orthop Belg 68:100-117, 2002.

Excellent review on the current status of total elbow arthroplasty with a discussion of prosthetic type, indication, surgical technique, results, complications, and survivorship. The author emphasizes that the results concerning pain relief and mobility are, for all properly placed prostheses, very satisfactory in the first years. A reliable account of long-term results (> 10 years of noninterrupted series of elbow prostheses) has so far been given only by a few authors. In cases with rheumatoid arthritis the survival rate at 10 years reaches 90%; the complication rate, however, is still definitely larger than other total joint arthroplasties. This is particularly true for post-traumatic and osteoarthritis cases. Aseptic loosening, infection, instability, and ulnar nerve lesions are at the fore and about twice as frequent as in rheumatoid arthritis, especially in patients younger than 60 years of age. The key to success as well as the facilitation of revision rests on the preservation or reconstruction of normal anatomy (e.g., condyle reconstruction) when implanting an elbow prosthesis.

18. Gschwend N, Scheier NH, Baehler AR: Long-term results of the GSB III elbow arthroplasty. J Bone Joint Surg Br 81:1005-1112, 1999.

The authors review the long-term results of the GSB III total elbow in 59 patients (six bilateral). Rheumatoid arthritis (RA) was the underlying cause in 51 of the patients and post-traumatic osteoarthritis (PTOA) in 8. Of these, 24 patients (28 prostheses) have since died; 2, both operated on bilaterally, had had their implants for more than 10 years and had already been assessed for inclusion in the long-term follow-up. The remaining 32 patients (28 RA, 4 PTOA) with 36 GSB III elbows were examined clinically and radiologically after a mean period of 13.5 years. Pain was considerably reduced in 91.6%. Mobility was increased by 37 degrees in those with RA and by 67 degrees in those with PTOA. There were three cases of aseptic loosening and three of deep infection. The main complication was disassembly of the prosthetic component in nine elbows (13.8%). This last group included 2 patients with postoperative fractures unrelated to the operative technique and 1 with neuropathic arthritis. Ulnar neuritis occurred in 2 patients. Eighty-eight percent of prostheses implanted in this period remained in situ, suggesting survivorship comparable to other total joint arthroplasties.

19. Gschwend N, Simmen BR, Matejovsky Z: Late complications in elbow arthroplasty. J Shoulder Elbow Surg 5(2 pt 1):86-96, 1996.

The authors discuss complications after total elbow arthroplasty. They indicate that the world literature complication rate of elbow arthroplasty amounts to 43%. Accordingly, a high revision rate (18% on average) and a considerable rate (15%) of permanent complications are also found. When complications are discussed, a clear distinction of the type of prosthesis is mandatory, because linked or nonlinked and nonconstrained or semiconstrained prostheses have specific complications. The following complications are discussed separately: loosening (radiologic and clinical), ulnar neuropathy, infection, dislocation and subluxation, uncoupling, intraoperative bone fractures, and failure of the implant. The possible causes are analyzed, and means to avoid or treat these complications are discussed.

21. Hildebrand KA, Patterson SD, Regan WD, et al: Functional outcome of semiconstrained total elbow arthroplasty. J Bone Joint Surg Am 82:1379-1386, 2000.

The authors review the results of primary total elbow arthroplasty with use of the Coonrad-Morrey prosthesis. Forty-seven consecutive patients (51 elbows) underwent total elbow arthroplasty, with 36 surviving patients (39 elbows) available for follow-up. The mean age at the time of the operation was 64 years. Eighteen patients (21 elbows) had inflammatory arthritis. Eighteen patients (18 elbows) had an acute fracture or post-traumatic condition. A review of the results showed that the mean score on the Mayo Elbow Performance Index for the group that had inflammatory arthritis was significantly higher than that for the group with a traumatic or post-traumatic condition (90 vs. 78 points) at the time of the latest follow-up. In both groups, the mean extensor torque of the involved elbow was significantly less than that of the contralateral elbow. No significant difference between the groups was found with respect to the flexion-extension arc of motion. Ten elbows had ulnar nerve dysfunction (a transient deficit in 6 and a permanent deficit in 4); 9, an intraoperative fracture (of the humeral diaphysis in 4, of the ulnar diaphysis in 4, and of the olecranon in 1); 3, a periprosthetic infection; 3, a triceps disruption; and 1, a revision because of a fracture of the ulnar component. There were no other revisions. Of the 34 elbows with complete radiographic follow-up, 23 had no change in the bone-cement interface. Progressive radiolucency was noted around the ulnar prosthesis in 8 elbows, around the humeral prosthesis in 1 elbow, and around both components in 2 elbows. The authors concluded that patients were generally satisfied. However, they emphasize that the rates of complications involving the ulnar nerve, intraoperative fracture, triceps disruption, deep infection, and periprosthetic radiolucency are of concern.

21a. Ikavalko M, Belt EA, et al: Revisions for aseptic loosening in Souter-Strathclyde elbow arthroplasty: Incidence of revisions of different components used in 522 consecutive cases. Acta Orthop Scand 73:257-263, 2002.

The authors present a large series of 522 primary Souter elbow replacements performed in the Rheumatism Foundation Hospital during the years 1982-1997. The mean duration of the disease at the time of operation was 25 (2 to 70) years. Elbows were often severely destroyed, and in one third of the joints essential bone structures were missing. Therefore, in 178 cases, the ulnar components were retentive and in the remaining 344 elbows with better bone stock they were nonretentive. Forty-seven patients had 51 operations for aseptic loosening up to the end of year 2000. In the survival analysis, the general cumulative success rates for the whole study cohort, without revision because of aseptic loosening 5 and 10 years after surgery, were 96% and 84%, respectively.

21b. Ikavalko M, Belt EA, et al: Souter arthroplasty for elbows with severe destruction. Clin Orthop (421):126-133, 2004.

The early results of 156 primary total elbow arthroplasties with the Souter elbow prosthesis were done on 132 patients with severe joint destruction (Larsen grade 5) or large bone defects or both. The mean age of the patients at the time of surgery was 57 years, and the mean disease duration was 27 years. Radiographically, severe bone defects were detected in 100 humeri and 134 ulnas. Retentive (snap-fit) ulnar components were implanted in 110 joints, and bone grafts were used

on 26 humeri and 14 ulnas. Major complications led to 5 early and 16 late reoperations in 19 patients. Four reoperations were done because of dislocation and 8 because of aseptic loosening. One reoperation was done because of early infection, and 5 were done because of late infection. In the survival analysis, the cumulative success rate without revision for aseptic loosening at 5 years follow-up was 97%. Despite the demanding nature of these arthroplasties, the primary results are encouraging. Technically, it is possible to do elbow replacement, even on elbows where the humeral condyles or olecranon or both are missing, if there is sufficient bone left on the diaphyseal areas for primary stem fixation.

21c. Ikavalko M, Lehto MU, et al: The Souter-Strathclyde elbow arthroplasty: A clinical and radiological study of 525 consecutive cases. J Bone Joint Surg Br 84:77-82, 2002.

This very large series describes the results of 525 primary Souter elbow arthroplasties. The mean age of the patients was 57 years; 119 patients had a bilateral procedure. The elbows were affected by chronic inflammatory disease—usually rheumatoid arthritis—which had been present for a mean of 24.7 years. In about 30% the joints were grossly destroyed with significant loss of bone. In 179 elbows the ulnar components were metal-backed and retentive; in the remaining 346, with better bone stock, they were nonretentive; all-polyethylene prostheses were used. During the early years the incidence of complications was higher. Complications necessitated 108 further operations in 82 patients. Dislocation was the indication for 30 further procedures in 26 patients. Thirty patients underwent 33 revision procedures for aseptic loosening; 12 had 29 operations because of deep infection, with 2 for superficial infection; and 14 further operations were done for other reasons. The cumulative rate of success, without aseptic loosening, 5 and 10 years after surgery, was 96% and 85%, respectively.

23. Kamineni S, Morrey BM: Distal humeral fractures treated with noncustom total elbow arthroplasty. J Bone Joint Surg Am 86:940-947, 2004.

This retrospective review supports the idea that total elbow arthroplasty is a reliable option for the treatment of elderly patients with a severe, comminuted fracture of the distal part of the humerus. Forty-three acute distal humeral fractures were treated with total elbow arthroplasty as the primary option and were followed for at least 2 years. The average age of the patients was 69 years, and the average duration of follow-up was 7 years. At the latest follow-up examination, the average flexion arc was 24 degrees to 131 degrees and the Mayo elbow performance score averaged 93 of a possible 100 points. Heterotopic ossification was present to some extent in 7 elbows, with radiographic abutment noted in 2. Thirty-two (65%) of the 49 elbows had neither a complication nor any further surgery from the time of the index arthroplasty to the most recent follow-up evaluation. Fourteen elbows (29%) had a single complication, and most of them did not require further surgery. Ten additional procedures, including five revision arthroplasties, were required in 9 elbows; five were related to soft tissue and five were related to the implant or bone. The authors conclude that complex distal humeral fractures should be assessed primarily for the reliability with which they can be reconstructed with osteosynthesis. When osteosynthesis is not considered to be feasible, especially in patients who are physiologically older and place lower demands on the joint, total elbow arthroplasty can be considered.

33. Mansat P, Morrey BF: Semiconstrained total elbow arthroplasty for ankylosed and stiff elbows. J Bone Joint Surg Am 82:1260-1268, 2000.

A semiconstrained total elbow arthroplasty was performed in 14 elbows with a preoperative range of elbow motion of 30 degrees or less owing to trauma or inflammatory arthritis. Nine elbows were ankylosed preoperatively. The mean age at the time of the surgery was 50 years. After a mean duration of follow-up of 63 months, the result was excellent for 4 elbows, good for 4, fair for 1, and poor for 5, according to the Mayo Elbow Performance Score. The mean arc of flexion improved from 7 degrees (range, 0 to 30 degrees) preoperatively to 67 degrees (range, 10 to 115 degrees) after the surgery. The most important factor that influenced the final result was the presence of ectopic bone surrounding the elbow joint. There were seven complications. Infection developed in 5 elbows. Three elbows had a superficial infection, which did not compromise the final result in 2 and which was treated with a myocutaneous flap in one with skin necrosis, with an excellent result. Deep infection developed in 2 other elbows. Both had an unsatisfactory result, 1 after implant removal and 1 after several débridements and retention of the prosthesis. Two patients sustained a fracture because of a loose component, and the prosthesis was revised. Four patients who lost motion within the first month after the surgery had a manipulation under anesthesia.

34. McKee MD, Pugh DM, Richards RR, et al: Effect of humeral condylar resection on strength and functional outcome after semiconstrained total elbow arthoplasty. J Bone Joint Surg Am 85:802-807, 2003.

The authors question whether excision of ununited humeral condyles during insertion of a semiconstrained total elbow prosthesis has a negative effect on strength, as the osseous origins of the common extensors and flexor-pronator muscles are lost. Sixteen matched pairs of patients were reviewed with use of standardized, objective testing of muscle strength of the elbow, forearm, wrist, and hand after total elbow arthroplasty. The normal, contralateral limb served as the control, and all strength values are given as a percentage of the normal side. The humeral condyles were intact in 16 patients and had been resected in the other 16. At follow-up, there were no significant differences between the two groups with regard to strength of pronation, supination, wrist flexion, wrist extension, or grip strength. There was also no difference between the two groups with regard to the Mayo Elbow Performance Score (79 points in the group with intact condyles compared with 77 points in the group with resection of the condyles; $P = .67$). The authors conclude that condylar resection has a minimal, clinically irrelevant effect on forearm, wrist, and hand strength and no effect on the Mayo Elbow Performance Score after total elbow arthroplasty. The findings of this study support the practice of condylar resection, which simplifies total elbow arthroplasty for many conditions.

37a. Morrey BF, Adams RA: Semiconstrained arthroplasty for the treatment of rheumatoid arthritis of the elbow. J Bone Joint Surg Am 74:479-490, 1992.

This study describes the early results of total elbow arthroplasty for rheumatoid arthritis at the Mayo Clinic. Fifty-four patients in whom a total of 58 semiconstrained modified Coonrad elbow implants had been inserted for rheumatoid arthritis were followed for a mean of 3.8 years (range, 2 to 8 years). At the latest follow-up, there was little or no pain in 53 elbows (91%). The arc of motion was on average increased 23 degrees in flexion-extension. An additional 10 patients who had had insertion of 10 modified Coonrad implants during the same period were followed for less than 2 years but were included in the assessment of complications. Fifteen (22%) of the 68 elbows had a complication: 4, infection; 8, acute or delayed condylar or ulnar fracture; and 1 each, ulnar neuritis, avulsion of the triceps, and fracture of the implant. Radiographic evaluation was performed for 54 of the 58 elbows; the other 4 were excluded from this evaluation because

of infection. A satisfactory radiographic appearance of the cement—its extent and the absence of skip areas—was noted for all of the ulnar components and for 51 (94%) of the humeral components. No patient had radiographic evidence of a loose implant. A reoperation was performed in 6 elbows: 4 were done for infection; 1, for insufficiency of the triceps; and 1, for a fractured ulnar component. Of the 58 elbows, 40 (69%) had an excellent result; 13 (22%), a good result; 4 (7%), a fair result; and 1, a poor result.

38. Morrey BF, Adams RA: Semiconstrained elbow replacement for distal humeral nonunion. J Bone Joint Surg Br 77:67-72, 1995.

The authors reviewed 36 of 39 consecutive patients with an average age of 68 years who had semiconstrained elbow replacement for distal humeral nonunion at an average follow-up of 50.4 months. Of these, 31 (86%) had satisfactory results, 3 (8%) had fair, and 2 (6%) had poor results; 32 patients (88%) had moderate or severe pain before, and 91% had no or only mild discomfort after the procedure. Motion had improved from a mean arc of 29 degrees to 103 degrees before operation to 16 degrees to 127 degrees after surgery. All five flail extremities were stable at last assessment. There were seven complications (18%): 2 patients had deep infection, 2 had particulate synovitis, 2 had ulnar neuropathy, and 1 had worn polyethylene bushes. Five of these 7, excluding the 2 with transient neuropathy, required reoperation (13%). Joint replacement arthroplasty can be a safe and reliable treatment for this difficult clinical condition, seen most commonly in elderly patients. This is a significant advance, because repeated osteosynthesis has been shown to be ineffective in most patients.

46a. Potter D, Claydon P, et al: Total elbow replacement using the Kudo prosthesis: Clinical and radiological review with five- to seven-year follow-up. J Bone Joint Surg Br 85:354-357, 2003.

This study reviews the results of the Kudo 5 total elbow arthroplasty in a total of 25 patients (29 procedures) with a mean follow-up of 6 years using the Mayo Elbow Performance Index. In addition, all patients were assessed for loosening using standard anteroposterior and lateral radiographs. At review, 19 elbows (65%) had either no pain or mild pain, 10 (35%) had moderate pain, and none had severe pain. The mean arc of flexion/extension was 94 degrees (35 to 130 degrees) and supination/pronation was 128 degrees (30 to 165 degrees). Postoperatively, there were no infections. One patient had a dislocation that was treated by closed reduction, and 5 had neurapraxia of the ulnar nerve. Radiologically, there was no evidence of loosening of the humeral component but two ulnar components had progressive radiolucent lines suggestive of loosening. Two other ulnar components had incomplete and nonprogressive radiolucent lines. This component may be the weak part of the Kudo prosthesis. With definite radiologic loosening as the end point, the probability of survival of the Kudo 5 prosthesis at 5 years using the Kaplan-Meier method was 89%. The results at 5 years are similar to those reported by other authors for other implant types.

49a. Redfern DR, Dunkley AB, et al: Revision total elbow replacement using the Souter-Strathclyde prosthesis. J Bone Joint Surg Br 83:635-639, 2001.

The Souter-Strathclyde prosthesis was used in 52 revisions of total elbow replacements (TERs) between August 1986 and May 1997. Of these, 50, carried out in 45 patients, were prospectively followed for a mean of 53 months (14 to 139 months). The procedure produced reliable relief of pain, and the range of movement was preserved. There was a considerable incidence of adverse events associated with revision (30%), and 12 further procedures have been required. Nonetheless, a revision is the preferred salvage procedure for failed primary arthroplasty in the absence of sepsis.

54. Rozing P: Souter-Strathclyde total elbow arthroplasty. J Bone Joint Surg Br 82:1129-1134, 2000.

We have reviewed 66 consecutive Souter-Strathclyde arthroplasties of the elbow implanted in 59 patients between 1982 and 1993. Thirteen patients (15 elbows) (19.6%) died. Sixteen elbows (24.2%) were revised, 6 for aseptic loosening (9%), 4 (6%) because of fracture or loosening after a fracture, 3 (4.5%) for infection, and 3 (4.5%) for dislocation. In 33 elbows with a follow-up of 93 months (60 to 167 months) complete relief of pain was achieved in 22 (67%) when seen at 1 year. After 10 years or more, 36% of the elbows were pain free and 64% had occasional slight pain especially under loading or stress. The mean gain in the arc of movement was 16 degrees, but a mean flexion contracture of 33 degrees remained. The main early complications were intraoperative fractures of the epicondyles (9%), postoperative dislocation (4.5%), and ulnar neuropathy. The incidence of ulnar neuropathy before operation was 19%. After operation, 20 patients (33%) had an ulnar neuropathy, in 7 of which it had been present before operation; and of these, weakness of the hypothenar muscle occurred in 2. The probability of survival of the Souter-Strathclyde elbow prosthesis based on the Kaplan-Meier calculation is 69% at 10 years. These somewhat poorer results contrast to the results reported by Ikavalko and coworkers in 2002.[21c]

55a. Samijo SK, Van den Berg ME, et al: Souter-Strathclyde total elbow arthroplasty: Medium-term results. Acta Orthop Belg 69:501-506, 2003.

The Souter-Strathclyde unconstrained elbow prosthesis was prospectively studied in 36 patients (45 prostheses) with rheumatoid arthritis. At 8.2 years' follow-up the authors' results were similar to other reports on the Souter-Strathclyde total elbow arthroplasty. The authors, however, underscore that loosening of the humeral component seems to be related to both the short humeral stem and a persistent extension deficit. This has implications for design modifications and post-operative rehabilitation for other patients undergoing total elbow arthroplasty.

57a. Schemitsch EH, Ewald FC, et al: Results of total elbow arthroplasty after excision of the radial head and synovectomy in patients who had rheumatoid arthritis. J Bone Joint Surg Am 78:1541-1547, 1996.

The authors compared the results of 23 consecutive capitellocondylar total elbow arthroplasties in 23 patients in whom an excision of the radial head and synovectomy for rheumatoid arthritis had failed with those of 23 nonconsecutive primary capitellocondylar total elbow arthroplasties in 23 patients who had rheumatoid arthritis. The average duration of follow-up was 4 years. At the most recent follow-up examination, use of a 100-point rating system demonstrated an improvement from an average preoperative score of 21 points to an average postoperative score of 87 points for the group in whom an excision of the radial head and synovectomy had failed. The group that had primary arthroplasty demonstrated an improvement from an average preoperative score of 22 points to an average postoperative score of 94 points. The group that had primary arthroplasty had a significantly greater improvement in terms of relief of pain, functional status, and the elbow-rating score than the other group. Four patients who had had failure of an excision of the radial head and synovectomy and none of those who had primary arthroplasty needed an additional operative procedure. Six of the patients who had had a failed excision and synovectomy and none of the patients who had primary arthroplasty had instability of the elbow components. The authors concluded that, although excision of the radial head and synovectomy is a conservative and effective method of treating a painful rheumatoid elbow, conversion to a capitellocondylar total elbow arthroplasty is more difficult after such an operation and the results at a minimum of 2 years are inferior to those for primary capitellocondylar total elbow arthroplasty. This article serves as an excellent complement to the conclusions gleaned by Fink and coworkers in 2002.[10a]

59a. Shah BM, Trail IA, et al: The effect of epidemiologic and intraoperative factors on survival of the standard Souter-Strathclyde total elbow arthroplasty. J Arthroplasty 15:994-998, 2000.

The authors review those patients who underwent revision of the standard Souter-Strathclyde total elbow arthroplasty in patients with rheumatoid arthritis. They note that of the 13% that were revised, 75% were due to loosening of the humeral component. The aim of this research was to specifically identify the specific epidemiologic and intraoperative factors that predisposed to this humeral loosening. Specifically, factors such as age, sex, radiologic staging of the disease, position of the implant in bone, and size of the implant inserted were evaluated. After analysis of 186 cases, they concluded that the position of the humeral component within the humerus is crucial for long-term survivorship. Specifically in the lateral plane, the stem should be aligned in the plane of the humerus and the implant inserted to the correct depth. The articular surface of the implant should lie at the level of the normal trochlea. In the anteroposterior plane, the implant should sit centrally and not be lateralized. Good surgical technique is crucial to the long-term effectiveness of this implant.

61. Spinner RJ, Morgenlander JC, Nunley JA: Ulnar nerve function following total elbow arthroplasty: A prospective study comparing preoperative and postoperative clinical and electrophysiologic evaluation in patients with rheumatoid arthritis. J Hand Surg [Am] 25:360-364, 2000.

This study was conducted to determine the incidence of ulnar and peripheral neuropathy in patients with rheumatoid arthritis undergoing total elbow arthroplasty and the effect it has on ulnar nerve function after surgery. Preoperative and postoperative clinical and electrodiagnostic examinations were completed in 10 patients. Before surgery 4 patients had clinical and electrophysiologic evidence of a neuropathy (2 each with a peripheral neuropathy and an ulnar neuropathy). One patient had subclinical evidence of a chronic T1 radiculopathy. After surgery, 2 patients showed neurologic improvement (1 had ulnar neuropathy and 1 had diabetic neuropathy). One patient who had normal test results before surgery developed transient ulnar sensory symptoms after surgery. An electrodiagnostic study confirmed an ulnar neuropathy that was not detected on physical examination; the electrodiagnostic findings improved 4 months later. A large percentage of patients (40%) with rheumatoid arthritis had evidence of ulnar or peripheral neuropathy before surgery. The presence of an ulnar or peripheral neuropathy did not predispose patients to develop postoperative ulnar nerve dysfunction either clinically or electrophysiologically. Preoperative and postoperative physical and electrodiagnostic examination results correlated in 9 of the 10 patients.

67a. van der Lugt JC, Geskus RB, et al: Primary Souter-Strathclyde total elbow prosthesis in rheumatoid arthritis. J Bone Joint Surg Am 86:465-473, 2004.

The authors present the results of the first prospective study of the Souter-Strathclyde total elbow prosthesis in 204 primary total elbow prostheses that were inserted in 166 patients with rheumatoid arthritis. No patient was lost to follow-up. The mean duration of follow-up was 6.4 years. All patients were examined preoperatively, at 1 and 2 years postoperatively, and at regular intervals thereafter. Six of the 204 elbows had pain at rest at the time of the latest follow-up. Ten patients (10 elbows) without previous neurologic symptoms had development of paresthesias in the distribution of the ulnar nerve postoperatively. Patients who had pain at rest or at night and those who had ulnar nerve symptoms preoperatively were found to have a significant chance of having the same complaints postoperatively. Pain at rest or at night and a decrease in function during the follow-up period were associated with humeral loosening. Twenty-four elbows had revision of the total elbow prosthesis because of loosening of the humeral component (10), loosening after fracture (6), dislocation (4), infection (2), restricted range of motion (1), or fracture of the middle part of the humeral shaft, proximal to the prosthesis (1). One prosthesis was removed because of humeral loosening, and eight were removed because of deep infection. Another five prostheses were radiographically loose at the time of the latest follow-up. The rate of implant survival, according to the method of Kaplan-Meier, was 77.4% after 10 years and 65.2% after 18 years. The authors highlight that, currently, the results associated with the Souter-Strathclyde total elbow prosthesis are comparable with the results associated with other prostheses but that loosening of the humeral component remains a concern.

69a. Wright TW, Wong AM, et al: Functional outcome comparison of semiconstrained and unconstrained total elbow arthroplasties. J Shoulder Elbow Surg 9:524-531, 2000.

This study highlights that for properly indicated patients both linked and unlinked total elbow arthroplasties, when properly performed, yield satisfactory functional results. The authors evaluated 26 patients, each of whom had undergone either a semiconstrained (linked Ewald total elbow) or an unconstrained (unlinked Mayo-Coonrad prosthesis) total elbow arthroplasty. The patients were examined specifically to evaluate the restoration of function with respect to activities of daily living. There were 14 elbows in 13 patients who had semiconstrained prostheses and 12 elbows in 10 patients who had unconstrained total prostheses. Average age at the time of elbow replacement surgery was 62.8 years for the semiconstrained group and 63.1 years for the unconstrained group. The semiconstrained group included 8 women and 6 men; the unconstrained group consisted of 10 women and 2 men. Follow-up averaged 35.5 months in the semiconstrained group and 73 months in the unconstrained group. Twenty-two operations were performed for rheumatoid arthritis, 3 for post-traumatic humeral nonunion, and 1 for post-traumatic degenerative arthritis. Two elbows required revision, one (in the semiconstrained group) for aseptic loosening and the other (in the unconstrained group) for metal synovitis and pain from a chronically dislocated prosthesis; both of these elbows were considered failures and excluded from the functional comparison. No significant differences in functional performance were found, and no elbows demonstrated progressive radiolucencies suggestive of loosening. With the exception of 1 patient (in addition to the patients who had revisions) with a dislocated unconstrained prosthesis, all patients were satisfied with the procedure.

70. Yamaguchi K, Adams RA, Morrey BF: Infection after total elbow arthroplasty. J Bone Joint Surg Am 80:481-491, 1998.

The purpose of this study was to review the experience with the treatment of 25 infections (in 25 patients) after total elbow arthroplasty and to examine indications for salvage of the prosthesis compared with those for resection arthroplasty. The patients were divided into three groups on the basis of treatment. Group I comprised 14 patients who were managed with multiple, extensive irrigation and débridement procedures with retention of the original components. The primary indication for retention of the prosthesis was evidence that it was well fixed as determined both radiographically and intraoperatively. Group II comprised 6 patients who had removal of the prosthesis and débridement followed by immediate or staged reimplantation. Group III comprised 5 patients who were managed with resection arthroplasty. The infection was successfully eradicated in 7 of the 14 elbows that had salvage of the prosthesis with irrigation and débridement. The results were strongly dependent on the causative organism; attempts at débridement failed in the four elbows that were infected with *Staphylococcus epidermidis* compared with 3 of the 10 that were infected with another organism. The authors concluded that salvage of the prosthesis with extensive irrigation and débridement in the presence of an infection about the elbow can be reasonably successful if the infecting organism is not *S. epidermidis* and if the components are well fixed. When removal of the components is warranted, staged reimplantation can also be highly successful when the infecting organism is not *S. epidermidis*. However, the repeated operations necessary to retain a prosthesis and the high rates of complications seen with this approach—and the relatively good rates of satisfaction obtained with resection arthroplasty—suggest that resection arthroplasty remains the procedure of choice in medically frail patients or in patients for whom function of the elbow is less of a concern.

73. Yanni ON, Fearn CB, et al: The Roper-Tuke total elbow arthroplasty: 4- to 10-year results of an unconstrained prosthesis. J Bone Joint Surg Br 82:705-710, 2000.

The authors report the results of a series of 59 unconstrained total arthroplasties of the elbow using the Rouper-Tuke total elbow arthroplasty after a mean follow-up of 6.5 years (4 to 10 years). All the patients had rheumatoid arthritis. Outcome was assessed by the Mayo Elbow Performance Index (MEPI). Of the 59 arthroplasties, 2 were lost to follow-up. Ten patients died, but because 2 of their arthroplasties were failures they were included in the results. The outcome in the remaining 49 was excellent in 26 (53%), good in 15 (31%), fair in 1 (2%), and poor or a failure in 7 (14%). There was an improvement in the pain score, movement, and function. Two patients developed instability, but neither required further surgery. There was a mean increase of 21 degrees in flexion and of 7 degrees in extension. The overall rate of complications was 33.9%. Lesions of the ulnar nerve, one of which did not recover, occurred in 4 patients, deep infection in 2, and stiffness in 5. The rates of complications were similar to those in recent reports of other elbow arthroplasties. A radiologic analysis was performed of 39 arthroplasties that showed radiolucent lines around the humeral component in 22 and around the ulnar component in 15. There were lower scores on the MEPI for those with radiolucent lines around the humeral component.

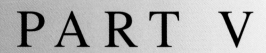

PART V

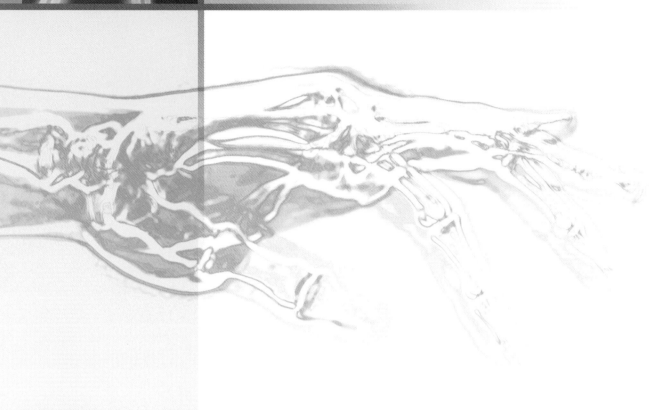

Nerve

CHAPTER 28

Compression Neuropathies

Susan E. Mackinnon • Christine B. Novak

Compression neuropathies in the upper extremity are common and are recognized with increasing frequency. The increasing prevalence of obesity in North America coupled with an aging population suggest that the problems of upper extremity compression neuropathy will likely increase in the next decade. The etiologic relationship between nerve compression disorders and occupation was extremely controversial in the 1990s.[23,46,47] The existence of multiple levels of nerve compression is now generally recognized, although the work-relatedness of these problems is still debated.[1,64] Except for significant exposure to vibration and some specific occupations with a high incidence of carpal tunnel syndrome, it is generally accepted that work is just one component of many factors that contribute to and aggravate compression neuropathy.[4,64] As compared with other compression neuropathies in the upper extremity, carpal tunnel syndrome is, in general, managed less successfully with nonoperative treatment.

The surgeon treating nerve compression in the upper extremity must be aware of other neurologic problems, such as brachial plexus neuritis, Parsonage-Turner syndrome, mononeuritis, and motor neuropathies that can mimic entrapment neuropathies and will not respond to surgical intervention. Similarly, there exists a group of individuals who are genetically sensitive to the development of nerve compression.[28] The prevalence of genetic predisposition is not known but, like systemic factors such as obesity, diabetes, and thyroid disease, may explain some patient presentations.

PATHOPHYSIOLOGY OF CHRONIC NERVE COMPRESSION

The clinical presentation of patients with chronic nerve compression is variable and reflects the broad spectrum of histopathologic changes that can occur in the nerve. Because of associated morbidity, neural tissue biopsy is not performed, and much of the information known about the histopathology of human nerve compression has been extrapolated from animal models. Some studies have suggested neural ischemia as contributing to compression neuropathies.[16-18,33,37,75,79] Many of these studies, however, reflect acute changes that occur with compression. Several animal models have been described that use different techniques to induce chronic nerve compression.[43,59] Although there is some concern about the potential for Silastic to induce reactive effects on a nerve, the histologic changes seen in the Silastic cuff model are essentially identical to those seen in the few histologic studies of chronic nerve compression that have been published. Dahlin and colleagues reported limited tissue reaction around the silicone tubes 1 year after human nerve repairs.[7]

The continuum of neural changes that occur will depend on the force of compression and the duration of compression. The histopathologic changes that occur with chronic nerve compression begin with breakdown in the blood-nerve barrier, followed by endoneurial edema and, subsequently, by perineurial thickening (Fig. 28-1).[43,59] Increased endoneurial pressure will result in changes in the microneural circulation and render the nerve susceptible to dynamic ischemia. With increased compression, there will be localized demyelination, followed by more diffuse demyelination and finally axonal degeneration. Neural changes may not occur uniformly across the nerve and may vary depending on the distribution of compressive forces across the nerve. Superficial fascicles will undergo changes sooner and may result in varying patient symptoms within a single nerve distribution.[32] For example, in early carpal tunnel syndrome the superficial fascicles to the long finger and ring finger are usually affected before the fascicles to the thumb and radial side of the index finger.

Patient sensory complaints will generally parallel the histopathologic neural changes and will progress from intermittent paresthesia to persistent numbness (see Fig. 28-1). Sensory testing will also vary with the degree of nerve compression. Initially, patients will have alteration in threshold measures and, with more severe nerve compression, will progress to deficits in two-point discrimination.

We would like to acknowledge **Robert M. Szabo, MD,** and **William W. Eversmann, Jr., MD,** for their contributions to the chapter on this subject in the previous editions of this textbook.

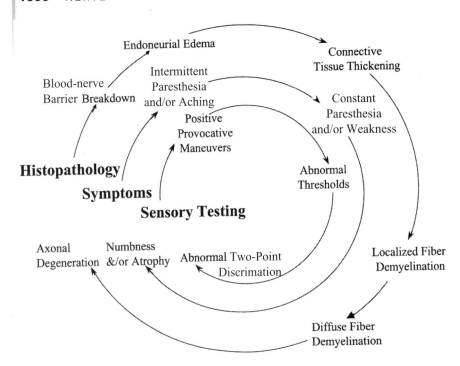

FIGURE 28-1. The histopathology of chronic nerve compression spans a spectrum of changes that begins with breakdown of the blood-nerve barrier and with continued compression will progress to axonal degeneration. The patient presentation and sensory testing will parallel the histopathologic changes occurring in the nerve.

Double Crush

First introduced by Upton and McComas,[81] the double crush mechanism is an important concept with nerve compression. In their clinical review of a series of 115 patients with median nerve or ulnar nerve compression there were 81 cases in which there was evidence of a cervical root lesion. They concluded that compression of a nerve at one level will make the nerve more susceptible to damage at another level, and they hypothesized that axoplasmic flow would be compromised by the proximal compression on the nerve and then further compromised by the distal compression site. The reverse double crush was described by Lundborg.[32] He hypothesized that a distal site of compression would decrease neurotrophic substances back to the neuron and thus decrease the production of substances to be transported distally. Other clinical studies have supported the double crush mechanism with associations between the cervical spine, thoracic outlet, and distal sites of compression, including the carpal and cubital tunnel.[2,24,40,60,61,88] Hurst and associates reported on 1000 cases of carpal tunnel syndrome in 888 patients and noted a significant relationship between bilateral carpal tunnel syndrome and those patients with cervical arthritis and diabetes.[24] Baba and coworkers reviewed the records of patients who had a cervical spine or peripheral nerve decompression (n = 768), and there were 65 surgical cases identified with both cervical radiculopathy and nerve entrapment in the arm.[2] Wood and colleagues reported on 165 cases of thoracic outlet syndrome, and in 73 cases the patients had a distal site of nerve compression that was confirmed with electrodiagnostic studies.[88]

Animal models to demonstrate the double crush mechanism have been described.[11,54] Using a canine model, Nemoto and colleagues placed compression clamps on the sciatic nerve and evaluated conduction velocity.[54] The placement of a second clamp at a proximal site reduced the motor conduction velocity as compared with both the normal and the clamped state. This study also evaluated the effect of removing the sequential compression clamps 3 weeks later. Removal of both clamps improved the motor conduction velocity to 65% of the original value and removal of only one clamp improved the conduction velocity to a lesser amount. Dellon and Mackinnon developed a rodent model that simulated sciatic nerve compression with Silastic tubes.[11] In one of three groups of animals, the Silastic tube was placed proximal to the sciatic nerve trifurcation. In the second group, the tube was placed on the tibial nerve distal to the trifurcation; and in the third group, tubes were placed simultaneously on the sciatic nerve and the peroneal nerve. In groups 1 and 2 after 7 months, a second tube was placed on the nerve (on the tibial nerve in group 1, and proximal to the sciatic nerve trifurcation in group 2) and no surgery was performed on the double band group. After 5 more months, the final electrodiagnostic studies were performed. The addition of a second band either proximally or distally resulted in a decrease in conduction velocity equal to the group that received the double bands initially. Because both the proximal and distal second band compromised the conduction velocity equally, this study supports the double crush and the reverse double crush mechanisms of nerve compression.

Systemic Conditions and Personal Factors

Other medical conditions and personal factors have been associated with carpal tunnel syndrome, including diabetes mellitus, hypothyroidism, excessive alcohol use, obesity, and tobacco use.[6,26,52,53,63,70-72] When compared with a control group without symptoms of carpal tunnel syndrome, the patients with carpal tunnel syndrome demonstrated a higher prevalence of hypothyroidism, diabetes, and obesity.[26] These findings supported previous reports of increased prevalence of these conditions in carpal tunnel syndrome.[3,6,63,70] In a retrospective case-control study, smoking history did not result in an increased incidence of carpal tunnel syndrome.[26]

A similar finding was noted in an experimental study of chronic nerve compression in a rodent study investigating the effect of cigarette smoke exposure and the severity of nerve compression.[12]

Hereditary motor-sensory neuropathy is a group of inherited disorders that affects the motor and sensory nerves of the peripheral nervous system and includes Charcot-Marie Tooth disease and hereditary neuropathy with liability to pressure palsies (HNPP). HNPP is an autosomal-dominant demyelinating motor-sensory neuropathy. It is characterized by an underexpression of the peripheral myelin protein-22 gene on chromosome 17 and presents as recurrent, multi-focal nerve compression.[28] Patients may present with rapid-onset neuropathies after minor trauma and with decreased nerve conduction studies (motor and sensory) in the affected and unaffected nerves. In most cases there is complete recovery without surgery. In the upper extremity the ulnar nerve is mostly commonly affected, and in the lower extremity the peroneal nerve is affected. The presence of HNPP should be considered in patients with multiple recurrent neuropathies.

Longitudinal Nerve Mobility

Longitudinal nerve mobility is important for normal nerve function. Whereas some longitudinal movement is permitted via the plexus formation within a nerve and via the loose attachment of its mesoneurium, damage may occur with excessive or prolonged traction. Venous flow blockage was shown with acute stretching of 8% of resting length, and ischemia occurred when the nerve was stretched 15% of its resting length.[38] Watanabe and colleagues investigated nerve strain in a rat model.[83] The authors used the same amount of strain in the continuous and the repetitive strain groups and reported abnormalities in the repetitive strain group as measured by histologic, electrophysiologic, and functional evaluation. They concluded that small repetitive strains on neural tissue may result in neural dysfunction, particularly in patients with subclinical pathology.

Byl and colleagues evaluated median and ulnar nerve strain during median and ulnar nerve tension tests.[5] They found that there was an increased strain on the median and ulnar nerve with neural tension tests. Nakamichi and Tachibana reported restriction of median nerve excursion in patients with carpal tunnel syndrome.[51] The authors theorize that nerve compression induces connective tissue and synovial thickening that may secondarily result in restriction of neural mobility with joint motion.[51,69,74]

Authors' Opinion

Much of the controversy associated with nerve compression is related to patients with diffuse symptoms and to the relationship of occupation to nerve compression disorders. Certain postures and positions may contribute to nerve compression. It is well accepted that wrist positions of moderate flexion and extension will increase pressures within the carpal canal, and this is hypothesized to contribute to carpal tunnel syndrome.[15,31,84] Similarly, elbow flexion will increase pressure within the cubital tunnel, thus compromising the ulnar nerve.[19,66] However, these postures and positions will not only impact the nerve but may also affect the surrounding musculature (Fig. 28-2).[45] We believe that abnormal postures or positions will affect the nerve and soft tissues in the upper extremity and cervicoscapular region and the resultant multiple sites of nerve compression and muscle imbalance will contribute to diffuse upper-quadrant patient symptoms.

EVALUATION

Different tests used for patient evaluation will yield important information at different stages of nerve compression (see Fig. 28-1). Not all tests will be positive at all stages; therefore, it is important to use the assessment tools that will give the most necessary information, to identify pathology or to grade severity. To develop an appropriate treatment

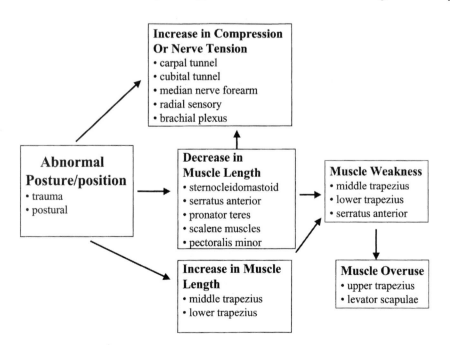

FIGURE 28-2. Abnormal postures and/or positions will have three main effects: (1) Nerves may be compressed or placed on tension and progress to chronic nerve compression; (2) muscles may be placed in shortened positions and then secondarily compress nerves; or (3) muscles in elongated or shortened positions will be weakened and thus underused. Other muscles will compensate for the weakness and be overused, establishing a pattern of muscle imbalance.

plan, it is important to identify all sites of nerve compression and musculoskeletal disorders that are contributing to patient symptomatology. A complete sensory and motor evaluation, including electrodiagnostic studies, can determine the severity of nerve compression. In cases of work-related symptoms, separate consideration should be given to determine the involvement of work as a contributing factor. The use of a subjective pain evaluation questionnaire is helpful to identify all symptomatic areas and other factors that may contribute to patient symptomatology.[27,30,49] We have found the use of a pain evaluation questionnaire utilizing a body diagram, a subjective questionnaire, and 0 to 10 visual analogue scales to be very useful in evaluating patients with nerve compression and/or diffuse symptoms (Fig. 28-3). For successful management, evaluation and treatment should be directed at all levels of nerve compression and soft tissue disorders that are present.[56]

Use of Provocation Tests

Many signs and provocation tests have been described to clinically evaluate carpal tunnel syndrome.* The concept of increasing tension or compression on a nerve to assess for

*See references 9, 13, 14, 20, 22, 39, 62, 67, 68, and 87.

Pain Questionnaire

Name:________________________ Date:__________________

Age:___ Sex: Male_ Female_ Dominant Hand: Right_ Left_ Diagnosis:__________

1. Pain is difficult to describe. Circle the words that best describe your symptoms:

Burning	Throbbing	Aching	Stabbing	Tingling	Twisting	Squeezing
Cramping	Cutting	Shooting	Numbing	Vague	Stinging	Indescribable
Pulling	Smarting	Pressure	Coldness	Dull	Other: ________	

Level of symptoms: place a mark through the line to indicate the level of your pain, if zero is no pain and the end of the line is the most severe pain you can imagine having.

For Example: No Pain ——|—— Most Severe Pain

2. Mark your average level of pain in the last month

No Pain ———— Most Severe Pain

3. Mark your worst level of pain in the last week

Right No Pain ———— Most Severe Pain

Left No Pain ———— Most Severe Pain

4. Where is your pain? (Draw on diagram)

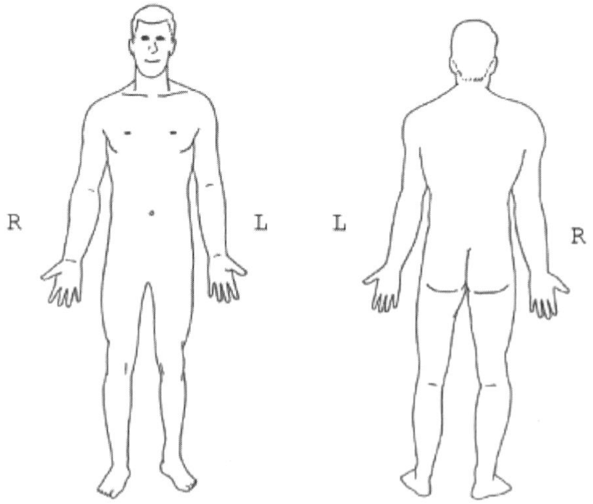

FIGURE 28-3. The pain evaluation questionnaire consists of pain adjectives, a body diagram, a questionnaire, and 0 to 10 visual analogue scales for pain, stress, and coping. Patients who select more than three adjectives, draw a pain pattern that does not follow a known anatomic pattern, or score more than 20 on the questionnaire are considered positive for that component. Patients who score positive in more than two components are considered for psychological or psychiatric evaluation before any surgical intervention. (Modified from Hendler N, Viernstein M, Gucer P, Long D: A preoperative screening test for chronic back pain patients. Psychosomatics 20:801-808, 1979; Mackinnon SE, Dellon AL: Surgery of the Peripheral Nerve. New York, Thieme Medical, 1988; and Melzack R: The McGill pain questionnaire: Major properties and scoring methods. Pain 1:277-299, 1975.) *Continued*

5. Mark your average level of stress in the last month.

at home |⎣_____⎦|
        0   10

at work |⎣_____⎦|
        0   10

6. How well are you able to cope with that stress?

at home |⎣_____⎦|
        Very Well   Not at all

at work |⎣_____⎦|
        Very Well   Not al all

7. How did the pain that you are now experiencing occur?
   a. Sudden onset with accident or definable event
   b. Slow progressive onset
   c. Slow progressive onset with acute exacerbation without an accident or definable event
   d. A sudden onset without an accident or definable event

8. How many surgical procedures have you had <u>in order to try to eliminate the cause of your pain</u>?
   a. None or one
   b. Two surgical procedures
   c. Three or four surgical procedures
   d. Greater than four surgical procedures

9. Does movement have any effect on your pain?
   a. The pain is always worsened by use or movement
   b. The pain is usually worsened by use and movement
   c. The pain is not altered by use and movement

10. Does weather have any effect on your pain?
   a. The pain is usually worse with damp or cold weather.
   b. The pain is occasionally worse with damp or cold weather.
   c. Damp or cold weather have no effect on the pain.

FIGURE 28-3—cont'd.

nerve compression at the carpal tunnel may be extrapolated to other sites of nerve compression in the upper extremity. The concept of the double crush mechanism is important in the assessment of patients with suspected nerve compression. Because one site of nerve compression may affect other sites of nerve compression, all potential entrapment sites of nerve compression should be assessed.

Provocation tests using direct pressure or joint movement to increase compression on the nerve can be used (Table 28-1). Beginning at the more distal sites, a Tinel's sign or a nerve percussion test is performed at each potential entrapment site by applying repeated digital percussion (carpal tunnel, median nerve forearm, cubital tunnel, radial sensory nerve, brachial plexus). The test is considered positive with radiation of a tingling sensation into the appropriate sensory neural distribution. In patients who are hyperresponsive to stimuli and/or have a positive nerve percussion testing at multiple entrapment sites, it is important to do a nerve percussion test at points where nerves are not anatomically located. Similarly, all provocative tests are done in both upper extremities in all patients, even with patients with only symptoms in one upper extremity.

Phalen's test that uses wrist flexion to increase pressure on the median nerve is a common provocation test used for assessment of carpal tunnel syndrome.[67,68] Since first described in 1966, a number of provocation tests using position and/or pressure to increase compression on the nerve have been reported.[9,13,14,20,22,39,62,87] Provocation tests should be maintained for 1 minute and are considered positive when patient symptoms are reproduced in the appropriate neural distribution. To correctly identify a site of chronic nerve compression, it is important to compress only one nerve entrapment site with each test. Pressure provocation can be performed to assess the median nerve at the carpal tunnel by placing the wrist in either wrist flexion or extension and then applying digital pressure just proximal to the carpal tunnel. In patients with restricted wrist movement, the pressure provocative test can be done with the wrist in a neutral position. Because the median nerve and the ulnar nerve can be compressed in this position, sensory alteration to the median and ulnar nerve distribution may be reported and should be documented. To evaluate the median nerve in the forearm, the patient's forearm is placed in full supination with full elbow extension and digital pressure is applied to the median nerve in the region of the pronator teres muscle. A positive response is noted with sensory alteration in the median nerve distribution. To evaluate the cubital tunnel, the elbow is placed in full flexion with neutral forearm rotation and the wrist in neutral. Digital pressure is placed on the ulnar nerve just proximal to the cubital tunnel.[55] The position of the ulnar nerve should also be evaluated because ulnar nerve subluxation over the medial epicondyle may occur in some patients. The radial sensory nerve is evaluated by placing the wrist in flexion and ulnar deviation and the forearm in a pronated position. Compression of the brachial plexus at the thoracic outlet should also be screened by having the patient raise both arms overhead and noting reproduction of patient symptoms

11. Do you ever have trouble falling asleep or awaken from sleep?
    a. No - Proceed to Question 12   **b.** Yes - Proceed to 11A & 11B

11A. How often do you have trouble falling asleep?
    a. Trouble falling asleep every night due to pain
    b. Trouble falling asleep due to pain most nights of the week
    c. Occasionally having difficulty falling asleep due to pain
    d. No trouble falling asleep due to pain
    e. Trouble falling asleep which is not related to pain

11B. How often do you awaken from sleep?
    a. Awakened by pain every night
    b. Awakened from sleep by pain more than 3 times per week
    c. Not usually awakened from sleep by pain
    d. Restless sleep or early morning awakening with or without being able to return to sleep, both unrelated to pain

12. Has your pain affected your intimate personal relationships?
    a. No   **b.** Yes

13. Are you involved in any legal action regarding your physical complaint?
    a. No   **b.** Yes

14. Is this a Workers' Compensation case?
    a. No   **b.** Yes

15. Are you presently receiving psychiatric treatment?
    a. No   **b.** Yes   **c.** Previous psychiatric treatment

16. Have you ever thought of suicide?
    a. No   **b.** Yes   **c.** Previous suicide attempts

17. Are you a victim of emotional abuse?
    a. No   **b.** Yes   **c.** No comment

18. Are you a victim of physical abuse?
    a. No   **b.** Yes   **c.** No comment

19. Are you a victim of sexual abuse?
    a. No   **b.** Yes   **c.** No comment

20. Are you presently a victim of abuse?
    a. No   **b.** Yes   **c.** No comment

FIGURE 28-3—cont'd.

in the hands.[57] Pain in the shoulder region is not considered predictive of brachial plexus nerve compression, and further evaluation of the shoulder is indicated.

Cervical nerve root impingement is assessed clinically with Spurling's test.[80] This foraminal nerve root encroachment test is performed by placing the patient's cervical spine in slight extension and lateral flexion. Axial compression is then applied to the patient's head, and if a "spray" of symptoms into the arm is reported, it is considered positive for nerve root compression. The test is repeated with lateral flexion to the contralateral side. Tong and colleagues evaluated 255 patients and found a 30% sensitivity and 93% specificity with Spurling's test.[80] This study would suggest that the test correctly identifies patients with no cervical radiculopathy, but it is not as effective in identifying patients with a cervical radiculopathy. Therefore, with a positive response to Spurling's test or symptoms suggesting involvement of the cervical spine, further cervical spine radiologic investigation is indicated.

Shoulder and Scapular Movement Examination

Examination of the shoulder and evaluation of scapular movement patterns are important components of the physical examination of patients complaining of upper extremity pain. Abnormal postures of the neck and shoulder and scapular region frequently result in muscle imbalance especially of the serratus anterior and middle and lower trapezius muscles. The patient is asked to forward flex the shoulders, raising the arms above the head. Scapular position and movement are noted. As the patient slowly lowers his or her arms, the examiner looks for any winging of the scapula to evaluate for serratus anterior strength. Similarly, to evaluate trapezius strength, the patient is asked to abduct the shoulders above the head and then slowly lower the arms as the examiner looks for winging of the scapula.

Compression of the nerves in the upper extremity will produce symptoms of paresthesia and numbness. By contrast, aching pain and arm fatigue symptoms are more associated with muscle imbalance. In patients presenting with these symptoms, examination of scapular position, and weakness of the serratus anterior and middle/lower trapezius muscles should be evaluated and treated. Similarly, if the patient has associated rotator cuff tendinitis or shoulder impingement, the symptoms will also be reflected in upper extremity discomfort. A shoulder examination for these problems is also important.

Sensory Evaluation

Whereas provocation of the nerve can help to identify the sites of nerve compression, it does not quantify sensory function. Many instruments and assessment devices have been described for evaluation of sensibility, but no one test

21. If you are retired, a student or homemaker, proceed to Question 21B.
  21A. Are you still working?
    a. Works every day at the same pre-pain job.
    b. Works every day but the job is not the same as the pre-pain job with reduced responsibility and physical activity
    c. Works occasionally.
    d. Not presently working.

  21B. Are you able to do your household chores?
    a. Does same level of household activities without discomfort.
    b. Does same level of household chores with discomfort.
    c. Does a reduced amount of household chores.
    d. Most household chores are now performed by others.

22. What medications have you used in the past month?
    a. No medications
    b. List medications:_____

    _____

    _____

23. If you had three wishes for anything in the world, what would you wish for?

    1. _____

    2. _____

    3. _____

0% |——————————————————————| 100%

FIGURE 28-3—cont'd.

has been accepted as the gold standard. This in part relates to the varying capacities of the sensory tests to evaluate different parameters of nerve function.

The four sensory receptors that are found in the glabrous skin of the hand are categorized by differing receptive field size and response qualities. The slowly adapting receptors (Merkel cell neurite complex and Ruffini end organs) respond to static touch, and the quickly adapting receptors (Meissner and Pacinian corpuscles) respond to moving touch. The threshold and tactile discrimination of the quickly and slowly adapting receptors can be evaluated. Threshold is the minimum stimulus required to elicit a response and is assessed with vibration thresholds (quickly adapting receptors) and with cutaneous pressure thresholds (slowly adapting receptors). Tactile discrimination reflects the number of innervated sensory receptors and is assessed with moving and static two-point discrimination. Vibration and cutaneous pressure thresholds will permit quantification of the early changes that occur with chronic nerve compression. Changes in the sensory receptor innervation density will occur in the later stages of chronic nerve compression, and therefore two-point discrimination measures will become abnormal only in the more severe stages of nerve compression.

Light Moving Touch

A quick screening of the large A-beta fibers can be performed using the ten test.[73] Introduced by Strauch and coworkers, the ten test allows the patient to rank his or her sensation of light moving touch on a scale from 0 to 10 as compared with the normal contralateral area.[73] Good reliability and validity were reported when compared with Semmes-Weinstein monofilament testing.[73] In patients with carpal tunnel syndrome, Patel and Bassini reported the ten test to be the most sensitive test as compared with the Weinstein Enhanced Sensory Test and two-point discrimination.[65] For assessment with the ten test, the examiner applies a light touch, moving the stimulus with his or her finger to an area of normal sensation on the contralateral digit. A similar stimulus is applied simultaneously to the affected area, and the patient is asked to rank the sensation on a scale from 0 to 10, with 10 being perfect sensation and 0 being no sensation. Whereas this has proved to be an excellent screening test, it has limited use in patients with systemic sensory neuropathy and bilateral upper extremity nerve compression.

Vibration Thresholds

Vibration can be used to assess the thresholds of the quickly adapting receptors. Qualitatively, vibration thresholds may be evaluated with a tuning fork. The tuning fork is applied to the affected and contralateral digit pulp, and the patient is asked to compare the stimuli. Limitations of this test include patient subjective assessment to recall the applied stimuli and a consistent application of the tuning fork by the examiner.

A number of fixed-frequency and variable-frequency vibrometers have been described to permit quantification of the vibration thresholds.[10,21,25,34-36] Although good reliability has been reported with single-frequency vibrometers, the greatest limitation is that only one frequency is assessed. In a study of 130 factory workers, Werner and colleagues did not find single-frequency vibrometry useful as a screening tool for median nerve pathology.[85] In nerve compression, it

PAIN EVALUATION SCORE SHEET

Name: _____   Date: _____

DOB: _____   Age: _____   Sex: M ___ F___   Dominant Hand: R ___ L___

Diagnosis: _____

1. Number of Descriptors: ____

2. Pain Level: on average ____   3. Pain Level: worst right _____ left ____

4. Body Diagram: _____

5. Stress Level: home _____ work _____   6. Coping Level: home _____ work _____

7	8	9	10		11	11A	11B
a. 0	a. 0	a. 0	a. 0		a. 3	a. 0	a. 0
b. 0	b. 2	b. 2	b. 2		b. 0	b. 1	b. 1
c. 3	c. 3	c. 3	c. 3			c. 2	c. 3
d. 4	d. 4					d. 3	d. 4
						e. 4	

12	13	14	15		16	17	18
a. 0	a. 0	a. 0	a. 0		a. 0	a. 0	a. 0
b. 2	b. 3	b. 2	b. 4		b. 2	b. 5	b. 5
			c. 2		c. 5	c. 3	c. 3

19	20	21A	21B	22		23	
a. 0	a. 0	a. 0	a. 0	a. 0		a. 0	No pain only wish
b. 5	b. 5	b. 0	b. 0	b. 1	Valium	b. 1	No pain one of wishes
c. 3	c. 3	c. 2	c. 2	c. 2	Narcotic	c. 2	Wishes only of personal nature
		d. 3	d. 3	d. 3	Psychotropic or antidepressant drugs	d. 3	Wishes of non-personal nature i.e. world peace

Total: _____

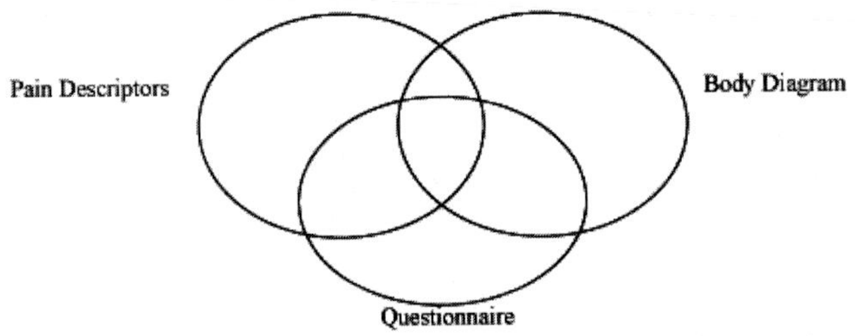

Pain Descriptors   Body Diagram

Questionnaire

FIGURE 28-3—cont'd.

is hypothesized that perception of the higher frequencies is affected earlier; therefore, evaluation at multiple frequencies may permit earlier identification of sensory loss.[35] In a study of patients with brachial plexus nerve compression, vibration thresholds measured at multiple frequencies were not useful in identifying these patients.[8]

Cutaneous Pressure Thresholds

Pressure thresholds of the slowly adapting receptors are commonly evaluated with Semmes-Weinstein monofilaments. These nylon monofilaments vary in diameter and thus differ in application force and produce different pressure thresholds. The set of Semmes-Weinstein monofilaments increases in diameter on a logarithmic scale (log_{10} force of 0.1 mg). The examiner applies pressure with each successive nylon filament until the filament just begins to bend. The smallest monofilament that the patient can perceive is documented as the pressure threshold. Consistency of monofilament diameter and of testing procedure is necessary to ensure reliability.[29,82] In a study evaluating normal subjects, variability of monofilament threshold was found with repeated testing.[48] Pressure thresholds have

been shown to be sensitive in testing for carpal tunnel syndrome.[75-78,160]

Two-Point Discrimination

Two-point discrimination more accurately reflects the number of innervated sensory receptors. Initially measured with a paper clip, other instruments such as the Disk-Criminator (Neuroregen, Baltimore, MD) have been described for the measurement of static and moving two-point discrimination.[42,50] Whereas good reliability has been shown with the Disk-Criminator,[57] alterations in two-point discrimination occur only with severe nerve compression.[77,78] Therefore, this is not a very sensitive test for patients with mild chronic nerve compression.

Electrodiagnostic Studies

Electrodiagnostic studies include electromyography (EMG) and nerve conduction studies. They are no substitute for a detailed clinical examination by an experienced clinician. Unfortunately, some physicians rely on these studies without recognizing the major limitations of the electrodiag-

Table 28-1
PROVOCATIVE TESTS FOR NERVE ENTRAPMENT

Nerve	Entrapment Site	Provocative Test	Conservative Management
Median	Carpal tunnel	Pressure proximal to carpal tunnel Phalen's test Reverse Phalen's test (hyperextension wrist)	Splint wrist in neutral position at night.
	Proximal forearm	Pressure over proximal forearm in region of pronator teres with forearm supination Resisted elbow flexion, pronation, and finger flexion	Use stretching exercises for pronator teres.
Ulnar	Guyon's canal	Pressure proximal to Guyon's canal Reverse Phalen's test	Splint wrist in neutral position at night.
	Cubital tunnel	Elbow flexion and pressure proximal to cubital tunnel	Educate about elbow pad, positioning in elbow extension and decreasing direct pressure on nerve.
Radial (posterior interosseous)	Arcade of Fröhse	Pressure over supinator Resisted supination Resisted long-finger and wrist extension	Position in supination and avoid repetitive pronation and supination activities.
Radial (sensory)	Forearm	Pressure over junction of brachioradialis/extensor carpi radialis tendon Forearm pronation with wrist ulnar flexion	Avoid repetitive pronation and supination activities.
Brachial plexus	Supraclavicular	Elevation of arms above head Pressure over brachial plexus in interscalene region	Avoid provocative positions. Stretch shortened muscles and strengthen weakened scapular stabilizers.

nostic examination.[86] A well-done study can complement the clinical evaluation by helping to localize the level and severity of the injury and in predicting the likelihood of spontaneous regeneration and recovery.

A major weakness of the *nerve conduction* portion of the electrodiagnostic study is that it evaluates only the large myelinated fibers. This will include motor axons and sensory axons relaying vibration and light touch but not the smaller axons conveying pain or temperature sensation. The determination of nerve latency reflects the conduction of the best myelinated fibers rather than the most severely affected axons, and normal latency may still be present even when many nerve fibers are affected. In chronic nerve compression, the first changes to occur in the nerve fiber population are changes to the unmyelinated nerve fibers, which cannot be evaluated with electrodiagnostic studies.[44] For example, symptoms of pain and paresthesia cannot be objectified by electrodiagnostic studies. Another limitation of nerve conduction studies relates to the location of the nerve injury in the extremity. Nerve problems occurring very distally in the extremity or very proximally in the extremity are difficult to assess. Dynamic changes in blood flow that may produce intermittent alterations in peripheral nerve function may not be detected with electrodiagnostic studies. The timing of the nerve conduction studies also influences their utility, because even complete nerve transection will not become apparent for 2 to 6 weeks after injury. In situations with more than one level of injury or when a systemic polyneuropathy is present, nerve conduction studies may be less reliable. Connective tissue changes, which would, for example, distinguish a second-degree from a third-degree injury,

would not be evaluated with electrodiagnostic studies. Although electrodiagnostic studies provide the surgeon with quantifiable values, they are extremely dependent on the expertise of the examiner who performs them.

Electromyography

For the EMG component of the study, needle-recording electrodes are inserted into muscles to evaluate either spontaneous or volitional electrical activity. Muscle response with needle insertion at rest and activation response is noted. A normal muscle will respond with a brief burst of electrical activity with needle insertion (insertional activity). Abnormal insertional activity can include insertional positive sharp waves, as seen in early denervation, or electrical silence, which is associated with chronic muscle degeneration without reinnervation. In the rest phase there will normally be electrical silence, but with nerve injury, spontaneous activity with fibrillation potentials is noted. Fibrillation potentials are the earliest sign of muscle denervation and are generated by muscles after denervation of at least 2 weeks. A single motor axon innervates hundreds to thousands of muscle fibers; thus, fibrillation potentials are the most sensitive indicator of motor axon loss and can be seen in nerve compression syndromes long before there is any clinical evidence of muscle weakness. During the muscle activation portion of the EMG, the patient is instructed to contract the muscle, causing voluntary motor unit potentials (MUPs). In a normal muscle, so many MUPs are activated that individual MUPs cannot be seen and a full interference pattern is noted. With nerve injury, incomplete MUP activation and reduced MUP recruitment is seen. Patients responding with pain, hysteria, or malingering can show incomplete MUP activation, but the rate will be slow to moderate. With reduced MUP recruitment due to a peripheral nerve problem, firing rate will be faster and the configuration will be of increased duration and amplitude. The neurologist doing the EMG will be able to determine chronic neurogenic MUP changes from incomplete MUP activation as seen with upper motor neuron disease or decreased patient effort. MUPs associated with reinnervation initially will be of very low amplitude and extremely polyphasic, firing at a slow to moderate rate. Eventually they will remodel so that the duration and number of phases decreases and the amplitude increases.

Nerve Conduction Studies

Nerve conduction studies can be used to study motor, sensory, and mixed nerves. Surface electrodes are used to stimulate and record from the nerve. During motor nerve conduction studies, electrodes are placed over the muscle and the motor axons are stimulated proximal to the surface electrode. Motor axons are indirectly assessed as the compound muscle action potentials (CMAPs) that are generated by the muscle fibers, not the motor nerve itself. This results in a large amplitude response as compared with sensory nerve conduction studies, in which the sensory axons themselves are directly assessed and the sensory nerve action potential (SNAP) is very small. Sensory nerve function can be assessed in antegrade (orthodromic) or retrograde (antidromic) fashion by placing the recording electrode either proximal or distal to the stimulating electrode, respectively. Because of their small size and low amplitude, SNAPs may be adversely affected by technical problems or by factors such as skin or room temperature. Nerve conduction studies evaluate amplitude, duration, latency, the area of the recorded response, and conduction velocity. Laboratories have their own set of normal values based on age. The best control for amplitude in individuals with unilateral neurologic problems will be an amplitude drop of more than 50% on the symptomatic side as compared with the normal extremity.

Latency is a measure of the speed of conduction expressed in milliseconds and measures transmission along the fastest conducting fibers. Sensory nerves are stimulated at only one point. The recorded latency is reported as an onset in peak latency. Motor nerves are generally stimulated at two points along their course.

Amplitude is the height of the action potential expressed in millivolts for motor nerve conduction studies and microvolts for sensory nerve conduction studies. The amplitude provides an assessment of the number of conducting axons. Amplitudes are more difficult to assess; but because they relatively reflect the number of functioning axons, they may give more information about symptoms of muscle weakness and paresthesias than do latency measurements, which reflect only the fastest conducting fibers. Conduction velocity is calculated by stimulating the nerve at two measured distances and determining the rate of conduction in meters per second between the two points. It is useful when comparing results between subjects with different limb lengths. However, it reflects the speed of the fastest conducting fibers and, unlike amplitude, does not give any information regarding the number of conducting axons. Area is a function of amplitude and duration of response and more accurately reflects the number of axons, but, like amplitude, is technically more difficult to assess.

Electrodiagnostic Studies and Nerve Compression

Electrodiagnostic studies give information about axon and myelin pathology, and each component is important to properly identify nerve pathology. Latency and conduction velocity should not be viewed in isolation, because the speed of conduction relates only to the healthiest surviving myelinated nerve fibers. In contrast, if amplitude is measured, then a drop in amplitude can reflect a loss of axons. The EMG studies will demonstrate scarce fibrillation potentials early on and, if the axonal problem is more severe, reduced MUP recruitment. Thus with mild injuries, the only abnormalities noted may be fibrillation potentials on the EMG, with maintenance of normal nerve conduction studies. With progression, the number of fibrillation potentials will increase and the nerve conduction study amplitudes will decrease. SNAP amplitudes are affected before the CMAP amplitudes. Eventually, MUP recruitment will decrease. With complete injury, nerve conduction motor and sensory responses will be absent, fibrillation potentials will be marked, and no MUPs will be identified.

The early stage of nerve compression is associated with dynamic ischemic events to the nerve. Thus, results of electrodiagnostic studies for the most part are normal. As the compression progresses, demyelination will occur and conduction velocity will slow across the site of compression. Axonal loss does not usually occur until late in the course of the neuropathy. With carpal tunnel syndrome, nerve conduction study latencies may be prolonged, but the EMG is usually normal until late in the disease. Demyelination and focal conduction slowing are typical of most cases of carpal tunnel syndrome and at least half of those of cubital tunnel syndrome, with axonal changes being found much later in the course of the disease.

Electrodiagnostic studies are useful in ruling out other associated problems such as cervical disk disease, motor neuron problems, or superimposed polyneuropathies. They are particularly useful in the investigation of symptoms relating to the ulnar nerve, which can sometimes herald the presence of other more sinister diagnoses. Patients presenting with isolated motor deficits and spared sensory function must have a motor neuropathy ruled out before diagnosing entrapment neuropathy. Electrodiagnostic studies can also help to rule out problems that are functional. Muscles that are weak or atrophic because of disuse will show no abnormalities on EMG other than poor voluntary MUP generation, in keeping with submaximal effort on the part of the patient. If the muscle is weak or atrophic because of a peripheral nerve problem, the CMAP will be of low amplitude, MUP recruitment will be reduced, and fibrillation potentials will be noted, unless the process is extremely chronic. Because of the proximal location at the brachial plexus and the often dynamic nature of the compression, electrodiagnostic studies are not generally helpful in confirming a diagnosis of thoracic outlet syndrome.

COMPRESSION OF THE MEDIAN NERVE

Median Nerve Compression at the Wrist: Carpal Tunnel Syndrome

Carpal tunnel syndrome is the term used to describe a group of symptoms associated with compression of the median nerve at the wrist and is the most commonly diagnosed site of nerve compression in the upper extremity.[94,135] Symptoms include paresthesia and/or numbness in the median nerve distribution of the hand (thumb, index, middle finger, and the radial side of the ring finger). Patients may describe aching in the thenar eminence, and, with severe nerve compression, weakness and atrophy of the abductor pollicis brevis and opponens pollicis. Carpal tunnel syndrome is a clinical diagnosis, based on a combination of symptom characteristics and characteristic physical findings; its presence may be subsequently confirmed with electrodiagnostic studies.[128,152]

 ## Anatomy

The carpal canal is defined by the flexor retinaculum, which spans from the hamate and triquetrum on the ulnar side to the scaphoid and trapezium on the radial side. The median nerve and flexor tendons (flexor pollicis longus, four flexor digitorum superficialis and four flexor digitorum profundus tendons) pass through this tunnel. Although the carpal tunnel is open at the proximal and distal ends, it maintains distinct tissue fluid pressure levels.[108] The carpal tunnel diameter is the most narrow at a point approximately 2 cm from its leading edge (Fig. 28-4),[109,154] and this corresponds to the site of morphologic changes in the nerve in patients with carpal tunnel syndrome.[95] The median nerve lies just beneath the flexor retinaculum. At the distal end of the flexor retinaculum, the median nerve gives off the recurrent motor branch to innervate the abductor pollicis brevis, the superficial head of the flexor pollicis brevis, and the opponens pollicis muscles and then divides into the digital nerves that provide sensation to the thumb, index, middle, and the radial half of the ring finger.

Knowledge of the variation in the branching of the median nerve is important particularly during surgical decompression.[140] Lanz has classified variations of the recurrent motor branch into four subgroups (Figs. 28-5 to 28-7).[132] In most cases, the motor branch divides from the median nerve distal to the flexor retinaculum in an extraligamentous pattern (46% to 90%). Less common variations include the subligamentous pattern (31%) or transligamentous pattern (23%).[164] There have been reports of the recurrent motor branch dividing from the medial side of the median nerve.[103,132] Amadio[93] and Szabo and Petty[161] described an unusual variation in which a separate compartment within the carpal tunnel contained half of a bifid median nerve. Variation in the branching pattern of the palmar cutaneous branch of the median nerve has also been reported.[113,115, 143,165] The palmar cutaneous nerve has been reported to branch through the palmaris tendon proximal to the palmar

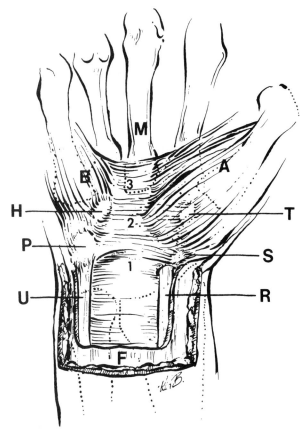

FIGURE 28-4. Anatomy of the three portions of the flexor retinaculum. The distal portion of the flexor retinaculum (3) consists of a thick aponeurosis between the thenar (A) and hypothenar (B) muscles. The thenar muscles attach to the radial half of the classic flexor retinaculum, which is composed of the distal portion of the flexor retinaculum (3) and the transverse carpal ligament (2). Bony attachments of the transverse carpal ligament—pisiform (P), hamate (H), tubercle of the trapezium (T), and tubercle of the scaphoid (S)—are also shown. The proximal portion of the flexor retinaculum (1) courses deep to the flexor carpi ulnaris (U) and the flexor carpi radialis (R). The flexor carpi radialis tendon is shown as it pierces the flexor retinaculum at the junction of the proximal and middle portions to enter its fibro-osseous canal. F, antebrachial fascia; M, third metacarpal. (From Cobb TK, Dalley BK, Posteraro RH, Lewis RC: Anatomy of flexor retinaculum. J Hand Surg [Am] 18:91-99, 1993.)

fascia[115] and also through the antebrachial fascia proximal to the wrist crease (Fig. 28-8).[113] To avoid injury to these anomalous branching patterns during surgical approach to the median nerve, Taleisnik recommended an incision ulnar to the axis of the flexed ring finger.[162] Although considerable variation in the length and location of the surgical incision used for carpal tunnel release exists among hand surgeons,[133] consideration of the anatomy of the palmar cutaneous and recurrent motor nerves is essential to avoid inadvertent injury.

Management

A number of nonoperative treatments for carpal tunnel syndrome have been described that vary from wrist splinting to corticosteroid injection.[104,120,125-127,166,167]

Wrist splinting is often recommended for nonoperative treatment of carpal tunnel syndrome.[104,167] Prefabricated

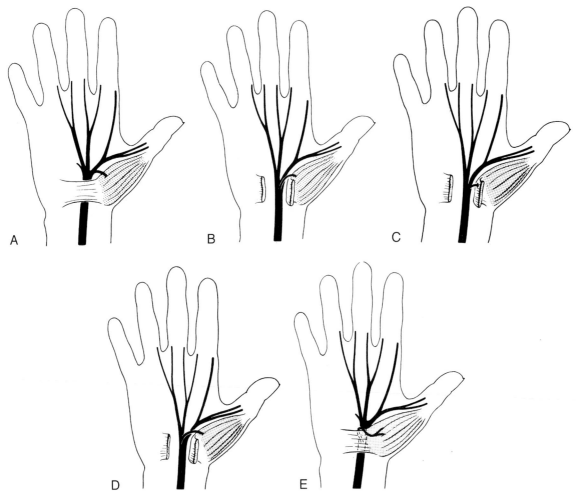

FIGURE 28-5. Variations in median nerve anatomy in the carpal tunnel. **A,** The most common pattern of the motor branch is extraligamentous and recurrent. **B,** Subligamentous branching of a recurrent median nerve. **C,** Transligamentous course of the recurrent branch of the median nerve. **D,** The motor branch can uncommonly originate from the ulnar border of the median nerve. **E,** The motor branch can lie on top of the transverse carpal ligament. (From Lanz U: Anatomical variations of the median nerve in the carpal tunnel. J Hand Surg [Am] 2:44-53, 1977.)

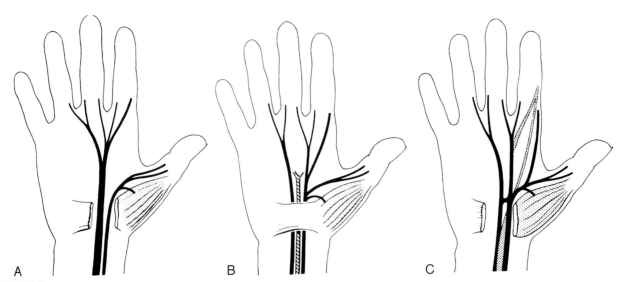

FIGURE 28-6. Variations in median nerve anatomy in the carpal tunnel. Group III variations include (**A**) high divisions of the median nerve that may be separated by (**B**) a persistent median artery of (**C**) an aberrant muscle. (From Lanz U: Anatomical variations of the median nerve in the carpal tunnel. J Hand Surg [Am] 2:44-53, 1977.)

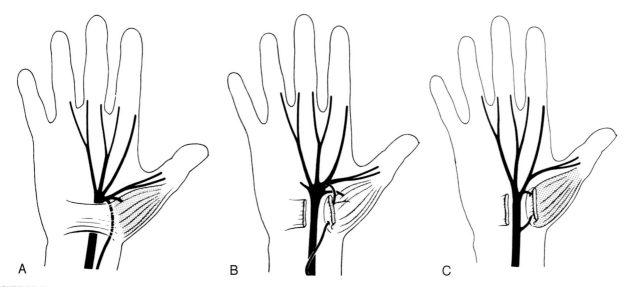

FIGURE 28-7. Variations in median nerve anatomy in the carpal tunnel. Group IV variations include those rare instances in which the thenar branch leaves the median nerve proximal to the carpal tunnel: (**A**) accessory branch; (**B**) accessory branch from the ulnar aspect of the median nerve; (**C**) accessory branch running directly into the thenar musculature. (From Lanz U: Anatomical variations of the median nerve in the carpal tunnel. J Hand Surg [Am] 2:44-53, 1977.)

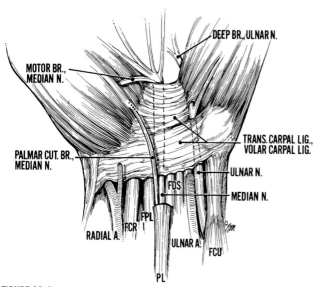

FIGURE 28-8. The palmar cutaneous branch of the median nerve lies radial to the median nerve and ulnar to the flexor carpi radialis tendon (FCR). It may pierce either the volar carpal or transverse carpal ligament or the antebrachial fascia before it becomes subcutaneous.

wrist splints are often used and can present a unique problem because these prefabricated splints are positioned in 30 degrees of extension. Carpal canal pressures have been shown to be elevated in patients with carpal tunnel syndrome, and pressure is further elevated in a position of wrist extension.[121,138,166] To control symptoms, wrist splints are most effective in a neutral position.[166] Maintaining the wrist in a neutral position will minimize the carpal canal pressures, but the functional position of the wrist is 30 degrees of extension. Because of the limitation of wrist movement

in a nonfunctional position, we do not recommend wrist splints during normal daily activity. We recommend splinting only at night to maintain the wrist in a neutral position.

Oral anti-inflammatory medications and corticosteroid injections have been used in the treatment of carpal tunnel syndrome with varying reported success.[104,120,125,127,167] Gonzalez and Bylak followed 30 patients with carpal tunnel syndrome for 18 months after corticosteroid injection and reported 11% with symptomatic relief at 12 and 18 months.[125] Celiker and colleagues reported a randomized controlled trial evaluating the efficacy of corticosteroid injection versus nonsteroidal anti-inflammatory drug and splinting.[104] They reported significant improvement in both methods of treatment; however, the brief follow-up time of only 8 weeks limited the applicability of the study. Edgell and coworkers[117] and Green[127] reported that relief from a carpal tunnel injection was an excellent prognostic factor for successful carpal tunnel surgery. Complications with steroid injections have been reported, including injury to the median nerve.[134,144] In a study evaluating the effects of steroid nerve injection in a rodent model, dexamethasone was found to have no deleterious effects on the nerve, even when injected directly into the nerve.[141] All other corticosteroids caused varying degrees of nerve injury when directly injected into the rodent sciatic nerve. However, given the temporary symptom relief in a small percentage of patients, corticosteroid injection is not indicated routinely. Vitamin B[6] has been reported as a nonoperative treatment for carpal tunnel syndrome, but its efficacy in one study was limited.[92]

More recently, nerve gliding exercises have been utilized to alleviate symptoms of nerve compression.[102,156,157] Rozmaryn and coworkers treated a group of patients with carpal tunnel syndrome with nerve and tendon gliding exercises and noted less surgical intervention in this group than a historical control group.[156] Seradge and associates reported good symptomatic relief and avoidance of surgery in patients treated with nerve gliding and stretching exercises.[157] Nathan and colleagues reported improvement in median nerve function after an aerobic exercise program.[150]

Operative Treatment

When a regimen of conservative treatment fails to relieve patient symptoms, surgical decompression of the median nerve is usually recommended. The first carpal tunnel release was reportedly performed by Herbert Galloway in 1924.[94] Numerous approaches to carpal tunnel release have been described, ranging from an open technique to small incision to endoscopic release.* Whereas release of the median nerve is the goal of treatment, injury to even a few fascicles of the nerve, although a known complication, can have devastating consequences for the patient.[99,114,147,159,163] Therefore, the surgeon should choose the surgical method that offers the best visualization of the median nerve to avoid injury to the nerve. It has been demonstrated that surgical release of the median nerve also has a salutary effect on symptoms of ulnar nerve compression in Guyon's canal.[158]

Endoscopic techniques were introduced to decrease the length of the incision and thus potentially decrease postoperative incisional discomfort. A number of endoscopic systems have been described, but the risk of complications, including iatrogenic nerve injury, poor visualization, inability to identify anatomic variations, incomplete release, and apparent beneficial cost savings, is still debated.† Those who support endoscopic carpal tunnel release also advocate specialized training in cadaveric courses before performance of endoscopic carpal tunnel release. Others have introduced surgical releases using smaller incisions termed "minimally invasive" to decrease postoperative incisional pain and thus minimize postoperative morbidity.[100,149,168]

Chow Two-Portal Endoscopic Technique. A two-portal endoscopic technique was introduced by Chow.[105-107] A tourniquet is placed but not inflated. Local anesthesia with 1% lidocaine without epinephrine is used in addition to intravenous sedation. The entry portal is located by drawing a line 1 to 1.5 cm radially from the proximal pole of the pisiform and a second line 0.5 cm proximally from the first line. A 1-cm transverse incision is made through the skin radially from the end of the second line (Fig. 28-9). A longitudinal incision is then made through the fascia. A curved dissector-obturator slotted cannula assembly is inserted through the distal edge of the entry portal incision following the long axis of the forearm. It is used to free synovial tissue from the inferior surface of the flexor retinaculum. The assembly tip touches the hook of the hamate, the hand is lifted off the table, and the wrist and fingers are hyperextended. At 1 cm proximal to a line drawn that bisects the angle formed by the distal border of the fully abducted thumb and the third web space, a 0.5-cm exit portal incision is made (Fig. 28-9). The slotted cannula assembly is distally advanced and the tip palpated at the exit portal in the palm. The assembly is passed through, and the hand is stabilized

in the holder (Fig. 28-9). The endoscope is inserted into the proximal tube opening, and a probe is inserted distally to identify the distal edge of the flexor retinaculum. The probe knife is used to release the distal edge of the flexor retinaculum in a distal-to-proximal direction. The triangle knife is then used to release the midsection of the flexor retinaculum, and then the retrograde knife is positioned in the second cut and drawn distally to join the first cut to release the distal part of the flexor retinaculum. The endoscope is placed in the distal tube opening, and the probe knife is used to release the proximal edge of the flexor retinaculum. The retrograde knife is inserted into the midsection and drawn proximally to complete the flexor retinaculum release. The trocar is reinserted and the cannula removed, and the skin is then sutured.

Agee Single-Portal Endoscopic Technique. A single incision technique was described by Agee.[89-91] A tourniquet is used for this procedure. Agee recommends that initially a general or regional anesthetic should be used and, with more surgeon experience, he recommends using local anesthesia. A 2- to 3-cm transverse skin incision is made in the distal wrist flexion crease between the flexor carpi radialis and flexor carpi ulnaris tendons (Fig. 28-10A). With the use of a spreading longitudinal dissection, the cutaneous nerves are protected and the forearm fascia is identified. A "U"-shaped, distally based flap of forearm fascia is incised and elevated in a palmar direction (see Fig. 28-10B). A probe is passed down the ulnar side of the carpal tunnel, radial to the hook of the hamate. The wrist is placed in slight extension, and the blade assembly is inserted with the viewing window toward the inner aspect of the flexor retinaculum. The blade assembly is palpated with the surgeon's contralateral hand (see Fig. 28-10C). The distal edge of the flexor retinaculum is located by video, ballottement, and light touch through the skin. When the correct position is ensured, the blade is elevated, the device is withdrawn, and the distal aspect of the flexor retinaculum is incised (see Fig. 28-10D). The blade assembly is reinserted, the flexor retinaculum division is inspected, and additional cuts are made to release the remaining flexor retinaculum. Using tenotomy scissors, the forearm fascia is released proximal to the skin incision (see Fig. 28-10E). The skin incision is closed, and splinting is at the discretion of the surgeon.[90] Agee strongly recommends that if complete visualization is not obtained then the endoscopic technique should be abandoned and the carpal tunnel released using an open technique.

Author's Preferred Technique: Open Carpal Tunnel Release

I (SEM) prefer the classic open carpal tunnel release with an intravenous regional anesthesia (Bier block) for treatment of carpal tunnel syndrome. General anesthesia is rarely indicated. Axillary blocks have been associated with nerve injection injuries; and although this complication is exceedingly rare, when it does occur, it is devastating for the patient. Many surgeons use simple local anesthesia, but I

---

*See references 89-91, 97, 98, 100, 101, 105-107, 122, 131, 139, 142, 146, 148, 149, 153, and 168.

†See references 96, 97, 99, 101, 114, 118, 129, 139, 147, 151, 155, and 159.

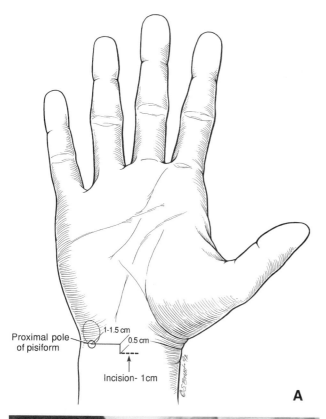

A

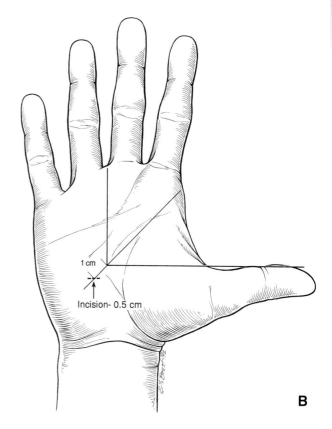

B

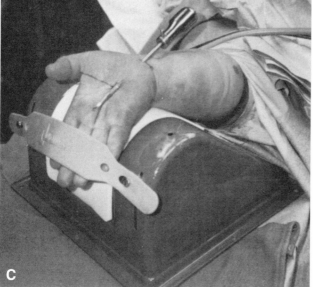

C

FIGURE 28-9. Chow two-portal endoscopic technique. **A,** Using the proximal pole of the pisiform as a landmark, the entry portal is made by drawing a line 1 to 1.5 cm radially and then a second line 0.5 cm proximally from the end of the first line. A third line is drawn approximately 1 cm radially from the end of the second line to indicate the entry portal. **B,** The exit portal is located by drawing a line that bisects the angle formed by the distal border of the fully abducted thumb and the third web space, approximately 1 cm proximal to the junction of these lines. **C,** Hand stabilized in a special hand holder. (From Chow JC: Endoscopic carpal tunnel release: Two-portal technique. Hand Clin 10:637-646, 1994.)

believe that patients are more comfortable with some sedation and tolerate the tourniquet better with an intravenous regional block (250 mm Hg). In the rare cases when the use of a tourniquet is contraindicated, the anesthetic nerve blocks of the median, radial, and ulnar nerves at the elbow can be used as an alternative to general anesthesia or brachial plexus blocks. As a preemptive strike against the sympathetic nervous system, bretylium is usually included with the intravenous regional anesthetic. A double tourniquet on the upper arm is used, changing the tourniquets at 10 minutes so that the patients do not experience tourniquet

pain. A forearm tourniquet is used in the obese patient because the upper arm tourniquet can sometimes be less reliable and result in a venous tourniquet. In thin patients with small hands when the tourniquet time is going to be exceedingly short, a forearm tourniquet is used. Less volume of anesthetic and no bretylium is used, and the tourniquet can be released earlier.

The incision is marked about 6 mm ulnar to the thenar crease to ensure that any scarring is away from the median nerve and that the incision is well ulnar to the palmar cutaneous branch of the median nerve, which is located in

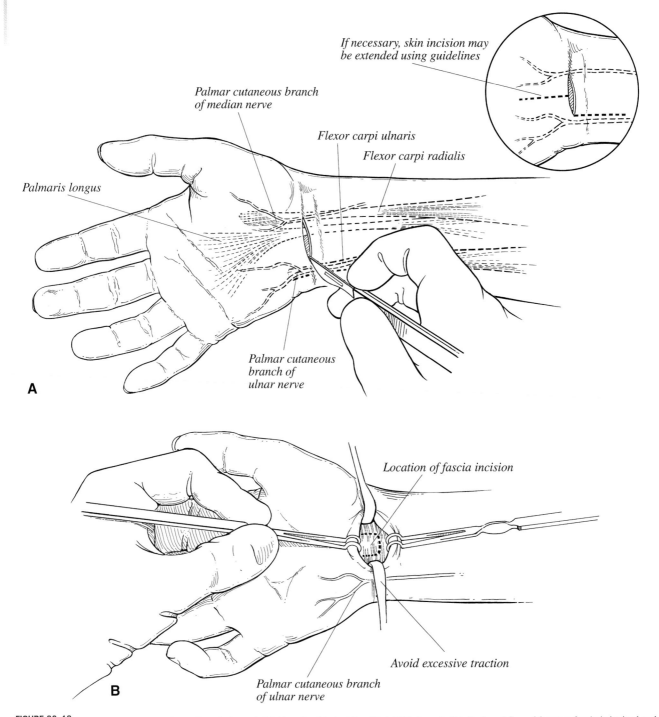

If necessary, skin incision may be extended using guidelines

Palmar cutaneous branch of median nerve

Flexor carpi ulnaris

Flexor carpi radialis

Palmaris longus

Palmar cutaneous branch of ulnar nerve

A

Location of fascia incision

Avoid excessive traction

Palmar cutaneous branch of ulnar nerve

B

FIGURE 28-10. Agee single-portal endoscopic technique. **A,** Making the skin incision. **B,** A "U"-shaped, distally based flap of forearm fascia is incised and elevated.(Courtesy of 3M Health Care, St. Paul, MN.)
Continued

the thenar crease (Fig. 28-11). A curvilinear incision is made paralleling the thenar crease, 2 or 3 cm in length, and ending just distal to the transverse wrist crease. If more exposure is necessary to release the antebrachial fascia, the incision is extended proximally in a zigzag fashion across the wrist in an ulnar direction. Two double hooks are used for retraction, and dissection is carried out through the soft tissue. About 15% of the time, a crossing cutaneous branch in the distal portion of the incision from the ulnar nerve will be identified

and protected. The down-curve portion of two Senn retractors is used to retract through the fatty tissue to expose the proximal portion of the flexor retinaculum and the distal portion of the antebrachial fascia. A No. 15 blade is used, and very carefully, slowly and with control, the proximal portion of the flexor retinaculum and distal portion of the antebrachial fascia are opened. A different color of the darker synovium around the flexor tendons will be seen once the ligament has been cut. The blunt end of a Freer

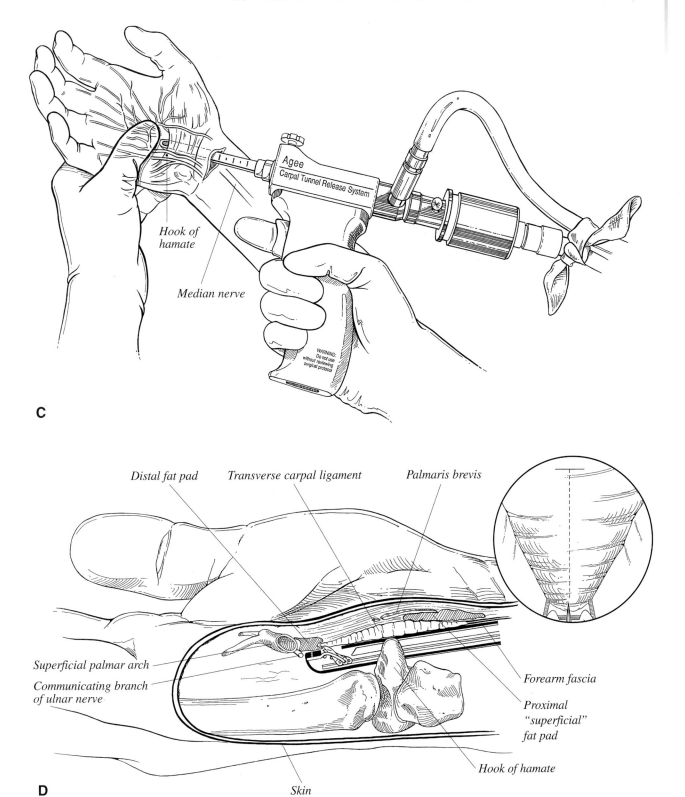

C

Hook of hamate

Median nerve

D

Distal fat pad

Transverse carpal ligament

Palmaris brevis

Superficial palmar arch

Communicating branch of ulnar nerve

Skin

Forearm fascia

Proximal "superficial" fat pad

Hook of hamate

FIGURE 28-10—cont'd. **C,** Introducing the blade assembly into the carpal canal. **D,** Incising the distal half of the transverse carpal ligament.

Continued

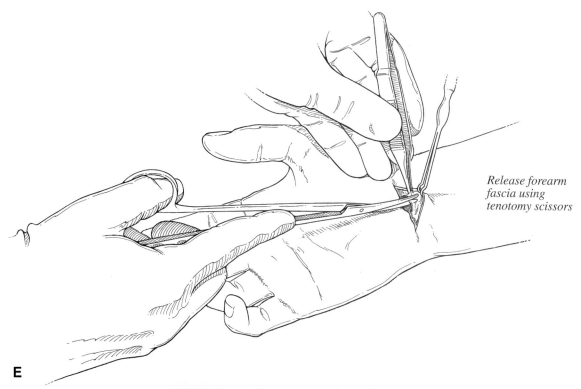

*Release forearm
fascia using
tenotomy scissors*

E

FIGURE 28-10—cont'd. E, Releasing the forearm fascia.

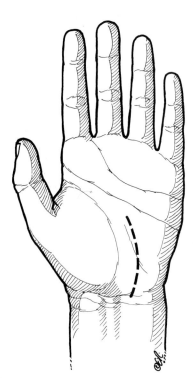

FIGURE 28-11. The author's (SEM) preferred carpal tunnel incision. A curved longitudinal incision is made paralleling the thenar crease and crossing the wrist crease obliquely in an ulnar direction at a point in line with the long axis of the flexed ring finger or just on the ulnar side of the palmaris longus tendon.

retractor can be gently placed into the carpal canal, if desired. The rake portion of the two Senn retractors is used to retract the soft tissue above the flexor retinaculum, and tenotomy scissors are used to spread the fatty tissue to identify the flexor retinaculum. The carpal ligament is carefully released along the ulnar side. The flexor retinaculum is released as far distally as the fat around the superficial arch. With observation of the fat, one is ensured that the distal ligament has been completely released. In obese individuals or people with very large hands, the incision may need to be extended more distally to ensure that the entire ligament has been released and to identify the fatty tissue signaling the end of the ligament. Proximally with the down-curved portion of two Senn retractors, the fatty tissue is retracted above the antebrachial fascia. I position myself at the end of the hand table to ensure excellent visualization. With the use of pick-ups, one edge of the antebrachial fascia is pulled distally. With slight volar wrist flexion, the median nerve will drop away from the antebrachial fascia. Under direct vision, the antebrachial fascia is released with the tenotomy scissors or a No. 15 blade. If difficulty releasing this antebrachial fascia under direct vision is encountered, the incision must be extended proximally above the wrist to ensure an adequate release of the antebrachial fascia and to ensure that there is no damage to the median nerve. The rake end of the Senn retractor is then used to retract the radial side of the divided flexor retinaculum up or anteriorly. The median nerve is then visualized. Rarely, some patients preoperatively will have deep, aching thenar pain and/or significant thenar wasting with minimal sensory complaints, indicating that a specific exploration of the recurrent motor branch of the median nerve is warranted. The rake end of the Senn retractor is used to pull up on the radial side of the divided ligament and then the median nerve is carefully retracted toward the surgeon. This will cause the recurrent motor branch of the median nerve to tent up as it enters the thenar muscle mass and allow identification of the recurrent motor branch as it curves toward the thenar muscle. In patients with a deep, aching thenar pain and/or thenar muscle wasting, the recurrent motor branch will often enter the thenar musculature through its own tendinous tunnel. (Similarly these patients may have the thenar motor branch coming off the ulnar side of the median nerve, thus exposing it to more compression as it travels across the top of the nerve and directly under the ligament.) This maneuver of pulling up on the flexor retinaculum and pulling the median nerve medially over toward the surgeon will help with easy identification of the recurrent motor branch. The floor of the carpal canal can be visualized by retracting the flexor tendons to evaluate for any pathology such as ganglions. I believe a neurolysis of the median nerve on a primary carpal tunnel release is not indicated.[111,122,130,136,137,142,153] Studies have also reported no benefit with epineurotomy.[98,119] Similarly, a synovectomy is not indicated on a primary carpal tunnel decompression. The tourniquet is deflated and bupivacaine (Marcaine) is injected into the incision under careful direct vision for postoperative comfort. Microbipolar cautery is used for hemostasis. The incision is closed with interrupted 4-0 nylon sutures and a bulky dressing is applied, keeping the wrist in neutral with fiberglass casting incorporated into the dressing. A sling may be used for the early postoperative period, but the patient is cautioned against unnecessary elbow flexion, which may flare an associated cubital tunnel syndrome, and against shoulder immobilization, which may stiffen the shoulder.

Postoperative Care

Immobilization after decompression of the carpal tunnel was historically used to protect the wound and to immobilize the wrist to prevent the flexor tendons from bowstringing. However, because of advancing knowledge in the importance of postoperative tendon and nerve gliding, this postoperative immobilization has been dramatically decreased. Das and Brown reported no problems with nerve or tendon bowstringing or nerve entrapment in the scar tissue.[112] Nathan and coworkers reported on a series of patients with carpal tunnel release who were treated with a short incision, no splinting, and early physical therapy.[149] They reported good results with no flexor tendon bowstringing. In a prospective randomized controlled trial, Cook and colleagues evaluated 50 patients who were randomly assigned to be splinted at the wrist for 2 weeks or no splinting after carpal tunnel decompression.[110] They reported no problems with tendon bowstringing or wound healing. However, prolonged splinting was associated with delay in return to work, return to activities of daily living, and pinch and grip strength. Duncan and associates in a survey of surgeons from the American Society for Surgery of the Hand reported that 81% splinted the wrist for 2 to 4 weeks after carpal tunnel decompression.[116] This survey, however, was published in 1987, and in a more recent review only

69% of hand surgeons immobilized the wrist postoperatively.[133] The initial dressing was removed a mean of 8 days after surgery (standard deviation, 9 days) and in many cases followed by only night splinting.

After carpal tunnel decompression, a bulky dressing is used to restrict wrist range of motion in the first 2 postoperative days for patient comfort. The bulky dressing is removed 2 days after surgery. The patient is instructed in

CRITICAL POINTS: CARPAL TUNNEL RELEASE

INDICATION
- Failed night splinting with wrist neutral

PREOPERATIVE EVALUATION
- Electrodiagnostic studies

PEARLS
- Document preoperative pain distribution.
- Document preoperative examination of entire upper extremity.
- Use bretylium in Bier block.
- Postoperatively, begin early movement.

TECHNICAL POINTS
- Make an incision ulnar to thenar crease.
- Avoid the ulnar cutaneous branch (15%) in the distal portion of the incision.
- Release the flexor retinaculum in a proximal-distal direction.
- Release the ligament distally to the fat pad.
- Release the antebrachial fascia under direct vision.
- Provide hemostasis after release of tourniquet.
- Use bupivacaine in the incision.

PITFALLS
- In obese patient, use forearm tourniquet.
- A failure to adequately release the distal ligament or the proximal antebrachial fascia may occur.

POSTOPERATIVE CARE
- Remove dressing on day 2 or 3.
- Use night splinting in neutral for 3 weeks.
- Begin range-of-movement exercises on day 2 or 3.
- Begin strengthening exercises in second month.
- There are no restrictions after the second month.

range-of-motion exercises for the fingers, wrist, and arm; and a splint in a wrist neutral position is used at night for 3 weeks for patient comfort. The sutures are removed 12 to 14 days postoperatively. At 1 month after surgery patients are allowed to return to work with a 2-lb weight restriction, and at 6 to 8 weeks after surgery they are allowed full activity without restrictions.

Median Nerve Compression in the Forearm

Compression of the median nerve in the forearm is less common than carpal tunnel syndrome. Gross and Jones reviewed EMG studies and found 0.2% of their patients had studies indicative of compression of the median nerve in the forearm.[175] Compression in the forearm can produce sensory disturbance in the median nerve distribution and/or motor dysfunction of the muscles innervated by the anterior interosseous nerve and median nerve. Parsonage and Turner described paralysis of the flexor pollicis longus and flexor digitorum profundus to the index finger, which they termed "neuralgic amyotrophy."[187,196] The pathology of this syndrome was related to the anterior horn cell. Kiloh and Nevin described two cases of isolated neuritis of the anterior interosseous nerve with partial recovery after 1 year.[180] The pathology was thought to be an isolated neuritis rather than compression of the median nerve in the forearm. Seyffarth described pronator syndrome and reported on 17 patients who were treated nonoperatively.[188] Johnson and colleagues reported their experience with median nerve compression in the forearm and described three levels of compression: the pronator teres, the flexor superficialis arch, and the lacertus fibrosus.[179]

Patients can present with spontaneous palsy secondary to a mononeuritis of the anterior interosseous nerve. Occasionally this can occur after a surgical procedure in the same upper extremity, which makes the etiology more confusing. There is almost always complete recovery without surgical intervention, although this may take many months.

Anatomy

The median nerve is formed from branches of the medial and lateral cords of the brachial plexus. It receives its sensory contribution from the lateral cord and its motor fibers from the medial cord. The median nerve crosses over the brachial artery to lie on the medial side in contact with the brachialis muscle. It continues distally between the brachialis muscle and the medial intermuscular septum and then passes through the antecubital fossa and under the lacertus fibrosus (bicipital aponeurosis). The nerve then travels between the deep and superficial heads of the pronator teres and in some cases passes posterior to the pronator teres (Fig. 28-12). Before the nerve divides into the main median nerve and the anterior interosseous nerve, the fascicles remain separate within the median nerve.[192] Before passing through the pronator teres, there are branches exiting to the palmaris longus, flexor carpi radialis, flexor

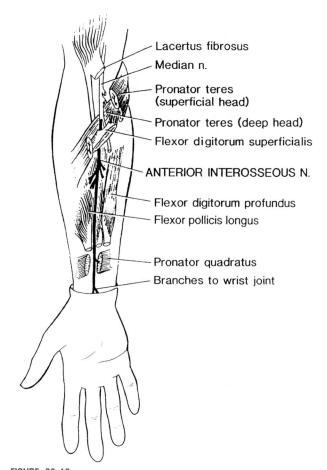

FIGURE 28-12. Schematic anatomy of the anterior interosseous nerve. (From Chidgey LK, Szabo RM: Anterior interosseous nerve compression syndrome. *In* Szabo RM [ed]: Nerve Compression Syndrome—Diagnosis and Treatment. Thorofare, NJ, Slack, 1989, pp 153-162.)

digitorum superficialis, and, rarely, to the flexor digitorum profundus muscle.[174] In a cadaveric anatomic study by Tung and Mackinnon, the pronator teres muscle received more than one branch in 73% of cases and the flexor digitorum superficialis received dual innervation in 94% of cases.[195] After exiting the pronator teres, the median nerve courses deep to the fibrous arch of the flexor digitorum superficialis and then becomes more superficial in the distal forearm. The most proximal site of median nerve compression in the upper extremity occurs under the ligament of Struthers in patients with a supracondylar process (Fig. 28-13).[170,189,193] A report by Spinner and colleagues identified an accessory bicipital aponeurosis that can cause an anterior interosseous nerve palsy.[191] Sensory disturbance to the median nerve by a snapping brachialis tendon has been reported.[169] Fibrous bands between the deep and superficial head of the pronator teres are frequently cited as the cause of compression in cases of anterior interosseous nerve palsy and pronator teres syndrome.[178,183,185,191,197] Compression may result from a fibrous arch between the two heads of the pronator teres, from a tendinous deep head of the pronator teres, from the flexor digitorum superficialis arch, or from other bands in the distal forearm.[174,177] Other accessory and anomalous muscles including the accessory head of the flexor pollicis longus (Gantzer's muscle), the palmaris profundus, and the

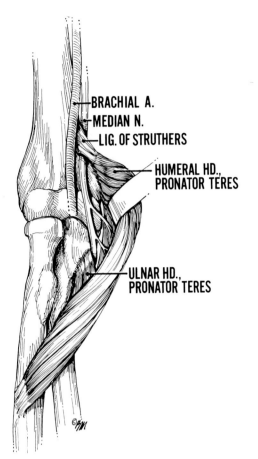

FIGURE 28-13. The median nerve lies deep and the brachial artery lies superficial to the ligament of Struthers, which forms an accessory origin for the pronator teres.

flexor carpi radialis brevis have been identified as compressive structures.[189] Gantzer's muscle was identified in one study to be present in 45% of cadavers.[172] Cadaveric dissections to identify the anatomic variations and fibrous arches that may contribute to compression in the forearm revealed that the superficial head of the pronator teres was always present, the flexor digitorum superficialis varied in origin size, and the median nerve may be crossed by one or two fibrous aponeurotic arches.[172] The fibrous arch of the pronator teres has been identified to be located 3 to 7.5 cm distal to the humeral epicondylar line and the fibrous arch of the flexor digitorum superficialis 6.5 cm distal to the humeral epicondylar line in its most proximal position.[174]

The anterior interosseous nerve provides innervation to the flexor digitorum profundus of the index and middle finger, the flexor pollicis longus, and the pronator quadratus, in addition to sensory fibers to the radiocarpal, intercarpal, carpometacarpal, and radioulnar joints. The anterior interosseous nerve is relatively tethered as it separates from the main median nerve, which makes it relatively more susceptible to traction injuries. A Martin-Gruber anastomosis (connection between the median and ulnar nerves in the forearm) is found in 15% of the population and in half of the cases the communicating branch originates from the anterior interosseous nerve.[194]

The palmar cutaneous nerve branches from the median nerve approximately 5 cm proximal to the proximal wrist crease. It separates from the median nerve and enters a tunnel immediately medial to the flexor carpi radialis tendon and then innervates the skin of the thenar eminence. Evaluation of this area of sensation is significant in differentiating median nerve compression at the carpal canal from more proximal sites of compression.

Pronator Syndrome

Pronator syndrome is defined as compression of the median nerve in the forearm that results in predominantly sensory alteration in the median nerve distribution of the hand and the palmar cutaneous distribution of the thenar eminence. This syndrome is much less common than carpal tunnel syndrome and has been reported in individuals who do repetitive upper extremity activity.[171,176] Provocation tests should reproduce symptoms in the median nerve distribution and include resisted forearm pronation, resisted elbow flexion with the forearm supinated, and resisted flexion of the middle finger flexor digitorum superficialis.[179,181] If the forearm is placed in maximum supination with the wrist in a neutral position, pressure over the leading edge of the pronator teres will reproduce symptoms in the median nerve distribution of the hand. In the majority of patients, electrodiagnostic testing is negative.[176] Mysiew and Colachis did not find that dynamic maneuvers improved the usefulness of electrodiagnostic testing in patients with pronator syndrome.[184] Olehnik and colleagues found electrodiagnostic studies to be a poor predictor of surgical intervention.[186] Radiographs of the distal humerus can identify the rare supracondylar process and alert the physician to the probability of a ligament of Struthers.

Anterior Interosseous Nerve Syndrome

Anterior interosseous nerve syndrome presents as weakness or motor loss of the flexor pollicis longus, the flexor digitorum profundus of the index finger and pronator quadratus, and, occasionally, the flexor digitorum profundus to the long finger.[190] In a true anterior interosseous nerve syndrome, weakness or loss of motor function usually occurs spontaneously. Patients may describe clumsiness with fine motor skills, such as writing and pinching. Because the anterior interosseous nerve does not innervate the skin, the syndrome is not associated with sensory loss.

Parsonage-Turner syndrome, or mononeuritis, should be considered in the differential diagnosis in patients presenting with an anterior interosseous nerve palsy. These patients typically have a history of severe pain for several weeks. The pain may follow a viral illness. High doses of corticosteroids and antiviral medications, such as acyclovir, are recommended if the neuritis is diagnosed early. In neuritis involving the anterior interosseous nerve, patients should be monitored for up to 1 year, because spontaneous recovery usually occurs. In patients with a spontaneous anterior interosseous nerve palsy and no electrodiagnostic evidence of reinnervation, consideration should be given for a nerve transfer at 7 to 10 months.[182] Local decompression in these cases will not accelerate the recovery. However, in cases of anterior interosseous nerve palsy caused by local compression of the median nerve in the forearm usually associated with some type of trauma or soft tissue tumor, the fibrous bands of the pronator teres are frequently the major compressive site.

Operative Technique

The operative technique for decompression of the median nerve in the forearm is the same for pronator syndrome and compression of the anterior interosseous nerve.

Author's (SEM) Preferred Technique

Preoperatively, significant compression points on the median nerve are determined by a physical examination, either with stress on a particular tendon or muscle unit or with the elicitation of pain with direct palpation. A tourniquet is used, and the incision begins at the antecubital fossa and continues distally in a lazy-"S" direction for about 10 cm (Fig. 28-14). The dissection is carried down through the soft tissue to identify and preserve any cutaneous sensory branches. The bicipital aponeurosis (lacertus fibrosus) is identified and divided (Fig. 28-15). The tendon of the superficial head of the pronator teres is identified. This is best identified in the distal portion of the surgical exposure

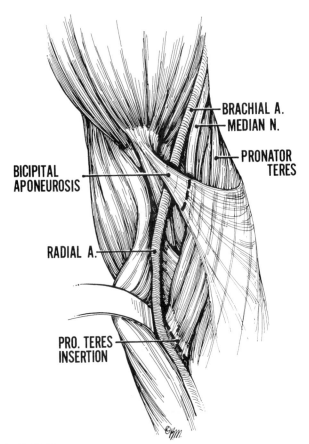

FIGURE 28-15. The bicipital aponeurosis may act as a compressive band across the flexor muscle in pronation; it should be divided during any exploration of the median nerve. A step-lengthening tenotomy of the tendon of the superficial head of the pronator teres is necessary to allow exposure of the median nerve.

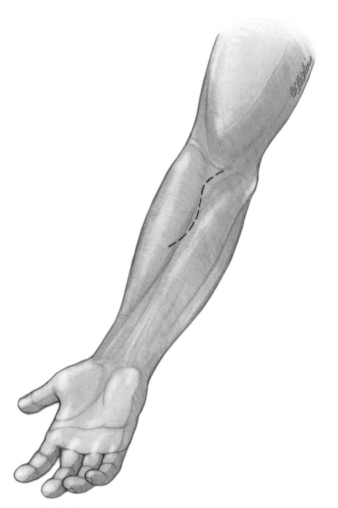

FIGURE 28-14. The incision to explore the median nerve and anterior interosseous nerve in the proximal forearm begins at least 5 cm above the elbow crease.

just radial to the radial vessels. A step-lengthening incision is made in the tendon of the superficial head of the pronator teres. The "up" cut on the tendon lengthening is done distally where visualization is more difficult. The "down" cut is done proximally (Fig. 28-16). Once this tendon lengthening is complete, this will take the tension off the superficial (radial) head of the pronator teres muscle and allow better identification of the median nerve. The median nerve is then identified proximally, just medial to the brachial artery and vein. The nerve is intimate with the pronator muscle and can be found just distal to the cubital crease adjacent to, if not just within, the flexor pronator muscle mass (Fig. 28-17). The median nerve is followed distally to identify the deep head of the pronator teres where it blends with the leading tendinous edge of the flexor superficialis. The proximal tendinous attachment of the deep head is about 2 cm in length. It arches around the median nerve and attaches as the deep ulnar head of the pronator teres onto the ulna. There is muscle attached to the tendinous tissue, and the tendinous portion is excised. The tendinous portion of the arch from the leading edge of the superficialis tendons is divided to completely release the median nerve. The surgeon can run a finger proximally along the median nerve, and if a ligament of Struthers is identified, the incision is extended above the elbow crease. During dissection, care is taken to obtain

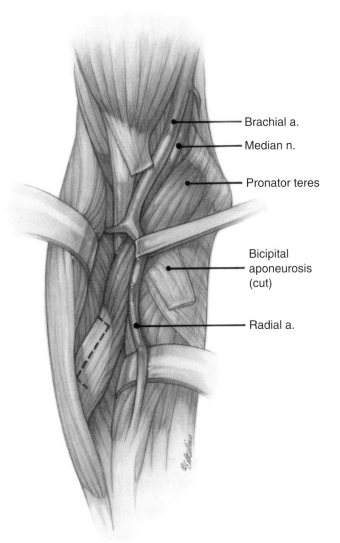

FIGURE 28-16. Exposure of the median nerve and anterior interosseous nerves by reflection of the humeral (superficial head of the pronator teres also exposes the arch of the superficialis and the deep head of the pronator teres (ulnar head). The step-lengthening tenotomy facilitates the exposure.

Brachial a.

Median n.

Pronator teres

Bicipital aponeurosis (cut)

Radial a.

fingers, wrist, and arm. A sling may be used at night for patient comfort to prevent full elbow extension. However, the patient is encouraged to begin exercises to regain full elbow extension with forearm supination. Patients are allowed full activity and can return to work without restrictions 6 to 8 weeks after surgery.

complete hemostasis. The vessels in this area are very thin walled and will "stain" the tissues if good hemostasis is not obtained with microbipolar cautery or ligature ties as necessary. Internal neurolysis or epineurotomy techniques are not indicated. There is no need to reconstruct the tendon lengthening of the pronator teres because the deep muscle has been left intact. The incision is closed with 3-0 absorbable suture in the subcutaneous tissue and a 4-0 subcuticular suture with adhesive strips. Bupivacaine is placed in the incision for postoperative comfort. In rare cases where the patient had extreme pain preoperatively, a bupivacaine infusion pump can be used. Fiberglass casting is incorporated into the dressing to keep the elbow slightly flexed and the wrist in a neutral position.

Postoperative Care

The bulky dressing is removed 2 days after surgery. The patient is instructed in range-of-motion exercises for the

CRITICAL POINTS: MEDIAN NERVE RELEASE, PROXIMAL FOREARM

INDICATIONS

- Rare as a pain syndrome
- Anterior interosseous nerve palsy localizing to the forearm
- A de novo anterior interosseous nerve palsy is most likely a neuritis and not due to mechanical decompression.
- Patients with median nerve sensory complaints localizing to the pronator teres are usually successfully treated with forearm flexor muscle stretching exercises.
- Patients with associated carpal tunnel syndrome usually require only a carpal tunnel release.

PREOPERATIVE EVALUATION

- Without motor findings, electrodiagnostic studies usually are normal.
- Persistent median nerve symptoms are reproduced with provocation at the forearm.

PEARLS

- The tendon of the superficial head of the pronator teres is located just *lateral* to the radial vessels in the distal part of the surgical exposure.
- The median nerve is located just *medial* to the vessels in the proximal portion of the surgical field and is intimate with the flexor pronator muscle mass.

TECHNICAL POINTS

- Use lazy-"S" incision in the proximal forearm.
- Release the lacertus fibrosus.
- Identify the superficial tendon of the pronator teres lateral to vessels.
- Use step-lengthening tenotomy of superficial tendon of the pronator teres.
- Identify the median nerve in the proximal forearm medial to vessels.
- Identify and excise the deep head of the pronator teres.

Continued

CRITICAL POINTS: MEDIAN NERVE RELEASE, PROXIMAL FOREARM—cont'd

TECHNICAL POINTS—cont'd

- Release the superficial tendinous arch of the flexor digitorum superficialis.
- Ensure no compressive bands proximally over the median nerve.

PITFALL

- Beware of inadequate release of the median nerve compression points of the arch of the pronator teres muscles and the flexor digitorum superficialis.

POSTOPERATIVE CARE

- Remove dressing at day 2 or 3.
- Begin early range-of-motion exercises at day 2 or 3.
- Begin strengthening exercises in the second month.

COMPRESSION OF THE ULNAR NERVE

The ulnar nerve is most commonly compressed at the elbow in the region of the cubital tunnel and less frequently at the wrist at Guyon's canal. With compression of the ulnar nerve, patient complaints will include paresthesia and/or numbness in the small finger and/or in the ring finger. In more severe cases, complaints resulting from ulnar nerve motor dysfunction will include weak pinch and grip and hand clumsiness.[229]

Guyon's Canal Compression

Guyon[247] first described the space in the hypothenar region of the wrist where the ulnar nerve divides and suggested that ulnar nerve compression could occur in this region. Compression in Guyon's canal may result from a number of causes, including acute trauma[250] or repetitive trauma, anomalous muscles,[243,244] or space-occupying lesions, including ganglia,[245] thrombosis, and pseudoaneurysms.

The unique anatomy of the region of Guyon's canal will influence the presenting symptoms.[242,246,248,249] Depending on the location of the compression on the ulnar nerve, presenting symptoms can include pure motor, pure sensory, or a mix of both motor and sensory loss. If the compression produces intrinsic weakness, the functional motor loss to the

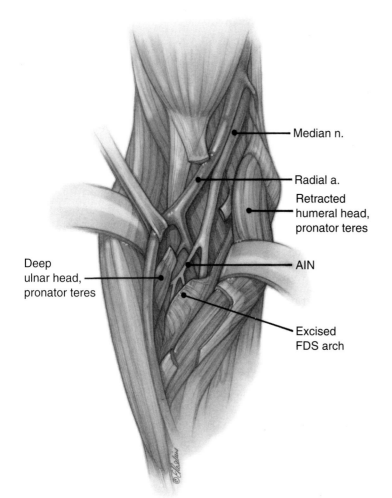

Deep ulnar head, pronator teres

Median n.

Radial a.

Retracted humeral head, pronator teres

AIN

Excised FDS arch

FIGURE 28-17. The proximal tendinous attachment of the deep head (ulnar) of the pronator teres and the proximal tendinous arch of the superficialis are excised to completely release the median nerve.

hand can be profound. Because of the propensity for space-occupying lesions within Guyon's canal, preoperative workup should include appropriate imaging studies in addition to electrodiagnostic studies, particularly when an isolated motor palsy is identified.

Anatomy

After passing anterior to the flexor retinaculum, the ulnar nerve divides into the superficial and deep branches. The superficial branch innervates the palmaris brevis muscle and then supplies sensory innervation to the small finger and the medial side of the ring finger. The deep branch of the ulnar nerve innervates the hypothenar muscle, the medial two lumbricals, the interossei muscles, and the adductor pollicis muscle (Fig. 28-18).

Operative Technique

Author's (SEM) Preferred Technique

The incision used for carpal tunnel release is appropriate for release of the ulnar nerve in Guyon's canal, except that it will need to be extended slightly more proximally and distally. Similar anesthetic and tourniquet techniques are used.

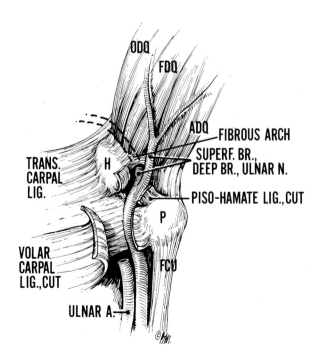

FIGURE 28-18. The ulnar nerve courses through Guyon's canal between the volar carpal ligament and the transverse carpal ligament. P, pisiform; H, hamate.

The incision is marked 6 mm ulnar to the thenar crease. A curvilinear incision (3 to 4 cm in length) is made paralleling the thenar crease. Two double hooks are used for retraction, and dissection is carried down through the soft tissue. A crossing cutaneous branch in the distal portion of the incision, running from the ulnar nerve up to the overlying skin, can be seen in about 15% of cases and needs to be identified and protected. Guyon's canal is opened, and the hook of the hamate is palpated. The neurovascular bundle is then dissected medially to identify the deep motor branch of the ulnar nerve. The technique for identifying the deep motor branch of the ulnar nerve is to note the oblique fascial pattern along the surface of the hypothenar muscles. At the proximal leading edge of the hypothenar muscles the surgeon will see just 1 or 2 mm of the deep motor branch of the ulnar nerve as it curves around the hook of the hamate. Tenotomy scissors are placed underneath the leading edge

CRITICAL POINTS: GUYON'S CANAL RELEASE

INDICATIONS

- Uncommon
- Ulnar nerve symptoms and signs localizing to Guyon's canal on physical examination

PREOPERATIVE EVALUATION

- Electrodiagnostic studies often are helpful in localizing compression point to Guyon's canal.
- Preoperative imaging studies are needed if space-occupying lesion is suspected.

PEARLS

- Only 1 or 2 mm of the deep motor branch can be seen diving beneath the hypothenar muscles.
- Look for the deep motor branch at the free edge of the hypothenar muscles.

TECHNICAL POINTS

- Make the same incision as for a carpal tunnel release, but extend it both proximally and distally.
- Avoid the ulnar cutaneous communicating branch in the distal portion of the incision.
- Open Guyon's canal.
- Palpate the hook of the hamate.
- Dissect the neurovascular bundle ulnarward along its length through Guyon's canal.
- Identify the leading tendinous edge of the hypothenar muscles.
- Release the deep motor branch of the ulnar nerve, which is located just below the leading tendinous edge of the hyperthenar muscle origin.

Continued

CRITICAL POINTS: GUYON'S CANAL RELEASE—cont'd

PITFALL

- Failure to identify and release the deep motor branch of the ulnar nerve

POSTOPERATIVE CARE

- Remove dressing at day 2 or 3.
- Splint wrist in neutral for 2 weeks at night.
- Begin range-of-motion exercises at day 2 or 3.
- Begin strengthening exercises in second month.
- If the carpal tunnel has also been released, then use a night splint in neutral for 3 weeks.

of the hypothenar muscles, and the muscle is divided to identify the deep motor branch of the ulnar nerve. It is released completely around the hook of the hamate, because there are often tendinous bands within the hypothenar muscles distally that can compress the ulnar nerve. There are also small, thin-walled vessels running with the deep motor branch of the ulnar nerve, which should be protected so that the surgeon does not need to obtain hemostasis with cautery near the deep motor branch. The ulnar nerve proper is released through Guyon's canal, and the incision is usually extended in a zigzag fashion proximal to the wrist to release the distal extent of the antebrachial fascia. The tourniquet is deflated, and microbipolar cautery is used for hemostasis. Infiltration of the incision with bupivacaine is used for postoperative comfort. The incision is closed with interrupted 4-0 nylon sutures and a bulky dressing is applied, keeping the wrist in a neutral position, with fiberglass casting incorporated into the dressing. If a carpal tunnel release has also been done, then night splinting with the wrist in neutral is done for 3 weeks; otherwise, night splinting is for patient comfort.

Postoperative Care

A bulky dressing is applied to maintain a wrist neutral position, and this dressing is removed 2 days after surgery. The patient is instructed in range-of-motion exercises for the fingers, wrist, and arm. A splint in a wrist neutral position is used at night for patient comfort. The sutures are removed 12 to 14 days postoperatively. Patients are allowed full activity and returned to work without restrictions 6 to 8 weeks after surgery.

Cubital Tunnel Syndrome

Chronic neuritis of the elbow was described by Buzzard in 1922.[202] In the 1930s and 1940s, Learmonth recognized ulnar nerve compression at the elbow and popularized techniques for decompression and transposition.[221] In 1958, Feindel and Stratford introduced the term *cubital tunnel syndrome* and focused on the anatomy in the region of the elbow and associated ulnar nerve compression.[208,209] At the

same time, Osborne described the tendinous leading edge of the flexor carpi ulnaris as an important compression point.[235] Chronic compression of the ulnar nerve at the cubital tunnel may occur through ischemia or mechanical compression with repeated elbow flexion or direct compression, although the exact etiology may be difficult to identify. The area within the cubital tunnel is decreased with elbow flexion, and this can increase the pressure on the cubital tunnel. Apfelberg and Larson[199] reported a 55% decrease in the cubital tunnel area with elbow flexion. Pechan and Julius reported increased pressure within the cubital tunnel with elbow flexion, and this pressure was further compromised with wrist extension and/or shoulder abduction.[66] Gelberman and colleagues reported with elbow flexion an increased intraneural ulnar nerve pressure and a decreased cubital tunnel volume with elbow flexion.[19] Ulnar nerve subluxation may also contribute to cubital tunnel syndrome. Acute trauma to the ulnar nerve as may occur with distal humeral fractures may compromise ulnar nerve function.

Compression of the ulnar nerve at the cubital tunnel is extremely common and second in incidence only to carpal tunnel syndrome. The diagnosis is a clinical one, because electrodiagnostic testing is often negative. Tinel's sign is usually positive over the nerve at or proximal to the cubital tunnel, but the test is overly sensitive and usually bilaterally positive. While the clinical diagnosis of cubital tunnel syndrome remains the gold standard, electrodiagnostic studies may be used to confirm the diagnosis. The nerve conduction studies and EMGs are useful in localizing the level of nerve compression in addition to identifying other sites of nerve compression or other disease processes (i.e., upper motor neuron disease, peripheral neuropathy) that may be present. To confirm the diagnosis of cubital tunnel syndrome with nerve conduction studies, many reports support the use of a decreased motor conduction velocity across the elbow.[207,224] Ulnar nerve motor conduction velocity across the elbow of less than 50 m/s is considered positive for cubital tunnel syndrome. Eversmann reported a motor conduction velocity decrease of 33% across the elbow to be indicative of cubital tunnel syndrome.[207] EMG changes in ulnar innervated muscles are more sensitive than nerve conduction studies in the early stages of cubital tunnel syndrome.

Provocative testing for cubital tunnel syndrome using combined elbow flexion with digital pressure placed on the ulnar nerve proximal to the cubital tunnel has good sensitivity and specificity.[55] McGowan described a classification system for ulnar neuropathy at the elbow, and it is based predominantly on the loss of ulnar nerve motor function and does not include sensory changes.[229] This classification system is widely quoted in the literature, although it is limited in clinical applicability. In McGowan's classification, grade I neuropathies have no muscle weakness, grade II have muscle weakness with no atrophy, and grade III have muscle atrophy.

Clinical evaluation is important to identity patients with cubital tunnel syndrome. Complaints often include paresthesia and numbness in the small and ring finger with aching in the medial elbow and forearm. With severe ulnar nerve compression, patients may present with clawing of the small and ring finger, atrophy of the ulnar nerve–innervated intrinsic muscles, and positive Froment and Wartenberg signs.

These motor changes will not identify the level of ulnar nerve compression. However, many patients present in the early stages of nerve compression and will have no obvious motor deficit. Careful sensory testing as outlined previously can help to quantify changes in sensibility. In the early stages of nerve compression, provocation testing may be the only positive sign, followed by alteration of threshold testing (vibration and Semmes-Weinstein monofilaments). In the later stages, two-point discrimination will become abnormal.

Cubital tunnel syndrome can often be managed conservatively, with education of the patient to avoid positions and activities that combine elbow flexion with pressure over the ulnar nerve, such as while driving, speaking on the telephone, or during sleep. Postural modifications may be necessary for several months before symptoms are resolved, and, occasionally, surgery will be necessary to relieve symptoms. Unfortunately, the incidence of poor outcomes after surgical management of cubital tunnel syndrome far exceeds that of carpal tunnel syndrome; and when surgery fails, the consequences for patients can be devastating.

Unlike carpal tunnel syndrome, there are other sinister diagnoses that can mimic cubital tunnel syndrome, such as motor neuron disease or Guillain-Barré syndrome. The surgeon must be alert for the common problem of cervical disk disease and the rare but devastating problem of amyotrophic lateral sclerosis, when evaluating patients with ulnar motor complaints, particularly when the motor findings exceed the sensory findings.

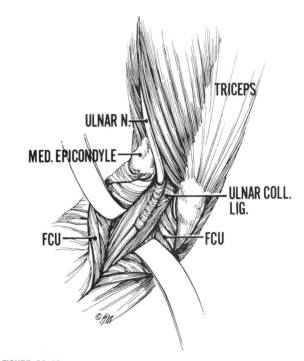

FIGURE 28-19. The ulnar nerve lies on the medial head of the triceps muscle, enters the cubital tunnel behind the medial epicondyle, and continues distally beneath the arcade of fascia joining the heads of the flexor carpi ulnaris.

 Anatomy

The ulnar nerve is derived from the C8 and T1 nerve roots and is a terminal branch of the medial cord. In the upper arm, the ulnar nerve is posteromedial to the brachial artery, posterior to the intermuscular septum, and anterior to the medial head of the triceps muscle (Fig. 28-19). The intermuscular septum is continuous from the humeral medial epicondyle to the coracobrachialis muscle. The arcade of Struthers is a band of deep brachial fascia that attaches to the intermuscular septum and covers the ulnar nerve approximately 8 cm proximal to the medial epicondyle (Fig. 28-20).[239] The medial antebrachial cutaneous nerve passes posterior to the ulnar nerve at or proximal to the epicondyle in 90% of cases.[226] The proximal branch of the medial antebrachial cutaneous nerve often runs with the medial intramuscular septum.[223] The ulnar nerve passes posterior to the medial epicondyle and medial to the olecranon. The ulnar nerve then enters the cubital tunnel, which is defined by a taut fascia layer extending from the flexor carpi ulnaris muscle and the arcuate ligament of Osborne. After passing through the cubital tunnel, the ulnar nerve travels deep into the forearm between the ulnar and humeral heads of the flexor carpi ulnaris muscle.

A number of sites within the region of the cubital tunnel can contribute to ulnar nerve compression, and the etiology is variable among affected individuals. The superficial position of the ulnar nerve at the cubital tunnel and the increase in tension and traction it experiences with elbow flexion

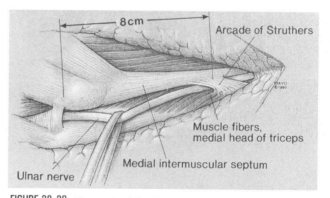

FIGURE 28-20. The arcade of Struthers arises 8 cm proximal to the medial humeral epicondyle. (From Spinner M: Nerve decompression. *In* Morrey BF [ed]: The Elbow. New York, Raven Press, 1994 and by permission of Mayo Foundation.)

likely combine to make it susceptible to compression neuropathy.

Nonoperative Treatment

Conservative treatment begins with patient education to avoid postures and positions that increase tension or compression of the ulnar nerve. A demonstration of the changes in skin tension can be useful in explaining the tightness that occurs to the ulnar nerve with elbow flexion (Fig. 28-21). Decreasing elbow flexion and direct pressure on the nerve may help to alleviate symptoms in patients with a mild or moderate degree of nerve compression. Recommendations for nonoperative treatment have included static night splinting of the elbow in extension. Rigid night splints are

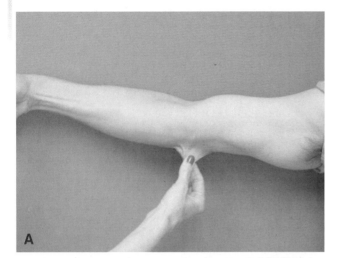

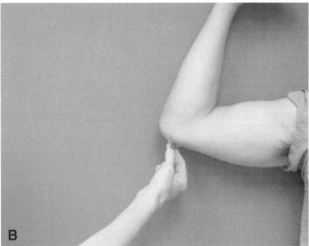

FIGURE 28-21. **A,** The effect of elbow flexion to increase tension on the ulnar nerve is illustrated to the patient by noting that when the elbow is extended, just like the skin is loose, the ulnar nerve is loose (A). **B,** By contrast, when the elbow is flexed, just like when the skin is tight, the nerve is stretched and tight.

often ineffective because of patient discomfort and noncompliance. Soft elbow pads can be used to protect the ulnar nerve from direct compression, and we recommend wearing these pads up to 24 hours per day. Because the ulnar nerve can be compressed between the two heads of the flexor carpi ulnaris muscle during hand and wrist activities, patients are instructed in specific stretching and nerve gliding exercises.

In our experience, many patients with mild cubital tunnel syndrome can successfully be managed with 2 to 4 months of nonoperative treatment. Padua and coworkers reported half of their patients with neurophysiologically positive cubital tunnel syndrome improved with nonoperative management.[237] We use motor conduction velocity across the elbow as a guide to management, and treat all patients with conduction velocity of 40 m/sec or greater with a minimum of 2 to 3 months of nonoperative treatment. If this is unsuccessful, or if initial conduction is less than 40 m/sec, the patient will likely require surgical intervention. A number of surgical approaches have been described for the treatment of cubital tunnel syndrome and include simple decompression, medial epicondylectomy, and anterior transposition of the

ulnar nerve in a subcutaneous, submuscular, intramuscular, or transmuscular position.

Operative Treatment

The fact that there are several techniques currently recommended by experienced hand surgeons for the management of cubital tunnel syndrome speaks to the ongoing controversy regarding the surgical management of cubital tunnel syndrome. Surgical options range from simple decompression to medial epicondylectomy to various anterior transposition techniques. The ideal operative technique should address the mechanism of cubital tunnel syndrome. The superficial position of the nerve at the elbow renders it susceptible to mechanical compression, and its position behind the medial epicondyle causes it to undergo increased tension with elbow flexion. In theory, only a transposition procedure would substantially change the tension on the nerve as the elbow is flexed. A comprehensive review concluded that with more advanced cubital tunnel syndrome simple decompression was unlikely to be successful.[204] In a meta-analysis of treatment for cubital tunnel syndrome that included 30 studies over five decades, Mowlavi and colleagues concluded that the recurrence rate was highest in nonoperated patients.[230] In patients with moderate nerve compression, relief was achieved most often with a submuscular transposition; and in severely affected patients, all treatments produced similarly poor results.[230] In contrast, a review by Bartels and coworkers determined that patients with severe compression had the best outcome with a subcutaneous transposition.[200] These authors recommended simple decompression for surgical treatment of cubital tunnel syndrome unless there is ulnar nerve subluxation, in which case an anterior subcutaneous transposition is employed.

Eversmann described the advantages of simple decompression as simple and safe because the intrinsic and extrinsic vascularity of the ulnar nerve is left undisturbed.[207] Osborne described the tendinous leading edge of the flexor carpi ulnaris as a significant compression point for cubital tunnel syndrome and in 1957 described favorable results with simple decompression of the ulnar nerve in 13 cases.[235] Foster and Edshage found no significant difference comparing 48 cases of cubital tunnel syndrome treated by either a simple decompression or an anterior transposition.[211] Macnicol documented success with the use of simple decompression in 110 cases, when the duration of the cubital tunnel syndrome was short.[225] In our opinion, the indications for in situ decompression of the ulnar nerve are limited, because mild cases of cubital tunnel syndrome in patients with a short duration of symptoms can usually be managed conservatively.[210] Furthermore, if a simple decompression fails to relieve symptoms, then secondary surgery needed to transpose the nerve will be significantly more difficult because of scar tissue formation.

Technique of In-Situ Decompression

An intravenous or regional anesthetic technique is used, and a 6- to 10-cm incision is made along the course of the ulnar nerve midway between the medial epicondyle and the olecranon.[240] Care is taken to avoid injury to the medial antebrachial cutaneous nerve. The intramuscular septum is palpated proximally, and the ulnar nerve is identified just below this septum. The ulnar nerve is decompressed distally through the cubital tunnel. The nerve is exposed between the two heads of the flexor carpi ulnaris muscle, and the leading tendinous edge of the flexor carpi ulnaris muscle is released. The ulnar nerve need not be disturbed in its bed, and a neurolysis is not performed. Care is taken to ensure that there is a good distal and proximal release of the ulnar nerve. The elbow is moved through a range of movement, and any points that might compress the ulnar nerve either proximally or distally are evaluated. The intramuscular septum and the brachial fascia where it might compress the ulnar nerve proximally are excised. If the ulnar nerve subluxes over the medial epicondyle when the elbow moves into flexion, consideration should be given for a medial epicondylectomy or anterior transposition to avoid postoperative discomfort. At the conclusion of the case, the tourniquet is deflated and hemostasis is obtained. Bupivacaine may be placed in the incision and the subcutaneous layer closed with a subcuticular skin closure. A bulky dressing with or without fiberglass support is applied. The postoperative dressing is removed at 2 to 3 days after surgery, and active range of motion is started at that time.

Medial Epicondylectomy

In 1950, King and Morgan described removal of the medial epicondyle in 16 patients with ulnar neuritis[217] and reported their late results in 1959.[218] Most patients in the series had post-traumatic injuries and were not typical of idiopathic cubital tunnel syndrome. Other surgeons have expanded this technique to treat nontraumatic causes of cubital tunnel syndrome and believe that it allows some degree of an anterior transposition with less dissection.[203,214,215,220] Hicks and Toby evaluated the strain on the ulnar nerve before and after a simple decompression and medial epicondylectomy using cadaver specimens.[216] They found significant reduction in ulnar nerve strain with medial epicondylectomy but not with in situ decompression. A potential complication of this technique is medial elbow instability, which can occur with "overzealous resection" of the epicondyle.[212] O'Driscoll demonstrated that only approximately 20% of the overall depth of the epicondyle can be removed without violating a portion of the anterior medial collateral ligament and described a safer plane for removal that would avoid the anteroinferior origin of the ligament from the epicondyle.[233]

An intravenous or regional anesthetic is used and the ulnar nerve is decompressed as with a simple decompression. The ulnar nerve is not disturbed in its bed. It is not necessary to perform an internal or an external neurolysis. The medial epicondyle is exposed subperiosteally, leaving the flexor/pronator origin in continuity with the periosteal sleeve (Fig. 28-22). A 2.5-cm osteotome is used to score the leading edge of epicondyle. To avoid detachment of the anterior medial band of the ulnar collateral ligament, a plane is chosen between the sagittal and coronal planes of the humerus, and not along the medial margin of the trochlea as traditionally described.[233] A portion of the epicondyle along with the attached medial intramuscular septum is removed (Fig. 28-23). Care should be taken to not enter the elbow joint or to detach the ulnar collateral ligament. After removal of the portion of the epicondyle, the raw bone edges are rasped smooth and the periosteal flaps with attached flexor/pronator origin are imbricated with a buried 3-0 non-

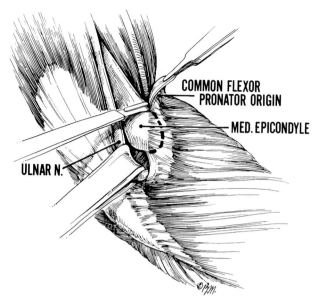

FIGURE 28-22. Medial epicondylectomy is begun by protecting the ulnar nerve and elevating the common flexor pronator origin from the medial epicondyle. The arcade of the flexor carpi ulnaris must be incised to the midportion of the proximal third of the forearm (not shown in the drawing).

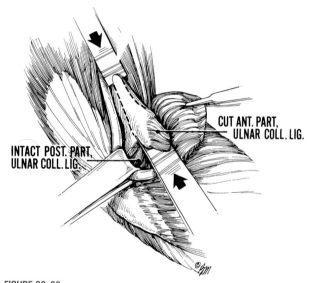

FIGURE 28-23. The guide for the proper plane of osteotomy for the medial epicondyle is the plane between the sagittal and coronal planes. The sharp posterior edge of the osteotomy must be smoothed and rounded.

absorbable suture (Fig. 28-24). The elbow is moved through a full range of movement to ensure that there is good gliding of the ulnar nerve and no compression of the nerve proximally or distally. Routine skin closure is used, and a bulky dressing is applied. The dressing is removed 2 to 3 days postoperatively, and range of motion is started.

Subcutaneous Anterior Transposition

Proponents of the subcutaneous anterior transposition believe that the procedure further reduces the tension on the ulnar nerve during elbow flexion.[236] However, some are concerned about compromise of flexor pronator muscle

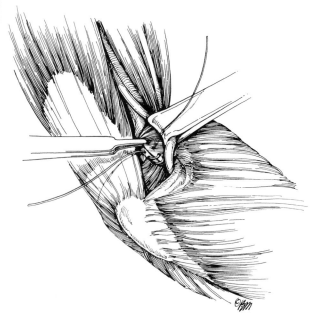

FIGURE 28-24. Repair of the flexor-pronator origin to the humerus. After repair of the muscles, the ulnar nerve is allowed to seek its own position. The arcade of the flexor carpi ulnaris must be opened sufficiently to prevent impingement on the nerve (not shown in the drawing).

strength and increased scarring associated with an intramuscular or submuscular transposition. Ogata and associates, using an experimental primate model, demonstrated that anterior transposition of the ulnar nerve was associated with a significant decrease in regional blood flow that was not noted with a simple decompression or medial epicondylectomy. Intraneural circulation was restored by the fourth to seventh postoperative day.[234]

Theoretically, an anterior transposition should adequately correct cubital tunnel symptoms as long as care is taken to ensure that new compression points are not created proximally and distally. Given the ulnar nerve's submuscular position above and below the cubital tunnel, an extensive proximal and distal exposure is needed to leave the nerve subcutaneous and to not produce kinking proximally or distally.

Intravenous or regional anesthesia is used and the procedure begins as a simple decompression. A longer incision is necessary (approximately 15 cm in length) to accommodate the transposition. The distal medial antebrachial cutaneous nerve crosses the incision about 3.5 cm distal to the medial epicondyle. The proximal branch of this nerve crosses the incision 1.5 cm proximal to the medial epicondyle and often runs with the medial intramuscular septum.[223] These sensory nerves are protected throughout the procedure. The ulnar nerve is identified below the medial intramuscular septum. After removal of the medial intramuscular septum, the ulnar nerve is released through the cubital tunnel and followed between the two heads of the flexor carpi ulnaris muscle. The motor branches to the flexor carpi ulnaris and the flexor digitorum profundus are preserved. The nerve is then carefully lifted from its bed with its accompanying longitudinal vascular supply intact, using a small Penrose drain to prevent constriction. Segmental feeding vessels are identified and ligated to

prevent tethering. A neurolysis can be used as necessary to separate the posterior motor branches from the main ulnar nerve to allow an adequate anterior transposition without tension.[221,241] These motor branches can also be followed into the flexor carpi ulnaris muscle to allow mobilization of the ulnar nerve and protection of these posterior motor branches. The ulnar nerve is then moved anteriorly to a subcutaneous position (Fig. 28-25). The ulnar nerve should be examined proximally and especially distally to ensure that it lies loosely with no proximal or distal compression points (Fig. 28-26). Even very thin fascial bands distally will compress the nerve and lead to a suboptimal result. To keep the ulnar nerve in its anterior position and prevent it from returning to its original position, some of the soft tissue of the anterior skin flap can be sutured to the fascia over the medial epicondyle. Care is taken not to include any branches of the medial antebrachial cutaneous nerve. Eaton has recommended the elevation of a 1- to 1.5-cm^2 flap of flexor-pronator fascia based on the medial epicondyle that is then sewn to the overlying dermis to create a barrier that maintains the nerve in its anterior transposed position.[205,206] Care must be taken to ensure that the fascial flap does not compress the ulnar nerve, causing a new compression point. Closure, dressing, and postoperative care are as previously described for the other cubital tunnel surgeries.

Intramuscular Transposition

In 1918, Adson[198] described an intramuscular transposition of the ulnar nerve. This is the technique also used by Kleinman.[219,238] Proponents of this method believe that it is an improvement over the subcutaneous transposition because the nerve lies in a straighter position as it moves

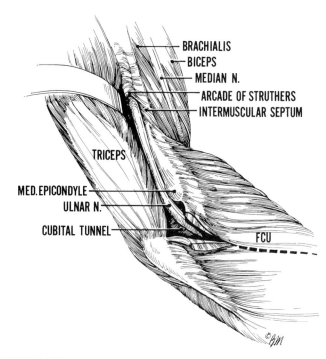

FIGURE 28-25. Mobilization of the ulnar nerve and any associated vessels necessitates decompression of the cubital tunnel, fasciotomy of the flexor carpi ulnaris, and dissection along the ulnar nerve, at least 8 cm proximal to the medial epicondyle.

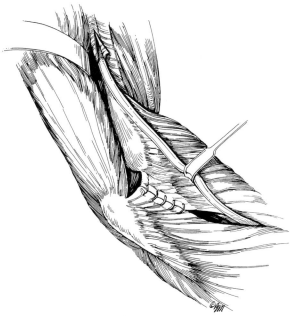

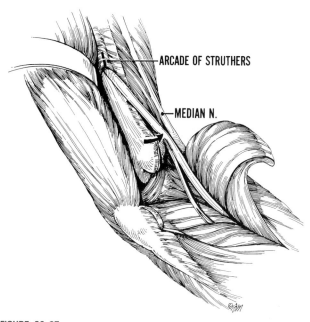

FIGURE 28-26. At the completion of a subcutaneous transposition, the arcade of Struthers does not bind the ulnar nerve and there is adequate release of the flexor carpi ulnaris for the ulnar nerve to reenter the forearm.

FIGURE 28-27. After submuscular transposition, care must be taken to prevent angulation of the ulnar nerve at the arcade of Struthers. The branches to the flexor carpi ulnaris should be preserved.

from the arm to the forearm and in a more protected position than the subcutaneous location.[219,238] Critics suggest that dissection into the muscle will cause more scarring.[201,222]

The procedure is the same as a subcutaneous transposition except that a groove is dissected in the muscle in line with the location of the ulnar nerve in its transposed position. Fibrous septa within the pronator muscle are removed to provide a soft vascularized muscle bed. A fascial flap or a subcutaneous flap is created as for a subcutaneous transposition to keep the nerve in its anterior location. Proponents of this procedure recommend 3 weeks of immobilization[219,238] and do not allow unrestricted activity until 10 weeks after this procedure.

Submuscular Transposition

In 1942 Learmonth described his classic submuscular transposition.[221] No follow-up results were given in this report. Proponents advocate the submuscular transposition as the "definitive" procedure and the procedure of choice in throwing athletes[240] and previously failed cubital tunnel surgery.[204] Critics cite the extensive dissection and concern for the longitudinal blood supply of the ulnar nerve, as well as the potential for new compression or heterotopic bone under the incised flexor-pronator muscle mass.

The ulnar nerve is exposed and transposed as described earlier for a subcutaneous anterior transposition. The incision, however, will be longer (15 to 20 cm). The extent of the flexor/pronator muscle mass is identified. A plane is developed distal to the medial epicondyle and beneath the flexor/pronator muscle mass. The flexor/pronator muscle mass is then incised 1 to 2 cm distal to the medial epicondyle, and a periosteal elevator is used to reflect the muscle distally. Care is taken to not disrupt the ulnar collateral ligament. The median nerve is exposed where it lies on the brachialis muscle, by dividing the lacertus fibrosus and dissecting lateral to the elevated flexor/pronator muscle

mass. The ulnar nerve is transposed anteriorly, adjacent and parallel to the median nerve (Fig. 28-27). The flexor/pronator muscle mass is then anatomically reattached with nonabsorbable sutures (Fig. 28-28). Alternatively, the flexor/pronator mass can be divided in a step-cut fashion and lengthened by 1 to 2 cm during closure to decrease compression on the transposed nerve. The elbow is then maintained at 90 degrees with a plaster-reinforced bulky dressing. Range of movement is started 5 to 10 days after surgery.

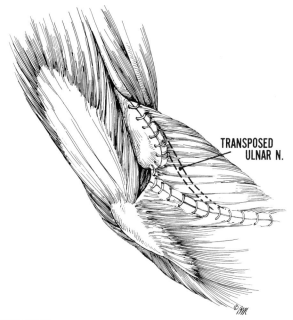

FIGURE 28-28. Completion of the submuscular transposition by repair of the flexor muscles to the medial epicondyle.

Author's (SEM) Preferred Technique

Optimal surgical management of cubital tunnel syndrome is controversial. Because the mechanism of cubital tunnel syndrome is related to the position of the nerve behind the axis of the elbow joint and elbow flexion increases tension on the nerve, procedures that do not transpose the nerve may not consistently correct the condition. A medial epicondylectomy goes partway toward decreasing the range through which the nerve must course with elbow flexion. A subcutaneous transposition should be effective as long as there is no kinking of the nerve in either the proximal or the distal transposition site, especially where the nerve moves from the subcutaneous to the intramuscular position distally. Associated epicondylitis cannot be adequately addressed with a subcutaneous transposition. The classic Learmonth submuscular transposition can result in compression of the nerve by remaining tendinous bands within the flexor/pronator muscle mass or at its distal transposition site. Associated medial epicondylitis is not addressed because the tension on the flexor/pronator muscle origin is actually increased as it is reset tighter when the flexor origin is reattached. Our preferred method is an anterior transposition of the nerve with a release of the flexor/pronator muscle origin and positioning of the nerve in a transmuscular location (Fig. 28-29).[224,227] The transposition through the muscle places no tension on the nerve in any direction and shortens the distance that the ulnar nerve must traverse in all ranges of elbow movement. Identification and removal of all potential tendons, bands, and fascial septum ensures no new compression points on the nerve. Release of the flexor/pronator muscle origin treats associated medial epicondylitis.[213] Leaving some flexor/pronator muscle intact facilitates earlier return of strength. The results of this procedure have been extremely satisfactory.[232]

The procedure is performed with the patient under general anesthesia using a single tourniquet, augmented by a Bier block with bretylium and lidocaine. The incision is placed behind the medial epicondyle (10 to 12 cm). Complete release of all points of ulnar nerve compression is performed as described earlier, and care is taken to identify and protect branches of the medial antebrachial cutaneous nerve.[223] The soft tissue above the flexor/pronator muscle origin is elevated, and then the fascial flaps are marked for elevation and transposition (see Fig. 28-29B and C). The flexor/pronator muscle origin is marked in half, and the first incision is made along this line. Distally the flap is connected to the incision that was made in the fascia of the flexor carpi ulnaris overlying the ulnar nerve. The proximal edge of the proximal flap is the free border of the flexor/pronator muscle fascia. The distal fascial flap is elevated with a sharp dissection. The proximal flap elevates easily with some muscle attached. The fascial bands are identified within the flexor/pronator muscle origin. The muscle attachments are released from proximal to distal to preserve muscle innervation. The "T"-shaped tendinous fascia (about 4-cm length) is removed. The ulnar nerve is identified as it courses through the proximal portion of the flexor carpi ulnaris muscle. There is another fascial septum here that needs to be removed. This septum is located between the median nerve–innervated flexor/pronator muscle and the ulnar nerve–innervated flexor carpi ulnaris muscle and curves around distally and over the ulnar nerve (see Fig. 28-29B). Just like the proximal medial intramuscular septum, if left intact, it will kink the ulnar nerve in the distal location of the transposition. Proximally, the flexor/pronator muscle is released for a short distance down to the level of the brachialis. Distally, the flexor/pronator muscle is released only as necessary to have the ulnar nerve transposed anteriorly with no tension on the ulnar nerve in the transposition site. It is important to ensure that the ulnar nerve, when transposed, lies in a straight line with no compression proximally or distally. Using loupe magnification and micro instrumentation, the posterior motor branch of the ulnar nerve will be neurolyzed from the main ulnar nerve so that the posterior motor branches remain intact and do not tether the ulnar nerve when it is moved anteriorly. The fascial flaps are closed loosely over the ulnar nerve with two nonabsorbable sutures. It should be possible to put at least a finger between the fascial flaps and the nerve below so that there is no pressure on the ulnar nerve from these flaps. The nerve should be evaluated again to ensure that there is no kinking of the nerve either proximally or distally. The more anterior the nerve is transposed, the possible "kinking" sites will be more distal in the forearm. Again, a final check should be done to ensure there is no kinking on the ulnar nerve at its proximal and distal transposition site. If inadvertently a branch of the medial antebrachial cutaneous nerve has been injured, the distal end should be cauterized and transposed well above the elbow and away from the scar. To assist with pain control, bupivacaine is placed in the incision and a continuous infusion pump can also be used. A Jackson-Pratt drain is placed. The incision is closed with 3-0 absorbable subcutaneous and 4-0 monofilament intradermal sutures with Steri-Strips. The arm is immobilized with a 4-inch light casting material in a padded dressing, keeping the wrist in neutral, the forearm pronated, and the elbow flexed.

Postoperative Care

The bulky dressing, bupivacaine infusion pump, and Jackson-Pratt drain are removed 2 days after surgery. The patient is instructed in range-of-motion exercises for the fingers, wrist, forearm, elbow, and shoulder. For patient comfort, a sling is used at night to limit elbow extension. The patient is restricted from heavy lifting for 1 month after surgery. Patients who do not regain full active range of motion within the first 2 to 3 weeks after surgery are referred for therapy. Most patients, however, begin therapy for strengthening exercises 4 weeks after surgery. Patients are allowed full activity and return to work without restrictions 8 weeks after surgery.

In a follow-up study of 119 operated cases at least 2 years after anterior transmuscular transposition of the ulnar nerve, 75% of patients who underwent unilateral procedures reported improvement and 68% of patients with bilateral surgery reported improvement.[232] There was no significant differences in patients with workers' compensation/litigation, obesity, concomitant carpal tunnel syndrome, or abnormal preoperative nerve conduction studies. However, nonsmokers had significantly better outcomes than smokers.

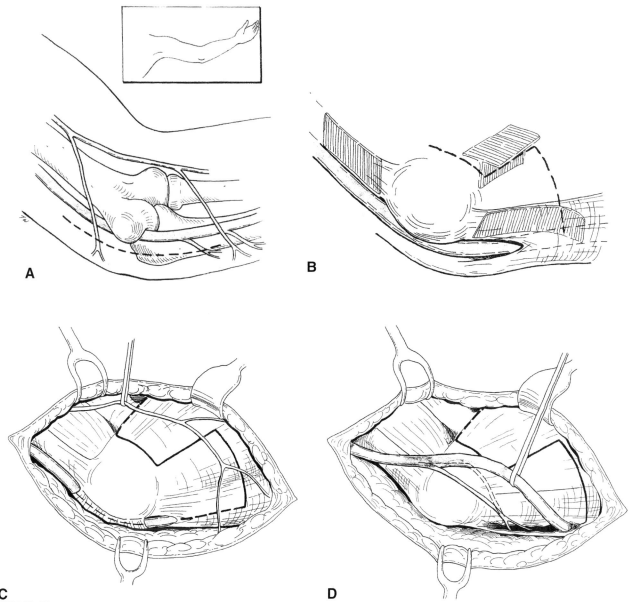

FIGURE 28-29. Author's (SEM) preferred technique of a transmuscular transposition of the ulnar nerve. **A,** The arm is positioned in shoulder external rotation and abduction and the forearm supinated. A 10- to 12-cm skin incision is made posterior to the medial epicondyle, and care is taken to avoid injury to the branches of the medial antebrachial cutaneous nerve (MABC). **B,** A series of three-dimensional fascial planes underlie the skin and subcutaneous tissues at the elbow, the intermuscular septum above the elbow, the cubital tunnel fascia overlying the ulnar nerve, the "T"-shaped fascia within the pronator teres muscle, the septum separating the pronator teres from the flexor carpi ulnaris muscle, and the leading edge of the flexor carpi ulnaris musculature. These structures must be released and/or excised to allow mobilization and transposition of the ulnar nerve. **C,** The MABC is mobilized and retracted laterally. The ulnar nerve is identified at the cubital tunnel and the superficial tissues are released. Working distally, the leading edge of the flexor carpi ulnaris (FCU) is identified and carefully divided above the nerve for 2 to 3 cm. The flexor/pronator origin is identified, and the fascia overlying the muscle incised in half along its obliquity. A perpendicular incision connects the fascia-splitting incision with the incision dividing the FCU leading edge to create a distal fascial flap. A second perpendicular incision connects the initial fascia-splitting incision with the free proximal border of the flexor/pronator muscle origin to create a proximal flap. **D,** Dissection is performed to allow complete mobilization of the ulnar nerve to avoid tethering during anterior transposition. Under loupe magnification, the posterior motor branch is neurolyzed proximally.

Continued

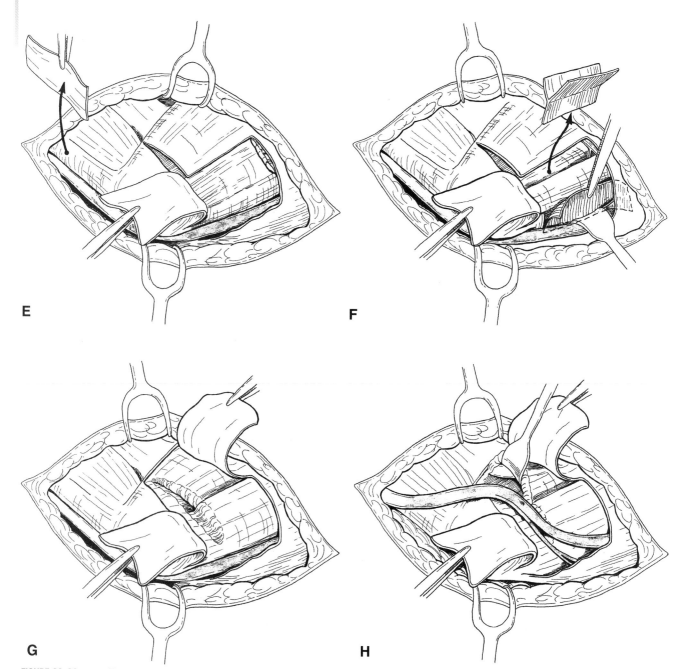

E

F

G

H

FIGURE 28-29—cont'd. **E,** The proximal segment of medial intermuscular septum is identified and excised to avoid kinking during anterior transposition. The previously defined distal flap of pronator fascia is then sharply elevated from distal to proximal. **F,** With elevation of the distal pronator fascia flap, a "T"-shaped fascial structure composed of a horizontal plate overlying a vertical plate, is exposed. The flexor/pronator muscle is dissected from these fascial edges. While protecting the ulnar nerve, a 4-cm piece of this fascial structure is sharply excised. With removal of the tendinous fascia, the fascial septum separating the pronator teres to the FCU is exposed, and this is also sharply excised. **G,** The previously defined proximal flap is then elevated from the flexor/pronator muscle. Scissors are used to make a shallow trough within the pronator muscle, perpendicular to the original pronator fascia-dividing incision. The proximal dissection is carried out to the level of the brachialis muscle, but distally some flexor/pronator muscle is left intact. This maneuver is carefully performed to avoid inadvertent injury to the median nerve, which is nearby but not typically visualized. **H,** The ulnar nerve is moved into the transmuscular position. There should be no tension on the transposed nerve and any points of tension either proximally or distally must be carefully released.

Continued

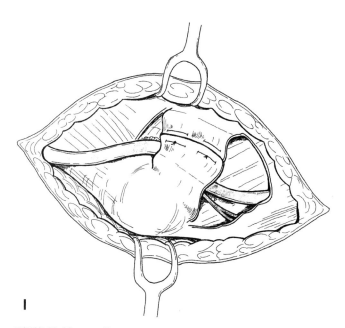

I

FIGURE 28-29—cont'd. **I,** The fascia flaps are sutured loosely over the transposed nerve. After adequate hemostasis, a Jackson-Pratt drain and bupivacaine (Marcaine) infusion pump are placed in the wound. The wound is closed in dermal and subcuticular layers.

CRITICAL POINTS: CUBITAL TUNNEL SURGERY

INDICATIONS

■ Failure to relieve symptoms with the use of elbow pad and avoidance of elbow flexion
■ Ulnar intrinsic wasting

PREOPERATIVE EVALUATION

■ Electrodiagnostic studies

PEARLS

■ Document preoperative pain distribution.
■ Document preoperative examination of entire upper extremity.
■ Use bretylium and Bier block.
■ Use bupivacaine (Marcaine) pain pump.
■ Begin early movement (postoperative day 2 or 3).

TECHNICAL POINTS

■ Avoid injury to all branches of the medial antebrachial cutaneous nerve.
■ Remove intermuscular septum.

CRITICAL POINTS: CUBITAL TUNNEL SURGERY—cont'd

TECHNICAL POINTS—cont'd

■ Elevate fascial flaps.
■ Remove tendinous bands in the flexor pronator muscle.
■ Dissect enough flexor/pronator muscle to allow the ulnar nerve to run in a straight line anterior to the medial epicondyle.
■ Close the fascial flaps above the ulnar nerve extremely loosely.
■ Most importantly, ensure that the ulnar nerve is not kinked at the distal transposition site.
■ Place bupivacaine in the incision.
■ Use a suction drain and an infusion pain pump.

PITFALLS

■ Kinking of the ulnar nerve may occur distally as it moves from its position within the flexor carpi ulnaris to its position anterior to the medial epicondyle.
■ Do not immobilize arm more than 2 or 3 days postoperatively.

POSTOPERATIVE CARE

■ Remove dressing at postoperative day 2 or 3.
■ Begin range-of-motion exercises within comfort starting on postoperative day 2 or 3.
■ Use sling at night for 3 weeks.
■ Begin strengthening exercises in second month.
■ Restrict weight lifting to 2 lb at 1 month.
■ There are no restrictions after second month.

COMPRESSION OF THE RADIAL NERVE

Superficial Radial Nerve Compression

In 1932, Wartenberg described five cases of compression neuropathy of the radial sensory nerve in the forearm and coined the term *cheiralgia paresthetica*.[295] The superficial location of the radial sensory nerve in the forearm renders it susceptible to external compression. Tight wristwatch bands[253,254,259,260,270] or handcuffs[258,262,276] have been implicated in this compression neuropathy. Work-related repetitive activity requiring significant pronation or supination of the forearm or ulnar wrist flexion has also been implicated, as has using a screwdriver, prolonged writing with a pen, or using a typewriter.[260,263] It has been suggested that anatomically the radial sensory nerve is relatively susceptible to increased compression and traction.[260] In pronation, the tendons of the brachioradialis and extensor carpi radialis longus come together to compress the nerve. As the wrist moves from radial extension to ulnar flexion, the nerve becomes stretched. Over time, edema and fibrosis can cause chronic nerve compression.[260] Histopathology in human cases has been studied to describe this compression neuropathy.[274]

Anatomy

The radial sensory nerve branches from the main radial nerve at the lateral humeral epicondyle, courses below the brachioradialis, and enters the subcutaneous tissue between the tendons of the brachioradialis and the extensor carpi radialis longus. In 3% to 10% of individuals, the superficial branch of the radial nerve will become subcutaneous by actually piercing the tendon of the brachioradialis.[251,293] It bifurcates into two main branches 5 cm proximal to the radial styloid, and the major palmar branch continues to innervate the dorsal radial aspect of the thumb. The major dorsal branch continues to innervate the dorsal ulnar aspect of the thumb and the dorsal radial aspect of the index finger. A third branch continues to become the dorsoulnar and dorsoradial digital nerve of the index and long fingers (Fig. 28-30).[251] The lateral antebrachial cutaneous nerve has a significant overlap pattern with the radial sensory nerve.[273]

Patients with radial sensory nerve compression typically describe paresthesia, pain, or numbness in the radial sensory nerve distribution. The diagnosis of radial sensory nerve entrapment is suspected with reproduction of symptoms with forearm pronation and ulnar wrist flexion and a positive nerve percussion sign where the radial sensory nerve exits the deep fascia in the forearm.[259,263] The differential diagnosis should include de Quervain's disease, and Finkelstein's sign can often be positive in patients with Wartenberg's syndrome. In fact, it has been suggested that inflammation of the first dorsal compartment sheath can cause scarring and entrapment of the distal branch of the superficial radial nerve.[284] Patients with de Quervain's disease should demonstrate normal sensory testing in the dorsal radial aspect of the hand as compared with patients with Wartenberg's syndrome in which sensation may be decreased. Patients with de Quervain's disease tend to have pain with percussion over the first extensor compartment but not the typical "Tinel-like" response. Electrodiagnostic studies are only occasionally useful in diagnosing this condition.[256,288]

Rarely, the lateral antebrachial cutaneous nerve, which partially or completely overlaps the sensory territory of the radial sensory nerve, may be entrapped.[252,273] Differential nerve blocks and positive nerve percussion testing will help distinguish these two nerve entrapments. Sprofkin suggested that Wartenberg's disease was second only to meralgia paresthetica in frequency among mononeuropathies.[290] In our experience, it is relatively rare. Patients who describe paresthesia, numbness, or pain in the radial sensory nerve distribution need to be examined to rule out cervical disk disease. If findings localize to the forearm and the cervical spine is excluded as a source of pathology, then the patient is instructed to modify inciting activities and to maintain the forearm in a more supinated position whenever possible. Modification of activities to avoid excessive pronation and supination and a local corticosteroid injection at the entrapment site between the tendons of the extensor carpi radialis longus and brachioradialis is usually successful, and surgical release is rarely necessary. Splinting is usually not successful because of the difficulty of splinting in forearm supination.

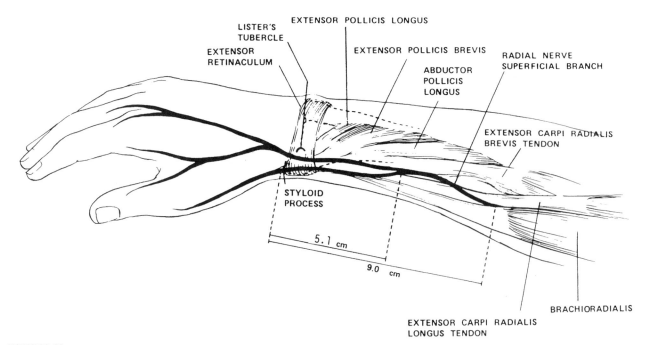

FIGURE 28-30. The most common pattern of the superficial branch of the radial nerve. (From Abrams RA, Brown RA, Botte MJ: The superficial branch of the radial nerve: An anatomic study with surgical implications. J Hand Surg [Am] 17:1037-1041, 1992.)

Radial Sensory Nerve Decompression

Author's (SEM) Preferred Technique

The radial sensory nerve is released at its point of compression between the tendons of the extensor carpi radialis longus and the brachioradialis (Fig. 28-31). Preoperatively the most intense site of Tinel's sign is determined. A longitudinal incision (2 to 3 cm) is marked just volar to the musculotendinous junction of the brachioradialis muscle. The radial sensory nerve will be identified just dorsal to this point between the tendon of the brachioradialis and the extensor carpi radialis longus. An intravenous regional technique is used with bretylium and lidocaine. Loupe magnification is used to identify and protect the crossing branches of the lateral antebrachial cutaneous nerve. The musculotendinous junction of the brachioradialis is identified, and the fascia between the tendons of the brachioradialis and the extensor carpi radialis longus is opened. The fascia above the radial sensory nerve is released to identify the radial sensory nerve. The nerve is followed proximally and distally for a distance of about 10 cm. A portion of the tendon of the brachioradialis can be resected to completely decompress the radial sensory nerve. With proximal and distal retraction, the radial sensory nerve can be released over a long distance. A neurolysis is not performed. The tourniquet is deflated, and good hemostasis is obtained.

Bupivacaine is placed in the incision. The incision is closed over a plastic angiocatheter, and 2 mL of dexamethasone is injected along the course of the radial sensory nerve through the angiocatheter, removing the angiocatheter when the wound is closed. A bulky dressing is applied, keeping the wrist in neutral.

Postoperative Care

The dressing is removed on the second postoperative day, and early movement of the upper extremity is encouraged. Desensitization of the radial sensory distribution on the dorsum of the hand is also started. Patients should avoid heavy lifting for the first month and then start strengthening exercises at the end of the first month.

Posterior Interosseous Nerve Syndrome and Radial Tunnel Syndrome

Compression of the radial nerve in the region of the proximal forearm can result in the posterior interosseous nerve syndrome or radial tunnel syndrome. In a posterior interosseous nerve palsy, the muscles innervated by the nerve are affected, including the extensor carpi radialis brevis, supinator, extensor carpi ulnaris, extensor digitorum communis, extensor digiti quinti, extensor indicis proprius, abductor pollicis longus, and extensor pollicis longus and brevis. The onset of symptoms may occur after trauma, or an insidious onset may be reported. Other causes can include proliferative rheumatoid synovitis and mononeuritis or Parsonage-Turner syndrome.[275,277] Rarely, iatrogenic injury can occur during elbow surgery for biceps reattachment, elbow arthroscopy, or radial head reconstruction. Tendon

---

CRITICAL POINTS: RADIAL SENSORY NERVE RELEASE

INDICATIONS

- Rare
- Failure of supination posture to relieve radial sensory symptoms

PREOPERATIVE EVALUATION

- Tinel's sign over entrapment point in forearm
- Electrodiagnostic studies

PEARLS

- Encouragement of a palm-up position and/or corticosteroid injection usually relieves symptoms without surgery.

TECHNICAL POINTS

- Preoperatively identify the muscle tendon junction of the brachioradialis.
- Make a longitudinal lazy-"S" incision just volar to the muscle tendon junction of the brachioradialis.
- Take care to avoid injury to the lateral antebrachial cutaneous nerve.
- Open the fascia between the brachioradialis and extensor carpi radialis longus.
- Remove a portion of the tendon of the brachioradialis to adequately release the radial sensory nerve.
- Release the radial sensory nerve proximally and distally to ensure no compressive fascial bands.
- Instill corticosteroid around nerve.
- Place bupivacaine in the incision.

PITFALLS

- Confusion with cervical disk disease
- Injury to the lateral antebrachial cutaneous nerve
- Failure to diagnose associated de Quervain's disease

POSTOPERATIVE CARE

- Remove dressing at day 2 or 3.
- Begin range-of-motion exercises at day 2 or 3.
- Begin strengthening exercises in the second month.

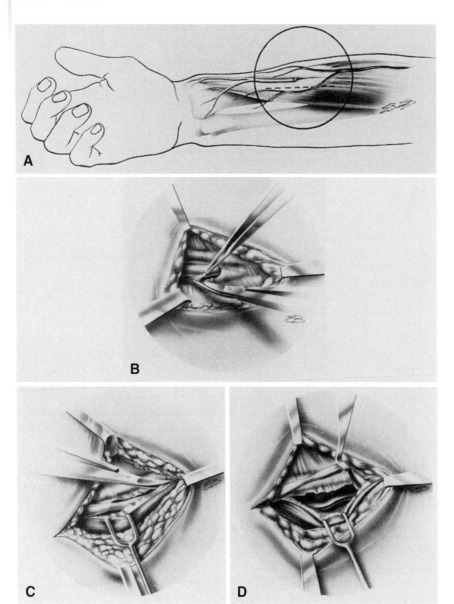

FIGURE 28-31. Radial sensory nerve decompression. **A,** The incision is on the flexor aspect of the forearm and centered on the radial sensory nerve. **B,** The fascia between the brachioradialis and extensor carpi radialis longus tendons is divided distally (**C**) and then proximally. **D,** The nerve is freed from its underlying bed. (From Dellon AL, Mackinnon SE: Radial sensory nerve entrapment in the forearm. J Hand Surg [Am] 11:199-205, 1986.)

rupture or masses at the elbow may also present as loss of posterior interosseous nerve function.[268,281,285] Because the extensor carpi radialis longus is innervated by the radial nerve proximal to the injury, active wrist extension with radial deviation is characteristic.

Radial tunnel syndrome is a more controversial diagnosis. Symptoms of pain and weakness may be reported by patients after activities of forceful elbow extension or forearm rotation.[269,286] Forearm pain typically localizes to the lateral aspect of the forearm, and weakness is often secondary to the pain. Lateral epicondylitis must be considered in the differential diagnosis. Both lateral epicondylitis and radial tunnel can occur simultaneously.[296] The tendinous origin of the extensor carpi radialis brevis can be implicated in both conditions.

The diagnosis is based on clinical examination, including tenderness over the radial tunnel, pain at the edge of the extensor carpi radialis brevis with resistance of middle finger extension, and pain with resisted forearm supination.[282] Electrodiagnostic studies are not particularly useful in this condition.[294] Because reproduction of pain with deep palpation is important in making this diagnosis, it is important to test the contralateral asymptomatic arm. Pressure is placed over the posterior interosseous nerve in the interval between the brachioradialis and the extensor carpi radialis brevis muscles, and the patient's response is compared between the two forearms. Pressure over the supinator may be quite painful. To determine if a concomitant problem exists over the radial nerve, pressure is exerted between the brachioradialis and the brachialis muscles just above the elbow. Because this is a subjective diagnosis, it is important to check the patient's pain response at nonentrapment sites and to re-examine the patient on a few occasions.

There is no specific nonoperative treatment for radial tunnel syndrome. However, nerve gliding exercises may be useful. In patients with concomitant lateral epicondylitis, therapy may ameliorate symptoms associated with the lateral epicondylitis. Tennis elbow straps are not recommended in patients with radial tunnel syndrome because of the increased pressure that may be placed on the radial nerve.

Anatomy

The radial nerve is one of two terminal branches of the posterior cord of the brachial plexus, splitting away from the axillary nerve just proximal to the quadrangular space. It lies behind the axillary artery and brachial artery anterior to the long head of the triceps muscle. The radial nerve then courses laterally and posteriorly deep to the long head of the triceps and lies deep to the lateral head and superficial to the medial head of the triceps near the spiral groove. After innervating the triceps, the nerve pierces the lateral intermuscular septum into the anterior compartment of the arm approximately 10 cm proximal to the lateral epicondyle (Fig. 28-32). The radial nerve sends one to three accessory branches to the brachialis muscle 3 to 9 cm proximal to the epicondylar line and a larger branch to the brachioradialis muscle. Occasionally this branch can arise from the superficial branch of the radial nerve distal to the epicondylar line.[265] The anconeus muscle is innervated proximal to the joint line, followed by the extensor carpi radialis longus. The radial nerve enters the forearm anterior to the lateral epicondyle and then divides into the superficial and deep branch (posterior interosseous nerve). The extensor carpi radialis brevis is generally innervated distal to the joint line from either the posterior interosseous nerve or the superficial radial nerve. The posterior interosseous nerve passes under the arcade of Fröhse before entering the interval between the two heads of the supinator. The arcade of Fröhse is a fibrous arch that originates from the lateral epicondyle and in a number of cases has a tendinous consistency.[289] Fibrous bands within the supinator muscle, or hypertrophy of the superficial head, may cause compression in this location.[255,261,268,291] After exiting the supinator muscle, the posterior interosseous nerve then divides into deep and superficial branches. The superficial branch innervates the extensor carpi ulnaris, extensor digitorum communis, and extensor digiti quinti muscles. The deep branch innervates the abductor pollicis longus, extensor pollicis longus, extensor pollicis brevis, and, lastly, the extensor indicis proprius muscles.

The radial tunnel begins anterior to the radiocapitellar joint and is approximately 5 cm in length. The tunnel is formed laterally by the extensor carpi radialis longus and brevis and the brachioradialis muscles, medially by the biceps tendon and brachialis, and posteriorly by the radiocapitellar joint capsule. The brachioradialis muscle passes over the nerve in a lateral to anterior direction, forming the tunnel roof.[271] Although the tunnel was originally described as ending at the arcade of Fröhse, compressive tendinous bands have been described that extend to the distal end of the supinator muscle.[283]

Operative Techniques

There have been several approaches described to release the posterior interosseous nerve based on the relationship of the incision to the brachioradialis muscle. An anterior approach has been described.[287] A posterior approach has been described by Henry[267] and Thompson,[292] and a transmuscular brachioradialis-splitting approach also has been described.[271]

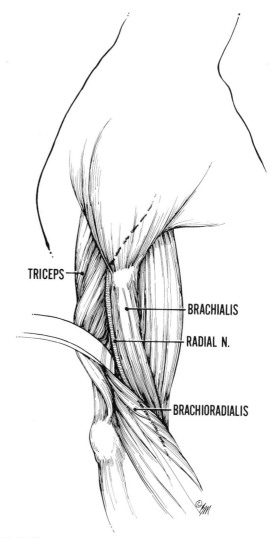

FIGURE 28-32. The radial nerve pierces the lateral intermuscular septum 10 cm above the lateral humeral condyle and courses in a groove between the brachialis and brachioradialis muscles.

Transmuscular Brachioradialis-Splitting Approach

With the use of regional or intravenous block anesthesia, a longitudinal or "S"-shaped incision is made, beginning proximal to the radial head and 3 cm lateral to the biceps tendon (Fig. 28-33). Lister has suggested a 4-cm transverse skin incision centered over the mobile wad in the forearm at a level just distal to the radial head.[271] The fascia over the brachioradialis muscle is incised and the muscle belly is split bluntly, aiming for the radial head until the fat overlying the radial nerve is seen. The brachioradialis muscle split is lengthened over the radial tunnel. Transverse vessels are coagulated, and the fibrous bands overlying the posterior interosseous nerve and the fibrous edge of the extensor carpi radialis brevis are divided. Recurrent radial vessels are ligated and the superficial head of the supinator muscle is completely divided.

Posterior (Henry or Thompson Approach)

The forearm is pronated and a 10-cm straight skin incision is made along an imaginary line extending from the lateral epicondyle to Lister's tubercle (Fig. 28-34). The incision

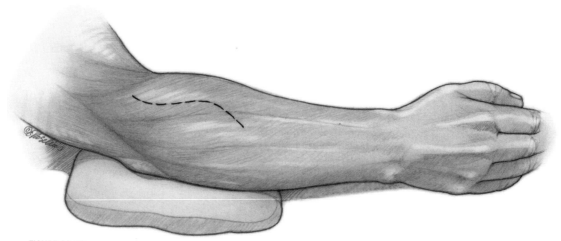

FIGURE 28-33. Extended approach to the posterior interosseous nerve through the brachioradialis-splitting approach.

can be extended proximally onto the lateral ridge of the epicondyle as necessary (Fig. 28-35). The posterior cutaneous nerve of the forearm is identified and protected. The forearm fascia is incised in the interval between the extensor digitorum communis and the radial wrist extensors. Dissection begins where the two tendons can be identified distally and is extended proximally to the lateral epicondyle. The extensor digitorum communis muscle can be partially detached from the lateral epicondyle as needed. The supinator is identified deep to the extensor muscles in the proximal third of the incision. The posterior interosseous nerve can then be found at the proximal edge of the supinator, and the fibrous leading edge of the extensor carpi radialis brevis and the tendinous leading edge of the supinator are released. The recurrent leash of Henry vessels is ligated. The superficial head of the supinator muscle should be released to its distal border.

Anterior (Modified Henry) Approach

A curvilinear incision is made, starting above the lateral humeral epicondyle and continuing distally between the biceps and brachioradialis muscles and then curving

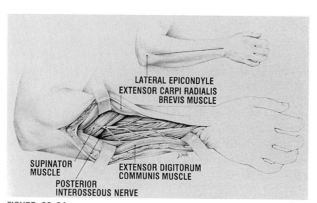

FIGURE 28-34. A straight longitudinal incision is used to expose the posterior interosseous nerve in the forearm in the posterior approach of Thompson. (From Siegel DB, Gelberman RH: Radial nerve: Applied anatomy and operative exposure. *In* Gelberman RH [ed]: Operative Nerve Repair and Reconstruction. Philadelphia, JB Lippincott, 1991, pp 393-407.)

laterally 2 cm above the elbow flexion crease, back over the mobile wad, and medial to the ulnar border of the brachioradialis muscle (Fig. 28-36). The cutaneous nerves are identified and protected and the fascia divided along the brachioradialis muscle, which is then retracted laterally while retracting the biceps and pronator teres in the distal wound medially. The radial nerve is identified in the interval between the brachialis and brachioradialis and then followed distally. Fibrous bands overlying the posterior interosseous nerve and the fibrous leading edge of the extensor carpi radialis brevis muscles are divided. The recurrent radial vessels of Henry are ligated and the arcade of Fröhse is released. The mobile wad is elevated and retracted to visualize the entire length of the supinator. The superficial head of the supinator is divided to expose the nerve to its terminal branches.

Author's (SEM) Preferred Technique

Decompression of the posterior interosseous nerve is done through the bloodless interval between the brachioradialis and the extensor carpi radialis longus.[266] This approach can easily be extended proximally to release the radial nerve in the interval between the brachialis and the brachioradialis and distally to decompress the posterior interosseous nerve through the supinator.

Preoperatively, it is important to identify the interval between the extensor carpi radialis longus and the brachioradialis muscles. The patient is instructed to resist elbow flexion and the planned incision is marked (10 cm) along the posterior border of the brachioradialis muscle (Fig. 28-37A). Intravenous regional or general anesthesia is used, as is loupe magnification and microbipolar cautery. The incision is made along the posterior border of the brachioradialis muscle. The posterior cutaneous nerve of the forearm is small, but it is always located exactly at the junction between the fascia of the brachioradialis muscle and the

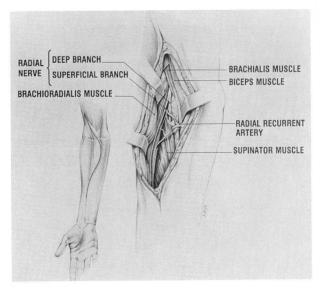

FIGURE 28-36. Operative incision and deep surgical dissection in the anterior approach to expose the posterior interosseous nerve in the proximal forearm. (From Siegel DB, Gelberman RH: Radial nerve: Applied anatomy and operative exposure. *In* Gelberman RH [ed]: Operative Nerve Repair and Reconstruction. Philadelphia, JB Lippincott, 1991, pp 393-407.)

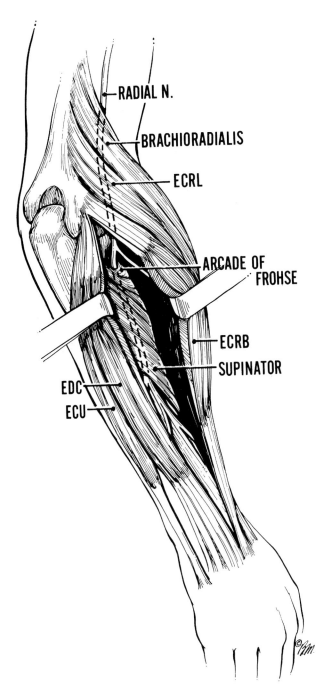

FIGURE 28-35. Extension of the posterior Thompson approach to the radial tunnel.

extensor carpi radialis longus muscle. There is a color distinction between the fascia of these two muscles. The brachioradialis muscle is a more intense red color because the fascia is thinner. By contrast, the fascia of the extensor carpi radialis longus is thicker and it appears as a lighter color. This fascial interval is then sharply divided with a No. 15 blade, and the dissection is deepened by blunt finger dissection down to the region of the arcade of Fröhse. If the dissection is not an easy finger dissection, then the surgeon is not in the correct plane. Deep down-curved retractors are then used to retract the brachioradialis muscle and the extensor carpi radialis longus muscles. The crossing vessels

are then identified and carefully ligated and divided. The surgeon can then easily identify the radial sensory nerve, the small nerve to the extensor carpi radialis brevis, and the posterior interosseous nerve. The tendon of the extensor carpi radialis brevis is then divided from its origin on the lateral epicondyle. This effectively treats any component of the symptoms that may have been attributed to lateral epicondylitis. Both the tendinous part and the underlying muscle of the superficial head of the supinator are divided to completely release the posterior interosseous nerve. Occasionally, there will be tendinous bands compressing the posterior interosseous nerve distally within the supinator, and thus the division should proceed to its distal edge. The surgeon should run a finger along the proximal portion of the posterior interosseous nerve above the elbow; and if any bands are encountered, then a second incision above the elbow along the anterior border of the brachioradialis muscle may be needed. Deep dissection is performed bluntly between the brachioradialis muscle and the brachialis muscles. If the dissection is difficult or through muscle fibers, then the surgeon is in the wrong plane. The radial nerve proper is easily identified and followed proximally to release any tendinous bands up to the level of the lateral intermuscular septum. Bupivacaine is placed in the incision(s). The tourniquet is deflated, and hemostasis is obtained with bipolar electrocautery. A drain is rarely needed. The incisions are closed in layers with absorbable suture. A bulky dressing immobilizes the arm with the wrist in neutral and the elbow flexed.

Postoperative Care

The dressing is removed 2 days postoperatively, and the patient is encouraged to begin full range-of-motion exercises. The sutures are removed 10 to 14 days after surgery. In the second month, strengthening exercises are begun. The patient could be released to light duty at the end of the first

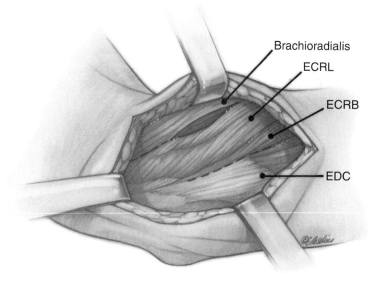

A

FIGURE 28-37. Extended approach to the posterior interosseous nerve through the brachioradialis/extensor carpi radialis longus interval. **A,** Superficial exposure. **B,** Deep exposure.

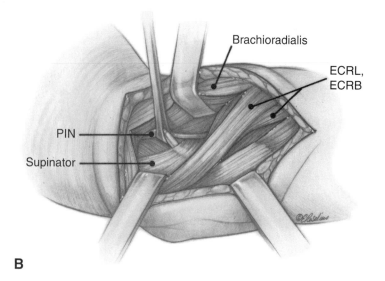

B

CRITICAL POINTS: POSTERIOR INTEROSSEOUS NERVE RELEASE

INDICATIONS

- Localized pain over the posterior interosseous nerve in the region of the arcade of Fröhse
- Failure to respond to physical therapy and treatment for possible concomitant lateral epicondylitis

PREOPERATIVE EVALUATION

- Document discrete significant pain at the brachioradialis/extensor carpi radialis longus junction.

PEARLS

- Preoperatively mark the incision just dorsal to the brachioradialis muscle.
- Use bretylium and Bier block.
- Note that the fascia of the brachioradialis is "redder" than the "lighter" fascia of the extensor carpi radialis longus.
- Release the tendon of the extensor carpi radialis brevis, thus treating for any potential associated lateral epicondylitis.
- Complete hemostasis.

CRITICAL POINTS: POSTERIOR INTEROSSEOUS NERVE RELEASE—cont'd

PEARLS—cont'd

- Begin early movement.
- If the patient preoperatively has localized pain over the radial nerve above the elbow, a second incision is made to decompress the main radial nerve above the elbow.

TECHNICAL POINTS

- Make an incision along the junction between the brachioradialis and extensor carpi radialis longus.
- Identify the posterior cutaneous nerve of the forearm.
- Use blunt dissection in the interval between the brachioradialis and the extensor carpi radialis longus down to the arcade of Fröhse.
- Preserve the nerve to the extensor carpi radialis brevis.
- Ligate the crossing vessels.
- Release the tendon of the extensor carpi radialis brevis over the posterior interosseous nerve.
- Release the superficial head of the supinator to completely decompress the posterior interosseous nerve.

- Use finger palpation proximally to feel for any fibrous bands over the radial head.
- Make a proximal incision above the elbow between the brachioradialis and brachialis if any fibrous bands are palpated from the distal incision.
- Place bupivacaine in the incision.

PITFALLS

- Failure to identify and protect the posterior cutaneous nerve of the forearm
- Failure to adequately excise the extensor carpi radialis brevis tendon and the entire superficial head of the supinator
- Failure to achieve meticulous hemostasis

POSTOPERATIVE CARE

- Remove dressing at postoperative day 2 or 3.
- Begin range-of-motion exercises at day 2 or 3.
- Continue range-of-motion exercises throughout the first month.
- Start strengthening exercises in the second month.
- If patient has had an associated procedure on the lateral epicondyle, then use a soft sling for 1 or 2 weeks.

month and released to full and unrestricted duty at the end of 2 months.

Proximal Radial Nerve Compression

Compression of the radial nerve proximal to the elbow is extremely uncommon. A fibrous arch from the lateral head of the triceps has been associated with radial nerve compression[279] and cases have been reported after strenuous muscular activities.[272,278,279] A bony exostosis of the humerus has also been associated with this problem.[257] Patients will present with a variable degree of radial nerve dysfunction. Typically it is not painful, and spontaneous recovery can be expected. Patients may provide a history of alcohol or drug abuse to suggest prolonged positioning with pressure over the radial nerve in the spiral groove. If there is no evidence clinically of recovery in 3 months, then electrodiagnostic studies should be done. If these do not show evidence of reinnervation, then surgical release of the radial nerve can be considered.

Operative Technique

With the patient under general anesthesia the entire arm is prepped and draped. Although distal dissection can be performed with the use of a sterile tourniquet, the case cannot be completed under tourniquet control because of the proximal exposure required. A long lateral incision is made between the deltoid and the lateral head of the triceps

muscle and extended distally along the lateral margin of the biceps, ending in the interval between the brachioradialis and the brachialis muscle just proximal to the cubital crease. The radial nerve is first identified by blunt dissection in the interval between the brachioradialis and the brachialis muscles. The nerve is then followed proximally and the lateral intermuscular septum divided to follow the nerve proximally under the lateral head of the triceps. Care is taken to protect the cutaneous radial branches. If necessary, intraoperative electrodiagnostic studies can be done to confirm the area of conduction block. If the long head of the triceps and the tendons of the teres major and latissimus dorsi are divided, these tendons must be reattached at the conclusion of the case. The incision is closed in layers, and a bulky dressing is applied using an arm sling.

Postoperative Care

The dressing is removed 2 days after surgery, and general range-of-motion exercises are started. The sling can be used at night for 3 weeks for comfort.

RECURRENT SURGERY FOR PREVIOUSLY FAILED PROCEDURES

In the carefully selected patient, well-performed surgery with good postoperative patient compliance should adequately decompress and/or take tension off a nerve such that symptoms from the compression neuropathy resolve and further surgery is not needed. As the extremity surgeon becomes experienced with the management of patients with compression neuropathies, he or she is likely to be referred patients who have had previous decompression surgeries with less than favorable results. The management of this patient population is much more challenging than that of patients with primary compressive neuropathies.[300] These patients often have a very significant pain component. Our pain evaluation form (see Fig. 28-3) is critical in helping to determine potential surgical candidates. The assistance of a pain management physician may also be required. Gabapentin (Neurontin) and/or nortriptyline can be recommended. If surgery is suggested, then informed consent will emphasize the possibility of not relieving pain and even decreasing neurologic function. In general, if the patient has had more than two surgical attempts to correct a nerve compression problem, it is less likely that a third operation to improve function will be helpful. In these situations with a motor deficit, nerve grafting, nerve transfer, or tendon transfers are considered. If pain is the primary problem, then a peripheral nerve stimulator or dorsal column stimulator should be considered.[302]

In general, after a failed procedure to treat a nerve compression, a patient's problems can be classified into three groups: (1) Patients may describe the *same symptoms* postoperatively as they had preoperatively with no relief of symptoms. (2) They may describe a period of relief of compression symptoms, followed at 6 months or later with *recurrence of the same symptoms.* (3) Finally, they may describe an entirely *new symptom-complex* after the decompression surgery. This last group is the most challenging to manage, because it typically includes patients with significant pain and nerve injury, either to the affected nerve or to a nearby cutaneous nerve.

Recurrent Carpal Tunnel

The most common reasons for persistent symptoms are failure to adequately decompress the carpal tunnel. Especially with the problem of increasing obesity, an incision of adequate length will be necessary to decompress the median nerve, especially at the proximal and distal sites of the surgical exposure.[298] Phalen's test will be positive in these patients, and no other significant sites of compression neuropathy along the course of the median nerve will be noted. Electrodiagnostic studies to evaluate recurrent carpal tunnel syndrome may not be particularly helpful, given the fact that patients with successful carpal tunnel surgery frequently will have persistent electrical changes.[301] A second common cause for persistent symptoms after primary carpal tunnel release is the likelihood that carpal tunnel syndrome was not the correct diagnosis or that it was causing an insignificant component of the patient's symptom complex, such that essentially a "wrong diagnosis" was made. These patients may demonstrate compression on the median nerve in the forearm or cervical disk disease or may have a sensory neuropathy resistant to surgical decompression. Patients with sensory complaints on the dorsal aspect of the thumb, index, and long finger obviously will not respond to carpal tunnel release.

Patients who have definite relief of symptoms for 6 months or longer and then have a recurrence of the same symptoms likely have developed a secondary traction neuritis of the median nerve due to scar formation. Incisions that are placed directly over the median nerve are susceptible to the development at a later period of time of scar between the median nerve and the overlying flexor retinaculum.[298] In these patients, Phalen's test is positive and there are no other sites of significant proximal median nerve compression.

The most challenging patient management group consists of those patients who develop completely new symptomatology after carpal tunnel release, and this is usually accompanied by very significant pain dysfunction. Whereas reflex sympathetic dystrophy or complex regional pain syndrome (CRPS) is uncommon after carpal tunnel release, minor injuries to the median nerve or the palmar cutaneous branch of the median nerve are unfortunately a well-recognized complication of a carpal tunnel release. A patient's history and physical examination will allow the surgeon to determine which component(s) of the median nerve or nearby cutaneous nerves have been injured. A proximal percussion test may help to determine this. Gentle digital percussion is made along the course of the median nerve and its palmar cutaneous branch 2 to 3 inches proximal to the surgical incision. At this level the patient will be able to describe painful paresthesia in the distribution of the involved nerve or nerve branches. By contrast, if digital percussion is done exactly over the area of nerve injury, it may be so painful as to not allow the patient to be specific about what components (fascicles) of the median nerve have been injured. Typically, the more superficial branch to the third web space (radial side of the ring finger and ulnar side of the long finger) is injured or caught up in scar tissue.

Patients are referred for therapy to decrease pain, increase range of motion, and increase strength. Medications such as gabapentin or nortriptyline may be helpful in decreasing neuropathic pain. In cases of nerve injury, nonoperative treatment will be unsuccessful. Revision surgery is recommended for patients with continued symptoms in the median nerve distribution that localizes to the level of the carpal tunnel or with identification of a partial median nerve injury or the palmar cutaneous branch of the median nerve.

Revision Surgery

The surgical management of persistent and recurrent carpal tunnel syndrome uses an incision well ulnar to the thenar crease regardless of the first incision and extends this proximal and distal to the area of the previous surgery. Dissection begins proximally to identify the median nerve and then is followed distally through the surgical site. The median nerve is usually found to be densely adherent to the underside of the flexor retinaculum. Micro internal neurolysis is almost always necessary in recurrent cases but is never indicated for primary carpal tunnel syndrome. Microsurgical instruments are used to perform a longitudinal epineurotomy. Frequently, however, there will be tension on the nerve both transversely and longitudinally, and thus a second epineurotomy going circumferentially around the nerve is also performed. The external epineurium is reflected and the neurolysis performed until bands of Fontana are noted in the fascicles. These bands represent redundancy in the peripheral nerves and thus are an "endpoint" for the neurolysis technique. Rarely, an abductor digiti minimi flap is used to provide soft tissue coverage over the nerve.[303] Occasionally, the nerve may be covered with fat from the neighboring Guyon canal; alternatively, a formal ulnar fat flap is transposed.[305] If the patient has a neuroma of the palmar cutaneous branch of the median nerve, then a neurolysis of the injured fascicle is performed well proximal from its branching point, and the transected nerve is transposed proximally to lie in the muscle interface between the deep and superficial flexors of the forearm. Injuries to the median nerve itself are treated as for the management of a neuroma in continuity; that is, injuries to the fascicles of the median nerve innervating the third web space can be reconstructed with a short nerve graft, or this fascicular group can be easily separated from the main median nerve for a very long distance and transposed proximally into the forearm between the two flexor masses.[304] The distal end of the third web space common digital nerve can be transferred in an end-to-side fashion to the second common digital nerve, to recover some sensibility in the third web space.[297,306]

Recurrent Cubital Tunnel Syndrome

Surgical failures are more frequent in cases of cubital tunnel syndrome than carpal tunnel syndrome, and the management of these cases is made exceedingly more difficult by the previous surgical procedure and resultant scarring of the nerve. Classification of failed cubital tunnel syndrome is similar to that for carpal tunnel syndrome. Patients may have persistence of the *same preoperative symptoms* with no change at all in their clinical status. They may have relief of symptoms for several months to years and then have *recurrent problems*. Finally, they may present with *new symptoms* of neurologic loss and/or pain after the cubital tunnel surgery.

Many conditions can mimic cubital tunnel surgery, and the surgeon needs to be well aware of these. Amyotrophic lateral sclerosis and Pancoast tumors can present as ulnar nerve symptoms. It is important to be alert for a situation in which sensory loss and motor loss are decidedly different. If the sensory loss far exceeds the motor complaints, then a sensory neuropathy should be considered. By contrast, if the motor complaints exceed the sensory complaints, compression in Guyon's canal should be considered, especially if the proximal extrinsic hand muscles are normal and there is no thenar atrophy. If there is additional thenar atrophy, then compression in the thoracic outlet with the very rare Gilliatt "true" neurogenic thoracic outlet syndrome should be considered.[297a] If the extrinsic motors are equally involved, then a brachial plexus neuritis can be considered, or an upper motor neuron disease if deep tendon reflexes are increased. Electrodiagnostic studies by an experienced examiner are critical in the differential diagnosis and localizing the level of compression.

Failure to relieve symptoms implies a poorly done primary surgical procedure or an incorrect diagnosis. Recurrent symptoms after a period of 6 months or more after relief of symptoms usually implies a new site of ulnar nerve compression in the previous surgical field. Severe causalgia-type pain at the elbow radiating into the medial aspect of the forearm suggests a neuroma of the medial antebrachial cutaneous nerve. Severe causalgia type pain into the ulnar nerve distribution suggests an injury to the ulnar nerve itself. The proximal percussion test above the area of the previous surgical site along the course of the basilic vein will result in pain and/or paresthesia in the distribution of the medial antebrachial cutaneous nerve if there is a neuroma of this nerve. Similarly, percussion along the course of the ulnar nerve above the area of the previous surgery will result in paresthesia and pain into the ulnar nerve distribution if there is a problem to the ulnar nerve itself. Palpation along the course of the ulnar nerve in the distal forearm progressing to the region of the surgical site will result in deep pain distal to the previous surgical site if there is a new compression point at the site of the distal surgical exposure. This finding is common if great care has not been taken to ensure a smooth transposition of the ulnar nerve from its position in the forearm underneath the flexor carpi ulnaris to the transposition site at the elbow.

Surgical management of a secondary cubital tunnel syndrome has been reviewed.[299] If the patient has previously had a simple decompression, the finding is usually scar around the ulnar nerve in the surgical site and/or a tendency for the ulnar nerve to sublux over the medial epicondyle. In either instance the ulnar nerve is mobilized and a transmuscular transposition is performed as described previously. Similar findings and management are utilized if the patient has previously had an unsuccessful medial epicondylectomy. If the patient has previously had a subcutaneous transposition, the nerve is usually found to be scarred along its course within the surgical site, either to the anterior surface of the medial epicondyle or distally where the ulnar nerve moves from its transposition site to the flexor carpi ulnaris muscle mass. Occasionally, a retained medial intermuscular septum will cause compression on the nerve proximally. In each of these instances, the ulnar nerve is mobilized, the distal and proximal compression sites dealt with, and a transmuscular procedure performed.

If the patient has previously had an intramuscular procedure, the nerve is usually scarred along its entire surgical course, or a tight fascial or suture band can be identified at the medial epicondyle, where the surgeon has created a sling to prevent subluxation. Typically, there is also compression of the ulnar nerve at the distal transposition site by fascia of the flexor carpi ulnaris muscle and the tendinous fascia between the pronator muscle and the flexor carpi ulnaris muscle. The ulnar nerve is mobilized, and fascial flaps are marked on the flexor/pronator muscle origin as described for a primary transmuscular transposition, except in this situation the flaps are based more anteriorly and just in front of the previous surgical intramuscular trough.

If the patient has had the classic Learmonth submuscular transposition, then the ulnar nerve may be found to be markedly compressed by the tendinous "T" fascia septum within the flexor/pronator muscle origin. The nerve typically takes a right-angled turn where it goes from its submuscular position in front of the medial epicondyle near the median nerve to its posterior location within the flexor carpi ulnaris muscle. The distal fascial septum between the pronator and the flexor carpi ulnaris is usually also intact and may compress the nerve. In these situations, the dissection starts proximally out of the area of the previous surgical site. The dissection carefully follows the ulnar nerve into the area of the previous surgery. The ulnar nerve is then found distal to the previous surgical site and followed proximally along its course into the region of the previous surgery. Because the patient has had a previous Learmonth submuscular transposition, it is usually possible to leave some overlying muscle intact and remove the tendinous fascial septa that are compressing the ulnar nerve. Thus, no fascial flaps are needed to prevent the ulnar nerve from relocating posteriorly, because the overlying flexor/pronator muscle accomplishes this. All tendinous bands and septa that are compressing the nerve are released under the muscle and proximally and distally.

When operating for recurrent cubital tunnel syndrome, and particularly in multiply operated cases, extreme care must be taken to preserve vascular supply to the nerve. The profound intrinsic blood supply of the normal ulnar nerve can change to be more extrinsic, and ischemia of the nerve can occur if too extensive a neurolysis is performed. An external epineurotomy and cautious external neurolysis are preferred only to ensure that ulnar nerve fascicles and bands of Fontana are visualized. Typically, in all situations of secondary cubital tunnel surgery, care must be taken to identify the medial antebrachial cutaneous nerve and follow the two main branches distally to make sure that they have been protected. If the branches have been injured, then the neuromas are excised and these nerves are transposed proximally to lie well away from the elbow and overlying scar. The distal end of the nerve is cauterized to "cap" the nerve endings with connective tissue and place them either in a muscular bed or in subcutaneous tissue, depending on the patient's body habitus.

Recurrent Guyon's Canal Release

Patients who have persistent ulnar intrinsic atrophy after release of Guyon's canal need to be evaluated to make sure that there is not another etiology for the ulnar intrinsic atrophy, as described previously. If not, then consideration for re-exploration can be given. In our experience, the majority of surgeons do not adequately release the deep motor branch as it curves around the hook of the hamate below the hypothenar muscles. Review of the previous operative note should provide insight as to whether that portion of the procedure has been performed.

Recurrent Posterior Interosseous Nerve Decompression

Patients who have forearm pain without motor weakness and have failed to respond to a posterior interosseous nerve decompression can be considered for re-exploration if other sources of forearm pain have been ruled out. These patients may demonstrate a positive pressure provocative response over the posterior interosseous nerve in the region of the arcade of Fröhse. Physical examination will also look for evidence of compression over the radial nerve proper above the cubital crease. Informed consent will emphasize the possibility of failure to relieve pain and the possibility of increasing neurologic deficit. Regardless of the previous approach used to decompress the posterior interosseous

nerve, we recommend the approach described earlier in this chapter but begin the incision and surgical exploration above the area of the previous surgical site. Intraoperative nerve stimulation with direct stimulation of the nerve will help to identify the small branch to the extensor carpi radialis brevis and the larger posterior interosseous nerve. There is typically a significant amount of scarring around the nerve in this area, and great care must be taken to protect the posterior interosseous nerve. Typically, the finding is an incomplete release of the posterior interosseous nerve through the supinator. Occasionally, however, the posterior interosseous nerve has not been explored at all, accounting for the obvious failure to release symptoms and attesting to the importance of understanding the anatomy of this region.

Median Nerve Compression in the Proximal Forearm

When this procedure has been done and the patient still has median nerve symptoms, care must be taken to evaluate for other sources of median nerve dysfunction. Regardless of the previous incision used, complete re-exploration using a lazy-"S" incision beginning above the cubital crease and extending into the mid forearm is necessary. Typically the median nerve has not been adequately released and the tendinous arch of the pronator teres is still compressing the nerve.

ANNOTATED REFERENCES

1. American Journal of Industrial Medicine, Special issue: Biobehavioral Mechanisms of Work-Related Upper Extremity Disorders. Am J Indust Med 41(5):293-455, 2002.

    This issue of this journal is devoted to the discussion of a variety of the controversial aspects of work-related upper extremity disorders with contributions from epidemiologists, psychologists, surgeons, and therapists. The articles will broaden the hand surgeon's understanding of how other very disparate specialties approach the same problem.

41. Mackinnon SE: Pathophysiology of nerve compression. Hand Clin 18:231-241, 2002.

    This article summarizes the current concepts about the pathophysiology of chronic nerve compression and provides a basis for understanding patient symptomatology, evaluation, and treatment; it includes a review of electrodiagnostic studies.

44. Mackinnon SE, Dellon AL, Hudson AR, Hunter DA: Histopathology of compression of the superficial radial nerve in the forearm. J Hand Surg [Am] 11:206-210, 1986.

    This is the best report to detail the histopathology of chronic nerve compression in the human.

56. Novak CB, Mackinnon SE: Thoracic outlet syndrome. Orthop Clin North Am 27:747-762, 1996.

    The authors of this monograph describe current evaluation and management of vascular and neurogenic thoracic outlet syndrome and relate this problem to upper extremity nerve compression neuropathies. The approach to the management of thoracic outlet syndrome with its associated muscle imbalance is critical in treating patients with associated distal compression neuropathies.

66. Pechan J, Julius I: The pressure measurement of the ulnar nerve: A contribution to the pathophysiology of the cubital tunnel syndrome. J Biomech 8:75-79, 1975.

This classic report emphasized the mechanism of cubital tunnel syndrome as relating to increased pressure and tension on the ulnar nerve at the elbow with elbow flexion. This was evidence for supporting transposition procedures to decrease pressure and tension on the ulnar nerve in patients with cubital tunnel syndrome.

75. Szabo RM, Gelberman RH: Peripheral nerve compression: Etiology, critical pressure threshold, and clinical assessment. Orthopedics 7:1461-1466, 1984.

This is an excellent summary article of a body of work performed by these authors in the early 1980s that helped to set the stage for understanding of the etiology, evaluation, and management of patients with compression neuropathy.

81. Upton ARM, McComas AJ: The double crush in nerve-entrapment syndromes. Lancet 2:359-362, 1973.

In this clinical review, Upton and McComas introduced the concept of the double crush mechanism.

86. Wilbourn AJ: The electrodiagnostic examination with peripheral nerve injuries. Clin Plast Surg 30:139-154, 2003.

This article is an outline of the information that every surgeon who operates on the upper extremity needs to know regarding the interpretation of electrodiagnostic studies, not only for patients with compression neuropathy but also for other nerve injuries.

128. Jablecki CK, Andary MT, So YT, et al: Literature review of the usefulness of nerve conduction studies and electromyography for the evaluation of patients with carpal tunnel syndrome. AAEM Quality Assurance Committee. Muscle Nerve 16:1392-1414, 1993.

This review of the literature examines the usefulness of nerve conduction studies (NCS) and electromyography in the diagnosis of carpal tunnel syndrome. The authors conclude the median sensory and motor NCS are valid, reproducible studies to confirm the clinical diagnosis of carpal tunnel syndrome.

139. MacDermid JC, Richards RS, Roth JH, et al: Endoscopic versus open carpal tunnel release: A randomized trial. J Hand Surg [Am] 28:475-480, 2003.

This randomized controlled trial evaluated patient outcome of endoscopic versus open carpal tunnel release. Both types of surgery improved all measures outcomes and there were no beneficial differences with endoscopic versus open surgery. No complications were reported.

142. Mackinnon SE, McCabe S, Murray JF, et al: Internal neurolysis fails to improve the results of primary carpal tunnel compression. J Hand Surg [Am] 16:211-218, 1991.

This prospective double-blind study concluded that internal neurolysis did not improve outcome in primary carpal tunnel decompression, suggesting that there is no role for neurolysis in primary surgery for carpal tunnel syndrome.

151. Palmer AK, Toivonen DA: Complications of endoscopic and open carpal tunnel release. J Hand Surg [Am] 24:561-565, 1999.

Although this survey study as the authors state has methodologic problems, it brings awareness to the fact that carpal tunnel release is not a simple surgery without complications, be it with endoscopic or open surgery.

152. Rempel D, Evanoff B, Amadio PC, et al: Consensus criteria for the classification of carpal tunnel syndrome in epidemiologic studies. Am J Public Health 88:1447-1451, 1998.

This consensus report on epidemiologic studies of carpal tunnel syndrome reviews the current status and debate of work-related upper extremity problems with emphasis on carpal tunnel syndrome.

162. Taleisnik J: The palmar cutaneous branch of the median nerve and the approach to the carpal tunnel: An anatomical study. J Bone Joint Surg Am 55:1212-1217, 1973.

The anatomy of the palmar cutaneous branch with respect to various incisions for the carpal tunnel stimulated Taleisnik to recommend a relatively ulnar incision in line with the fourth ray.

221. Learmonth JR: A technique for transplanting the ulnar nerve. Surg Gynecol Obstet 75:792-793, 1942.

This publication is a charming description of Learmonth's procedure for ulnar nerve transposition. This description is detailed with 11 illustrations and one paragraph of his classic technique. Interestingly, no patient reports are provided.

230. Mowlavi A, Andrews K, Lille S, et al: The management of cubital tunnel syndrome: A meta-analysis of clinical studies. Plast Reconstr Surg 106:327-334, 2000.

A meta-analysis of 30 clinical studies between 1945 and 1995 was performed and provides a good overview of the outcome after treatment for cubital tunnel syndrome.

239. Spinner M: Injuries to the Major Branches of Peripheral Nerves of the Forearm. Philadelphia, WB Saunders, 1978.

If you can find this textbook, it is a classic book with excellent drawings by Thomas and insights by Spinner on the peripheral nerves and critical compression points in the upper extremity.

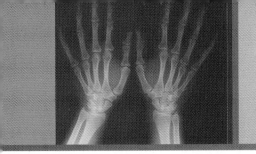

CHAPTER 29

Thoracic Outlet Compression Syndrome

Karen Johnston Jones

Peripheral nerve compression in the upper extremity keeps hand surgeons busy. Fortunately, however, carpal and cubital tunnel syndromes are relatively simple to diagnose and treat. Well-established techniques of diagnosis based on reproducible physical findings and common presenting history are learned early in our training. We use objective electrodiagnostic studies to confirm our clinical suspicions, refute them, or stage the disease. Thoracic outlet compression syndrome (TOCS), unfortunately, does not share any of the characteristics of the other compressive neuropathies. For most surgeons who operate on the upper extremity there are few disorders as difficult to diagnose or as frustrating to treat as TOCS. This is especially true in the instance of a patient with global upper extremity symptoms and a workers' compensation claim or lawsuit pending. In the overwhelming majority of these patients the diagnosis is one of exclusion and often is based on clinical diagnostic criteria alone.

Although we will see a number of patients in our clinics with vague upper extremity pain or symptoms, it is rare that hand surgeons have received comprehensive training in recognition and treatment of TOCS. It is well known that a large number of these patients will not be rendered pain free with either surgical or nonsurgical treatment, and most will never return to their "preinjury" level of function. There are some fortunate patients, however, who have access to experienced surgeons and therapists that are highly experienced in treatment of this disorder. Most upper extremity surgeons do not treat TOCS surgically without a vascular or thoracic surgeon present. In a recent e-mail survey of the American Society for Surgery of the Hand (ASSH) membership regarding TOCS, whereas 60% of respondents reported that they treat patients with TOCS, only 19% actually perform surgery for TOCS and only 10 of the 255 hand surgeons who responded perform more than 10 cases per year. Thirty-three percent of respondents operate with a vascular or thoracic surgeon present. This is appropriate when one considers that the complications of surgical treatment for this disorder can be life or limb threatening and represent risks that the typical fellowship-trained hand surgeon rarely encounters.[291]

Most surgeons do not like taking care of patients with TOCS, and the reasons are self-evident. The surgical treat-ment of TOCS is the most litigated single procedure in surgery.[33] Although much progress has been made in the past several decades to understand the pathophysiology of nerve compression and the complex interrelation between muscle imbalance, postural problems, and cumulative trauma, application of this knowledge to the treatment of patients with the clinical stigmata of TOCS still remains difficult. Because of ever-increasing concerns about cost containment, both from health maintenance organizations and employers, little is likely to ever be done in terms of preventive medicine for this condition. Perhaps this is why TOCS has been likened to reflex sympathetic dystrophy or low back pain.

HISTORY

Historically significant events in the early recognition of TOCS as a clinical entity are well detailed in Sanders and Haug's text *Thoracic Outlet Syndrome: A Common Sequela of Neck Injuries.*[233] From that text, three periods of history are notable (Table 29-1). The reader is referred to the text for more detailed discussion of the individual historical events. A second excellent source of historical information and state-of-the-art treatment is available as a monograph published as an edition of *Hand Clinics.*[290]

CLASSIFICATION

Wilbourn's Classification

There are two basic types of TOCS and four subtypes. The two basic types are vascular and neurogenic. The vascular type is further divided into arterial and venous subtypes, whereas the neurogenic type has been subdivided into "true" neurogenic and "disputed" neurogenic subtypes. The sub-classification and distinction of true versus disputed neurogenic TOCS are attributed to Wilbourn.[293]

In general, classification schemes for most pathologic conditions attempt to group and organize similar conditions, but this does not seem to be true when it comes to the four

Table 29-1

SIGNIFICANT EVENTS IN THE EARLY RECOGNITION OF THORACIC OUTLET COMPRESSION SYNDROME

Period I—The Cervical Rib: 1740-1927
Anatomic Descriptions

- Galen, Vesalius first recognition of cervical rib
- Hunald, 1740—First description of extra ribs
- Gruber, 1842—Classified cervical ribs into four groups

Embryology

- Todd, 1912—Descent of limb theory
- Jones, 1913—Elongation of vertebrae theory

Clinical Description

- Cooper, 1821—First description of vascular compression from cervical rib

Surgical Resection

- Coote, 1861—First resection of cervical rib for vascular TOCS

Physiology of Subclavian Aneurysms

Period II—The Cervical Rib Syndrome Without Cervical Ribs: 1920-1956
Congenital Ligaments and Bands

- Law, 1920—First description of ligaments of cervical rib to first rib, sternum

Scalenus Anticus Syndrome

- Adson and Coffey, 1927—Determined scalene was cause of rib symptoms or not
- Ochsner, Gage, and DeBakey, 1935—Trauma and muscle hypertrophy
- Naffziger and Grant, 1938—Coined term scalenus anticus syndrome

Costoclavicular Syndrome

- Eden, 1939—Described costoclavicular syndrome
- Falconer and Wendell, 1943—Coined term costoclavicular syndrome

Normal First Rib

- Bramwell, 1903—TOCS from a normal first rib
- Tom Murphy, 1910—First normal first rib excision for TOCS

- Stopford, 1919—10 Cases of normal first rib excision, noted traumatic cause

Abnormal or Rudimentary First Rib

- Keen, 1907—Symptoms from abnormal first rib
- Thorburn, 1908—First abnormal first rib excision for TOCS
- Brickner and Milch, 1925—Normal and abnormal first rib, same clinical picture

Middle Scalene Muscle Variations

- Stiles, 1929—Middle scalene can cause TOCS
- Kirgus and Reed, 1948—Recommended anterior and middle scalenotomy for TOCS patients

Pectoralis Minor Syndrome (Hyperabduction Syndrome)

- Wright, 1945—Reported subclavian artery compression from hyperabduction

Period III—Current Era of TOCS: 1956-Present
The Name: Thoracic Outlet Syndrome

- Peet, 1956—Term thoracic outlet syndrome coined
- Rob and Standeven, 1958—First use of thoracic outlet compression syndrome

Approaches to First Rib Resection

- Clagett, 1962—Posterior approach
- Roos, 1966—Transaxillary approach
- Gol, 1968—Infraclavicular approach

Objective Diagnostic Tests

- Adson, 1927—Adson maneuver
- Lang, 1962—Arteriography
- Winsor, 1966—Plethysmography
- Caldwell, 1971—Ulnar nerve conduction velocity
- Hongladarom, 1976—F-wave abnormalities
- Glover, 1981—Somatosensory evoked potentials

Histochemical Microscopy

- Machleder, 1986—First sampled scalenes and noted abnormalities
- Sanders, 1990—Fiber changes and scar tissue in anterior and middle scalenes

Modified from Sanders RJ, Haug CE: Thoracic Outlet Syndrome: A Common Sequela of Neck Injuries. Philadelphia, JB Lippincott, 1991, pp 12-17.

subtypes of TOCS. Whereas three of the four subtypes (arterial, venous, and "true" neurogenic) can be relatively easily diagnosed by physical examination and routine diagnostic imaging or testing, the fourth subtype ("disputed" neurogenic) is difficult to diagnose and even more difficult to treat. Perhaps this is why the fourth subclassification is referred to as the "disputed" subtype.

The "disputed" neurogenic type of TOCS alone accounts for all the controversy regarding TOCS. This subgroup of patients accounts for up to 97% of all patients diagnosed and treated for TOCS and is a unique entity for surgeons accustomed to objective diagnostic studies or imaging. In fact, there are no set diagnostic criteria or objective means by which one can make the diagnosis. Although several

experienced authors have their own established algorithms to determine which patients with normal diagnostic studies have TOCS, in general the routine patient with "disputed" type of TOCS remains a diagnostic dilemma for most upper extremity surgeons. In one survey of ASSH members it was reported that 19% of respondents did not believe that TOCS exists as a diagnosis.[291]

Patients with the other three subtypes (arterial, venous, and "true" neurogenic TOCS) present with obvious mechanical obstruction to blood flow or nerve conduction and rarely have secondary issues (workers' compensation issues, litigation) that cloud the diagnostic picture. Diagnosis is straightforward, and surgical treatment, when indicated, is relatively successful.

Arterial TOCS

Arterial TOCS is uncommon, accounting for only 1% to 2% of all cases of TOCS. It is further classified into major or minor subtypes. The major subtype is associated with osseous anomalies in proximity to the vertebral column and the rib cage and occasionally presents as a limb-threatening situation. The minor subtype is more indolent and can present as a history that suggests intermittent complete or partial arterial occlusion. Symptoms are induced by sports activities that place the upper extremity in the extended and hyperabducted position. Clavicular nonunion, malunion, or post-traumatic subluxation of the sternoclavicular joint has also been identified as an inciting cause.[40,70,93] The patho-anatomy of the minor type of arterial TOCS can usually be localized to the anatomic area of the pectoralis minor muscle. The clinical features of an acute or acute-on-chronic arterial TOCS are usually quite dramatic. The four classic "P's" of ischemia (pain, pallor, pulselessness, and paresthesias) are noted in cases of acute proximal thrombosis or thrombosis with embolism. More indolent cases have fingertip ulcerations, unilateral Raynaud's phenomenon, or claudication. A fully developed cervical rib has been reported in 50% of patients with arterial TOCS, whereas the remaining 50% are thought to have some other type of bony anomaly causing the compression (Fig. 29-1).[100,124]

Venous

Venous TOCS is slightly more common than the arterial type and represents 2% to 3% of all cases. These patients may have a sudden, effort-induced thrombosis (Paget-Schroetter syndrome) or, less commonly, a thrombosis that occurs at rest with the extremity in a compromised position for a prolonged time. There may be intermittent venous compression alone or intermittent compression that precedes a sudden event. With time, large venous collaterals about the shoulder, chest, or breast are present or develop (Fig. 29-2).

In acute thrombosis, pain, edema, and cyanosis are dramatic. This contrasts to patients who have a history of intermittent compression, in whom collateral venous drainage minimizes signs of distal swelling and cyanosis. In the latter group, however, fullness in the supraclavicular and infra-clavicular areas makes the clavicle hard to discern (see Fig. 29-2). Most venous TOCS is seen in muscular young males with symptoms that develop after vigorous exercise or physical exertion. Throwing athletes and swimmers have been acknowledged as "at risk" athletes owing to repetitive extremity positioning in postures that occlude the subclavian vein.[55,211]

"True" Neurogenic

"True" or classic neurogenic TOCS is also quite rare and occurs in 1:1 million patients.[72,294] These patients have objective physical evidence of chronic nerve compression such as hypothenar atrophy, decreased grip, and sensory deficits, usually in the C8/T1 distribution (Fig. 29-3). The pain and paresthesias seen in the other subtypes are also typical. In "true" neurogenic TOCS, as described by Wilbourn, there is always a bony anomaly causing the compression, such as a rudimentary or fully developed cervical rib (Fig. 29-4).

"Disputed" Neurogenic

The "disputed" neurogenic type of TOCS is the subtype most commonly encountered by a hand or upper extremity surgeon. These patients have a wide variety of upper extremity complaints and usually no objective findings on electrodiagnostic testing, Doppler imaging, pulse volume recordings, or radiographs. Vagueness and ambiguity of reported symptoms are typical. The consensus seems to be that physical complaints reproduced by provocative testing alone, in the absence of another explanation for the patient's complaints, are sufficient to justify a working diagnosis of TOCS.

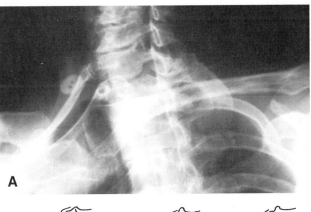

A

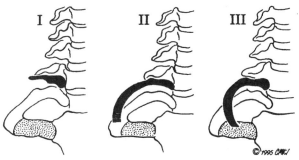

B

FIGURE 29-1. **A,** An oblique radiograph of the cervical spine of a patient with a complete right cervical rib and true TOCS *(button marks on the rib).* **B,** Three common variants of cervical ribs: I, rudimentary; II, fused with first thoracic rib; and III, fully developed. (From the Christine M. Kleinert Institute for Hand and Microsurgery, Inc., with permission.)

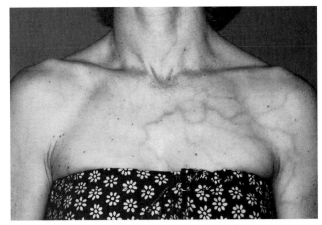

FIGURE 29-2. Photograph of venous collaterals in left anterior chest in a patient with subclavian thrombosis (Paget-Schroetter syndrome).

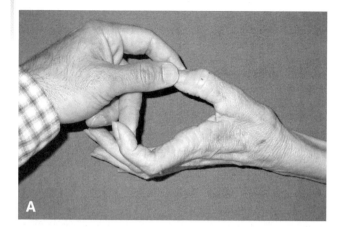

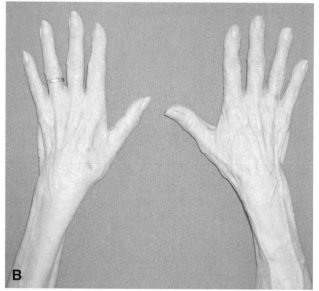

FIGURE 29-3. A and **B,** Photographs of a patient with "true" TOCS demonstrating intrinsic atrophy of the left hand.

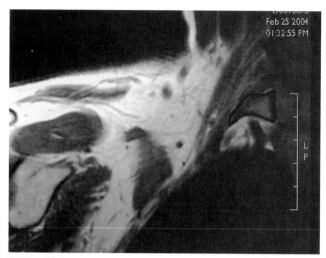

FIGURE 29-4. Coronal MRI of the patient pictured in Figure 29-3 demonstrating superior displacement of the lower trunk of the plexus by a cervical rib.

Roos' Classification

Roos has also classified TOCS according to the segment of brachial plexus involved.[217] Categories of compression include upper trunk compression, lower trunk compression, and combined compression. Symptoms attributable to the lower trunk and combined compression groups are found in 85% to 90% of all patients with TOCS. This classification scheme is less popular than that described by Wilbourn, presumably because most patients have only subjective complaints, so that objective localization is not possible.

EPIDEMIOLOGY

Although epidemiologic reports are few, the five most frequently cited predisposing factors for TOCS are sex, age, occupation, geographic location, and insurance status.

TOCS is diagnosed in women three and one-half to four times as often as in men and most frequently in adults of working age. Occupational risk factors for TOCS have been suggested. From 1987 to 1989, according to the Bureau of Labor Statistics, there was a 100% increase in the reported number of cases of cumulative trauma disorder. Diagnoses

reported in the shoulder region, including TOCS, ranked second only to lower back and neck complaints in frequency.[3,248] Awkward or static upper extremity positioning, including holding the arm in 45 degrees of abduction, has been found to increase the prevalence of symptoms of TOCS.[227] Hairdressers, painters, heavy construction workers, grocery clerks, switchboard operators, nurses, and secretaries have an increased incidence of TOCS when compared with the general public. These occupations have in common repetitive lifting and/or repetitive, uninterrupted arm movements with the hand at or above the shoulder level, and awkward or static posture of the extremity.[119,178,210,227,248]

In the United States, TOCS is being diagnosed with increasing frequency, especially in patients with workers' compensation or personal injury cases. Because the criteria to make a diagnosis of the disputed type of TOCS are so poorly defined, TOCS is being diagnosed with increasing frequency by practitioners with little training or knowledge of the condition in patients whose upper extremity pain is otherwise unexplained.

This phenomenon should be contrasted to the almost negligible rate of TOCS in countries where the entities of cumulative trauma disorder and repetitive stress injury are not recognized as legitimate work-related conditions, such as Australia and England. A study by Cherington and Cherington that was based on data accumulated from the 1989 Colorado Hospital Association records stands out in the literature.[32] In 1 year alone, 280 patients were discharged from the hospital with a principal diagnosis of TOCS. Of the 280, 174 patients had surgery. These data sharply contrast to records from the Mayo Clinic, where only 120 procedures were performed over a 32-year period.[32,294]

Other interesting findings in the Cherington and Cherington study include the fact that women outnumbered men by 3 to 1 for both the incidence and surgical treatment of TOCS. The typical patient for both diagnosis and surgical treatment of TOCS was female, aged 37, with private health insurance. Only one patient with Medicaid insurance underwent surgery, whereas 30% of the patients treated nonoperatively had Medicaid insurance.

In the Colorado study, TOCS was rarely diagnosed in patients without private insurance or workers' compensation, and the Medicaid group was the smallest. Similarly, in the same study, patients undergoing surgery were almost always insured or covered by workers' compensation.

The reported incidence of TOCS in the general population is 0.3% to 0.7%.[115] Others believe that the incidence should be more like 1% to 2%, thus implying that TOCS is underdiagnosed and undertreated.[8,219] From Cherington and Cherington's findings it is probably most accurate to say that the true incidence of the "disputed" neurogenic type of TOCS is unknown.

Anatomy

The anatomy of the thoracic outlet and brachial plexus is familiar to all surgeons who operate on the upper extremity, even those who do not operate on the brachial plexus. Whereas the neuroanatomy of the brachial plexus and the vascular components of the thoracic outlet are relatively constant, the bony and muscular anatomy is not. Fibrous or fascial bands, as well as developmental or acquired variations, are not uncommon, especially in the dynamic situation created with movement or positioning of the neck, thorax, and shoulder girdle. The upper extremity surgeon must listen carefully to the patient's history when trying to determine a cause for the patient's symptoms, thoroughly examine the patient with provocative testing, and then order and review appropriate imaging or testing before labeling the patient with a diagnosis or embarking on any type of treatment.

Despite attempts to rename the various anatomic territories as well as the clinical disorder, *thoracic outlet* remains the preferred term for the various sites of compression.[203] This anatomic corridor has been partitioned into three sections: the interscalene triangle, the costoclavicular triangle, and the subcoracoid or pectoralis minor space (Fig. 29-5).

The *interscalene triangle* is defined anteriorly by the anterior scalene, posteriorly by the middle scalene, and inferiorly by the first rib. The subclavian vein passes anterior to the anterior scalene and just inferior and lateral to the costocoracoid or costoclavicular ligament.[159] The subclavian artery passes with the plexus between the anterior and middle scalenes. The anterior scalene originates from the anterior tubercles of the transverse processes of C3 to C6. The middle scalene originates from the posterior tubercles of the transverse processes of C2 to C7.[193] A wide range of anatomic variation can predispose to pathology. The distance between the scalenes at the base of the triangle ranges from 0 to 2.2 cm with an average of 1.1 cm.[8,159,193] Actual crossing, or "intercostalization," of the insertions has been found in 15% of cadaver dissections.[260] This produces a "V"-shaped deformity at the base that can have a scissoring effect on the neural and vascular structures. Alternatively, a "U"-shaped formation can occur and create a sling effect that places pressure on the structures from below (Fig. 29-6).[8] The scalenus minimus arises from C6 to

C7 and inserts on the deep fascia between the subclavian artery and lower trunk, where it can produce a wedge effect on the latter.[8,157] The downward slope of the first rib, when increased (more commonly seen in women), may drive the neurovascular structures into the angle formed by the lateral edge of the anterior scalene tendon and the first rib.[193]

Cervical ribs, a commonly cited etiology for TOCS, have been identified in 0.5% to 0.6% of the population and are bilateral in 50% to 80% of those affected.[8] Cervical rib growth is developmentally suppressed by a full contribution of the lower spinal nerve root (T1) to the plexus; thus there is an association between cervical ribs and a prefixed plexus.[159] Many cervical ribs will be incomplete but have a taut fibrous band or "anlagen" connecting the bony tip to the first rib or deep fascia. Such a fibrous band represents only one of many types or locations of fibrous bands that represent the most common cause of nerve compression in TOCS patients.[270] Roos described nine different patterns of fibrous bands seen in clinical and cadaveric specimens, and three additional types of bands were reported by Poitevin a decade later (Fig. 29-7).[199,217,233,290] As one would expect, obvious bony compression of the nerve and vascular structures is an accepted, credible cause of TOCS, yet there is much dispute as to whether fascial or fibrous bands can or do cause TOCS. Part of the controversy is attributed to a cadaveric study in which only 10% of 98 cadaveric dissections had "normal" anatomy bilaterally (without bone, muscular, or fibrous/fascial bands).[101] The most frequently found bands were those seen to bowstring across the anterior concavity of the first rib, the "scalenus minimus" muscle band, and fascial attachments between the anterior and middle scalene muscle groups, crossing the nerve roots of the brachial plexus in either an oblique or perpendicular fashion.[101]

The volume of literature describing findings in the interscalene triangle should not obscure the importance of compression occurring at the two more distal regions. The costoclavicular space is bounded anteriorly by the clavicle, subclavius muscle, and costocoracoid ligament; posteromedially by the first rib; and posterolaterally by the superior border of the scapula (see Fig. 29-5).[92] Physiologic narrowing of this space with limb movement is enhanced by the mobility of joints at both ends of the space's boundaries.[193] A hypertrophied subclavius tendon insertion can apply compression specifically to the subclavian vein as in Paget-Schroetter syndrome.[8]

The subcoracoid space allows compression via three mechanisms. With arm abduction, the neurovascular bundle stretches around the coracoid, and external rotation of the scapula accentuates this pulley effect. Abduction also tenses the pectoralis minor tendon, further increasing compression (Fig. 29-8).[193]

The incidence of these findings may vary widely, but in one series of 200 consecutive transaxillary surgical approaches for TOCS, cervical ribs were encountered in 8.5%, scalenus minimus in 10%, subclavius tendon anomalies in 19.5%, and anomalies of scalene muscle development or insertion in 43%.[159,205] In another study of 250 cadavers (500 thoracic outlets) anatomic anomalies were noted in 46%. Histologic study of operative specimens has demonstrated an increased amount of connective tissue in the scalene muscles, thus supporting muscle imbalance or developmental abnormality as an inciting problem.[235] The

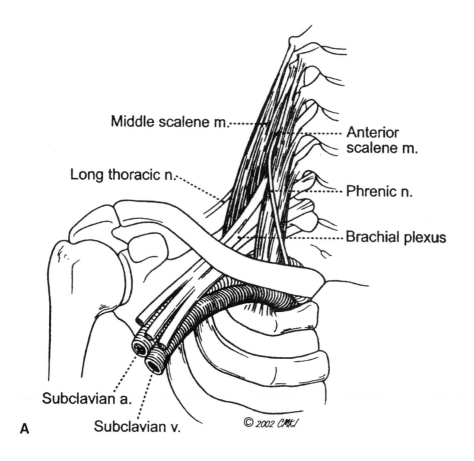

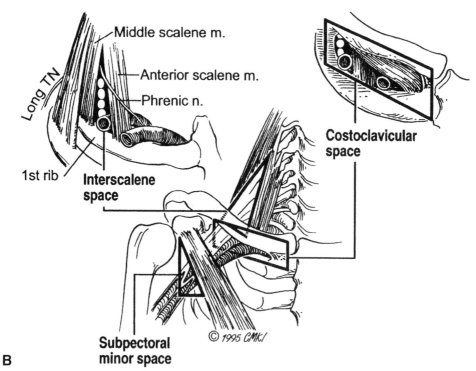

FIGURE 29-5. **A,** Line drawing of essential thoracic outlet anatomy demonstrating anatomic relationships between the plexus, bony anatomy, and musculature of the area (scalenes). **B,** The three anatomic triangles of the thoracic outlet. (From the Christine M. Kleinert Institute for Hand and Microsurgery, Inc., with permission.)

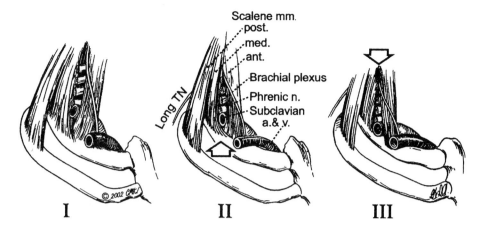

FIGURE 29-6. Common scalene muscle abnormalities: (I) "V" pattern where the anterior and middle scalene muscles cross over one another at the insertion to the first thoracic rib. (II) "U" pattern where the anterior and middle scalenes meet under the plexus forming a sling. (III) Proximal or superior compression of the plexus secondary to fascial bands, adhesions, or common muscle origin. (From the Christine M. Kleinert Institute for Hand and Microsurgery, Inc, with permission.)

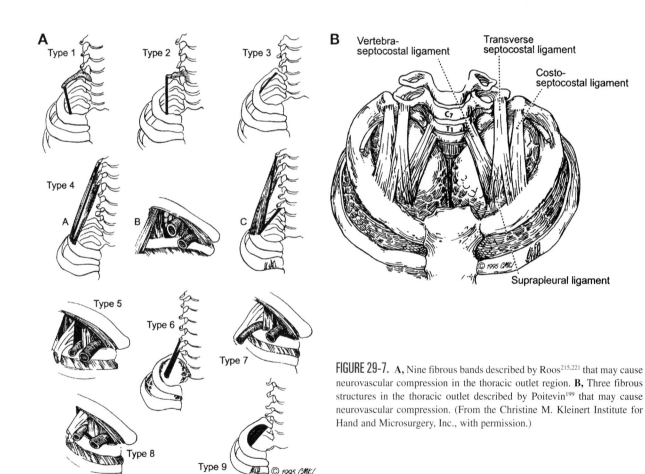

FIGURE 29-7. **A,** Nine fibrous bands described by Roos[215,221] that may cause neurovascular compression in the thoracic outlet region. **B,** Three fibrous structures in the thoracic outlet described by Poitevin[199] that may cause neurovascular compression. (From the Christine M. Kleinert Institute for Hand and Microsurgery, Inc., with permission.)

influence of awkward posture, repetitive strain, muscle imbalance, and eccentric muscle contraction have been extensively studied, and objective effects on muscle strength, endurance, and decreased sarcomere length have been documented.[6,64,67-69,90,179-181,224] It should be reemphasized that the presence of these abnormalities must be correlated with an individual's growth and development, body habitus, and patterns of limb usage to define the particular pathoanatomy.

CLINICAL FINDINGS

Because most symptomatic patients would be classified as the "disputed" neurogenic type, the diagnosis of TOCS is usually made by physical examination and provocative maneuvers. There is no substitute for experience in evaluating these patients. Although clinical symptoms are highly variable, there are certain commonalities that deserve description.

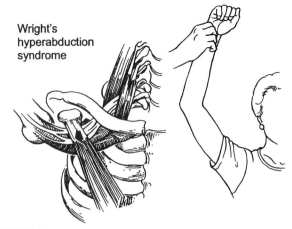

Wright's
hyperabduction
syndrome

FIGURE 29-8. Depiction of clinical and anatomic compression and stretch of the plexus with hyperabduction and external rotation of the upper extremity. (From the Christine M. Kleinert Institute for Hand and Microsurgery, Inc., with permission.)

The most commonly reported complaints are chronic pain of insidious onset involving the shoulder girdle, neck, and upper back in association with paresthesias into the upper extremity. Paresthesias are present in up to 95% of patients with TOCS and are the most common initial complaint.[283] Although the paresthesias usually involve the inside of the arm (ring and small finger), paresthesias involving the median nerve distribution or even the entire hand or arm are not uncommon. A patient's description of pain may be dull, nagging, and/or throbbing. Easy fatigability of the extremity when used in a provocative position is typical. As in carpal tunnel syndrome, symptoms while driving and grooming are common. Nocturnal complaints are frequent but different from those associated with carpal tunnel syndrome.[256] Some patients require narcotics, tricyclic antidepressants, neurotropics, or benzodiazepines to sleep. The clinician should exercise considerable caution when prescribing these medications so as to avoid drug dependence.

An association between distal nerve compression and TOCS, the so-called double crush phenomenon, has been made.[132,137,149,165,175,270,272] Although the *concept* of the double crush phenomenon was first introduced by Lishman and Russell in 1961,[132] the *clinical syndrome* of double crush was not introduced until 1973, when it was described by Upton and McComas.[272] The theory is that proximal nerve compression with resultant mild physiologic changes, while insufficient to cause clinical symptoms, may make the nerve more susceptible to a more distal peripheral entrapment.

Although the idea and theory of the "double" or even "multiple" crush syndrome[149] are accepted by many prominent peripheral nerve surgeons,[118,149,175,176,272,301,306] others strongly debate its existence.[13,26] Advocates of the "double crush" theory have described carpal tunnel syndrome in 21% to 45% of patients with TOCS; cubital tunnel syndrome occurring in up 10%; and, more rarely, radial tunnel syndrome, pronator syndrome, and cervical radiculopathy.[45,135,149,175,176,300,301,306,307] Critics believe that these "associations" are not actually separate areas of pathology but rather misdiagnoses. Carroll and Hurst[26] were the first to publish a large patient series with variable symptoms that they attributed to nerve compression at only one site. Although in their series patients did have multiple areas of surgery, in-depth review of the patients' symptoms revealed that relief was obtained by one procedure only in each instance. The authors emphasize the difficulty of diagnosing carpal tunnel syndrome and differentiating it from TOCS in patients with a primary complaint of shoulder pain. They also emphasize the importance of diagnosing and treating distal compression neuropathies in patients suspected of having TOCS. These distal sites of compression are typically more simple and economical to treat with little risk of morbidity to the patient.[156] Others characterize TOCS as a great mimicker and cite patients in whom the diagnosis of TOCS is delayed because of multiple prior surgeries on distal nerves without relief.[26,200] A more thorough discussion of the "double crush phenomena" is presented in the section on controversies later in this chapter.

Vague vascular complaints are very common in the "disputed" neurogenic type, including a sense of swelling and differential coolness of the hand, with a blue or purple discoloration. More variable complaints include headaches, vertigo, memory loss, syncope, chest pain "pseudoangina," conjunctival swelling, and facial pain or numbness.*

Psychological issues can be secondary to chronic pain and the stress of being examined and treated by multiple practitioners, undergoing multiple tests without a definitive diagnosis, and unremitting symptoms.[95,96,141,261] Depression, anger, and frustration, especially when dealing with medical personnel, become more prevalent the longer the symptoms persist. For this reason, the concept of multispecialty treatment, including psychological testing and therapy is very important in dealing with these patients. I have had several patients initially resistant to such intervention who only later were able to deal with their discomfort and anger and participate in rehabilitation and life-style modification after intensive psychotherapy.

PHYSICAL EXAMINATION

As in most conditions, a thorough physical examination with the patient in a gown and all concealing or constricting clothing, jewelry, or hair out of the way is essential. Because the history tends to be nonspecific and the clinical diagnosis in 97% of patients is made by physical examination alone, the initial patient evaluation tends to be time consuming. A pain questionnaire is essential and helps the patient focus on his or her symptoms. There are many unspoken issues that can be gleaned from analysis of a patient's written response to a pain questionnaire and an anatomic pain diagram (Fig. 29-9). One must carefully look for other possible causes of the patient's complaints, as well as for stigmata of TOCS.

The general appearance of the patient both standing and sitting should be noted. Does the patient slouch with the head in a forward position? Is the female patient particularly large breasted? Are there thick grooves in the shoulder from an "industrial-strength" brassiere? Is the neck held to one

---

*See references 8, 18, 47, 119, 151, 152, 154, 161, 186, 189, 193, and 218.

Appendix D
Pain Questionnaire: Pain Rating Scale

PREOPERATIVE ASSESSMENT OF PATIENTS WITH HAND PAIN

NAME: _____ HISTORY # _____ DATE: _____

A. Pain Descriptors

Is your pain like: (circle as many as you wish)

BURNING	THROBBING	ACHING	STABBING	TINGLING	DULL
TWISTING	CRAMPING	CUTTING	SHOOTING	NUMBING	VAGUE
STINGING	SQUEEZING	PULLING	SMARTING	PRESSURE	COLDNESS
INDESCRIBABLE		OTHER: _____			

How is your pain now? (mark on any part of the line below)

No
Pain |—————————————————————————| Severe
Pain

How is your mood now? (Mark on any part of the line below)

Worse
Mood |—————————————————————————| Best
Mood

B. Body Diagram

Where is your pain? (Please indicate on the diagram, may use color pen)

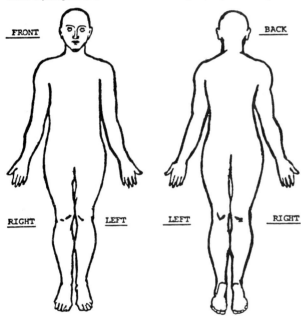

FRONT   BACK

RIGHT   LEFT   LEFT   RIGHT

FIGURE 29-9. Example of pain question-naire. (From MacKinnon SE, Dellon AL: Surgery of the Peripheral Nerve. New York, Thieme Medical Publishers, 1988, with permission.)

side? Is one shoulder drooping? These are very important clues regarding muscle imbalance (Fig. 29-10). The skin and contour of the anterior and posterior chest wall should be inspected. Masses, fullness in the supraclavicular and infraclavicular area, and venous engorgement or collaterals are noted (see Fig. 29-2). The tone and bulk of the muscles of the neck, upper back, shoulder, arm, forearm, and hand are inspected by palpation and against resistance. Circumferential measurements of the arm and forearm at designated levels above and below the antecubital fossae are recorded comparing the symptomatic and asymptomatic side. Unilateral swelling or atrophy identified in this fashion indicates chronicity. Sensory abnormalities in dermatomal distribution and by moving and static two-point discrimination and Semmes-Weinstein monofilaments are noted. Reflexes are evaluated. Areas of tenderness from the neck to the fingertips are observed, with special attention paid to the scalenes, clavicular area, and brachial plexus.

Before provocative testing for TOCS is performed, provocative maneuvers for distal sites of compression should be conducted (Table 29-2). This practice has evolved from the observation that frequently once provocative TOCS testing is conducted, the patient complains of symptoms with just about every maneuver from that point forward during the examination. Start distal and work proximal. Look for carpal tunnel syndrome, tendinitis, cubital tunnel syndrome, rotator cuff problems, and cervical radiculopathy before testing for TOCS.

Provocative Tests for Thoracic Outlet Compression Syndrome

There are several standard provocative maneuvers. In general, the patient's symptoms must be reproduced and/or the radial pulse diminished or obliterated for a test to be considered positive.

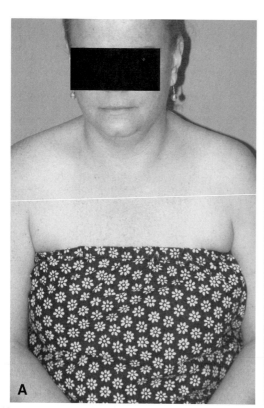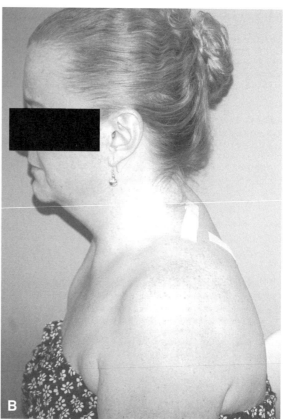

FIGURE 29-10. Frontal (**A**) and lateral (**B**) views demonstrating common posture in a patient with TOCS: neck flexed forward, shoulders forward and internally rotated, clavicle not visible. This patient had botulinum chemodenervation injections for pain control (bandaids).

Table 29-2
PROVOCATIVE TESTS AND RECOMMENDED MANAGEMENT FOR DISTAL NERVE ENTRAPMENT SYNDROMES

Nerve	Entrapment Site	Provocative Test	Management
Median nerve	Carpal tunnel	Pressure proximal to carpal tunnel Phalen's test Reverse Phalen's test (hyperextension of the wrist)	Night splint wrist in neutral
	Proximal forearm	Pressure over proximal forearm in region of pronator teres Resisted elbow flexion, pronation, and long finger flexion	Stretch pronator teres Rest periods in supination
Ulnar nerve	Guyon's canal Cubital tunnel	Pressure proximal to Guyon's canal Elbow flexion and pressure proximal to cubital tunnel	Night splint wrist in neutral Elbow pad Education to decrease direct pressure on nerve and avoid elbow flexion
Radial nerve	Forearm	Pressure over junction of brachioradialis/extensor carpi radialis tendon	Positioning in supination and avoidance of repetitive pronation and supination activities
Brachial plexus	Supraclavicular and infraclavicular	Arm elevation above head Pressure over brachial plexus in interscalene region	Avoid arm-elevated positions Postural correction Stretch shortened muscles and strengthen weakened scapular stabilizers

From Mackinnon SE, Novak CB: Evaluation of the patient with thoracic outlet syndrome. Semin Thorac Cardiovasc Surg 8:190-200, 1996.

Adson's Test

Also known as the scalene test, Adson and Coffey first described this test in 1927, and it has been used in patient evaluation ever since. With the arm at the side, the patient hyperextends the neck, turns the face *toward* the affected side, and inhales deeply (Fig. 29-11).[2] Some authors believe that this test is more valuable if the patient turns the head away from the affected side.[100]

The Halstead Maneuver

This test is more commonly known as the costoclavicular test or the military brace test. With both arms at the side, the patient moves the shoulders downward and backward with the chest protruding to draw the clavicle closer to the first rib, thus narrowing the thoracic outlet (Fig. 29-12).[256] The costoclavicular compression test is easily performed after the Halstead test by applying downward compression of the clavicle with longitudinal traction on the affected extremity.

Wright's Hyperabduction Maneuver

In this elevated arm test, the arm is externally rotated and abducted 180 degrees and the patient inhales deeply. This maneuver was originally described with the elbow flexed 90 degrees, but MacKinnon and others[141,152] have modified it so that the elbow is only slightly flexed to maintain external

rotation. By doing so, provocation of cubital tunnel syndrome symptoms is minimized. Although Wright originally described this test as positive only if the pulse was diminished or obliterated, in general most clinicians consider the test significant if it reproduces clinical symptoms at or before 1 minute of testing (Fig. 29-13).

Roos' Test

Roos' test is also called the 90-degree abduction external rotation test, or stick-up test. The patient holds the arm(s) in the abducted, externally rotated position and pumps the hands open and closed quickly and repetitively for 3 minutes. A positive test requires reproduction of symptoms or rapid fatigue of the extremity (Fig. 29-14). Some clinicians believe that patients with positional nerve compression will tolerate this position for 1 minute or less. This maneuver, also referred to as the elevated arm stress test (EAST) test is thought by many to be the most sensitive and reproducible provocative maneuver in the patient with TOCS.[216,220]

Cervical Rotation Lateral Flexion Test

A more recent addition to the standard four tests just presented, the cervical rotation lateral flexion test has been found to be reproducible between different examiners.[128]

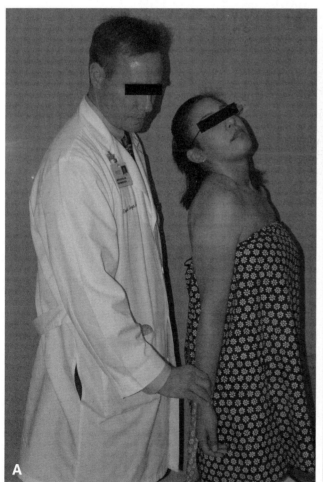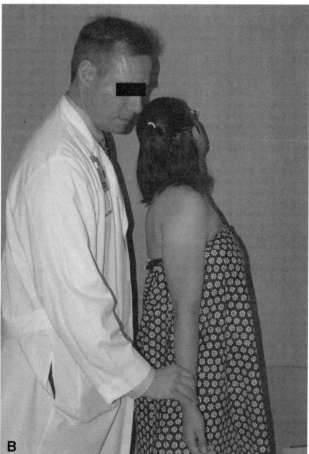

FIGURE 29-11. Demonstration of Adson's maneuver. With both arms at the side, the patient turns her head toward (**A**) the symptomatic extremity, while inhaling deeply (inflating the lung). Diminution or obliteration of a radial pulse is considered a positive test. The maneuver may also be performed turning the head to the opposite side (**B**), which stretches and tighten the scalenes.

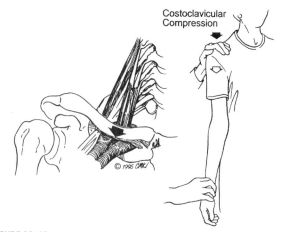

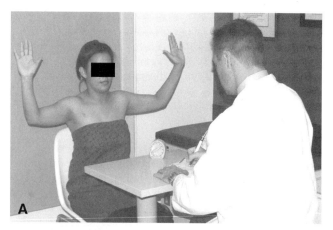

FIGURE 29-12. Depiction of the costoclavicular compression test (Halstead maneuver with compression of the clavicle). (From the Christine M. Kleinert Institute for Hand and Microsurgery, Inc., with permission.)

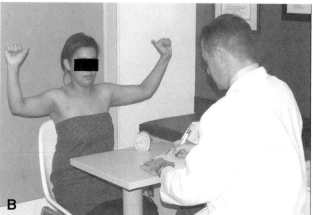

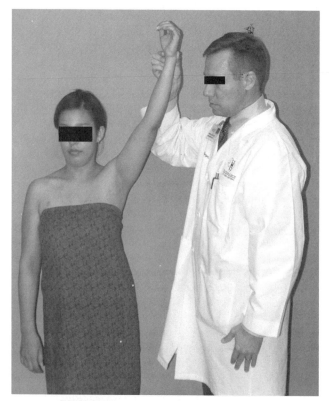

FIGURE 29-13. Wright's hyperabduction maneuver.

FIGURE 29-14. **A** and **B,** Demonstration of Roos' test with the patient making a tight fist and then relaxing repetitively for 3 minutes. The arm should be elevated to the shoulder level and the elbow should be slightly more extended than in this photograph to eliminate conflicting ulnar nerve compression at the elbow.

Office Doppler Examination

As a final office-based diagnostic test, a pencil Doppler probe can be used to listen to the signals over the subclavian, axillary, and brachial artery and vein. Small recorders that connect to the pencil Doppler are also available as a way of quantifying differences in Doppler signals and generate pulse volume (waveform) recordings. Bruits, differences in pitch, or significant diminution or obliteration of signal with provocative maneuvers should be noted (Fig. 29-16). I recommend evaluation of the patient in the sitting position at rest first, listening both above and below the clavicle before testing the patient standing and in different positions that might provoke findings.

Scalene Injection

Although some physicians advocate diagnostic injection of the scalene(s)[235] with lidocaine during one of the initial encounters, this technique is not universally practiced. Lidocaine injection alone is thought by most to be too nonspecific and variable in terms of technique and interpretation to be conclusive. Scalene injection with a long-acting anesthetic and corticosteroid has also been advocated for the patient with palpable spasm of the scalenes as an adjuvant to physical therapy. More recent clinical reports

The test evaluates the patient for subluxation of the first rib, which has been shown to limit cervical rotation combined with lateral flexion.[130] The test begins with the patient's neck in neutral position. The neck is maximally rotated *away from* the affected side and then flexed forward as far as possible so that the ear moves toward the chest. The test is considered positive if there is a bony block to lateral flexion and asymmetry in comparison to the "normal" side. Physical findings may also be reproduced as the subluxated rib irritates the C8 and T1 nerve roots (Fig. 29-15).

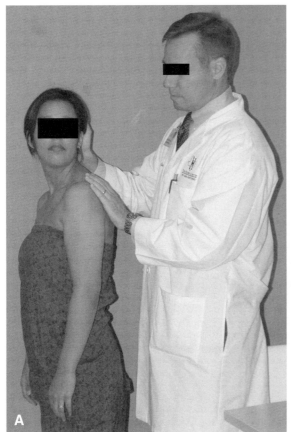
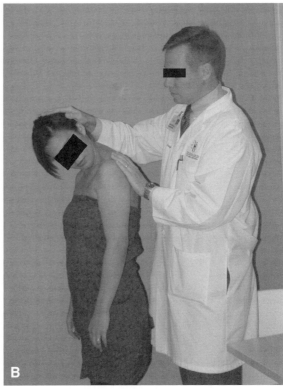

FIGURE 29-15. **A** and **B,** Demonstration of the cervical rotation lateral flexion test.

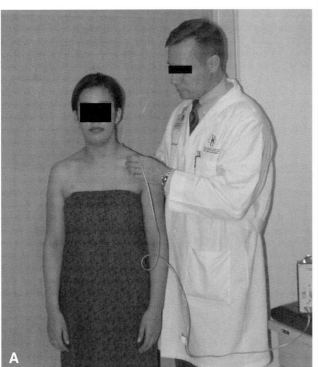
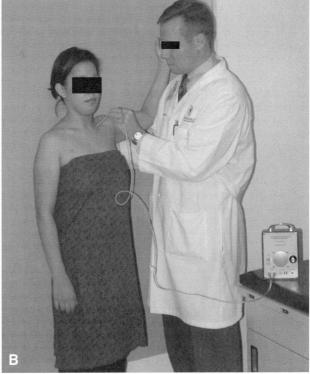

FIGURE 29-16. Demonstration of use of the pencil Doppler probe to evaluate subclavian blood flow. A, Baseline examination. **B,** Provocative arm positioning. The probe is employed above and below the clavicle.

indicate that botulinum toxin injections provide improved relief of painful muscle co-contraction for up to 3 months.[98] Microscopic analysis of operative specimens from the involved scalene muscle(s) has demonstrated pathology at the cellular level in the afflicted scalene muscle. The use of botulinum toxin injections in patients with muscle rigidity due to co-contraction is becoming more popular with a high degree of patient satisfaction. Because of cost, however, many insurers will not authorize this treatment. The best results in my practice have been with patients with symptoms of less than 6 months' duration, when performed as a series of two or three injections spaced several months apart and when combined with an immediate postinjection stretching program.

The real challenge comes in interpretation of the clinical findings. Although the clinical tests are the best we have, there remains the question of the tests' accuracy in diagnosis of the condition. A study by Warrens and Heaton[289] was performed to evaluate the prevalence of positive provocative testing in a random series of 64 volunteers. Adson's test, Wright's test, the Halstead maneuver, and supine hyperabduction were tested. In 58% of the volunteers at least one of the four tests was positive, whereas only 17% had any TOCS symptoms on a detailed questionnaire. Only 2% of the group had more than two tests positive. From this we can conclude that although a single positive test is probably meaningless, more than two positive responses may be important. Confirmatory clinical maneuvers, when combined with the history, and lack of findings on other elements of the physical examination, may lead the examiner to a working diagnosis of TOCS.

DIAGNOSTIC STUDIES

Radiologic Evaluation

Radiographs of the cervical spine and chest should be part of the initial evaluation. Other extremity films may be warranted by results of the physical examination.

Invasive vascular testing is indicated only for those patients with physical evidence of acute vascular compromise. Otherwise, noninvasive testing using color duplex sonography and waveform analysis should be used initially. Color duplex sonography can visualize stenosis, thrombosis, or flow problems in the arterial and venous system.[287] It has been found to be 92% sensitive and 95% specific in the diagnosis of vascular compromise in patients with TOCS.[134] Photoplethysmography or pulse volume recordings can suggest arterial compression, which then can be followed by magnetic resonance angiography or arteriography if the clinical situation so warrants.[58]

Angiography remains the "gold standard" in the evaluation of arterial TOCS and provides the best visualization of arterial anatomy as well as the potential for therapeutic thrombolysis in the acute situation. Special attention should be given to evaluation of the bony structures in the thoracic outlet in any patient with suspected arterial compression, because these patients will universally have a bony anomaly as the cause of the compression. Clavicular nonunions and malunions have been implicated in arterial TOCS. If no anomaly is visible on plain radiographs, computed tomog-raphy (CT) should be performed. In a study by Bilbey and coworkers,[17] CT identified bony anomalies in 8 of 12 patients with TOCS and "normal" plain radiographs; CT identified impingement of the C7 transverse process on the scalene triangle or anteromedial aspect of the middle scalene muscle in those 8 patients. Helical CT angiography is perhaps the best test for the rare arterial TOCS.[156,207] In patients with "disputed" neurogenic TOCS, CT has been found to be of low yield and not recommended as part of the initial diagnostic evaluation.[152,188] CT is, however, very helpful in defining posterior rib remnants or regrowth of cervical or thoracic ribs in the "failed" or "recurrent" group of patients who have undergone surgical decompression (Fig. 29-17). For suspected venous compression or occlusion, although venous Doppler has a role, venography is the "gold standard" (Fig. 29-18). Venography with the extremity in provocative positions can be diagnostic in patients with intermittent and exercise-induced venous symptoms and normal baseline venograms.[1,146,166] The late phase of these studies may document a vast network of collaterals, which will support the diagnosis and illustrate chronicity.

Magnetic resonance imaging (MRI) of the brachial plexus has not been found to be beneficial in the routine evaluation of patients with "disputed" neurogenic TOCS. Multiple case reports describing MR techniques used to evaluate patients with TOCS have been published in the past decade.[37,61,192] Improvements in software and magnet technology have helped our ability to identify pathologic anatomy. Although the sensitivity of MRI is 79% in terms of detecting "distortions" of the brachial plexus from mass lesions (tumors, aneurysms), the false-positive rate is 10% and the studies were not specific in terms of determining the cause or exact site of the distortion.[192] MR angiography has also been described in isolated case reports[61,191] and may, at some point, replace standard angiography in the evaluation of patients with suspected arterial compression. Techniques have not been standardized, and availability is not widespread. MRI of the cervical spine and cervicothoracic junction has yielded diagnoses of syringomyelia and multiple sclerosis as well as cervical disk disease. A clinical index of suspicion should guide the surgeon when imaging studies beyond standard radiographs are necessary.

Thermography[254] has been described as a diagnostic tool in patients with nonspecific upper extremity pain, but in itself thermography is a very nonspecific test that most clinicians do not know how to interpret. Neurography[259] has also been described for the evaluation of neurogenic TOCS, but it is an invasive technique that has not gained wide acceptance.

Electrodiagnostic Evaluation

Although the typical patient with "disputed" neurogenic TOCS has normal electrodiagnostic studies,[110,286] these studies are still recommended as part of the initial work-up. The consensus is that these patients may have a distal nerve compression syndrome such as carpal tunnel or cubital tunnel syndrome as a primary diagnosis or may have a "double crush" syndrome. Treatment of the distal compression may alleviate some of the complaints or at least make the remaining symptoms manageable by nonoperative means.

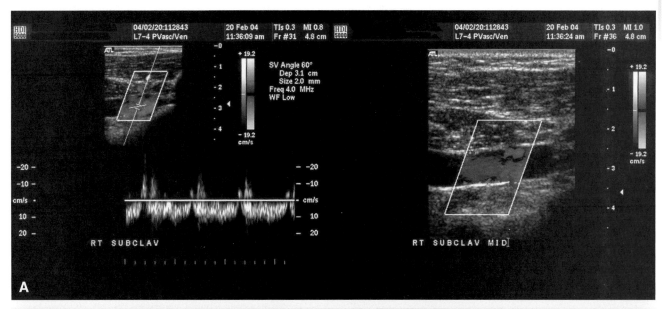

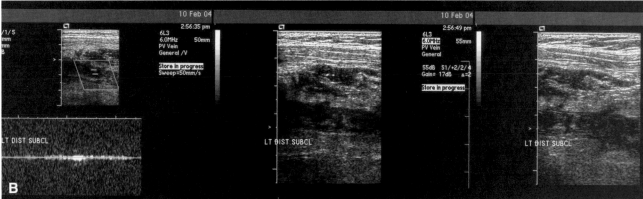

FIGURE 29-17. Color duplex sonography evaluation of two patients with Paget-Schroetter syndrome demonstrating (**A**) a patent subclavian vein after first rib removal and (**B**) a patient with thrombosis of the subclavian vein. Note the pulse volume recording *(lower left)* in both cases.

Whereas some authors advocate performing somatosensory evoked potentials (SEPs) on all patients with suspected TOCS,[142,148] others disagree.[110,257,285,286,312] Machleder and associates[142,148] have correlated an improvement in SEP with clinical improvement after transaxillary first rib resection. Other reports are more subjective. In one study testing of the conduction velocity of the C8 nerve root from its origin to the supraclavicular fossa[196] in all patients was discussed. A conduction time greater than 1.3 msec was found in all patients with clinical evidence of TOCS. It is fair to conclude that there is no consensus in the literature on whether SEP testing is necessary or helpful.

Whereas in patients with "true" neurogenic TOCS, no reproducible sequence of electrodiagnostic abnormalities is described, a few recent reports deserve mention. A study by Passero and colleagues[195] reported on 30 patients with "true" neurogenic TOCS as determined by bony anomalies in the thoracic outlet and consistent physical findings, all of whom underwent extensive electrodiagnostic testing. They found that electromyographic (EMG) abnormalities were the first changes to be seen, followed by changes in F waves and SEPs. Nerve conduction velocity changes were only seen late in patients with long-standing anomalies and severe muscle atrophy. The "classic" electrodiagnostic picture of chronic partial denervation of the hand, reduced amplitude/prolongation of the ulnar SEP latency, delay in F-wave latency, and changes in median nerve motor action potential (MAP) and ulnar nerve sensory nerve action potential (SNAP) is only seen very late. EMG evidence of chronic denervation of the intrinsic muscles of the hand was found in all patients with obvious neurologic findings clinically, but also in 23% of patients with only subjective symptoms.

A report by Smith and Trojaborg[246] found similar trends. In 10 patients with cervical ribs or other bony anomalies and obvious clinical evidence of "true" neurogenic TOCS, abnormalities on EMGs documenting chronic partial denervation and an abnormal SNAP in the fifth digit after stimulation at the wrist were the most common findings and occurred in 80%. Despite the abnormal SNAP distally in the small finger, the median and ulnar SNAP and MAP were normal in the patients tested in this study.

Another report, by Nishida and associates,[184] described four patients with known cervical ribs who also underwent extensive testing. The medial antebrachial cutaneous (MABC) nerve amplitude was also tested and found to be the most sensitive evidence of TOCS in their small series. It was found to be reduced to 64% to 100% as compared with

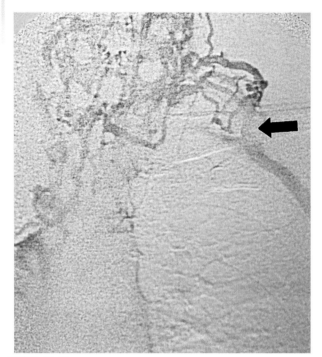

FIGURE 29-18. Venography of a patient with acute thrombosis of the subclavian and internal jugular *(arrow)*. Note the vast network of collateral veins, an indicator of long-standing compression.

the asymptomatic side. This compared with a maximum of 32% side-to-side difference in normal volunteers. Although all four patients had abnormalities in MABC amplitude, only one patient had EMG abnormalities.

From these studies one may conclude that abnormalities in MABC amplitude or distal SNAP from the wrist to the digits in patients with lower trunk compression may be useful early findings in "true" neurogenic TOCS. EMG findings in the intrinsic muscles of the hand may be the earliest findings in these patients. Extensive testing and EMGs should be performed as part of the electrodiagnostic profile in the rare patient with "true" neurogenic TOCS.

In a patient who has what appears to be "disputed" neurogenic TOCS, routine electrodiagnostic testing, including EMGs but not specifically SEP, MABC amplitude, C8 testing, or distal SNAPs, still remains the standard of care. Further testing may be conducted if routine screening is revealing.

TREATMENT

Nonoperative Treatment

There is universal agreement in the literature that nonoperative treatment is the first line of treatment for all patients with "disputed" neurogenic TOCS. As noted previously, the disputed neurogenic group of patients represents up to 97% of all patients in whom TOCS is diagnosed and, therefore, nearly all of the patients who will be referred to an upper extremity surgeon for evaluation and treatment.

Much has been written on the necessary physical assessment of these patients at the outset of the therapy program.[31,105,125,174,185,255,288] Increased risk factors for failure of nonoperative treatment include obesity (based on body mass index [BMI]),[280] poor cardiovascular condition, and failure to institute a multimodality treatment program that addresses poor posture and exacerbating activities both at work and at home.[185] These patients must commit themselves to significant life style and workplace modifications to have any hope of a good outcome. Nutritional counseling, diet, and exercise programs must start simultaneously with stage I treatment (below).

Although some authors have reported excellent results after inpatient therapy programs,[125] the cost of such programs makes them prohibitive in most instances. Whether inpatient or outpatient, most therapy programs consist of a four-staged program. The first goal is to relieve pain and control progression of symptoms. Stage 1 focuses on identification and treatment of myofascial trigger points, local areas of spasm, tendinitis, and/or bursitis. The use of muscle relaxants, mild narcotics, antidepressants, anti-inflammatories, or sleeping aids may be necessary. Some advocate the use of centrally acting "nerve" medication such as amitriptyline (Elavil), carbamazepine (Tegretol), or gabapentin (Neurontin). Most therapists advocate the use of moist heat and/or ice, transcutaneous electrical nerve stimulation (TENS), ultrasound, and other modalities at this stage, but Novak[185] argues that overuse of these modalities may encourage dependence on therapy. Trigger point injections, scalene muscle injection, botulinum toxin, and epidural corticosteroids can be beneficial in the appropriate clinical scenario.

Stage II is usually instituted concurrently and consists of using stretching, relaxation, breathing, and myofascial manipulation to restore normal mobility and a balanced posture to the cervical spine, shoulder girdle, and cervicothoracic region. Cardiovascular conditions and weight-loss programs are important to institute at this stage, and are continued throughout the program. Pathologic postures, such as the head-forward position, lead to decreased overall flexibility of the cervicothoracic unit and compensatory cervical lordosis, thoracic flexion, shoulder internal rotation, and scapular abduction. Such postures are thought to lead to tightening of the anterior muscle groups and compensatory elongation of the posterior muscles. This pathologic muscle imbalance has been cited by MacKinnon, Novak, and others* as being one of the key pathologic entities to identify and correct. Attention to lumbar lordosis, leg-length discrepancy, and other dysfunctional postures is necessary. Brachial plexus gliding[269] and peripheral nerve mobilization[24] may also be included at this stage.

Stage III consists of muscle strengthening, increasing endurance, and restoration of the patient to presymptomatic levels of function both at work and at home. The therapist must undertake this stage carefully, because too vigorous an exercise or aerobic conditioning program can exacerbate symptoms.[276] It is important to establish realistic goals and understand that all patients will not be rendered pain free.

If a patient graduates through the first three stages of treatment, stage IV consists of establishing a home program and returning the patient to the workplace. Analysis of the job site is frequently beneficial before return to work.

---

*See references 152, 154, 185, 187, 188, 197, 208, 209, 226, and 292.

CRITICAL POINTS: INITIAL PHYSICAL EXAMINATION, DIAGNOSIS, AND TREATMENT

INITIAL PHYSICAL EXAMINATION

- Initial physical examination, history, and counseling take at least 30 minutes.
- Patient must be undressed from the waist up (to search for atrophy, swelling, venous engorgement).

Sequence of Examination

- Observation
- Peripheral nerve examination first (include measurements for muscle atrophy)
- Cervical spine second
- TOCS examination last (symptom overlay)

Equipment Needed

- Pencil Doppler device (for vascular assessment including provocative testing)
- Reflex hammer
- Tape measure (to measure for girth, atrophy)
- Two-point discriminator (± Semmes-Weinstein monofilaments)
- Grip dynamometer
- Pinch gauge
- Stopwatch or wristwatch with a second hand for elevated arm stress test (EAST)

INITIAL DIAGNOSTIC EVALUATION

- Radiographs of cervical spine and other areas as indicated by history and physical examination
- Vascular symptoms and signs: venography (stress/abduction), arteriography, duplex ultrasonography
- Nerve tests with electromyograms as determined by clinical examination (motor or sensory deficits) including medial antebrachial cutaneous (MABC) nerve amplitude

INITIAL TREATMENT

Disputed and Early or Mild True Neurogenic TOCS

- Initiate physical therapy and postural and activity modification.
- Refer for psychological, social, and nutritional counseling as indicated.

Vascular

- Provide prompt surgical/thrombolytic treatment for acute arterial cases with first rib resection and vascular reconstruction (sympathectomy).
- Begin anticoagulation with subsequent first rib resection for nonurgent vascular symptoms (Paget-Schroetter syndrome, post-stenotic arterial dilatation).

Life-style changes and proper "work hygiene" consisting of taking breaks as necessary for stretching, breathing, and relaxation are important in the maintenance program. Necessary ingredients of the home exercise program include scalene stretching, cervical protraction and retraction, diaphragmatic exercises, pectoralis stretching, and shoulder circumduction exercises. The exercises are done 10 times each, 3 times per day.[89,197,245,288]

The use of custom-made scapular retraction harnesses has been advocated by some,[157] but the consensus is that orthotics cannot substitute for a staged therapy protocol and correction of postural and muscular imbalances. Dependence on orthotics and splints may weaken the same muscles that the therapy program is working to strengthen.

The results of nonoperative treatment are variable and hard to compare. This is not surprising since patients with the "disputed" type of TOCS do not have objective findings by which to standardize results of treatment. Reports of successful treatment range from 50% to 100%. Success is usually defined as avoidance of surgery, return to work, and satisfactory pain relief.[3,92,105,117,125,226,288]

Operative Treatment

Operative treatment of TOCS has evolved significantly in the past 70 years. Although Coote excised a cervical rib in 1860,[42] it was not until the next century that surgical management of TOCS became popular. In 1927, Adson and Coffey[2] described the diagnostic maneuver for scalenus anticus syndrome and recommended anterior scalenotomy as a means of operative treatment. In 1962, Clagett[35] documented a high failure rate with scalenotomy alone and advocated first rib resection via a posterior approach for patients with TOCS. The transaxillary approach to first rib resection was introduced by Roos in 1966.[214] In the 1980s, a combined transaxillary and supraclavicular approach was introduced as a means of resecting the first rib and releasing the scalenes.[201] Current approaches differ between surgeons and their subspecialty of surgery. Atasoy recommends transaxillary resection of the first rib followed by immediate transcervical anterior and middle scalenectomy. Others use this technique for the "failed" or "recurrent" TOCS patient. Isolated supraclavicular approach for anterior and middle scalenectomy without first rib resection has been advocated as well.[28,206,230] Although some surgeons prefer more limited procedures,[52] the most widely performed procedure for TOCS in 2004 includes (1) excision or release of anomalous anatomy, (2) resection of the first rib, (3) release or excision of the anterior and middle scalene muscles, and (4) neurolysis of the brachial plexus as indicated.

The two most popular surgical approaches are the transaxillary approach (Fig. 29-19) and the supraclavicular approach (Fig. 29-20). Because complications and benefits have been reported with both approaches, it seems that it is

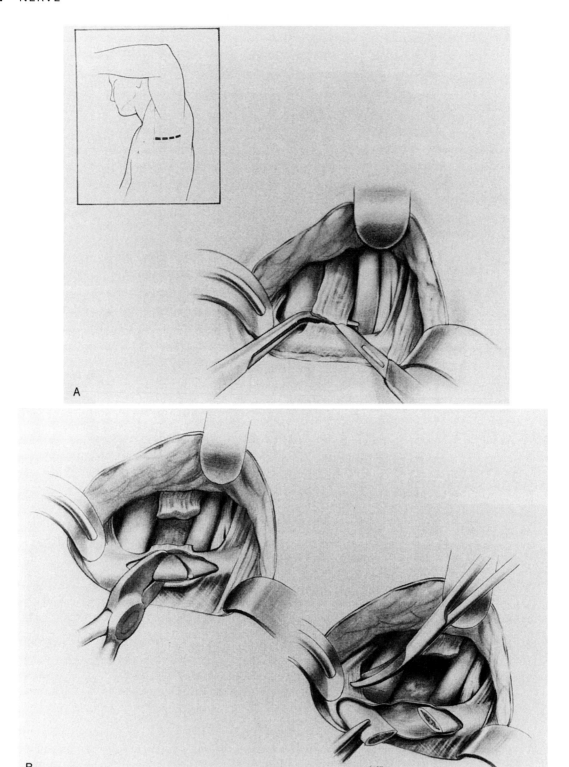

FIGURE 29-19. Operative technique for transaxillary first rib resection. **A,** The incision is transaxillary below the hairline and transverse between the pectoralis major muscle anteriorly and the latissimus dorsi muscle posteriorly. The incision is carried directly to the chest wall without angling up toward the first rib. When the chest wall is encountered, the dissection is carried superiorly to the first rib and the intercostobrachial nerve is identified as it exits between the first and second ribs. It is preserved by retracting it anteriorly or posteriorly. (Division produces 6 months to 1 year of paresthesias on the inner surface of the upper arm.) The first rib is dissected subperiosteally with a Shaw-Paulson periosteal elevator and the scalenus anticus muscle is identified. A right-angled clamp is placed behind the muscle while being careful to not injure the subclavian artery or vein. The scalenus anticus muscle is divided near its insertion on the first rib. (This avoids injury to the phrenic nerve, which courses away from the muscle at this level.) **B,** After dividing the scalenus anticus muscle, the first rib is dissected free subperiosteally and separated from the pleura. A triangular piece of the rib is removed in the avascular area. The vortex of the triangle is at the scalenus tubercle. The anterior part of the rib is removed by dividing the costoclavicular ligament and resecting the rib subperiosteally back to the costocartilage of the sternum. (From Urschel HC Jr: The transaxillary approach for treatment of thoracic outlet. Semin Thorac Cardiovasc Surg 8:214-220, 1996.)

Continued

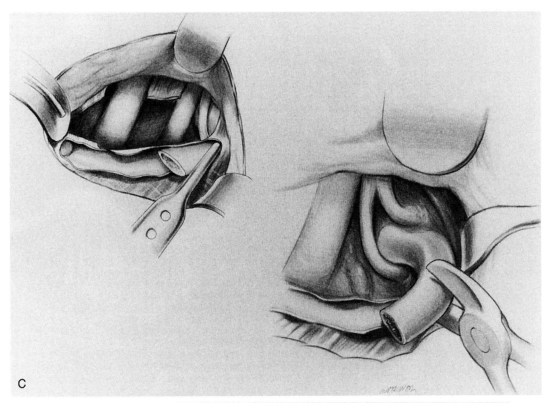

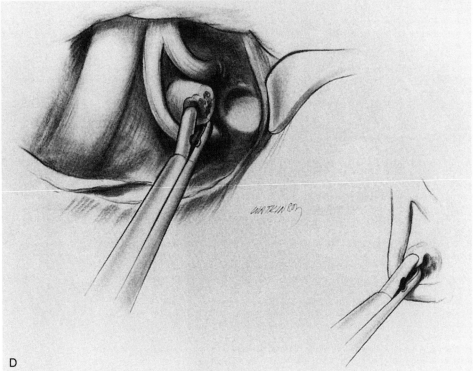

FIGURE 29-19—cont'd. C, The posterior part of the rib is dissected subperiosteally to the transverse process, where it is divided by a pair of rib shears. The rib may be resected posteriorly with an Urschel-Leskell reinforced rongeur. Care is taken to avoid injury to the C8 and T1 nerve roots as the scalenus medius muscle is dissected from the rib. **D,** After visualization of the transverse process articulation, the head and neck of the rib are removed with an Urschel reinforced pituitary rongeur. It is important to completely remove the head and neck of the rib to minimize regeneration. Care is taken to avoid injury to the T1 nerve root below or the C8 nerve root above. After complete removal of the first rib, neurolysis of the C7, C8, and T1 nerve roots as well as the middle and lower trunks of the brachial plexus is performed. A video-thoracoscope is used for this purpose because of its magnification and light. The scalenus medius and scalenus anticus muscles are resected up into the neck so that they will not reattach to Sibson's fascia or the pleura. Bands and adhesions are removed from the axillary-subclavian artery and axillary-subclavian vein so that they are completely free. Hemostasis is secured.

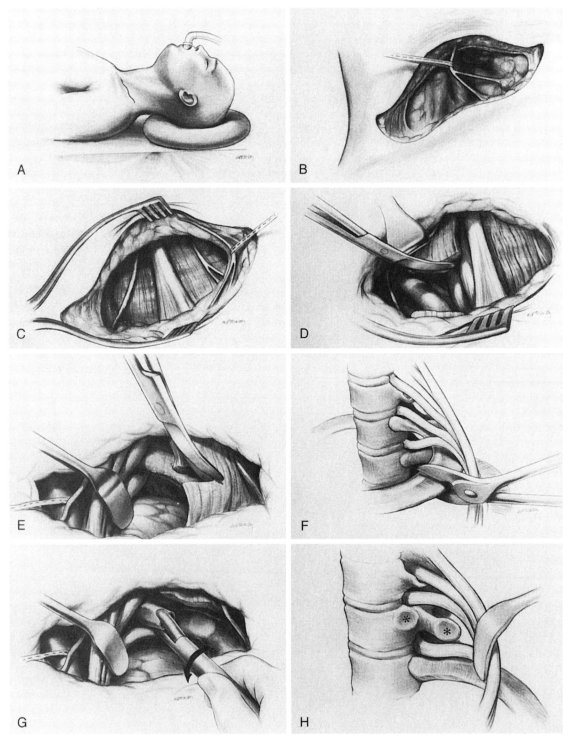

FIGURE 29-20. Operative technique for supraclavicular first rib resection and scalenectomy. **A,** The surgical incision is parallel to the clavicle. A slightly lazy "S" incision will be closed later in a subcuticular fashion for an optimum cosmetic result. **B,** The supraclavicular nerves are identified just below the platysma muscle and mobilized. A vessel loop facilitates retraction. **C,** The brachial plexus is noted in its position between the scalenus anticus and medius muscles. The phrenic nerve is seen coursing in a lateral-to-medial direction across the anterior surface of the scalenus anticus muscle. The supraclavicular nerves are being retracted. Also shown is the long thoracic nerve exiting from the posterior border of the scalenus medius. **D,** Division of the scalenus anticus insertion from the first rib. The subclavian artery will be directly behind the scalenus anticus muscle. **E,** The scalenus medius is divided from the first rib. **F,** The first rib is divided with a rib cutter. **G,** With rongeurs, the posterior aspect of the rib is removed with a twisting motion. **H,** The entire posterior portion of the first rib is removed so that there is no residual first rib left to produce new bone and subsequent recurrence of symptoms. The articular facets of the costovertebral and costotransverse joints are noted with *asterisks.* (From Mackinnon SE, Patterson GA: Thoracic outlet syndrome: Supraclavicular first rib resection and brachial plexus decompression. *In* Neurosurgical Operative Atlas. Baltimore, Williams & Wilkins, 1993, vol 3.)

CRITICAL POINTS: OPERATIVE INTERVENTION

INDICATIONS

- True neurogenic TOCS with intrinsic wasting
- Vascular symptoms (compression of the subclavian artery or vein)
- "Disputed neurogenic" TOCS having failed an extensive course of physical therapy and appropriate treatment of distal sites of peripheral nerve compression

PREOPERATIVE EVALUATION

- Radiographs of the cervical spine (MRI of cervical spine if clinically indicated)
- Electrodiagnostic studies, with EMGs including MABC
- Venography, duplex ultrasonography, or arteriography for vascular symptoms

TECHNICAL POINTS

- Supraclavicular approach:
  - Preferred procedure for disputed neurogenic TOCS: scalenotomy only; cervical rib excision, if present; occasional first rib resection (pathological fracture).
  - True neurogenic, vascular: scalenotomy, excision of cervical and first rib, vascular reconstruction as indicated (by a vascular or cardiovascular surgeon) and sympathectomy
  - Brachial plexus neurolysis: reserve for revision surgery and possibly for post-traumatic cases due to scarring.
- Perform surgical dissection under 4.3× (or similar) loupe magnification.
- Place patient supine with a sandbag between the scapulae and neck in slight extension.
- Avoid long-acting paralytic agents to allow for intraoperative nerve stimulation.
- Make an incision 2 cm above and parallel to the clavicle.
- Mobilize and retract the supraclavicular nerves with vessel loop.
- Divide omohyoid, mobilize supraclavicular fat pad, and divide lateral portion of sternocleidomastoid muscle (repaired at closure).
- Identify scalenes and palpate brachial plexus.
- Identify phrenic nerve on the anterior scalene.
- Identify long thoracic nerve on or in middle scalene.
- Release anterior and middle scalene insertions; check and divide any fibrous bands associated with scalene insertions.
- Mobilize upper, middle, and lower trunks of the brachial plexus without neurolysis unless indicated (trauma, reoperation) to allow for retraction and first rib resection.
- Identify first rib (C8 above, T1 below) and any cervical ribs.
- Use rib cutter to divide first rib in area of best exposure (midportion).
- Remove entire first rib (posterior portion in pieces with ronguer).
- Confirm adequate resection by identifying articular cartilage from costotransverse and costovertebral joints.
- Remove any cervical ribs and prominent cervical transverse processes in pieces.
- Insert a small drain, maintain maximum lung inflation by anesthesiologist after closure, and place arm in sling.

PITFALLS

- Injury to the supraclavicular (cutaneous) nerves during exposure or surgery: recognize, resect nerve, perform neurolysis, and bury ends deep in innervated muscle.
- Pneumothorax: obtain chest radiograph in operating room after closure and lung inflation.
- Injury to phrenic or long thoracic nerve during exposure: perform direct repair. Diaphragmatic function is unlikely to recover owing to distance from level of injury and diaphragm.
- Brachial plexus injury: perform a direct repair, and consider distal nerve transfers.
- Vascular injury or bleeding: obtain a type and screen on all patients. Consider crossmatch for revision cases or vascular reconstruction.

POSTOPERATIVE CARE

- Procedure requires a 23-hour overnight stay.
- Drain is removed the morning after surgery.
- Active and gentle active-assisted range-of-motion neck and shoulder exercises are begun on day 3 postoperatively; start desensitization.
- Work toward full active range of motion by 2 to 3 weeks.
- Strengthening and more vigorous desensitization is done along with ultrasound and transcutaneous electrical nerve stimulation at 6 weeks as necessary.

RETURN TO ACTIVITIES

- Return to unrestricted activity is acceptable at 3 months as pain and strength allow.

a matter of personal preference. Surgical results are similar as long as the entire first rib is removed, the scalenes are divided, and any anomalies are adequately decompressed. Some advocate the transaxillary approach for safety because the brachial plexus and vessels are not manipulated. Injuries to the long thoracic and phrenic nerves from retraction have been recognized after the supraclavicular approach. Others advocate the supraclavicular approach, even though the plexus and vessels have to be retracted, because they believe that the posterior aspect of the first rib is poorly visualized in the transaxillary approach and access to the plexus is incomplete. A combined approach probably allows the safest, most thorough identification and removal of pathologic anatomy.

For patients with vascular TOCS and arterial compression, early or urgent decompression is favored through a combined approach, with removal of the offending bony anomaly and arterial reconstruction as necessary. In patients with venous compression or Paget-Schroetter syndrome, early thrombolysis followed by first rib resection is recommended. Once the area is decompressed, long-term anticoagulation is not thought to be necessary unless the patient has a hematologic predisposition for thrombosis. In patients with "true" neurogenic TOCS, the goals are to decompress the plexus by removing any bony or fibrous anomalies, release or remove the anterior and middle scalenes, and remove the first rib.

The real controversy revolves around the indications for surgery in the "disputed" neurogenic group of patients. In *Seminars in Thoracic and Cardiovascular Surgery* in 1996, the diversity of opinions among leaders in the field was obvious. Whereas Urschel[279] stated that it is "absolutely essential to have the objective reliability and reproducibility of ulnar and median nerve conduction velocities" to manage a patient with TOCS and severe pain, in the same issue, MacKinnon and Patterson disagreed. Their indications for surgery in this group of patients included failure of 3 months of supervised nonoperative management and patients with a double crush situation that have failed surgical management of the other entity.[153] More recently, other leaders in the field have adopted Urschel's approach.[33,282]

Although thoracic outlet surgery is usually performed by a vascular or thoracic surgeon, in some instances a combined surgical team is advantageous. MacKinnon and Patterson[110] advocate this approach. The peripheral nerve surgeon explores the brachial plexus, whereas the thoracic or vascular surgeon removes the first rib and performs whatever vascular intervention is necessary. The combined approach especially makes sense in a patient with recurrent symptoms because a peripheral nerve specialist is needed to neurolyse or mobilize the brachial plexus.[110]

Author's Preferred Treatment

Although few hand surgeons will participate in the surgical treatment of a patient with TOCS, all upper extremity surgeons will see and treat patients with this condition on a nonsurgical basis. Fortunately, most of these patients (with disputed neurogenic TOCS) will improve without surgery.

For those patients who fail nonoperative treatment, have true neurologic compression, or have vascular compromise, the hand/peripheral nerve surgeon should have an association with a vascular or cardiothoracic surgeon to provide appropriate surgical care. The literature supports a combined approach to the treatment of these patients. Because there are neurologic and vascular components to the approach and pathology, a two-surgeon/specialist approach is prudent in most cases. There are a few large centers in the United States and Europe where a large number of surgical procedures for TOCS are performed. In these centers, there are individual peripheral nerve surgeons and vascular surgeons with the experience and resources readily available to perform thoracic outlet surgery without a second specialist present. Before surgery, the patient is extensively counseled regarding the inherent potential risks and complications of the surgery, including injury to the brachial plexus, spinal cord, major vessels, and apex of the lung. Fully informed consent is imperative. There should be documentation about potential for transfusion, death, and irreversible neurologic injury.

For patients without vascular compromise, the supraclavicular approach to thoracic outlet decompression is preferred (Fig. 29-20). For cases with the disrupted neurogenic subtype, anterior and medial scalenectomy alone is performed; for all other patients, the first rib and any other bony abnormalities must also be excised. Surgery is performed under high-power loupe magnification with the patient in a supine position. A sandbag or roll between the medial border of the scapula and the spine facilitates exposure of the outlet. Long-acting paralytic agents should be avoided to allow for intraoperative nerve stimulation. The incision is made parallel and 2 cm above the clavicle. The platysma is divided and elevated with the skin flaps, which are widely mobilized to maximize exposure. Supraclavicular nerves are identified and retracted with vessel loops. The lateral border of the sternocleidomastoid and the external jugular vein are identified and retracted, and exposure can be facilitated by dividing the lateral border of the sternocleidomastoid muscle from the clavicle. Care must be taken at this stage to avoid injury to the underlying subclavian vein. The supraclavicular fat pad is mobilized and retracted laterally, and the omohyoid muscle is ligated and divided with stay sutures. The large transverse cervical artery and vein overlie C7, and may require ligation for full exposure. The plexus is identified between the anterior and middle scalenes, and the phrenic nerve mobilized with a vessel loop off the anterior surface of the anterior scalene. Careful inferior dissection is performed to release the anterior and middle scalenes, together with any anomalous fibrous bands, from the first rib. The three trunks of the brachial plexus will require gentle mobilization to complete the scalenectomy and expose the first rib. The first rib is subperiosteally exposed in its midportion, and a rib cutter is used to divide it. Careful subperiosteal dissection is carried out anteriorly and posteriorly to separate the first rib from the underlying pleura, and the anterior and posterior portions are resected with a rongeur. A cervical rib, as well as any prominent cervical transverse processes, must be removed piecemeal to complete the decompresson. Meticulous hemostasis is attained, and the wound closed over suction drains. The arm is placed in a sling, and the patient kept overnight for observation. A chest radiograph is important to rule out a pneumothorax. Active and active-assisted range of motion exercises are begun on day 3 and advanced to full mobility within three weeks of surgery.

A combined referral resource should be established for treatment failures. Because of the inherent risks involved when one operates around the cervical spine, brachial plexus, and cardiothoracic cage, the best situation would be to send the patient to a vascular or thoracic surgeon who is comfortable not only with the anatomic area but also with the management of complications inherent to surgery in this area, which include pneumothorax and injury to the great vessels and potentially to the thoracic duct. In this scenario, the upper extremity surgeon participates in the surgical treatment as an assistant, to mobilize and/or protect the brachial plexus and perform nerve repair in the unfortunate event of injury. For this reason, the surgical treatment of this condition, in general, is outside the realm of this text. The standard of care in most centers would place the surgical treatment of these patients in another specialties area.

Complications

Complications of nonoperative treatment are few and relatively minor, except in the rare case of a patient with "true" neurogenic TOCS or vascular TOCS who refuses surgical intervention and suffers from progression of the disease. Some patients report exacerbations of their symptoms from an inappropriate physical therapy regimen or too vigorous a strengthening program. In most instances, these flares of increased symptoms resolve. There is also a risk of drug dependency, severe depression, and/or other psychiatric disorders if care is not taken to manage the patient's chronic pain syndrome and associated psychosocial issues.

In contrast, the complications of surgical treatment for TOCS can be devastating. Complications related to surgery for TOCS were recognized as early as the late 1800s, as recorded by Keen in his 1907 review of the subject.[103] The first brachial plexus injury was recorded by de Quervain,[51] who performed one of the first cervical rib excisions in 1895 and described temporary hand numbness thereafter that was attributed to a traction injury. More significant brachial plexus injuries were recorded in 1899 by Gordon,[77] who had the first patient to have a temporary, but complete motor paralysis of the arm, and also in 1900 by Borchardt,[19] who noted complete arm paralysis and severe arm pain. By the time of Keen's article in 1907, brachial plexus injuries had been recognized in 17% of the first 42 cases of cervical rib surgery.[103]

It is interesting to note that few surgical complications were reported for the first two decades after the introduction of transaxillary first rib resection in 1966. There had been some 5000 operations performed in the United States by 1984,[66] but brachial plexus injuries were "purportedly nonexistent."[88] Although there had been a few scattered reports of nerve injury during this period,[49,78,96,104,137,138,222,249,306] those few cases were much downplayed. In a textbook written in 1985, the incidence of permanent brachial plexus injury in TOCS surgery was reported as 0%.[56]

It was not until a review by Dale[50] in 1982 that some representation of the true incidence and extent of brachial plexus injuries was recognized. His survey of the members of the International Cardiovascular Society revealed that 52% of the surgeons responding had seen some sort of brachial plexus injury and that the numbers reflected that 273 injuries of varying degree had occurred. From this point forward it seems that clinicians began to take a more serious look at their indications for surgery and technique. Although surgery for TOCS is still popular, more recent reports reflect a more conservative approach to the consideration of surgery and a trend toward nonoperative management.

Although surgical treatment is deemed "successful" in approximately 80% of cases when careful patient selection is used, 20% of all cases end up with unsatisfactory outcomes.[273,275] Reported surgical complications include injuries to the subclavian artery and/or vein that have led to exsanguination and subsequent death; transection of phrenic or long thoracic nerves; and division of the medial cord or C8 nerve root.[108] Additional surgical complications include hemothorax, pneumothorax, chylothorax, causalgia, and traction injuries to the plexus, including total paralysis and complete sensory loss. Although many brachial plexus injuries are transient, some require re-exploration and repair or grafting.[88] Cutaneous nerve dysesthesias have also been noted to occur almost universally and involve the intercostobrachial, posterior cutaneous nerves, and supraclavicular nerves. Although these dysesthesias usually resolve within 6 months, occasionally they are permanent.[120]

Although the aforementioned complications account for some of the surgical failures, other patients have unsatisfactory outcomes without surgical complications. Some believe that one of the largest reasons for "failed" surgery for TOCS is an incorrect diagnosis. A report by Kostic and Kulka[111] analyzed reasons for failed TOCS surgery in 142 operations on 124 patients. Missed diagnoses included glenohumeral or cervical arthritis and cervical disk herniation. Another patient had a Pancoast tumor that was missed during the initial evaluation. Thirteen reoperations were necessary because of inadequate or failed first rib resection.

The practitioner considering surgery for TOCS should be aware of the unusually high rate of litigation associated with transaxillary first rib resection. A study by the National Association of Insurance Commissioners[65] from 1975 to 1978[304] revealed that transaxillary first rib resection accounted for the greatest number of malpractice claims in the general thoracic surgery subspecialty. Retrospectively speaking, this study followed the great popularity of that particular procedure in the early 1970s, and it has since become more selectively performed.

More recently, as experience with the surgical treatment of patients with TOCS of all types increases, complications have decreased and careful analysis of complications, failed surgery, and recurrent or persistent symptoms have been recognized and investigated. For patients who have TOCS, whether "true" or "disputed," the consensus is that carefully selected patients do well after surgical treatment.

Recurrent Symptoms After Surgical Treatment

Failure of surgical decompression of the thoracic outlet should be carefully scrutinized to determine whether there was a symptom-free interval. Failure to improve after adequate decompression and first rib resection implies either incorrect diagnosis or other "issues," including the potential for secondary gain. The rate of true recurrent symptoms is reported to be between 5% and 25%,* and the symptoms tend to occur within 4 to 6 months postoperatively.[243] Although patients undergoing anterior scalenotomy alone have a higher likelihood of recurrent symptoms, the recurrence rate for patients undergoing combined anterior and middle scalenotomies (14%) is similar to that of transaxillary first rib resection alone (19%). Patients undergoing a combined first rib resection and scalenotomy have the lowest recurrence rate (6%).[223,231]

In several reviews, the cause of recurrent symptoms was most frequently due to scar tissue around the brachial plexus or due to a retained or unstable segment of the first rib (Fig. 29-21).[29,127,223,231,243] The supraclavicular approach seems to be the most popular approach for revision surgery because it allows better access to the brachial plexus. It also allows access to the supraclavicular fat, which can be used to wrap the plexus after neurolysis in an attempt to prevent recurrence of adhesions between the plexus and the scalenes.

The complication rate for secondary procedures is slightly higher than that of primary procedures, with the incidence of pleural tears or pneumothorax as high as 62% in one series.[29] Results of reoperation for recurrent symptoms demonstrate "improvement" or "success" in 74% to 90% of patients early after surgery (3 months). Recurrence of symptoms and "surgical failure," however, occur in up to 59% of patients after 10 to 15 years. Surgical results correlate directly with the identification of residual anomalous anatomy, such as retained bone, periosteum, or an unstable residual rib, and are worse in patients in whom only scar tissue around the brachial plexus is found at the time of

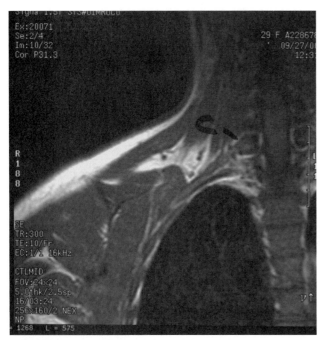

FIGURE 29-21. Coronal MR image of a patient with persistent symptoms after transaxillary first rib resection. Note remaining posterior portion of first thoracic rib fused with a cervical rib that was not removed. This is a case of "missing middle rib" and inadequate resection of the posterior 2 cm of the first rib.

reoperation. Sympathectomy has been suggested at the time of reoperation to improve results but is not commonly performed.[216] Comparative analysis of techniques of reoperation is impossible because of small patient numbers and lack of a standardized objective means of preoperative or postoperative assessment.

Results

The results of operative and nonoperative treatment of TOCS are difficult to objectively assess, because there is no standardized means of patient assessment or sufficient patient follow-up. Many patients in the "disputed" neurogenic category of TOCS have short-term symptoms precipitated by an isolated event, activity, or accident. These patients have symptoms that are self-limited and improve with short courses of physical therapy, activity modification, medication, and self-management of their symptoms.

For patients with more persistent or severe symptoms, nonoperative treatment such as the four-stage rehabilitation program advocated by Novak and colleagues[187] is recommended and successful, at least in the short term. In one study, 44 patients with symptoms of TOCS were followed for 12 months, and none was reported to be worse in terms of symptoms, lifestyle, or work activities. Four of 44 were "not improved," and 3 of 44 were "completely" better. Most of the patients (35/44) were either "partially" or "almost completely" better. Another report detailed 100% complete relief of symptoms in the short term with a multimodality therapy program.[262] The long-term fate of these patients is not known and requires further study.

The literature reviewing surgical treatment is abundant and demonstrates a high degree of variability, with good to excellent results achieved in 24% to 100%.† This variability may be attributed to many factors, including the lack of objective outcome measures, diagnostic criteria, follow-up periods, and widely variable surgical techniques and training. Early results (3 months) tend to be better, with a 90% or better success rate, and long-term results (>5 years) indicate an approximately 70% success rate. A review by Sanders[235] provides the most extensive summary of the literature to date (Tables 29-3 to 29-5). This paper demonstrates that the combination of anterior and middle scalenectomies and first rib resection yields the best results (99% good) whereas scalenotomy alone yields inferior results (57% good). In Sanders' own series in which subtotal scalenectomy alone was compared with first rib resection and combined scalenectomy and rib resection, no difference between early and long-term results was noted (Fig. 29-22).[233,235] Despite this, Sanders' more current surgical technique includes a "complete" scalenectomy, and he acknowledges that the combination of rib resection and scalenectomy yields "slightly" better results than either procedure alone.[163]

There is a consensus that patients with vascular or true neurogenic TOCS have a better outcome with surgical

*See references 9, 12, 34, 127, 164, 168, 170, 177, 178, 198, 223, 229, 231, 235, 244, 264, 273, 275, 281, and 299.
†See references 18, 21, 39, 80, 94, 112, 129, 131, 168, 176, 189, 202, 231, 235, 271, and 305.

Table 29-3
SUMMARY OF RESULTS OF ALL OPERATIONS FOR THORACIC OUTLET SYNDROME*

Technique	No. of Operations	% Good	% Fair	% Failed
Anterior scalenotomy	241	57	13	30
Anterior scalenectomy	338	79	9	12
Transaxillary first rib	3097	83	5	12
Supraclavicular first rib	715	83	13	4
Infraclavicular first rib	44	82	9	9
Posterior first rib	175	86	9	5
Transpleural first rib	18	75		25
Combined transaxillary[†] and scalenectomy[‡]	94	99		1

*The length of follow-up varied greatly within each study from 3 months to more than 10 years. With the exception of transpleural first rib resection, all operations, including anterior scalenectomy, were significantly superior to anterior scalenotomy (P < .01 to < .001).

[†]Transaxillary first rib resection.

[‡]Anterior and middle scalenectomy.

Modified from Sanders RJ, Haug CE: Thoracic Outlet Syndrome: A Common Sequela of Neck Injuries. Philadelphia, JB Lippincott, 1991.

Table 29-4
RESULTS OF TRANSAXILLARY FIRST RIB RESECTION

Author	Year	No. of Operations	No. (%) Good	No. (%) Fair	No. (%) Failed	Length of Follow-Up (mo)
Hoofer	1973	135	135 (100)		0	Not stated
McGough	1979	113	90 (80)	15 (13)	8 (7)	6-60
Youmans	1980	258	193 (75)	42 (16)	23 (9)	3-96 (average, 34)
Roos	1982	1315	1210 (92)		105 (8)	Presumed 3-180
Batt	1983	94	76 (80)		18 (20)	
Qvarfordt	1984	97	77 (79)		20 (21)	4-48
Davies	1988	115	103 (89)		12 (11)	6-180
Selke	1988	460	363 (79)	64 (14)	33 (7)	6-240
Stanton	1988	87	74 (85)	4 (4)	10 (11)	12-144
Lindgren	1989	175	103 (59)		72 (41)	24
Lepantalo	1989	112	56 (52)	27 (25)	29 (23)	1
Green	1991	136	107 (79)		29 (21)	60 mean ± 7
Totals		3097	2587 (83)	152 (5)	361 (12)	
Range		3444	37-100	(0-14)	(0-41)	

Modified from Sanders RJ, Haug CE: Thoracic Outlet Syndrome: A Common Sequela of Neck Injuries. Philadelphia, JB Lippincott, 1991.

treatment than do those with the "disputed" neurogenic type of TOCS. Similarly, there are supportive data to demonstrate that patients with work-related claims or litigation do worse than other patients, whether treated surgically or non-surgically.[21,60,80,200,235] In one study, patients with compensable injuries improved only 48% of the time as compared with 95% in the non–workers' compensation patients.[200] Another study gives figures of only a 28% improvement rate in compensation cases versus 50% in others,[21,80] and Sanders' recent report notes that patients with workers' compensation claims had 13% to 15% lower rates of success than all other patients.[235]

Table 29-5

RESULTS OF SUPRACLAVICULAR FIRST RIB RESECTION (INCLUDES ANTERIOR AND MIDDLE SCALENECTOMY)

Author	Year	Operations	No. (%) Good	Fair	Failed	Length of Follow-Up (mo)
Graham	1973	78	71 (91)	4 (5)	3 (4)	4-84
Thompson	1979	15	13 (87)		2 (13)	Not stated
Hempel	1981	433	366 (84)	55 (13)	12 (3)	Not stated
Thomas	1983	128	106 (83)	17 (13)	5 (4)	Not stated
Reilly	1988	39	23 (59)	13 (33)	3 (8)	1-30
Loh	1989	22	15 (68)	5 (23)	2 (9)	4-72
Total		715	594 (83)	94 (13)	27 (4)	
Range		715	(59-91)	(5-33)	(3-13)	

Modified from Sanders RJ, Haug CE: Thoracic Outlet Syndrome: A Common Sequela of Neck Injuries. Philadelphia, JB Lippincott, 1991.

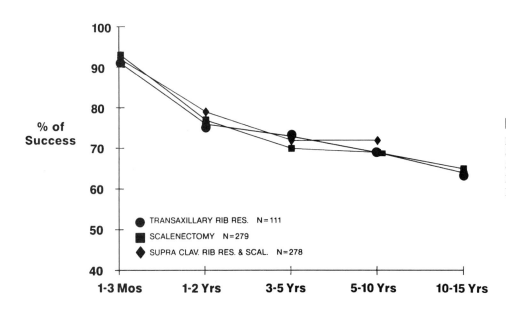

FIGURE 29-22. Results of three primary operations for TOCS. (From Sanders RJ, Haug C: Thoracic Outlet Syndrome: A Common Sequela of Neck Injuries. Philadelphia, JB Lippincott, 1991, with permission.)

CONCLUSION

Most upper extremity surgeons will perform few, if any, surgical procedures for TOCS, but the prevalence of these patients in one's practice will probably continue to increase. Careful attention to details about the patient's history and physical examination is the key to diagnosis. The practitioner must recognize this and schedule appropriate time for the initial examination. Patients who demonstrate vascular or true neurogenic TOCS should be considered for early surgery or referred for operative consultation. For patients without obvious vascular compromise or neurologic findings, conservative treatment can be successful in controlling symptoms in nearly all patients, at least in the short term. Psychological assessment and support are essential early on, as are lifestyle and workplace modifications. Persistent symptoms warrant thorough radiographic evaluation, elec-

trodiagnostic studies, and specialized diagnostic testing to identify bony or soft tissue anomalies and to rule out other treatable afflictions.

Selected patients who have failed several months of nonoperative treatment and continue to have significant or progressive symptoms may warrant surgical decompression. Great care should be exercised in patient selection, especially in workers' compensation cases. A combined approach that enables first rib resection and anterior/middle scalenectomy should be considered to minimize operative morbidity and reduce the likelihood of recurrence.

For those patients who require operative treatment, careful consideration should be given to referral of the patient to a surgeon or surgical team that routinely performs TOCS surgery. There are several major centers in the United States that perform TOCS surgery, and results of treatment of patients in those centers are predictably superior to the results of surgeons performing fewer than 10 procedures per year. Those surgeons who do perform operative treatment should have hands-on individual training in the procedure, including management of potential complications (which could require thoracotomy). Even with the assistance of a vascular or thoracic surgeon, extensive experience in brachial plexus surgery is imperative.

ANNOTATED REFERENCES

14. Barker WF: An historical look at the thoracic outlet compression syndrome. Ann Vasc Surg 3:293-298, 1989.

    A thorough review of historical aspects of TOCS, including initial identification of offending anatomic structures: the cervical rib, first rib, and the scalenes.

31. Cherington M: A conservative point of view of the thoracic outlet syndrome. Am J Surg 158:394-395, 1989.

    An editorial article by an author skeptical about the existence of disputed neurogenic TOCS and the surgical treatment of the same. This is a useful review of the literature (at that time) regarding risks of complications of surgical procedures in patients with normal preoperative electro-diagnostic and noninvasive vascular studies. It was written by the same author who subsequently published data suggesting that the incidence of the diagnosis and surgical treatment of patients with disputed neurogenic TOCS was related to reimbursement in a series of patients in Colorado in 1989.

156. MacKinnon SE, Novak CB: Thoracic outlet syndrome. Curr Prob Surg 39:1070-1145, 2002.

    This recent monograph written by one of the world's most experienced and respected peripheral nerve surgeons, details her experience and current thoughts about the pathophysiology and treatment of patients with TOCS. Detailed text, drawings, and figures provide the reader with specific "how to" techniques for treatment, especially regarding physical examination, conservative treatment, and surgical technique.

233. Sanders RJ, Haug CE: Thoracic Outlet Syndrome: A Common Sequela of Neck Injuries. Philadelphia, JB Lippincott, 1991.

    The authors' experience and knowledge of this subject were unequaled at the time of publication. It is required reading for any physician who treats patients with TOCS. In fewer than 350 pages are all the pertinent historical data, thorough reviews of pathoanatomy, clinical pearls, reviews of diagnostic issues, and guidelines for both surgical and non-surgical treatment for TOCS. Detailed reports of complications, results, and approaches are included as well as an impressive annotated bibliography in historical order.

236. Sanders RJ, Hammond SL: Management of cervical ribs and anomalous first ribs causing neurogenic thoracic outlet syndrome. J Vasc Surg 36:51-56, 2002.

    This report documents the necessity of excision of both any cervical ribs and the first rib in patients with true neurogenic TOCS. In 54 patients presenting with true neurogenic TOCS trauma is identified as the most common cause of symptoms in patients with abnormal cervical and/or anomalous first ribs. Results of the operative treatment document that both cervical and first rib resection are necessary for complete decompression. Failure rate without first rib resection was 75% in the work-related group and 38% in the non–work-related group. With first rib resection, rates were 25% in the work-related group and 20% in the non–work-related group.

205. Redenbach DM, Nelems B: A comparative study of the structures comprising the thoracic outlet in 250 human cadavers and 72 surgical cases of thoracic outlet syndrome. Eur J Cardiothorac Surg 13:353-360, 1998.

    A large series is presented of anatomic findings in cadavers, catalogued by both an anatomist and a thoracic surgeon with comparison to surgical findings in 72 patients who underwent surgery for TOCS by the same thoracic surgeon. Significant anatomic variants were noted in 46% of cadavers and 100% of surgical patients as verified by a second surgeon. Anomalies posterior to the brachial plexus were prevalent in the surgical group. Females in the surgical group had anterior and posterior anomalies in 73% that created a "scissors-like" pattern of neural entrapment.

215. Roos DB: Congenital anomalies associated with thoracic outlet syndrome: Anatomy, symptoms, diagnosis and treatment. Am J Surg 132:771-778, 1976.

    Classic article detailing anatomic findings in 980 trans-axillary first rib resections in 776 patients and findings in another 58 cadaveric dissections. Description is presented of the seven types of anomalous bands in the thoracic outlet seen commonly in patients with TOCS.

220. Roos DB: Thoracic outlet syndrome is underdiagnosed. Muscle Nerve 22:126-129; discussion 136-137, 1999.

296. Wilbourn AJ: Thoracic outlet syndrome is overdiagnosed. Arch Neurol 47:328-330, 1990.

    Consecutive articles providing a lively review of current standards of diagnosis and treatment of patients with disputed neurogenic TOCS. Debate type style of text summarizes the literature to date from both sides of this controversy.

281. Urschel HC Jr, Razzuk MA: Neurovascular compression in the thoracic outlet: Changing management over 50 years. Ann Surg 228:609-617, 1998.

    Largest patient group (>15,000) evaluated for TOCS with largest number of surgical cases (3914 primary, 1221 for recurrent) treated by nine surgeons and three physiatrists. Analysis of cases revealed breast implantation and median sternotomy as potential causes of TOCS. Recommendations are made for surgical treatment of all types of patients. Thrombolysis followed by prompt first rib resection for Paget-Schroetter syndrome produces the best results for venous TOS. Complete first rib resection at the initial surgical procedure markedly reduced the incidence of recurrent symptoms and secondary surgery. Dorsal sympathectomy for patients with sympathetically mediated pain syndrome or those recurrent symptoms who underwent a second procedure improved results.

290. Wehbe MA (ed): Thoracic Outlet Syndrome. Hand Clin 20:1-130, 2004.

    This issue of *Hand Clinics* is a valuable resource for any upper extremity surgeon and is a must-have for any surgeon treating patients with TOCS. Nineteen concise articles written by experts in the field address all current pertinent diagnostic and treatment issues. Authors include physical therapists, vascular and thoracic surgeons, radiologists, and hand/peripheral nerve surgeons, each of whom addresses the most up-to-date techniques in his or her area of specialty, offering different perspectives on the subject. Historical information, diagnostic issues, recommendations for conservative and surgical treatment, and current outcomes and complications of accepted treatments are detailed. The issue is well organized, is well illustrated, and has complete and valuable references.

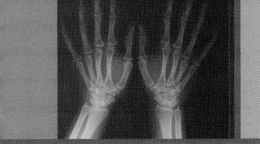

CHAPTER 30

Nerve Repair

Rolfe Birch

Although the decision to operate on a nerve is usually straightforward, in the acute case of an open wound or when the nerve injury is associated with damage to long bones, to joints, and to blood vessels it is not always as easy. The primary reasons for operating include (1) to confirm or establish diagnosis, (2) to restore continuity to a severed or ruptured nerve, and (3) to relieve a nerve of an agent that is compressing, distorting, or occupying it.

INDICATIONS

The indications for operating on nerves after an injury include the following:

- Deep paralysis after a wound over the course of a major nerve or after an injection close to the course of that nerve
- Deep paralysis after a closed injury, especially high-energy injuries, with severe damage to soft tissues and skeleton
- Deep paralysis after closed traction injury of the brachial plexus
- A nerve lesion associated with an arterial injury
- A nerve lesion associated with fracture or dislocation requiring urgent open reduction and internal fixation
- Worsening of nerve injury while under observation
- Failure to progress toward recovery in the expected time after a closed injury
- Failure to recover from conduction block within 6 weeks of injury
- Persistent pain
- Treatment of the painful neuroma

The aim of the operation is to preserve or restore function. This is achieved by preserving or restoring the innervation of the skin, muscle, soft tissues, skeleton, and other target organs. When a nerve is severed, repair offers the only chance of doing this. That repair may be done by suture or by graft. If the proximal stump is hopelessly damaged or if there is no continuity between that proximal stump and the spinal cord, then transfer of other nerves to the distal stump may be possible. If the distal stump is hopelessly damaged, then direct implantation of nerves into the muscle (muscular neurotization) may be possible. When the neurologic injury is, by whatever means, irreparable, then palliation may be achieved by musculotendinous transfer or other "reconstruction."

The sooner the distal segment is reconnected to the cell body and to the proximal segment, the better the result will be. In the extreme case of replantation after traumatic amputation O'Brien[116] showed that primary suture of nerves gave the only hope of recovery. Merle and coworkers,[104] Leclercq and colleagues,[89] and Birch and Raji[21] have shown the harm from delay and repair of median and ulnar nerves. A degree of experience and special equipment, surgical skill, and a good supporting staff are necessary for worthwhile results. Uncomplicated open wounds and nerves can be left for 24 hours to receive attention from an experienced surgeon. When, however, a nerve injury is associated with damage to a major blood vessel, with an impending threat of peripheral ischemia, or with increasing pressure within a fascial compartment, then delay is not permissible. The case is an emergency, as it is with cases of open fracture or fracture-dislocation.

The reasons not to proceed to repair of a transected nerve include the following:

- The general condition of the patient. After having saved a life or limb by means of successful arterial repair, the patient, the anesthetist, and the surgeon may well have had enough.
- The attributes and skills of the operating team and the availability of specialized equipment
- Uncertainty about the viability or the state of the nerve trunks. This is particularly valid when the nerve has been torn by a saw or by a bullet.
- The risk of local or systemic sepsis. If local soft tissue damage and contamination from an open fracture or high-velocity gunshot wound is severe, it is critical to wait until the soft tissue bed is stabilized before proceeding with nerve repair.
- When the condition of the nerve is such that function will more surely and more rapidly be restored by musculo-tendinous transfer

Anatomy

The nervous system is a mechanism through which the organism is kept in touch with its internal structures and external environments and reacts to changes in them. The peripheral nervous system connects the central nervous system to the periphery. It includes the cranial nerves, the spinal nerves with their roots and rami, the peripheral nerves, and the peripheral components of the autonomic nervous system. Peripheral nerves contain motor fibers to end plates of skeletal muscle; sensory fibers from organs in endings in skin, muscle, tendon, and joint; and autonomic fibers to blood vessels, sweat glands, and hair follicle musculature. The concentration of functional capacity is unmatched by any other system. Severance in an adult's arm of a median nerve of about 5 mm in diameter effectively ruins the function of the hand and forearm.

The essential component of the system is the cell body with its dendrites and its prolongation of the axons. This is a column of neuronal cytoplasm enclosed by a cell membrane, the *axolemma*. Thomas and associates[149] described the axoplasm as a "fluid cytosol in which are suspended formed elements." The cytoskeleton contains microtubules, neurofilaments, and matrix; it provides the apparatus for axoplasmic transport.

The axons are closely associated with Schwann cells. Larger axons are wrapped along their length by a continuous series of Schwann cells into which they are invaginated. The nodes of Ranvier represent the points of contiguity of adjacent Schwann cells. Smaller fibers are contained in bundles by similar columns of Schwann cells.

Larger axons are enveloped in a myelin sheath, which is laid down in spiral layers by the surface of the Schwann cell, moving around the axon.[156] The nerve fiber is the axon and its enveloping Schwann cell sheath with or without myelin, contained within a basal lamina or basement membrane (Fig. 30-1).

The caliber of nonmyelinated axons varies from 0.4 to 1.25 μm. Myelinated fibers range from 2 to 22 μm in diameter. The largest and fastest conducting elements are myelinated fibers around 20 μm in diameter concerned with somatic afferent and efferent activity. The smallest and slowest conducting are approximately 1 μm in diameter and subserve autonomic activity and delayed pain sensibility. The specialized property of nerve fibers is their ability to propagate action potentials. In the unmyelinated fibers, a wave of depolarization spreads continuously along the axon and is attenuated by the large capacitance of the axolemma, so that the velocity of conduction is restricted to about 1 m/sec. In the myelinated fiber, myelin restricts electrical activity to the nodes of Ranvier, so that the impulse has to travel in leaps from one node to the next by saltatory conduction. The speed of conduction is very much greater. Demyelination leads to a decrease of conduction velocity and, if severe, to a complete conduction block.

Axonal Transport

Young[163] described the genesis of the idea of axonal transport. The axon functions as part of a neuron as a whole in transporting materials to and from the cell body. Two forms of transport are recognized: fast and slow.[117] Fast transport may be centrifugal or centripetal. Membranous elements are conveyed centrifugally from the cell to the terminal as membrane proteins, secretory proteins, and peptides. The centripetal or retrograde fast component conveys membranes from the terminal by endocytosis and conveys this to the cell body as multifascicular bodies. Nerve growth factor and other neurotrophins are conveyed to the cell body from

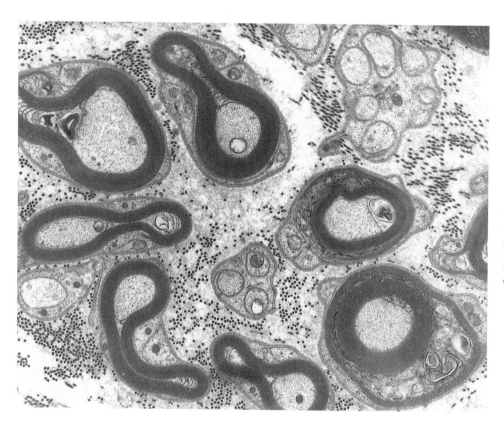

FIGURE 30-1. Proximal stump of fifth cervical nerve 24 hours after traction rupture showing nonmyelinated fibers that are enveloped into clusters by Schwann cell cytoplasm. Numerous mitochondria are seen in the axons and in the Schwann cell cytoplasm. Large myelinated fibers contain neurofilaments and neurotubules. (Original magnification, ×19,500.)

the periphery by this system. The rates of fast transport are from 200 to 400 mm/day.

Slow transport is centrifugal and is associated with the transport of elements of the cytoskeleton. Rates of transport are from 1 to 4 mm/day, about the same as the rate of peripheral regeneration after axonotomy.

Axonal transport is oxygen dependent, and it is sensitive to temperature. Interference with the process leads to marked slowing or cessation of conduction and, when prolonged, to degeneration of the nerve cells.

The Schwann cells, the skin, and other target organs are rich sources of nerve growth factor and other neurotrophins that are essential for the development, the maturation, and the maintenance of the cell bodies. Deprivation of this supply by transection of a peripheral nerve can lead to central cell death. This is most apparent when the injury is violent and close to the neuraxis and even more so in the immature central nervous system This matter is very well reviewed by Terenghi[146] and by Frostick and coworkers.[51]

Connective Tissue Elements

Nerve fibers are embedded in the endoneurium, which contains longitudinally orientated cells, abundant collagen fibrils, and blood vessels. Nerve fibers are aggregated into fascicles by the perineurium, which is composed of flattened cell processes alternating with layers of collagen. The perineurium is a diffusion barrier and is a strong membrane with high resistance to compression from without, distention from within, and longitudinal traction.[91]

Groups of fascicles are aggregated within the nerve trunk by epineurium. This is the most abundant of all of the connective tissue elements of a nerve trunk and occupies between 60% and 85% of its cross-sectional area.[143] It is looser than the perineurium and contains numerous longitudinally orientated blood vessels. It is condensed at its surface as a glistening, translucent membrane; and in the uninjured nerve, individual fascicles can be seen within, surrounded by an opaque pearly white membrane, the perineurium. Jabaley[72] describes the epineurium as internal and external. Epineurium ensheaths the entire nerve and lies between the fascicles, where it blends with the perineurium and aggregates a numbers of these into discrete bundles. Jabaley cautions: "In both dissection and suturing the principle reason for avoiding perineurial injury is to avoid injury to the internal milieu, the conducting portion of the nerve."

There is one further connective tissue structure that is of great clinical significance, the adventitial "paraneurium" or "mesoneurium." This is loose areolar tissue that permits gliding of the nerve; at intervals, vascular pedicles pass through this layer to the nerve trunk. Lundborg[92] describes a rich blood supply; the *intrinsic* epineurial, perineurial, and endoneurial plexus; and the extrinsic regional vessels that course through the mesoneurium. These two systems form "separate but extensively interconnected microvascular systems." Some of these extrinsic pedicles are so well formed, such as those arising from the superior ulnar collateral vessels, that they provide the basis for free vascularized nerve grafts. The subject is thoroughly reviewed by McManis and coworkers.[101]

Wilgis and Murphy[158] found that the brachial plexus had an excursion of at least 15 mm in relation to the position of the arm and that the median and ulnar nerves at the elbow moved through an average distance of 7.3 and 9.8 mm with full motion. The greatest excursion of peripheral nerves occurred at the wrist, proximal to the carpal tunnel; here the median and ulnar nerves had 15.5 and 14.8 mm of longitudinal gliding, respectively. Wilgis[157] commented on the effects of injury on gliding: "In other words, the length of the nerve substance has been shortened because of the injury. Because of this overall shortening, excursion cannot take place."

It is the mesoneurium that permits normal nerve gliding. Injury or surgical intervention that compromises the gliding of the nerve will impair function. Tethering or entrapment of a nerve may cause severe neuropathic pain (Fig. 30-2).

The importance of retaining or restoring gliding of peripheral nerves, and of preventing their tethering or entrapment, cannot be overemphasized. Lundborg[91] describes the connective tissue of a nerve trunk as a collection of sliding interphase zones that permit considerable excursion of the epineurium within the adventitial mesoneurium and of the individual bundles within the deep layer of the epineurium. Among the most important of Millesi's many contributions is his recognition of the importance of this function.[107] He argues for the preservation of the "gliding apparatus" in a paper that should be widely read.

Functional Segregation

Sunderland[140] wrote a highly detailed work that describes the arrangement of fascicles and of bundles of fascicles along the course of nerve trunks, showing branching, fusion, and changes in number. These findings have been interpreted to cast a doubt on the possibility of achieving accurate coaptation of the ends of divided nerves. In fact, Sunderland demonstrated a degree of topographic segregation of nerve fibers according to function over considerable lengths of the trunks. Microneurographic studies have confirmed these findings.[124]

Narakas,[108] Slingluff and coworkers,[133] and Bonnel and Canovas[23] have made an extensive analysis of the distribution of nerve fibers within bundles within the nerves of the brachial plexus. The segregation of nerve fibers is

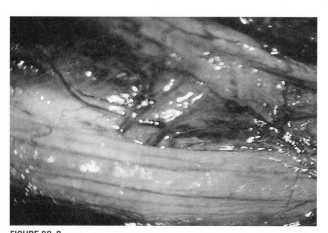

FIGURE 30-2. Blood supply of ulnar nerve seen at operation. The nerve lies in a foamy, glistening adventitia, containing longitudinal vessels running in the external epineurium. Deeper vessels run in the epineurium between individual fascicles. (Original magnification, ×40.)

FEATURES OF CONNECTIVE TISSUE

1. The *endoneurium* provides connective tissue support for the nerve fibers. The resistance of the nerve trunk to stretching injury is granted by the undulating course of nerve fibers within the fascicles. As Tupper[152] states, "individual fascicles are identified by the spiral bands of Fontana located in the perineurium. If longitudinal tension is applied to the perineurium, these bands disappear, indicating that they are tension wrinkles, probably affording some protection from stretch deformation." Resistance to stretch is further provided by the connective tissue sheaths, most especially the perineurium.

2. The *perineurium* is responsible for maintaining the physiologic milieu of the conducting elements. It is a diffusion barrier. It is strong. Breaching the perineurium interferes with conduction and provokes demyelination of underlying nerve fibers. Section of the perineurium leads to "pouting out" of the endoneurium and of the nerve fibers.

3. The *epineurium* contains many blood vessels. It protects the nerve against compression. It occupies between 60% and 85% of the cross-sectional area of the nerve, and it is most abundant where the nerve traverses joints. It is the connective tissue sheath of particular surgical interest.

4. The adventitial *mesoneurium* conveys extrinsic segmental blood vessels to the nerve trunks. It enables gliding of the nerve.

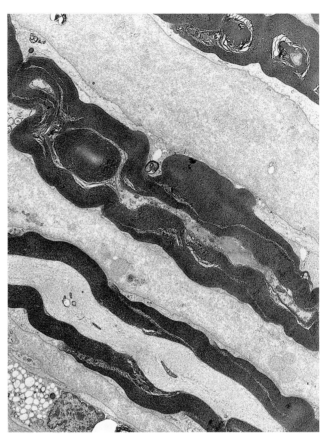

FIGURE 30-3. Wallerian degeneration. Appearance of the distal stump of ulnar nerve 3 weeks after transection. The myelin sheaths have collapsed. The endoneurium is swollen. There is opening of Schmidt-Lantermann incisures. Axoplasm and neurofilaments are seen in the lower fibers. (Original magnification, ×3,400.)

established more proximally so that the suprascapular nerve can be traced to an anterior bundle within C5 at the level of the anterior tubercle. One bundle, controlling the radial extensors of the wrist, can be consistently displayed by stimulation within the posterior division of the upper trunk, when exploration is performed within 36 to 48 hours after transection. It is this segregation that permits such transfers as Oberlin's,[115] in which one bundle of the ulnar nerve destined for the flexor muscles of the forearm is anastomosed to a nerve in the biceps.

RESPONSES TO INJURY

Wallerian Degeneration

A lesion deep enough to interrupt the axon leads to wallerian degeneration.[155] This process extends beyond the axon to the cell body, to the Schwann cell envelope and myelin sheath, to the endoneurial cells, and, ultimately, to the motor and sensory end organs. My colleagues and I have found that the interval between injury and the failure of neuromuscular conduction ranges from 48 to 160 hours. Many misdiag-

noses of neurapraxia could be avoided by the simple procedure of demonstrating whether there is or is not conduction within the peripheral nerve segments (Fig. 30-3).

When there is no regeneration of axons into the distal stump, changes occur in target organs that, over time, become irreversible. Motor end plates disappear, and the denervated muscle becomes fibrosed. Brushart[28] thought that ideal reinnervation could be expected before 1 to 3 months of degeneration, functional reinnervation could be expected for up to 1 year, and no reinnervation could be expected after 3 years. The reaction of muscle spindles and of cutaneous sensory organs is rather slower.

The proximal consequences are every bit as significant as those distal to the level of section. Within days of axonotomy there is reduction in the caliber of the proximal axon that may atrophy. The velocity of conduction in the proximal segment drops. There are changes in the cell bodies. Dyck and associates[47] examined the spinal cord of two patients years after amputation of the lower limb and found that loss of the target tissue by axonotomy led to atrophy and then loss of motor neurons. There should be no disagreement about the trophic support for the motor neuron. Carlstedt and Cullheim[32] collate persuasive evidence about this and about the harmfulness of delay in reconnection between the motor neuron and the peripheral axon (Figs. 30-4 and 30-5). Neurons within the immature nervous system are even more vulnerable to axonotomy.

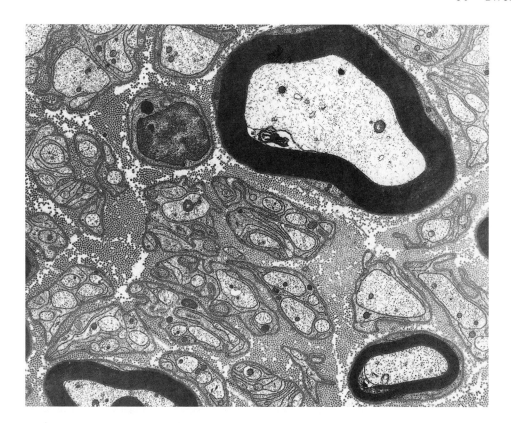

FIGURE 30-4. Nerve regeneration. Proximal stump of sciatic nerve 3 months after thermal injury from extruded cement used in total hip arthroplasty. Large numbers of both axonal sprouts and Schwann cell processes are seen. Three healthy myelinated nerve fibers are evident. This biopsy was taken 10 mm proximal to the site of injury (Original magnification × 4600.)

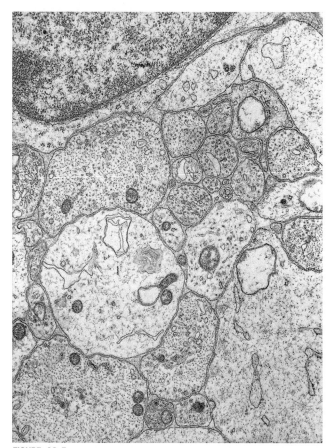

FIGURE 30-5. Nerve regeneration. Proximal stump of median nerve 6 weeks after section. Numerous axonal sprouts lie within Schwann cell cytoplasm. There is remyelination of axons. Numerous mitochondria are apparent. (Original magnification, ×31,000.)

Alvares and Fitzgerald[4] described changes in the behavior of neurotrophins, neurotransmitters, ion channels, and receptors in the course of maturation from the embryo to the adult. They comment: "The developing nervous system is more vulnerable to peripheral injury than the adult, presumably due to its greater dependence upon retrograde signals from the periphery for survival."

These central changes are more extreme in more proximal, more extensive, and more violent injuries. They are a fundamental factor in prognosis after repair and an important explanation for harmfulness of delay of nerve repair after such a lesion. A recent and outstanding review about peripheral nerve degeneration and regeneration comes from Stoll and associates.[137]

Stretch Injury

Peripheral nerves outside the spinal canal have considerable tensile strength, but function is damaged by elongation of 12% or more. Lundborg and Rydevik[95] showed that venous flow was blocked when a nerve was stretched by 8% of its resting length and that stretching by 16% produced ischemia. In the early stages of stretching of a nerve, elongation is enabled by stretching of the epineurium and straightening of the irregular course of the fibers within the fascicles. Haftek[63] observed, "Before rupture of the epineurium the damage to the nerve fibers is either neurapraxia or axonotmesis, because the endoneurial sheath and Schwann fibers remain intact." With continued traction, the caliber of the fibers is diminished, endoneurial space narrows, and myelin is disrupted.[34] Finally, rupture occurs when all elements, including the epineurium, are torn. I have exposed traction injuries, however, wherein the bundles within the epineurium have ruptured and had withdrawn even though there was continuity of the external epineurium. The shock wave from bullets or other missiles passing through the limb in the immediate vicinity of a nerve may produce a comparable injury.

CLASSIFICATION OF NERVE INJURIES

Seddon distinguished between three types of nerve injury[131]:

1. *Neurapraxia* (nerve not working). There is a physiologic block to conduction but no anatomic disturbance of the nerve.
2. *Axonotmesis* (axon cutting). The axon is severed, its distal portion degenerates, and the basal lamina of the Schwann cell remains intact.
3. *Neurotmesis* (nerve cutting). There is interruption of continuity of all elements of a nerve.

In neurapraxia, distal conduction persists, the axon has not been cut, and it does not degenerate. On the other hand, wallerian degeneration occurs in both axonotmesis and neurotmesis. Thus, in two of the subtypes (neurapraxia and axonotmesis), the prognosis is favorable *if the cause is removed,* but with neurotmesis, recovery can occur only if the nerve is repaired. Clinicians must always remember that a favorable lesion may progress to a much less favorable one if the original cause is not dealt with. Recovery is likely for the nerve accidentally encircled by a suture or crushed under a plate if the cause is urgently removed. If that cause remains for days or weeks, then a much more unfavorable lesion develops. Nerves crushed in a swollen ischemic limb or in a tense compartment progress from conduction block to much deeper and much less favorable degenerative lesions.

Sunderland[141] introduced a rather more elaborate system of classifying injuries. Five degrees of severity were recognized, ranging from simple conduction block to loss of continuity. Some clinicians may find this classification of more practical use than Seddon's earlier classification, espe-

Table 30-1
CLASSIFICATION OF FOCAL MECHANICAL NERVE INJURY

I. Focal Conduction Block
  A. Transient
    1. Ischemic
    2. Other
  B. More persistent
    1. Demyelinating
    2. Axonal constriction

II. Axonal Degeneration
  A. With preservation of basal laminal sheaths of nerve fibers
  B. With partial section of nerve
  C. With complete transection of nerve

Modified from Thomas PK, Holdorff B: Neuropathy due to physical agents. *In* Dyck PJ, Thomas PK, Griffin JW, et al (eds): Peripheral Neuropathy, 3rd ed. Philadelphia, WB Saunders, 1993.

cially in the analysis of stretch lesions. Distinctions between the intermediate subtypes within the Sunderland classification, however, cannot be made without histologic analysis of a resected portion of the nerve. My colleagues and I have tended toward a further simplification to classification as *degenerative* (axonal discontinuity) and *nondegenerative* (conduction block) and suggest that this is the manner in which clinicians should regard nerve injuries.[11] Thomas and Holdorff[150] develop this concept in a very useful manner (Table 30-1).

CLINICAL DIAGNOSIS

When a nerve has stopped working and there is a wound over the course of a nerve, then the diagnosis is nerve transection until proved otherwise. The extent of the lesion is shown by weakness or paralysis of muscle and by the extent of loss of cutaneous sensation. There are pitfalls: there is considerable variation in the cutaneous innervation of the skin of the hand by the median and the ulnar nerves and considerable compensatory activity of uninvolved muscles, such that trick movements may mislead the examiner. I have seen instances in which elbow flexion from the brachioradialis muscle has led to delay in diagnosis of transection of the musculocutaneous nerve. Sympathetic paralysis, however, is a sure sign of interruption of axons. The skin in the territory of the affected nerve becomes red and dry. Severe pain indicates continuing damage, scarcely consistent with the diagnosis of nondegenerative conduction block (neurapraxia).

Analysis of the force expended on the limb is particularly important in the diagnosis of nerve injury that results from closed fractures or fracture-dislocations. The extent of force expended on the nerve trunk can be estimated by the velocity at impact or the height of the fall. Local bruising at the tip of the shoulder or linear abrasions in the neck indicate that there has been violent separation of the forequarter from the neck. Linear bruising of skin is indicative of rupture of axial structures. Radiographs are useful in showing the

---

CRITICAL POINTS: CLASSIFICATION

- The most useful clinical classification of nerve lesions distinguishes conduction block (neurapraxia) from degeneration (axonotmesis and neurotmesis). In the former, the axon is intact; in the latter, the axon is divided and the process of wallerian degeneration ensues.

- Conduction block (neurapraxia) is uncommon in surgical practice and a diagnosis should not be used if (1) the nerve palsy is complete, (2) there is vasomotor and sudomotor paralysis in the territory of the nerve, and (3) there is a Tinel sign at the level of lesion.

- Conduction block (neurapraxia) is unlikely if (1) there is neuropathic pain and (2) there is a wound over the course of the nerve.

extent of displacement of bone fragments, and imperfect reduction or a block to reduction implies interposition of soft tissues. Concerning nerves injured in the arm or the elbow, Seddon[126] thought that recovery could be awaited if two conditions were met: (1) reasonable apposition of bony fragments and (2) complete certainty that there is no threat of ischemia of the forearm muscles.

Physical Examination of Nerve Injury

The Tinel Sign

Elicitation of this important clinical feature is simple enough. The examiner lightly percusses along the course of the affected nerve from distal to proximal. When the finger percusses over the zone of regenerating fibers the patient will announce the sensation of pins and needles, which may be quite painful, into the cutaneous distribution of the nerve. The clinical significance of the Tinel sign might be summarized as follows:

1. A strongly positive Tinel sign over a lesion soon after injury indicates rupture or severance. I regularly find this on the day of injury, most especially in closed traction rupture.
2. After repair that is going to be successful, the centrifugally moving Tinel sign is persistently stronger than that at the suture line.
3. After repair that is going to fail, the Tinel sign at the suture line remains stronger than that at the growing point.
4. Failure of distal progression of the Tinel sign in a closed lesion indicates rupture or other lesion impeding regeneration.

CRITICAL POINT: THE TINEL SIGN

- The Tinel sign should be reserved for traumatic neuropathy. Tinel himself made a clear distinction between this and the sensitivity of the nerve trunk in cases of "neuralgia."

Wound Inspection

The single most important determinant of outcome is the violence of injury to the nerve and the limb, and the extent of destruction of nerve tissue is a reflection of this. For the past 30 years nerve injuries have been classed into three groups.

1. *The tidy wound:* caused by knife or glass or the surgeon's scalpel. Damage is confined to the wound. Primary repair of all divided structures is desirable.
2. *The untidy wound:* commonly caused by open fractures or by penetrating missile injury. There is extensive tissue damage with a high risk of sepsis. Arterial injury is common. The contaminated wound from close-range shotgun injury is one example in which urgent repair cannot be entertained. There is the risk of sepsis from dead or devitalized tissue or from unnoted small fragments of foreign material; the extent of intraneural longitudinal damage cannot easily be ascertained in the freshly exposed case. Sepsis greatly compounds the problem, causing even more longitudinal destruction within the nerve. The International Red Cross Wound Classification set out by Coupland[39] will be of particular interest to those treating penetrating missile injuries.
3. *The closed traction injury:* these are very destructive of nerves and of axial vessels. There is wide retraction of ruptured nerves and of vessels, and there is considerable longitudinal damage within the ruptured trunk. The outcome after nerve repair in this pattern of injury, when complicated by arterial lesion, is the worst of all groups.

Neurologic Examination

A complete assessment of the innervation of all muscles distal to the injury site is imperative on the day of injury and at subsequent examinations. The record of a table of manual muscle strength in the patient's record is useful in following progression or absence of nerve recovery. I use the Medical Research Council grading system (see Table 30-4) to chart recovery of denervated muscle after injury or repair. Similarly, a careful sensory examination of the affected and surrounding dermatomes, using both threshold and density assessments, is important in the evaluation and management of closed nerve injuries. Most patients are able to describe, with accuracy, the boundary between skin with normal sensation and diminished or abnormal sensation and also the boundary between abnormal sensation and complete loss of sensation. I ask patients to mark out these areas with a colored skin pencil for anesthetic skin and then with a red marker pencil for skin with abnormal sensation and the limb is then photographed. The photograph is kept with the patient's files. These areas of loss or impairment of sensation may be marked out on standard charts of the hand, the upper limb, and the lower limb and this, too, provides a useful permanent record.

Neurophysiologic Investigations: Electrodiagnosis

According to Smith, "Nerve conduction studies and electromyography should be considered as an extension of the clinical examination of nerve, muscle, and the neuromuscular junction."[134] The study of nerve conduction advises the clinician about the health of axons, about their myelination, and, when applied to the proximal stump of a nerve, whether there is continuity between the exposed nerve and the spinal cord.

After transection of a nerve, axons become inexcitable and neuromuscular transmission fails. Direct stimulation of the nerve distal to the level of lesion elicits no response. However, some conduction is maintained for some days after nerve transection.

Fibrillation potentials appear as muscles are denervated, but their onset depends on the distance between the site of nerve lesion and the muscle so that there may be an interval of 10 to 14 days before fibrillations are seen.

The reappearance of voluntary motor unit potential activity indicates that reinnervation is taking place, and the electromyographic evidence of this usually precedes clinical evidence of recovery. The finding of a few motor units showing reinnervation even at early stage after injury does not imply that full recovery of a nerve will take place.

Table 30-2

ELECTRODIAGNOSTIC FEATURES OF NERVE INJURY

Nerve Injury Type	SAP	CMAP	Conduction Velocity	EMG
Neurapraxia	Reduced amplitude proximal to block. Normal amplitude distal to block		Usually preserved	No or sparse fibrillations Characteristic IP of normal MUPs firing Rapid rates with reduced interference pattern
Axonotmesis	↓	↓	Normal/reduced to a degree dependent on severity of axonal degeneration and fiber type involved	Fibrillations Reduced IP, ↓ firing rate of MUPs Evidence of reinnervation dependent on age of lesion (see Table 30-1)
Neurotmesis	A	A	Unmeasurable	Profuse fibrillations No voluntary MUPs

SAP, Sensory action potential; CMAP, compound muscle action potential; ↓, decreased; ↑, increased; A, absent; IP, interference pattern; MUP, motor unit potential.

From Smith SJM: Electrodiagnosis. *In* Birch R, Bonney G, Wynn Parry CB: Surgical Disorders of the Peripheral Nerves. London, Churchill Livingstone, 1998.

Electrodiagnostic work needs to be done and interpreted by an expert and further considered by an informed surgeon. The findings of these investigations must be interpreted with very great care in the first 10 to 14 days after transection of a nerve. In analysis of incomplete lesions of large nerve trunks (like those seen in the sciatic nerve after arthroplasty of the hip) the clinician may be lulled into a sense of false security by electrodiagnostic evidence of an incomplete lesion. Such evidence should not be taken to imply that full recovery can be anticipated. Unless the nerve has been wholly transected it is likely that there will be mixed elements of neurotmesis, of axonotmesis, and of prolonged conduction block.

The subject is comprehensively reviewed by Smith,[134] from whose work Tables 30-2 and 30-3 are taken. This correlates electrodiagnostic findings with Seddon's classification of nerve injury. As Smith says, however, "the distinction between neurapraxia and axonal degeneration of partial or complete degree is difficult in the acute stages of nerve injury, prior to evidence of denervation in the form of fibrillation potentials on EMG. Therefore, electrodiagnostic tests cannot reliably differentiate a neurapraxic lesion from one with Wallerian degeneration in the first few days after nerve injury."

Dellon[43] emphasizes that the study is not a substitute for obtaining a careful history and physical examination, that normal values do not necessarily indicate absence of neurologic abnormality, and that an abnormal electrodiagnostic study does not mean that the patient requires operative treatment!

It is within the operating theater that electrodiagnostic work is of particular value. Bonney and Gilliatt[25] demonstrated persisting conduction in sensory fibers when the dorsal root ganglion has become separated from the dorsal horn of the spinal cord in traction injuries of the brachial plexus. This principle was extended to intraoperative investigation. Landi and associates[86] recorded cortical evoked potentials through scalp electrodes from nerve stumps stimulated at operation. I have used intraoperative evoked potential studies since 1977.

Kline and Hudson[78] relate extensive experience in the use of electrodiagnostic work for the analysis of injured peripheral nerves. Compound nerve action potentials are used to measure regeneration into the distal nerve by stimulating and recording across the site of lesion. The outcome of the investigation, related to the clinical outcome, is described in nearly 1000 nerves with serious lesions in continuity in both upper and lower limbs. Four hundred and thirty-eight nerves showed a recordable nerve action potential traversing the lesion. Neurolysis was done; and of these, 404 nerves (92%) went on to at least useful functional outcome. In another 428 nerves no nerve action potential could be recorded and repair was done. Of these, 240 (56%) went on to regain useful functional recovery. Other important data are assembled about nerves where partial repair was done, preserving

Table 30-3

EMG FINDINGS IN DENERVATION AND REINNERVATION

Denervation	Spontaneous activity (fibrillations, positive sharp waves in acute denervation; fasciculations and complex repetitive discharges in chronic denervation)
Reinnervation	
Early	Normal motor units with increased duration because of late potentials (satellite fibers incorporated through collateral sprouting)
Ongoing	Moderate amplitude polyphasic motor units of long duration, unstable firing due to variable conduction along unmyelinated sprouts and low safety margin of neuromuscular transmission
Late	Large amplitude polyphasic motor units with stable transmission

From Smith SJM: Electrodiagnosis. *In* Birch R, Bonney G, Wynn Parry CB: Surgical Disorders of the Peripheral Nerves. London, Churchill Livingstone, 1998.

those individual bundles with recordable nerve action potentials.

As Kline and Hudson[79] have written, the objective in operative recording is to measure a nerve action potential distal to the lesion. In the initial 9 months after injury the nerve action potential's amplitude and conduction velocity are not as important as the simple presence or absence of the response. The presence of a nerve action potential indicates axons of sufficient number, caliber, and maturation to presage useful recovery of function for at least a portion of the injured cross section of the nerve. Absence of a nerve action potential indicates that recovery will not occur without resection and repair.

THE LESION IN CONTINUITY

Whether to leave alone a lesion in continuity or whether to resect and bridge the gap is a most difficult decision, made more so when there is clinical evidence of some recovery. The decision is easier when some intact fascicles can be shown traversing the lesion. The consistency and the diameter of the neuroma is helpful. The harder and the larger, indeed the more florid, the neuroma, the less likely that recovery will be good.

Most informative is to stimulate above the lesion and to record from the nerve or from individual fascicles below it: a response of good amplitude may well indicate a good prognosis. A response in individual fascicles may allow separation of an intact part of a nerve from the damaged portion.

I have rarely regretted resection and repair and have often regretted not so acting. *Patients must be warned that there may be a falling off of function—that there must be one step back to take two steps forward.*

CRITICAL POINTS: NEUROPHYSIOLOGIC DIAGNOSIS

- Neurophysiologic investigations distinguish between conduction block and degenerative lesions.
- Neurophysiologic investigations cannot distinguish between a favorable degenerative lesion (axonotmesis) and nonfavorable degenerative lesion (neurotmesis). This distinction can be made only by the passage of time or by exposure of the nerve.

CONSIDERATIONS BEFORE SURGICAL INTERVENTION

1. Lifesaving or limb-saving measures come first. The surgeon has a duty to assess a patient's ability to go through a prolonged intervention.
2. In late cases, indolent wounds and infections must be cleared. The texture of the skin may require massage and

oiling. Nonunion of a long bone can be dealt with at the same time as the nerve repair. A torn rotator cuff is repaired either at the same time as the circumflex nerve or after nerve repair.
3. Deep scars from penetrating missile injury or from burns offer a most hostile bed to nerve grafts. These will need replacement by healthy full-thickness skin flaps, pedicle or free, before nerve repair.
4. The timing of treatment of severe fixed deformity from uncorrected paralysis or ischemic fibrosis is adapted to the individual patient's needs. When possible, I operate for these at the same time as the nerve repair. Serial plaster of Paris splinting is particularly useful in overcoming fixed flexion deformity of the wrist, of the proximal interphalangeal joints, and of the elbow.[70]
5. Is it worthwhile? Are other, simpler measures available? "By the time the changes of degeneration are present the patient is a better candidate for the examination halls than for restorative treatment. The object of the clinician must be to make the diagnosis before the signs of peripheral degeneration have appeared: that is, before the best time for intervention has passed."[12] The paralysis of neglected high radial, high ulnar, or common peroneal nerve lesions may be better treated by the appropriate musculo-tendinous transfer.
6. Static or dynamic splinting is helpful to patients by diminishing their disability, by giving an indication of what is hoped to be achieved, and, of course, by ensuring that these are ready during the course of postoperative treatment.
7. Patients appreciate a clear statement of what has happened, what can be done, and when it can be done. It is helpful for them to know for how long they must plan to be away from work and curtail daily activities and driving. One fourth of all of my patients have suffered iatrogenic nerve injuries. I think that the clinician responsible for retrieving the situation should take charge, give clear advice, set out a clear plan of action, and avoid a partisan approach. I advise patients that appropriate records of operative findings will be released promptly to their legal advisors but that I will not, myself, prepare a medicolegal report.

THE CONSULTATION AND OPERATIVE RECORD

I hope to establish diagnosis and set out a plan of action at the first consultation with the patient. This information is sent, in a letter of opinion, to the referring consultant and the family practitioner. Many patients are already working with a physiotherapist or occupational therapist, and letters are sent to them at the patient's own address. I find this particularly useful when treating children. Communication with other colleagues is essential, and it is the basis of adequate continuing care for those patients who come from afar. Necessary dynamic or static splints are made at that first consultation.

The operative record should be carefully maintained and supplemented with a diagram and photographs (Fig. 30-6).

1. *Preoperative evaluation:* includes information about the limb dominance, the nature of the patient's work, the cause

ROYAL NATIONAL ORTHOPAEDIC HOSPITAL, STANMORE
PERIPHERAL NERVE INJURY UNIT

Operation Note

Name:

Hospital No:

Ward:

Operation:
Code:

Surgeons:

Anaesthetist:
Duration of GA:
Tourniquet Time:
Blood Loss:

Operation Date:

Pre-operatively:

Position:
Incision:

Findings

Procedure:

Repair:

Summary of Abnormalities:

Closure:

Records/Specimens:

Post-operatively:

Comments

Signature

Copies: Outpatient Department, coding person (in Unit), operating surgeons, referring surgeon,
genereal practitioner, operation file, case notes

FIGURE 30-6. Operative record of a peripheral nerve injury unit. (Courtesy of the Royal National Orthopaedic Hospital, Stanmore, United Kingdom.)

and date of injury, associated injuries, summary of pre-operative neurologic defect and the consequences of that, and relevant information from ancillary investigations.
2. *Findings:* include information about electrodiagnostic work as well as description of the lesions.
3. *Repair:* the state of the stumps after resection and the gap after resection must always be included.
4. *Records:* relate to the findings from electrodiagnostic work and to material taken for histologic examination or for research purposes.

5. *Postoperative care:* is particularly important, setting out timing of removal of sutures, of duration and of changing of splinting, of timing and method of work with physiotherapists or occupational therapists, of treatment of neuropathic pain together with an indication of later reconstructive operations.
6. *Comment:* summing up of the lesion, of action taken, of indications for expected outcome, and of later necessary work. The record is factual, avoiding criticism of other colleagues. Facts can speak for themselves.

This record is sent to the referring surgeon and to the family practitioner, and a separate letter is sent to both of them, setting out the time and course and indicating how long the patient must wait to return to normal daily activities. If work with physiotherapists or occupational therapists needs to be done in another unit, then a letter is sent to that person, via the patient's own address. Copies of *all* correspondence go to the family practitioner, who is the "conductor of the orchestra."

NERVE RESECTION AND NEUROLYSIS

Exposure

The surgical exposure must be adequate to secure proximal control of damaged blood vessels, the nerve trunks, and, if need be, the underlying skeleton. There are a number of excellent monographs and texts that discuss such exposure of the peripheral nerves, and the one from Kline, Hudson, and Kim[81] is particularly impressive. One exposure that has been found extremely useful is that developed by Fiolle and Delmas[49] because it is the method of choice for an exposure of the neurovascular axis from the second part of the subclavian artery to the terminal part of the axillary artery. Full display of supraclavicular, retroclavicular, and infraclavicular plexus, of the second part of the subclavian to the terminal axillary artery, and of the axillary and subclavian vein deep to the clavicle is achieved. It is most valuable in fresh cases of laceration or rupture of the great vessels deep to or below the clavicle and in later cases of false aneurysm or for repair of the nerves after primary vascular repair. It is the exposure of choice in the closed traction lesion in infraclavicular rupture of both vessels and nerves.[14] I infiltrate the line of the incision with local anesthetic (levobupivacaine 0.25%) before cutting the skin. Nerves of cutaneous sensation require attention during exposure—patients do not take kindly to unexpected nerve lesions! Exposure of the nerve trunk is more easily done in unscarred tissue planes, proximal and distal to the site of the lesion. Short incisions are long on difficulty.

Resection of Damaged Nerve

The extent of resection of a damaged stump is easy enough in a tidy wound from a knife or from glass. Resection is minimal, 1 mm or less. In closed traction rupture remarkably little resection is needed, sufficient to display an orderly and recognizable architecture of bundles. When the procedure is performed within 72 hours of injury, stimulation of distal stumps can provide information about the level where the nerve is still physiologically active. In the proximal stump it may be possible to demonstrate the point along the nerve where conduction is preserved. In acute closed traction rupture I suggest the following: nerves are resected back until discrete pouting bundles become evident. I have found that the amount of nerve resected will be no more than 1 cm from either end.

Diagnosis is usually easier the earlier the exploration is done. Not only is the field free from scar tissue, but the axons of the distal stump continue to conduct so that bundles with predominantly motor function can be identified. With early operation it is possible to match fascicular arrangements of the stumps; as time goes by, the matching becomes progressively difficult. With delay there is progressive intraneural collagenization.

In late cases, the distinction between motor and sensory fascicles, and the matching of the bundle patterns are more difficult. A most practical contribution comes from Gschmeissner and colleagues,[61] who developed a 2-minute assessment of the stumps by frozen section. Brushart[29] related his experience in histochemical studies of nerve stumps in late repair, using stains for acetylcholinesterase.

Technical Aspects

General anesthesia is usually necessary because of the duration of the operation and because of the need for incisions in other parts of the limb or in another limb for elevation of grafts. Muscle relaxants are avoided, to permit nerve stimulation and recording. When possible, display of the nerves of limbs is more easily done in a bloodless field. One must remember the effect of tourniquet ischemia on conduction, which will have an onset in about 15 minutes and result in temporary complete conduction block within 30 minutes.

These operations are time consuming, often unpredictably so, and it is especially important to protect pressure points at the knee, elbow, and elsewhere. Operations on nerves of the neck carry the risk of air embolism.

Apparatus and Instruments

1. Simple stimulators are available when no more than a straightforward motor response is sought.
2. A more elaborate apparatus is required for simulation and recording from nerve and muscle. The stimulator I prefer is bipolar with platinum electrodes. Recording is from a bipolar electrode on the surface of the nerve fascicle or from a concentric needle electrode in the muscles. For stimulation and recording of sensory evoked potentials from the neck and scalp the settings are as follows: filter, 20 Hz to 2 KHz; time base, 1, 2, 3 or 5 msec; volts/division, 20 to 50 µV; duration, 0.2 single; stimulation intensity, 1 to 50 volts.
3. For magnification I use loupes and the operating microscope. The microscopes are OPMI 6SD FC and OPMI 6 (Karl Zeiss, Oberkochen). The stand is the universal S3B (Karl Zeiss, Oberkochen).
4. In addition to a fine soft tissue set, special requirements include instruments for internal fixation of bone and a fine vascular instrument; De Bakey scissors and forceps are useful for handling nerves.
5. A range of sutures is used: 6-0 and 7-0 nylon on an 8-mm vascular needle is useful for epineurial suture. Finer sutures of 8-0, 9-0, and 10-0 are used for perineurial suture, for nerve transfer, and in grafting.
6. The appropriate needle holders, fine forceps, and scissors for work under the microscope should be available.
7. Fine skin hooks, plastic slings, light clips, and malleable retractors are necessary.
8. Fibrin clot glue[162] was regularly used in the Royal National Orthopaedic Hospital (RNOH) and St. Mary's Hospital until the early 1980s. The raw material then

became unavailable. A commercial product was reintroduced. I now use Tisseel (Immuno, Ltd., Arctic House, Rye Lane, Dunton Green, SevenOaks TN14 5HB-UK). The aprotinin solution must be diluted with sterile water; otherwise there is a risk of inducing fibrosis. The undiluted preparation is reserved for hemostasis. The tip of the needle attached to the prepared syringe should be directed away from the junction between the grafts and stump or the level of nerve repair, or otherwise there may be displacement at the line of repair. A steady gentle pressure is exerted so that a film of the fluid bathes the repair thus sealing it. Fibrin clot glue acts as an envelope around the nerve but offers no resistance to tension. Careful closure of the tissue layers over the nerve repair is important in enhancing the security of the repair, and careful and appropriately maintained splinting of the limb is as essential as after conventional suturing methods. A particularly good review comes from Narakas,[109] who thought his results were improved by 15%.

9. All tissues must be treated gently. The healing of the wound without infection and the recovery of the nerve lesion depends on tissue viability. Avoidance of infection by tender handling of the tissues and accurate hemostasis are more important than antibiotics.

10. The operating field should be kept as free of blood as possible but kept moist by regular saline irrigation.

11. Nerves are handled with extreme care. They should be retracted with very fine skin hooks in the epineurium or with plastic slings. They should not be mobilized over such a length as to impair blood supply.

Neurolysis

There has been confusion about the meaning of this term, most especially in the distinction between "external" and "internal" neurolysis. Frykman and colleagues[52] have greatly helped by clarifying terminology. External neurolysis means to free the nerve from a constricting or a distorting agent, and in this procedure the epineurium is not breached. Decompression of the median nerve at the wrist or at the lower trunk of the brachial plexus in the neurogenic thoracic outlet syndrome are examples of external neurolysis. Extrication of a nerve trunk from within a fracture or a joint or liberation by dissection of a nerve from a bed of scar tissue are other examples. External neurolysis is certainly valuable when it is used to free a nerve from an external distorting or compressing agent so long as that agent will not recur. Removal of a nerve from a bed of scar tissue will succeed only if the nerve can be replaced in a bed free of scar tissue. Even then there is bound to be some regrowth of scar tissue.

Internal neurolysis is the exposure of fascicles by epineurotomy with partial removal of the epineurium and separation of individual fascicles if necessary by the removal of interfascicular scar tissue. For this procedure Frykman and colleagues[52] recommend the term *interfascicular* neurolysis. The procedure involves division and removal of the interfascicular epineurium.

The indications for internal neurolysis are narrow:

1. The separation of intact from damaged fascicles in nerves that have suffered partial transection (neuroma in continuity)

2. Separation of individual fascicle from a nerve for the purposes of transfer as in Oberlin's operation[115]

3. Separation of the intact fascicles during removal of benign but infiltrative tumor

4. During the preparation of a stump for the reception of nerve grafts in delayed repair

Methods of Suture

Much has been written about the relative advantages of perineurial (fascicular) and epineurial sutures. Tupper[152] summarized the general experience that there was no demonstrable difference between the results of epineurial and fascicular sutures. Orgell[120] described a modified fascicular suture, "group fascicular suture," and concluded that epineurial suture was "the technique of choice for most acute nerve lacerations." He pointed out that it was easier and faster and entailed less manipulation of the internal structure of the nerve than did fascicular suture. Kline and Hudson[77] suggest that fascicular suture be reserved for "some oligofascicular nerves."

Millesi[106] thought that the epineurium was the main source of the infiltration of the suture line by fibroblasts. In his technique of fascicular suture, epineurium is resected from the proximal and the distal nerve stumps and the trunk is divided into clusters of bundles. The suture line is shielded by grafts of healthy muscle and fat. Kato and coworkers[75] present a careful study of 51 low median and ulnar nerves repaired by intraneural dissection and electrical fascicular orientation: this combination appeared to improve anatomic matching. Hall[64] gives an exceptionally valuable review providing a neurobiologist's view of nerve repair.

I continue to use bundle suture for primary repair of clean transection of most trunk nerves and expect to use group fascicular suture in delayed cases. I think that repair of the epineurium is important by adding strength to the repair, by sealing off the nerve trunk from adjacent tissue, and by restoring, as much as possible, a gliding plane between the nerve trunks and adjacent tissue.

Much has been written about techniques of nerve suture. I think that the operating surgeon will use his or her own judgment about what is appropriate, always bearing in mind the primary aim in repair, which is to coapt, as accurately as possible, healthy nerve without undue interference of the perineurium and blood supply without undue (nonphysiological) tension.

Protection of the repair by carefully regulated flexion of adjacent joints is essential. The surgeon should use that technique with which he or she is most confident and is most appropriate. Within the general principles set out earlier, I find it hard to say that there is a "right" or a "wrong" way of doing things. As Brushart[30] says, in commenting on the timing of repair, "In peripheral nerve surgery, the first repair must be the best repair possible."

Direct Suture or Graft?

End-to-end suture is preferable as long as the gap after resection is small, little mobilization of the nerve is needed to close that gap, and the repaired nerve lies without tension and without excessive flexion of the adjacent joints. Clark and colleagues[36] demonstrated very clearly the detrimental effects of tension on a nerve repair.

I do not think that end-to-end suture of the nerves of the brachial plexus above the clavicle or of the accessory nerve is ever practicable and prefer always to use interposed grafts even if these are short.

There is an elastic recoil of nerve stumps once the trunk has been severed, and it is very much easier to overcome this without undue tension on the nerve when the operation is performed within days of injury. The longer the delay, the more likely it is that grafting will be required, because the stumps become embedded in scar tissue and because there has been increasing collagenization within the nerve stumps.

Direct observation shows that anterior transposition of such nerves as the ulnar or the radial gains, at most, 3 cm. I found it necessary to use grafts for all delayed repairs of the median nerve in the forearm and for all repairs where 1 cm of the nerve has been lost.

One simple test about the advisability of direct suture of a nerve trunk at the wrist or in the forearm involves passing an epineurial suture of 7-0 nylon, with the wrist flexed to no more than 30 degrees. If this suture will draw the stumps together without tearing the epineurium and without causing blanching of the epineurial vessels, then suture is reasonable. Failing that, grafting is necessary.

I have found it necessary to use graft in all cases of closed traction rupture of the supraclavicular brachial plexus, in virtually all cases of compound nerve injury caused by fracture, and in a great majority of nerves transected in "untidy" wounds. My colleagues and I used grafts in about 80% of our cases, a figure that seems rather high but that may reflect the pattern of cases of nerve injury referred to our unit. Seddon's[127] rather sanguine views of the effect on the blood supply are not confirmed by the later injection studies of Bell and Weddell in 1984[8]; indeed, later clinical experience has shown that it is preferable to bridge a gap by interposition rather than by mobilization.[31]

Direct Suture

I use the terms *primary suture* when the operation is performed within 5 days of injury and *delayed primary suture* when up to 3 weeks has passed. Some resection, of a millimeter or so of the nerve stump, is always necessary after the passage of a few days, even in cases of clean section with a knife or razor. *Secondary suture* is used for repairs done after 3 weeks from injury, and it involves resection of a neuroma proximally and of glioma distally.

The median and ulnar nerves are commonly sectioned at the wrist in "tidy wounds." This is the ideal case for primary suture.

1. The limb is prepared with aqueous antimicrobial solution. Iodine- and alcohol-based preparations are avoided.
2. A tourniquet cuff is placed about the arm, but it is not inflated until the limb has been prepared and exposure can be begun. The cuff remains inflated for the exposure and identification of all divided structures, and ideally for the repair of the flexor tendons, their synovium, and the radial and ulnar artery, but I always release the tourniquet at 1 hour. In all operations the tourniquet is released before nerve repair or graft. Repair of the nerve trunks is done last after repair of other tissues. Bleeding from epineurial vessels along the surface of the median nerve or even within its substance can be troublesome, and if this fails to respond to gentle pressure, then careful use of the bipolar diathermy set at low amplitude is necessary.

3. The incision is extended so that all divided structures can be displayed. In a deep wound with damage to the arteries of the wrist, I open the carpal tunnel to help identify injured structures and to diminish the risk of later compression of the median nerve within the tunnel (Fig. 30-7).
4. The tendons are repaired by core and epitendinous suture. Repair of the synovium around each tendon is, I think, an essential step to diminish adhesions between the tendon and the nerve repair. The nerve must be permitted to glide between synovial layers. Arteries are repaired with interrupted sutures with 8-0 nylon.
5. The adventitial mesoneurium tissue is pushed back from each stump to expose the true epineurium (Fig. 30-8). Matching of the nerve stumps is aided by the varying size of the fascicles and by the orientation of epineurial blood vessels. A sketch of each nerve face helps in planning suture placing. Matched bundles, identified by their size and by their position in the nerve, are drawn together by

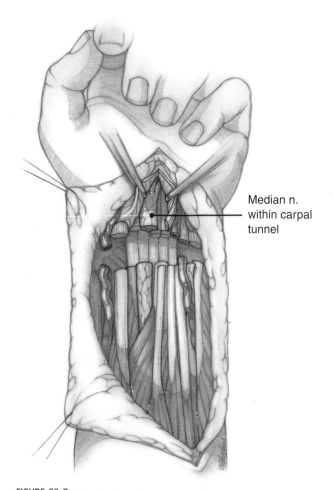

Median n. within carpal tunnel

FIGURE 30-7. Identification is not always easy. I have seen the median nerve sutured to the tendon. Note the extension of the incision so that normal tissues are exposed, enabling accurate definition of what is and what is not damaged.

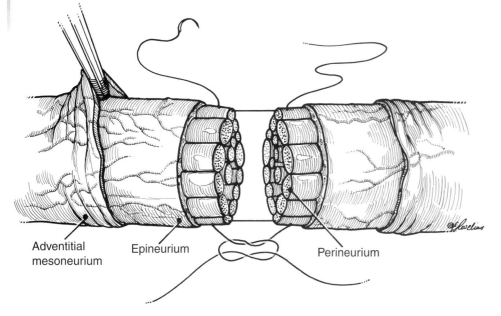

FIGURE 30-8. Note the retraction of the flimsy and loose adventitia exposing the true epineurium and fine sutures passing through the condensed internal epineurium and perineurium of selected bundles.

Adventitial
mesoneurium

Epineurium

Perineurium

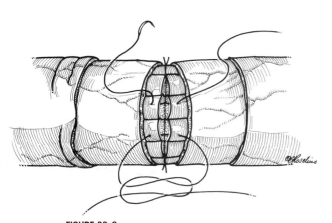

FIGURE 30-9. Completion of the bundle sutures.

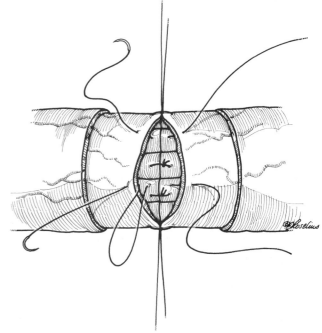

FIGURE 30-10. Finally, sutures of the epineurium proper ensure a strong repair.

perineurial sutures of 10-0 nylon (Fig. 30-9). For the median nerve, between six and eight key bundles will be sutured in this manner to coapt the nerve faces as accurately as possible. The repair is then completed by passing sutures of 9-0 nylon through the perineurium and epineurium (Fig. 30-10). The nerve can be rotated on a saline-soaked dental swab, first from one side and then from the other so that the whole circumference of the nerve is accessible. By this method between 18 and 25 sutures are necessary to repair the adult median nerve at the wrist.

Epineurial Repair

Orientation of the bundles is achieved as well as is possible, and the epineurium is united with two lateral sutures of 8-0 nylon, the ends of which are left long. The repair of the anterior face is completed with three or four more sutures of 7-0 nylon. The nerve is then rotated by manipulation of the lateral sutures so that the posterior epineurium can be united.

It is in the fresh wound that the disadvantages of epineurial repair are best shown. The bundles may twist around within the epineurium.

Delayed Suture

It is preferable to raise a flap rather than reopen the old scar (Fig. 30-11).

There will be considerable thickening of the external epineurium and of the perifascicular epineurium. This layer is now robust enough to take a suture. The mobility of the

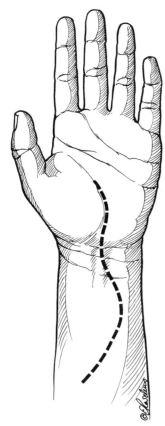

FIGURE 30-11. Transverse scar at the crease overlies divided median nerve. The incision is placed to allow elevation of a flap over the nerve.

bundles of the fascicles within the epineurium is very much less.

The nerve may have formed two bulbs, separated by a gap, or one bulb, a neuroma "in continuity" (Fig. 30-12).

1. The first stage of the operation requires resection of the terminal bulbs until a recognizable pattern of healthy pouting fascicles is reached. The temptation to resect as little as possible so to minimize the gap between the prepared nerve face must be resisted. Palpation of the nerve stump is very helpful in determining the fibrous or firm scarred segment from the softer, more pliable, and

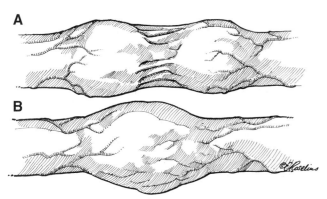

FIGURE 30-12. The nerve lesion may present as double bulbs, neuroma proximally and glioma distally (**A**) or as a neuroma "in continuity" (**B**).

less fibrosed part. I use a fresh scalpel blade and section at 2- to 3-mm intervals until a soft nerve face with recognizable bundle architecture is reached.

2. A trial of drawing the two stumps together with 6-0 or 7-0 nylon is done, with elbow extended and wrist in neutral.

3. Once the nerve faces have been prepared, a sketch of the surfaces is useful as a memory aid. Adventitia, and external epineurium, should be trimmed away. The ideal placing for the suture is through the internal epineurium about individual fascicles or bundles of fascicles. Sutures of 8-0 nylon are used (Fig. 30-13).

I think that the technical aspects of delayed or secondary suture are somewhat easier than primary suture.

Use of Fibrin Clot Glue in Suturing

I modify the technique of suture when using fibrin clot glue. Fewer sutures are used. The most important are those that draw together, as accurately as possible, the larger bundles, securing as best as one can topographic orientation. Some six or eight of the larger bundles will be drawn together in this manner, and there will then be another six or so epineurial sutures used to complete the repair. Fibrin clot glue is then applied, avoiding injection of the fluid into the suture line.

Preparation of the Nerve Bed

Preparation of the bed for the nerve repair is of the utmost importance. The nerve must not be left to lie against a naked tendon; synovium must be drawn together. Similarly, lacerated muscle belly is a very unfavorable bed for a nerve repair, and rotation of either adjacent synovium or undamaged fat should be done.

Closure and Postoperative Care

A patient and careful assistant is invaluable at this stage—to see an elegant repair torn apart by careless handling of the limb is, to say the least, disheartening!

1. Local anesthetic (levobupivacaine 0.5%) instilled around the proximal, median, and ulnar stumps will do much to ease postoperative pain. I use antibiotics for prolonged operations or where arterial repair has been done, giving a bolus dose of cefuroxime, 750 mg. The skin is sutured with interrupted sutures.

2. The elbow, the wrist, and the joints of the hand must now be restricted so that the flexor tendon and the nerve repairs are protected. Extremes of joint positioning must be avoided.

3. The splint used will hold the elbow to 90 degrees of flexion, the wrist at between 30 and 40 degrees of flexion, the metacarpophalangeal (MCP) joints at about 70 degrees of flexion, and the proximal interphalangeal (PIP) joints at no more than 30 degrees of flexion. The dorsal splint extends to the tips of the fingers and the palmar splint to the PIP joints only. The splints are bandaged so that there is restriction but not rigid immobilization. Gentle, active flexion of the fingers and the

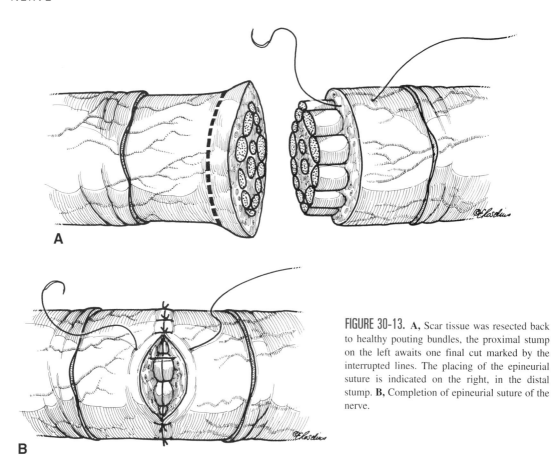

FIGURE 30-13. **A,** Scar tissue was resected back to healthy pouting bundles, the proximal stump on the left awaits one final cut marked by the interrupted lines. The placing of the epineurial suture is indicated on the right, in the distal stump. **B,** Completion of epineurial suture of the nerve.

thumb is encouraged from the outset. The arm is supported in a sling, but there should be encouragement of gentle active lateral rotation and of elevation of the shoulder to 90 degrees from the first postoperative day.

4. At 3 weeks the splints and the sutures are removed.
5. The next splint does not restrict the elbow. The wrist is splinted to prevent extension beyond 20 degrees. The dorsal hood, which again extends to the tips of the fingers, blocks the MCP joints to 30 degrees of flexion and the PIP joints to 30 degrees of flexion. Increasingly, vigorous active flexion of the fingers and the thumb is now permitted and gentle active flexion at the wrist is also encouraged within the confines of the splint, bandaged as it is to the forearm and hand. In direct sutures of nerves in the elbow region a hinged splint is applied at 3 weeks from operation. This permits active flexion but blocks extension. The range of permitted movement is increased at weekly intervals by adjusting the hinge.
6. By 6 weeks, splints are discarded and vigorous active flexion work against resistance is introduced. Now, gentle passive stretching work can be introduced for the fingers and the thumb.
7. Some protection must be given to the suture line of the nerve for a minimum of 6 weeks, and the key to this is to modify the range of excursion of the wrist joint. It is also important, however, to encourage gentle, early active movements within the confines of the splint and the bandages to diminish the risk of the nerve becoming rigidly embedded within scar tissue.

NERVE GRAFTING

Choice of Graft

After an extensive analysis of fascicle arrangement, connective tissue content, and nerve fiber size, Sunderland[140] concluded that "the two outstanding (choices for nerve graft) are the superficial radial and the sural nerve. Next in order of suitability are in turn the medial cutaneous nerve of forearm, the lateral cutaneous nerve of the forearm and the lateral cutaneous nerve of the thigh, but these have only slender claims to selection." The superficial radial nerve should never be used unless the parent nerve is irreparably damaged. We reserve it for cases of avulsion of the fifth and the sixth cervical nerves or in irreparable high injuries of the posterior cord or radial nerve. I agree with Magalon and colleagues,[98] who expose the sural nerve through a long posterior midline incision because of the variability in communication with branches of the common peroneal nerve. They showed that neural tissue amounted to less than 30% of the total surface of the nerve and that internal topographic arrangement of fascicles varied considerably along the course of the nerve. Narakas[112] described the medial cutaneous nerve of forearm. The interconnections between the medical cutaneous nerve of the forearm and the medial cutaneous nerve of arm in the axilla call for careful dissection.

I prefer to use grafts from the damaged upper limb wherever possible. When harvesting the sural nerve, the patient may be placed prone, although I prefer that an assistant holds one leg up, with the patient supine.

The *sural nerve* is approached through a posterior midline longitudinal incision, preserving the short saphenous veins. The nerve is best identified at the lateral malleolus and then traced back as it lies lateral to the short saphenous vein to where it perforates the deep fascia of the leg, generally at the junction of the upper two thirds and the lower one third of the limb. Gentle traction on the nerve here with a phrenic hook will identify the branches of the nerve, which can be cut cleanly with fine vascular scissors at equivalent level. The nerve can now be demonstrated where it arises from the tibial nerve in the popliteal fossa, and gentle traction here will confirm whether there is a communicating branch coming down from the common peroneal nerve (Fig. 30-14). It is possible to deliver the nerve into the popliteal fossa, which has the advantage of stripping it of much of its adventitia. Avoid traction on the tibial or common peroneal nerves! Respect the short saphenous vein; it may be needed later.

The *medial cutaneous nerve* requires a longitudinal exposure and is best identified lying adjacent to the axillary vein within the brachial sheath. The nerve is picked up with a light nerve hook and traced proximally into the axilla, avoiding damage to adjacent branches of the medial cutaneous nerve of the arm. In the middle part of the arm the medial cutaneous nerve divides into an anterior and a posterior branch. It perforates the deep fascia shortly after this. Both of the divisions are used and traced down to the level of the elbow (Fig. 30-15). About 25 cm of nerve can be obtained. Do not confuse the medial cutaneous nerve with the ulnar nerve! Stimulate it if you are in doubt.

The *superficial radial nerve* is delivered through separate incisions—first at the wrist, identifying the trunk where it emerges from deep to brachioradialis, following the branches down, and dividing them at equivalent levels. The radial trunk is displayed between brachioradialis and brachialis. The superficial radial nerve component is identified by light traction on the nerve, which enables its delivery into the elbow wound, a maneuver that has the advantage of stripping it of much of its adventitia. Twenty-five to 30 cm of nerve is available. Do not confuse it with the posterior interosseous nerve! Use gentle traction.

The *lateral cutaneous nerve* of the forearm is used when the musculocutaneous nerve is irretrievably damaged, when repair of that nerve is confined to restoration of elbow flexion, or when a short length of graft is needed for an adjacent major nerve. The nerve passes just lateral to the biceps tendon, and it can be displayed in the plane between the biceps and brachialis in the lower part of the arm. About 15 cm of useful nerve can be retrieved.

The trunk to be grafted is prepared. It is extremely important that the bed into which the grafts must lie is as healthy as possible. Unscarred synovium, or fat, is best—"raw" muscle is not a good bed; bone or metal implants are hopeless.

The gap between the nerve faces is measured with the elbow extended and the wrist in neutral. The length of the graft must exceed this by at least 15% because of the inevitable shrinking of the prepared graft from elastic recoil.

At all times the graft is handled with care and kept in a blood-stained swab or one soaked with lactated Ringer's solution. Adventitia is cleared by gentle dissection with a fresh scalpel or microscissors: nerves exposed for grafting must be handled as tenderly as any other nerve.

The grafts are placed to permit as accurate topographic matching as possible. The greater the defect in the nerve trunk, the more difficult this will be. One of the advantages of primary grafting in an acute injury is that nerve stimulation enables some understanding of the orientation of bundles distally, by observing muscular response (Fig. 30-16).

The grafts are cut into lengths with either a fresh scalpel blade or a pair of vascular scissors. Two to three millimeters at the end of the graft must be scrupulously cleared of adventitia and of superficial epineurium, so that fascicles protrude. The grafts are sewn into place, and because the individual strands of graft are likely to be around the same size as an individual fascicle or a bundle of fascicles, the

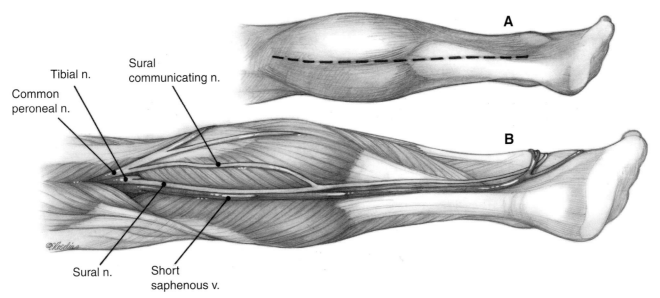

FIGURE 30-14. This shows the course of the sural nerve. It is easier to identify this nerve in the distal part of the wound just lateral to the Achilles tendon. The communicating branch arising from the common peroneal nerve is very variable but is usually present.

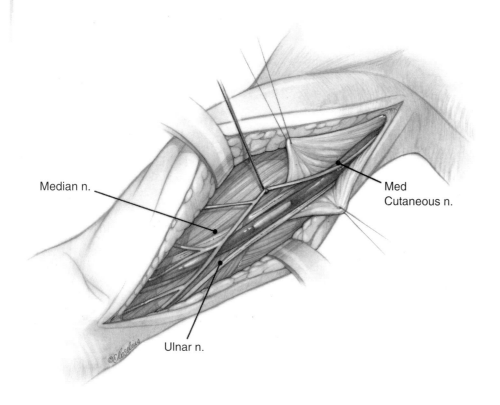

Median n.

Med
Cutaneous n.

Ulnar n.

FIGURE 30-15. The medial cutaneous nerve of the forearm is in close relation to the axillary and brachial vein. It must not be confused with the ulnar nerve!

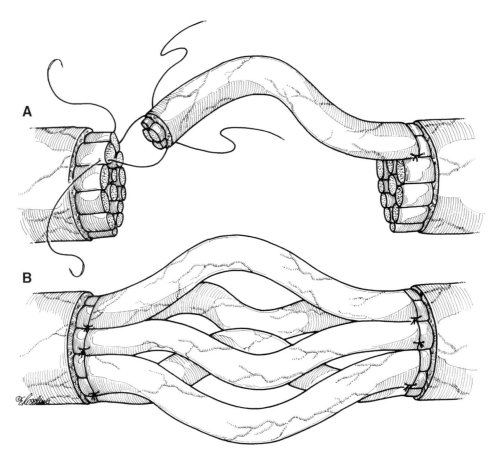

A

B

FIGURE 30-16. A and **B,** Suturing of grafts. Note that they lie really quite loosely. Suture is passed through the epineurium of the graft and through the perineurium and condensed internal epineurium about the individual bundles of the nerve trunk itself.

suture joins epineurium of the graft to perineurium of the bundle. Two lateral sutures of 9-0 nylon are used for each graft. When a large number of grafts need to be done it is possible to use two or three grafts as a foundation for the others. As much as possible of each graft is led from a fascicle to a matching fascicle in the other stump. It is very important once the repair has been completed at both ends to inspect the grafts and the suture lines to make certain that one or other junction line has not been disturbed.

Further security for the grafts can be provided by using tiny pieces of absorbable sponge to act as a buttress while grafts are being placed and sutured. In many situations of repair of deep seated nerves at the elbow or in the proximal forearm, careful apposition of the overlying muscle planes enfolds the grafts and undoubtedly enhances the security of the arrangement but at the same time tends to congregate them into one mass.

Millesi[106] begins his dissection of the fascicle roots in the healthy nerve above and below the lesion and makes the section at the point at which each group loses its healthy appearance. In the distal stump, the fascicle groups are traced back from the point of identification of their destination to the level just distal to the lesion. Fascicular patterns of distal and proximal stumps are matched, and individual grafts are used to unite the fascicular group. Millesi resects fascicular groups at different levels and then uses very fine sutures through interfascicular epineurium or perineurium for coaptation, resulting in grafts interdigitating with the fascicles of the stump. Fryckman and Cally[53] discussed the use of interfascicular grafting and found results were better than those of direct suture.

Seddon's[128] term *cable grafting* is misleading: It did not imply that segments of graft were closely bundled up to replace the lost trunk nerve; in practice they were spread about across healthy unscarred tissue to ensure their prompt revascularization.

Postoperative Care

One of the main principles in grafting is that tension on the nerve repair is avoided and for this reason splinting need not be so prolonged as it is after suture of the nerve. For grafting of the median and the ulnar nerve at the wrist the forearm and hand will be splinted as for primary suture for the first 3 weeks. At that time, the fingers and the thumb will be set free and a simple "door stop" plaster of Paris splint is applied that blocks extension of the wrist beyond 30 degrees but permits full flexion. The extension block splint is discarded at 6 weeks from the day of operation.

OTHER METHODS OF GRAFTING AND ALTERNATIVE METHODS OF REPAIR

For many years surgeons have endeavored to improve the results of grafting or even to replace nerve by alternative material. Some methods, grounded in considerable experimental work, have gone as far as careful clinical studies.

The Vascularized Nerve Graft

Survival of a graft depends on its revascularization. Seddon[128] summarized the work done by himself and his colleagues in the 1940s and 1950s in which studies were made of the survival and the usefulness of dispensable trunk nerves and concluded "there is a critical diameter for survival of a graft taken from normal nerve: the radial nerve falls within the limit, the common peroneal nerve beyond it." Pedicle grafting was introduced to enhance the viability of such trunk nerves as the ulnar.[138] This led to the development of the free vascularized ulnar nerve, supplied by the ulnar vessels by Jamieson and Bonney in the 1970s and reported by them in 1984.[24] Later the ulnar nerve was used based on ulnar collateral vessels.[20,103,147] My colleagues and I used this in 68 cases of traction injury to the supraclavicular brachial plexus when the eighth cervical and the first thoracic nerve had been avulsed from the spinal cord so that the prognosis for ulnar nerve function was hopeless. We aimed to restore useful function within the hand by reinnervation of the median nerve. Potentially useful hand function was regained in three cases; two were in young adults operated on within 4 days of injury and one was in a 3-year-old child operated on at 8 weeks from injury. Our aim only rarely was achieved.

CRITICAL POINTS: NERVE GRAFTING

- Prepare the whole limb for access to grafts.
- Use the tourniquet for as short a time as possible
- Exposures must be adequate.
- It should be possible to repair the radial and ulnar artery and the flexor tendons with the tourniquet in place.
- Gliding planes *must* be restored; the synovium should be repaired about the tendons and between the tendons and the nerve.
- Nerve repair should always be done after release of the tourniquet.
- Direct suture is difficult in the arm and probably impossible above the collar bone, or when more than about 1 cm of the nerve trunk has been lost. The situation for the great nerves in the lower limb is different because of the paucity of available graft.
- One can never have too much graft. Allow for retraction of the repaired nerves and of the graft itself. The graft should be cut in the wound, allowing 15% to 20% of excess, after laying the whole graft loosely in place.
- Prolonged and careful protection of nerve repair is important, and this will be about 6 weeks in the upper limb and for as long as 12 weeks in the lower limb.
- The clinician must be aware constantly of the risks of fixed deformity, of disuse atrophy, and of neuropathic pain.
- The best rehabilitation is return to normal life and activity.

The first free vascularized nerve graft was described by Taylor and Ham in 1976.[145] The subject is thoroughly reviewed by Breidenbach,[26] Gilbert,[55] Doi and associates,[45] and Frey and Gruber.[50]

The evidence accumulated is not decisively in favor of the vascularized nerve graft, although there may be indications when the gap is a long one and when the bed is particularly badly scarred. We were not able to demonstrate an overwhelming improvement in results with the vascularized ulnar nerve graft compared with lesions of the brachial plexus repaired by cutaneous nerve grafts.

Freeze-Thawed Muscle Graft

Experimental and clinical work on the use of freeze-thawed muscle grafts is provided by Gatusso and colleagues[54] and Lawson and Glasby.[88]

The technique for a long defect in large trunk nerves has not, on the whole, been met with the anticipated recovery of function. A definitive review of axonal regeneration through acellular muscle graft comes from Hall.[65]

Entubulation

There was considerable interest in the use of synthetic tubes or vein grafts for the repair of nerves during World War I, and the relative failure of these methods probably brought about a degree of prejudice against the use of nerve grafting. In 1997, Lundborg and associates[94] presented significant work in a prospective randomized trial comparing silicone entubulation and suture of median and of ulnar nerves in 18 patients. Seven nerves were sutured; in 11 others, the nerve stumps were placed within a silicone tube. Each nerve stump was sutured within the tube with one fine suture, leaving a gap of 3 to 4 mm. Assessment of recovery was done with very great care. No significant difference in outcome between the two groups could be demonstrated.

The possible advantages from placing of nerve stumps within a silicone tube is that a chamber is provided separate from surrounding tissues so that there may be a local accumulation of neurotrophic factors, longitudinal orientation of fibrin matrix within the tube, and the possibility that regenerating axons are better guided into distal Schwann tubes. In one case the tube was removed at 11 weeks and these workers relate "it was found that the former empty space was now occupied by newly formed nerve tissue in direct continuity with the proximal and distal nerve ends. There was macroscopically spontaneous reconstitution of the original nerve trunk. It was not possible to define the exact level of the previous nerve injury."

This is impressive work and offers a potential alternative to nerve suture and possibly to short grafts. I have no personal experience with this method.

Nerve Transfer

The idea of transferring an uninjured nerve to the distal stump of an injured nerve is not new. Narakas[110,111] describes early work, pointing out that the principles for operations now performed were recognized decades ago. The literature on this subject is extensive and is well summarized by Narakas and his colleagues.[2-4] Oberlin[115] pioneered and suc-

cessfully employed one or two fascicles of the ulnar nerve to reinnervate the motor branch of the biceps in brachial plexus palsies, with outstanding restoration of muscle strength. Gu and his colleagues[62] have used the contralateral seventh cervical nerve to reinnervate the limb after complete lesion of the brachial plexus. I was able to review some of Professor Gu's patients in Shanghai, and the results in one of these in particular were extremely impressive. Chen and Gu[35] confirmed that the contralateral seventh cervical nerve was a more effective donor than the phrenic nerve and that the vascularized ulnar nerve graft was superior to a nonvascularized graft as an interposed graft between the donor C7 and the recipient trunk within the damaged limb.

My colleagues' and my experience with 403 nerve transfers done between 1986 and 1992 is summarized elsewhere.[15]

I have little experience of nerve transfer within the distal upper limb apart from some cases of transfer of the dorsal branch of the ulnar cutaneous nerve onto the median nerve for restoration of sensation. Battiston and Blanzetta[7] reported seven cases of unfavorable high ulnar nerve palsies treated by transfer of palmar cutaneous branch of the median and of the anterior interosseous nerve before it entered the quadratus into the ulnar nerve at the wrist. Good results were achieved in six. Ozkan and coworkers[121] relate impressive results from transfer of digital nerves in irreparable median or ulnar nerve lesions. Eighteen of 20 patients experienced improvement after transferring nerves from inner to outer digits: sensory retraining was used.

Direct Muscular Neurotization

Brunelli and Monini[27] showed that a nerve avulsed from muscle could be implanted back into that muscle and that it could secure reinnervation with a development of new end plates. This method works in clinical practice. I have used it in cases of avulsion of the circumflex nerve from the deltoid muscle and for avulsion of the musculocutaneous nerve from the elbow flexor muscles. I am unaware of clinical applications for this technique within the forearm and hand.

Allograft

Mackinnon[97] revitalized the use of allografts in a case of extensive loss of the tibial nerve in a 12-year-old boy. A 20-cm gap was bridged by eight allografts. Immunosuppression was with cyclosporine and prednisone and continued for over 4 months. Mackinnon gives a qualified recommendation: "in the carefully selected patient with an otherwise irreparable nerve injury, consideration for nerve transplantation should be given."

RECOVERY AFTER REPAIR

The quality of recovery after repair depends chiefly on the number of axons reaching their correct targets and on the later development and myelination of those axons. Some factors influencing this process of regeneration include the following:

- Delay between injury and repair
- The quality of the apposed nerve ends

- The quality and accuracy of fascicular matching
- The degree of damage to the nerve ends during the operation of repair
- The length of gap after resection of damaged nerve stumps
- The number of channels provided by the interposed graft for regenerating columns
- The extent of fibroblastic infiltration of the stumps and of the interposed graft
- The rate of regeneration. The speed of axonal regeneration is variable and is estimated to be about 1 mm a day, which corresponds to the rate of slow transport of the neurofilament protein. That rate is substantially faster in children, and it is almost certainly faster after primary than after secondary repair.[21] Lundborg[93] suggested that regeneration is faster proximally than distally. I suggest a rate of 2 mm/day after suture of clean wounds of nerves in the infraclavicular fossa and in the proximal part of the lower limb. Such wounds are nearer to the nerve cell than are more distal injuries.

Lundborg[90] reviews the symbiosis between experimental and clinical studies in a balanced and informative manner.

Assessment of Recovery of Function

Seddon[129] developed a system for measurement of outcome that classified results of nerve repair as good, fair, poor, and bad, based on the Medical Research Council (MRC) system. Seddon and his colleagues fully recognized the defects and limitations of the MRC system, but it has stood the test of time. My colleagues and I have simplified this into good, fair, and poor (Tables 30-4 and 30-5).[16] In some nerves, muscular function is a good deal more important than recovery of sensation. For the spinal accessory, suprascapular, axillary, musculocutaneous, and radial nerves little significance is attached to the extent of recovery of cutaneous sensation except when recovery was complicated by severe pain (in this case, the result is considered poor regardless of motor return). Recovery of sensation has been given equal importance to muscle function in the description of results of median and ulnar nerves: indeed it is probable that sensibility is the most important function of the median nerve. Kline and Hudson[79] described the Louisiana State University Medical Center grading system for motor and sensory function and for the whole nerve. This valuable method is based on great clinical experience.

Rosen and Lundborg[122,123] refined a detailed method of describing outcome after repair of median and ulnar nerves at the wrist or in the distal forearm. They describe three "domains" of function: sensory, motor, and pain/discomfort. The last domain refers to hypersensitivity and cold intolerance. A total score is developed in this system, which correlated well with the patient's own estimate of global function and also with the MRC sensory system.

Quantitative sensory and autonomic testing provides information about small myelinated and unmyelinated nerve fibers as well as large fiber function. These methods were used to demonstrate remarkable aspects of restoration of cutaneous sensation in children suffering particularly severe injuries of the brachial plexus at birth.[5]

Table 30-4
THE MEDICAL RESEARCH COUNCIL SYSTEM

Motor Recovery	
M0	No contraction
M1	Return of perceptible contraction in the proximal muscles
M2	Return of perceptible contraction in both proximal and distal muscles
M3	Return of perceptible contraction in both proximal and distal muscles of such degree that all *important* muscles are sufficiently powerful to act against resistance
M4	Return of function as in stage 3 with the addition that all *synergic* and independent movements are possible
M5	Complete recovery

Sensory Recovery	
S0	Absence of sensibility in the *autonomous area*
S1	Recovery of deep cutaneous pain sensibility within the *autonomous area* of the nerve
S2	Return of some degree of cutaneous pain and tactile sensibility within the autonomous area
S3	Return of some degree of superficial cutaneous pain and tactile sensibility within the *autonomous area* with disappearance of any previous overreaction
S3+	Return of sensibility as in stage 3 with the addition that there is some recovery of two-point discrimination within the *autonomous area*
S4	Complete recovery

From Results. *In* Birch R, Bonney G, Wynn Parry CB: Surgical Disorders of the Peripheral Nerves. London, Churchill Livingstone, 1998.

Table 30-5
GRADING OF RESULTS

Motor Recovery	Sensory Recovery
M4 or better	Good
M3	Fair
M2	Poor
M1 and 0	Bad
S4 (normal) or S3+	Good
S3	Fair
S2	Poor
S1 and 0	Bad

Note: The Peripheral Nerve Injury Unit of the Royal National Orthopaedic Hospital groups "poor" and "bad" together. Rarely the grade "excellent" is used for results where function is almost indistinguishable from normal.

From Results. *In* Birch R, Bonney G, Wynn Parry CB: Surgical Disorders of the Peripheral Nerves. London, Churchill Livingstone, 1998.

Factors in Prognosis

The MRC Special Report[102] defined a number of factors that determine outcome after repair of nerves. Five of these are particularly important: age, level of lesion, the nature of the nerve injury, delay from injury to repair, and the cause of the injury.

Age

A properly performed urgent repair of median and ulnar nerves at the wrist will be followed by function indistinguishable from normal in infancy or young children, a result scarcely seen in adults. However, children are not at all immune from the deleterious effect of delay nor from a depression of regeneration in violent proximal injuries. Furthermore, the risk of progressive deformity in the growing limb from uncorrected muscular imbalance can be extremely severe.

Level of Lesion

The effect of level of injury is most evident in those nerves of longest course—the radial, median, and ulnar. A properly executed urgent repair of the ulnar nerve at the wrist will usually result in useful function within the small muscles of the hand, but this is exceptional even in excellent primary sutures for tidy wounds of the ulnar nerve in the axilla. Repair of the posterior interosseous nerve is usually successful in restoring extension of fingers and thumb, but this is unusual after repair of the radial nerve proximal to the spiral groove. However, urgent repair of stab wounds or even of closed traction ruptures of C5, C6, and C7 or of the upper and middle trunks often achieves results as good as or even better than those seen after repair of combined injuries to the terminal nerve branches of the plexus in more distal lesions.

Nature of the Nerve Injury

There is no such thing as a pure motor or pure sensory peripheral nerve. The palmar digital cutaneous nerves contain within them many postganglionic sympathetic efferent fibers. Nerves, such as the spinal accessory or the suprascapular, which have no cutaneous innervation contain within them large numbers of afferent fibers. In the spinal accessory nerve these are nociceptors. In the suprascapular nerve they are afferent fibers from muscle spindles and from joint structures. However, it is the case that nerves innervating one or two muscles (the accessory, nerve to serratus anterior, musculocutaneous) fare better than those with extensive territories of cutaneous and muscle innervation, such as the median, radial, and ulnar. The ill reputation of the superficial radial and the medial cutaneous nerve of forearm is well deserved. Accidental damage to these nerves, especially in their terminal parts, regularly produces severe neuropathic pain.

Delay From Injury to Repair

The evidence for the harmfulness of delay is overwhelming. The long and wearisome debate about the timing of nerve repair should be assigned to the dustbin of history. The passage of every week sees progressive atrophy of target tissues distally and a progressive deterioration of the capacity within the central nervous system for regeneration. Local changes include retraction of the divided nerve stumps, from elastic recoil and increasing fibrosis within those stumps so that the gap between healthy nerve faces increases.

Omer[118] confirmed the findings of Woodhall and Beebe[159]: "delay in suture induces a loss of, on average, about 1% of maximal performance for every six days of delay."

The Cause of Injury

There are two aspects to this. First, one must consider the extent of damage to the nerve and loss of neural substance. The length of the defect between nerve stumps is a material factor in outcome after repair. The outlook for a nerve repaired after the extensive destruction of a close-range shotgun blast or deep burn is far worse than after severance by knife. The second factor to consider is the extent of injury to the tissues of the limb as a whole. Neglected peripheral ischemia is the most serious. It is almost inconceivable that a complacent attitude is still taken, from time to time, to the treatment of the pulseless upper or lower limb.

CRITICAL POINTS: PROGNOSIS

- The single most important factor in prognosis after injury to a nerve is the violence of that injury and the extent of the damage to the limb as a whole.
- Associated arterial injury is particularly important.
- The most important factor relating to prognosis that is within the control of the clinician is delay between injury and repair.

Results

I shall describe results for the median, the ulnar, the radial, and the digital nerves. Because these were primarily acute low median and ulnar injuries with short reinnervation distances, an "excellent" category is included for near-normal function and sensation (Table 30-6).

The Median and Ulnar Nerves

Four factors are particularly striking for the three great trunk nerves: age, level of injury, the cause of injury, and the delay between injury and repair. Birch and Raji[21] discussed the results of 108 repairs of median and ulnar nerves injured in tidy wounds in patients ranging in age from 15 to 55 years. Results were clearly better after primary repair, although there were rather more arterial, tendon, and muscle injuries in these patients. Tables 30-7 and 30-8 set out the results for 299 median and ulnar nerve repairs done between 1977 and 1999. There is no significant difference between the delayed suture and the delayed grafts. The gap after resection was certainly greater in the latter, suggesting that these nerve injuries were somewhat more severe.

A less demanding system of assessment is used for repair of nerves damaged in the axilla and arm, because the results after repair of high median and ulnar nerve lesions are, on the whole, much more modest than those after distal repairs.

Table 30-6

METHODS OF GRADING RESULTS OF MEDIAN AND ULNAR NERVES

Grade	Motor	Sensory	Equivalent on Seddon's Grading
Excellent	Power MRC 5 No wasting or deformity No trophic changes	Function indistinguishable from normal hand. Good stereognosis, no hypersensitivity. Two-point discrimination equivalent to uninjured digits.	Good M5, S4
Good	Power MRC 4 to 5. Abolition of paralytic deformity Minimal pulp wasting	Accurate speedy localization. Can recognize texture or objects. Minor cold sensitivity and hypersensitivity. Two-point discrimination < 8 mm at tips of fingers.	Good M5, S3+
Fair	MRC 3 or more. Some sweating. Pulp wasted	Accurate localization to digit. No stereognosis. Two-point discrimination > 8 mm. Significant cold sensitivity and hypersensitivity.	Fair M3, S3
Poor and bad	MRC 3 or less. No sweating, trophic changes	No sensation or severe cold sensitivity and hypersensitivity.	Bad M1 or S2 or less

From Birch R, Raji A: Repair of median and ulnar nerves. J Bone Joint Surg Br 73:154-157, 1991.

Table 30-7

REPAIR OF 165 ULNAR NERVES IN ADULTS (AGE 16 TO 65 YEARS) IN TIDY WOUNDS FROM DISTAL WRIST CREASE TO ELBOW CREASE

	Primary Repair	Delayed Suture	Graft	Total
Excellent	8	1	2	11
Good	26	7	25	58
Fair	14	19	30	63
Poor or bad	2	10	21	33
Total	50	37	78	165

Note: All but one of the excellent results were seen in patients aged 21 or younger.

Table 30-8

REPAIR OF 134 MEDIAN NERVES IN ADULTS (AGE 16 TO 65 YEARS) IN TIDY WOUNDS FROM DISTAL WRIST CREASE TO ELBOW CREASE

	Primary Repair	Delayed Suture	Graft	Total
Excellent	5	1	0	6
Good	29	11	13	53
Fair	14	16	27	57
Poor or bad	3	8	7	18
Total	51	36	47	

Note: Five of the six excellent results were seen in patients aged 21 or younger.

Using the strict criteria of Birch and Raji's original assessment, scarcely any of the high median and ulnar repairs could be graded as good, save for a few occurring in children or where repair was done of clean transections within 48 hours of injury. The method of assessment is set out in Table 30-9, and the results of 216 median and ulnar nerve repairs in the axilla and arm in adults and in children are set out in Tables 30-10 and 30-11.

Cavanagh[33] analyzed results of the complex infraclavicular injury in which several nerve trunks were ruptured or torn by knife or missile and complicated by rupture of the axillary artery in over one third of cases. Results in this particular serious group of injuries were generally poor. "Useful" function was restored in about one third of cases of closed traction ruptures. Only 1 of 22 cases of median and ulnar nerves achieved a good result in the delayed repair group. Results were particularly poor when there was a two-level lesion with associated damage to the supraclavicular brachial plexus: they were better in open wounds, especially in tidy wounds. In a number of cases where a ruptured artery had not been repaired, or when a vascular prosthesis had been used, nerve repair was abandoned so poor were the tissues. The harmful effect of delay is particularly evident in this group.

Cooney[38] provides a very careful review of six series totaling over 400 cases of repair of median nerve. Recovery of muscle to M3 to M4 (useful) ranged from 40% to 90% within the series; recovery of sensation from S2+ to S4 (useful or good) ranged from 53% to 100%. Cooney comments "whilst thenar motor strength is regained in 50% of patients, recovery of two point discrimination is not generally obtained."

Strickland[139] reviewed eight series totaling over 500 cases of repair of ulnar nerves and found that functional motor recovery was noted in 35% of cases (M4) and functional sensory recovery in 30% to 68% (S3).

Vastamaki and colleagues[154] found useful results in 52% of 110 cases of secondary microsurgical repair of the ulnar

Table 30-9

GRADING OF RESULTS IN HIGH MEDIAN AND ULNAR NERVE REPAIR

	Median
Good	Long flexor muscles MRC 4 or better Localization to digit, without hypersensitivity Return of sweating
Fair	Long flexor muscles MRC 3 or 3+ "Protective sensation"; moderate or no hypersensitivity Sweating diminished or absent
Poor or bad	Long flexor muscles MRC 2 or less "Protective sensation" but severe hypersensitivity *or* no sensation

	Ulnar
Good	FCU and FDP little and ring MRC 4 or better Intrinsic muscles MRC 2 or better Localization to little and ring fingers; no hypersensitivity Return of sweating
Fair	FCU and FDP little and ring fingers MRC 3 or 3+ No intrinsic muscle function "Protective" sensation little and ring fingers Moderate hypersensitivity Little or no sweating
Poor or bad	FCU and FDP little and ring fingers MRC 2 No intrinsic muscle function "Protective" sensation with severe hypersensitivity *or* no sensation No sweating

From Birch R, Bonney G, Wynn Parry CB: Surgical Disorders of the Peripheral Nerves. London, Churchill Livingstone, 1998.

nerve and demonstrated four unfavorable factors: age, width of contusion, delay, and level.

The same unit found excellent or good results in 49% of 132 late repairs of the median nerve.[74] The outcome was better in the 21 children: it was worse in relation to the length of lesion, delay before repair, and level of lesion.

Table 30-10

RESULTS IN 117 REPAIRS BY CAUSE IN ADULTS AND CHILDREN OF MEDIAN NERVE: INFRACLAVICULAR—AXILLA—ARM

	Tidy	Untidy	Traction	Total
Good	8	6	3	17
Fair	10	16	22	48
Poor	4	15	33	52
Total	22	37	58	117

Note: This includes 28 repairs of either lateral or medial root of nerve in the axilla: 13 of the 17 good results followed repair within 5 days of injury and 4 of them were in children.

Table 30-11

RESULTS OF 99 REPAIRS BY CAUSE IN ADULTS AND CHILDREN OF ULNAR NERVE OR MEDIAL CORD: INFRACLAVICULAR—AXILLA—ARM

	Open	Untidy	Traction	Total
Good	5	5	0	10
Fair	7	16	24	47
Poor	3	14	25	42
Total	15	35	49	99

Note: Seven of the good results followed repair within 48 hours of injury, three in children. Results of repair with a delay of 3 months or more were almost all poor in the untidy and traction group.

Barrios and coworkers[6] followed 44 secondary repairs of ulnar nerves showing a clear deterioration with delay and severity of associated injury. Their nine patients did well.

Trevett and associates[151] gave clear indications for supplementary tendon transfers in their study of 50 patients with ulnar palsy. Early tendon transfers are advised for manual laborers with high lesions.

Digital Nerves

The results for adults and children are set out in Table 30-12. Coates and associates[37] made a very detailed study in 27 adults. Thirty nerves were repaired, all but one by primary repair using sutures, for I did not have access to fibrin clot glue at that time. The digital artery was repaired if

Table 30-12

DIGITAL NERVE REPAIR

74 Adult Digital Nerves Repaired Within 48 Hours of Injury*	
Excellent	1
Good	33
Fair	24
Poor or bad	16

28 Adult Digital Nerves Repaired 2 Weeks or More From Injury	
Excellent	0
Good	9
Fair	11
Poor or bad	8

27 Children's Digital Nerves Repaired at Varying Intervals From Injury (Age ≤ 15 Years)	
Excellent	17
Good	8
Fair	2
Poor or bad	0

*Fourteen digital arteries repaired at primary operation; 17 flexor tendons repaired at primary operation.

Table 30-13
GRADING OF RESULTS—RADIAL NERVE

	Good	Fair	Poor
High—above nerves to triceps: 21 cases	Elbow extension M4 Wrist extension M3 or better	Elbow extension M4	Less than this
Intermediate—proximal to PIN: 221 cases. Useful triceps function	Wrist extension M4 Finger and thumb extension M3 or better	Wrist extension M3 or better	Less
PIN: 18 cases	Finger and thumb extension M4	Finger and thumb extension M3	Less

PIN, posterior interosseous nerve.
From Shergill G, Birch R, Bonney G, Munshi P: The radial and posterior interosseous nerves. J Bone Joint Surg Br 83:646-649, 2001.

necessary. Results were surprisingly poor. It seems that the more scrupulously one examines outcome of a nerve repair, the more one will find something wrong. Forty percent of my patients complained of persistent hyperesthesia for up to 2 years. Coates and associates concluded "following repair of the divided digital nerve, normal sensation will never be regained. Hyperesthesia may be present for months or for years but will ultimately resolve. The final result will take two or three years to achieve." Fortunately, results do seem to be a good deal better in children.

Gould[59] described an extensive experience of 169 nerves repaired in a 3-year period. Sixty-eight nerves were in replanted digits or in a finger with severe vascular injury. Fifty-three nerves were repaired within 7 days of injury. The results are good: delay did not appear important, but age did. Results are shown to be better with microscopic repair using finest sutures.

Kallio[73] used a range of sensitive methods to analyze outcome in 254 secondary repairs of digital nerves in 95 patients: temperature and electrical resistance of skin was measured, and threshold to heat and cold recorded. Eighty percent of sutures reached "useful" levels; 56% of grafts did so. Four of 26 grafts for defects in excess of 5 cm gained "useful" sensation. All 33 nerves repaired in children aged 15 years or younger reached S3 or S4 in the MRC scale.

It does seem odd that recovery of sensation after a well-executed primary repair of the median nerve at the wrist is regularly better than that from repair of digital nerves more distally. A number of patients do report striking improvement in sensation with loss of cold sensitivity and hypersensitivity to touch some years after recovery. Recovery of sensation and improvement in sensitivity is a very prolonged business.

The Radial Nerve

The radial nerve is the largest terminal branch of the brachial plexus, and Sunderland[142] showed that it was the most commonly injured nerve, reported in 16,500 cases of war wounds. In civilian practice, injury to the radial nerve comes third after that to the median and ulnar nerves.

Zachary[164] studied 113 cases of repair by direct suture done within 6 months of injury. The maximum amount of nerve resected was 5 cm. All of these nerves were sutured. Good or fair results were achieved in over 60% of cases. In Seddon's own series[130] of 63 nerve sutures, over 75% of results were so graded. Kline and Hudson[80] related the outcome of 171 cases of repair of the radial nerve. Results

were better in the more distal lesions, and the outcome after repair of "lacerated" nerves was better than that of nerves damaged by fractures or gunshot wounds. The best results were gained after primary repair, followed by secondary suture; the worst were in cases that required grafting.

Shergill and coworkers[132] presented the results of 260 repairs of the radial and the posterior interosseous nerves. Of the 18 repairs of the posterior interosseous nerve, 16 achieved a good result. Results of the radial nerve itself were not so good: 30% had good results, and 42% of the repairs failed. The violence of injury was the most important factor in determining outcome. Seventy-nine percent of open tidy repairs achieved a good or fair result. Thirty-six percent of cases with arterial injury reached this level. Most repairs failed when the defect in the nerve trunk exceeds 10 cm. Forty-nine percent of all repairs carried out within 14 days of injury achieved a good result; 28% of later repairs did so. All repairs undertaken after 12 months failed (Tables 30-13 and 30-14).

These results suggest that results for repair of the radial nerve have not improved during the past 50 years. This may be because of the higher incidence of closed traction injury and the associated arterial damage in this series. On the other hand, 77 repairs were carried out within 14 days, a higher proportion than that seen in other series.

Early flexor to extensor transfer is indicated when the prognosis for recovery is poor, for example, in a high traction rupture, above the spiral groove, with a defect between the prepared stumps exceeding 10 cm, or when the interval from injury exceeds 12 months.

NERVE INJURIES IN CHILDREN

In writing about nerve injuries in children Seddon[129] stated "it is firmly established that recovery in children is far better than in adults and there should, therefore, be no hesitation in embarking on the repair of proximally situated lesions in the young."

There are factors that work against the successful outcome in repair of children's nerves:

1. There are profound biological differences between the immature and the mature peripheral nervous systems. The developing nervous system is more vulnerable to injury than that of the adult. This is, of course, particularly important in the study of obstetric brachial plexus

Table 30-14

RESULTS OF REPAIR OF 242 RADIAL NERVES BY CAUSE AND BY NUMBER (PERCENTAGE)

Cause	No. of Nerves Repaired	Results		
		Good	Fair	Poor
Open tidy	73	28 (38)	30 (41)	15 (21)
Closed traction	62	19 (31)	17 (27)	26 (42)
Open untidy	52	13 (25)	13 (25)	26 (50)
Associated vascular injury	55	12 (22)	8 (14)	35 (64)
Total	242	72 (30)	68 (28)	102 (42)

From Shergill G, Birch R, Bonney G, Munshi P: The radial and posterior interosseous nerves: Results of 260 repairs. J Bone Joint Surg Br 83:646-649, 2001.

palsy. Myelination is not complete in the neonate, and conduction velocity at term is about one half of that found in the normal adult. Motor conduction velocity reaches adult levels at about 3 years of age, sensory conduction velocity perhaps a little earlier.

2. Dissociation of the insensate hand from function is a remarkably constant finding in young children. If a child cannot feel a part, that part is ignored; it may even be mutilated. The slow course to recovery after repair of severe lesion of the brachial plexus in the young child is, perhaps, a reflection of the importance of maturation of the afferent pathways. The hand is drawn back into function long after electromyographic evidence confirms copious reinnervation of the affected muscles.

3. Denervation of the limb in the growing child causes disturbance of growth. In the lower limb this may cause severe impairment of function.

4. The muscular imbalance consequent on neurologic injury in a growing child may provoke severe and progressive deformity. The outstanding example of this in the upper limb is the medial rotation contracture at the shoulder complicating obstetric brachial plexus palsy. The effect on the posture of the foot after irreparable tibial or common peroneal lesion is severe, and that deformity superimposed on the limb and foot shortened after injury to the lumbosacral plexus or the divisions of the sciatic nerve is crippling.

There is, however, much clinical evidence showing that recovery of sensibility in children is very much better than it is in adults and that sensibility is rarely attended by neuropathic pain. Perhaps the most extreme example of this is the finding of remarkably high levels of restoration of cutaneous sensation in the hands of children suffering particularly severe injuries of the brachial plexus in whom reinnervation was achieved by means of transfer of the intercostals from remote segments of the spinal cord.[5]

There have been relatively few articles on the study of outcome in children's nerves. Bolitho and colleagues[22] showed very good results after primary epineurial repair in 19 ulnar nerves in children aged 13 years or younger. All of these gained good function to intrinsic muscles and an average two-point discrimination to 6 mm.

From this same group[69] came a similarly detailed study of the results of primary epineurial repair of the median nerve in children. The authors stated, "Our series supports the contention that primary repair should always be performed where possible," and it is interesting that they use epineurial suture for all of these cases.

Slightly less optimistic perhaps is the paper from Duteille and associates[46] that compares the outcome of 38 median and ulnar nerve injuries at the wrist. There were 15 adults and 15 children. While the children showed better sensory recovery, a number demonstrated persistent motor defects. Nerve conduction studies were similar in both adults and children. These workers found that about 25% of children remained with significant defect in motor function compared with about 50% of adults with a similar level of defect. They comment that nerve regeneration may be slightly better than it is in adults but that cerebral plasticity probably accounts for the gain in sensation.

Gilbert and Kaaden[56] followed 34 repairs of ulnar nerves damaged at the elbow and in the proximal forearm in children. A minimum of 3 years was necessary to take a view of final outcome, and in eight of their children palliative tendon transfer was found to be necessary. In not one case was there significant cold sensitivity or vasomotor disturbance. Results were rather better in tidy wounds. Delay of up to 3 months did not seem to reflect on outcome. A particularly interesting finding from this work is that results were better in the dominant hand, and the authors suggest that the hand remained in daily functional use because of the intact median nerve, so, in effect, the children were doing their own physiotherapy.

Birch and Achan[10] related their experience from 359 operations for nerve injuries in children aged 6 months to 15 years. Two hundred and seven nerves were repaired. Eighteen cases of severe postischemic Volkmann's contracture were described. Some findings from this study include the following:

1. A nerve entrapped within a fracture or within a dislocated elbow joint will proceed to full recovery *if* it is extricated within days of injury. If intervention is delayed, then the nerve lesion will progress from a conduction block to a very much less favorable degenerative lesion and,

ultimately, to neurotmesis. In three late cases, resection and grafting was not done when the nerve was extricated and I was forced to rectify this omission at a second intervention.

2. Nerve trunks are more resistant to ischemia than are muscles. In cases of Volkmann's contracture, late decompression of median and ulnar nerve was usually followed by useful recovery of sensation and of the small muscle function within the hand, even though the flexor muscles themselves were irredeemably fibrosed. In a child with loss of peripheral pulses after injury at the elbow, the surgeon must be ready to observe the situation with meticulous care on an hourly basis if the decision is made not to operate and must be ready to change that policy if there is increasing pain, if there is development of nerve palsy, and if there is any hint at all of impending ischemia of the flexor muscles of the forearm. It is almost inconceivable that a complacent attitude can be adopted to a pulseless upper limb.

3. As Klink and Kleinart[82] say, "upper extremity vascular injuries in children have a high association with (injuries to) nerves and tendons. Early and aggressive surgical intervention and repair are warranted to prevent long term sequelae. Because the surgeon cannot predict what the future will hold when treating children, all vessels should be repaired."

REHABILITATION

Rehabilitation is the staged withdrawal of support while the patient reintegrates himself or herself into normal daily life. Repair of the nerve is but the first step in the rehabilitation for the patient. The prognosis is now clear, the time to recovery is prolonged, and the implications for employment can be severe. Cold sensitivity is the reason why many skilled workers in such trades as butchery, fishery, or outdoor engineering are unable to return to work. The surgeon must involve himself or herself in the process of reintegration for the patient and act to support and encourage and to intervene if the occasion arises. The surgeon is in a good position to advise occupational health physicians and others and, from time to time, to act as an advocate for the patient in any, at times, difficult and depressing dealings with the government, the agents of the government, or corporations.

The aims of rehabilitation are as follows:

1. The objective assessment of disability and the accurate measurement of outcome
2. The reduction of degree of disability by physical and other therapies
3. The return of the patient to his or her original work, to that work modified, or to suitable other work for the restoration of the patient's ability to live in his or her home, to enjoy recreation and social activities, and to be independently mobile

The approach is, of course, multidisciplinary, and the field has been reviewed.[9,17,160]

Specific treatment may be indicated for the following:

1. Fixed deformity, weakness, loss of endurance, loss of balance, and loss of confidence. Planned and graduated physiotherapy, combined with serial splinting, is useful here, but it must be structured and with clear goals, and I very much prefer a system of short, sharp bursts of treatment with clearly defined objectives. It does a patient no good at all to be preoccupied with dilatory attendance at hospital outpatient departments for months or years.

2. Neuropathic pain, as opposed to the pain of regeneration and cold sensitivity. This is a rare complication after properly conducted repair. It must be treated vigorously by physical measures, including massage, transcutaneous electrical nerve stimulation, percussion, and use of the part. A strictly supervised use of drugs that act to stabilize nerve membranes such as antiepileptic agents may be necessary. Omer[119] wrote, "there are only two principles in the treatment of established pain syndrome involving the upper extremity: to relieve the subjective pain experience and to institute active function of the involved extremity...." The best functional activity occurs when the patient returns to daily work. Patients who continue functional activities will ultimately 'cure' themselves."

3. Functional training and functional splinting. The restoration of function for return to unsupported daily life and to work can be helped by occupational therapy and by functional splinting. In a fully equipped rehabilitation unit, appropriate facilities are available for simulation and stimulation of actions used in the patient's work and daily life. The simplest splints can greatly aid a patient with partial paralysis of the lower limb or improve function of the hand.

4. Return to work. Professional occupational counselors are available to advise on the possibilities of return to work, and liaison between them and the surgeon can be very helpful to the patient. In 1969, Brewerton introduced, at the Royal National Orthopaedic Hospital, the concept and the practice of a hospital employment advisor who is available to help patients who, because of their disability, are likely to experience problems in returning to work. The patient is seen while he or she is in hospital. Problems can be discussed and in the favorable case difficulties can be resolved before discharge. The advisor can, with the patient's agreement, make contact with the employer and discuss job prospects. When permanent disability is so severe as to prevent a return to anything like the original work, the question of retraining may be raised. The advisor can arrange for such patients to be seen at one of numerous employment assessment centers, which may lead to specialized training courses. The employment advisor and the occupational therapist can help in the matter of transport and mobility. Patients with serious disability of one upper limb are able to handle a car fitted with an automatic gear box and adjustments for the steering wheel and hand brake.

Recovery of sensibility in the adult depends on reestablishing the central analysis of input of new patterns, and much can be done to aid recovery by retraining that central perception. Wynn Parry and Salter[161] record our early experience, which was, at that time, largely based on residential retraining. My colleagues and I have expanded on this experience.[18] Dellon[42] argues persuasively that such retraining is an essential part of rehabilitation after nerve suture. Imai and associates[71] measured the improvement in hand function after sensory re-education, showing a substantial improvement in the ability of the patient to recognize small objects and considerable improvement in recognition of moving two-point discrimination. Training is started as soon as the patient can recognize stimuli at the fingertips, and it aims to improve function by improvement of the qualities of localization and of recognition. An hour's transcutaneous stimulation before the start of the session may ease hypersensitivity or even allodynia.

Dahlin and colleagues[41] provide an excellent review of central plasticity in relation to hand surgery, describing the functional reorganization of the somatosensory cortex. Impressive work with sense substitution by this group shows how "sleeping sensibility" can be awakened and some stereognosis regained.[96]

The quality of reinnervation is not necessarily related to function. For the purpose of research, both academic tests of sensory restoration and tests of function need to be used.

CRITICAL POINTS: REHABILITATION

- Rehabilitation is the staged withdrawal of support.
- The process must be supervised by the clinician from start to finish.
- Further operation, such as palliative musculotendinous transfers, should be seen as an integral part of the process of rehabilitation.

THE PERIPHERAL NEUROMA

Unlike a successful peripheral nerve repair, the neuroma is the inevitable, unavoidable, and biologic response of the proximal stump after it has been divided in situations where regenerating axons are impeded from reentering the distal stump. The swelling of the terminal bulb of the proximal stump that ensues contains Schwann cells, fibroblasts, blood vessels, and, above all, numerous regenerating axons that are partially myelinated or not at all myelinated.

Severe and persisting pain arising from a neuroma is unusual: most clean transections of major nerves do not provoke severe neuropathic pain. Two processes provoke severe pain in relation to neuromas. The first is persistent mechanical or chemical irritation of the axons within the neuroma. The second is the development of spontaneous and disturbing sensory symptoms, caused by persistent stimulation of the axons within the neuroma and accompanied by the development of spontaneous activity of neurons within the dorsal root ganglion, the dorsal horn of the spinal cord, and at even more proximal levels within the central nervous system. Severe pain from neuromas is more likely after partial injuries of nerve trunks, and it is a particularly severe problem after injuries to the terminal branches of nerves of cutaneous sensation, including the medial cutaneous nerve of the forearm, the superficial radial nerve, the sural nerve, and the long saphenous nerve. It is a remarkable and unexplained fact that the clean removal of these nerve trunks for the purpose of repairing a major nerve is very rarely attended by severe pain, whereas significant pain is really quite common after accidental damage to the terminal branches of those same cutaneous nerves.

In complete or terminal neuromas, the nerve trunk has been divided. The term *partial neuroma* or *neuroma-in-continuity* is applied to those nerves where some bundles are intact, and it is in these that the possibility of resecting the damaged portion and repairing it seems logical. Neuromas in amputation stumps present a particular problem because there is no possibility of reconnecting the divided nerves with the peripheral stumps.

CRITICAL POINTS: DIAGNOSIS OF NEUROPATHIC PAIN

- Distinguish between spontaneous symptoms, painful or otherwise, from evoked pain such as allodynia.
- Note extension of pain beyond the proper territory of the nerve.
- Close analysis of the patient's own description allied with physical examination enables the clinician to recognize distinct patterns or syndromes of neuropathic pain.

Pathophysiology

Terms in common use include:

- *Paresthesia,* or a spontaneous abnormal sensation
- *Dysesthesia,* or an unpleasant spontaneous normal sensation
- *Hyperesthesia,* or an increased sensitivity to a stimulus that would not normally be painful
- *Hyperalgesia,* or an increased response to a stimulus that is normally painful
- *Allodynia,* or a perception of a nonpainful stimulus as painful
- *Hyperpathia,* or a state of exaggerated and a very painful response to stimulation

Sood and Elliot[136] treated 10 painful neuromas within the hand and wrist by relocation of the damaged nerve into the pronator quadratus muscle. They defined four types of characteristic neuroma pain: (1) spontaneous pain, (2) painful cutaneous "hyperesthesia," which is a reflection of spontaneous activity, (3) "pressure" pain from mechanical stimulation of the neuroma, and (4) evocation of pain by movement of adjacent joints, which is a reflection of mechanical stimulation of nerve fibers within the neuroma.

Pain from a neuroma is one subtype of neuropathic pain, which is caused by a lesion of the nervous system, usually of peripheral nerves. Some neuropathic pain states are exceptionally severe, and they are characterized by persistence; intractability; disproportion between the extent of lesion and the severity of the pain; and the fact that the pain is no longer necessary for the survival of the organism.

Neuropathic pain is usually associated with sensory or motor disturbance and quite often with sympathetic dysfunction. The sensory symptoms described by patients are sometimes so clear that diagnosis of the cause and some understanding of the subsequent pattern of physiologic events are possible from the history alone. (For a detailed discussion of diagnosis and treatment of neuropathic pain and complex regional pain syndrome, see Chapter 57.)

The spontaneous symptoms of neuropathic pain indicate that there is spontaneous firing of nerve fibers within the neuroma itself and/or within the proximal neurons of the dorsal root ganglion, the dorsal horn of the spinal cord, or higher. The nervous system is responding inappropriately to a nonexistent stimulus. In some cases of mechanical allodynia it seems that neurons within the dorsal root ganglion or the dorsal horn are sensitized by catecholamines. As Koltzenburg says, "an explanation consistent with these findings is that primary afferents acquire a sensitivity to catecholamines that permits an abnormal excitation by adrenaline."[83] Such stimulation may occur at the postganglionic sympathetic fibers or may occur owing to circulating epinephrine. A particularly important observation from Michaelis and coworkers[105] provides an understanding of the deep-seated pain of *hyperpathia,* most especially the deep-seated poorly localized nature of that pain. In experiments on rats the nerve to the gastrocnemius muscle and the sural nerve were sectioned. Section of the motor nerve induced bursting spontaneous discharges in the relevant dorsal root ganglia, corresponding to nonmyelinated sensory afferents. The authors conclude that these findings provide the first evidence that after peripheral nerve injury both axotomized as well as intact afferent neurons supplying skeletal muscle generate ongoing activity within the dorsal root ganglion, probably because of a yet unknown signal in the ganglion triggered by axotomy. Nathan noted that "it is a general and essential feature of the behavior of the central nervous system to preserve the effects of stimulating after stimulation has ceased." Evidently, injury to a relatively unimportant peripheral nerve may act to accentuate this general and essential behavior.[113]

Whether the sympathetic nervous system is involved in the propagation of neuropathic pain states secondary to peripheral nerve injury is a point of some controversy. Lowe and Nathan[89a] related a particularly significant study in 45 patients with chronic neuropathic pain. Peripheral nerves were damaged by partial section, compression, amputation, or herpes in 23 and lasting relief of pain followed sympathetic block in 11 of these. Loh and Nathan[89a] emphasized that the presence of hyperpathia suggested that blocks were more likely to succeed. The clinical evidence of disturbance of sympathetic function, of itself, was not an indication for success or failure. They proposed that such pain states were brought about by abnormal firing of peripheral nerve fibers (in particular, the mechanoreceptors) that alter the behavior of neurons in the substantia gelatinosa and lamina 2, either by diminishing their inhibition, by facilitating their activity, or by both. "Thus, stopping the emission of the normal sympathetic transmission stops the firing of peripheral nerve fibers and that stops the abnormal function within the central nervous system. The abnormal state is kept going by mechanoreceptors and the large afferent fibers. The sympathetic outflow is acting on these fibers or receptors to cause

the input to the spinal cord which causes a state of disinhibition or facilitation spreading from the original site of input."[89a]

On the other hand, Schott[125] firmly questioned the role of sympathetic blockade, reviewing series that show no difference between placebo and guanethidine and stating that interrupting the sympathetic outflow is "a futile procedure for many patients."

Pain states that are attributed to iatrogenic injuries of cutaneous nerves are rarely dependent on sympathetic activity and have proved resistant to all forms of treatment. Piling of treatment on treatment in pain clinics usually made them worse. The cause is both central and peripheral. Centrally, there is an alteration of the mechanisms of analysis and modification of impulses. Peripherally, there is alteration of incoming impulses due to a loss of the normal pattern of cutaneous innervation. Axonal sprouting from adjacent cutaneous nerves may cause further confusion of the pattern of innervation. An excellent review from Gold[57] outlines some of these mechanisms. The model studied was ligation of spinal nerves in mammals. Gold summarizes evidence that allodynia, hyperalgesia, and spontaneous pain occur because of the changes in primary afferent neurons in the dorsal root ganglion. The allodynia and hyperalgesia arise from uninjured afferent fibers; the constant spontaneous pain arises from injured afferents. Repair seems to be particularly appropriate when pain spreads beyond the territory of the nerve, with allodynia and even hyperpathia in adjacent skin. Here the only possible way to rectify this situation is to restore volleys of afferent impulses from reinnervated skin and so hope to reverse the changes in the dorsal horn.

Treatment

A painful neuroma may not be the sole explanation for a patient's loss of function and, of itself, is not an indication for operation. The clinician should take time to establish the diagnosis and elicit important background information about the cause of injury, as well as contributing factors including litigation and compensation.

Occupational therapists can be asked to see these patients and provide a measure of functional disturbance. Advice can be given about how to maintain the part within the activities of daily function. Simple padded finger stalls can ease the situation of a hypersensitive or tender digit. Custom-made padded straps can protect a neuroma of superficial radial nerve or palm or cutaneous or median nerve from mechanical irritation.

A trial of transcutaneous nerve stimulation (TENS) will do no harm. I have found it only occasionally useful, but quite a number of symptoms of painful neuromas are in fact exacerbated by the technique. I am not aware of controlled studies that prove the effectiveness of nonoperative techniques such as taping, percussion, massage, ultrasound, or TENS.

Wynn Parry[160] describes extensive experience in the treatment of painful neuromas by a vigorous program of desensitization and functional retraining, which is supplemented by blocking of the affected nerve by local anesthetic or guanethidine (a sympatholytic drug). Gergis and Wynn Parry related their experience in the treatment of 78 patients with severe pain after injury to nerves in the distal parts of limbs by serial guanethidine blockade.[19] A total of 696 guanethidine blocks were given, with the total for each patient ranging from 4 to 39. All patients had transient relief of pain. In successful blocks, pain relief lasted for some hours, and this interval tended to increase with further blocks. The treatment is given on an inpatient basis as injections two to three times a week. Intensive physiotherapy was given with the aim of improving stiffness, swelling, and skin sensibility; and occupational therapy was used to enhance function and to help patients learn techniques of adaptation while continuing to use the hands. Simple protective splints were, on occasion, useful. Twenty-three of 78 patients obtained complete relief of pain. Twenty-eight experienced partial relief. Twenty-seven experienced no improvement at all. There was a significant rate of recurrence of pain at between 6 and 12 months from discharge. In addition, three groups of patients were identified that did particularly badly: those with pain after operations on the ulnar nerve at the elbow, those with iatrogenic injury to the superficial radial nerve, and those with pain from damaged sensory nerves in the foot.

Chemical Methods

A number of sclerosing agents have been tried to suppress axonal regeneration. Sunderland came to the conclusion that they were of no real value in preventing the formation of neuromas.[140]

Smith and Gomez[135] injected triamcinolone with local anesthetic directly into the neuroma and surrounding tissues. The treatments were successful in half of patients with a single injection and in 80% of patients after multiple injections. Thirty-four neuromas in 22 patients were treated. The technique was less successful when used for the deeper neuromas in the palm and in the wrist; it seemed to be most effective for digital neuromas.

I have no personal experience of this technique. Some patients referred to me after a trial of it found the method too painful to persist.

Prevention

The treatment of the painful neuroma is deeply unsatisfactory. The number of operative techniques described is so large that it is clear that not one is wholly reliable. Prevention is best. A painful neuroma is a rare occurrence after a well-executed suture of a transected nerve particularly when attention has been paid to restoring the gliding plane for the nerve and the repair of damaged adjacent tissue. Tupper and Booth[153] found that a well-sealed epineural repair of a severed nerve rarely resulted in a painful neuroma, and Herndon and Hess[66] believed "when operating on or near nerves, prevention of injury in neuroma formation should be foremost in the surgeons' mind....great care is taken when working around nerves to prevent the iatrogenic injury during exploration. This is especially true for such operative procedures as ganglion excisions at the wrist or the release of the first dorsal compartment in de Quervain's tenosynovitis." This advice should be remembered by all clinicians during operations and applied during operation at the elbow, the knee, the ankle, and the foot.

Operations

General Principles

Tables 30-15 and 30-16 set out the numbers of operations performed for injuries to nerves of cutaneous sensibility. Over one half were for nerves damaged in the course of operation or other interventions. The consequences of iatrogenic damage to tiny cutaneous nerves can be particularly severe. In most of these cases the nerves were cut, although sometimes they were ligated and then cut. These patients experienced spontaneous or induced pain, hyperesthesia and hyperalgesia, and even allodynia and hyperpathia. I have seen one patient who went on to amputation of an upper limb for persistent pain after damage to the superficial radial nerve at the wrist. In that particular case the refusal of the defendants to accept a reasonable early settlement was a significant factor in prolonging and magnifying the patient's complaints.

The partial neuroma is a common and difficult problem. I usually advise neurolysis with a 24- to 48-hour infusion of local anesthetic, during which time the patient is encouraged to move the part, with the aim of restoring gliding of the nerve. This can be very effective for nerves tethered by a focus of scar. If the procedure fails, consideration is given to resection and repair or repair and translocation. Gould[60] described a very logical and systematic algorithmic approach, which includes nonoperative methods. The nerve is blocked with local anesthetic, followed by a course of anti-inflammatory and membrane-stabilizing agents, combined with desensitization and other therapy techniques. If this fails, operation is done, which combines neurolysis with wrapping of the nerve by vein or vascularized fascia. Gould evaluated implanted nerve stimulators in a helpful manner. Excision of the nerve is reserved for those with recalcitrant nerve pain.

 ## Author's Preferred Technique

The primary aim of surgery is to reconnect, where possible, the central and the distal stumps of the damaged nerve so that regenerating axons can grow to their proper targets. Surgical repair offers the chance for restoration of normal afferent volleys of impulses and so restores the normal inhibitory effects of these impulses on central neurons. If reconnection is impossible, then the damaged proximal stump must be moved to a less hostile and a less exposed place. Translocation of the proximal stump into other tissues such as muscle may permit a new connection between regenerating axons and the host tissue.

The principles of operation on nerves have been described earlier in this chapter. These steps apply in the exposure and treatment of a neuroma. The tourniquet is useful. Particular care is needed in the display of the damaged nerve, and I find it better to expose that trunk proximally, in healthy tissue, and then work distally to the site of lesion. The nerve must be handled with exquisite care, avoiding traction. Particular attention must be paid to the bed of the nerve, and wherever possible the quality of that

Table 30-15
OPERATIONS FOR PAINFUL NEUROMAS OF CUTANEOUS (SENSORY) NERVES: 1975-2000

	No.	Neurolysis	Repair	Resection ± Translocation
Upper Limb				
Supraclavicular and cervical plexus	16	4	7	5
Medial cutaneous of forearm	49	12	16	21
Medial cutaneous of arm—internal brachial	3	2	1	
Superficial radial nerve	136	18	82	36
Lateral cutaneous nerve of forearm	6	2	2	2
Palmar digital	185	20	128	37
Palmar median	12	2	10	
Dorsal cutaneous ulnar	13	5	5	3
Total	420	61	244	115
Lower Limb				
Lateral cutaneous nerve of thigh	11	5	2	4
Sural	35	8	13	14
Saphenous (including infrapatellar branches)	31	11	10	10
Plantar cutaneous	26	4	17	5
Terminal branches common peroneal	24	4	10	10
Total	127	32	52	43

Table 30-16
OPERATIONS FOR IATROPATHIC INJURIES TO NERVES OF CUTANEOUS SENSIBILITY

Nerve	No. of Nerves
Neck and Upper Limb	
Supraclavicular and cervical plexus	11
Medial cutaneous nerve of forearm	15
Superficial radial	92
Palmar including palmar cutaneous of median	42
Dorsal branch of ulnar	11
Total	171
Lower Limb	
Lateral cutaneous nerve of thigh	8
Saphenous, including infrapatellar branch	21
Sural	24
Plantar	21
Terminal branches of common peroneal nerve	16
Total	90

bed should be improved by excision of scar so that the repaired nerve can lie on healthy tissue, preferably synovium or fat. If the bed is unsuitable or the distal stump beyond salvage, the affected nerve is ligated with a suture and the neuroma excised; the nerve is then transposed well proximal to the zone of injury and buried deep within a muscle belly.

It has been my practice, for a number of years, to infiltrate the line of the incision with local anesthetic before cutting the skin. This is extended in the treatment of the painful neuroma by leaving an indwelling catheter adjacent to the proximal stump, permitting the infusion of local anesthetic for a minimum of 24 hours after operation. I use an epidural catheter that is taped securely to the skin. Infusion of local anesthetic (0.25% levobupivacaine) is given by top-up bolus injections at 4-hour intervals or by continual infusion. It is essential that the part is used and worked from the outset, and postoperative splinting must do no more than protect the repaired or transfer nerve. The patient should be encouraged to move the fingers, to massage them, and to work them in the very early postoperative phase.

Operations for Terminal Neuroma
The many techniques described can be contained within four groups: (1) resection of the neuroma, (2) containment of the neuroma, (3) translocation of the neuroma, and (4) repair.

Resection of the Neuroma

My colleagues and I[13] outlined the indications for resection of a terminal neuroma and thought this operation was justifiable when:

1. There is persistent pain and dysesthesia.
2. There is no hope of reuniting the damaged nerve.
3. There is a palpable tender neuroma in the line of the damaged nerve.
4. That neuroma is, or may be, irritated within by adherence to moving muscle or tendon.
5. There is no suggestion of distortion of symptoms or signs by the patient.
6. There has been no previous excision of neuroma.

It is best to excise the neuroma with the terminal 10 cm of the nerve so that the distal end of the proximal stump lies in more or less unscarred tissue, and if possible, in unscarred muscle. A new neuroma is, of course, bound to develop; one can only hope that it will not grow in such a site or to such a size as to cause trouble.

Containment of a Neuroma

A number of methods have been described to contain the fascicles within the nerve trunk thus reducing cellular and axonal proliferation or seeking to provide a barrier of nerve sheath between that proliferating tissue and surrounding tissues. Kline and Hudson[76] suggest sealing the ends of the fascicles with bipolar diathermy. Herndon[67] reviews methods of ligature and of epineurial closure. Tupper and Booth[153] described resection of fascicles within a sleeve of epineurium that is ligated. Forty-five neuromas in 28 patients were so treated, and there was considerable improvement in symptoms in 81% of patients. Tupper and Booth thought that this method was better than a simple neurectomy, but they stated that the number of cases was too small for the results to be conclusive.

Swanson and associates[144] reported a series of 18 patients with 38 neuromas treated with placement of a silicone cap over the excised nerve. In 15 patients, symptoms were relieved but the authors found that 2 patients had developed causalgia. They have shown that several factors are important in inhibiting axonal growth and resultant neuroma formation:

- The length-to-diameter ratio should be a minimum of 5:1, that is, the shorter the cap, the more likely a neuroma will form.
- The nerve cap should only be slightly larger than the nerve. It should not fit too loosely, because this might allow axons to grow back proximally between the cap and the epineurium.

Technique

Epineurial Sleeve. With the use of the microscope, the nerve is transected proximal to the neuroma. The epineurium is then carefully peeled back over the nerve trunk. Each fascicle is identified and individually sectioned 1 cm proximally. The empty epineurial tube is then double ligated with 6-0 nylon. The nerve end is then placed in adjacent healthy tissue (Fig. 30-17).[67]

Martini and Fromm[99] also create an epineurial sleeve and then seal it with histoacryl glue (butyl-2-cynoacrylate). They compared this method with others, including simple nerve ligation and epineurial ligation, and found that the fewest neuromas formed in subjects in whom the glue was used.

Silastic Cap. In Swanson's technique, the first step is to resect the neuroma. A silicone cap slightly larger than the nerve, but not too tight, is chosen (Fig. 30-18). It is trimmed to the approximate length (5 to 10 times the nerve diameter). With the use of a 5-0 nonabsorbable Bunnell-type suture,

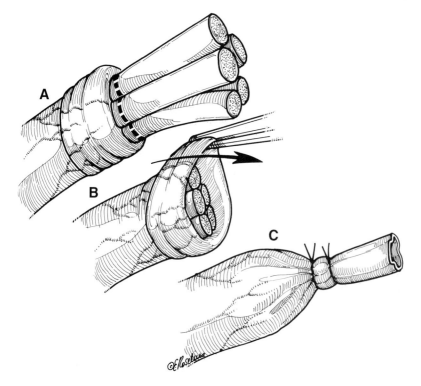

FIGURE 30-17. The neuroma has been excised (**A**) having pushed back epineurium. This is then drawn over the freshly cut bundles (**B**) and then the epineurial sleeve is ligated (**C**).

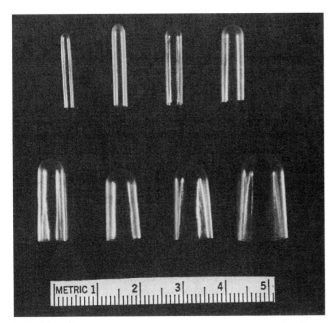

FIGURE 30-18. Silicone caps (Swanson design) are available in several sizes. A cap only slightly larger than the diameter of the nerve should be used.

Silicone Tubes. Dahlin and Lundborg[40] review the use of tubes in peripheral nerve repair. They also related preliminary experience in using silicone tubes for the treatment of painful neuromas. The concept was based on observations from experimental morphologic studies. They indicated that when a proximal nerve end is introduced into the silicone tube or a mesothelial tube, exceeding a critical length and lacking a distal nerve segment, no or limited axonal regeneration occurs inside the tube. The proximal nerve end extends only a few millimeters into the tube and forms a cone-shaped structure without forming a true neuroma. This nerve structure does not show typical neurophysiologic characteristics of a painful neuroma such as spontaneous activity. The neurons growing in such tubes are quiet.

A number of painful neuromas have been treated using this method, with silicone tubes of at least 20 mm in length. Dahlin and Lundborg relate that most of their patients describe improvement or, in some cases, substantial pain relief from neuroma pain. This is a very interesting development, and of all of the methods that I have encountered it seems to be that which comes closest to suppression of neuroma formation. Undoubtedly, this concept will be the subject of further detailed clinical study.

Translocation of the Nerve

Without Excision of the Neuroma. This method was introduced by Littler in 1967,[68] and Herndon, in the last edition of this work, recommended this method when the distal portion of the severed nerve was absent or irreparable so that repair could not be performed. Every effort is made to keep the neuroma intact with its mature encapsulating scar while transposing it en bloc to another area free of scar and not subjecting it to repeated trauma.

The neuroma with its fibrous capsule is carefully isolated. A proximal area that is free of scar and away from

the cap is secured over the freshly amputated nerve stump (Fig. 30-19). The nerve stump is transferred to healthy tissue.[67]

Tupper and Booth[153] reported a series of 32 neuromas in 17 patients in whom they used two types of silicone caps. The first was a silicone rubber Ducker-Hayes tube, and the second was a Frackleton cap that fitted snugly over the nerve ends. No clear advantage followed capping over simple excisional neurectomy.

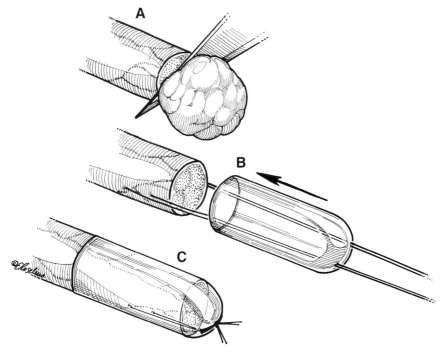

FIGURE 30-19. Silastic capping. **A,** The neuroma is excised, and **(B)** the Silastic cap is drawn over the nerve stump, but not too tight! **C,** The Silastic cap is secured by the suture.

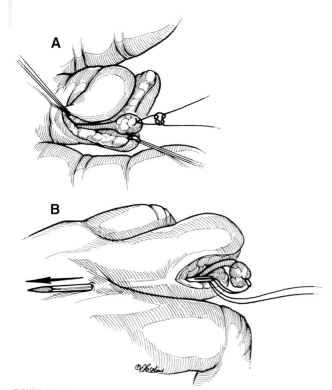

FIGURE 30-20. Translocation of neuroma. In this technique the neuroma is not excised, it is mobilized with the nerve (**A**) and then drawn backward into proximal healthy and unscarred tissue (**B**). *The nerve must lie loosely, Avoid tension!*

local trauma is selected, preferably deep to a muscle, in a web space, or between the shafts of adjacent metacarpals. The dorsal site is preferable to a palmar location that might lead to pressure on the neuroma with manual activity such as the gripping of tools (Figs. 30-20 and 30-21).

The neuroma with its nerve is then carefully dissected proximally until the neuroma bulb can be transferred to its new location without tension on the nerve. A fine absorbable suture is then placed through the capsule (not the neuroma) and tied. Another knot is tied 3 to 4 mm away from the neuroma. The free ends of the suture are then channeled subcutaneously and passed through the skin proximal to the location selected for the neuroma. This suture is drawn through the skin and tied, maintaining a 3- to 4-mm separation between the dermis and the neuroma. The nerve trunk is carefully examined to make certain no tension or twisting exists along its path. A similar technique is used when the neuroma is buried in the muscles. For neuromas in the finger stumps, it is preferred to transfer the nerve end into the web space; for neuromas in the palm, the nerve ends are transferred to the dorsum of the hand between the metacarpals.

I have not used this method, but I can see that it is logical in cases where the pain from the neuroma is obviously related to compression or to mechanical stimulation. The technique avoids the risk of igniting further neurophysiologic changes by inflicting another lesion on the damaged peripheral nerve. Success is less probable when there is spontaneous pain in the skin beyond the proper territory of the damaged nerve.

With Excision of Neuroma. The nerve end may be implanted within the medullary canal of bone. A high rate of success was achieved by Mass and colleagues[100] and by Goldstein and Sturim.[58]

This operation aims to contain the nerve stump within a compartment, thus restricting the size of the neuroma, and also to protect the neuroma from direct trauma. These authors emphasize some important technical details:

- There should be adequate mobilization of the nerve.
- There should be absence of tension on the transferred nerve.
- The nerve should not be angulated where it enters bone.

It is unwise to implant the nerve just distal to a joint that will inevitably subject it to traction. Elliot (personal communication, 2002) has considerable experience with this method in the treatment of digital neuromas. His current practice is to relocate nerves into metacarpals except in cases of very distal injury, because this reduces the risk of traction on the transferred nerve.

Translocation of Nerve into Muscle

Results of this method when the nerve is transferred into the small muscles of the hand have not been good.[85] More promising work comes from Dellon and Mackinnon,[44] who found that relocating the superficial radial nerve into the undersurface of the brachioradialis was an effective way of treating neuromas. Evans and Dellon[48] successfully treated

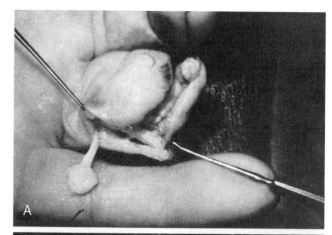

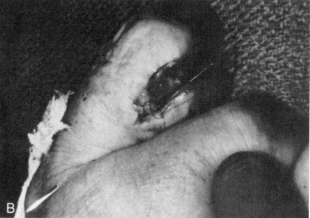

FIGURE 30-21. Clinical photographs showing relocation of an intact neuroma. **A,** The neuroma dissected free. **B,** Transposition of the neuroma.

13 end-neuromas of the palmar cutaneous branch of the median nerve by translocation into the pronator quadratus, and Sood and Elliot[136] translocated 13 end-neuromas into the muscle. Results were good, but Elliot points out that all patients require immobilization of the wrist for several weeks, and some for several months. Pain at the extremes of extension of the wrist or supination of the forearm was induced in most patients. However, for most patients there was disappearance of spontaneous pain, and pressure pain was abolished and, thus, the end result was a great improvement.

I translocate the injured nerve stump into muscle in those cases where repair is not possible because there is no distal stump or where the site of repair would be so close to the skin that mechanical sensitivity would persist. The method has been used in over 30 cases of terminal neuromas of the superficial radial and of the palmar cutaneous nerve of median, of the infrapatellar branch of saphenous nerve, and of branches of the sural and the superficial division of the common peroneal nerve close to the ankle. No patient has been made worse. Most experienced useful improvement.

The nerve is exposed. The neuroma is resected. The parent trunk is displayed for about 10 cm proximally. The nerve is mobilized, gently avoiding traction. It is sectioned so that a healthy face with pouting bundles is seen.

The sheath of an adjacent muscle is incised. The nerve trunk is then drawn into a tunnel within the muscle, using a plastic vascular sling. The nerve must lie very loosely before it enters muscle, and the excursion of that muscle is tested by putting the adjacent joint through full range of movement. There must be no traction on the translocated nerve. No sutures are put through the nerve; it is held in place by combining fine absorbable sutures to close the incision within the muscle sheath and also bathing the entry point in fibrin clot glue.

Wherever possible, nerves are implanted into muscle with relatively limited excursion. The brachioradialis is suitable for the superficial radial nerve; the pronator quadratus is used for the palmar cutaneous branch of the median nerve. Implanting nerves into the deep flexor muscles of the forearm or into the muscles of the deep flexor compartment of the leg may subject that nerve to traction during normal movement (Fig. 30-22).

An epidural catheter is placed adjacent to the proximal stump of the nerve, permitting the infusion of local anesthetic for up to 48 hours after operation.

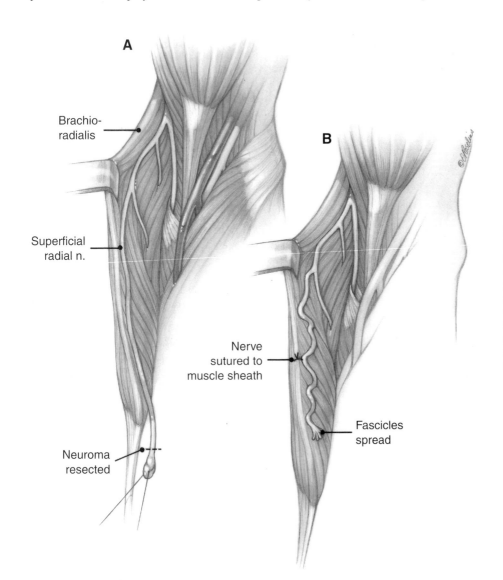

FIGURE 30-22. Implantation of nerve into muscle. **A,** In this case, the superficial radial nerve is exposed and mobilized. **B,** The neuroma is resected and the individual fascicles are gently eased apart. The nerve is implanted within the brachioradialis muscle, in a tunnel, and very lightly sutured to the muscle sheath. *Avoid any tension. The nerve must lie very loosely by this technique.*

The part is not immobilized; rather, it is protected with a padded bandage and the patient is encouraged to move the part, the fingers, and wrist, or the ankle and toes, on the same day as the operation.

Most patients are improved by this procedure, but I reserve it for those cases in which the problem is largely one of mechanical irritation of a nerve. When spontaneous symptoms indicate firing of central neurons and when there is hyperalgesia of the skin within the area supplied by adjacent nerves of cutaneous sensation then the outlook is more uncertain. In these cases it is our practice to begin a course of agents that stabilize the nerve membrane, such as gabapentin, and this is continued for at least 3 months after the operation is done.

Repair of the Nerve

Langley and Anderson[87] may have approached a state of inhibition of regeneration in their proposal to suture one nerve trunk to another in amputation stumps. Kon and Bloem[84] applied this to palmar digital nerves by suturing one to another or, when the injury was unilateral, by suturing the dorsal to the palmar branches. The principle of these operations is to sequester regenerating axons within the epineurial sheath. My limited experience with this technique has not been successful.

Repair of the Damaged Nerve

I agree with Herndon when he emphasizes that repair, when possible, is desirable because no method of translocation can succeed in altering spontaneous activity of neurons within the dorsal root ganglion or within the central nervous system.

To inflict damage on another nerve of cutaneous sensation for the sake of one damaged, which is already painful, seems to me illogical; and it carries with it the risk, in my opinion, of leaving the patient with two neuromas instead of one. Norris and coworkers[114] have shown that the matrix of skeletal muscle can provide a conduit for regenerating axons. My colleagues and I have used the freeze-thawed muscle graft in the treatment of painful neuromas in 62 patients. Preliminary results with this technique were reported by Thomas and colleagues[148] in 22 neuromas in 20 patients. Fifteen of these were in the upper limb, and 7 were in the lower limb. Pain was improved in 11 of the 15 in the upper limb and in 2 of the 7 lower-limb neuromas. The authors believed that this was because the gap or the defect in the nerve in the lower limb was higher. In 6 of the 15 neuromas in the upper limb there was some restoration of sensation. Thus the authors say, "There is much circumstantial evidence for suggesting that 5 cm is the maximum safe length to use."

After exposure of the nerve the adjacent muscle is exposed. A block of muscle is cut parallel to the fibers; in the upper limb, the palmaris longus and flexor carpi radialis are suitable. The muscle graft is measured at least two-and-a-half times the length of the nerve defect. It is wrapped in aluminum foil and placed in liquid nitrogen until effervescence has ceased (about 45 seconds). The package is then placed in sterile water at room temperature for at least 3 minutes. The graft always contracts to about half its fresh length, and fragmentation is a problem in grafts more than 3 cm in length. The graft is now cut to size, allowing 20% excess in length and diameter and sutured into position. The nerve repair is protected as for a graft (Fig. 30-23).

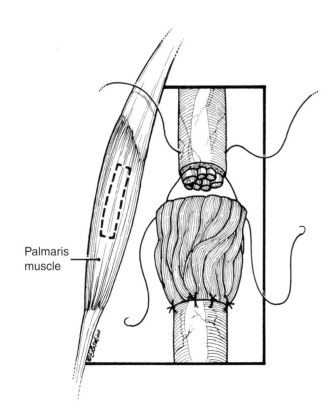

Palmaris
muscle

FIGURE 30-23. Free-thawed muscle graft. The neuroma has been resected so that healthy, pouting faces are displayed. A block of muscle has been taken from the palmaris longus, and I aim for a length of muscle at least three times as long as the defect in the nerve, thus allowing for shrinkage. After freezing and thawing, the block of muscle tissue is lightly sutured between the nerve faces. The diameter of the muscle block is greater than that of the recipient nerve. As always, tension must be avoided.

CONCLUSION

Successful treatment of a neuroma requires the following:

- Analysis of the extent of the disability
- From time to time use of membrane-stabilizing drugs or other agents
- Operation that includes postoperative infusion of local anesthetic
- An urgent program of rehabilitation for the part and the patient

Prevention is best. The steady increase in iatrogenic lesions must be a source of concern for those responsible for the training of surgeons.

CRITICAL POINTS: SUMMARY OF MANAGEMENT OF NEUROMA

- Avoidance is best. Far too many painful neuromas are caused by surgeons. Respect nerves of cutaneous sensation.
- Swift action is best.
- The nerve should be repaired if that is possible.
- Translocation is next best method.
- Infusion of local anesthetic is an integral part of any operation on a painful neuroma.
- The operation must be seen as an integral part of rehabilitation.
- Work with a colleague particularly interested in neuropathic pain. Should be seen as a collaborative venture. Clinicians should not transfer patients to pain clinics without making a clear diagnosis of the cause of the pain.

ANNOTATED REFERENCES

10. Birch R, Achan P: Peripheral nerve repairs and their results in children. Hand Clin 16:579-597, 2000.

   This is quite a large series of nerve injuries in children that clarifies the factors determining prognosis and contains useful sections on Volkmann's ischemic contracture.

11. Birch R, Bonney G, Wynn Parry CB: Reactions to injury. *In* Surgical Disorders of the Peripheral Nerves. London, Churchill Livingstone, 1998, pp 37-55.

150. Thomas PK, Holdorff B: Neuropathy due to physical agents. *In* Dyck PJ, Thomas PK (eds): Peripheral Neuropathy, 3rd ed. Philadelphia, WB Saunders, 1993, pp 990-1014.

   These two works discuss the response of nerve to injury in a very helpful manner and explain the difference between conduction block and degenerative lesions, thus providing a framework for modern clinical practice.

16a. Birch R, Bonney G, Wynn Parry CB: Classification of pain. *In* Surgical Disorders of the Peripheral Nerves. London, Churchill Livingstone, 1998, p 388.

   This describes a classification of neuropathic pain states that has proven remarkably robust in clinical practice.

28. Brushart TM: Nerve repair. *In* Green DP, Hotchkiss RN, Pederson WC (eds): Green's Operative Hand Surgery, 4th ed. New York, Churchill Livingstone, 1999, pp 1384-1385.

   An excellent work that is particularly helpful in understanding biologic factors.

32. Carlstedt T, Cullheim S: Spinal cord motoneuron maintenance, injury and repair. Prog Brain Res 127:501-514, 2000.

47. Dyck PJ, Nukada H, Lais CA, Karnes J: Permanent axotomy: A model of chronic neuronal degeneration produced by axonal atrophy, myelin remodelling and regeneration. *In* Dyck PJ, Thomas PK, Lambert EH, Bunge R (eds): Peripheral Neuropathy, 2nd ed. Philadelphia, WB Saunders, 1984, pp 660-690.

   These two extremely important contributions demonstrate profound effect upon the central nervous system of transection of peripheral nerves.

36. Clark WL, Trumble TE, Swiontowski MF, Tencer AF: Nerve tension and blood flow in a model of immediate and delayed repairs. J Hand Surg [Am] 17:677-687, 1992.

   A valuable study of the effects of tension on blood supply to the repaired nerve.

42. Dellon AL: Evaluation of Sensibility and Re-education of Sensation in the Hand. Baltimore, Williams & Wilkins, 1981.

   This fascinating text provides essential reading in analysis of recovery of sensation.

44. Dellon AL, Mackinnon SE: Treatment of the painful neuroma by neuroma resection and muscle implantation. Plast Reconstr Surg 77:427-438, 1986.

   This valuable paper sets out very clearly the indications for and the results of transposition of a nerve of cutaneous sensation into muscle.

44a. Dobyns JH: Pain dysfunction syndrome. *In* Gelberman RH (ed): Operative Nerve Repair and Reconstruction. Philadelphia, JB Lippincott, 1991, pp 1489-1495.

   This is a particularly thoughtful, indeed scholarly approach to the treatment of neuropathic pain.

52. Frykman GK, Adams J, Bowen WW: Neurolysis. Orthop Clin North Am 12:325-342, 1981.

   This is an excellent review of the concepts of, and indications for, neurolysis.

54a. Gelberman RH (ed): Operative Nerve Repair and Reconstruction. Philadelphia, JB Lippincott, 1991.

   This is an excellent, excellently referenced, two-volume work covering clinical and surgical aspects of nerve injury and repair.

60. Gould JS: Treatment of the painful injured nerve in continuity. *In* Gelberman RH (ed): Operative Nerve Repair and Reconstruction. Philadelphia, JB Lippincott, 1991, pp 1541-1550.

   This is a valuable review of great personal experience in the treatment of lesions in continuity with reference to the experience with the indwelling nerve stimulator.

64. Hall S: Nerve repair: A neurobiologist's view. J Hand Surg [Br] 26:129-136, 2001.

90. Lundborg G: A 25-year perspective of peripheral nerve surgery; evolving neuroscientific concepts of clinical significance. J Hand Surg [Am] 25:391-414, 2000.

   These two articles provide excellent and critical reviews of the biological factors underlying the healing of nerves.

65a. Hazari A, Elliot D: Treatment of end-neuromas, neuromas-in-continuity and scarred nerves of the digits by proximal relocation. J Hand Surg [Br] 29:338-350, 2004.

A paper from Elliot's team that is of great importance, describing results of relocation for the painful nerve. The description of the method is outstanding, and this is essential reading.

67. Herndon JH: Neuromas. *In* Green DP, Hotchkiss RN, Pederson WC (eds): Green's Operative Hand Surgery, 4th ed. Amsterdam, Elsevier Science, 1999, pp 1469-1480.

This is a detailed and critical review of different methods of treatment of a painful neuroma and is based on great experience.

76. Kline DG, Hudson AR: Nerve Injuries. Philadelphia, WB Saunders, 1995.

This is outstanding work. The chapter on intraoperative neurophysiologic studies is essential reading.

81. Kline DG, Hudson AR, Kim DH: Atlas of Peripheral Nerve Surgery. Philadelphia, WB Saunders, 2001.

This is probably the best surgical atlas, and I consider this, with the work of Fiolle and Delmas, as essential reading.

91-93. Lundborg G: Nerve Injury and Repair. New York, Churchill Livingstone, 1988.

This is a gem. The sections on the blood supply of the nerves and on the connective tissue envelopes are especially illuminating.

107. Millesi H, Zoch G, Rath T: The gliding apparatus of peripheral nerves: Its clinical significance. Ann Hand Surg 9:87-97, 1990.

This is a particularly valuable contribution from a surgeon whose writings have been prolific and influential. Millesi and his colleagues emphasize the importance of the gliding of the nerve and of the anatomic features that permit this.

110. Narakas AO: Thoughts on neurotisation of nerve transfers in irreparable nerve lesions. *In* Tertzis JK (ed): Microreconstruction of Nerve Injuries. Philadelphia, WB Saunders, 1987, pp 447-454.

The contributions of Algimentas Narakas were of immense importance. He was a polymath, and study of all of his works is worthwhile. This contribution to Julie Tertzis' book provides a thoughtful, conceptual background to the concepts of nerve transfer.

118. Omer GE: Injuries to nerves of the upper extremity. J Bone Joint Surg Am 56:1615-1624, 1974.

119. Omer GE: The management of pain. *In* Lamb DW (ed): The Paralysed Hand. Edinburgh, Churchill Livingstone, 1987, pp 216-231.

Both of these papers contain a distillation of vast clinical knowledge.

134. Smith SJM: Electrodiagnosis. *In* Birch R, Bonney G, Wynn Parry CB (eds): Surgical Disorders of the Peripheral Nerves. London, Churchill Livingstone, 1998, pp 467-490.

This is probably the clearest exposition of the role of neurophysiologic investigations in clinical practice.

136. Sood MK, Elliot D: Treatment of painful neuromas of the hand and wrist by re-location into the pronator quadratus. J Hand Surg [Br] 23:214-219, 1998.

An important contribution describing a method of treatment for painful neuromas at the wrist and within the palm of the hand.

157. Wilgis EFS: Longitudinal excursion of nerves: Nerve repair and grafting. *In* Green DP (ed): Operative Hand Surgery, 2nd ed. New York, Churchill Livingstone, 1988, pp 1377-1378.

This paper is a valuable contribution to understanding the gliding properties of nerves and the extent of their excursion across joints.

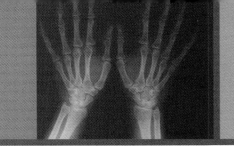

CHAPTER 31

Radial Nerve Palsy

David P. Green

Loss of radial nerve function in the hand creates a significant disability. The patient cannot extend the fingers and thumb and therefore has great difficulty in grasping objects. Perhaps more importantly, the loss of active wrist extension robs the patient of the mechanical advantage that wrist extension provides for grasp and power grip.[40] Tendon transfers to restore function in radial nerve palsy are among the best and most predictable transfers in the upper extremity, but, as Riordan[67] has pointed out, "in muscle tendon surgery there is very little hope that errors in technique can be overcome by local adaptation. The success or failure of an operation depends upon the technical competence of the operator and his painstaking after-care." Riordan[68] also noted that "there is usually only one chance to obtain good restoration of function in such a paralyzed hand."

Trauma to the upper extremity is such that most injuries of the radial nerve occur distal to the branches to the triceps in the upper arm. For this reason, transfers to restore triceps function are not included in this chapter.

It is imperative that the surgeon make the important distinction between complete radial nerve palsy (excluding the triceps) and posterior interosseous nerve palsy. The radial nerve innervates the BR and ECRL* before it divides into its two terminal branches, the posterior interosseous (motor) and superficial (sensory) branches. Clinically, I believe that it is extremely difficult, if not impossible, to determine the integrity of the ECRB in the presence of an intact ECRL, and the presence of the ECRB is variable in posterior interosseous nerve palsy. Spinner[75] has noted that the ECRB receives its innervation in the majority of limbs (58%) from the superficial radial nerve rather than from the posterior interosseous nerve. In any case, patients with posterior interosseous nerve palsy have at least one strong radial wrist extensor intact, resulting in radial deviation of the wrist with extension, which may be rather marked in some patients (Fig. 31-1). This clinical finding has significant implications in the choice of appropriate tendon transfers, as discussed later in the chapter.

---

*For simplicity, the abbreviations used throughout this chapter are listed in Table 31-1.

Table 31-1
ABBREVIATIONS USED IN THIS CHAPTER

APL	Abductor pollicis brevis
BR	Brachioradialis
ECRB	Extensor carpi radialis brevis
ECRL	Extensor carpi radialis longus
ECU	Extensor carpi ulnaris
EDC	Extensor digitorum communis
EDM	Extensor digiti minimi
EIP	Extensor indicis proprius
EPB	Extensor pollicis brevis
EPL	Extensor pollicis longus
FCR	Flexor carpi radialis
FCU	Flexor carpi ulnaris
FDP	Flexor digitorum profundus
FDS	Flexor digitorum sublimis (superficialis)
FPL	Flexor pollicis longus
PL	Palmaris longus
PT	Pronator teres
II	Index finger
III	Long finger
IV	Ring finger
V	Small finger

Anatomy

As it emerges from the supinator about 8 cm distal to the elbow joint, the posterior interosseous nerve splays out into multiple branches, which Spinner[75] has likened to the cauda equina. The difficulty in repairing an untidy laceration of the nerve at this level[63] often has an important influence on the timing of tendon transfers.

Abrams and associates[1] produced the best reference on the innervation order and location of motor branches of the radial nerve (Table 31-2). Although they found innervation order to be variable, knowledge of the general patterns and variations is important for the surgeon in following recovery from radial nerve injuries.

The surgeon who plans to perform transfers for radial nerve palsy must have a comprehensive three-dimensional understanding of the anatomy of the flexor and extensor muscles of the forearm. This is a complex area of anatomy

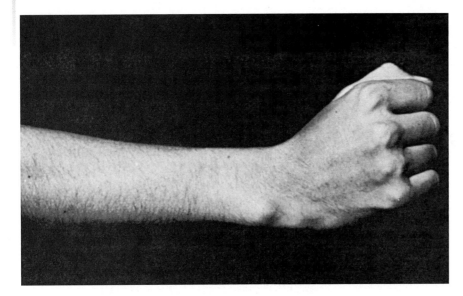

FIGURE 31-1. In a patient with posterior interosseous nerve palsy the ECRL is intact, resulting in radial deviation of the wrist in extension.

that is difficult to master, and continual review is mandatory. I find that the best sources for augmenting my knowledge of forearm anatomy are actual dissections in the laboratory, Henry's classic book,[34] the superb *Color Atlas of Human Anatomy* by McMinn and Hutchings,[50] and Doyle and Botte's new book on upper extremity anatomy.[27]

REQUIREMENTS IN THE PATIENT WITH RADIAL NERVE PALSY

The patient with irreparable radial nerve palsy needs to be provided with (1) wrist extension, (2) finger (metacarpophalangeal [MP] joint) extension, and (3) a combination of thumb extension and abduction. The motors available for transfer in a patient with an isolated radial nerve palsy include all the extrinsic muscles innervated by the median and ulnar nerves. This multitude of available motors provides the surgeon with an almost limitless number of possible combinations of transfers. Indeed, almost every conceivable combination has been tried, and a careful historical review of transfers for radial nerve palsy (see page 1118) will save the surgeon from some of the errors of the past.

Table 31-2
INNERVATION ORDER OF MUSCLES: RADIAL NERVE
BR
ECRL
Supinator*
ECRB
EDC
ECU
EDM
APL
EPL
EPB
EIP

*The supinator is included for completeness but cannot be tested clinically.

Unless the patient has a painful neuroma, the sensory part of the radial nerve can usually be ignored. Loss of sensibility on the radial side of the dorsum of the hand is perhaps bothersome but rarely a disability. Occasionally, the patient with a complete radial nerve palsy has no demonstrable sensory deficit, because in some patients the superficial branch of the radial nerve is absent and its function is preempted by the lateral antebrachial cutaneous nerve.[48,75]

NONOPERATIVE TREATMENT

By far the most important aspects of nonoperative management of the patient with radial nerve palsy are maintenance of full passive range of motion in all joints of the wrist and hand and prevention of contractures, including that of the thumb-index web. In most patients, the constant supervision of a therapist is not required, but the patient must be taught very soon after the original nerve injury how to carry out an appropriate exercise program to keep the joints supple. It is the patient's responsibility to do the exercises, and the role of the therapist at this point is to teach the patient and to monitor progress to be certain that the exercise program is carried out correctly.

Many types of splints have been described for patients with radial nerve palsy.[5,25,60,80] Most of these incorporate some type of dynamic outriggers to extend the fingers and thumb with elastic traction while allowing full mobility for active flexion. Not all patients with radial nerve palsy need this much elaborate splinting, and each patient's individual needs should dictate the type of splinting used; the same orthosis should not be prescribed for every patient. For example, a person who does data entry and wishes to continue working might be able to do so with the dynamic finger and thumb extension splint shown in Figure 31-2. However, an insurance salesman who is more concerned about appearance would probably be content with only a small, inconspicuous volar cock-up wrist splint, even though this does not provide nearly as much functional improvement as the dynamic splint.[33] In some patients, merely stabilizing the wrist in extension imparts remarkably good

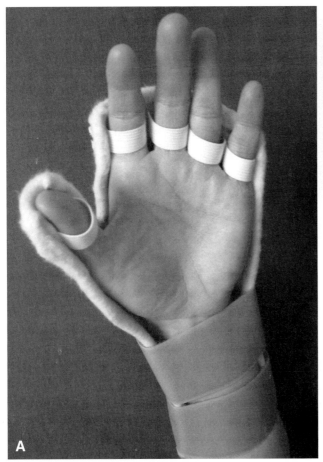

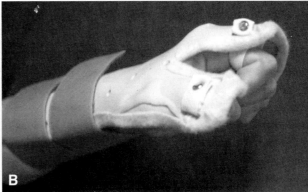

FIGURE 31-2. Many types of splints have been designed for patients with radial nerve palsy, most of which offer some type of extension assist. **A,** In one of the less cumbersome designs, passive MP extension is provided by simple elastic webbing beneath the proximal phalanges. **B,** Active flexion of the PIP joints is not impeded.

temporary function. Burkhalter[22] observed that grip strength may be increased three to five times by simply stabilizing the wrist with a splint. Brand[17] recommended that if a wrist splint is only worn during the day, the patient should alternate this with a night splint that holds the wrist and fingers in extension. This is because the disturbed balance of the wrist in radial nerve palsy can result in loss of fiber length of the flexor muscles, making it more difficult to achieve normal balance after the final nerve recovery or operation.[17]

Early Transfers ("Internal Splint")

It may seem to be a contradiction in terms to discuss early tendon transfer under nonoperative treatment, but this is to stress the concept of early transfers to provide a temporary "internal splint" and not as definitive treatment of the radial nerve palsy.

Burkhalter[22] believed that the greatest functional loss in the patient with radial nerve injury is weakness of power grip. Consequently, he was perhaps the strongest advocate of an early PT to ECRB transfer to eliminate the need for an external splint and, at the same time, to restore a significant amount of power grip to the patient's hand. In advocating early tendon transfer, Burkhalter was careful to emphasize what he called three indications and three important principles. The indications are that the transfer (1) works as a substitute during regeneration of the nerve to eliminate the need for splintage; (2) works as a helper after reinnervation

by adding the power of a normal muscle to the reinnervated muscles; and (3) acts as a substitute in cases in which the results of nerve repair are statistically poor (e.g., elderly patients, chronic injuries, crush injuries). The important principles are that the transfer should (1) not significantly decrease the remaining function in the hand; (2) not create a deformity if significant return occurs following nerve repair; and (3) be a phasic transfer or one capable of phase conversion.

Burkhalter believed that the PT to ECRB transfer fulfills all of these indications and principles, and he therefore suggested that the operation be done at the time of radial nerve repair or as soon as possible thereafter. The tendon juncture is done end-to-side, and the continuity of ECRB is not disrupted so that it may regain its own function if reinnervation should occur.

I have no personal experience with the use of this transfer as an internal splint, but its use was also supported by Omer[56] and Brand.[15]

OPERATIVE TREATMENT

Nerve Repair/Grafting Versus Tendon Transfers

The first decision to make in a patient with an established radial nerve palsy is whether to attempt late repair of the nerve or to restore lost function with tendon transfers. Obviously the time since injury is a critical factor (see page 1117), but late repair of the radial nerve can produce reasonably good results at least in part because the nerve is almost entirely motor and the motor branches are often reasonably close to the site of injury.[79] As discussed later under Timing of Tendon Transfers, if the prognosis for return after nerve repair is poor, it would appear prudent to forego an attempt at repair and proceed directly to tendon transfers.

When attempting late repair, the surgeon must be prepared to do nerve grafts if the gap is too great to overcome by direct epineurial repair without tension. Several authors[9,38,52,93,113] have shown reasonable results with late grafting of the radial nerve. Samardzic and colleagues[113] grafted gaps of 2 to 10 cm, but Kallio and coworkers[38] concluded that results were better if the grafts were less than 5 cm (see Chapter 30).

In patients with late radial nerve injuries, the surgeon should be fairly confident of successful repair before choosing that alternative over tendon transfers. If the nerve repair should fail, that costs the patient an additional 4 to 6 months of waiting for function to return before resorting to tendon transfers.

Principles of Tendon Transfers

The application of certain fundamental principles is essential for successful transfer of muscle tendon units. These important concepts were established by such masters as Mayer,[49] Steindler,[77] and Bunnell[13] and were re-emphasized by Littler,[44] Boyes,[10] Curtis,[26] White,[87] and Brand.[15] They have in fact been repeated so often that their significance may sometimes be obscured by familiarity, but they remain essential elements in successful tendon transfers.

Correction of Contracture

From the outset in the management of any patient with peripheral nerve palsy, it is imperative that all joints be kept supple, because soft tissue contracture is far easier to prevent than to correct. The essential principle here, of course, is that maximum passive motion of all joints must be present before a tendon transfer is performed, because no tendon transfer can move a stiff joint, and it is impossible for a joint to have more active motion postoperatively than it had passively preoperatively.

Adequate Strength

The tendon chosen as a donor for transfer must be sufficiently strong to perform its new function in its altered position. An appreciation of the relative strengths of the forearm muscles is important to the surgeon in selecting an appropriate motor (Table 31-3). Brand[16,18] has done elaborate anatomic dissections and biomechanical studies in an

effort to apply more scientific principles to tendon transfers, and his work should be read by every hand surgeon. Brand has noted that work capacity of a muscle is related to its volume and that excursion is related to its fiber length.[18] Lieber and colleagues[41] have further noted that the architectural features of individual muscles are highly specialized for function, and they have done extensive studies to determine how surgeons can make donor choices based on those features. In working toward this goal, they devised an intraoperative laser diffraction method, although this does not yet appear to be user (surgeon) friendly.[42,43]

Perhaps even more important than the theoretical strength of a given motor is its actual strength at the time of tendon transfer; and, in general, a muscle should not be used for transfer unless it can be graded as being at least good (Steindler recommended 85% of normal). If at all possible, I try to avoid using a muscle that has been previously denervated and now has returned to function. Omer[55,57] noted that a muscle will usually lose one grade of strength (on Highet's clinical scale) after transfer.

Amplitude of Motion

The surgeon must also have some appreciation of the amplitude of tendon excursion for each muscle. Although more precise values of these have been determined,[14,86,89] Boyes[12] suggested the use of the following values for practical purposes:

> Wrist flexors and extensors: 33 mm
> Finger extensors and EPL: 50 mm
> Finger flexors: 70 mm

These numbers have practical significance, because it is obviously impossible for a wrist flexor with an excursion of 33 mm to substitute fully for a finger extensor that requires an amplitude of 50 mm. Although the true amplitude of tendon excursion cannot be increased, two things can be done to augment its effective amplitude. First, a muscle can be converted from monarticular to biarticular or multiarticular, thereby effectively utilizing the natural tenodesis effect. For example, when an FCU or FCR is transferred to the EDC, it is converted to a multiarticular muscle and the effective amplitude of the tendon is increased significantly by active volar flexion of the wrist, thereby allowing the transferred wrist flexor to extend the fingers fully (Fig. 31-3). The second factor that can increase amplitude is extensive dissection of the muscle from its surrounding fascial attachments. This is particularly true of the BR.

Straight Line of Pull

The pioneers of tendon transfer surgery repeatedly emphasized that the most efficient transfer is one that passes in a direct line from its own origin to the insertion of the tendon being substituted. Although this is not always possible (e.g., in an opponensplasty), it is a desirable goal to seek and is particularly important in the FCU to EDC transfer, which is described later in this chapter.

One Tendon—One Function

It is obvious that a single tendon cannot be expected to perform two diametrically opposing actions simultaneously, for example, to flex and extend the same joint. It is perhaps not quite so obvious that the effectiveness of a tendon

Table 31-3
WORK CAPACITY OF FOREARM MUSCLES

Donor Muscles (Mkg)		Recipient Muscles (Mkg)	
BR	1.9	EPL	0.1
PT	1.2	APL	0.1
FCR	0.8	EPB	0.1
FCU	2.0	EDC	1.7
PL	0.1	EIP	0.5
FDS	4.8	ECRL	1.1
FDP	4.5	ECRB	0.9
FPL	1.2	ECU	1.1

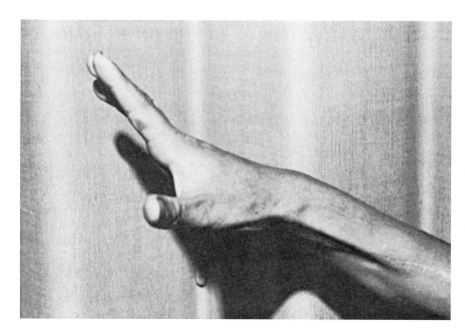

FIGURE 31-3. A wrist flexor transferred to the finger extensors does not have sufficient amplitude of excursion to simultaneously extend the wrist and fingers. In this patient after FCU to EDC transfer, note that he uses the tenodesis effect created by active volar flexion of the wrist to enhance the effective excursion of the tendon and thereby achieve excellent active extension of the fingers (compare with Figure 31-12).

transfer is reduced when it is expected to produce two dissimilar functions even when they are not direct opposites. If a muscle is inserted into two tendons having separate functions, the force and amplitude of the donor tendon will be dissipated and less effective than it would be if it motored only a single tendon.[71] At the very least, if a single tendon is transferred into two separate tendons, the excursion of the two should be the same.[17]

Synergism

There is debate among hand surgeons as to the importance of synergistic motion in the hand, that is, finger flexors acting in concert with wrist extensors and finger extensors acting with wrist flexors. Littler[44] was a major advocate of the use of synergistic muscles for transfer whenever possible, and I believe that it is easier to retrain muscle function after synergistic muscle transfers. A possible exception to this rule is the use of the superficialis (sublimis) tendons, which have more independent cortical control than other muscles in the hand.

Expendable Donor

Removal of a tendon for transfer must not result in unacceptable loss of function; there must be sufficient muscle remaining to substitute for the donor muscle. The classic example of this is the necessity of retaining one strong wrist flexor (PL is not adequate) in any combination of transfers for radial nerve palsy (see page 1118).

Tissue Equilibrium

The timing of tendon transfers is somewhat controversial, but all authors agree that no transfer should be done until the local tissues are in optimal condition. Steindler's classic expression "tissue equilibrium" (quoted by Boyes[10]) is a good one; it implies that soft tissue induration is gone, the wounds are mature, the joints are supple, and the scars are as soft as they are likely to become. To perform tendon transfers or any elective operation before tissue equilibrium has been reached is to invite disaster. If scar tissue remains after maximum recovery has been achieved, the surgeon must

consider providing new skin coverage with flaps before transfer or, alternatively, devise transfers that will avoid the scarred areas. Tendon transfers work best when passed between the subcutaneous fat and deep fascial layer; they are not likely to work at all in a pathway of scar. Brand[17] emphasized the concept of gentle tunneling, using a blunt-tipped instrument and probing natural tissue planes to find the path of least resistance. When performing tendon transfers, the surgeon should think in terms of trying to minimize scar formation, and skin incisions should be planned so as to place tendon junctures beneath flaps rather than directly beneath incisions.[55]

Timing of Tendon Transfers

The appropriate time to perform transfers for radial nerve palsy is a somewhat controversial subject. As noted previously, several authors[15,17,22,56,63] advocate only a limited transfer (PT to ECRB) almost immediately after injury to act as an internal splint and also to supplement any return in the reinnervated extensor muscles. Brown[21] suggested that it is advisable to proceed with the full component of tendon transfers early when there is a questionable or poor prognosis from the nerve repair. For example, if there is a nerve gap of more than 4 cm or if there is a large wound or extensive scarring or skin loss over the nerve, he recommended ignoring the nerve and proceeding directly to the tendon transfers. I basically agree with Brown: if the chances of nerve regeneration are poor, there is no point in waiting before doing the transfers. However, if a good repair of the nerve has been accomplished, it is my practice to wait a sufficient period of time before considering transfer. In my opinion, "sufficient time" is determined by using Seddon's[73] figures for nerve regeneration (i.e., approximately 1 mm/day). This means that it may take as long as 5 or 6 months before one sees return in the most proximal muscles (BR and ECRL) after nerve repair in the middle third of the arm (see Fig. 38-13). The remaining muscles should return in orderly progression at the same rate of 1 mm/day (Table 31-4).

Table 31-4

DISTANCES (CM) FROM THE DISTAL END OF SUPINATOR TO THE POINT OF INNERVATION

ECU	1.25
EDC	1.25-1.8
EDM	1.8
APL	5.6
EPB	6.5
EIP	6.8
EPL	7.5

From Spinner M: The radial nerve. *In* Injuries to the Major Branches of Peripheral Nerves of the Forearm. Philadelphia, WB Saunders, 1972, pp 28-65.

Table 31-5

JONES TRANSFERS

1916[35]
PT to ECRL and ECRB
FCU to EDC III-V
FCR to EIP, EDC II, and EPL

1921[37]
PT to ECRL and ECRB
FCU to EDC III-V
FCR to EIP, EDC II, EPL, EPB, and APL

To my knowledge, there is little popular support for the concept offered by Bevin[6] of never repairing the radial nerve and proceeding directly to tendon transfers. Although he demonstrated impressive differences in disability times (8 weeks after tendon transfers, 7.5 months after nerve repair), I believe that most surgeons would agree that the results of radial nerve repair are sufficiently good to warrant routine repair in all cases except perhaps in those identified by Brown as having a poor prognosis.

There does not appear to be any time limit as to how long a delay can be tolerated before transfers are done after nerve injury. Brodman[19] reported successful transfers 24 years after radial nerve injury, despite what he described as "gelatinous degeneration" (i.e., translucent appearance) of the paralyzed tendons at the time of operation.

Historical Review

As with the management of peripheral nerve injuries, the development of operative procedures for treatment of irreparable radial nerve palsy mainly evolved during the two world wars. Most of the important articles that established the fundamentals of transfers for radial nerve palsy are to be found in the immediate postwar years. The tragedies of the wars enabled a few individuals to accumulate a lifetime of experience in a very short period of time. For example, Scuderi[71] reported 45 patients with radial nerve palsy in whom he performed transfers during a 12.5-month period.

Sir Robert Jones is credited with being the major innovator of radial nerve transfers, and all the articles in the post–World War I era acknowledged his fundamental contributions. However, the "classic" Jones transfer has been quoted and misquoted so many times in articles and texts that it is worthwhile to review his original articles[35-37] to see exactly what he did advocate. Part of the confusion arises from the fact that Jones did describe at least two slightly different combinations of transfers, as outlined in Table 31-5.

Although the Jones transfers came to be one of the more popular operations for radial nerve palsy, they were by no means universally accepted. Virtually every conceivable combination of transfers for radial nerve palsy has been reported,[4,7,20,28,36,59,61,67,78] and the reader interested in this fascinating aspect of medical history is referred to Boyes' superb article,[11] which outlines the multitude of procedures described between 1897 and 1959. For the purpose of this discussion, it is pertinent to mention some of the more important highlights in the development of transfers for radial nerve palsy.

The only part of the classic Jones transfer that has become universally accepted is the use of the PT to provide active wrist extension; however, even this acceptance came relatively recently. Saikku[70] pointed out that at the onset of World War II there were two schools of thought regarding the best method of restoring wrist extension in the patient with radial nerve palsy. The British and Americans tended to favor Jones' transfer of the PT to the radial wrist extensors, whereas the Germans were influenced by the recommendation of Perthes, who advocated a tenodesis or arthrodesis to maintain a dorsiflexed attitude of the wrist. Saikku reviewed a large series comparing the two methods and concluded that the Jones transfer was superior, noting a high failure rate with tenodesis due to loosening. A few authors have favored wrist arthrodesis,[58,77] but most believe that it is important to maintain wrist motion in a patient with radial nerve palsy.[5,10,12,44,64,66,70,90]

The only current controversy regarding the pronator transfer centers around the optimal insertion of the PT[16,17,20,44,51,54,56] (see page 1123).

Major disagreement arises concerning the optimal method of restoring finger extension and thumb extension and abduction. It is clear that Jones advocated transferring both strong wrist flexors (FCU and FCR), a practice apparently not questioned by most of his contemporaries. Although Starr,[76] in 1922, was the first to transfer the PL and leave one of the strong wrist flexors intact, his article leads the reader to wonder if he fully appreciated the significance of his contribution. Indeed, it was not until 1946 that Zachary[91] documented and convincingly illustrated the concept that it is desirable to leave one wrist flexor intact. He showed that the PL is not adequate to provide satisfactory wrist flexion if both the FCU and FCR are transferred. As recently as 1996, Gaur and Swarup[31] used both the FCR and FCU, but they reaffirmed the principle that improved functional results were achieved if the FCU was spared to maintain flexion and ulnar deviation of the wrist.

In 1949, Scuderi[71] refined the PL to rerouted EPL transfer, emphasizing the important principle that function is better when the transfer is done into only one tendon (note in Table 31-5 that by 1921 Jones was suturing the FCR into four tendons with separate functions!).

The results of these and other studies gradually evolved into what has been referred to by some as the "standard" set of tendon transfers for radial nerve palsy:

PT to ECRB
FCU to EDC II-V
PL to rerouted EPL

In France, a slightly modified version of this set (FCU to EDC and EPL; PL to EPB and APL) is known as the Merle d'Aubigné procedure[39] for the renowned orthopedic surgeon who first described it in 1946.

However, there is still not total agreement on the best combination of transfers. In 1960, Boyes[11] offered a reasonable alternative to the standard set of transfers that seems to have withstood the test of time.[24] Boyes reasoned that the FCU is a more important wrist flexor to preserve than the FCR because the normal axis of wrist motion is from dorsoradial to volar-ulnar. Brand's extensive biomechanical and clinical studies have led him to the firm conviction that the FCU should not be used as a tendon transfer for two reasons[16,17]: (1) the FCU is too strong and its excursion too short for transfer to the finger extensors; and (2) its function as the prime ulnar stabilizer of the wrist is too important to sacrifice. Despite these theoretical concerns, some recent studies have shown no functional loss of power grip with the FCU set.[29,62]

Another reason for not using the FCU set of transfers is that it cannot provide simultaneous wrist dorsiflexion and finger extension. Because the amplitude of the wrist flexors is only about 33 mm and that of the finger extensors is 50 mm, full active extension of the fingers with an FCU or FCR transfer can be achieved only by simultaneous volar flexion of the wrist, relying on the tenodesis effect of the transfer (see Fig. 31-3). Boyes thus concluded that, because of their greater excursion (70 mm), the superficialis (sublimis) tendons would be ideal motors for finger extensors. Yet another reason for his new combination of transfers was to provide more independent control of the thumb and index finger. The combination of transfers he described is as follows:

PT to ECRL and ECRB
FCR to EPB and APL
FDS III to EDC (via interosseous membrane)
FDS IV to EPL and EIP (via interosseous membrane)

Tendon Transfers

Although there are almost an infinite number of possible combinations of transfers for radial nerve palsy, I believe it is safe to say that there are three sets of transfers that are currently considered to be the most reasonable alternatives (Table 31-6). In the past, the most widely used set of transfers was probably that using FCU. Boyes' procedure that utilizes the superficialis tendons for finger extension has also proved to be quite satisfactory. The third combination is that first proposed by Starr[76] in 1922 and more recently described in detail by Brand,[15] which utilizes the FCR instead of the FCU. The operative techniques for these three procedures are described in detail below.

It is of course obvious that in a patient with posterior interosseous palsy the PT transfer is not necessary to restore wrist extension. In addition, the isolated posterior interosseous nerve palsy provides perhaps the most compelling indication for the FCR transfer; static radial deviation postural deformity may occur when the only remaining ulnar deviator is transferred.

Table 31-6

BEST COMBINATIONS OF TENDON TRANSFERS FOR RADIAL NERVE PALSY

FCR Transfer (Starr,[76] Brand,[15] Tsuge and Adachi[84])
PT to ECRB
FCR to EDC
PL to rerouted EPL

Superficialis Transfer (Boyes[11]; Chuinard et al[24])
PT to ECRL and ECRB
FDS III to EDC
FDS IV to EIP and EPL
FCR to APL and EPB

FCU Transfer
PT to ECRB
FCU to EDC
PL to reroute EPL

FCU Transfer

The first incision (Fig. 31-4) is directed longitudinally over the FCU in the distal half of the forearm. Its distal end is "J" shaped, with the transverse extension being long enough to reach the PL tendon. The FCU tendon is transected just proximal to the pisiform and freed up as far proximally as the incision will allow. Separation of this muscle from its particularly dense fascial attachments is facilitated by a special tendon stripper designed by Carroll (Fig. 31-5); however, if this tendon stripper is not available, the dissection of the FCU can be done under direct vision by extending the first incision more proximally. The muscle belly of the FCU is very long, extending usually to within a few centimeters of the insertion of the tendon. I prefer to excise rather generously that part of the muscle belly that is attached to the distal half of the tendon, because this will later facilitate the transfer and cause a less bulky appearance of the muscle in its new position around the ulnar border of the forearm.

The second incision begins 2 inches below the medial epicondyle and angles across the dorsum of the proximal forearm, aimed directly toward Lister's tubercle. The deep fascia overlying the FCU muscle belly is excised, and the remainder of the fascial attachments to the muscle is incised. It is imperative that the FCU be completely freed up so that the entire muscle belly and tendon can be displaced into the proximal wound to redirect the muscle. The limiting factor in the dissection is the innervation of the FCU, which enters the muscle in its proximal 2 inches, and the dissection must not extend this far proximally.

The third incision begins on the volar-radial aspect of the mid forearm, passes dorsally around the radial border of the forearm in the region of the insertion of the PT, and then angles back on the dorsum of the distal forearm toward Lister's tubercle. The tendon of the PT is identified in the volar aspect of the wound and followed to its insertion on the radius. It is important to free up the insertion with an intact long strip of periosteum to ensure that the length will be sufficient for a strong tendon juncture later (Fig. 31-6). Tubiana and colleagues[85] emphasized that the PT muscle-tendon unit must be freed up proximally to divide adhesions

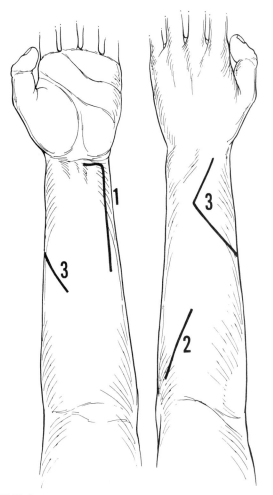

FIGURE 31-4. Incisions used in the FCU combination of transfers (see text).

to improve subsequent excursion. The PT muscle and tendon are then passed subcutaneously around the radial border of the forearm, superficial to the BR and ECRL, to be inserted into the ECRB just distal to its musculotendinous junction.

A tendon passer or large Kelly clamp is then passed from the dorsal wound (third incision) subcutaneously around the ulnar border of the forearm, and the tendon of the FCU is pulled into the dorsal wound (Fig. 31-7). At this point, if there is still excessive bulk of muscle overlying the ulnar border, the FCU muscle belly can be trimmed a bit more. It is imperative that the line of pull of the FCU be as straight as possible from the medial epicondyle to the EDC tendon

just proximal to the dorsal retinaculum. If the previous dissection has not freed up all the fascial attachments of FCU, it will be impossible to achieve this important direct pull.

The EPL muscle is then identified in the dorsal wound; it is divided at its musculotendinous junction and rerouted out of Lister's canal toward the volar aspect of the wrist across the anatomic snuffbox (Fig. 31-8). The PL tendon is transected at the wrist, and the muscle-tendon unit is freed up proximally enough to allow a straight line of pull between the PL and the rerouted EPL tendon. The PL tendon is delivered into the dorsal wound in the region of the snuffbox.

A variation in technique recommended by Moberg and Nachemson[53] is to open the dorsal retinaculum "to prevent ischemic necrosis of the tendons secondary to postoperative edema." I am not aware of this being a common problem, but their modification does provide a straighter line of pull.

At this point, I prefer to release the tourniquet, establish hemostasis, and close the first and second incisions before doing the final tendon junctures.

Setting the proper tension in the transfers is a somewhat tricky task but is very critical to the outcome of the operation. It is difficult to describe precisely how to adjust tension in tendon transfers, and a certain amount of experience is essential in being able to "feel" the proper tension. In general, however, one should probably err on the side of suturing extensor tendon transfers too tightly rather than too loosely because the extensors tend to stretch out with time.[74] The tendons must be tight enough to provide full extension of the wrist, fingers, and thumb, yet not so tight as to limit flexion of the digits. I usually suture the PT to ECRB (*not* including the ECRL) just distal to the musculotendinous junction. The long tongue of periosteum at the end of the PT tendon is woven through the tendon of the ECRB and secured with multiple 4-0 nonabsorbable sutures. (Omer[55] prefers larger [2-0 or 3-0] material.) Even if a tongue of periosteum has been harvested with the PT insertion, I have found that this often provides a rather insecure tendon juncture, and I now routinely reinforce this juncture with a short strip of free tendon graft taken from the ECRL. The transfer is sutured with the PT in maximum tension and the wrist in moderate (45 degrees) extension.

The FCU transfer is then sutured. I generally use the technique described by Omer[54] (and depicted in Figure 31-7), weaving the FCU tendon through the EDC tendons at a 45-degree angle just proximal to the dorsal retinaculum. Moberg and Nachemson[53] have suggested that better results can be achieved if 4 to 5 cm of inactivated EDC muscle-tendon is resected just proximal to the intended site of suture. Although I have not used this technique, it does

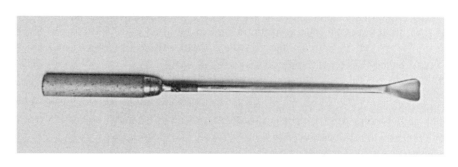

FIGURE 31-5. This instrument designed by Carroll facilitates division of the extensive fascial attachments of the muscle belly of the FCU.

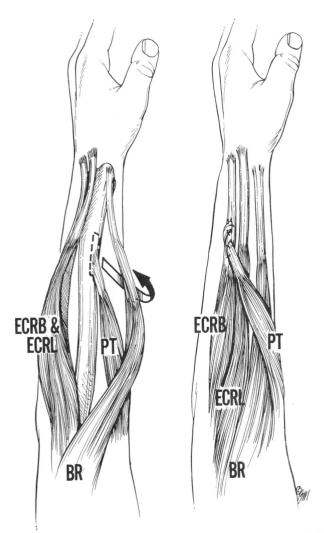

FIGURE 31-6. PT to ECRB transfer. It is important to take a strip of periosteum in continuity with the PT insertion to ensure adequate length for the transfer.

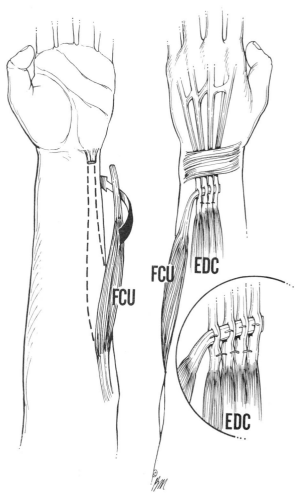

FIGURE 31-7. FCU to EDC transfer. The FCU must be freed up extensively to create a direct line of pull from its origin to the new insertion into the EDC tendons just proximal to the dorsal retinaculum. End-to-side juncture is shown here. Moberg and Nachemson[53] have suggested that 4 to 5 cm of the paralyzed EDC tendons be resected proximal to the juncture, allowing an end-to-end suture and a more direct line of pull.

provide a more direct line of pull because the tendon juncture is end-to-end rather than end-to-side.[30]

Most authors do not include the EDM in the transfer for fear of creating excessive tension in the small finger. I determine whether to include it by pulling on the EDC tendons with an Allis clamp (proximal to the intended site of juncture); if the small finger extends adequately, the EDM is not included, but if there is an extensor lag in the small finger (signifying an inadequate slip of EDC to the small finger), I include the EDM among the recipient tendons. It is important to suture the FCU tendon into each EDC slip separately and to adjust the tension in the EDC tendons individually so that all four MP joints extend synchronously and evenly. I prefer 4-0 nonabsorbable suture, and the tension I use is with the wrist and MP joints in neutral (0 degrees) and the FCU under maximum tension. A good assistant is very helpful at this point to aid in holding the tension while the tendons are sutured.

Retraction on the distal end of the third incision will allow the third and final juncture (PL to rerouted EPL) to be made in the region of the anatomic snuffbox superficial to the dorsal retinaculum. The direction of the tendons is

essentially in line with the first metacarpal (Fig. 31-9). My preferred tension is with the wrist in neutral and with maximum tension on both the EPL and PL tendons.

The tension must be tested by passively moving the wrist to demonstrate the synergistic action of the new transfer; with the wrist in extension, it should be possible to easily flex the fingers completely into the palm, and with the wrist in volar flexion, the MP joints should pull into full extension but not hyperextension.

The third incision is then closed while an assistant stabilizes the position of the wrist and hand to protect the transfers. I prefer to close all three wounds with subcuticular sutures to avoid unattractive crosshatches in the scars.

Postoperative Management

In the operating room, a long-arm splint is applied that immobilizes the forearm in 15 to 30 degrees of pronation, the wrist in approximately 45 degrees of extension, the MP joints in slight (10 to 15 degrees) flexion, and the thumb in maximum extension and abduction. The proximal interpha-

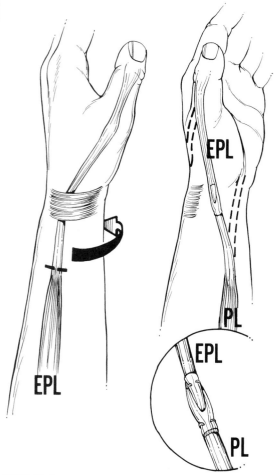

FIGURE 31-8. PL to rerouted EPL transfer. By rerouting the EPL out of the dorsal retinaculum, the transfer creates a combination of abduction and extension force on the thumb.

CRITICAL POINTS: FCU TO EDC

- Do not use for tendon transfer in posterior interosseous palsy.
- The FCU must be freed up extensively, requiring a long incision.
- Generously excise muscle from the distal half of the tendon to reduce bulk.
- Free up the muscle sufficiently to allow it to be redirected obliquely across the forearm.
- Protect the muscle's innervation in the proximal muscle belly.
- Create a line of pull from the medial epicondyle to the EDC as straight as possible.
- Tendon juncture: weave the FCU through the EDC tendons at a 45-degree angle just proximal to the dorsal retinaculum.
- Include the EDM only if there is a lag in extension of the small finger.
- Tension:
  - Wrist in neutral (0 degrees)
  - MP joints in neutral (0 degrees)
  - FCU under maximum tension

langeal (PIP) joints of the fingers are left free. Because limited elbow motion will not cause undue tension on the suture lines, a single sugar tong splint is a satisfactory alternative to the long-arm splint. The splint and sutures are removed at 10 to 14 days, and a Munster-type long-arm cast is applied in the same position as noted previously. The cast is removed 4 weeks postoperatively; removable short-arm splints to hold the wrist, fingers, and thumb in extension are made, which the patient wears for an additional 2 weeks, removing them only for exercise.

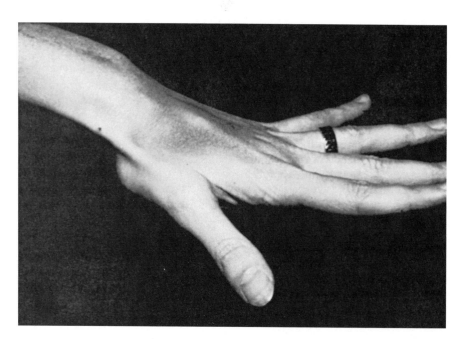

FIGURE 31-9. PL to rerouted EPL transfer. Note that the line of pull is essentially in line with the thumb metacarpal.

CRITICAL POINTS: PL TO REROUTED EPL

- EPL is transected at its musculotendinous junction.
- EPL tendon is rerouted to pass along the radial border of the thumb metacarpal.
- Tendon juncture of PL to EPL is in the snuffbox superficial to dorsal retinaculum in line with thumb metacarpal.
- Tension:
  • Wrist in neutral (0 degrees)
  • Maximum tension on distal stump of EPL
  • PL under maximum tension

CRITICAL POINTS: PT TO ECRB

- Take a strip of periosteum from the radius in continuity with the PT insertion.
- Free up the muscle proximally to gain maximum excursion.
- Pass the tendon around the radial border of forearm superficial to the BR and ECRL.
- Suture only into ECRB—do not include ECRL—just distal to musculotendinous junction.
- Tension:
  • Wrist in 45 degrees of extension
  • PT under maximum tension
- Reinforce juncture with strip of free tendon graft.

A planned exercise program, begun at 4 weeks, under the guidance of an experienced hand therapist is very beneficial to achieve the optimal results from this procedure. After these transfers, I find it particularly useful to instruct the patient in synergistic movements. A well-motivated patient should have good control of function by 3 months, although many patients take as long as 6 months to reach maximum recovery.

Potential Problems

Excessive Radial Deviation. Removing the FCU (an important wrist flexor and the only remaining ulnar deviator) from the wrist in a patient with radial nerve palsy may contribute to radial deviation of the hand. This is likely to be further aggravated if the PT is inserted into the ECRL, which Youm and coworkers[89] have shown to be mainly a radial deviator rather than an extensor of the wrist. Even if the transfer is into the more centrally located ECRB, there may be some radial deviation because the ECRB, although more centrally located than the ECRL, still imparts some radial deviation.[15] Also, significant intercommunication between the ECRL and ECRB has been identified by Albright and Linburg.[3] The problem is particularly severe in patients with posterior interosseous nerve palsy who have a normally functioning, strong ECRL; in my experience, removing the FCU in these patients can seriously aggravate the radial deviation problem.

Several solutions to the problem have been suggested and are listed below.

Avoidance. I consider significant preoperative radial deviation (e.g., the patient with posterior interosseous nerve palsy) to be a contraindication to the FCU transfer. In such cases, I prefer to use Boyes' superficialis transfers or the FCR transfer.

Alter the Insertion. Although avoidance of the problem is preferable (by not doing the FCU transfer), it is also possible to reduce radial deviation by altering the insertion of the radial wrist extensors at the time of PT transfer. The simplest way to do this is to resect the distal 2 to 3 cm of the ECRL tendon and suture the tendon more proximally into the adjacent ECRB, thereby eliminating any possibility of pull through the ECRL insertion. A more radical approach is to shift the distal end of the ECRB into the tendon of the ECU[84] or to cut the ECU at its musculotendinous junction, transpose the proximal end across the forearm, and include it in the PT to ECRB transfer, as suggested by Said.[69] Brand[16] said that this is not a good idea because the ECU has a very small moment for extension and such an altered insertion would limit the total extension moment of the PT. His preference was to attach PT to the ECRL and ECRB together proximally and then detach the insertion of ECRL and reinsert it into the base of the fourth metacarpal. Tubiana and colleagues[85] also preferred to centralize the insertion of the ECRL. In addition to the different moment arms of ECRL and ECRB for wrist extension and radial deviation, they were also concerned about adhesions between the two tendons. Therefore, they sutured the PT to only the ECRB but also rerouted the insertion of the ECRL. The ECRL tendon is divided at its insertion into the base of the second metacarpal, freed up proximally to its musculotendinous junction, rerouted beneath the dorsal retinaculum in the fourth (EDC) compartment, and fixed to the base of the third and fourth metacarpals with sutures and staples (Fig. 31-10).

Absence of the PL. Absence of the PL compromises the FCU set of transfers because it obviously eliminates the important PL to rerouted EPL transfer. In this situation, several authors suggest simply including the EPL into the FCU to EDC transfer, although this significantly limits the abduction component of the transfer's effect on the thumb. Bevin[6] suggested including all of the thumb extrinsics (EPL, EPB, and APL) in the FCU to EDC transfer, but this seriously violates the one tendon–one function principle. Milford[51] advocated the use of the BR, which is of course possible only in posterior interosseous nerve palsy and not in complete radial nerve palsy. If the BR is used as a transfer, extensive freeing up of the muscle belly is necessary to augment its excursion, and Beasley[5] has commented that the BR is more difficult to re-educate in the rehabilitation program. Tsuge[84] and Goldner[32] substituted the FDS III or IV for an absent PL.

Not being totally satisfied with any of these alternatives, I generally do Boyes' superficialis transfers when the PL is absent.

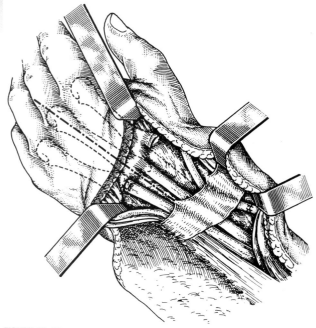

FIGURE 31-10. Tubiana's method of reinserting the ECRL into the base of the third and fourth metacarpals (see text for details). (From Tubiana R, Miller HW IV, Reed S: Restoration of wrist extension after paralysis. Hand Clin 5:53-67, 1989.)

Bowstringing of the EPL. Tsuge[84] noted a relatively minor problem of bowstringing of the rerouted EPL tendon across the radial aspect of the wrist. He reported that this may be prevented by hooking the EPL around the insertion of the APL at the time of the tendon transfer. I have not seen this problem and therefore have no experience with this modification.

Superficialis Transfer (Boyes[11,24])

Through a long incision on the volar side of the radial aspect of the mid forearm, the tendons of PT, ECRL, and ECRB are exposed. The insertion of the PT is removed with a 2- to 3-cm strip of periosteum, and this tendinous portion is interwoven through the ECRB just distal to the musculotendinous junction. As noted on page 1120, I prefer to reinforce the tendon juncture with a short strip of free tendon graft taken from the ECRL if the periosteal strip of PT is not substantial enough to provide secure fixation. In the original descriptions of this transfer,[11,24] the PT was sutured to both the ECRL and ECRB, but for the reasons noted previously, I use only the ECRB.

The superficialis (sublimis) tendons of the long and ring fingers are exposed through a transverse incision in the distal palm or through separate transverse incisions at the base of each finger. The tendons are divided proximal to the chiasma, freed up, and delivered into the forearm wound. At a level just proximal to the pronator quadratus, two 1 × 2-cm openings are excised from the interosseous membrane, one on each side of the anterior interosseous artery. Care is taken to protect both the anterior and posterior interosseous vessels. Numerous authors,[2,5] including Boyes,[13] have recommended that the muscle bellies of the transferred muscles be passed through the interosseous space to minimize adhesions. This may necessitate a larger opening in the interosseous membrane than that recommended by Chuinard and coworkers.[24] Others[82] prefer to route the superficialis tendons around the radial and ulnar borders of the forearm, respectively, in an effort to avoid tendon adherence, although ulnar nerve compression can occur when the FDS is transferred around the ulnar border.[83] Care should be taken to route the transfer deep to the ulnar bundle and immediately superficial to the periosteum of the ulna to avoid this complication.

A "J"-shaped incision is then made on the dorsum of the distal forearm; the transverse limb runs from the radial styloid to the ulnar styloid, and the longitudinal limb extends proximally along the ulna. The flexor tendons are passed to the dorsum through the openings in the interosseous membrane, with the FDS III routed to the radial side of the profundus mass, between the FDP and FPL, and the FDS IV routed to the ulnar side of the profundus muscle mass. Care must be taken to avoid kinking the median nerve as the muscles are passed into the opening. O'Brien (O'Brien ET, personal communication, 1982) has noted kinking of the nerve by a band of fascia on the superficialis muscle belly. The FDS III is interwoven into the tendons of the EIP and EPL, and the FDS IV into EDC. (Chotigavanich[23] modified the Boyes technique by using only the FDS IV to power the finger extensors.) The EDM is not included, and the recipient tendons are not divided proximal to the tendon juncture. The suture lines are placed proximal to the dorsal retinaculum, which may be narrowed if there is danger of impingement by the tendon junctures.

Reid[63] described Raffety's technique for setting the tension in this set of transfers. An assistant clenches the patient's fingers and thumb into a fist and brings the wrist into 20 degrees of extension. This position is maintained until all the transferred tendons are attached to their new insertions under "considerable tension."

Through a transverse incision at the base of the thumb, the FCR tendon is divided and freed up sufficiently to allow it to be turned dorsally and passed through the multiple slips of the APL, where it is sutured in place. Boyes' original description included insertion into the EPB, but I prefer to follow the one tendon–one function rule (see page 1116) and therefore do not include the EPB.

CRITICAL POINTS: FDS TO EDC AND EPL

- Divide the FDS tendons to III and IV in the distal palm proximal to the chiasma.
- To minimize adhesions in passing through the interosseous membrane (IOM), excise a large opening in the IOM and pass the muscle bellies through.
- Tension:
  - Wrist in 20 degrees of extension
  - Fingers and thumb held in a fist by an assistant
  - FDS under maximum tension

Milford[51] and Omer[57] stressed the importance of deflating the tourniquet before wound closure because of possible damage to the interosseous vessels.

Postoperative Management

Postoperative splints similar to those described on page 1121 are applied and worn for 4 weeks, at which time the sutures are removed and a splint is worn day and night for the next 2 weeks, except during exercise periods. All external support is then discontinued at 6 weeks postoperatively. The exercise program should emphasize specific control of the superficialis muscles to try to take advantage of the greater excursion of these tendons. It should not use the tenodesis techniques that are useful after the synergistic (FCU and FCR) transfers.

FCR Transfer (Starr[76]; Brand[15,17]; Tsuge[84])

The PT to ECRB transfer, when required, is performed as described previously with the other transfers.

A straight longitudinal incision is made in the distal half of the volar radial aspect of the forearm between the FCR and PL. Both tendons are identified, transected near their insertions, and freed up to the middle of the forearm to allow redirection of the tendons to their new insertions. A second longitudinal incision is made on the dorsum, extending from just distal to the dorsal retinaculum to the mid forearm. The FCR is passed around the radial border of the forearm through a subcutaneous tunnel, which is created with a blunt-nosed instrument that probes natural tissue planes to find the path of least resistance.[17] The juncture between the FCR and EDC can be made by leaving the EDC in continuity (similar to the FCU transfer depicted in Figure 31-7), but Brand recommended that the EDC tendons be divided so that a formal end-to-end suture can be done between the FCR and EDC, as shown in Figure 31-11. To avoid the problem of multiple exposed raw tendon ends, Brand suggested burying each cut tendon end. The finger extensor tendons are all tested for extension of the MP joint, and "four good tendons are chosen."[15] These are divided at their musculotendinous junctions, withdrawn distally, superficial to the intact dorsal retinaculum, and redirected to a point over the distal radius, where they can meet the FCR tendon in a straight line. A preliminary suture between the EDC tendons before sectioning can be helpful to maintain correct balance of tension between the tendons. The tendons are then retested for effective pull-through at the MP joints in case the change of direction has placed some cross connection under tension. Brand left the two best tendons long to join the FCR, suturing the other two to their neighbors more distally. The tendon juncture is done as shown in Figure 31-11, passing the two slips of the EDC into slits in the FCR and burying their ends in a second slit. With the tendons left long, care is taken to ensure appropriate tension on each of the four tendons before making the final cut of the tendons and burying their ends. I would recommend suturing the tendons with the wrist and MP joints in neutral and the FCR tendon under maximum tension. Tsuge[84] modified the FCR transfer by passing it through the interosseous membrane to obtain a straighter line of pull.

The PL to rerouted EPL transfer is performed as described on page 1121. If the PL is absent, the EPL is joined with the EDC to the FCR transfer.[15] Postoperative management is the same as that described on page 1121.

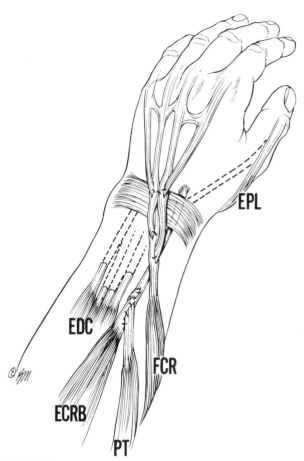

FIGURE 31-11. FCR to EDC transfer. Brand[15] suggested that the EDC tendons be transected and transposed superficial to the dorsal retinaculum to create a straight-line end-to-end juncture with the FCR. (Adapted from Brand PW: Tendon transfers in the forearm. *In* Flynn JE [ed]: Hand Surgery, 2nd ed. Baltimore, Williams & Wilkins, 1975, pp 189-200.)

CRITICAL POINTS: FCR TO EDC

- Divide the FCR near its insertion and pass it subcutaneously around the radial border of forearm.
- Divide the EDC tendons just proximal to the retinaculum and reposition the stumps superficial to the retinaculum.
- Tension:
  - Wrist in neutral (0 degrees)
  - MP joints in neutral (0 degrees)
  - FCR under maximum tension

 Author's Preferred Method of Treatment

I believe it is important for the hand surgeon to be well versed in at least two of the previously described transfers, because it is preferable to choose an operation for the individual patient rather than to try to adapt all patients to a single procedure.

I strongly prefer the FCR set of transfers for most patients with radial or posterior interosseous nerve palsy. The operation is considerably easier than the FCU set and has the major advantage of leaving the FCU in its very important position as the prime ulnar stabilizer of the wrist.

Boyes' superficialis set of transfers is also an excellent operation and is probably the only way to achieve simultaneous active extension of the wrist and fingers, although in my experience this goal is more likely to be achieved in children than in adults (Fig. 31-12). The Boyes' set is the best choice in a patient with no PL.

The FCU set of transfers is definitely contraindicated in patients with posterior interosseous nerve palsy; and even in complete radial nerve palsy the FCU transfer may result in some radial deviation of the wrist. I have not used the FCU set in more than 10 years.

Direct Nerve Transfers

Direct transfer of intact nerves to denervated muscles has proven to be a reasonable way to restore function in patients with brachial plexus palsy when no other option is available. Recently that concept has been investigated for treatment of radial nerve palsy by MacKinnon and associates.[45,46] These authors, who have an exceptional understanding of the topographic and cross-sectional anatomy of peripheral nerves, have discovered that the median nerve supplies several redundant branches to the FDS, which are therefore expendable and available for transfer. Branches to the PL and FCR are also available if those muscles are not required for future tendon transfers. In a very limited number of patients, they have done direct transfers of these branches to the posterior interosseous nerve and to the individual motor nerves of the denervated muscles.

These authors stress that future refinements in the technique are required before it can be recommended for general use, but this is a most exciting possibility in the future treatment of patients with radial nerve palsy, particularly in those patients whose proximal nerve cannot be repaired because of avulsion, segmental loss, or local soft tissue damage.

RADIAL NERVE PALSY ASSOCIATED WITH FRACTURES OF THE HUMERUS

Few topics generate more heated or emotional discussion in a fracture conference than radial nerve palsy associated with fractures of the humerus. The literature dealing with this topic over the past 50 years serves only to add to the controversy, because one can find at least one article to support virtually any plan of management. It is therefore important to review this entire spectrum of contradictory articles and consider each in its proper context and perspective.

The reported incidence of radial nerve palsy associated with humeral fractures has varied from 1.8% to 18%,[100,106,108,110] although some of these studies were selected or referred series and probably do not reflect an accurate incidence. When data are used from a consecutive series of humeral shaft fractures in a major trauma center,[111] the actual incidence is probably less than 10%.

There are basically three ways in which radial nerve palsy seen with a humeral shaft fracture can be managed; a discussion of each follows.

Early Exploration of the Nerve

Some authors[101,109,119] have advocated that all radial nerve injuries associated with humeral shaft fractures should be treated with early exploration. They cite the following theoretical advantages to support this position:

1. The status of the nerve (i.e., is it intact, contused, entrapped in the fracture site, impaled on a fragment, or lacerated) can be ascertained at the time of injury, thereby facilitating decisions regarding nerve repair or tendon transfers.
2. Stabilization of the fracture by internal fixation protects the radial nerve from further damage.
3. Early operation is technically easier and safer.

Several aspects of these arguments require closer scrutiny. The first question has to do with how many of these patients have a "surgically correctable" lesion. Foster and coworkers[100] encountered nerve laceration or entrapment in 9 of 14 open

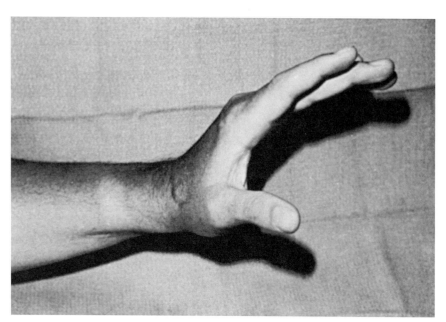

FIGURE 31-12. Simultaneous extension of the fingers and wrist is not possible after transfer of a wrist flexor (FCR or FCU) to the finger extensors because of limited tendon excursion. It is possible to achieve this, however, with the Boyes superficialis transfer, as shown in this patient (compare with Figure 31-3).

humeral shaft fractures they treated operatively. Sim and associates[119] stated that "remediable lesions were encountered too frequently to ignore early exploration," but considerable evidence exists to support the opposite conclusion. Kettelkamp and Alexander[105] found *no* surgically correctable lesions in any of the 16 radial nerves that they explored. Sonneveld and colleagues[120] explored 14 cases and found the nerve to be contused in 1 and visibly normal in the other 13. Dabezies and coworkers[97] encountered only one lacerated nerve in 15 patients with radial nerve palsy associated with fractures of the humerus. No nerves were entrapped, and all intact nerves recovered.

One of the reasons for these widely divergent observations may be that, with early exploration, an accurate assessment of the degree and extent of nerve injury cannot be ascertained.[107] This is particularly true if the nerve is in continuity and not entrapped in the fracture site. In the past, no nonoperative methods were available to help make this determination, but Bodner and coworkers[95] said that they were able to distinguish between severe nerve damage and minor damage (fascicular hematoma) with ultrasound. Although it has not yet been reported, perhaps magnetic resonance imaging may offer a way to evaluate the status of the nerve without exploration.

Holstein-Lewis Fracture

In a paper published in 1963 that has since been frequently quoted, Holstein and Lewis[104] described a fracture of the distal humerus in which the radial nerve is in particular jeopardy. The proximal spike of this spiral fracture breaks through the lateral cortex of the humerus at or near the point where the nerve is most closely apposed to the bone as it passes through the lateral intermuscular septum from the posterior to the anterior compartment of the arm. Their findings in seven patients with this particular lesion led Holstein and Lewis to the conclusion that early operative intervention was indicated in all such patients. However, in a more recent and larger collection of Holstein-Lewis fractures with radial nerve palsy, Szalay and Rockwood[122] concluded that early operative treatment is not necessary. Of their 15 patients with this combination of injuries, all 11 who were treated without exploration had complete nerve recovery, and in the 4 patients in whom exploration was carried out, the nerve was found to be in continuity and all had full recovery of nerve function.

Secondary Palsy

Another point regarding early exploration deals with those patients who develop "secondary" radial nerve paralysis in conjunction with a fractured humerus, that is, where the nerve is intact when the patient is first seen and subsequently goes out, usually after fracture reduction. In several articles,[98,101,118] this situation was cited as an absolute indication for immediate nerve exploration, although more than one study[96,117] has offered convincing evidence that even secondary radial nerve paralysis can be treated nonoperatively with good expectation for full recovery in most cases.

Finally, the source of the clinical material for each of these studies must be examined. Those who have most strongly advocated early exploration based their conclusions on series of patients treated in referral centers (The New York Orthopaedic Hospital[101,109] and the Mayo Clinic,[119]

where the percentage of complicated problems and failures from other treatment facilities is unusually high). Sim and associates,[119] in fact, acknowledged that their series from the Mayo Clinic was difficult to evaluate because most of the patients were referred. Conversely, in those studies drawn from major trauma centers where consecutive series of patients with humeral shaft fractures complicated by radial nerve palsy were evaluated, the authors[94,96,111,117,122] virtually all agree that nonoperative management of the radial nerve palsy is the treatment of choice.

Nerve Exploration at 6 to 8 Weeks If No Return

Shaw and Sakellarides[118] reviewed a series of patients from the Massachusetts General Hospital in 1967 and concluded that the nerve should be explored at 7 to 8 weeks if there is no evidence of return of function. They offered the following reasons for this decision:

1. All patients in their series showed some signs of recovery of nerve function within the first 2 months.
2. An unnecessary operation will be avoided in most patients, in whom spontaneous nerve recovery will occur.
3. There is no interference with fracture healing.
4. The waiting period allows the neuroma to become well delineated and hence to be adequately resected but is short enough to minimize nerve retraction.

Goldner and Kelley[102] advocated a similar position, but they considered the absence of an advancing Tinel sign to be an important added indication for exploration at 6 to 8 weeks. However, they went on to say that "a longer waiting period could not be criticized, because some of the patients in this group recovered completely without sign of motor recovery for 20 weeks." Amillo and associates[93] recommended surgical exploration at 3 months if there are no clinical or electrophysiologic signs of nerve recovery. However, in Mast and colleagues' study,[108] fewer than half of the nerves that recovered spontaneously did so in less than 12 weeks.

Nerve Exploration If No Return After a Longer Waiting Period

Because it is well documented that the initial signs of motor recovery may not appear until 4 or 5 months after a radial nerve palsy associated with a fractured humerus, a third option is available. This plan of management is based on the work of Seddon[114,116] regarding nerve regeneration and is best summarized in the abstract by Szalay and Rockwood.[122] Assuming that a nerve regenerates at the rate of approximately 1 mm/day and adding 30 days for an initial latent period as Seddon has suggested,[114] the maximum length of time that may be required for motor recovery to first manifest itself can easily be calculated by measuring the distance on the x-ray from the fracture site to the point of innervation of the brachioradialis muscle (approximately 2 cm above the lateral epicondyle[116]). In most midshaft humerus fractures, this distance is 90 to 120 mm (Fig. 31-13).

Although electromyographic evidence of reinnervation may precede clinical appearance of motor function by approximately 4 weeks,[112] it may take 4 to 5 months for evidence of function to be seen in the brachioradialis or

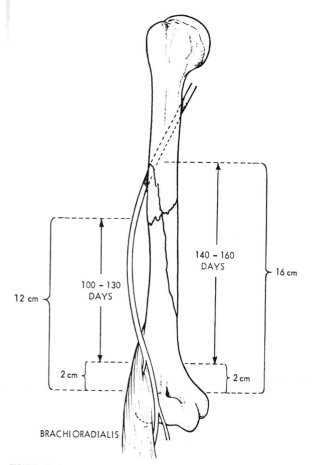

FIGURE 31-13. Calculation of the time that must elapse before signs of recovery can be expected after fractures of the shaft of the humerus, causing a degenerative lesion of the radial nerve. The information on the left is for a transverse fracture; on the right, it is provided for an oblique fracture. (From Seddon H: Surgical Disorders of the Peripheral Nerves, 2nd ed. Edinburgh, Churchill Livingstone, 1975.)

radial wrist extensors. Therefore, it is altogether logical to wait this long before proceeding with exploration if there is no return of nerve function. The major advantages of this plan of management are (1) unnecessary operative intervention is avoided in the large majority of patients; (2) most of these patients will achieve full recovery of the radial nerve without surgical treatment; and (3) the humerus fracture will usually be healed.

A question that must be raised, of course, is whether the delay in nerve repair for those very few patients in whom neurorrhaphy becomes necessary is excessive and will lessen the chances for good functional recovery. According to Sunderland,[121] a delay of 12 months or even longer is not likely to jeopardize functional motor return after nerve repair. Seddon[72,114,116] reported that prognosis for good recovery worsens only after a 12-month delay, quoting Zachary's[92] conclusions that the radial nerve can be repaired successfully 9 to 16 months after injury, depending on the level of injury. He also quoted Zachary as showing that prospects for recovery when repair is performed within 6 months of injury are better than after 6 months.

Author's Preferred Method of Treatment

It has long been my policy to treat most patients with radial nerve palsy associated with humeral shaft fractures nonoperatively, considering exploration of the nerve only after a realistic waiting time as outlined in the third option described in the previous section and illustrated in Figure 31-13.

There are, however, certain specific indications for early operative treatment of humeral shaft fractures, which include the following: (1) open fractures[100]; (2) fractures in which satisfactory alignment cannot be achieved by closed reduction techniques; (3) fractures with associated vascular injuries; and (4) patients with multiple trauma.[103] In all such cases, I believe that it is imperative to expose and visualize the radial nerve at the time of operative intervention. Closed intramedullary nailing is probably *not* a good option in such patients, because further damage to the nerve could occur if the nerve is entrapped.[123]

Based on studies previously cited, I do not consider a secondary nerve radial nerve palsy (i.e., occurring after fracture manipulation) to be in itself an absolute indication for early nerve exploration. Rather, I would still rely on the four indications just listed for early nerve exploration.

Following these indications, it must be acknowledged that there will be a very few patients in whom spontaneous return of function will not occur, but my experience is similar to that of others who have shown that these patients will be so few that routine exploration of all radial nerve injuries is not justified.

Finally, although I favor the third option for management, I find less objection to early exploration than to exploration at 6 to 8 weeks, or even 3 months. There may be some valid arguments for early exploration, but in my opinion there is no sound rationale for exploring the nerve at 6 to 12 weeks. If the decision has been made to await spontaneous return of function, I believe that it is only reasonable to wait an appropriate period of time.

ANNOTATED REFERENCES

11. Boyes JH: Tendon transfers for radial palsy. Bull Hosp Jt Dis 21:97-105, 1960.

   A "classic" article that describes in great detail all of the various combinations of tendon transfers that have been used in the treatment of radial nerve palsy. This is by far the best historical reference on this subject.

16. Brand PW: Operations to restore muscle balance to the hand. *In* Clinical Mechanics of the Hand. St. Louis, CV Mosby, 1985, pp 127-165.

   Perhaps one reason that the FCR set of transfers took a long time to be fully accepted is that there was no well recognized article in which it was described. However, in this chapter, the master biomechanic of the hand, Paul Brand, explains why he favored this over the FCU set.

26. Curtis RM: Fundamental principles of tendon transfer. Orthop Clin North Am 5:231-242, 1974.

   Tendon transfers are not done as often as they were 30 years ago, and thus the principles of these operations are not stressed as much as they were in training programs of that era. In this article, these principles are described by one of the masters.

91. Zachary RB: Tendon transplantation for radial paralysis. Br J Surg 23:358-364, 1946.

Zachary was the first to emphasize the importance of leaving one wrist flexor (FCU or FCR) intact.

Radial Nerve Palsy Associated With Fractures of the Humerus

116. Seddon HJ: Surgical Disorders of the Peripheral Nerves, 2nd ed. Edinburgh, Churchill Livingstone, 1975.

In the post–World War II era, the recognized guru of nerve injuries was Professor Seddon. His explanation of how and at what pace nerves regenerate is fundamental to rational treatment of radial nerve palsy associated with fractures of the humerus.

117. Shah JJ, Bhatti NA: Radial nerve paralysis associated with fractures of the humerus. Clin Orthop 172:171-176, 1983.

It had long been taught that secondary radial nerve palsy (i.e., that occurring after closed reduction of the fracture) was an absolute indication for immediate exploration of the nerve. This article, since supported by others, showed evidence that operative intervention is not necessarily indicated in all such patients.

122. Szalay EA, Rockwood CA Jr: The Holstein-Lewis fracture revisited. Orthop Trans 7:516, 1983.

This series disputed the previously held belief that fractures of the distal third of the humerus with a radial nerve palsy required exploration.

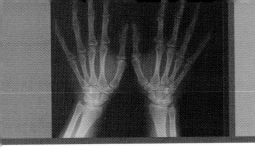

CHAPTER 32

Median Nerve Palsy

Timothy R. C. Davis

The aim of reconstructive surgery in median nerve palsy is to restore lost motor function, in particular, thumb opposition and flexor pollicis longus (FPL) and index finger profundus function. Attempts to restore sensibility in the hand, specifically to the thumb tip, with neurovascular island skin flaps have now generally been abandoned.[13] The benefits of reconstructive surgery are, to a large degree, determined by the quality of hand sensation,[8] contralateral hand function, the patient's motivation,[59] and the ability to adapt to any sensory loss.

Median nerve injuries are classified as "high" or "low," depending on whether the lesion is proximal or distal to the origin of the anterior interosseous nerve in the proximal forearm. In "low" injuries, the thenar intrinsic muscles innervated by the median nerve, usually the abductor pollicis brevis (APB), opponens pollicis, and superficial head of the flexor pollicis brevis (FPB), are paralyzed. In "high" injuries, the pronator teres, the flexor carpi radialis (FCR), all the finger superficiales, the index and middle finger profundi, the FPL, and the pronator quadratus muscles are also paralyzed.

LOW MEDIAN NERVE PALSY

Polio, a disease now on the verge of eradication, was the predominant cause of thenar muscle intrinsic paralysis in the first half of the 20th century. Because this disease causes a pure motor deficit, it provided an ideal indication for opponensplasty. The two world wars also produced a large number of median nerve injuries that were frequently complex and occurred in conjunction with other nerve and severe soft tissue injuries. The present indications for restoration of thumb opposition include compression and traumatic division of the median nerve; leprosy; neurologic diseases such as Charcot-Marie-Tooth disease, spinal muscular atrophy, and syringomyelia; and congenital absence of the thenar muscles.

Biomechanics of Thumb Opposition

Thumb opposition is a complex movement requiring trapeziometacarpal joint abduction, flexion, and pronation. Retroposition, the opposite movement, is a combination of trapeziometacarpal joint adduction, extension, and supination. Axial thumb rotation, usually 90 degrees of pronation and 60 degrees of supination, occurs on the spheroid area of the saddle-shaped trapezial articular surface.[78] Pronation is probably an obligatory passive movement[22] that occurs during circumduction toward the palm as a result of the force-couple produced by thumb intrinsic muscle contraction and passive tension within the dorsal trapeziometacarpal ligament.[78] Retroposition also probably occurs passively during thumb extension as a result of the force-couple produced by contraction of the extensor pollicis longus (EPL) and brevis (EPB) and the abductor pollicis longus (APL) muscles and passive tension within the radiopalmar (anterior oblique) ligament. Although these force-couples may be the prime mechanism of axial rotation, other mechanisms must exist inasmuch as thumb pronation is preserved after trapeziectomy.

It is now generally accepted that the prime muscle of thumb opposition is the APB, although both the opponens pollicis and FPB also produce some opposition.[22] The adductor pollicis and the two extrinsic thumb extensors cause thumb retroposition, whereas the FPL can act as either an opposer or a retroposer, depending on the position of the thumb.[78]

The classic description of thumb intrinsic muscle innervation is that the APB, the opponens pollicis, and the FPB are supplied by the motor branch of the median nerve whereas the adductor pollicis is supplied by the deep branch of the ulnar nerve. However, there is considerable diversity in the pattern of innervation, and clinical studies suggest that all the thenar muscles are innervated, in part at least, by either the ulnar (2%) or the median (2%) nerve in a few instances. Furthermore, the FPB remains functional in 73% of complete median and 58% of complete ulnar nerve injuries, thus demonstrating that this muscle frequently has a dual median and ulnar innervation.[66] Anatomic dissection suggests that the median nerve supplies the APB, the opponens pollicis, and the superficial head of the FPB in 63%, but only the APB and the opponens pollicis in 30% of hands.[58] Zancolli and Cozzi[78] believe that the superficial head of the FPB has dual median and ulnar innervation in 30% of hands, whereas its deep head has dual innervation in 79% of cases and is exclusively supplied by the ulnar nerve in 19%. They also believe that the oblique head of the adductor pollicis has dual ulnar and median innervation in 35% of cases, whereas its transverse head is practically always (96%) innervated by the ulnar nerve. Although some of these findings are contradictory, the variability of thenar muscle innervation explains why thumb abduction and opposition are frequently retained after complete median nerve injuries.[6,43]

The Deficit and the Deformity

Thumb abduction and opposition are frequently retained after isolated median nerve injury as a result of preserved ulnar nerve function. Jensen[35] believed that opponensplasty was required in only 14% of median nerve injuries, and it is my experience that reasonable opposition is commonly retained in this situation. Furthermore, even in the presence of significant thenar wasting, I find that satisfactory thumb opposition is usually retained in severe carpal tunnel syndrome, although 6.6% of the patients of Foucher and colleagues[26] had absent or inadequate thumb opposition. All the thenar intrinsic muscles are paralyzed after combined median and ulnar nerve injuries; in this situation, thumb opposition is absent and the patient is only able to flex the thumb across the palm by using the FPL. In combined ulnar and high median nerve injuries, the thumb is extended and supinated by the unopposed extrinsic extensor muscles.

Tendon Transfers to Restore Thumb Opposition

History

Steindler is credited with performing the first opponensplasty in 1917. He attached a radial slip of the FPL tendon onto the dorsum of the base of the thumb proximal phalanx.[71] Shortly afterward, Cook used the extensor digiti minimi (EDM) for an opponensplasty[73] and Ney attached either the palmaris longus or FCR to the EPB tendon, which was rerouted through the carpal tunnel.[53] Huber,[32] in 1921, and Nicolaysen,[54] in 1922, described the abductor digiti minimi (ADM) opponensplasty. Then Bunnell,[16] in 1924, and Camitz,[20] in 1929, both reported that the palmaris longus tendon could be satisfactorily elongated with a strip of palmar aponeurosis so that it could be used in an opponensplasty without the need for a tendon graft. To maximize thumb opposition, Bunnell recommended passing the transferred tendon through a pulley on the ulnar border of the wrist so that it runs subcutaneously across the palm to its thumb insertion.[16,17] Thompson[75] used the ulnar border of the palmar aponeurosis as a pulley for Royle's superficialis transfer.[67] Aguirre and Caplan,[1] in 1956, first described the extensor indicis proprius (EIP) opponensplasty, which can be used for both high and low median nerve palsies and does not require a pulley or a tendon graft. A theoretical alternative to opponensplasty is neurotization, joining the anterior interosseous nerve in the distal forearm to the thenar branch of the median nerve, possibly with an intervening nerve graft.[75a]

Patient Counseling

Although the indication for an opponensplasty is loss of opposition, the need for surgery is loss of function due to loss of opposition. If the loss of opposition is unilateral, especially if affecting the nondominant hand, then the loss of function that it is causing may be minimal and insufficient to warrant surgery. Additionally, if there is also loss of, or absent, sensation in the median nerve territory, this may reduce any potential benefit of an opponensplasty because the loss of function is primarily due to the loss of sensation. Careful patient counseling about the possible functional benefit, the rehabilitation process, and the likely outcome of surgery (this may be rather less than the published success rates for restoration of opposition movement) is mandatory. The surgeon must have a clear picture of the functional disability and be confident that this is due to the loss of opposition and not to other factors, such as sensory impairment or joint stiffness.

General Principles of Tendon Transfer With Reference to Opponensplasty

The principles of tendon transfer surgery[4] are frequently reiterated but often forgotten. Failure to remember the following principles is a common cause of unsatisfactory results, and all must be considered carefully before embarking on an opponensplasty:

1. An elective tendon transfer should never be performed in the presence of unhealed wounds.
2. Full passive joint motion must be restored before tendon transfer.
3. The transfer must not pass through areas of scar tissue or under skin grafts. Furthermore, surgical incisions should not be placed directly over the transfer.
4. Whenever possible, cutaneous sensibility should be restored before tendon transfer.
5. The normal function of the transferred muscle must be expendable.
6. The transferred muscle must be under voluntary control and must have an independent action.
7. The transferred muscle must have sufficient amplitude and power to perform its new function; thus, reinnervated muscles should be used only in exceptional circumstances.
8. If the transfer cannot perform its new function with a straight line of pull from its origin to its insertion, it should pass through no more than one pulley. Acute angulation of the transfer at the pulley should be avoided.
9. Synergism between the muscle's original and new actions facilitates rehabilitation.

Prevention and Preoperative Treatment of Contractures

It is always easier to prevent a soft tissue contracture than to correct an established one. In median nerve palsy and complete thumb intrinsic paralysis, the thumb may adopt a supinated and adducted position, and a first web space contracture may develop. This, however, is usually readily prevented by passive thumb abduction and opposition exercises and by abduction splints. When there are associated severe thenar or first web space soft tissue injuries and thus a high risk of first web space contracture, temporary internal splintage of the thumb metacarpal in abduction with a Kirschner wire may be indicated.

Established soft tissue contractures must be corrected either before or during opponensplasty because no opponensplasty has sufficient strength to improve the preoperative passive range of opposition. Failure to detect and correct contractures preoperatively is a common cause of failure.[12] First web space contractures are generally due to contractures of the skin and deep fascia on its extensor surface[8] and are usually readily detected. However, contracture of the dorsal capsule of the trapeziometacarpal joint, which restricts opposition but permits abduction, is detected only by careful clinical examination.[47] If supervised physiotherapy and splintage[2,3] fail to correct a contracture, surgical release is indicated. In the absence of any injury to the thenar muscles or the base of the thumb, first web contractures can usually be released satisfactorily through a dorsal web space incision. The fascia over the adductor pollicis and the first dorsal interosseous muscles is released and the dorsal web space skin widened with a skin graft or flap (Fig. 32-1).[8,52] Isolated capsular contractures of the trapeziometacarpal joint should be released through a small incision over the base of this joint.[47] In severe contractures, both rotational osteotomy at the base of the thumb metacarpal[67] and trapeziectomy[29] have been recommended. An osteotomy modifies rather than improves the range of thumb movement. For a more comprehensive discussion of thumb web contractures, see Chapter 53.

Selection of Motor for Transfer

The normal function of the muscle selected for opponensplasty must be expendable, and this muscle must have strength and potential excursion similar to that of the APB and opponens pollicis muscles, whose functions it is to replace. The strength of a muscle is proportional to its cross-sectional area and is expressed as a tension fraction, whereas potential excursion is determined by muscle fiber length.[9,22] Thus the ideal opponensplasty motor should have a tension fraction similar to that of the combined APB and opponens pollicis tension (1.1 + 1.9 = 3.0) and a muscle fiber length that is at least as long as that of the APB (Table 32-1). The

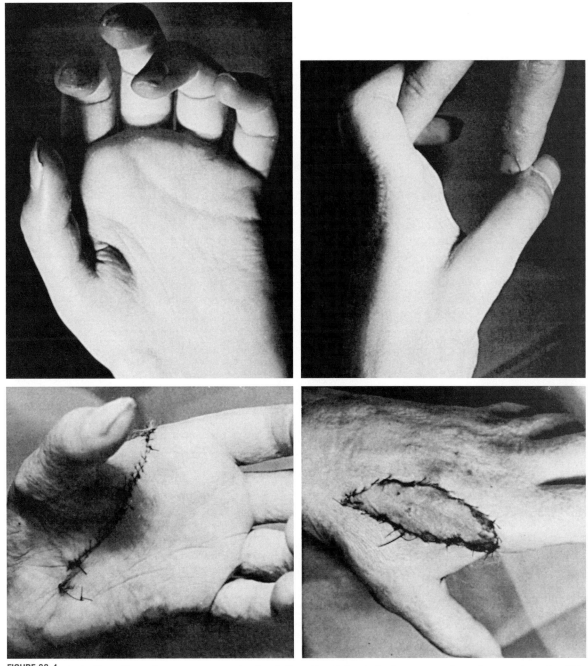

FIGURE 32-1. A significant first web space contracture developed after a direct injury to the thenar area and a median nerve laceration. This was released before opponensplasty by using a dorsal rotation flap and skin graft. Postoperatively, the position of the thumb was maintained with a threaded Steinmann pin.

Table 32-1

RESTING MUSCLE FIBER LENGTHS AND TENSION FRACTIONS OF THE MEDIAN-INNERVATED THUMB INTRINSIC MUSCLES AND POTENTIAL OPPOSITION TRANSFER MOTORS

	Resting Muscle Fiber Length (cm)	Tension Fraction (%)
Paralyzed Muscles		
Abductor pollicis brevis	3.7	1.1
Flexor pollicis brevis	3.6	1.3
Opponens pollicis	2.4	1.9
Median		
Palmaris longus	5.0	1.2
Flexor carpi radialis	5.2	4.1
Flexor digitorum superficialis, middle	7.0	3.4
Flexor digitorum superficialis, ring	7.3	3.0
Flexor pollicis longus	5.9	2.7
Ulnar		
Abductor digiti minimi	4.0	1.4
Flexor carpi ulnaris	4.2	6.7
Radial		
Extensor carpi radialis brevis	6.1	4.2
Extensor carpi radialis longus	9.3	3.5
Extensor carpi ulnaris	4.5	4.5
Extensor pollicis longus	5.7	1.3
Extensor indicis proprius	5.5	1
Extensor digiti minimi	5.9	1

From Brand PW: Tendon transfers for median and ulnar nerve paralysis. Orthop Clin North Am 1:447-454, 1970.

greater the potential excursion of the transfer, the greater the margin of error when setting the transfer's tension.

It is also advantageous to select a motor with a tendon that is long enough to reach the thumb metacarpophalangeal (MP) joint and thus avoid the need for a tendon graft. This makes the operation simpler and reduces the likelihood of troublesome adhesions. All transferred muscles lose one grade of power as a result of altered muscle tension and inevitable soft tissue adhesions, so reinnervated muscles should be considered only when no normal muscles are available for transfer.[6]

Finally, rehabilitation is simpler if the selected motor acts synergistically with the APB, although Omer[59] and Brand[8] both believe that any transfer can be re-educated to fulfill its new function, especially in children, provided that the restored function is of benefit to the patient.

Pulley Design

If a tendon transfer does not run in a straight line, increased force is expended to overcome friction with the surrounding soft tissues and the transfer will try to migrate so that it does run in a straight line. Because thumb opposition is best restored by transfers that run subcutaneously across the palm, parallel to the APB muscle, all true extrinsic opponensplasties (as opposed to the Camitz procedure) must pass

around a stout fixed pulley in the region of the pisiform on the ulnar border of the wrist.[17] Opponens transfers from the forearm extensor compartment generally use the distal ulna as the pulley, and most of these transfers are simply passed through a wide subcutaneous tunnel on the ulnar border of the distal forearm. Alternatively, some extensor muscle opponensplasties pass through and use a window in the interosseous membrane as the pulley,[48,51] in which case it is important to make a very large window.

If a forearm flexor compartment muscle is used for opponensplasty, a pulley has to be manufactured on the ulnar border of the wrist. Numerous designs have been described, and these are discussed later in the chapter in the section on superficialis transfers (see page 1137).

Opponensplasty Insertions

Many insertions have been described (Fig. 32-2),[23] and these can be broadly divided into single- and dual-insertion techniques. Dual insertion aims to allow the tendon transfer to perform two functions, usually active opposition and either passive stabilization of the MP joint or restriction of interphalangeal (IP) joint flexion, which is beneficial in combined median and ulnar nerve palsies. Tendon transfers are most efficient when they perform only one active function; if a transfer has two insertions that perform different functions, it will act predominantly on the tighter insertion. Bunnell[17] recommended and others[75] used a drill hole in the dorsoulnar aspect of the base of the thumb proximal phalanx as their opponensplasty insertion (Fig. 32-3) to produce thumb pronation as well as abduction. However, pronation occurs passively when the thumb is abducted and flexed,[78] and biomechanical studies suggest that attaching the opponensplasty to the APB insertion on the radial aspect of the thumb MP joint produces as good opposition as the Bunnell and other commonly used insertions.[22] Thus the APB insertion is now widely used in isolated median nerve palsies.[11,18,43,46,51,70] Dual insertions into the APB insertion and either the dorsal MP joint capsule or the thumb extensor expansion[2,18,35,65] are probably unnecessary in isolated median nerve palsy, although they may be useful in a completely intrinsic-minus thumb.[21] Use of the EPB tendon and its insertion is reserved for complex cases when either the palmaris longus or a wrist flexor or extensor muscle is selected as the opponensplasty motor.[63] The EPL[7,28,36,48,51,65] and FPL[45,57] tendon insertions are sometimes used in complex cases.

Results

The majority of papers on opponensplasty report a high percentage of excellent and good results and attribute most failures to persistent contractures or technical problems. There is no universally accepted method of classifying the results of opponensplasty, but recent papers are probably more stringent than earlier articles in their assessment of outcome. Unfortunately, it is impossible to compare the results and complication rates of different opponensplasties because of multiple variables: (1) the underlying disease process (polio, leprosy, nerve injury); (2) the neurologic deficit (low median, high median, or combined median and ulnar); (3) the sensory defect; and (4) the potential for spontaneous recovery. For example, if transfers are performed early when there is still potential for recovery, restoration of

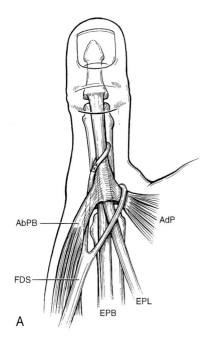

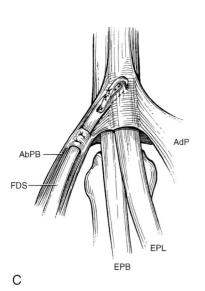

A

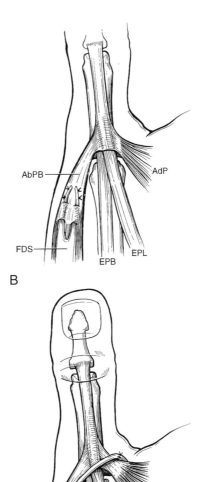

B

AbPB

FDS

EPL

EPB

AdP

FIGURE 32-2. A to **D,** Techniques of distal attachment as described by Brand, Littler, Riordan, and Royle-Thompson. AbPB, Abductor pollicis brevis; FDS, flexor digitorum superficialis; AdP, adductor pollicis brevis; EPB, extensor pollicis brevis; EPL, extensor pollicis longus.

AbPB

FDS

EPL

EPB

AdP

C

AbPB

FDS

EPB

EPL

AdP

D

excellent opposition may be incorrectly attributed to the opponensplasty instead of nerve regeneration. Sixty-six percent of patients regain or never lose good opposition after median nerve repair,[17] and thenar muscle function can recover after carpal tunnel release.[27,55]

Many papers classify an excellent result as one in which strong opposition with full mobility is restored. A fair result is one with either full but weak opposition or limited but strong opposition.[34] Sundararaj and Mani[72] graded their results in leprosy according to the range of opposition and the position of the thumb IP joint (Table 32-2). In contrast, Foucher and colleagues[26] objectively measured active thumb abduction, opposition, and rotation occurring on movement of the thumb from full active retroposition to opposition.

Although a patient may demonstrate good muscle opposition to the surgeon in the clinic and be convincing that the opponensplasty is of functional benefit, the patient may not use the newly restored opposition in everyday life. This is

especially the case with combined median and ulnar nerve palsies, where the patient frequently finds it easier and quicker to hold objects between the sides of the thumb and hand (lateral pinch) by using the EPL to adduct and supinate the thumb.[8]

Four Standard Opponensplasties

There are four widely used, reliable opponensplasties, at least one of which will be appropriate for the vast majority of clinical situations:

1. Flexor digitorum superficialis (FDS) opponensplasty
   a. Royle-Thompson technique
   b. Bunnell technique
2. EIP opponensplasty
3. Huber transfer (ADM)
4. Camitz procedure (palmaris longus)

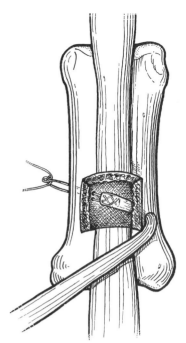

FIGURE 32-3. Method of bony attachment of a tendon transfer using internal sutures rather than external pull-out techniques. This technique may require an additional skin incision for exposure of the opposite cortex and tying of the suture and is being superceded by the use of bone anchors.

Superficialis Opponensplasties

There is no universally accepted "best technique" of superficialis transfer, and a wide variety of different harvest techniques, pulley constructions, and transfer insertions are used. The ring finger superficialis is widely used as the opponensplasty motor. However, because this may weaken power grip, some surgeons prefer to use the middle finger superficialis if this is available. Potential transfer insertions have been discussed earlier in this chapter.

Superficialis Tendon Harvest

Royle[67] and Thompson[75] both divided the ring finger superficialis tendon at its insertion onto the middle phalanx through a transverse insertion within the basal finger crease. How-

> ## CRITICAL POINTS: MANAGEMENT PRINCIPLES IN OPPONENSPLASTY
>
> - Surgery is needed when loss of opposition causes a meaningful functional deficit for the patient.
> - The surgeon should adhere to all general principles of tendon transfer.
> - Established soft tissue contractures must be corrected before or during opponensplasty; careful preoperative evaluation is essential.
> - The ideal opponensplasty motor should have a tension fraction of around 3.0 and a muscle fiber length at least as long as the APB.
> - Tendon grafts should be avoided.
> - Rehabilitation is simpler if the selected motor acts synergistically with the APB.
> - When possible, a single insertion of the transferred tendon is preferred.

ever, it has subsequently been recognized that several superficialis harvest techniques, including division at its insertion, can cause donor digit proximal interphalangeal (PIP) joint flexion contractures or, especially in the supple Asian hand, swan neck and other deformities.

North and Littler[56] suggested that division of the superficialis tendon at its insertion destroys the vincula and disrupts the blood supply to the profundus tendon; furthermore, surgical trauma may create scar tissue within the flexor sheath and PIP joint capsule and thus cause deformity. They recommended division of the superficialis tendon proximal to its bifurcation through a window between the A1 and A2 pulleys with the finger fully flexed. This avoids injury to the flexor sheath at the level of the PIP joint and leaves behind a 3-cm length of superficialis tendon that glides freely within the flexor sheath. With this technique, 8 of those authors' 16 patients experienced no problems in the donor digit and the

Table 32-2

TWO METHODS OF ASSESSMENT OF OPPONENSPLASTY SURGERY

Sundararaj and Mani,[72] 1984		Jacobs and Thompson,[34*] 1960
Excellent	Opposition to ring or little finger tip with interphalangeal joint extended	75% of function of opposite thumb when normal *or*
Good	Opposition to index or middle finger tip with interphalangeal joint extended	Less than 20° difference between the planes of the opposed thumb nail and the palm with good power
Fair	Thumb interphalangeal joint flexes during opposition	Full, though weak, opposition *or* Restricted, but strong, opposition
Poor	No opposition restored	No opposition restored

*Jacobs and Thompson did not subdivide excellent and good results.

remainder only lost an average of 8 degrees extension of the PIP joint. None experienced any major disability or deformity. Other surgeons have recommended that the distal tags of the donor superficialis tendon are left long and sutured across the palmar plate to reinforce it and prevent hyperextension.[35]

In a series of 116 superficialis opponensplasties performed by Anderson and associates,[3] the ring finger superficialis tendon was harvested through either a midlateral approach or a Bruner incision on the flexor surface of the finger. Extension lag at the distal interphalangeal (DIP) joint and fixed flexion deformities at the PIP joint occurred in 44% and 8% of cases, respectively, when the lateral approach was used but in only 8% and 0% of cases, respectively, when the Bruner incision was used. Anderson and associates believed that the high complication rates associated with the lateral approach were due to scar tissue and adhesion formation around the lateral bands of the extensor hood, which are retracted during this exposure. However, in another series of 100 leprosy patients with ulnar, median, or combined nerve palsies, no correlation was found between harvest technique and donor digit morbidity and deformity.[10] Swan neck deformities and DIP joint extension lags occurred in 15% and 29% of the donor fingers, respectively. The DIP joint extension lags were usually less than 20 degrees, unless associated with a swan neck deformity, in which case they could be as much as 80 degrees. In addition, 26% of the cases in this study had check-rein PIP joint deformities (50 to 70 degrees), and PIP joint flexion was reduced in 16%. These authors concluded that postoperative deformity in superficialis donor digits is multifactorial and depends on the preoperative condition of the PIP joint, the method of superficialis harvest, the surgeon's skill, postoperative rehabilitation, the expertise of the therapist, and the patient's motivation.

Many surgeons believe that division of the superficialis tendon at its insertion increases the risk of swan neck deformity. Furthermore, this technique usually requires an additional palmar incision to split the distal superficialis tendon and free it from the profundus tendon. Because sufficient superficialis tendon length for opponensplasty is provided by harvesting the superficialis tendon through an incision in the distal aspect of the palm,[56] there seems little point in risking a more distal division.

The Pulley

Passing the superficialis tendon around the flexor carpi ulnaris (FCU) tendon in the distal forearm was a popular and simple pulley design,[6,41,46] but this has fallen out of favor because the pulley is not fixed and migrates proximally. Thus the transfer gradually adopts an increasingly longitudinal line of action and becomes less efficient with time (Fig. 32-4). Another simple pulley design is to pass the transfer through a subcutaneous tunnel in the hypothenar eminence and use the fibrous raphe, which pass vertically between the deep

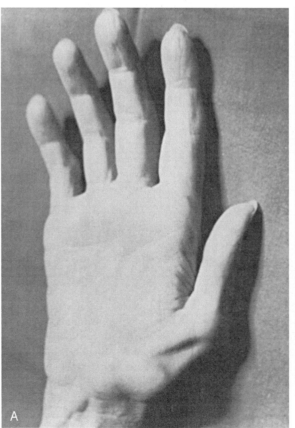
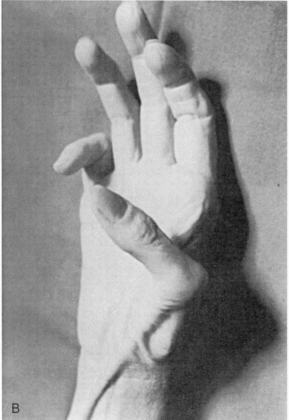

FIGURE 32-4. **A** and **B,** A poor Bunnell superficialis (flexor digitorum superficialis) transfer. There was no fixed pulley at the pisiform. The transfer has migrated and is now acting more as a flexor of the metacarpophalangeal joint than as a real abductor/opposer. Satisfactory opposition needs a fixed pulley near the pisiform.

fascia and the overlying skin, as the pulley. Although many surgeons think that these raphae are not sufficiently strong to prevent radial migration of this pulley (thus reducing the effectiveness of the opponensplasty), it is still used in the United Kingdom and may be reinforced by also passing the transfer through a slit in the palmar aponeurosis.

Bunnell[17] described several pulley designs for use with superficialis and other forearm flexor opponensplasties. These included looping a free tendon graft around the FCU tendon as it passes between the pisiform and the base of the fifth metacarpal and using a strip of the FCU tendon based on its attachment to the pisiform. Although the use of a distally based strip of FCU as a pulley is popular, its raw surface may encourage adhesion formation, and radial migration of this pulley has been observed over a period of years. To prevent this migration, the distally based slip of FCU tendon can be attached to the extensor carpi ulnaris (ECU) tendon.[68] The angle between the distal edge of the flexor retinaculum and the ulnar border of the palmar aponeurosis is used effectively as a pulley in the Thompson-Royle transfer,[34,75] and good opposition is also restored when a window in the flexor retinaculum is used as the pulley.[5,49,70] Guyon's canal can also be used as a pulley,[7,62] and although radial migration may occur, this does not necessarily reduce the effectiveness of the opponensplasty.[3]

Biomechanical studies[22] have shown that the function of an opponensplasty can be modified to an individual patient's requirements by altering the position of the pulley. Placing the pulley so that the transfer's line of action passes toward the pisiform produces maximal thumb abduction and opposition but only a small amount of flexion at the thumb MP joint. Positioning the pulley so that the transfer's line of pull passes distal to the pisiform produces more thumb MP joint flexion but less abduction. Thus, a distally placed pulley may benefit patients with combined ulnar and median nerve palsies and paralyzed FPB muscles.

Royle-Thompson Opponensplasty[67,75]

Technique. A 3-cm longitudinal incision is made at the base of the palm on the radial border of the hypothenar eminence. The ulnar border of the palmar aponeurosis is exposed and retracted radially, and the ring finger superficialis tendon is identified as it emerges from the carpal tunnel. This tendon is then divided distally through a transverse incision at the base of the digit and is delivered into the palmar wound so that it passes ulnar to the palmar aponeurosis. A third incision is made over the dorsum of the thumb MP joint, and a wide subcutaneous tunnel is created between this and the palmar incision. The superficialis tendon is passed through this tunnel, with the angle created by the distal edge of the flexor retinaculum and the ulnar border of the palmar aponeurosis acting as the pulley. The transfer is then attached to the thumb by one of the many insertion techniques. Thompson originally used a dual insertion that stabilized the thumb MP joint and is thus useful in combined median and ulnar palsies. However, the technique of insertion is not critical, and Thompson himself subsequently used the APB insertion.[34]

The tourniquet is released and hemostasis is obtained before the incisions in the palm and at the base of the ring finger are closed. The superficialis transfer attachment to the thumb is then sutured while the thumb is held in full opposition. Because the ring finger superficialis tendon has a large potential excursion and crosses the wrist joint, adjusting the tension is not as critical as with other transfers and there is a considerable margin for error. However, the transfer's tension should be adjusted so that it is tight when the thumb is fully opposed and the wrist is in neutral. Postoperatively, Thompson held the thumb in opposition for 4 to 6 weeks with spiral adhesive strapping that allowed some active thumb movement. However, most surgeons immobilize the thumb in full opposition with a cast for several weeks.

Results. Some surgeons believe that this opponensplasty does not produce as wide thumb abduction as some other transfers because it runs along the path of the superficial head of the FPB and not that of the APB muscle. However the results were excellent or good in 8 of Thompson's 10 original opponensplasties,[75] and a subsequent report found excellent or good results in 78% of 94 opponensplasties.[34]

Bunnell's Opponensplasty

Bunnell's precept for restoration of full thumb opposition was that the transfer should run in line with the fibers of the APB to an insertion on the dorsoulnar aspect of the thumb proximal phalanx. Because his transfer passes distal to the axis of rotation of the MP joint, it also flexes this joint.

Technique. The ring finger superficialis tendon is divided at the base of this digit by using one of the previously described techniques (see page 1136). An incision is then made over the ulnar neurovascular bundle, just proximal to the wrist crease, and the ring finger superficialis tendon is identified. The distal portion of the FCU tendon is then exposed and cut halfway across, 4 cm proximal to its insertion on the pisiform. The tendon is then split into two equal halves up to its pisiform insertion, thus creating a distally based strip of tendon tissue. The free end of this tendon slip is sutured back onto its base at the pisiform to create a fixed pulley through which the superficialis tendon can pass easily. Care should be taken to not make this loop too tight. An incision is then made on the dorsum of the thumb, and a wide subcutaneous tunnel is created across the palm between the two incisions. A hole large enough to accommodate the superficialis tendon is then drilled from the dorsoulnar cortex to the radial cortex of the base of the proximal phalanx. The ring finger superficialis is delivered into the wrist incision and passed through the pulley and then along the subcutaneous tunnel into the dorsal thumb incision. Next, the tourniquet is released, hemostasis is achieved, and the skin incisions at the base of the ring finger and at the wrist are closed. The superficialis tendon is then passed superficial to the EPL tendon, across the dorsum of the thumb MP joint. It is then passed through the drill hole in the base of the proximal phalanx in a dorsoulnar-to-radiopalmar direction. Once the tendon has been passed through this drill hole, the transfer's tension is set so that the thumb lies in full opposition with the wrist in neutral. The transfer is then sutured back onto itself or to the radial border periosteum. Alternatively, it may be held with a pull-out suture tied over a dental roll or attached to the proximal phalanx by using the technique shown in Figure 32-3.

Results. Jensen used the Bunnell opponensplasty and reported good opposition in 22 of his 27 superficialis transfers.[35]

EIP Opponensplasty

The EIP opponensplasty (Fig. 32-5) was favored by Burkhalter, who wrote earlier editions of this chapter, and is popular in high median nerve palsy and other instances when the ring and middle finger FDS tendons are unavailable. It has been increasingly used in preference to the superficialis transfer in low median nerve palsies because it does not weaken grip and causes no functional disability.[18]

Technique. A short incision is made over the index finger MP joint, and the EIP tendon is divided immediately proximal to the extensor hood. Some surgeons recommend that a contiguous slip of the extensor hood be harvested with the tendon to lengthen the transfer.[18] However, this is unnecessary, and if the extensor hood is not properly repaired its radial and ulnar halves may subluxate palmarly and cause an extensor lag.[15] A long incision is then made on the dorsoulnar aspect of the distal forearm, the extensor indicis tendon is delivered into this wound, and it and its muscle are freed of soft tissue attachments in the distal third of the forearm. It is important to retrieve the tendon proximal to the extensor retinaculum for adequate tendon length and line of pull. Sometimes this is only possible after soft tissue connections between the extensor indicis and index communis tendons have been divided through a small incision on the back of

the hand. Next, small incisions are made in the pisiform area and on the dorsoradial aspect of the thumb MP. A wide subcutaneous tunnel is then developed from the extensor surface of the forearm to the thumb incision, passing around the ulnar border of the wrist and across the palm. The extensor indicis tendon is passed through this tunnel while making certain that the tendon goes superficial to the FCU tendon; inadvertently passing it beneath the FCU tendon may later result in compression of the ulnar nerve. The tourniquet is then released and hemostasis obtained before the wrist and index finger incisions are closed. The distal attachment of this transfer depends on the clinical setting. In isolated median nerve palsies, it is simply attached to the APB tendon with the wrist in 30 degrees of flexion and the thumb in maximum opposition. In combined median and ulnar nerve palsies with an intrinsic-minus thumb, the transfer is attached in sequence to the APB tendon, the MP joint capsule, and the EPL tendon over the proximal phalanx, as described by Riordan.[65] The transferred tendon will reach this new origin if the thumb is fully opposed and the wrist is flexed. This attachment restricts IP joint flexion and thus allows the FPL to flex the MP joint more effectively and substitute for the paralyzed FPB.[18] Postoperatively, the hand is immobilized with the wrist in flexion and the thumb in full opposition for 3 to 4 weeks.

Results. Burkhalter and colleagues[18] reported the results of extensor indicis opponensplasty in 65 trauma cases, which included 32 combined ulnar and median nerve, 13 high

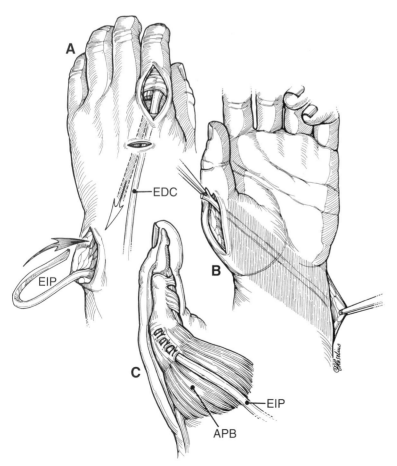

FIGURE 32-5. EIP transfer. **A,** The tendon is divided and delivered into a large dorsoulnar wrist incision; this may require an additional incision on the dorsum of the hand immediately distal to the extensor retinaculum, where the EIP and index extensor digitorum communis tendons may be attached to each other. **B,** The muscle belly of the EIP is mobilized and placed on the ulnar aspect of the wrist and its tendon is passed through a subcutaneous tunnel around the wrist to an incision over the thumb MP joint. **C,** The transfer is then sutured to the APB tendon.

median nerve, and 2 brachial plexus injuries. Eighty-eight percent of the patients achieved excellent results, with powerful opposition to within 20 degrees of the plane of the palm of the hand. Perceived additional benefits of this transfer included ease of surgery (performed satisfactorily by residents) and rehabilitation (its excursion is naturally augmented by a wrist tenodesis effect). A disadvantage is that extensor indicis muscle fiber length is shorter than that of the abductor pollicis brevis and the ring finger superficialis, so thumb extension may be restricted.

Anderson and associates[2] used this transfer in 12 high and 28 low median nerve palsies caused by leprosy, trauma, and other conditions. In contrast to Burkhalter's description, they attached the transfer to the thumb with the wrist in neutral and the thumb fully abducted and extended. Excellent or good results were seen in 88% of the cases monitored for more than a year. These workers subsequently compared these results with those achieved by superficialis transfer and concluded that the EIP transfer should only be used in supple hands.[3]

ADM (Huber) Opponensplasty

The ADM opponensplasty (Fig. 32-6), described independently by Huber[32] and Nicolaysen,[54] was popularized by Littler and Cooley,[42] who considered the ADM a close substitute for the APB. This transfer also improves the hand's appearance by increasing the bulk of the thenar eminence.

Technique. A midlateral incision is made on the ulnar border of the little finger proximal phalanx and extended proximally and radially to the distal palmar crease. It then runs along the radial border of the hypothenar eminence and curves ulnarly as it crosses the distal wrist crease. The two ADM insertions (base of the proximal phalanx and extensor apparatus) are divided, and this muscle is then freed of soft tissue attachments by retrograde dissection toward its pisiform origin. When mobilizing the proximal portion of the ADM, great care must be taken to not damage its thin neurovascular pedicle, which is on its dorsoradial aspect. Alternatively, this pedicle can be identified by exposing the ulnar nerve and artery proximally at the wrist and tracing them distally. Once the neurovascular bundle has been isolated, the transfer's length is increased by elevating the abductor origin from the pisiform while carefully retaining an attachment on the FCU tendon by dissecting a tendinous slip proximally. The transfer's only remaining soft tissue attachments are then its neurovascular pedicle and the FCU tendon. Next, a dorsoradial incision is made over the thumb MP joint and a wide subcutaneous tunnel is created between this incision and the area immediately proximal to the pisiform; this is easier if a third skin incision is made in the thenar crease at the base of the thenar eminence (not shown in Fig. 32-6). The ADM muscle is then turned through 180 degrees on its long axis to reduce the tension on its neurovascular bundle (as if turning the page of a book), passed

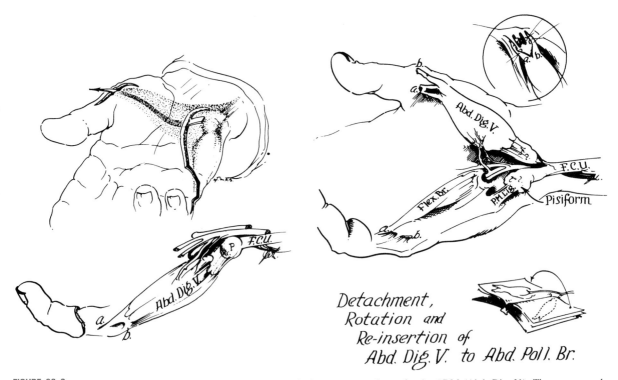

Detachment, Rotation and Re-insertion of Abd. Dig. V. to Abd. Poll. Br.

FIGURE 32-6. Huber ADM opponensplasty. Two incisions are required to expose and transfer the ADM (Abd. Dig. V.). The neurovascular structures enter the muscle proximally on its deep and radial aspect. The muscle is freed from the other hypothenar muscles, and its origin on the pisiform (P) is elevated while preserving a tendinous attachment to the tendon of the flexor carpi ulnaris (F.C.U.). The ADM is then rotated 180 degrees on its long axis and passed subcutaneously to the area of the thumb MP joint. The distal attachment is to the APB (Abd. Poll. Br.) muscle. (P.M. Lig., pisometacarpal ligament; Flex. Br., flexor digiti minimi brevis.) (From Littler JW, Cooley SGE: Opposition of the thumb and its restoration by abductor digiti quinti transfer. J Bone Joint Surg Am 45:1389-1484, 1963.)

through the subcutaneous tunnel, and attached to the APB insertion. Because the ADM muscle has only sufficient length to just reach the APB insertion, it is invariably attached under adequate tension.

Postoperatively, the thumb is immobilized in a cast in full opposition for 4 weeks. The position of the wrist is not critical inasmuch as the transfer does not cross this joint.

Results. Littler and Cooley[42] performed four Huber transfers, one of which failed and became fibrotic, probably as a result of vascular insufficiency. They considered this transfer difficult and recommended that it be performed only when simpler opponensplasties are contraindicated. Furthermore, primate studies have highlighted this transfer's precarious blood supply, which is significantly reduced by dividing its pisiform insertion.[25] In light of these concerns, many surgeons[39] retain the pisiform origin and lengthen the transfer with a short tendon graft when necessary. Wissinger and Singsen[76] preserved the pisiform origin in 15 Huber transfers and reported one failure as a result of transfer fibrosis. Twelve of their cases achieved excellent results with no donor site morbidity (Fig. 32-7). Their two fair results were caused by dehiscence of the thenar insertion and recurrent contracture.

Palmaris Longus Opponensplasty (Camitz)

The Camitz palmaris longus opponensplasty (Fig. 32-8) is a simple transfer that is usually performed for loss of abduction and opposition occurring as a complication of severe carpal tunnel syndrome. The procedure, which can be performed under regional anesthesia at the same time as carpal tunnel release, restores palmar abduction rather than opposition. Even though thumb opposition and abduction may recover after carpal tunnel release,[27] this will probably take many months and thus it is reasonable to perform a Camitz procedure at the same time as carpal tunnel release in patients with functional disability.[43] This transfer is not recommended for traumatic median nerve injuries because the palmaris longus, which lies directly over the median nerve, and the overlying skin are usually also scarred and damaged.

Technique. Preoperatively, the presence of the palmaris longus tendon is confirmed by opposing the thumb to the little finger with the wrist flexed. A longitudinal skin incision starting 2 cm proximal to the distal wrist crease and running to the proximal palmar crease is made in line with the ring finger. Care is taken to identify and avoid injury to the palmar cutaneous branch of the median nerve, which lies just radial to the palmaris longus tendon. The palmaris longus tendon is freed up in the forearm and into the palm, where a 1-cm-wide strip of palmar aponeurosis is dissected out in continuity with the tendon. The carpal tunnel is decompressed, and a second incision is made over the dorsoradial aspect of the thumb MP joint. A wide subcutaneous tunnel is then developed between this joint and the distal forearm incision, through which the palmaris longus tendon and its aponeurotic extension are passed. The palmar skin incision is then closed and the tendon transfer is usually attached to the APB insertion.[11,43,74] (Foucher and coworkers[26] favor attachment to either the EPB tendon or the dorsal capsule of the MP joint in an effort to restore opposition as well as abduction.) Whichever distal attachment is used, it is sutured

with the thumb in full opposition, the MP joint extended, and the wrist in neutral. The thumb incision is then closed, and a light cast holding the wrist in neutral and the thumb opposed is worn for 4 weeks. A night splint is then worn for another week.

Results. In a series of 73 Camitz procedures performed for severe carpal tunnel syndrome by Foucher and coworkers,[26] 50% of the patients regained good opposition within 1 year and 91% regained good thumb abduction and satisfactory opposition by 16 to 102 months. Attaching the palmaris longus to the dorsal capsule of the MP joint or the EPB tendon slightly restricted (15 to 25 degrees) MP joint movement in 20% of the patients in this series. Braun[11] successfully used the Camitz procedure to re-establish thumb abduction in 28 cases, whereas Terrono and colleagues[74] improved thumb function in 27 of 29 cases and believed that formal physiotherapy was unnecessary (Fig. 32-9).

What we call the Camitz transfer was actually first described by Bunnell,[16] who also suggested passing the palmaris longus tendon through a pulley close to the pisiform to create a more oblique line of pull and restore opposition. Passage of the transfer through a window in the flexor retinaculum has also been suggested.[44] If the superficial head of the FPB muscle is innervated by the ulnar nerve, this may provide pronation and thus allow a standard Camitz procedure to restore good opposition.

Other Opponensplasties

Other opponensplasties include the ECU, extensor carpi radialis longus (ECRL), and EDM opponensplasties.

ECU Opponensplasty

The ECU opponensplasty described by Phalen and Miller[63] allows the ECU to be used as an opponensplasty without the need for a free tendon graft.[37,53]

Technique. A short incision is made on the dorsoradial border of the distal forearm, and the EPB tendon is divided at its musculotendinous junction, just proximal to the first extensor compartment. An incision is then made on the extensor surface of the thumb MP joint, and the EPB tendon is delivered into this wound while preserving its insertion on the proximal phalanx. Next, an "L"-shaped incision is made on the ulnar border of the wrist, its short arm passing transversely along the flexor wrist crease toward the palmaris longus insertion. A wide subcutaneous tunnel running from the thumb MP joint to the pisiform area is then created across the palm. The EPB tendon is passed proximally through this tunnel, and the ECU tendon is then divided close to its insertion on the base of the fifth metacarpal. This tendon is withdrawn back under the extensor retinaculum and freed of soft tissue attachments throughout the distal third of the forearm. It is then passed around the ulnar border of the distal forearm and sutured to the EPB tendon while the thumb is opposed to the base of the middle finger with its MP and IP joints extended. Postoperatively, the thumb is immobilized in opposition with the wrist in neutral for 3 to 4 weeks.

Results. Wood and Adams[77] performed this procedure on 12 complex cases with few available motors, and in four

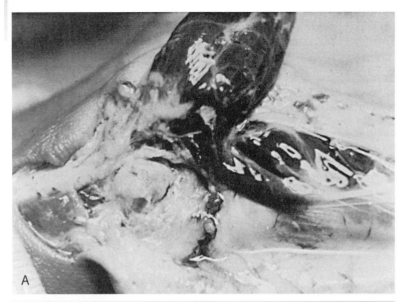

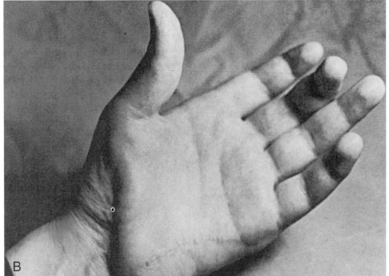

FIGURE 32-7. Huber ADM opponensplasty. **A,** Freeing of the ADM from the pisiform, which leaves the FCU and the neurovascular bundle as its only remaining attachments. **B** and **C,** Satisfactory function has been restored, at least partly because the direction of pull is really from the pisiform.

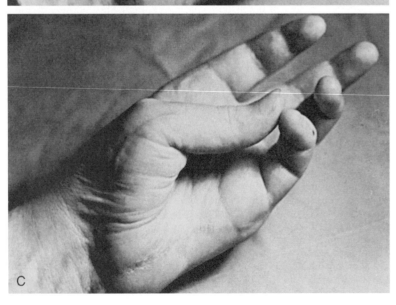

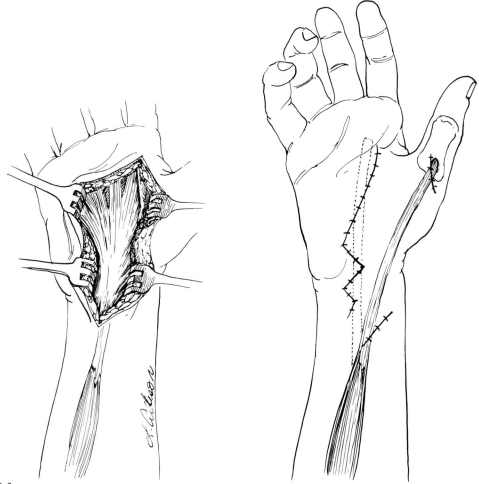

FIGURE 32-8. Camitz transfer. The palmaris longus is elongated with a strip of palmar aponeurosis and attached to the APB insertion.

instances they observed radial deviation wrist deformities that caused severe grip weakness. This may have occurred as a result of FCU paresis or paralysis, but an anomalous ECRL insertion onto the radial rather than the dorsal border of the index metacarpal was also implicated. In two patients the radial deviation deformity was corrected by transferring the ECRL tendon to the distal ECU stump. There are three other problems with this transfer.[38,77] First, the EPB tendon is sometimes nonexistent. Second, an MP joint flexion deformity may occur if the EPB tendon is dissected out from the extensor hood right up to its insertion; in contrast, if it is not dissected out sufficiently distally, it can cause MP joint hyperextension. Third, a tendinous slip sometimes connects the EPB and EPL tendons; if this is present, it must be divided because the transfer may otherwise cause unwanted extension of the IP joint.

ECRL Opponensplasty

The tendon of the ECRL muscle can be lengthened with a standard tendon graft.[31] Alternatively the ECRL (or ECRB) tendon may be detached distally at its insertion onto the index metacarpal, brought out into a wound in the dorsal forearm, and carefully split longitudinally in half, such that one strip remains attached to the muscle and the other half

is free. The free strip of tendon is then sutured to the distal end of attached strip to lengthen the tendon. The transfer is then passed through a wide subcutaneous tunnel around the ulna, just proximal to the pisiform, and inserted into the APB attachment and EPL.[3a] Alternatively, Kaplan and coworkers[36] elongated the ECRL tendon with the EPL tendon in four patients with isolated median or combined median and ulnar nerve injuries.

Technique. A skin incision is made over the dorsum of the distal radius, and the EPL tendon is divided at its musculotendinous junction. The ECRL tendon is then divided close to its insertion and freed of soft tissue attachments in the distal forearm. Next, the EPL tendon is delivered into a second incision on the extensor surface of the thumb MP joint and a third skin incision is made on the ulnar border of the wrist at the level of the ulnar styloid process. Wide subcutaneous tunnels are then created across the palm and around the ulnar border of the wrist/distal forearm. The EPL tendon is passed through the palmar tunnel to the ulnar border of the wrist, where it is sutured to the ECRL tendon with the wrist flexed and the thumb abducted and opposed. Postoperatively, the hand is immobilized with the wrist flexed and the thumb opposed in a below-elbow cast for 3 weeks.

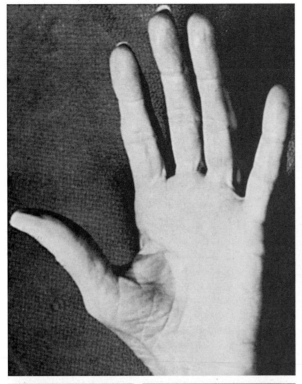

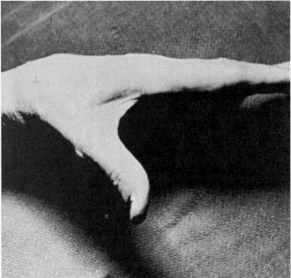

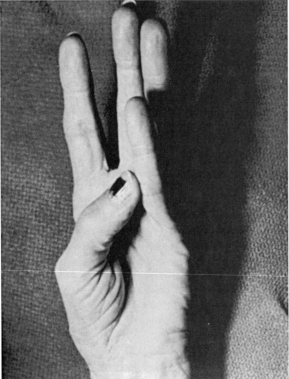

FIGURE 32-9. A patient presented with long-standing carpal tunnel syndrome and thenar muscle atrophy with loss of abduction and opposition. A Camitz transfer was performed at the same time as a carpal tunnel release, and excellent thumb abduction was restored. Thumb pronation was provided by the weak FPB.

Results. In the small series of Kaplan and coworkers,[36] all thumbs regained abduction and opposition and thumb IP joint flexion and extension were preserved. Henderson[31] also used the ECRL in five patients, all of whom regained satisfactory opposition. Baek and colleagues,[3a] who prefer this transfer to the use of the EIP which they consider only allows weak opposition, achieved excellent results in 10 of 11 cases.

EDM Opponensplasty

The EDM may be used for an opponensplasty,[69] particularly when the EIP is not available, usually because it has been used or will be used for another transfer. It is important that the surgeon has an alternate transfer in mind, in the event that the EDM is determined to be insufficient or absent.

Technique. An incision is made over the little finger MP joint, and the EDM tendons (there are usually two tendons) are identified on the ulnar side of the little finger common extensor tendon. These tendons and, in continuity with them distally, a central slip of the extensor hood are freed distally and withdrawn proximally into a large incision on the dorsoulnar aspect of the distal forearm. The tendons are then freed of soft tissue attachments in the distal third of the forearm, and the little finger extensor hood is carefully repaired with interrupted, nonabsorbable sutures. The transfer is then passed outside of the extensor retinaculum, around the ulnar border of the wrist, and subcutaneously across the palm by using the technique described for EIP transfer (see page 1139). In the original description of this transfer, it was attached to the APB, the extensor expansion, and the EPL tendon over the base of the proximal phalanx. Postoperatively, the thumb is immobilized in opposition with the wrist in neutral for 3 weeks.

Results. Schneider[69] reported good opposition in 8 of 10 cases, most of which were combined median and ulnar nerve injuries (Fig. 32-10). The donor tendon is not long enough on its own, so a portion of the extensor hood must be taken to ensure adequate length. Despite careful repair of the hood, the authors have encountered extension lag of the little finger after this transfer.

Tendon Transfers ("Compromise Opponensplasty") for Severe Nerve Deficits

In a complete or nearly complete intrinsic-minus thumb, such as occurs in combined median and ulnar nerve palsies, the FPL and EPL muscles both adduct and supinate the thumb. Furthermore, the combined overactivity of these two extrinsic muscles causes the IP joint to hyperflex and the MP joint to extend. The hyperflexed IP joint prevents the thumb pulp

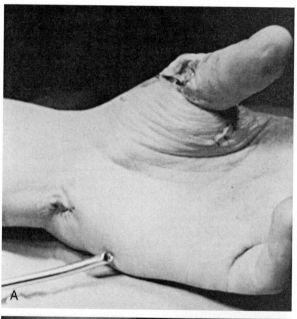

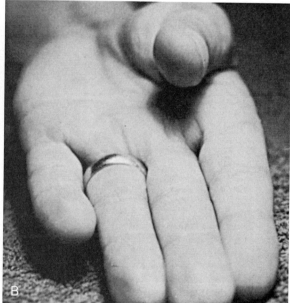

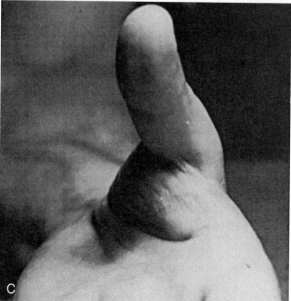

FIGURE 32-10. EDM transfer for opposition of the thumb. Note the position at the time of surgery (**A**) and postoperative active abduction and rotation of the thumb (**B** and **C**), even with an immobile wrist.

from meeting the index finger properly in either pulp or key pinch, and the fingers tend to strike the nail or the dorsum of the thumb, which is disabling and causes thumb supination (Fig. 32-11). However, the patient can usually hold objects between the adjacent sides of the thumb and hand (lateral squeeze) and often prefers this "pinch" to that provided by an opponensplasty, which the patient therefore does not use.[8] It is thus an attractive concept, which stems from the days of poliomyelitis, to use one of these extrinsic thumb muscles for an opponensplasty.

In progressive severe paralysis, a combination of two tendon transfers, one to provide opposition and the other to restore FPB function, is a luxury and the hand may not have sufficient function to benefit from true opposition.[50] In these instances, restoration of short flexor action alone often provides adequate thumb function. This can be produced by a single tendon transfer and thumb joint fusion or, less commonly, IP joint tenodesis.[46]

FPL Opponensplasty

A FPL transfer only provides limited pronation and is used for patients with severe hand paralysis in whom pinch of the thumb pulp to the sides of the index or long fingers is more important than pinch to the pulp. The desired end result is a single-axis thumb that can clear the fingers and oppose the fingertips and their sides with considerable power.

Technique. The distal attachment of the FPL is exposed and divided through a zigzag incision on the flexor surface of the interphalangeal joint. A "Y" incision is then made over the dorsum of that joint, and the EPL tendon is divided at its insertion and retracted proximally. Next, the IP joint is fused in extension. The FPL tendon is delivered into an incision on the radiopalmar aspect of the wrist. Sometimes this is possible only after adhesions between the tendon and the radial palmar bursa have been divided through a further

incision at the level of the A1 pulley. The FPL is then passed around a pulley on the ulnar border of the hand; any of the superficialis transfer pulleys described earlier in this chapter may be used. If the Thompson pulley is chosen, a palmar incision is made in line with the ulnar border of the ring finger. Next, the FPL tendon is passed through the carpal tunnel, between the superficialis and profundus flexor tendons, and is delivered into the palmar incision. An incision is then made over the dorsoradial aspect of the thumb MP joint, and the FPL tendon is passed through a wide subcutaneous tunnel into this incision. After the tourniquet has been released and hemostasis obtained, all but the last incisions are closed.

The FPL tendon is usually attached to the superficial head of the FPB rather than the APB. This allows the transfer to stabilize the MP joint in slight flexion as well as abduct and to a lesser extent pronate the thumb. Furthermore, if the APB is used as the insertion, thumb opposition and flexion will be much weaker. Because the FPL muscle has a large potential excursion, setting the tension in this transfer is relatively easy and the thumb should rest in almost full opposition at the end of the procedure.

The hand is immobilized postoperatively with the wrist in 40 degrees of flexion and the thumb in full opposition for 3 weeks. Rehabilitation is then begun by using active wrist extension to bring the thumb into opposition. This is followed by exercises to increase power of the transfer.

Results. Burkhalter believed that this transfer had distinct advantages for the completely intrinsic-minus thumb, in which case short flexor action is more important than opposition. He found that EPL overactivity tended to disappear, and his patients quickly realized that they had a functional short flexor muscle and no longer needed to use the EPL as a secondary thumb adductor (Fig. 32-12). After this transfer, the patient uses the EPL to move the thumb away from the fingers and the FPL opponensplasty for prehension activity.

Alternative FPL Opponensplasties

Makin[45] transferred the FPL "in continuity," without dividing the tendon or its insertion, by passing it through an oblique osteotomy in the proximal phalanx. The "transfer" then spirals around the proximal phalanx and the MP joint. The osteotomy is stabilized with a longitudinal Kirschner wire, which also holds the IP joint in extension. Makin used this procedure on 14 patients in whom no standard muscles were available for transfer and reported that it restored strong active opposition in all. Four osteotomies failed to unite, and this was attributed to the initial use of a transverse rather than an oblique osteotomy. Oberlin and Alnot[57] used a similar technique in 11 intrinsic-minus thumbs and reported very good results in eight of the nine cases reviewed. Rather than passing the FPL tendon through an osteotomy, they passed it through either the IP or the MP joint, which was then fused. They stressed that the transfer must pass over the extensor surface of the MP joint and not over the dorsum of the proximal phalanx, which may cause a flexion deformity of the MP joint. These authors recommended this transfer for completely intrinsic-minus thumbs in high nerve injuries but favored EIP opponensplasty and MP joint arthrodesis if there were no fixed deformity of the IP joint.

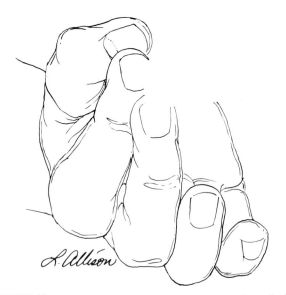

FIGURE 32-11. With hyperflexion of the IP joint, a moment for supination of the thumb occurs if the index finger contacts the thumb with power. Brand calls this the crank handle effect.

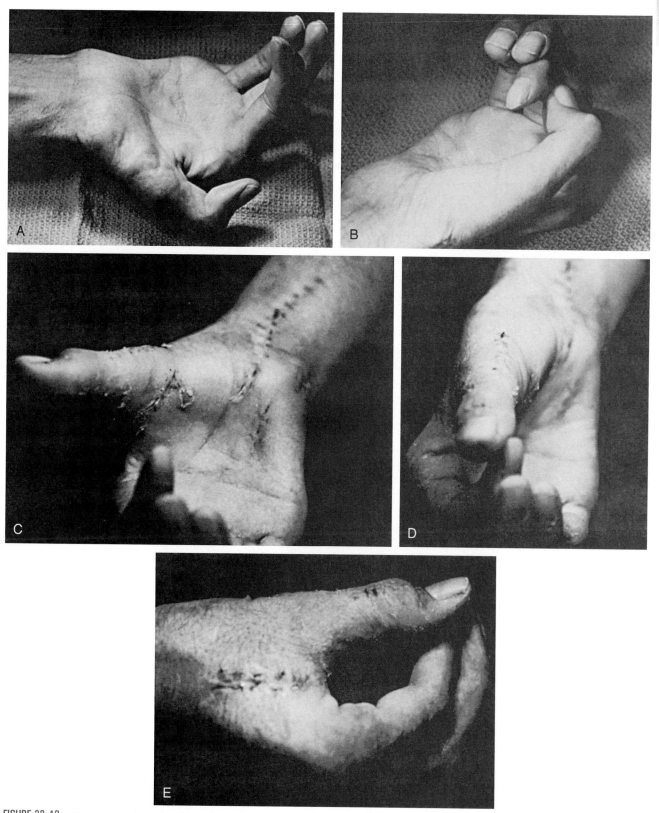

FIGURE 32-12. FPL opponensplasty. **A** and **B,** A 25-year-old man presented with a brachial plexus injury and the equivalent of an intrinsic-minus thumb. The thumb extrinsic muscles were causing MP joint extension and IP joint hyperflexion. An FPL opponensplasty and thumb IP arthrodesis restored short thumb flexor and EPL function. **C** to **E,** Improved thumb function was apparent as soon as the cast was removed. The EPL now functions not as an adductor but as an extensor, and the FPL now functions as a short flexor replacement. The pulley for the transfer was at the pisiform, and its distal attachment was the APB tendon.

EPL Opponensplasty

In some cases of peripheral nerve disease or spastic paralysis, when the only functioning thumb extrinsic or intrinsic motors are the EPL, EPB, and the APL, an IP joint flexion contracture may occur even though the FPL is weak or totally paralyzed. This is due to a tenodesis effect of the FPL, which occurs as the functioning thumb muscles extend and supinate the trapeziometacarpal and MP joints. In this situation, the extension and supination deformity at the base of the thumb may be corrected by an intermetacarpal bone block (static correction) or an EPL opponensplasty (Fig. 32-13) if this muscle is under voluntary control. If a spastic EPL is transferred, the thumb will lie in front of (and get in

the way of) the fingers because the APL on its own is not sufficiently strong to hold the thumb out of the palm.

Technique. An incision is made on the extensor surface of the proximal phalanx and MP joint of the thumb. The EPL tendon, with a contiguous central portion of the extensor expansion, is then freed from its insertion on the distal phalanx while preserving the lateral portions of the extensor hood over the proximal phalanx and the MP joint. This tendon is then withdrawn into an incision on the extensor surface of the wrist and distal forearm, and a further incision is made near the pisiform. The EPL tendon is passed through a wide subcutaneous tunnel that runs around the ulnar border

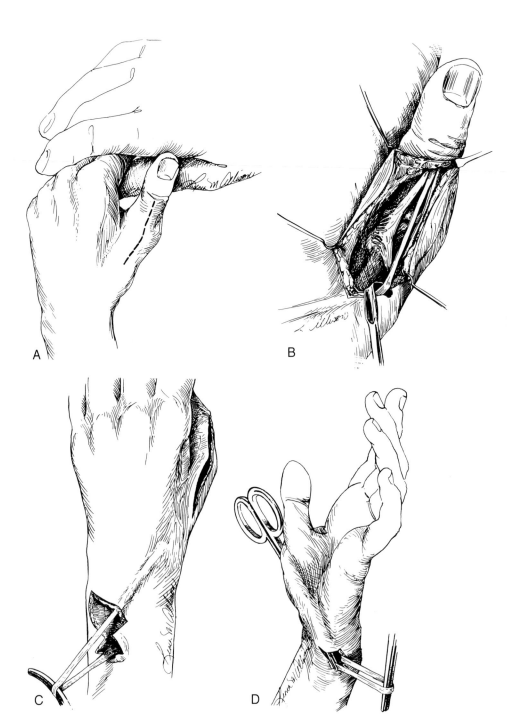

FIGURE 32-13. EPL opponensplasty. **A** and **B**, The middle portion of the EPL tendon is exposed over the proximal phalanx and removed in continuity with the main EPL tendon proximal to the MP joint. **C** to **E**, The transfer is then passed around the ulnar border of the wrist, and the thumb MP joint is fused.

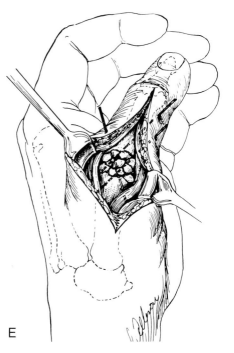

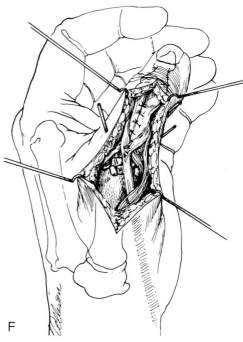

E

F

FIGURE 32-13—cont'd. F, The two lateral portions of the EPL tendon over the proximal phalanx are sutured together, and the transfer is sutured around them. The IP joint is temporarily pinned in extension to protect the transfer while it heals. (From Riley WB, Mann RJ, Burkhalter WE: Extensor pollicis longus opponensplasty. J Hand Surg 5:217-220, 1980.)

of the wrist and across the palm to the initial thumb incision. Next, the thumb MP joint is fused in almost full extension and some pronation (Figs. 32-14 and 32-15). The transferred EPL tendon is then looped around the lateral portions of the extensor hood at the level of the MP joint and sutured back onto itself. The two lateral portions of the extensor hood over the proximal phalanx are sutured together, thereby restoring continuity of the EPL and preserving extension of the IP joint. The IP joint is then held in extension with Kirschner wires, and the hand is immobilized with the thumb in full opposition and the wrist in 40 degrees of flexion. It is most important that the fixation of the MP arthrodesis is secure so that this transfer can be mobilized actively within 4 weeks, when the arthrodesis is not yet solid. At that stage the patient should be taught to differentiate between EPL

and APL function. It is also important that after completion of the transfer it is possible for the fingers to clear the thumb with the wrist in neutral, because, after this transfer, only the EPB and APL extend the thumb.

Results. Riley and colleagues[64] used this transfer in 11 patients with progressive neurologic disease, such as syringomyelia and Charcot-Marie-Tooth disease, or traumatic high median or combined median and ulnar nerve intrinsic paralyses. They reported satisfactory results in view of the severity of the original motor deficit and found that the APL and EPB muscles were always able to extend the thumb sufficiently to clear the palm and not impede finger flexion (Fig. 32-16). However, all the patients had a diminished range of retroposition.

Alternative EPL Opponensplasties

Moutet and associates[51] and Mennen[48] have used EPL opponensplasties more routinely, both for isolated and combined median nerve injuries. However, instead of transferring the EPL tendon around the ulnar border of the wrist, they both passed it through a window in the interosseous membrane. Moutet and associates then passed it around either the FCR (isolated median nerve injury) or FCU (combined median and ulnar nerve injury) tendon, and both sutured the transfer back onto the divided distal end of the EPL. Neither fused the MP joint.

Mennen's Technique of EPL Opponensplasty.[48] The EPL tendon is exposed through an incision on the extensor surface of the MP joint and divided 1 cm proximal to this joint. This tendon is then delivered into a second incision on the extensor surface of the forearm. The tendon and its muscle are freed of soft tissue attachments throughout the distal half of the forearm. An incision is made on the flexor surface of the forearm, 3 cm proximal to the wrist crease and just radial to the ulnar artery. The interosseous membrane is then exposed

FIGURE 32-14. If the thumb MP joint is fused in flexion, the index finger exerts a powerful supinatory effect on the thumb during pinch. The moment arm is the entire length of the distal and proximal phalanges of the thumb. This is the same crank handle effect as seen in Figure 32-11, but with an even longer moment arm.

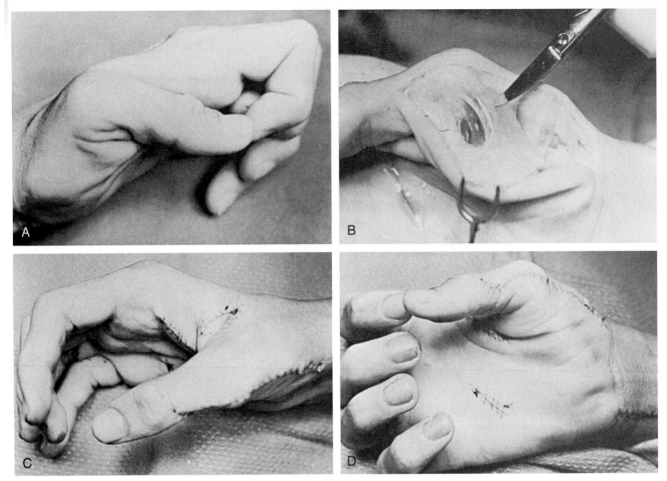

FIGURE 32-15. **A** and **B,** A completely intrinsic-minus thumb in which only a single motor was used to reconstruct thumb function. In spite of adequate release (**C**), this patient needs either an MP joint arthrodesis in full extension or a second transfer to restore short flexor-adductor function. As the patient attempts to pinch the thumb and the index finger together (**D**), thumb MP joint flexion will produce a tremendous crank handle action.

between the ulnar neurovascular bundle and the finger flexor tendons, and a window is made that is large enough to accommodate the distal portion of the EPL muscle easily. A subcutaneous tunnel is then created between the incisions on the anterior of the forearm and back of the thumb, and the EPL tendon is passed through the interosseous membrane and subcutaneously along the thenar eminence to the extensor surface of the thumb MP joint. Here it is passed under the EPB tendon and reattached to its own distal stump with a 1-cm overlap. The thumb is immobilized in a short-arm thumb spica cast for 4 weeks, and a dynamic opposition splint is then used for another 4 weeks.

Results. By using this technique, Mennen regained normal opposition between the thumb and little finger pulp in 26 of 35 cases and also found that normal power of extension of the IP joint of the thumb was retained. In the series by Moutet and associates, 14 of 16 patients recovered functional opposition[51] and the results remained satisfactory 13 years later.[28]

Adductor Pollicis and FPB Opponensplasties

DeVecchi[24] transferred the adductor pollicis to the insertion of the superficial head of the FPB. This transfer requires an extensive palmar incision that extends from the adductor

insertion across the palm toward the middle finger metacarpal and then proximally toward the base of the thumb. The carpal tunnel is opened, and the median nerve and its branches are protected. The adductor tendon is then divided at its insertion and freed from the FPB. It is passed superficial to the index finger flexor tendons, the index/middle common digital neurovascular bundle, and the FPL tendon and attached to the superficial head of the FPB. This transfer restores FPB function and provides some thumb pronation but does not produce true opposition.

Orticochea[61] transferred the ulnar-innervated deep head of the FPB around the extensor surface of the thumb and attached it to the aponeurosis of the adductor tendon.

Postoperative Management of Opponensplasty

The thumb is immobilized in opposition for 3 weeks after most opponensplasties, and the wrist should also be immobilized if the tendon transfer crosses the flexor surface of this joint. Transfers of muscles with relatively short excursions, such as the EIP, should be relaxed by immobilizing the wrist in 30 degrees of flexion and the thumb in full opposition. However, after transfer of muscles with larger excursions, such as the superficialis, the wrist can be immobilized in neutral with the thumb in full opposition. If the

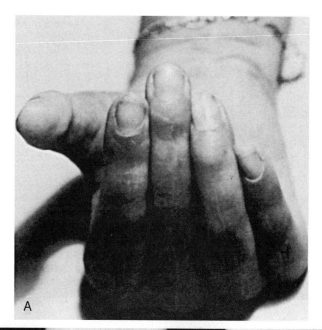

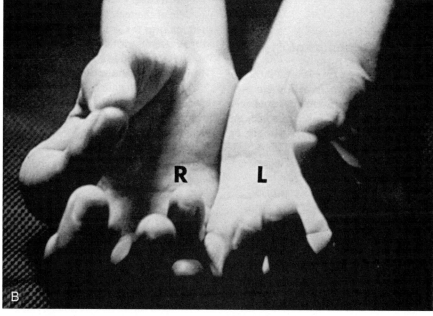

FIGURE 32-16. This patient with Charcot-Marie-Tooth disease has undergone arthrodesis of the thumb MP joint as well as an EPL opponensplasty. **A,** The APL can move the thumb clear of the fingers so that it does not interfere with power grip. **B,** In addition, notice that the MP joint of the left thumb has been arthrodesed in hyperpronation whereas on the right it has been fused in an almost neutral position. The crank handle effect is much less obvious in the left thumb, which suggests that fusion of the MP joint in hyperpronation, as well as full extension, is preferable for patients with combined median and ulnar nerve palsy.

transfer is attached to either the extensor mechanism or the APB insertion, the IP joint of the thumb should also probably be immobilized in full extension. I find it useful to maintain thumb opposition postoperatively by using cyanoacrylate glue to stick the skin of the thumb tip to the little finger at the end of the operation, before the transfer's tension is set. With desquamation, the thumb is spontaneously released from the little finger after 2 to 3 weeks. After 3 weeks, all splintage can usually be discarded and most patients quickly regain thumb control. The emphasis should be on early restoration of wrist movement, which will alternately relax and tighten the opponensplasty. However, in certain conditions, such as high combined median and ulnar nerve palsies and diseases such as Charcot-Marie-Tooth disease and leprosy, the thumb extensors are strong and unbalanced and the sensory loss is profound; in these conditions the patient may stretch the transfer if the thumb

is mobilized after 3 weeks, and it is advisable to protect the opponensplasty for 3 months with splints that prevent full adduction, supination, and extension of the thumb.

Author's Preferred Method of Treatment: Low Median Nerve Palsy

My enthusiasm for reconstructive surgery in median nerve palsy is tempered by my belief that sensation is the prime determinant of hand function in this situation, so I believe that isolated injuries to the motor branch of the median nerve and focal pure motor deficits caused by nonprogressive or slowly progressive neurologic disease are the best indications for opponensplasty. The more severe the sensory deficit, the less likely that the patient will benefit from reconstructive surgery. Thus, I believe that opponensplasty is rarely indicated in combined complete median and ulnar nerve injuries in adults because the permanent sensory deficit is often severe even after careful nerve repair.

In my practice, few patients require or request an opponensplasty after isolated traumatic division of the median nerve; in fact, many never lose opposition, presumably because of anomalous thenar muscle innervation.

In combined nerve deficits it is imperative that both the patient and the surgeon consider whether the loss of opposition, taken in isolation from the rest of the neurologic deficit, is causing sufficient disability to justify further surgery and rehabilitation. Many of my patients, especially those with unilateral loss of opposition and in times of job insecurity, adapt well and minimize their disability so that an opponensplasty is not indicated.

My favored transfers are the Camitz procedure and the EIP transfer. I used to favor the Royle-Thompson superficialis transfer but was converted to the EIP transfer after writing this chapter for the fourth edition by the papers of Burkhalter (who wrote previous editions of this chapter) and discussions with Nicholas Barton (my coauthors for that chapter). I use the Camitz procedure in patients with loss of opposition secondary to carpal tunnel syndrome and perform this transfer at the same time as carpal tunnel release, even though I believe that thenar muscle function will recover in a considerable number of cases. I do this because the procedure has low morbidity and complication rates and requires little rehabilitation and also because the recovery of thenar muscle function is unpredictable and may not occur for over a year. It does require general or regional anesthesia, whereas most of my carpal tunnel releases are done under local infiltration anesthesia. Restoration of thumb abduction in these patients may produce immediate improvement in hand function if median nerve sensation has not been completely lost and there is a reasonable prospect for sensory regeneration.

In other instances, I now favor the EIP transfer, which rarely causes any donor site morbidity, provided that the index finger extensor hood is not damaged. Furthermore, this transfer uses a natural pulley (the ulnar border of the wrist), which is resilient and cannot migrate. In isolated median nerve transfers, this transfer is inserted into the APB tendon. I have not experienced significant loss of thumb extension after this transfer and have found rehabilitation and re-education straightforward.

With more complex upper limb paralyses it is important to assess the disability carefully, ascertain which musculotendinous units are available for transfer, and consider the probable effects of loss of the transfer's normal function before making any decision.

Expectations/Patient Counseling: Low Median Nerve Palsy

What I tell the patient about the expected outcome depends on (1) whether the underlying neurologic pathology is progressive (progressive neurologic disease) or static (nerve injury after regeneration period); (2) the functional disability attributable to the isolated loss of opposition; and (3) the functional disability attributable to other problems in the hand, such as sensory loss and loss of other motor functions. I would advise a motivated patient with an otherwise normal hand (e.g., isolated injury to the motor branch of the median nerve) that restoration of opposition with either an EIP, FDS, or ADM transfer should restore useful opposition and improve hand function considerably in 7 or 8 of every 10 cases. I tell patients with loss of opposition due to severe carpal tunnel syndrome that they will regain thumb abduction in a similar number of instances but that the functional benefit of this depends to a great extent on the recovery of lost sensation in the thumb and index and middle fingers after the carpal tunnel release. For more complex cases, such as loss of opposition after combined median and ulnar nerve injuries, I tell patients that opposition can be restored in 7 or 8 of every 10 cases but I stress that their lost opposition is (usually) only causing a small amount of their total hand disability and that they may not gain any significant functional benefit from a successful opponensplasty: in my opinion there has to be convincing evidence that the loss of opposition, rather than loss of sensation or other motor deficits, is causing loss of function before recommending surgery. When dealing with progressive neurologic disease, it is vital to have the opinion of the treating neurologist regarding the likely course and speed of progression of the condition and to be aware of whether the deficit is/will be purely motor or combined sensory and motor. I then carefully discuss the likely short- and long-term benefits of an opponensplasty with the patient so he or she can make an informed decision on its likely impact, both in the short and the long term, on the hand function.

CRITICAL POINTS: MANAGEMENT OF LOW MEDIAN NERVE PALSY

- The more severe the sensory deficit, the less likely the patient will benefit from reconstructive surgery.
- Expected patient outcomes depend on the underlying neurologic pathology (progressive or static), the functional disability attributed to the isolated loss of opposition, and the functional disability attributable to other problems in the hand (e.g., sensory loss, other motor functions).

HIGH MEDIAN NERVE PALSY

In high median nerve paralysis, all the flexor compartment forearm muscles apart from the ulnar-innervated FCU and the profundi to the little and ring fingers are paralyzed. However, the working part of the profundus muscle often provides a full, although weak range of middle finger flexion.

The prime aim of tendon transfers in high median nerve palsy is to restore flexion of the index finger and thumb, as well as opposition. Only the brachioradialis, ECRL, and ECU are available and suitable for transfer to the extrinsic flexors, and the ECU may be required for an opponensplasty. Because these three muscles all have less potential excursion than the index profundus and FPL (Table 32-3), satisfactory results are obtained only if the patient can amplify the transfer's excursion by actively flexing and extending the wrist. Full finger and thumb flexion and extension are then achieved by the tenodesis effect of extending and flexing the wrist, respectively.

The brachioradialis is usually used to restore FPL function and the ECRL to restore index finger profundus function (Fig. 32-17). If these transfers are performed before the anticipated regeneration period after a nerve repair or graft, they should be attached in an end-to-side fashion so that the patient can benefit from any subsequent motor recovery. In fact, inasmuch as extremely late recovery of motor function is sometimes observed, end-to-end tendon transfer attachments are only exceptionally performed after nerve injuries without any prospect of recovery.

Table 32-3
THE RESTING MUSCLE FIBER LENGTHS AND TENSION FRACTIONS OF THE EXTRINSIC MUSCLES WHOSE FUNCTION IS COMMONLY RESTORED IN HIGH MEDIAN INJURY AND THEIR REPLACEMENTS

	Resting Muscle Fiber Length (cm)	Tension Fraction (%)
Paralyzed Muscles		
Flexor pollicis longus	5.9	2.7
Flexor digitorum profundus, index	6.6	2.7
Flexor digitorum profundus, middle	6.6	3.4
Potential Motors for Transfer		
Brachioradialis	16.1 (10.9–21.3)	2.4
Extensor carpi radialis longus	9.3	3.5
Extensor carpi ulnaris	4.5	4.5

From Brand PW: Tendon transfers for median and ulnar nerve paralysis. Orthop Clin North Am 1:447-454, 1970.

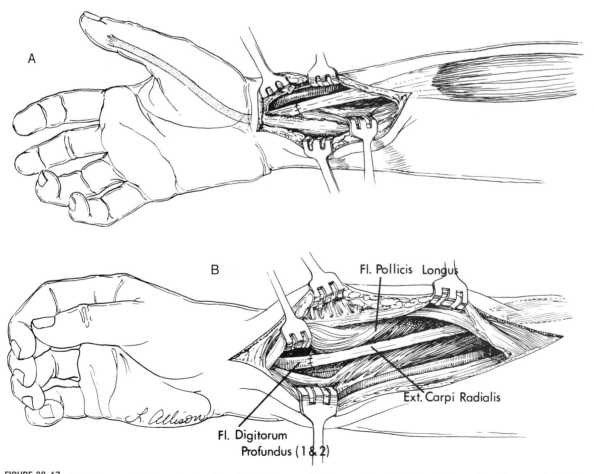

FIGURE 32-17. Extrinsic reconstruction using brachioradialis-to-flexor pollicis longus (**A**) and ECRL-to-index and long finger profundi (**B**) transfers. The transfers shown here are end-to-end transfers but should be done in an end-to-side fashion if there is to be any chance of recovery.

Timing and Selection of Extrinsic Transfers

The selection and timing of tendon transfers for both intrinsic and extrinsic paralysis in high median nerve lesions depend on the prognosis for the median nerve injury, as well as the surgeon's assessment and the patient's perception of the functional disability.

In patients with median nerve palsy, the sensory loss is probably the most important single disability, and this dramatically reduces the functional benefit of tendon transfers. Although some surgeons believe that the severe sensory loss is a strong contraindication to tendon transfers, others argue that eyesight can provide sensory input and some hand function remains; thus they believe that a mobile, opposable thumb is probably more useful than one that cannot reach the remaining areas of the hand with normal sensation.[19]

The functional deficit associated with a high median lesion is so profound that some surgeons advocate early tendon transfers in selected patients to restore either opposition alone or opposition and extrinsic muscle function.[19] These early transfers maintain motor function during nerve regeneration and act as an internal splint, thereby preventing contractures and eliminating the need for cumbersome external splints that may severely limit the patient's ability to use the hand. Thus early transfers can be of considerable benefit in the rehabilitation of some patients. If the patient ultimately regains only partial function in the muscles involved, the transfers will act in synergy and provide additional power, whereas if no recovery occurs, the transfers act as a permanent substitute.

Extrinsic Transfers

Good extrinsic muscle function is usually restored after repair of a high median nerve laceration, in which case transfers to restore flexion of the thumb and index finger are not required. However, these should be considered if there is no evidence of extrinsic muscle recovery several months after a nerve repair. For practical purposes, extrinsic tendon transfers are indicated only when a high median nerve injury is not repaired or is grafted. As mentioned previously, if there is any hope of subsequent motor recovery, these transfers should be performed in an end-to-side fashion. If one decides to not perform early extrinsic tendon transfers, it is essential that mobility of the thumb and index finger are maintained until recovery occurs. Because the potential excursions of the muscles available for extrinsic transfer are restricted, it is also necessary that the wrist have a full range of motion at the time of extrinsic tendon transfer.

Restoration of Thumb Opposition

As previously mentioned, many patients retain thumb opposition after median nerve injury and do not require an opposition transfer. Burkhalter, who had a wealth of expertise[14,40] and wrote this chapter in previous editions, believed that those who lost opposition should undergo an opposition transfer soon after neurorrhaphy or grafting and before sensory recovery. His rationale was that the likelihood of recovery of thumb intrinsic muscle function after high median nerve injury is low.

Patients who have lost thumb opposition and abduction use the APL and the extrinsic extensor muscles to position

their thumb when picking up an article from a table. Although the thumb index web is open, the thumb is supinated and extended because all these muscles are supinators. With the thumb in this position, the patient can pick up objects from a flat surface only by fully pronating the hand, either by pronating the forearm or internally rotating the shoulder (Fig. 32-18). Thus the patient cannot see the palm of the hand and cannot use sight as a substitute for the median nerve sensory loss, which renders motor function of little use to the patient. For this reason, some surgeons recommend early opposition transfer to allow the patient to pick up objects with the forearm in any position of rotation. If a patient is able to use a paralyzed hand to pick up articles and transfer objects from hand to hand in a position other than full pronation, the FPB is probably still functioning and an opponensplasty is not needed.

Restoration of Opposition in High Median Nerve Palsy

In high median nerve palsy, the EPL, EIP, and EDM are most readily available for opposition transfer. They position the thumb well, do not create significant donor morbidity, and do not require lengthening with a tendon graft. Although strong opposition can be restored with the FCU (which may be elongated with a paralyzed superficialis tendon),[30,33] this eliminates the only functioning wrist flexor. Moreover, strong thumb opposition is not required as long as there are functioning intrinsic muscles capable of acting as a short flexor or short flexor substitute.

ECRL-to-Index Profundus Transfer

An ECRL-to-index profundus transfer is performed only in patients who need strength on the radial side of the hand and are unlikely to obtain significant reinnervation after nerve repair. Usually, index finger range of flexion but not strength is restored by side-to-side suturing of the index and the conjoint middle, ring, and little finger profundus tendons in the distal forearm. If an ECRL transfer is indicated, its tension is adjusted so that the finger is virtually fully extended when the wrist is flexed 30 degrees and is fully flexed when the wrist is extended 30 to 45 degrees. If this transfer is placed in excessive tension, flexion contractures will result and cause considerable disability.

Brachioradialis-to-FPL Transfer

To achieve 30-mm excursion, the brachioradialis muscle must be freed of all soft tissue and fascial attachments throughout the distal two thirds of the forearm. This involves dissection well proximal to the musculotendinous junction because the peripheral fibers of this muscle insert onto the deep fascia of the forearm.[8] The transfer's tension is set so that all three thumb joints can be fully passively extended when the wrist is flexed 30 degrees; again, and for the same reason mentioned for the ECRL to index profundus transfer, excessive tension must be avoided. Although this tension will not allow full IP joint flexion, it will stabilize this joint, improve thumb strength, and prevent a disabling flexion contracture from developing (Fig. 32-19). Most precision pinch activities are performed with the thumb IP joint fully extended.

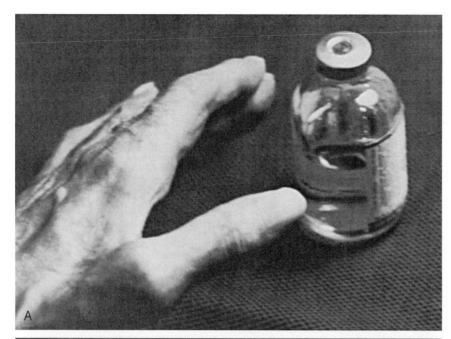

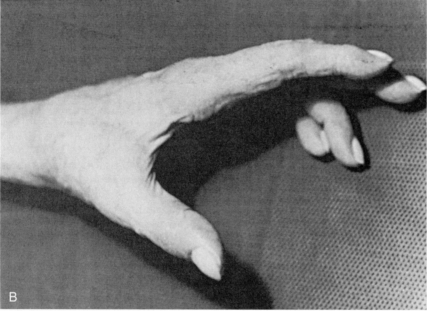

FIGURE 32-18. **A,** A patient with a brachial plexus injury is attempting to pick up a bottle by positioning his hand in full pronation. This is a substitute maneuver for absent APB and FPB function. **B,** After opponensplasty it is possible to position the hand for grasp with the forearm in neutral, and the patient can now see the palmar surface of his hand.

Because the prime function of the brachioradialis is elbow flexion, its usefulness as a transfer depends on elbow position. When the elbow is extended, reasonably powerful thumb flexion is usually provided, but thumb flexion is much weaker when the elbow is flexed. For this reason, Brand and others have considered fixing the brachioradialis origin distal to the elbow,[8,60] but this practice is not widely performed.

Complications

Swan neck deformities can develop in patients with hyperextensible PIP joints after high median paralysis. These usually develop gradually as the PIP palmar plates stretch and may cause disability with locking of these joints in extension. Because tendon transfers to restore index and middle finger profundus function may aggravate preexisting swan

neck deformities, consideration should be given in patients with hyperextensible joints to modified transfers such as the following:

1. Transfer of the ECRL to the index and middle superficialis tendons. The profundus tendons of both these digits are then used to tenodese their DIP joints in 30 degrees of flexion.
2. Transfer of the ECRL to the index and middle profundus tendons. The flexor digitorum profundus tendons of these fingers are then sutured to the A4 pulleys with nonabsorbable sutures so that they tenodese the DIP joints in 30 degrees of flexion and primarily flex the PIP joints.
3. Transfer of the ECRL to the index and middle profundus tendons with DIP joint arthrodeses.

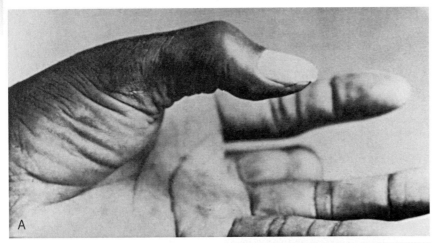

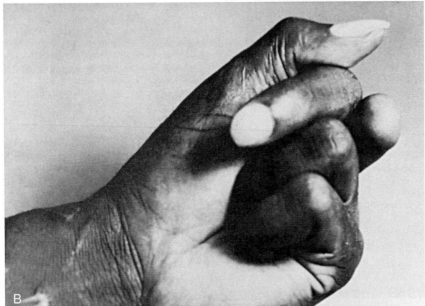

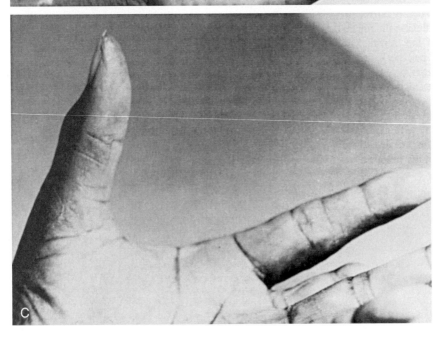

FIGURE 32-19. High median nerve palsy treated with brachioradialis-to-FPL and ECRL-to-index finger profundus tendon transfers. **A** and **B,** There is good FPL power but a limited range of active IP joint flexion when the wrist is held still. **C,** Note the absence of either thumb or index finger flexion contractures.

Summary of High Median Nerve Palsy

In a high median nerve injury, the surgeon should consider performing an opposition transfer if forearm pronation is used as a substitute motion. If the nerve has been repaired, extrinsic transfers are seldom required because satisfactory extrinsic muscle function is usually regained. If the patient needs a nerve graft, especially if this is done late or under unfavorable conditions (e.g., a long graft or a poor bed), useful extrinsic functional recovery is unlikely and one should consider performing early extrinsic end-to-side transfers and/or a side-to-side transfer of the index and conjoint profundus tendons. All these intrinsic and extrinsic transfers can be performed at the same time.

Author's Preferred Method of Treatment: High Median Nerve Palsy

Again, my enthusiasm for reconstructive surgery is tempered by my belief that sensation is the prime determinant of hand function and because I believe that sensory recovery after a high median nerve repair in adults is always poor and is even worse if a nerve graft is required. Furthermore, I believe that nerve repair hardly ever restores lost opposition, although useful reinnervation of the forearm flexor muscles undoubtedly occurs. For these reasons, I do not favor early extrinsic tendon transfers and only restore opposition if, after maximal recovery has occurred, both the patient and the surgeon believe that this will improve hand function. Most patients will adapt and increasingly use their normal arm (even if this is the nondominant arm) for precision func-

tion; I thus rarely attempt to restore opposition when there is a combined median sensory and motor deficit. If an opposition transfer is indicated, I favor EIP transfer.

I use the brachioradialis transfer for restoration of thumb flexion, especially in conditions in which there is relative sensory sparing, and use an end-to-side attachment unless there is no prospect of later reinnervation. I do not believe that an ECRL transfer to restore index finger flexion is often needed and prefer to join the index and the common (middle, ring, and little) profundi tendons in a "side-to-side" fashion. Although this does not restore power to the index finger, I believe that the condition of the hand is usually too poor to benefit from an ECRL transfer, especially if there is a marked sensory deficit.

Expectations/Patient Counseling: High Median Nerve Palsy

It is imperative to stress to patients with high median nerve injury that they have suffered a severe injury and will never regain normal hand sensation, strength, or function. They should be aware that the aim of all surgery is to create the best possible "helper hand," although this will always have rudimentary function when compared with their normal contralateral hand. I thus do not enthusiastically recommend opponensplasty in the presence of severe sensory loss in the median nerve distribution because most patients will use their other hand for fine pinching tasks, even after a "successful" opponensplasty. In contrast, I do recommend tendon transfers for persistent loss of the thumb and finger extrinsic flexor function. However, I stress that the restored thumb and finger flexion will be weak, although with sensory input provided by the eyes, should allow rudimentary use of the hand to hold and steady light objects.

CONCLUSION

Tendon transfers (Table 32-4) can restore selected motor functions after high and low median nerve palsy, but their ability to improve function is restricted by the severity of any associated sensory loss. Numerous opposition transfers have been described, and almost every possible motor has been used. Many pulleys are available, and there are numerous methods of distal attachment. The main reasons for failure of opposition transfers are persistent thumb contractures (recognized or unrecognized) and selection of a poor motor. Early opposition transfer has been recommended in patients who use forearm pronation as a substitute for the paralyzed APB. Extrinsic tendon transfers in high median nerve palsy are usually required only when the nerve injury is bridged with a nerve graft or left untreated.

CRITICAL POINTS: MANAGEMENT OPTIONS IN HIGH MEDIAN NERVE PALSY

- Because worthwhile sensory recovery is so unlikely in these cases, opponensplasty is typically not beneficial.
- The goal of any repair is to create the best possible "helper" hand; precision function must be assumed by the other hand.

Table 32-4
SUMMARY OF POSSIBLE OPPONENSPLASTIES

Motor	Pulley	Reference
Ring finger superficialis	Angle between flexor retinaculum and palmar aponeurosis	Jacobs and Thompson, 1960; Thompson, 1942
	FCU tendon	Beasley, 1970; Littler, 1949
	FCU loop	Bunnell, 1938; Jensen, 1978
	FCU/ECU sling	Groves and Goldner, 1975; Sakellarides, 1970
	Flexor retinaculum window	Bohr, 1953; Michelinakis and Vourexakis, 1981; Snow and Fink, 1971
	Guyon's canal	Anderson et al., 1992; Brand, 1970; Palande, 1975
Extensor indicis proprius	Ulnar border of wrist/forearm	Aguirre and Caplan, 1956; Anderson et al., 1991; Anderson et al., 1992; Burkhalter et al., 1973
Abductor digiti minimi	None	Huber, 1921; Littler and Cooley, 1963; Nicolaysen, 1922; Wissinger and Singsen, 1977
Palmaris longus	None	Braun, 1978; Camitz, 1929; Foucher et al., 1991; Littler and Li, 1967; Terrono et al., 1993
	Window in flexor retinaculum	MacDougal, 1995
	Near pisiform	Bunnell, 1924
Extensor carpi ulnaris	Ulnar border of wrist/forearm	Kessler, 1969; Kirklin and Thomas, 1948; Ney, 1921; Phalen and Miller, 1947; Wood and Adams, 1984
Extensor carpi radialis longus	Ulnar border of wrist/forearm	Baek et al., 1999; Henderson, 1962; Kaplan et al., 1976
Extensor digiti minimi	Ulnar border of wrist/forearm	Schneider, 1969
Extensor pollicis longus	Ulnar border of wrist/forearm	Riley et al., 1980
	Intraosseous membrane	Gerard et al., 1994; Mennen, 1992; Moutet et al., 1986
Flexor pollicis longus	Thumb proximal phalanx/MP joint	Makin, 1967; Oberlin and Alnot, 1988

ANNOTATED REFERENCES

2. Anderson GA, Lee V, Sundararaj GD: Opponensplasty by extensor indicis and flexor digitorum superficialis tendon transfer. J Hand Surg [Br] 17:611-614, 1992.

   This study reports a large experience of two opponensplasties, performed for leprosy in an Asian population.

9. Brand PW, Beach RB, Thompson DE: Relative tension and potential excursion of muscles in the forearm and hand. J Hand Surg 6:209-219, 1981.

   In this classic paper the authors assess the relative strengths and potential excursions of muscles whose function one wishes to restore (e.g., APL), as well as those of muscles that can be transferred to restore the lost function. In addition all hand surgeons should read and understand: Brand PW: Clinical Mechanics of the Hand. St. Louis, CV Mosby, 1985 or its recent second edition. The original edition is one of the pillars of hand surgery. It is clearly and simply written by an author with great experience of tendon transfers and contains much common sense (which is all too often forgotten), distinguishes between deficit and disability, and remains completely pertinent and relevant 19 years after publication.

10. Brandsma JW, Ottenhoff-De Jonge MW: Flexor digitorum superficialis tendon transfer for intrinsic replacement: Long-term results and the effect on donor fingers. J Hand Surg [Br] 17:625-628, 1992.

    This describes, better than any other paper, the potential morbidity of FDS harvest on the donor finger in Asian patients, who are generally perceived to have supple finger joints.

18. Burkhalter W, Christensen RC, Brown P: Extensor indicis proprius opponensplasty. J Bone Joint Surg Am 55:725-732, 1973.

    Burkhalter, who wrote this chapter in previous editions of the book, was the champion of the EIP. Here he reports his results in a substantial series of cases.

20. Camitz H: Uber die Behandlung der Oppositionslahmung. Acta Chir Scand 65:77-81, 1929.

    The original description of the palmaris longus opponensplasty—often referenced but rarely read.

26. Foucher G, Malizos C, Sammut D, et al: Primary palmaris longus transfer as an opponensplasty in carpal tunnel release: A series of 73 cases. J Hand Surg [Br] 16:56-60, 1991.

    One of the few papers to attempt objective measurement of opposition. The paper describes several techniques for measuring opposition, and these should be considered by all surgeons wishing to audit or report their results: ideally these measurements should be performed both preoperatively and postoperatively.

32. Huber E: Hilfsoperation bei median Uhlahmung. Dtsch Arch Klin Med 136:271, 1921.

The original description of the ADM opponensplasty—often referenced but rarely read.

66. Rowntree T: Anomalous innervation of the hand muscles. J Bone Joint Surg Br 31:505-510, 1949.

This relatively obscure article, rarely quoted, is nonetheless important because it was the first to point out that the intrinsic muscles of the hand can have any conceivable combination or variation of innervation patterns from the median and ulnar nerves.

75. Thompson TC: A modified operation for opponens paralysis. J Bone Joint Surg 26:632-640, 1942.

Although Royle first used the FDS as an opponensplasty, this article describes the prototype of the modern FDS opponensplasty with a pulley on the ulnar border of the hand. The pulley used is "naturally occurring" (angle between the distal edge of the flexor retinaculum and the palmar aponeurosis), has stood the test of time, and, in my view, is simple and effective.

INDEX

Note: Page numbers followed by the letter f refer to figures; those followed by the letter t refer to tables.